TARGET HIGH™ Next

NURSING DECODE

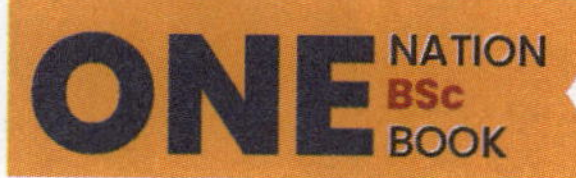

for BSc Nursing University Exams

TARGET HIGH™ Next

NURSING DECODE

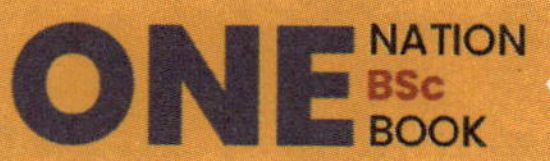

for BSc Nursing University Exams

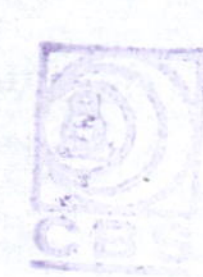

1st Year
BSc Nursing
Semester I & II

Muthuvenkatachalam Srinivasan
PhD (INC Consortium), MSc Nursing (AIIMS, New Delhi), D Pharma
RN (NMBA Australia)
Assistant Professor
Institute of Human Behaviour and Allied Sciences (IHBAS)
Govt. of NCT
New Delhi

Ambili M Venugopal
MSc Pediatric Nursing (AIIMS), BSc (Hons) Nursing (AIIMS)
Tutor/Clinical Instructor
All India Institute of Medical Sciences
New Delhi

Edited by
Swati Mehra

Published by

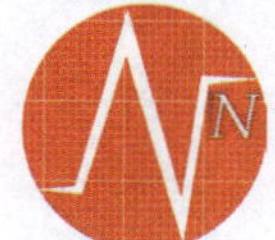

Nursing Next Exam Prep Pvt Ltd

2nd Floor, AMCO Tower A-5,6,7 Amaltash Marg A Block, Sector 9, Noida, Uttar Pradesh 201301

Marketing & Distribution

CBS Publishers & Distributors Pvt Ltd

4819/XI, Prahlad Street, 24 Ansari Road, Daryaganj, New Delhi 110002, India: **E-mail:** delhi@cbspd.com, cbspubs@airtelmail.in: **Website:** www.cbspd.com

• New Delhi • Bengaluru • Chennai • Kochi • Kolkata • Lucknow • Mumbai • Hyderabad • Jharkhand • Nagpur • Patna • Pune • Uttarakhand

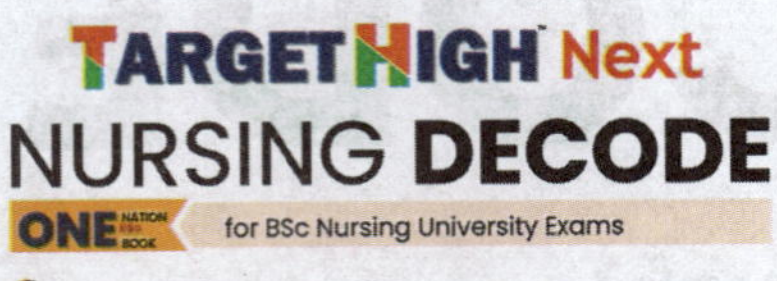

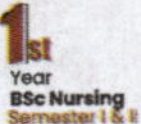

ISBN: 978-93-94630-60-4

First Edition: 2024

Published by **Nursing Next Live A unit of Nursing Next Exam Prep Pvt. Ltd**

Corporate Office: 2nd Floor, 204 FIE, Industrial Area, Patparganj, Delhi 110092

Ph: +91-11-4934 4934 Fax: 4934 4935

e-mail: admin@nursingnextlive.in Website: www.nursingnextlive.in

Distribution by **CBS Publishers & Distributors Pvt Ltd**

4819/XI Prahlad Street, 24 Ansari Road, Daryaganj, New Delhi 110 002, India.

Ph: +91-11-23289259, 23266861, 23266867 Website: www.cbspd.com

Fax: 011-23243014

e-mail: delhi@cbspd.com; cbspubs@airtelmail.in.

Corporate Office: 204 FIE, Industrial Area, Patparganj, Delhi 110 092

Ph: +91-11-4934 4934 Fax: 4934 4935

e-mail: feedback@cbspd.com; bhupesharora@cbspd.com

Printed at : Goyal Offset Works Pvt. Ltd. Haryana (INDIA)

The Team Behind

About the Authors

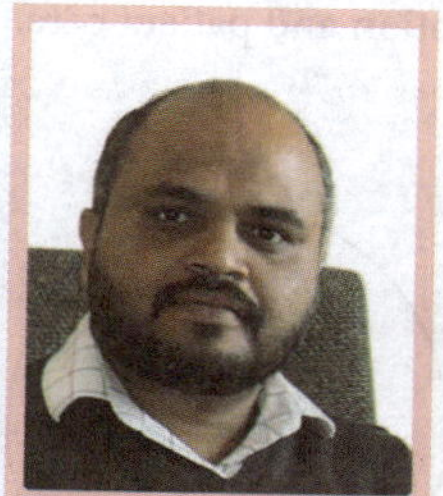

Muthuvenkatachalam Srinivasan
PhD (INC Consortium), MSc Nursing (AIIMS, New Delhi), D Pharma, RN (NMBA Australia)
Assistant Professor
Institute of Human Behaviour and Allied Sciences (IHBAS)
Govt. of NCT
New Delhi

Muthuvenkatachalam Srinivasan, PhD (INC Consortium), MSc (AIIMS), D Pharma, RN (NMBA Australia), is a highly qualified professional with a rich academic background. Currently, he is serving in the capacity of Assistant Professor at IHBAS, New Delhi. His prior experience as an Associate Professor at AIIMS, and his considerable expertise in the field of Nursing contribute significantly to the field of healthcare and nursing education.

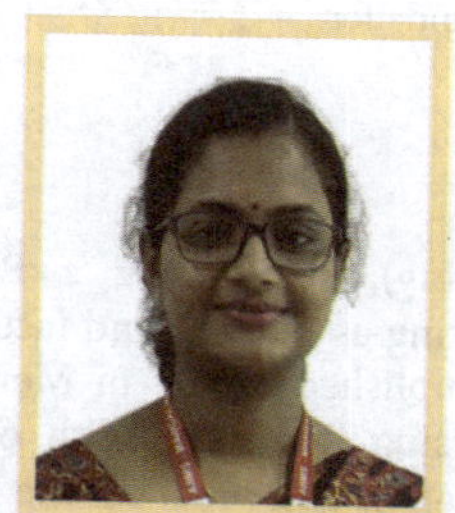

Ambili M Venugopal
MSc Pediatric Nursing (AIIMS), BSc (Hons) Nursing (AIIMS)
Tutor/Clinical Instructor
All India Institute of Medical Sciences
New Delhi

Ambili M Venugopal, MSc (Pediatric Nursing), BSc (Hons) in Nursing from AIIMS is an aspiring scholar pursuing a PhD in Pediatric Nursing through the National Consortium. Presently, she is serving as a Tutor at the College of Nursing, All India Institute of Medical Sciences in Mangalagiri, Andhra Pradesh, and contributing to the advancement of nursing education and practice.

About the Editor

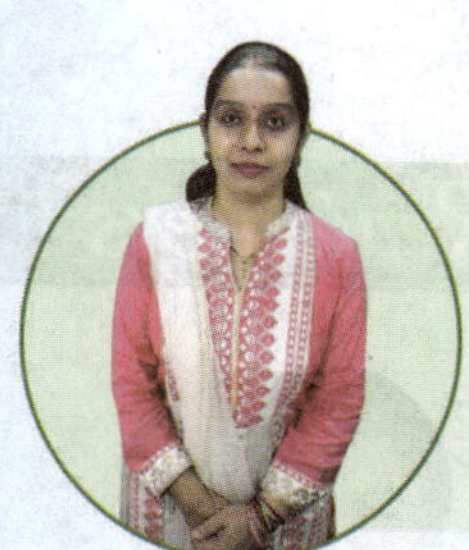

Swati Mehra
BDS, MDS (Oral Pathology and Microbiology)
Senior Content Strategist
Nursing Next Live

Swati Mehra, BDS, MDS (Oral Pathology and Microbiology), is a highly proficient healthcare expert with almost a decade of experience in publishing, editing and academics. She brings her expertise to her role as Senior Content Strategist at Nursing Next Live. Prior to this, she performed multiple roles of content strategist, senior dental associate, senior lecturer and many more. Her dedicated career path reflects a commitment to excellence and continuous growth in her field.

About the Contributors

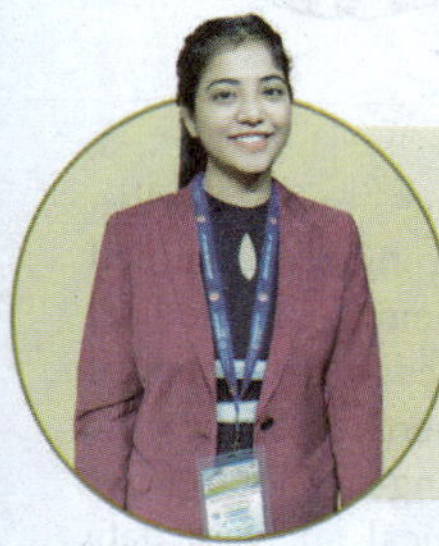

Deep Shikha
BSc (N) (Hons), AIIMS, Bhubaneswar
MSc Medical Physiology, AIIMS, Jodhpur
PhD Physiology (Pursuing), AIIMS, New Delhi
Applied Anatomy and
Applied Physiology

Deep Shikha, BSc Hons. (Nursing) from AIIMS Bhubaneswar, MSc (Medical Physiology) from AIIMS Jodhpur, is currently pursuing her PhD at AIIMS, New Delhi in Applied Anatomy and Applied Physiology. Her academic journey reflects a strong commitment to advancing knowledge in the field of Physiology.

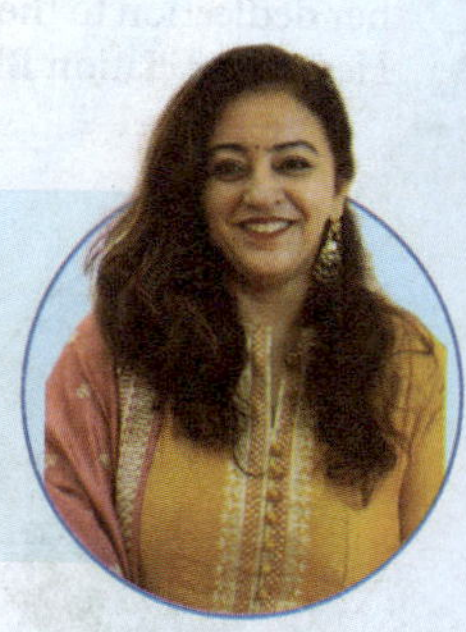

Neha Sethi
MDS, MBA
Content Strategist
Nursing Next Live
[Applied Biochemistry and Nutrition & Dietetics]

Neha Sethi a highly skilled and accomplished professional with more than 12 years of experience, is currently working as a Content Strategist in Nursing Next Live. She has specialization in Periodontology and Implantology, Dental Implants and Pre-implant procedures. She is proficient in General Dentistry, Endodontics and Cosmetic Dentistry. Moreover, she has over 6 years of experience in managing hospitals, overseeing clinical operations, ensuring quality assurance, and procuring equipment. Her commitment to healthcare was recognized with an 'Award of Appreciation' during the COVID-19 vaccination campaign.

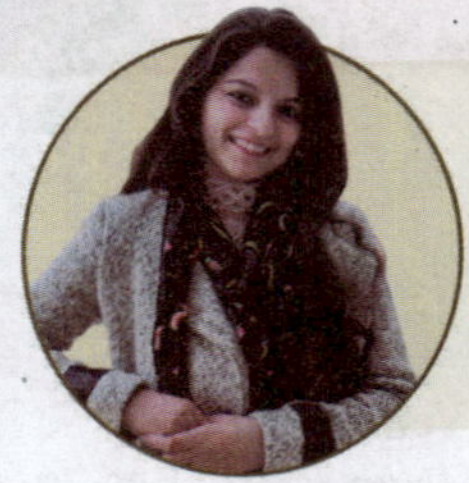

Anjali Arora
MSc (N) (MSN)
Tutor
Holy Family College of Nursing
New Delhi
[Nursing Foundation]

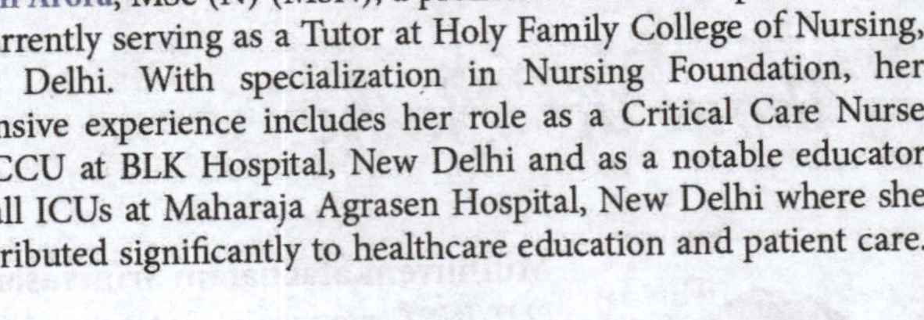

Anjali Arora, MSc (N) (MSN), a proficient healthcare professional, is currently serving as a Tutor at Holy Family College of Nursing, New Delhi. With specialization in Nursing Foundation, her extensive experience includes her role as a Critical Care Nurse in ICCU at BLK Hospital, New Delhi and as a notable educator for all ICUs at Maharaja Agrasen Hospital, New Delhi where she contributed significantly to healthcare education and patient care.

Chetana, MSc (Mental Health Nursing) is pursuing a PhD in the same field, and is currently working as Mastermind faculty at Nursing Next Live. She is an accomplished expert in Mental Health Nursing, Psychology, and Nursing Research. With over 15 years of experience in nursing education and practice, she has an impressive background of participation in various conferences, workshops, and holds notable research contributions.

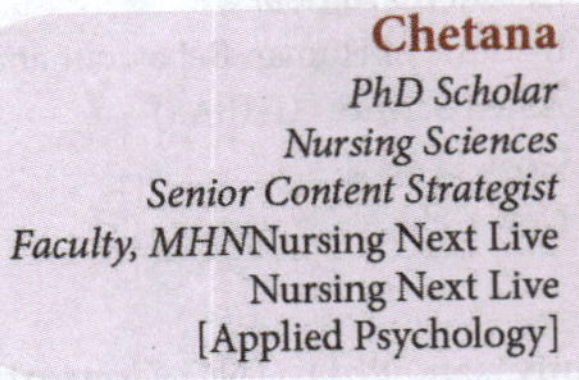

Chetana
PhD Scholar
Nursing Sciences
Senior Content Strategist
*Faculty, MHN*Nursing Next Live
Nursing Next Live
[Applied Psychology]

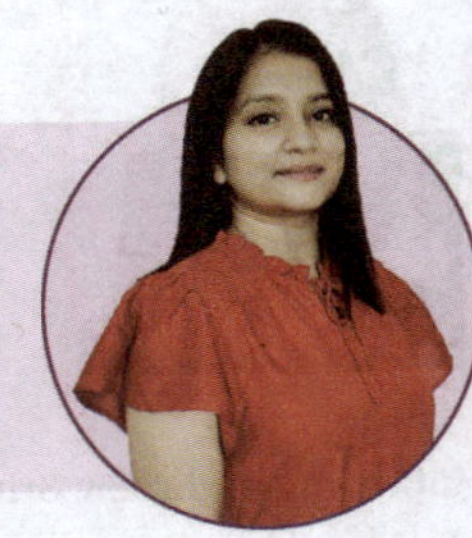

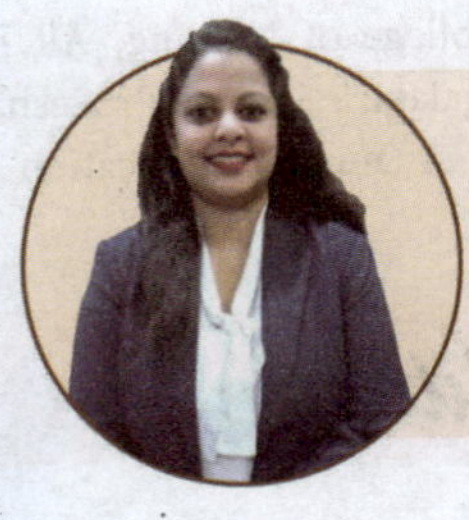

Priyanka Randhir
MSc (N) (Pediatrics), MA (Sociology)
Senior Content Strategist
Nursing Next Live
[Applied Sociology]

Priyanka Randhir, BSc (N), RN, RM and MA (Sociology) is currently serving as a Senior Content Strategist at Nursing Next Live, contributing her knowledge and experience to enrich the nursing profession. Earlier, she worked as a Nursing Tutor at Khalsa College of Nursing for three years, enriching her knowledge and practical expertise. She is a highly skilled healthcare professional with over a decade of experience in the field.

About the Reviewers

Sabina Ali, BSc (N) and MSc (MSN), is currently working as a Mastermind faculty in Nursing Next Live. She is a highly accomplished and skilled professional with a background in Nursing Foundation and ENT. With over seven years of experience in nursing education, her impressive academic record, expertise and participation in national and international conferences show her dedication to the field. Furthermore, she is a certified American Heart Association BLS and ACLS instructor.

Sabina Ali
RN, RM Critical Care Nurse
Senior Content Strategist and
Quality Check
Nursing Next Live

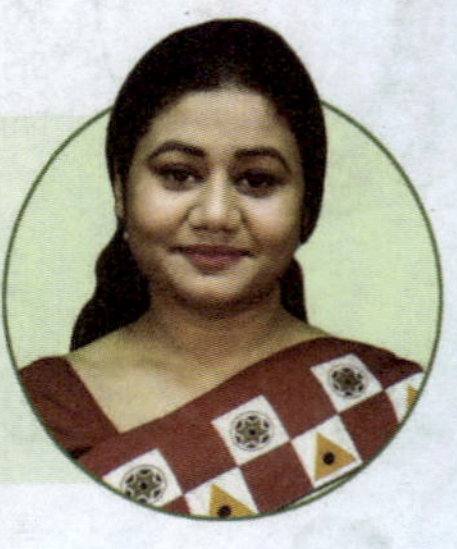

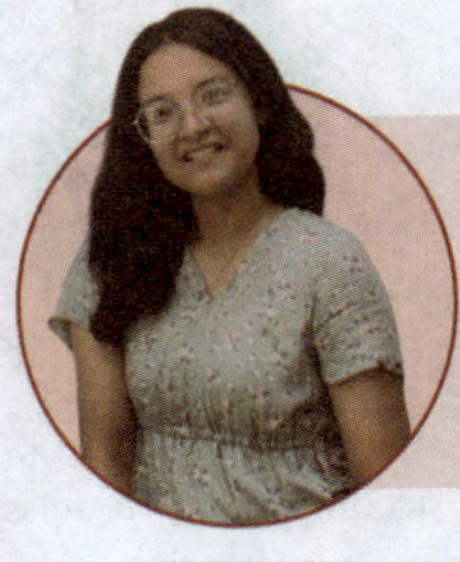

Rishika Rawat
BSc (Hons) Nursing, English (Hons), DU
Senior Guidance and Counsellor cum
Mentor

Rishika Rawat, BSc (Hons.) in Nursing and English (Hons.) from the University of Delhi, is a highly qualified healthcare professional. With prior experience in medical setups, she seamlessly blends her knowledge in medical writing, analytical skills and clinical expertise. Since the beginning of her career, she has been focusing on honing her proficiency in clinical documentation, statistical analysis, data interpretation and presentation. This reflects her dedication to excellence in the field.

Sumaira Ayaz Ali, is currently working as a Content Strategist at Nursing Next Live. She started her career as a Tutor at Skylark Paramedical College to add valuable insights into the field. She has a solid foundation in BSc Nursing from the Government College of Nursing in Srinagar. Her dedication to professional growth is evident through her active participation in various management programs, seminars and research activities.

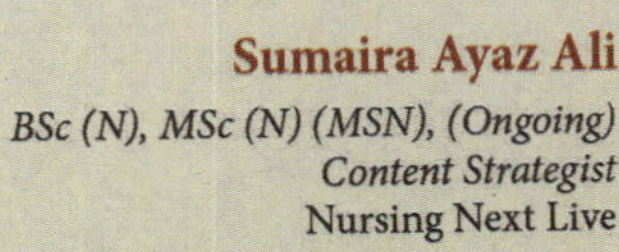

Sumaira Ayaz Ali
BSc (N), MSc (N) (MSN), (Ongoing)
Content Strategist
Nursing Next Live

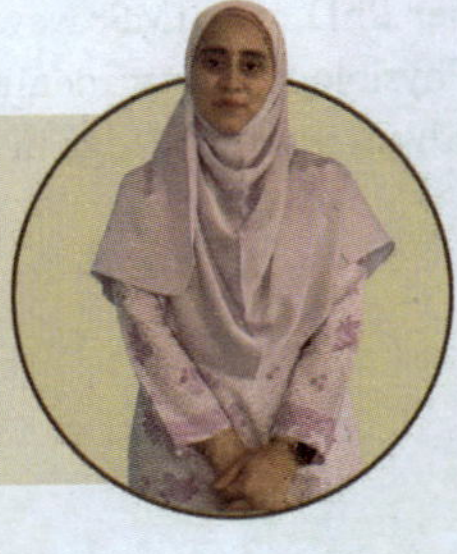

Preface

Every student wants to study hard and pass the exams with flying colors, but not all of them score well in the exams. How do you approach your examination becomes a deciding factor as far as your scores are concerned. Flurry of questions haunt a student's mind when he/she appears for an exam, like—How to start writing the answer? What should be the length of answer and so on and so forth.

The above-mentioned issues have inspired us to design and conceive the idea of **"Target High Next Nursing DECODE"** Series for **Nursing Undergraduate students**.

In this book, our focus is on seven subjects—Applied Anatomy, Applied Physiology, Applied Biochemistry, Applied Nutrition & Dietetics, Nursing Foundation, Applied Psychology and Applied Sociology.

The book provides conceptual clarity in the form of **conceptual theory, conceptual exercises** and **conceptual revision** leaving no aspect of learning untouched. **Conceptual theory** provides **comprehensive and concise summary** of important/high-yield topics asked in university examinations with **important terminologies** providing rapid review of entire topic/chapter.

Conceptual exercises are the perfect blend of topic-wise important/high-yield **Long Answer Questions, Short Notes** and **Short Answer Questions** asked in various university exams, like **Tamil Nadu Dr. M.G.R. Medical University, Delhi University, Kerala University of Health Sciences, Rajasthan University of Health Sciences and many more**. We have spent good amount of time in brainstorming session to make the answers authentic and accurate. The answers given here have been checked and cross-checked several times by the subject experts, and finally, reviewed and edited for the authenticity of content.

Apart from the solved questions of the last 10 years, **Multiple Choice Questions** and **Golden Points** under conceptual revision have been added to give a boost to revision and practice, and also to help students in self-evaluation before examination. Integration of **Nursing Care Plans** on important topics provides a 360-degree approach for enhancing the practical and clinical knowledge and skills.

Content is backed with various pedagogical features, like tables, images, flowcharts to help students understand the concepts and memorize the facts and figures with less time and effort. The flowcharts and line diagrams are easy to draw and reproduce. The images provide a real-time environment with easy and quick understanding of the concepts.

For quick revision, recall and practice, important and repeatedly asked topics/questions are highlighted adding an extra value to your last-minute preparation. A special section on color plates for practice has been added for the digram practice before examination. Integration of color plates related to important anatomical images, illustrations and flowcharts enhances the visualization and photomicrographic memory which is highly important for last-minute preparation as well.

Use this book very smartly and strategically to achieve your ultimate goal. We are pretty sure that this book will prove quite handy and very useful in developing your skills, approach and style of answer writing.

All the Best!

Director's Message

Dear Nursing Students/Future Nursing Officers,

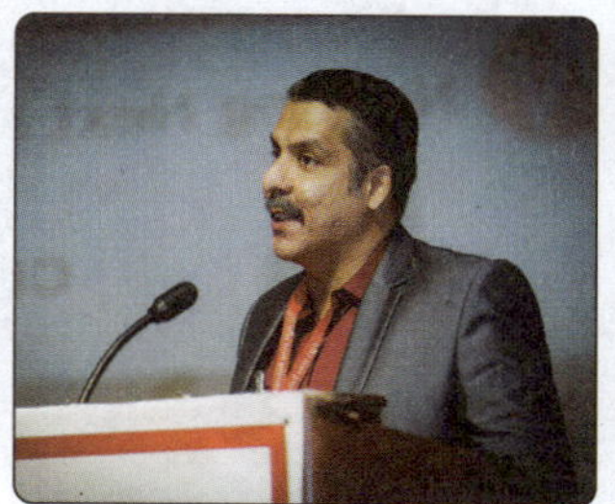

First and foremost, I would like to congratulate all of you on choosing this noble career of Nursing. This is the first step toward service to mankind. After completing the 12th examination, the two most sought-after medical professions are of Doctors and Nurses. Both the professions are considered equally significant for strengthening any country's health system. A noble profession, like Nursing not only demands knowledge and skills but also empathy, compassion, and a strong commitment to the well-being of others. As future nurses, you have chosen a path that will allow you to make a significant impact on the lives of individuals and community as a whole.

Nursing is not just a job; it is a service beyond self-interest. The journey you are about to embark upon is both challenging and rewarding, and it is my privilege to guide you through this transformative experience.

Always remember, for every good work or big achievement, you need to follow certain principles and imbibe certain traits within you, like:

- You must love the profession you join
- You must be hardworking
- You must be sincere
- You must have faith in yourself

And, of course, you have all these traits; that's why you are here. It is just the beginning of your Nursing journey as you all have miles to go.

During the last three years, we have revolutionized digital education in Nursing across India. Our initiatives have been well recognized and accepted by Nursing Students preparing for Nursing competitive examinations, like NORCET and other Nursing Officers' examinations of national repute. And now we have introduced Digital Learning to graduates in the form of "Plan UG".

To complement Digital Learning along with preparation for university exams, we have designed and created comprehensive, concept-oriented and student-friendly study material specifically tailored for nursing undergraduates under the banner of most trusted study companion "Target High" with a goal to create an unparalleled source of flawless and complete information for students.

This book is a complete package of very carefully, clearly and concisely designed concepts along with a collection of solved exercises and revision exercises that will help you practice and apply your understanding. The meticulous selection of questions in the book coupled with their comprehensive explanations and solutions will help you grasp the underlying principles and reasoning.

With this invaluable resource, focus your energy on mastering the concepts and honing your critical thinking skills.

We believe in the saying, "One Day or Day One." If you believe that One Day will come, and then you will start the preparation for your university examination, that day will never come, so why not from Day One? Always remember, your success as a nursing professional begins with a solid foundation built during your undergraduate years.

We believe, no matter how good a book is, there is always a scope for improvement. And that is why we request you to keep sharing your valuable feedback on a regular basis so that we could provide you with the best possible content.

I wish you all the best in your studies and future endeavors as nurses. May you find fulfillment, purpose, and endless opportunities to make a difference in the lives of those you serve!

Bhupesh Aarora
Director
Nursing Next Live
Sr. Vice President – Health Sciences Division (Publishing & Marketing)
CBS Publishers and Distributors Pvt Ltd

Special Features of the Book

TARGET HIGH™ Next NURSING DECODE

Covering:

- **225+** Long Answer Questions
- **540+** Short Answer Questions
- **11030+** MCQs
- **600+** Short Notes
- **15400+** Golden Points

An Innovative Study Companion for BSc Nursing First Year that combines traditional content with digital resources to empower BSc Nursing First Year students with a comprehensive and exam-centric learning experience. A detailed Subject-wise cum Topic-wise coverage of content with **3-Way Approach "Conceptual Theory–Conceptual Exercises–Conceptual Revision"** along with tables, figures, and flowcharts makes it unique in its own way.

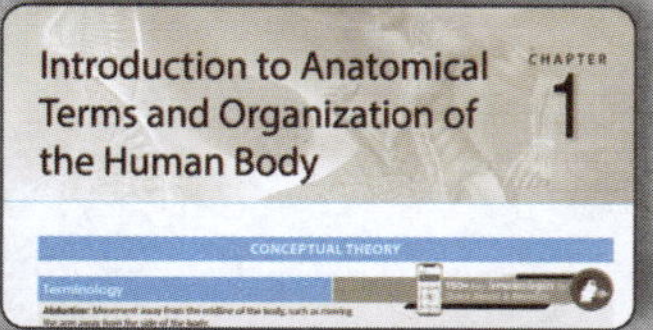

CONCEPTUAL THEORY

Important synopses of all the chapters have been covered in a nutshell referring to the frequently asked Topics in the previous year examinations for brief overview in one go.

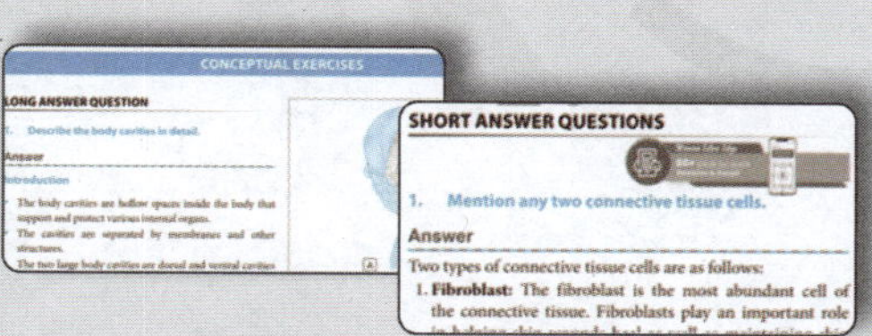

CONCEPTUAL EXERCISES

***225+** Long Answer Qs and **500+** Short Answer Qs have been included after referring to all the important universities previous examination papers of last 10 Years.*

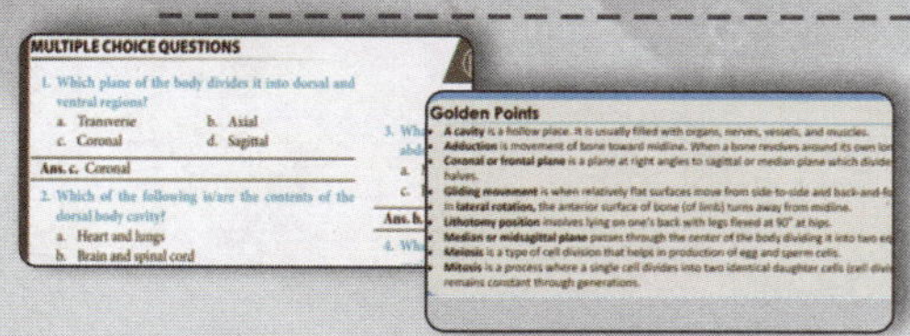

CONCEPTUAL REVISION

*This section covers **15K+** Golden Points and **11K+** Multiple Choice Qs for last-minute revision.*

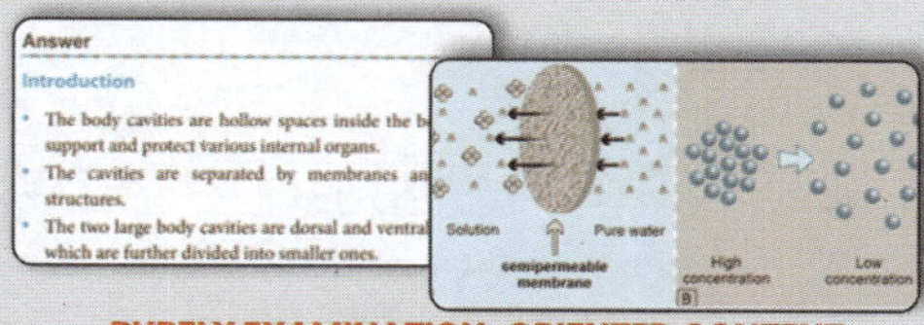

PURELY EXAMINATION-ORIENTED CONTENT

Each answer has been solved keeping the latest marking scheme criteria in mind which gives a complete visualization of real-time examination and also supplemented by Figures, Flowchart, Tables for helping students in grasping the core idea of the topic discussed in chapters.

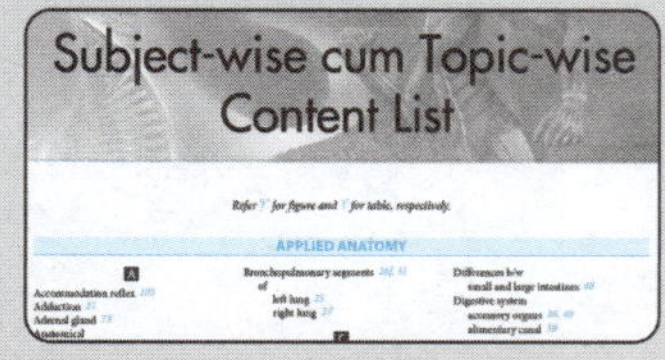

SUBJECT-WISE CUM TOPIC-WISE CONTENT

In the beginning of the book detailed Subject-wise cum Topic-wise TOC have been provided for quick access to respective Topic Qs which makes the book useful with dual approach.

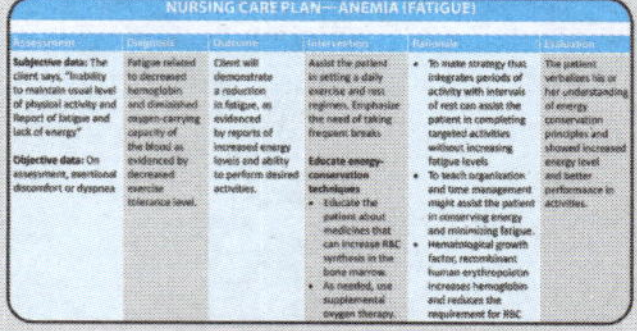

NURSING CARE PLAN

Includes nursing care plan According to NANDA Diagnosis which is frequently asked in examination.

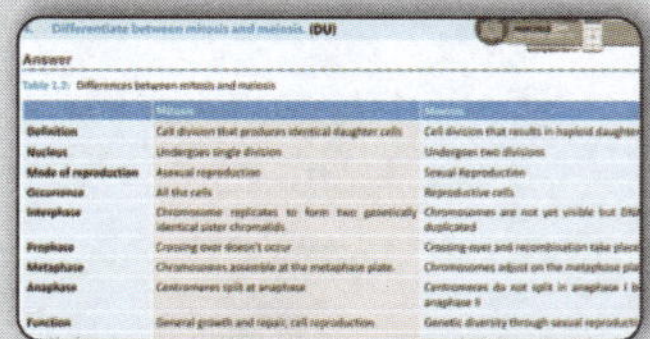

RECENT UPDATES/ADDON

Content is enriched with all the recent and latest updates giving up-to-date information of the respective topic.

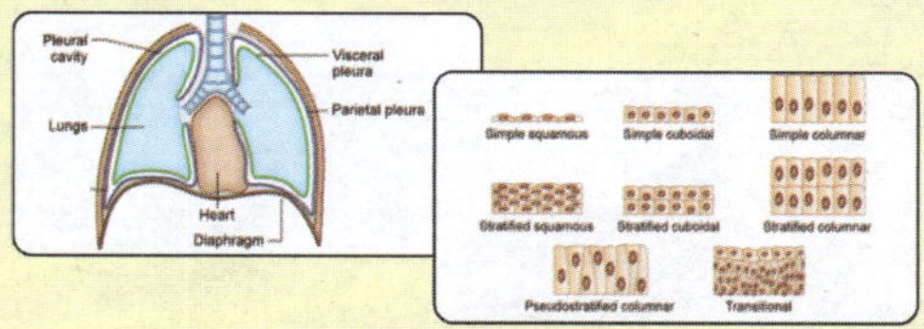

PICTORIAL WORKSHEETS

Covering 60 colored images, figures and flowcharts related to Anatomy, Physiology and Biochemistry to enhance the visualization and recall feature from the practice point of view.

Contents

APPLIED BIOCHEMISTRY

APPLIED NUTRITION AND DIETETICS

NURSING FOUNDATION

APPLIED PSYCHOLOGY

APPLIED SOCIOLOGY

Detailed Table of Contents

APPLIED ANATOMY

Abbreviations: GP, Golden Points; LAQs, Long Answer Questions; MCQs, Multiple Choice Questions; SAQs, Short Answer Questions; SN, Short Notes.

APPLIED PHYSIOLOGY

CHAPTERS		CONCEPTUAL THEORY	CONCEPTUAL EXERCISES			CONCEPTUAL REVISION		PAGES
Number	**Title**	**Pages**	**LAQs**	**SN**	**SAQs**	**MCQs**	**GP**	
CHAPTER 1	General Physiology—Basic Concepts	3	1	9	6	100+	200+	187–199
CHAPTER 2	Respiratory System	4	1	4	10	100+	200+	200–208
CHAPTER 3	Digestive System	5	3	6	12	100+	200+	209–224
CHAPTER 4	Circulatory and Lymphatic System	6	4	4	9	100+	200+	225–241
CHAPTER 5	Blood	3	6	2	8	100+	200+	242–256
CHAPTER 6	Endocrine System	4	3	5	11	100+	200+	257–269
CHAPTER 7	Sensory Organs	3	1	5	5	100+	200+	270–278
CHAPTER 8	Musculoskeletal System	3	1	5	5	100+	200+	279–287
CHAPTER 9	Renal System	3	1	3	7	100+	200+	288–295
CHAPTER 10	Reproductive System	3	1	9	5	100+	200+	296–307
CHAPTER 11	Nervous System	4	2	3	8	100+	200+	308–317
	Total	**41**	**24**	**55**	**86**	**1100+**	**2200+**	**131**

APPLIED BIOCHEMISTRY

APPLIED NUTRITION AND DIETETICS

CHAPTERS		CONCEPTUAL THEORY	CONCEPTUAL EXERCISES			CONCEPTUAL REVISION		PAGES
Number	**Title**	**Pages**	**LAQs**	**SN**	**SAQs**	**MCQs**	**GP**	
CHAPTER 1	Introduction to Nutrition	3	1	3	4	120+	120+	429–433
CHAPTER 2	Carbohydrates	3	1	3	6	120+	120+	434–439
CHAPTER 3	Proteins	2	1	2	–	120+	120+	440–444
CHAPTER 4	Fats	2	–	2	10	120+	120+	445–449
CHAPTER 5	Vitamins	1	5	7	8	120+	120+	450–461
CHAPTER 6	Minerals	2	2	7	8	120+	120+	462–470
CHAPTER 7	Balanced Diet	4	6	19	8	120+	120+	471–491
CHAPTER 8	Nutritional Deficiency Disorder	2	1	13	16	120+	120+	492–504
CHAPTER 9	Therapeutic Diet	2	3	10	7	120+	100+	505–512
CHAPTER 10	Cookery Rules and Preservation of Nutrients	3	4	10	10	120+	120+	513–526
CHAPTER 11	Nutritional Assessment and Nutrition Education	2	2	5	10	120+	120+	527–533
CHAPTER 12	National Nutritional Program and Role of Nurse	1	2	7	3	120+	100+	534–544
CHAPTER 13	Food Safety	1	–	1	–	120+	120+	545–546
	Total	**28**	**28**	**89**	**90**	**1560+**	**1520+**	**118**

NURSING FOUNDATION

Contd...

CHAPTERS		CONCEPTUAL THEORY	CONCEPTUAL EXERCISES			CONCEPTUAL REVISION		PAGES
Number	**Title**	**Pages**	**LAQs**	**SN**	**SAQs**	**MCQs**	**GP**	
CHAPTER 15	Health Assessment	8	2	7	5	200+	250+	718–737
CHAPTER 16	Nursing Process	3	2	4	4	200+	200+	738–745
CHAPTER 17	Nutritional Needs	3	4	4	4	200+	100+	746–755
CHAPTER 18	Hygiene	5	1	8	5	200+	300+	756–765
CHAPTER 19	Elimination Needs	4	2	14	6	200+	150+	766–780
CHAPTER 20	Diagnostic Testing	3	1	4	2	200+	300+	781–788
CHAPTER 21	Oxygenation Needs	4	2	2	4	200+	300+	789–798
CHAPTER 22	Fluid and Electrolyte Imbalance	3	1	4	2	200+	300+	799–808
CHAPTER 23	Administration of Medications	7	5	5	5	200+	300+	809–826
CHAPTER 24	Sensory Needs	4	1	2	1	200+	300+	827–835
CHAPTER 25	Care of Terminally Ill Patient	5	1	4	5	200+	300+	836–844
CHAPTER 26	Psychosocial Needs	5	1	4	3	200+	300+	845–854
CHAPTER 27	Nursing Theories	4	1	3	2	200+	200+	855–863
CHAPTER 28	Nursing Care Plan	–	–	–	–	–	–	864–873
	Total	**111**	**56**	**182**	**107**	**5400+**	**7300+**	**325**

APPLIED PSYCHOLOGY

APPLIED SOCIOLOGY

CHAPTERS		CONCEPTUAL THEORY	CONCEPTUAL EXERCISES			CONCEPTUAL REVISION		PAGES
Number	**Title**	**Pages**	**LAQs**	**SN**	**SAQs**	**MCQs**	**GP**	
CHAPTER 1	Introduction to Sociology	3	5	2	3	50+	70+	1001–1010
CHAPTER 2	Social Structure	10	7	13	5	50+	70+	1011–1032
CHAPTER 3	Culture	5	3	5	5	50+	70+	1033–1043
CHAPTER 4	Family and Marriage	7	4	2	5	50+	70+	1044–1057
CHAPTER 5	Social Stratification	7	3	1	5	50+	70+	1058–1071
CHAPTER 6	Social Organization and Disorganization	22	4	4	6	50+	70+	1072–1101
CHAPTER 7	Clinical Sociology	4	3	2	4	50+	50+	1102–1110
	Total	**58**	**29**	**29**	**33**	**350+**	**470+**	**110**

Subject-wise cum Topic-wise Content List

This content list will give a quick glance over the important topics; all the terms have been arranged alphabetically subject-wise

Refer 'f' for figure and 't' for table, respectively.

APPLIED ANATOMY

APPLIED PHYSIOLOGY

APPLIED BIOCHEMISTRY

APPLIED NUTRITION AND DIETETICS

NURSING FOUNDATION

APPLIED PSYCHOLOGY

APPLIED SOCIOLOGY

Pictorial Worksheets

These worksheets cover **60 colored images, figures and flowcharts** related to Anatomy, Physiology and Biochemistry. These illustrations are highly important which enhance the visualization and recall feature from the practice point of view. All the illustrations have been provided with vacant spaces for students to memorize and reproduce the same in the examination with ease.

APPLIED ANATOMY

Color Plates	Get Yourself Practice

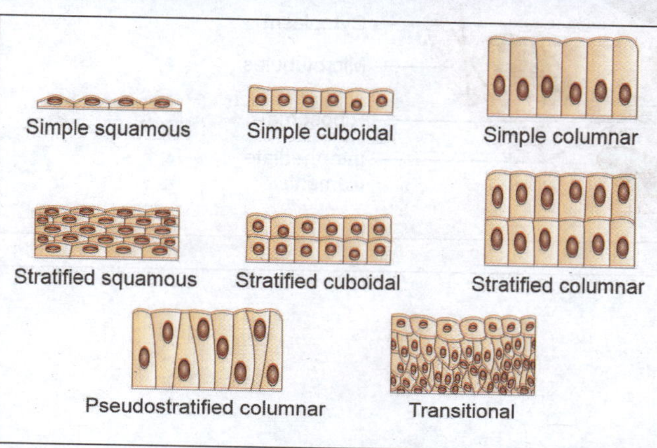

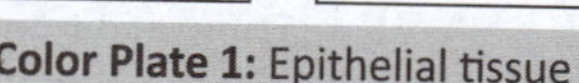
Color Plate 1: Epithelial tissue

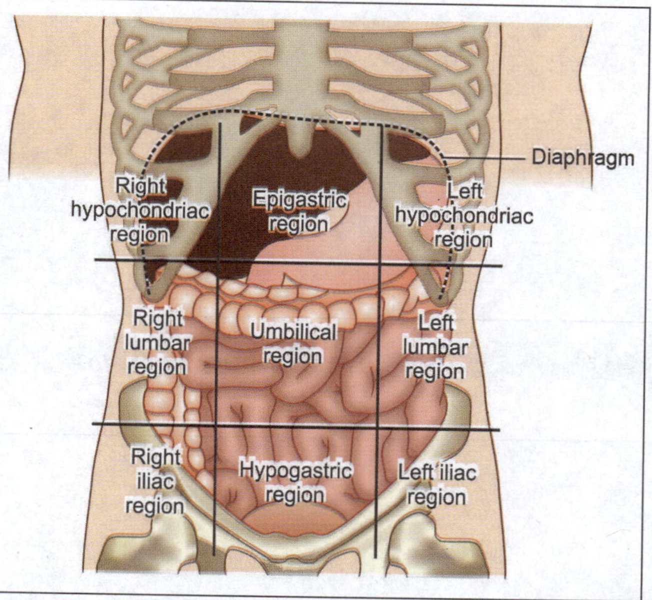

Color Plate 2: Regions of stomach

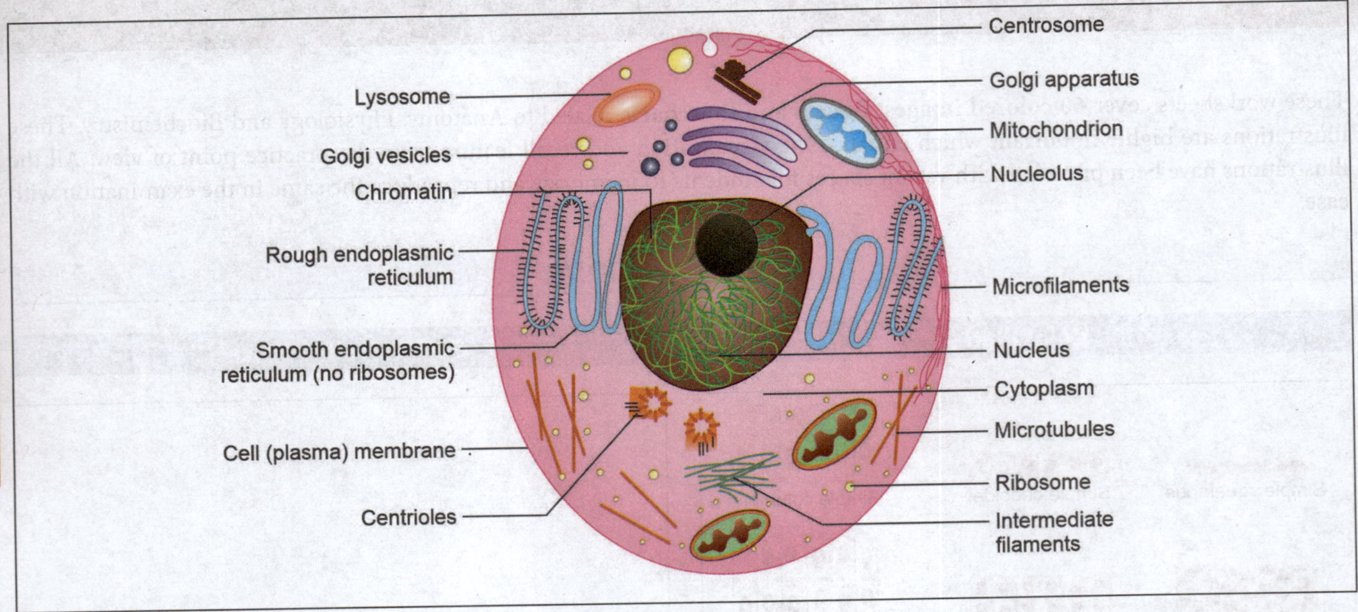

Color Plate 3: Cell

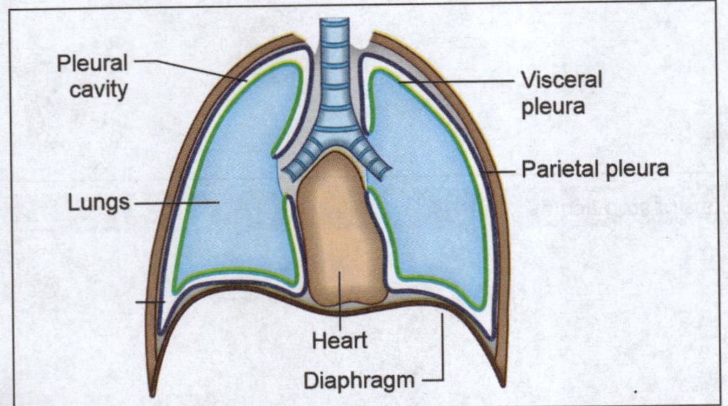

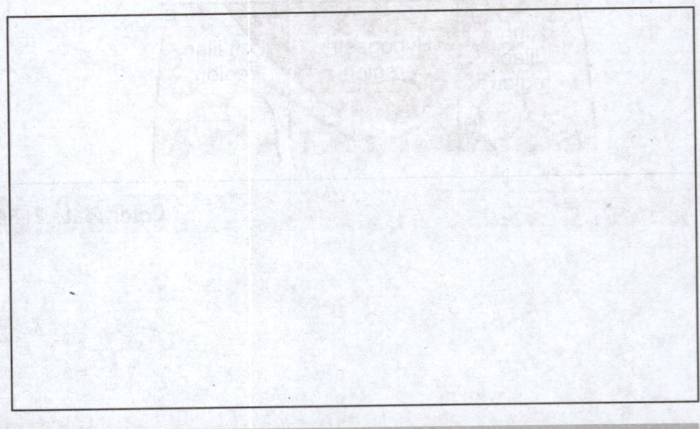

Color Plate 4: Pleural cavity

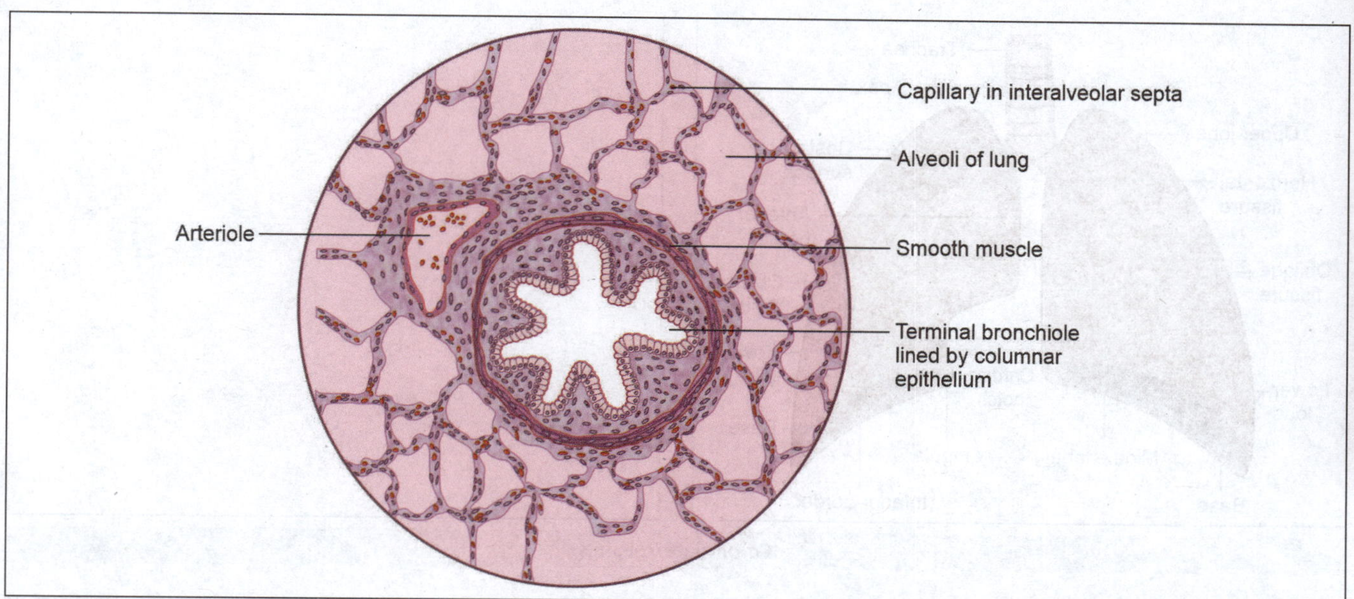

Color Plate 5: Lung histology

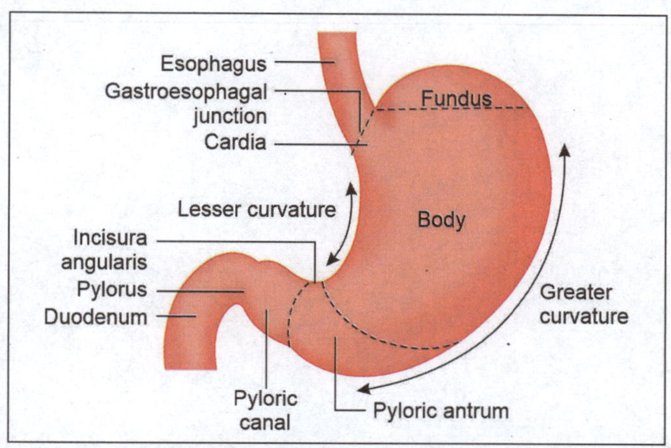

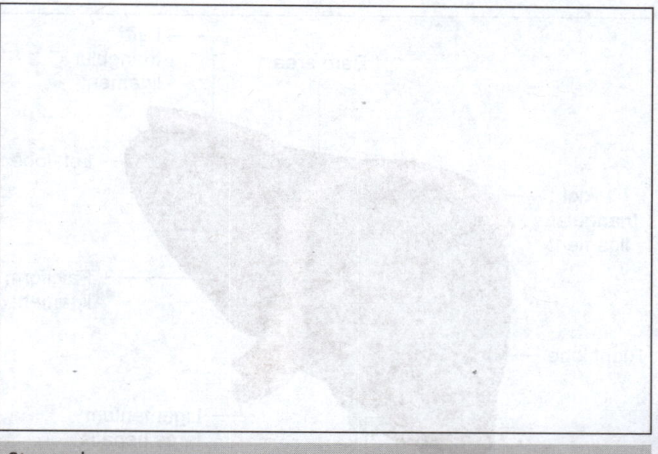

Color Plate 6: Stomach

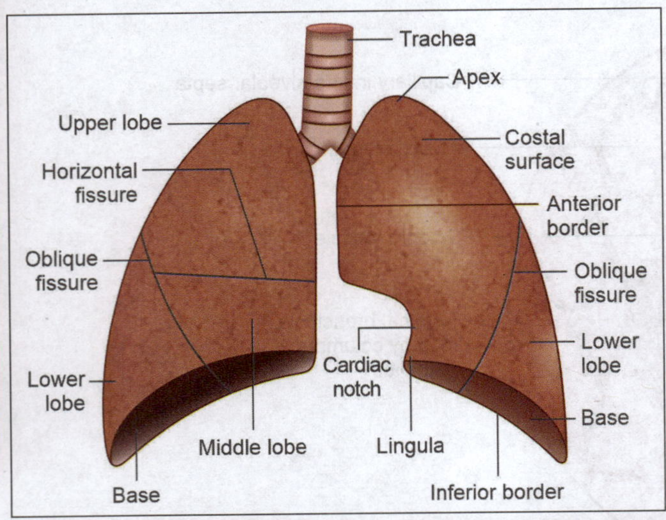

Color Plate 7: Lungs

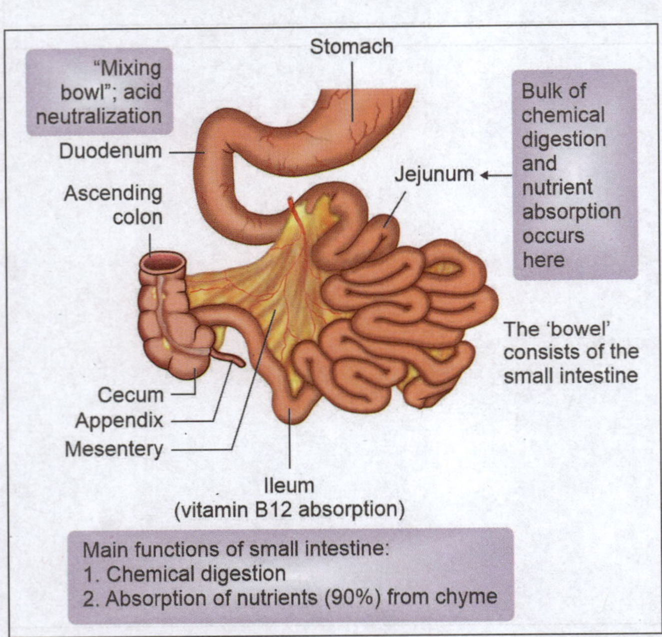

Color Plate 8: Small intestine

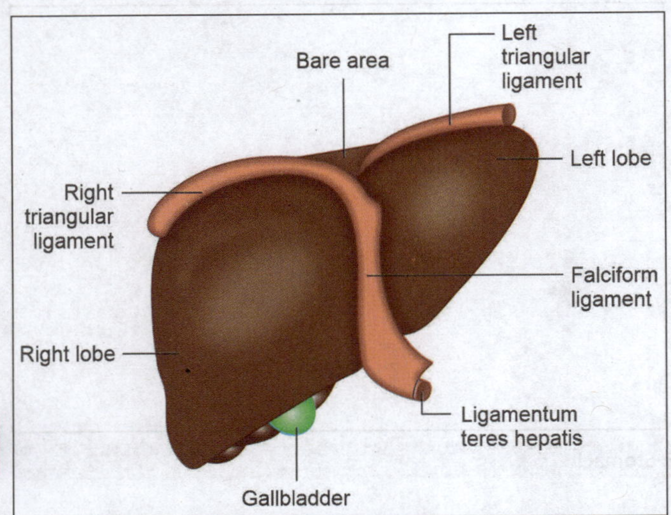

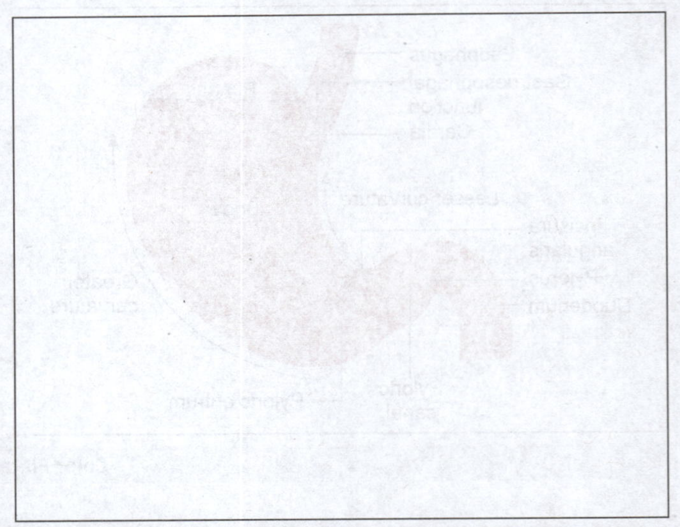

Color Plate 9: Ligaments of liver

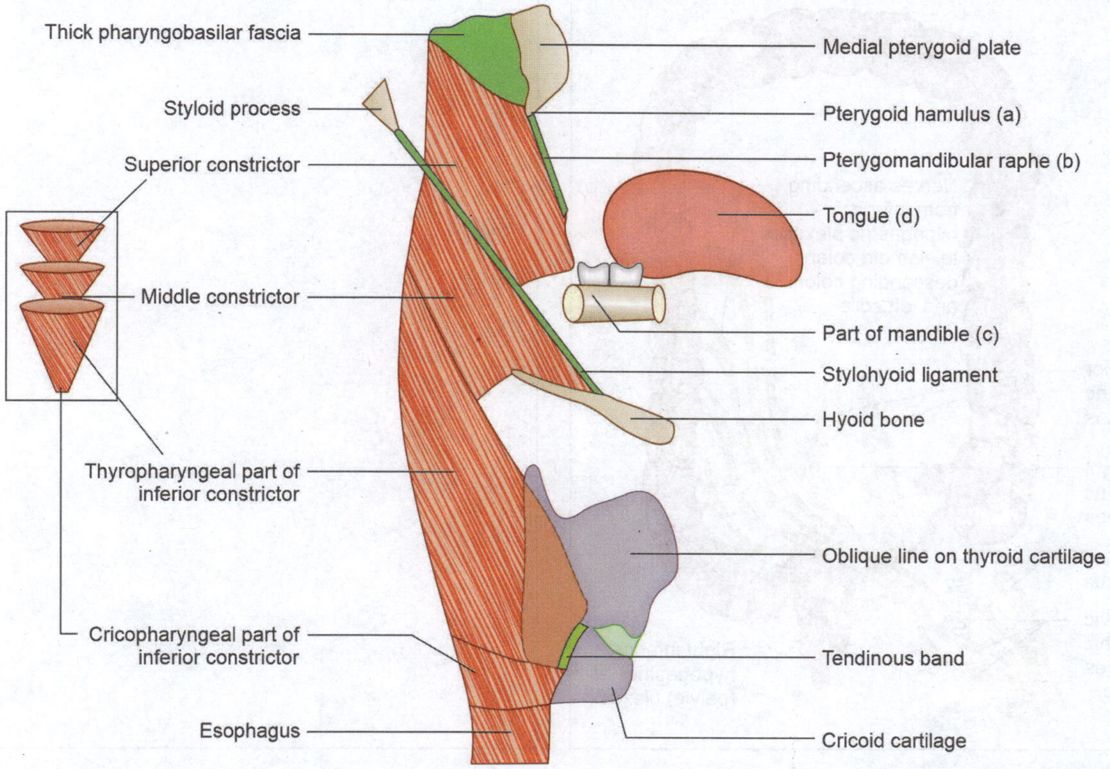

Color Plate 10: Muscles of pharynx

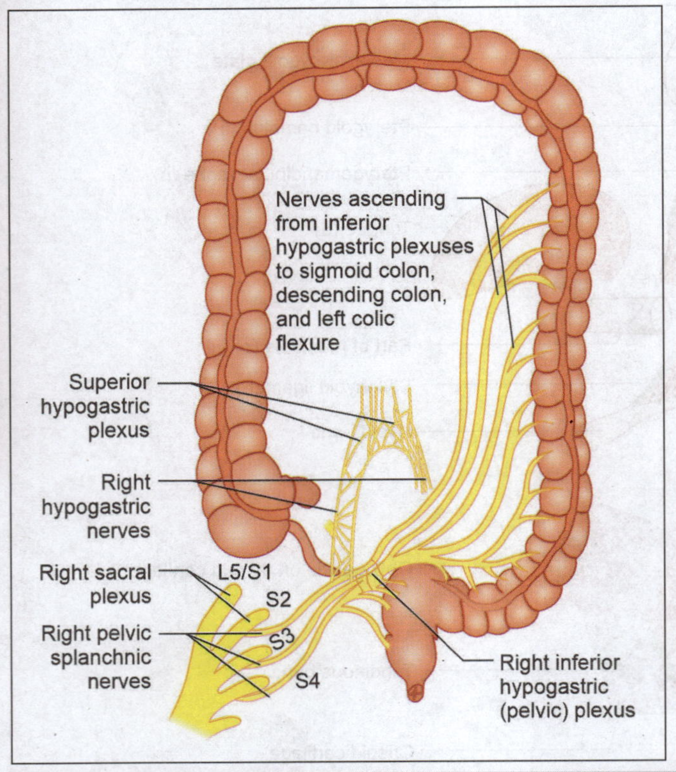

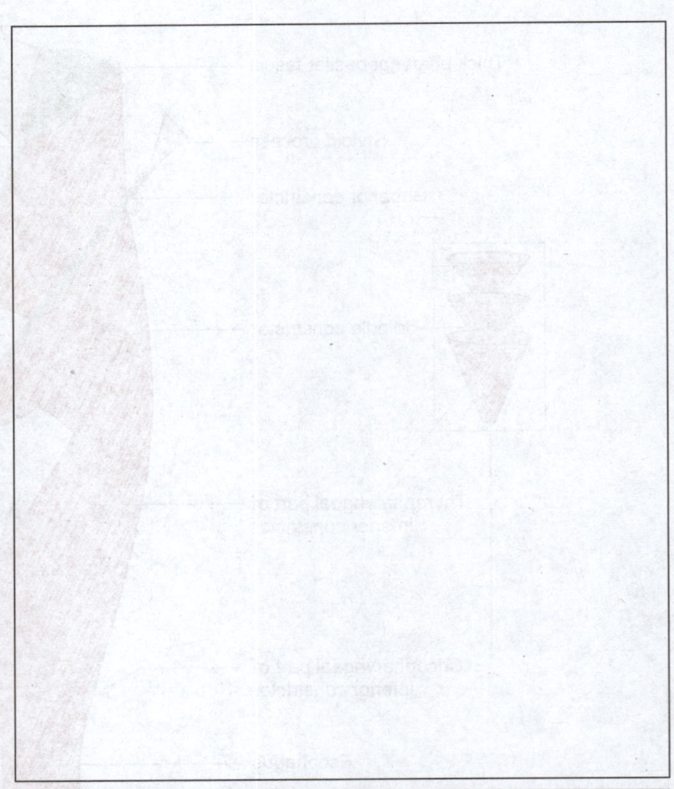

Color Plate 11: Large intestine

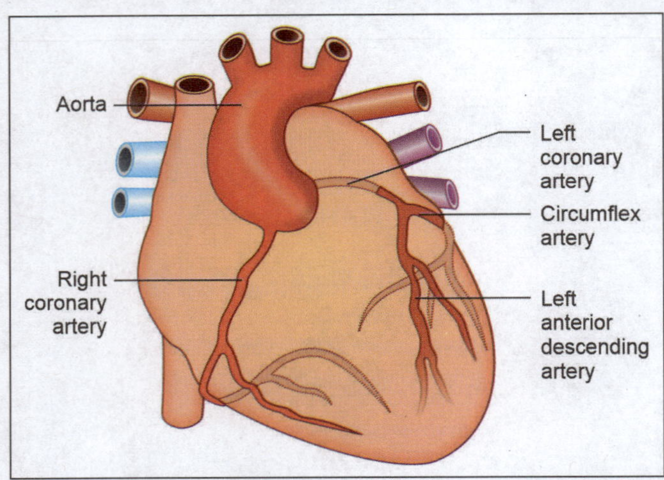

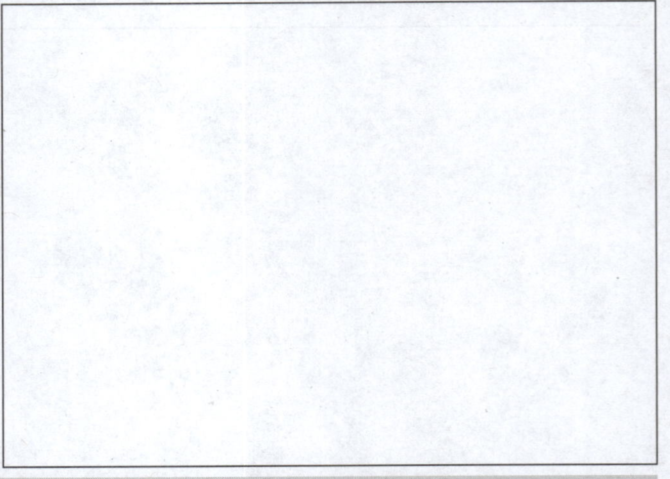

Color Plate 12: Coronary arteries

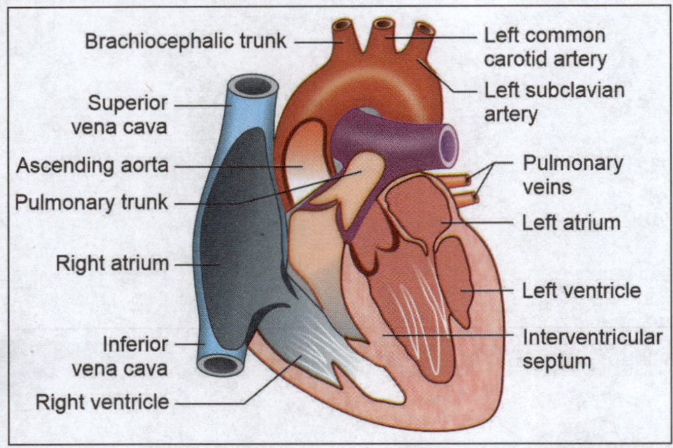

Color Plate 13: Coronal section of heart

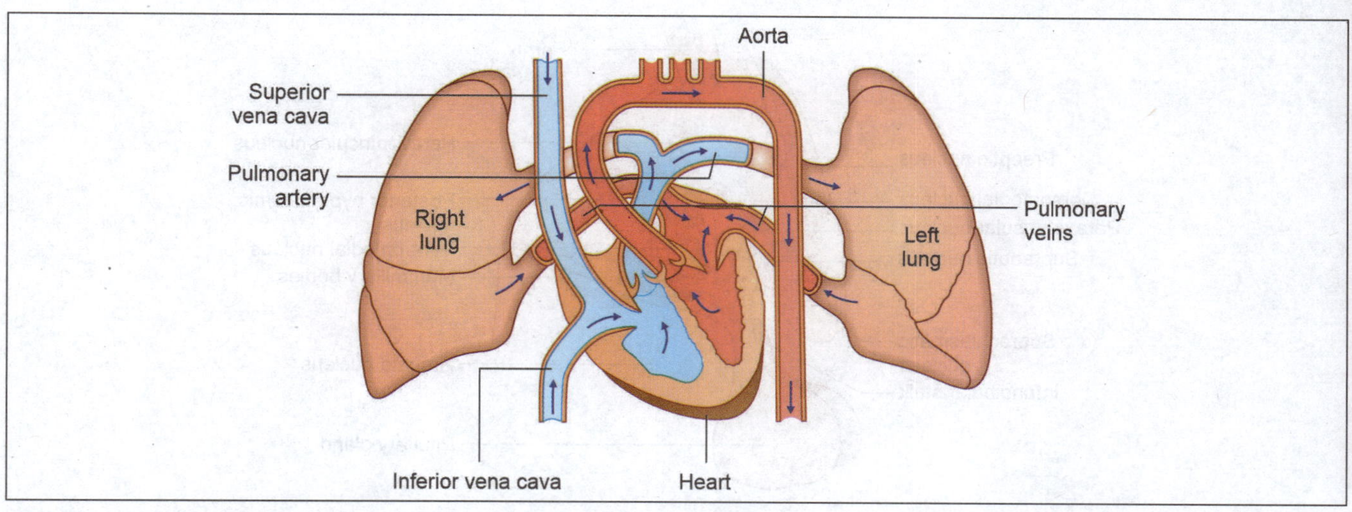

Color Plate 14: Pulmonary circulation

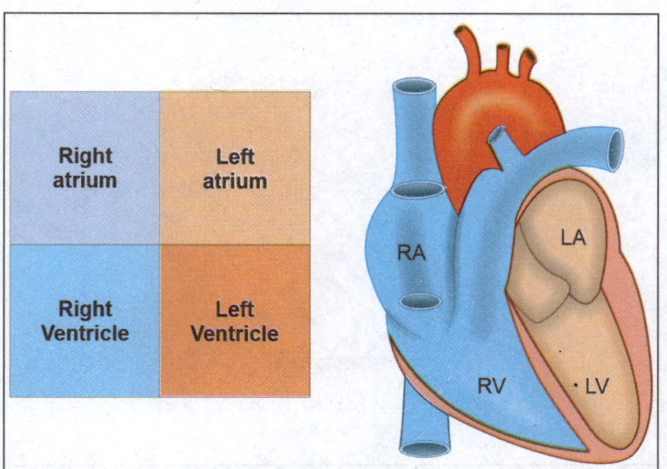

Color Plate 15: Chambers of heart

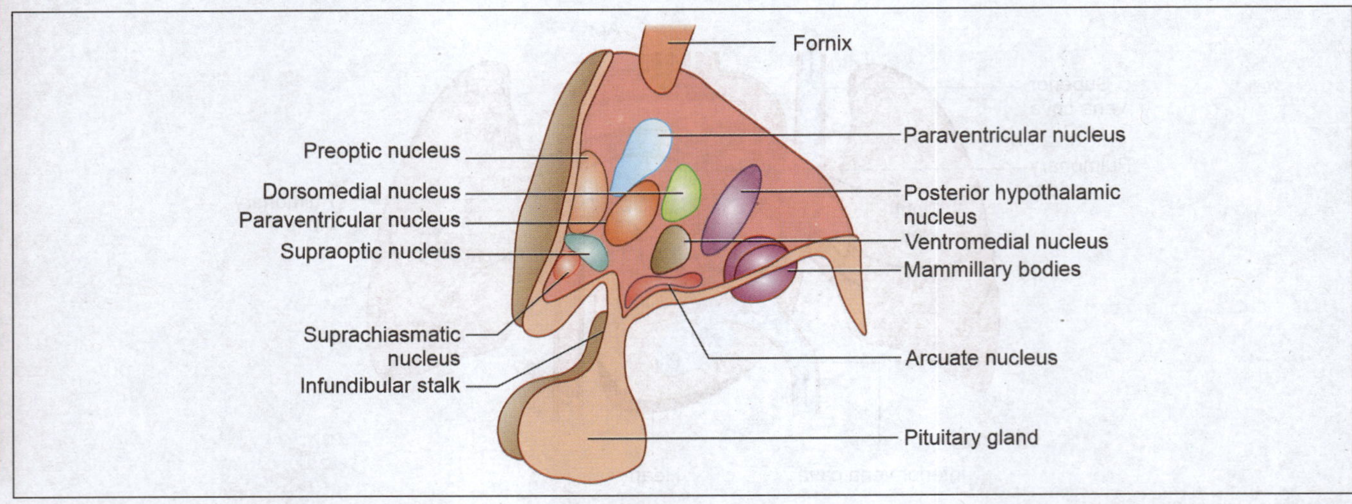

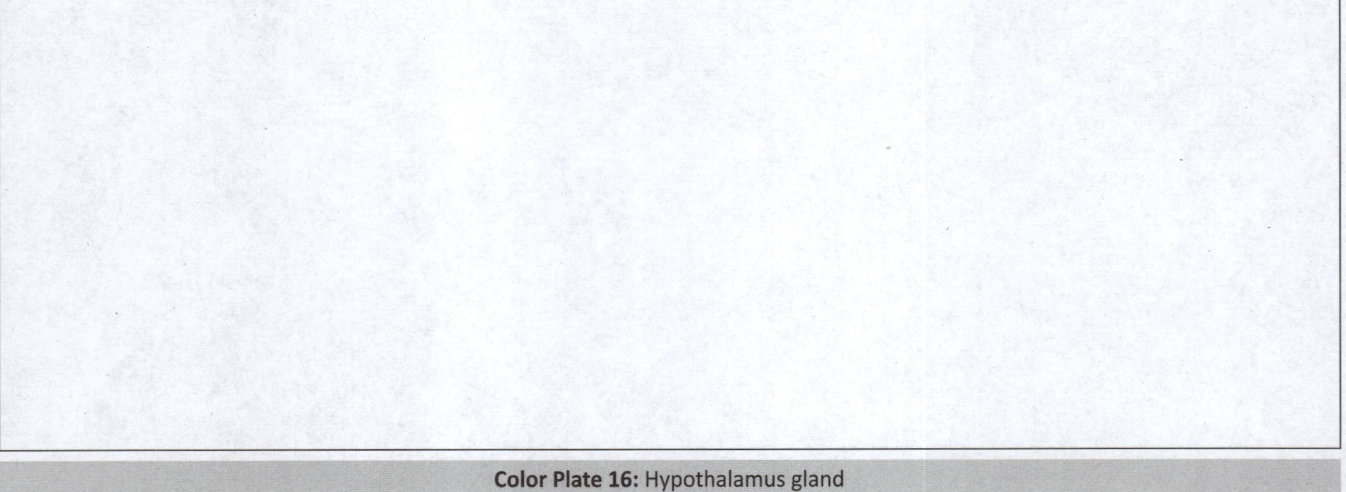

Color Plate 16: Hypothalamus gland

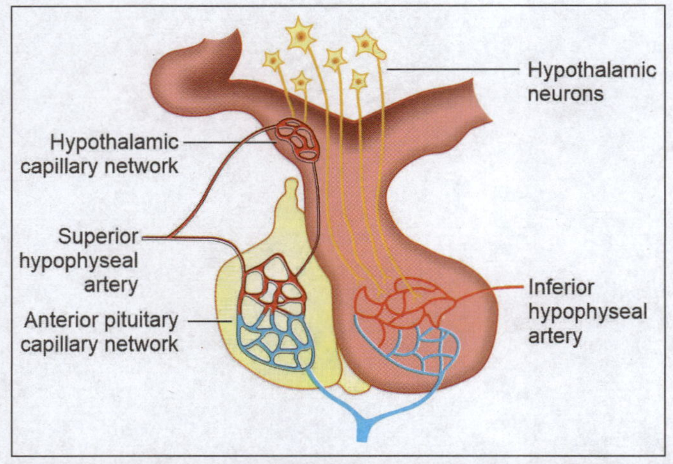

Color Plate 17: Pituitary gland

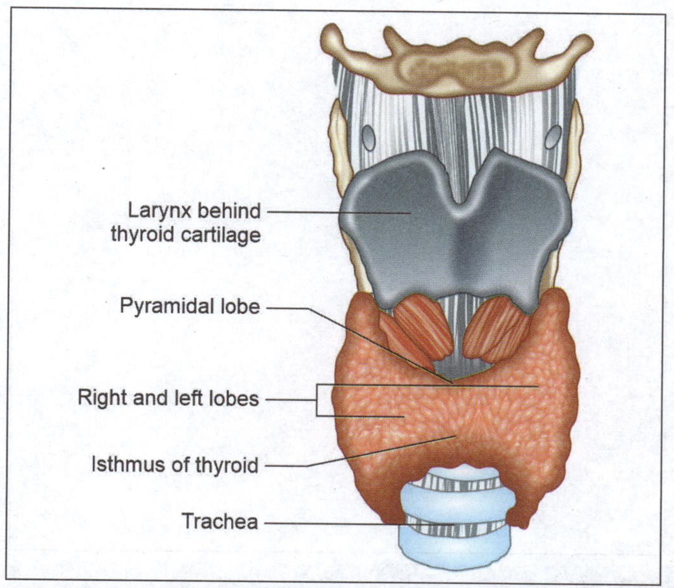

Color Plate 18: Thyroid gland

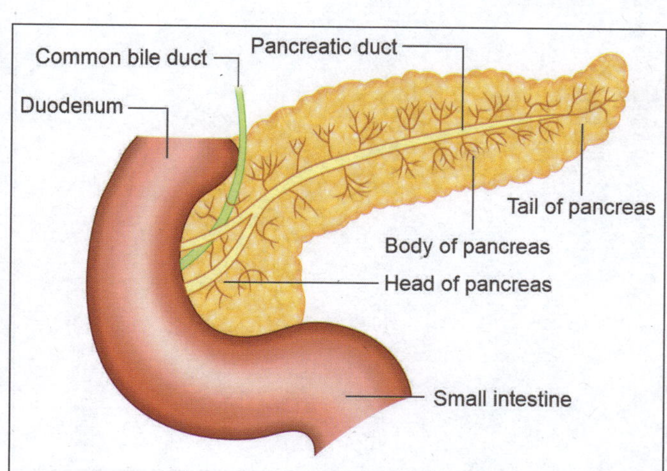

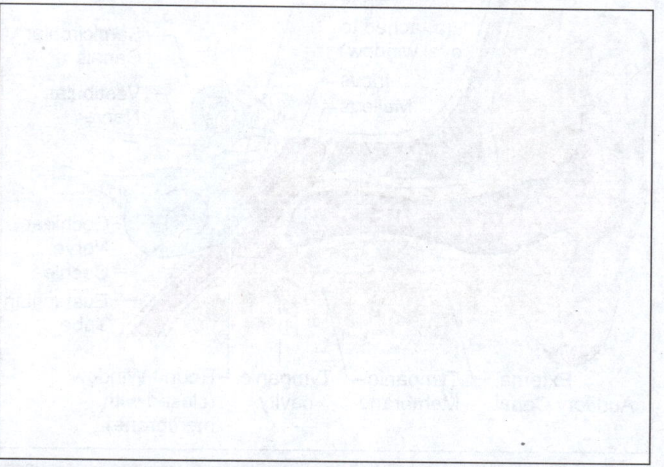

Color Plate 19: Pancreas

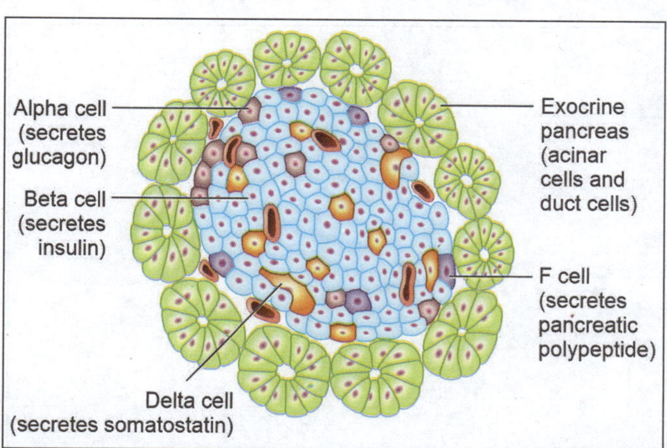

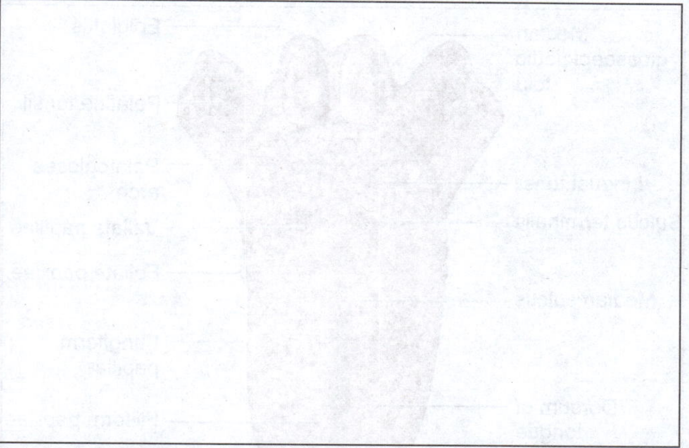

Color Plate 20: Islets of Langerhans

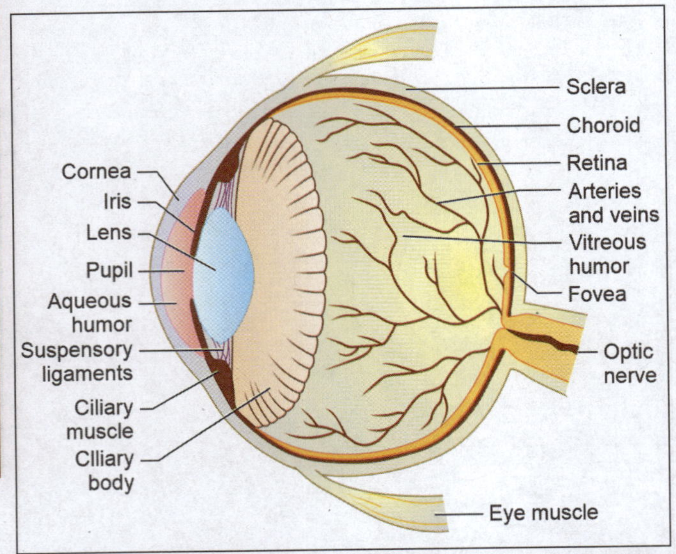

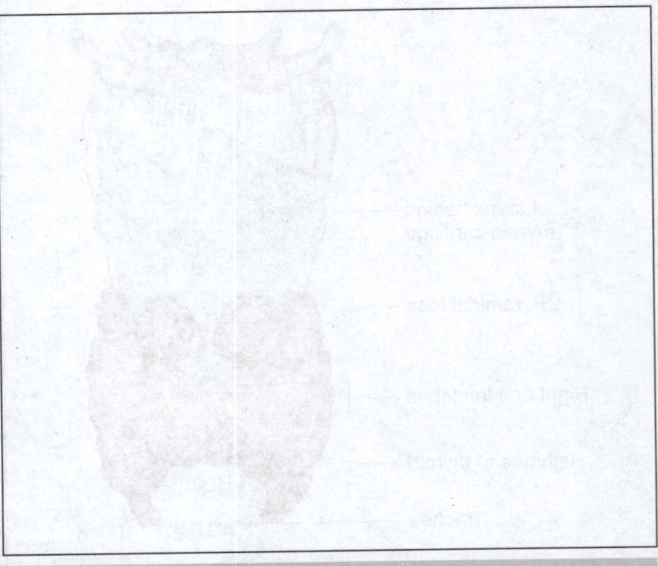

Color Plate 21: Structure of eye

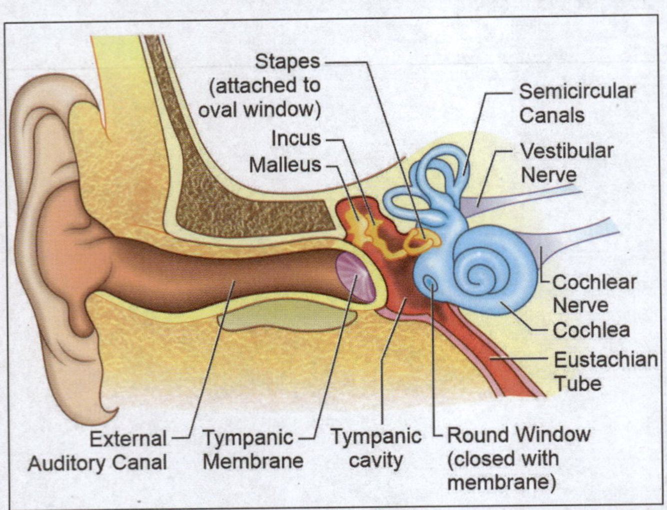

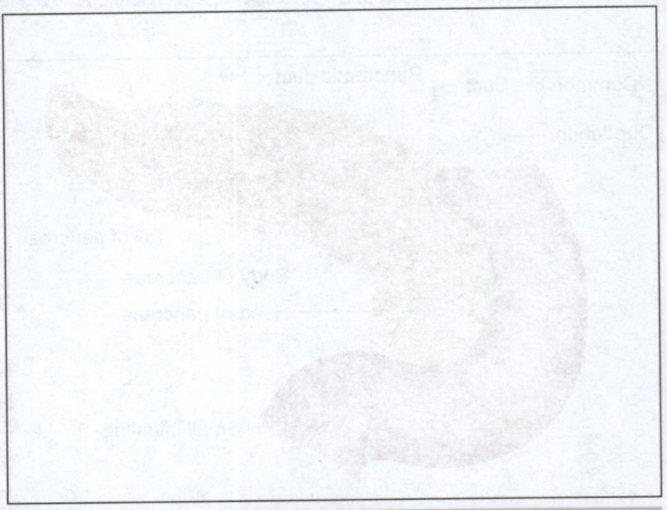

Color Plate 22: Structure of ear

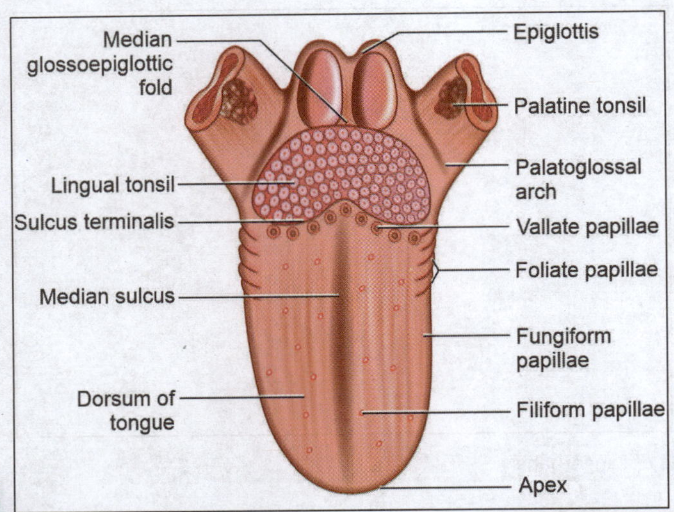

Color Plate 23: Structure of tongue

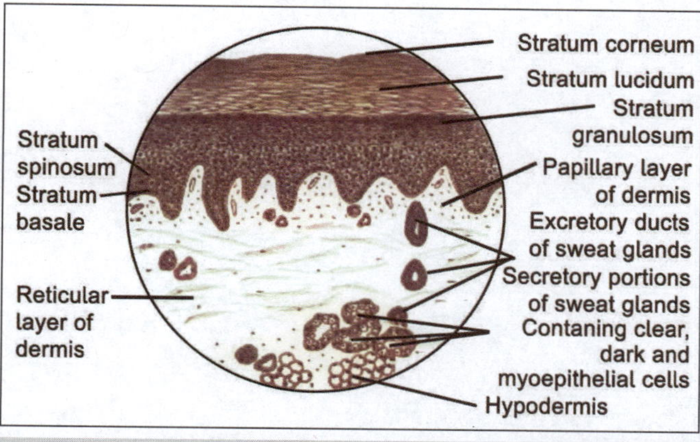

Color Plate 24: Microanatomy of skin

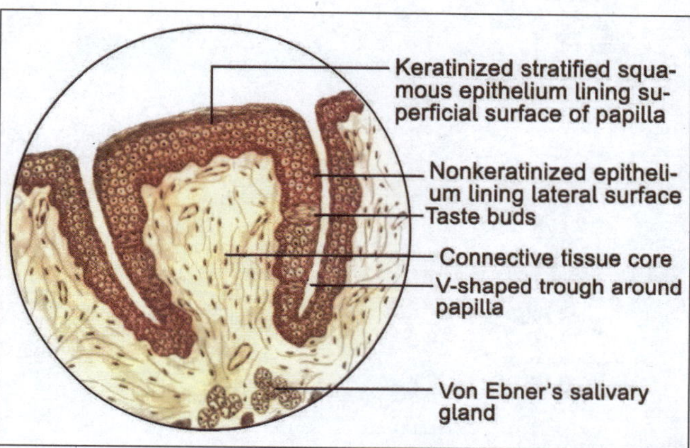

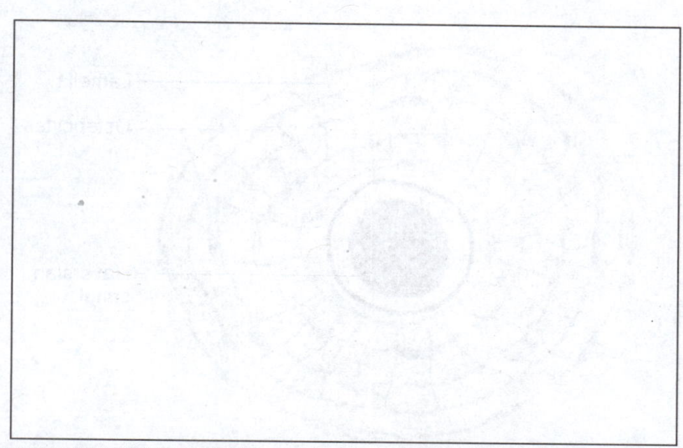

Color Plate 25: Circumvallate papillae

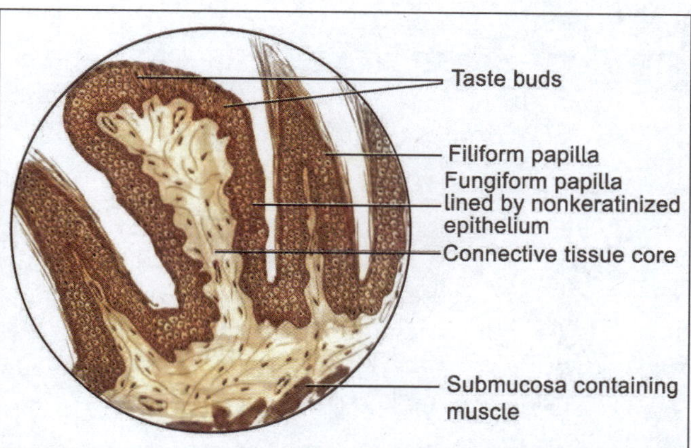

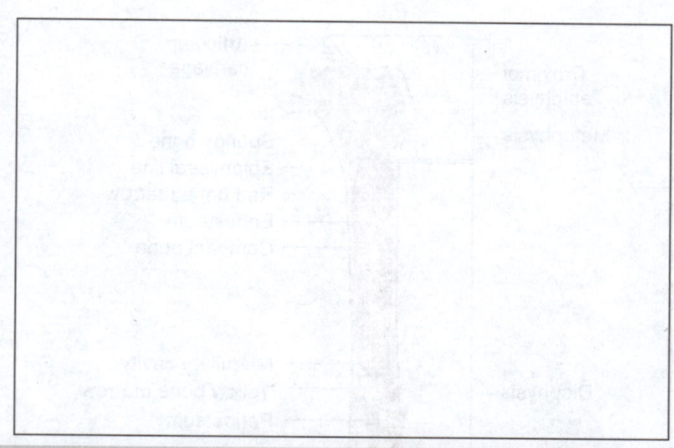

Color Plate 26: Fungiform and filiform papillae

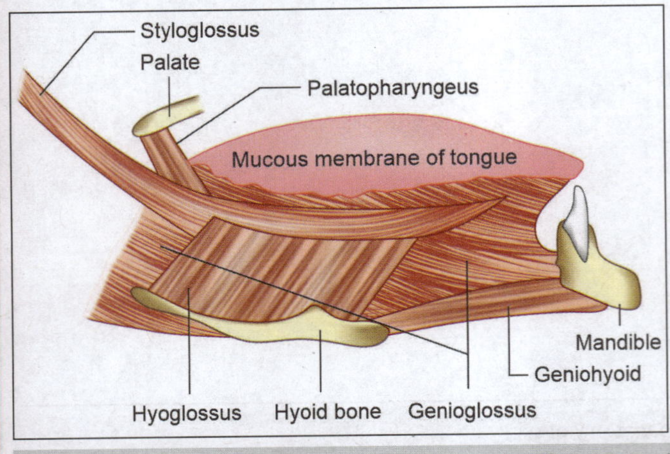

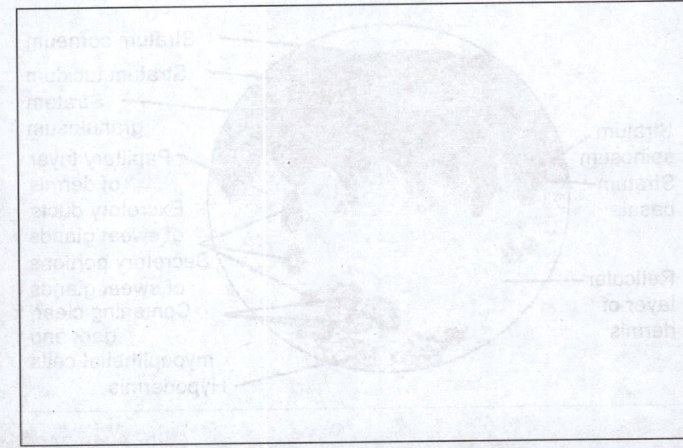

Color Plate 27: Extrinsic muscles of tongue

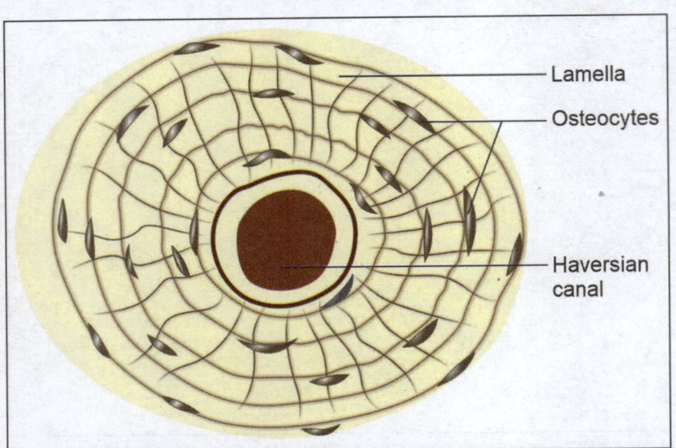

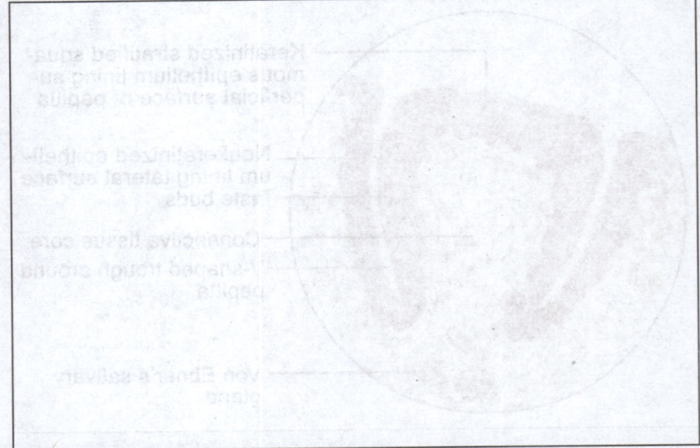

Color Plate 28: Haversian canal with osteocytes and lacuna

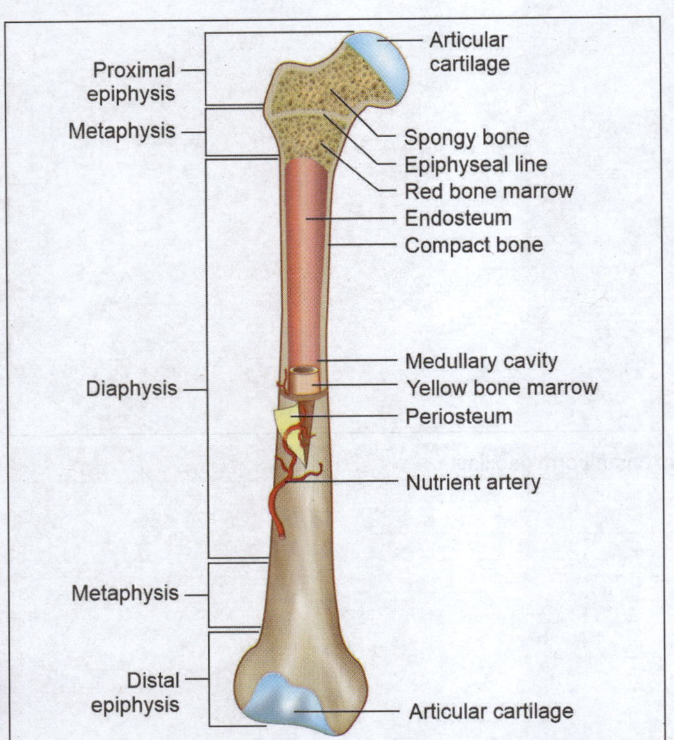

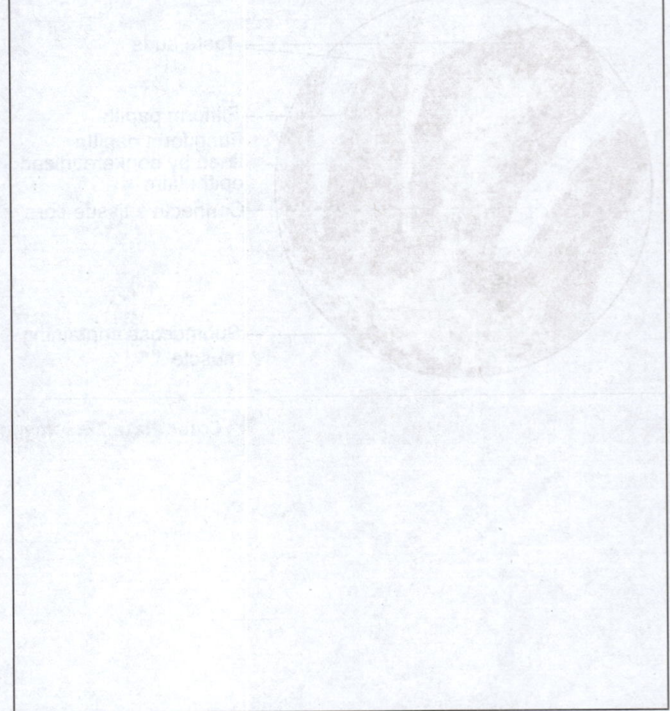

Color Plate 29: Structure of long bone

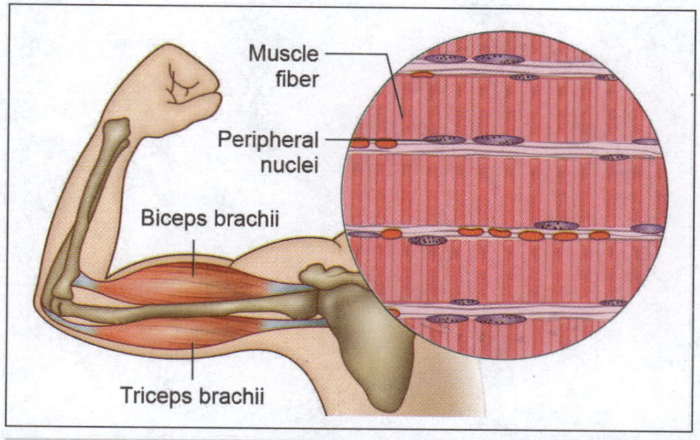

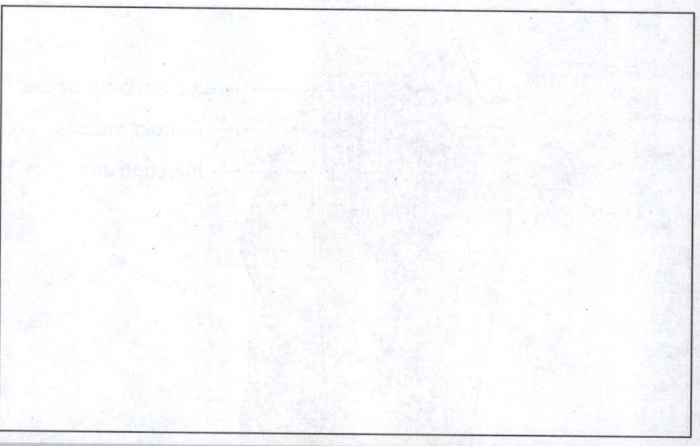

Color Plate 30: Striated muscle

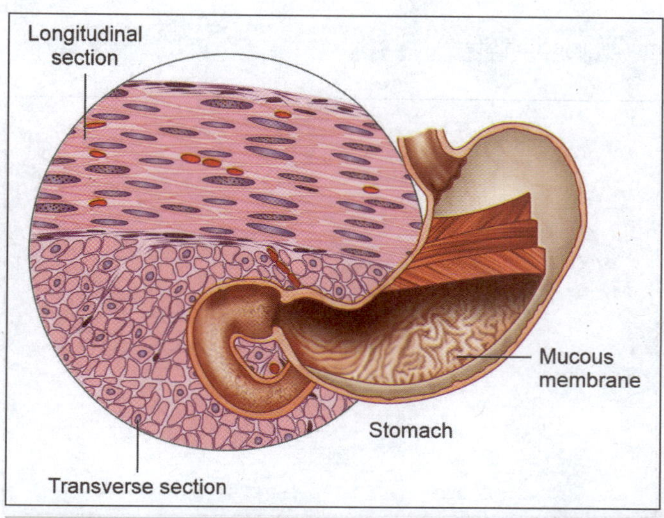

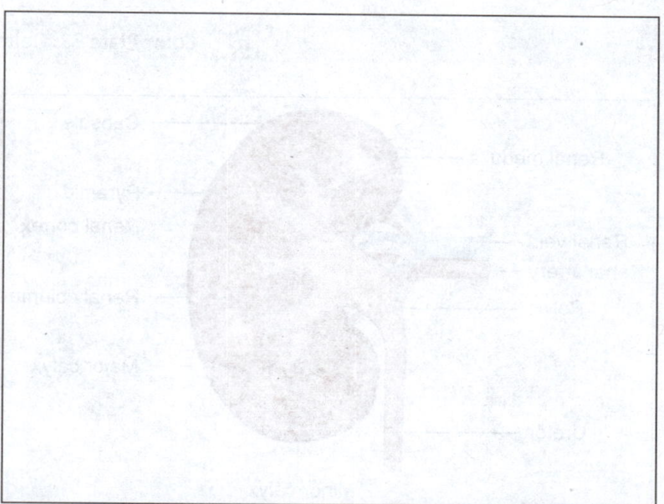

Color Plate 31: Smooth muscle

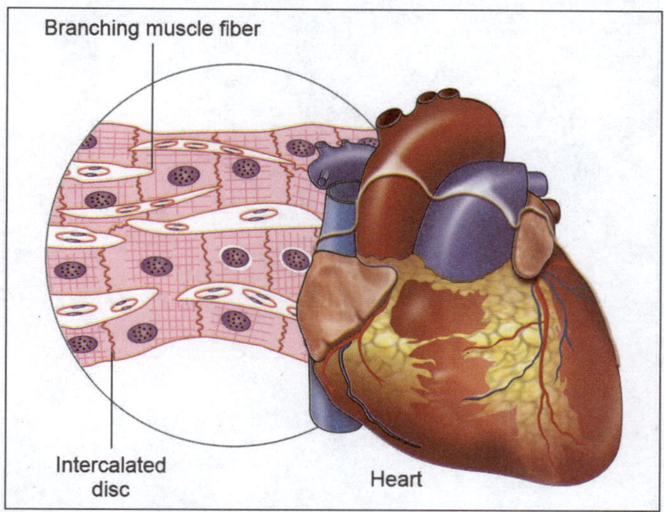

Color Plate 32: Cardiac muscle

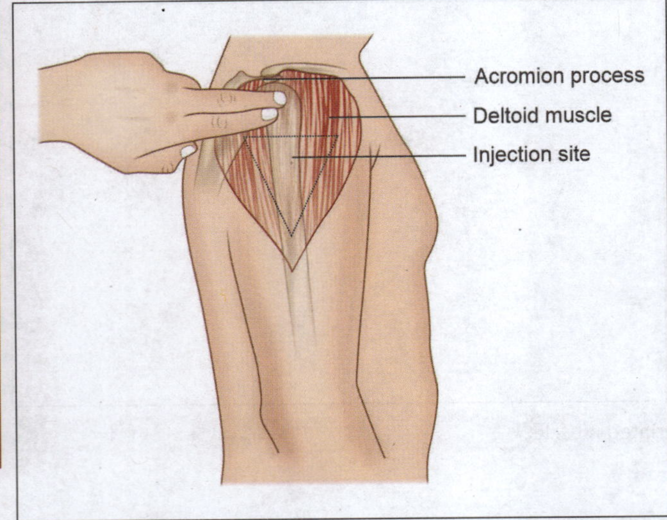

Color Plate 33: Deltoid muscle injection site

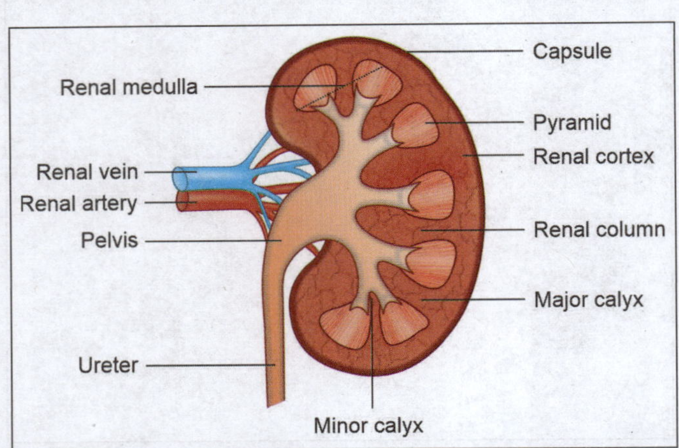

Color Plate 34: Structure of kidney

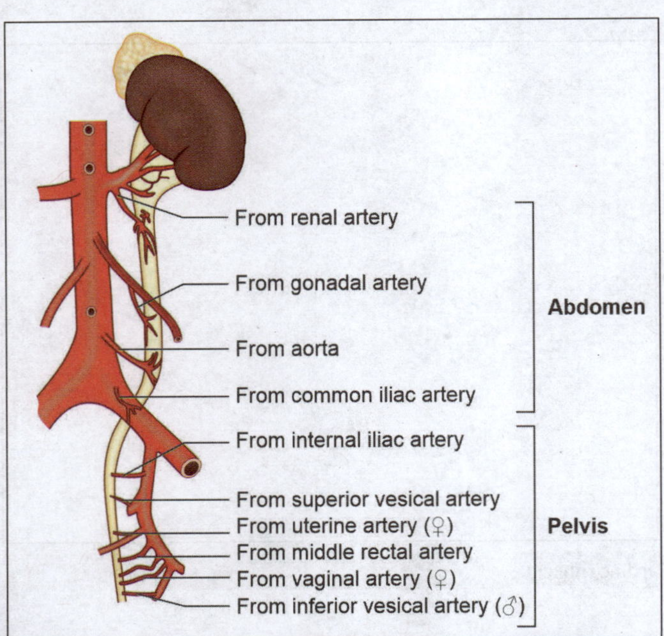

Color Plate 35: Blood supply of urinary bladder

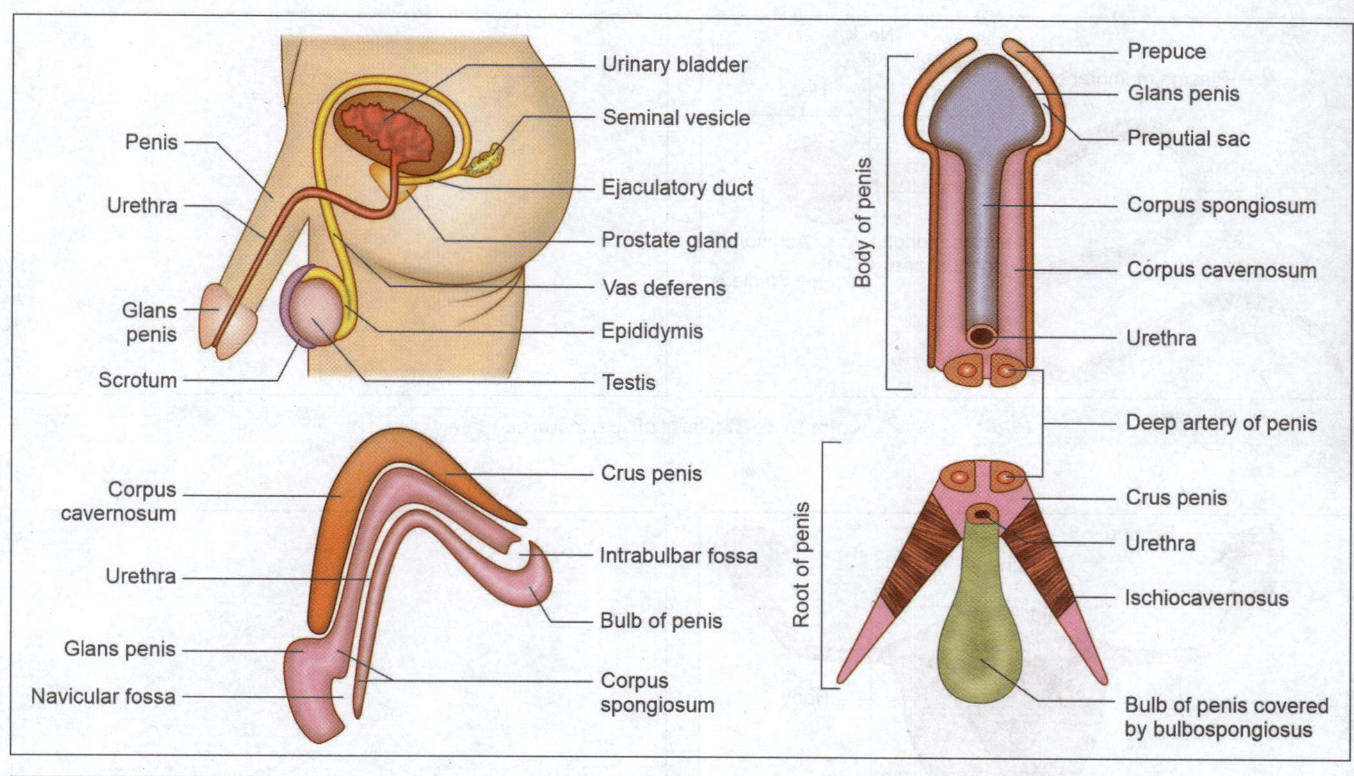

Color Plate 36: Male genital organs

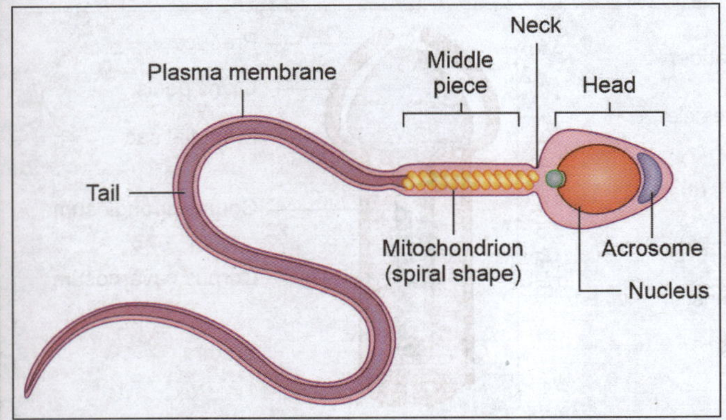

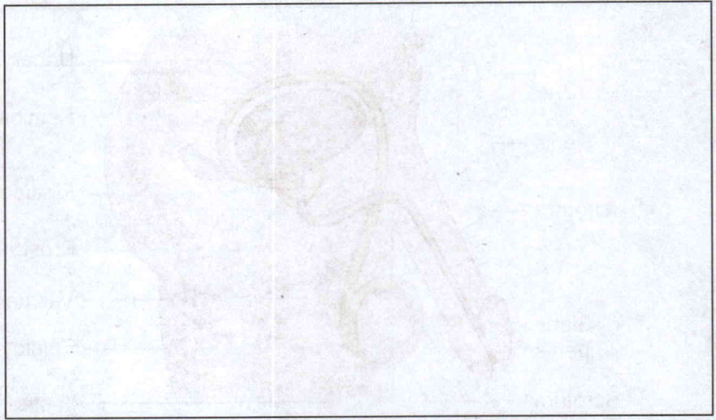

Color Plate 37: Parts of spermatozoa

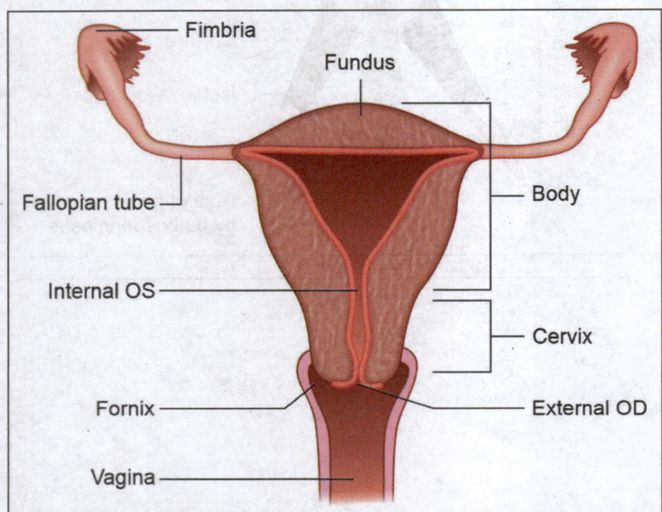

Color Plate 38: Female genital organs

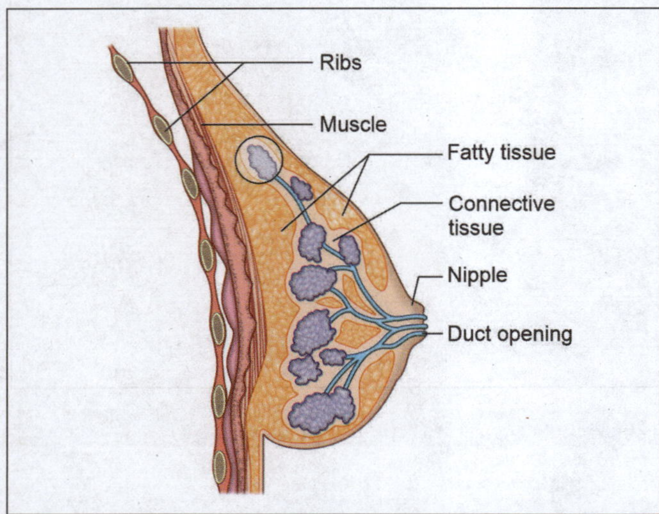

Color Plate 39: Structure of breast

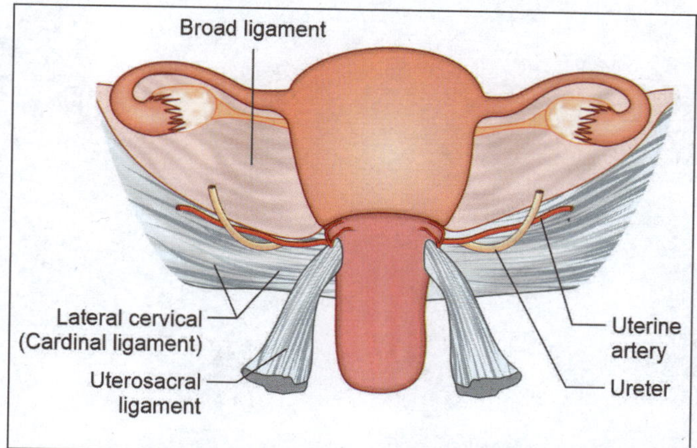

Color Plate 40: Ligament supports of uterus

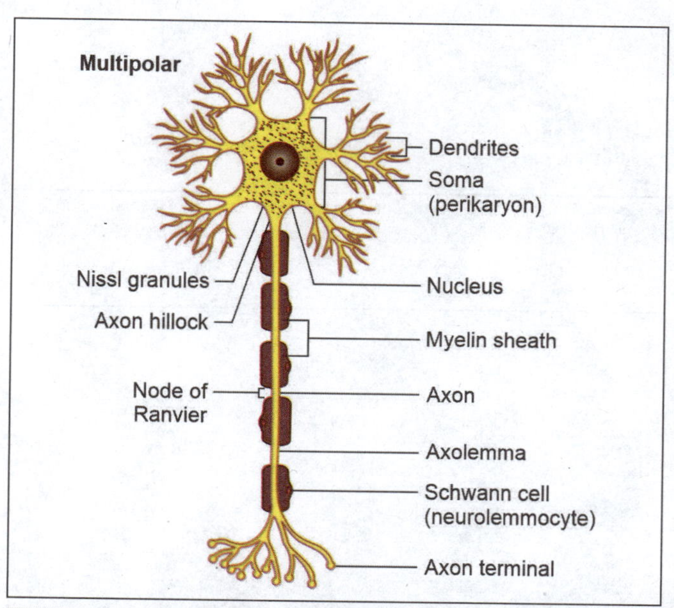

Color Plate 41: Multipolar neuron

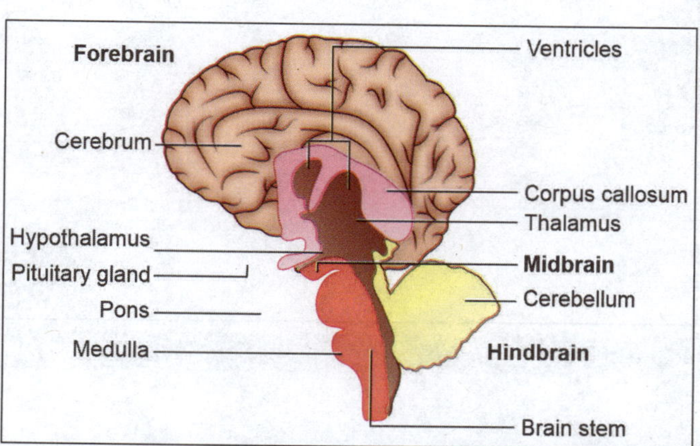

Color Plate 42: Transverse section of cerebrum

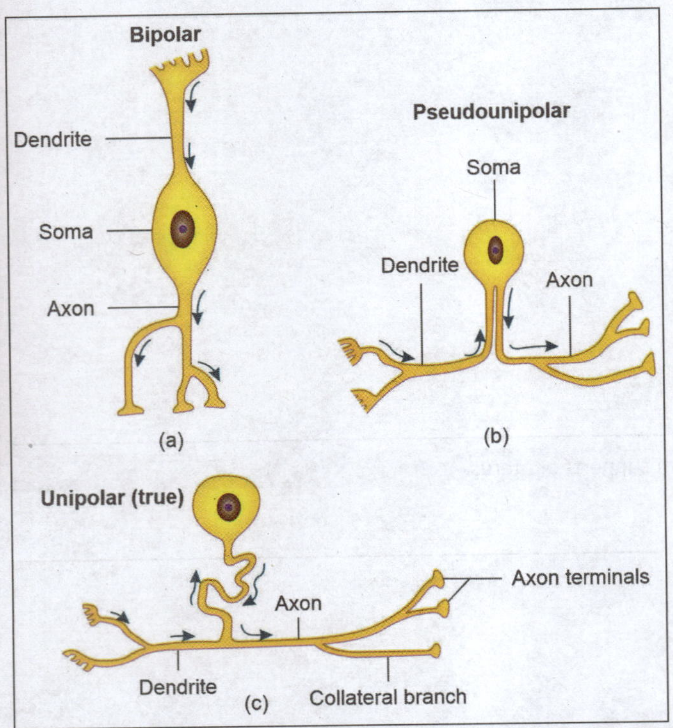

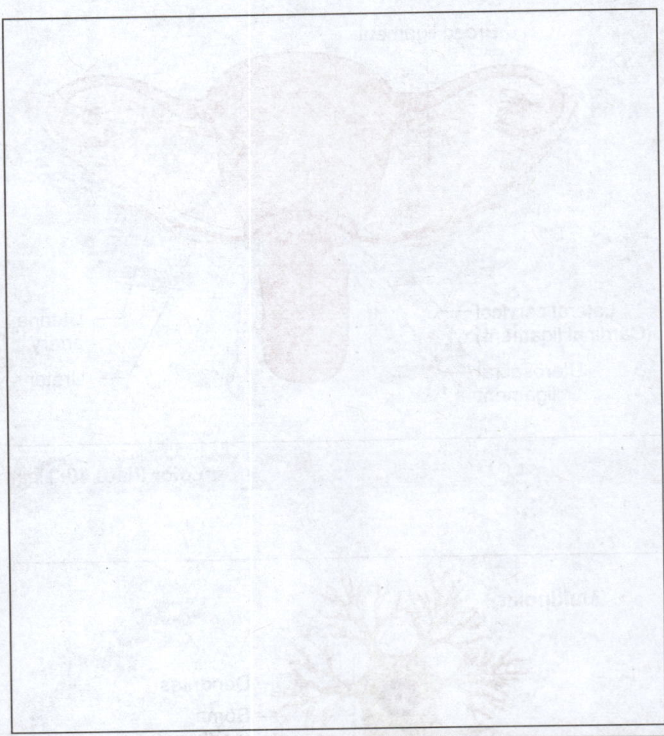

Color Plate 43: Types of neurons

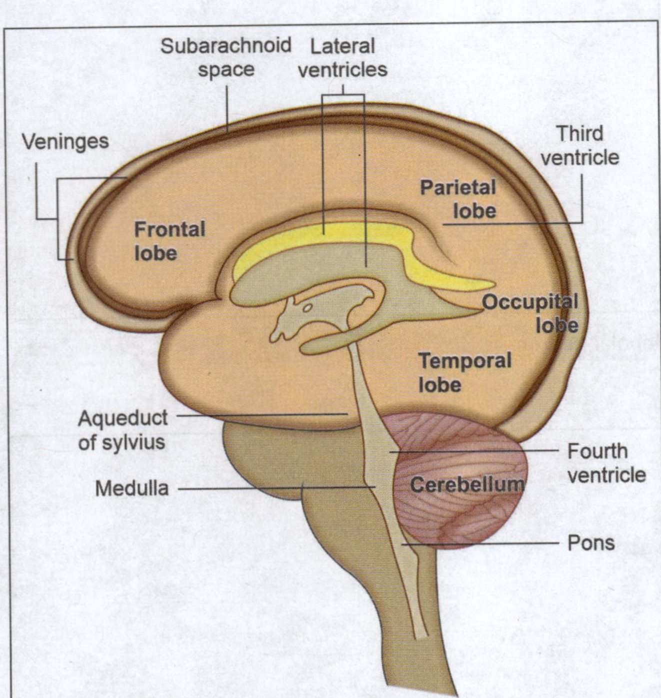

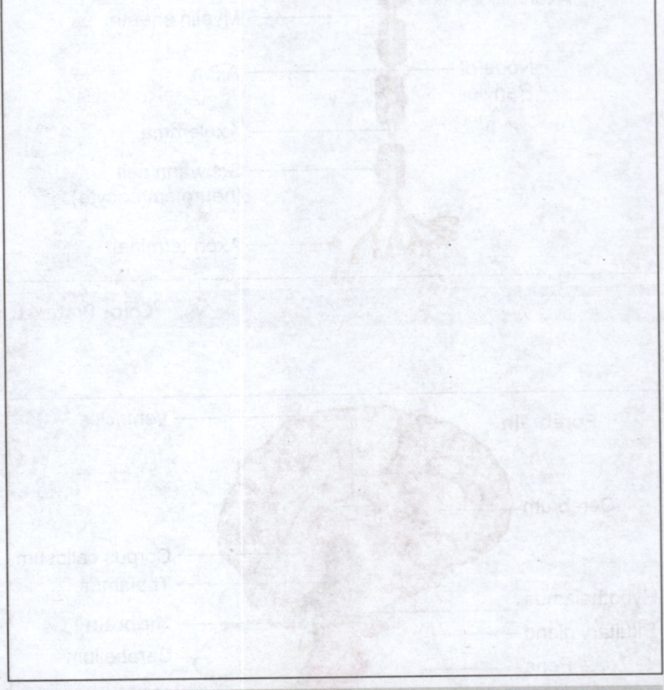

Color Plate 44: Structure of brain

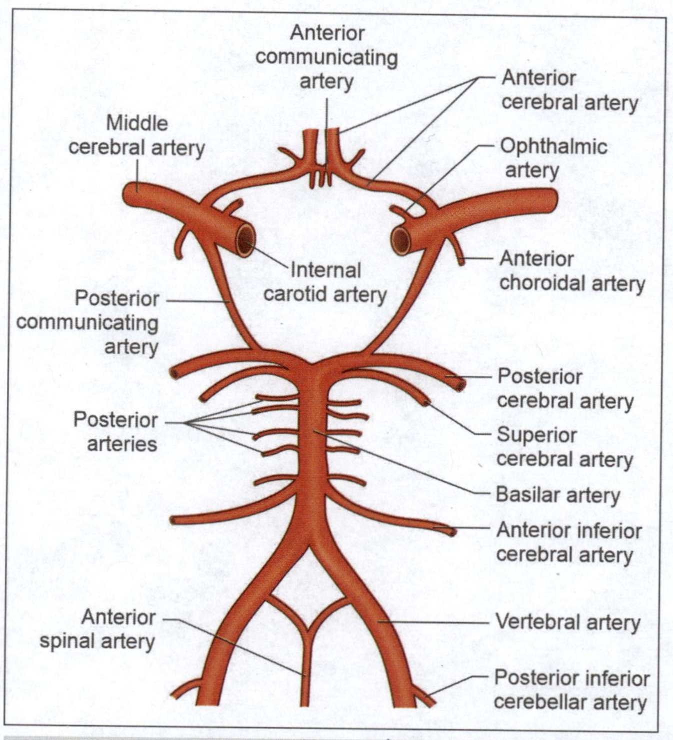

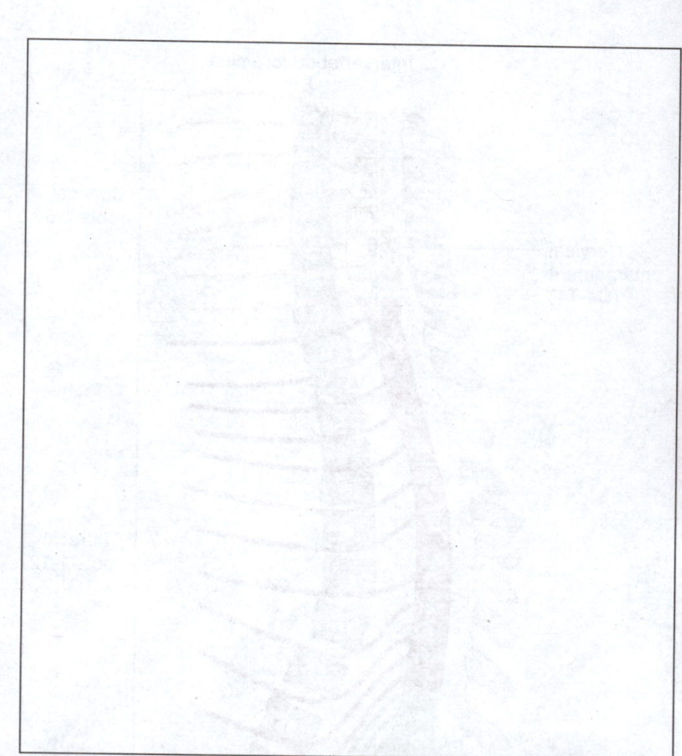

Color Plate 45: Circle of Willis

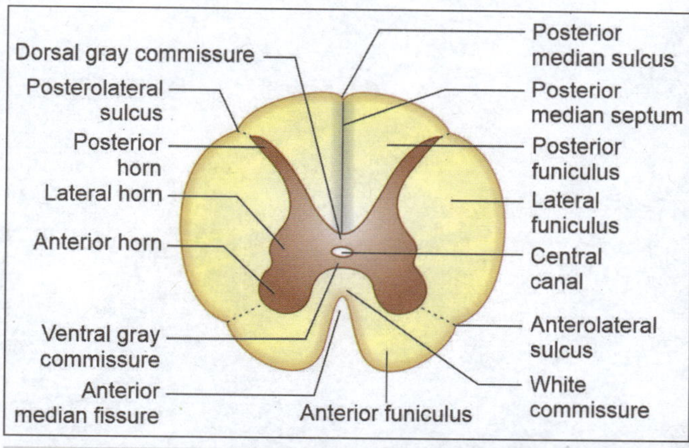

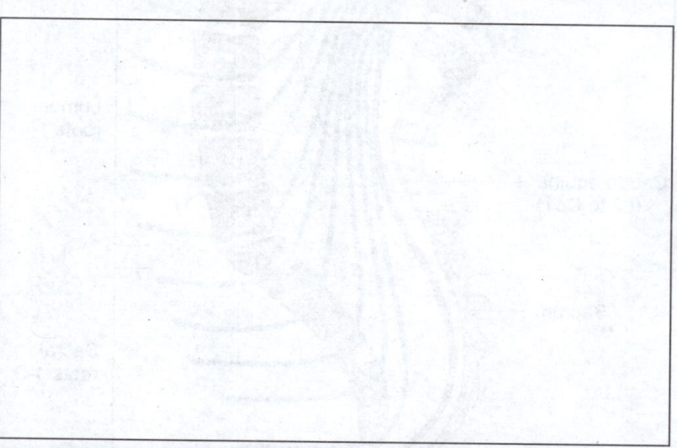

Color Plate 46: Microscopic structure of spinal cord

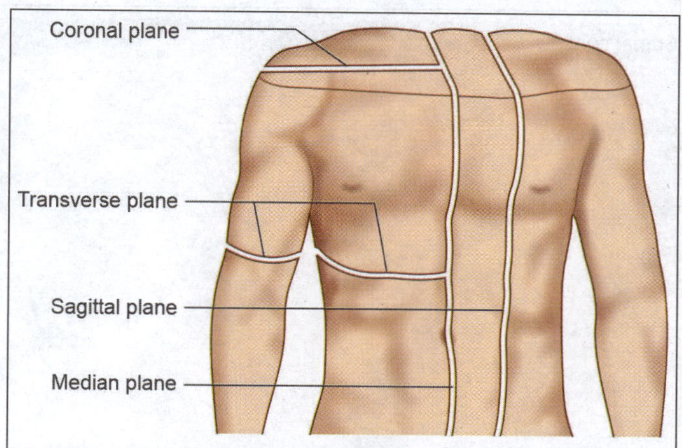

Color Plate 47: Anatomical planes

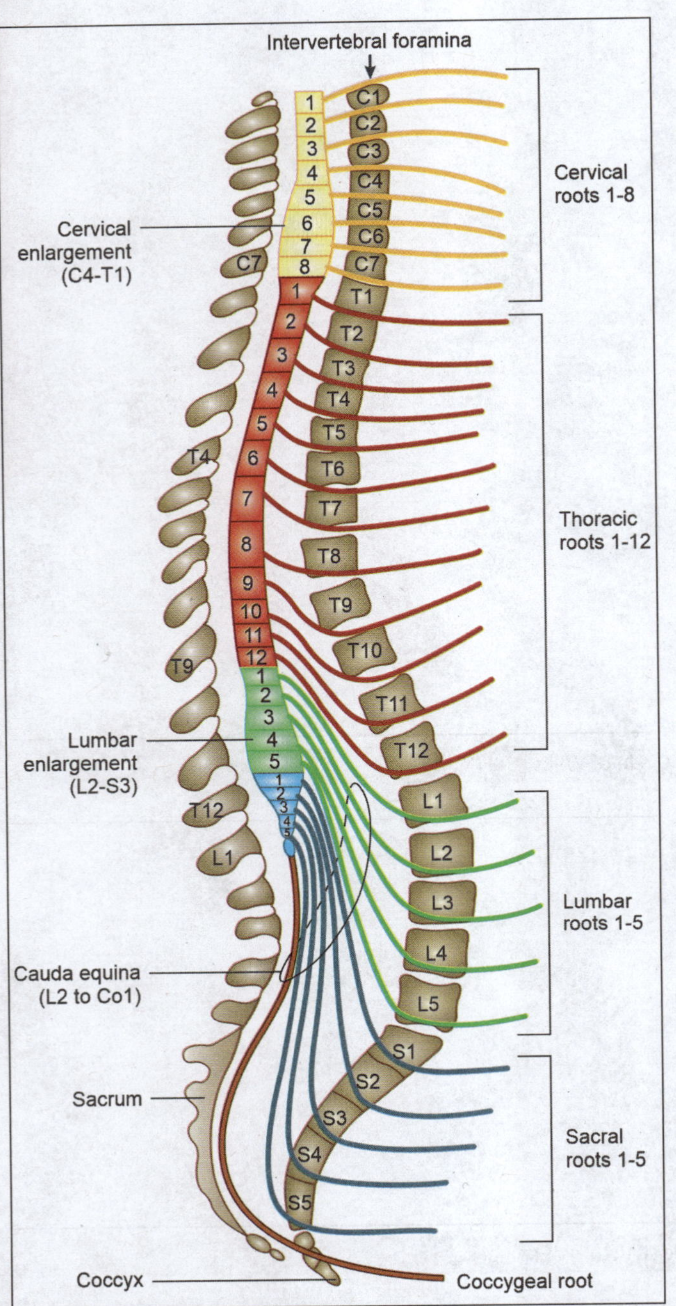

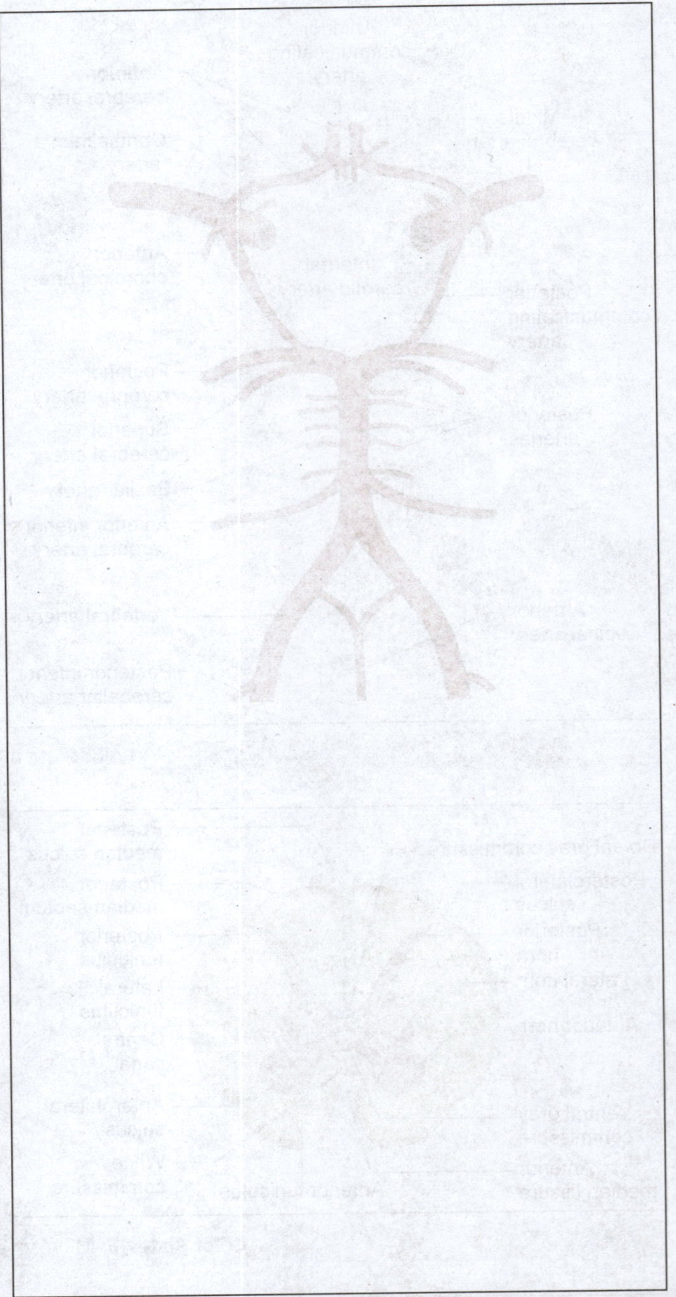

Color Plate 48: Spinal cord

APPLIED PHYSIOLOGY

Color Plates	Get Yourself Practice

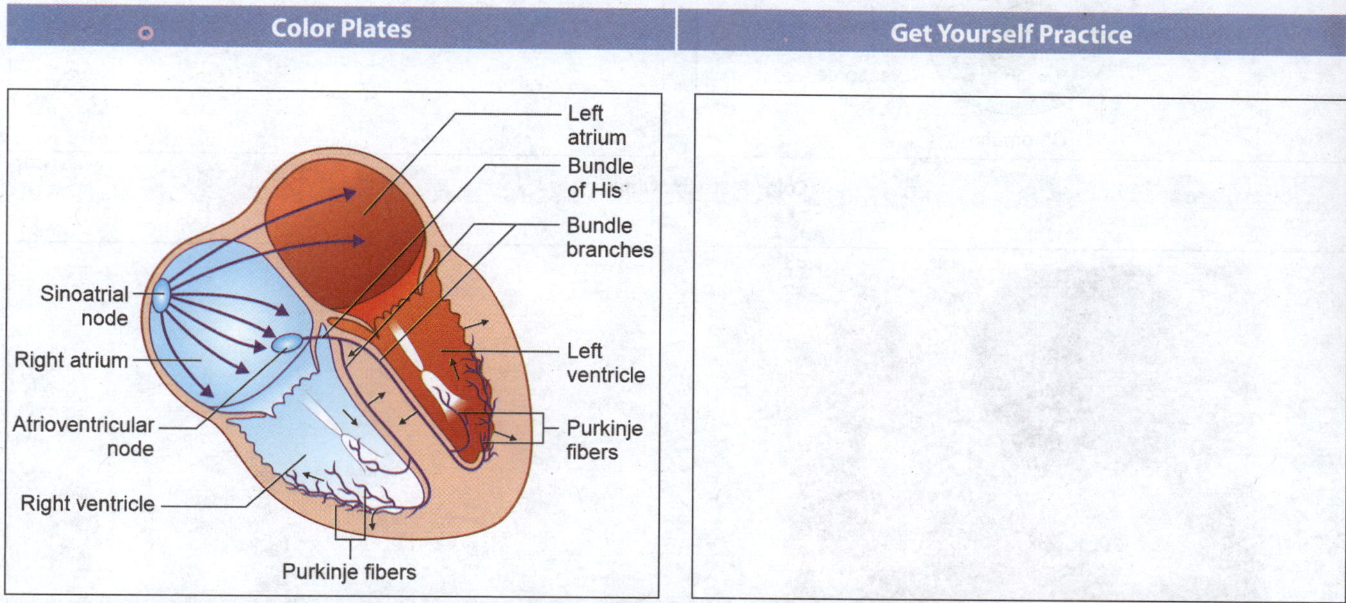

Color Plate 49: Conduction system of the heart and spread of impulse

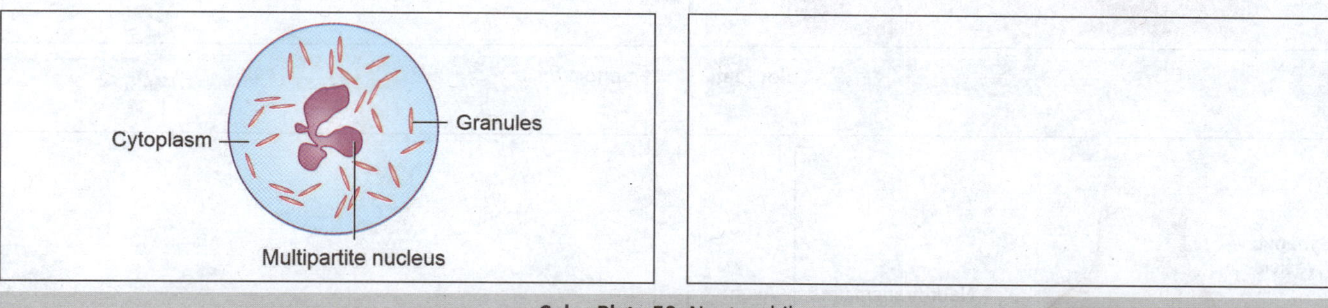

Color Plate 50: Neutrophils

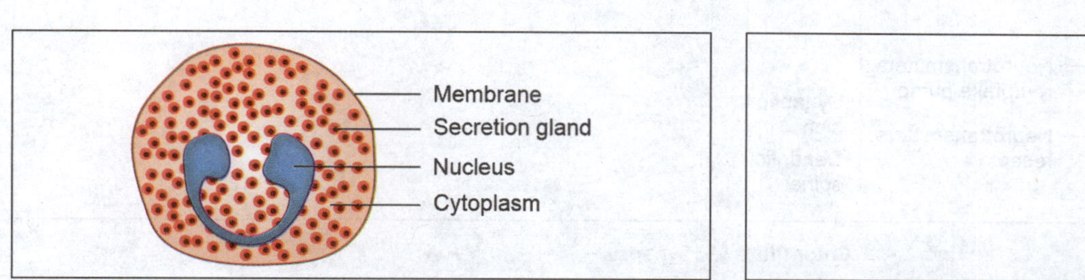

Color Plate 51: Eosinophils

Color Plate 52: Basophils

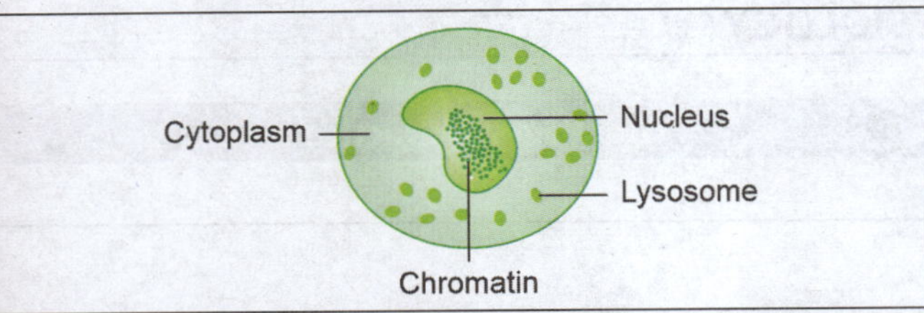

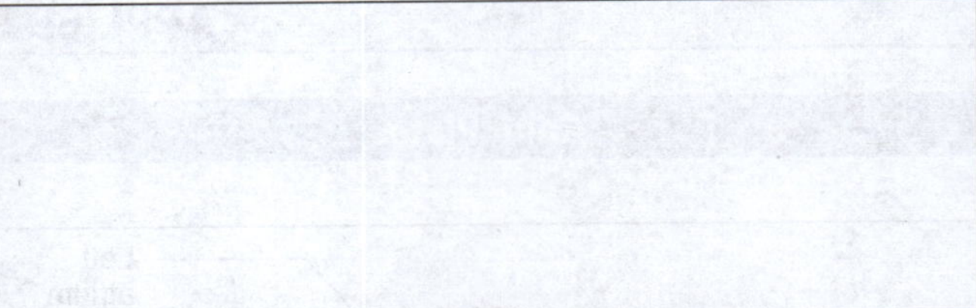

Color Plate 53: Monocytes

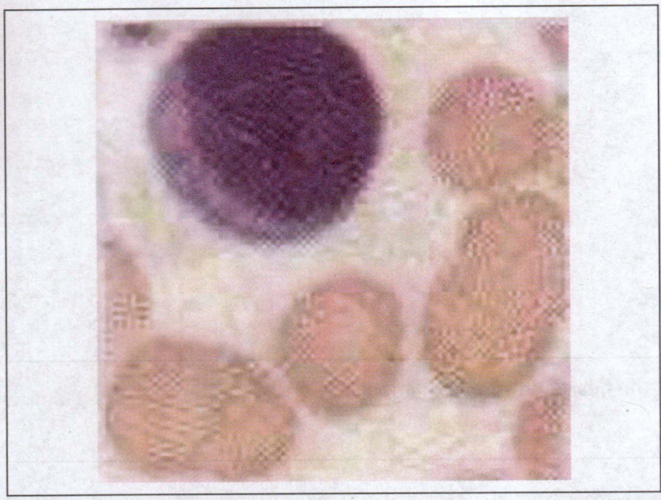

Color Plate 54: Lymphocytes

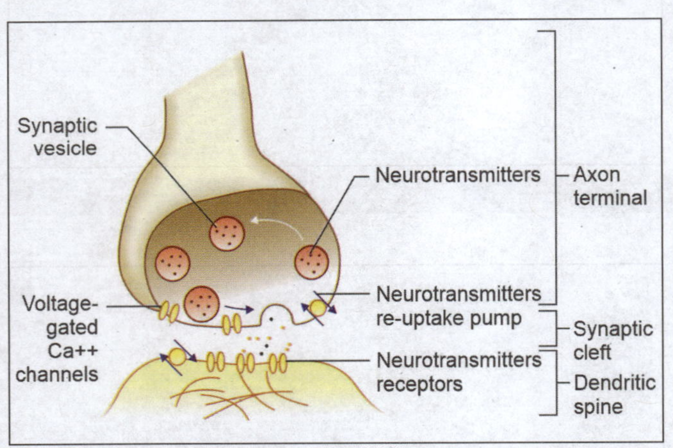

Color Plate 55: Synapse

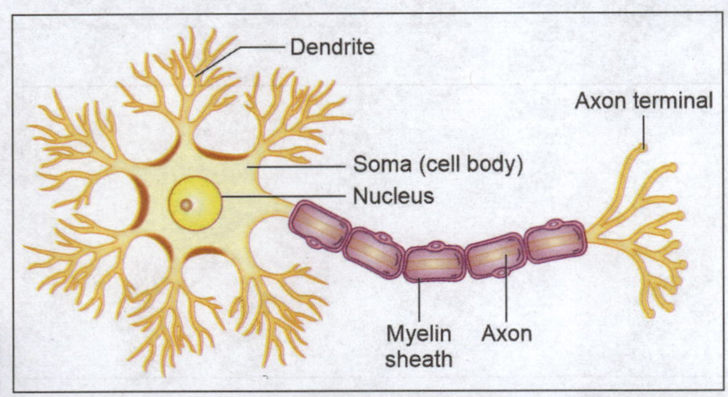

Color Plate 56: Structure of neuron

APPLIED BIOCHEMISTRY

Color Plates	Get Yourself Practice

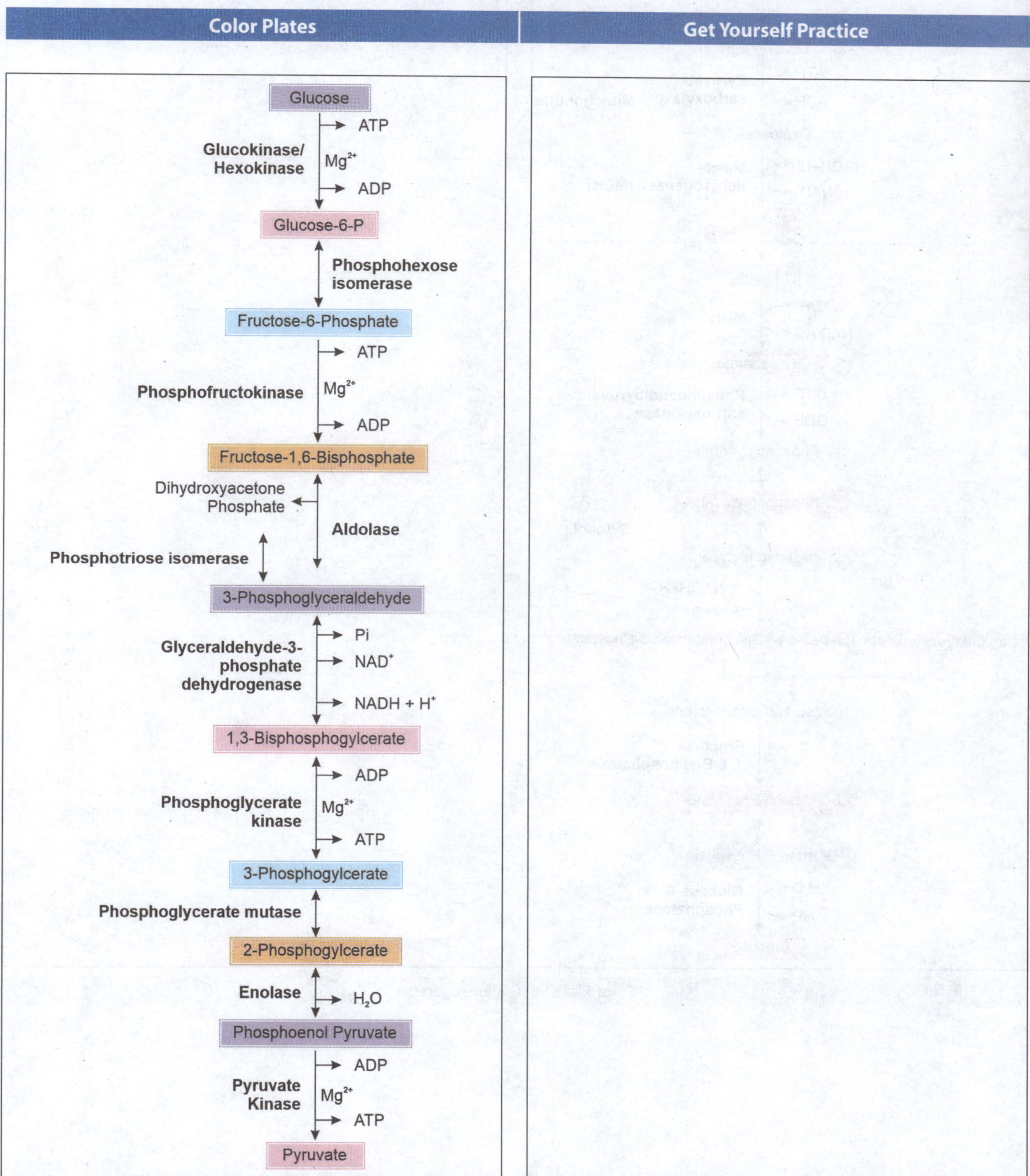

Color Plate 57: Metabolism of glucose via aerobic glycolysis

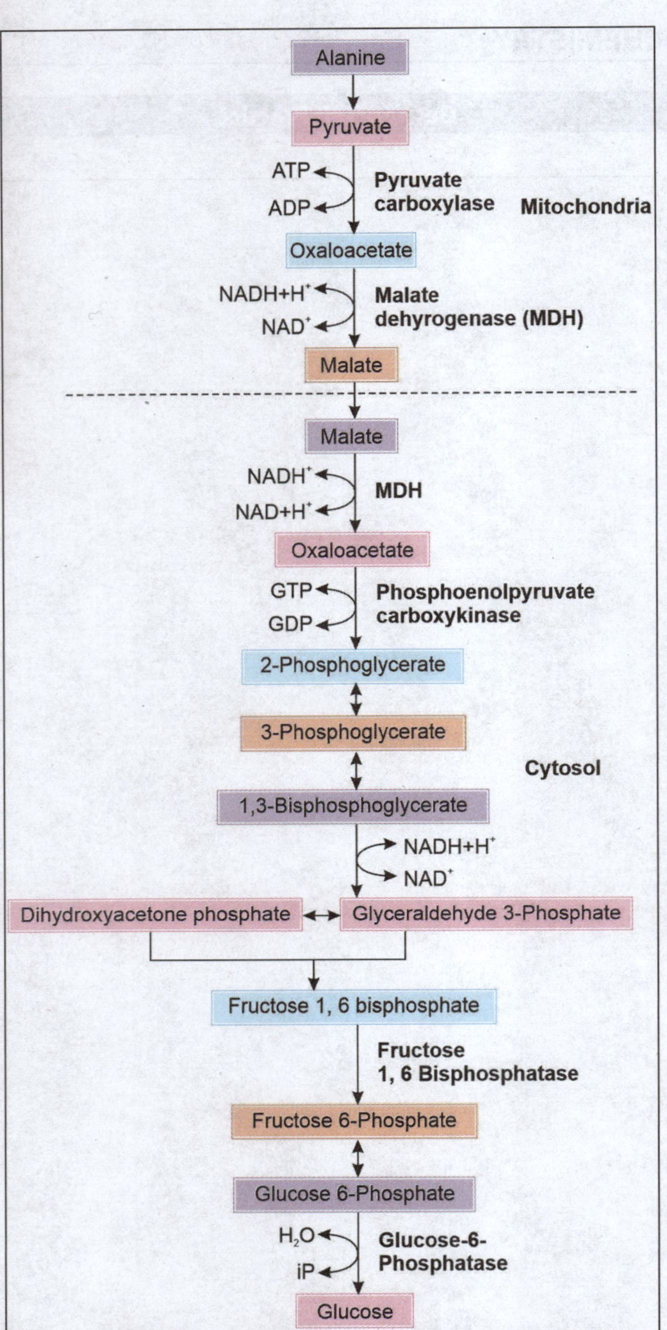

Color Plate 58: Gluconeogenesis

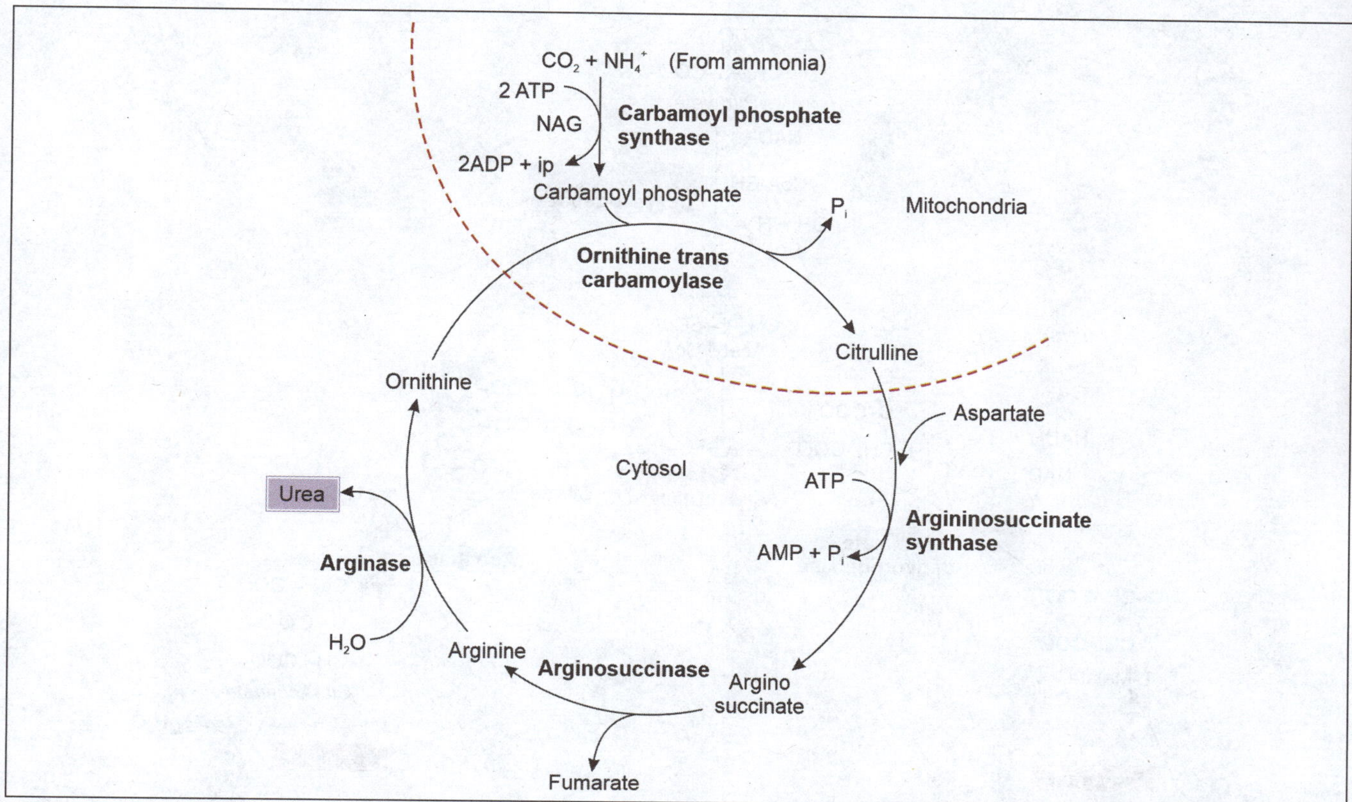

Color Plate 59: Urea cycle

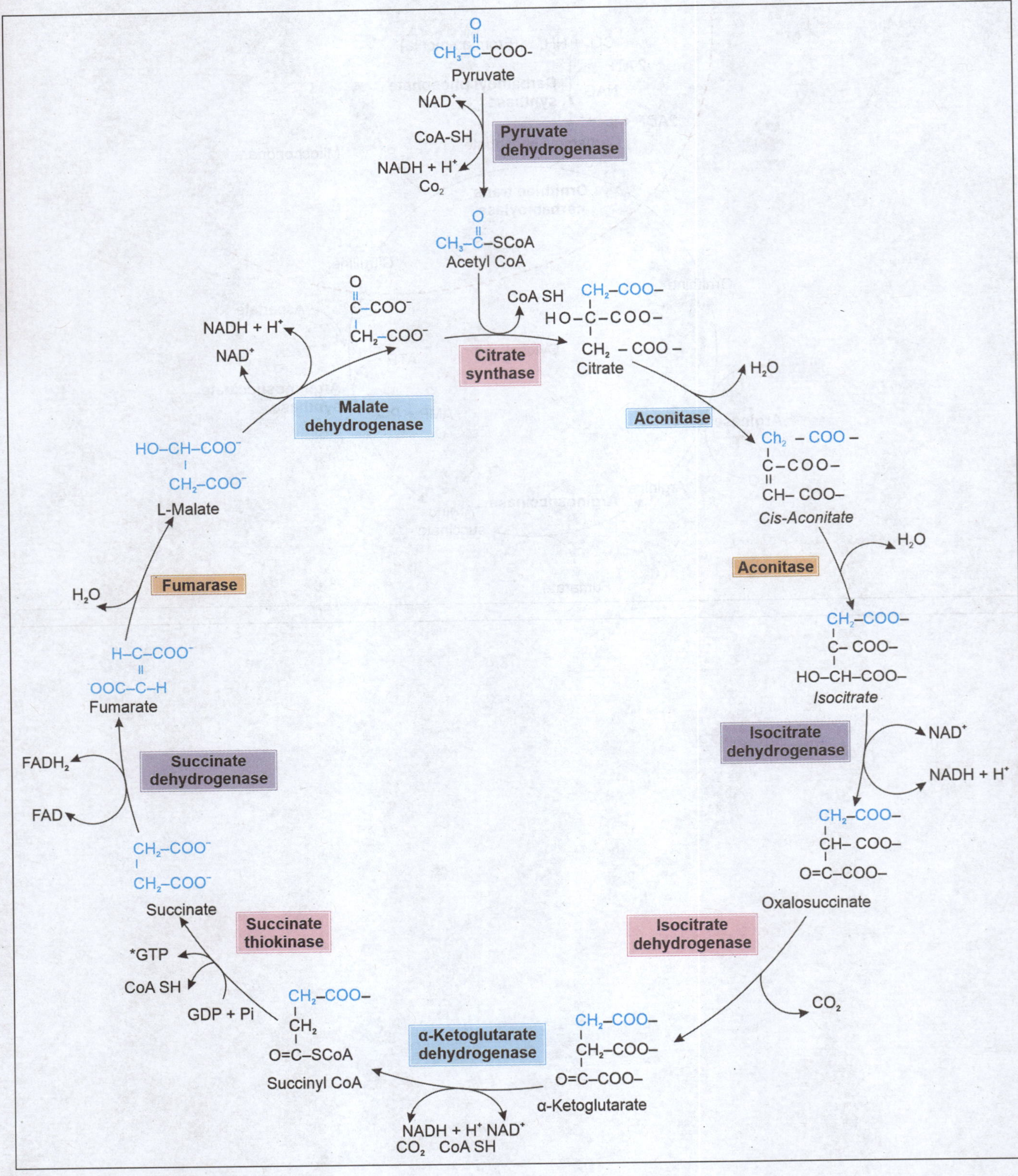

Pyruvate
NAD+
CoA-SH
NADH + H+
Co2
Pyruvate dehydrogenase
Acetyl CoA
CoA SH
Citrate synthase
Citrate
H2O
Aconitase
Cis-Aconitate
H2O
Aconitase
Isocitrate
Isocitrate dehydrogenase
NAD+
NADH + H+
Oxalosuccinate
Isocitrate dehydrogenase
CO2
α-Ketoglutarate
α-Ketoglutarate dehydrogenase
NADH + H+ NAD+
CO2 CoA SH
Succinyl CoA
GDP + Pi
CoA SH
*GTP
Succinate thiokinase
Succinate
FAD
FADH2
Succinate dehydrogenase
Fumarate
H2O
Fumarase
L-Malate
Malate dehydrogenase
NAD+
NADH + H+

Color Plate 60: Citric acid cycle or Krebs cycle

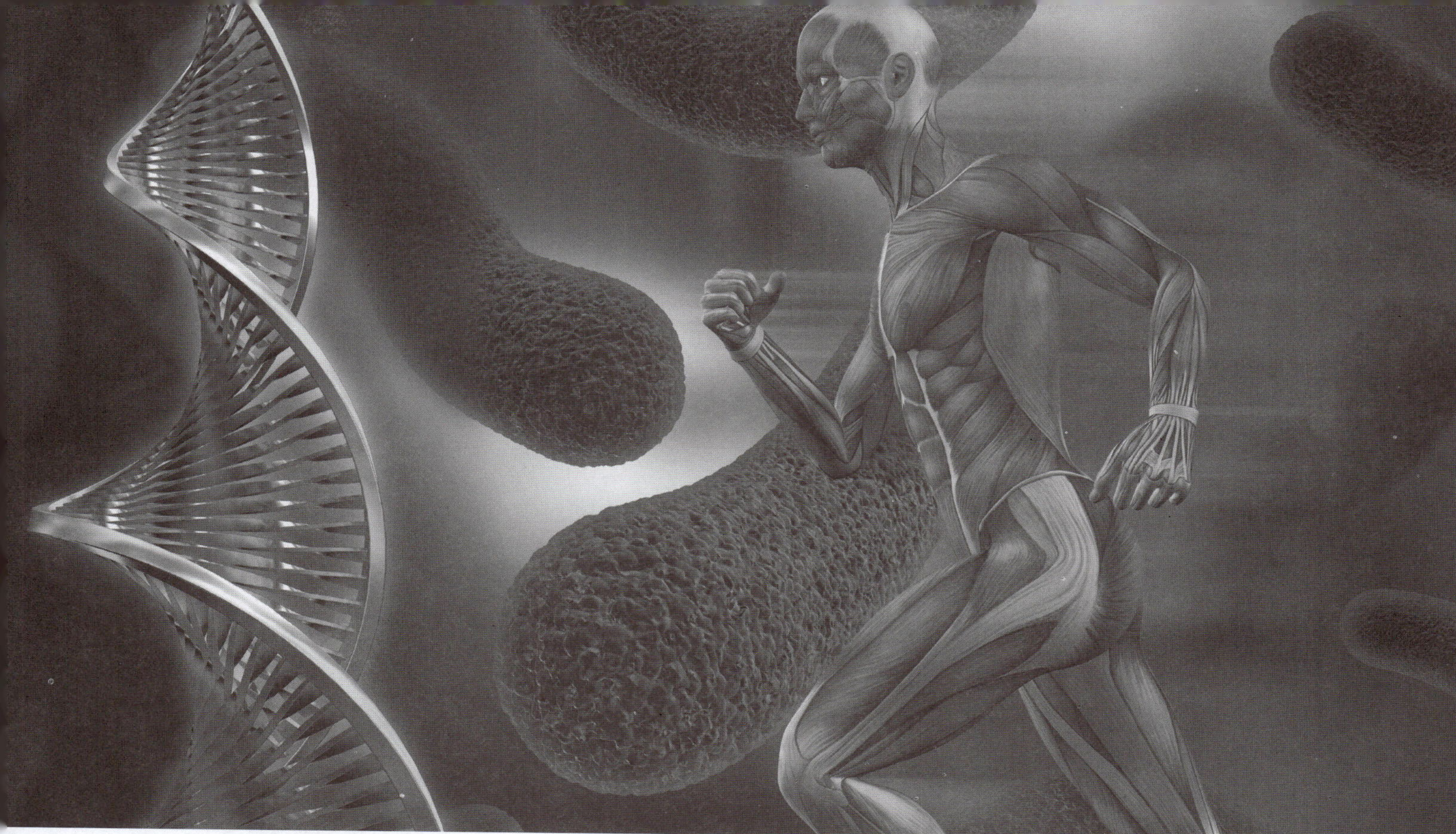

Applied Anatomy

Unit Outline

Introduction to Anatomical Terms and Organization of the Human Body

CHAPTER 1

CONCEPTUAL THEORY

Terminology

Abduction: Movement away from the midline of the body, such as moving the arm away from the side of the body.
Adduction: Movement toward the midline of the body, such as bringing the arm back to the side of the body.
Anatomical position: Person standing erect, eyes looking forward, feet together and forearms supinated with palms facing forward.
Circumduction: The circular motion of a joint with the distal end free to move in a circle and the proximal end fixed is known as circumduction.
Coronal plane: Divides the body into anterior and posterior halves.
Eversion: When foot is moved to face the sole outward and its lateral border is moved upward.
Inversion: When foot is moved to face the sole inward and medial border of foot is raised.
Lithotomy position: Person lies on the back in this position. Legs are strapped up so that the perineal area is clearly visible for delivery of the baby or surgery in the perineal area.
Midsagittal plane: Divides the body into exactly right and left halves from anterior to posterior sides.
Pronation: When the palm faces backwards or downwards.
Prone position: Person lies on his/her abdomen with hands on sides and feet together.
Protraction: Lower jaw/mandible is pulled forward beyond the upper jaw.
Retraction: Lower jaw pulled backward behind and below the maxilla.
Supination: When the palm is facing forward and upward.
Supine position: Person is lying on his/her back with hands on the sides and feet together.
Tissues: Cells of different types form tissues. Different tissues form organs. Organs serving similar functions form a system.
Transverse plane: Divides the body or limb into upper/proximal and lower/distal parts.

ANATOMICAL TERMS

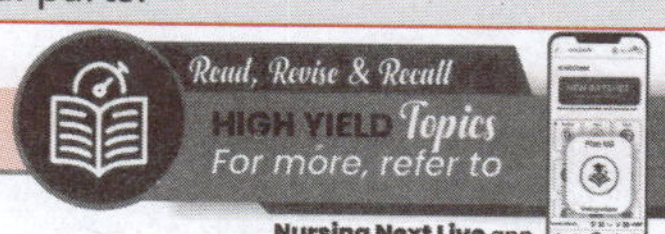

Anatomical Position

Anatomical position	Description
Anterior or ventral	Refers to the front or forward-facing part of the body or a structure. In anatomical terms, it is often used synonymously with "ventral".
Posterior or dorsal	Describes the back or rear-facing part of the body or a structure. It is often used interchangeably with "dorsal".
Superior	Describes a structure that is located above or higher than another structure in the body. It refers to a structure being closer to the head or further away from the feet when the body is in an upright position.
Inferior	The term "inferior" describes a structure that is located below or lower than another structure. It refers to a structure being closer to the feet or further away from the head when the body is in an upright position.
Medial	Structure that is located closer to the midline of the body.
Lateral	Structure that is located farther away from the midline of the body.
Proximal	Position closer to the point of reference or the center of the body.
Distal	Position farther away from the point of reference or the center of the body.

Contd...

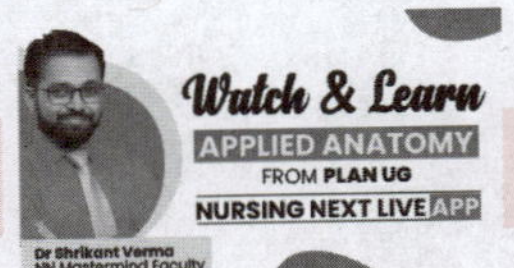

Anatomical position	Description
Superficial	Superficial refers to a position closer to the surface of the body or a specific structure.
Deep	Deep describes a position farther away from the surface of the body or a specific structure.
Supine	Lying face upward on the back.
Prone	Lying face downward on the front.
Plantar	The plantar surface refers to the inferior (bottom) surface of the foot.
Palmar	The palmar surface refers to the anterior (front) surface of the hand, specifically the palm.

Anatomical Planes

Anatomical plane	Description
Axial/Transverse/ Horizontal	The transverse plane is a horizontal plane that divides the body into upper (superior) and lower (inferior) sections.
Saggital/Vertical	The sagittal plane is a vertical plane that divides the body into left and right halves.
Coronal/Frontal	The frontal plane is a vertical plane that divides the body into front (anterior) and back (posterior) sections.
Oblique	Plane that can be any angle other than horizontal or vertical.

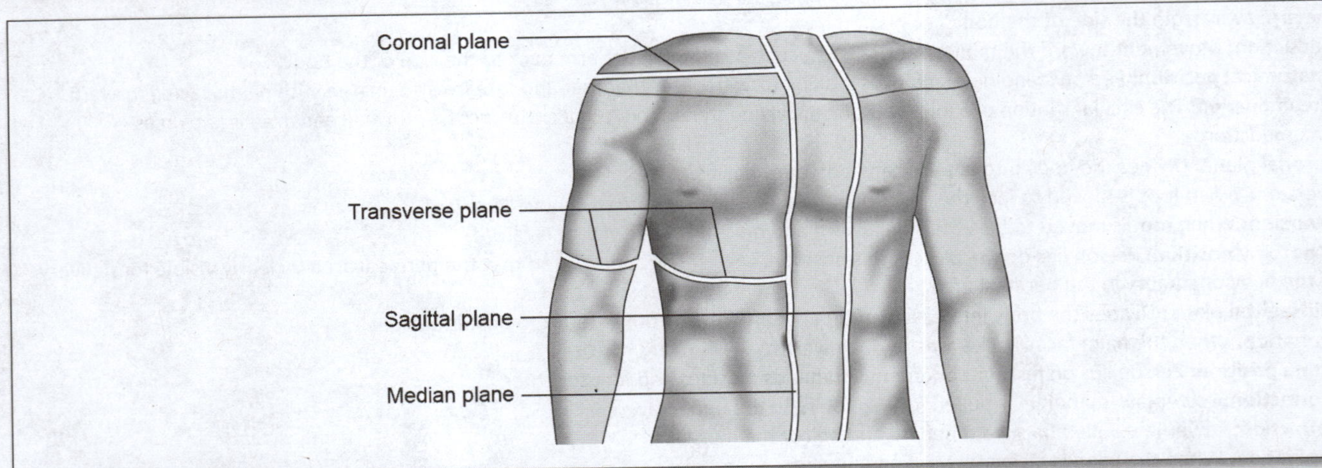

Anatomical Movements

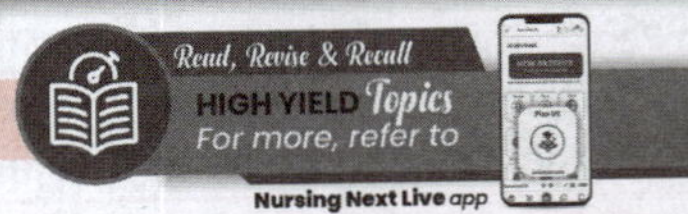

Anatomical movement	Description
Dorsiflexion	Flexion of the foot and ankle joint, bringing the top of the foot toward the anterior tibia.
Plantar flexion	Extension of the foot and ankle joint, pointing the toes downward away from the tibia.
Flexion	Bending or decreasing the angle between two body parts, such as bending the elbow.
Extension	Straightening or increasing the angle between two body parts, such as straightening the elbow.
Abduction	Movement away from the midline of the body, such as moving the arm away from the side of the body.
Adduction	Movement toward the midline of the body, such as bringing the arm back to the side of the body.
Pronation	Rotation of the forearm where the palm faces downward or backward.
Supination	Rotation of the forearm where the palm faces upward or forward.
Eversion	Outward turning of the foot at the ankle joint, resulting in the sole facing laterally.
Inversion	Inward turning of the foot at the ankle joint, resulting in the sole facing medially.
Cirumduction	The circular motion of a joint with the distal end free to move in a circle and the proximal end fixed is known as circumduction.
Medial rotation	Medial rotation refers to inward rotation toward the midline.
Lateral rotation	Lateral rotation refers to outward rotation away from the midline.

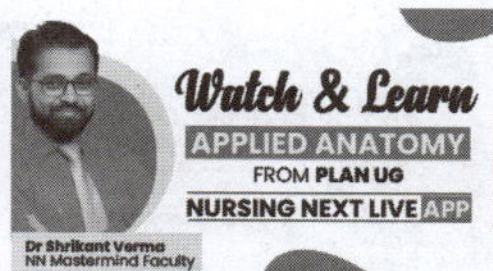

ORGANIZATION OF HUMAN BODY

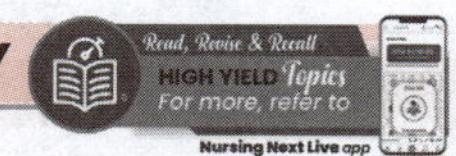

Cell Structure

Cell structure refers to the organization and components within a cell. Cells are the basic building blocks of life, and they exhibit a variety of structures that enable them to carry out their functions. Here is a more detailed overview of cell structure:

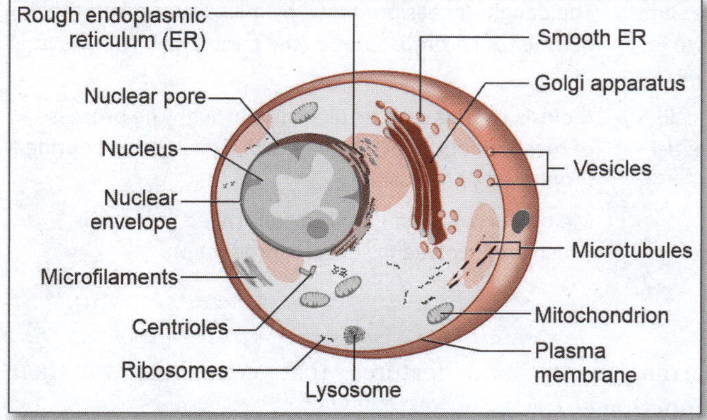

- **Cell membrane/plasma membrane:** The cell membrane is a thin, flexible barrier that surrounds the cell. It consists of a phospholipid bilayer with embedded proteins.
- **Nucleus:** The nucleus houses the cell's genetic material, which is organized into chromosomes. It is surrounded by a nuclear envelope and contains a nucleolus.
- **Cytoplasm:** The cytoplasm is the jelly-like fluid that fills the cell. It contains various organelles, cytosol (the liquid component), and other cellular components.
- **Mitochondria:** Mitochondria are often referred to as the "powerhouses" of the cell because they produce energy in the form of ATP through cellular respiration.
- **Endoplasmic reticulum (ER):** The endoplasmic reticulum is a network of membranes that is involved in protein and lipid synthesis and transport. The rough ER has ribosomes attached to its surface, while the smooth ER lacks ribosomes and is involved in lipid metabolism and detoxification.
- **Golgi apparatus:** The Golgi apparatus processes, modifies, sorts, and packages proteins and lipids for transport within the cell or secretion outside the cell.
- **Lysosomes:** Lysosomes are membrane-bound organelles containing digestive enzymes. They break down cellular waste, worn-out organelles, and foreign materials.
- **Peroxisomes:** Peroxisomes are involved in various metabolic processes, including the breakdown of fatty acids and the detoxification of harmful substances.
- **Cytoskeleton:** The cytoskeleton provides structural support and maintains the shape of the cell. It is composed of protein filaments, including microtubules, microfilaments, and intermediate filaments.
- **Vacuoles:** Vacuoles are fluid-filled sacs found in plant and fungal cells. They store water, nutrients, ions, and waste products, and contribute to turgor pressure in plant cells.

Cell Division

Cell division is the process by which a parent cell divides into two or more daughter cells. It is a fundamental process in all living organisms which plays a crucial role in growth, development, and tissue repair. There are two primary methods of cell division:

1. **Mitosis:** Mitosis is a type of cell division that results in the production of two daughter cells that are genetically identical to the parent cell.
2. **Meiosis:** Meiosis is a specialized form of cell division that occurs in sexually reproducing organisms to produce gametes (sperm and eggs).

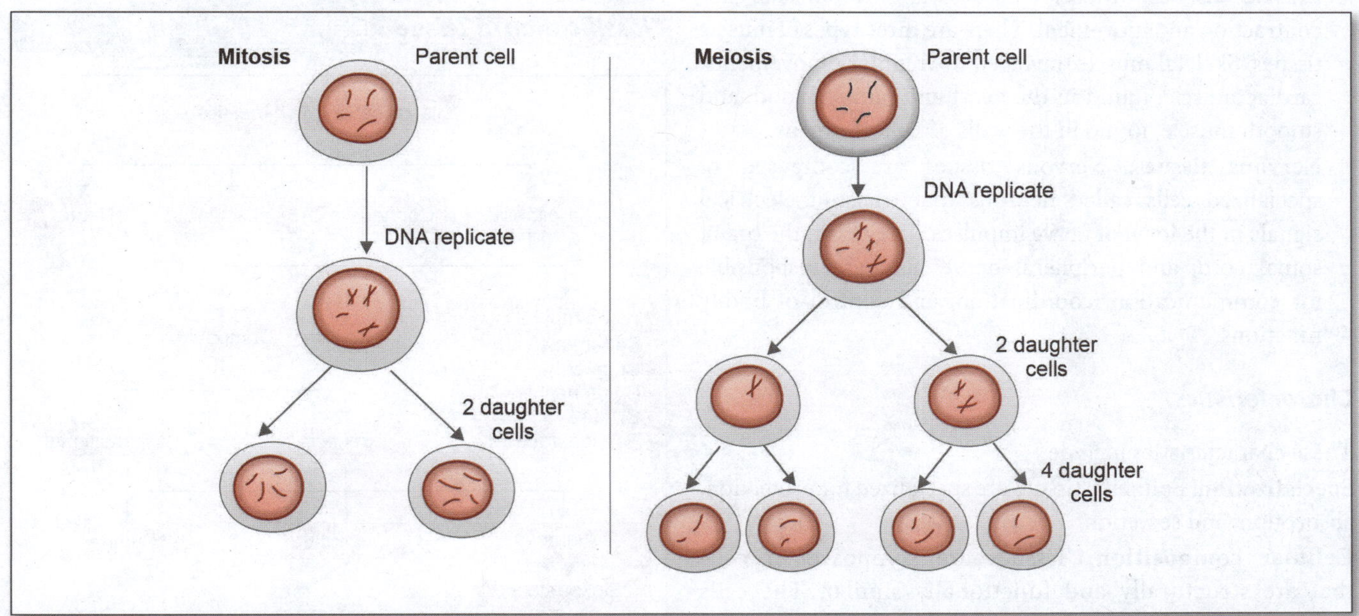

Description	Mitosis	Meiosis
1. Purpose	The primary purpose of mitosis is the growth, development, and maintenance of multicellular organisms.	Meiosis is specifically involved in the production of gametes (sperm and eggs) for sexual reproduction.
2. No. of divisions	Mitosis involves a single round of cell division, resulting in the production of two daughter cells.	Meiosis consists of two rounds of cell division, called Meiosis I and Meiosis II, resulting in the production of four daughter cells.
3. Chromosome number	The daughter cells produced by mitosis have the same number of chromosomes as the parent cell, which is typically diploid.	The daughter cells produced by meiosis have half the number of chromosomes as the parent cell.
4. Genetic diversity	Mitosis produces genetically identical daughter cells, as there is no exchange or recombination of genetic material between the chromosomes.	Meiosis creates genetic diversity through the process of recombination, or crossing over, which occurs during Prophase I of Meiosis I.
5. Occurrence	Mitosis occurs in somatic (non-reproductive) cells throughout the body for growth, repair, and maintenance.	Meiosis occurs in specialized cells called germ cells, which are involved in sexual reproduction.

Tissues

Tissues are a group or collection of specialized cells that work together to perform a specific function or functions within an organism.

Types

- **Epithelial tissues:** Epithelial tissues line the surfaces of organs, cavities, and tubes, both internally and externally. They act as a protective barrier, aid in absorption and secretion.
- **Connective tissues:** Connective tissues support and connect different structures and organs in the body. They include various types of tissues, such as bone, cartilage, adipose (fat) tissues, blood, and loose or dense fibrous connective tissues.
- **Muscle tissues:** Muscle tissues are responsible for contraction and movement. There are three types of muscle tissues: Skeletal muscle, involved in voluntary movements; cardiac muscle, found in the heart and pumps blood; and smooth muscle, found in the walls of hollow organs.
- **Nervous tissues:** Nervous tissues are composed of specialized cells called neurons that transmit electrical signals in the form of nerve impulses. They form the brain, spinal cord, and peripheral nerves and are responsible for communication, coordination, and control of bodily functions.

Characteristics

These characteristics include:

Specialization: Epithelial tissues are specialized for protection, absorption, and secretion.

Cellular composition: Tissues are composed of cells that are structurally and functionally similar. The cells within a particular tissue type often have specific shapes, arrangements, and features that contribute to their function.

Extracellular matrix: Many tissues have an extracellular matrix (ECM), which is a complex mixture of proteins, fibers, and other substances secreted by the cells. The ECM provides structural support, facilitates communication between cells, and influences cell behavior and tissue function.

Organization: Tissues are organized into higher levels of structural complexity, such as organs and organ systems.

Vascularization: Blood vessels deliver oxygen, nutrients, and hormones to the cells of these tissues and remove waste products.

Regeneration and repair: Tissues have varying capacities for regeneration and repair. Some tissues, like epithelial and liver tissue, have a high regenerative capacity and can rapidly replace damaged or lost cells.

Classification of Tissue

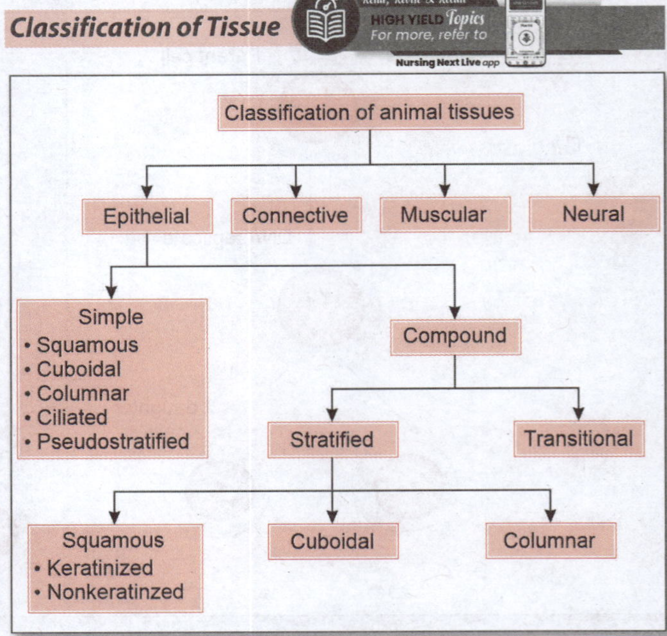

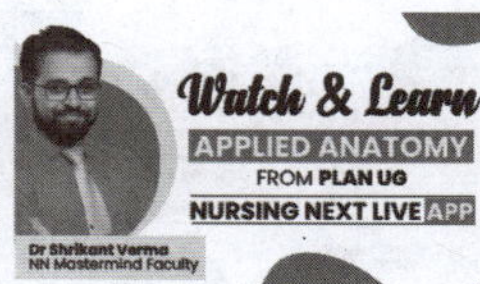

Location of Tissues

- **Epithelial tissues:**
  - Surface epithelium lines the outer surfaces of the body, such as the skin (epidermis).
  - Mucous membranes consist of epithelial tissues and line the respiratory tract, digestive tract, and reproductive tract.
  - Glandular epithelium forms the glands of the body, such as the salivary glands, sweat glands, and endocrine glands.
- **Connective tissues:**
  - Loose connective tissues are found beneath the skin, surrounding blood vessels and organs, and between muscles.
  - Dense connective tissues form tendons, ligaments, and the dermis of the skin.
  - Bone tissues form the skeletal system.
  - Cartilage is located in areas such as the nose, ears, joints, and respiratory tract.
  - Blood and lymphatic vessels contain connective tissue elements.
- **Muscle tissues:**
  - Skeletal muscle tissues are attached to bones and enable voluntary movement.
  - Cardiac muscle tissues are found in the heart.
  - Smooth muscle tissues line the walls of hollow organs, such as the digestive tract, blood vessels, and uterus.
- **Nervous tissues:**
  - The brain and spinal cord are primarily composed of nervous tissues.
  - Peripheral nerves extend throughout the body, connecting the central nervous system to various organs and tissues.

Membrane, Glands — Classification and Structure

Membranes are thin layers or sheets of tissues that cover surfaces, line cavities, or separate compartments within the body. They serve various functions, including protection, secretion, absorption, and lubrication. Here are some examples of different types of membranes found in the human body:

- **Epithelial membranes:**
  - **Mucous membranes:** Also known as mucosae, these membranes line the internal surfaces of organs and body cavities that are open to the external environment.
  - **Serous membranes:** Serous membranes line the body cavities that do not open to the external environment and cover the organs within those cavities.
- **Synovial membranes:** Synovial membranes line the cavities of joints (synovial joints). They secrete synovial fluid, which lubricates the joints and reduces friction.
- **Cutaneous membrane:** The cutaneous membrane is the skin, which covers the external surface of the body. It consists of an outer layer of stratified squamous epithelium (epidermis) and an underlying layer of connective tissues (dermis).
- **Meninges:** The meninges are a set of membranes that surround and protect the brain and spinal cord. They consist of three layers: The dura mater, arachnoid mater, and pia mater.

Glands

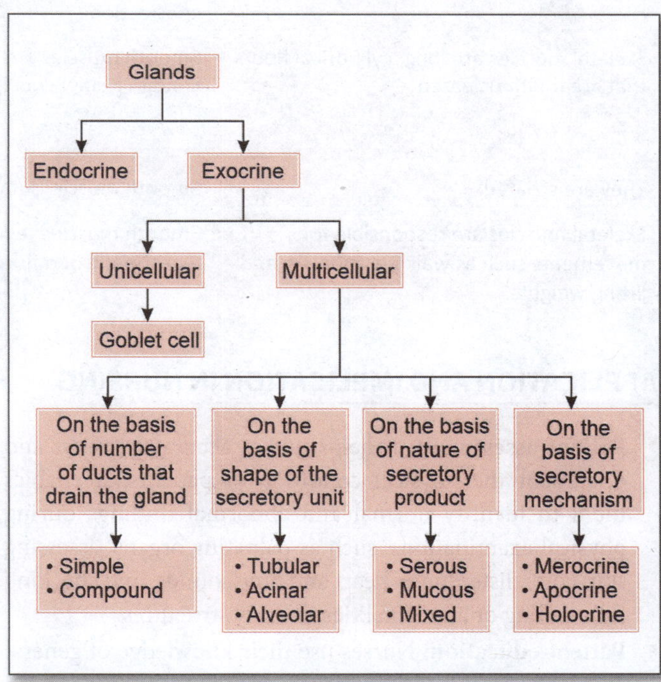

Hyaline, Fibro Cartilage, Elastic Cartilage

Parameters	Hyaline cartilage	Fibro cartilage	Elastic cartilage
Structure	Hyaline cartilage is the most common type of cartilage. It has a glassy, translucent appearance and is composed of a dense network of collagen fibers embedded in a gel-like matrix.	Fibrocartilage is characterized by a combination of dense collagen fibers and cartilage matrix.	Elastic cartilage contains a dense network of elastic fibers in addition to collagen fibers. It is more flexible and elastic compared to hyaline cartilage.

Contd...

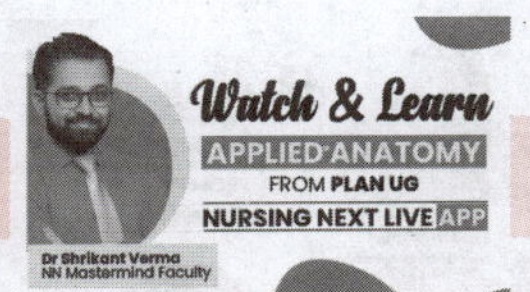

Parameters	Hyaline cartilage	Fibro cartilage	Elastic cartilage
Composition	It primarily consists of collagen fibers (mainly type II collagen) and proteoglycans, which provide strength and resilience.	It contains a high concentration of collagen fibers, predominantly type I collagen, which provides tensile strength.	It consists of elastin fibers, collagen fibers (primarily type II collagen), and proteoglycans.
Function	Hyaline cartilage provides a smooth surface for joint movement, reduces friction between bones, and acts as a shock absorber.	Fibrocartilage is found in areas that require both support and the ability to withstand tension and compression.	Elastic cartilage provides both structural support and elasticity. It is found in structures that require flexibility and recoil, such as the external ear (pinna), the epiglottis, and the Eustachian tube.

Features of Skeletal, Smooth and Cardiac Muscle

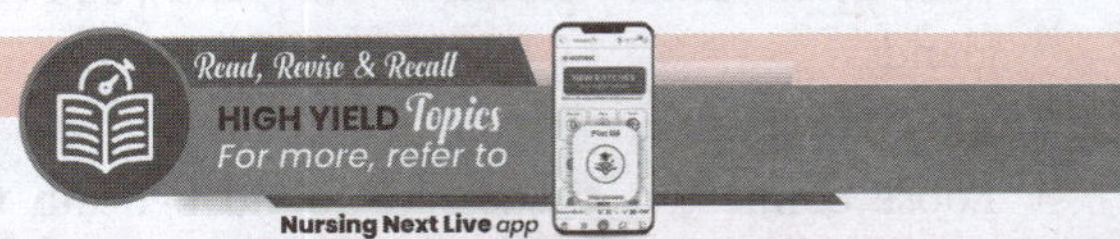

Skeletal muscle	Smooth muscle	Cardiac muscle
Skeletal muscle is a type of muscle tissue that is attached to the skeleton and allows movement of the body.	Smooth muscle is found on the walls of various organs and structures throughout the body, such as the digestive tract, blood vessels, and respiratory airways.	Cardiac muscle is found exclusively in the heart and is responsible for its contraction.
It is under voluntary control, meaning we can consciously control its activation.	It is not under voluntary control and is responsible for involuntary movements and contractions.	It is also an involuntary muscle, meaning it functions automatically without conscious control.
Skeletal muscles are long, cylindrical fibers that are multinucleated	Smooth muscles are spindle-shaped and contain a single nucleus per cell.	Cardiac muscle cells are branched and interconnected, forming a network that allows the heart to contract in a coordinated manner.
They are striated	Smooth muscle is not striated	Cardiac muscle is striated
Skeletal muscles are responsible for movements such as walking, running, and lifting weights.	Smooth muscles regulate processes like digestion, blood flow, and breathing.	The rhythmic contractions of cardiac muscle pump blood throughout the body, providing oxygen and nutrients to tissues.

APPLICATION AND IMPLICATION IN NURSING

- **Patient assessment:** It helps nurses accurately assess and document the physical condition of patients. It enables them to identify normal and abnormal findings during physical examinations, such as palpating organs, assessing skin color, listening to heart and lung sounds, and checking for swelling or abnormalities in body structures.
- **Patient education:** Nurses use their knowledge of general anatomy to educate patients about their conditions, procedures, and treatments. By explaining anatomical structures and their functions, nurses can help patients understand the underlying causes of their health issues and the importance of following prescribed treatments.
- **Medication administration:** Administering medications safely and effectively require knowledge of anatomy. Nurses need to understand anatomical landmarks to administer injections or intravenous medications accurately. They also need to be aware of potential anatomical variations in patients that could impact drug absorption, distribution, and metabolism.
- **Surgical care:** Nurses who work in surgical settings need a solid understanding of anatomy to assist surgeons during procedures. They must be able to anticipate the surgeon's needs, identify anatomical structures, and provide appropriate surgical instruments and supplies.
- **Patient safety:** Knowledge of anatomy helps nurses prevent complications and promote patient safety. For example, understanding the anatomy of blood vessels and nerves helps prevent inadvertent injury during procedures such as venipuncture or catheter insertions.
- **Patient advocacy:** Nurses advocate for their patients by understanding and communicating their anatomical concerns to other health care professionals.

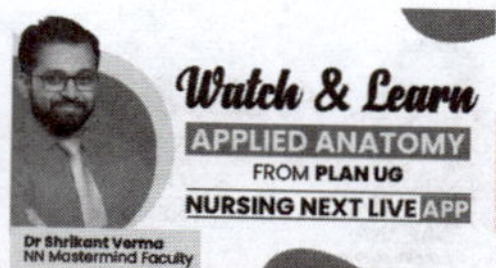

CONCEPTUAL EXERCISES

LONG ANSWER QUESTION

1. Describe the body cavities in detail.

Answer

Introduction

- The body cavities are hollow spaces inside the body that support and protect various internal organs.
- The cavities are separated by membranes and other structures.
- The two large body cavities are dorsal and ventral cavities which are further divided into smaller ones.

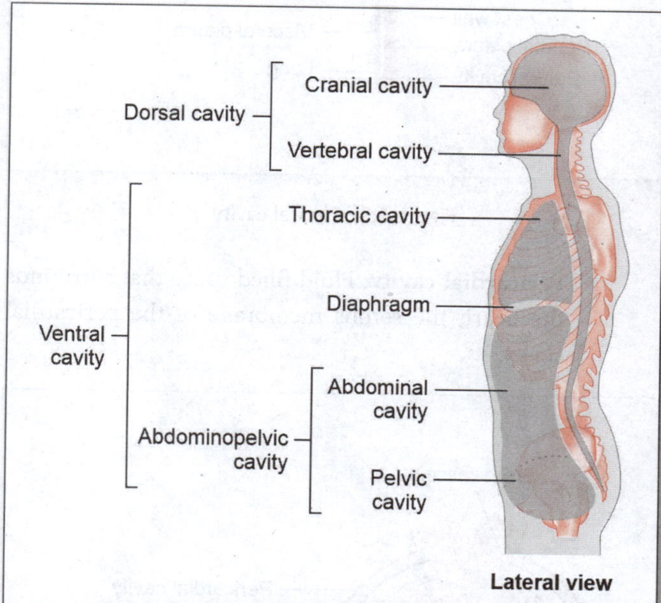

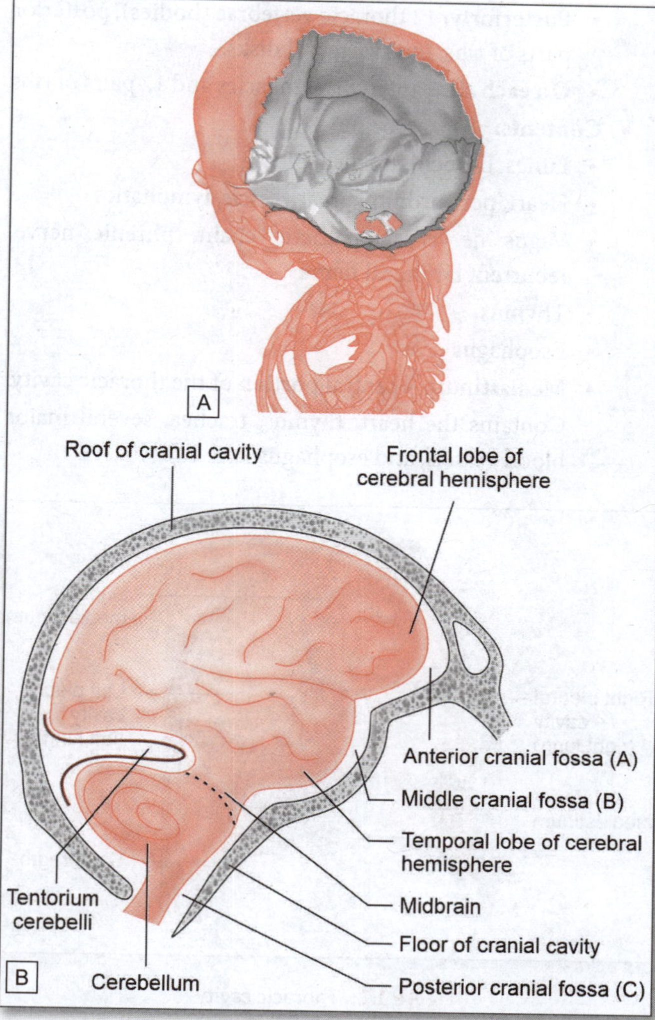

Figures 1.1A and B: Cranial cavity

Body Cavities

Dorsal cavity: Present at the back of the body (posteriorly) and divided into two cavities:

1. **Cranial cavity:**
   - Formed by the fusion of eight bones.
   - **They are:**
     - **Anteriorly:** Frontal bone
     - **Posteriorly:** Occipital bone
     - **Inferiorly:** Sphenoid and ethmoid bone
     - **Superiorly:** Paired parietal bone
     - **Laterally:** Paired temporal bones
   - Contains the meninges, brain, venous sinuses, endocrine glands (pineal and pituitary gland) and CSF
2. **Vertebral cavity:**
   - Formed by the vertebrae and contains the spinal cord with meninges and CSF

Ventral cavity:

- Present ventrally or anteriorly to the spine. This cavity is a true coelom formed from mesoderm. The cavity is divided into two cavities:
  1. **Thoracic cavity:** Further divided into one pericardial and two pleural cavities
  2. **Abdominopelvic cavity:** Divided into:
     - Abdominal cavity
     - Pelvic cavity

1. **Thoracic cavity**
   - One of the major cavities of the body.
   - **Boundaries:**
     - **Superiorly:** Structures that form root of neck

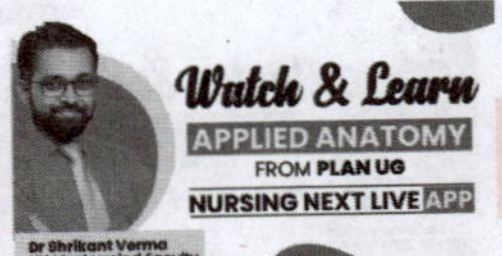

- **Inferiorly:** Diaphragm (muscular sheet)
- **Anteriorly:** Sternum, anterior parts of ribs and their costal cartilages
- **Posteriorly:** 12 thoracic vertebrae (bodies), posterior parts of ribs, intervertebral disks.
- **On each side:** Intercostal muscles and 12 pairs of ribs

- **Contents:**
  - Lungs, bronchi, trachea, pleura
  - Heart, pericardium, great vessels, lymphatics
  - Vagus nerve, sympathetic chain, phrenic nerve, recurrent laryngeal nerve
  - Thymus
  - Esophagus
  - Mediastinum – central portion of the thoracic cavity. Contains the heart, thymus, trachea, several major blood vessels, and esophagus.

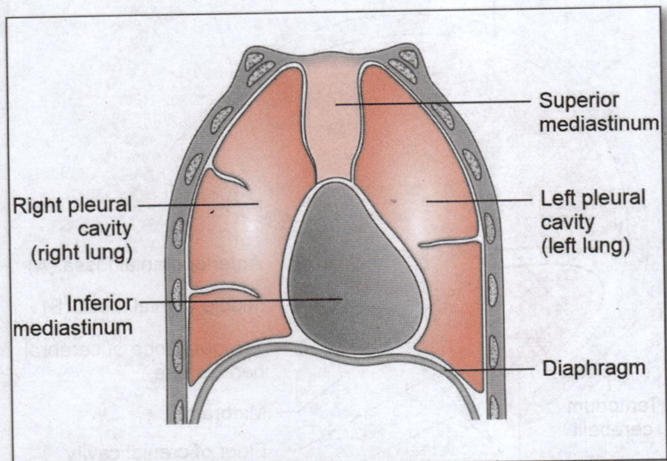

Figure 1.2: Thoracic cavity

Table 1.1: Major structures of the thoracic cavity

	Superior mediastinum		Thymus, great vessels, trachea, esophagus, and thoracic duct
Mediastinum	Inferior mediastinum	Anterior	Thymus
		Middle	Heart, pericardium, and roots of great vessels
		Posterior	Thoracic aorta, thoracic duct, esophagus, and azygos venous system
Pleural cavities	Right pleural cavity		Right lung
	Left pleural cavity		Left lung

- **Pleural cavity:** Fluid-filled space that surrounds each lungs.

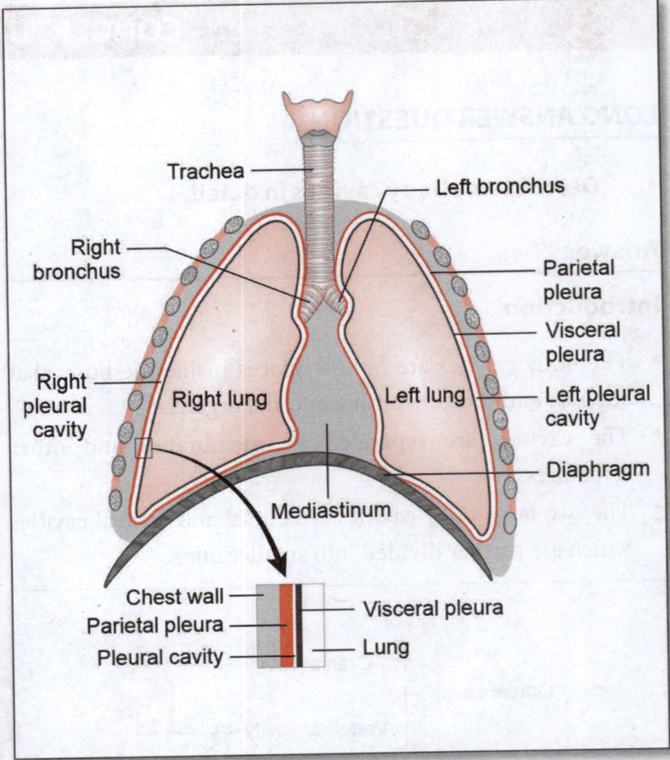

Figure 1.3: Pleural cavity

- **Pericardial cavity:** Fluid filled space that surrounds the heart, the serous membrane of the pericardial cavity.

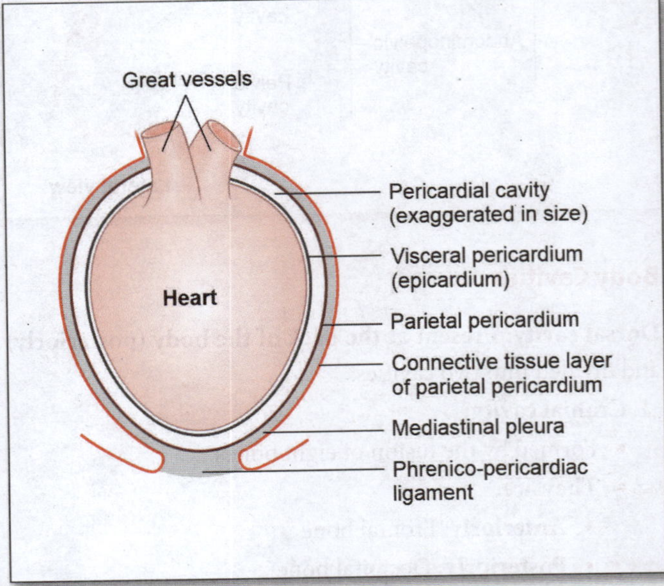

Figure 1.4: Pericardial cavity

2. **Abdominopelvic cavity**

- **Abdominal cavity**
  - Largest cavity of the body

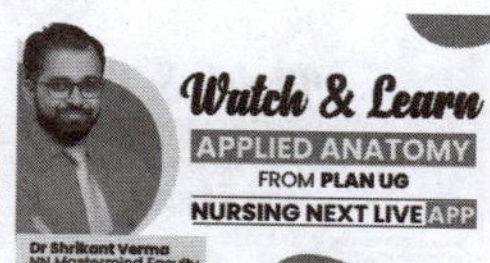

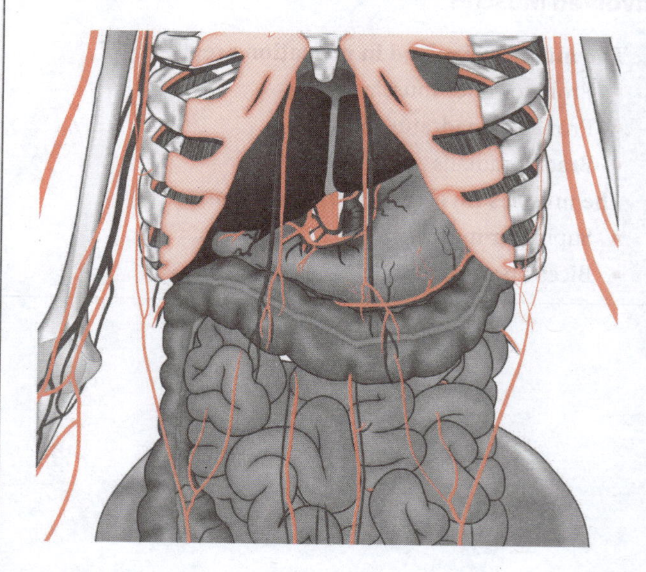

Figure 1.5: Abdominal cavity

- Divided into nine regions by two vertical planes (lateral) and two horizontal planes.
- Nine regions of abdomen:
  i. Epigastrium
  ii. Right hypochondrium
  iii. Left hypochondrium
  iv. Umbilical
  v. Right lumbar
  vi. Left lumbar
  vii. Suprapubic or hypogastrium
  viii. Right iliac fossa or right inguinal region
  ix. Left iliac fossa or left inguinal region

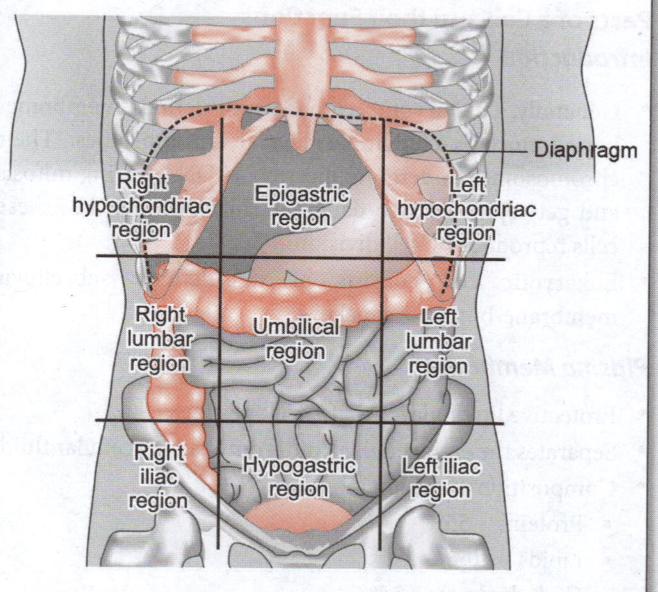

- **Boundaries**
  - **Anteriorly:** Anterior abdominal wall
  - **Posteriorly:** Posterior abdominal wall and lumbar vertebra
  - **Superiorly:** Diaphragm (separates it from thoracic cavity)
  - **Inferiorly:** Pelvic cavity
  - **Laterally:** Muscles of abdominal wall and lower limbs
- **Contents**
  - Contains vital organs
  - Stomach, the small intestine (jejunum and ileum), large intestine
  - Liver, spleen, gall bladder, pancreas
  - Uterus, fallopian tubes, ovaries
  - Kidneys, ureters, bladder
  - Many blood vessels (arteries, veins)

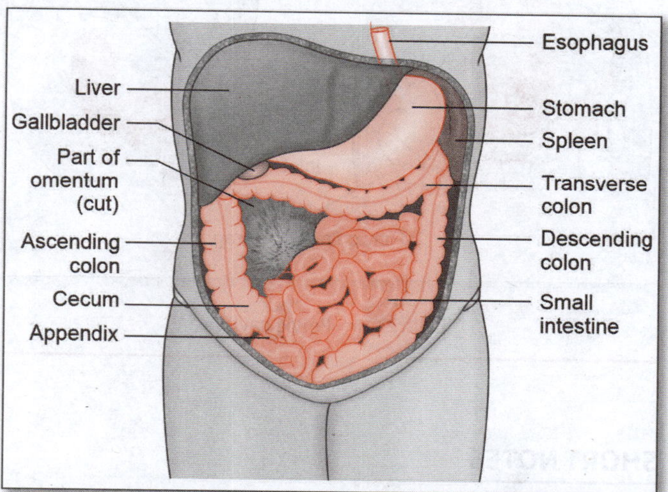

Abdominal cavity (anterior part)

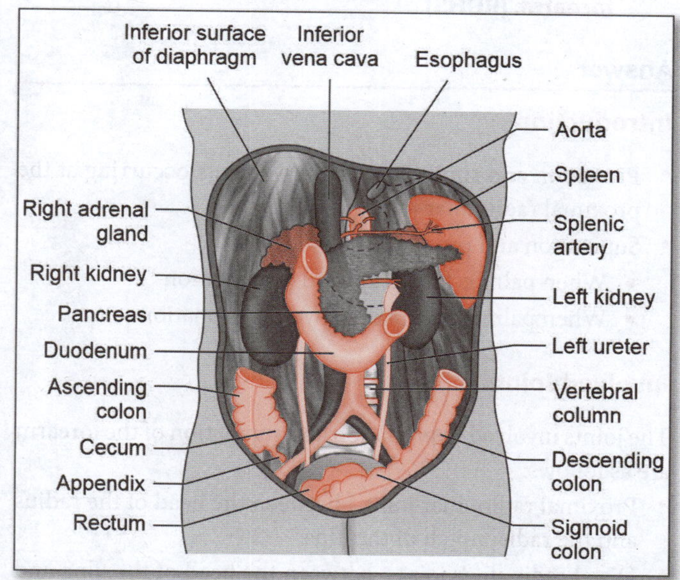

Abdomial cavity (posterior part)

- **Pelvic cavity:**
  - Extends from the lower end of the abdominal cavity
  - **Boundaries:**
    - **Anteriorly:** Pubic bones
    - **Posteriorly:** Coccyx and sacrum
    - **Superiorly:** Continuous with abdominal cavity
    - **Inferiorly:** Pelvic floor
    - **Laterally:** Hip bones
  - **Contents:**
    - Reproductive organs
    - Urinary bladder, distal ureters, urethra
    - Terminal sigmoid colon
    - Rectum and anal canal

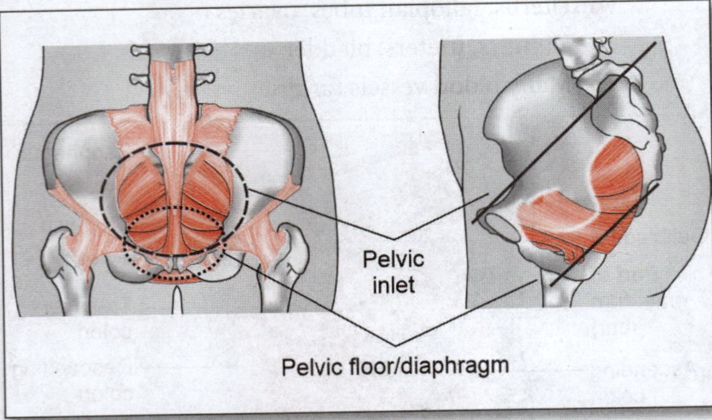

Figure 1.6: Pelvic cavity

SHORT NOTES

1. Write a short note on pronation and supination of forearm. (RUHS)

Answer

Introduction

- Pronation and supination are movements occurring at the proximal radioulnar joints.
- Supination and pronation
  - When palm is facing upward—supination
  - When palm is facing downward—pronation

Involved Joints

The joints involved in pronation and supination of the forearm are as follows:

- Proximal radioulnar joint—between the head of the radius and the radial notch of the ulna
- Distal radioulnar joint—between the head of the ulna and the ulnar notch of the radius

Involved Muscles

- **The muscles involved in pronation are:**
  - Pronator teres muscle
  - Pronator quadratus muscle
  - Brachioradialis
- **The muscles involved in supination are:**
  - Supinator muscle
  - Biceps brachii muscle

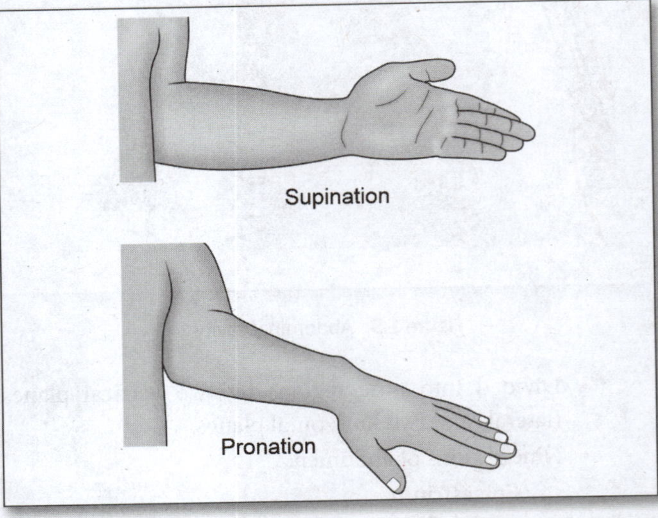

Figure 1.7: Supination and pronation

2. Write a short note on the parts of a cell and their functions. (KUHS)

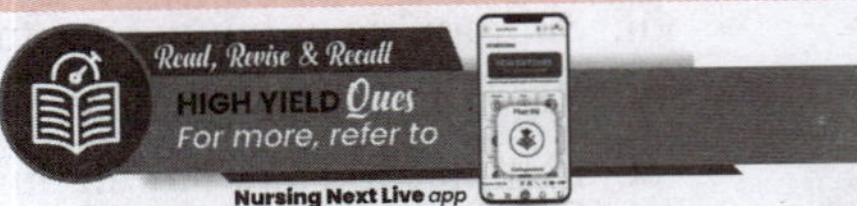

Answer

Parts of a Cell and their Functions

Introduction

- Generally, a eukaryotic cell has a well-defined membrane-bound nucleus containing several chromosomes. Their chromosomes undergo replication of DNA during mitosis and get separated into daughter chromosomes, i.e., these cells reproduce by cell division.
- Eukaryotic cell consists of well-defined subcellular membrane-bound organelles.

Plasma Membrane

- Protective lipid bilayer that envelopes the cell.
- Separates the extracellular fluid from the intracellular fluid.
- Composition of cell membrane
  - Proteins – 55%
  - Lipids – 40%
  - Carbohydrates – 5%

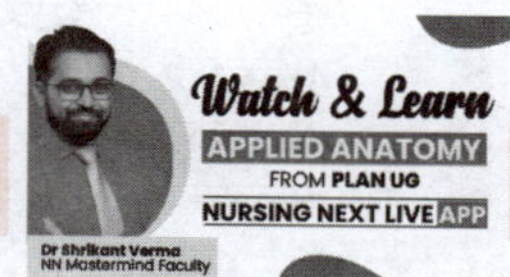

- Functions of plasma membrane
  - Protection of the cellular organelles and content
  - Semipermeability
  - Absorptive function
  - Maintenance of size and shape of the cell
  - Acts as a medium for exchange of gases

Subcellular Organelles

Nucleus

- Largest organelle
- Contains DNA—repository of genetic information
- Surrounded by a nuclear membrane

Endoplasmic Reticulum

- Large intracellular membranous organelle
- Made of membranous sheets and tubules
- Accounts for >50% of the total lipid bilayer of cell
- Two types—Rough endoplasmic reticulum (RER) and smooth endoplasmic reticulum (SER)
- Functions of endoplasmic reticulum
  - **Cisternae:**
    - Associated with lipid metabolism
    - Important in maintaining calcium balance intercellularly
- *Protein synthesis and folding*—occurs in RER
- *Lipid synthesis*—occurs in SER
- SER—site of storage and release of Ca^{2+} ions

Mitochondria

- Membrane-bound organelle, 0.5–1 micron in diameter and 5–10 micron in length.
- Relatively solid bodies, granular, sausage-shaped in form and remain scattered throughout the cytoplasm.
- Thread-like appearance under a light microscope
- Called the powerhouse of cell-presence of enzymes

Functions

- Potent site of aerobic respiration
- Oxidative phosphorylation and ATP formation: Inner membrane houses the enzymes for Krebs cycle. Production of energy rich compound that is ATP – powerhouse or power plant of cell.
- **Cell replication:** Mitochondria possess some amount of circular DNA that controls the replication of cells of mitochondrion.

Golgi Apparatus

- Complex structure of interconnecting tubules, vesicles, and cisternae
- Concerned with synthetic process of cell, especially secretions
- Involved in modification, sorting and packaging of proteins
- Involved in the transport of lipids
- Produces secretory granules which store hormones and enzymes.

Lysosomes

- Spherical vesicles enveloped by a single membrane
- Contain digestive enzymes
- Contain enzymes – hydrolases
- Hydrolytic enzymes are potent to digest their own content – suicidal bags
- Responsible for maintaining the cellular compounds in a dynamic state
- Primary function is intracellular digestion and cell necrosis or autolysis.

Peroxisomes

- Oxidative organelles
- Contain enzymes oxidases
- Protect the cells from the toxic effects of peroxides.

Cilia and Flagella

- Fine, hair-like extensions on the free surface of some cells
- Help in movement

Microfilaments

- Provide structural support
- Maintain the shape of cell

Microtubules

Help in the movement of cell and organelles within cell.

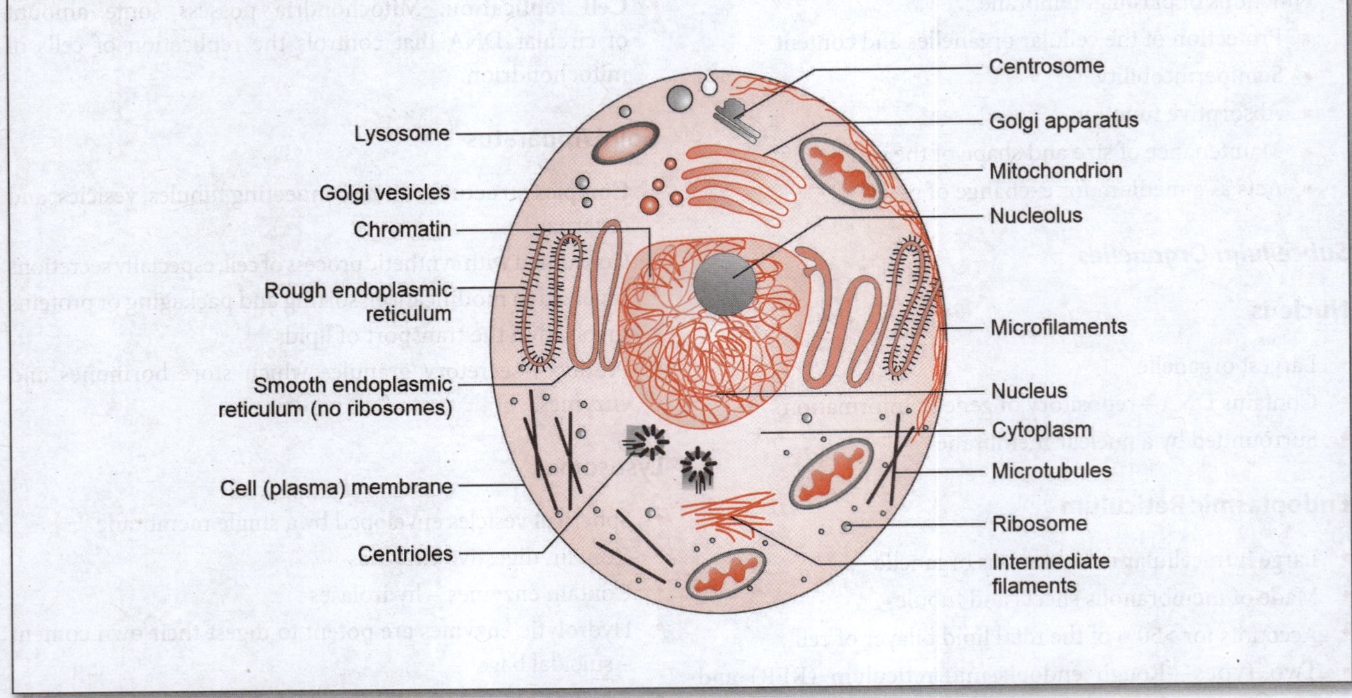

Figure 1.8: Cell organelles

3. Write a short note on tissues. (MGR)

Answer

Introduction

Organized group of cells lying in close proximity and performing one or more specific functions.

Types of Tissues

Epithelial Tissues

- Highly cellular tissues that overlie body surfaces and form a protective barrier.
- These form glands and specialized junctions to create a barrier between connective tissues and free surfaces.

Connective Tissues

- Most abundant tissues in the body.
- Contain cells, fibers and extracellular matrix.
- Mesenchymal in origin

Muscle Tissues

- Elastic, extensible and contractile
- This contraction is a result of sliding actin and myosin filaments.

Nervous Tissues

- Cells of the nervous system are highly specialized to transmit electrical impulses around the body.

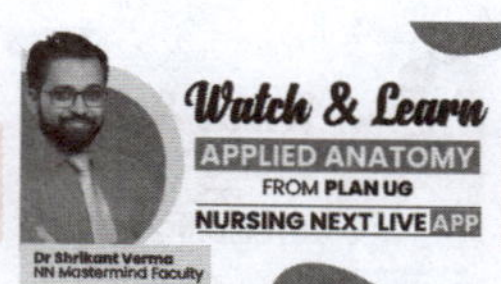

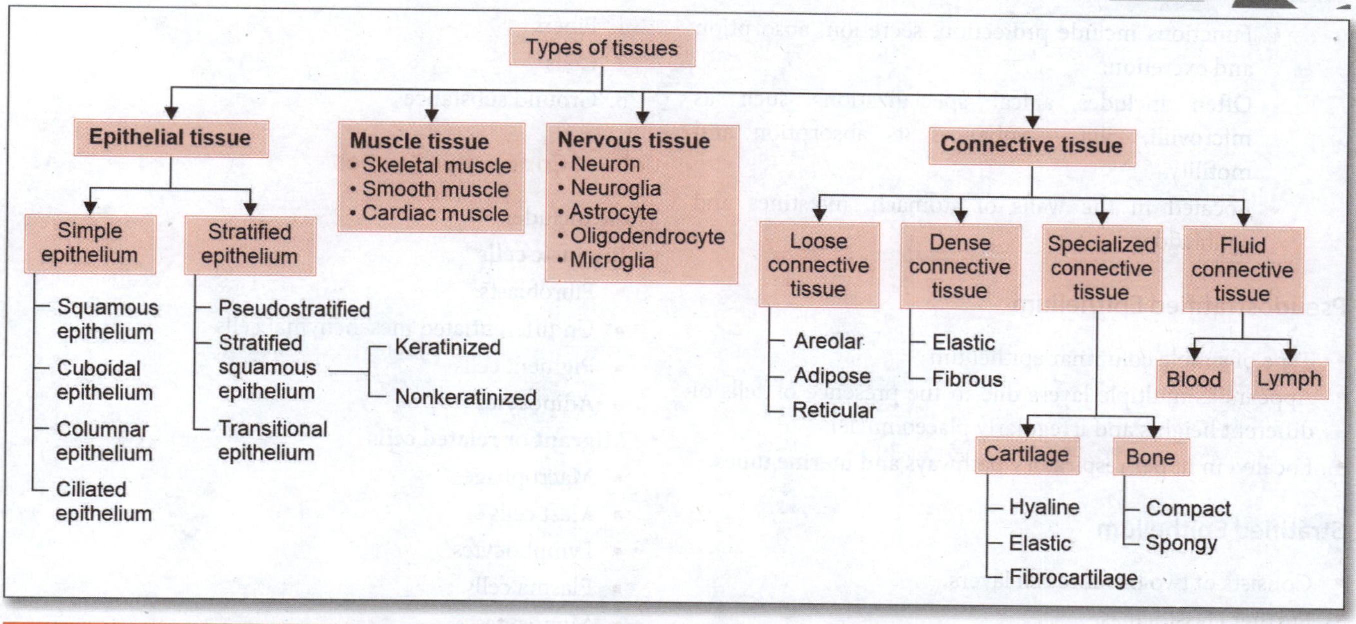

4. Write a short note on epithelial tissues. (MGR)

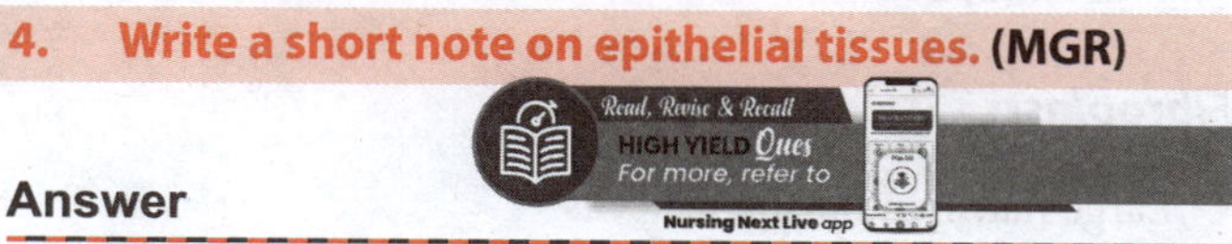

Answer

Epithelial Tissues

- Highly cellular tissues that overlie body surfaces and form a protective barrier
- These form glands and specialized junctions to create a barrier between connective tissues and free surfaces.
- Epithelial cells are the building blocks of the epithelial tissues.

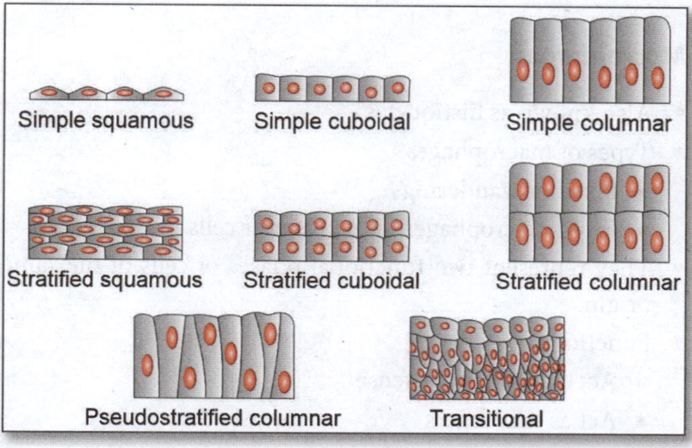

Types of Epithelial Tissues

- **Based on the type of cells:**

Squamous	Cells are flattened. Can be keratinized or nonkeratinized	Functions: Protection and Diffusion
Cuboidal	Cube shaped cells	Functions: Secretion and absorption
Columnar	Cells are rectangular in shape Cilia are present	Functions: Absorption, secretion, protection and lubrication

Contd...

- **Based on the number of layers**
  - **Simple:** One layer of cell
  - **Stratified:** Two or more layers of cells
  - **Pseudostratified:** Single layer of cells that appear stratified in appearance
- **Specialized**
  - This includes transitional epithelium, keratinized or nonkeratinized squamous epithelium.

Simple Epithelial Tissues

- Consist of one layer of epithelial cells lying on basement membrane
- Cells may be squamous, cuboidal and columnar
  - Simple squamous epithelium
    - One layer of thin flattened cells
    - **Functions:** Diffusion, filtration
    - **Location:** Capillaries, blood vessels, alveoli of lungs, glomeruli of kidney.
  - Simple cuboidal epithelium
    - Contains single layer of cuboidal cells.
    - Functions include secretory, absorptive and excretory properties.
  - **Simple columnar epithelium**
    - Single layer of columnar cells

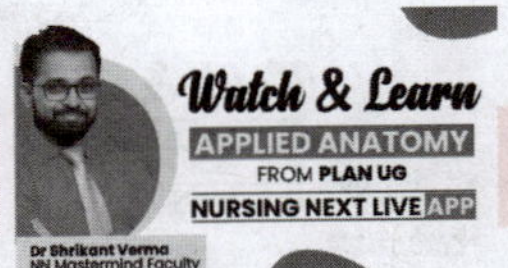

- Functions include protection, secretion, absorption and excretion.
- Often includes apical specializations such as microvilli, cilia – enhances its absorption and motility.
- Located in the walls of stomach, intestines and gallbladder.

Pseudostratified Epithelium

- Type of simple columnar epithelium
- Appears as multiple layers due to the presence of cells of different heights and irregularly placed nuclei.
- Located in upper respiratory pathways and uterine tubes.

Stratified Epithelium

- Consists of two or more cell layers.
- Further classified as:
  - Stratified squamous epithelium
    - Contains multiple layers of flat squamous epithelium
    - Major function – protection against abrasion and dehydration.
    - Further divided into keratinized and nonkeratinized epithelium.
  - Stratified columnar epithelium
    - Protective and secretory role
    - Lines the excretory ducts of various glands and ovarian follicles.
  - Transitional epithelium
    - Present in organs that distend.
    - On stretching, the cuboidal cells change to squamous cells.
    - Present in the urinary tract, renal calyces, urinary bladder
- **Functions**
  - Secretion
  - Absorption
  - Transportation
  - Protection
  - Receptor function

---

5. Write a short note on connective tissues. (KUHS)

Answer

Introduction

- Connective tissues fills the spaces between the more specified tissues.
- They are is basically made-up of three elements:

1. Fibers
2. Cells
3. Ground substance

Cells of Connective Tissues

These include:

- **Intrinsic cells**
  - Fibroblasts
  - Undifferentiated mesenchymal cells
  - Pigment cells
  - Adipocytes
- **Migrant or related cells**
  - Macrophages
  - Mast cells
  - Lymphocytes
  - Plasma cells
  - Monocytes
  - Eosinophils

Fibroblasts

- Large flat, spindle-shaped cells
- Present in large numbers in the connective tissue
- Functions
  - Responsible for the production of fibers and ground substances
  - Contribute to the formation of connective tissues.
  - Secrete collagen proteins — help in maintaining the structural framework of tissues.
  - Role in wound healing

Macrophages

- Also known as histiocytes
- Types of macrophages
  - Fixed or wandering
  - Fixed macrophages – e.g., Kupffer cells
- They represent two functional phases of cells of the same origin.
- Functions
  - Act as agents of defense
  - Act as scavengers
  - Secrete important substances such as lysosomes, elastase and collagenase.

Fat Cells

- Large cells seen in groups.
- When seen in large groups, the tissue is called adipose tissue.

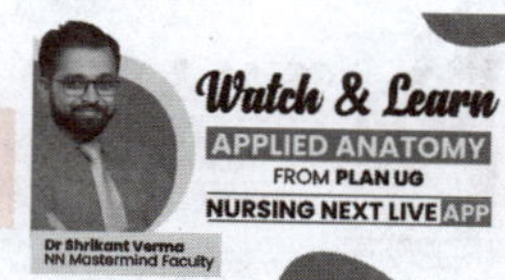

- Each cell has a large glistening droplet of fat, surrounded by a thin rim of cytoplasm.
- Nucleus is pushed to one side and flattened.

Undifferentiated Mesenchymal Cells

- Pluripotent cells
- Develop from mesoderm
- Mainly seen around the blood vessels

Pigment Cells

- Main pigment present is melanin
- Present in:
  - Skin
  - Choroid coat of eye
  - Pia mater
- Functions
  - Protection from UV radiation
  - Prevention of light from reaching deeper tissues.

Mast Cells

- Irregularly oval
- Contain cytoplasmic granules
- Occur in groups in relation to blood vessels.
- Functions:
  - Secrete heparin, histamine and serotonin.
  - Mediate immediate hypersensitivity reactions.

Plasma Cells or Plasmatocytes

- Small cells with round basophilic cytoplasm.
- Function
  - Produce antibodies

6. Write a short note on the two glands lined by cuboidal epithelium. (MGR)

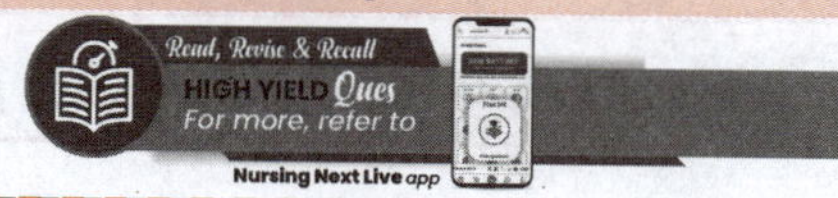

Answer

Cuboidal Epithelium

- Short cuboidal cells having roughly similar thickness and width.
- Appears hexagonal in cross-section.
- Located in the ducts of glands that perform secretion, absorption or both.
- Glands lined by cuboidal epithelium are:
  - Thyroid gland
    - The thyroid gland is a butterfly-shaped gland located in the neck, just below the Adam's apple.
    - It is composed of small spherical structures called thyroid follicles.
    - The follicular cells that line the thyroid follicles are **cuboidal epithelial cells**. These cells secrete thyroid hormones, primarily thyroxine (T4) and triiodothyronine (T3), which are essential for regulating metabolism, growth, and development in the body.
  - Gonads
    - The simple cuboidal epithelium of the gonads that aid in the formation of gametes by undergoing meiosis are called germinal cuboidal epithelial cells.
    - Line the seminiferous tubules of the testes and also line the ovaries.
  - Salivary glands
    - Cuboidal epithelium lines the salivary glands and ducts.

7. Write a short note on salivary glands. (RUHS)

Answer

Salivary Glands

- Exocrine glands that produce saliva.
- Salivary glands can be classified as major/minor or serous/mucous/mixed.
- Three pairs of salivary glands are present:
  1. Parotid glands:
     - Largest salivary glands
     - Situated on each side of face just below the external acoustic meatus
     - Mainly serous
     - Duct of the parotid gland — Stensen's duct opens in the buccal vestibule opposite to the maxillary 2nd molar.
     - Mumps – viral infection of the parotid gland
  2. Submandibular glands:
     - Lie on each side of face under the mandible.
     - Mixed gland
     - Duct of submandibular gland — Wharton's duct opens on the side of the lingual frenum
  3. Sublingual glands
     - Lie on the floor of the mouth in front of the submandibular glands
     - Mainly mucous
     - Bartholin's duct — duct of the sublingual glands – 8–10 in number, open in the floor of the mouth.

Nerve Supply

- Innervated either directly or indirectly by the parasympathetic or sympathetic nerves.
- Parotid gland — receives parasympathetic supply by the glossopharyngeal nerve *via* the otic ganglion.

- Submandibular and sublingual glands receive the parasympathetic innervation by the facial nerve *via* the submandibular ganglion.

Structure of the Salivary Gland

- The gland is divided into lobules. Blood vessels and nerves enter the glands at the hilum and gradually branch into the lobules.
- Acini
  - Group of secretory cells.
  - Located at the terminal part of the gland.
  - Connects to the ductal system of the gland.
- Ducts
  - Lumina of the ducts is formed by the intercalated ducts, which in turn join to form striated ducts.
  - Found in both major and minor glands.

Functions

- Lubrication and Protection
- Buffering action
- Pellicle formation
- Antimicrobial action
- Digestion
- Taste

8. Write a short note on types of cartilage. (MGR, DU)

Answer

Types of Cartilage

Hyaline Cartilage

- Hyaline cartilage is a type of connective tissues which are found in areas such as the nose, ears, and trachea of the human body.
- The word "hyaline" means "glass-like", and it is a glossy, grayish-white tissue with a uniform appearance.
- Hyaline cartilage is the most abundant type of cartilage in the body.
- **Microscopic findings**
  - When a thin slice of hyaline cartilage is examined under the microscope, it appears to consist of cells (chondrocytes) of a rounded or angular form, lying in groups of two or more in a granular or almost homogeneous matrix. The cells are contained in cavities in the matrix, called cartilage lacuna.
- **Distribution**
  - Present at the epiphyseal ends of bone in children.
  - Present in articular cartilage, thyroid cartilage, tracheal rings, costal, bronchial and nasal cartilages.

Elastic Cartilage

- In this cartilage, the matrix is traversed by yellow elastic fibers which anastomose and branch in all directions.
- Extracellular matrix is metachromatic – due to the presence of glycosaminoglycans.
- Outer covering is known as perichondrium.
- Distribution
  - Pinna of external ear
  - Epiglottis
  - Cuneiform cartilage
  - Apex of arytenoid cartilage
  - Auditory tube
  - External auditory meatus

Fibrocartilage

- Also known as the white cartilage.
- Macroscopically, it is a dense fibrous tissue.
- Microscopically, it is made-up of large bundles of type I collagen fibers.
- The fibers merge with fibers of surrounding connective tissues.
- It has great tensile strength and high elasticity.
- **Distribution:**
  - Intervertebral disk
  - Interpubic disk
  - Menisci of knee joint
  - Articular disks of temporomandibular joint

9. Write a short note on hyaline cartilage. (KUHS)

Answer

For answer, refer to Short Notes no. 8, pg. no. 18

10. Write any two characteristic features of cardiac muscle. (DU, KUHS)

Answer

Two Characteristic features of Cardiac Muscle

Autorhythmicity

- Due to constant alterations in membrane permeability, pacemaker tissues exhibit an unstable resting membrane potential.

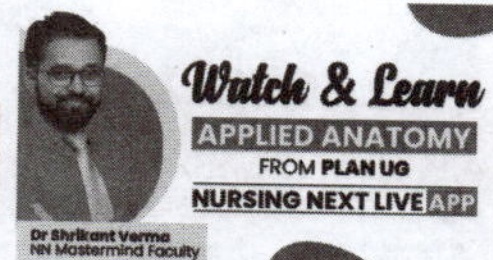

- Therefore, there is a gradual decrease in the membrane potential after each action potential unless it reaches firing level, and another action potential gets generated.
- This sluggish depolarization between action potential is referred to as pacemaker potential or diastolic depolarization.

Conductivity

- Depolarization begins in the SA node and spreads to the AV node at the rate of 1 m/sec.
- Conduction of AV node is minimum due to small fiber diameter and slow action potential.
- Due to slow conduction of AV node viz. 0.05 m/sec, there is an approximate delay of 0.1 second before excitation spreads to the ventricles referred to as A-V nodal delay.
- AV nodal delay= 0.09 seconds; AV bundle delay = .04 seconds
- This delay is due to less number of gap junctions and allows the atria to empty blood into ventricles before ventricular contraction begins.
- Affects the efficacy of pumping action of heart due to long refractory period of AV node cells, which limits the impulse conduction to 180 beats/min.
- AV nodal delay increases by excitation of parasympathetic nerves and decreases by stimulation of sympathetic nerves.

11. Enumerate the structural differences between skeletal, cardiac and smooth muscles. (MGR)

Answer

Table 1.2: Structural differences between skeletal, cardiac and smooth muscles

Characteristic	Skeletal muscle	Cardiac muscle	Smooth muscle
Location	Attached to the bones of the body	Found only in the heart	Line the walls of organs
Nervous Control	• Voluntarily controlled by somatic nervous system • Requires nerve or hormonal stimulation to generate action potential which results in movement • Resting membrane potential of skeletal muscle is -80 mV	• Involuntarily controlled by autonomic nervous system • Requires stimulation by pacemaker cells for contraction • Resting membrane potential of cardiac muscle is -90 mV	• Involuntary movements • Regulation by the somatic nervous system, endocrine system, hormones and various chemical messengers.
Function	Responsible for the movement of bones and cartilage	Responsible for pumping of the heart	Responsible for the movement of internal organs to facilitate their function.
Refractory period	Short	Long	
Speed of conduction impulse	3–5 m/s	< 1 m/s	< 1 m/s
Muscle fiber length	100 micrometer	10 micrometer	200 micrometer
Muscle diameter	200 millimeter	50 micrometer	5 micrometer
Structure	Skeletal muscle is a striated muscle attached to a bone by collagen fibers known as tendons. It contains actin and myosin, and the muscle fibers are formed by the coalition of myoblasts present.	Cardiac muscle is a striated muscle with alternate thin and thick striations along with intercalated disks and T-tubules. The striations consist of proteins. The thin striations are known as I-bands, while the thick ones are known as A-bands. The T-tubules form the triads, and the intercalated disks connect the cardiac myocyte to syncytium.	Comprise single, tapering non-nucleated cells. Non-striated, fewer myofibrils are found.
Fatigability	Do not fatigue	Easily fatigue	Do not fatigue

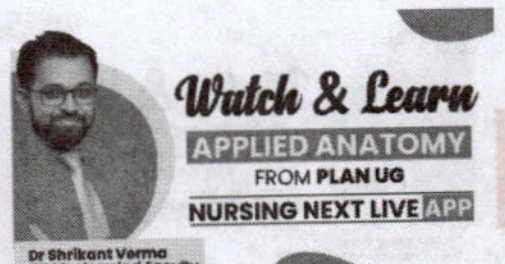

SHORT ANSWER QUESTIONS

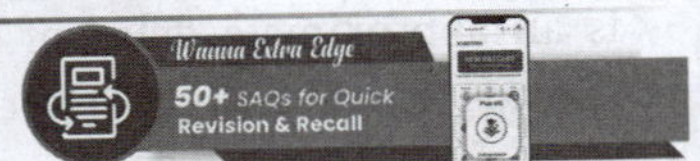

1. Mention any two connective tissue cells.

Answer

Two types of connective tissue cells are as follows:

1. **Fibroblast:** The fibroblast is the most abundant cell of the connective tissue. Fibroblasts play an important role in helping skin wounds heal as well as maintaining skin firmness and tightness.
2. **Cartilage:** Specialized connective tissues where chondrocytes and fibers are embedded in a firm gel like matrix.

2. Name two organs lined by columnar epithelium.

Answer

The lining of the stomach and the lining of the uterus are composed of a layer of columnar epithelial cells.

3. Name two glands lined by cuboidal epithelium.

Answer

Sweat glands are exocrine glands and thyroid gland is an endocrine gland. They are lined by cuboidal epithelial cells.

4. What is transitional epithelium.

Answer

Transitional epithelium is a type of stratified epithelium that is composed of several layers of cells and is found lining the urinary tract, including the bladder, ureters, and parts of the urethra.

5. Mention the layers of the epidermis of the skin.

Answer

The skin is composed of four main layers:

The four layers of the skin from outermost to innermost:

1. Stratum corneum:
2. Stratum granulosum
3. Stratum spinosum
4. Stratum basale (also known as the basal cell layer):

CONCEPTUAL REVISION

MULTIPLE CHOICE QUESTIONS

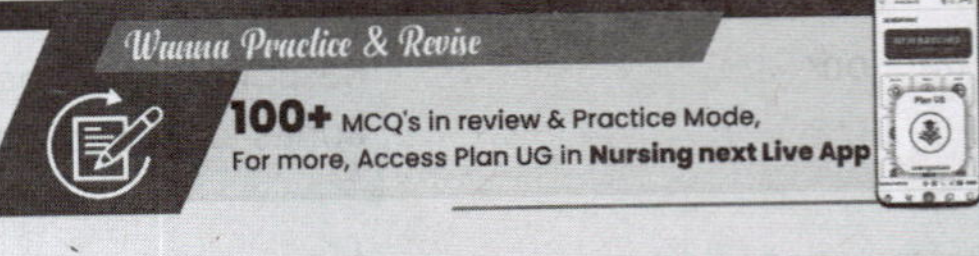

1. Which plane of the body divides it into dorsal and ventral regions?

a. Transverse b. Axial
c. Coronal d. Sagittal

Ans. c. Coronal

2. Which of the following is/are the contents of the dorsal body cavity?

a. Heart and lungs
b. Brain and spinal cord
c. Viscera
d. Gut, kidneys, liver, pancreas, spleen, bladder, internal reproductive organs

Ans. b. Brain and spinal cord

3. What structure separates the thoracic cavity from the abdominal cavity?

a. Mediastinum b. Diaphragm
c. Peritoneum d. Pylorus

Ans. b. Diaphragm

4. What body part is able to perform pronation and supination?

a. Forearm b. Foot
c. Thigh d. Wrist

Ans. a. Forearm

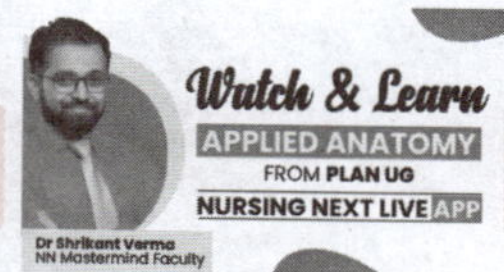

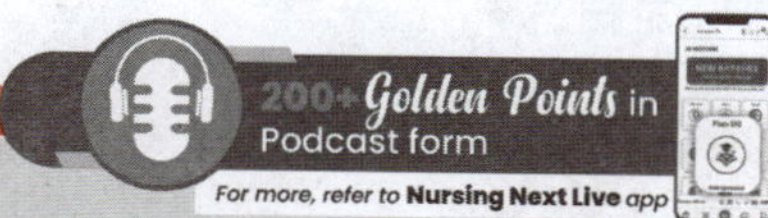

Golden Points

- **A cavity** is a hollow place. It is usually filled with organs, nerves, vessels, and muscles.
- **Adduction** is movement of bone toward midline. When a bone revolves around its own longitudinal axis, it is known as **rotation.**
- **Coronal or frontal plane** is a plane at right angles to sagittal or median plane which divides the body into anterior and posterior halves.
- **Gliding movement** is when relatively flat surfaces move from side-to-side and back-and-forth with respect to one another.
- In **lateral rotation,** the anterior surface of bone (of limb) turns away from midline.
- **Lithotomy position** involves lying on one's back with legs flexed at 90° at hips.
- **Median or midsagittal plane** passes through the center of the body dividing it into two equal right and left halves.
- **Meiosis** is a type of cell division that helps in production of egg and sperm cells.
- **Mitosis** is a process where a single cell divides into two identical daughter cells (cell division). Here the number of chromosomes remains constant through generations.

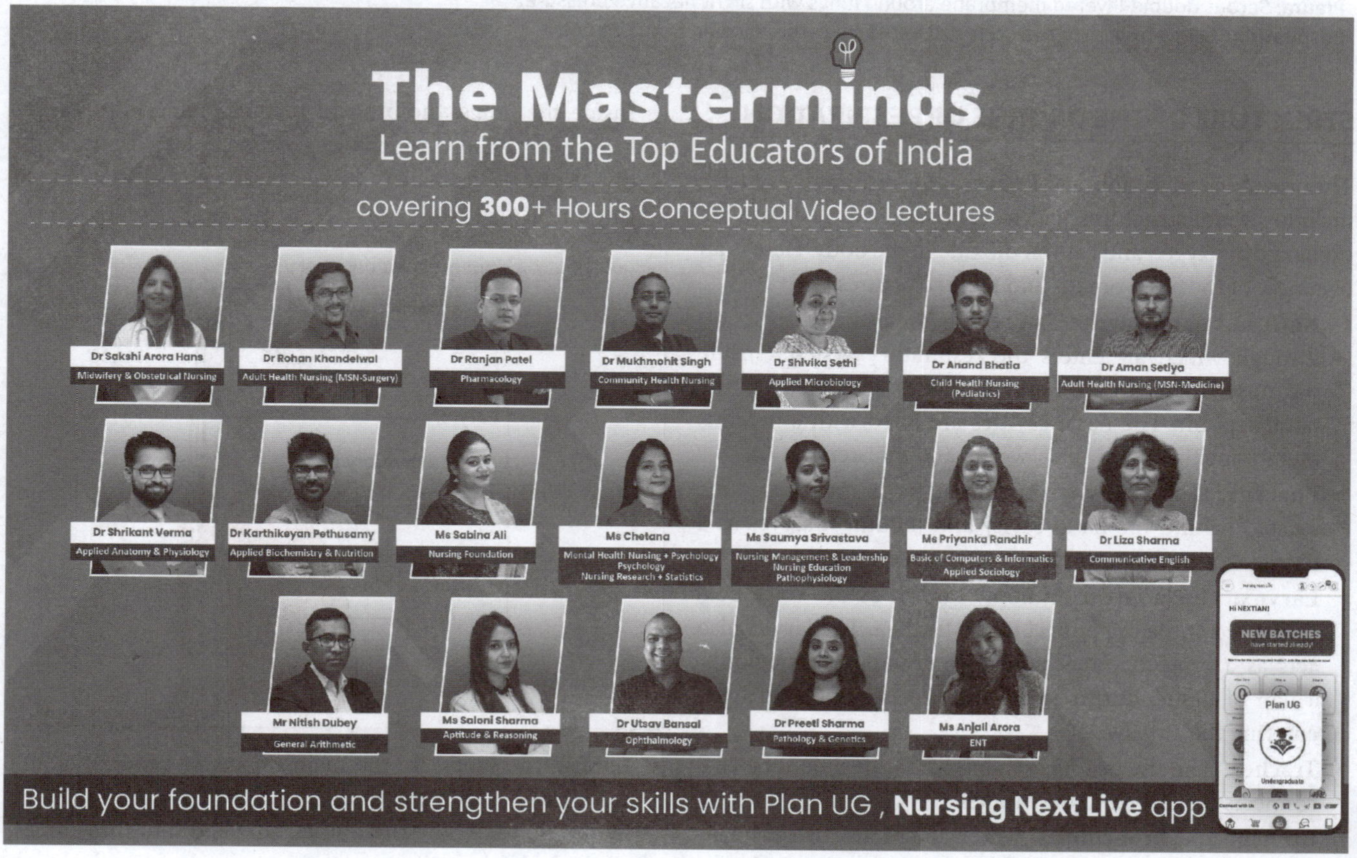

CHAPTER 2

Respiratory System

CONCEPTUAL THEORY

Terminology

150+ key terminologies for Quick Recall & Revision

Diaphragm: The diaphragm is a dome-shaped muscle located at the base of the lungs, separating the thoracic cavity from the abdominal cavity.

Intercostal muscles: The intercostal muscles are located between the ribs and assist in the process of breathing.

Larynx: Also called voice box. Muscles move the vocal cords to produce sounds/vowels. Safety muscle of larynx is posterior cricoarytenoid as it is the only abductor of vocal cord.

Nasopharynx: Part of pharynx posterior to the posterior nasal apertures. Few lymph nodules lie in this area.

Olfactory epithelium: Lines the uppermost part of nasal cavity. The impulses carry the sense of smell.

Paranasal sinus: Air spaces between the two tables of some of the skull bones. Paranasal sinus lightens the weight of the head, humidifies and heats up or cools down the inhaled inspired air.

Pleura: Serous double-layered membrane around lungs with slight negative pressure.

Respiration: Taking oxygen in the body and expelling carbondioxide from the body.

STRUCTURE OF THE ORGANS OF RESPIRATION

The organs of respiration, also known as the respiratory system, include several structures that work together to facilitate the exchange of oxygen and carbon dioxide in the body. Here is an overview of the main organs and their structures:

- **Nose and nasal cavity:** The nose is the external structure through which air enters the respiratory system. Inside the nose, there are two nasal cavities separated by the nasal septum. The nasal cavities are lined with a mucous membrane that helps filter, warm, and moisten the air.
- **Pharynx:** The pharynx, or throat, is a muscular tube located behind the nasal cavity and mouth. It serves as a passage for both air and food.
- **Larynx:** The larynx, commonly known as the voice box, is situated at the upper part of the trachea. The larynx also acts as a protective mechanism by closing the epiglottis, a flap of tissue, during swallowing to prevent food from entering the airway.
- **Trachea:** The trachea, or windpipe, is a flexible tube that connects the larynx to the bronchi.
- **Bronchi and bronchioles:** The bronchi are two primary branches of the trachea that enter the left and right lungs. Inside the lungs, the bronchi further divide into smaller branches called bronchioles. Bronchioles continue to divide into even smaller passageways, eventually leading to tiny air sacs called alveoli.

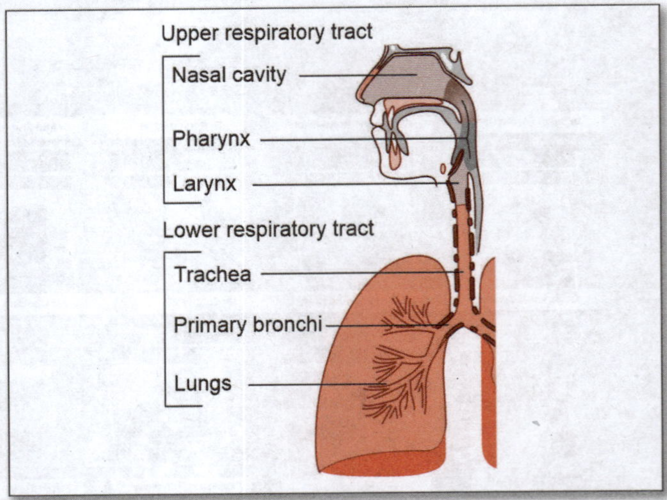

- **Lungs:** The lungs are the main organs of respiration and are located within the thoracic cavity. They are protected by the rib cage. The right lung is divided into three lobes, while the left lung has two lobes to accommodate the heart.

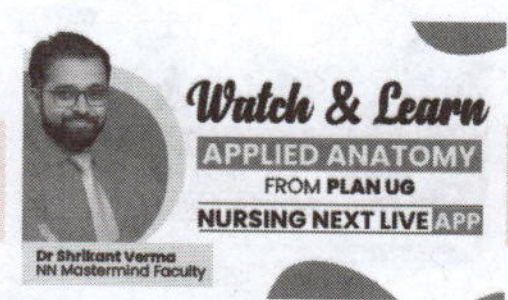

It contains alveoli, which are responsible for the exchange of oxygen and carbon dioxide with the bloodstream.

- **Diaphragm:** The diaphragm is a dome-shaped muscle located at the base of the lungs, separating the thoracic cavity from the abdominal cavity.

MUSCLES OF RESPIRATION

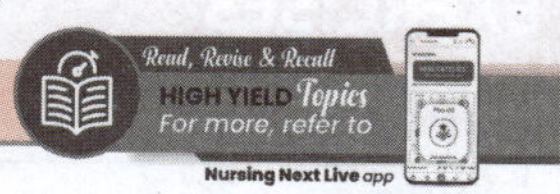

The process of respiration involves the contraction and relaxation of various muscles to facilitate inhalation and exhalation.

Here are the main muscles of respiration:

- **Diaphragm:** The diaphragm is a dome-shaped muscle located at the base of the lungs, separating the thoracic cavity from the abdominal cavity. It is the primary muscle of respiration. During inhalation, the diaphragm contracts and moves downward, increasing the volume of the thoracic cavity and causing air to enter the lungs. During exhalation, the diaphragm relaxes and moves upward, decreasing the volume of the thoracic cavity and helping to expel air from the lungs.
- **Intercostal muscles:** The intercostal muscles are located between the ribs and assist in the process of breathing. There are two sets of intercostal muscles:
    i. **External intercostal muscles:** These muscles are involved in inhalation. When they contract, they elevate the ribcage, expanding the thoracic cavity and aiding in the intake of air.
    ii. **Internal intercostal muscles:** These muscles are involved in forced exhalation. When they contract, they depress the ribcage, decreasing the volume of the thoracic cavity and assisting in the expulsion of air.
- **Accessory muscles of inhalation:** In certain situations, such as during exercise or respiratory distress, additional muscles are recruited to aid in inhalation.
    - **Sternocleidomastoid:** These muscles are located in the neck. When they contract, they lift the sternum and clavicles, increasing the size of the thoracic cavity and facilitating inhalation.
    - **Scalene muscles:** There are three sets of scalene muscles: anterior, middle, and posterior. When these muscles contract, they elevate the upper ribs, aiding in inhalation.
    - **Pectoralis minor:** This muscle is located in the chest. When it contracts, it helps elevate the ribs, contributing to inhalation.
- **Abdominal muscles:** Although primarily involved in core stabilization and trunk movement, the abdominal muscles also play a role in respiration, particularly during forced exhalation:
    - **Rectus abdominis:** This is the central abdominal muscle commonly referred to as the "six-pack." When it contracts, it increases intra-abdominal pressure, assisting in forced exhalation.
    - **External and internal obliques:** These muscles are located on the sides of the abdomen. Contraction of these muscles also increases intra-abdominal pressure, aiding in forced exhalation.

APPLICATION AND IMPLICATION IN NURSING

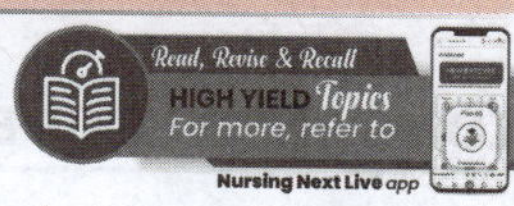

The respiratory system plays a vital role in nursing practice, and understanding its application and implications is crucial for nurses. Here are some key areas where the respiratory system is relevant in nursing:

- **Assessment and monitoring:** Nurses regularly assess and monitor patients respiratory status, including their breathing pattern, lung sounds, oxygen saturation levels, and respiratory rate. This information helps nurses identify respiratory problems, such as respiratory distress, respiratory infections, or compromised lung function.
- **Oxygen administration:** Nurses are responsible for administering oxygen therapy to patients who require supplemental oxygen. Monitoring oxygen saturation levels and assessing patients response to therapy is also essential.
- **Airway management:** Nurses assist with airway management techniques to maintain a patent airway and ensure adequate oxygenation. This includes techniques such as positioning, suctioning, and the use of airway adjuncts like oropharyngeal or nasopharyngeal airways.
- **Medication administration:** Nurses administer various respiratory medications, such as bronchodilators, corticosteroids, or antibiotics, to manage respiratory conditions like asthma, chronic obstructive pulmonary disease (COPD), or pneumonia. They need to understand the proper administration techniques, dosage calculations, potential side effects, and patient education regarding these medications.
- **Respiratory rehabilitation:** Nurses play a vital role in respiratory rehabilitation programs for patients with lung diseases. They educate patients about breathing exercises, use of incentive spirometers, and techniques to improve lung function and promote airway clearance.
- **Infection prevention:** Nurses are responsible for implementing infection prevention strategies to minimize the risk of respiratory infections, particularly in healthcare settings.
- **Patient education and health promotion:** Nurses educate patients about maintaining optimal respiratory health, recognizing early signs of respiratory problems, and managing chronic respiratory conditions. They provide smoking cessation counseling, teach proper inhaler technique, and emphasize the importance of vaccination (e.g., influenza and pneumococcal vaccines) for respiratory health.
- **Emergency response:** Nurses are often at the forefront of emergency response situations, including respiratory

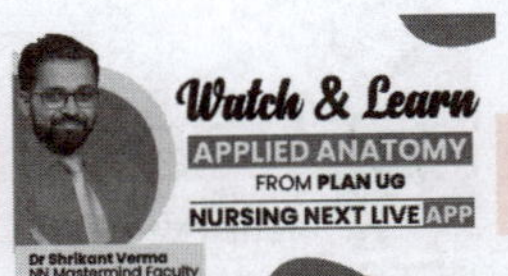

emergencies such as choking, respiratory distress, or respiratory arrest. They are trained to initiate life-saving interventions, like cardiopulmonary resuscitation (CPR), airway management, and use of emergency equipment like bag-valve-mask devices.

CONCEPTUAL EXERCISES

LONG ANSWER QUESTIONS

1. Enumerate the parts of respiratory system and write in detail about the lung. (MGR)

Answer

Parts of Respiratory System

- **Nose and nasal cavity:** The nose is the external structure through which air enters the respiratory system.
- **Pharynx:** The pharynx, or throat, is a muscular tube located behind the nasal cavity and mouth. Divided into three parts
  i. Nasopharynx—nasal part—transmits only air
  ii. Oropharynx—oral part—transmits both air and food
  iii. Laryngopharynx—laryngeal part—allows only food
- **Larynx:** The larynx, commonly known as the voice box, is situated at the upper part of the trachea. It is a passage of air that connects laryngopharynx and the trachea. It consists of nine cartilages, of which three are unpaired and three are paired.
  - 1 thyroid cartilage
  - 1 cricoid cartilage
  - 2 arytenoid cartilages
  - 1 epiglottis
- **Trachea:** The trachea, or windpipe, is a flexible tube that connects the larynx to the bronchi. Composed of three layers of tissue, and is held open by incomplete C shaped rings (16–20 in number) of hyaline cartilage. Patency is maintained due to the presence of C shaped cartilaginous rings in its walls.
- **Bronchi and bronchioles:** The bronchi are two primary branches of the trachea that enter the left and right lungs. Inside the lungs, the bronchi further divides into smaller branches called bronchioles. Bronchioles continue to divide into even smaller passageways, eventually leading to tiny air sacs called alveoli.
- **Lungs:** The lungs are the main organs of respiration and are located within the thoracic cavity. They are protected by the rib cage.
- **Diaphragm:** The diaphragm is a dome-shaped muscle located at the base of the lungs, separating the thoracic cavity from the abdominal cavity.

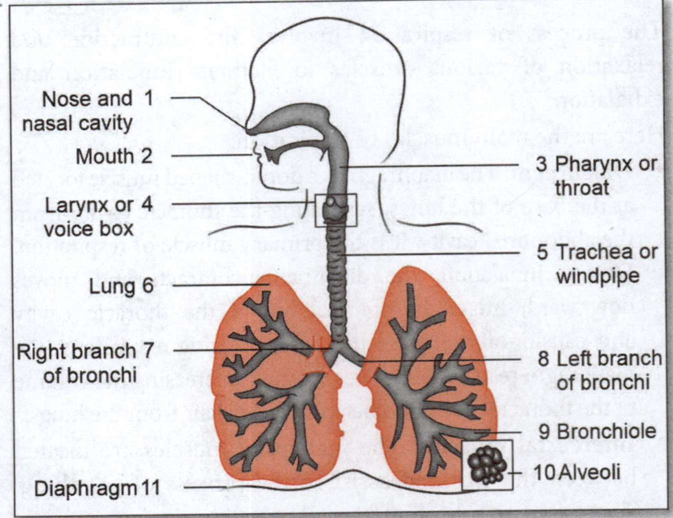

Lungs

- Cone-shaped lungs, one lying on each side of midline in the thoracic cavity.
- Each has an apex, a base, a costal surface and a medial surface.
- Most important organ of respiratory system.
- Voluminous cone-shaped organ occupying most of the thoracic cavity.
- Made-up of two portions

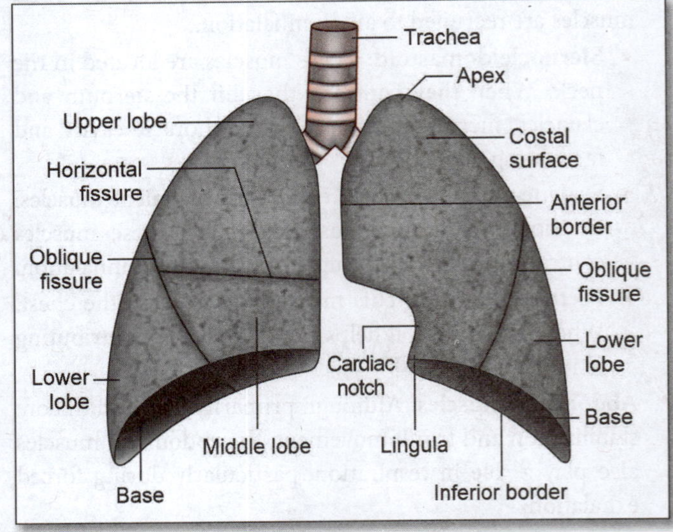

Figure 2.1: Lungs

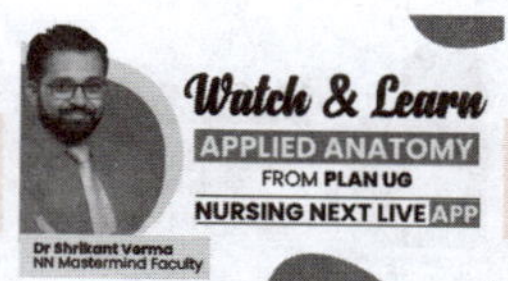

i. Conducting portion
ii. Respiratory portion

Pleura

- It is a closed serous sac which encloses the lung.
- It has two layers:
  i. **Parietal pleura:** Lines the inner surface of the chest wall and the thoracic surface of diaphragm.Its parts are cervical, costal, mediastinal and diaphragmatic pleura.
  ii. **Visceral pleura:** Lines the outer surface of the lung and its fissures.
- **Pleural cavity**
  - Space between the two pleura
  - Separated by a thin layer of serous fluid.

Conducting Portion of Lungs

- The primary bronchus enters the lung at the hilum.
- The right and left lungs are further divided into smaller lobes.
- The left lung is smaller than the right and contains two lobes, whereas right lobe contains three lobes.
- In general, each lung has ten segments:
  - Upper lobes—3 segments
  - Middle lobe/Lingula—2 segments
  - Lower lobes—5 segments
- Each segmental bronchus divides repeatedly into smaller ones till its diameter becomes 1.0 mm, when they are known as terminal bronchioles.
- **Respiratory Portion**
  - These are the main sites where gaseous exchange occurs.
  - Terminal bronchiole divides further and forms respiratory bronchiole, alveolar sac and finally the alveoli.
- **Bronchopulmonary Segments**
  - Bronchopulmonary segmental anatomy describes the division of the lungs into segments based on the tertiary or segmental bronchi.
  - The trachea divides into the right and left main bronchi at the carina, which enters the lungs and divides further.
  - The initial division is into lobar bronchi. Subsequent divisions give rise to smaller bronchi and bronchioles till the terminal respiratory bronchioles and alveoli.
  - Each segment has its own arterial supply—bronchopulmonary segment is formed by the bronchus and its artery.

Bronchopulmonary Segments of Right Lung

- The superior lobe of right has three bronchopulmonary segments.
  i. Topmost is the apical segment or segment I (SI).
  ii. Below and posterior to it is the posterior segment (S II). This segment is limited inferiorly by the posterosuperior part of the right oblique fissure and posterior part of the horizontal fissure.
  iii. Anterior segment (S III) is anteroinferior to the apical segment. It is limited inferiorly by the horizontal fissure.
- The middle lobe lies between the horizontal and anteroinferior part of the oblique fissures.
  - It is divided into lateral (S IV) and medial (S V) bronchopulmonary segments.
  - The lateral segment is seen on the costal surface of the lung, while the superficial boundary of the medial segment wraps around the anterior border of lung.
  - It tapers off at the hilum and is superiorly related to the oblique fissure.
- The inferior lobe has five bronchopulmonary segments.
  - The superior segment (S IV) is present on both costal and mediastinal surfaces of right lung, as the segment also includes a portion of the posterior border of the right lung.
  - The medial basal segment present on the mediastinal surface of the lung, lies below the hilum.
  - It is anteriorly related to the posterior basal segment (S X), which abuts the lateral basal segment (S IX) around the posterior border of the lung.
  - The anterior basal segment (S VIII) is limited anteriorly by the caudal part of the oblique fissure and is juxtaposed with the lateral basal segment posteriorly.

Bronchopulmonary Segments of Left Lung

The left lung is subdivided into two lobes and thereby, into eight segments.

The notation in brackets refers to the Boyden classification of bronchi.

1. Left upper lobe
   - Apicoposterior segment (B1/2)
   - Anterior segment (B3)
   - Posterior
   - Lingula
   - Superior segment (B4)
   - Lingula inferior segment (B5)
2. Left lower lobe
   - Superior segment (B6)
   - Medial basal
   - Anteromedial basal (B8)
   - Lateral basal (B9)
   - Posterior basal (B10)

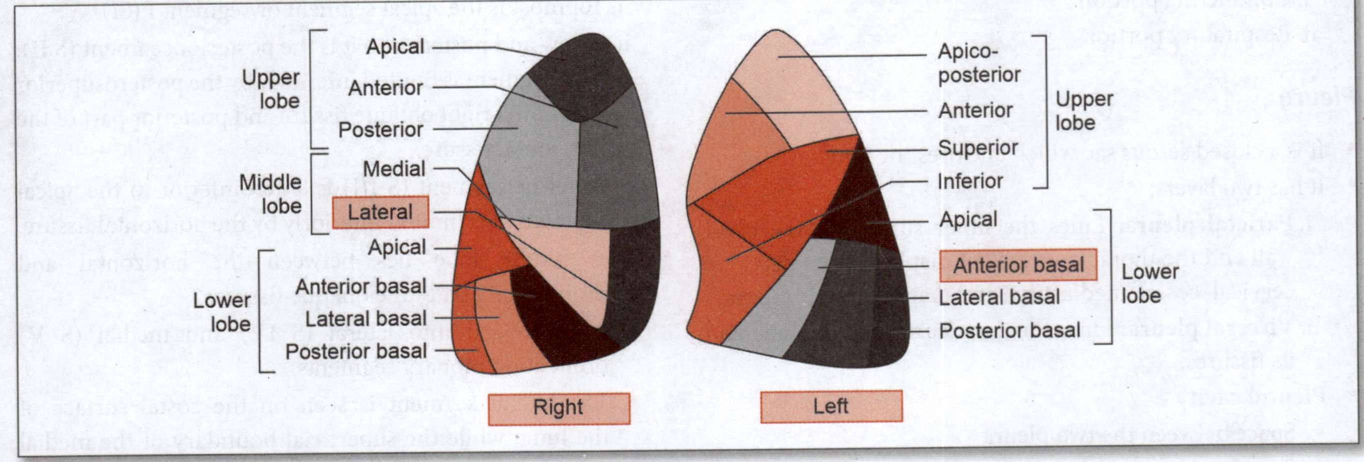

Figure 2.2: Bronchopulmonary segments

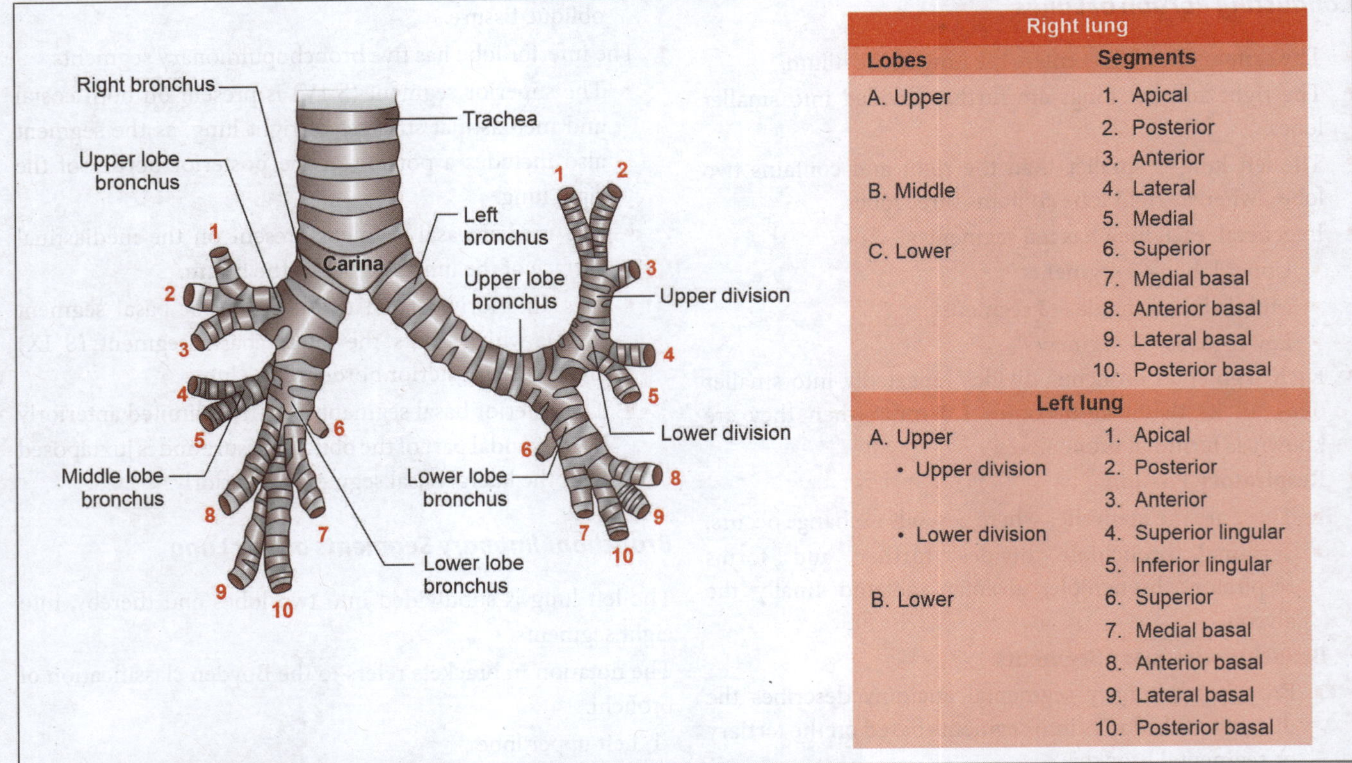

Right lung	
Lobes	**Segments**
A. Upper	1. Apical
	2. Posterior
	3. Anterior
B. Middle	4. Lateral
	5. Medial
C. Lower	6. Superior
	7. Medial basal
	8. Anterior basal
	9. Lateral basal
	10. Posterior basal
Left lung	
A. Upper	1. Apical
• Upper division	2. Posterior
	3. Anterior
• Lower division	4. Superior lingular
	5. Inferior lingular
B. Lower	6. Superior
	7. Medial basal
	8. Anterior basal
	9. Lateral basal
	10. Posterior basal

Figure 2.3: Bronchopulmonary segments

Hilum of Lung

- The mediastinal surface of the lung is concave and has the hilum.
- It is triangular in shape and surrounded by a pleura.
- It is located at the region between T5 and T7.
- It acts as a space/channel from where structures can enter or leave the lungs.
- It provides the attachment to the root of the lung.
- Also it is the only point where the visceral and parietal pleura meet.
- **Structures which leave and enter the hilum are:**
  - Bronchus/bronchi
  - Pulmonary artery
  - Pulmonary veins
  - Bronchial artery and bronchial vein
  - Lymphatic vessels
  - Nerves
  - Areolar tissue

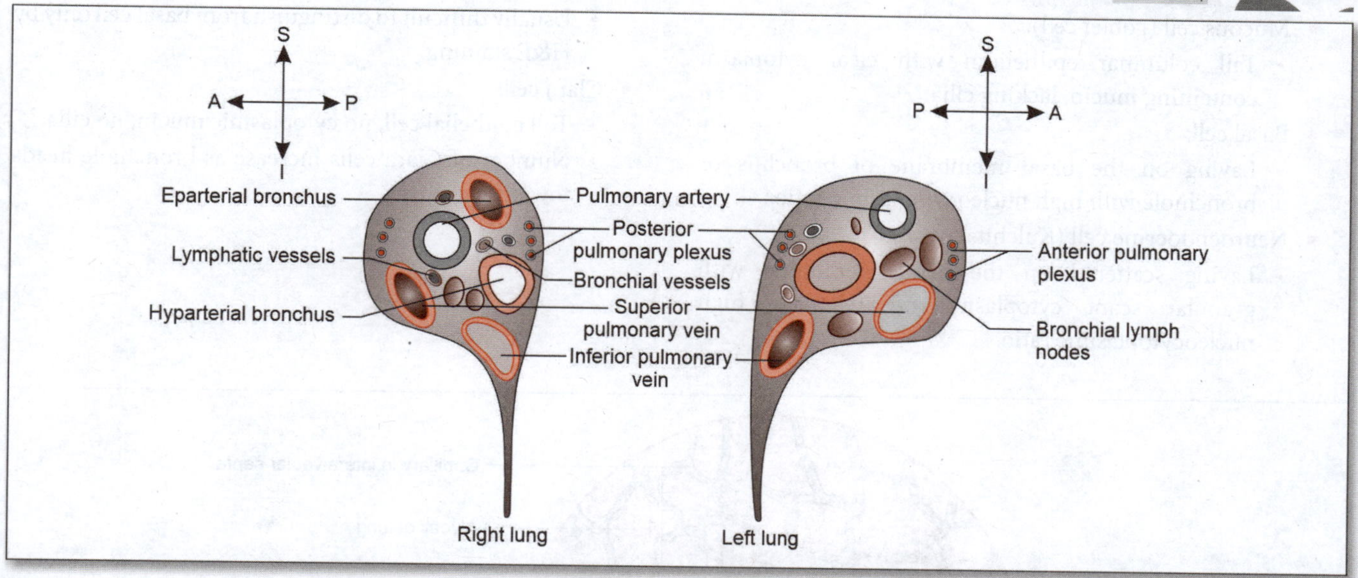

Figure 2.4: Structures passing through the hilum of right lung

Blood Supply of Lung

- The lungs are supplied with deoxygenated blood by the paired pulmonary arteries. Once the blood has received oxygenation, it leaves the lungs *via* four pulmonary veins (two for each lung).
- The bronchi, lung roots, visceral pleura and supporting lung tissues require an extra nutritive blood supply. This is delivered by the bronchial arteries, which arise from the descending aorta.
- The bronchial veins provide venous drainage. The right bronchial vein drains into the azygos vein, whilst the left drains into the accessory hemiazygos vein.

Histology of Lung

- Lung is characterized by the presence of numerous thin walled alveoli. These are mostly lined by a single layer of squamous cells, type I pneumocytes. Some cuboidal cells are present, these are type II pneumocytes.
- Alveolar duct:
  - Terminal airway opening to alveolus, of which alveolar entrance rings constitute the walls.
  - Alveolar entrance rings contain elastic fibers and smooth muscles.
- Alveolus:
  - Sac-like structure lined by alveolar epithelium.
  - Alveolar septum contains pulmonary capillaries.
  - Strictly speaking, alveolar structure is not sac-shaped but is a polyhedral architecture.
- Type I alveolar epithelium (pneumocyte):
  - Thin flat epithelium covering about 90–95% of alveolar lumen in area, about 40% of all alveolar epithelia in number.
- Type II alveolar epithelium (pneumocyte):
  - Cuboid epithelium covering 5 – 10% of the alveolar lumen in area, about 60% of all alveolar epithelia in number.
  - Type II cells produce serous fluid surfactant, which prevents the alveoli from collapsing by decreasing the surface tension.
- Between the alveoli are fine capillaries for exchange of gases. CO_2 is taken from the blood and oxygen is given to the blood, thus oxygenating it.
- Besides the alveoli and capillaries there are intrapulmonary bronchi and bronchioles.
- Bronchus:
  - Airway lined by pseudostratified ciliated epithelium
  - Mucosal and submucosal layer are separated by elastic membrane.
  - Bronchial glands exist in the submucosa; cartilage and annular muscular layer exist in the wall between submucosa and adventitia.
  - Cartilage is seen as small plates with smooth muscle fibres in between, outermost is thin connective tissue layer.
- Bronchiole:
  - Bronchioles are dilated spaces lined by columnar epithelium with no cartilage or gland, only smooth muscle fibers are present.
  - Lacks bronchial glands and cartilage.
- Special cells in lungs are:
  - Ciliated cell:
    - Tall columnar epithelium, with cilia on the edge of airway side.
    - Height becomes shorter as bronchiole heads toward periphery.

- Mucous cell (goblet cell):
  - Tall columnar epithelium with clear cytoplasm containing mucin, lacking cilia.
- Basal cell:
  - Laying on the basal membrane of bronchus or bronchiole with high nucleocytoplasmic ratio.
- Neuroendocrine cell (Kulchitsky cell):
  - Laying scattered on the basal membrane with granular scant cytoplasm and relatively high nucleocytoplasmic ratio.
  - Usually difficult to distinguish from basal cell only by H&E staining.
- Clara cell:
  - Toll epithelial cell, no cytoplasmic mucin, no cilia
  - Number of Clara cells increase as bronchiole heads toward periphery.

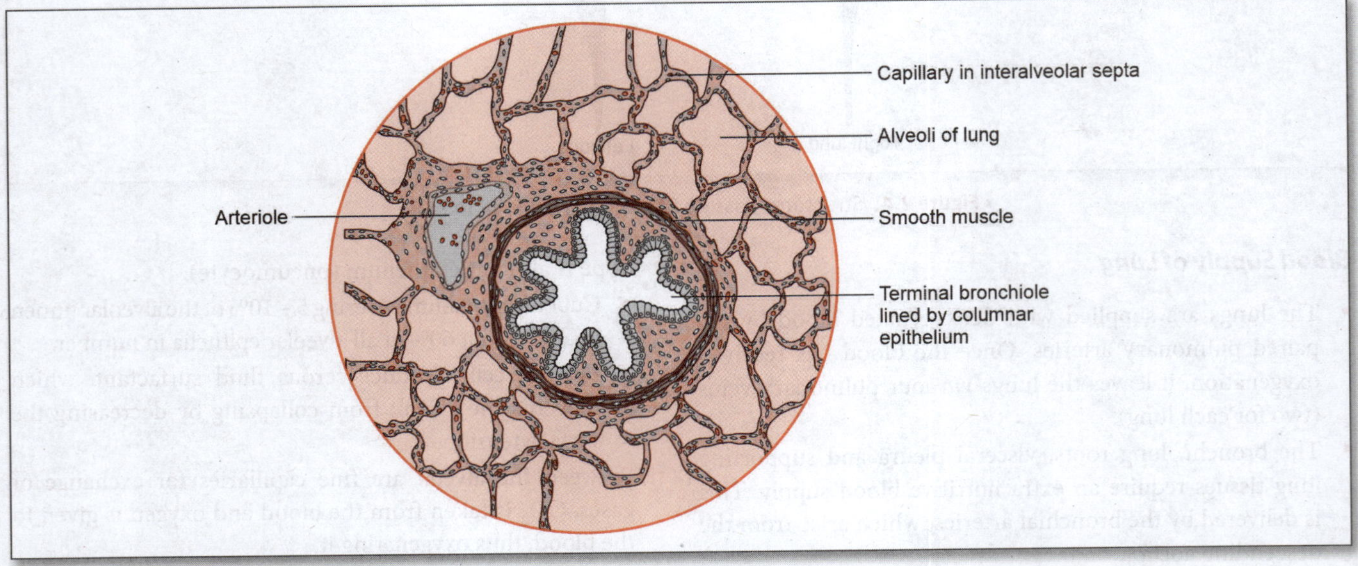

Figure 2.5: Lung histology

Functions

- Exchange of gases
  - External respiration: In the lungs
  - Internal respiration: In the tissues
- Pulmonary Ventilation
- Immunity
  - Due to the presence of lymphocytes, plasma cells and alveolar macrophages.

2. Describe in detail muscles of respiration, intercostals and diaphragm.

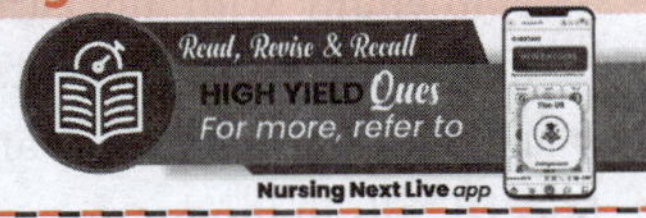

Answer

Muscles of Respiration

For Quiet Respiration

- Diaphragm
- External costal muscles

For Deep Inspiration

- Erector spinae
- Scalene muscles
- Pectoral muscles

For Expiration

Passive process

Forced Expiration

Muscles of anterior abdominal wall

Characteristic Features of Respiratory Muscles

- Fatigue resistant
- Under both voluntary and involuntary control.

Inspiratory and Expiratory Muscles

- Muscles that expand the thoracic cavity are known as inspiratory muscles. These muscles aid in inhalation.

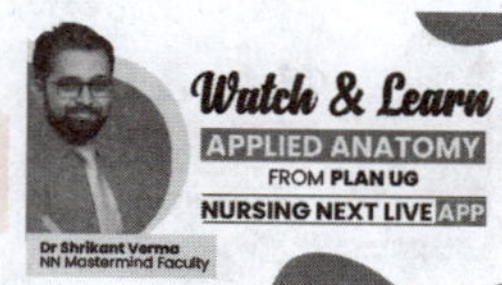

- Muscles that compress the thoracic cavity are known as expiratory muscles. These muscles aid in exhalation.
- The muscles of inspiration elevate the ribs and sternum.
- Primary muscles—diaphragm and the external intercostals.

Muscles of Exhalation

- Quiet expiration is a passive process, no muscle is involved in exhalation.
- This process is driven by the elastic recoil of the lungs.
- During forced expiration, or conditions where the elasticity of the lungs is compromised, the accessory expiratory muscles play a role.
- These muscles push the abdominal muscles into the thoracic cavity, thus reducing the volume of the thoracic cavity.
- The internal intercostal muscles have fibers that run obliquely downward and backward from rib to rib.

These muscles assist in lowering the rib cage and aid in exhalation.

- The thoraco-abdominal diaphragm is a dome-shaped muscle that separates the thoracic and the abdominal cavity.
- It gives passage to a number of structures passing in both the directions.
- It forms the roof of the abdominal cavity.

Intercostal Muscles

Three types:

1. External
2. Internal
3. Innermost

- The external intercostal muscles are the most important.
- Their fibers run obliquely downward and forward from rib to rib. These muscles contract to raise each rib toward the above, with an overall effect of raising the rib cage assisting in inhalation.
- Accessory muscles have no definite role. Their effect depends on the effort of respiration. Overall, the accessory muscles help to elevate the rib cage to assist in inhalation.

Diaphragm

- Double dome muscle separating the thoracic and the abdominal cavity.
- It is the main inspiratory muscle.
- During inspiration, it contracts and moves in an inferior direction that increases the vertical diameter of the lung.
- Lung expands, decreasing the pressure inside the lungs, causing it to draw the air in.
- **Sternal part**
  - Originates from the posterior aspect of xiphoid process.
- **Costal part**
  - Arises from the inner surface of the cartilages of lower six ribs, interdigitating with transversus abdominis muscle.
- **Lumbar part**
  - Originates from the median arcuate ligament. It is a tendinous arch across the aorta at the level of L1 vertebrae.
  - Medial arcuate ligament is a tendinous arch in fascia covering upper part of psoas major.
  - Lateral lumbosacral arch or lateral arcuate ligament.

Insertion

- All muscles of diaphragm are inserted into the central tendon of diaphragm. It lies below the pericardium and is fused with the pericardium.

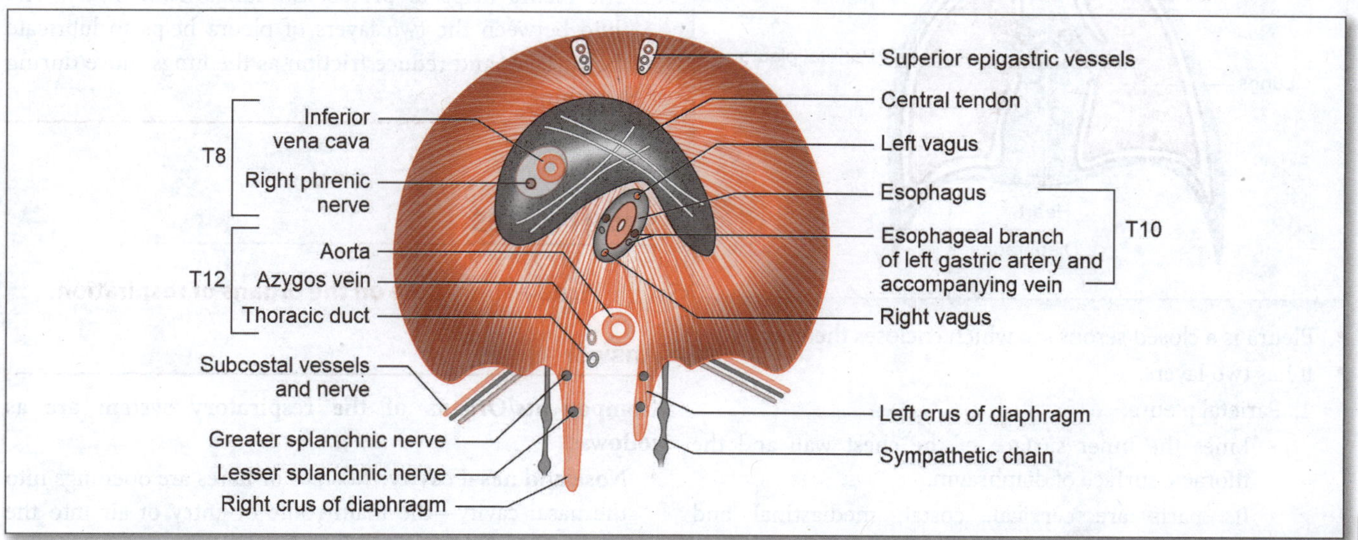

Figure 2.6: Diaphragm-nerve and blood supply

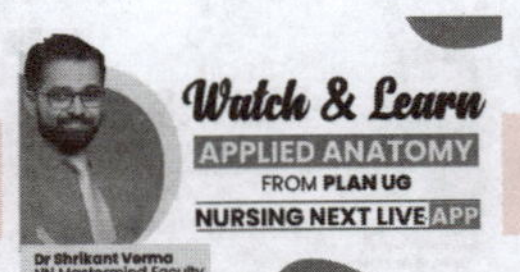

- The tendon is trilobar in shape made-up of three leaflets
  - Left and right are tongue shaped, left narrower than right
  - Middle is triangular.

Nerve Supply

- Motor nerve:
  - Phrenic nerve
- Sensory nerve
  - The phrenic nerves are sensory to the central and lower six thoracic nerves are sensory to the peripheral part of the diaphragm.

Actions

- Principal muscle of inspiration
  - On contraction of diaphragm, vertical diameter of the thorax increases.
- Acts in all expulsive acts to give additional power to each effort.
- Right crus of diaphragm has a sphincteric action on the lower end of esophagus.

3. What is pleura and its importance? Mention its arrangement in relation with the lung.

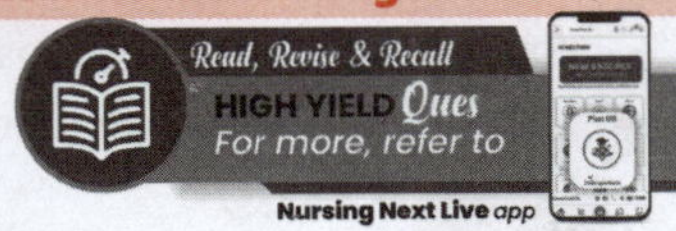

Answer

Pleura

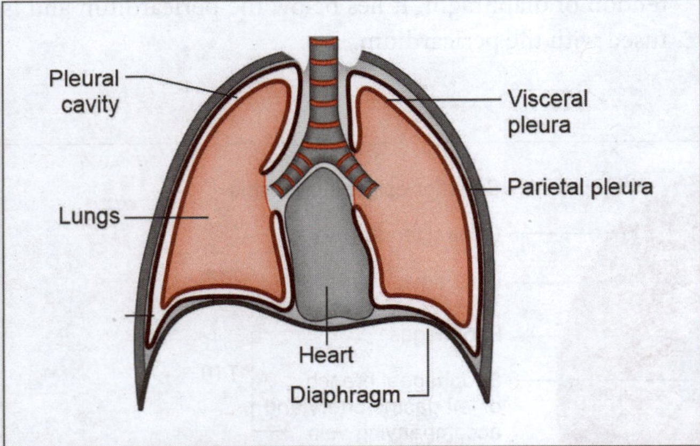

- Pleura is a closed serous sac which encloses the lung.
- It has two layers:
  1. Parietal pleura:
     - Lines the inner surface of the chest wall and the thoracic surface of diaphragm.
     - Its parts are cervical, costal, mediastinal and diaphragmatic pleura.
     - It is reflected at the hilum to become the visceral pleura.
  2. Visceral pleura:
     - Lines the outer surface of the lung and its fissures.
- Pleural cavity
  - Space between the two pleura
  - Separated by a thin layer of serous fluid.

The arrangement of the pleura in relation to the lung is as follows:

- The visceral pleura covers the entire surface of the lungs, including the lobes and fissures.
- The parietal pleura lines the inside of the thoracic cavity, including the mediastinum, the diaphragm, and the ribs.
- The two layers of pleura are separated by a small amount of fluid.

Functions

- The structure of the pleura is essential for respiration, providing the lungs with lubrication and cushioning needed to inhale and exhale.
- Interpleural space
  - Contains four cubic centimeters of pleural fluid
  - Reduces friction between the lungs
- Pleural fluid creates the surface tension that helps maintain the position of the lungs against the chest wall.
- The pleurae serves as a division between other organs in the body, preventing them from interfering with lung function and vice versa.

Clinical Importance

- Pleura is self-contained, it can help prevent the spread of infection to and from the lungs.
- The pleura helps to protect the lungs from injury. The fluid between the two layers of pleura helps to lubricate the surfaces and reduce friction as the lungs move during breathing.

SHORT NOTES

1. Write a short note on the organs of respiration.

Answer

Components/Organs of the respiratory system are as follows:

- **Nose and nasal cavity:** Nostrils or nares are openings into the nasal cavity—the main route of entry of air into the respiratory system.

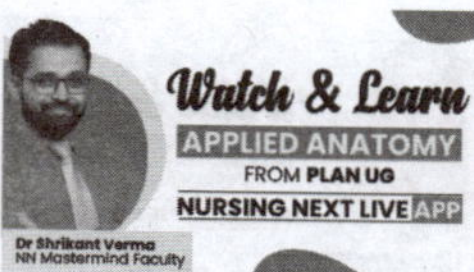

- **Paranasal sinuses**
  - Air-filled spaces present within the bones around the nasal cavity.
  - Includes frontal, maxillary, sphenoidal and ethmoidal.
  - Open into the nasal cavity through lateral wall.
  - Functions:
    - Warm and humidify the inhaled air.
    - Make the skull lighter.
    - Add resonance to the voice.
- **Pharynx:** Wide muscular tube situated behind the nose, mouth and larynx. Also known as throat.
- **Larynx:**
  - It is a passage of air that connects the laryngopharynx and trachea.
  - Functions:
    - Acts as voice box—contains special structures known as vocal folds that produce sound.
    - Acts as a sphincter for lower respiratory passages.
    - Protection of the lower respiratory tract during swallowing—due to the epiglottis.
    - Humidifies, filters and warms inhaled air.
- **Trachea:**
  - 10 – 11 cm long noncollapsible wide tube forming the beginning of the lower respiratory passages.
  - Also known as the windpipe.
  - Functions:
    - The soft posterior wall allows expansion of the esophagus during the passage of food.
    - Ciliary escalator action helps to remove mucus and foreign particles from the laryngopharynx.
    - Aids in cough reflex.
- **Lungs:**
  - Cone-shaped lungs, one lying on each side of midline in the thoracic cavity.
  - Each has an apex, a base, a costal surface and a medial surface.
  - Most important organ of the respiratory system.
  - Voluminous cone-shaped organ occupying most of the thoracic cavity.
  - Made-up of two portions:

i. Conducting portion
ii. Respiratory portion

  - Functions
    - Purification of air and distribution of oxygen

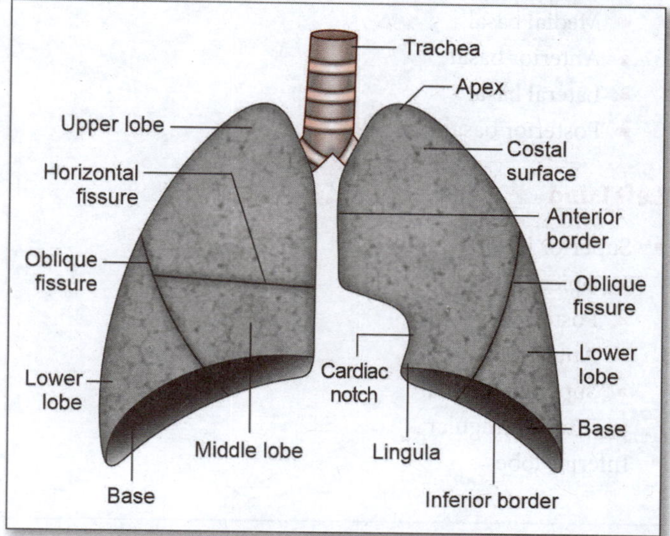

Figure 2.7: Lungs

2. Write a short note on bronchopulmonary segments.

Answer

Bronchopulmonary Segment

- Trachea divides into principal bronchi which subsequently give rise to lobar branches.
- Each lobar bronchus on the right and left side of the lung divides into several segmental bronchi.
- The lung tissue aerated by each segmental bronchus is a distinct structural and functional entity known as the bronchopulmonary segment.
- The segmental bronchus and the pulmonary arteries occupy a central position within a bronchopulmonary segment; whereas the pulmonary veins and their tributaries run in the connective tissue septa adjoining two segments (intersegmental drainage).
- There are ten bronchopulmonary segments on each side.

Right Lung

- Superior lobe
  - Apical
  - Posterior
  - Anterior
- Middle lobe
  - Lateral
  - Medial
- Inferior lobe
  - Superior

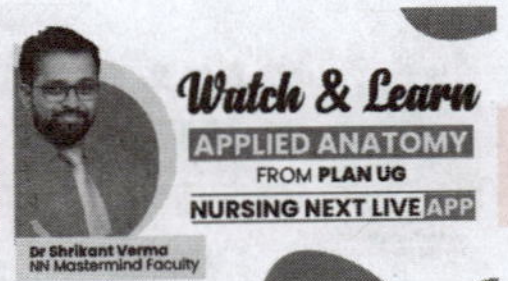

- Medial basal
- Anterior basal
- Lateral basal
- Posterior basal

Left Lung

- Superior lobe
  - Apical
  - Posterior
  - Anterior
  - Superior lingular
  - Inferior lingular
- Inferior lobe
  - Superior
  - Medial basal
  - Anterior basal
  - Lateral basal
  - Posterior basal

Applied Anatomy

- During surgical resection, the anatomy of bronchopulmonary segments is essential in defining the lung tissue to be resected.
- Surgeon plans along the intersegmental planes and ligates the segmental bronchus to demarcate the boundaries of the segment to be removed.

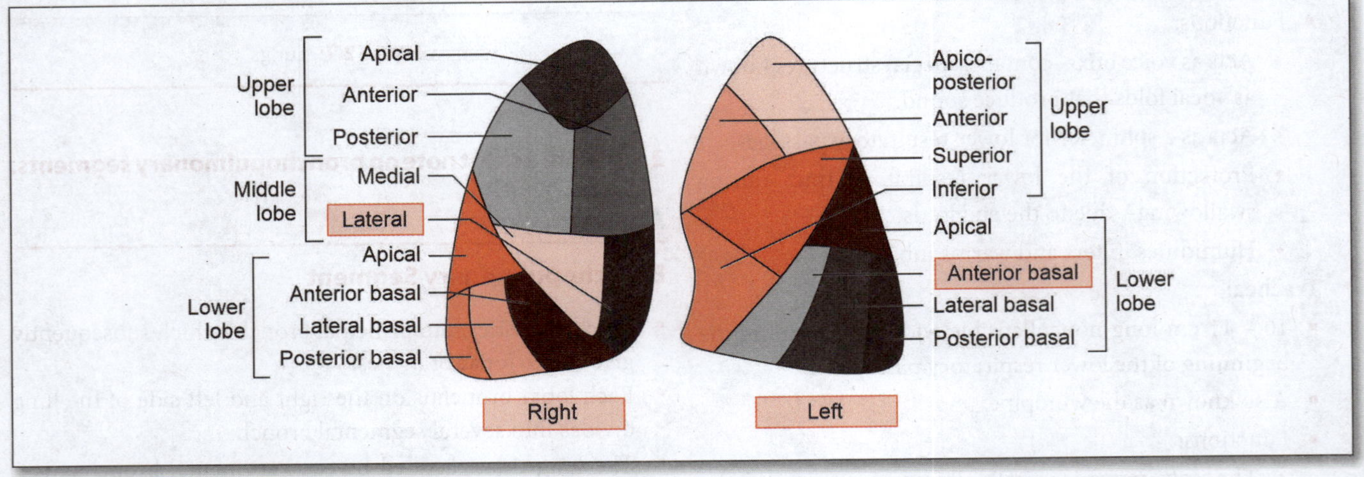

Figure 2.8: Bronchopulmonary segments

3. Write a short note on diaphragm and major openings in it.

Answer

Diaphragm

- The thoraco-abdominal diaphragm is a dome-shaped muscle that separates the thoracic and the abdominal cavity.
- It gives passage to a number of structures passing in both directions.
- It forms the roof of the abdominal cavity.

Diaphragm Openings

- **Caval (T8):**
  - Inferior vena cava and right phrenic nerve
- **Left muscular dome (T8):**
  - Left phrenic nerve
- **Anterior hiatus (T9):**
  - Superior epigastric artery and vein
- **Esophageal (T10):**
  - Esophagus
  - Left and right vagus nerves
  - Esophageal branches of left gastric artery/vein
  - Lymphatics
- **Aortic (T12) (Strictly behind diaphragm):**
  - Aorta
  - Azygos vein and hemiazygos vein (may pass *via* left crus)
  - Thoracic duct
- **Crura (T12):**
  - Greater, lesser and least splanchnic nerves
- Behind medial arcuate ligament:
  - Sympathetic chain
- Behind lateral arcuate ligament:
  - Subcostal nerve (T12), artery and vein

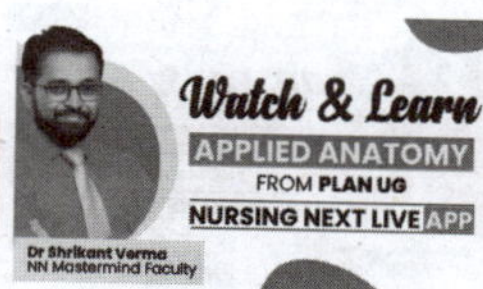

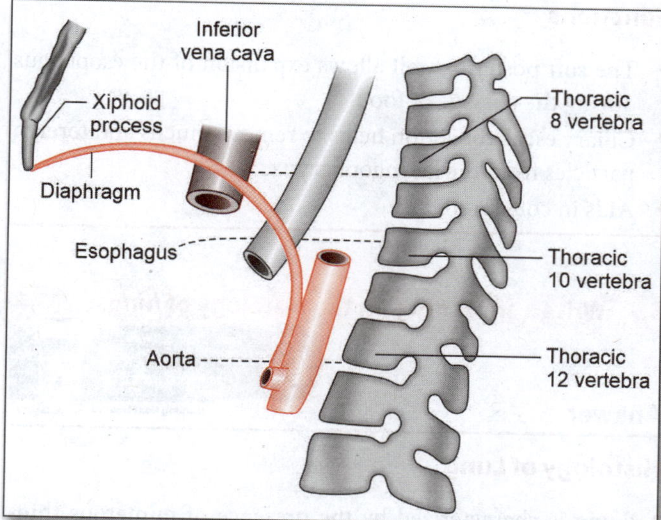

Figure 2.9: Openings in the diaphragm

4. Write a short note on lungs.

Answer

Lungs

- Cone-shaped lungs, one lying on each side of midline in the thoracic cavity.
- Each has an apex, a base, a costal surface and a medial surface.
- Most important organ of the respiratory system.
- Voluminous cone-shaped organ occupying most of the thoracic cavity.
- Made-up of two portions:
  1. Conducting portion
  2. Respiratory portion

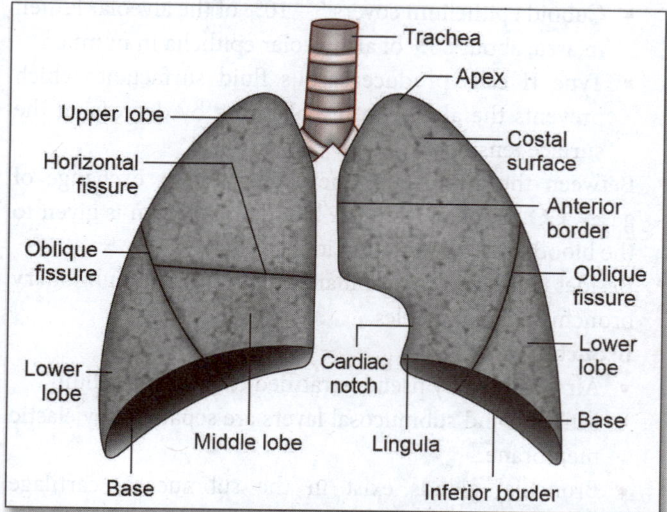

Figure 2.10: Lungs

Pleura

- Pleura is a closed serous sac which encloses the lung.
- It has two layers:
  1. Parietal pleura
  2. Visceral pleura
- Pleural cavity:
  - Space between the two pleura.
  - Separated by a thin layer of serous fluid.

Conducting Portion of Lungs

- The primary bronchus enters the lung at the hilum.
- The right and left lungs are further divided into smaller lobes.
- The left lung is smaller than the right and contains two lobes, whereas right lobe contains three lobes.

Respiratory Portion

- These are the main sites where gaseous exchange occurs.
- Terminal bronchiole divides further and forms respiratory bronchiole, alveolar sac and finally the alveoli.

Blood Supply of Lung

- **Pulmonary arteries:** The lungs are supplied with deoxygenated blood by the paired pulmonary arteries.
- Once the blood has received oxygenation, it leaves the lungs *via* four pulmonary veins (two for each lung).
- **Bronchial arteries:** The bronchi, lung roots, visceral pleura and supporting lung tissues require an extra nutritive blood supply. This is delivered by the bronchial arteries, which arise from the descending aorta.
- The bronchial veins provide venous drainage.

Functions

- Exchange of gases
  - **External respiration:** In the lungs
  - **Internal respiration:** In the tissues
- Pulmonary ventilation
- **Immunity:** Due to the presence of lymphocytes, plasma cells and alveolar macrophages.

5. Write a short note on trachea – length, histology and divisions.

Answer

Trachea

- Trachea is a 10–15 cm long noncollapsible wide tube forming the beginning of the lower respiratory passages.

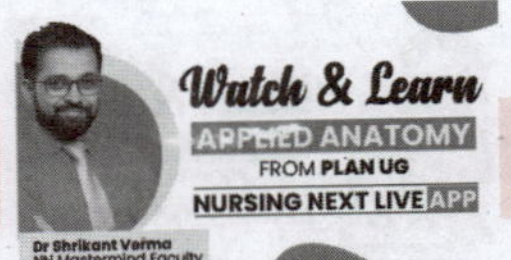

- Also known as the windpipe.
- Composed of three layers of tissue, and is held open by incomplete C-shaped rings (16–20 in number) of hyaline cartilage.
- Patency is maintained due to the presence of C-shaped cartilaginous rings in its walls.
- Begins at the lower border of the cricoid cartilage opposite the lower border of vertebra C6.

Dimensions

- About 10–15 cm long
- Its upper half lies in the neck and its lower half in the superior mediastinum.
- The external diameter measures 2 cm in males and 1.5 cm in females.
- The lumen is about 3 mm at 1 year of age, and corresponds to the age in years during childhood, with a maximum of 12 mm at puberty.

Histology of Trachea

- Consists of 16–20 C-shaped cartilaginous rings with fibrous tissues, smooth muscle fibers and mucous membrane. It is made of hyaline cartilage to keep it permanently patent.
- It is lined by pseudostratified ciliated columnar epithelium. The cells are of varying height, giving a false appearance of more than one layer of cells. Deep to the epithelium are mucus and serous glands.
- **Carina**
  - Last tracheal ring
  - It is thick and broad.
  - Hook-like process that curves downward and backward between the bronchi.

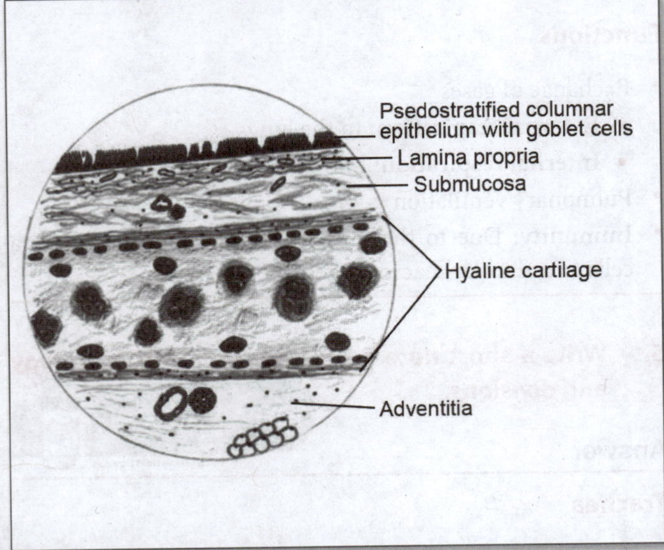

Figure 2.11: Microanatomy of trachea

Functions

- The soft posterior wall allows expansion of the esophagus during the passage of food.
- Ciliary escalator action helps to remove mucus and foreign particles from the laryngopharynx.
- Aids in cough reflex.

6. Write a short note on the histology of lungs.

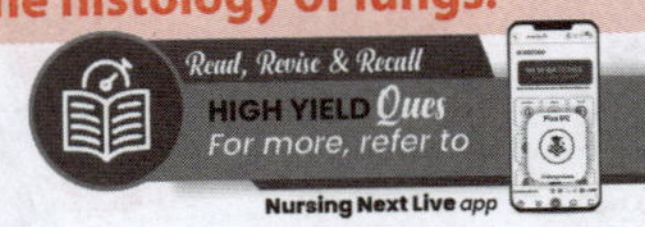

Answer

Histology of Lung

- Lung is characterized by the presence of numerous thin-walled alveoli. These are mostly lined by a single layer of squamous cells known as type I pneumocytes.
- Some cuboidal cells are present, which are known as type II pneumocytes.
- **Alveolar duct:**
  - Terminal airway opening to alveolus, of which alveolar entrance rings constitute the walls.
  - Alveolar entrance rings contain elastic fibers and smooth muscles.
- **Alveolus:**
  - Sac-like structure lined by alveolar epithelium.
  - Alveolar septum contains pulmonary capillaries.
  - Strictly speaking, the alveolar structure is not sac-shaped but is a polyhedral architecture.
- **Type I alveolar epithelium (pneumocyte):**
  - Thin flat epithelium covers about 90 – 95% of alveolar lumen in area, about 40% of all alveolar epithelia in number.
- **Type II alveolar epithelium (pneumocyte):**
  - Cuboid epithelium covers 5 – 10% of the alveolar lumen in area, about 60% of all alveolar epithelia in number.
  - Type II cells produce serous fluid surfactant, which prevents the alveoli from collapsing by decreasing the surface tension.
- Between the alveoli are fine capillaries for exchange of gases. CO_2 is taken from the blood and oxygen is given to the blood, thus oxygenating it.
- Besides the alveoli and capillaries, there are intrapulmonary bronchi and bronchioles.
- **Bronchus:**
  - Airway lined by pseudostratified ciliated epithelium
  - Mucosal and submucosal layers are separated by elastic membrane.
  - Bronchial glands exist in the submucosa; cartilage and annular muscular layer exist in the wall between submucosa and adventitia.

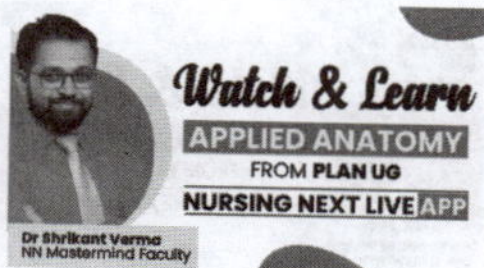

- Cartilage is seen as small plates with smooth muscle fibers in between, outermost is thin connective tissue layer.
- **Bronchiole:**
  - Bronchioles are dilated spaces lined by columnar epithelium with no cartilage or gland, only smooth muscle fibers are present.
  - Lacks bronchial glands and cartilage.
- **Special cells in lungs are as follows:**
  - **Ciliated cell:**
    - Tall columnar epithelium, with cilia on the edge of airway side.
    - Height becomes shorter as bronchiole heads toward periphery.
  - **Mucous cell (goblet cell):**
    - Tall columnar epithelium with clear cytoplasm containing mucin, lacking cilia.
  - **Basal cell:**
    - Lay on the basal membrane of bronchus or bronchiole with high nucleocytoplasmic ratio.
  - **Neuroendocrine cell (Kulchitsky cell):**
    - Lay scattered on the basal membrane with granular scant cytoplasm and relatively high nucleocytoplasmic ratio.
    - Usually difficult to distinguish from basal cell only by H&E staining.
  - **Clara cell:**
    - Tall epithelial cell, no cytoplasmic mucin, no cilia.
    - The number of Clara cells increases as bronchiole heads toward periphery.

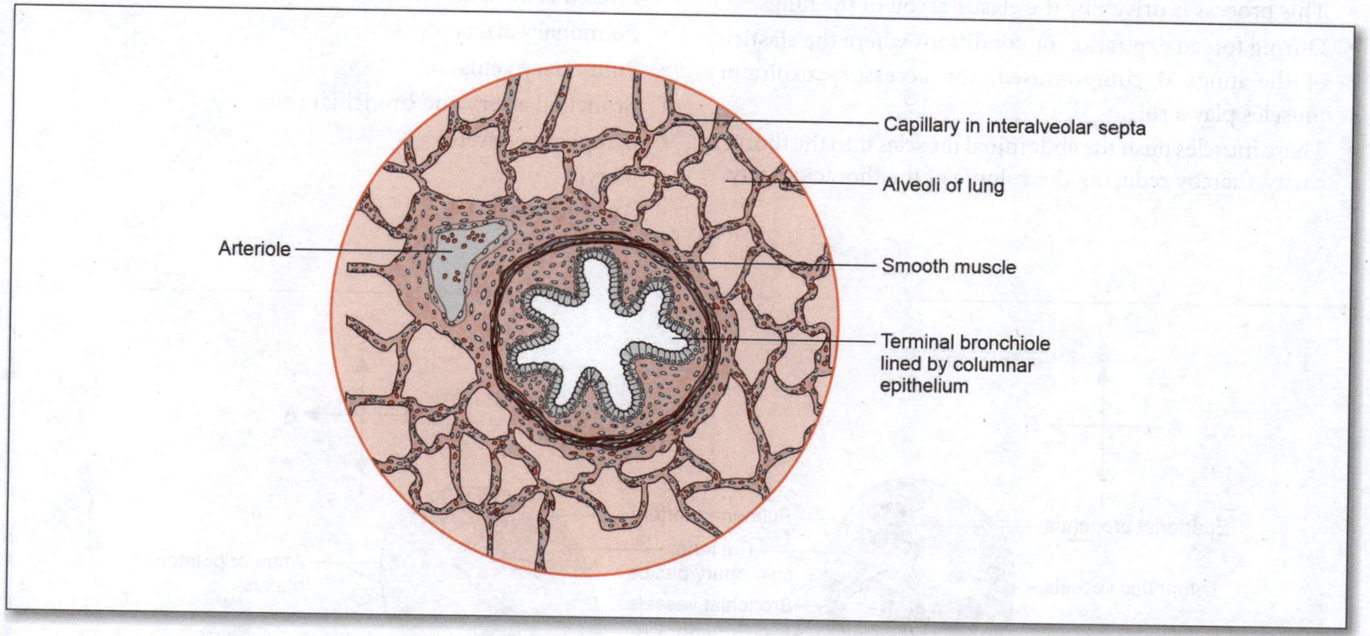

Figure 2.12: Lung histology

7. Write a short note on muscles of respiration.

Answer

Muscles of Respiration

- **For quiet respiration:** Diaphragm and external costal muscles
- **For deep inspiration:**
  - Erector spinae
  - Scalene muscles
  - Pectoral muscles
- **For quiet expiration:** A passive process
- **Forced expiration:** Muscles of anterior abdominal wall

Inspiratory Muscles

- The muscles of inspiration elevate the ribs and sternum.
- **Primary muscles:** Diaphragm and the external intercostals.
- Diaphragm
  - Double dome muscle separating the thoracic and the abdominal cavity.
  - It is the main inspiratory muscle.

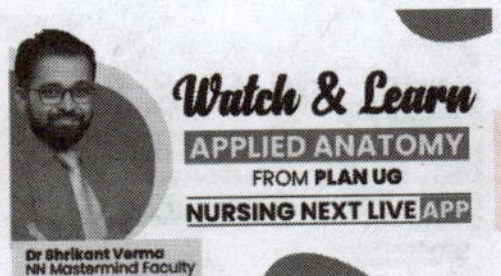

- During inspiration, it contracts and moves in an inferior direction that increases the vertical diameter of the lung.
- Lung expands, decreasing the pressure inside the lungs, causing it to draw the air in.

- Intercostal muscles
  - Three types:
    1. External
    2. Internal
    3. Innermost
- Accessory muscles have no definite role. Their effect depends on the effort of respiration. Overall, the accessory muscles help to elevate the rib cage to assist in inhalation.

Muscles of Exhalation

- Quiet expiration is a passive process; no muscle is involved in exhalation.
- This process is driven by the elastic recoil of the lungs.
- During forced expiration or conditions where the elasticity of the lungs is compromised, the accessory expiratory muscles play a role.
- These muscles push the abdominal muscles into the thoracic cavity, thereby reducing the volume of the thoracic cavity.
- The internal intercostal muscles have fibers that run obliquely downward and backward from rib to rib.
  - These muscles assist in lowering the rib cage and aid in exhalation.

8. Name the structures passing through the hilum of right lung.

Answer

Hilum of Lung

- The mediastinal surface of the lung is concave and has the hilum.
- It is triangular in shape and surrounded by a pleura.
- It is located at the region between T5 and T7.

The structures which leave and enter the hilum are:

- Bronchus/bronchi
- Pulmonary artery
- Pulmonary veins
- Bronchial artery and bronchial vein
- Lymphatic vessels
- Nerves
- Areolar tissue

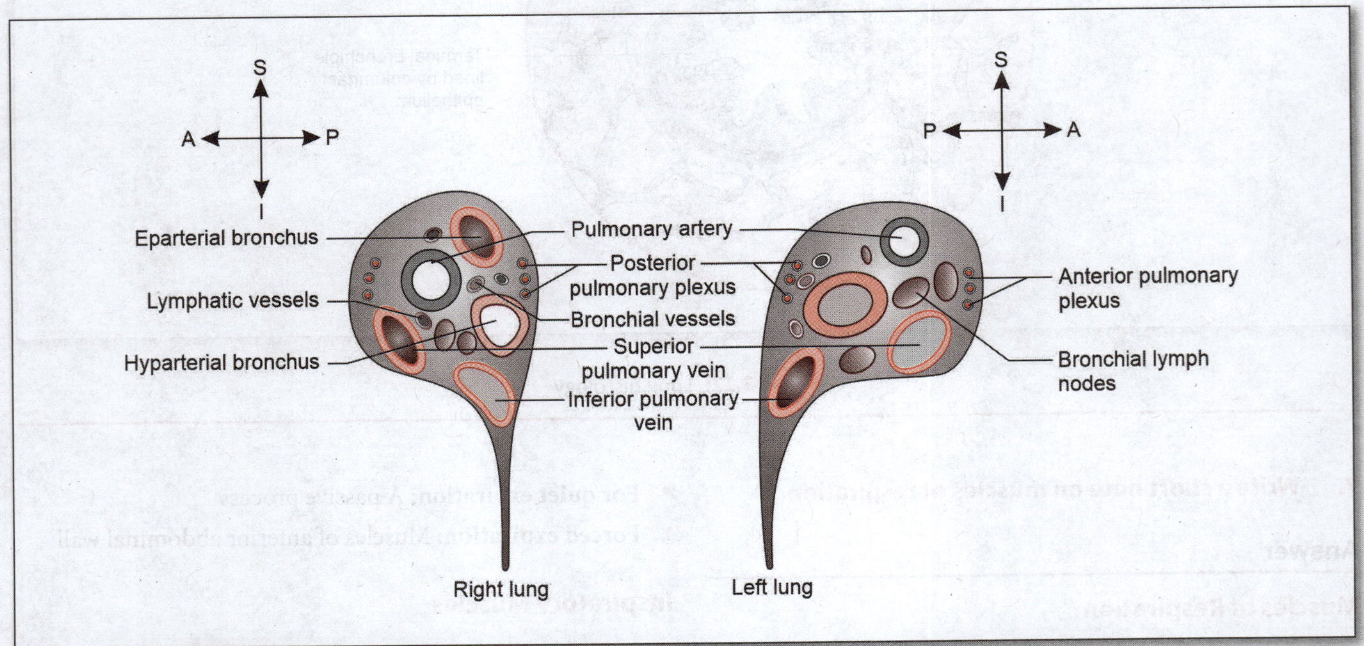

Figure 2.13: Structures passing through the hilum of right lung

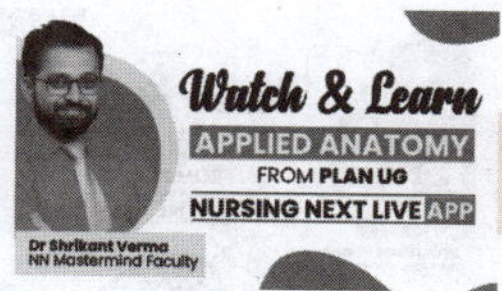

SHORT ANSWER QUESTIONS

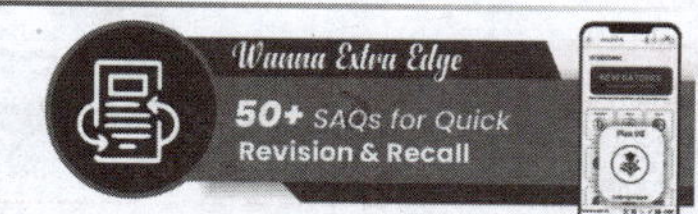

1. Name the organs involved in respiratory system.

Answer

- Nose and nasal cavity
- Pharynx
- Larynx
- Trachea
- Bronchi and bronchioles
- Lungs
- Diaphragm

2. Name the fissures and lobes of the right and left lung.

Answer

- The right lung is divided into three lobes (superior, middle and inferior lobes) by two fissures (oblique and horizontal fissures)
- The left lung is divided into two lobes (Superior and inferior lobes) by one fissure (Obliques fissure).

3. Name the major muscles involved in respiration.

Answer

- Diaphragm
- External Intercostal Muscles
- Internal Intercostal Muscles
- Accessory muscles of inhalation
- Sternocleidomastoid
- Scalene muscles
- Pectoralis minor
- Abdominal muscles (Rectus abdominis, External and internal obliques)

4. Define Pleural recesses.

Answer

Pleural recesses are potential spaces in the pleural cavity where the lung does not normally extend fully. There are two pleural recesses: Costodiaphragmatic recess and Costomediastinal recess.

5. Define pleuritis.

Answer

Pleuritis is a medical condition in which the pleura, the thin membrane that lines the lungs and chest wall, becomes inflamed with a sharp chest pain and difficulty in breathing.

CONCEPTUAL REVISION

MULTIPLE CHOICE QUESTIONS

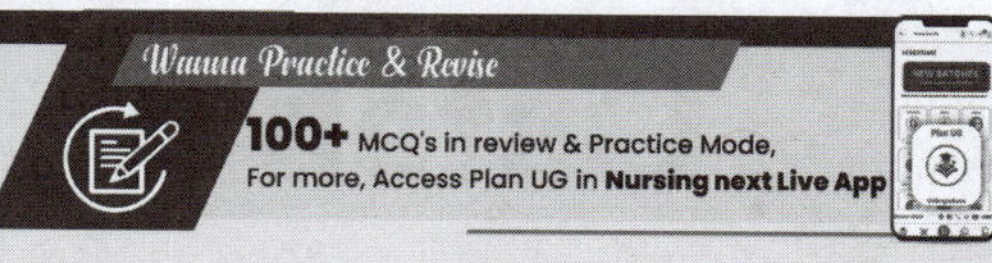

1. How is the diaphragm innervated?

a. By the parasympathetic division arising from the sacral region
b. By the spinal nerves arising from T5 to T10
c. By the phrenic nerves arising from C5 to C7
d. By the phrenic nerves arising from C3 to C5

Ans. d. By the phrenic nerves arising from C3 to C5

2. What distinguishes bronchioles from the larger bronchi?

a. Bronchioles have no cartilage in their walls
b. Bronchioles have smooth muscle in their walls
c. Bronchioles collapse between exhalation and inhalation
d. The alveoli open onto these air passages

Ans. a. Bronchioles have no cartilage in their walls

3. The walls of the trachea are held open by which of the following?

a. Nerve impulses
b. Rings of cartilage
c. Fine bones
d. Smooth muscle contractions

Ans. b. Rings of cartilage

4. What are the main muscles involved in normal inspiration?

a. Muscles of the neck
b. Abdominal muscles
c. Intercostal muscles
d. Intercostals and the diaphragm

Ans. d. Intercostals and the diaphragm

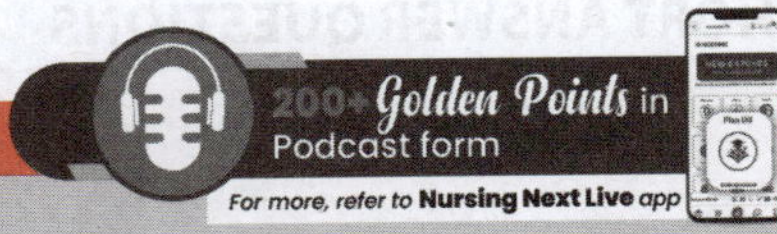

Golden Points

- Aggregations of lymphoid tissue constitute Waldeyer's lymphatic ring and is involved in the antibody production.
- For quiet inspiration-diaphragm and external intercostal muscles are responsible.
- Hilum of lung contains bronchus/bronchi, one pulmonary artery, two pulmonary veins, nerve plexuses, lymph vessels and lymph nodes.
- Larynx acts as sphincter for lower respiratory passages.
- Lungs are made-up of two portions, a conducting portion and a respiratory portion.
- Paranasal sinuses are air-filled spaces around the nasal cavities. These are *frontal*, *maxillary*, *sphenoidal* and *ethmoidal*. They open into the nasal cavity.
- Pleura is a closed serous sac enclosing the lungs and preventing lungs against friction during breathing.
- Respiration involves exchange of gases and is a two fold process of external and internal respiration.
- Respiratory muscles are superior constrictor, middle constrictor and inferior constrictor.
- The external nose has *nasal septum* with a median osseocartilaginous partition between the two halves of the nasal cavity. On each side, it is covered by mucous membrane and forms the medial wall of both nasal cavitie.
- The organs of respiration include nose, paranasal sinuses, nasopharynx, larynx, trachea and bronchi and lungs.
- The *pharynx* is a part of the upper respiratory passage and also gives characteristic note to the voice.
- The respiratory center is formed by groups of nerve cells and these control the rate and depth of respiration.
- Trachea is a non-collapsible, wide tube and is kept patent because of the presence of C-shaped cartilaginous "rings" in its wall.

CHAPTER

3

Digestive System

CONCEPTUAL THEORY

Terminology

Components of digestive system: (i) The alimentary canal or gastrointestinal tract (GIT) beginning at mouth and ending at anus. It runs through neck, thorax, abdomen and pelvis, (ii) Accessory glands, e.g., three pairs of salivary glands, liver, gallbladder, pancreas and biliary tract.

Esophagus: 25 cm long passage with course in neck, thorax and abdomen. Lower end of esophagus has portacaval anastomoses which may rupture in cirrhosis of liver leading to hematemesis.

Large intestine (Colon): It consists of the cecum, colon (ascending, transverse, descending, and sigmoid), rectum, and anus.

Layers of GIT: Mucosa, submucosa, muscularis externa and serosa/adventitia.

Liver: The liver is the largest internal organ located in the upper right abdomen and produces bile.

Pharynx: Comprises upper nasopharynx; middle oropharynx and lower laryngopharynx. Food passage and air passage cross each other in the region of oropharynx.

Salivary glands: Parotid glands are purely serous innervated by glossopharyngeal nerves. Duct opens in vestibule. Submandibular glands are mixed, innervated by chorda tympani nerve. Duct opens at submandibular papilla on the floor of mouth. Sublingual glands are purely mucus glands, innervated by chorda tympani nerve, 8–10 ducts open on sublingual papilla on the floor of mouth.

Small Intestine: The small intestine is the longest part of the alimentary canal and is divided into three sections: the duodenum, jejunum, and ileum.

Stomach: Has three layers of smooth muscles fibers. Peptic ulcer is seen along its lesser curvature.

Vestibule of mouth: Vestibule is the space between soft tissues and the tooth and gums. Space on each side of the oral cavity is bounded by several structures.

STRUCTURE OF ALIMENTARY CANAL AND ACCESSORY ORGANS OF DIGESTION

The alimentary canal is a long muscular tube that extends from the mouth to the anus and is responsible for the digestion and absorption of food. It consists of the following structures:

- **Mouth (Oral cavity):** The mouth is the initial site of digestion. It contains the teeth for mechanical breakdown of food and the tongue for manipulation and swallowing of food. Salivary glands produce saliva, which contains enzymes that begin the process of breaking down carbohydrates.
- **Pharynx:** The pharynx is a muscular tube that serves as a common pathway for both air and food. It connects the mouth and nasal cavity to the esophagus and larynx.
- **Esophagus:** The esophagus is a muscular tube that carries food from the pharynx to the stomach through peristaltic contractions.
- **Stomach:** The stomach is a J-shaped muscular organ located in the upper abdomen. It stores and mixes food with gastric juices, which contain enzymes and hydrochloric acid for the breakdown of proteins. The stomach also helps to regulate the release of partially digested food (chyme) into the small intestine.
- **Small intestine:** The small intestine is the longest part of the alimentary canal and is divided into three sections: the duodenum, jejunum, and ileum. It is the primary site for digestion and absorption of nutrients. The inner surface of the small intestine is covered with finger-like projections called villi, which increase the surface area for absorption.
- **Large intestine (Colon):** The large intestine is responsible for the absorption of water, electrolytes, and vitamins from undigested food residues. It consists of the cecum, colon (ascending, transverse, descending, and sigmoid), rectum, and anus.

Accessory Organs

The accessory organs of digestion are responsible for producing and secreting various substances that aid in the digestive process. These include:

- **Salivary glands:** The salivary glands, including the parotid, submandibular, and sublingual glands, produce saliva. Saliva contains enzymes (such as amylase) that initiate the breakdown of carbohydrates.
- **Liver:** The liver is the largest internal organ and is located in the upper right abdomen. It produces bile, which is stored and concentrated in the gallbladder. Bile aids in the digestion and absorption of fats.
- **Gallbladder:** The gallbladder is a small pear-shaped organ located beneath the liver. It stores and releases bile into the small intestine in response to the presence of fatty food.
- **Pancreas:** The pancreas is an elongated organ located behind the stomach. It produces digestive enzymes (such as pancreatic amylase, lipase, and proteases) that are released into the small intestine.

APPLICATION AND IMPLICATIONS IN NURSING

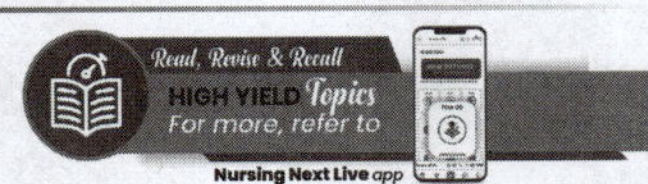

- **Nutritional assessment:** Nurses assess patients' nutritional status by evaluating their dietary intake, weight changes, and signs of malnutrition. Understanding the digestive system helps nurses identify potential nutritional deficiencies and develop appropriate care plans to address them.
- **Enteral nutrition:** Nurses are involved in the administration and management of enteral nutrition, which involves providing nutrients directly into the gastrointestinal tract.
- **Medication administration:** Nurses administer medications orally, which requires an understanding of the digestive system.
- **Gastrointestinal disorders:** Nurses care for patients with various gastrointestinal disorders, such as gastroesophageal reflux disease (GERD), peptic ulcers, inflammatory bowel disease (IBD), and liver diseases.
- **Bowel management:** Nurses assess and manage patients with bowel dysfunction, including constipation, diarrhea, and fecal incontinence.
- **Ostomy care:** Nurses care for patients with ostomies, which are surgically created openings in the abdomen to divert urine or feces. They educate patients about ostomy care, assess the stoma for signs of complications, and provide support and guidance in adjusting to life with an ostomy.
- **Infection control:** Nurses play a crucial role in preventing health care-associated infections related to the digestive system. This includes implementing hand hygiene practices, adhering to infection prevention protocols during procedures like insertion and maintenance of feeding tubes, and monitoring patients for signs of infection.
- **Patient education:** Nurses educate patients about maintaining a healthy digestive system and promoting good nutrition. They provide information on dietary modifications, portion control, and the importance of a balanced diet for overall health.

CONCEPTUAL EXERCISES

LONG ANSWER QUESTIONS

1. **Enumerate the organs of digestion including accessory organs of digestion. Describe stomach in detail under the following headings: (MGR, KUHS, RUHS)**

   a. Situation b. Parts c. Relation d. Blood supply e. Nerve supply f. Applied anatomy

Answer

Introduction

- Digestive tract/alimentary tube—the main component of the digestive system.
- **Parts of the digestive tube:**
  - **Mouth:** The mouth is where food is chewed and mixed with saliva. Saliva helps to moisten the food and make it easier to swallow.
  - **Pharynx:** The pharynx is a muscular tube that connects the mouth to the esophagus.
  - **Esophagus:** It is a muscular tube that carries food from the pharynx to the stomach.
  - **Stomach:** The stomach is a muscular sac that stir and mixes food with gastric juices.
  - **Small intestine:** It is a long, coiled tube that is responsible for most of the digestion and absorption of nutrients. The small intestine is divided into three parts: the duodenum, the jejunum, and the ileum.
  - **Large intestine:** is a shorter, wider tube that absorbs water and salts from food. The large intestine is divided into three parts: The cecum, the colon, and the rectum.
  - **Rectum and anus:** is a short, muscular tube that stores waste products before they are eliminated from the body. The anus is the opening at the end of the rectum through which waste products are eliminated.

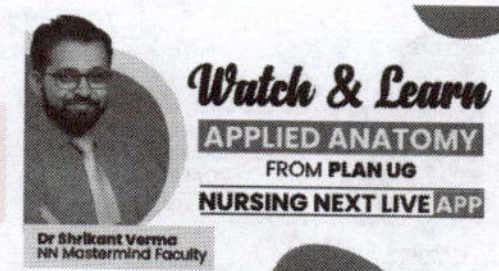

- **Accessory glands include:**
  - **Salivary glands:** The salivary glands produce saliva, which helps to moisten food and make it easier to swallow.
  - **Liver:** The liver produces bile, which helps to break down fats.
  - **Gallbladder:** The gallbladder stores bile, which is released into the small intestine when food is present.
  - **Pancreas:** The pancreas produces digestive enzymes that help to break down carbohydrates, proteins, and fats.
  - **Intestinal glands:** The intestinal glands produce mucus and enzymes, which helps to protect the lining of the small intestine.

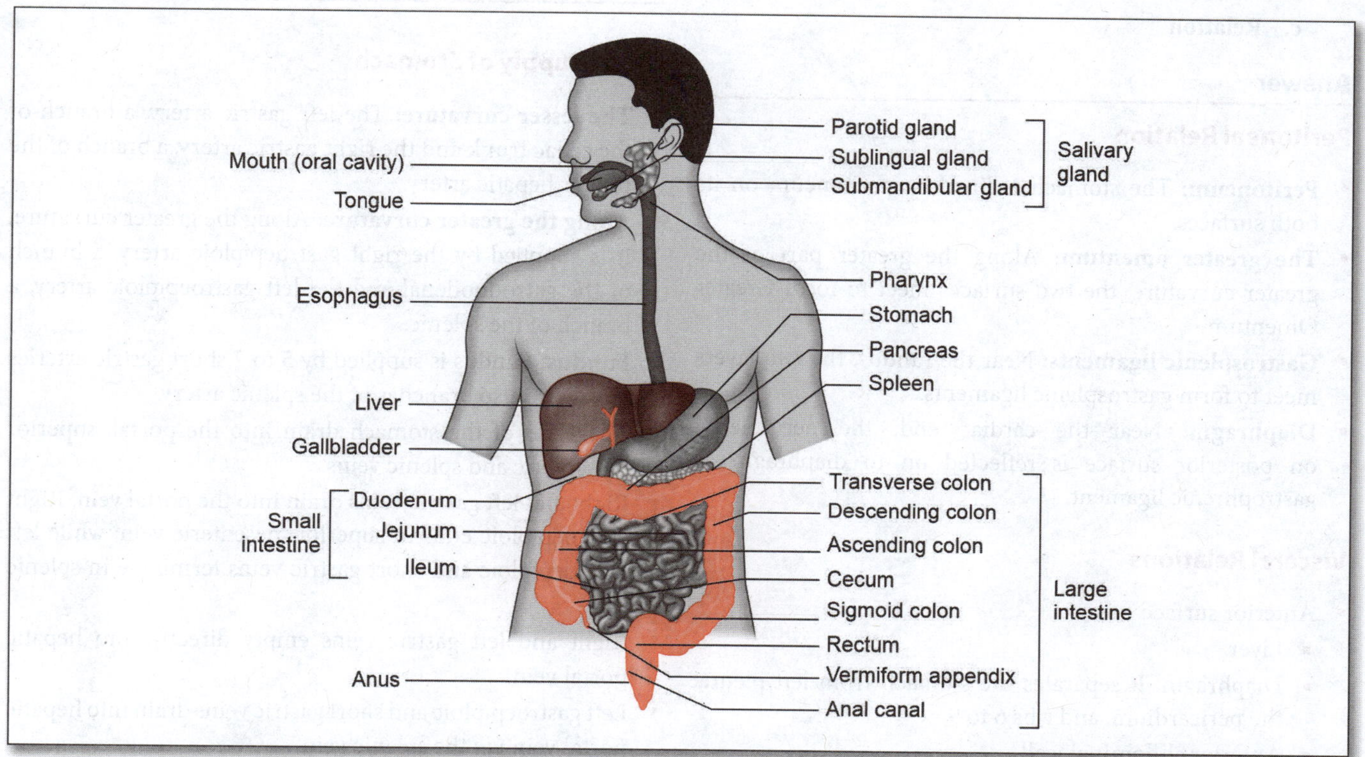

Figure 3.1: Digestive system

Stomach

- The stomach is a muscular organ located on the left side of the upper abdomen.

  a. **Situation**

Answer

Situation

- **Stomach is J shaped with two surfaces:** Anterior and posterior.
- **Two openings:** Cardia and pyloric orifice (Pyloric sphincter)

  b. **Parts**

Answer

- **Parts:** Stomach has five parts:

1. **Cardia:** The first part is closest to the esophagus.

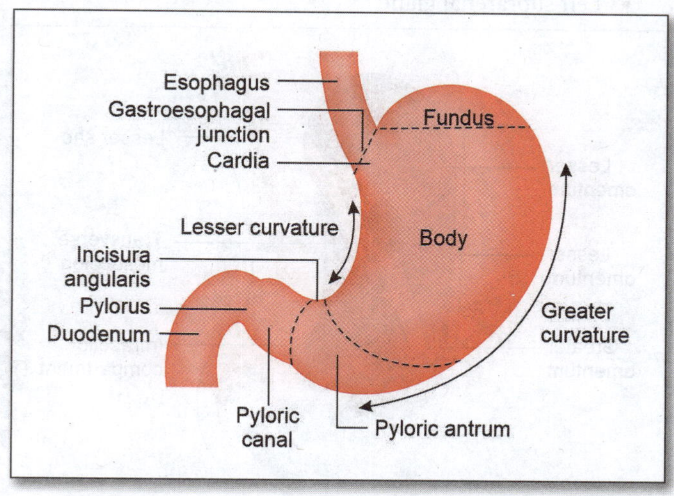

Figure 3.2: Stomach

2. **Fundus:** The upper part of the stomach next to the cardia.

3. **Body (corpus):** The main part of the stomach, between the upper and lower parts.
4. **Antrum:** The lower portion (near the intestine), where the food mixes with gastric juice.
5. **Pylorus:** The last part of the stomach, which acts as a valve to control emptying of the stomach contents into the small intestine.

c. **Relation**

Answer

Peritoneal Relation

- **Peritoneum:** The stomach is lined by peritoneum on its both surfaces.
- **The greater omentum:** Along the greater part of the greater curvature, the two surfaces meet to form Greater Omentum.
- **Gastrosplenic ligaments:** Near the fundus, the two layers meet to form gastrosplenic ligaments.
- **Diaphragm:** Near the cardiac end, the peritoneum on posterior surface is reflected on to diaphragm as gastrophrenic ligament.

Visceral Relations

- Anterior surface
  - Liver
  - Diaphragm: It separates the stomach from left pleura, the pericardium, and ribs 6 to 9.
  - Anterior abdominal wall
- Posterior surface
  - Diaphragm
  - Left Kidney
  - Left suprarenal gland
  - Pancreas
  - Transverse mesocolon
  - Splenic of colon
  - Splenic artery

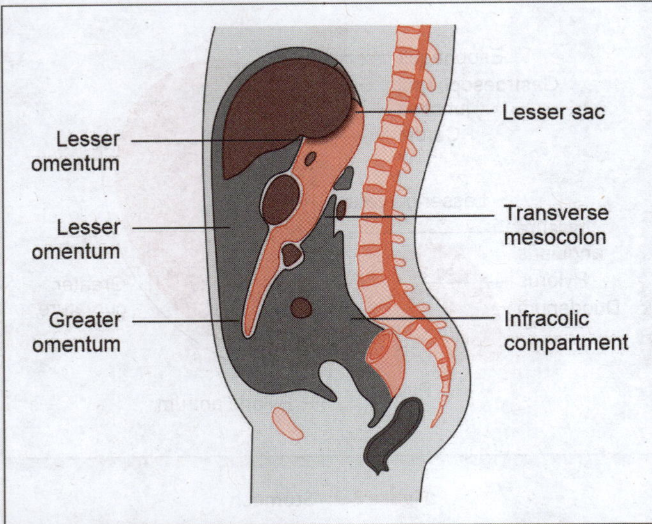

Figure 3.3: Relations of stomach

d. **Blood supply**

Answer

Blood Supply of Stomach

- **The lesser curvature:** The left gastric artery, a branch of the celiac trunk and the right gastric artery, a branch of the proper hepatic artery.
- **Along the greater curvature:** Along the greater curvature, it is supplied by the right gastroepiploic artery, a branch of the gatroduodenal and the left gastroepiploic artery, a branch of the splenic.
- **Fundus:** Fundus is supplied by 5 to 7 short gastric arteries which are also branches of the splenic artery.
- The veins of the stomach drain into the portal, superior mesenteric and splenic veins.
- Right and left gastric veins drain into the portal vein. Right gastroepiploic ends in superior mesenteric vein; while left gastroepiploic and short gastric veins terminate in splenic vein.
- Right and left gastric veins empty directly into hepatic portal vein.
- Left gastroepiploic and short gastric veins drain into hepatic portal vein *via* the splenic vein.
- Right gastroepiploic vein drains into superior mesenteric vein.

There are four lymphatic drainage points:

1. Pancreatosplenic area (area 3) drains into pancreatosplenic nodes.
2. Area (1) drains into left gastric nodes.
3. Area (2) drains into right gastroepiploic nodes.
4. Lymph from area (4) drains in different directions into pyloric, hepatic and left gastric nodes and passes from all these nodes into celiac nodes.

e. **Nerve supply**

Answer

Nerve Supply

Sympathetic nerves: Supply the blood vessels and also carry the pain impulses.

Vagus nerve: Secretory to the glands, causes peristalsis and inhibit pyloric sphincter.

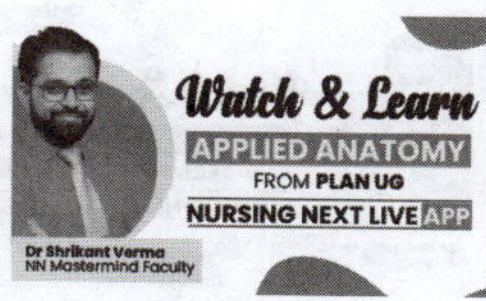

f. **Applied anatomy**

Answer

Applied Anatomy

- **Peptic ulcer:** It occurs in the sites of pepsin and HCl, i.e., in the stomach, first part of duodenum, lower end of esophagus and Meckel's diverticulum.
- **Gastric carcinoma:** It occurs along the greater curvature. Metastasis occurs through the thoracic duct to the left supraclavicular lymph node (Troisier's sign), also known as signal nodes.
- **Pyloric obstruction:** It may be congenital or acquired. It causes peristalsis in the epigastrium and vomiting after meals.
- **Gastric pain:** It is felt in the epigastrium because the stomach is supplied from segments T6 to T10 of the spinal cord. Pain either occurs by spasm of muscle or by over distension.

2. Describe structure of liver in detail. (RUHS)

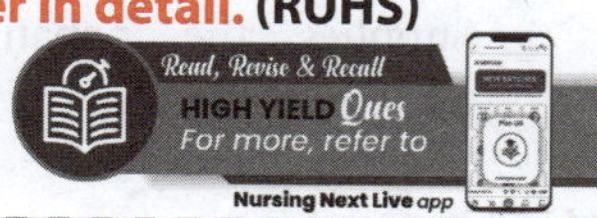

Answer

Liver

- The liver is a peritoneal organ positioned in the right upper quadrant of the abdomen. It is the largest visceral structure in the abdominal cavity, and the largest gland in the human body.
- Largest gland in the body weighing about 1500 g that filters 1500 cc of blood per minute.

Location

- The liver is predominantly located in the right hypochondrium and epigastric areas and extends into the left hypochondrium.
- Liver is divided into four lobes:
  i. Right lobe—largest
  ii. Left lobe
  iii. Caudate lobe
  iv. Quadrate lobe

Ligaments of Liver

- The ligaments that attach the liver to the surrounding structures are formed by a double layer of peritoneum.
- Ligaments of liver
  - **Falciform ligament:** This ligament attaches the anterior surface of the liver to the anterior abdominal wall and leads to division of the left and right lobes of the liver. The ligamentum teres is present at the free edge of this ligament.
  - Coronary ligament (anterior and posterior folds): The superior surface of the liver and the inferior surface of the diaphragm are attached by the coronary ligament and it separates the bare area of the liver.
  - Triangular ligaments (left and right):
    - Left: The left triangular ligament is made-up by the union of the anterior and posterior layers of the coronary ligament at the apex of the liver. It attaches the left lobe of the liver to the diaphragm.
    - Right: The right triangular ligament lies adjacent to the bare area. It attaches the right lobe of the liver to the diaphragm.
  - **Lesser omentum:** Attaches the liver to the lesser curvature of the stomach and first part of the duodenum. It consists of the hepatoduodenal ligament (extends from the duodenum to the liver) and the hepatogastric ligament (extends from the stomach to the liver). The hepatoduodenal ligament surrounds the portal triad.
  - In addition to these supporting ligaments, the posterior surface of the liver is secured by the inferior vena cava by hepatic veins and fibrous tissue.

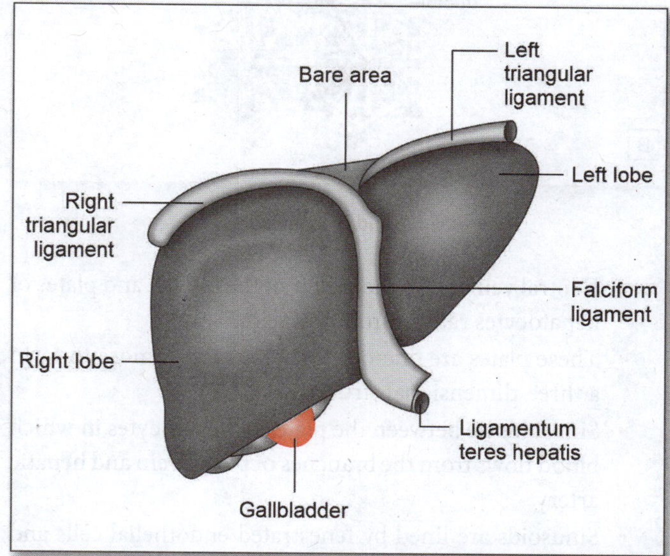

Figure 3.4: Ligaments of liver

Histology of Liver

- Liver is covered by a thin connective tissue capsule (Glisson's capsule).
- Capsule is thick at porta hepatis.
- In cross-section:
  - The shape of the lobule is hexagonal.
  - At the angles of hexagons, small triangular areas containing portal triads are found.

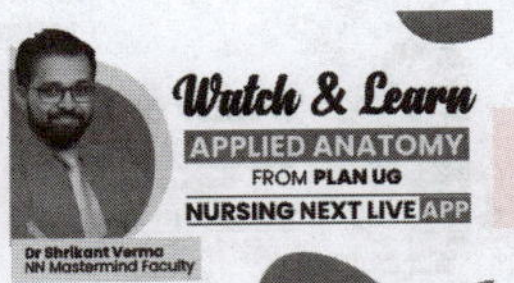

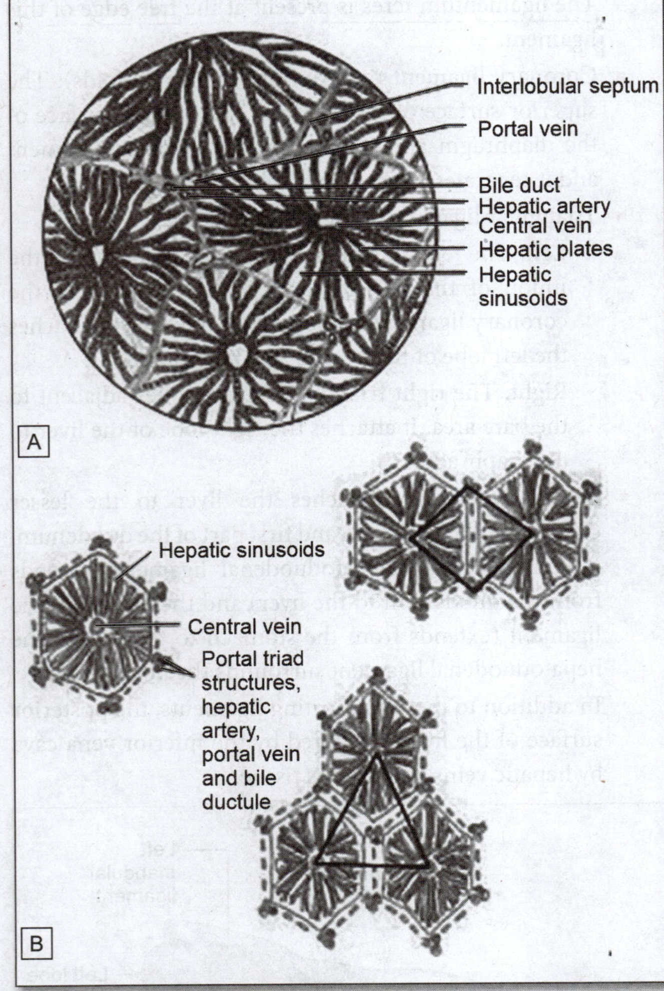

Figures 3.5A and B: Histology of liver

- Central vein lies in the center of the lobule, and plates of hepatocytes radiate from the vein.
- These plates are one-cell thick and anastomose to form a three-dimensional structure.
- Sinusoids lie between the plates of hepatocytes in which blood flows from the branches of portal vein and hepatic artery.
- Sinusoids are lined by fenestrated endothelial cells and phagocytic Kupffer cells.
- Kupffer cells either lie by the side of endothelial cells or lie over its surface.

- Space between the endothelium and the plates is known as perisinusoidal space or space of Disse.
  - This space contains short microvilli of hepatocytes, reticular fibers, lipocytes and occasional nonmyelinated nerve fibers.
  - The structural framework of liver is formed by a delicate network of reticular fibers embedded in extracellular matrix.
  - This network of reticular fibers is continuous with Glisson's capsule at the periphery.
  - Space between the surrounding wall and the portal triad is known as space of Mall.

Bare Area of Liver

- The bare area of the liver is a large triangular area on the diaphragmatic surface of the liver, devoid of peritoneal covering.
- The bare area of the liver is clinically important because of the portacaval anastomosis, and it represents a site where infection can spread from the abdominal cavity to the thoracic cavity. It is important because it encloses the right extra peritoneal subphrenic space.

Blood Supply

- Hepatic artery proper
  - Branch of the celiac trunk
  - Supplies the nonparenchymal structures of liver
- Hepatic portal vein
  - Supplies the hepatic parenchyma with partially deoxygenated blood.

Venous Drainage

Hepatic veins which drain into the inferior vena cava.

Nerve Supply

- Hepatic parenchyma is innervated by the hepatic plexus
- Glisson's capsule is innervated by the branches of the lower intercostal nerves.

Lymphatic Drainage

- From the anterior aspect—drain into the hepatic lymph nodes.
- From the posterior aspect—drain into the phrenic and posterior mediastinal nodes.

Functions of Liver

- Converts glucose into glycogen for the storage of insulin.
- Carbohydrate metabolism: liver maintains the plasma glucose levels by converting glucose to glycogen and back with variations in blood glucose levels.
- Protein metabolism: amino acids and nucleic acids are broken down to urea and uric acid in liver.
- Fat metabolism: fat stored is metabolized to release energy
- Liver secretes bile that contains the bile pigments, bile salts and cholesterol. Also stores iron and vitamins like B12, A, D, E, K.

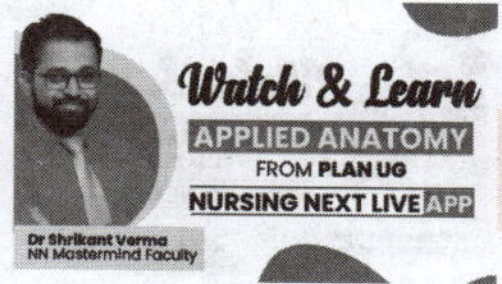

- Site for detoxification of toxic substances
- Site for metabolism of thyroid hormones, alcohol and steroids.
- Site for protein synthesis.

3. Describe lobes of Liver. (RUHS)

Answer

Lobes of Liver

- Anatomically liver has four main lobes
- Smaller left lobe and larger right lobe are separated by the falciform ligament.
- Caudate and quadrate lobes are anatomically parts of the right lobes.

Functional Division of Liver

Eight hepatic segments are as follows:

1. Segment I—the caudate lobe—is the posterosuperior part of the left medial sector.
2. Segment II is the posterosuperior segment of the left lateral sector.
3. Segment III is the anteroinferior part of the left lateral sector.
4. Segment IV includes the entire left medial lobe anteriorly, and the quadrate lobe viscerally. It is further subdivided into segments IVa and IVb. Segment IVa lies superiorly, while IVb lies inferiorly and corresponds with the location of the quadrate lobe.
5. Segment V forms the inferior part of the right medial sector.
6. Segment VI is the inferior part of the right lateral sector.
7. Sector VII is the superior aspect of the right lateral sector.
8. Sector VIII is the superior aspect of the right medial sector.

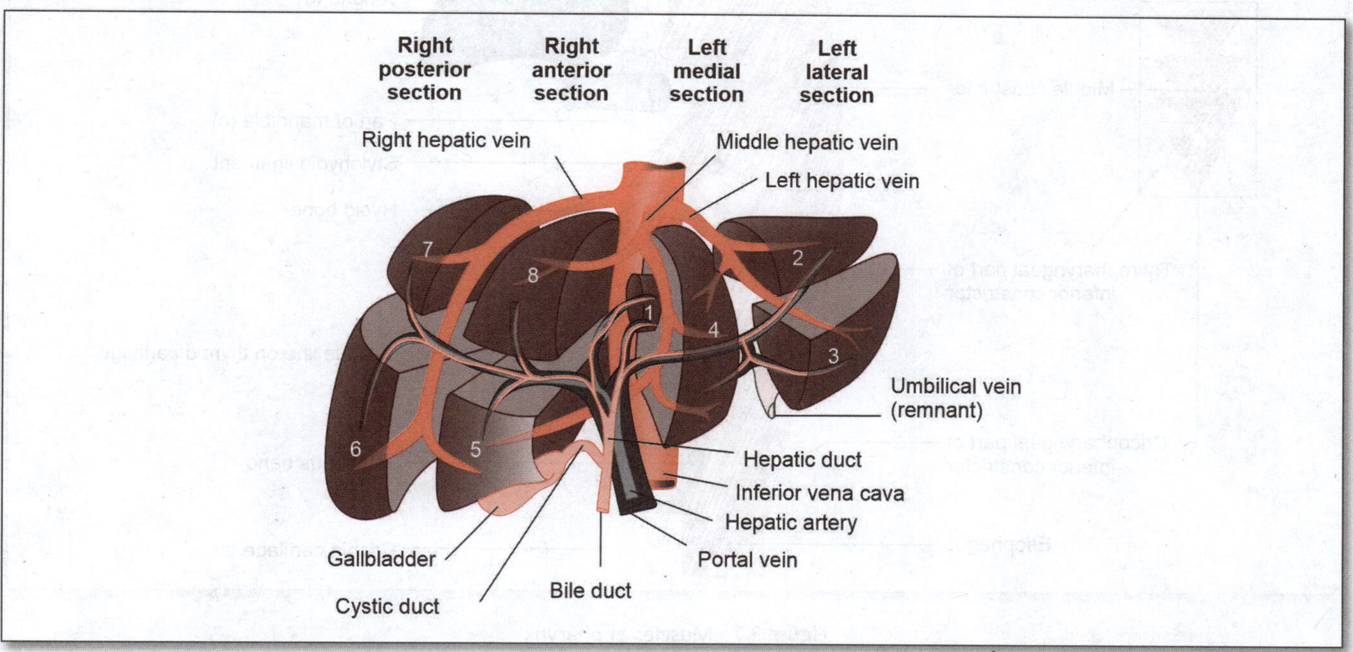

Figure 3.6: Segmental division of liver

SHORT NOTES

1. Write a short note on Pharynx. (MGR)

Answer

Pharynx

- Wide muscular tube situated behind the nose, mouth and larynx.

- Also known as throat.
- It is about 13 cm long and 3.5 cm wide in the upper part
- Divided into three parts
  1. Nasopharynx—nasal part—transmits only air
  2. Oropharynx—oral part—transmits both air and food
  3. Laryngopharynx—laryngeal part—allows only food.

Functions of Pharynx

- Passage for food and air
- Warms/cools and humidifies the air
- Aids in hearing and speech
- Provides immunity due to the presence of Waldeyer's ring.

Muscles of Pharynx

- Superior constrictor muscle
- Middle constrictor muscle
- Inferior constrictor muscle
- Other muscles include:
  - Palatopharyngeus
  - Stylopharyngeus
  - Salpingopharyngeus

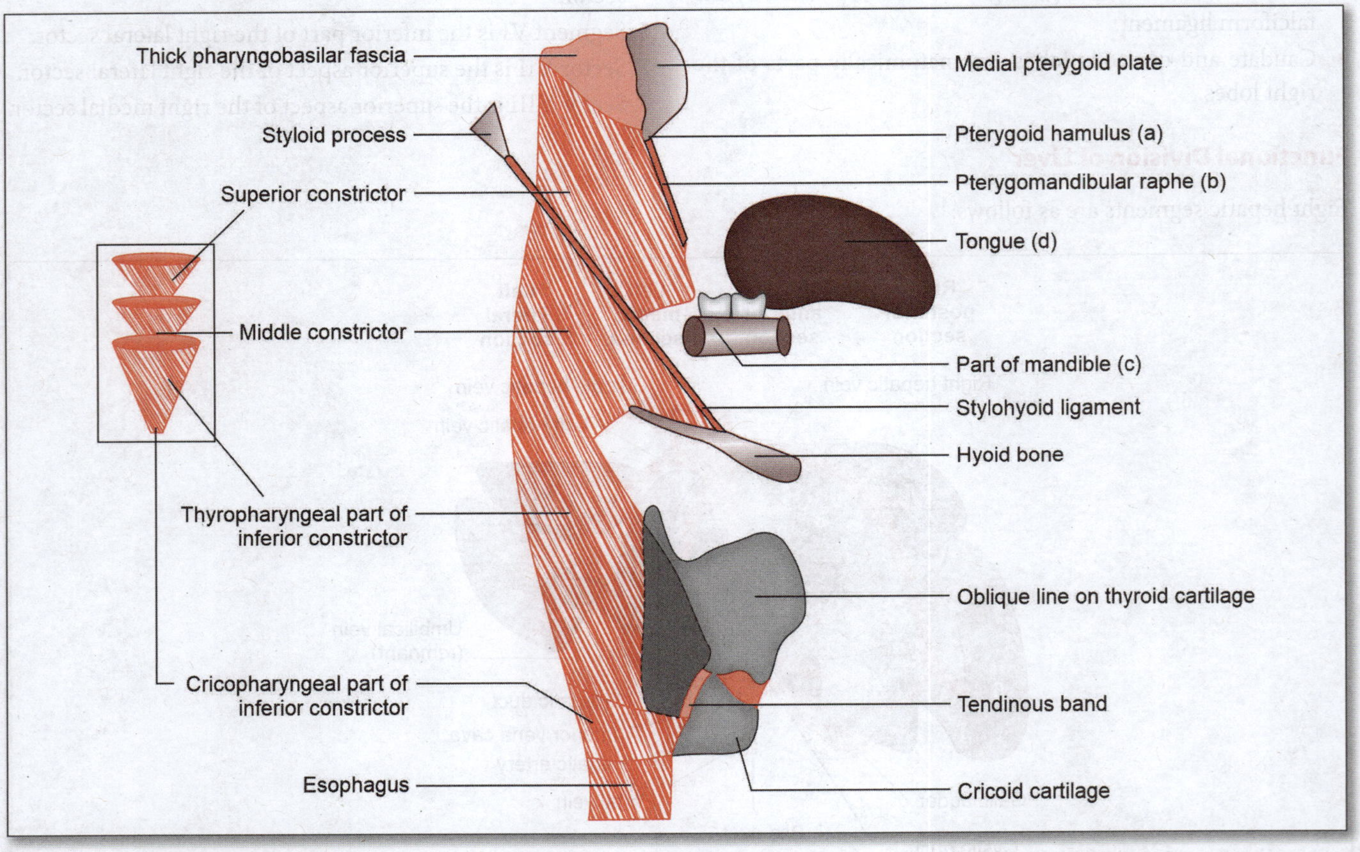

Figure 3.7: Muscles of pharynx

Blood Supply of Pharynx

- Ascending pharyngeal branch of the external carotid artery
- Ascending palatine and tonsillar branches of the facial artery
- Dorsal lingual branches of the lingual artery
- Venous drainage is into the internal jugular and facial vein

Nerve Supply

Pharyngeal plexus formed by the vagoaccessory complex.

2. Write a short note on Stomach. (MGR)

Answer

Stomach

- The stomach is a muscular organ located on the left side of the upper abdomen.
  - **Stomach is J shaped with two surfaces:** Anterior and posterior.
  - **Two openings:** Cardia and pyloric orifice (Pyloric sphincter)

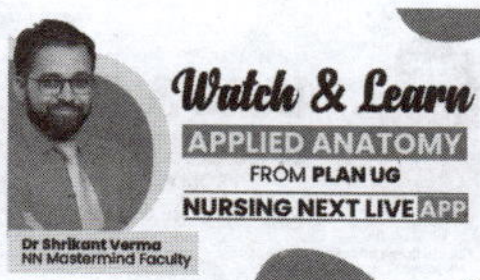

- **Parts:** Stomach has five parts:
  i. **Cardia:** The first part is closest to the esophagus
  ii. **Fundus:** The upper part of the stomach next to the cardia
  iii. **Body (corpus):** The main part of the stomach, between the upper and lower parts
  iv. **Antrum:** The lower portion (near the intestine), where the food mixes with gastric juice
  v. **Pylorus:** The last part of the stomach, which acts as a valve to control emptying of the stomach contents into the small intestine.

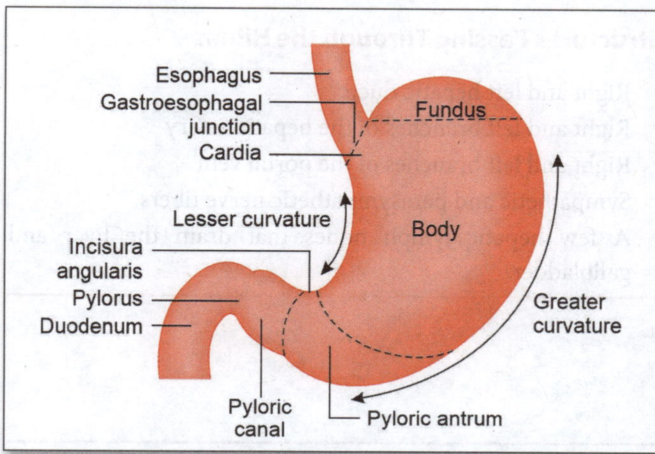

Figure 3.8: Stomach

Peritoneal Relation

- Peritoneum
- The greater omentum
- Gastrosplenic ligaments
- Diaphragm

Visceral Relations

- Anterior surface
  - Liver
  - Diaphragm: It separates the stomach from left pleura, the pericardium, and ribs 6 to 9.
  - Anterior Abdominal wall
- Posterior surface
  - Diaphragm
  - Left kidney
  - Left suprarenal gland
- Pancreas
- Transverse mesocolon
- Splenic of colon
- Splenic artery

Lymphatic Drainage

There are four lymphatic drainage points:

1. Pancreatosplenic area (area 3) drains into pancreatosplenic nodes.
2. Area (1) drains into left gastric nodes.
3. Area (2) drains into right gastroepiploic nodes.
4. Lymph from area (4) drains in different directions into pyloric, hepatic and left gastric nodes and passes from all these nodes into celiac nodes.

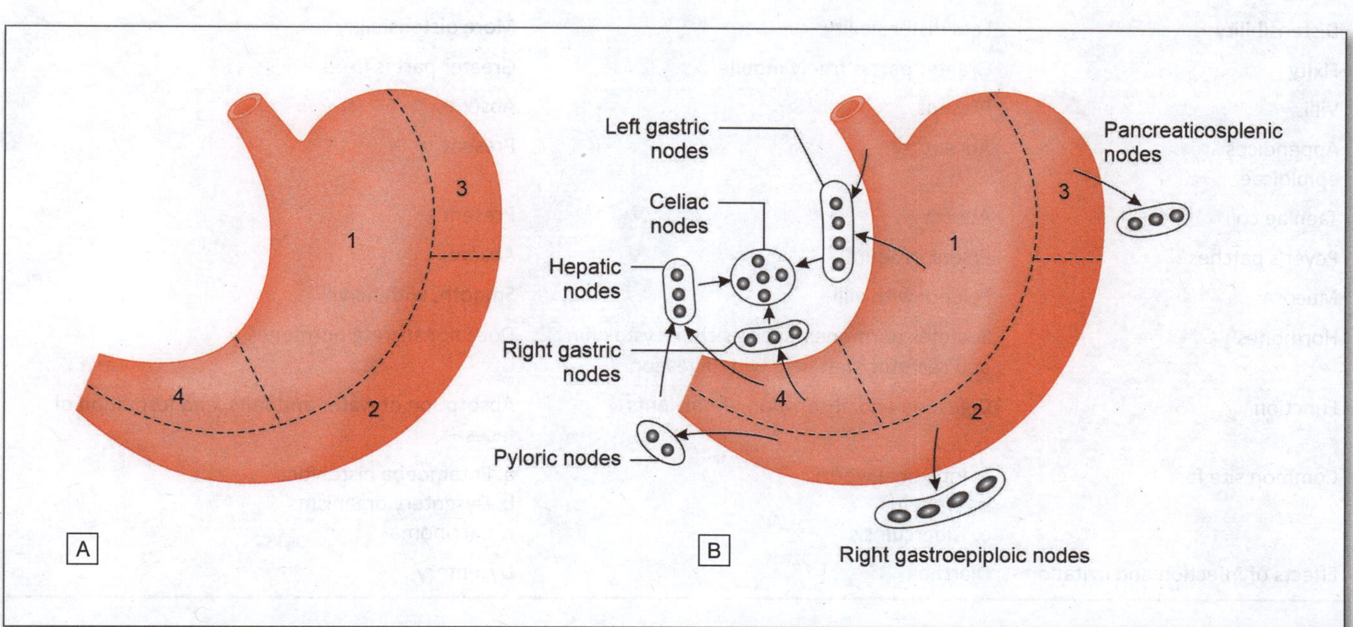

Figures 3.9A and B: Lymphatic drainage of stomach

Applied Anatomy

- **Peptic ulcer:** It occurs in the sites of pepsin and HCl, i.e., in the stomach, first part of duodenum, lower end of esophagus and Meckel's diverticulum.
- **Gastric carcinoma:** It occurs along the greater curvature. Metastasis occurs through the thoracic duct to the left supraclavicular lymph node (Troisier's sign), also known as signal nodes.
- **Pyloric obstruction:** It may be congenital or acquired. It causes peristalsis in the epigastrium and vomiting after meals.
- **Gastric pain:** It is felt in the epigastrium because the stomach is supplied from segments T6 to T10 of the spinal cord.
- Pain either occurs by spasm of muscle or by over distension.

3. Write a short note on structures present in the hilum of the liver.

Answer

Hilum of the Liver

- Liver hilum or the porta hepatis separates the quadrate lobe and the caudate lobe of the liver.
- This is the area where the portal vein and the hepatic artery enter the liver and the hepatic duct leaves the liver.

Structures Passing Through the Hilum

- Right and left hepatic ducts
- Right and left branches of the hepatic artery
- Right and left branches of the portal vein
- Sympathetic and parasympathetic nerve fibers.
- A few hepatic lymph nodes that drain the liver and gallbladder.

4. Differences between small and large intestines. (MGR)

Answer

Table 3.1: Differences between the small intestine and the large intestine

Features	Small intestine	Large intestine
Length	20–25 feet (6–7.6 m)	5–6 feet (1.5–2 m)
Diameter	1–2 inches (2.5–5 cm)	2–3 inches (5–7.6 cm)
Layers	Four layers: Mucosa, submucosa, muscularis externa, and serosa	Four layers: Mucosa, submucosa, muscularis externa, and serosa
Distensibility	Less distensibility	More distensibility
Fixity	Greater part is freely mobile	Greater part is fixed
Villi	Present	Absent
Appendices epiploicae	Absent	Present
Taeniae coli	Absent	Present
Peyer's patches	Prsent in ileum	Absent
Mucosa	Folded, with villi	Smooth, with no villi
Hormones	Secretes hormones, such as cholecystokinin and secretin, that help with digestion	Does not secrete hormones
Function	Digestion and absorption of nutrients	Absorption of water and salts, and formation of feces
Common site for	a. Intestinal worms b. Typhoid c. Tuberculosis	a. Entamoeba histolytica b. Dysentery organisms c. Carcinoma
Effects of infection and irritation	Diarrhea	Dysentery

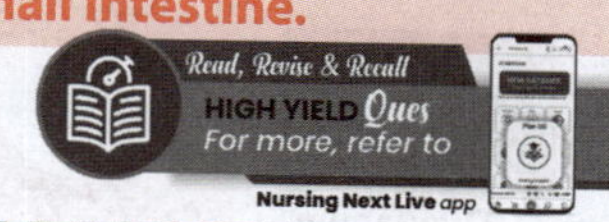

5. Write a short note on Vermiform appendix. (MGR)

Answer

Vermiform Appendix

- Narrow, hollow muscular tube suspended from the terminal ileum by small mesentery.
- It opens into the posteromedial wall of the cecum.
- It contains aggregations of lymphoid tissue.

Dimensions

It is about 2 cm, may vary from 2–20 cm.

Location

- It is located in the right lower quadrant of abdomen, more specifically in the right iliac fossa.
- Base – lies at the McBurney's point (junction of lateral one third and medial two thirds of the line joining the umbilicus to the right anterior superior iliac spine.).
- Appendicular orifice is guarded by the valve of Gerlach.

Clock Positions of Appendix

Position	Percentage	Clock position
Subcecal	2% cases	11 o'clock
Retrocecal	60% cases	12 o'clock
Splenic	1 – 2% cases	2 o'clock
Promontoric	Very rare	3 o'clock
Pelvic	30% cases	4 o'clock
Midinguinal	Very rare	6 o'clock

Most common is the retrocecal position.

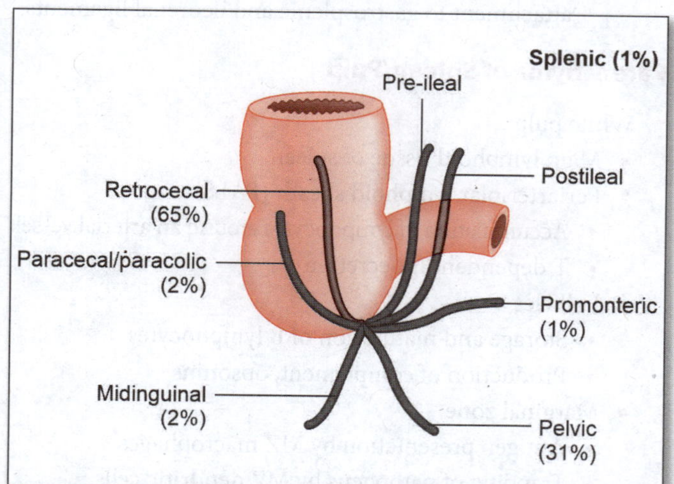

Figure 3.10: Positions of appendix

6. Write a short note on small intestine.

Read, Revise & Recall
HIGH YIELD Ques
For more, refer to
Nursing Next Live app

Answer

Introduction

- Small intestine is the longest part of digestive system
- Small intestine extends form the pylorus to the ileocecal junction and is approx. 6 meters long.

Parts of Small Intestine

Duodenum

- It is the first part of the small intestine
- It extends from the pyloric sphincter of the stomach, and ends at duodenojejunal flexure.
- It is "C" shaped with head of pancreas lying in its concavity.
- The bile duct and pancreatic duct open into duodenum by a common opening at major duodenal papilla, 10 cm from the pylorus.
- Duodenum is divided into four parts – superior (duodenal bulb/ampulla), descending, horizontal and ascending.

Jejunum and Ileum

- Most of the part of small intestine is formed by jejunum and ileum.
- Ileum and jejunum are suspended from the posterior abdominal wall by mesentery.
- Jejunum begins at the duodenojejunal flexure and is found in the upper left quadrant of the abdomen and it is entirely intraperitoneal.
- Wall of the jejunum is thicker and its lumen is wider than in ileum.
- Ileum is the last and longest part of the small intestine and found in the lower right quadrant of the abdomen.

Blood Supply of Small Intestine

- **Arteries:** Celiac trunk, superior mesenteric arteries.
- **Veins:** Hepatic portal vein, superior mesenteric vein.

Nerve Supply of Small Intestine

- **Parasympathetic:** Vagus nerve (CN X) (Through the submucosal (Meissner's) and myenteric (Auerbach's) nervous plexuses).
- **Sympathetic:** Thoracic splanchnic nerves.

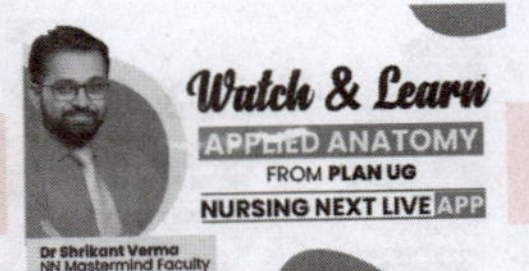

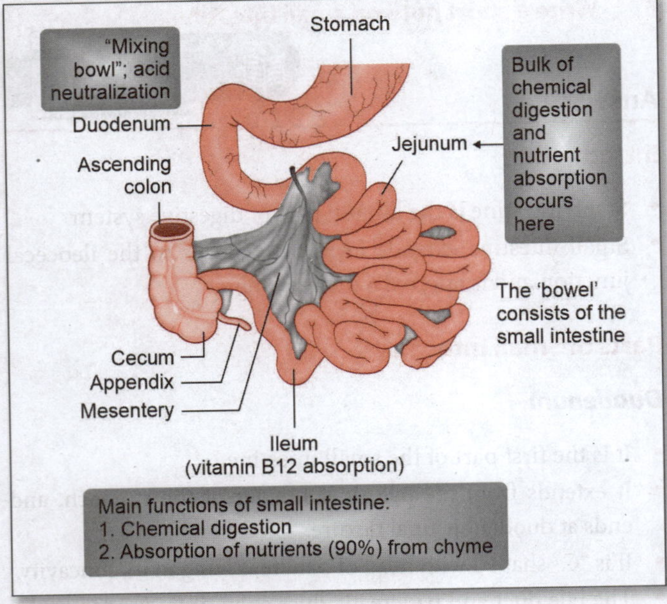

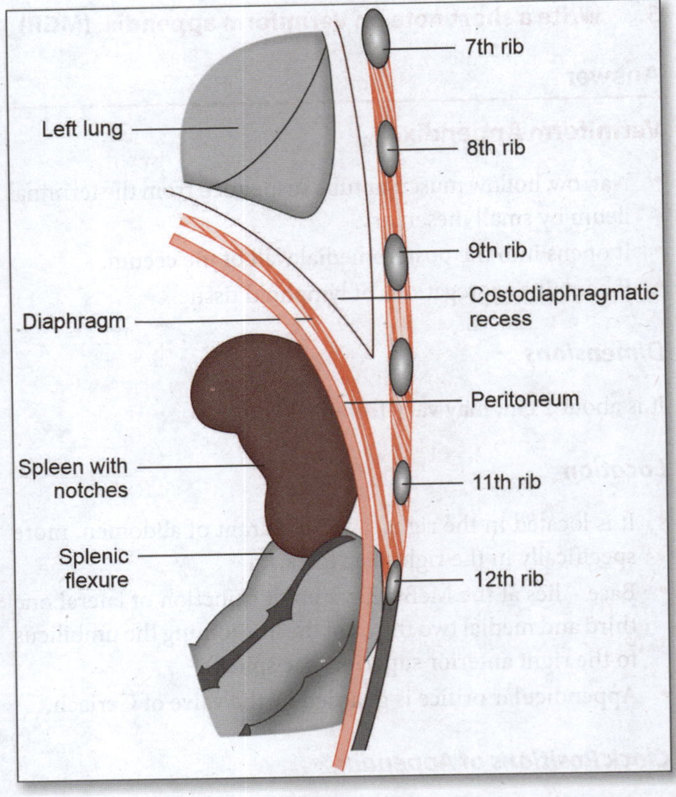

Figure 3.11: Spleen with its ends and borders

7. Write a short note on Spleen. (RUHS)

Answer

Spleen

- Largest lymphoid organ which is covered by a dense connective tissue capsule.
- Functions of spleen include phagocytosis, storage of blood, immunity, erythropoiesis, storage of platelets, circulating pool of lymphocytes.
- Soft and friable, largest single mass of lymphoid tissue in body.
- Red – brown in color, wedge shaped.

Location

- Located in the left hypochondriac region opposite to the 9th, 10th and 11th ribs.
- Its long axis is parallel to the 10th rib.

External Features

- Has two ends, three borders and two surfaces
  - Anterior or lateral end – expanded
  - Posterior or medial end – rounded and directed backward and medially
  - Inferior border – rounded
  - Superior border – notched and indicates lobulated origin of spleen
  - Intermediate border – rounded and directed to right
  - Outer diaphragmatic surface – convex and smooth
  - Visceral surface – irregular, has various impressions:
    - Gastric impression: created by the fundus of stomach. It is the largest visceral impression.
    - Renal impression: due to left kidney
    - Colic impression: due to splenic flexure of colon
    - Pancreatic impression: due to tail of pancreas.
  - Hilum:
    - Cleft present along the long axis of spleen that transmits splenic vessels and nerves and also provides attachment to gastrosplenic and ileorenal ligaments.

Parenchyma of Spleen/Pulp

- White pulp
  - Main lymphoid tissue of spleen.
  - Periarteriolar lymphoid sheath (PALS)
    - Accumulation of lymphocytes around an arterial vessel.
    - T dependent Ig secretion
  - Follicles
    - Storage and maturation of B lymphocytes
    - Production of complement, opsonins
  - Marginal zone
    - Antigen presentation by MZ macrophages
    - Trapping of pathogens by MZ dendritic cells
  - **Red pulp**
    - Consists of
      - splenic venous sinuses

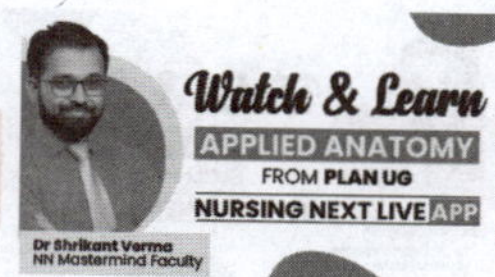

- Cords of Billroth
- Linings of splenic macrophages around the sinuses.
- Functions
  - Filtering of bloodborne pathogens
  - Storage and destruction of RBCs
  - Rapid antibody release *via* B cells and plasma cells.

Blood Supply

- **Arterial supply:** Splenic artery – largest branch of celiac trunk.
- **Venous drainage:** Splenic vein that emerges from the hilum of spleen and joins with the superior mesenteric vein behind the neck of the pancreas to form portal vein.

Lymphatic Drainage

Splenic lymph nodes that finally drain into the celiac lymph nodes.

Nerve Supply

Autonomic nerves from the celiac plexus.

Functions of Spleen

- Immune response
- Destruction of RBCs
- Production of all blood cells
  - Spleen acts as a site for fetal erythropoiesis
  - In adults, only lymphocytes are produced
- Storage of blood
  - Storage of RBCs
  - Stores 1/3rd of platelets

Nursing Implications

- Splenomegaly – the enlarged spleen can be palpated under the left costal margin.
- Splenic infarction – occurs due to infarction of spleen. Results in referred pain to the left shoulder (Kehr's sign)
- Splenic rupture – occurs due to blunt injuries to the stomach. Results in massive hemorrhage. Management involves splenectomy.

8. Write a short note on parts of large intestine. (KUHS, MGR)

Answer

Large Intestine

- 1.5 meter long extending from the ileocecal junction to the anus
- It is divided into the:
  - Right colic flexure
  - Transverse colon
  - Left colic flexure
  - Descending colon
  - Sigmoid colon
  - Rectum
  - Anus
- **Appendix (vermiform appendix):** Narrow, hollow, muscular tube with aggregations of lymphoid tissue. Suspended from the terminal ileum by small mesentery containing the appendicular vessels.
- **Rectum:** Starts at the middle of sacrum and 15 cm long. It follows forward curvature of sacrum and coccyx and ends 2.5 cm below and in front of coccyx where it continues as anal canal.
- **Anal canal:** Last part of digestive tube.
  - About 4 cm long
  - From the anorectal junction, it passes downward and backward to the anus.
- **Functions of large intestine:**
  - Absorption of carbohydrates, proteins and fats that have been acted upon by the gastric juices and intestinal and pancreatic secretions.
  - **Absorption of water:** Most of the water is absorbed in the small intestine, remaining is absorbed in large intestine.

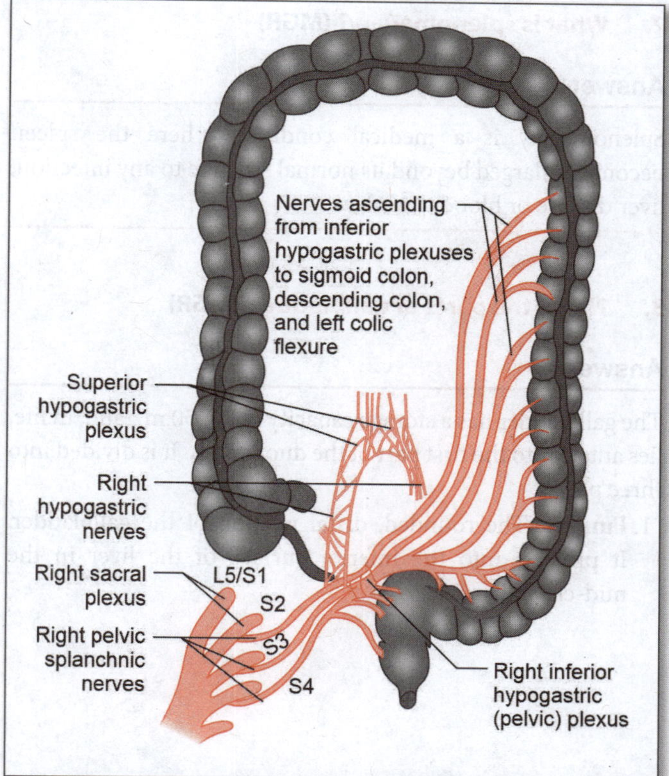

Figure 3.12: Large intestine

  - **Defecation:** Defecation is associated with voluntary contraction of abdominal muscles, descent of diaphragm and peristalsis of colon and relaxation of internal and external anal sphincters.

- **Sensory function:** The microvilli of some cells serve the sensory function.
- **Synthesis of vitamins:** Certain bacteria in the large intestine synthesize vitamin K.

SHORT ANSWER QUESTIONS

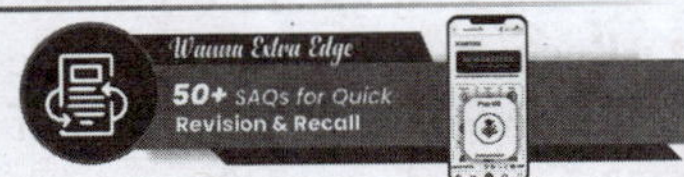

1. Name the parts of pancreas. (MGR)

Answer

Pancreas is divided into three parts:

1. **Head:** The head of the pancreas is the widest part and is situated on the right side of the abdomen.
2. **Body:** The body of the pancreas is the middle portion, extending horizontally across the abdomen behind the stomach.
3. **Tail:** The tail of the pancreas is the narrowest part and extends toward the left side of the abdomen, adjacent to the spleen.

2. What is splenomegaly? (MGR)

Answer

Splenomegaly is a medical condition where the spleen becomes enlarged beyond its normal size due to any infection, liver disease or blood disorders.

3. Name the parts of gallbladder. (MGR)

Answer

The gallbladder has a storage capacity of 30–50 mL and, in life, lies anterior to the first part of the duodenum. It is divided into three parts:

1. **Fundus:** The rounded, distal portion of the gallbladder. It projects into the inferior surface of the liver in the mid-clavicular line.
2. **Body:** The largest part of the gallbladder. It lies adjacent to the posteroinferior aspect of the liver, transverse colon and superior part of the duodenum.
3. **Neck:** The gallbladder tapers to become continuous with the cystic duct, leading into the biliary tree.

4. Write four differences between small intestine and large intestine. (MGR)

Answer

Small intestine	Large intestine
It is longer and has small width.	It is shorter and has broad width.
It is in between the stomach and large intestine.	It is the last part of the digestive system.
It helps in digestion and absorption.	It helps in reabsorption of food and elimination of waste.
It has three parts – duodenum, jejunum and ileum.	It has four parts – cecum, colon, rectum and anal canal.

5. Name the parts of esophagus. (MGR)

Answer

The esophagus is a fibromuscular tube, approximately 25 cm in length that transports food from the pharynx to the stomach.

Level of origin: It originates at the inferior border of the cricoid cartilage (C6) and extends to the cardiac orifice of the stomach (T11).

Parts of Esophagus

The esophagus has been subdivided into three portions:

1. **The cervical** portion extends from the cricopharyngeus to the suprasternal notch.
2. **The thoracic** portion extends from the suprasternal notch to the diaphragm.
3. **The abdominal** portion extends from the diaphragm to the cardiac portion of the stomach.

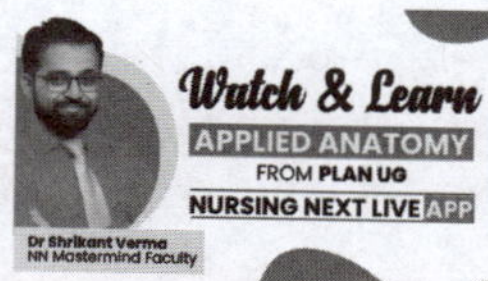

CONCEPTUAL REVISION

MULTIPLE CHOICE QUESTIONS

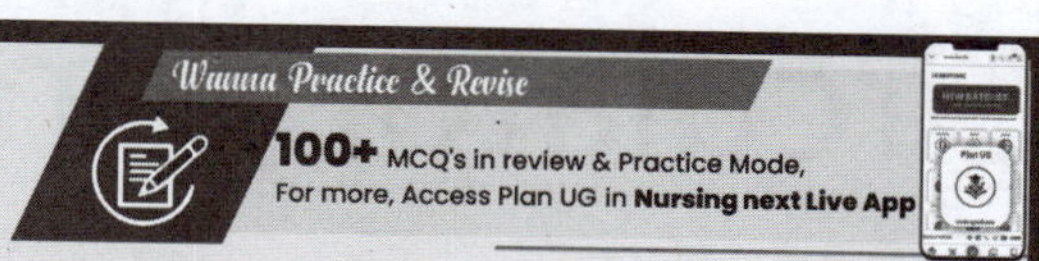

1. Posterior gastric artery is a branch of:

a. Left gastric artery b. Right gastric artery
c. Splenic artery d. Hepatic artery

Ans. c. Splenic artery

2. The gastroduodenal artery is derived from:

a. Celiac artery b. Hepatic artery
c. Splenic artery d. Cystic artery

Ans. b. Hepatic artery

3. Stomach is supplied by:

a. Celiac trunk b. Splenic artery
c. Gastroduodenal artery d. All of these

Ans. d. All of these

4. Valvulae conniventes are seen in:

a. Jejunum b. Ileum
c. Stomach d. Colon

Ans. a. Jejunum

Golden Points

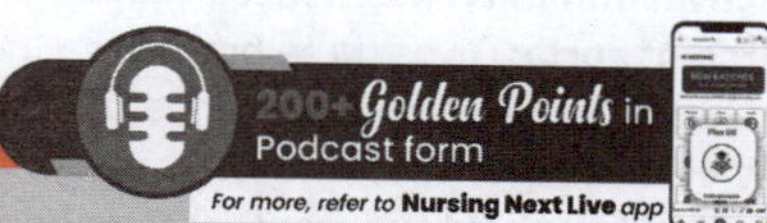

- Abdominal cavity is subdivided into nine regions.
- Digestive system is a group of organs that help in the breakdown of food and liquids into simpler substances.
- Duodenum is 'C' shaped with **head of pancreas** lying in its concavity.
- Esophagus is a 25 cm long muscular tube. It starts at the level of **6th cervical vertebra**, runs the most of its part through the thoracic cavity.
- Gallbladder is pyriform organ, 7 cm long with a capacity of 50 mL
- Large intestine is divided into the cecum, the ascending colon, right colic flexure, the transverse colon, left colic flexure, the descending colon, the sigmoid colon, the rectum and the anal canal.
- Liver is divided into **four lobes**—right lobe (largest), left lobe, caudate lobe and quadrate lobe.
- **McBurney point** occurs at the junction of lateral 1/3rd and medial 2/3rd of a line between right anterior superior iliac spine and umbilicus. It is the site of maximum tenderness.
- Pancreas is 15 cm long, and consists of a **head**, **neck**, **body** and **tail**.
- Part of the stomach above the gastroesophageal junction is called the **fundus** of the stomach. The main part is the **body** and the distal part is the **pyloric part.**

CHAPTER

4

Circulatory and Lymphatic System

CONCEPTUAL THEORY

Terminology

150+ key terminologies for Quick Recall & Revision

Active immunity: Resistance acquired due to antigenic stimulus.

Arch of aorta: Gives three branches. One branch divides into two. So, there are two arteries each for right side and two for the left side of head, neck, brain, upper limbs and thorax.

AV valves: Right atrioventricular valve has three cusps while left AV valve has two stronger cusps.

Central lymphoid tissues: These are bone marrow and thymus.

Circulatory system: Comprises heart enveloped in pericardium with arteries, capillaries and veins.

Coronary arteries: These are the first arteries to arise from the ascending aorta. These are functional end arteries and are likely to be partially/completely blocked.

Endocardium: The endocardium is the innermost layer of the heart wall.

Epicardium: The epicardium is the outermost layer of the heart wall and is also known as the visceral pericardium.

Immunity: Resistance to diseases due to biological defenses.

Innate or nonspecific immunity: It occurs due to genetic, mechanical barriers, biochemical factors and cellular factors.

Lymph nodes: These are present in neck, axilla, posterior thoracic and abdominal wall, inguinal region.

Lymphocytes: These are of two types: 'T' and 'B' lymphocytes.

Myocardium: The myocardium is the middle and thickest layer of the heart wall. It is made-up of specialized cardiac muscle cells called cardiomyocytes.

Passive immunity: Resistance provided passively.

Pericardium: Consists of an outer fibrous pericardium and inner double layered serous pericardium; made of an outer parietal and an inner visceral layer, most important content of pericardium is the heart with vessels entering and leaving it.

Peripheral lymphoid organs: These are numerous lymph nodes and spleen.

Semilunar valves: Aortic valve contains one anterior and one right posterior and one left posterior cusps. Pulmonary valve shows one posterior and two anterior cusps.

Specific immunity: It is due to types of T cells, i.e., helper, suppressor and cytotoxic and B cells, i.e., memory B cells and plasma cells.

STRUCTURE OF BLOOD COMPONENTS, BLOOD VESSELS — ARTERIAL AND VENOUS SYSTEM

- **Red blood cells (RBCs)**
  - Small, biconcave disks containing hemoglobin for oxygen transport.
  - Lack a nucleus and most organelles.
  - Flexible and can change shape to pass through narrow vessels.
- **White blood cells (WBCs)**
  - Various types, including neutrophils, lymphocytes, monocytes, etc.
  - Contain a nucleus and other cellular organelles.
  - Play a role in immune responses and defense against infections.
- **Platelets**
  - Fragments of larger cells called megakaryocytes.
  - Aid in blood clotting and formation of blood clots.
- **Plasma**
  - Liquid component of blood, constituting about 55% of blood volume.
  - Contains water, proteins (such as albumin and fibrinogen), ions, nutrients, hormones, etc.

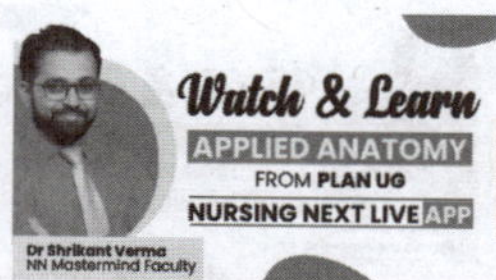

Aspect	Arterial system	Venous system
Function	Carries oxygenated blood away from the heart	Returns deoxygenated blood back to the heart
Blood flow	Blood flows under higher pressure	Blood flows under lower pressure
Blood composition	Oxygen-rich blood (except for pulmonary artery)	Oxygen-poor blood (except for pulmonary vein)
Blood vessels	Arteries, arterioles, and capillaries	Veins, venules, and capillaries
Structure	Thicker, more muscular walls	Thinner, less muscular walls
Elasticity	More elastic, allowing for pressure regulation	Less elastic, accommodating blood volume
Valves	Absent	Present in most veins
Direction of flow	Away from the heart	Toward the heart
Pulmonary circulation	Carries blood to the lungs for oxygenation	Carries oxygenated blood from the lungs
Systemic circulation	Supplies oxygenated blood to body tissues	Collects deoxygenated blood from body tissues
Blood pressure	Higher systolic and diastolic pressures	Lower systolic and diastolic pressures
Blood color	Bright red (oxygenated)	Dark red (deoxygenated)
Exceptions	Pulmonary artery carries deoxygenated blood	Pulmonary vein carries oxygenated blood
Examples	Aorta, coronary arteries, brachial artery	Superior vena cava, femoral vein, hepatic vein

Position of Heart Related to the Associated Structures

Base of the heart: The base of the heart is also called its posterior surface. It is formed mainly by the left atrium and by a small part of the right atrium.

Borders of the Heart

- The upper border is slightly oblique, and is formed by the two atria, chiefly the left atrium.
- The right border is more or less vertical and is formed by the right atrium. It extends from superior vena cava to inferior vena cava (IVC).
- The inferior border is nearly horizontal and is formed mainly by the right ventricle. A small part of it near the apex is formed by left ventricle. It extends from IVC to apex.
- The left border is oblique and curved. It is formed mainly by the left ventricle, and partly by the left auricle. It separates the anterior and left surfaces of the heart. It extends from apex to left auricle.

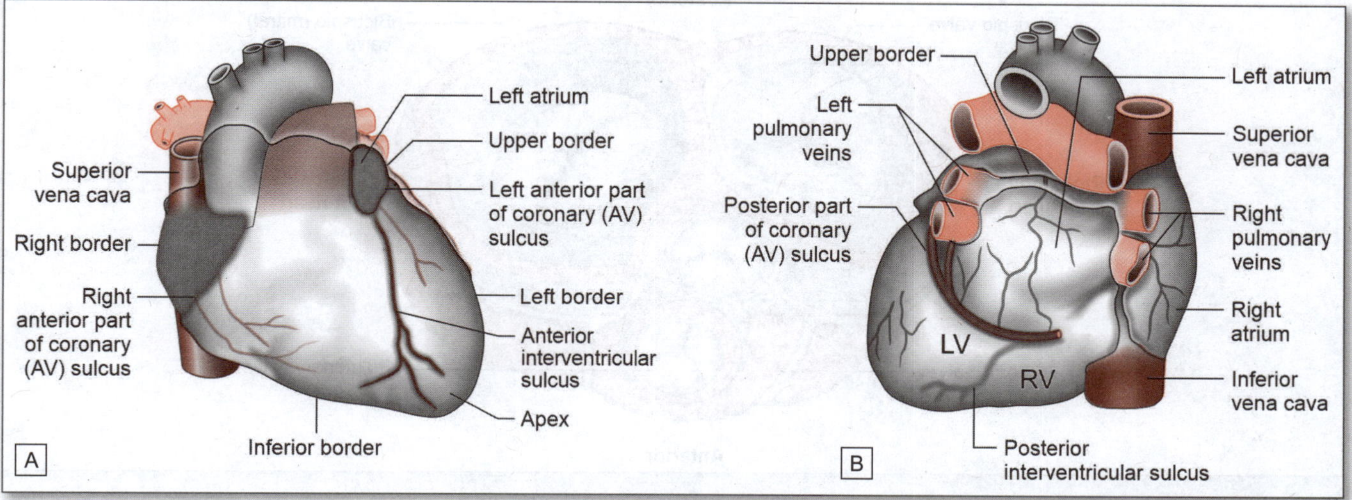

Figures 4.1A and B: The posterior base and inferior surface of the heart

Chambers of Heart

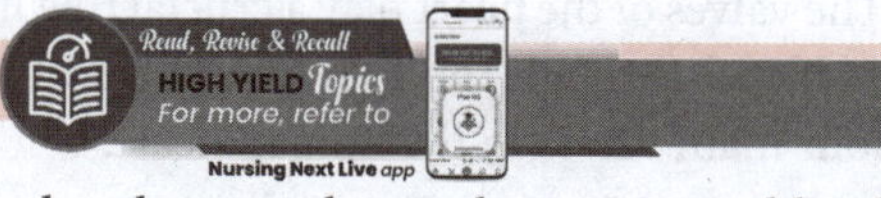

The human heart consists of four chambers: Two atria and two ventricles. These chambers work together to pump blood throughout the body.

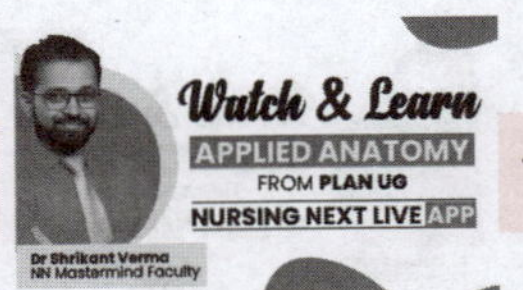

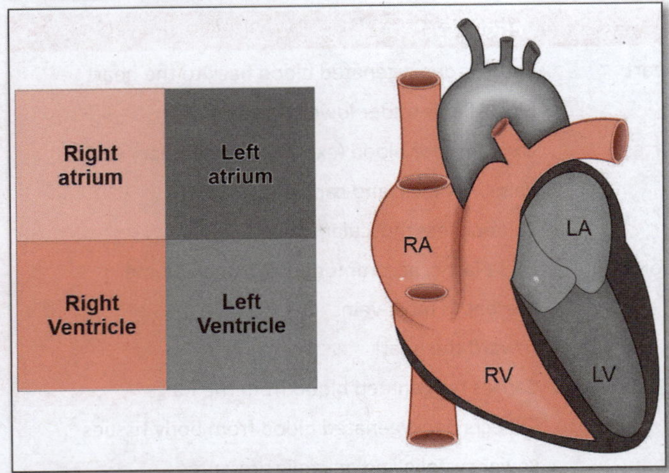

Figure 4.2: Chambers of heart

1. **Right atrium:** The right atrium is the upper chamber on the right side of the heart. It receives deoxygenated blood from the body through two large veins called the superior vena cava and inferior vena cava.
2. **Right ventricle:** The right ventricle is the lower chamber on the right side of the heart. When the right atrium contracts, it pushes blood into the right ventricle. The right ventricle then contracts, pumping the deoxygenated blood into the pulmonary artery, which carries it to the lungs for oxygenation.
3. **Left atrium:** The left atrium is the upper chamber on the left side of the heart. It receives oxygenated blood from the lungs through four pulmonary veins. The left atrium contracts, forcing the blood into the left ventricle.
4. **Left ventricle:** The left ventricle is the lower chamber on the left side of the heart and is the thickest and most powerful chamber. When the left atrium contracts, it pushes blood into the left ventricle. The left ventricle then contracts, pumping the oxygenated blood out of the heart through the aorta, which delivers it to the rest of the body.

Layers of Heart

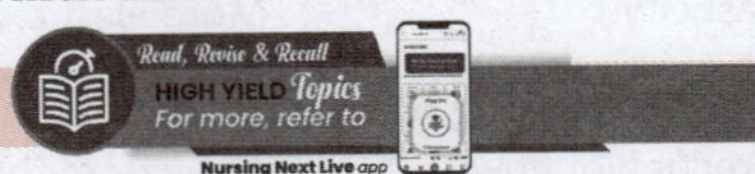

The heart is composed of three main layers, known as the heart wall. From the innermost layer to the outermost layer, these layers are:

1. **Endocardium:** The endocardium is the innermost layer of the heart wall. It is a thin, smooth layer composed of endothelial cells that line the chambers of the heart and the valves. The endocardium provides a smooth surface for blood to flow through the heart.
2. **Myocardium:** The myocardium is the middle and thickest layer of the heart wall. It is made-up of specialized cardiac muscle cells called cardiomyocytes. The myocardium is responsible for powerful contractions of the heart that pump blood throughout the body.
3. **Epicardium:** The epicardium is the outermost layer of the heart wall and is also known as the visceral pericardium. It is a thin, protective layer composed of connective tissue and a layer of mesothelial cells.

Heart Valves

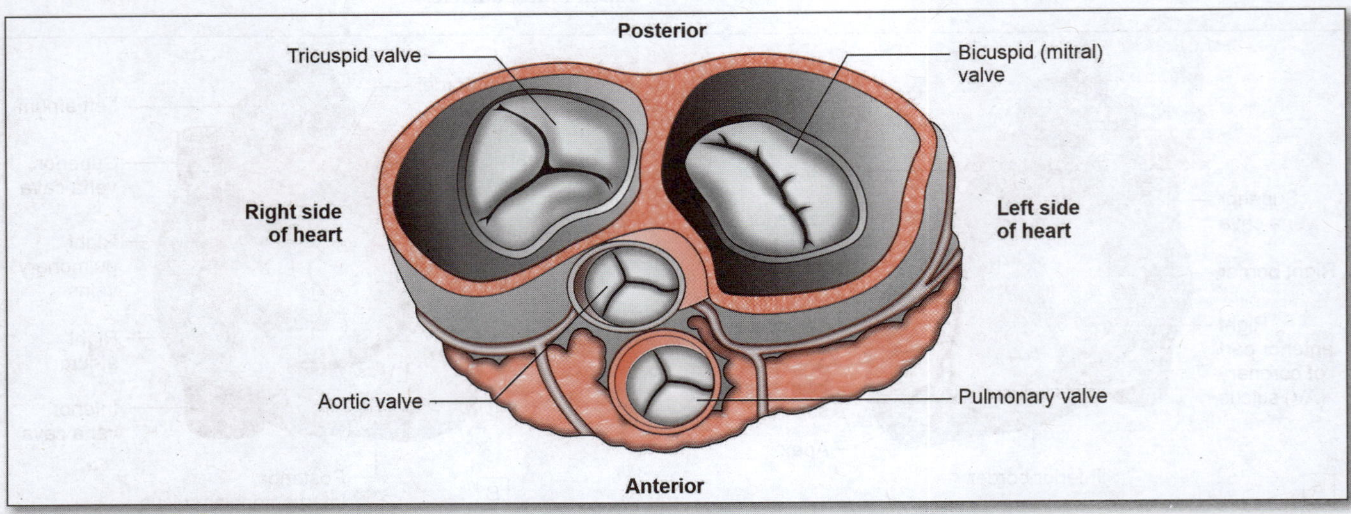

Figure 4.3: Heart valves

The valves of the heart play a crucial role in regulating the flow of blood through the four chambers of the heart. There are four main valves in the human heart:

1. **Tricuspid valve:** This valve is located between the right atrium and the right ventricle. It consists of three leaflets or cusps that open to allow blood to flow from the right atrium to the right ventricle and close to prevent backflow when the right ventricle contracts.
2. **Pulmonary valve:** Found between the right ventricle and the pulmonary artery, this valve has three semilunar cusps.

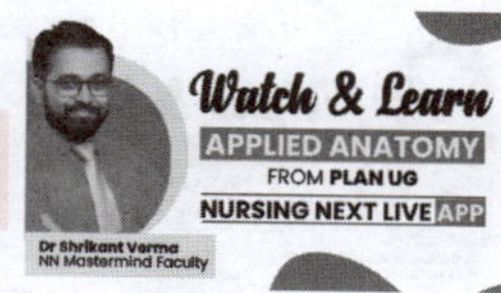

It opens when the right ventricle contracts to allow blood to be pumped into the pulmonary artery and closes to prevent blood from flowing back into the right ventricle during relaxation.

3. **Mitral valve (Bicuspid valve):** Positioned between the left atrium and the left ventricle, the mitral valve has two leaflets. It permits blood to flow from the left atrium to the left ventricle during relaxation and prevents backflow when the left ventricle contracts.
4. **Aortic valve:** Situated between the left ventricle and the aorta, the aortic valve also consists of three semilunar cusps. It opens when the left ventricle contracts, allowing blood to be pumped into the aorta (the main artery of the body), and closes to prevent blood from returning to the left ventricle.

Coronary Arteries

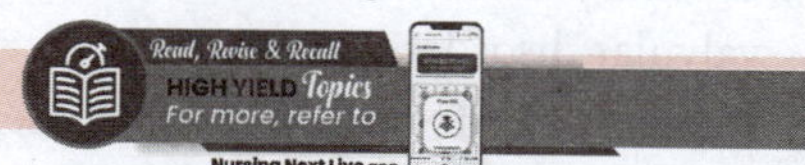

Coronary arteries are blood vessels that supply oxygenated blood to the heart muscle (myocardium). They branch off from the aorta, the main artery that carries oxygenated blood from the heart to the rest of the body.

There are two main coronary arteries:

1. **Left coronary artery (LCA):** The left coronary artery originates from the aorta and divides into two main branches:
   i. **Left anterior descending artery (LAD):** This artery supplies blood to the front and left side of the heart, including the majority of the septum and the anterior wall of the left ventricle.
   ii. **Left circumflex artery (LCX):** The LCX supplies blood to the left atrium and the back of the left ventricle.
2. **Right coronary artery (RCA):** The right coronary artery also arises from the aorta and travels along the surface of the heart. It supplies blood to the right atrium, right ventricle, and a portion of the back of the left ventricle. Additionally, it gives rise to branches called marginal arteries, which supply blood to the outer wall of the right ventricle.

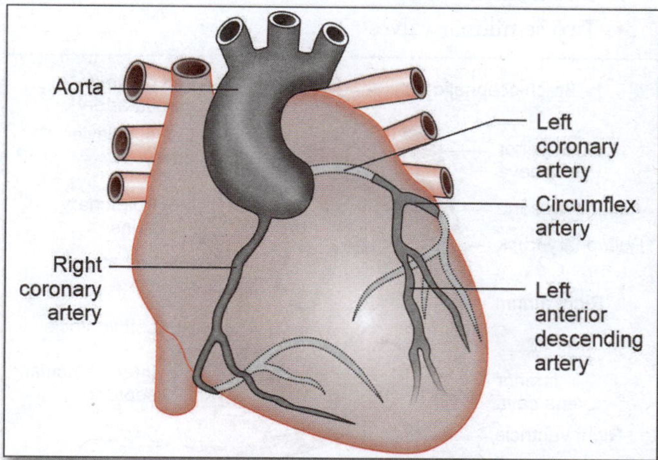

Figure 4.4: Coronary arteries

Nerve and Blood Supply to Heart

Nerve supply to the heart: The nerve supply to the heart is controlled by the autonomic nervous system, which consists of two main divisions: The sympathetic nervous system and the parasympathetic nervous system.

- **Sympathetic nervous system:** Sympathetic nerves originate from the upper thoracic segments of the spinal cord. They innervate the heart and release norepinephrine (noradrenaline), which increases heart rate, contractility, and the force of cardiac muscle contraction. Sympathetic stimulation prepares the heart for physical activity or stressful situations, commonly known as the "fight-or-flight" response.
- **Parasympathetic nervous system:** Parasympathetic nerves originate from the vagus nerve (cranial nerve X) and reach the heart. These nerves release acetylcholine, which slows down the heart rate and decreases contractility. Parasympathetic stimulation helps to restore normal heart rate and function during periods of rest and relaxation.

LYMPHATIC TISSUE

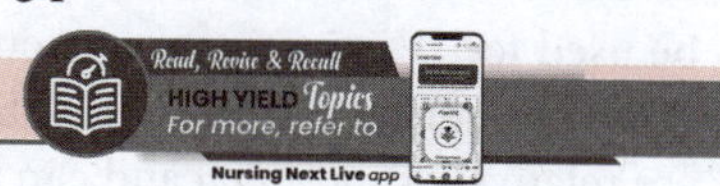

- Lymphatic tissue is a part of the lymphatic system, which is a network of vessels, nodes, and organs involved in the body's immune response and fluid balance.
- The lymphatic system works alongside the circulatory system to help remove waste products, toxins, and foreign substances from the body and fight against infections.
- Lymphatic tissue is composed of various types of specialized cells, including lymphocytes, which are a type of white blood cell involved in the immune response. It is found throughout the body, with higher concentrations in certain areas such as lymph nodes, tonsils, adenoids, and the spleen.
- The main function of lymphatic tissue is to produce and store lymphocytes and other immune cells. These cells help identify and eliminate pathogens, such as bacteria and viruses, as well as abnormal cells, such as cancer cells.
- Lymphatic tissue also filters and purifies lymph, a fluid that circulates through the lymphatic system, by trapping and removing foreign particles and cellular debris.
- Lymph nodes are the primary sites of lymphatic tissue, acting as filters along the lymphatic vessels.
- They contain specialized compartments where immune cells interact and respond to foreign substances.
- When an infection or inflammation occurs nearby, lymph nodes may become swollen and tender as immune cells accumulate to fight off the invaders.

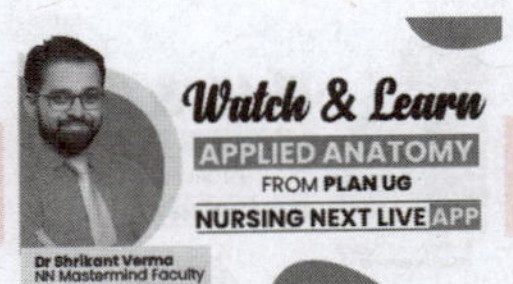

Veins Used for IV Injections

Intravenous (IV) injections involve the administration of fluids, medications, or blood products directly into a vein.

- **Cephalic vein:** The cephalic vein is located in the upper arm and forearm on the lateral (outer) side. It is often visible and easily accessible, making it a common choice for IV injections and cannulation.
- **Basilic vein:** The basilic vein is located in the upper arm and forearm on the medial (inner) side. It is often larger than the cephalic vein and can be used for IV injections when the cephalic vein is not accessible or suitable.
- **Median cubital vein:** The median cubital vein is a superficial vein located in the antecubital fossa, which is the bend of the elbow. It is often the preferred vein for IV injections, blood draws, and venipuncture because it is usually prominent and easily accessible.
- **Radial vein:** The radial vein runs along the radial bone of the forearm. It can be used for IV injections, especially in situations where other veins are not accessible or suitable.
- **Dorsal hand veins:** The veins on the back of the hand can be used for IV injections, particularly in cases where other veins are not accessible or suitable. The dorsal hand veins are relatively superficial and can be visible and accessible.

Application and Implication in Nursing

- **Assessment and monitoring:** Nurses assess and monitor patients' circulatory and lymphatic systems to identify abnormalities and changes in their cardiovascular and lymphatic status.
- **Medication administration:** Nurses administer various medications related to the circulatory system, such as anticoagulants, antiplatelet agents, vasopressors, and cardiac medications.
- **Intravenous therapy:** Nurses play a crucial role in administering intravenous (IV) fluids and medications, ensuring the correct rate of infusion, monitoring potential complications, and maintaining the patency and integrity of IV access devices.
- **Cardiovascular disorders:** Nurses care for patients with various cardiovascular conditions, such as hypertension, coronary artery disease, heart failure, arrhythmias, and valvular disorders.
- **Hemodynamic monitoring:** Nurses utilize hemodynamic monitoring techniques, such as central venous pressure (CVP), arterial blood pressure monitoring, and pulmonary artery catheterization, to assess patients' cardiovascular status and response to treatment.
- **Lymphedema management:** Nurses provide care for patients with lymphatic system disorders, such as lymphedema. They assess and measure limb swelling, implement compression therapy, teach self-care techniques, and promote skin integrity and infection prevention.

CONCEPTUAL EXERCISES

LONG ANSWER QUESTIONS

1. Describe anatomy of heart. (RUHS)

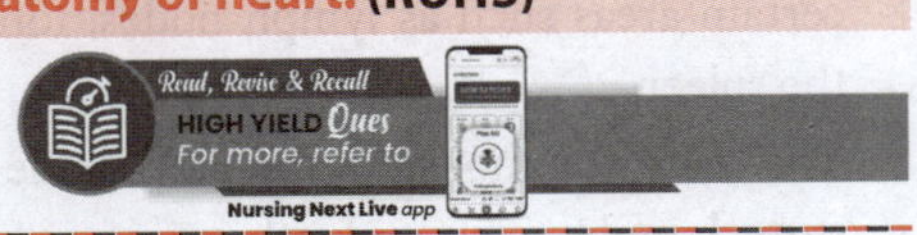

Answer

Gross Anatomy of the Heart

- **Size and shape:** The heart measures:
  - Anterioposteriorly — 6 cm
  - Widest transverse diameter — 8 to 9 cm
  - Length — 12 cm
  - Weight — more in males than females – average 230–340 g
- **Location**
  - The heart is located in the middle mediastinum with apex facing downward, forward and toward the left just medial to the midclavicular line in the 5th intercostal space.
  - Base of the heart lies upward and backward on the right side extending to the right 3rd costal cartilage.
- Heart has four chambers – two atria and two ventricles.
- The interior of the heart consists of:
  - Left and right atria
  - Left and right ventricles
  - Interventricular septum
  - Two atrioventricular valves
  - Two semilunar valves

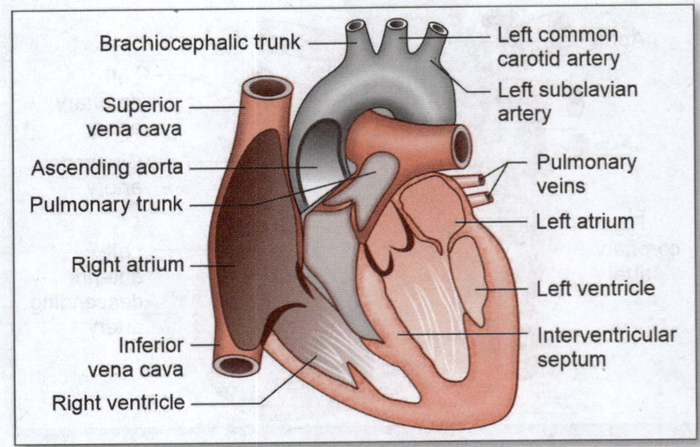

Figure 4.5: Coronal section of heart

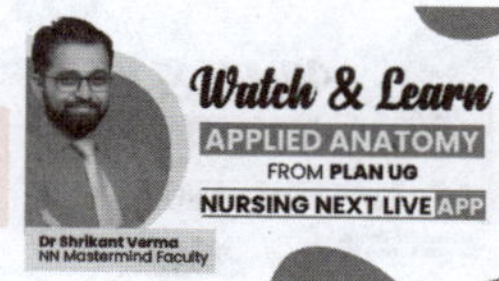

Layers of Heart

Heart is enveloped by pericardium, a fibroserous sac that encloses the heart and the roots of the great vessels. It is situated in the middle mediastinum.

Pericardium consists of two layers:

1. **Fibrous pericardium:** The outer fibrous layer
2. **Serous pericardium:** Inner double serous membrane layer

Pericardial Cavity

Potential space between the parietal pericardium and the visceral pericardium.

Contents of the Pericardium

- Heart
- Cardiac vessels and nerves
- Ascending aorta
- Lower half of the superior vena cava
- Terminal part of the inferior vena cava
- Pulmonary trunk
- Terminal parts of the pulmonary veins

Sinuses with in the Pericardial Cavity

- Two sinuses are present within the pericardial cavity
- Oblique pericardial sinus
  - Space behind the heart between the pulmonary veins
- Transverse pericardial sinus
  - Space above the heart behind the aorta and pulmonary trunk
  - Used to clamp the aorta during the cardiac surgery.

Relations of the Heart

- Superiorly
  - Aorta, superior vena cava, pulmonary artery and pulmonary veins
- Inferiorly
  - Apex rests on the central tendon of the diaphragm
- Anteriorly
  - Ribs and intercostal muscles
- Posteriorly
  - Esophagus, trachea, left and right bronchus, descending aorta, inferior vena cava and thoracic vertebrae.
- Laterally
  - Lungs

Surfaces of Heart

- **Base:** Directed backward
- **Apex:** Directed downward, forward and to the left
- **Sternocostal surface:** Anterior
  - Formed by the right ventricle and partly by right atrium, left ventricle and left auricle.
- **Diaphragmatic surface:** Inferior
  - Formed by both the ventricles, mainly left one.
  - Posterior interventricular groove divides this surface into right one-third and left two-thirds.
- **Pulmonary surface:** Left lateral
  - Formed mainly by the left ventricle, which occupies the cardiac notch of the left lung.

Borders

- **Right border:** Formed by right atrium
- **Inferior border:** Mainly by right ventricle
- **Left border:** Mainly by left ventricle, partly by left auricle.
- **Superior border:** Left atria mainly

Right Atrium

- Right atrium is the upper right chamber of heart and receives venous blood from all parts of the body.
- It forms the right and upper border of the heart, sternocostal surface and base of the heart.
- It is the first to receive the deoxygenated blood from the body through the superior and inferior venae cavae.
- It plays an important role in originating and regulating the coordination of the heart.

Interior of Right Atrium

Divided into three parts: Anterior part, posterior part and septal wall (also called the central wall of the posterior wall)

1. **Anterior part:**
   - Also called rough part or the pectinate part
   - Internal muscular ridge forms the crista terminalis
2. **Posterior part:**
   - Also called smooth part or sinus venorum
   - Contains the opening of superior vena cava
   - Contains openings of venae cordis minimae or the Thebesian veins
   - Coronary sinus opens here which is guarded by a valve.
3. **Septal wall:**
   - Fossa ovalis is present
   - Limbus fossa ovalis: Prominent margin of fossa ovalis; anterior edge is continuous with left end of valve of inferior vena cava.

Right Ventricle

- Right inferior chamber of the heart
- Triangular in shape.

- It receives deoxygenated blood from the right atrium and pumps it to the lung through the pulmonary trunk and pulmonary arteries.

Interior of Right Ventricle

- It has two openings
  1. Right atrioventricular opening or orifice – guarded by the tricuspid valve.
  2. Pulmonary opening or orifice – guarded by the pulmonary valve.
- Thickness of the wall of the right ventricle is less than that of the left ventricle.
- The cavity of the right ventricle is crescentric in shape, due to the forward bulge of the interventricular septum.

Left Atrium

- Upper left part of the heart.
- Forms the left two thirds of the base of heart.
- Quadrangular in shape.
- It receives oxygenated blood from the lungs through the pulmonary veins.
- It pumps the blood to the left ventricle through the left atrioventricular or biscuspid orifice.

Left Ventricle

- Left ventricular cavity is circular in shape.
- It receives the oxygenated blood from the left atrium and pumps it into the aorta.
- Forms the apex of the heart.

Interior of the Left Ventricle

The interior of the left ventricle shows two orifices:

1. Left atrioventricular or bicuspid or mitral orifice – which is guarded by the mitral valve
2. The aortic orifice – which is guarded by the aortic valve.

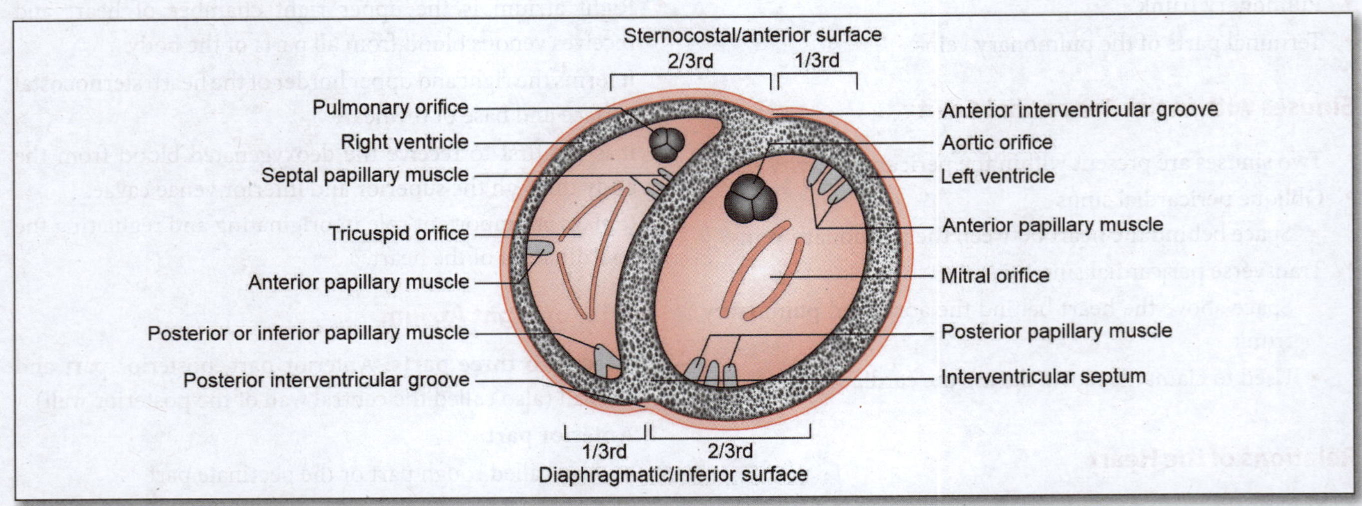

Figure 4.6: Transverse section through the ventricles of the heart

Valves of Heart

- Valves maintain unidirectional blood flow and prevent its backflow in the opposite direction.
- Two types of valves:
  1. Pair of atrioventricular valves
  2. Pair of semilunar valves
- Right atrioventricular valve
  - Tricuspid valve as it has three cusps – anterior, posterior and septal.
- Left atrioventricular valve
  - Bicuspid valve – as it has two cusps – large anterior cusp and small posterior one.
  - Also known as mitral valve.
  - Attached to the chordae tendinae.
- Aortic valves
  - Has one anterior and two posterior – right and left cusps.
- Pulmonary valves
  - Has three semilunar cusps – one posterior and two anterior.

Sulci

- Visible grooves on the surface of the heart
- Mark the boundaries of four chambers

Blood Supply of Heart

- The heart receives its own supply of blood from the coronary arteries.
- Right coronary artery: Its branches include:
  - The sinoatrial nodal branch

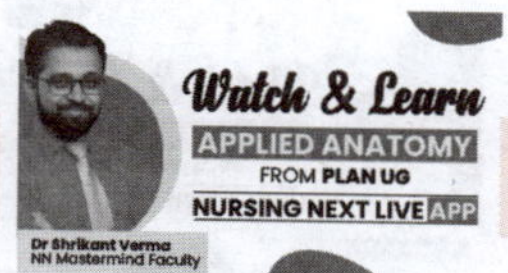

- The right marginal branch
- The atrioventricular nodal branch
- The posterior interventricular branch

- These branches supply the right atrium, the majority of the right ventricle, the diaphragmatic surface of the left ventricle, part of the intraventricular and interatrial septa, the sinoatrial node and the atrioventricular node.
- Left coronary artery: The left coronary artery runs between the left auricle and the pulmonary trunk. It gives rise to the following branches:
  - Circumflex branch
  - Anterior interventricular branch
- Venous drainage into coronary sinus

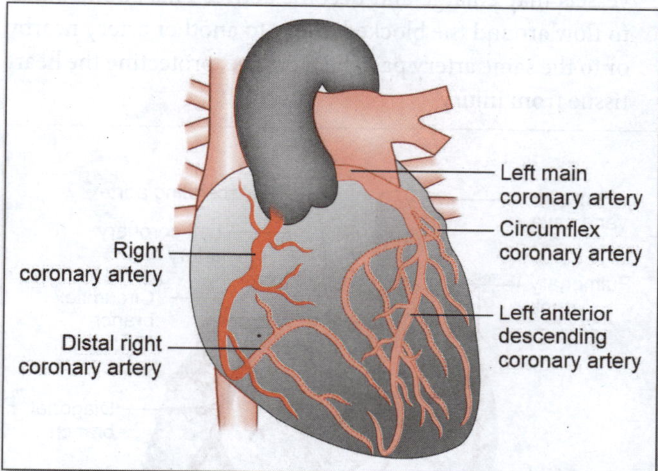

Figure 4.7: Arterial supply of heart

Nerve Supply of the Heart

- The heart receives its nervous innervation by the sympathetic and the parasympathetic fibers of the autonomic nervous system.
- The fibrous and parietal pericardia are supplied by the phrenic nerves. They are sensitive to pain. The epicardium is supplied by autonomic nerves of the heart and is not sensitive to pain.

2. Name the types of circulation. Describe in detail the blood supply of heart along with its applied anatomy. (MGR)

Answer

Types of Circulation

The cardiovascular system is composed of two circulatory systems:

1. **Pulmonary circulation:** Path through the lungs where blood is oxygenated.
2. **Systemic circulation:** Circulation through the rest of the body to provide oxygenated blood.

The two systems are linked to each other through the heart, creating a continuous cycle of blood through the body.

Pulmonary Circulation

- Pulmonary circulation is the movement of blood from the heart to the lungs for oxygenation, then back to the heart again.
- Oxygen-deficit blood from the body leaves the systemic circulation when it enters the right atrium through the superior and inferior venae cavae.
- The blood is then pumped into the right ventricle through tricuspid valve. From there, blood is pumped through the pulmonary valve and into the pulmonary artery.
- The oxygenated blood leaves the lungs through pulmonary veins, which returns it to the left atrium, completing the pulmonary circuit. As the pulmonary circuit ends, the systemic circuit begins.

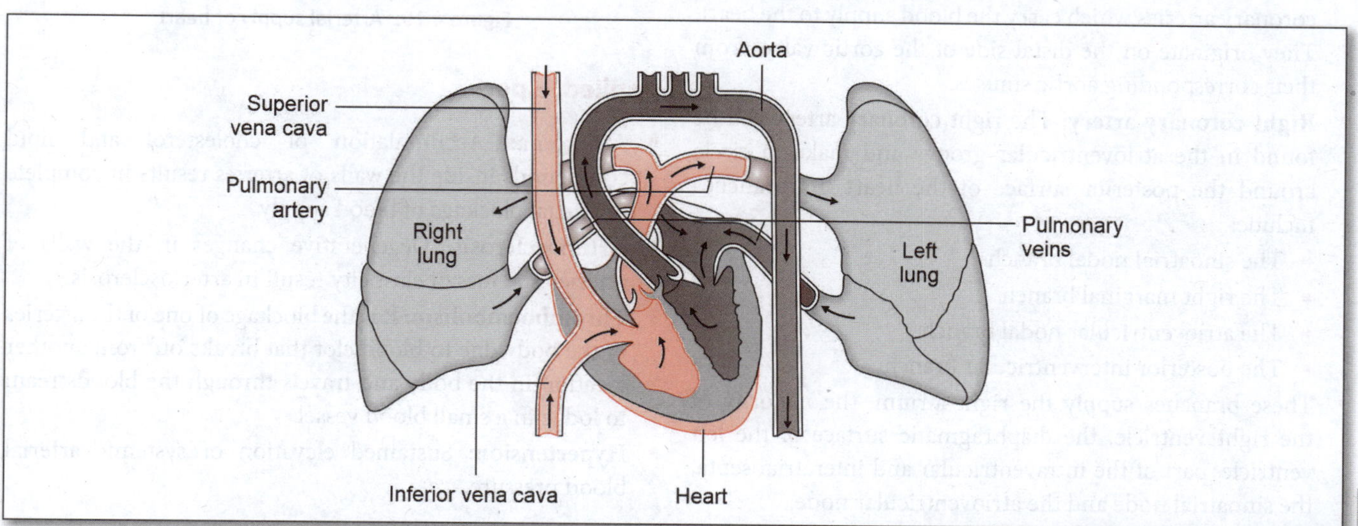

Figure 4.8: Pulmonary circulation

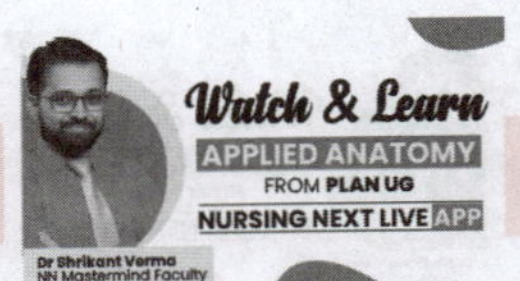

Systemic Circulation

Systemic circulation refers to the movement of blood from the heart through the body to provide oxygen and nutrients to the tissues of the body while bringing deoxygenated blood back to the heart.

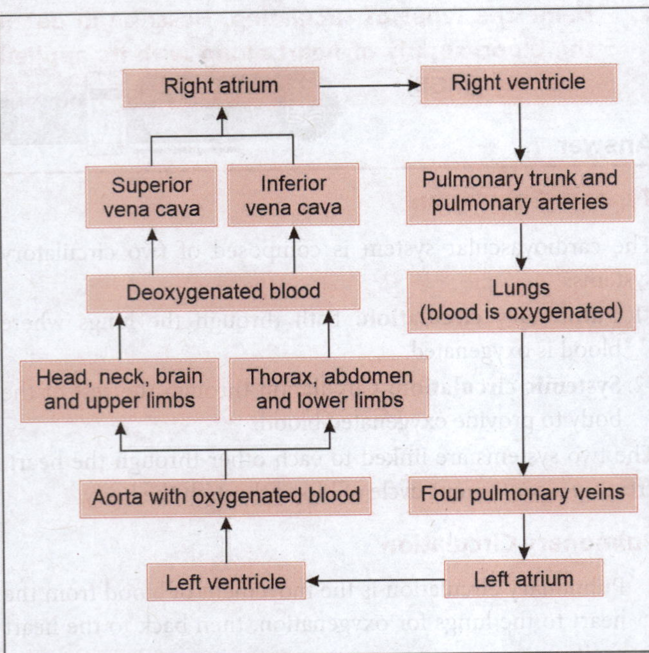

Figure 4.9: Circulation of blood

Blood Supply of Heart

- The heart receives its own supply of blood from the coronary arteries. Two major coronary arteries branch off from the aorta near the point where the aorta and the left ventricle meet. Left main coronary artery is also called the left main trunk.
- The first branches of the aorta are the right and left coronary arteries which carry the blood supply to the heart. They originate on the distal side of the aortic valve, from their corresponding aortic sinuses.
- **Right coronary artery:** The right coronary artery can be found in the atrioventricular groove and makes a circle around the posterior surface of the heart. Its branches include:
  - The sinoatrial nodal branch
  - The right marginal branch
  - The atrioventricular nodal branch
  - The posterior interventricular branch
- These branches supply the right atrium, the majority of the right ventricle, the diaphragmatic surface of the left ventricle, part of the intraventricular and interatrial septa, the sinoatrial node and the atrioventricular node.
- **Left coronary artery:** The left coronary artery runs between the left auricle and the pulmonary trunk. It gives rise to the following branches:
  - **Circumflex branch:** It sometimes branches further to give a sinoatrial nodal branch.
  - **Anterior interventricular branch:** The areas supplied by these branches are the left atrium, most of the left ventricle, a small area of the right ventricle, the interventricular septum and the sinoatrial node.
- Collateral circulation is a network of tiny blood vessels, and, under normal conditions, not open. When the coronary arteries narrow to the point that blood flow to the heart muscle is limited (coronary artery disease), collateral vessels may enlarge and become active. This allows blood to flow around the blocked artery to another artery nearby or to the same artery past the blockage, protecting the heart tissue from injury.

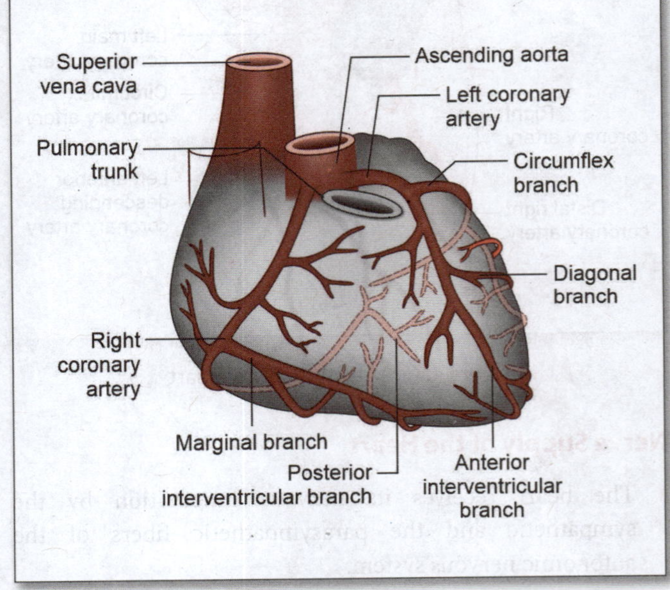

Figure 4.10: Arterial supply of heart

Applied Aspect

- **Atheroma:** Accumulation of cholesterol and lipid compounds inside the walls of arteries results in complete or partial blockage of blood supply.
- **Arteriosclerosis:** Degenerative changes in the walls of arteries and loss of elasticity result in arteriosclerosis.
- **Thromboembolism:** It is the blockage of one of the arteries of the body due to blood clot that breaks off from another location in the body and travels through the bloodstream to lodge in a small blood vessel.
- **Hypertension:** Sustained elevation of systemic arterial blood pressure.

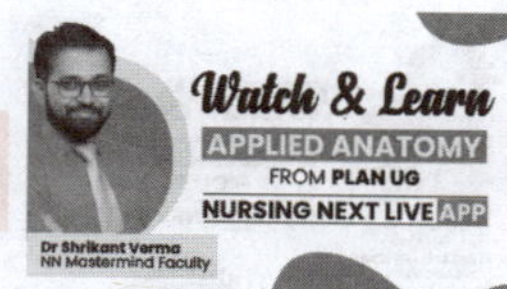

- **Superficial thrombophlebitis:** Inflammation of the superficial veins of the limbs due to intravenous fluid infusion and results in thrombosis.
- **Deep vein thrombosis:** Clotting of venous blood in the deep veins due to damage to vessel wall or change in blood viscosity.
- **Varicose veins:** Occur in lower limb due to incompetent valves of the superficial veins or of the perforators.

SHORT NOTES

1. Write a short note on cardiac muscle. (RUHS)

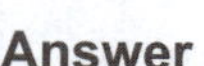

Answer

Cardiac Muscle

- Cardiac muscle (also called heart muscle or myocardium) is an involuntary, striated muscle that comprises the main tissue of the walls of the heart.
- Each muscle fiber has striations and one central nucleus.
- Cardiac muscle fibers are interconnected through intercalated disks which consist of gap.
- Requires stimulation by pacemaker cells for contraction.
- Auto rhythmicity is an inherent property of cardiac muscle and rate is controlled by autonomic nerves, hormones, local metabolites, and other metabolites.
- **Histology**
  - **Cardiac muscle cells:** Cardiac muscle cells or cardio-myocytes are the contracting cells which allow the heart to pump.
  - Cardiomyocytes contain T-tubules, pouches of membrane that run from the surface to the cell's interior which help to improve the efficiency of contraction. Most of these cells contain only one nucleus.
  - **Intercalated disks:** The cardiac syncytium is a network of cardiomyocytes connected to each other by intercalated disks that enable the rapid transmission of electrical impulses through the network, which enable the syncytium to act in a coordinated contraction of the myocardium.
  - **Fibroblasts:** Cardiac fibroblasts are vital supporting cells within cardiac muscle. They are unable to provide forceful contractions like cardiomyocytes, but instead are largely responsible for creating and maintaining the extracellular matrix which forms the mortar in which cardiomyocyte bricks are embedded.
  - **Extracellular matrix:** The matrix is composed of proteins such as collagen and elastin along with polysaccharides (sugar chains) known as glycosaminoglycans. The matrix in immediate contact with the muscle cells is referred to as the basement membrane, mainly composed of type IV collagen and laminin.

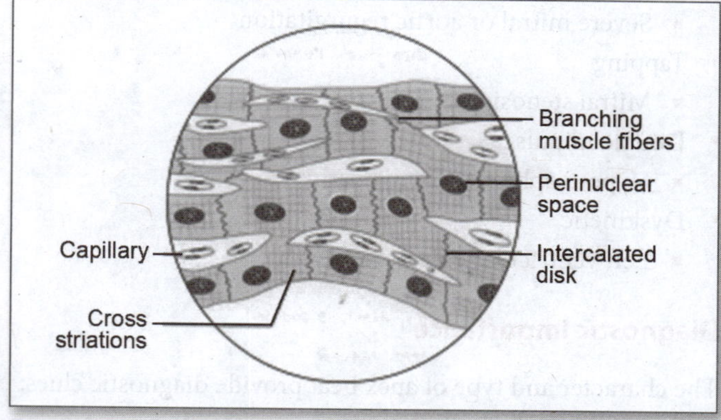

Figure 4.11: Histology of cardiac muscle

2. Write a short note on apex beat. (DU)

Answer

Introduction

- Apex beat is the point of maximum impulse.
- It is the furthermost point laterally and inferiorly from the sternum at which the cardiac impulse can be felt.
- Cardiac impulse results due to rotation of the heart, and its movement against the chest wall during systole.

Location

- The apex beat can be felt or palpated in the:
  - **Adults:** 5th left intercostal space at the point of intersection with the left midclavicular line.
  - **Children:** 4th intercostal space medial to the nipple.
- Abnormal locations:
  - **In case of dextrocardia:** Apex beat may be felt on the right side.

Types of Apex beat

- Normal apex beat
  - Seen in healthy individuals
- Normal but shifted
  - Normal character but abnormal position due to mediastinal shift
- Impalpable:
  - Hyperinflated lungs
  - Pericardial effusion
  - High BMI

- Pressure loaded
  - Left ventricular hypertrophy
  - Aortic stenosis
- Volume loaded
  - Severe mitral or aortic regurgitation
- Tapping
  - Mitral stenosis
- Double impulse
  - Hypertrophic cardiomyopathy
- Dyskinetic
  - Left ventricular apical aneurysm

Diagnostic Importance

The character and type of apex beat provide diagnostic clues:

- Forceful impulse indicates pressure overload – hypertension
- Uncoordinated apex beat – dyskinetic beat – indicates ventricular dysfunction.

Nursing Implications

- Displacement of the apex beat laterally or inferiorly usually indicates:
  - Cardiomegaly
  - Pleural or pulmonary diseases
  - Deformities of the chest wall
- Absent apex beat is seen in:
  - Cases of reduced stroke volume
  - Ventricular tachycardia
  - Shock

3. Write a short note on the interior of the heart.

Answer

- The interior of the heart consists of:
  - Left and right atria
  - Left and right ventricles
  - Interventricular septum
  - Two atrioventricular valves
  - Two semilunar valves

Interior of Right Atrium

Divided into three parts: Anterior part, posterior part and septal wall (also called the central wall of the posterior wall)

1. **Anterior part:**
   Also called rough part or the pectinate part
2. **Posterior part:**
   - Also called smooth part or sinus venorum
   - Contains the opening of superior vena cava
   - Contains openings of venae cordis minimae or the Thebesian veins
   - Coronary sinus opens here which is guarded by a valve.
3. **Septal wall:**
   - Fossa ovalis is present here which is a shallow saucer-shaped depression and is derived from septum primum.

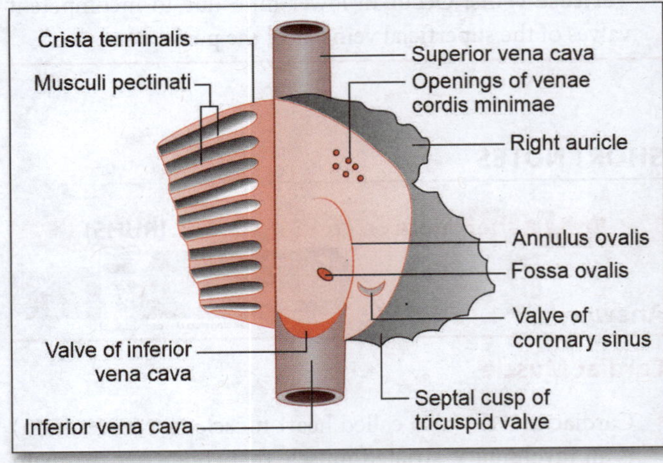

Figure 4.12: Interior of right atrium (Cut along sulcus terminalis)

Interior of Right Ventricle

- It has two openings.
  1. Right atrioventricular opening or orifice — guarded by the tricuspid valve.
  2. Pulmonary opening or orifice — guarded by the pulmonary valve.
- Thickness of the wall of the right ventricle is less than that of the left ventricle.
- The cavity of the right ventricle is crescent-shaped due to the forward bulge of the interventricular septum.

Interventricular Septum

The interventricular septum is the stout wall separating the ventricles, the lower chambers of the heart, from one another.

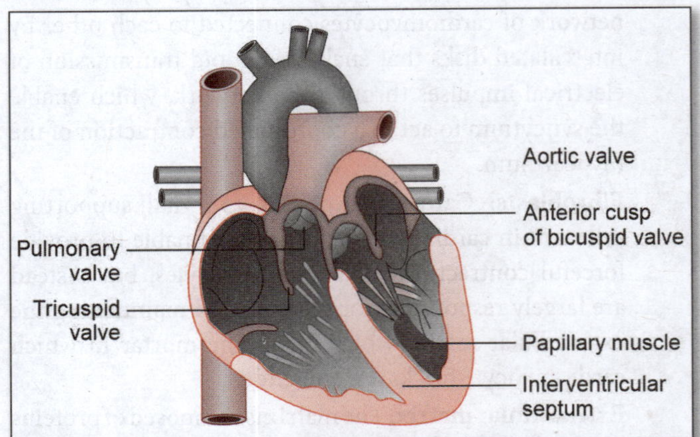

Figure 4.13: Interventricular septum

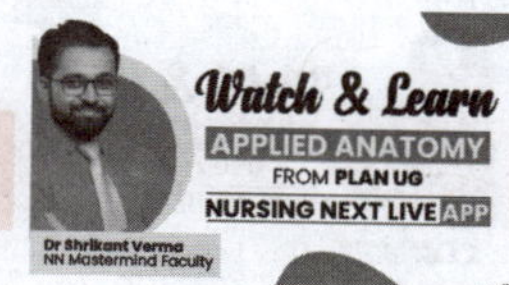

Left Atrium

- Upper left part of the heart.
- Forms the left two-thirds of the base of heart
- Quadrangular in shape.
- It receives oxygenated blood from the lungs through the pulmonary veins.
- It pumps the blood to the left ventricle through the left atrioventricular or bicuspid orifice.
- The appendage of the left atrium, the left auricle projects anteriorly to overlap the infundibulum of the right ventricle.

Interior of the Left Ventricle

- The interior of the left ventricle shows two orifices:
  1. Left atrioventricular or bicuspid or mitral orifice – which is guarded by the mitral valve
  2. The aortic orifice — which is guarded by the aortic valve.

Valves of Heart

- Two types of valves:
  1. Pair of atrioventricular valves
  2. Pair of semilunar valves
- Right atrioventricular valve
  - Tricuspid valve as it has three cusps – anterior, posterior and septal.
- Left atrioventricular valve
  - Bicuspid valve — as it has two cusps – large anterior cusp and small posterior one
  - Also known as mitral valve.
  - Attached to the chordae tendineae.
- Aortic valves
  - Has one anterior and two posterior – right and left cusps.
- Pulmonary valves
  - Has three semilunar cusps — one posterior and two anterior.

4. Write a short note on the right atrium. (MGR)

Answer

Right Atrium

- Heart has four chambers – two atria and two ventricles.
- Right atrium is the upper right chamber of heart and receives venous blood from all parts of the body.
- It forms the right and upper border of the heart, sternocostal surface and base of the heart.
- It is the first to receive the deoxygenated blood from the body through the superior and inferior venae cavae.
- It plays an important role in originating and regulating the coordination of the heart.

Gross Anatomy

- It is ellipsoid in shape except the right atrial appendage that arises anteriorly. It overlies the aortic root and proximal right coronary artery.
- It receives the deoxygenated blood from:
  - Superior vena cava
  - Inferior vena cava
  - Coronary sinus
  - Thebesian veins
- It is separated from the left atrium by the interatrial septum and from the right ventricle by the tricuspid valves.
- Right atrium has the following boundaries:
  - **Superiorly:** Orifice of superior vena cava
  - **Inferiorly:** Orifice of inferior vena cava
  - **Posteriorly:** Interatrial septum
  - **Anteriorly and right lateral wall:** Cardiac wall
  - **Left laterally:** Right atrioventricular ostium
- It is related to the right ventricle, aortic root and valve on the left lateral surface and to the right lung and pleura, phrenic nerve, pericardiophrenic artery and vein on the right lateral surface. Posteriorly, it is related to the left atrium and the pulmonary veins.

Interior of Right Atrium

Divided into three parts: Anterior part, posterior part and septal wall (also called the central wall of the posterior wall).

Refer Figure 4.12 pg. 64

Blood Supply of Right Atrium

- The heart receives its own supply of blood from the coronary arteries.
- Venous drainage of atrium is into the atrial walls and the Thebesian veins.

Nerve Supply

- SA node (sinoatrial node)
- AV node (atrioventricular node)

5. Write a short note on coronary circulation. (MGR)

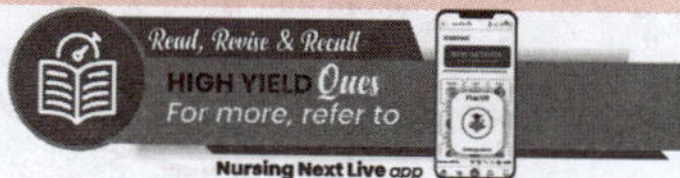

Answer

Coronary Circulation

- Arterial supply
  - The cardiac muscle is supplied by two coronary arteries, i.e., the right and left coronary arteries.

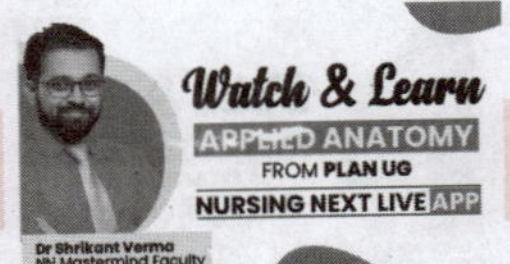

- Both arteries arise from sinuses behind the cusps of aortic valves at the root of aorta.
- Venous drainage of heart
  - Coronary sinus
  - Anterior cardiac veins
  - Great cardiac vein
- Lymphatics of heart
  - Lymphatics of heart accompany the coronary arteries and form two trunks.
  - Right trunk ends in brachiocephalic nodes and left trunk into tracheobronchial lymph nodes.

Peculiar Features of Coronary Circulation

- Normal coronary blood flow of both arteries is 60–80 mL/100 g/min
- The oxygen consumed by the myocardium is high during coronary blood flow; for instance, resting VO_2 is 250 mL/min and left ventricle VO_2 is 8–10 mL/100 g/min
- With each cardiac cycle, there is fluctuation in coronary blood flow, 80% of coronary blood flow occurs in the left ventricle during diastole and 20% during systole.

Phasic Changes in Coronary Circulation

- Variations in coronary blood flow occur due to variation in blood flow to an organ that is determined by either pressure head or extravascular pressure.
- Coronary blood flow during systole is less than that during diastole.
- During isovolumetric contraction phase, there is minimal blood flow due to compression of coronary blood vessels with low aortic pressure.
- During diastole, coronary blood flow is more.
- During isovolumetric relaxation phase, there is maximal blood flow due to dilated blood vessels with high aortic pressure.

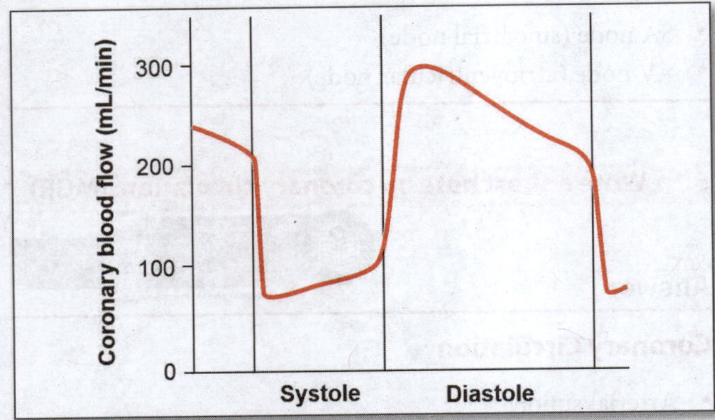

Figure 4.14: Coronary blood flow-phasic variations during systole and diastole

Ascending Aorta

- Arises from the upper end of the left ventricle.
- It provides major supply to the heart musculature through its branches – left and right coronary arteries.

Left coronary artery: The left coronary artery is an artery that arises from the aorta above the left cusp of the aortic valve and feeds blood to the left side of the heart.

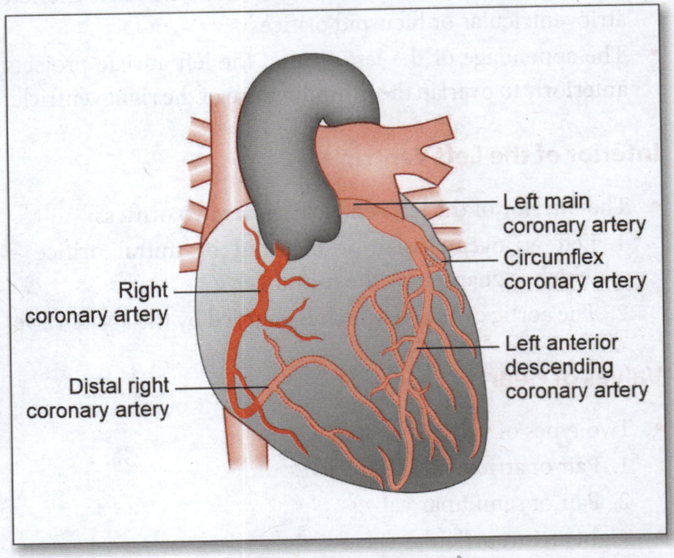

Figure 4.15: Coronary artery

Right Coronary Artery

The right coronary artery is an artery that arises from the anterior aortic sinus of the ascending aorta and feeds blood to the right side of the heart.

6. Write a short note on the arch of aorta. (MGR)

Answer

Arch of Aorta

- The arch of aorta begins at the level of the right 2nd costal cartilage and runs upward, backward, and to the left, in front of the bifurcation of the trachea.
- The arch of aorta arches over the root of the left lung.
- It begins and ends at the same level, i.e., at sternal angle.
- It begins anteriorly and ends posteriorly.

Posterior and to the Right

- Trachea
- Esophagus
- Left recurrent laryngeal nerve
- Thoracic duct
- Vertebral column

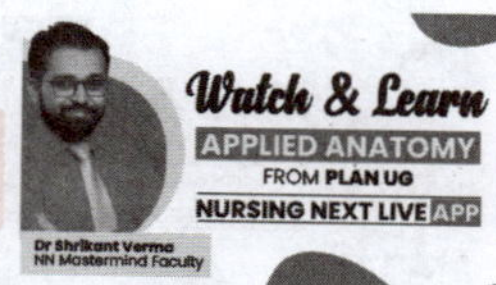

Anterior and to the Left

- Left lung and pleura
- Left phrenic nerve
- Left vagus nerve

Inferior

- Left bronchus
- Bifurcation of pulmonary trunk
- Ligamentum arteriosum
- Left recurrent laryngeal nerve
- Superficial cardiac plexus

Superior

- Brachiocephalic trunk
- Left common carotid artery
- Left subclavian artery
- Left brachiocephalic vein
- Thymus

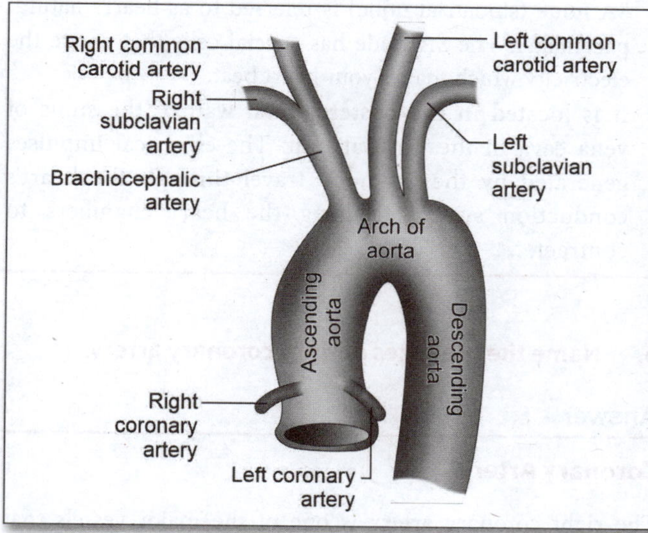

Figure 4.16: Aorta

Branches

- Brachiocephalic (innominate) artery.
- Left common carotid artery.
- Left subclavian artery.
- Occasionally, a fourth branch referred to as thyroidea ima artery may originate from the arch of aorta.

Clinical Significance

- Aortic knuckle in X-ray chest (PA view), the shadow of the arch of aorta appears as a small bulb-like projection in the upper end of the left margin of the cardiac shadow termed the aortic knuckle. The aortic knuckle is visible in old age because of undue folding of the arch caused by atherosclerosis.
- **Coarctation of aorta:** It is congenital narrowing of the aorta just proximal or distal to the entrance of the ductus arteriosus.

7. Write a short note on the blood supply of heart.

Answer

For answer, refer to Long Question no. 2, pg. no. 61

8. Write a short note on the nerve supply of the heart.

Answer

Nerve Supply of the Heart

- The nerve supply to the heart is responsible for its functioning.
- The heart receives its nervous innervation by the sympathetic and the parasympathetic fibers of the autonomic nervous system.
- These form the cardiac plexus, which receives contributions from the sympathetic trunk and the vagus nerve.
- The fibrous and parietal pericardia are supplied by the phrenic nerves. They are sensitive to pain. The epicardium is supplied by autonomic nerves of the heart and is not sensitive to pain.
- Pain of pericarditis originates in the parietal pericardium alone. On the other hand, cardiac pain or angina pectoris originates in the cardiac muscle or in the vessels of the heart.

Influence of Autonomic Nerves

- The vagal nerves supply the SA node, AV node and atrial muscle.
- Parasympathetic stimulation
  - Efferent fibers
    - Derive from the vagus nerve.
    - Decrease the heart rate by influencing the heart rate.
    - Decrease the conduction velocity of impulse through AV node.
    - Decrease the force of contraction of atrial muscle fibers.
    - Cause vasoconstriction of the coronary arteries.
  - Afferent fibers
    - Derived from the vagal cardiac nerves.
    - Regulate the blood pressure.

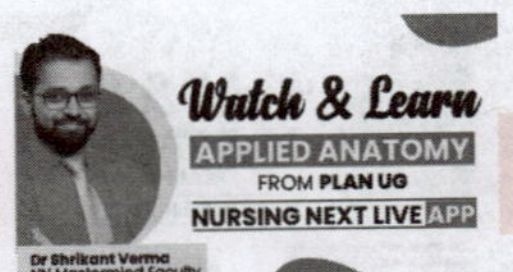

- Sympathetic stimulation
  - Efferent fibers
    - Derived from the lower cervical and upper thoracic ganglia
    - Increase the heart rate by influencing the activity of SA node
    - Increase the speed of impulse
    - Increase the force of contraction of the myocardium
    - Fight-or-flight response
  - Afferent fibers
    - Afferent to the upper thoracic and lower cervical ganglia
    - Regulate blood pressure
    - Regulate pain sensation

Nursing Implications

- **Cardiac plexus injury**
  - Vagus nerve injury results in tachycardia.
  - Injury to the sympathetic fibers causes bradycardia.

SHORT ANSWER QUESTIONS

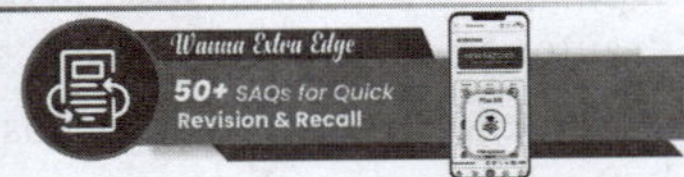

1. Median cubital vein — position and clinical importance. (MGR)

Answer

The median cubital vein is a vein located in the antecubital fossa (bend of the elbow) of the arm. It is a common site for collecting blood samples for laboratory tests, administering medications, fluids or blood products.

2. Name the branches of arch of aorta. (MGR)

Answer

The arch of aorta begins at the level of the right 2nd costal cartilage and runs upward, backward, and to the left, in front of the bifurcation of the trachea.

Branches

- Brachiocephalic (innominate) artery.
- Left common carotid artery.
- Left subclavian artery.
- Occasionally, a fourth branch referred to as thyroidea ima artery may originate from the arch of aorta.

3. Varicose veins.

Answer

Varicose Veins

- Common, abnormal, dilated superficial blood vessels caused by weakening in the vessel wall.
- Appearance — swollen, twisted clusters of blue or purple veins.
- Most commonly occur on the legs and pelvic areas.
- More prevalent in females than males.

4. Define pacemaker of heart.

Answer

- SA node (sinoatrial node) is referred to as heart's natural pacemaker. The SA node has special cells that create the electricity which makes your heart beat.
- It is located in the posterolateral wall of the sinus of vena cava in the right atrium. The electrical impulses generated by the SA node travel through the heart's conduction system, causing the heart chambers to contract.

5. Name the branches of right coronary artery.

Answer

Coronary Artery

The right coronary artery is one of the major vessels that provides blood to the heart.

Branches

- Right conus artery
- Anterior ventricular branches: 2–3 numbers
- Marginal branch
- Posterior ventricular branches, which give a branch to atrioventricular artery
- Posterior interventricular artery
- Atrial branches and artery of the sinoatrial node which also supply atria.

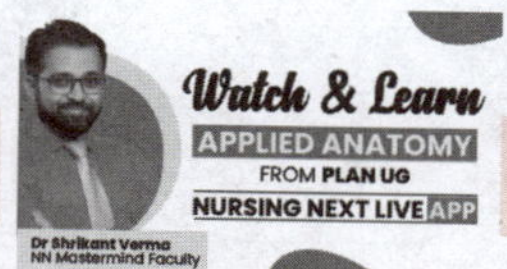

CONCEPTUAL REVISION

MULTIPLE CHOICE QUESTIONS

1. What describes the SA node's ability to discharge an electrical impulse spontaneously?

a. Excitability
b. Contractility
c. Conductivity
d. Automaticity

Ans. d. Automaticity

2. Which of the following arteries primarily feeds the anterior wall of the heart?

a. Left anterior descending artery
b. Circumflex artery
c. Right coronary artery
d. Internal mammary artery

Ans. a. Left anterior descending artery

3. Right coronary artery supplies all of the following parts of conducting system in the heart; EXCEPT:

a. SA node
b. AV node
c. AV bundle
d. Right bundle branch

Ans. d. Right bundle branch

4. Blood from the heart flows through the blood vessels in which order?

a. Veins, arterioles, capillaries, venules, arteries
b. Capillaries, arterioles, arteries, venules, veins
c. Arteries, arterioles, capillaries, venules, veins
d. Arteries, capillaries, arterioles, venules, veins

Ans. c. Arteries, arterioles, capillaries, venules, veins

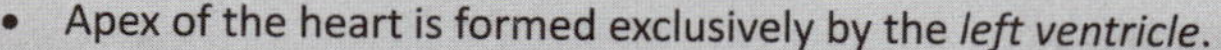

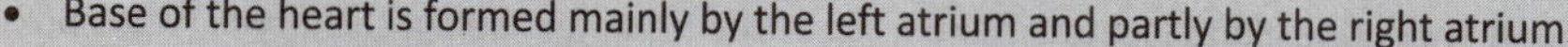

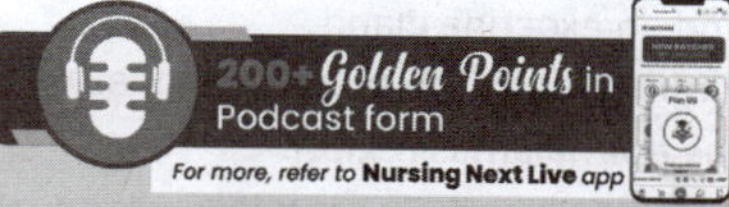

Golden Points

- Apex of the heart is formed exclusively by the *left ventricle*.
- Base of the heart is formed mainly by the left atrium and partly by the right atrium.
- Coronary arteries are blood vessels that supply oxygenated blood to the heart muscle (myocardium). They branch off from the aorta, the main artery that carries oxygenated blood from the heart to the rest of the body.
- Heart is enveloped by pericardium.
- Lymphatic tissue is a part of the lymphatic system, which is a network of vessels, nodes, and organs involved in the body's immune response and fluid balance.
- Right atrium receives the entire systemic blood.

CHAPTER

5

Endocrine System

CONCEPTUAL THEORY

Terminology

Hypothalamus: Hypothalamus is a part of diencephalon. It is present below the thalamus and extends downward from the brain into a stalk known as the pituitary stalk (or infundibular stalk), which connects it to the pituitary gland.

Pancreas: The pancreas is an elongated, flattened gland located in the upper abdomen, behind the stomach. It is both an endocrine gland and an exocrine gland.

Pineal gland: The pineal gland, also known as the pineal body or epiphysis, is a small endocrine gland located deep within the brain, in the epithalamus region.

Pituitary gland: The pituitary gland, also known as the hypophysis, is a small, pea-sized gland located at the base of the brain within a bony cavity called the sella turcica. It is often referred to as the "master gland".

Thyroid gland: The thyroid gland is a butterfly-shaped endocrine gland located in the front of the neck, just below the larynx (voice box).

INTRODUCTION

The endocrine system is a system of glands that produce hormones.

Hormones are chemical messengers that travel through the bloodstream and control many of the body's functions.

The endocrine system is made-up of the following glands:

- Hypothalamus
- Pineal gland
- Pituitary gland
- Thyroid gland
- Parathyroid glands
- Adrenal glands
- Pancreas (mixed endocrine and exocrine gland)
- Ovaries
- Testes

HYPOTHALAMUS

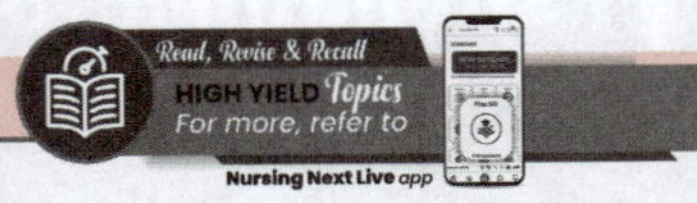

- Hypothalamus is a part of diencephalon. It is present below the thalamus and extends downward from the brain into a stalk known as the pituitary stalk (or infundibular stalk), which connects it to the pituitary gland.
- It forms floor and lower part of lateral wall of third ventricle.
- It is also known as "head ganglion" of the autonomic nervous system and it weighs about 4 grams.

Table 5.1: Regions and nuclei

Region	Nuclei
Preoptic region	**Preoptic nucleus**
Anterior or supraoptic region	Supraoptic nucleus Anterior nucleus Paraventricular nucleus
Middle or tuberal region	Arcuate nucleus Ventromedial nucleus Dorsomedial nucleus Lateral nucleus
Posterior or mammillary region	Posterior nucleus Mammillary nucleus

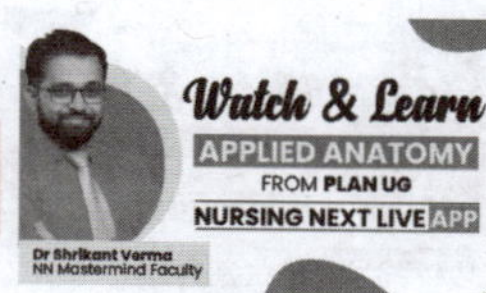

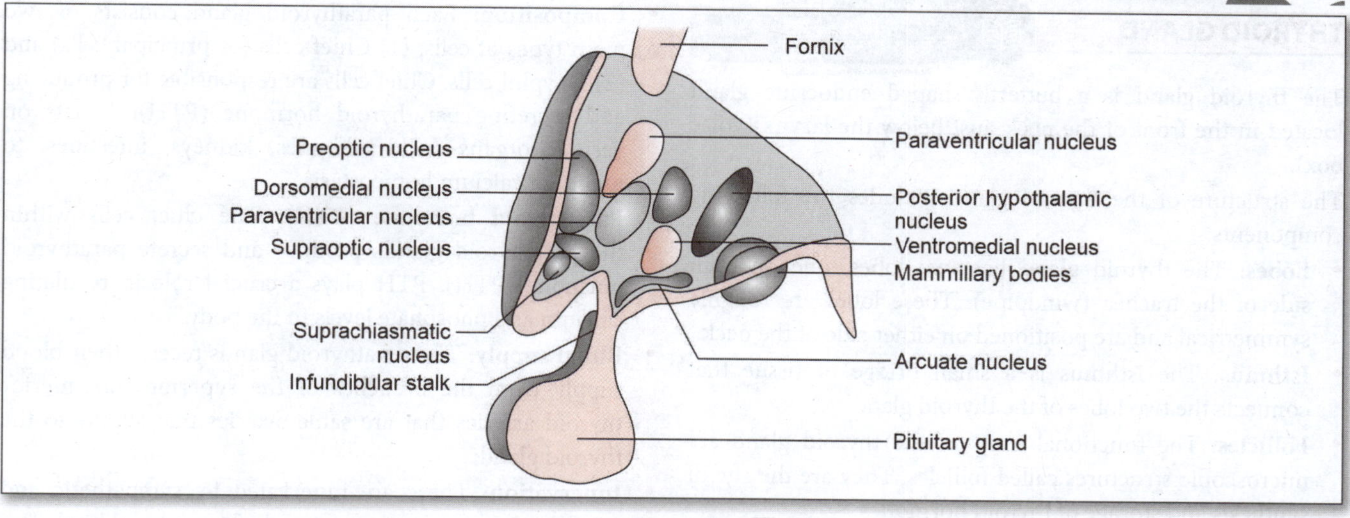

Figure 5.1: Hypothalamus gland

PINEAL GLAND

- The pineal gland, also known as the pineal body or epiphysis, is a small endocrine gland located deep within the brain, in the epithalamus region.
- It is shaped like a pine cone, hence its name.
- The pineal gland plays a crucial role in the regulation of various biological rhythms and the production of the hormone melatonin.
- The pineal gland is responsive to light and darkness.
- The pineal gland receives input from the visual pathways and the suprachiasmatic nucleus (SCN) of the hypothalamus.

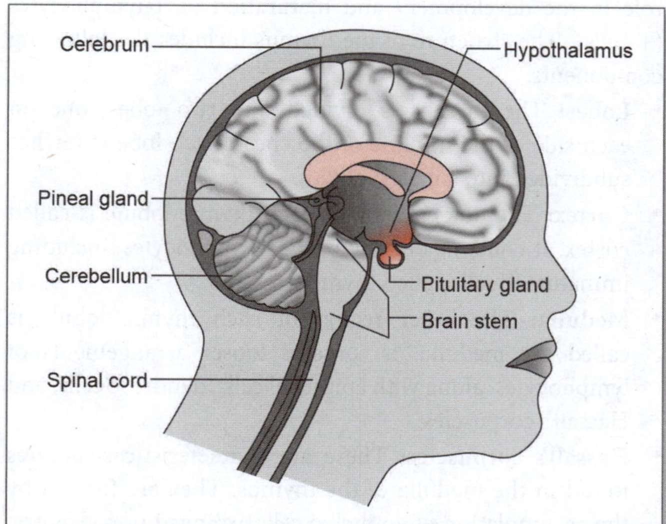

Figure 5.2: Pineal gland

PITUITARY GLAND

The pituitary gland, also known as the hypophysis, is a small, pea-sized gland located at the base of the brain within a bony cavity called the sella turcica. It is often referred to as the "master gland" because it plays a crucial role in regulating and controlling various hormonal functions in the body.

The pituitary gland is divided into two main parts:

1. **Anterior Pituitary (Adenohypophysis):**
   - The anterior pituitary comprises about 75% of the total weight of the pituitary gland. It is composed of glandular tissue and is connected to the hypothalamus by a network of blood vessels known as the hypothalamic-hypophyseal portal system.
   - It secretes several important hormones, including growth hormone (GH), adrenocorticotropic hormone (ACTH), thyroid-stimulating hormone (TSH), follicle-stimulating hormone (FSH), luteinizing hormone (LH), prolactin and melanocyte-stimulating hormone (MSH).
2. **Posterior Pituitary (Neurohypophysis):**
   - The posterior pituitary makes up the remaining 25% of the pituitary gland and consists of neural tissue.
   - Posterior pituitary does not produce hormones but it acts as a storage and releases site for two hormones synthesized by the hypothalamus: (i) Antidiuretic hormone (ADH) or Vasopressin and (ii) Oxytocin.

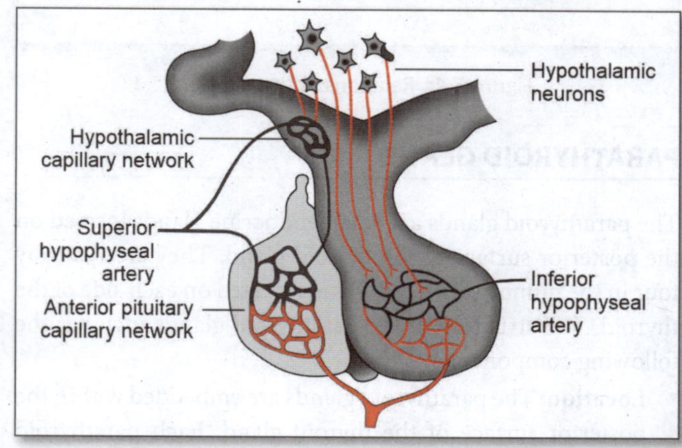

Figure 5.3: Pituitary gland

THYROID GLAND

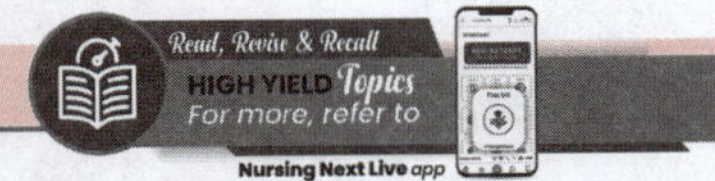

The thyroid gland is a butterfly-shaped endocrine gland located in the front of the neck, just below the larynx (voice box).

The structure of the thyroid gland includes the following components:

- **Lobes:** The thyroid gland has two lobes, one on each side of the trachea (windpipe). These lobes are roughly symmetrical and are positioned on either side of the neck.
- **Isthmus:** The isthmus is a small bridge of tissue that connects the two lobes of the thyroid gland.
- **Follicles:** The functional units of the thyroid gland are microscopic structures called follicles. They are the site of synthesis and storage of thyroid hormones.
- **Blood supply:** The thyroid gland is highly vascularized, receiving a rich blood supply from the superior and inferior thyroid arteries.
- **Nerve supply:** The thyroid gland is innervated by branches of the autonomic nervous system, including sympathetic and parasympathetic fibers.

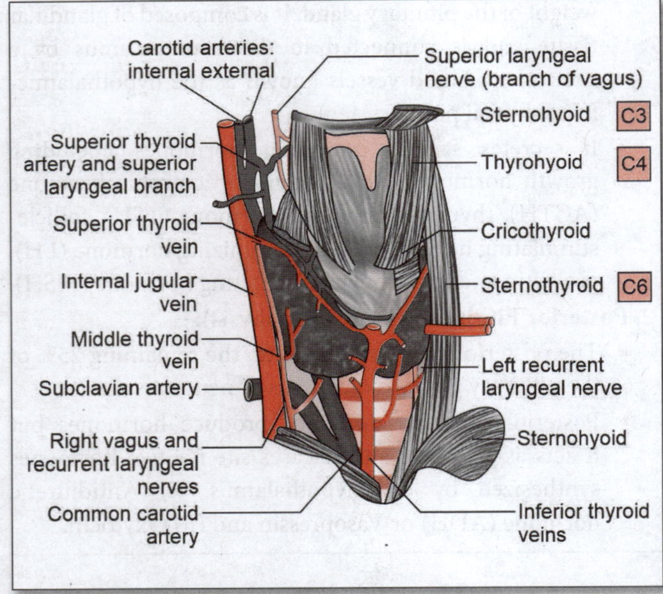

Figure 5.4: Relations of thyroid gland

PARATHYROID GLAND

The parathyroid glands are small endocrine glands located on the posterior surface of the thyroid gland. They are typically four in the number, with two glands located on each side of the thyroid. The structure of the parathyroid glands includes the following components:

- **Location:** The parathyroid glands are embedded within the posterior surface of the thyroid gland. Each parathyroid gland is about the size of grain rice.
- **Composition:** Each parathyroid gland consists of two main types of cells: (1) Chief cells (or principal cells) and (2) Oxyphil cells. Chief cells are responsible for producing and secreting parathyroid hormone (PTH). It acts on various organs such as bones, kidneys, intestines, to maintain calcium homeostasis.
- **Parathyroid hormone (PTH):** The chief cells within the parathyroid glands produce and secrete parathyroid hormone (PTH). PTH plays a crucial role in regulating calcium and phosphate levels in the body.
- **Blood supply:** The parathyroid glands receive their blood supply from the branches of the superior and inferior thyroid arteries that are same arteries that supply to the thyroid gland.
- **Innervation:** These are innervated by sympathetic and parasympathetic nerve fibers, which regulate blood flow and glandular activity.

It is important to note that the parathyroid glands are separate from the thyroid gland although they are located in close proximity. While the thyroid gland produces hormones involved in metabolism, the parathyroid glands play a crucial role in regulating calcium and phosphate levels in the body through the secretion of parathyroid hormone.

THYMUS GLAND

Thymus is a specialized lymphoid organ located in the upper chest, behind the sternum and in front of the heart. It is an essential part of the immune system and plays a crucial role in the development and maturation of T-lymphocytes (T-cells). The structure of the thymus includes the following components:

- **Lobes:** The thymus is divided into two lobes, one on each side of the midline of the chest. Each lobe is further subdivided into smaller lobules.
- **Cortex:** The outer region of each thymic lobule is called cortex. It contains densely packed lymphocytes, including immature T cells called thymocytes.
- **Medulla:** The inner region of each thymic lobule is called the medulla. It contains looser arrangements of lymphocytes, along with epithelial cells, dendritic cells, and Hassall's corpuscles.
- **Hassall's corpuscles:** These are characteristic structures found in the medulla of the thymus. They are formed by the accumulation of epithelial cells arranged in concentric layers.
- **Epithelial cells:** The thymus contains two types of epithelial cells: (1) Cortical epithelial cells (found in the cortex) and (2) Medullary epithelial cells (found in the medulla). These epithelial cells play a vital role in the development and selection of T cells, providing them with necessary signals for maturation and tolerance induction.

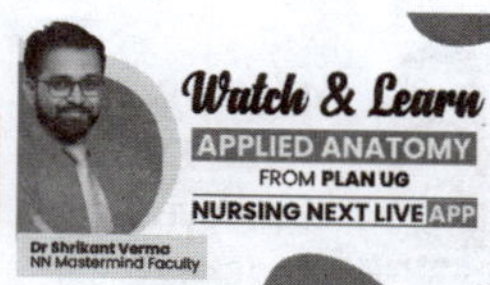

- **Blood supply:** The thymus receives its blood supply from branches of the internal thoracic arteries. Veins carry the blood away from the thymus, eventually draining into the brachiocephalic veins.
- **Lymphatic drainage:** The thymus has its own network of lymphatic vessels that allow the transport of lymphatic fluid containing immune cells.

PANCREAS

The pancreas is an elongated, flattened gland located in the upper abdomen, behind the stomach. It is both an endocrine gland and an exocrine gland, meaning it has functions related to hormone secretion and digestive enzyme production. The structure of the pancreas includes the following components:

- **Head:** The head of the pancreas is the widest part and is situated on the right side of the abdomen. It lies within the curve of the duodenum (the first part of the small intestine).
- **Body:** The body of the pancreas is the middle portion, extending horizontally across the abdomen behind the stomach.

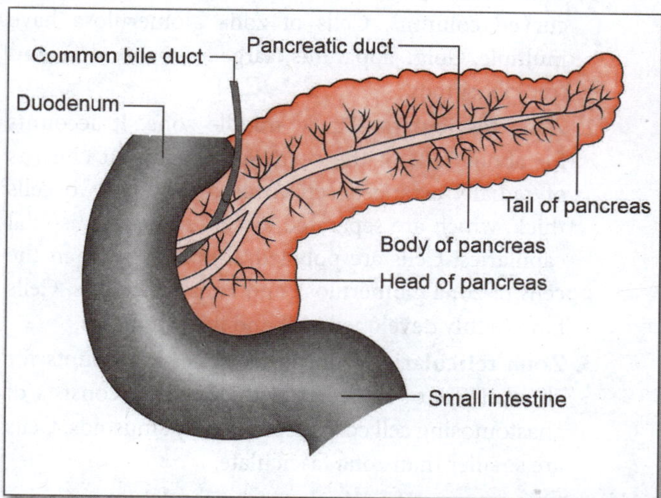

Figure 5.5: Pancreas

- **Tail:** The tail of the pancreas is the narrowest part and extends toward the left side of the abdomen, adjacent to the spleen.
- **Ducts:** The pancreas has two main ducts that traverse its length. The larger duct, called the pancreatic duct, runs through the center of the pancreas and carries pancreatic juice, a mixture of digestive enzymes, into the duodenum. The smaller duct, called the accessory pancreatic duct, may also exist in some individuals and provides an additional route for pancreatic juice to enter the duodenum.
- **Islets of Langerhans:** Scattered throughout the pancreas, particularly in the body and tail regions, are clusters of specialized endocrine cells called the islets of Langerhans. These islets contain several types of hormone-secreting cells, including alpha cells that produce glucagon, beta cells that produce insulin, delta cells that produce somatostatin, and others.
- **Acinar cells:** The majority of the pancreas is composed of exocrine cells called acinar cells. These cells produce and secrete digestive enzymes into the pancreatic ducts. The enzymes include amylase (for carbohydrate digestion), lipase (for fat digestion), and various proteases (for protein digestion).
- **Blood supply:** The pancreas receives its blood supply from branches of the celiac trunk, which is a major branch of the abdominal aorta. Blood flows through a network of arteries and veins within the pancreas, providing oxygen and nutrients while carrying away waste products.
- **Nerve supply:** The pancreas is innervated by sympathetic and parasympathetic nerve fibers, which regulate its functions. Nerves from the autonomic nervous system control the secretion of pancreatic enzymes and the release of hormones.

ADRENAL GLAND

- Adrenal gland is also known as suprarenal gland. It is two in number and situated on the upper pole of each kidney.
- Each gland is about 4 cm long and 2–3 cm in width.
- The gland weighs about 3.5–5 g.
- The gland is roughly triangular or semilunar flattened gland at the cranial pole of each kidney.
- Each gland consists of outer yellow cortex and inner dark brown medulla surrounded by outer cortex.

Cortex

The cortex has three zones:

1. **Zona glomerulosa:** The outermost zone and the cells of this zone secrete mineralocorticoids – the most important being aldosterone. Aldosterone is responsible for increased reabsorption of sodium from distal convoluted tubules of kidney.
2. **Zona fasciculata:** It is the middle thick layer or zone and responsible for secretion of glucocorticoids the cortisol and cortisone. The secretion of glucocorticoids is stimulated by ACTH secreted from anterior pituitary.
3. **Zona reticularis:** Moderately thick inner layer continuous with medulla and secretes small amount of androgens (male sex hormones).

Medulla

- The adrenal medulla is under the direct control of hypothalamus.
- Medulla consists of chromaffin cells and these cells produce adrenaline and noradrenaline to help fright, flight or fight reactions.
- Adrenaline consists of approximately 80% of total secretion of the gland.

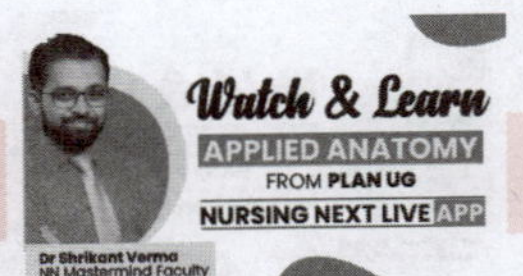

Blood Supply

- The gland is supplied by superior, middle and inferior suprarenal arteries.
- The venous drainage is by suprarenal veins.

CONCEPTUAL EXERCISES

LONG ANSWER QUESTIONS

1. Name the important endocrine glands of the body. Give a brief description of suprarenal glands. (RUHS)

Answer

Endocrine Glands

Endocrine glands and certain organs secrete hormones/secretions into the bloodstream to travel to the distant targets and exert their effect.

Important Endocrine Glands

- Pituitary gland
- Thyroid gland
- Parathyroid gland
- Adrenal glands/Suprarenal glands
- Pancreas
- Gonads
- Pineal gland

Suprarenal/Adrenal Glands

- The adrenal glands (also known as suprarenal glands) are endocrine glands that produce a variety of hormones including adrenaline and the steroids aldosterone and cortisol.

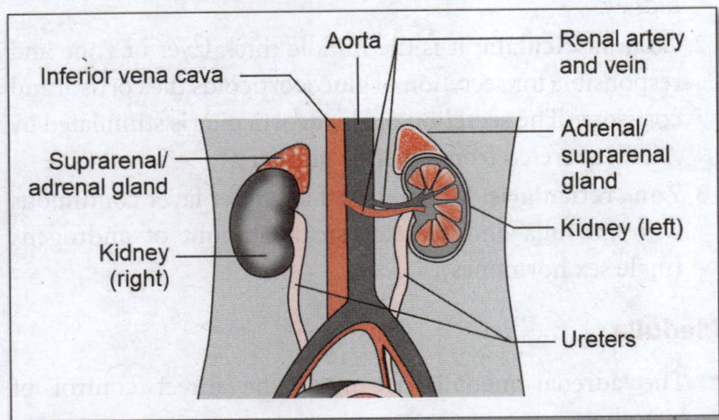

Figure 5.6: Suprarenal glands

- They are present above the kidneys.
- Each gland has an outer cortex which produces steroid hormones and an inner medulla.

Microscopic Anatomy

- The adrenal gland is enclosed in a connective tissue capsule that extends septae into the substance of the gland.
- It is richly vascularized; and capsular blood vessels, nerves and lymphatics penetrate along with the connective tissue septae.
- The adrenal is divided into cortex and medulla.
  - Three concentric zones can be distinguished in the cortex:
    1. **Zona glomerulosa:** Thin, outermost zone. It accounts for about 15% of the cortical thickness. Cells are organized into small rounded groups or curved columns. Cells of zona glomerulosa have multiple Golgi apparatus, large mitochondria and free ribosomes.
    2. **Zona fasciculata:** Thick, middle zone. It accounts for about 75% of the cortical thickness. It consists of radially arranged cell cords of one or two cells thick, which are separated by fenestrated sinusoidal capillaries. Cells are polyhedral and larger than the cells of zona glomerulosa and zona reticularis. Cells have highly developed SER and mitochondria.
    3. **Zona reticularis:** Thin, inner zone. It accounts for about 5–7% of the cortical thickness. It consists of anastomosing cell cords separated by sinusoids. Cells are smaller than zona fasciculate.
- Histologic examination reveals a rich vasculature.

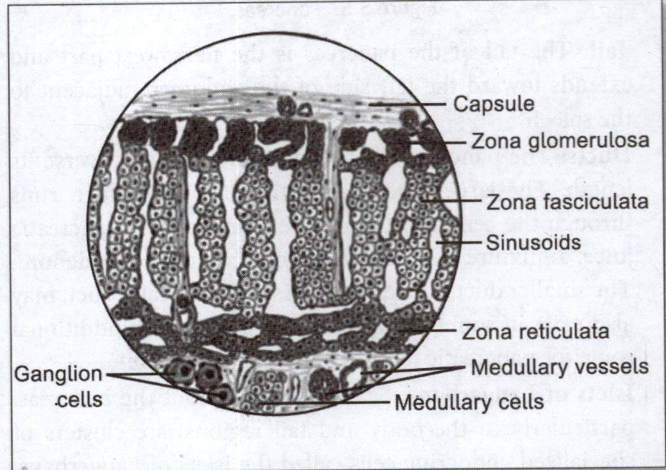

Figure 5.7: Histology of suprarenal gland

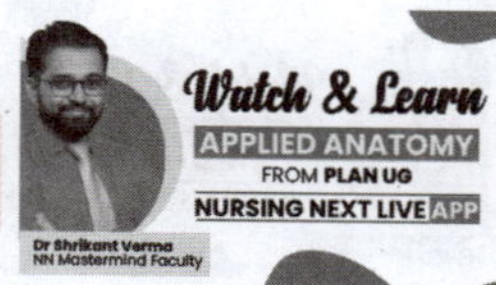

Functions

The medulla consists of chromaffin cells which produce adrenaline and noradrenaline. The noradrenaline is the chemical transmitter of the sympathetic nervous system. Its major function is regulation of the blood pressure by way of vasoconstriction.

Other functions of adrenaline and noradrenaline are:

- Cutaneous vasoconstriction
- Increasing the heart rate and force of contraction
- Conversion of glycogen to glucose.
- Dilation of pupils
- Dilatation of bronchi and bronchioles.

Hormones produced by the adrenal cortex are:

- **Glucocorticoids**
  - Secreted by the zona glomerulosa (outer zone)
  - Include cortisol, corticosterone and cortisone.
  - Their secretion is under the control of ACTH
  - Functions include:
    - Regulation of carbohydrate metabolism
    - Sodium and water reabsorption from renal tubules
    - Storage of glycogen
    - Maintenance of blood glucose levels
    - Role in stress
- **Mineralocorticoids**
  - Secreted by the middle zone – zona fasciculata
  - Aldosterone – main mineralocorticoid
  - Functions include:
    - Stimulate the reabsorption of water and sodium
    - Promote the excretion of potassium by the kidneys
    - Role in renin-angiotensin system
- **Androgens**
  - Secreted by zona reticularis
  - Effects include:
    - Deposition of proteins in muscles
    - Retention of nitrogen

Applied Anatomy

- **Cushing syndrome**
  Pathologies of the suprarenal gland originate from either the cortex or the medulla. Pituitary adenomas can result in a hypersecretion of ACTH. Excess ACTH will overstimulate the adrenal cortex resulting in hypercortisolism or Cushing syndrome. The disease is more prevalent in women in the young adult age group. Immunosuppression, muscular atrophy, weight gain and hyperglycemia are some of the clinical manifestations of the disease. Both medical and surgical options can be implemented to correct this disorder.
- **Pheochromocytoma**
  Pheochromocytoma (PCC) is the primary neoplasm of the adrenal medulla. These tumors are rare and may cause life-threatening hypertension. The neoplasms can also affect extra-adrenal chromaffin tissue. The lesion results in a hyperproduction of catecholamines, which eventually result in an overactive sympathetic response.

2. Enumerate the endocrine glands. Briefly indicate their location and secretion.

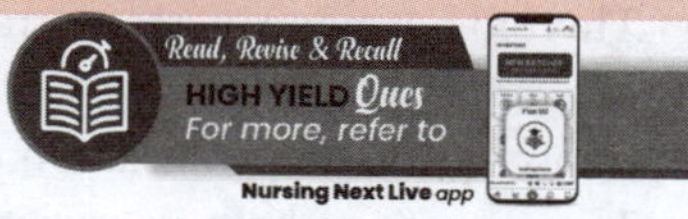

Answer

Important Endocrine Glands

- Pituitary gland
- Thyroid gland
- Parathyroid gland
- Adrenal glands/Suprarenal glands
- Pancreas
- Gonads
- Pineal gland

Pituitary Gland

- Pituitary gland—small ovoid structure attached to the base of brain.
- Lies in the hypophyseal fossa located on the superior surface of the body of sphenoid bone.
- Also known as hypophysis cerebri
- Divided into three parts:
  1. Anterior pituitary
  2. Posterior pituitary
  3. Pars media

1. **Anterior pituitary**
   - Constitutes major part of the pituitary
   - Linked to the hypothalamus by the hypothalamohypophyseal portal vessels.
   - Various hormones secreted by the anterior pituitary are:
     - **Growth hormone:**
       - Important for growth and development in the body.
     - **Thyroid-stimulating hormone:**
       - Stimulation and regulation of thyroid gland activity.
       - Secretion of T3 and T4 hormones.
     - **Adrenocorticotropic hormone (ACTH)**
       - Regulates the secretion of steroid hormones
     - **Prolactin**
       - Stimulates lactation
     - **Gonadotropins**

2. **Posterior pituitary**
   - Constitutes about 20% of the pituitary gland.
   - Consists of nervous tissues and blood vessels.
   - Linked with neural hypothalamohypophyseal tract
   - Secretes oxytoxin and ADH

Thyroid Gland

- Highly vascular gland situated infront of larynx and trachea at the level of 5th, 6th and 7th cervical and 1st thoracic vertebra.
- Thyroid hormone increases transcription of a large number of genes by binding on nuclear receptors. Thus, initiation of transcription and translation of large number of proteins. These proteins help in growth and development of CNS along with various systems in body and metabolism.

Parathyroid Gland

- The parathyroid glands consist of four small glands that are located behind the thyroids in the neck.
- It secretes parathormone. Its secretion is regulated by low plasma Ca^{2+} concentration
- Primarily involved in increasing plasma Ca^{2+} levels.
- Action of PTH on bone
  - Increased osteoclastic activity, leading to demineralization of bones
- Action on kidney and intestine:
  - PTH increases the synthesis of calcitriol, thus decreasing the excretion and increasing the absorption of calcium and phosphorus.

Adrenal Glands

- The adrenal glands (also known as suprarenal glands) are endocrine glands that produce a variety of hormones including adrenaline and the steroids aldosterone and cortisol.
- They are present above the kidneys.
- Each gland has an outer cortex which produces steroid hormones and an inner medulla.
- **Hormones produced by the adrenal cortex are:**
  - Glucocorticoids
    - Secreted by the zona glomerulosa (outer zone)
    - Include cortisol, corticosterone and cortisone.
    - Functions include:
      - Regulation of carbohydrate metabolism
      - Sodium and water reabsorption from renal tubules
  - Mineralocorticoids
    - Secreted by the middle zone—zona fasciculata
    - Aldosterone—main mineralocorticoid
    - Function include:
      - Stimulate reabsorption of the water and sodium
        - Role in renin-angiotensin system
- Androgens
  - Secreted by zona reticularis
  - Effects include:
    - Deposition of proteins in muscles
    - Retention of nitrogen

Pancreas

- Gland presents across the upper part of posterior abdominal wall from right to left side.
- Pancreas is a mixed gland, both exocrine and endocrine; it lies transversally across the posterior abdominal wall.
- It is 'J' shaped and secretes the digestive pancreatic juice, and the endocrine part secretes hormones, e.g., insulin.
- Contains both exocrine secretion for digestion of carbohydrates, fats and proteins; and endocrine secretion from islets of Langerhans, which act in the carbohydrate metabolism.

Gonads

- Some glands are specific to males or females. For instance, the ovaries are specific to females and are located in the pelvic cavity. While the testes are specific to males. Ovaries produce estrogen that is important for reproduction and female sex characteristics. Testes produce testosterone that is responsible for male sex characteristics. Also, they result in increased muscle mass and body hair.
- The ovaries and testes are found in females and males, respectfully and are responsible for creating the sex hormones. These hormones regulate the entire reproductive process and enable procreation to occur.

Pineal Gland

- Pineal gland is composed of two types of cells, pinealocytes and neuroglial cells, with a rich network of blood vessels and sympathetic fibers. It was regarded as a vestigial organ for long. It produces hormones that have an important regulatory influence on other endocrine glands.
- Hormones secreted by pineal gland are:
  - Melatonin
    - Causes changes in skin color
    - Synthesis and discharge are influenced by exposure to light. The secretion increases with increase in darkness.
    - It aids in coordination of circadian and diurnal rhythms of many tissue
    - It affects the mood of the person.

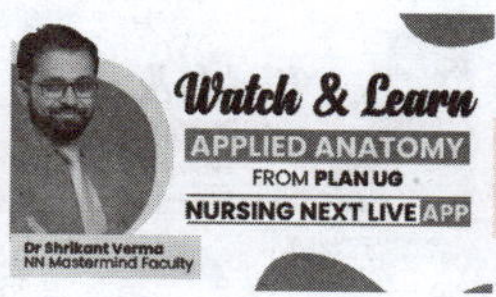

- It inhibits the growth and development of sex organs for puberty.

Hypothalamus

- Hypothalamus is a part of diencephalon, lies in the floor and lateral wall of the third ventricle. Hypothalamus controls pituitary gland with releasing and inhibiting hormones. It serves as a major integrating link between nervous and endocrine systems.
- Endocrinal function: Secretion of releasing and inhibitory hormones like:
  - Gonadotropin-releasing hormone (GnRH)
  - Prolactin-releasing hormone (PRH)
  - Growth hormone-releasing hormone (GHRH)
  - Thyrotropin-releasing hormone (TRH)
  - Corticotropin-releasing hormone (CRH)
  - Prolactin-inhibiting hormone (PIH)
  - Growth hormone-inhibiting hormone (somatostatin)

3. Name the endocrine glands present in our body and describe in detail the thyroid gland. (MGR)

Answer

Important Endocrine Glands

- Pituitary gland
- Thyroid gland
- Parathyroid gland
- Adrenal glands/Suprarenal glands
- Pancreas
- Gonads
- Pineal gland

Thyroid Gland

Introduction

Highly vascular gland situated in front of the larynx and trachea at the level of 5th, 6th and 7th cervical and 1st thoracic vertebra.

Anatomy of Gland

- Weight of gland—25 g
- Butterfly in shape, consists of two lobes, one on either side of the thyroid cartilage and upper cartilaginous rings of the trachea.
- The lobes are joined by a narrow isthmus, lying in front of the trachea.
- The lobes are roughly cone-shaped and are about 5 cm long and 3 cm wide.

Location

- The thyroid gland is located in the anterior neck, situated between the C5 and T1 vertebrae.
- It is an endocrine gland, divided into two lobes which are connected by an isthmus.
- It is located behind the sternohyoid and sternothyroid muscles, wrapping around the cricoid cartilage and superior tracheal rings.
- It lies inferior to the thyroid cartilage of the larynx. The gland is in the visceral compartment of the neck, along with the trachea, esophagus and pharynx. The compartment is bound by pretracheal fascia.
- During development, the thyroid gland initially forms in the floor of the primitive pharynx, near the base of the tongue. It then descends down the neck to lie in its adult anatomical position.

Parts

- It consists of three lobes:
  i. Right and left lobes which are joined by the isthmus.
  ii. The third is pyramidal lobe, projects upward from the isthmus.
  iii. A fibrous or fibromuscular band descends from the body of the hyoid bone to the isthmus or pyramidal lobe.

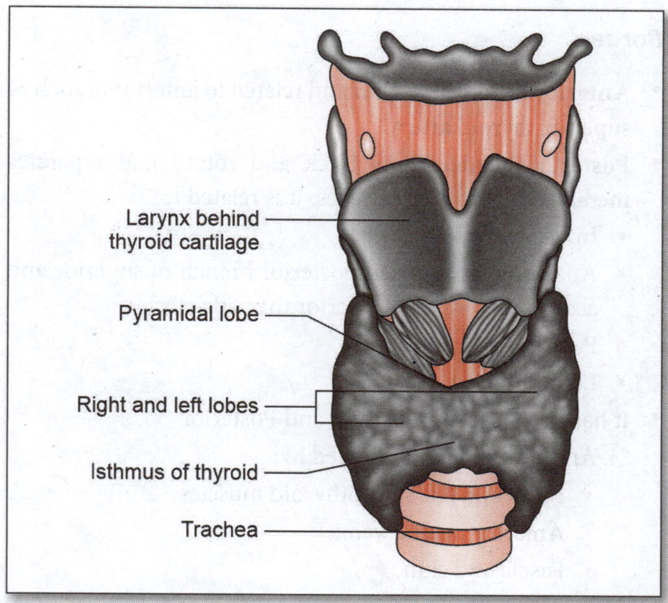

Figure 5.8: Thyroid gland

Coverings

- **Two capsules:**
  1. **True capsule:** It is the peripheral condensation of the connective tissue of the gland.

2. **False capsule:** It is derived from the pretracheal layer of the deep cervical fascia. It is thinner on the posterior border of the lobes, and thick on the inner surface of the gland, where it forms the suspensory ligament which connects the lobe to the cricoid cartilage.

- The lobes are conical in shape and each lobe has:
  - **An apex:** It is directed upward and laterally. It is related to the superior thyroid artery and the external laryngeal nerve.
  - **A base:** It is at level with fourth and fifth tracheal rings. It is related to inferior thyroid artery and recurrent laryngeal nerve.

Three Surfaces

1. **Lateral surface:** It is convex and is covered by:
   - The sternohyoid
   - The superior belly of omohyoid
   - The sternothyroid
   - The anterior border of sternocleidomastoid
2. **Medial surface:** It is related to:
   - Two tubes, trachea, esophagus
   - Two muscles, inferior constrictor, cricothyroid
   - Two nerves, external laryngeal and recurrent laryngeal
3. **Posterior surface:** It is related to carotid sheath and overlaps the common carotid artery.

Borders

- **Anterior border:** It is thin and related to anterior branch of superior thyroid artery.
- **Posterior border:** It is thick and round and separates medial and posterior surfaces. It is related to:
  - Inferior thyroid artery
  - Anastomosis between posterior branch of superior and ascending branch of inferior thyroid arteries
  - Parathyroid glands
  - Left thoracic duct
- It has two surfaces: Anterior and Posterior
  i. Anterior surface is covered by:
    - Right and left sternothyroid muscles
    - Anterior jugular veins
    - Fascia and skin

  ii. Posterior surface is related to two and four tracheal rings.
    - Upper border is related to anterior branches of the right and left superior thyroid arteries which anastomose here.
    - Lower border: Inferior thyroid veins leave the gland here.

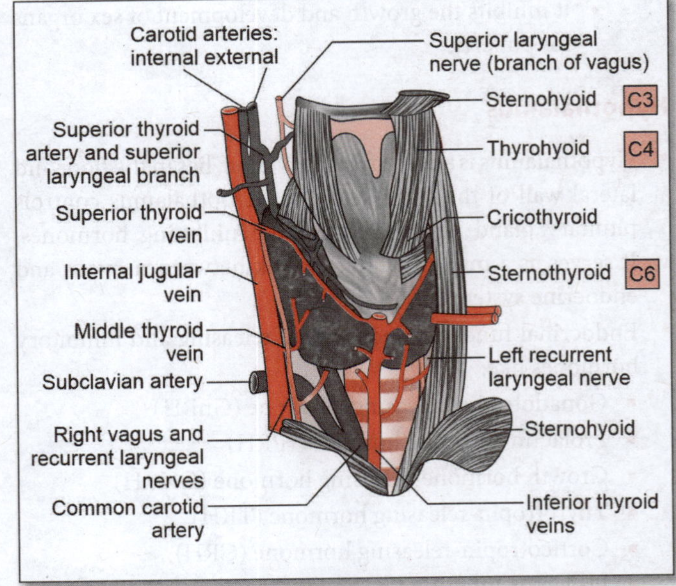

Figure 5.9: Relations of thyroid gland

Blood Supply

- Blood supply to the thyroid gland is achieved by two main arteries: (1) The superior and (2) Inferior thyroid arteries.
- The superior thyroid artery is the first branch of the external carotid artery and supplies the superior and anterior portions of the gland.
- The inferior thyroid artery arises from the thyrocervical trunk. It tends to supply the posteroinferior aspect.
- In a small proportion of people (around 10%), there is an additional artery present: The thyroid ima artery. It comes from the brachiocephalic trunk of the arch of aorta, supplying the anterior surface and isthmus.

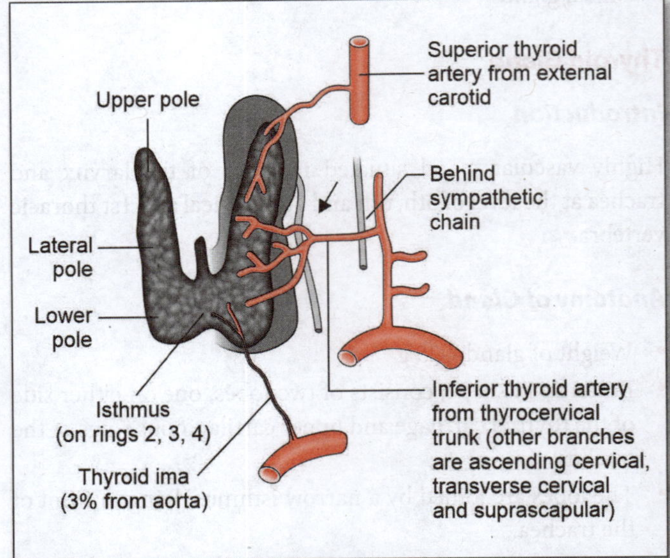

Figure 5.10: Arterial supply of thyroid gland

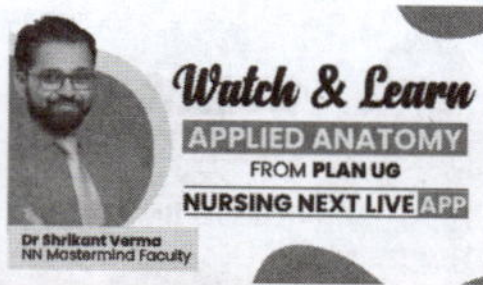

Venous drainage is carried out by the superior, middle and inferior thyroid veins, which form a venous plexus.

Histology

- Thyroid gland is made-up of two types of secretory cells.
  1. **Follicular cells:** Line the follicles of the gland, they secrete triiodothyronine and tetraiodothyronine which stimulates the basal metabolic rate and is responsible for somatic and psychic growth of the individual.
  2. **Parafollicular cells:** Also known as C cells, these are light and few, and lie between the follicles. They secrete thyrocalcitonin which promotes deposition of calcium salts in skeletal and other tissues, and causes hypocalcemia.

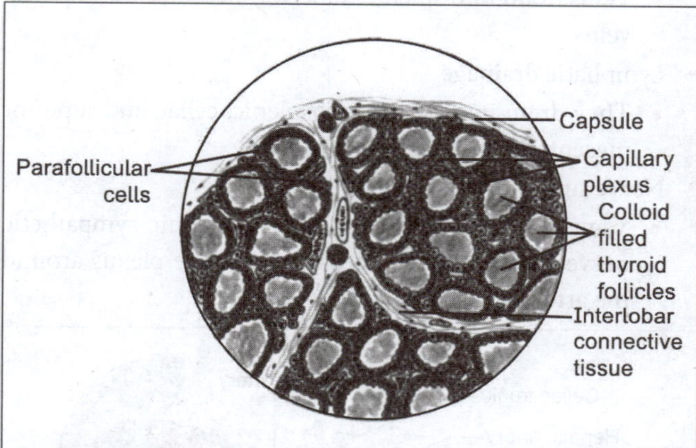

Figure 5.11: Histology of thyroid gland

Applied Anatomy

- Goiter or swelling of thyroid gland is palpated from behind.
- **Hyperthyroidectomy:** Removal of thyroid with true capsule is done in hyperthyroidism.
- Cretinism in infants and myxedema in adults.
- Benign tumors
- **Hashimoto's disease:** An autoimmune thyroid disorder characterized by the production of antibodies in response to thyroid antigens. It is 20 times more common in women than men.

SHORT NOTES

1. Write a short note on the adrenal glands/suprarenal glands. (DU)

Answer

For answer, refer to Long Question no. 1, pg. no. 74

2. Describe pancreas with the help of a diagram. (MGR)

Read, Revise & Recall HIGH YIELD Topics For more, refer to Nursing Next Live app

Answer

Pancreas

- Pancreas is a mixed gland, both exocrine and endocrine; it lies transversally across the posterior abdominal wall.
- It is 'J' shaped and secretes the digestive pancreatic juice, and the endocrine part secretes hormones, e.g., insulin.
- Contains both exocrine secretion for digestion of carbohydrates, fats and proteins; and endocrine secretion from islets of Langerhans, which act in the carbohydrate metabolism.
- Pancreas is 15 cm long consisting of:
  - **Head:** Lies in the C portion of the duodenum. Bile duct runs behind the head of pancreas.
  - **Neck:** Small segment behind which superior mesenteric vein and splenic vein join to form the portal vein.
  - **Body:** Triangular in shape and is related to the splenic artery along the upper border, transverse mesocolon along the anterior border.
  - **Tail:** Part lying anterior to left kidney reaching up to hilum of spleen.

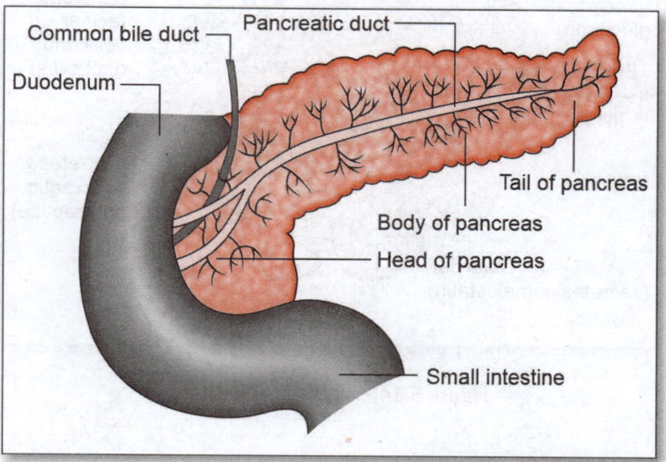

Figure 5.12: Pancreas

Histology

- The exocrine part is a serous gland made of tubular acini lined by pyramidal cells, with basal round nuclei, and contains zymogen granules, it secretes digestive pancreatic juice.
- The endocrine part is made of pancreatic islets of Langerhans.
  - They are most numerous in the tail. B cells are most important, these are granular and basophilic and produce insulin.

- Others are alpha cells, with subtypes A1 and A2. These are granular and acidophilic.
  - A1 cells belong to the enterochromaffin group and secrete pancreatic gastrin and serotonin.
  - A2 cells secrete glucagon.

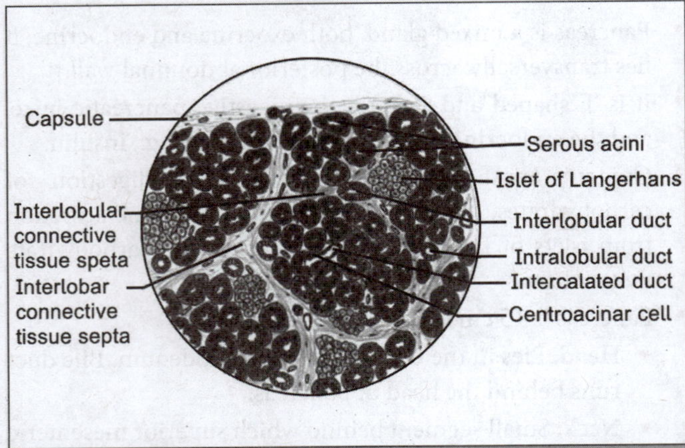

Figure 5.13: Microanatomy of pancreas

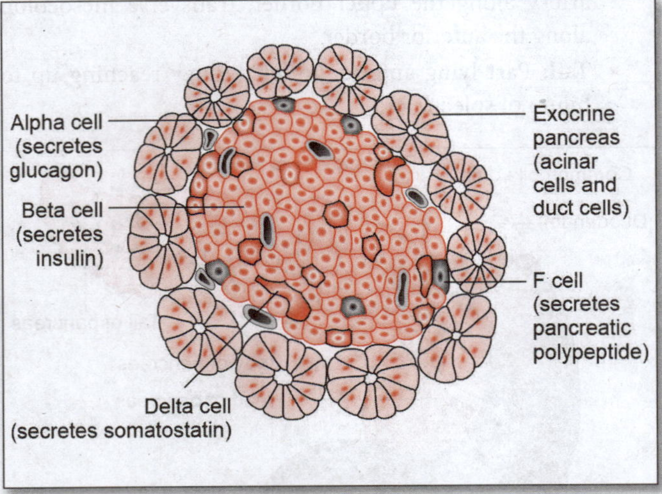

Figure 5.14: Islets of Langerhans

Functions

Pancreas consists of two major types of secretory tissues which reflect its dual function.

1. Exocrine gland
   - Localized in acinar cells
     - Various enzymes such as amylase, lipase and proteases are secreted which aid in the digestion of carbohydrates, lipids and proteins.
     - Presence of acidic chyme from stomach in duodenum stimulates the production of secretin and cholecystokinin hormones from endocrine cells in the wall of duodenum. These hormones in turn stimulate the production of pancreatic juice.
2. Endocrine gland
   - Localized in islets of Langerhans
   - Releases hormones

Blood Supply

- Arterial supply
  - Pancreatic branches of splenic artery
  - Superior pancreaticoduodenal artery
  - Inferior pancreaticoduodenal artery
- Venous drainage
  - Veins drain into splenic, superior mesenteric and portal veins.
- Lymphatic drainage
  - They drain into pancreaticosplenic, celiac and superior mesenteric group of lymph nodes.
- Nerve supply
  - Vagus or parasympathetic and splanchnic sympathetic nerves supply the pancreas through the plexus around the arteries.

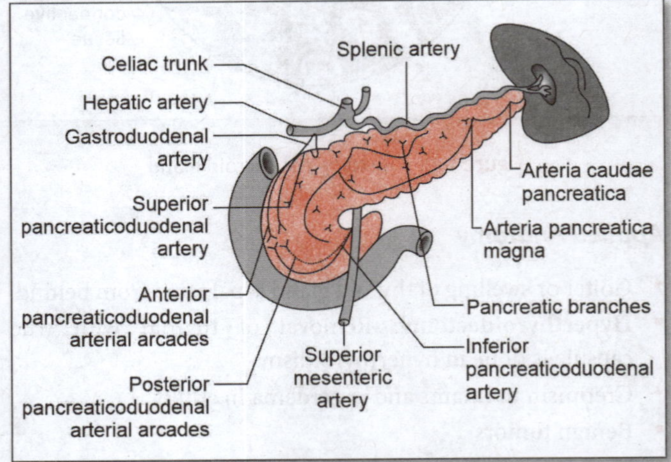

Figure 5.15: Blood supply of pancreas

3. Write a short note on the parts of pituitary gland. (RUHS)

Answer

Anterior Pituitary

- It constitutes a major part of the pituitary.
- Linked to the hypothalamus by the hypothalamohypophyseal portal vessels.

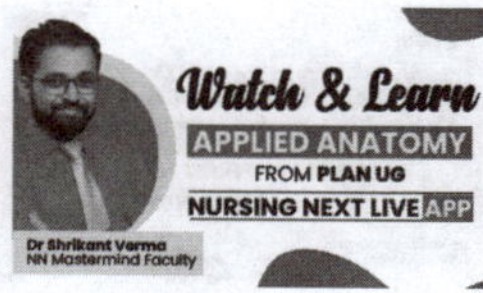

Table 5.2: Hormones secreted by different parts of pituitary gland

Cell type	Releasing hormone	Hormone secreted	Physiological actions
Adenohypophysis			
Acidophil:			
Somatotrope	Somatotropin-releasing hormone	Somatotropin	Stimulates growth of long bones, uptake of amino acids and protein synthesis
Mammatrope	Prolactin-releasing hormone	Prolactin	Stimulates secretion of milk
Basophil:			
Thyrotrope	Thyrotropin-releasing hormone	Thyrotropin	Stimulates thyroid hormone synthesis and its release
Corticotrope	Corticotropin-releasing hormone	Corticotropin	Stimulates release of hormone of adrenal cortex
Gonadotrope	Gonadotropin-releasing hormone	Follicle-stimulating hormone (FSH) and Luteinizing hormone (LH)	Stimulates development of ovarian follicles in females and spermatogenesis in males
Pars intermedia:			
Cells	Melanocyte-stimulating hormone in amphibians and fishes. Pars intermedia is not developed in human	—	Increases pigmentation of skin
Neurohypophysis			
Cells		Vasopressin or antidiuretic hormone	Increases permeability of collecting ducts and reabsorbs water
Cells		Oxytocin	Increases contraction of smooth muscle fibers of uterus during parturition. During suckling also, this hormone causes contraction of myoepithelial cells around secretory acini of mammary gland

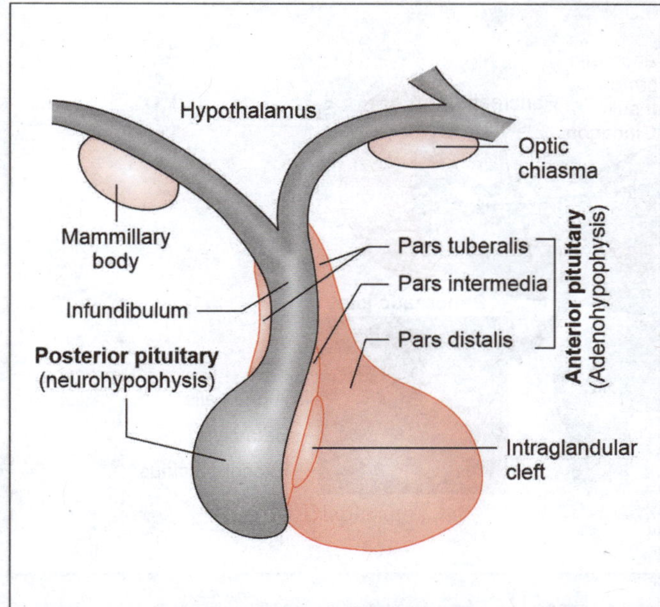

Figure 5.16: Anatomy of pituitary gland

4. Write a short note on pancreas along with applied anatomy. (RUHS)

Answer

Pancreas

For answer, refer to Short Notes Q. 2, pg. no. 79

Applied Anatomy

Pancreas plays a major role in the regulation of blood sugar levels.

- Insulin and glucagon play a significant role in the regulation of blood sugar levels.
- Insulin promotes a decrease in blood glucose.
- Glucagon promotes an increase in blood glucose.
- Glucagon increases blood glucose concentration partly by breaking down glycogen in the liver.
- Excess glucose is kept as glycogen in the liver. Stored glycogen, via glucagon, is converted into glucose by a pathway referred to as glycogenolysis.

- Glucose is also produced in liver via fat (fatty acids) and proteins (amino acids) through the process of gluconeogenesis.
- Both glycogenolysis and gluconeogenesis help in rise of blood glucose levels.
- Thus, glycemia is regulated via a complex interaction between the gastrointestinal tract, the pancreas, and the liver.
- Insulin promotes the entry of glucose into cells of the body and controls the rate of carbohydrate metabolism.
- Glucose can then be used immediately for energy or it will be stored in the form of glycogen or fat.
- **Diabetes mellitus**
  - A chronic disorder in which the body cannot produce its own insulin which is normally produced in the pancreas.
  - Diabetes occurs due to either an absolute (type 1) or a relative (type 2) deficiency of insulin.

5. Write a short note on exocrine pancreas. (RUHS)

Answer

Exocrine Part of Pancreas

- It constitutes a major portion of pancreas—approximately 85%.
- It has the major function of secretion of digestive enzymes, water and bicarbonates.
- It aids in the digestion of food and helps in neutralizing stomach acid.

Structure

- The functional unit of the exocrine pancreas includes the acinus and the ducts.
- These are specialized cells that are involved in the synthesis of enzymes, their storage and secretion.
- The duct system modifies the aqueous secretions. These are under the control of the parasympathetic nervous system and inhibited by the sympathetic system.
- Anatomically, the main pancreatic duct merges with the bile duct, which leads to the **Ampulla of Vater**. It is here that these secretions pour into the duodenum and help neutralize and digest chyme.

Functions of Exocrine Pancreas

- Major role in digestion
- Enzymes secreted are proteases, pancreatic lipases, amylase, ribonucleases and other enzymes such as gelatinase and elastase.
- Bicarbonate secretion
  - For neutralization of stomach acid
  - Activation of proenzymes

The functional unit of the exocrine pancreas includes the acinus and its duct system.

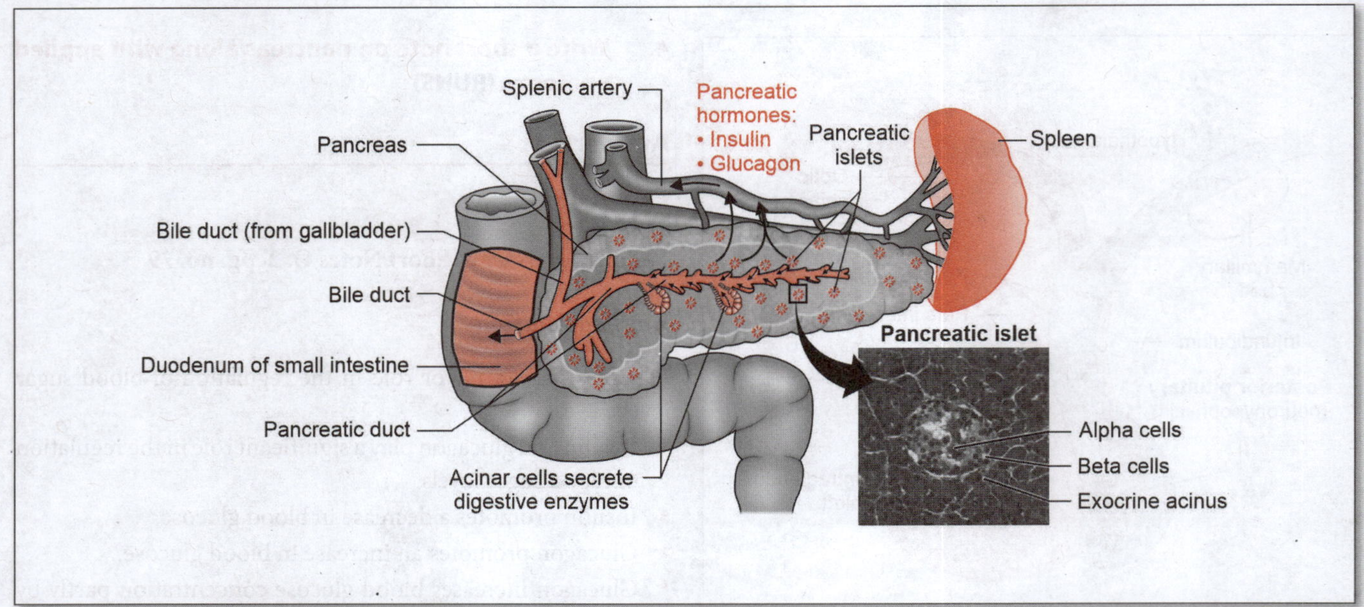

Figure 5.17: Anatomical structure of pancreas

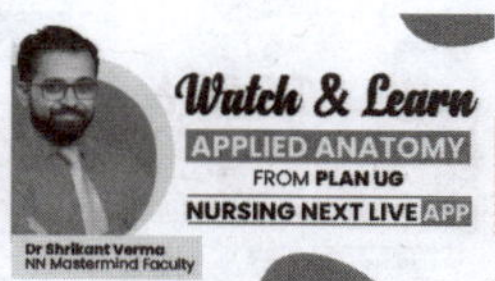

6. Write a short note on thymus gland. (DU)

Answer

Introduction

- The thymus is a specialized primary lymphoid organ of the immune system.
- The thymus is an encapsulated primary lymphoid organ.

Location

Present between the thyroid gland (superiorly) and fourth costal cartilage (inferiorly) within the superior mediastinum and anterior part of inferior mediastinum.

Structure

- Thymus gland consists of two lobes interconnected by an isthmus.
- Encapsulated structure

Blood Supply

- Internal thoracic artery
- Thyroid arteries (superior, inferior)

Venous Drainage

- Left innominate vein
- Superior inferior thyroid veins
- Middle thyroid veins
- Inferior thyroid veins

Nerve Supply

- Vagus nerve
- Sympathetic trunk

Lymphatics

Lymph drains to the thymic lymph nodes, i.e., internal mammary-parasternal, hilar and mediastinal lymph nodes.

Functions

- Hematopoietic precursor cells mature T cells via positive and negative selection.
- A process known as positive selection that checks developing T cell is able to differentiate self from foreign cells.
- Negative selection—T cells undergo the process of interaction with the thymic dendritic cells. Those cells with high level of autoreactivity are eliminated to reduce the likelihood of autoimmune reactions.
- T cells are further differentiated into T helper cells and T killer cells.

SHORT ANSWER QUESTIONS

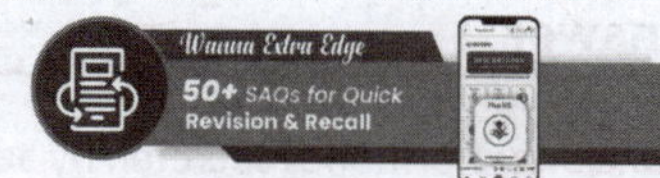

1. Name the endocrine glands. (MGR)

Answer

- Pituitary gland
- Thyroid gland
- Parathyroid gland
- Adrenal glands
- Pancreas
- Pineal gland
- Thymus gland
- Ovaries (in females)
- Testes (in males)

2. Enumerate parts of pituitary gland. (MGR)

Answer

Parts of pituitary gland are as follows:

Anterior Pituitary

- Constitutes major part of the pituitary.
- Linked to the hypothalamus by the hypothalamohypophyseal portal vessels.

Posterior Pituitary

- Constitutes about 20% of the pituitary gland.
- ADH and oxytocin are synthesized in hypothalamus and transported by the neural tracts to posterior pituitary and are released from there.

3. What are the effects of mineralocorticoids? (MGR)

Answer

Mineralocorticoids

- Aldosterone is the main mineralocorticoid. It maintains the electrolyte balance in the body.
- Effects/Functions
  - It maintains the electrolyte balance in the body.
  - Stimulates the reabsorption of sodium by the renal tubules. Increased amount of sodium reabsorption results in increased potassium excretion
  - Role in renin-angiotensin system

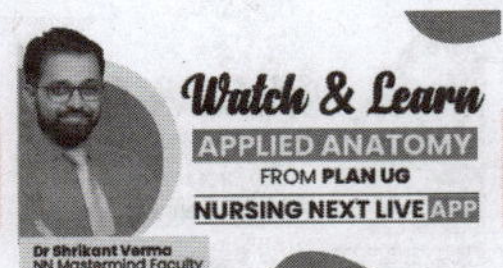

4. Enumerate hormones secreted by adenohypophysis. (MGR)

Answer

Table 5.3: Hormones secreted by adenohypophysis

Cell type	Releasing hormone	Hormone secreted
Acidophils:		
Somatotrope	Somatotropin-releasing hormone	Somatotropin
Mammatrope	Prolactin-releasing hormone	Prolactin
Basophil:		
Thyrotrope	Thyrotropin-releasing hormone	Thyrotropin
Corticotrope	Corticotropin-releasing hormone	Corticotropin
Gonadotrope	Gonadotropin-releasing hormone	Follicle-stimulating hormone (FSH) and Luteinizing hormone (LH)

5. Define tetany. (MGR)

Answer

Tetany is a condition characterized by muscle spasms and cramps. It is caused by a decrease in the blood levels of calcium, which is essential for muscle function. Tetany may be caused by hypoparathyroidism.

CONCEPTUAL REVISION

MULTIPLE CHOICE QUESTIONS

1. **Endocrine gland that is situated in the brain is:**
   a. Pituitary gland b. Hypothalamus
   c. Adrenal gland d. Thyroid gland

Ans. a. Pituitary gland

2. **Which one of the following is not a part of the endocrine system?**
   a. Islets of Langerhans (pancreatic islets)
   b. Thyroid gland
   c. Acini cells of the pancreas
   d. Parathyroid glands

Ans. c. Acini cells of the pancreas

3. **Where is hypothalamus located in the body?**
   a. On the inferior surface of the brain
   b. In the cortex of the adrenal gland
   c. In the anterior pituitary gland
   d. On the dorsal surface of the thyroid gland

Ans. a. On the inferior surface of the brain

4. **What hormone is produced by the parafollicular cells of the thyroid gland?**
   a. Parathyroid hormone
   b. Calcitonin
   c. Thyroid hormone
   d. Thyroxine

Ans. b. Calcitonin

5. **Which endocrine gland secretes cortisol?**
   a. Ovaries b. Thyroid
   c. Adrenal cortex d. Adrenal medulla

Ans. c. Adrenal cortex

6. **Which hormone has the element iodine as part of its molecule?**
   a. Calcitonin b. Hemoglobin
   c. Thyroxine d. Parathyroid hormone

Ans. c. Thyroxine

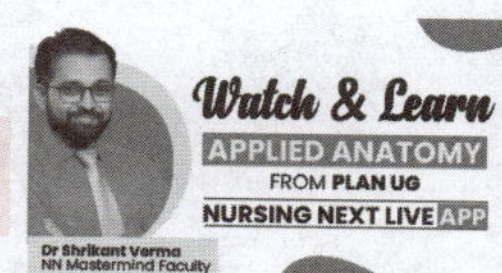

Golden Points

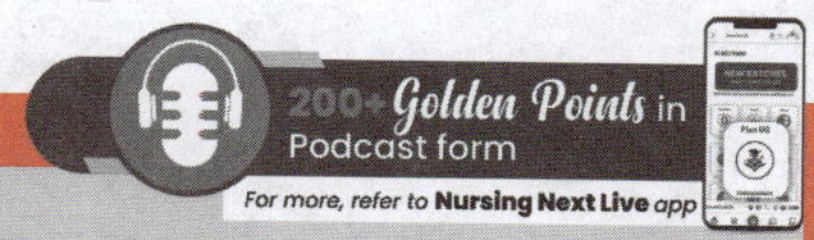

- Adrenal gland is also known as suprarenal gland. It is two in number and situated on the upper pole of each kidney. Each gland consists of outer yellow cortex and inner dark brown medulla surrounded by outer cortex.
- **Anterior pituitary** is the first part of pituitary gland and it constitutes 80% of pituitary gland.
- Hypothalamus is a part of diencephalon. It is present below the thalamus and extends downward from the brain into a stalk known as the pituitary stalk (or infundibular stalk), which connects it to the pituitary gland.
- It is shaped like a pine cone, hence its name.
- **Posterior pituitary** is second part of pituitary gland. It constitutes 20% of pituitary gland.
- The cortex of suprarenal gland shows three zones, outermost—*zona glomerulosa*, a thick middle layer—*zona fasciculata*, and moderately thick inner layer - zona *reticularis* which is continuous with the medulla.
- The endocrine glands are devoid of ducts and the secretions are poured directly into the blood. through the capillaries and numerous sinusoids draining and irrigating the gland.
- The endocrine glands have rich blood supply.
- The Intermediate lobe of pituitary gland produces melanocyte—stimulating hormone to synthesize melanin.
- The lumen of the follicles contains colloid and its main constituents are *thyroglobulin* and *iodothyroglobulin*.
- The pancreas is an elongated, flattened gland located in the upper abdomen, behind the stomach. It is both an endocrine gland and an exocrine gland.

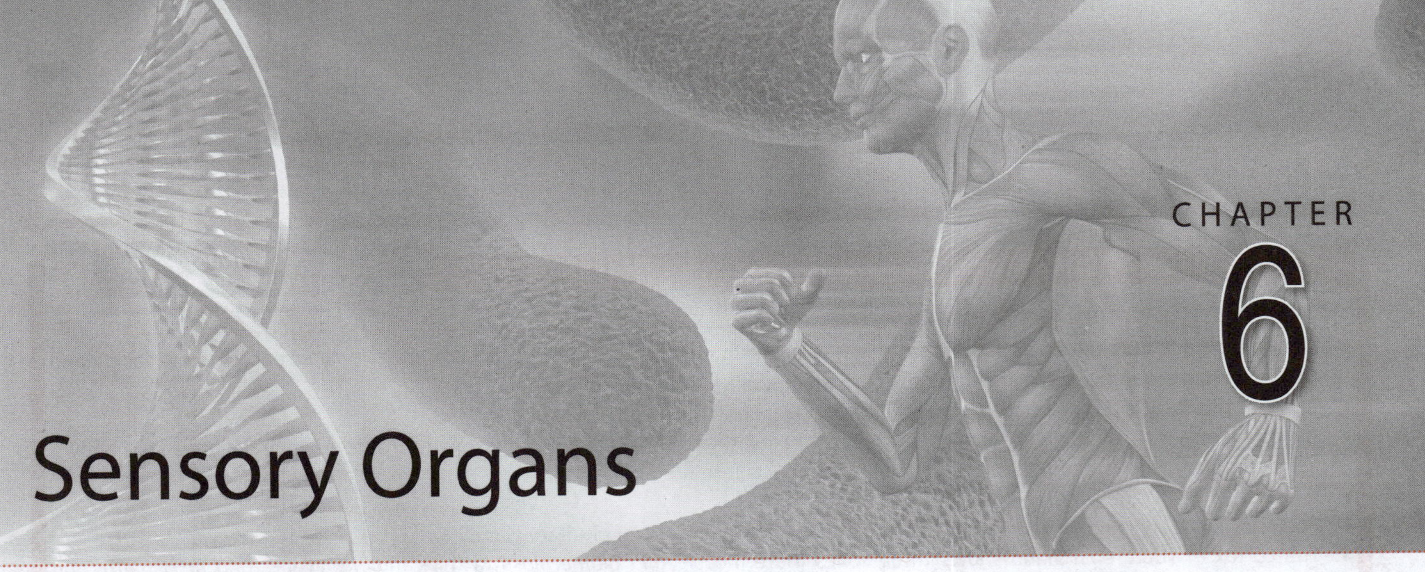

CHAPTER 6

Sensory Organs

CONCEPTUAL THEORY

Terminology

150+ key terminologies for Quick Recall & Revision

Appendages of skin: They are sweat glands, sebaceous gland, hair follicle arrector pilorum muscle and nails
Area of taste: Area of taste is in the lowest part of postcentral gyrus.
Basic tastes: Sweet, sour, salt, bitter and umami.
Blind spot: Lies at the optic disk of retina. There are no rods/cones at this spot.
Bones of internal ear bony ossicles: Malleus, incus and smallest is stapes.
Center for sight: Lies on occipital lobe of the cerebrum, above and below calcarine sulcus.
Center of hearing: Lies in the posterior part of superior temporal gyrus.
Extraocular muscles: Part of levator palpebrae superioris (LPS), superior rectus, medial rectus, inferior rectus, inferior oblique and intraocular muscles, e.g., ciliaris muscles and sphincter pupillae muscle.
Layers of dermis: These are outer reticular layer and inner papillary layer.
Layers of epidermis: These are stratum basale, stratum spinosum, stratum granulosum, stratum lucidum and stratum corneum.
Olfactory epithelium: Comprises supporting cells and olfactory receptor cells.
Parts of ear: External, middle and internal ears.
Sebaceous glands: They are holocrine glands present in the angle between hair follicle and the arrector pilorum muscle.
Sense of olfaction: Limited to 5–7 mm area on the uppermost part of lateral walls and both sides of septum of nose.
Special senses: Senses of taste, smell, sight, hearing, balance and touch are the special senses.

INTRODUCTION

Sensory organs are specialized cells or tissues that detect stimuli from the environment and transmit them to the brain. There are five main types of sensory organs:

1. Skin
2. Eyes
3. Ears
4. Nose
5. Tongue

SKIN

- The skin is the largest organ of the human body which serves as a protective barrier between the internal organs and the external environment.
- It consists of three primary layers and various specialized structures.
- The structure of the skin includes the following components:

Epidermis

- The epidermis is the outermost layer of the skin and is primarily composed of epithelial cells.
- It acts as a waterproof barrier and protects the underlying layers from environmental damage.
- The epidermis contains several sublayers, including:
  - **Stratum corneum:** The outermost layer of the epidermis is composed of dead skin cells (keratinocytes) that are constantly shed and replaced.
  - **Stratum granulosum:** A layer of flattened cells that produce a protein called keratin, which provides strength and waterproofing to the skin.
  - **Stratum spinosum:** A layer of living cells that help support the epidermis and provide strength and elasticity.
  - **Stratum basale (also known as the basal cell layer):** The innermost layer of the epidermis that contains actively dividing cells called basal cells. These cells

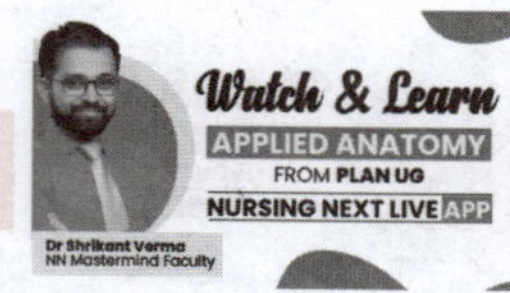

produce new keratinocytes and melanocytes (pigment-producing cells).

Dermis

- The dermis is the middle layer of the skin, located beneath the epidermis.
- It consists of connective tissue, blood vessels, nerves, hair follicles, sweat glands, and sebaceous glands.
- The dermis provides structural support, flexibility, and elasticity to the skin. It is composed of two main layers—the thin layers is called papillary dermis and the thick layer is known as reticular dermis.

Hypodermis (Subcutaneous Tissue)

- The hypodermis is the deepest layer of the skin, located beneath the dermis.
- It consists of adipose (fat) tissue and connective tissue, providing insulation, cushioning, and energy storage.
- The hypodermis also contains blood vessels and nerves.

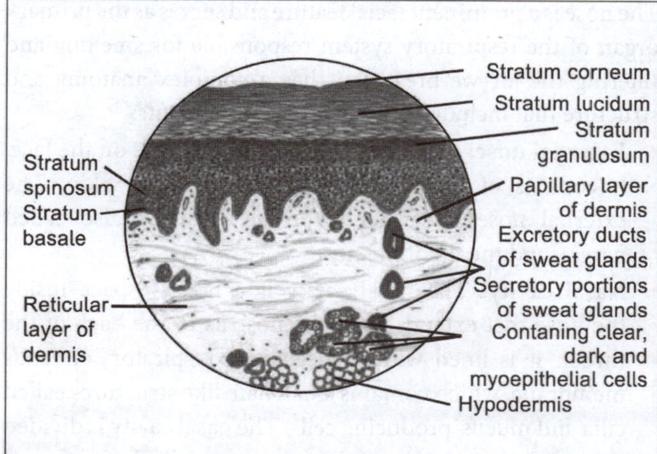

Figure 6.1: Microanatomy of skin

EYE

The eye is a complex sensory organ that allows us to perceive visual information about the world around us. The major anatomical structures of the eye include:

- The sclera is the tough, white, outermost layer of the eye. It provides shape, protection, and structural support for the internal components of the eye.
- The cornea is the transparent, dome-shaped front surface of the eye. It allows light to enter the eye and helps focus incoming light onto the retina.
- The iris is the colored part of the eye located behind the cornea. It controls the size of the pupil, which regulates the amount of light entering the eye. The iris gives the eye its distinctive color.
- The pupil is the dark circular opening in the center of the iris. It adjusts in size based on the amount of light presents in the environment.
- The lens is a clear, flexible structure located behind the iris and the pupil. It helps focus light onto the retina by changing its shape through a process called accommodation.
- The retina is a thin, light-sensitive layer that lines the back of the eye. It contains specialized photoreceptor cells called rods and cones, which convert light into electrical signals.
- The macula is a small, specialized area in the central part of the retina. It is responsible for central vision and contains a high density of cone cells, which are essential for color vision and detailed visual acuity.
- The optic nerve is a bundle of nerve fibers that carry visual information from the retina to the brain.
- The vitreous humor is a gel-like substance that fills the central cavity of the eye, known as the vitreous chamber. It helps maintain the shape of the eye and support the internal structures.
- The aqueous humor is a clear fluid that fills the front part of the eye, between the cornea and the lens. It nourishes and provides oxygen to the cornea and the lens, while also helping maintain the eye's shape.
- The ciliary body is a ring-shaped structure located behind the iris. It contains muscles that control the shape of the lens during accommodation, enabling the eye to focus on objects at different distances.

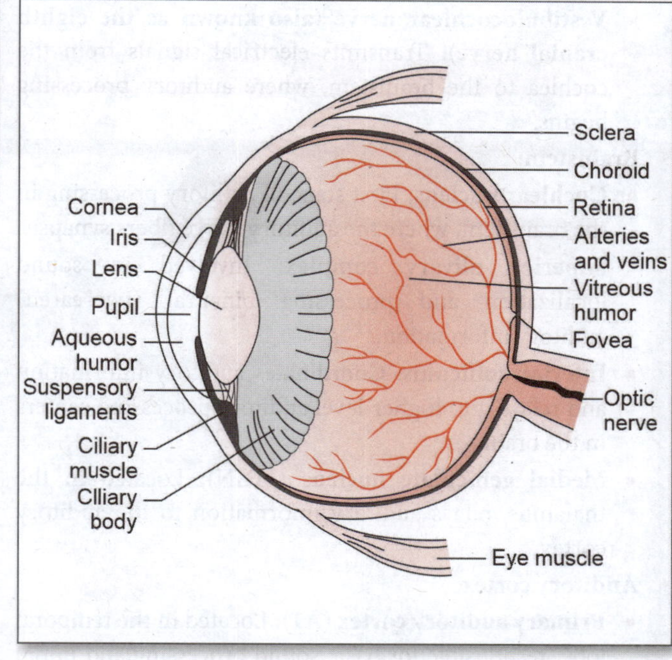

Figure 6.2: Structure of eye

- The eyelids protect the front of the eye and help distribute tears over the surface. The eyelashes help shield the eyes from dust and foreign particles.

- The lacrimal glands are located above the outer corner of each eye and produce tears that keep the surface of the eye moist and lubricated.

EAR

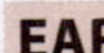

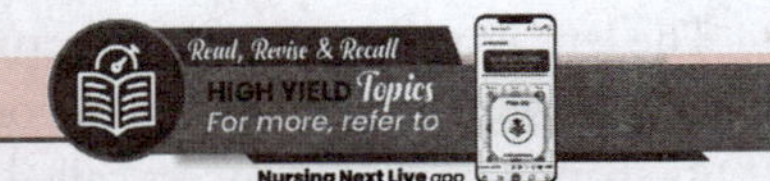

The main divisions of the auditory system and their functions are as follows:

- **Outer ear:**
  - **Pinna (auricle):** Collects sound waves from the environment and funnels them into the ear canal.
  - **Ear canal:** Directs sound waves toward the middle ear.
- **Middle ear:**
  - **Tympanic membrane (eardrum):** Vibrates in response to sound waves and transmits the vibrations to the ossicles.
  - **Ossicles (malleus, incus, and stapes):** Three small bones that amplify and transmit sound vibrations from the eardrum to the inner ear.
- **Inner ear:**
  - **Cochlea:** Spiral-shaped structure responsible for converting sound vibrations into electrical signals that can be interpreted by the brain.
  - **Vestibular system:** Consists of the semicircular canals and otolith organs, which contribute to the sense of balance and spatial orientation.
- **Auditory nerve:**
  - **Vestibulocochlear nerve (also known as the eighth cranial nerve):** Transmits electrical signals from the cochlea to the brainstem, where auditory processing begins.
- **Brainstem:**
  - **Cochlear nucleus:** First stage of auditory processing in the brainstem, where the auditory nerve fibers synapse.
  - **Superior olivary complex:** Involved in sound localization and processing binaural (two-eared) auditory information.
  - **Inferior colliculus:** Coordinates auditory information and relays it to higher-level auditory processing centers in the brain.
  - **Medial geniculate nucleus (MGN):** Located in the thalamus, relays auditory information to the auditory cortex.
- **Auditory cortex:**
  - **Primary auditory cortex (A1):** Located in the temporal lobe, responsible for basic sound processing and initial interpretation of auditory information.
  - **Auditory association areas:** Higher-level regions involved in complex sound analysis, speech perception, and sound recognition.

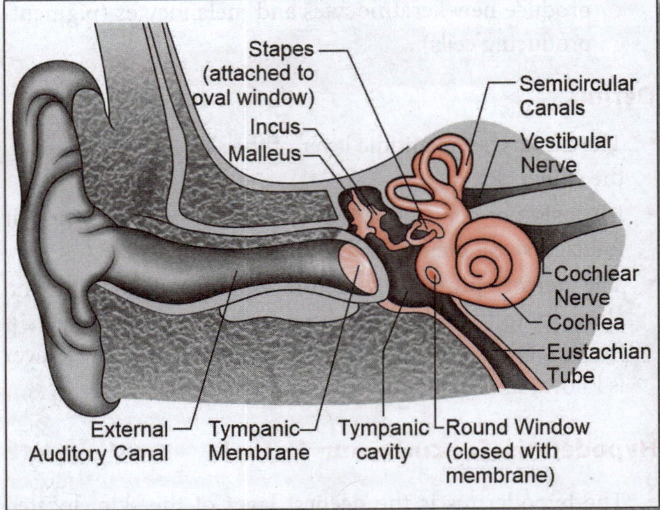

Figure 6.3: Structure of ear

NOSE

The nose is a prominent facial feature and serves as the primary organ of the respiratory system responsible for smelling and filtering the air we breathe. It has a complex anatomy and structure that includes the following components:

- **External nose:** It is the visible part of the nose on the face. It consists of cartilage and bone covered by skin. The external nose includes the bridge, nostrils (also called nares), and the tip of the nose.
- **Nasal cavity:** The nasal cavity is a hollow space inside the nose that extends from the nostrils to the back of the throat. It is lined with a specialized respiratory mucous membrane, which contains small hair-like structures called cilia and mucus-producing cells. The nasal cavity is divided into two halves by the nasal septum, composed of bone and cartilage.
- **Nasal septum:** It is a partition that separates the two sides of the nasal cavity. It is composed of the perpendicular plate of the ethmoid bone in the upper part, the vomer bone in the lower part, and cartilage in the anterior portion.
- **Turbinates (Nasal Conchae):** The nasal cavity contains three bony shelves called turbinates or nasal conchae (superior, middle, and inferior). These structures help in increase the surface area of the nasal cavity and create turbulence in the inhaled air, which aids in humidification, filtering, and warming of the air.
- **Olfactory epithelium:** Located high up in the nasal cavity, the olfactory epithelium is responsible for the sense of smell. It contains specialized olfactory receptor cells that detect and transmit odor signals to the brain.
- **Sinuses:** Nose is connected to four pairs of air-filled cavities called sinuses, which are located in the skull bones

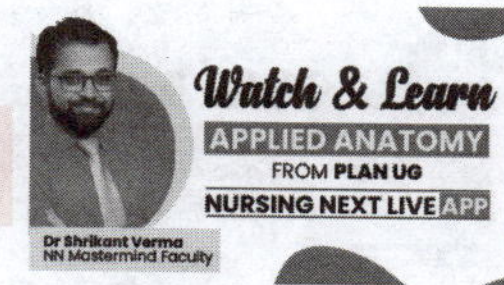

surrounding the nasal cavity. The sinuses include the frontal sinuses (in the forehead), ethmoid sinuses (between the eyes), sphenoid sinuses (behind the nose), and maxillary sinuses (in the cheekbones). The sinuses help lighten the skull, produce mucus, and resonate the voice.

- **Blood supply and innervation:** The nose receives its blood supply from branches of the maxillary artery and ophthalmic artery. It is innervated by branches of the trigeminal nerve (cranial nerve V), including the ophthalmic, maxillary, and mandibular divisions.

TONGUE

The tongue is a muscular organ located in the oral cavity and is involved in various functions, including taste, chewing, swallowing, and speech production. It is composed of several anatomical structures that contribute to its unique structure and functions.

The anatomy and structure of the tongue include the following components:

- **Papillae:** The surface of the tongue contains small structures called papillae, which give the tongue its rough texture. There are four types of papillae:
  1. **Filiform papillae:** These are the most numerous and have a thread-like appearance. They cover most of the tongue's surface and are responsible for tactile sensation.
  2. **Fungiform papillae:** These mushroom-shaped papillae are scattered among the filiform papillae, primarily at the tip and sides of the tongue. They contain taste buds and play a role in taste perception.
  3. **Foliate papillae:** These papillae are located on the sides of the tongue and are arranged in parallel ridges. They contain taste buds, especially during infancy and childhood.
  4. **Circumvallate papillae:** These are the largest papillae and are positioned in a V-shaped row at the back of the tongue. They also contain taste buds and help detect bitter tastes.
- **Taste buds:** They are specialized sensory organs located on the papillae of the tongue. They contain taste receptor cells that are responsible for detecting and transmitting taste sensations to the brain. Taste buds are particularly concentrated on fungiform and circumvallate papillae.
- **Lingual frenulum:** It is a thin fold of tissue that anchors the tongue to the floor of the mouth. It helps stabilize the tongue's movement and prevents excessive posterior displacement.
- **Intrinsic and extrinsic muscles:** The tongue is composed of various intrinsic and extrinsic muscles that allow for its movement and manipulation. The intrinsic muscles are responsible for fine motor control, altering the shape of the tongue during speech and swallowing. The extrinsic muscles are larger and provide broader movements, allowing the tongue to protrude, retract, elevate, depress, and move from side to side.
- **Salivary glands:** The tongue is moistened by saliva produced by the salivary glands. The sublingual glands, located beneath the tongue, secrete saliva that keeps the tongue and oral cavity lubricated.
- **Blood supply and innervation:** The tongue receives its blood supply from branches of the lingual artery, which is a branch of the external carotid artery. The tongue is innervated by several cranial nerves, including the hypoglossal nerve (cranial nerve XII), which controls the majority of the tongue's motor functions, and the glossopharyngeal nerve (cranial nerve IX), which carries taste sensations from the posterior part of the tongue.

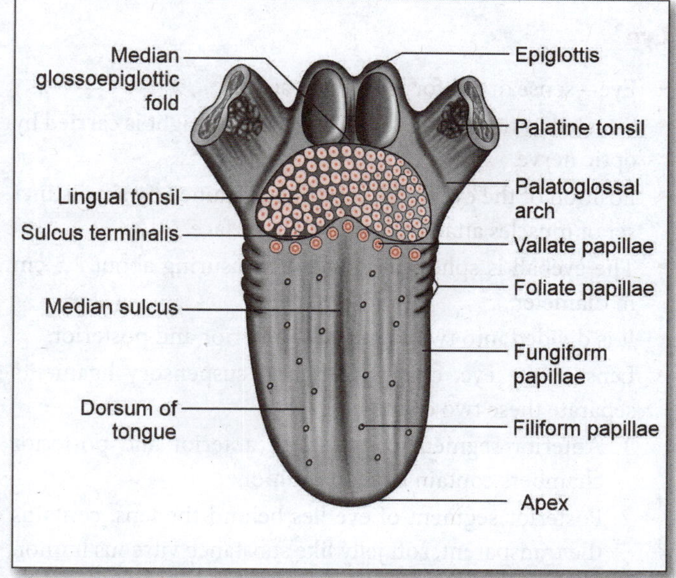

Figure 6.4: Structure of tongue

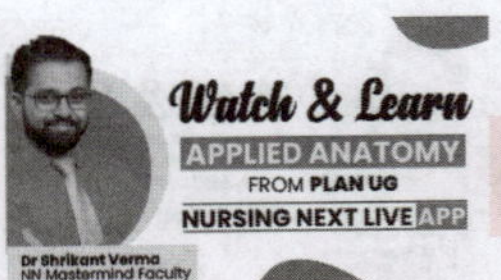

CONCEPTUAL EXERCISES

LONG ANSWER QUESTIONS

1. Enumerate the different special sensory organs of the human body. Describe in detail about eye. (MGR)

Answer

Sense Organs

- Specialized organs that help to sense the surroundings. They help in perceiving the world around us.
- The sense organs have specialized receptors on them that relay information through the sensory neurons within the brain.
- Five sense organs are:
  1. **Eyes:** Visual sensory organs
  2. **Ears:** Auditory sense organs
  3. **Nose:** Responsible for smell and olfaction
  4. **Tongue:** Responsible for taste or gustaoception.
  5. **Skin:** Responsible for touch

Eye

- Eye—sense organ for vision and sight.
- Situated in the orbital cavity and sense of sight is carried by optic nerve.
- Position of the eye in the orbit is maintained by six distinct set of muscles attached to its outer surface.
- The eyeball is spherical in shape measuring about 2.5 cm in diameter.
- It is divided into two segments—anterior and posterior.
- Lens of the eye, ciliary body and suspensory ligaments separate these two chambers.
  1. Anterior segment of eye, with anterior and posterior chambers contain aqueous humor.
  2. Posterior segment of eye lies behind the lens, contains the transparent, soft jelly like substance vitreous humor.
- Three layers in the wall of eye are as follows:
  1. **The outer supporting layer:** Consisting of the sclera and cornea.
  2. **The middle vascular layer:** Uveal tract made of choroid, ciliary body and the iris
  3. **The inner retinal layer:** Consists of retina

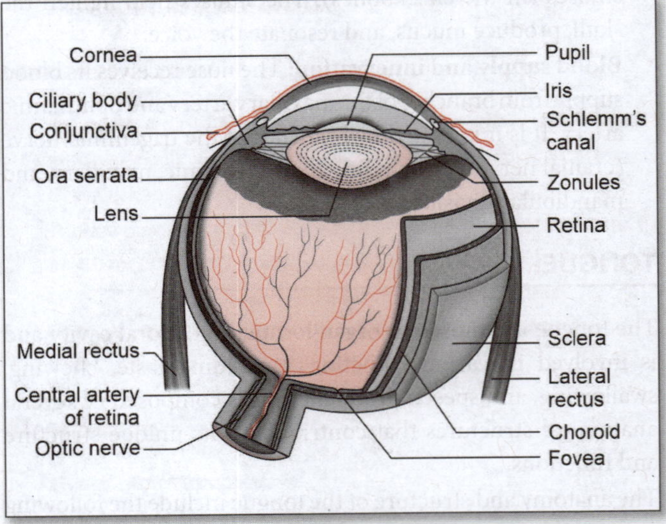

Figure 6.5: Cross-section of human eye

Outer Layer of the Eyeball

- **Sclera**
  - Firm, fibrous membrane
  - Maintains the shape of the eye
  - It is white in color and forms about 5/6th of the eyeball.
  - It is the site for insertion of eye muscles.
  - Functions
    - Resists intraocular pressure and maintains the shape of the eyeball
    - Allows smooth movements of the eye
    - Forms a fibrous tunic and protects the delicate structures of the eye.
- **Cornea**
  - White portion of eye
  - It is transparent
  - Forms the anterior 1/6th of the eye
  - It is avascular portion of the eye. It receives its nourishment from the peripheral vessels by diffusion.
  - Function
    - Refracts the light rays to focus on the retina.

Vascular Layer of Eyeball

- The vascular layer of the eye, also known as the uvea or uveal tract.

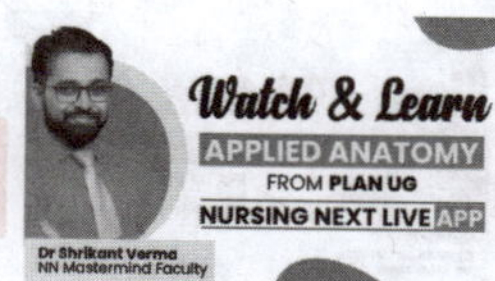

- **It consists of three layers:** Choroid, ciliary body and iris (from posterior to anterior).
- It has blood vessels to supply blood and oxygen and is made up of connective tissue.
- It is situated between sclera and retina.
- This layer consists of various parts:
  - **Choroid:**
    - Thin, vascular and pigmented membrane
    - Accounts for 90% of total blood flow in eye.
    - Outer surface of choroid is firmly attached to inner surface of sclera and inner surface is attached to retina.
    - The choroid is divided into three layers:
      - Vessel layer
      - Capillary layer
      - Bruch's membrane
  - **Ciliary body:**
    - It is a thickened vascular layer in the anterior portion of the eyeball.
    - It consists of ciliary muscle and secretory epithelial cells.
    - These muscles help lens to focus by either increasing or decreasing tension on **suspensory ligament** of lens.
    - Ciliary muscles are supplied by the parasympathetic nerves through oculomotor nerve.
    - It also produces aqueous humor and some elements of vitreous humor.
  - **Ciliary processes:**
    These are inward extensions (muscles) of ciliary body that hold the lens in place.
  - **Iris:**
    - This is the colored part of eye, an anterior extension of the choroid layer which lies behind the cornea in front of lens.
    - It is thin and muscular.
    - Contraction and relaxation of iris regulate the size of the pupil.
  - **Lens:**
    - It is elastic, colorless and transparent biconvex body made up of epithelial cells lying posterior to iris.
    - The lens can accommodate and change its shape, focusing on different objects at different distances, i.e., the lens is adjustable.
    - This accommodation is brought about by ciliary muscles.

Inner Layer

- **Retina**
  - Innermost layer having the photosensitive layers composed of the sensory receptor cells
    - Rods—for night vision
    - Cones—for day vision and colors
    - Bipolar cell layer
    - Ganglionic cell layer
  - It is thin, delicate layer and is continuous with optic nerve.
  - Its outer surface is attached to choroid and inner surface is in contact with hyaloid membrane of the vitreous.

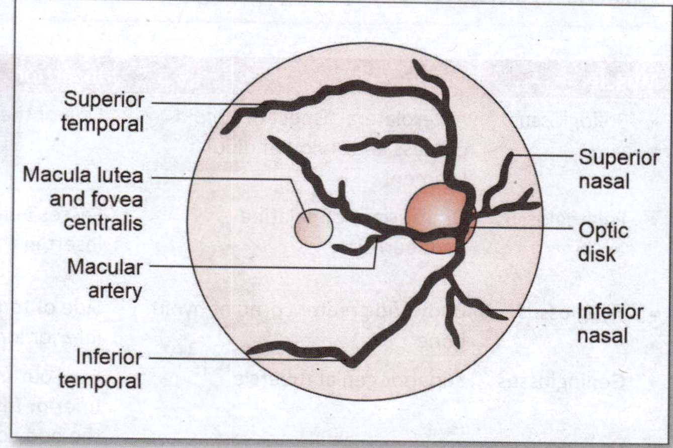

Figure 6.6: Retina and its blood supply

2. Write in detail about the tongue. (MGR)

Answer

Tongue

The tongue is a muscular organ in the mouth. The tongue is covered with moist, pink tissue called mucosa. Tiny bumps called papillae give the tongue its rough texture. Thousands of taste buds cover the surfaces of the papillae. Taste buds are collections of nerve-like cells that connect to nerves running into the brain.

Parts

It has three main parts:

1. The tip or apex of the tongue is the most anterior and most movable aspect of the organ.
2. The tip is followed by the body of the tongue. It has a rough dorsal (superior) surface that abuts the palate and is populated with taste buds and lingual papillae, and a smooth ventral (inferior) surface that is attached to the floor of the oral cavity by the lingual frenulum.
3. The base of the tongue is the most posterior part of the organ. It is populated by numerous lymphoid aggregates known as the lingual tonsils along with foliate papillae along the posterolateral surface.

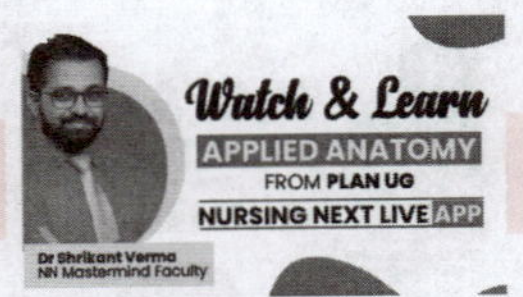

Relations of Tongue

- Anterior and lateral—teeth
- Superior—hard and soft palates
- Inferior—mucosa of the floor of the oral cavity, sublingual salivary glands, posterior wall of oropharynx
- Posterior—epiglottis, pharyngeal inlet
- Lateral—palatoglossal and palatopharyngeal arches

Muscles

- Mainly a muscular organ with small amounts of fats and fibrous tissue.
- All muscles are paired structures.
- Two types:
  1. Intrinsic muscles
  2. Extrinsic muscles

Muscle	Origin	Insertion	Actions
• Styloglossus	Anterolateral aspect of styloid process and stylomandibular ligament	Side of the tongue	Pulls the tongue upward and backward
• Palatoglossus	Oral surface of palatine aponeurosis	Passes beneath the palatoglossal arch to insert in the dorsum and sides of tongue	Elevation of tongue Closes off oropharyngeal isthmus
• Hyoglossus	Body and greater cornu of hyoid bone	Side of tongue between styloglossus and inferior longitudinal	Depresses the tongue
• Genioglossus	Superior genial tubercle	Fans out upward and backward. **Inferior fibers:** Upper anterior surface of the body of hyoid **Intermediate fibers:** Posterior part of the tongue **Superior fibers:** Ascend forward to enter the whole length of ventral surface of tongue	**Forward traction of the tongue:** To protrude the apex. **Acting B/L:** Depress the central part of tongue **Acting U/L:** Deviates tongue to opposite side
• Inferior longitudinal	Above the ventral lingual surface. Extends from root	To apex of tongue	Shorten the tongue Dorsum convex
• Superior longitudinal	Beneath mucosa of dorsum of tongue. From the submucous fibrous tissue near epiglottis and the median lingual septum	Lingual margins	Shorten the tongue Dorsum concave
• Transverse	Median fibrous septum	Submucous fibrous tissue of lingual margins	Narrows and elongates the tongue
• Vertical	Dorsal aspect	Ventral aspect	Flattens and broadens the tongue

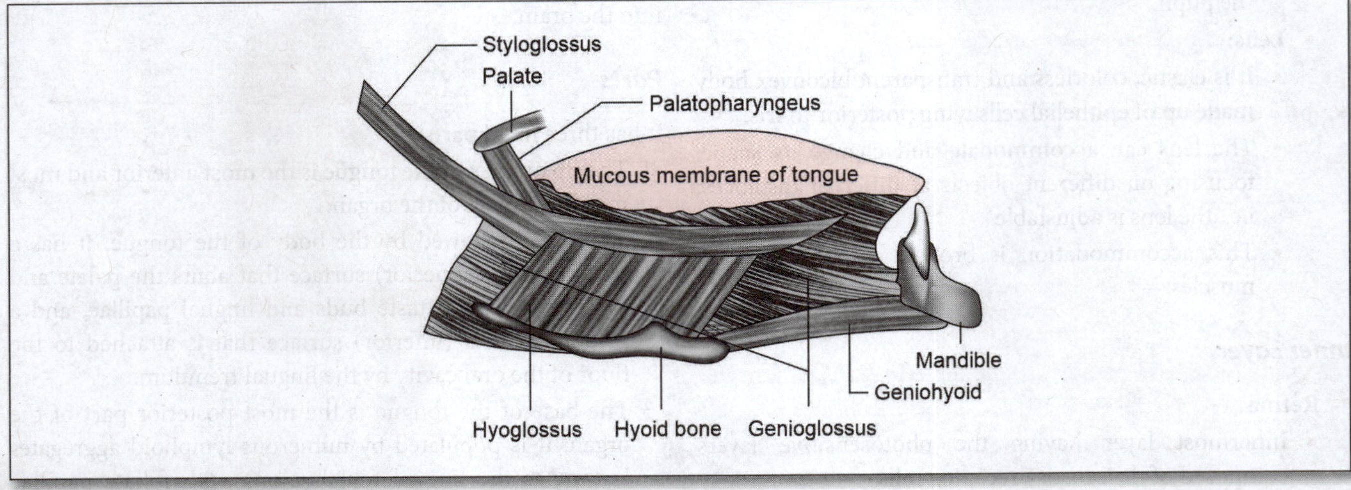

Figure 6.7: Extrinsic muscles of tongue

Microstructure of Tongue

The dorsal mucosa of the oral tongue is characterized by numerous raised structures known as lingual papillae. They give the characteristic rough appearance of the dorsal surface. The pharyngeal tongue also has raised dome-like structures throughout the mucosa.

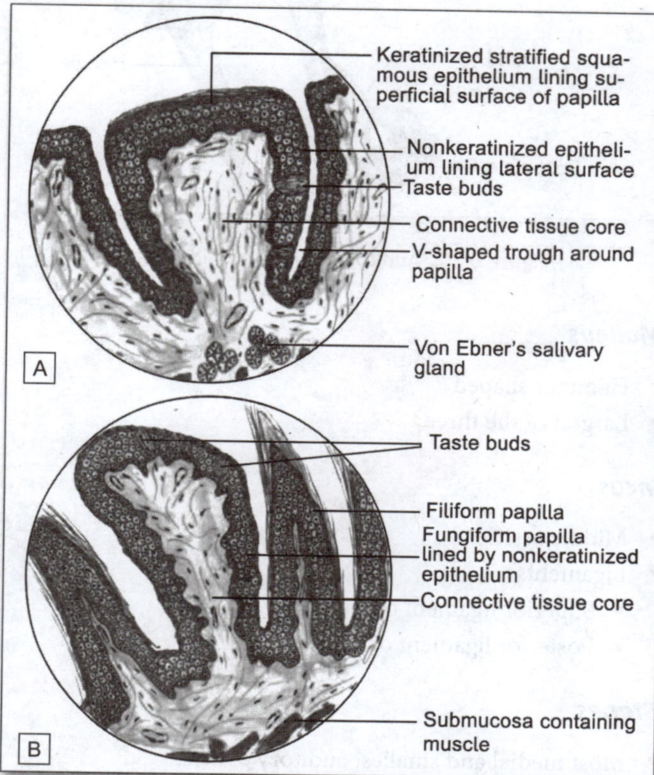

Figures 6.8A and B: **A** Circumvallate papillae; **B.** Fungiform and filiform papillae

Lingual Papillae

- There are four types of lingual papillae found on the surface of the human tongue. These include:
  1. **Filiform papillae**
     - Most abundant among the four types of papillae.
     - Stretched, conical, gray white papillae that are covered in a heavy coat of keratinized squamous epithelium.
     - They make the dorsal surface of the tongue rough and provide friction to allow movement of the food bolus during chewing.
     - Do not possess taste buds.
  2. **Fungiform papillae**
     - Weakly keratinized, highly vascular, mushroom-shaped papillae
     - Less abundant than the filiform papillae.
     - They are scattered across the entire dorsal surface of the tongue.
     - Contain a few taste buds on the apical aspect.
  3. **Foliate papillae**
     - Bilaterally paired, parallel, longitudinal slits on the posterolateral margin of the tongue, near the sulcus terminalis.
     - Nonkeratinized
     - Populated with numerous taste buds.
  4. **Circumvallate (Vallate) papillae**
     - Present linearly, as a set of four to six large papillae anterior to each limb of the sulcus terminalis (i.e., eight to twelve papillae in total).
     - In longitudinal section, the characteristic furrow found within the papillae can be appreciated.
     - These moats facilitate the drainage of serous salivary von Ebner's glands that empty into the structure.
     - Persistent lubrication creates a favorable environment for gustatory particles to dissolve so that they can be detected by the taste buds.

Blood Supply

- **Arterial supply**
  - Lingual artery, branch of external carotid artery, further branches into:
    - Dorsal lingual arteries to the dorsal mucosa of the tongue, palatoglossus, soft palate, palatine tonsils and epiglottis.
    - Sublingual arteries
    - Deep lingual artery
  - **Ascending palatine** and **tonsillar arteries**, branch of facial artery.
  - Ascending pharyngeal artery, branch of the external carotid
- **Venous drainage**

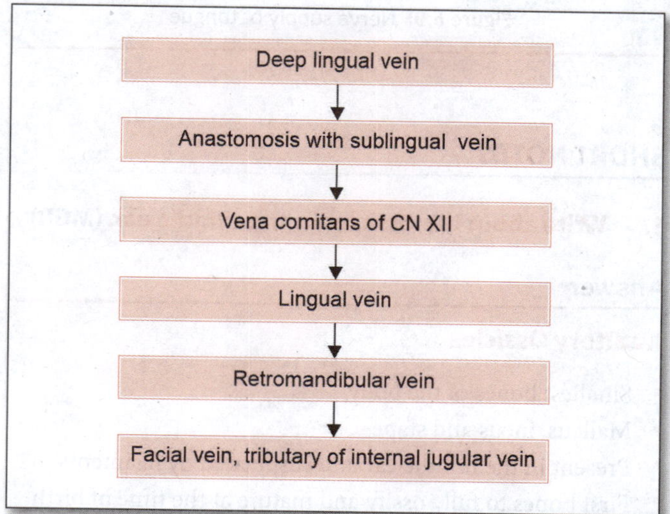

  - Dorsal lingual veins drain the lateral margins and dorsal surface of the tongue and join the internal jugular vein.

- **Lymphatic drainage**
  - Anterior parts of tongue drain into marginal and central lymph vessels, which drain into the submandibular or the jugulo-omohyoid lymph nodes.
  - Posterior one-third drains into the dorsal lymph vessels, which drain into the jugulo-omohyoid and jugulodigastric lymph nodes.

Innervation

- In the anterior two-thirds, general sensation is supplied by the trigeminal nerve (CN V). Especially lingual nerve which is a branch of the mandibular nerve (CN V3).
- Taste in the anterior two-thirds is supplied from the facial nerve (CN VII).
- The posterior one-third of the tongue is supplied by the glossopharyngeal nerve (CN IX).

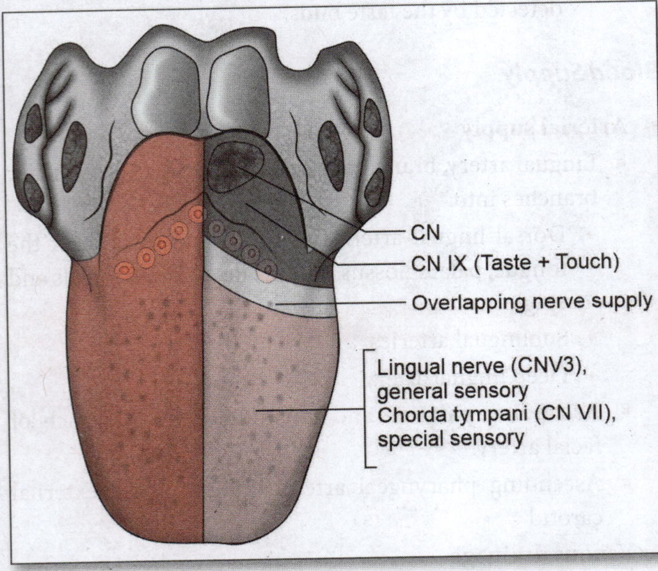

Figure 6.9: Nerve supply of tongue

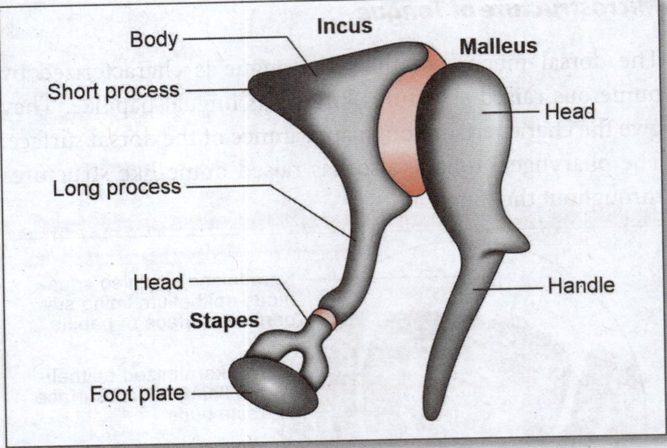

Figure 6.10: Auditory ossicles of middle ear

Malleus

- Hammer shaped
- Largest of the three

Incus

- Middle ossicle.
- Ligaments
  - Superior ligament of incus
  - Posterior ligament of incus

Stapes

- Most medial and smallest auditory ossicle.
- Ligaments
  - Stapedial membrane
  - Annular ligament

Function of Auditory Ossicles

Transmit the sound vibrations of the tympanic membrane to the internal ear (oval window).

SHORT NOTES

1. **Write about the ossicles in the middle ear. (MGR)**

Answer

Auditory Ossicles

- Smallest bones of the body
- Malleus, incus and stapes
- Present in the middle ear and suspended by ligaments
- First bones to fully ossify and mature at the time of birth.
- Articulate with each other by synovial joints.

2. **Mention the layers of the epidermis of the skin. (MGR)**

Answer

Layers of Epidermis

Five layers of the epidermis are easily appreciable in thick skin as compared to thin skin. Going from superficial to deep, the layers are:

1. Stratum corneum—Cornified layer
2. Stratum lucidum—Clear layer

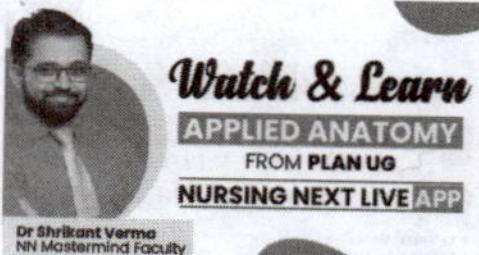

3. Stratum granulosum—Granular layer
4. Stratum spinosum—Prickle cell layer
5. Stratum basale/germinativum—Basal layer

Stratum Corneum

- Topmost layer
- Contains dead cells filled with keratohyaline filaments
- Enucleated
- Main function is the protection of deeper layers.

Stratum Lucidum

- Presents only in palms and soles
- Contains translucent cells filled with keratohyaline granules.
- Cells are devoid of nuclei and organelles.

Stratum Granulosum

- Flattened polygonal pyknotic cells
- Contains keratohyaline granules and Odland bodies
- This layer contributes to the selective permeability of skin, making it relatively waterproof.

Stratum Spinosum

- Contains post-mitotic cells from the basal layer
- Approximately 4–6 layers of cuboidal or slightly flattened cells in this region
- Adjacent cells are attached to each other via desmosomes.
- Prickled appearance of cells gives them the name.
- Contains keratin fibrils, melanosomes and Langerhans cells

Stratum Germinativum

- Stem cells continuously undergoing mitosis to regenerate other layers
- Consists of a mixture of simple cuboidal to columnar epithelium.
- Large euchromatic cells with prominent nucleoli.

Cells in Epidermis

- Keratinocytes—squamous epithelial cells that form in the basal layer and mature gradually toward the corneum layer.
- Melanocytes—melanin-producing cells
- Langerhans cells—antigen-presenting cells
- Merkel cells—mechanoreceptors

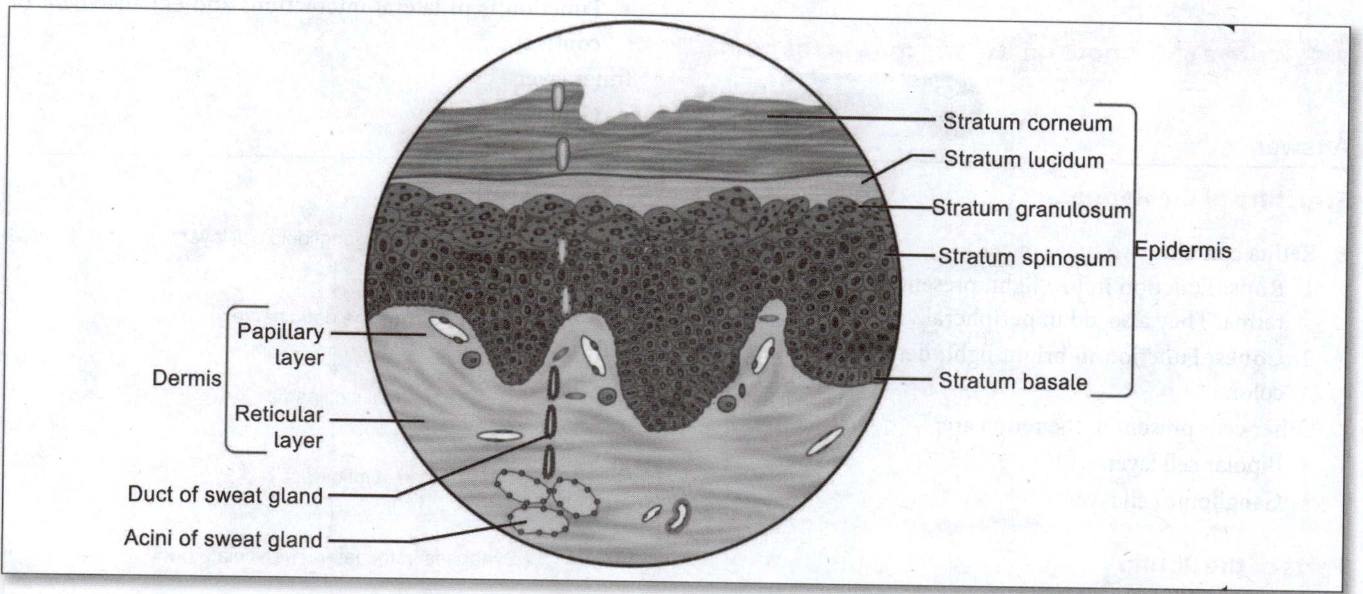

Figure 6.11: Histology of thick skin

3. Write a short note on appendages of skin. (DU)

Answer

Appendages of Skin

These include hair, nail and glands.

Hair

- Hairs are keratinous filaments derived from invaginations of the germinative layer of the epidermis into the dermis.
- Help in the conservation of their body heat.
- They grow at the rate of 1.5–2 mm/week.
- Color of hair depends on the amount and type of melanin.

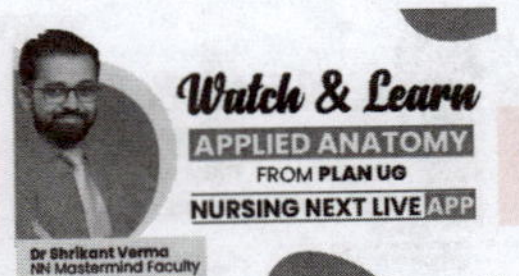

Nails

- Ectodermal modification of skin
- Function: protection of the dorsal aspect of tip of digits and esthetics
- Hardened keratin plates (cornified zone) on the dorsal surface of the tips of fingers and toes. Each nail has the following parts:
  - **Root:** Proximal hidden part
  - **Body:** Exposed part of the nail that is adherent to the underlying skin, root and body.
  - **Free border:**
    - Free end of the nail
    - Attached to the under surface by the hyponychium.

Glands

- **Sweat glands:**
  - Distributed all over the skin, except lips, nail bed and glans penis.
  - Two types—eccrine and apocrine
  - These glands help in the regulation of body temperature and excretion of body salts.

4. Write a short note on the structure of the retina.

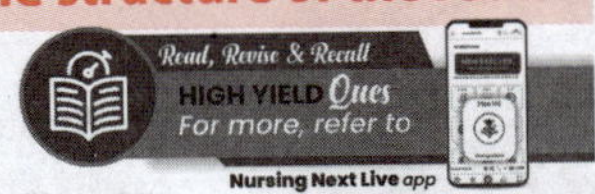

Answer

Structure of the Retina

- Retina contains two types of cells:
  1. **Rods:** Function in low light, present at the periphery of retina. They also aid in peripheral vision.
  2. **Cones:** Function in bright light, detect fine details and color.
- Other cells present in the retina are:
  - Bipolar cell layer
  - Ganglionic cell layer

Parts of the Retina

- Optic part:
  - Sensitive to light
  - Consists of:
    - Nervous tissues
    - Optic
    - Ciliary
    - Iridial
  - Extends from the optic disc to the posterior end of the ciliary body.
- Optic disk
  - Absence of rods and cones
  - Insensitive to light
  - Also known as the blind spot.
- Macula lutea
  - Presents in the posterior part of the retina.
  - Known as the yellow spot or fovea centralis.
  - Contains only cone cells

Retinal Cells

- Outer layer
  - Photoreceptors are present in this layer. These are rods and cones.
  - Rods – for night or low light vision
  - Cones – for day vision, color and perception of density
- Middle layer
  - Bipolar neurons – horizontal cells
  - Amacrine cells – lie deeper to the bipolar neurons.
  - Function is in lateral interactions and enhancement of contrast.
- Inner layer
  - Ganglionic cells

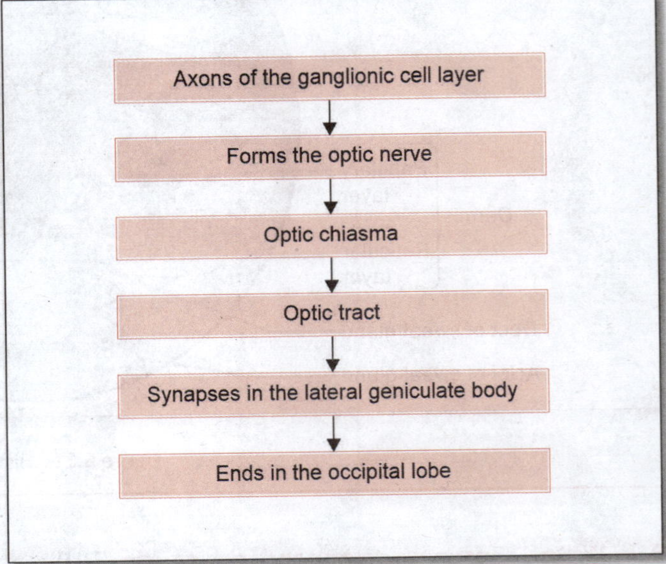

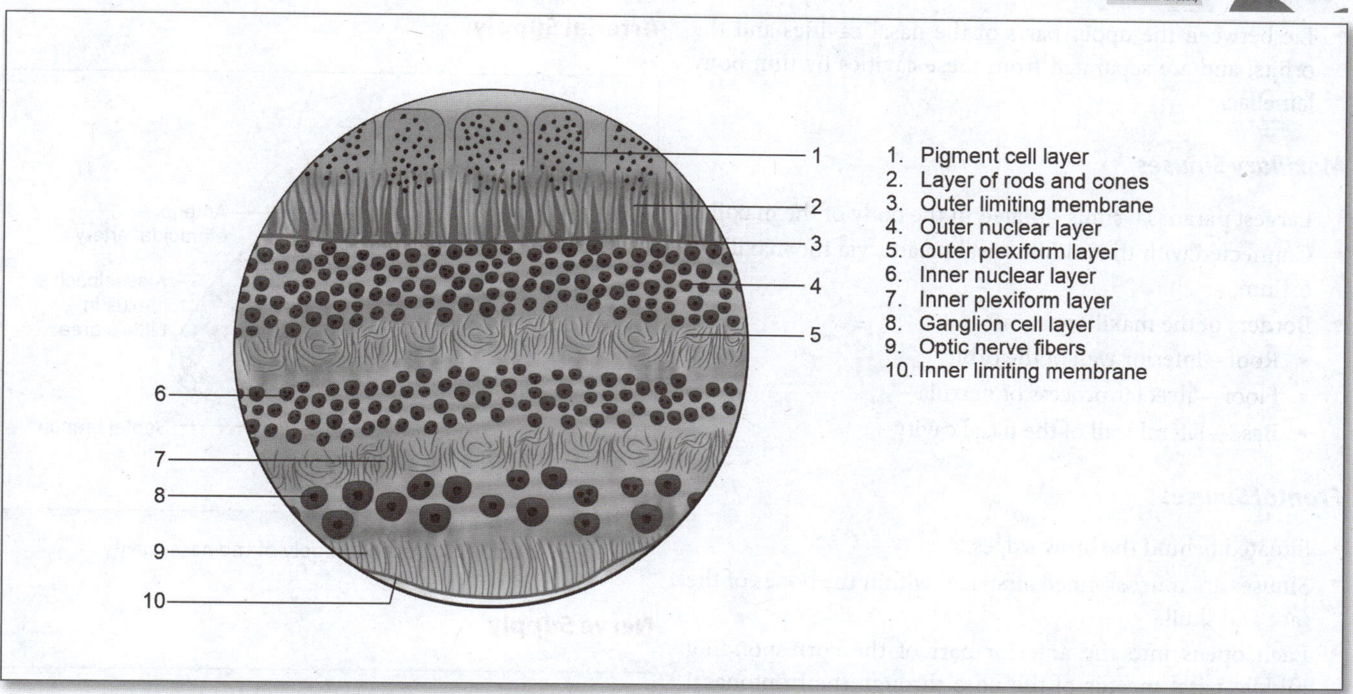

Figure 6.12: Histology of retina

Blood Supply

- Central artery of retina, branch of the ophthalmic artery.
- It divides into superior and inferior nasal branches.

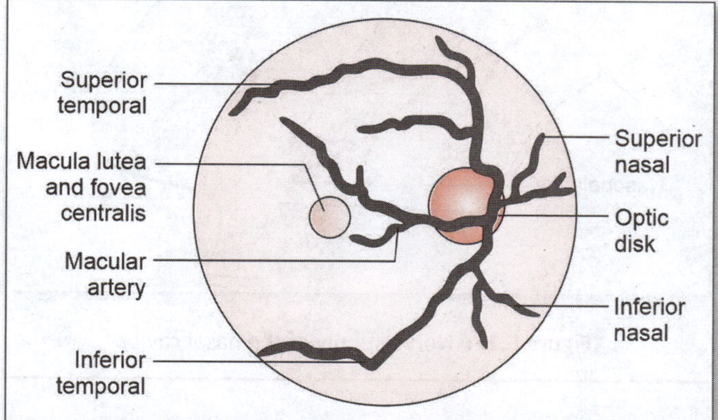

Figure 6.13: Retina and its blood supply

5. Enumerate air sinuses open in the middle meatus.

OR

Write short notes on paranasal sinuses. (RUHS)

Answer

Middle Meatus

- The middle meatus is an air passage of the lateral nasal cavity located between the middle nasal concha and lateral nasal wall. The anterior ethmoid air cells, maxillary and frontal sinuses all drain into the middle meatus.

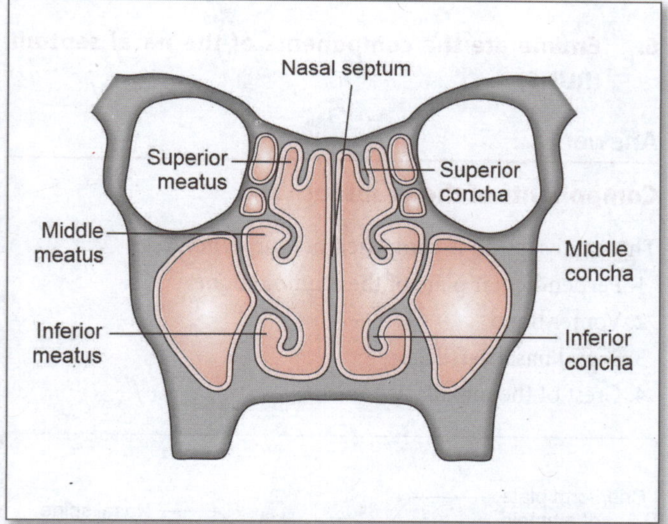

Figure 6.14: Nasal meatuses

Anterior Ethmoid Air Cells

- One of the four paired paranasal sinuses.
- Cells are variable in both size and number.
- Divided into anterior and posterior groups.
- Ethmoid air cells are numerous thin-walled cavities situated in the ethmoidal labyrinth and completed by the frontal, maxilla, lacrimal, sphenoidal and palatine bones.

- Lie between the upper parts of the nasal cavities and the orbits, and are separated from these cavities by thin bony lamellae.

Maxillary Sinuses

- Largest paranasal sinus situated in the body of the maxilla.
- Connected with the middle nasal meatus via the maxillary ostium.
- Borders of the maxillary sinus:
  - Roof—inferior wall of the orbit
  - Floor—alveolar process of maxilla
  - Base—lateral wall of the nasal cavity

Frontal Sinuses

- Situated behind the brow ridges.
- Sinuses are mucosa-lined airspaces within the bones of the face and skull.
- Each opens into the anterior part of the corresponding middle nasal meatus of the nose through the frontonasal duct which traverses the anterior part of the labyrinth of the ethmoid.
- These structures then open into the semilunar hiatus in the middle meatus.

6. Enumerate the components of the nasal septum. (RUHS)

Answer

Components of the Nasal Septum

The nasal septum is composed of four structures:

1. Perpendicular plate of the ethmoid bone
2. Vomer bone
3. Septal nasal cartilage
4. Crest of the maxillary bone

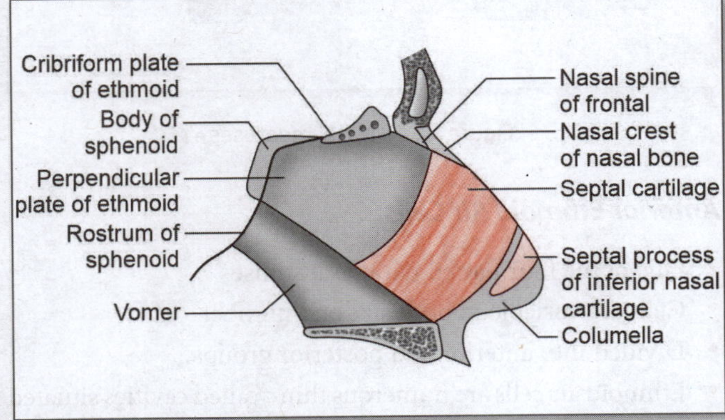

Figure 6.15: Components of the nasal cavity

Arterial Supply

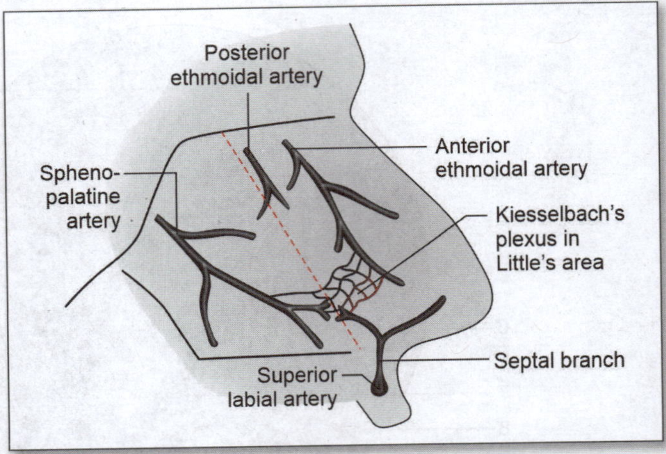

Figure 6.16: Arterial supply of the nasal cavity

Nerve Supply

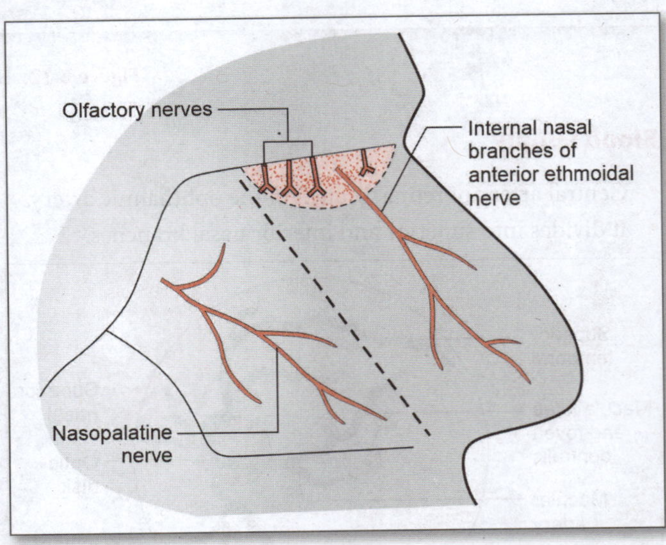

Figure 6.17: Nerve supply of the nasal cavity

7. Write a short note on coverings of eyeball. (MGR, RUHS)

Answer

Coverings of Eyeball

- Three layers in the wall of eye are:
  - **The outer supporting layer:** Consists of the sclera and cornea.
  - **The middle vascular layer:** Uveal tract made of the choroid, ciliary body and iris.
  - **The inner retinal layer:** Consists of the retina.

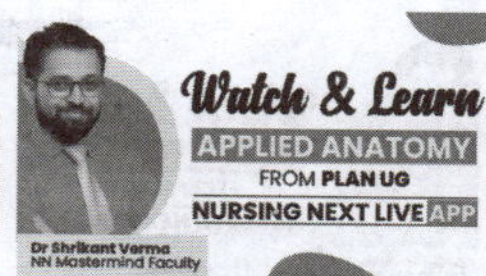

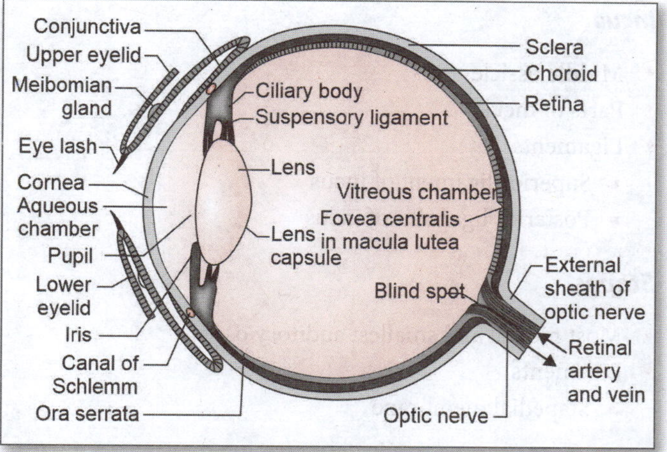

Figure 6.18: Structure of human eye

Outer Layer of the Eyeball

- **Sclera**
  - Firm, fibrous membrane
  - Maintains the shape of the eye
  - It is white in color and forms about 5/6th of the eyeball.
  - It is the site for the insertion of eye muscles.
- **Cornea**
  - White portion of eye
  - It is transparent
  - It is avascular portion of the eye. It receives its nourishment from the peripheral vessels by diffusion.
  - Function
    - Refracts the light rays to focus on the retina.

Vascular Layer of the Eyeball

- The vascular layer of the eye, also known as the uvea or uveal tract.
- It consists of three layers: choroid, ciliary body and iris (from posterior to anterior).
- It has blood vessels to supply blood and oxygen and is made up of connective tissue.
- It is situated between the sclera and retina.

Inner Layer

- Retina
  - Innermost layer having the photosensitive layers composed of the sensory receptor cells
    - Rods—for night vision
    - Cones—for day vision and colors
    - Bipolar cell layer
    - Ganglionic cell layer
  - It is a thin, delicate layer and is continuous with the optic nerve.
  - Its outer surface is attached to the choroid and inner surface is in contact with the hyaloid membrane of the vitreous.

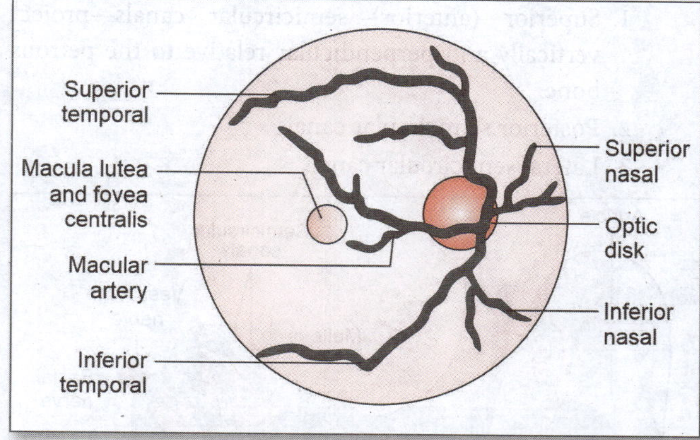

Figure 6.19: Retina and its blood supply

8. Draw the labeled diagram of eyeball.

Answer

For answer, refer to Short Notes Q. no. 7, Figure no. 6.18 pg. no. 99

9. Describe the structure of the inner ear. (MGR)

Answer

Structure of the Inner Ear

- **Cochlear component:**
  - Concerned with hearing
  - Spirally coiled like snail's shell.
  - Thickest at the base, gradually thinning with each coil and terminates at the cochlear cupula.
  - Consists of basilar and Reissner's membrane.
  - Scala vestibuli lies above the Reissner's membrane.
  - Scala tympani lies below the basal membrane.
- The organ of Corti consists of stereocilia suspended in supporting cells that are covered by the tectorial membrane.
- **Vestibular component**
  - Hollow cavity is located between the cochlea and the semicircular canals.
  - Consists of utricle and saccule
  - Concerned with static balance
  - Contains three recesses:
    1. Elliptical recess
    2. Cochlear recess
    3. Spherical recess

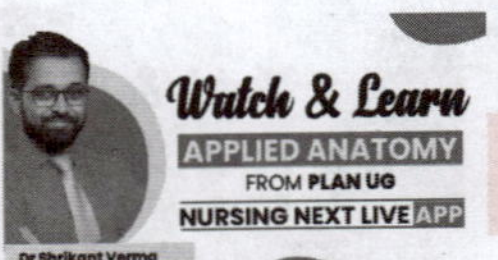

- **Semicircular component**
  - Regulates balance while in motion.
  - Three semicircular bony structures are present:
    1. Superior (anterior) semicircular canals—project vertically and perpendicular relative to the petrous bone.
    2. Posterior semicircular canals
    3. Lateral semicircular canals

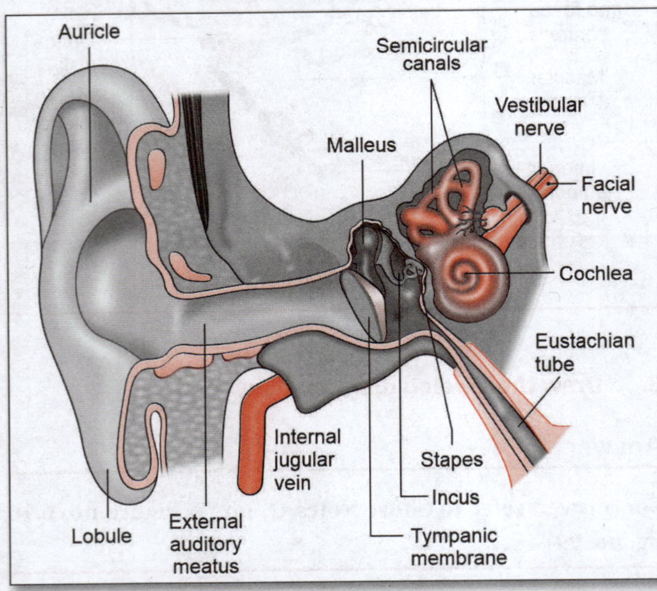

Figure 6.20: Anatomy

Blood Supply

- Arterial supply is by the labyrinthine artery, a branch of the basilar artery.
- The stylomastoid artery supplies the inner ear.
- Venous drainage is by labyrinthine veins that drain into the inferior and superior petrosal sinus.

Nerve Supply

- Sensory innervation is by vestibulocochlear nerve.

10. Name the contents of the middle ear cavity. (MGR)

Answer

Contents of Middle Ear

Malleus

- Hammer shaped
- Largest of the three
- Ligaments of malleus
  - Anterior ligament
  - Superior ligament
  - Lateral ligament

Incus

- Middle ossicle
- Parts of incus
- Ligaments
  - Superior ligament of incus
  - Posterior ligament of incus

Stapes

- Most medial and smallest auditory ossicle.
- Ligaments
  - Stapedial membrane

Muscles of Middle Ear

- Tensor tympani
  - Arises from the cartilaginous part of the auditory tube and forms the base of the skull.
  - Inserted into the handle of the malleus.
  - Functions:
    - Tenses the tympanic membrane
    - Reduces the amplitude of oscillations
  - Nerve supply:
    - Mandibular nerve
- Stapedius
  - Lies on the posterior wall of the middle ear
  - Insertion is in the neck of the stapes.
  - Nerve supply:
    - Branch of facial nerve.

11. Describe papillae of tongue with the help of a diagram. (DU)

Answer

Papillae of Tongue

- There are four types of lingual papillae found on the surface of the human tongue. These include:
  1. **Filiform papillae**
     - Most abundant of the four types of papillae.
     - Stretched, conical, gray-white papillae that are covered in a heavy coat of keratinized squamous epithelium.
     - They make the dorsal surface of the tongue rough and provide friction to allow movement of the food bolus during chewing.
     - Do not possess taste buds.
  2. **Fungiform papillae**
     - Weakly keratinized, highly vascular, mushroom-shaped papillae

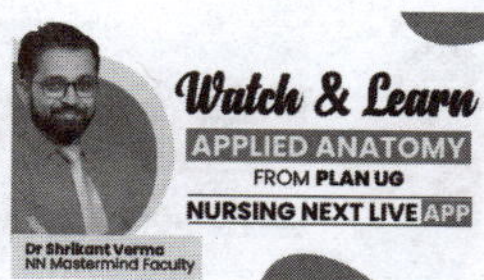

- Less abundant than the filiform papillae.
- They are scattered across the entire dorsal surface of the tongue.
- Contain a few taste buds on the apical aspect.

3. **Foliate papillae**
   - Bilaterally paired, parallel, longitudinal slits on the posterolateral margin of the tongue, near the sulcus terminalis.
   - Nonkeratinized
   - Populated with numerous taste buds.
4. **Circumvallate (Vallate) papillae**
   - Present linearly, as a set of four to six large papillae anterior to each limb of the sulcus terminalis (i.e., eight to twelve papillae in total).
   - In the longitudinal section, the characteristic furrow found within the papillae can be appreciated.
   - These moats facilitate the drainage of serous salivary von Ebner's glands that empty into the structure.
   - The persistent lubrication creates a favorable environment for gustatory particles to dissolve so that they can be detected by the taste buds.

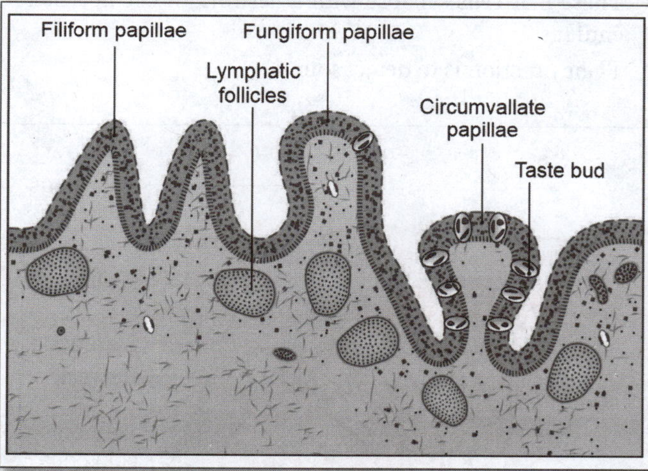

Figure 6.21: Papillae of tongue

12. Write a short note on the tympanic membrane. (DU)

Answer

Tympanic Membrane

- The tympanic membrane is also known as eardrum.
- It is a thin, oval and semitransparent structure.
- It is situated at the medial end of the external auditory meatus and the tympanic cavity of the middle ear.

Parts

- The tympanic membrane is divided into two parts:
  1. Pars tensa:
     - Major part of the tympanic membrane
     - Forms the fibrocartilaginous ring, known as the tympanic ring.
  2. Pars flaccida
     - Also known as Shrapnell's membrane.
     - Small triangular portion of the membrane located between the anterior and posterior malleolar folds.

Surfaces

- Two surfaces:
  1. Lateral (external) surface
     - Concave toward the external auditory meatus
     - Directed anteriorly and inferolaterally.
  2. Medial surface
     - Convex toward the tympanic cavity
     - Point of maximum convexity of membrane is known as umbo.

Blood Supply

- Has dual blood supply
- Deep auricular artery supplies the outer part
- Anterior and posterior tympanic artery supplies the medial part

Nerve Supply

- Anterior portion of lateral surface is innervated by the auriculotemporal nerve of the mandibular nerve.
- Posterior portion of the lateral surface is innervated by the vagus nerve.
- Medial surface is innervated by the glossopharyngeal nerve.

Functions

- Serves as a physical barrier between the middle and outer ear
- Protects the middle and inner ear
- Plays a role in sound transmission from the outer ear to the auditory ossicles.

13. Write a short note on the iris of the eye.

Answer

Iris of the Eye

- This is the colored part of the eye, an anterior extension of the choroid layer which lies behind the cornea in front of lens.
- The color of the eye is dependent on the pigment in the iris.

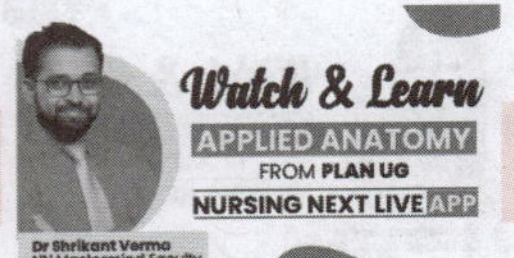

- It is thin and muscular.
- Contraction and relaxation of the iris regulate the size of the pupil.

Layers of the Iris

- The layers of the iris are:
  - Anterior limiting layer
  - **Stroma:** Front pigmented fibrovascular layer
  - Iris sphincter muscle
  - Iris dilator muscle
  - Pigmented epithelial layer
    - Divided into anterior and posterior layers.
- The stroma is connected to sphincter pupillae and dilator pupillae which contracts and dilates the pupil, respectively.

Region of the Iris

The iris is divided into two parts:

1. Ciliary zone:
   - Outer zone
   - The iris arises from the margin of the ciliary body and forms a diaphragm.
2. Pupillary zone
   - Inner zone whose edge forms the boundary of the pupil.

Muscles of the Iris

- Sphincter pupillae—causes constriction of the pupil when it contracts.
- Dilator pupillae—ill-defined sheet of radially arranged fibers. Causes dilation of the pupil.
- Both are smooth involuntary muscles.
- Iris receives innervation from both parasympathetic and sympathetic nerves.
  - Parasympathetic—causes constriction
  - Sympathetic—causes dilation

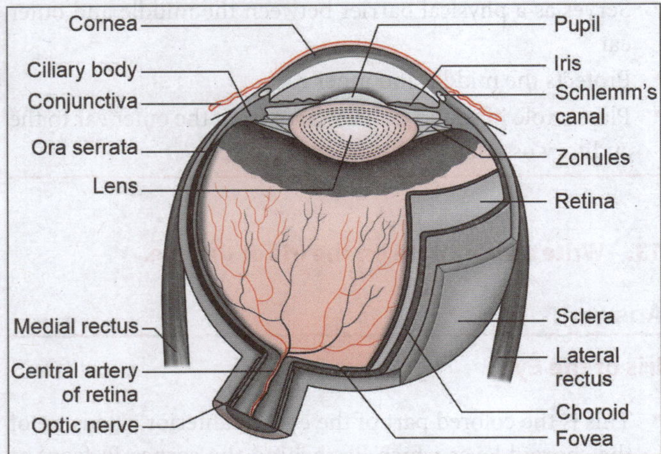

Figure 6.22: Cross section of human eye

14. Write a short note on the organ of Corti. (DU)

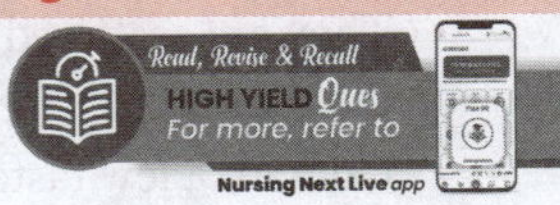

Answer

Organ of Corti

- Organ of the inner ear
- Receptor organ that generates nerve impulses in response to basilar membrane vibration.
- It is located on the surface of the basilar fibers and basilar membrane within the cochlea.

Structure of the Organ of Corti

- Consists of two specialized types of nerve cells
  - Internal hair cells
    - Single layer
    - Approximately 3,500 in number
  - External hair cells
    - 3–4 layers
    - Approximately 12,000 in number.
- These hair cells synapse with a network of cochlear nerve endings.
- Their function is to detect sound.

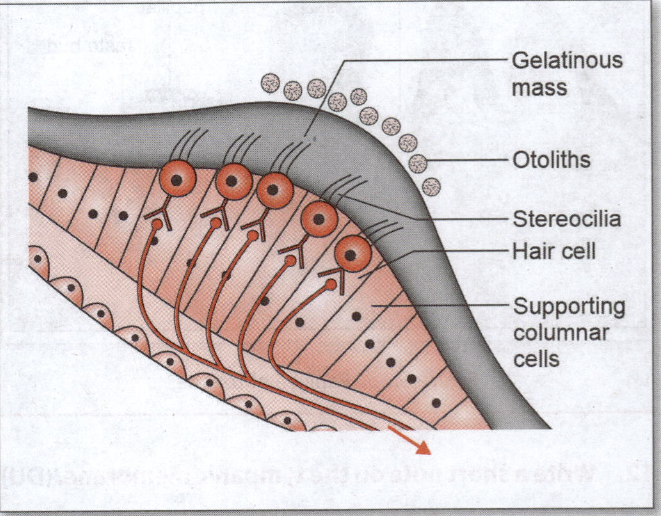

Figure 6.23: Organ of Corti

Functions of the Organ of Corti

- The primary function is the transduction of auditory signals.
- Responsible for the conversion of mechanical energy into chemical energy that can be read by the nerves.

SHORT ANSWER QUESTIONS

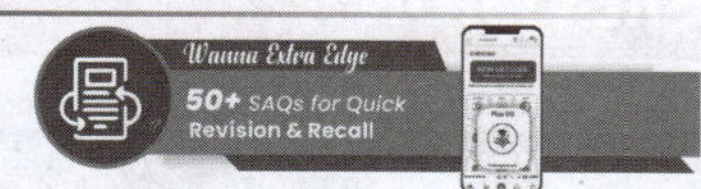

1. Name the muscles of tongue. (MGR)

Answer

The muscles of the tongue include mainly intrinsic and extrinsic muscles.

- **Intrinsic muscles:**
  - Superior longitudinal muscle
  - Inferior longitudinal muscle
  - Transverse muscle
  - Vertical muscle
- **Extrinsic muscles:**
  - Genioglossus muscle
  - Styloglossus muscle
  - Hyoglossus muscle
  - Palatoglossus muscle

2. Enumerate parts of lacrimal apparatus. (MGR)

Answer

- The components of lacrimal apparatus include:
- **Lacrimal gland:**
  - Produces the aqueous component of tear film with antimicrobial substances, like Lysozyme, Lactoferrin, and Immunoglobulin A.
  - Parts of lacrimal gland
    - Orbital part
    - Palpebral part
- **Lacrimal ducts/canals:** Small channels or ducts, present in each eyelid that drain the lacrimal sac.
- **Lacrimal sac:** Lacrimal canaliculi join together to open into lacrimal sac.
- **Nasolacrimal duct:** Nasolacrimal duct connects the lacrimal sac to the inferior meatus of the nose.
- **Meibomian glands:** Specialized sebaceous glands that form the tear film.

3. Trace the pathway of accommodation reflex. (MGR)

Answer

Accommodation Reflex

- This is the process by which the curvature of lens is increased to see an object close to eye.

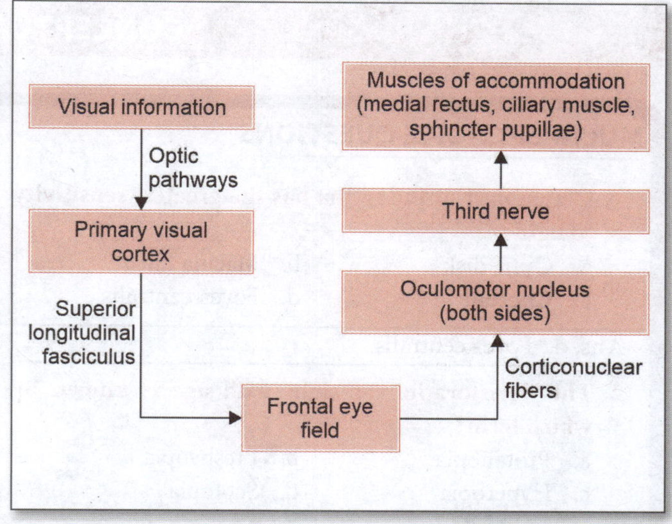

4. Name the bones of middle ear. (MGR)

Answer

- **Malleus:** It is the largest and most lateral of the ear bone
- **Incus:** The body articulates with the malleus and the stapes.
- **Stapes:** It is the smallest bone in the human body. Articulates with the incus and oval window.

5. Name the extraocular muscles. (MGR)

Answer

Extraocular Muscles of Eye

The extraocular muscles are the six muscles that control movement of the eye and one muscle that controls eyelid elevation (levator palpebrae).

There are seven extraocular muscles:

1. The levator palpebrae superior is
2. Superior rectus
3. Inferior rectus
4. Medial rectus
5. Lateral rectus
6. Inferior oblique
7. Superior oblique.

Functionally, they can be divided into two groups:

1. **Responsible for eye movement:** Recti and oblique muscles.
2. **Responsible for superior eyelid movement:** Levator palpebrae superioris.

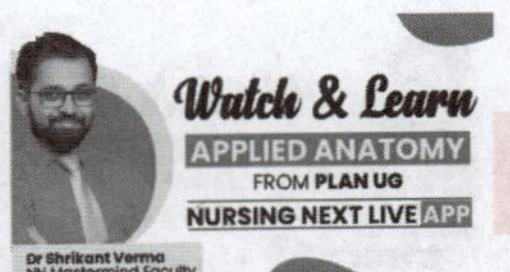

CONCEPTUAL REVISION

MULTIPLE CHOICE QUESTIONS

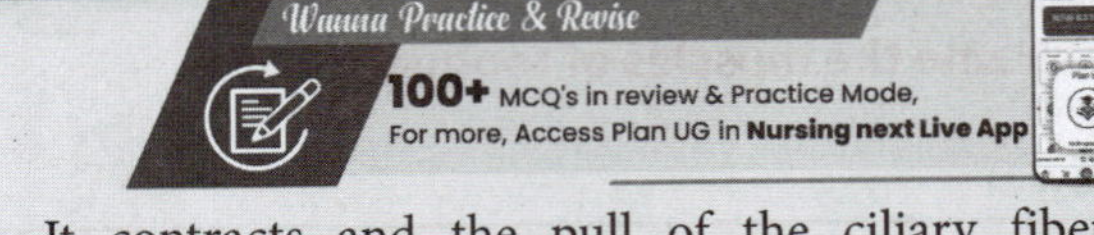

1. Which part of the retina has the greatest sensitivity to light?

a. Optic disk
b. Macula lutea
c. Choroid
d. Fovea centralis

Ans. d. Fovea centralis

2. The deterioration of sight with age is known by which term?

a. Protanopia
b. Presbyopia
c. Hyperopia
d. Scotopia

Ans. b. Presbyopia

3. What is the place where the blood vessels and nerve fibers come together and leave the posterior chamber of the eye called?

a. Macula lutea
b. Optic disk
c. Fovea centralis
d. Choroid

Ans. b. Optic disk

4. What does the ciliary muscle do when accommodation (focusing) in the eye occurs?

a. It contracts and the tension on the ciliary fibers increases making the eye lens less convex.
b. It relaxes and the tension on the ciliary fibers decreases allowing the eye lens to become more convex.
c. It contracts and the pull of the ciliary fibers decreases allowing the lens to become more convex.
d. It relaxes and the pull of the ciliary fibers increases to make the lens less convex.

Ans. c. It contracts and the pull of the ciliary fibers decreases allowing the lens to become more convex.

5. What is the purpose of the optic chiasma?

a. To allow images from each eye to cross over to the other side of the brain prior to crossing back at the decussation of pyramids.
b. To allow fibers from the medial aspect of one eye to join fibers from the lateral aspect of the other eye to form an optic tract.
c. To allow the fibers from the lateral aspect of each eye to come together as an optic tract.
d. To allow light entering the left eye to be interpreted by the right hand side of the occipital lobe (and vice versa).

Ans. b. To allow fibers from the medial aspect of one eye to join fibers from the lateral aspect of the other eye to form an optic tract.

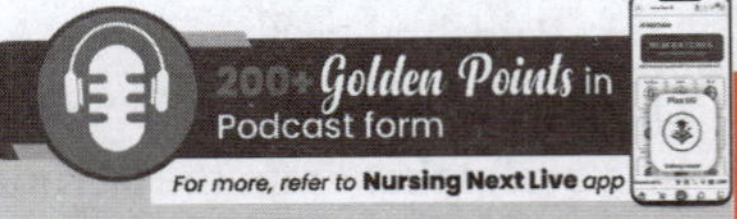

Golden Points

- Anterior segment of eye, with anterior and posterior chambers contain aqueous humor.
- Behind the lens, filling the posterior segment is vitreous humor, which is a transparent, soft jelly-like substance.
- Blood supply of the eye is from ophthalmic artery, and branch of internal carotid.
- Ciliary body consists of ciliary muscle
- External ear consists of pinna or auricle and external auditory meatus.
- Eye consists of the eyeball including muscles and nerves related to the eyeball and lacrimal apparatus.
- Eye is the sense organ for the sense of sight.
- Fluids present in the eye are: Aqueous humor and vitreous humor
- Internal ear is made up of two parts, one within the other.
- Iris lies behind cornea in front of lens.
- Lens is circular biconvex elastic structure lying behind the pupil.

CHAPTER 7

Musculoskeletal System

CONCEPTUAL THEORY

Terminology

150+ key terminologies for Quick Recall & Revision

Joint: As a junction of two or more bones or cartilages. It is a device to permit movements.
Muscle: It is a contractile tissue which causes movements. These are like motors of the body.
Parts of a young long bone: Diaphysis, metaphysis, growth plate, in center, epiphyses and articular cartilage at each end.
Periosteum: Outer covering of bone is made of fibrous and an osteogenic layer. Richly supplied by blood and nerves.
Skeletal/striped/somatic/voluntary muscles: These are maximum in amount; present on the external aspect of various regions of the body.
Types of cartilages: Hyaline, e.g., costal cartilages, white fibro, e.g., intervertebral disk, yellow elastic, e.g., epiglottis.
Types of ossification: Intramembranous, i.e., membrane bone. Intracartilaginous, i.e., membrane cartilage replaced by bone.
Visceral/unstriped/involuntary muscles: They are present inside the body cavity, e.g., digestive system, genitourinary system and all blood vessels.

BONES – TYPES, STRUCTURE, GROWTH AND OSSIFICATION

Bone type	Anatomical structure	Growth and ossification	Examples
Long bones	Long, cylindrical shape with expanded ends (epiphyses)	Growth occurs at the epiphyseal plates, which are made of cartilage that ossifies over time	Femur, Humerus, Tibia, Fibula
Short bones	Cuboidal shape with a spongy interior	Growth occurs through appositional growth (outer layer of bone thickens)	Carpals (Wrist Bones), Tarsals (Ankle Bones)
Flat bones	Thin, flat shape with two layers of compact bone enclosing spongy bone	Growth occurs through appositional growth	Skull Bones, Scapula, Sternum
Irregular bones	Complex, irregular shape with varying amounts of compact and spongy bone	Growth occurs through appositional growth	Vertebrae, Hip Bones, Facial Bones
Sesamoid bones	Small, rounded bones embedded within tendons or joint capsules	Formed in response to stress or friction on tendons	Patella (Kneecap)
Pneumatized bones	Contain air-filled spaces or sinuses	Formed by the extension of air-filled cavities into the bone	Ethmoid Bone (within the skull), Maxillary Sinuses (within the facial bones)

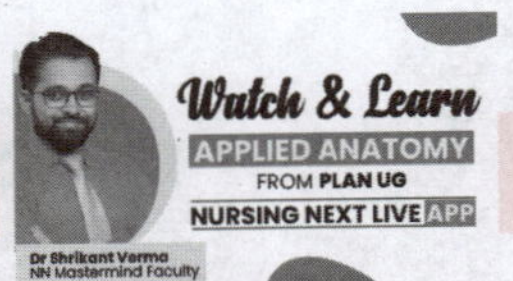

AXIAL AND APPENDICULAR SKELETON

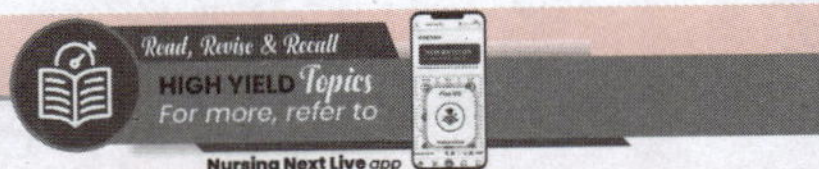

Skeleton component	Characteristics	Anatomy and structure	Examples
Axial skeleton	• Forms the central axis of the body	• Composed of bones along the midline of the body, including the skull, vertebral column, and rib cage	Skull, Vertebral Column, Rib Cage
	• Protects vital organs and supports body weight	• Skull: Comprises cranial bones and facial bones, enclosing and protecting the brain and sensory organs	Cranial Bones (Frontal, Occipital), Facial Bones
		• Vertebral column: Made up of individual vertebrae, providing structural support, flexibility, and protecting the spinal cord	Cervical Vertebrae, Thoracic Vertebrae
		• Rib cage: Consists of ribs and sternum, forming the ribcage that protects the heart and lungs	True Ribs, Sternum
		• Hyoid bone: A U-shaped bone located in the neck, supporting the tongue and facilitating swallowing	Hyoid Bone
		• Sacrum and coccyx: Fused bones at the base of the vertebral column, providing stability and support	Sacrum, Coccyx
Appendicular skeleton	• Supports and facilitates movement	• Composed of bones of the upper and lower limbs, as well as the girdles that connect them to the axial skeleton	Upper Limbs (Arm, Forearm, Hand), Lower Limbs (Thigh, Leg, Foot)
		• Pectoral girdle: Consists of the scapula and clavicle, attaching the upper limbs to the axial skeleton	Scapula, Clavicle
		• Pelvic girdle: Formed by the hip bones (coxal bones), connecting the lower limbs to the axial skeleton	Hip Bones (Ilium, Ischium, Pubis)
		• Upper limbs: Comprises the humerus, radius, ulna, carpals, metacarpals, and phalanges, facilitating arm and hand movement	Humerus, Radius, Ulna, Carpals, Metacarpals, Phalanges
		• Lower limbs: Consists of the femur, tibia, fibula, tarsals, metatarsals, and phalanges, supporting walking and running	Femur, Tibia, Fibula, Tarsals, Metatarsals, Phalanges

JOINTS – CLASSIFICATION, MAJOR JOINTS AND STRUCTURE

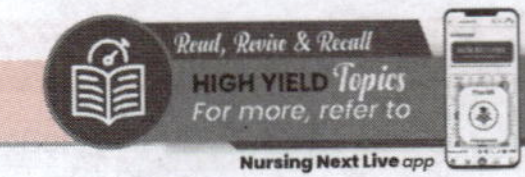

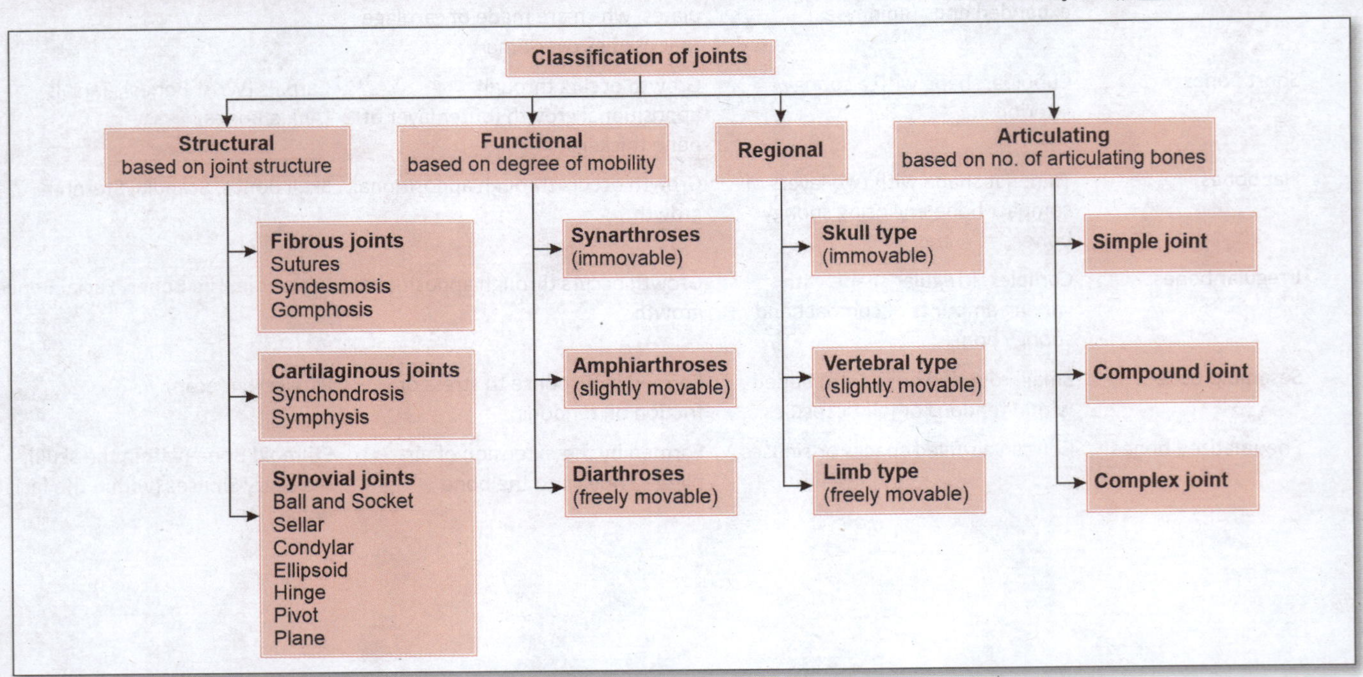

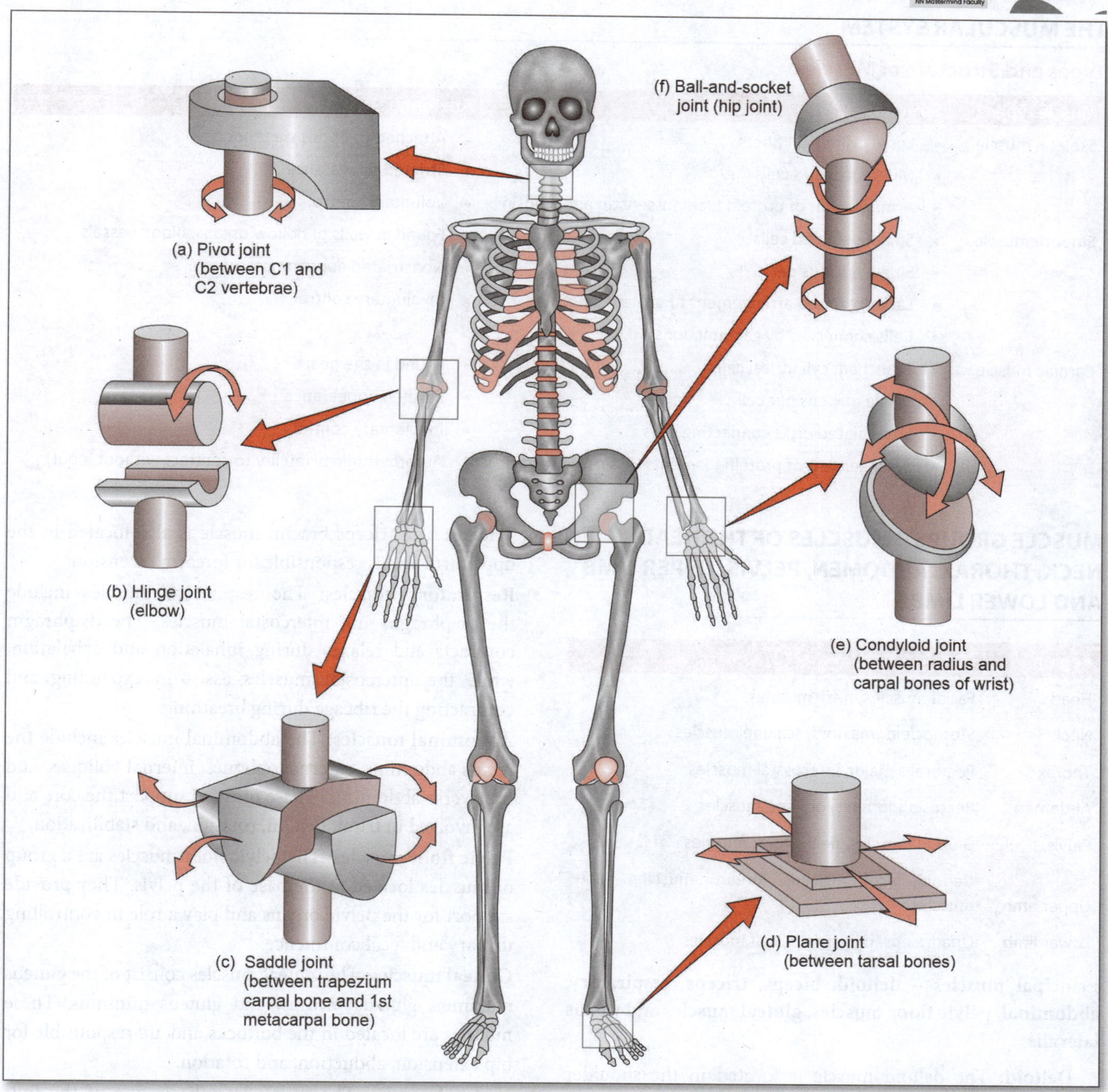

Figure 7.1: Types of synovial joints

APPLICATIONS AND IMPLICATIONS IN NURSING

- **Patient assessment:** Nurses use their understanding of musculoskeletal anatomy to conduct comprehensive physical assessments of patients. They assess the range of motion, muscle strength, joint stability, and overall musculoskeletal health to identify abnormalities, injuries, or potential complications.
- **Injury and fracture management:** Nurses play a crucial role in the management of musculoskeletal injuries and fractures. They assist in immobilization techniques, such as splinting or casting, to support the affected area and promote proper healing.
- **Safe patient handling and mobility:** Understanding the anatomy of bones, joints, and muscles helps nurses determine the appropriate techniques and assistive devices to minimize the risk of injury and ensure patient comfort.

THE MUSCULAR SYSTEM

Types and Structure of Muscles

Muscle type	Structure	Anatomy
Skeletal muscle	• Long, cylindrical fibers	• Attached to bones via tendons
	• Multinucleated cells	• Striated appearance
	• Arrangement of protein filaments: Actin and myosin	• Voluntary control
Smooth muscle	• Spindle-shaped cells	• Found in walls of hollow organs, blood vessels
	• Single nucleus per cell	• Nonstriated appearance
	• Lack organized arrangement of protein filaments	• Involuntary control
	• Cells connected by gap junctions	
Cardiac muscle	• Branched, cylindrical cells	• Found in the heart
	• Single nucleus per cell	• Striated appearance
	• Intercalated disks connecting cells	• Involuntary control
	• Arrangement of protein filaments: Actin and myosin	• Autorhythmicity (ability to contract without input)

MUSCLE GROUPS – MUSCLES OF THE HEAD, NECK, THORAX, ABDOMEN, PELVIS, UPPER LIMB AND LOWER LIMBS

Region	Muscle groups
Head	Facial muscles, neck muscles
Neck	Sternocleidomastoid, scalene muscles
Thorax	Pectoralis major, intercostal muscles
Abdomen	Rectus abdominis, oblique muscles
Pelvis	Gluteal muscles, pelvic floor muscles
Upper limb	Deltoid, biceps, triceps, forearm muscles, hand muscles
Lower limb	Quadriceps, hamstrings, calf muscles

Principal muscles – deltoid, biceps, triceps, respiratory, abdominal, pelvic floor muscles, gluteal muscles and vastus lateralis

- **Deltoid:** The deltoid muscle is located in the shoulder region and is responsible for shoulder abduction, flexion, and extension.
- **Biceps:** The biceps brachii muscle is located in the upper arm and is responsible for forearm flexion and supination.
- **Triceps:** The triceps brachii muscle is also located in the upper arm and is responsible for forearm extension.
- **Respiratory muscles:** The respiratory muscles include the diaphragm and intercostal muscles. The diaphragm contracts and relaxes during inhalation and exhalation, while the intercostal muscles assist in expanding and contracting the ribcage during breathing.
- **Abdominal muscles:** The abdominal muscles include the rectus abdominis, external obliques, internal obliques, and transverse abdominis. These muscles support the core and are involved in trunk flexion, rotation, and stabilization.
- **Pelvic floor muscles:** The pelvic floor muscles are a group of muscles located at the base of the pelvis. They provide support for the pelvic organs and play a role in controlling urinary and fecal continence.
- **Gluteal muscles:** The gluteal muscles consist of the gluteus maximus, gluteus medius, and gluteus minimus. These muscles are located in the buttocks and are responsible for hip extension, abduction, and rotation.
- **Vastus lateralis:** The vastus lateralis is one of the four muscles that makes up the quadriceps muscle group. It is located on the front and outer side of the thigh and is responsible for knee extension.

Major Muscles Involved in Nursing Procedures

Nursing procedure	Major muscles involved
Moving and positioning patients	Deltoids, biceps, triceps, gluteal muscles, quadriceps, hamstrings
Assisting with ambulation	Quadriceps, hamstrings, gluteal muscles, calf muscles
Lifting and transferring patients	Deltoids, biceps, triceps, gluteal muscles, quadriceps, hamstrings
Performing CPR	Pectoralis major, trapezius, deltoids, intercostal muscles

Contd...

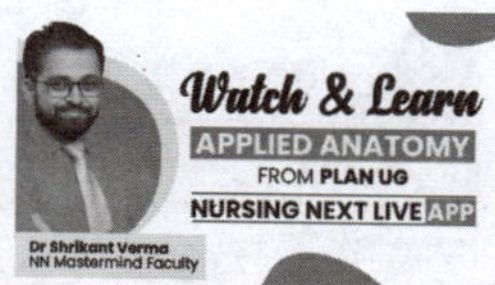

Nursing procedure	Major muscles involved
Administering injections	Deltoids, gluteal muscles, vastus lateralis
Assisting with range of motion (ROM)	Various muscle groups depending on the joint and movement needed
Assisting with Wound Care	Various muscle groups depending on the location of the wound
Assisting with Breathing Exercises	Diaphragm, intercostal muscles
Assisting with Urinary Catheterization	Pelvic floor muscles

CONCEPTUAL EXERCISES

LONG ANSWER QUESTIONS

1. Write origin, insertion, nerve supply and actions of temporalis. (RUHS)

Answer

Introduction

- Temporalis is thin, fan shaped muscle involved with mastication.
- It is situated within the temporal fossa of the skull.
  - **Origin:** Temporal fossa
  - **Insertion:** Coronoid process of the mandible, anterior margin of the ramus of the mandible
  - **Innervation:** Deep temporal nerves (branches of the mandibular nerve)
  - **Action:** Elevation and retraction of the mandible
- It is divided into anterior and posterior parts.
  - Anterior fibers run inferiorly in an almost vertical direction
  - Posterior fibers run almost horizontally

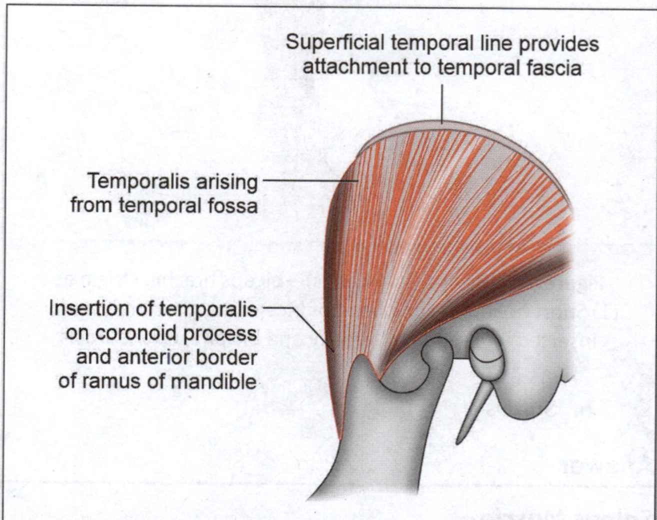

Figure 7.2: Temporalis muscles-insertion and origin

- Anterior and posterior fibers converge on a narrow tendon and run medial to the zygomatic arch. The tendon inserts onto the apex and medial surface of the coronoid process of mandible.
- **Inferiorly:** Temporal fossa
- **Superficially:** Temporal fascia, masseter, subcutaneous tissue and skin.
- Also related to the superficial aspect of temporalis muscle are the auriculotemporal, facial and zygomaticotemporal nerves.

Innervation

Anterior, middle and posterior deep temporal branches of the anterior trunk of mandibular nerve.

Blood Supply

- Deep temporal branches of the maxillary artery
- Temporal branches of the superficial temporal artery.

Function

- Strongest muscle of the temporomandibular joint and the primary retractor of the mandible.
- Contraction of
  - Anterior fibers—causes elevation of the mandible
  - Posterior fibers—causes retrusion of the mandible
- Together they result in closure of the mouth.
- Unilateral contraction of the temporalis muscle plays an important role in the side to side movements of the jaw.

Applied Anatomy

Tension of the temporal muscles can induce in the temporal area. Common causes include:

- Misalignment of the teeth
- Traumatic injuries
- Prolonged immobilization
- Prolonged opening due to dental innervation.

2. Write origin, insertion, nerve supply and actions of the following muscles. (RUHS)

a. **Biceps brachial.**
b. **Soleus.**

Answer

Biceps Brachial

- Chief muscle of arm
- It is involved in few movements of arm
- It originates at the scapula and inserts into the radius, thus, acts on both the shoulder and elbow joint.
- It is large, thick muscle of the arm consisting of two heads:
  - Long head
    - Supraglenoid tubercle above the glenoid cavity of the scapula.
    - Lies within the intracapsular space
    - Long biceps tendon makes a sharp turn at the humeral head and continues its course in the bicipital groove (intertubercular sulcus)
  - Short head
    - Arises at the apex of the coracoid process of the scapula.

Origin

- **Short head:** Apex of the Coracoid process of the scapula
- **Long head:** Supraglenoid tubercle of the scapula
- Both heads unite to one large muscle belly at the anterior side of the humerus and attach to the radial tuberosity.
- **Inferiorly:** Brachialis and coracobrachialis muscle
- Both its origin tendons are covered by the deltoid, its insertion tendon can be easily seen.
- The space between the biceps and triceps forms the medial and lateral bicipital grooves.
- The medial bicipital grooves contain the brachial artery and both the ulnar and median nerves.
- The lateral bicipital groove contains the radial nerve.

Insertion

- Radial tuberosity of the radius
- Deep fascia of forearm

Nervous Innervation

Musculocutaneous nerve (C5–C6), branch of brachial plexus.

Blood Supply

Brachial artery

Function

- Muscles of two joints:
  1. **Shoulder joint:** Both muscle heads partially enforce the opposite movements
     - The long head pulls the arm away from the trunk (abduction) and causes inward rotation.
     - The short head causes adduction.
     - When both heads contract together, it causes flexion of arm.
  2. **Elbow joint:** Flexion and supination of the forearm at the elbow joint.
- Weak flexor of the arm at the glenohumeral joint
- The biceps also functions to support the head of the humerus within the shoulder joint.

Applied Anatomy

- Helps in the measurement of the brachial pulse.
- Serves as a reference muscle for the nerve roots C5 and C6 (testing of the biceps reflex)
- Biceps tendinitis – inflammation of the long biceps tendon – often caused by bursitis or tendinitis involving the rotator cuff.
- Biceps tendon ruptures in severe injuries to this region.

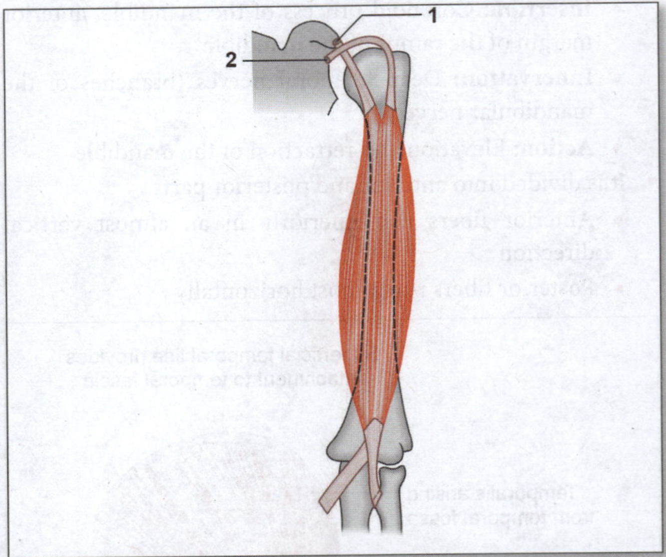

Figure 7.3: Biceps (two heads)—biceps brachii: Origin as (1) Short head, (2) Long head of biceps brachii with its belly. Inserted into radial tuberosity and bicipital aponeurosis

b. **Soleus**

Answer

Soleus Muscle

- Wide flat leg muscle found on the posterior leg.

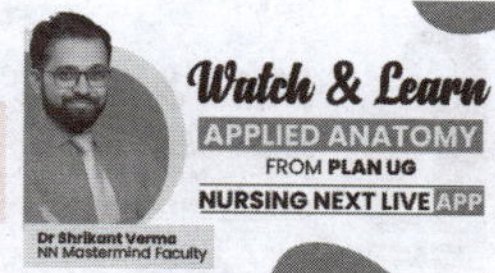

- Originates below the knee and continues till the heel.
- It lies immediately deep into the gastrocnemius.
- Forms the superficial posterior compartment of the calf muscles along with the gastrocnemius and plantaris muscle.
- Results in strong plantar flexion.
- It helps in maintaining an upright posture – antigravity muscle.

Origin

- Soleal line
- Medial border of the tibia
- Head of fibula
- Posterior border of fibula
- Also from the tendinous arch of the soleus.

Insertion

- Posterior surface of calcaneus (via calcaneal tendon)
- It runs along the gastrocnemius muscle and inserts into the posterior surface of the calcaneus via the calcaneal tendon. This is the strongest tendon in humans – easily visible and palpable at the heel.

Innervation

Tibial nerve (S1–S2)

Blood Supply

- Arterial supply
  - Superior branch—popliteal artery
  - Inferior branch—peroneal artery (fibular artery) or the posterior tibial artery.
  - Minor accessory arteries arise from peroneal, posterior tibial and lateral sural arteries.
- Venous drainage
  - Venous plexus formed by the popliteal vein.

Function

- Talocrural joint
- Foot plantar flexion—enabling the lifting the heel against gravity when walking or jumping.
- Part of the anti-gravity muscles—maintains the upright posture.

Clinical Relations

- Soleus tear
  - Results from overuse or sports injuries
  - Causes lateral calf pain on either side of soleus
- Soleus pain
  - May or may not be a symptom of soleus tear.

3. Write Origin, insertion, nerve supply, applied anatomy of gluteus maximus. (MGR, RUHS)

Answer

Gluteus Maximus Muscle

- Most superficial gluteal muscle
- Forms the prominence of the gluteal region.
- Belongs to the gluteal group of hip muscles.
- Other muscles of this group are:
  - Gluteus medius
  - Gluteus minimus
  - Tensor fasciae latae
- Extends from the pelvis to the gluteal tuberosity of femur.
- Innervated by the inferior gluteal nerve (L5–S2).
- Its main functions include extension and external rotation of the thigh at the hip joint.

Origin

- The gluteus maximus muscle originates from the
  - Lateroposterior surface of sacrum and coccyx
  - Gluteal surface of ilium (behind the posterior gluteal line)
  - Thoracolumbar fascia
  - Sacrotuberous ligament
- The muscle fibers take an inferolateral course, overhanging the femur.

Insertion

- The most superficial three quarters of the muscle form a tendinous lamina that inserts between the two layers of the fascia lata. The deeper part of the muscle inserts into the gluteal tuberosity of femur via a broad aponeurosis.
- It is enveloped in a thin fascia that separates it from the adjacent subcutaneous tissue.

Structures Under the Cover of Gluteus Maximus

- Ilium
- Sacrum
- Coccyx
- Ischial tuberosity
- Greater trochanter of femur
- Sacrotuberous and sacrospinous ligaments
- Gluteus medius
- Piriformis
- Superior and inferior gemelli
- Obturator internus and externus
- Quadratus femoris

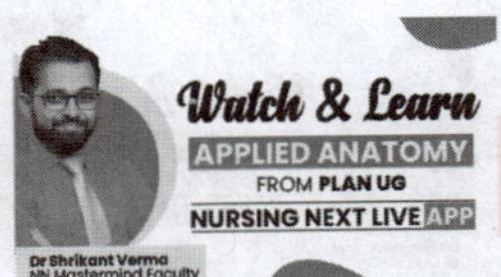

- Origin of Biceps (Long head)
- Semitendinosus
- Semimembranosus
- Adductor magnus

Structures Passing through Greater Sciatic Foramen

- Superior to piriformis
  - Superior gluteal vein and nerve.
- Inferior to Piriformis
  - Inferior Gluteal vein and nerve.
  - Sciatic nerve
  - Posterior cutaneous nerve of thigh
  - Pudendal nerve
  - Internal pudendal vein
  - Nerve to obturator internus
  - Nerve to quadratus femoris
  - Terminal branch of medial circumflex artery
  - Ist perforating artery

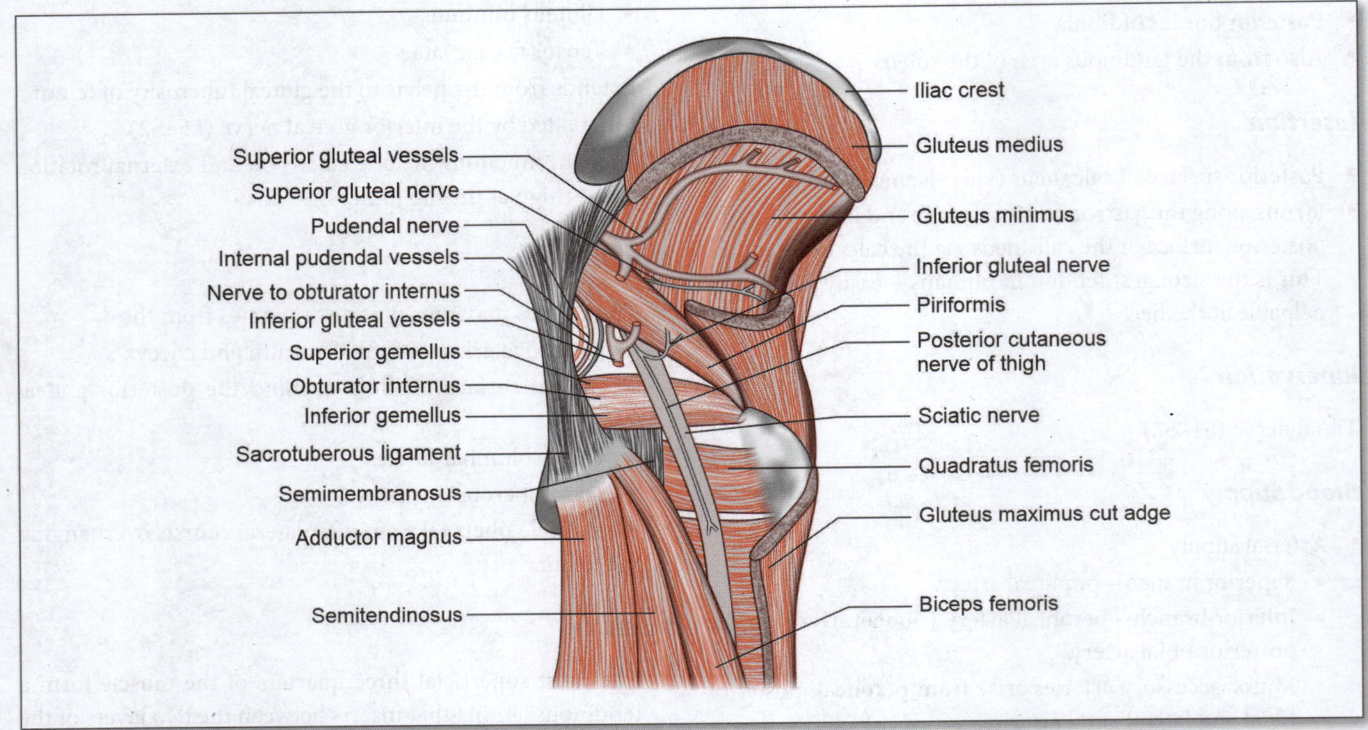

Figure 7.4: Structures under the cover of gluteus maximus

Nerve Supply

Inferior gluteal nerve (L5, S1, S2)

Blood Supply

Inferior gluteal and superior gluteal arteries, branches of internal iliac artery.

Functions

- The gluteus maximus muscle exhibits four actions on the hip joint:
  - Extension of thigh
  - External rotation of thigh
  - Abduction of thigh (superior part)
  - Adduction of thigh (inferior part)

4. Define a joint. Explain the features of synovial joints. Classify various types of synovial joints with suitable examples and applied anatomy. (MGR)

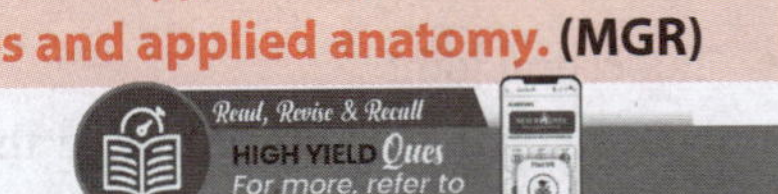

Answer

Definition

A joint is formed where one or more bones articulate together. Joints may or may not allow movement.

Classification of Joints

Based on the tissue they unite:

- Fibrous joints
- Cartilaginous joints
- Synovial joints

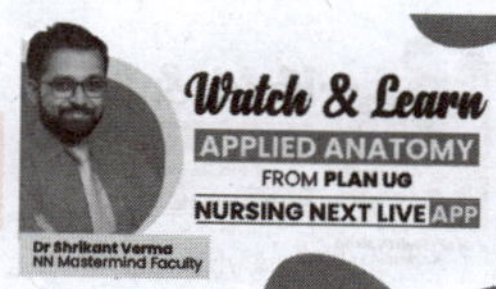

Synovial Joints

- Most common joints in body
- Provide free movement
- These joints are lined by synovial membrane and contain synovial fluid
- The synovial fluid lubricates the joint cavity.

Characteristic Features of Synovial Joints

- Joint cavity covered by capsule
- An articular cartilage
- An articular capsule lined internally by a synovial membrane.

Components of Synovial Joints

- Articular surface:
  - Consists of corresponding ends of articulating bones
- Articular cartilage:
  - Covers the articular surfaces of the articulating bones.
  - Made of hyaline cartilage
  - It has no perichondrium and no regenerative power.
  - This provides a smooth gliding surface and reduces the forces of compression during weight bearing.
  - It is porous and absorbs fluid.
- Synovial fluid
  - Clear pale yellow viscous alkaline fluid
  - Dialysate of blood plasma with hyaluronic acid, sulfate free glycosaminoglycans.
  - Functions
    - Provides nutrition to articular cartilage
    - Provides lubrication to the joint cavity
    - Prevents wear and tear of the joint
- Synovial membrane
  - Cellular connective tissue membrane
  - Pink in color, smooth and shiny
  - Mesenchymal in origin
  - Articular cartilage and menisci are not lined by smooth membrane.
  - Functions:
    - Secretes synovial fluid
    - Liberates hyaluronic acid
    - Removes particulate matter from synovial fluid.
- Joint cavity
  - It is enclosed within a fibrous capsule.
  - It is lubricated by the synovial fluid.
- Articular capsule
  - Consists of fibrous capsule lined by synovial membrane.
  - Formed by bundles of collagen fibers arranged in irregular pattern.
- Articular disk or meniscus
  - Made of fibrocartilage and divides the joint into two incomplete or complete joint cavities.
  - Helps in increasing the range of movement
- Labrum
  - Made of fibrocartilage
  - Increases the depth of the cavity
  - Provides stability to the joint
- Ligaments
  - Two types – true and accessory
  - Provide stability to the joint

Classification of Synovial Joints

Type	Axes of movements	Example
• **Plane or gliding**	All axes	Intercarpal joints
• **Uniaxial joints**		
▪ Hinge joint	Transverse	Elbow joint, ankle joint
▪ Pivot joint	Vertical	Superior and inferior radioulnar joints
• **Biaxial joints**		
▪ Condylar joint	Transverse and vertical	Knee joint
▪ Ellipsoid joint	Transverse and antero-posterior axes	Wrist joint
• **Multiaxial joints**		
▪ Ball-and-socket joint	Transverse, antero-posterior and vertical axes	Shoulder and hip joints
▪ Saddle joint	Transverse and antero-posterior axes with rotation	1st carpometacarpal joint

Applied Anatomy

- **Sprain and strain:** Forcible movement of joints results in ligament tear leading to sprain. Partial tearing of the ligament causes strain.
- **Dislocation and subluxation:** Dislocation is displacement of a bone from a joint resulting in tear of ligament, tendons and capsule. The most commonly dislocated joint in adult is shoulder joint. Subluxation is the partial or incomplete dislocation.
- **Rheumatoid arthritis:** Chronic inflammatory autoimmune disease associated with the primary involvement of synovial membrane but heart, blood vessels and skin are also affected. More common in females.
- **Osteoarthritis:** Degenerative non-inflammatory disease of joints associated with gradual thinning of articular cartilage. It is due to aging and affects large weight bearing joints, like knees, hips and spine.

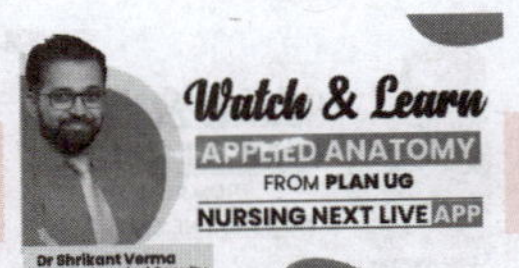

- **Ankylosing spondylitis:** An autoimmune inflammatory arthritis. Usually, sacroiliac joint, spine and bigger joints like hip and shoulder are affected.
- **Acute septic arthritis:** Joints affected by bacterial infection. More common in children. Usually spread by blood.
- **Gout:** Inflammatory disorder usually caused due to deposition of sodium urate crystal in joints and tendons.

Other conditions like:
- Fracture into the joint space
- Stiffness of joints
- Neuropathic joint

SHORT NOTES

1. Write a short note on the Haversian system of bones. (KUHS)

Answer

Introduction

- The Haversian system of bones refers to the arrangement of osteons and lamellae.
- Seen in compact bone.

Structure and Function

- An osteon comprises a long, hollow central canal that is surrounded by concentric layers called lamellae.
- This hollow central canal is known as Haversian canal.
- The long axis of the osteon is parallel to the long axis of the bone.
- Each osteon has a cylindrical structure that is composed of:
  - Haversian canals are present in the center. Small blood vessels that are present in the central canal perform the function of supplying blood to the osteocytes.
  - It also contains nerve fibers or filaments.
  - Volkmann's canals connect these Haversian canals to each other. Volkmann's canals are transverse vessels that run perpendicular to the long axis.
  - These also connect the blood vessels present in the Haversian canals to the periosteum.
  - Volkmann's canals are not surrounded by the concentric lamellae.
- The Haversian canal system is formed by:
  - Lamellae—concentric rings of strong bone matrix. Mineral salts and collagen fibers lend strength to the matrix.
  - The lamellae consist of collagen fibers that run in different directions—this provides strength to the osteon.
  - Mineral salts such as calcium and phosphates are present in the matrix of the bone.
  - Lacunae are small spaces present between the lamellae. They contain osteocytes.
  - Nutrient canals or canaliculi connect the lacunae. These canals function to provide nutrients to the osteocytes and carry waste products from them.
  - Interstitial lamellae are seen between the osteons. These are remnants of the previous concentric lamellae.

Functions

- The Haversian system plays a vital role as it facilitates the supply of oxygenated blood and nutrients to the bones.
- The canaliculi network also facilitates the passage of substances between the blood vessels and the mature bone cells.

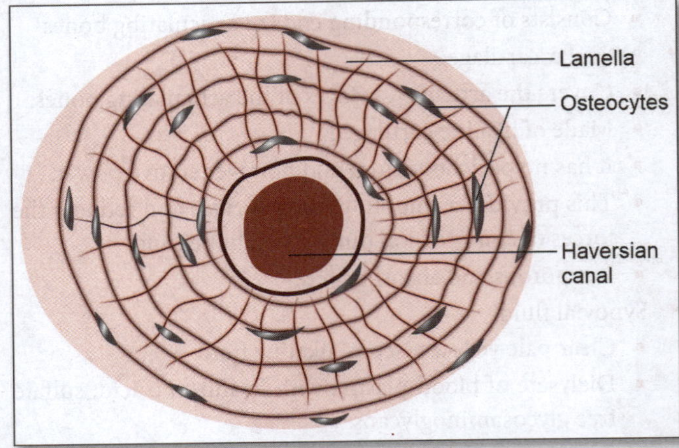

Figure 7.5: Haversian canal with osteocytes and lacuna

2. Write origin, insertion, nerve supply and applied anatomy of deltoid muscle. (RUHS)

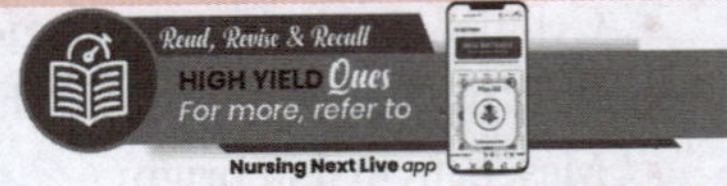

Answer

Introduction

- Deltoid muscle is a thick, triangular shoulder muscle.
- It has a wide origin spanning the clavicle, acromion and spine of scapula.
- It passes inferiorly surrounding the glenohumeral joint on all sides and inserts onto the humerus.
- It is formed by
  - Acromial part (middle fibers)
    - Abducts the arms
  - Clavicular part (anterior fibers)
    - Acts as a flexor and internal rotator of the arm
  - Scapular spinal part (posterior fibers)
    - Extends and externally rotates the arm.

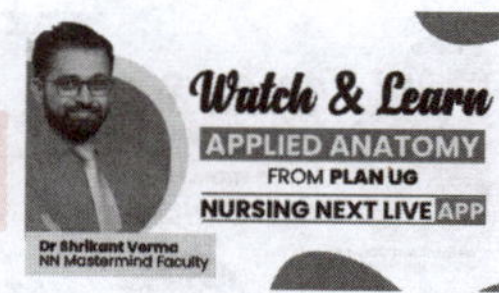

- Clavicular and scapular spinal parts play a significant role in stabilization, ensuring a steady plane of abduction.

Origin and Insertion

- The deltoid has three functionally and anatomically distinct parts. The origin of deltoid is from:
  1. Clavicular part—superior surface and anterior border of lateral 1/3rd of clavicle
  2. Acromial part—lateral margin and superior surface of acromion
  3. Spinal part—lateral 1/3rd of spine of scapula
- The muscle fibers then run inferiorly toward the humeral shaft and converge to a narrow strong tendon to insert into the deltoid tuberosity of humerus.
- The **acromial part**, sometimes also known as the middle or central, is the largest and the strongest. It is a multipennate muscle. It arises as four intramuscular septa, which interdigitate with the three tendons at the insertion site (one each for the anterior, posterior and middle parts). The four septa are connected by short and strong muscle fibers.
- The **clavicular** (anterior) and **scapular spinal** (posterior) **parts** are both unipennate and converge directly onto the inserting tendon.

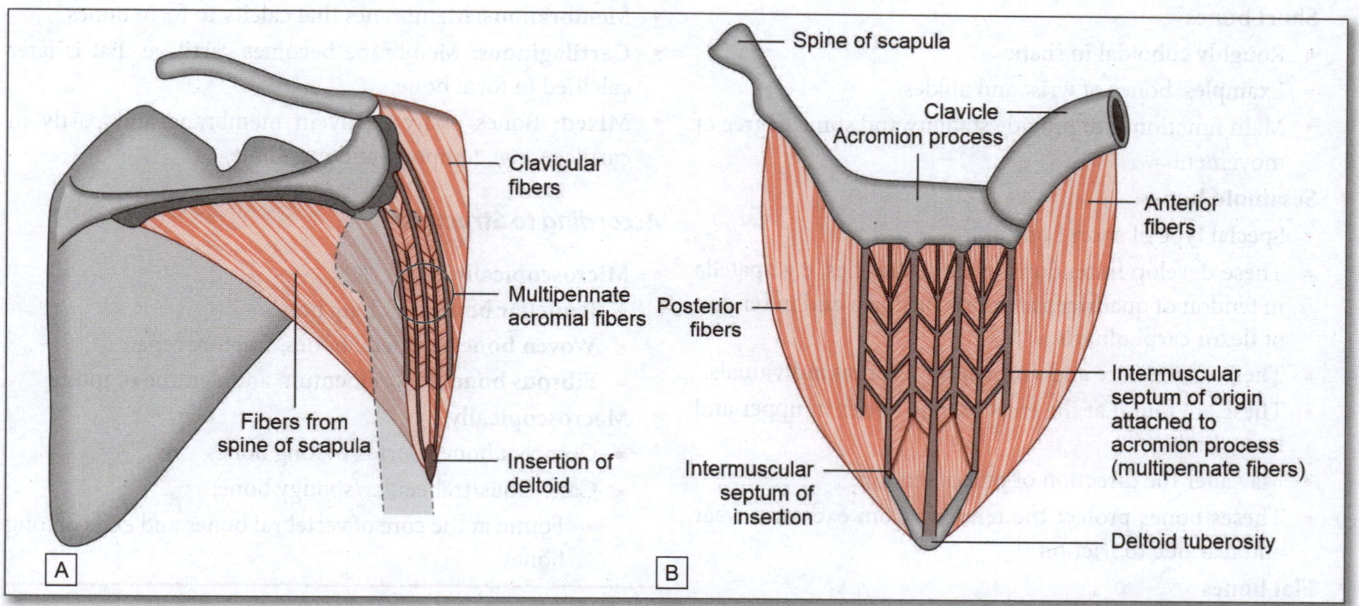

Figures 7.6A and B: Origin and insertion of the deltoid muscle

Nerve Supply

Axillary nerve (C5, C6), branch of brachial plexus

Blood Supply

- Deltoid and acromial branches of thoracoacromial artery
- Subscapular artery, branch of axillary artery
- Anterior and posterior circumflex humeral arteries
- Deltoid branch of deep brachial artery

Applied Anatomy

- **Axillary nerve palsy:** Damage to axillary nerve results in symptoms such as shoulder or arm muscle weakness, pain, numbness, arm muscle wasting, etc.
- **Rotator cuff tears:** Partial or complete tear of tendons results in deltoid strain leading to recurrent pain, muscle weakness, cracking or grating sound, etc.
- **Vascular injuries:** Damage to cephalic vein results in peripheral edema leading to nerve damage and the loss of muscle strength. Injury to the deltoid muscle can also damage the thoracoacromial artery, resulting in nerve injury, pain, spasms, and muscle atrophy.
- **Strains and overuse injuries:** Overstretching of the fibers results in pain and difficulty in moving the arms.
- **Tendonitis:** When the tendons in the shoulder get inflamed, it results in shoulder tendonitis. Symptoms may include pain and tenderness in the shoulder.

3. Write a short note on the classification of bones with examples. (MGR)

Answer

Classification of Bones

Bones are classified according to shape, position, ossification and structure.

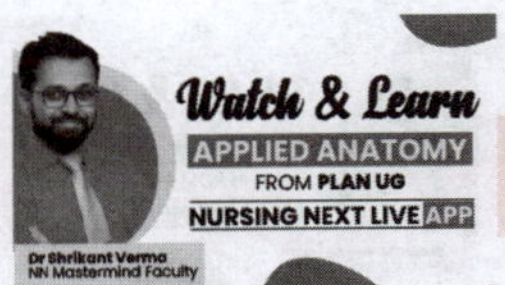

According to shape, bones may be classified into long, short, irregular, flat and sesamoid.

- **Long bones**
  - Length exceeds the width
  - Consist of shaft and two extremities. Shaft is made up of compact bone that encloses the medullary cavity.
  - Long bones ossify in cartilage—endochondral ossification.
  - These serve as weight bearers and provide attachments to muscles
  - Found in limbs, such as fibula, tibia, femur, radius, ulna, humerus
- **Short bones**
  - Roughly cuboidal in shape
  - Examples: bones of wrist and ankles.
  - Main function is to provide stability and some degree of movement.
- **Sesamoid bones**
  - Special type of short bone.
  - These develop in tendons of some muscles, e.g., patella in tendon of quadriceps femoris pisiform and in tendon of flexor carpi ulnaris.
  - These vary in size and number in different individuals.
  - These are found at the ends of long bones in upper and lower limbs.
  - May alter the direction of pull of tendon.
  - Theses bones protect the tendons from excessive wear and tear due to friction.
- **Flat bones**
  - Thin, flattened and usually bit curved
  - Made up of two plates of compact bone with spongy bone in between.
  - Formed by endochondral ossification
  - **Examples:** Sternum, scapula, ribs, most skull bones.
  - Main function is protection of organs such as brain, heart, etc.
- **Irregular bones**
  - Have irregular and variable shapes
  - In it, a thin layer of compact bone covers a mass of spongy bone.
  - Examples: vertebra and hip bones.
  - Its main function is to protect the internal structures such as spine and pelvic organs.

According to position, bones may be classified into axial and appendicular skeleton.

- **Axial skeleton**
  - The axial skeleton forms the central axis of the body. It transmits the weight from the upper extremities down to the lower extremities at the hip joints.
  - It is responsible for the upright position of the human body.
  - Axial skeleton includes:
    - Skull including mandible and ear ossicles
    - Hyoid bone
    - Sternum
    - 12 pairs of ribs
    - Vertebral column
- **Appendicular skeleton**
  - It consists of bones of upper and lower limbs.

According to ossification, bones may be classified into membranous, cartilaginous, and mixed.

- **Membranous:** Membranes that calcify to form bones.
- **Cartilaginous:** Membrane becomes cartilage that is later calcified to form bone.
- **Mixed:** Bones ossify partly in membrane and partly in cartilage, e.g., temporal and mandible.

According to Structure

- **Microscopically,**
  - **Lamellar bone:** e.g., long bones
  - **Woven bone:** e.g., fetal bones, fracture repair
  - **Fibrous bone:** e.g., cementum and dentine of tooth.
- **Macroscopically,**
  - Compact bone: Cortex of long bones
  - Cancellous/trabecular/spongy bone:
    - Found at the core of vertebral bones and ends of long bones.

4. Write a short note on sesamoid bones. (MGR)

Answer

Introduction

- Sesamoid bones are small round or ovoid bones embedded in certain tendons.
- Small nodular foci of bone or cartilage or both.
- Have a shape similar to sesame seeds—thus the name.
- They act to hold the tendon further away from the joint; thus, the angle of the tendon is increased—increasing the force of muscle.

Location

- The most common sesamoid bones are found in
  - Foot
    - Hallucal sesamoids
    - Lesser metatarsal sesamoids
    - Interphalangeal joints

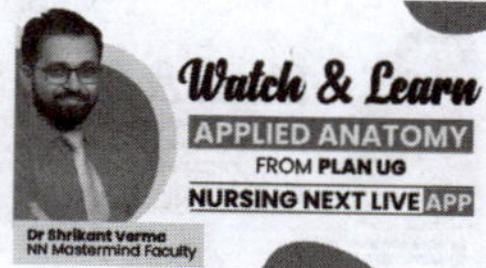

- Sesamoids of great toe
- Hand
  - Pollicis sesamoids
  - Second and fifth metacarpal
  - Interphalangeal joint of thumb
  - Pisiform
- Patella
- Fabella

Functions of Sesamoid Bones

- Protection of the tendons from damage
- Increase the mechanical advantage of the associated muscle.
- They modify pressure and decrease friction at the joint.

Types of Sesamoid Bones

- Type A and Type B
- **Type A:**
  - Located adjacent to an articulation with its tendon incorporated into the joint capsule
  - E.g., patella, halluces and pollicis
- **Type B:**
  - Located at sites where tendons are angled and separated from the underlying bone by a bursa
  - E.g., sesamoid of the peroneus longus tendon

5. Write a short note on parts of a long bone. (MGR)

Answer

Parts of Growing Lone Bone

- The growing long bone or a young bone consists of four regions:
  1. Diaphysis – shaft or the primary ossification center
  2. Metaphysis
  3. Epiphysis
  4. Epiphyseal growth plate

Diaphysis

- Largest part of bone.
- Also known as shaft of bone.
- Enveloped by periosteum.
- Within the shaft is the compact bone and medullary cavity.
- The cavity contains red bone marrow during childhood.
- At puberty it is replaced by yellow (fat) bone marrow, except at its ends.

Epiphysis

- Two ends of the bone are known as epiphysis.
- Between diaphysis and both the ends is the epiphyseal plate (growth plate) which causes an increase in the length of bone.

Metaphysis

- Epiphyseal end of diaphysis is metaphysis.
- At the age of puberty, growth of bone stops and metaphysis becomes a part of diaphysis.

Growth Plate

- Growth plate becomes bone; and diaphysis and epiphysis fuse.
- Made of hyaline cartilage
- Responsible for the growth of bone—increase in length.

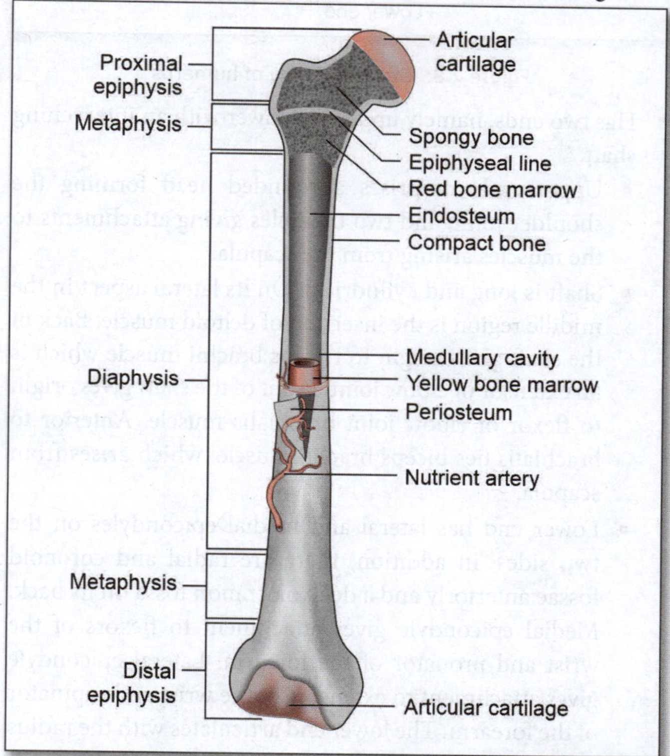

Figure 7.7: Structure of Long Bone

6. Write a short note on humerus. (RUHS)

Answer

Humerus

- Largest bone of upper limb.

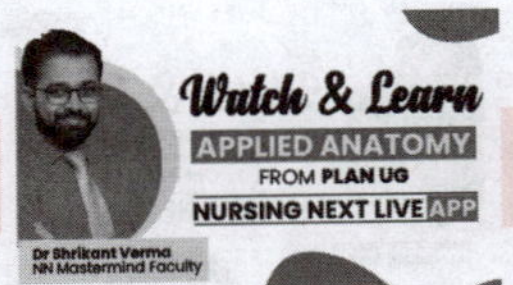

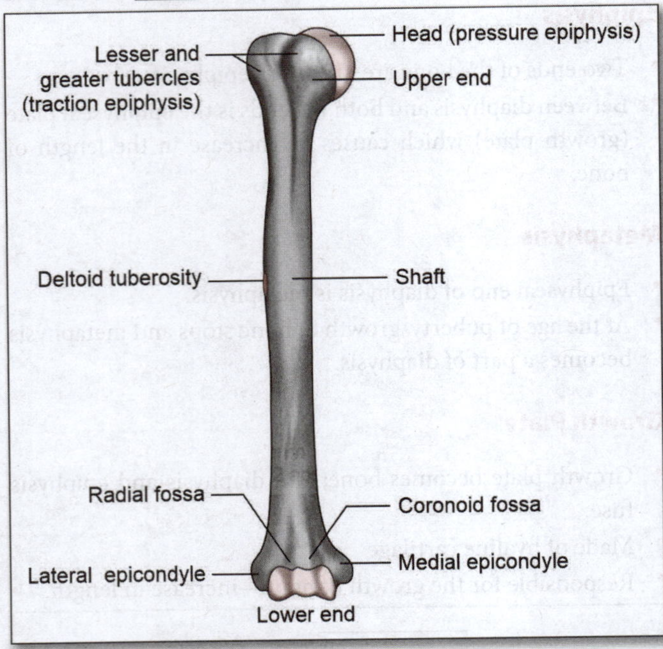

Figure 7.8: Gross anatomy of humerus

- Has two ends, namely upper and lower with an intervening shaft.
  - Upper end comprises a rounded head forming the shoulder joint, and two tubercles giving attachments to the muscles arising from the scapula.
  - Shaft is long and cylindrical. On its lateral aspect in the middle region is the insertion of deltoid muscle. Back of the shaft gives origin to triceps brachii muscle which is an extensor of elbow joint. Front of the shaft gives origin to flexor of elbow joint brachialis muscle. Anterior to brachialis lies biceps brachii muscle, which arises from scapula.
  - Lower end has lateral and medial epicondyles on the two sides; in addition, there are radial and coronoid fossae anteriorly and a deep olecranon fossa on its back. Medial epicondyle gives attachment to flexors of the wrist and pronator of the forearm. Lateral epicondyle gives attachment to extensors of the wrist and supinator of the forearm. The lower end articulates with the radius and ulna to form the elbow joint.
- Characteristic feature:
  - The head of the humerus articulates with scapula to form a ball and socket joint or shoulder joint.

Lower End of Humerus

The lower end of the humerus forms the condyle which is expanded from side to side and shows lateral supracondylar ridge; and medial supracondylar ridge is a similar ridge on the medial side.

The lower end of the humerus provides the following features:

Articular Part

- Trochlea, a medial pulley-shaped structure.
- Capitulum, a lateral rounded convex projection.
- Radial fossa, a small fossa above the capitulum.

Trochlea

The trochlea is pulley and it covers the anterior, posterior and inferior surfaces of the medial condyle of the humerus. It is in articulation with the ulna at the trochlear notch. During the extension of elbow, the posterior and inferior aspects are linked with the ulna. Whereas during the flexion of the elbow, the posterior part is no longer in contact, because the trochlear notch slides toward the anterior aspect of the humerus.

Capitulum

The capitulum is a convex and round projection, which covers the anterior and inferior surfaces of the lateral condyle of the humerus. It articulates with the head of the radius. During extension, the inferior surface is in contact with the radius; whereas during flexion, the radial head slides toward the anterior aspect of the humerus.

Nonarticular Part

- Coronoid fossa, a small fossa above the trochlea
- Medial epicondyle, a prominent projection on the medial side
- Lateral epicondyle, a prominent projection on the lateral side but less than the medial epicondyle
- Olecranon fossa, a big, deep hollow on the posterior aspect above the trochlea
- Distally, at the elbow joint, the capitulum of the humerus articulates with the head of the radius and the trochlea of the humerus articulates with the trochlear notch of the ulna.

Medial Epicondyle

Medial epicondyle is a projection superomedially present to the medial condyle, and forms at the termination of the medial border of the humerus. The ulnar nerve crosses its posterior surface. The superficial muscles of the anterior compartment of the forearm arise from the anterior surface of the medial epicondyle.

The muscles are the:

- Flexor carpi ulnaris
- Palmaris longus
- Flexor carpi radialis
- Pronator teres

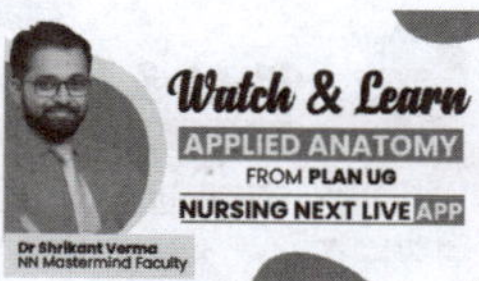

Lateral Epicondyle

- The lateral border of the humerus terminates at the lateral epicondyle.
- The muscles forming the epicondyle are:
  - Brachioradialis
  - Extensor carpi radialis longus
  - Extensor carpi radialis brevis
  - Extensor digitorum
  - Extensor digiti minimi
  - Extensor carpi ulnaris
  - Anconeus
- **Olecranon fossa**
  - The olecranon fossa is a deep hollow area on the posterior surface, superior to the trochlea. During extension of elbow, the tip of the ulnar olecranon process lodges into this fossa.
- **Coronoid fossa**
  - The coronoid fossa is a small hollow area located superior to the trochlea, but anteriorly. During flexion of the elbow, the coronoid process of the ulna lodges into the coronoid fossa. The radial fossa is present lateral to the coronoid fossa and superior to the capitulum.

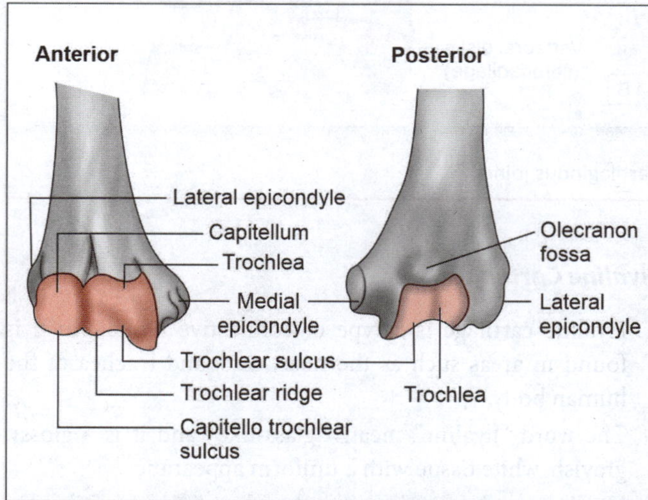

Figure 7.9: Lower end of humerus

Nursing Implication

The following nerves are located on the following aspects of the humerus:

- The axillary nerve: Surgical neck
- The radial nerve: Radial groove
- The median nerve: Distal humerus
- The ulnar nerve: Medial epicondyle
- If any of these aspects of the humerus is fractured, there may be damage to these nerves.

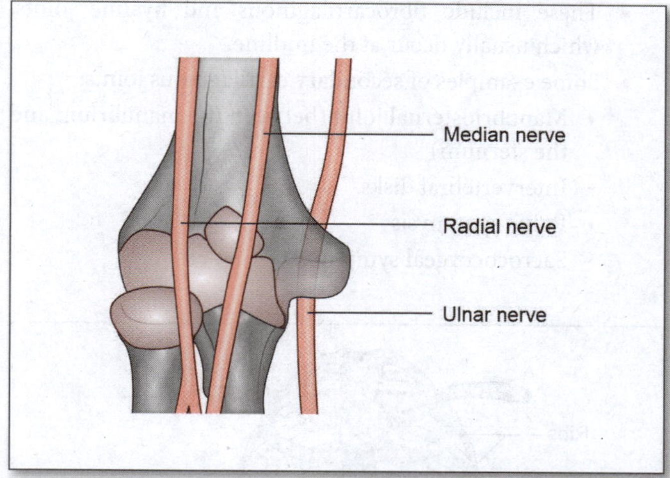

Intercondylar Fracture

An intercondylar fracture can occur due to a fall on the elbow while it is in flexion. This results in separation of one or both of the condyles from the shaft of the humerus.

7. Write a short note on cartilaginous joints. (DU)

Answer

Cartilaginous Joints

- Cartilaginous joints are connected entirely by the cartilage.
- These joints allow more movement between the joints than the fibrous joints but less than the highly mobile synovial joints.
- These joints form the growth regions of immature long bones and the intervertebral disks of the spinal column.

Types of Cartilaginous joints

- There are two types of joints
  1. Primary cartilaginous joints
  2. Secondary cartilaginous joint
- **Primary:**
  - Primary cartilaginous joints are known as "synchondrosis".
  - These joints are connected by hyaline cartilage and sometimes occur between ossification centers.
  - Examples of primary cartilaginous joints in humans:
    - "Growth plates" between ossification centers in long bones.
    - First sternocostal joint
    - Neurocentral joints of vertebrae
    - Petrobasilar synchondrosis
    - Spheno-occipital synchondrosis
  - These joints here allow for only a little movement, such as in the spine or ribs.
- **Secondary:**
  - These joints are known as "symphysis".

- These include fibrocartilaginous and hyaline joints, which usually occur at the midline.
- Some examples of secondary cartilaginous joints:
  - Manubriosternal joint (between the manubrium and the sternum)
  - Intervertebral disks
  - Pubic symphysis
  - Sacrococcygeal symphysis

Features of Cartilaginous Joints

- Lack a joint cavity
- Slightly movable joints
- These joints are united by cartilage
- They are mainly limited to axial skeleton, such as the vertebral column
- Provide stability and strength to the joints.

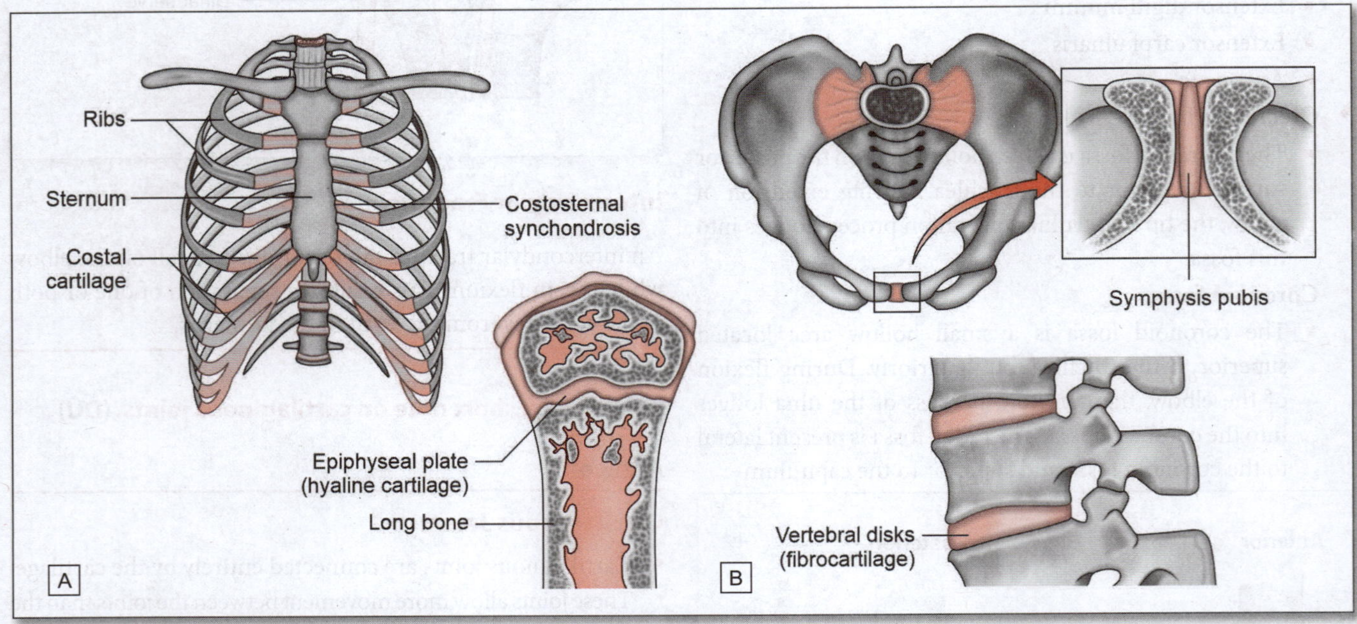

Figures 7.10A and B: Cartilaginous joints

8. Write a short note on types of cartilages. (DU)

Answer

Introduction

- Cartilage is a specialized connective tissue which provides strength and elasticity.
- Composed of cells and fibers embedded in a firm gel-like matrix which is rich in mucopolysaccharides.
- Characteristic features of cartilage are:
  - It is avascular
  - Has no nerve supply
  - Grows by appositional growth as well as interstitial growth
  - Has low antigenicity

Types of Cartilage

- Hyaline cartilage
- Elastic cartilage
- Fibrocartilage

Hyaline Cartilage

- Hyaline cartilage is a type of connective tissue which is found in areas such as the nose, ears, and trachea of the human body.
- The word "hyaline" means "glass-like", and it is a glossy, grayish-white tissue with a uniform appearance.
- Hyaline cartilage is the most abundant type of cartilage in the body.
- Microscopic Findings
  - When a thin slice of hyaline cartilage is examined under the microscope, it appears to consist of cells (chondrocytes) of a rounded or angular form, lying in groups of two or more in a granular or almost homogeneous matrix. The cells are contained in cavities in the matrix, called cartilage lacuna.
- Distribution
  - Present at the epiphyseal ends of bone in children
  - Present in articular cartilage, thyroid cartilage, tracheal rings, costal, bronchial and nasal cartilages.

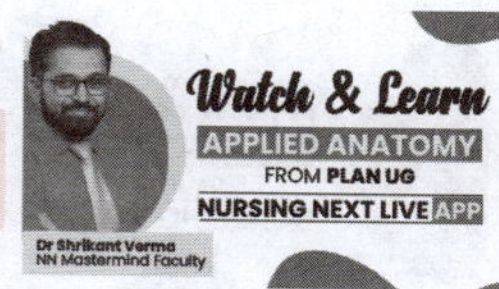

Elastic Cartilage

- In this, the matrix is traversed by yellow elastic fibers which anastomose and branch in all directions.
- Extracellular matrix is metachromatic—due to the presence of glycosaminoglycans
- Outer covering is known as perichondrium
- Distribution
  - Pinna of external ear
  - Epiglottis
  - Cuneiform cartilage
  - Apex of arytenoid cartilage
  - Auditory tube
  - External auditory meatus

Fibrocartilage

- Also known as the white cartilage.
- Macroscopically, it is dense fibrous tissue.
- Microscopically, it is made up of large bundles of type I collagen fibers.
- The fibers merge with fibers of surrounding connective tissues.
- It has great tensile strength and high elasticity.
- Distribution:
  - Intervertebral disc
  - Interpubic disk
  - Menisci of knee joint
  - Articular discks of temporomandibular joint

9. Write a short note on types of joints with examples. (MGR)

Answer

Introduction

A joint is formed where one or more bones articulate together. Joints may or may not allow movement.

Classification of Joints

Based on the tissue they unite:

- Fibrous joints
- Cartilaginous joints
- Synovial joints

Fibrous Joints

- Articulating surfaces connected by fibrous tissue.
- Types of fibrous joints
  - Sutures - E.g., frontal and parietal
  - Syndesmosis - E.g., interosseous membrane connects the radius and ulna.
  - Gomphosis- Present between the tooth and its socket

Cartilaginous Joints

- Cartilaginous joints are connected entirely by the cartilage.

Primary (Synchondrosis/hyaline cartilage joint)	Growth plate, Spheno-occipital joint, first chondrosternal joint, Costochondral joint
Secondary (Symphyses or fibrocartilaginous joint)	Symphysis pubis, Manubriosternal joint, intervertebral joint, Sacrococcygeal joint, Acromioclavicular joint

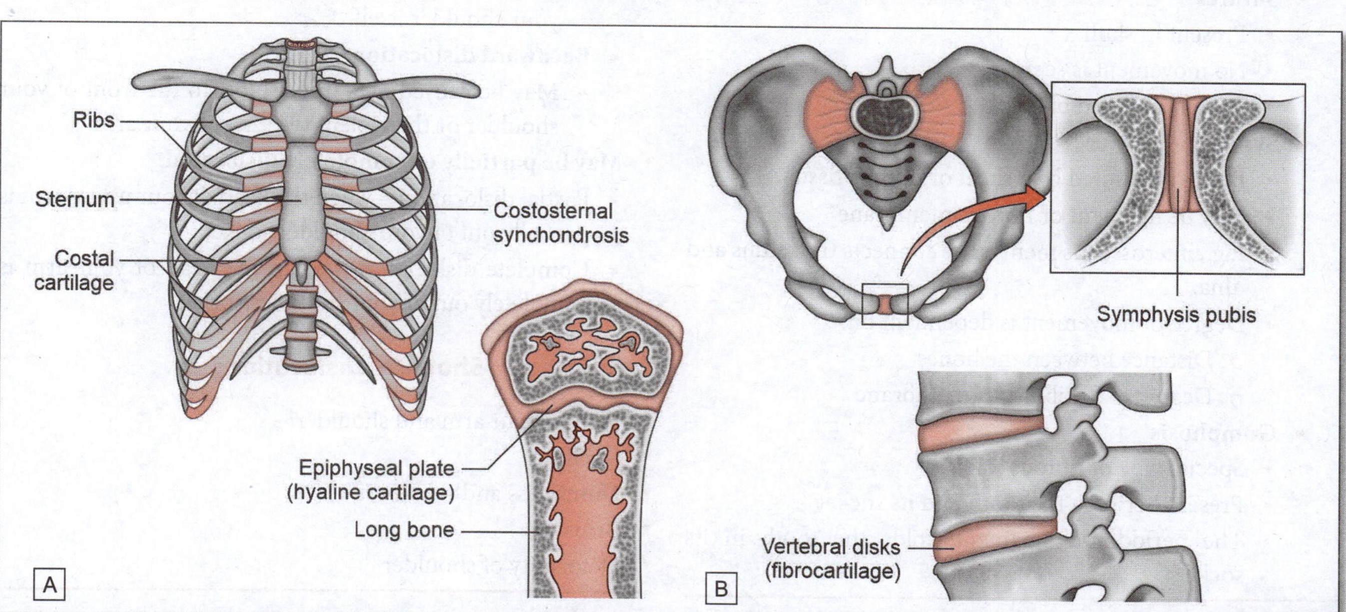

Figures 7.11A and B: Cartilaginous joints

Synovial Joints

- Most common joints in body
- Provide free movement

Classification of Synovial Joints

Type	Axes of movements	Example
• **Plane or gliding**	All axes	Intercarpal joints
• **Uniaxial joints** ▪ Hinge joint ▪ Pivot joint	 Transverse Vertical	 Elbow joint, ankle joint Superior and inferior radioulnar joints
• **Biaxial joints** ▪ Condylar joint ▪ Ellipsoid joint	 Transverse and vertical Transverse and antero-posterior axes	 Knee joint Wrist joint
• **Multiaxial joints** ▪ Ball-and-socket joint Saddle joint	 Transverse, antero-posterior and vertical axes Transverse and antero-posterior axes with rotation	 Shoulder and hip joints 1st carpometacarpal joint

10. Write a short note on fibrous joints. (RUHS)

Answer

Introduction

A joint is formed where one or more bones articulate together. Joints may or may not allow movement.

Fibrous Joints

- Articulating surfaces connected by fibrous tissue.
- Types of fibrous joints
  - **Sutures**
    - Present in skull
    - No movement is seen
    - E.g., frontal and parietal
  - **Syndesmosis**
    - Bones are united by a sheet of fibrous tissue.
    - May be ligament or fibrous membrane
    - E.g., interosseous membrane connects the radius and ulna.
    - Degree of movement is dependent on:
      - Distance between the bones
      - Degree of flexibility of membrane
  - **Gomphosis**
    - Special type of fibrous joint
    - Present between the tooth and its socket
    - The periodontal ligament holds the tooth in its socket.

11. Write a short note on the dislocation of shoulder joint. (MGR)

Answer

Introduction

- Dislocation is caused by significant force that separates your shoulder joint from the joint's socket.
- Can occur:
  - **Forward and downward dislocation**
    - Most common
    - Results from falling on your outstretched hand or on your shoulder itself.
  - **Backward dislocation**
    - May be caused by a direct blow to the front of your shoulder or the violent twisting of your arm.
- **May be partially or completely dislocated.**
  - Partial dislocation – when the head of your upper arm is partially out of your shoulder socket.
  - Complete dislocation – when the head of your arm is completely out of your shoulder socket.

Symptoms of Shoulder Dislocation

- Pain in your arm and shoulder
- Swelling
- Numbness and weakness
- Bruising
- Deformity of shoulder

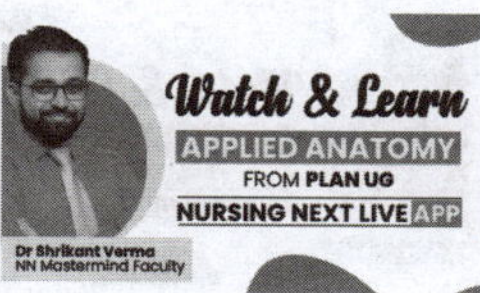

12. Write a note on locking and unlocking of knee joint. (RUHS)

Answer

Locking and Unlocking of Knee Joint

- **Locking:** It is the terminal stage of full extension of the knee joint.
- **Unlocking:** It is the early stage of flexion of the knee joint.

Mechanism of Locking

- The leg (the tibia) is laterally rotated and the thigh (the femur) is medially rotated.
- This rotator movement locks the joint (which means that the joint cannot be fixed unless it is unlocked by the reverse rotation.)
- In full extension with the locked knee, all the ligaments are stretched and the joint is stable.
- Produced by biceps femoris muscle.

Mechanism of Unlocking

The leg is medially rotated and the thigh is laterally rotated.

Movements

- **Locking of knee**
  - Lateral rotation of tibia, at the end of extension.
  - Results mainly by tension of anterior cruciate ligaments.
  - In locked knee, all ligaments become tight.
- **Unlocking of knee**
  - Medial rotation of tibia, at the beginning of flexion.
  - Performed by popliteus to relax ligaments and allow easy flexion.

13. Write a short note on the types of muscles. (MGR)

Answer

Introduction

- Muscles are contractile tissues which cause movements. These are like motors of the body.
- These movements may be voluntary or involuntary.
- Involve the use of energy.

Types of Muscles

- Skeletal muscles
  - Attached mainly to the skeletal bones and other structures.
  - Striated muscle – presence of banding pattern
- Cardiac muscles
  - Responsible for the rhythmic contractions of heart.
  - Cause involuntary movements
  - Presence of intercalated disks.
- Smooth muscles
  - Line the walls of organs

Skeletal Muscles

- Each muscle is made of numerous subunits or bundles called fascicles that are surrounded by connective tissue called the perimysium.
- Each fascicle is composed of numerous muscle fibers.
- Muscle cells are enclosed by endomysium and are made up of myofibrils.
- These myofibrils are composed of long protein molecules called myofilaments.

Two Ends

1. Origin
   - One end of the muscle remains fixed during contraction
2. Insertion
   - Other end moves during its contraction.
   - In the limb muscles, origin is usually proximal to insertion.

Two Parts

1. Fleshy part
   - Contractile and called the belly
2. Fibrous part
   - Noncontractile and nonelastic

Cardiac Muscles

- Cardiac muscle (also called heart muscle or myocardium) is one of the three types of vertebrate muscles, the other two being skeletal and smooth muscles. It is an involuntary, striated muscle that comprises the main tissues of the walls of the heart.
- Cardiac muscle fibers are interconnected through intercalated disks which consist of gap junctions that conduct electrical current throughout the cardiac muscle and it acts as functional syncytium.
- The cardiac muscle fibers form long loops which are attached to the fibrous skeleton. Upon contraction, the blood from the cardiac chambers is wrung out like water from a wet cloth. The atrial fibers are arranged in a superficial transverse layer and a deep anteroposterior layer.

Smooth Muscles

- Smooth muscles are spindle-shaped and have a single nucleus
- They lack striations.

- They contain actin and myosin and thick and thin filaments.
- Thin filaments are anchored by dense bodies.
- They line the hollow organs in the body.

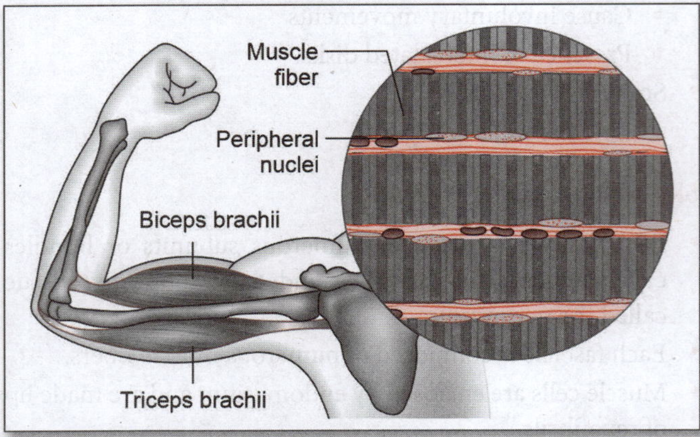

Figure. 7.12: Striated muscle (longitudinal section); biceps brachii and triceps brachii (upper arm)

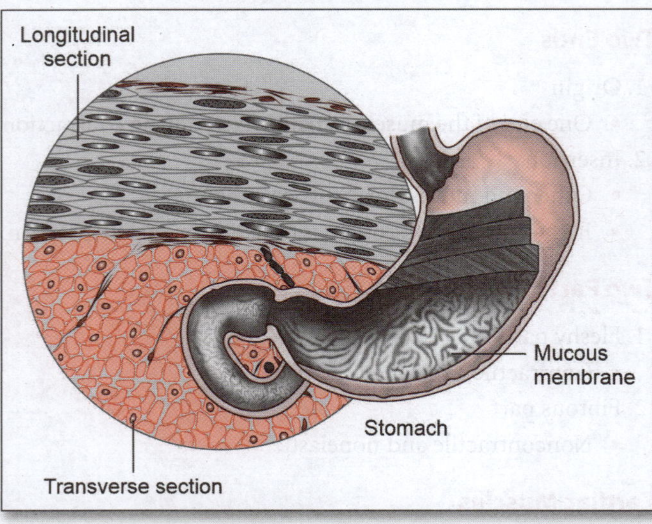

Figure 7.13: Smooth muscle

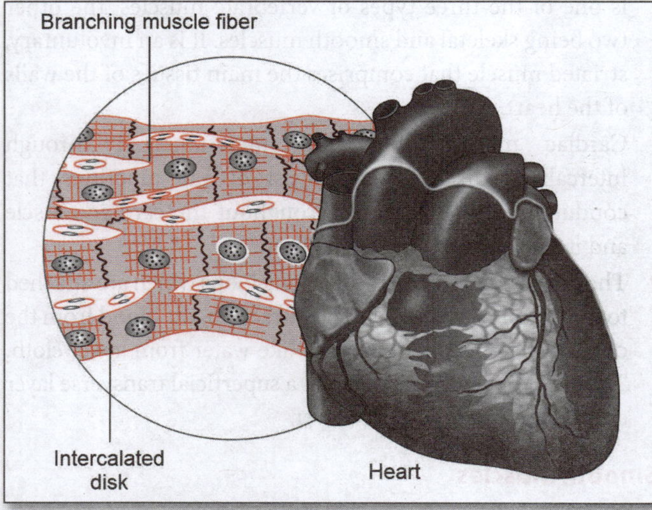

Figure 7.14: Cardiac muscle: Heart

14. Write a short note on quadriceps femoris muscle. (MGR)

Answer

Introduction

- The quadriceps femoris is a group of muscles located in front of the thigh.
- The group contains four separate muscles:
  1. Vastus lateralis
  2. Vastus medialis
  3. Vastus intermedius
  4. Rectus femoris

Origin and Insertion

The parts of the quadriceps femoris get their origin from:

- Vastus lateralis
  - Intertrochanteric line
  - Greater trochanter
  - Gluteal tuberosity
  - Linea aspera of femur
- Vastus medialis
  - Intertrochanteric line
  - Pectineal line of femur
  - Linea aspera
  - Medial supracondylar line of femur
- Vastus intermedius
  - Anterior surface of femoral shaft
- Rectus femoris
  - Anterior iliac spine
  - Supra-acetabular groove
- The rectus femoris and vastus intermedius insert into the tibial tuberosity (via patellar ligament) and patella
- The vastus lateralis inserts into the tibial tuberosity, patella and the lateral condyle of tibia.
- The vastus medialis inserts into the tibial tuberosity via the patellar ligament, patella and the medial condyle of tibia.

Innervation

By the femoral nerve (L2–L4)

Blood Supply

- Rectus femoris
  - Femoral artery
  - Lateral femoral circumflex artery
  - Superficial circumflex iliac arteries
- Vastus medialis
  - Femoral artery

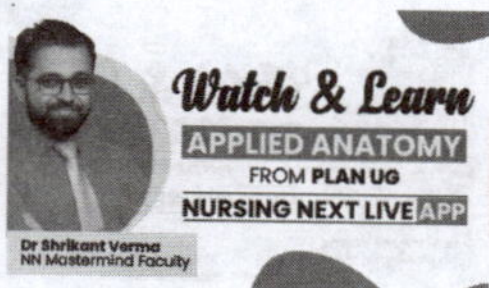

  - Deep femoral artery
  - Descending genicular artery
- Vastus lateralis
  - Lateral circumflex artery
  - Femoral and deep femoral arteries
  - Artery to quadriceps
- Vastus intermedius
  - Artery to quadriceps
  - Deep femoral arteries

Functions

- Flexion of the thigh at the hip joint
- Extension of the leg at the knee joint

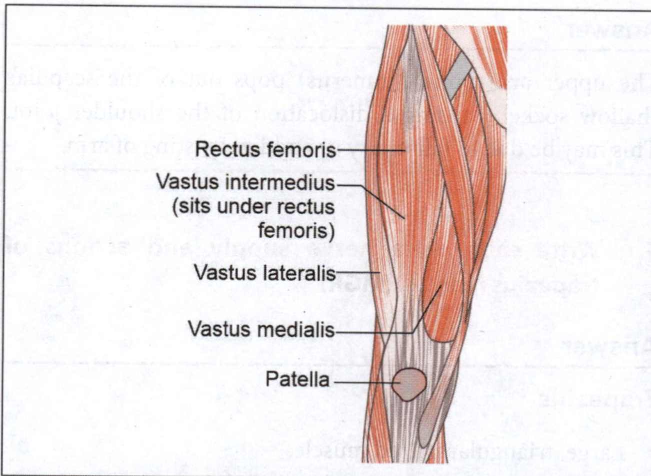

Figure 7.15: Quadriceps muscles

15. Write a note on major muscles involved in IM injections. (MGR)

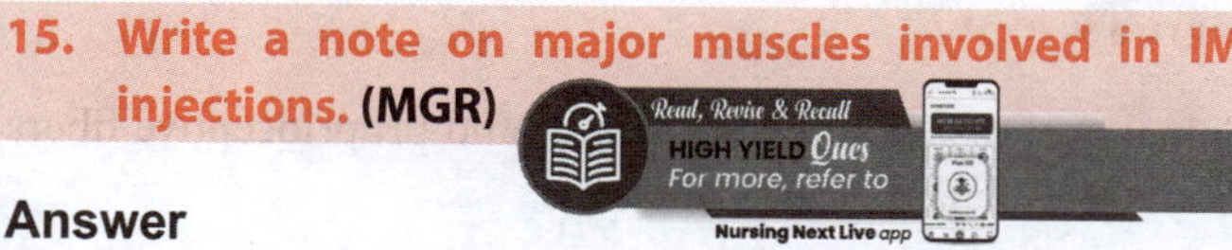

Answer

Introduction

- An intramuscular injection is a technique used to deliver a drug deep into the muscles.
- This allows the drug to get absorbed into blood faster.

Advantages

- Faster absorption due to greater blood supply in muscles.
- Can hold a larger volume of drug as compared to subcutaneous route.

Muscles Involved in IM Injections

- Deltoid muscle of arm
  - Most common muscle for administration of vaccines.
  - Located on the top of upper arm, below the acromion process.
  - Not used for self-injection or when the volume of drug to be delivered is more than 1 mL.

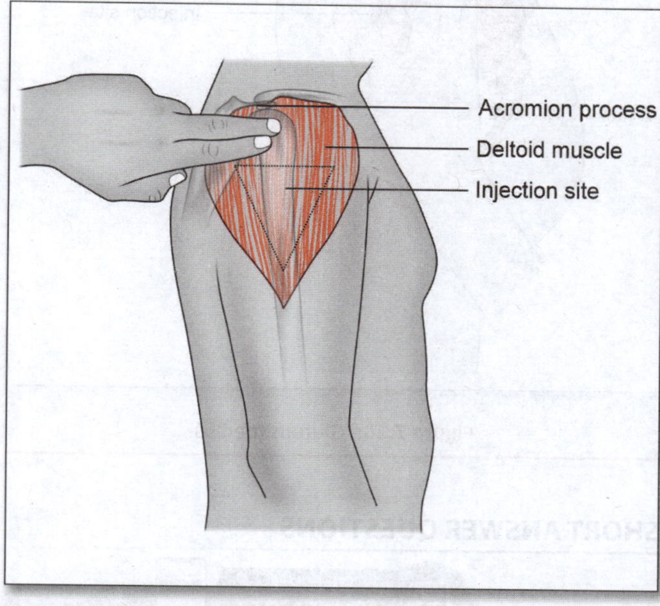

Figure 7.16: Deltoid muscle injection site

- Vastus lateralis muscle of thigh
  - Can be used for self-injection

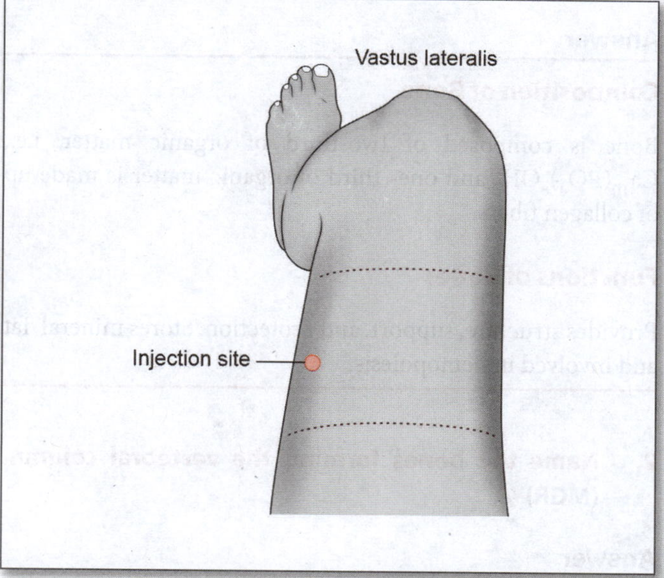

Figure 7.17: Vastus lateralis muscle injection site

- Gluteus medius muscle of the hip
  - Safest site for adults and children above 7 years of age.
  - Deeply situated and not close to any major blood vessel and nerve.
  - Least associated with any adverse effects.
  - Difficult for self-administration

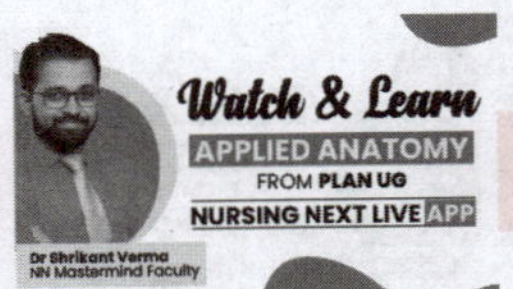

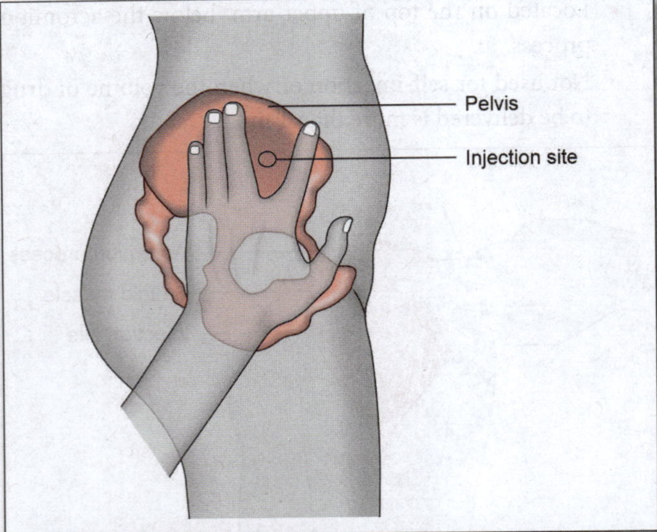

Figure 7.18: Gluteus medius

SHORT ANSWER QUESTIONS

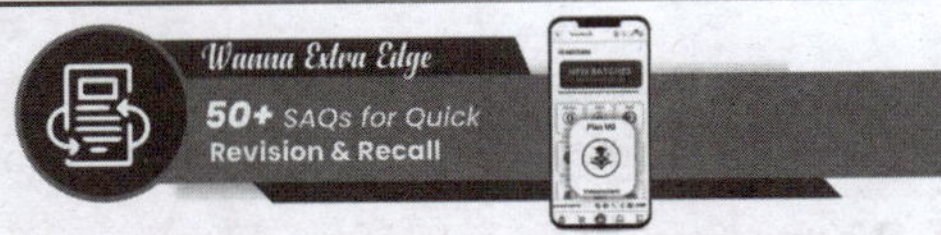

1. Provide the composition and functions of the bones. (MGR)

Answer

Composition of Bone

Bone is composed of two-third of organic matter, i.e., $Ca_{10}(PO_4)_6OH_2$ and one- third of organic matter is made up of collagen fibers.

Functions of Bones

Provides structure, support, and protection. Stores mineral, fat and involved in hemopoiesis.

2. Name the bones forming the vertebral column. (MGR)

Answer

The vertebral column is made up of 33 individual vertebrae that are cervical vertebrae (seven bones), Thoracic vertebrae (12 bones), Lumbar vertebrae (five bones), sacral vertebrae (five fused bones) and coccygeal vertebrae (four fused bones).

3. Movements taking place at 1st carpometacarpal joint. (MGR)

Answer

Movements at First Carpometacarpal Joint

Movements	Muscles responsible
• Flexion with medial rotation	Flexor pollicis brevis
• Extension with lateral rotation	Extensor pollicis brevis
• Abduction	Abductor pollicis brevis
• Adduction	Adductor pollicis
• Opposition	Opponens pollicis

4. Define dislocation of shoulder joint. (MGR)

Answer

The upper arm bone (humerus) pops out of the scapula's shallow socket, causing a dislocation of the shoulder joint. This may be due to fall injury or sudden twisting of arm.

5. Write short note nerve supply and actions of trapezius muscle. (MGR)

Answer

Trapezius

- Large, triangular paired muscle.
- Present on the upper side of neck and thorax.
- This muscle lifts the shoulder joint and scapula upward, so it is called "Shrugging muscle".

Nerve Supply

Spinal root of XI (accessory nerve) and proprioceptive fibers from C3, C4 via the cervical plexus.

Actions

- Superior fibers/Descending part
  - Shrugging of shoulder
  - Extension of head and neck
  - Lateral flexion of head and neck (ipsilateral)
  - Rotation of head
- Middle fibers/Transverse part
  - Retraction of scapula
  - Draws scapula medially
- Lower fibers/Ascending part
  - Upward and lateral rotation of glenoid cavity as in overhead abduction.
  - Draws scapula inferomedially

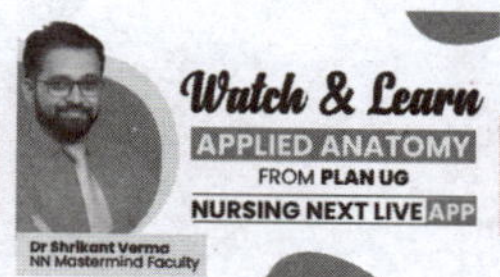

6. Give two examples of a ball and socket joint. (MGR)

Answer

Two examples of a ball and socket joint are:

- Shoulder joint
- Hip joint

CONCEPTUAL REVISION

MULTIPLE CHOICE QUESTIONS

1. The directional term "superior" in anatomy means which of the following?

a. Cephalic b. Ventral
c. Caudal d. Dorsal

Ans. a. Cephalic

2. Which of the listed bones is superior to the rest?

a. Manubrium b. Xiphoid process
c. Coccyx d. Femur

Ans. a. Manubrium

3. Which cells do not originate from osteogenic cells?

a. Osteoblasts b. Osteocytes
c. Osteoclasts d. Osteoprogenitor cells

Ans. d. Osteoprogenitor cells

4. Hardest bone of the body is?

a. Calcaneum b. Osseous labyrinths
c. Head of humerus d. Tibial condyle

Ans. b. Osseous labyrinth

5. What is depicted by the arrow in the figure?

a. Inion b. Stephanion
c. Pterion d. Bregma

Ans. c. Pterion

6. Which of the following is the last fontanel to close?

a. A b. B
c. C d. D

Ans. a. A

7. The type of joint between the sacrum and the coccyx is a:

a. Symphysis
b. Synostosis
c. Synchondrosis
d. Syndesmosis

Ans. a. Symphysis

8. Which of the following joint is seen between the carpal and metacarpal bones of thumb?

a. Ball and socket
b. Ellipsoid joint
c. Pivot joint
d. Saddle joint

Ans. d. Saddle joint

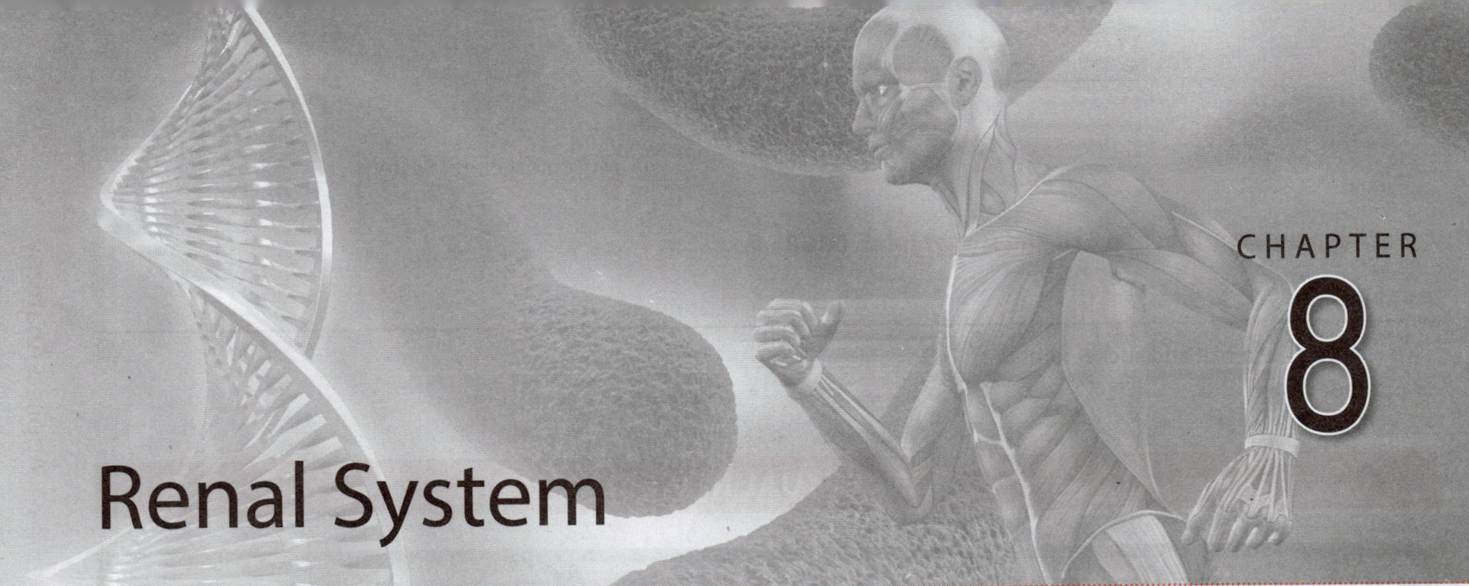

CHAPTER

8

Renal System

CONCEPTUAL THEORY

Terminology

150+ key terminologies for Quick Recall & Revision

Cortical arches/lobules: Part of the cortex arching over the pyramid of kidney.
Hilum of kidney: Middle of medial border of kidney shows a depression, this depression is hilum of kidney and structure seen at hilum are renal vein, renal artery and renal pelvis from before backwards.
Lobe of kidney: One pyramid with its overlying cortex is called lobe of kidney.
Parts of empty bladder: Apex, base—directed backwards; neck–lowest and fixed part; three surfaces—superior, right and left inferolateral. Four borders—anterior, posterior and two lateral.
Renal column: Part of the cortex of kidney lying in between the pyramids of kidney.
Renal pyramid: These are 10–12 conical masses present in the medulla of kidney. Their apices form renal papillae which indent the minor calyces.
Ureter: Ureter lies 2 cm lateral to supravaginal part of the cervix

STRUCTURE OF KIDNEY

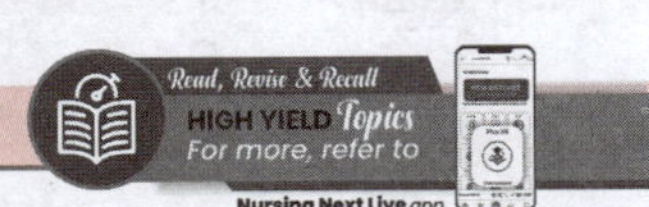

Kidneys are the vital organs of urinary system responsible for filtering waste products and excess fluid from the blood to produce urine. They also help regulate electrolyte balance, blood pressure, and the production of red blood cells. The anatomy and structure of the kidneys include the following components:

- **Renal capsule:** The kidneys are surrounded by a thin, fibrous layer called the renal capsule, which provides protection and maintains the kidney's shape.
- **Renal cortex:** The renal cortex is the outer region of the kidney. It contains millions of filtering units called nephrons, which are responsible for filtering blood and producing urine. The renal cortex also houses the glomeruli (networks of tiny blood vessels) and the convoluted tubules of the nephrons.
- **Renal medulla:** The renal medulla is the inner region of the kidney, located deep to the renal cortex. It consists of cone-shaped structures called renal pyramids, which contain tubules that transport and concentrate urine. The renal medulla also contains collecting ducts that carry urine to the renal pelvis.
- **Renal pelvis:** The renal pelvis is a funnel-shaped structure in the center of the kidney. It collects urine produced by the nephrons and transports it to the ureter, which carries urine from the kidneys to the bladder.
- **Renal artery and vein:** The renal artery supplies oxygenated blood to the kidneys, branching into smaller arteries within the renal cortex. The deoxygenated blood is then carried away from the kidneys by the renal veins, which merge to form the inferior vena cava.
- **Nephrons:** Nephrons are the functional units of the kidneys responsible for urine formation. Each kidney contains millions of nephrons, each composed of a renal corpuscle and a renal tubule. The renal corpuscle consists of a cluster of capillaries called the glomerulus and a surrounding structure called the Bowman's capsule. The renal tubule consists of several segments, including the proximal convoluted tubule, loop of Henle, and distal convoluted tubule.
- **Renal blood supply:** The kidneys receive a significant blood supply to support their functions. The renal artery branches into smaller arteries, arterioles, and eventually into the glomerular capillaries within the nephrons. Blood is then drained from the nephrons into venules, which merge to form the renal vein.

URETER

- The ureters are long, muscular tubes that connect the kidneys to the urinary bladder. They transport urine

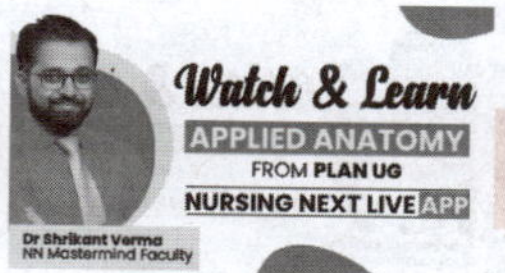

from the kidneys to the bladder through peristaltic contractions.

- The complex anatomy and structure of the kidneys allow them to perform crucial functions in maintaining fluid and electrolyte balance, regulating blood pressure, and eliminating waste products from the body. The nephrons, located within the renal cortex and medulla, play a central role in the filtration and reabsorption processes involved in urine production.
- Each human has two ureter, one for each kidney.

The anatomy and structure of the ureter include the following components:

- **Length and location:** The ureters are approximately 25–30 centimeters long in adults. They originate from the renal pelvis, which is the expanded upper part of the kidney's collecting system. From there, they descend downward along the back of the abdominal cavity and enter the pelvis, where they continue toward the urinary bladder.
- **Muscular walls:** The walls of the ureters are composed of smooth muscle tissue, allowing them to contract and propel urine toward the bladder through peristalsis. The muscular layer consists of an inner longitudinal layer and an outer circular layer, which work together to facilitate urine transport.
- **Ureteral orifices:** The lower ends of the ureters have openings known as ureteral orifices. These orifices are located within the urinary bladder and serve as the entry points for urine to enter the bladder. The ureteral orifices are equipped with a valve-like mechanism that prevents urine from flowing backward into the ureters, helping to maintain one-way flow.
- **Blood supply and innervation:** The ureters receive their blood supply from branches of the renal artery and the common iliac artery. The blood vessels form a network around the ureters, ensuring they receive oxygen and nutrients. Innervation of the ureters includes sympathetic, parasympathetic, and sensory nerve fibers, which help regulate the contraction and relaxation of the smooth muscle walls.
- **Ureterovesical junction:** The point where each ureter enters the urinary bladder is known as the ureterovesical junction. This junction is anatomically important as it ensures the proper flow of urine into the bladder and prevents the reflux of urine back into the ureters.

The ureters play a crucial role in the urinary system, facilitating the transport of urine from the kidneys to the urinary bladder. The muscular walls of the ureters contract to propel urine forward through peristaltic movements. The ureteral orifices and the ureterovesical junction helps maintain the one-way flow of urine and prevent backflow.

URINARY BLADDER

The urinary bladder is a hollow organ located in the pelvis that functions as a temporary storage reservoir for urine before it is eliminated from the body. It has a unique anatomy and structure that enables its storage capacity and controlled release of urine.

The anatomy and structure of the bladder include the following components:

- **Trigone:** The trigone is a triangular area located at the base of the bladder, defined by three openings—two ureteral openings (where the ureters enter the bladder) and the urethral opening (where the urethra exits the bladder). The trigone plays a role in maintaining continence and preventing urine reflux.
- **Detrusor muscle:** The detrusor muscle is a layer of smooth muscle that forms the main muscular wall of the bladder. It contracts to squeeze and expel urine during urination. The detrusor muscle is under the control of the autonomic nervous system, with parasympathetic stimulation causing its contraction and sympathetic stimulation causing its relaxation.
- **Epithelial lining:** The inner lining of the bladder is composed of a specialized epithelial tissue called transitional epithelium. This lining allows the bladder to stretch and accommodate increasing volumes of urine without leakage. It also helps protect the underlying tissues from the potentially harmful effects of urine.
- **Ureteral openings:** The ureteral openings are two small openings in the trigone region where the ureters, which carry urine from the kidneys to the bladder, enter the bladder. The openings are guarded by flap-like valves called ureterovesical valves (also known as the ureteral orifices) that prevent backflow of urine from the bladder into the ureters.
- **Urethral opening:** The urethral opening is the exit point of the bladder, where the urethra begins. It allows urine to be expelled from the bladder during urination. In males, the urethra is longer and also serves as a passage for semen during ejaculation.
- **Blood supply and innervation:** The bladder receives its blood supply from branches of the internal iliac artery, specifically the superior vesical artery in males and the vaginal artery in females. The bladder is innervated by both the sympathetic and parasympathetic divisions of the autonomic nervous system, which control the bladder's contraction and relaxation, as well as the sensation of bladder fullness.

The unique structure of the bladder allows it to accommodate and store urine until an appropriate time for voluntary urination. The detrusor muscle contracts to expel urine, while the ureteral openings and urethral opening play crucial roles in the controlled flow of urine. The bladder's epithelial lining and muscular walls ensure its integrity and function, allowing for efficient urine storage and elimination.

URETHRA

Male Urethra

- Preprostatic part is 1–1.5 cm in length and extends vertically from bladder neck to verumontanum(superior aspect) in prostatic urethra.
- Prostatic part is 3–4 cm in length. It tunnels through the substance of prostate closer to anterior than the posterior surface of gland.
- Anterior part is called bulbar urethra surrounded by bulbospongiosus and is the wide part of urethra.
- External urethral orifice is the narrowest part of urethra.

Female Urethra

- Female urethra is 4 cm long and 6 mm in diameter.
- It begins at the internal urethral orifice of bladder and runs anteroinferiorly behind the symphysis pubis and ends at external urethral.

CONCEPTUAL EXERCISES

LONG ANSWER QUESTIONS

1. Draw and label a neat diagram of urinary system. Write in detail about the kidney. (MGR)

Answer

Urinary System

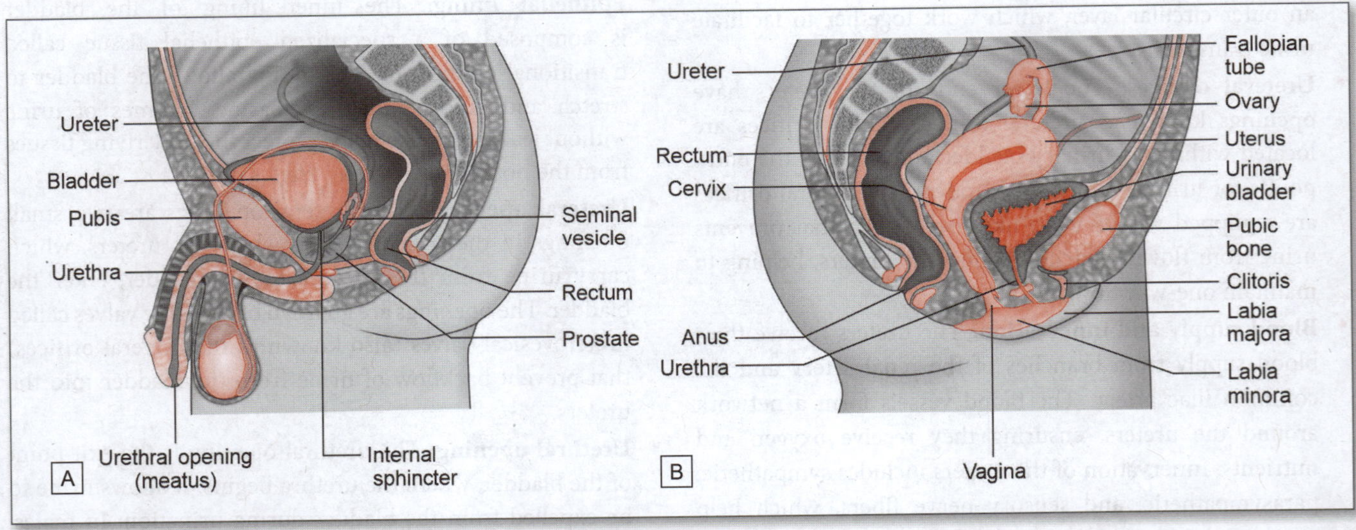

Figures 8.1A and B: Urinary system: **A.** Male; **B.** Female

Kidney

The kidneys are two bean-shaped organs, each about the size of a fist. They are located just below the rib cage, one on each side of your spine.

Location

The kidneys are located on the posterior abdominal wall, one on each side of the vertebral column, behind the peritoneum, opposite 12th thoracic (T12) and upper third lumbar (L3) vertebrae. They reside in epigastric, hypochondriac, lumbar and umbilical regions.

Anatomy of Kidney

- **Shape:** Legume-shaped
- Measurements:
  - **Length:** 11 cm. (Left kidney is somewhat longer and narrower).
  - **Width:** 6 cm.
  - **Thickness:** (anteroposterior) 3 cm.
  - **Weight:** 150 g in men; 135 g in females.

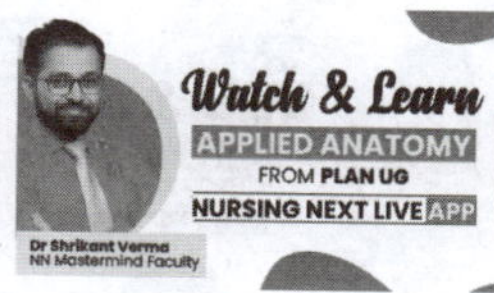

Structure

- The right kidney is generally slightly smaller and lower than the left one to make space for the liver.
- A tough, fibrous renal capsule surrounds each kidney. Beyond that, two layers of fat serve as protection. The adrenal glands lie on top of the kidneys.
- Blood enters the kidneys through the renal arteries and leaves through the renal veins. The kidneys are relatively small organs but receive 20–25% of the heart's output.
- Each kidney excretes urine through a tube called the ureter that leads to the bladder.

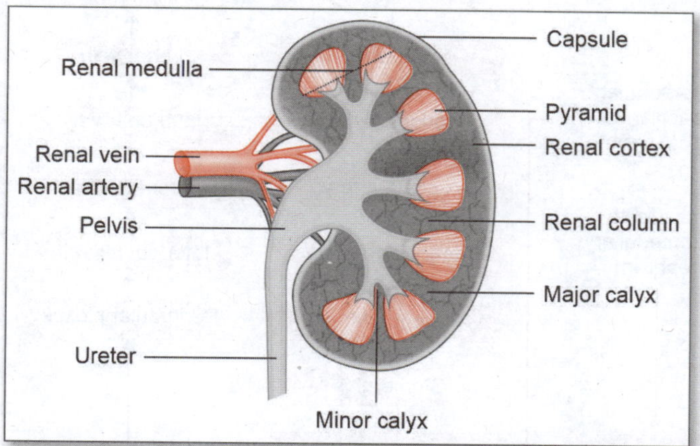

Figure 8.2: Structure of kidney

Vascular Segments of Kidney

- The renal artery gives five segmental branches, four from its anterior division and one from its posterior division.
- The segments are as follows:
  - On anterior aspect
    - Apical
    - Upper
    - Middle
    - Lower
  - On the posterior aspect

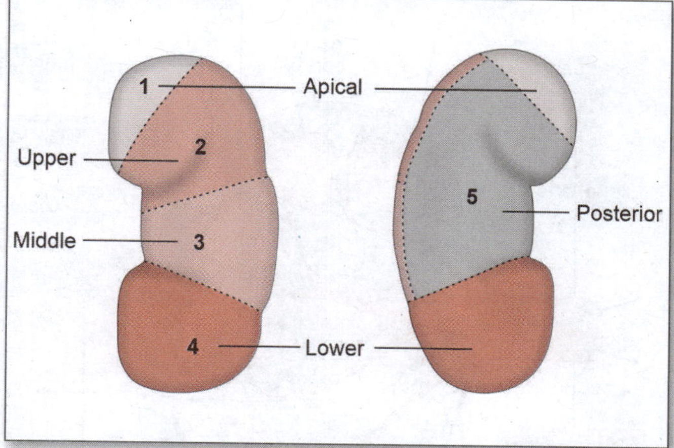

Figure 8.3: Vascular segment of kidney

Internal Anatomy

- A frontal section through the kidney reveals an outer region called the renal cortex and an inner region called the medulla.
- The renal columns are connective tissue extensions that radiate downward from the cortex through the medulla to separate the renal pyramids and renal papillae.
- The papillae are bundles of collecting ducts that transport urine made by nephrons to the calyces of the kidney for excretion.
- The renal columns also serve to divide the kidney into 6–8 lobes and provide a supportive framework for vessels that enter and exit the cortex. The pyramids and renal columns taken together constitute the kidney lobes.

Relations of Kidney

Anterior Relations

Anterior relation of right kidney	Anterior relations of left kidney
Right suprarenal gland (not covered with peritoneum)	Left suprarenal gland (not covered with peritoneum)
Second part of duodenum (not covered with peritoneum)	Spleen (covered with peritoneum)
Right colic flexure (not covered with peritoneum)	Pancreas (not covered with peritoneum)
Right lobe of liver (covered with peritoneum)	Left colic flexure (not covered with peritoneum)
Jejunum (covered with peritoneum)	Stomach (covered with peritoneum)

Posterior Relations

Muscles	Nerves	Vessels	Ribs/bones
Quadratus lumborum transversus abdominis diaphragm, Psoas major	Iliohypogastric subcostal ilioinginal	Subcostal vessels forth lumber artery only on right side	12th rib (only on right) 11th and 12th rib on left side

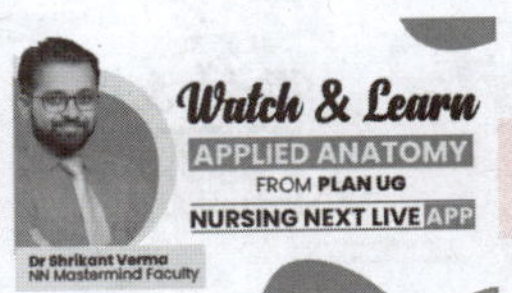

Blood Supply

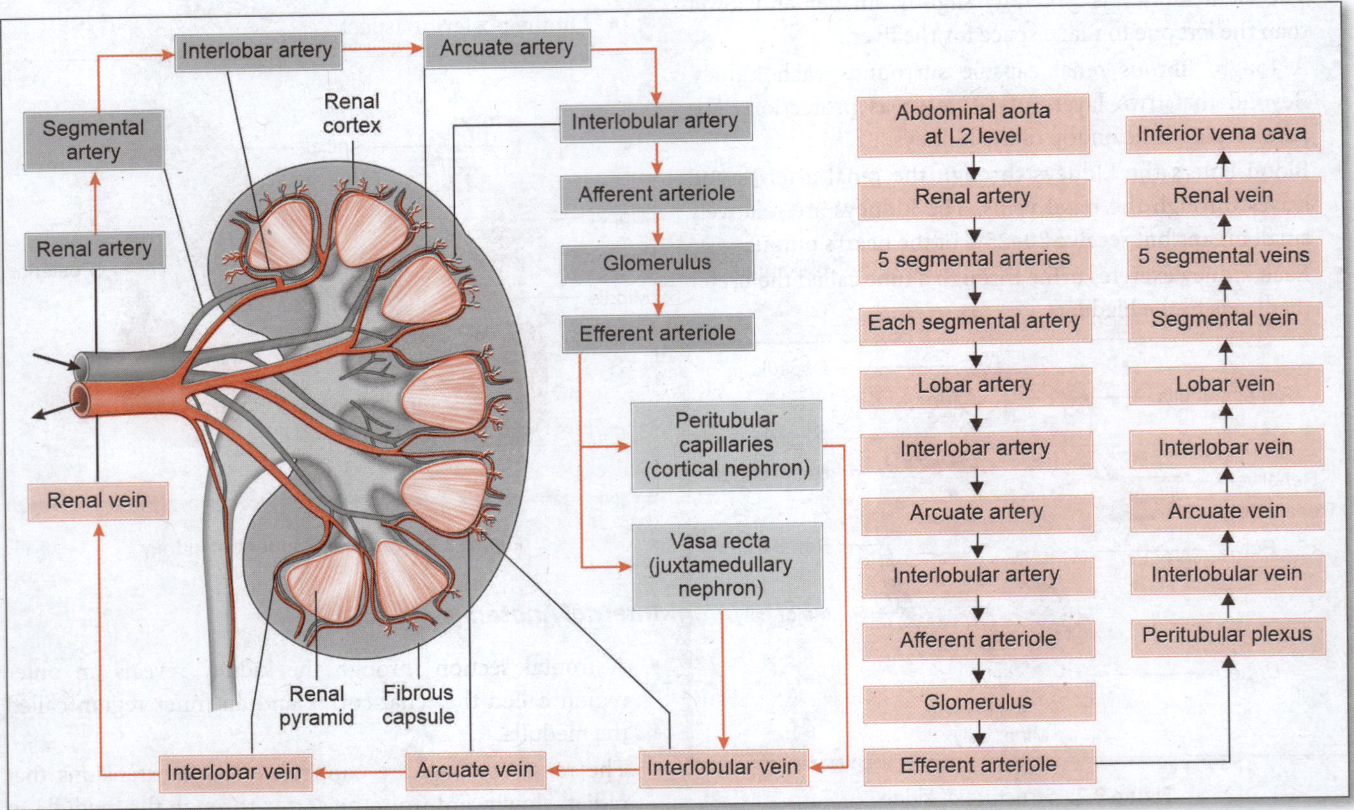

Figure 8.4: Blood supply of kidney

Nerve Supply

- Sympathetic supply is through the renal plexus, a branch of the celiac plexus.
- These are chiefly vasomotor.
- Afferent supply is through segments T10–T12.

SHORT NOTES

1. Write a short note on Structure of Nephron. (MGR)

Answer

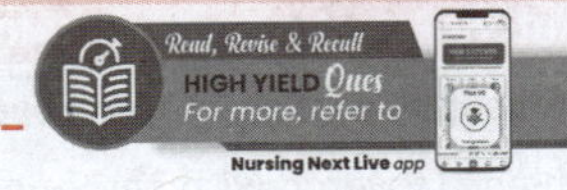

Structure of Nephron

- Kidney consists of 1–3 millions of uriniferous tubules/ nephrons.
- Nephron is the structural and functional unit of kidney.
- Nephron is the excretory part and consists of
  - **Renal corpuscle or Malpighian corpuscle:** Made up of glomerulus surrounded by Bowman's capsule and responsible for filtration of substances from the plasma.
  - **Renal tubule:**
    - Renal tubule is a long and convoluted structure emerges from the glomerulus and responsible for selective resorption of substances from the glomerular filtrate. It is divided into three parts:
      1. The first part is proximal convoluted tubule (PCT) present in the renal cortex due to its proximity to the glomerulus
      2. The second part is loop of Henle, also known as nephritic loop because it forms a loop (with descending and ascending limbs) that goes through the renal medulla.
      3. The third part of the renal tubule is distal convoluted tubule (DCT) and this part is also restricted to the renal cortex
- Collecting part starts from the distal convoluted tubule as a junctional tubule.
- Tubules unite to form the ducts of Bellini that opens into the minor calyces through renal papillae.
- Juxtaglomerular apparatus is formed at the vascular pole of glomerulus. It consists of:
  - **Macula densa:** Formed by altered cells of distal convoluted tubule
  - **Juxtaglomerular cells:** Consist of epithelioid cells in the media of the afferent arteriole
  - **Agranular cells:** Present between macula densa and the granular proper.

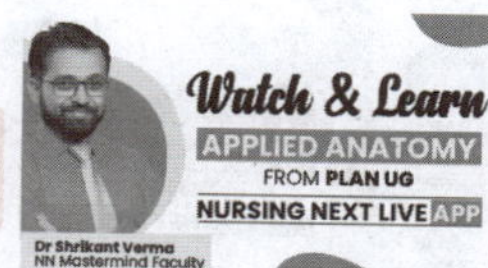

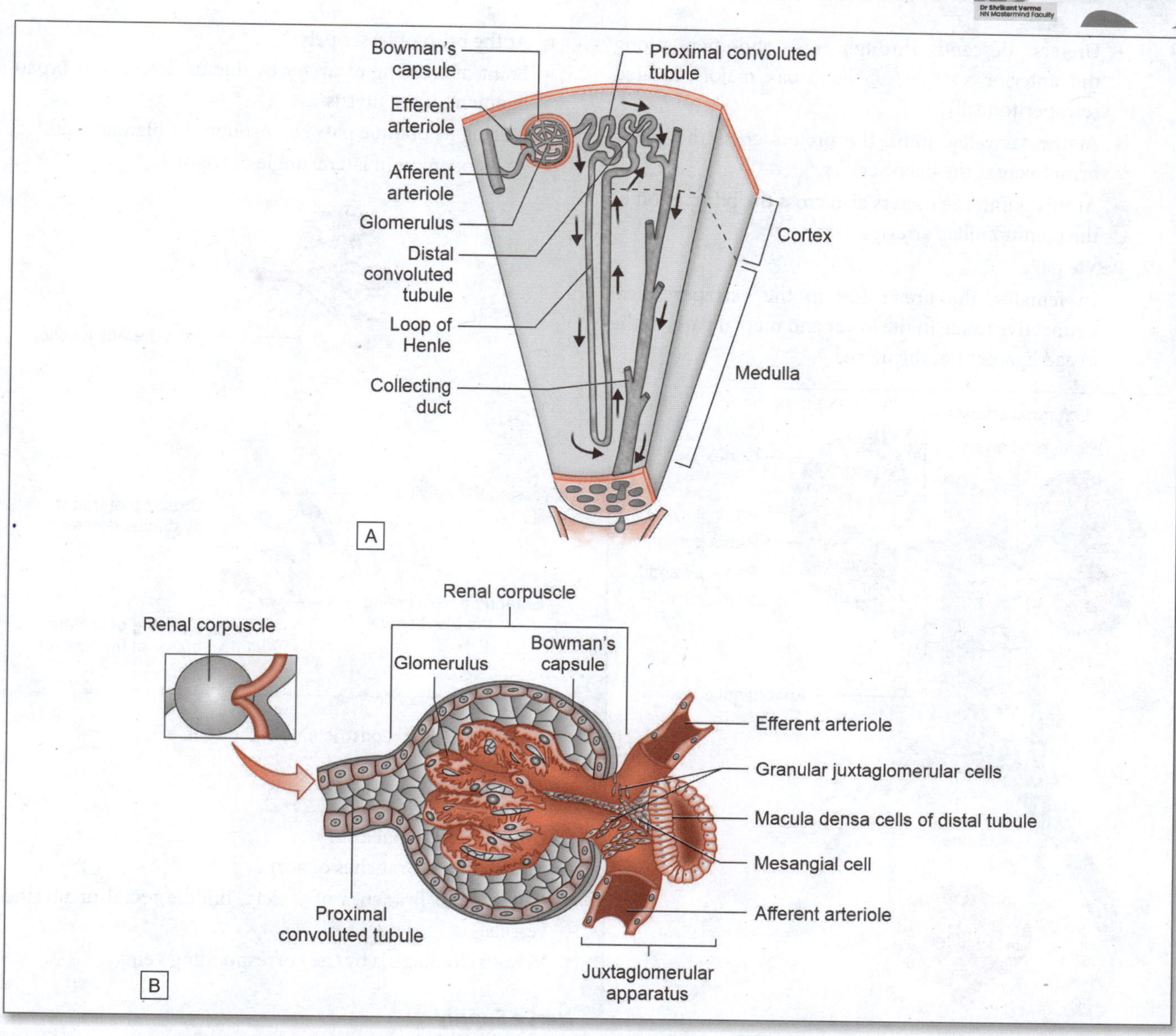

Figures 8.5A and B: **A.** Placement of the uriniferous tubule/nephron in various zones of kidney; **B.** Renal corpuscle with juxtaglomerular apparatus

2. Write about the parts of the ureter. (MGR)

Answer

Ureter

- The ureters are a pair of narrow, thick walled muscular tubes which convey urine from the kidneys to the urinary bladder.
- Lie deep to the peritoneum, in close proximity to the posterior abdominal wall in the upper part and to the lateral wall in the lower part.
- Measures about 25 cm in length and has varying widths.

Course

- It begins at the renal pelvis and descends along its medial margin or partly behind it.
- Gradually it narrows till the lower end of the kidney where it becomes the ureter proper.

Parts of Ureter

- Ureters arise in the abdomen as a continuation of the renal pelvis and terminate in the pelvic cavity.
- Thus, the ureter can be divided into two parts:
  1. **Abdominal part**
     - Ureters arise from the ureteropelvic junction within the kidney hilum.

- Ureters descend through the abdomen along the anterior surface of the psoas major—located retroperitoneally.
- At the sacroiliac joint, the ureters cross the pelvic brim to enter the pelvic cavity.
- At this point, the ureters also cross the bifurcation of the common iliac arteries.

2. **Pelvic part**
   - In females, the ureter lies in the extraperitoneal connective tissue in the lower and medial parts of the broad ligament of the uterus.

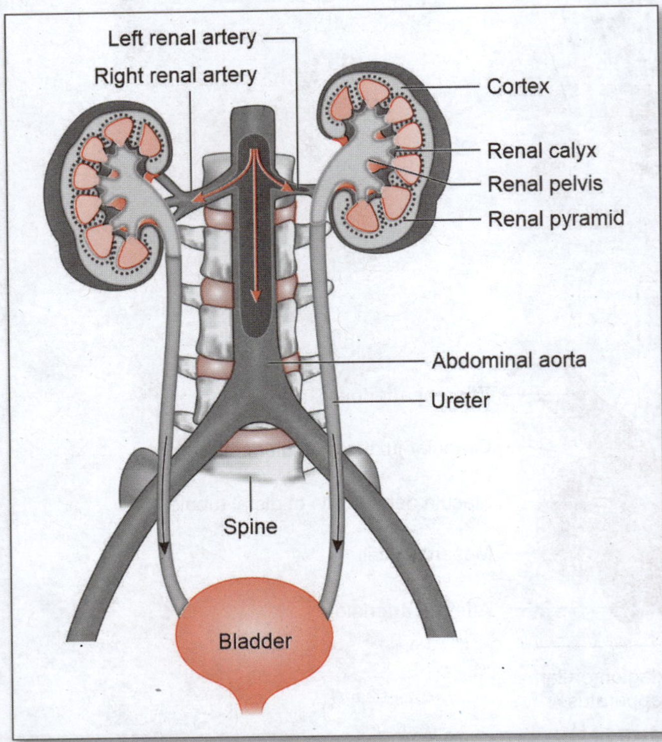

Figure 8.6: cut section of kidney with ureter and urinary bladder

   - Uterine artery lies first above and in front of the ureter for a distance of about 2.5 cm and then crosses it superiorly from lateral to medial side.
   - The ureter lies about 2 cm lateral to the supravaginal portion of the cervix. It runs slightly above the lateral fornix of the vagina.
   - The terminal portion of the ureter lies anterior to the vagina.
   - The ureters enter the bladder in an oblique manner—to prevent the back flow of urine.

Constrictions of Ureter

- The ureter is slightly constricted at five places as given below:
  - At the pelvi-ureteric junction
  - At the brim of lesser pelvis
  - Point of crossing of ureter by ductus deferens or broad ligament of the uterus
  - During its oblique passage through the bladder wall.
  - At its opening in lateral angle of trigone.

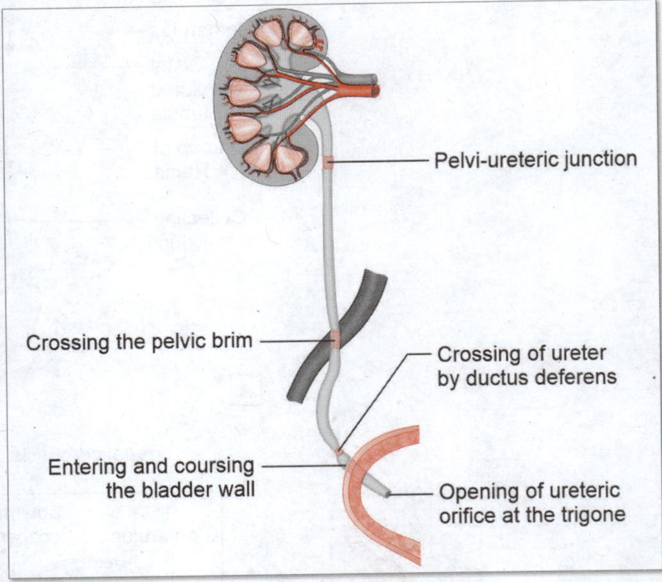

Figure 8.7: Constrictions in the course of ureter

Blood Supply

- **Upper part:** Renal artery
- **Middle part:** Branches of aorta
- **Pelvic part:** Branches of vesicle, middle rectal or uterine vessels.
- Venous drainage is by the corresponding veins

Nerve Supply

- Via the renal, testicular/ovarian and hypogastric plexuses.
- Sensory supply is through the segments T11–T12, with the ureteric pain being referred to the corresponding dermatomal areas.

3. Write a short note on urinary bladder. (MGR)

Answer

Introduction

- The urinary bladder is a muscular sac in the pelvis, just above and behind the pubic bone. When empty, the bladder is about the size and shape of a pear. Urine is formed in the kidneys and travels down two tubes called ureters to the bladder. The bladder stores urine, allowing urination to be infrequent and controlled.

External Features

- The appearance of the bladder varies depending on the amount of urine stored. When full, it exhibits an oval shape, and when empty, it is flattened by the overlying bowel. The external features of the bladder are as follows:
  - **Apex:** Located superiorly, pointing toward the pubic symphysis. It is connected to the umbilicus by the median umbilical ligament (a remnant of the urachus).
  - **Body:** Main part of the bladder, located between the apex and the fundus
  - **Fundus (or base):** Located posteriorly. It is triangular-shaped, with the tip of the triangle pointing backward.
  - **Neck:** Formed by the convergence of the fundus and two inferolateral surfaces. It is continuous with the urethra.

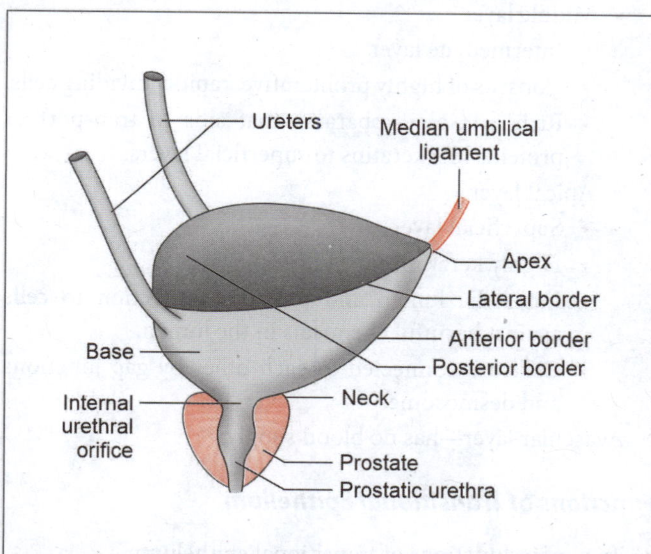

Figure 8.8: Shape of the urinary bladder

Relations

- Relations of the male urinary bladder
  - Superiorly with the peritoneal cavity and the small bowel within.
  - Inferiorly with the prostate gland and the periprostatic venous plexus.
  - Laterally with smooth bowel (if distended) and the obturator internus muscle in the pelvis
  - Posteriorly with the rectovesical pouch and rectum (superiorly), with the seminal glands intervening more inferiorly
  - Anteriorly with the anterior abdominal wall and the pubic symphysis.
  - **Apex:** It is connected to the umbilicus by the median umbilical ligament.
  - **Base**
    - **Female:** It is related to the uterine cervix and vagina.
    - **Male:** Upper part of the base is separated from the rectum by the rectovesical pouch and the contained coils of intestine; and the lower part is related to the seminal vesical and termination of vas deferens.
  - **Neck:** It is present three to four centimeters behind the lower part of pubic symphysis, just a little above the plane of pelvic outlet.
    - **Males:** Bundles of smooth muscles surround the bladder neck and preprostatic urethra. This is devoid of parasympathetic cholinergic nerves.
    - **Females:** Neck is related to pelvic fascia which surrounds the upper part of urethra.
  - Superior surface
    - **Males:** It is covered by peritoneum and is in contact with sigmoid colon and coils of terminal ileum.
    - **Females:** Peritoneum covers most of the superior surface except for a small area near the posterior border which is related to supravaginal part of the uterine cervix.
  - Inferolateral
    - **Male:** Each surface is related to pubis, puboprostatic ligaments, retro pubic fat, levator ani and the obturator internus.
    - **Female:** Here the puboprostatic ligaments are replaced by pubovesical.

Blood Supply

- The bladder is supplied by the vesical arteries and drained by the vesical veins.

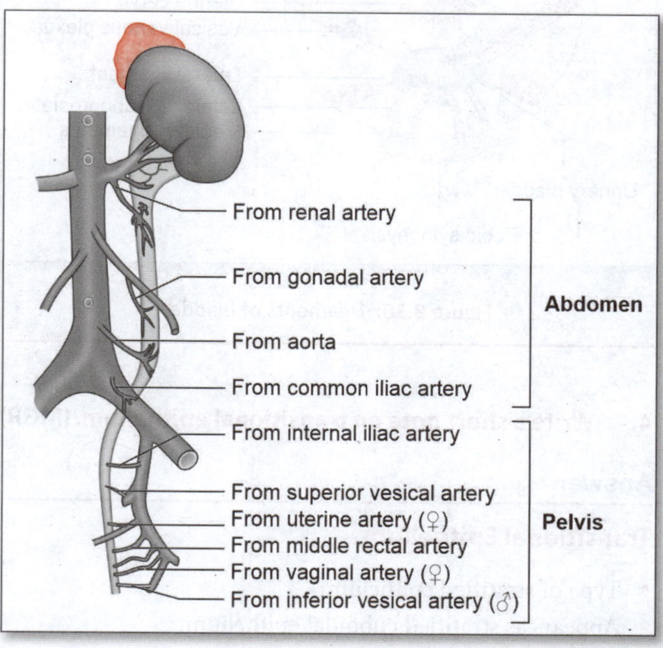

Figure 8.9: Blood supply

- The lymph drained from the bladder begins in a series of networks throughout the mucosal, muscular and serosal layers
- A majority of these vessels drain into the external iliac lymph nodes.

Ligaments

- **True ligaments**
  - **Lateral true ligament:**
    - It extends from the side of the bladder to the tendinous arch of the pelvic fascia.
  - **The medial umbilical ligament is the remnant of urachus.**
    - Posterior ligament of the bladder: It is directed backward and upward along the vesical plexus of the veins. It extends on each side from the base of the bladder to the wall of the pelvis.
- **False ligaments**
  - These include:
    - Median umbilical fold
    - Medial umbilical fold
    - Lateral false ligament formed by peritoneum of the paravesical fossa.
    - Posterior false ligament formed by peritoneum of sacrogenital fold

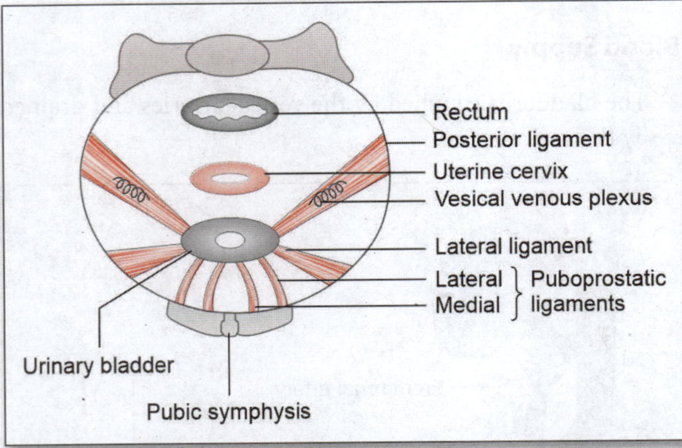

Figure 8.10: Ligaments of bladder

4. Write a short note on transitional epithelium. (MGR)

Answer

Transitional Epithelium

- Type of stratified epithelium.
- Appears as stratified cuboidal epithelium.
- It lines the urinary tract.
- The uppermost layers are not flattened but dome-shaped.
- The lower layers are pear-shaped and columnar.
- This epithelium allows distension of the organ.

Structure of Transitional Epithelium

- The cells are pear-shaped or round, while the cells in the basal layer appear cuboidal or columnar.
- The layers of transitional epithelium are as follows:
  - Basal layer
  - Lowermost layer
  - Directly attached to the basement membrane
  - It is responsible for providing constant renewal of cells
  - Rich in cytoplasmic proteins that bind to form tonofibrils and mitochondria.
  - Attached to basement membrane by hemidesmosomes.
  - Middle layer
    - Intermediate layer
    - Consists of highly proliferative, rapidly dividing cells.
    - Rich in Golgi apparatus that aids in transport of proteins like keratins to superficial layers.
  - Apical layer
    - Superficial layer
    - Highly keratinized
    - Lines the lumen and provides protection to cells against harmful chemicals in the lumen.
    - Cells are connected to each other by gap junctions and desmosomes.
- Avascular layer—has no blood supply

Functions of Transitional Epithelium

- Two main functions of transitional epithelium
  1. Permeability barrier
     - This is due to the presence of large amounts of keratin in the cells.
     - These cells are highly resistant against osmotic pressure; so, they provide protection against desiccation even when cells are fully stretched.

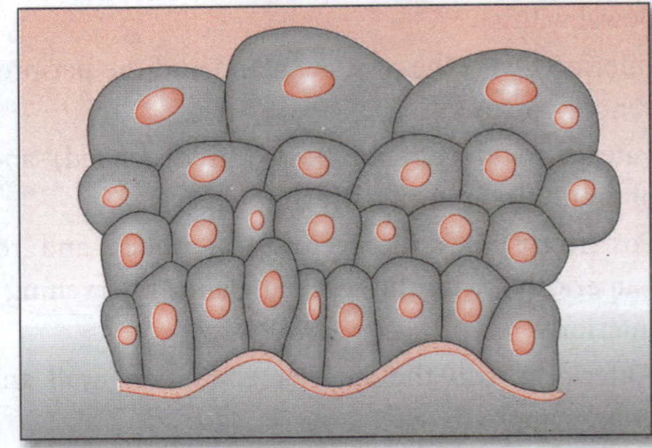

Figure 8.11: Transitional epithelium

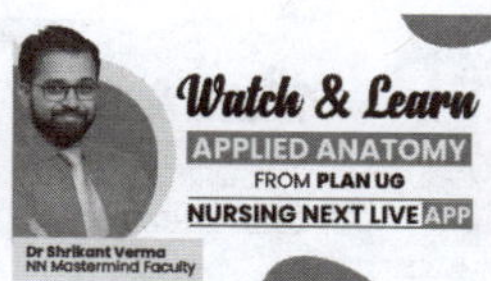

2. Flexibility

- The important function of transitional epithelium is its ability to allow changes in shape and size by stretching with change in pressure.

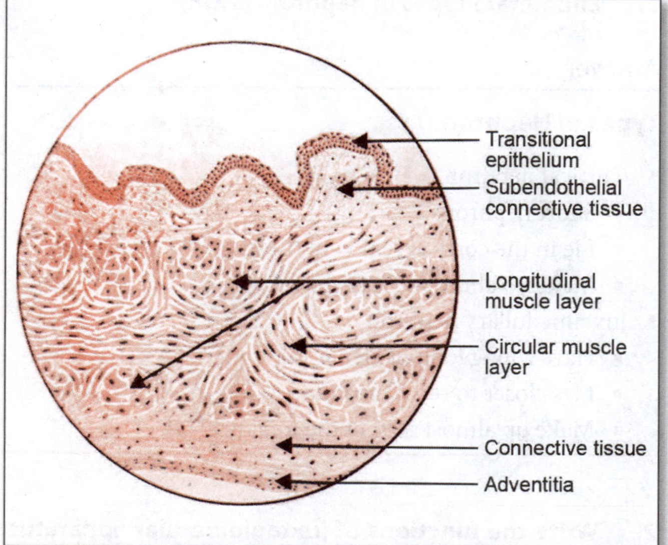

Figure 8.12: Histology of urinary bladder demonstrating transitional epithelium

5. Write a short note on kidney. (MGR)

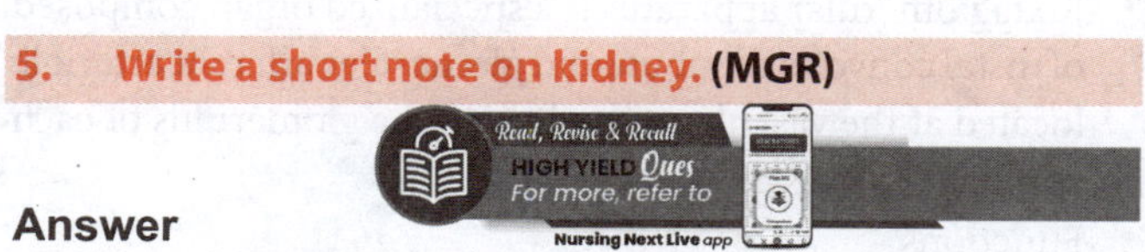

Answer

Kidney

The kidneys are two bean-shaped organs, each about the size of a fist. They are located just below the rib cage, one on each side of your spine.

Location

The kidneys are located on the posterior abdominal wall, one on each side of the vertebral column, behind the peritoneum, opposite 12th thoracic (T_{12}) and upper third lumbar (L3) vertebrae. They reside in epigastric, hypochondriac, lumbar and umbilical regions.

Anatomy of Kidney

- **Shape:** Legume-shaped
- **Measurements:**
  - **Length:** 11 cm (Left kidney is somewhat longer and narrower).
  - **Width:** 6 cm
  - **Thickness:** (Anteroposterior) 3 cm.
  - **Weight:** 150 grams in men; 135 grams in females.

Structure

- The right kidney is generally slightly smaller and lower than the left, to make space for the liver.
- A tough, fibrous renal capsule surrounds each kidney. Beyond that, two layers of fat provide protection. The adrenal glands lie on top of the kidneys.
- Blood enters the kidneys through the renal arteries and leaves through the renal veins. The kidneys are relatively small organs but receive 20–25% of the heart's output.
- Each kidney excretes urine through a tube called the ureter that leads to the bladder.

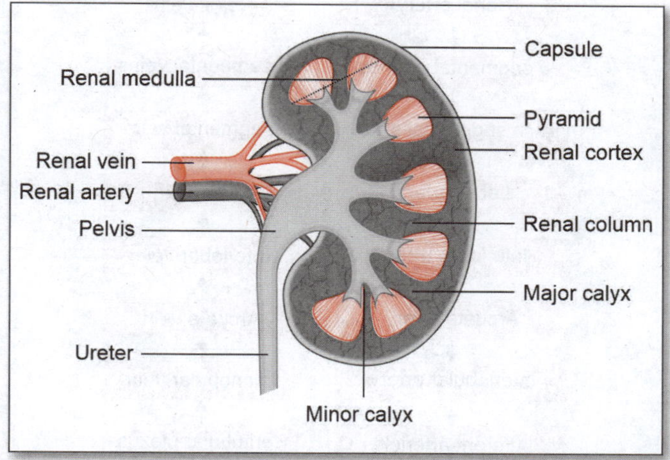

Figure 8.13: Structure of kidney

Vascular Segments of Kidney

- The renal artery gives five segmental branches, four from its anterior division and one from its posterior division.
- These segments are as follows:
  - On anterior aspect
    - Apical
    - Upper
    - Middle
    - Lower
  - On the posterior aspect

Internal Anatomy

- A frontal section through the kidney reveals an outer region called the renal cortex and an inner region called the medulla.
- The renal columns are connective tissue extensions that radiate downward from the cortex through the medulla to separate the renal pyramids and renal papillae.
- The papillae are bundles of collecting ducts that transport urine made by nephrons to the calyces of the kidney for excretion.

- The renal columns also serve to divide the kidney into 6–8 lobes and provide a supportive framework for vessels that enter and exit the cortex. The pyramids and renal columns taken together constitute the kidney lobes.

Blood Supply

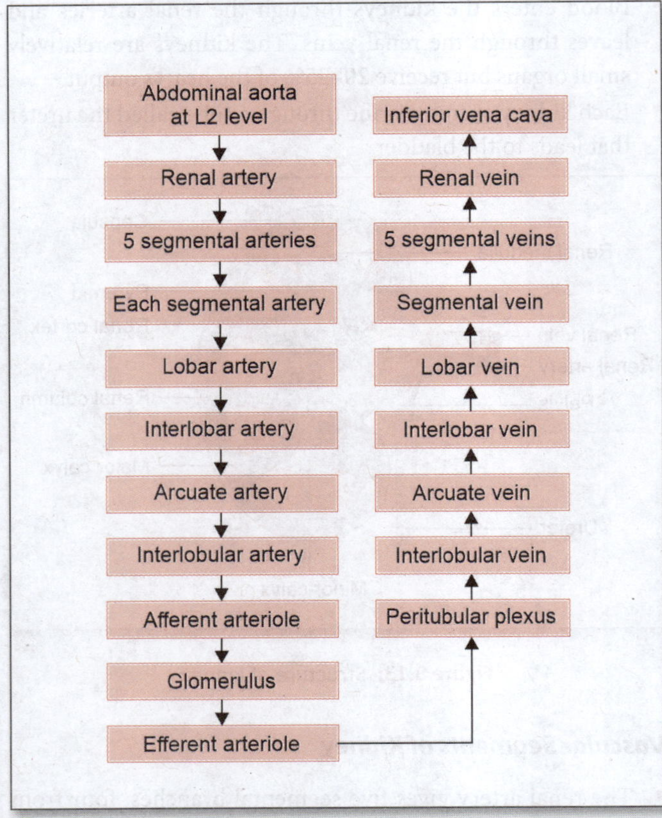

Nerve Supply

- Sympathetic supply is through the renal plexus, a branch of the celiac plexus.
- These are chiefly vasomotor.
- Afferent supply is through segments T10–T12.

Applied Anatomy

- Glomerulonephritis
- Acute nephritis
- Nephrotic syndrome
- Hypertension
- Diabetic nephropathy
- Pyelonephritis
- Renal calculi
- Acute renal failure
- Polycystic kidney disease

SHORT ANSWER QUESTIONS

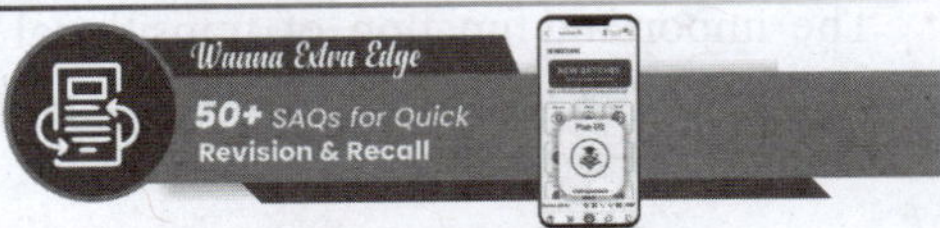

1. Enumerate types of nephron. (MGR)

Answer

Types of Nephron

- Cortical nephron
  - Short nephrons
  - Lie in the cortical region of the kidney.
  - Make up almost 80% of the total
- Juxtamedullary nephron
  - Have a long loop of Henle
  - Lies closer to renal medulla
  - Make up almost 20% of the total

2. Write the functions of juxtaglomerular apparatus. (MGR)

Answer

- Juxtaglomerular apparatus is a specialized organ composed of distal convoluted tubule and glomerular afferent arteriole located at the vascular pole close to the glomerulus of each nephron. (juxta = near).
- Functions
  - Regulates Blood pressure
  - Regulates filtration rate of glomerulus
  - Secretion of hormones viz renin and prostaglandin.

3. Name the vascular segments of kidney. (MGR)

Answer

The renal artery gives five segmental branches, four from its anterior division and one from its posterior division.

These segments are as follows:

- Apical
- Upper
- Middle
- Lower
- Posterior

4. What is automatic urinary bladder? (MGR)

Answer

Automatic Urinary Bladder

- Occurs in injuries at or below S2.

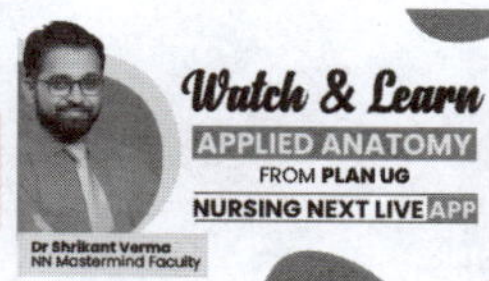

- The bladder reflex center is destroyed.
- If sensory neurogenic bladder is present, the affected individual may not be able to sense when the bladder is full.
- If motor neurogenic bladder, the individual will sense the bladder is full, but detrusor may not contract—this condition is known as detrusor areflexia.
- It may lead to urinary incontinence.
- Typical causes are as follows:
  - Sacral cord tumor
  - Herniated disk
  - Pelvic injuries
  - Lumbar laminectomy

5. Enumerate the sites of constrictions of the ureter. (MGR)

Answer

- The ureter is a pair of narrow, thick walled muscular tubes which convey urine from the kidneys to the urinary bladder.

Constrictions of Ureter

- The ureter is slightly constricted at five places as given:
  1. At the pelvi-ureteric junction
  2. At the brim of lesser pelvis
  3. Point of crossing of ureter by ductus deferens or broad ligament of ureter
  4. During its oblique passage through the bladder wall.
  5. At its opening in lateral angle of trigone.

CONCEPTUAL REVISION

MULTIPLE CHOICE QUESTIONS

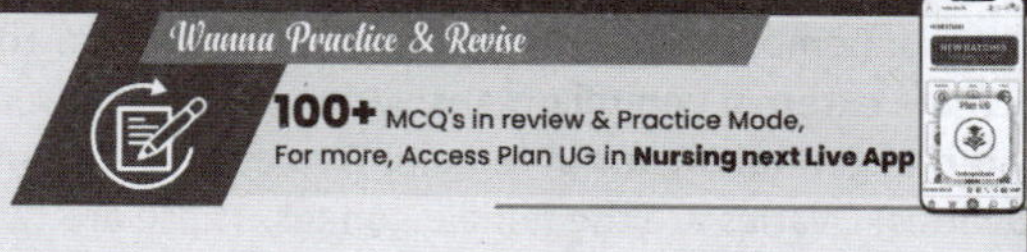

1. What is the name for the entry point to the kidney for nerves, blood vessels, ureters and lymphatics?

a. Calyx
b. Hilus
c. Pelvis
d. Pyramid

Ans. b. Hilus

2. What structure does the blood from the afferent arteriole enter?

a. The peritubular capillaries
b. The vasa recta
c. The glomerulus
d. Bowman's capsule

Ans. c. The glomerulus

3. What is the collective term applied to the proximal and distal convoluted tubules, the loop of Henle (i.e., the nephron loop) and the glomerular capsule?

a. The renal corpuscle
b. The renal tubule
c. The nephron
d. The renal capsule

Ans. b. The renal tubule

4. What is the name of the tube that connects the bladder to the kidney?

a. Renal tubule
b. Ureter
c. Urethra
d. Collecting duct

Ans. b. Ureter

5. The renal tubule of the nephron includes which of the following structures?

a. Proximal convoluted tubule, vasa recta, Bowman's capsule, collecting duct
b. Distal convoluted tubule, ascending limb of Loop of Henle, Bowman's capsule, proximal convoluted tubule
c. Descending limb of Loop of Henle, collecting duct, distal convoluted tubule, ascending limb of Loop of Henle
d. Glomerulus, proximal convoluted tubule, distal convoluted tubule, Bowman's capsule

Ans. b. Distal convoluted tubule, ascending limb of Loop of Henle, Bowman's capsule, proximal convoluted tubule

6. Which one of the following is part of the renal tubule?

a. Glomerulus
b. Vasa recta
c. Collecting duct
d. Macula densa

Ans. d. Macula densa

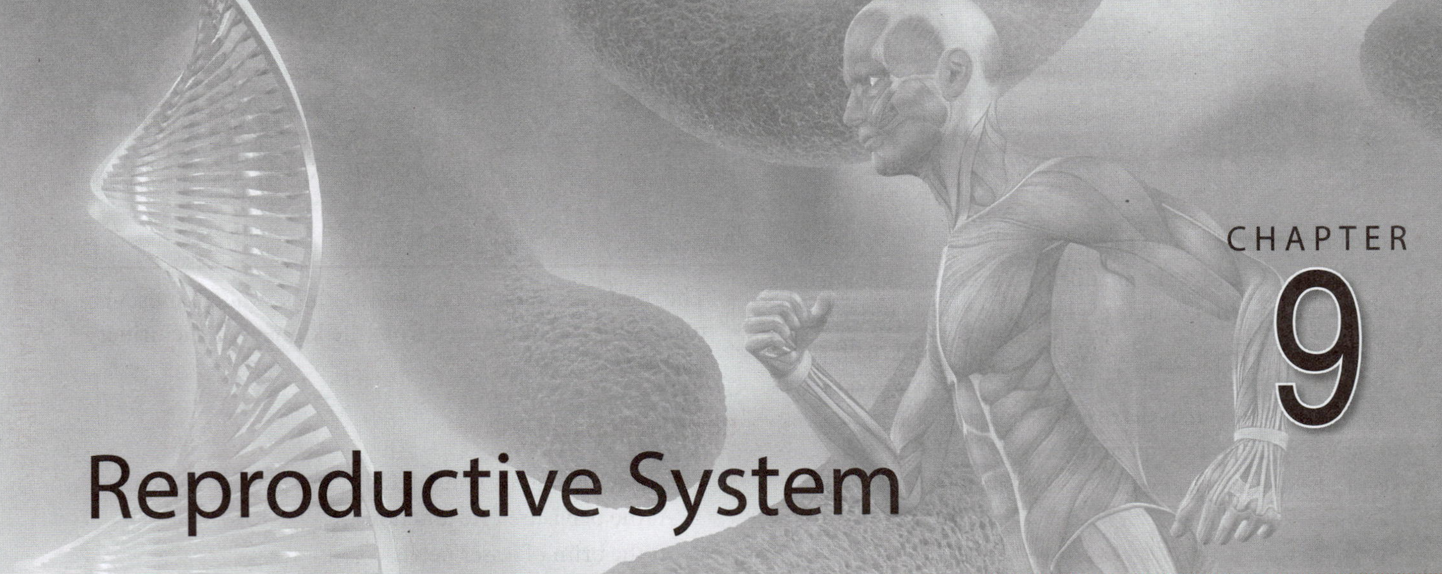

Reproductive System

CONCEPTUAL THEORY

Terminology

150+ key terminologies for Quick Recall & Revision

Cells present in the testis: Spermatogenic series of cells, Leydig's cells which secrete testosterone and cells of Sertoli.
Clitoris: Composed of only two corpora cavernosa. There is no corpus spongiosum and no urethra in the clitoris.
Female external genital organs: Mons pubis, labia majora, labia minora, clitoris, vestibule and greater vestibular glands.
Internal genital organs in female: Two ovaries, one uterus, two fallopian tubes and one vagina.
Ovaries: Ovaries are the female gonads. These are two almond-shaped structures in the lateral wall of true pelvis.
Parts of uterus: Fundus, body and cervix. Cervix has internal os cervical canal and external os.
Semen: It is a viscous white fluid containing sperms and seminal fluid.
Spermatozoa: It is the male gamete (22 + Y/22 + X chromosomes). It consists of a head with acrosome and nucleus, middle piece with mitochondria; tail piece with flagellum and an end piece.
Uterine tube: Also called oviduct/fallopian tube. It is 10 cm long on each side of uterus and runs tortuously because of lack of space. Its parts are infundibulum with fimbriae, ampulla, isthmus and intramural parts. Fertilization usually occurs in its ampulla.

STRUCTURE OF MALE REPRODUCTIVE ORGANS

Component	Structure	Anatomy	Function
Testes	Two oval-shaped organs located in the scrotum	Composed of seminiferous tubules, Leydigs cells, and connective tissue	Production of sperm and testosterone
Epididymis	Coiled tube located on the back of each testis	Head, body, and tail segments; lined with cilia	Sperm maturation, storage, and transportation
Vas deferens	Muscular tube connecting the epididymis to the ejaculatory duct	Extends from the epididymis to the ejaculatory duct	Transports of mature sperm from the epididymis during ejaculation
Seminal vesicles	Glandular structures located behind the bladder	Paired, with ducts connecting to the ejaculatory ducts	Production of seminal fluid containing fructose and prostaglandins
Prostate gland	Gland located below the bladder, surrounding the urethra	Composed of glandular and muscular tissue	Secretion of alkaline fluid to nourish and protect sperm
Bulbourethral glands	Small glands located below the prostate gland	Paired, located on either side of the urethra	Production of pre-ejaculatory fluid for lubrication
Penis	External organ composed of erectile tissue	Shaft, glans, and urethra	Sexual intercourse and ejaculation
Urethra	Tube connecting the bladder to the external urethral orifice	Extends through the penis	Passage for urine and semen during ejaculation

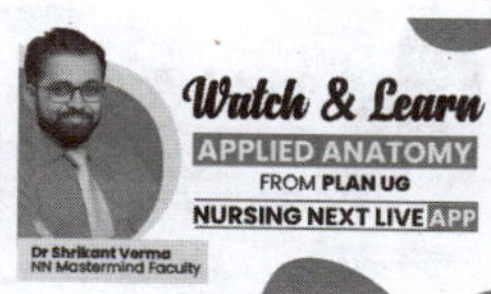

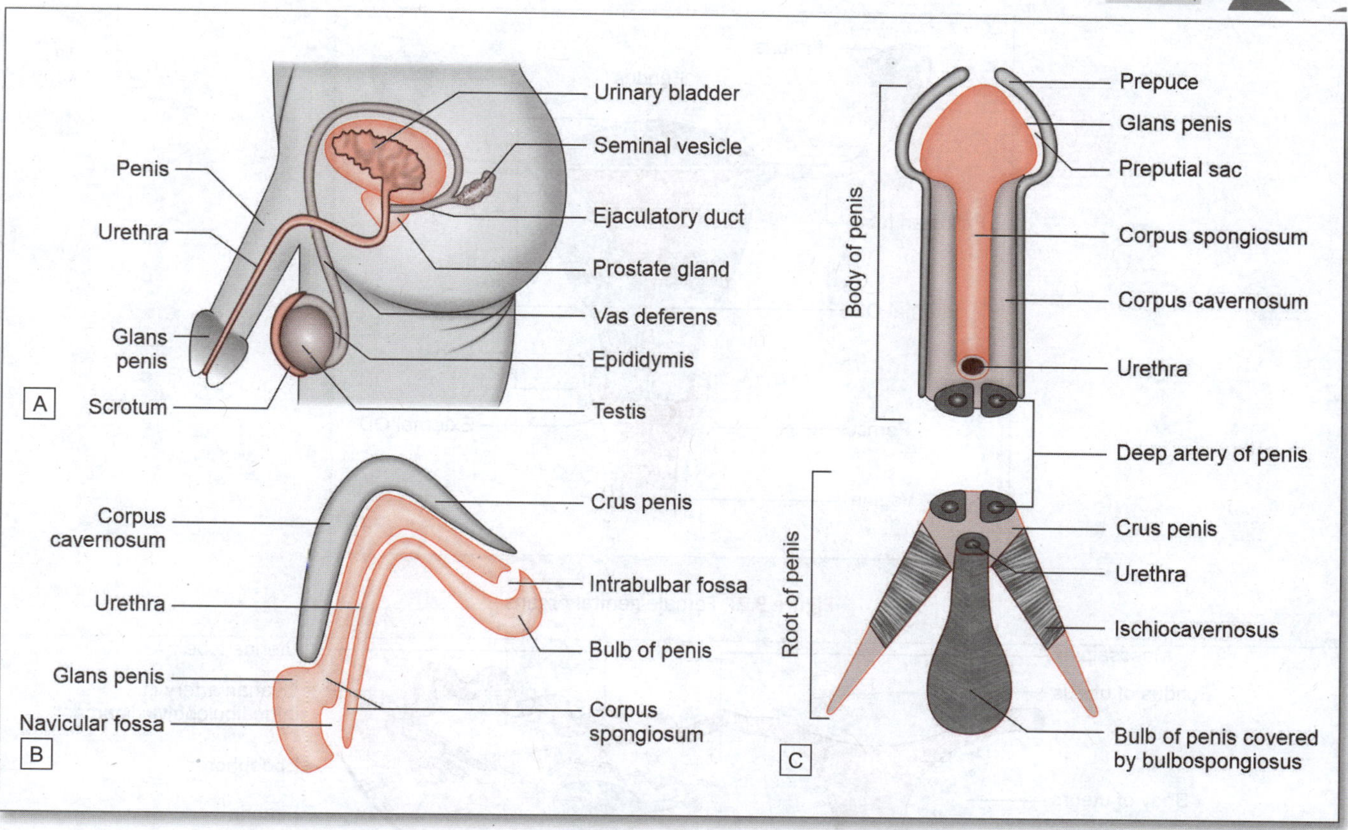

Figures 9.1A to C: **A.** Male genital organs; (B and C) parts of penis, **B.** ventral view, and **C.** Sagittal section

STRUCTURE OF FEMALE REPRODUCTIVE ORGANS

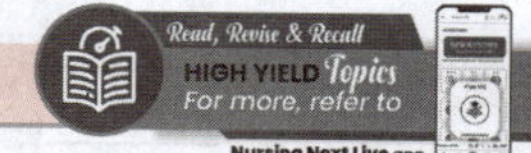

Structure	Anatomy	Function
Ovaries	Two almond-shaped organs located in pelvis	Produce eggs (ova) and female sex hormones (estrogen and progesterone)
Fallopian tubes	Narrow tubes extending from ovaries	Transport eggs from ovaries to the uterus, provide the site for fertilization
Uterus	Muscular organ in the pelvis	Provides a site for implantation of a fertilized egg, supports embryo/fetus during development, expels the fetus
Cervix	Lower part of the uterus	Acts as a passageway between the uterus and vagina, secretes mucus to protect the uterus from infections
Vagina	Muscular tube connecting cervix and external genitalia	Receives the penis during sexual intercourse, serves as a birth canal during childbirth, allows menstrual flow
Labia majora	Outer folds of skin surrounding vaginal opening	Protects the internal reproductive organs and other structures, contains sweat and oil glands
Labia minora	Inner folds of skin inside the labia majora	Protects the clitoris and vaginal opening, helps to keep the area moist
Clitoris	Sensitive organ located at the front of the vulva	Contains erectile tissue, plays a role in sexual pleasure
Mammary glands	Located in the breasts	Produce milk to nourish newborns

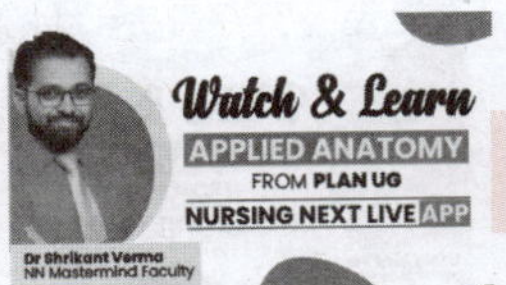

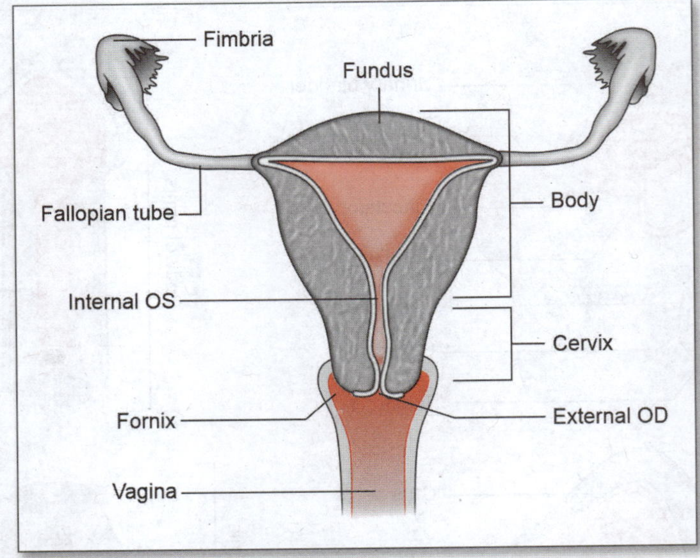

Figure 9.2: Female genital organs

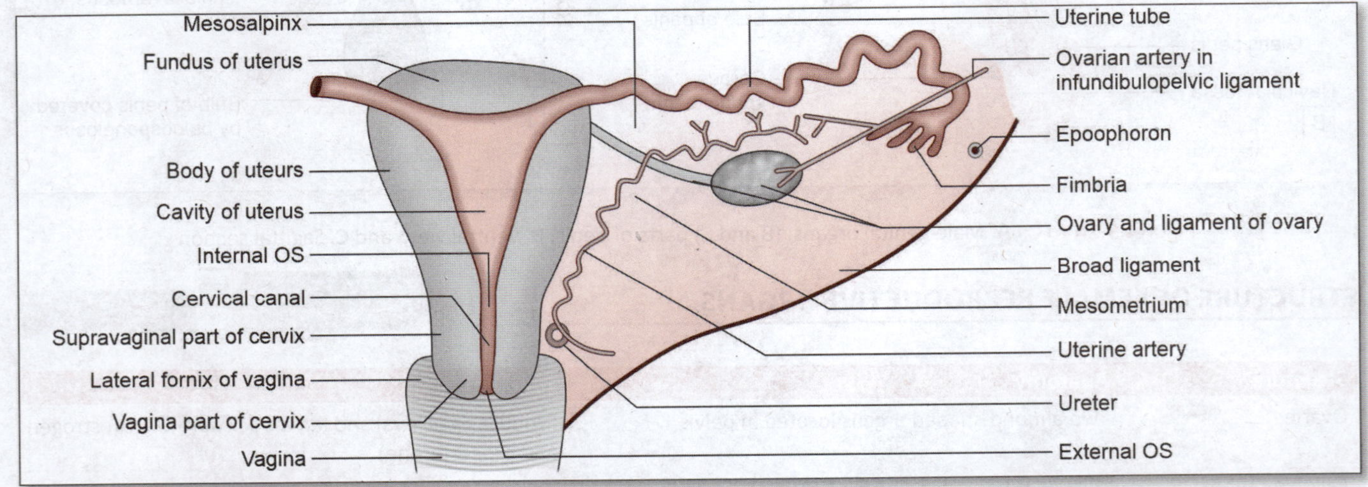

Figure 9.3: Posterosuperior view of the uterus and the right broad ligament

STRUCTURE OF BREAST

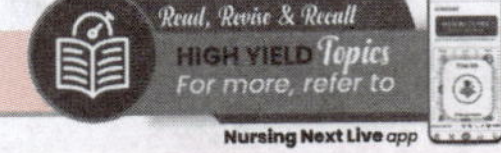

Aspect	Anatomy	Function
Location	Situated between the second and sixth ribs	Produces milk, facilitates breastfeeding
Shape	Tends to be conical in shape	Provides esthetic appearance
Size	Influenced by genetics, hormones, and body weight	Accommodates glandular tissue and fat
Nipple	Composed of erectile tissue and lactiferous ducts	Releases milk during breastfeeding
Areola	Contains Montgomery glands and pigmented skin	Protects the nipple and aids in breastfeeding
Glandular tissue	Contains milk-producing cells	Produces and secretes milk
Duct system	Transports milk from lobules to the nipple	Facilitates milk flow during breastfeeding
Fatty tissue	Surrounds and supports the glandular and ductal tissue	Provides shape, protection, and cushioning
Blood supply	Supplied by branches of the internal mammary arteries	Delivers oxygen and nutrients to breast tissues
Lymphatic system	Includes axillary, internal mammary, and other nodes	Drains excess fluid, filters waste, and fights infection
Hormonal influence	Affects breast development, growth, and milk production	Regulates menstrual cycle and lactation

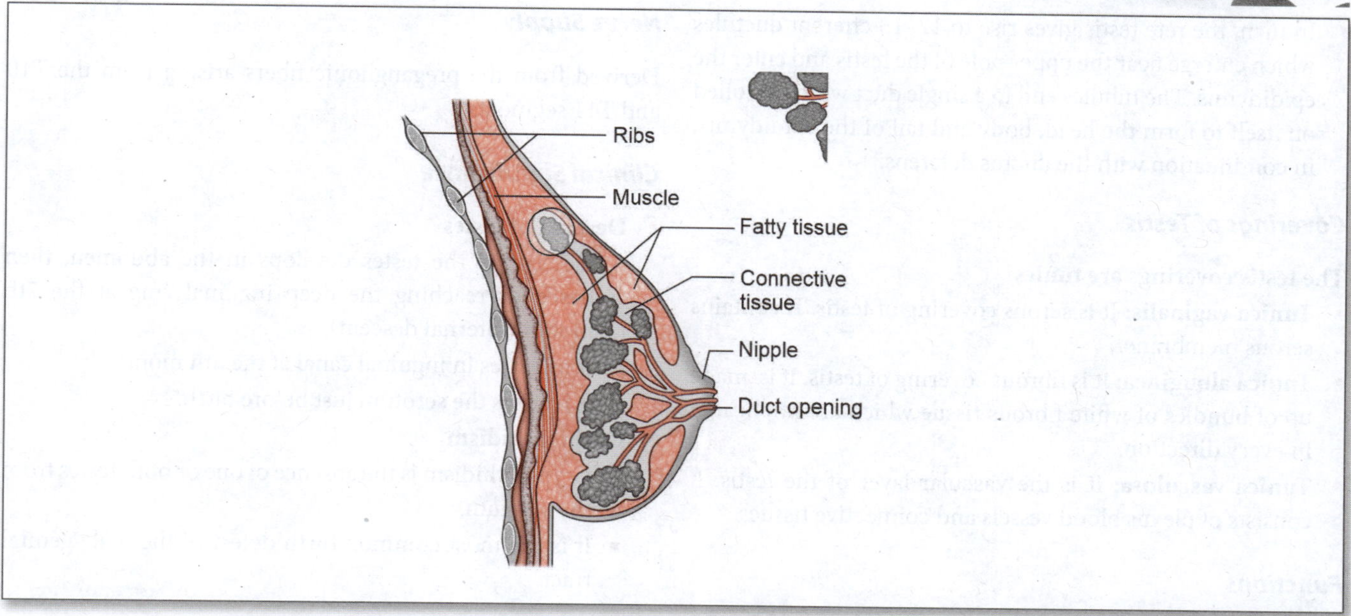

Figure 9.4: Structure of breast

CONCEPTUAL EXERCISES

LONG ANSWER QUESTIONS

1. Give a brief description of male sex gland—testes. What is epididymis and what is its importance? (DU)

Answer

Testes

- Testes, also known as testicles, are the male gonads
- Suspended in the scrotum by the spermatic cord.
- Oval in shape, and is compressed from side to side.
- It is 3.75 cm long, 2.5 cm broad and 1.8 cm thick and weighs about 10–15 g.
- A typical male has two testes approximately 5 cm long, 3 cm wide and 2.5 cm thick. Weighing 10–15 g each, the testes are suspended outside the body in a fleshy sac called the scrotum.
- The scrotum attaches to the body between the base of the penis and anus. The left testis lies slightly lower than the right.

External Features

- Two poles—upper and lower
- Two borders—anterior and posterior
- Two surfaces—medial and lateral

Histology

- The glandular part of the testis consists of 200–300 lobules.
- Each lobule contains two to three seminiferous tubules.
- Each tubule is highly coiled on itself. The tubules are lined by cells which represent stages in the formation of spermatozoa.

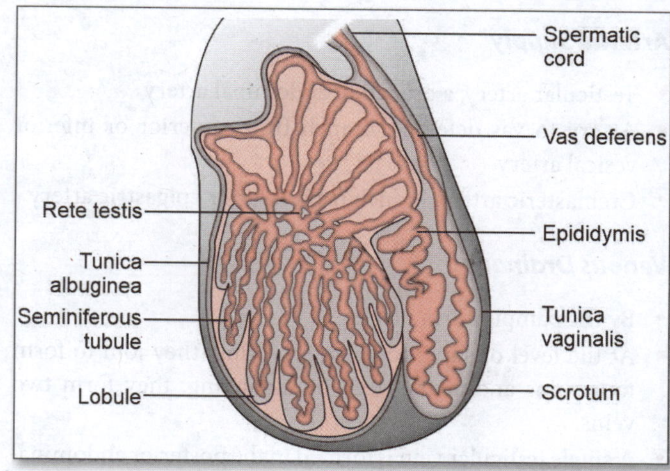

Figure 9.5: Cross-section of testes

- The seminiferous tubules join together at the apices of lobules to form 20 to 30 straight tubules which enter the mediastinum. Here, they anastomose with each other to form a network of tubules, called rete testis.

- In turn, the rete testis gives rise to 12–13 efferent ductules which emerge near the upper pole of the testis and enter the epididymis. The tubules end in a single duct which is coiled on itself to form the head, body and tail of the epididymis, in continuation with the ductus deferens.

Coverings of Testis

The testis coverings are tunics:

- **Tunica vaginalis:** It is serous covering of testis. It contains serous membrane.
- **Tunica albuginea:** It is fibrous covering of testis. It is made up of bundles of white fibrous tissue which are implicated in every direction.
- **Tunica vasculosa:** It is the vascular layer of the testis. It consists of plexus blood vessels and connective tissues.

Functions

- **Spermatogenesis**
  - The primary function of the testes is to produce sperms and the main components of the testes which play a role in sperm production are the seminiferous tubules, Sertoli and Leydig's cells.
  - There are also a series of ducts and tissues within the testis which play an accessory role in producing and/or transporting sperm from the testes.
- **Secretion of testosterone**
  - The testes consist of a series of tubules containing testosterone and sperm-producing cells, which are covered by a multi-layered tunica.
- **Descent of testes**

Arterial Supply

- Testicular artery, a branch of abdominal artery
- Artery to vas deferens, branch from superior or inferior vesical artery
- Cremasteric artery, branch from inferior epigastric artery.

Venous Drainage

- By the pampiniform plexus.
- At the level of superficial inguinal ring, they join to form four veins and at the deep inguinal ring, they form two veins.
- A single testicular vein is formed in the posterior abdominal wall.
- Right testicular vein drains into inferior vena cava
- Left testicular vein drains into left renal vein.

Lymphatic Drainage

Drains into the pre-aortic and the para-aortic lymph nodes.

Nerve Supply

Derived from the preganglionic fibers arising from the T10 and T11 segments.

Clinical Significance

- **Descent of testes**
  - Descent of the testes develops in the abdomen, then descends reaching the deep inguinal ring at the 7th month (internal descent).
  - It migrates in inguinal canal at the 8th month.
  - It reaches the scrotum just before birth.
- **Cryptorchidism**
  - Cryptorchidism is the absence of one or both testes from the scrotum.
  - It is the most common birth defect of the male genital tract.

Epididymis

Comma-shaped body made up of highly coiled tubes situated along the lateral part of the posterior border of the testis.

Parts of Epididymis

The epididymis consists of the following parts:

- **Head:**
  - Formed by coiling of efferent ductules from testis.
  - Receives the spermatozoa via the efferent ducts of mediastinum of testis.
  - Is made up of thick epithelium with long stereocilia and little smooth muscles.
- **Body:** Middle part
  - Has intermediate epithelium and smooth muscle thickness.
- **Tail:**
  - Lower part
  - Continues with vas deferens
  - Has the thinnest epithelial layer
  - Smooth muscle thickness is maximum.
- Body and tail of the epididymis are made up of single coiled epididymal duct. The canal of epididymis is 20 feet long when uncoiled.

Importance of Epididymis (functions)

- It plays an important role in the storage of sperms and the ejaculant.
- Spermatozoa formed in the testis are incomplete when they enter the caput epididymis. They lack motility and ability to fertilize the egg.
- Maturation of sperms takes place in epididymis.

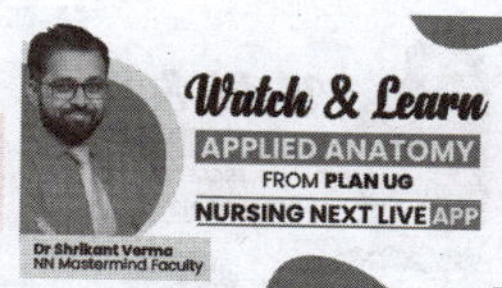

- Epididymal transit takes about two to six days in humans. During this transit, sperms acquire the motility and fertility.
- Final maturation takes place in the female reproductive tract.
- It is involved in absorption of fluid from the sperm to make it more concentrated. This process takes place in the head of the epididymis.
- Also secretes immobilin, a large glycoprotein responsible for creating the viscoelastic luminal environment – it serves to mechanically immobilize spermatozoa until ejaculation.
- Immobilin is predominantly secreted into the proximal caput epididymis prior to the acquisition of sperm motility.

Nursing Implications

- Epididymitis
  - Inflammation of the epididymis.
  - Epididymectomy is performed as a permanent contraceptive method.

2. Describe the structures belonging to the male genital system of the body. (DU)

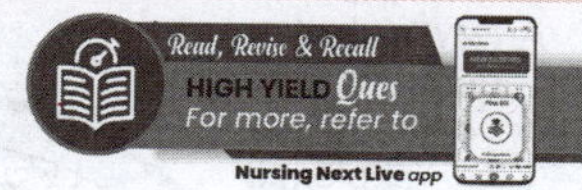

Answer

Introduction

- The male reproductive system is responsible for sexual function and urination.
- Mainly located outside of the body.
- The external organs include penis, scrotum and testicles.
- Internal organs include:
  - Two gonads—Testes
  - Duct system—epididymis, head, body, tail, ductus deferens, ejaculatory duct, and associated glands
  - Prostate, pair of seminal vesicles, urethra

External Genital Organs

- **Penis**
- Male organ of copulation
- Made up of:
  - **Root or attached portion:**
    - Composed of three masses of erectile tissue, namely the two crura and one bulb.
    - Each crura is covered by the ischiocavernosus muscles.
    - The bulb is covered by the bulbospongiosus muscles.
  - **Body or free portion:**
    - The free portion of the penis is completely enveloped by skin.
    - It is composed of three elongated masses of erectile tissue. These masses are the right and left corpora cavernosa and a median corpus spongiosum.
    - The two corpora cavernosa are forward continuations of the crura. They are in close apposition with each other throughout their length. They terminate under cover of the glans penis in a blunt conical extremity. They are surrounded by a strong fibrous envelope called the tunica albuginea.
    - The corpus spongiosum is the forward continuation of the bulb of the penis. Its terminal part is expanded to form a conical enlargement, called the glans penis. Throughout its whole length, it is traversed by the urethra.
    - The base of the glans penis has a projecting margin, the corona glandis, which overhangs an obliquely grooved constriction, known as the neck of the penis. Within the glans, the urethra shows a dilatation called the navicular fossa.
    - The skin covering the penis is very thin and dark in color. It is loosely connected with the fascial sheath of the organ. At the neck, it is folded to form the prepuce or foreskin, which covers the glans to a varying extent and can be retracted backward to expose the glans. On the undersurface of the glans, there is a median fold of skin called the frenulum

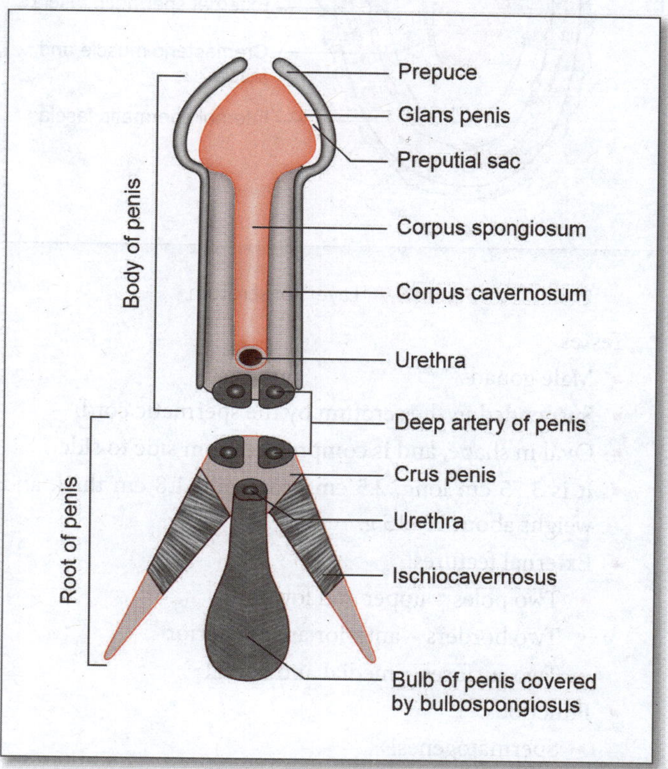

Figure 9.6: Constituent parts of penis

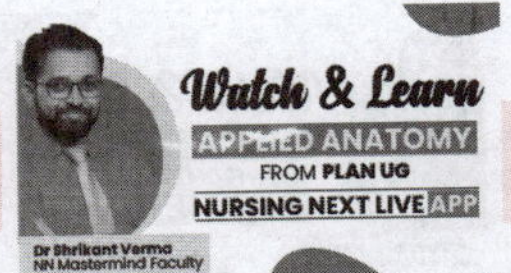

- Arteries of penis
  - The internal pudendal artery gives off three branches which supply the penis.
    1. Deep artery of penis
    2. Dorsal artery of penis
    3. Artery of the bulb
- **Scrotum**
  - Cutaneous bag containing the right and left testes, epididymis and the lower parts of the spermatic cords.
  - Externally divided into right and left parts by a ridge or raphae.
  - Dartos – subcutaneous muscle of scrotum – helps in the regulation of temperature within the scrotum.
  - Layers of scrotum (from without inward):
    - Skin
    - Dartos muscle
    - External spermatic fascia
    - Cremasteric muscle and fascia
    - Internal spermatic fascia

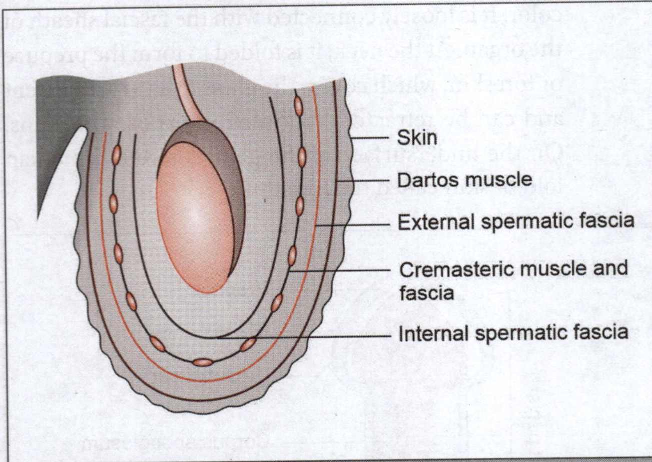

Figure 9.7: Layers of scrotum

- **Testes**
  - Male gonads
  - Suspended in the scrotum by the spermatic cord.
  - Oval in shape, and is compressed from side to side.
  - It is 3.75 cm long, 2.5 cm broad and 1.8 cm thick and weighs about 10–15 g.
  - External features:
    - Two poles – upper and lower
    - Two borders – anterior and posterior
    - Two surfaces – medial and lateral
  - Functions:
    - Spermatogenesis
    - Secretion of testosterone
    - Descent of testes

- **Spermatic cord**
  - The spermatic cord is a cord-like structure in males formed by the vas deferens (ductus deferens) and surrounding tissue that runs from the deep inguinal ring down to each testicle.
  - The anatomical course of the spermatic cord is relatively short, beginning in the inferior abdomen and ending in the scrotum.
  - Constituents of the spermatic cord are:
    - Ductus deferens
    - Testicular and cremasteric arteries
    - Pampiniform plexus of veins
    - Lymph vessels from testes
    - Genital branch of the genitofemoral nerve
    - Plexus of sympathetic nerves around the artery to ductus deferens
    - Remains of processus vaginalis
  - Coverings of spermatic cord (from within outward)
    - Internal spermatic fascia
    - Cremasteric fascia
    - External cremasteric fascia

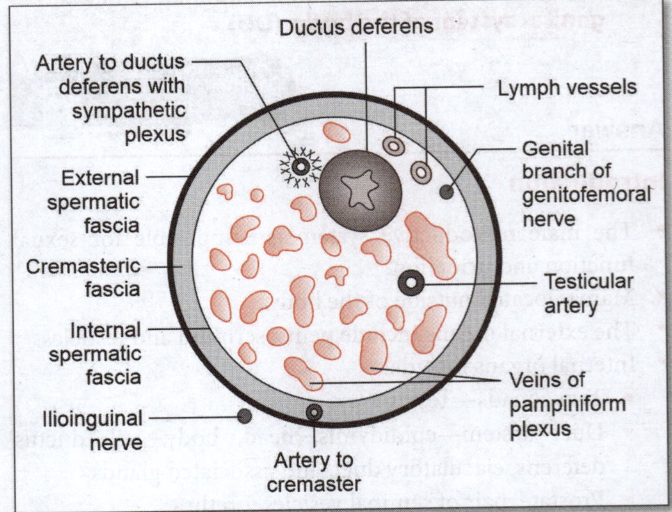

Figure 9.8: Transverse section through the spermatic cord

Internal Genital Organs

- **Ductus deferens**
  - 45 cm long, thick walled, muscular tube which transmits spermatozoa from the epididymis to the ejaculatory duct.
  - At the base of the prostate, the ductus deferens is joined at an acute angle by the duct of the seminal vesicle to form the ejaculatory duct.
  - Supplied by the terminal branches of the superior vesicle artery.
  - Drained by the vesicle venous plexus that opens into the internal iliac vein.

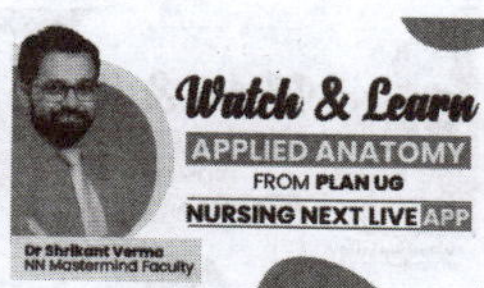

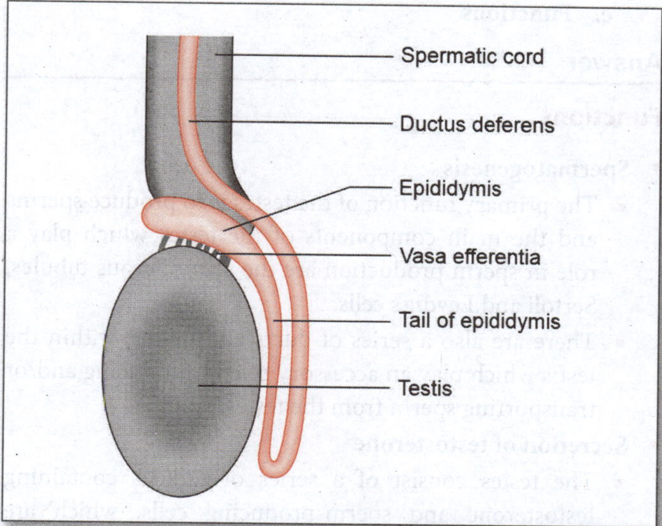

Figure 9.9: Relationship of the ductus deferens to the testis and the spermatic cord

- **Seminal vesicles**
  - Two in number
  - Lobulated sacs present between the bladder and rectum
  - The lower narrow end forms the duct of the seminal vesicle which joins the ductus deferens to form the ejaculatory duct.

3. Enumerate the organs of male reproductive system. Describe the testis in detail under the following headings:

a. Structure, b. Coverings, c. Blood supply, nerve supply and lymphatic drainage d. Clinical significance, e. Functions (MGR, RUHS)

Answer

Organs of Male Reproductive System

The male reproductive system is responsible for sexual function and urination.

- Mainly located outside of the body.
- The external organs include penis, scrotum and testicles.
- Internal organs include:
  - Two gonads—testes
  - Duct system—epididymis, head, body, tail, ductus deferens, ejaculatory duct and associated glands
  - Prostate, pair of seminal vesicles and urethra

a. Structure

Answer

Structure of Testis

- Male gonads
- Suspended in the scrotum by the spermatic cord.
- Oval in shape, and is compressed from side to side.
- It is 3.75 cm long, 2.5 cm broad and 1.8 cm thick and weighs about 10–15 g.
- A typical male has two testes approximately 5 cm long, 3 cm wide and 2.5 cm thick. Weighing 10–15 g each, the testes are suspended outside the body in a fleshy sac called the scrotum.
- The scrotum attaches to the body between the base of the penis and anus. The left testis lies slightly lower than the right.
- **External features**
  - Two poles—upper and lower
  - Two borders—anterior and posterior
  - Two surfaces—medial and lateral
- The glandular part of the testis consists of 200–300 lobules. Each lobule contains two to three seminiferous tubules. Each tubule is highly coiled on itself. The tubules are lined by cells which represent stages in the formation of spermatozoa.

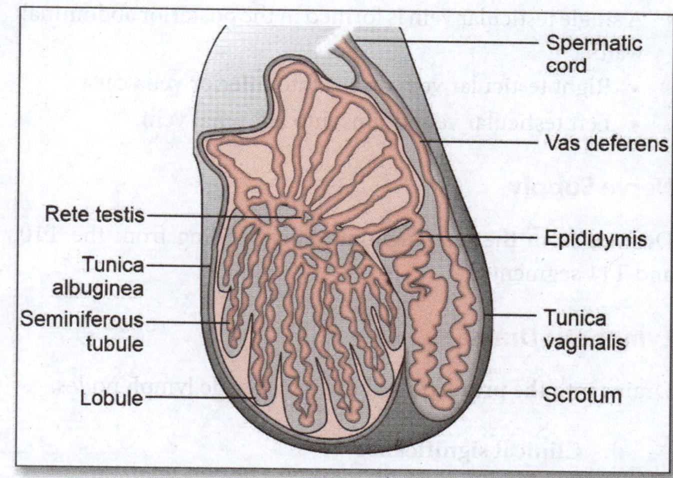

Figure 9.10: Cross-section of testes

- The seminiferous tubules join together at the apices of lobules to form 20 to 30 straight tubules which enter the mediastinum. Here, they anastomose with each other to form a network of tubules, called rete testis.
- The rete testis gives rise to 12–13 efferent ductules which emerge near the upper pole of the testis and enter the epididymis.

b. Coverings

Answer

Coverings of Testis

- **The testis coverings are tunics:**
  - **Tunica vaginalis:** It is serous covering of testis. It contains serous membrane.

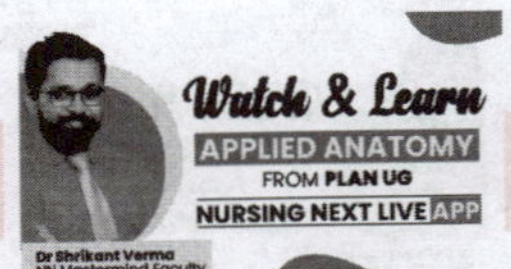

- **Tunica albuginea:** It is fibrous covering of testis. It is made up of bundles of white fibrous tissue which are implicated in every direction.
- **Tunica vasculosa:** It is the vascular layer of the testis. It consists of plexus blood vessels and connective tissues.

c. **Blood supply, nerve supply and lympahtic drainage**

Answer

Arterial Supply

- Testicular artery, a branch of abdominal artery
- Artery to vas deferens, branch from superior or inferior vesical artery
- Cremasteric artery, branch from inferior epigastric artery.

Venous Drainage

- By the pampiniform plexus.
- At the level of superficial inguinal ring, they join to form four veins and at the deep inguinal ring, they form two veins.
- A single testicular vein is formed in the posterior abdominal wall.
  - Right testicular vein drains into inferior vena cava
  - Left testicular vein drains into left renal vein.

Nerve Supply

Derived from the preganglionic fibers arising from the T10 and T11 segments.

Lymphatic Drainage

Drains into the preaortic and the para-aortic lymph nodes.

d. **Clinical significance**

Answer

Clinical Significance

- **Testicular torsion:** Twisting of spermatic cord and obstruction of blood supply to testis. This results in sudden urgent pain and requires emergency treatment.
- **Testicular carcinoma:** Common in undescended or ectopic testis
- **Undescended testis (Cryptorchidism):** If testis does not descend and remain in lumbar or inguinal region and there is reduced fertility and increased risk of testicular carcinoma. It is the most common birth defect of the male genital tract.
- **Varicocele:** Dilatation and tortuosity of veins of pampiniform plexus.
- **Hydrocele:** Accumulation of fluid in the tunica vaginalis of testis.

e. **Functions**

Answer

Functions

- **Spermatogenesis**
  - The primary function of the testes is to produce sperms and the main components of the testes which play a role in sperm production are the seminiferous tubules, Sertoli and Leydig's cells.
  - There are also a series of ducts and tissues within the testis which play an accessory role in producing and/or transporting sperm from the testes.
- **Secretion of testosterone**
  - The testes consist of a series of tubules containing testosterone and sperm-producing cells, which are covered by a multilayered tunica.
- **Descent of testes**

4. Describe in detail the supports of uterus. (MGR)

Answer

Supports of the Uterus

The uterus is a mobile organ, which undergoes extensive changes in size and shape during the reproductive period of life. It is supported and prevented from sagging down by a number of factors which are chiefly muscular and fibromuscular.

Classification of the Supports of Uterus

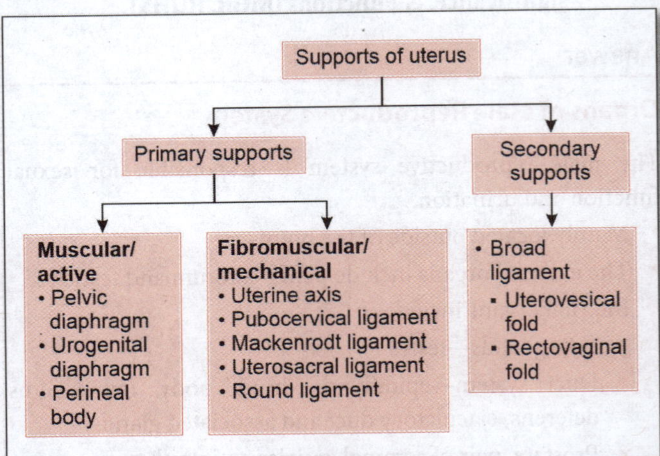

Primary Supports

Muscular/Active Supports

- **Pelvic diaphragm:**
  - Supports the pelvic viscera and resists any rise in the intra-abdominal pressure

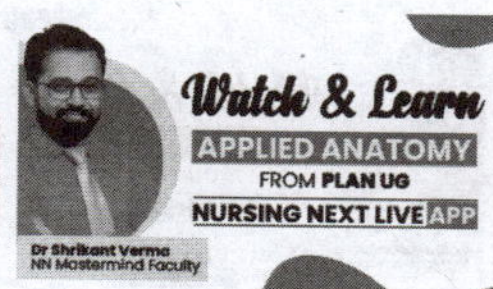

- Pubococcygeus part of levator ani supports uterus from below. It is inserted into the perineal body between the vagina and rectum.
- Pubovaginalis part forms a sling
- **Perineal body:**
  - The perineal body is a fibromuscular mass, and irregular in shape. It is present at the junction of the urogenital and anal triangles. This structure comprises skeletal muscle, smooth muscle and collagenous and elastic fibers.
  - Anatomy:
    - Anatomically, the perineal body lies deep to the skin. This is a point of attachment for muscle fibers from the pelvic floor and the perineum itself.
    - Fibromuscular node into which ten muscles attach.
    - Maintains the integrity of the pelvic floor.
  - **The muscles are:**
    - Two superficial transverse perinei
    - Two deep transverse perinei
    - Two pubococcygeus part of levator ani
    - Two bulbospongiosus
    - Single sphincter ani externus and unstriped fibers of longitudinal muscle coat of the anal canal.
    - In women, it is a tear resistant body between the vagina and the external anal sphincter, supports the posterior part of the vaginal wall against prolapse. In males, it presents between the bulb of penis and the anus.

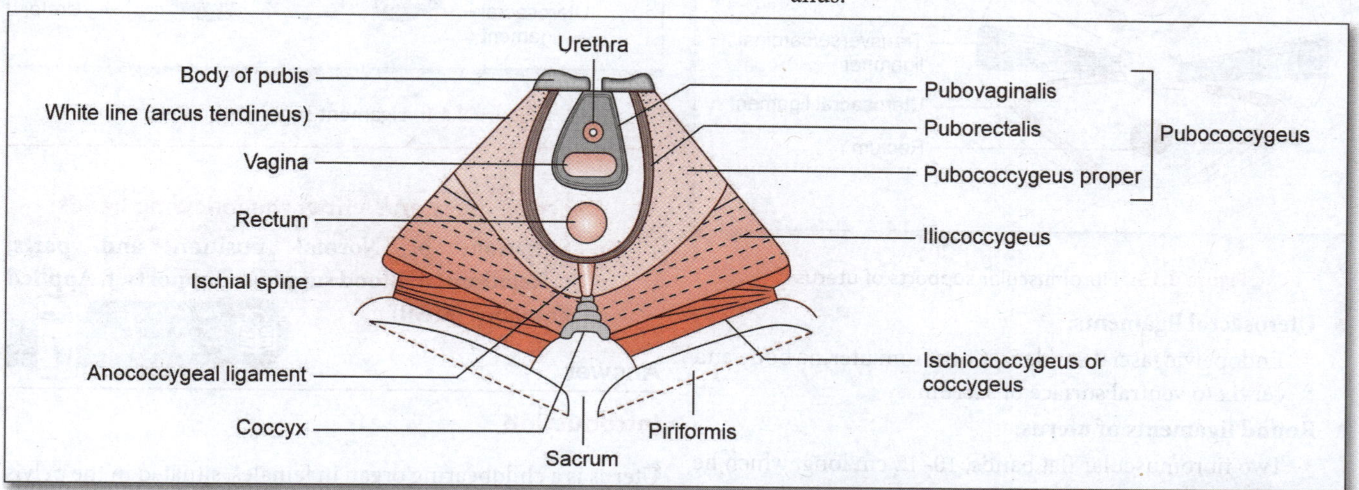

Figure 9.11: Pelvic diaphragm

- Childbirth can lead to damage (stretching/tearing) of the perineal body, thereby leading to the prolapse of pelvic viscera.
- **Distal urethral sphincter mechanism:**
  - Controls the exit of urine through urethra.
  - There are compressor urethrae and sphincter urethrae vaginalis.
  - As these are inserted into the vagina, they support the uterus indirectly.

Fibromuscular/Mechanical Supports

- **Fibromuscular uterine axis:**
  - Anteverted uterus prevents its prolapse.
- **Pubocervical ligaments:**
  - Endopelvic fascial condensations from ventral surface cervix around the urethra to the posterior surface of the pubic bones.

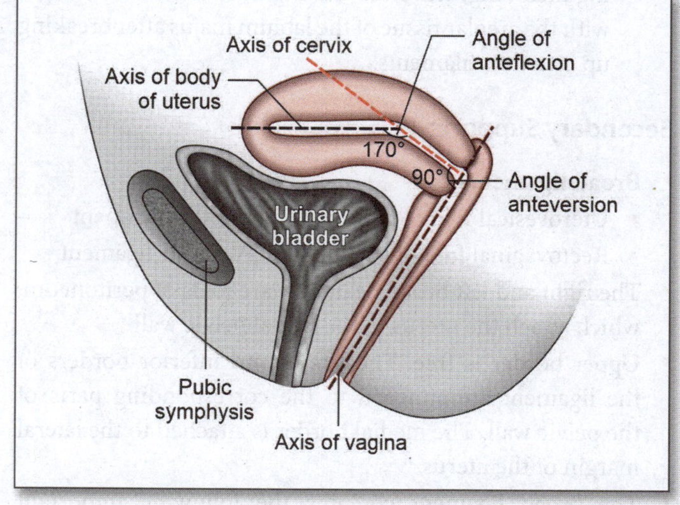

Figure 9.12: Angulation of uterus, vagina and cervix with body of uterus

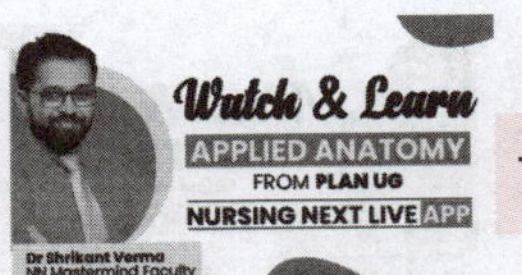

- **Transverse cervical ligaments of Mackenrodt/cardinal ligaments:**
  - Endopelvic fascial condensations from cervix and lateral fornix of vagina to the lateral pelvic walls.
  - They connect the lateral aspects of the cervix and of the upper vaginal wall to the lateral pelvic wall, about 2.5 cm ventral to the ischial spine.
  - They form a "hammock" that supports the uterus.

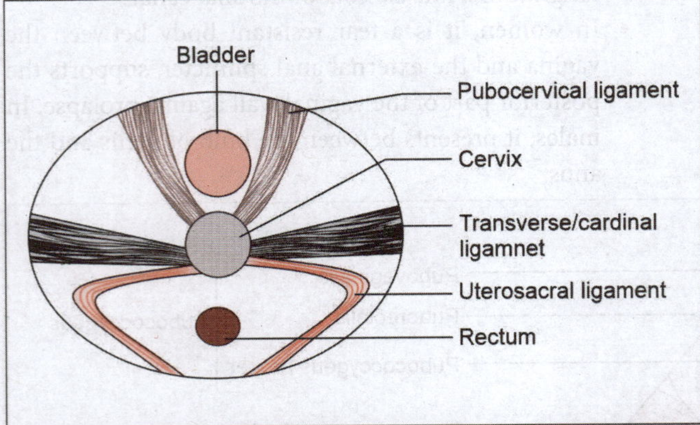

Figure 9.13: Fibromuscular supports of uterus

- **Uterosacral ligaments:**
  - Endopelvic fascial condensations from uterine body and cervix to ventral surface of sacrum.
- **Round ligaments of uterus:**
  - Two fibromuscular flat bands, 10–12 cm long, which lie between the two layers of the broad ligament.
  - Each ligament begins at the lateral angle of the uterus, runs forward and laterally, passes through the deep inguinal ring, traverses the inguinal canal and merges with the areolar tissue of the labium majus after breaking up into thin filaments.

Secondary Supports

- **Broad ligaments:**
  - Uterovesical fold of peritoneum/Anterior ligament
  - Rectovaginal fold of peritoneum/Posterior ligament
- The right and left broad ligaments are folds of peritoneum, which attach the uterus to the lateral pelvic wall.
- Upper border is free. The lateral and inferior borders of the ligament are attached to the corresponding parts of the pelvic wall. The medial border is attached to the lateral margin of the uterus.
- The broad ligament contains the following important structures:
  - The uterine tube
  - The round ligament of the uterus
  - The ligament of the ovary
  - Uterine vessels near its attachment to the uterus
  - Ovarian vessels in the infundibulopelvic ligament
  - The uterovaginal and ovarian nerve plexuses

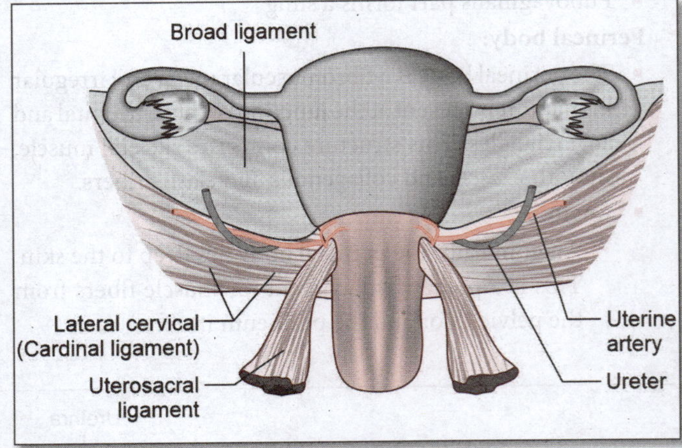

Figure 9.14: Ligament supports of uterus

5. Describe the uterus under the following heads:

a. Situation, b. Normal position and parts, c. Relations, d. Blood supply, e. Supports, f. Applied anatomy. (MGR)

Answer

Introduction

Uterus is a childbearing organ in females, situated in the pelvis between the bladder and rectum. Though hollow, it is thick walled and firm, and can be palpated bimanually during the per vaginal examination.

a. Situation

Answer

Situation

- It is pyriform in shape, and is divisible into an upper expanded part called the body and a lower cylindrical part called the cervix.
- Part of the uterus above the opening of the fallopian tubes is called the fundus.
- It protects and provides nutrition to a fertilized ovum, enabling it to grow into a fully formed fetus.

b. Normal position and parts

Answer

Position

- The anatomical location of the uterus varies with the degree of distension of the bladder. In a normal adult uterus, it can

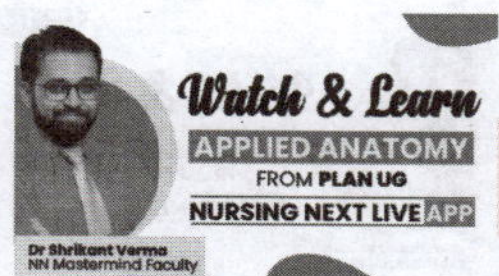

be described as anteverted with respect to the vagina, and anteflexed with respect to the cervix.

- **Anteverted:** Rotated forward, toward the anterior surface of the body.
- **Anteflexed:** Flexed, toward the anterior surface of the body.

- Thus, the uterus normally lies immediately posterosuperior to the bladder, and anterior to the rectum.

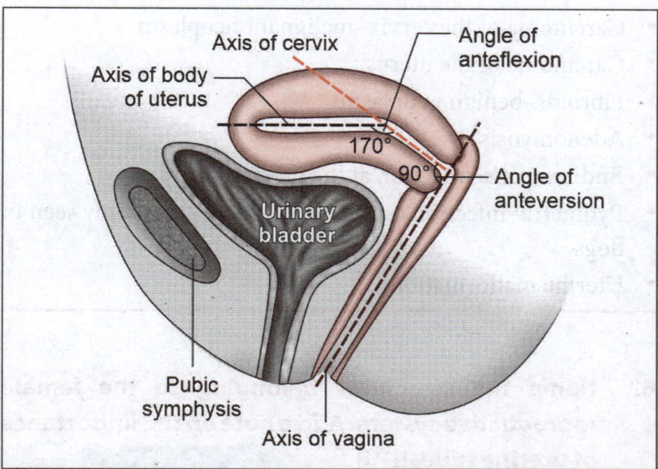

Figure 9.15: Position of uterus

Parts

- **Fundus**
  - Fundus is broad and curved in shape. It is the upper part of the uterus. The fallopian tubes attach to the uterus just below the fundus.
- **Corpus**
  - Corpus is muscular and stretchable to accommodate a developing fetus. During labor, the muscular walls of the corpus contract to help push the baby through the cervix and vagina. The corpus is the main body of the uterus.
  - The corpus is lined by a mucous membrane known as the endometrium. The endometrium changes its thickness during each menstrual cycle in order to respond to reproductive hormones. The fertilized egg is attached to the endometrium. If there is no fertilization, the endometrium sheds its outer layer of cells, which is shed off during menstruation.
- **Isthmus**
  - The position of the uterus between the corpus and the cervix is called the isthmus. The walls of the uterus begin to narrow toward the cervix here.
- **Cervix**
  - It is the lowest part of the uterus. It is lined with a smooth mucous membrane and connects the uterus to the vagina. The cervical glands mostly produce a thick mucus. But during ovulation, the mucus becomes thinner to allow sperm to easily pass into the uterus.
  - **The cervix has three main parts:**
    1. **Endocervix:** It is the inner part of the cervix which leads to the uterus.
    2. **Cervical canal:** The cervical canal is the link between the uterus and vagina.
    3. **Exocervix:** The exocervix is the outer part of the cervix that invaginates into the vagina.
  - During childbirth, the cervix widens to allow the baby pass through the birth canal.

c. **Relations**

Answer

Relations

- **Anteriorly:** The body of uterus is associated with the uterovesical pouch and the superior surface of urinary bladder.
  - The supravaginal portion of cervix is associated with the posterior surface of urinary bladder.
- **Posteriorly:** The body of uterus is linked to the rectouterine pouch with coils of ileum and sigmoid colon in it.
  - The supravaginal portion of cervix is associated with the rectouterine pouch with coils of ileum and sigmoid colon in it.

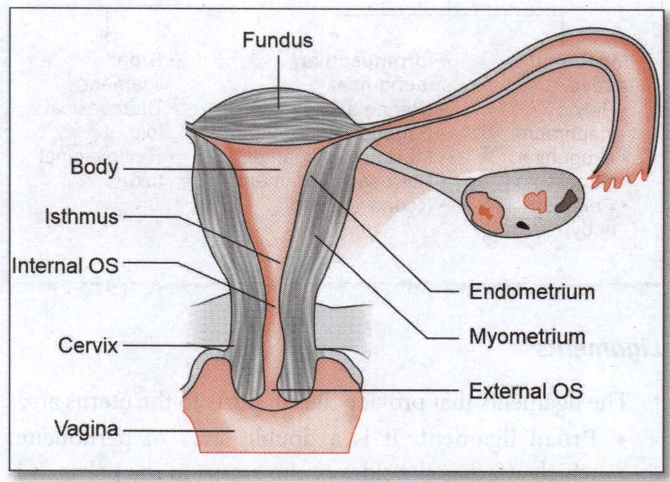

Figure 9.16: Ovaries and their relationships to uterine tube and uterus

  - Vaginal portion of cervix is related to posterior fornix.
- **Laterally:** The body of uterus is related to the broad ligament and uterine artery and vein.
  - The supravaginal portion of cervix is linked to the ureter and uterine artery.
  - The vaginal portion of cervix is linked to the lateral fornices of the vagina.

d. **Blood supply**

Answer

Blood Supply

- Blood supply to the uterus is via the uterine artery.
- Venous drainage is via a plexus in the broad ligament that drains into the uterine veins.
- Lymphatic drainage of the uterus is via the iliac, sacral, aortic and inguinal lymph nodes.

e. **Supports**

Answer

Supports of Uterus

The uterus is a mobile organ, which undergoes extensive changes in size and shape during the reproductive period of life. It is supported and prevented from sagging down by a number of factors which are chiefly muscular and fibromuscular.

Classification of the Supports of Uterus

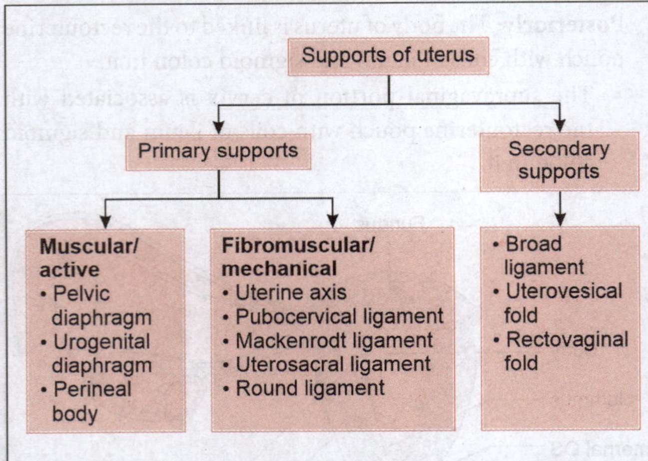

Ligaments

- The ligaments that provide the supports to the uterus are:
  - **Broad ligament:** It is a double layer of peritoneum which attaches the sides of the uterus to the pelvis. It is like a mesentery for the uterus and helps in maintaining it in position.
  - **Round ligament:** It is a remnant of the gubernaculum which extends from the uterine horns to the labia majora through the inguinal canal. It helps in maintaining the anteverted position of the uterus.
  - **Ovarian ligament:** It joins the ovaries to the uterus.
  - **Cardinal ligament:** It is present at the base of the broad ligament and extends from the cervix to the lateral pelvic walls.
  - **Uterosacral ligament:** It extends from the cervix to the sacrum and provides support to the uterus.

f. **Applied anatomy**

Answer

Applied Anatomy

- Prolapse of the uterus
- Carcinoma of the cervix–malignant neoplasm
- Carcinoma of the uterus
- Fibroids–benign neoplasms
- Adenomyosis
- Endometritis, infection at the uterine cavity
- Pyometra–infection of the uterus, most commonly seen in dogs
- Uterine malformations

6. Name the structures belonging to the female reproductive system. Add a note on the importance of uterine tube. (DU)

Read, Revise & Recall HIGH YIELD Ques For more, refer to Nursing Next Live app

Answer

Introduction

The female reproductive system is comprised of the external and internal sex organs. These organs play a role in reproduction.

The functions of the female reproductive system are:

- Formation of ova
- Reception of spermatozoa
- Provision of suitable environment for fertilization and fetal development
- Parturition
- Lactation

Parts of Female Reproductive System

Female reproductive organs or genitalia include both external and internal organs.

External Genitalia (Vulva)

- It consists of:
  - Mons pubis
  - Labia majora
  - Labia minora
  - Clitoris
  - Vaginal orifice
  - Vestibule

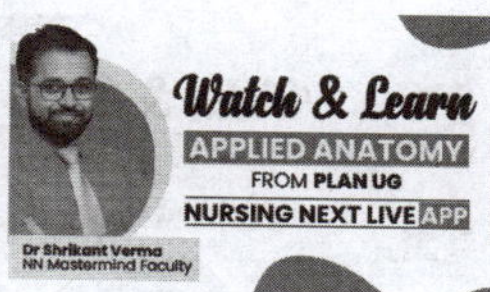

- Hymen
- Vestibular glands (Bartholin's glands)

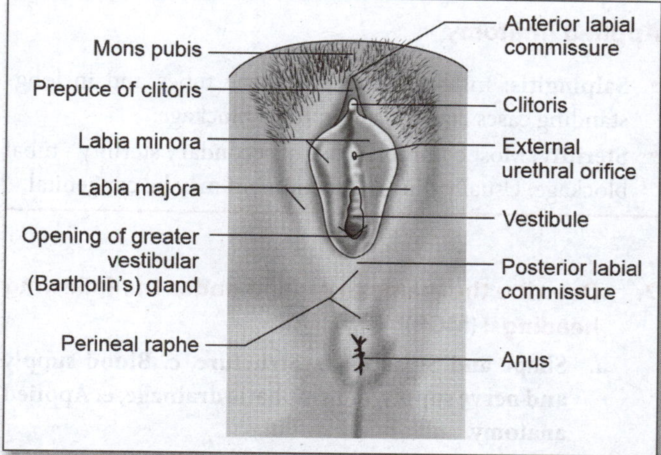

Figure 9.17: External genital organs in females

Mons Pubis

- Rounded eminence presents in front of the pubic symphysis.
- Formed by accumulation of subcutaneous fat.
- Covered by pubic hair.

Labia Majora

- Two large folds forming the boundary of pudendal cleft.
- Outer surfaces are covered with hair and inner surfaces with large sebaceous glands.

Internal Genitalia

- Internal reproductive system lies in the pelvic cavity and consists of:
  - Vagina
  - Uterus
  - Two uterine tubes
  - Two ovaries

Uterus

- Uterus is a childbearing organ in female, situated in the pelvis between the bladder and rectum.
- It is pyriform in shape, and is divisible into an upper expanded part called the body and a lower cylindrical part called the cervix.
- Part of the uterus above the opening of the fallopian tubes is called the fundus.

Ovaries

- Ovaries are female gonads.
- Paired almond-shaped structure.
- Located in the lateral wall of the pelvis.
- Ovaries secrete estrogen under the effect of FSH of anterior pituitary and progesterone under the effect of LH of anterior pituitary.
- Ovaries show many types of follicles in their cortex.

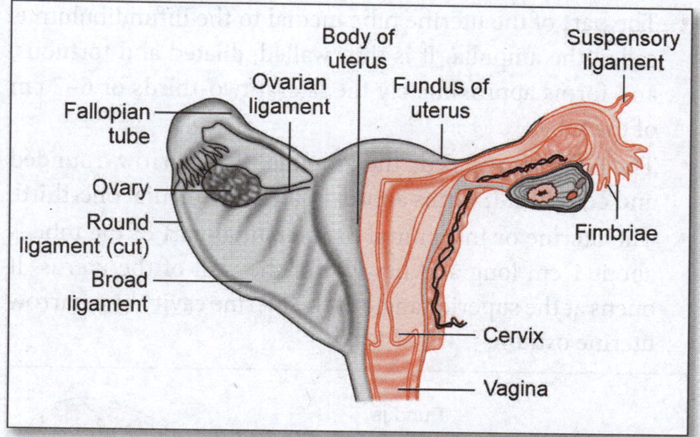

Figure 9.18: Structure of ovary

Uterine Tubes/Fallopian Tubes

- Tortuous ducts that convey oocyte from the ovary to the uterus.
- Also known as uterine tubes/salpinx.
- Spermatozoa reach the ovum through the fallopian tubes, where the fertilization takes place.
- Each tube is about 10 cm long.

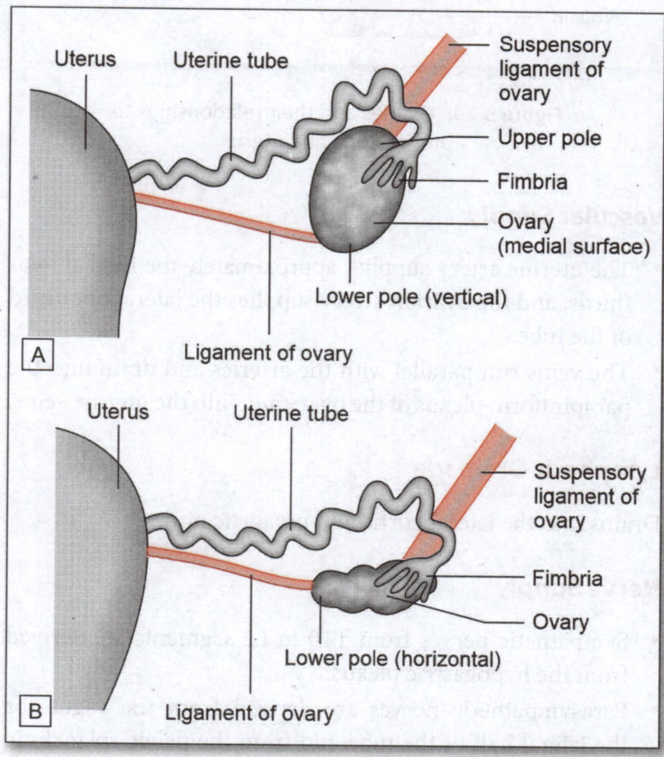

Figures 9.19 Positions of the ovary: **A.** Mullipara-vertical; **B.** Multipara - horizontal

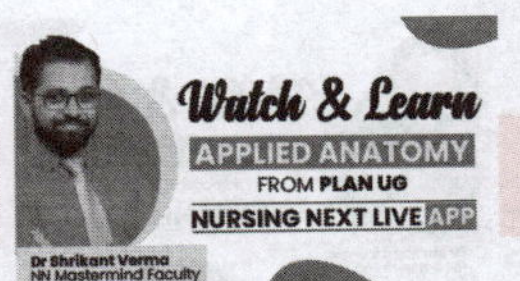

Parts of Fallopian Tube

- The lateral end of the uterine tube is shaped like a funnel and is, therefore, called the infundibulum. It bears a number of finger-like processes called fimbriae and is, therefore, called the fimbriated end.
- The part of the uterine tube medial to the infundibulum is called the ampulla. It is thin walled, dilated and tortuous, and forms approximately the lateral two-thirds or 6–7 cm of the tube.
- The isthmus succeeds the ampulla. It is narrow, rounded and cord like. It forms approximately the medial one-third.
- The uterine or intramural or interstitial part of the tube is about 1 cm long and lies within the wall of the uterus. It opens at the superior angle of the uterine cavity by a narrow uterine ostium.

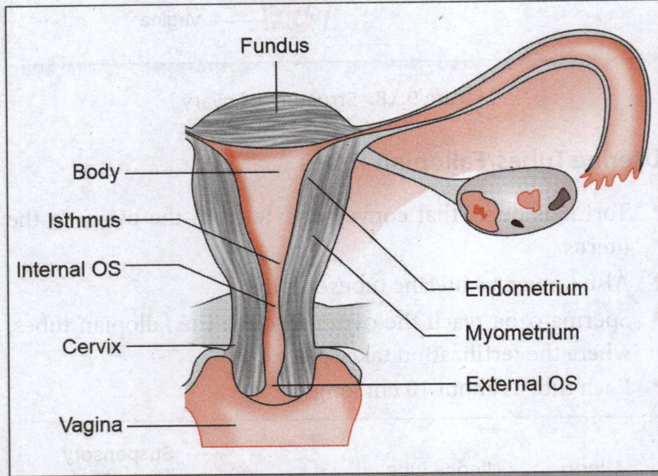

Figure 9.20: Ovaries and their relationships to uterine tube and uterus

Vascular Supply

- The uterine artery supplies approximately the medial two-thirds, and the ovarian artery supplies the lateral one-third of the tube.
- The veins run parallel with the arteries and drain into the pampiniform plexus of the ovary and into the uterine veins.

Lymphatic Drainage

Drains into the lateral aortic and preaortic nodes.

Nerve Supply

- Sympathetic nerves from T10 to L2 segments are derived from the hypogastric plexus.
- Parasympathetic nerves are derived from the vagus for the lateral half of the tube and from the pelvic splanchnic nerves from S2-S4 segments of spinal cord for the medial-half.

Applied Anatomy

- **Salpingitis:** Inflammation of uterine tubes and in long-standing cases could result in tubal blockage.
- **Sterility:** Most common cause of secondary sterility - tubal blockage. Usually due to infection but may be congenital.

7. Describe the mammary gland under the following headings: (MGR)

a. Shape and Surfaces, b. Structure, c. Blood supply and nerve supply, d. Lymphatic drainage, e. Applied anatomy.

Answer

Introduction

- Commonly known as breast.
- Exocrine gland present bilaterally in the pectoral region
- Present in both males and females, but female breasts are more developed after puberty.
- It is a modified sweat gland.

a. Shape and surfaces

Answer

Shape

- External features of human adult breast are:
  - Base
    - Circular, vertically extends from the 2nd to 6th rib in the midclavicular line.
    - Rests on the pectoralis major muscle.
  - Nipple
    - Conical projection below the center of breast
    - Pierced by 15–20 lactiferous ducts.
    - Contains circular and longitudinal muscles.
    - Circular muscles cause the erection of nipple and longitudinal muscles help in its retraction.
  - Areola
    - Pigmented circular area of skin around the base of nipple.
    - Modified sebaceous gland
    - Provides lubrication during lactation.
  - Axillary tail
    - Tail-like projection from upper outer quadrant of the breast into the axilla.

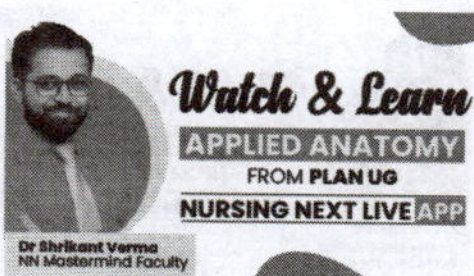

b. Structure

Answer

Structure

Consists of three components:

1. **Glandular tissue:**
   - Alveoli
     - Lined with milk-secreting cuboidal cells and myoepithelial cells.
     - Alveoli join to form lobules.
     - The breast consists of 15–20 pyramidal lobes. Each lobe is connected to a lactiferous duct that drains into the nipple.
     - The myoepithelial cells contract under the stimulation of oxytocin to excrete the milk secreted by alveolar units into the lobule.
2. **Fibrous tissue**
   - To protect and maintain the morphology of alveoli, extracellular matrix along with adipocytes and fibroblast—that form the stroma—are essential.
   - Mammary epithelial ECM contains the myoepithelial basement membrane and connective tissue.
   - It serves as a communicating bridge between mammary epithelia and the external environment.
3. Interlobar fatty tissue makes the breast rounded in contour. Fat is absent beneath the nipple and areola.

c. Blood supply and nerve supply

Answer

Blood Supply

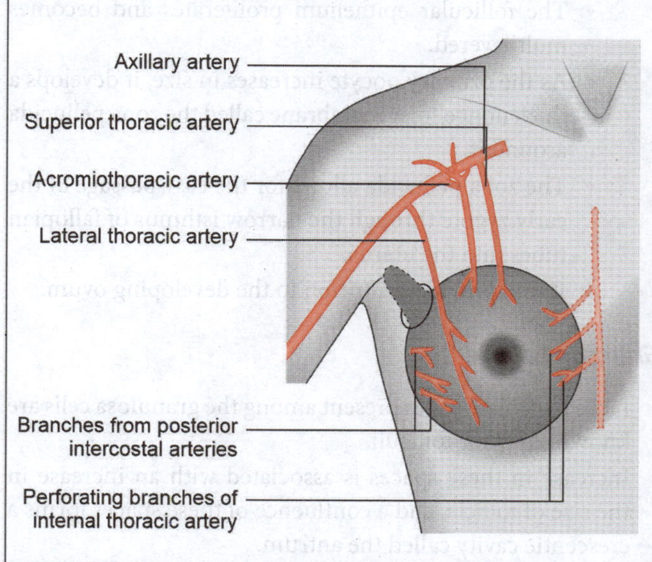

Figure 9.21: Blood supply of the mammary gland

- **Supplied by the:**
  - Lateral mammary branches of axillary artery
  - Perforating branches from 2nd, 3rd and 4th intercostals arteries (internal thoracic artery)
  - Superior thoracic artery
- **Venous drainages into:**
  - Axillary veins
  - Internal thoracic veins
  - Intercostal veins

Nerve Supply

- Intercostal nerves
- Sympathetic fibers provide the sensory supply

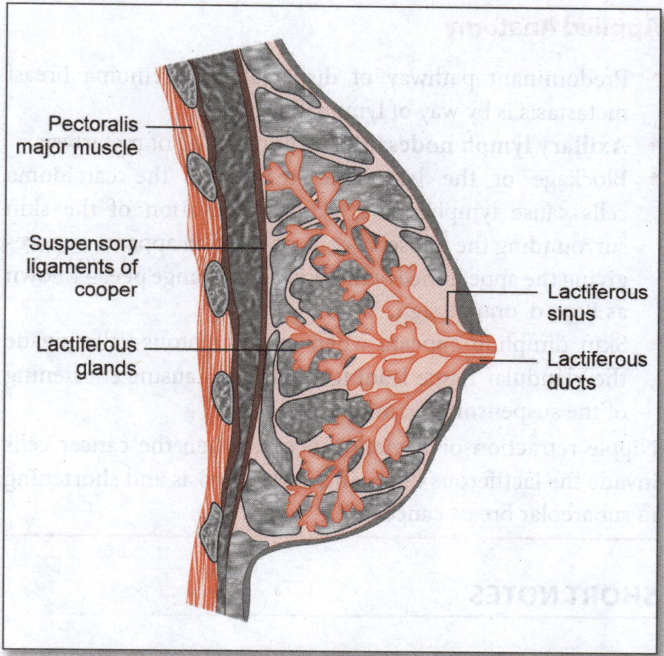

Figure 9.22: Mammary glands of female

d. Lymphatic drainage

Answer

Lymphatic Drainage of Breast

- **Dermal network:** Drain skin over the breast except that from nipple and areola pass radially.
- **Lateral aspect:** Drain into axillary lymph nodes
- **Superior aspect:** Supraclavicular nodes, few may reach nodes along cephalic vein in deltopectoral triangle
- **Medial aspect:** Drain into internal mammary nodes/ parasternal nodes
- **Inferior aspect:** Form a subperitoneal plexus and drain into subdiaphragmatic nodes. Crosses midline and communicates with contralateral lymphatics
- Lymphatics from parenchyma of breast:

- **From areola:** Subareolar plexus of Sappey communicates with breast lymphatics
- Axillary lymph nodes drain 75% of breast parenchymal lymphatics.
- Lymphatics from the parenchyma pass laterally toward the axillary tail receiving tributaries on their way: Mostly drain into anterior group and few into posterior group – finally drain into central and apical groups.
- Lymphatics from deep parts of breast pierce pectoralis major to drain into axillary and parasternal nodes.

e. **Applied anatomy**

Answer

Applied Anatomy

- Predominant pathway of dispersal of carcinoma breast metastasis is by way of lymphatic spread.
- **Axillary lymph nodes:** Most common site of metastasis.
- Blockage of the lymphatic vessels by the carcinoma cells cause lymphedema: Causing elevation of the skin surrounding the pilosebaceous unit which appears as pores giving the appearance of the skin of an orange peel—known as Peau d' orange sign.
- Skin dimpling appears when carcinomatous cells invade the glandular tissue leading to fibrosis causing shortening of the suspensory ligaments.

Nipple retraction or deviation occurs when the cancer cells invade the lactiferous ducts and cause fibrosis and shortening in subareolar breast cancer.

SHORT NOTES

1. Write a short note on histology of ovary. (RUHS)

Answer

Introduction

- Internal genital organ in females.
- Situated in the ovarian fossa on the lateral pelvic wall.

Histology

- Ovary is composed of the following parts from outside to inside.
  - Germinal epithelium
    - Cubical cells derived from peritoneum
  - Tunica albuginea
    - Thin layer of connective tissue
  - Cortex
    - Contains ovarian follicles at various stages of development
    - Each follicle contains one oocyte.
    - After the oocytes are liberated, the Graafian follicle gets converted into corpus luteum.

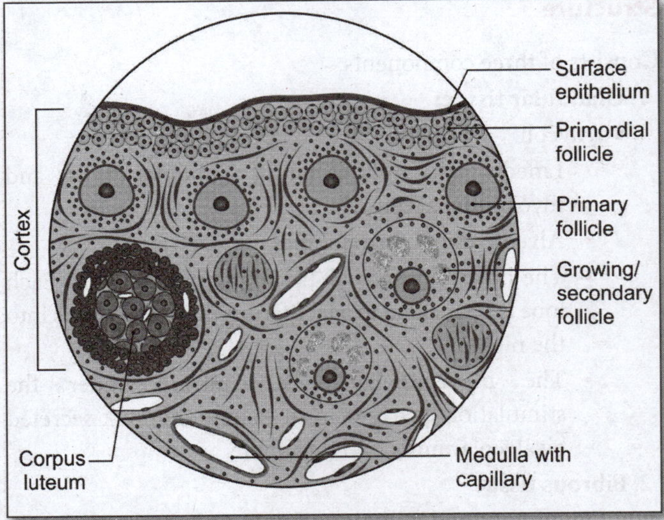

Figure 9.23 : Histology of ovary

Ovarian Follicles

- Seen in the cortex of ovary after puberty and are classified as:
  - Primordial follicle
    - It consists of primary oocyte surrounded by a single layer of flattened cells.
  - Primary follicle
    - It has a primary oocyte surrounded by the cuboidal cells.
    - The primary oocyte has a large nucleus, prominent nucleolus and pale chromatin.
  - Secondary follicle
    - The follicular epithelium proliferates and becomes multilayered.
    - As the primary oocyte increases in size, it develops a thick noncellular membrane called the zona pellucida around it.
    - The zona pellucida allows for the easy passage of the early zygote through the narrow isthmus of fallopian tubes into the uterus.
    - It also provides nutrition to the developing ovum.

Graafian Follicle

- Little irregular spaces present among the granulosa cells are known as liquor folliculi.
- Increase in these spaces is associated with an increase in the size of follicle, and a confluence of these spaces forms a crescentic cavity called the antrum.
- At this stage, the primary oocyte lies on one side of cavity.

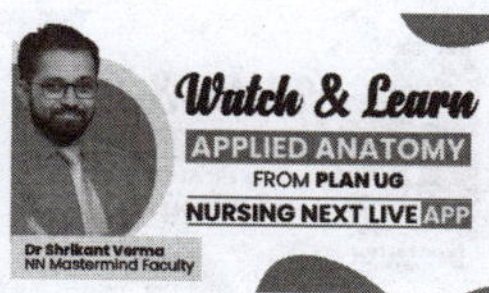

- Follicular cells surrounding the ovum are known as cumulus oophorus.
- The stroma around the follicle arranges itself into an inner theca interna that is vascular and cellular and outer theca externa that is fibrous.
- The theca interna secretes estrogen.
- The follicle bulges onto the surface of the ovary to form the mature Graafian follicle.
- The primary oocyte undergoes first meiotic division and becomes the secondary oocytes and bursts from the follicle.
- Corona radiata cells surround the follicular cells in secondary oocyte.
- The rupture of follicle to release the secondary oocyte is known as ovulation.
- **Functions of Graafian follicle:**
  - Forms mature ova
  - Secretes estrogen
  - Provides a medium for the growth of corpus luteum.
    - Atretic follicle
      - Many follicles undergo degeneration and are called atretic follicle. These secrete estrogen.
    - Corpus luteum
      - After the rupture of follicle and liberation of secondary oocyte, the granulosa and theca interna cells get thrown into folds.
      - The granulosa cells become enlarged, accumulate lipid and are transformed into pale staining polygonal cells called the lutein cells.
      - Theca interna cells
    - Smaller and fewer
      - Stain dark
      - Also known as prolutein cells.
      - Secrete progesterone and estrogen
      - Changes involving the formation of ovarian follicles till the degeneration of corpus luteum constitute the ovarian cycle.

2. Write a short note on ovary. (RUHS)

Answer

Introduction

- Internal genital organ in females.
- Situated in the ovarian fossa on the lateral pelvic wall.

Gross Anatomy of Ovary

- Before the onset of ovulation, the ovaries have smooth surfaces and are grayish-pink in color.
- After puberty, the surface becomes uneven and the color changes from pink to gray.

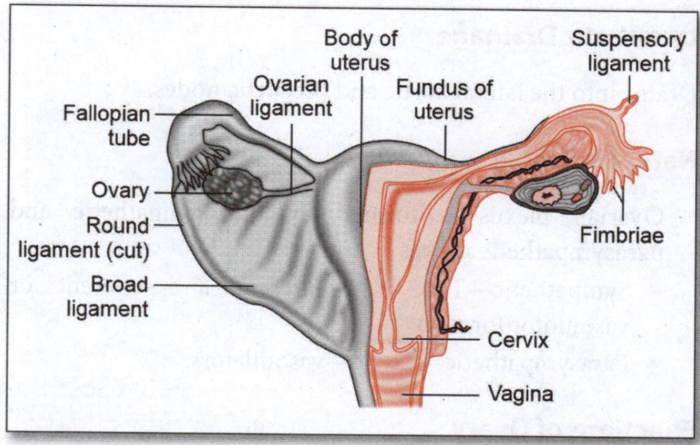

Figure 9.24: Structure of Ovary

Relations

- **Peritoneal relations**
  - Ovary is covered by the peritoneum.
  - It is connected to the posterior layer of the broad ligament by a short fold of peritoneum called mesovarium.
  - The mesovarium transmits the vessels and nerves.
  - Suspensory ligament of the ovary – formed by the lateral segment of the broad ligament. Also known as infundibulopelvic ligament. It contains the ovarian nerves and vessels.
- **Visceral relations**
  - Upper or tubal pole
    - Broader than lower pole.
    - Related to the fallopian tubes and the external iliac veins.
    - May or may not be related to the appendix (right ovary).
  - Lower or uterine pole
    - Narrower
    - Related to the pelvic floor
  - Anterior or mesovarian border
    - Straight and related to the fallopian tubes.

Arterial Supply

- Ovarian artery, branch of abdominal aorta
  - Enters the ovaries through the suspensory ligament.
  - Also supplies the uterine tubes, side of uterus and ureter.

Venous Drainage

- Pampiniform plexus—the plexus condenses into a single ovarian vein near the pelvic inlet.

- Drains into the inferior vena cava on the right side and left renal vein on the left side.

Lymphatic Drainage

Drains into the lateral aortic and preaortic nodes.

Nervous Supply

- Ovarian plexus is formed by the sympathetic and parasympathetic nerves
  - Sympathetic—T10, T11—afferent and efferent or vasomotor for pain
  - Parasympathetic—S2-S4—vasodilators.

Functions of Ovary

- Production of oocytes
  - During the reproductive life, ovaries produce one secondary oocyte alternatively each month. Liberation of oocyte from the ovary is called ovulation.
- Production of hormones
  - Ovary controls the whole reproductive life of females.
  - Two main functions of ovary are exocrine and endocrine secretions.
  - Exocrine secretion:
    - Aids in oogenesis in fetal life
    - Maturation of ova
  - Endocrine secretion: It secretes four hormones
    - Estrogen
      - Secreted by the Graafian follicles (membrane granulosa or theca interna)
    - Progesterone
      - Secreted by the corpus callosum
    - Androgen
    - Relaxin
- Functions of ovarian hormones
  - Changes during puberty
    - Growth and development of uterus
    - Growth and development of fallopian tubes and vagina
    - Menstrual changes
    - Appearance of secondary sexual characteristics such as growth of mammary glands and pubic hair
  - Pregnancy and changes associated with it.
    - Embedding of ovum
    - Development of placenta
    - Growth of mammary glands
    - Relaxin – plays a role in parturition

3. Write about contents of spermatic cord. (RUHS)

Answer

Introduction

The spermatic cord is a cord-like structure in males formed by the vas deferens (ductus deferens) and surrounding tissue that runs from the deep inguinal ring down to each testicle.

Contents of Spermatic Cord

The spermatic cord consists of vessels, nerves and ducts that run to and from the testes. They are surrounded by fascia, which forms a cord-like structure.

- Via the Deep Inguinal Ring
  - Vas
  - Artery to vas (inferior vesical)
  - Testicular artery (aorta)
  - Cremasteric artery (inferior epigastric)
  - Cremasteric vein (inferior epigastric)
  - Testicular vein (IVC/left renal)
  - Obliterated processus vaginalis
  - Lymphatics
  - Sympathetics
  - Genital branch of genitofemoral nerve (L2)
- In Canal
  - Internal spermatic fascia
  - Cremasteric fascia
  - Cremasteric muscle
  - Ilioinguinal nerve
- Outside Superficial Ring
  - External spermatic fascia

Anatomical Course of Spermatic Cord

- The anatomical course of the spermatic cord is relatively short, beginning in the inferior abdomen and ending in the scrotum.
- The spermatic cord is formed at the opening of the inguinal canal, known as the deep inguinal ring. This opening is located laterally to the inferior epigastric vessels.
- The cord passes through the inguinal canal, entering the scrotum via the superficial inguinal ring. It continues into the scrotum, ending at the posterior border of the testes.

Arteries of the Spermatic Cord

- Testicular artery–branch of the aorta that arises just inferiorly to the renal arteries.
- Cremasteric artery and vein–supply the cremasteric fascia and muscle.

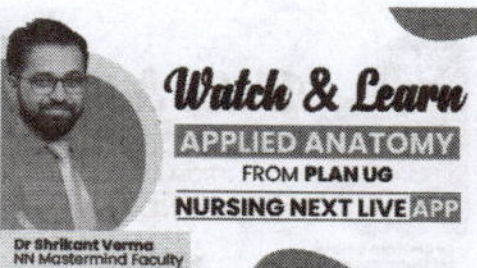

- Artery to the vas deferens–branch of the inferior vesicle artery, which arises from the internal iliac.
- Pampiniform plexus of testicular veins–drains venous blood from the testes into the testicular vein.

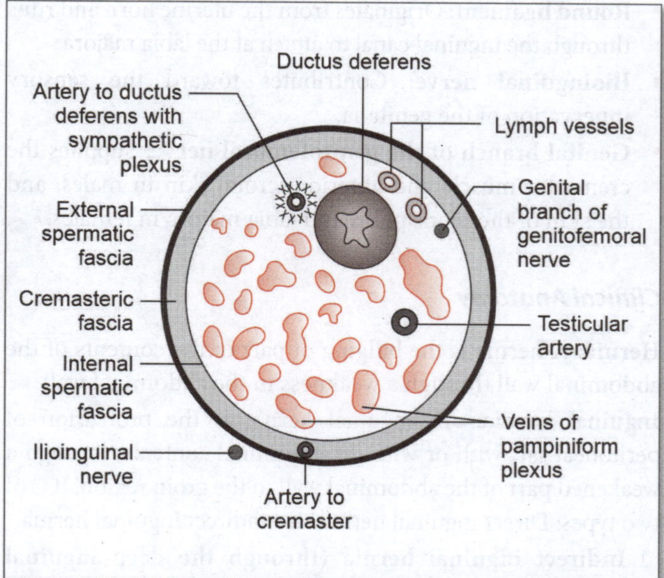

Figure 9.25: Transverse Section through the spermatic cord

4. Write a short note on Graafian follicle. (RUHS)

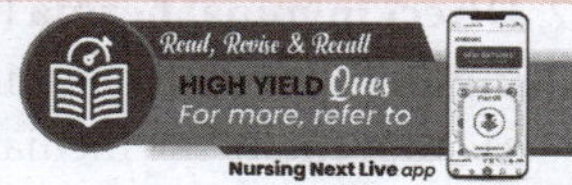

Answer

Graafian Follicle

- Little irregular spaces present among the granulosa cells are known as liquor folliculi.
- Increase in these spaces is associated with increase in size of follicle, and a confluence of these spaces form a crescenteric cavity called the antrum.
- At this stage, the primary oocyte lies on one side of cavity.
- Follicular cells surrounding the ovum are known as cumulus oophorus.
- The stroma around the the follicle arranges itself into an inner theca interna that is vascular and cellular and outer theca externa that is fibrous.
- The theca interna secretes estrogen.
- The follicle bulges onto the surface of the ovary to form the mature Graafian follicle.
- The primary oocyte undergoes first meiotic division and becomes the secondary oocytes and bursts from the follicle.
- Corona radiata cells surround the follicular cells in secondary oocyte.
- The rupture of follicle to release the secondary oocyte is known as ovulation.

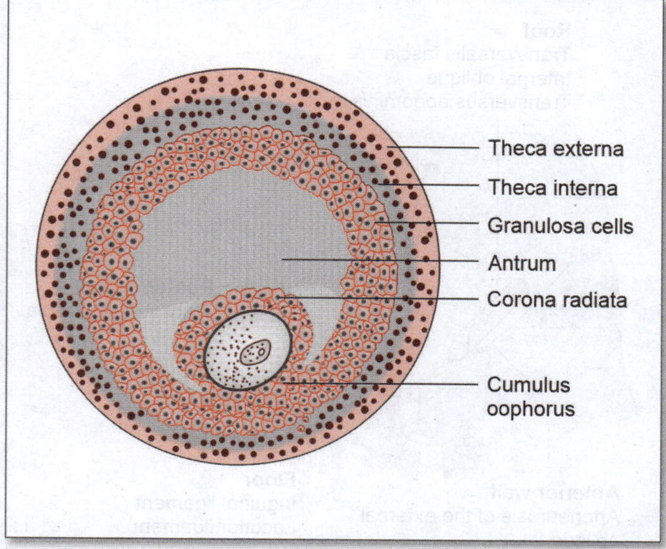

Figure 9.26: Graafian follicle

Functions of Graafian Follicle

- Forms mature ova
- Secretes estrogen
- Provides a medium for the growth of corpus luteum.

5. Write a short note on Inguinal canal (MGR)

Answer

Inguinal Canal

- The inguinal canal is a short passage that extends inferiorly and medially through the inferior part of the abdominal wall.
- It is superior and parallel to the inguinal ligament.
- The canal serves as a pathway by which structures can pass from the abdominal wall to the external genitalia.

Boundaries

- **The inguinal canal has four walls:** Anterior, posterior, superior (roof) and inferior (floor).
- **It has two openings:** The superficial and deep rings.

Walls

- **Anterior wall:** Aponeurosis of the external oblique, reinforced by the internal oblique muscle laterally.
- **Posterior wall:** Transversalis fascia.
- **Roof:** Transversalis fascia, internal oblique, and transversus abdominis.
- **Floor:** Inguinal ligament

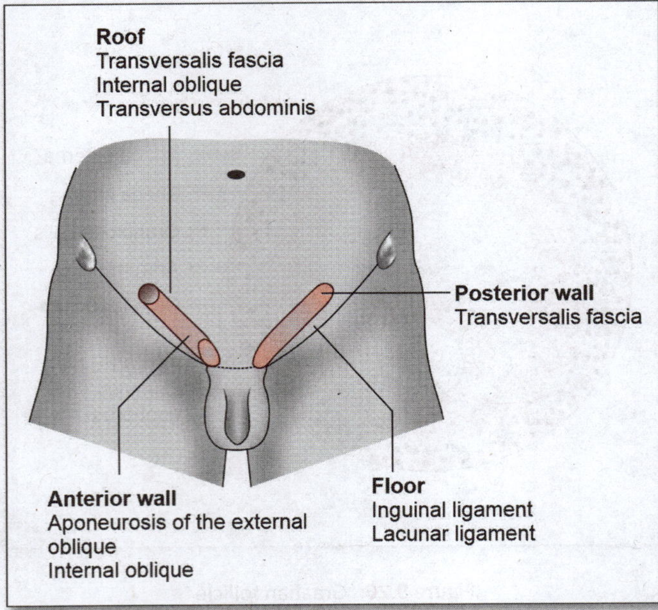

Figure 9.27: Walls of inguinal canal

Rings

The two openings to the inguinal canal are known as rings. The **deep (internal) ring** lies at the midpoint of the inguinal ligament. Which is lateral to the epigastric vessels.

The ring is created by the transversalis fascia, which invaginates to form a covering of the contents of the inguinal canal. The **superficial (external) ring** is the end of the inguinal canal and lies just superior to the pubic tubercle.

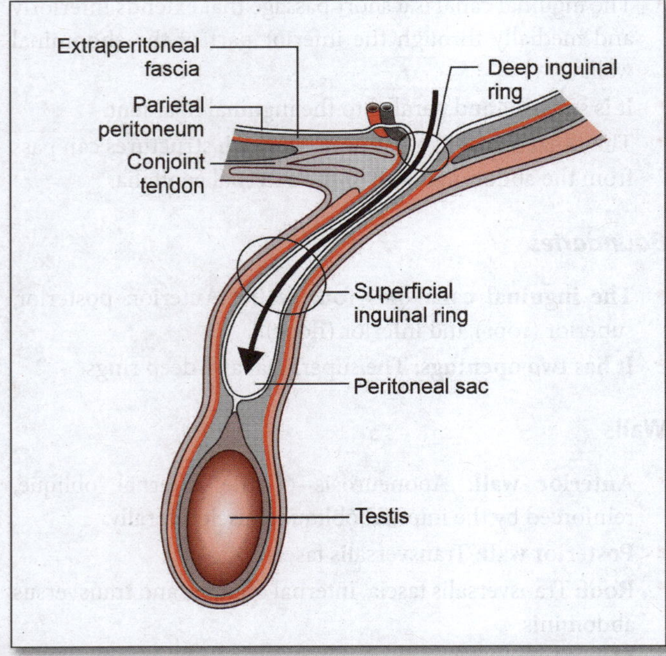

Figure 9.28: Rings of inguinal canal

Contents

The contents of the inguinal canal include:

- **Spermatic cord:** Contains neurovascular and reproductive structures that supply and drain the testes.
- **Round ligament:** Originates from the uterine horn and runs through the inguinal canal to attach at the labia majora.
- **Ilioinguinal nerve:** Contributes toward the sensory innervation of the genitalia.
- **Genital branch of the genitofemoral nerve:** Supplies the cremaster muscle and anterior scrotal skin in males, and the skin of the mons pubis and labia majora in females.

Clinical Anatomy

Hernia: A hernia is the bulging of part of the contents of the abdominal wall through a weakness in the abdominal wall.

Inguinal hernia: An inguinal hernia is the protrusion of peritoneal sac, with or without abdominal contents, through a weakened part of the abdominal wall in the groin region. It is of two types: Direct inguinal hernia and indirect inguinal hernia.

1. **Indirect inguinal hernia (through the deep inguinal ring):** The indirect inguinal hernia is of two types and is much more common in men than in women. The protruding peritoneal sac enters the inguinal canal by passing through the deep inguinal ring, just lateral to the inferior epigastric vessels.
2. **Direct inguinal hernia (through the posterior wall of the inguinal canal):** The direct inguinal hernia is peritoneal sac that enters the medial end of the inguinal canal directly through a weakened posterior wall. A hernia is medial to the inferior epigastric vessels.

6. Write a short note on pouch of douglas. (RUHS)

Answer

Pouch of Douglas

- Also known as rectouterine pouch.
- It is an extension of the peritoneal cavity between the rectum and the posterior wall of the uterus in the female human body.

Structure

- In women, it is the deepest point of the peritoneal cavity, posterior to (behind) the uterus and anterior to (in front of) the rectum. (The pouch on the other side of the uterus is the vesicouterine pouch.) It is near the posterior fornix of the vagina.
- It is normal to have approximately 1–3 mL of fluid in the rectouterine pouch throughout the menstrual cycle. After

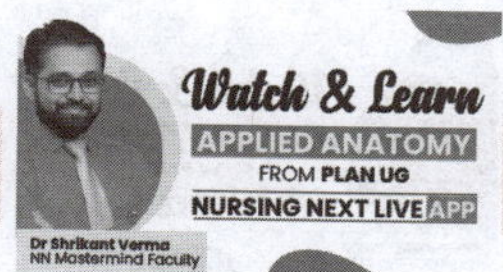

ovulation, there is between 4 and 5 mL of fluid in the rectouterine pouch.

- In men, the region corresponding to the rectouterine pouch is the rectovesical pouch, which lies between the urinary bladder and rectum. The rectouterine pouch, also known as the rectovaginal pouch, cul-de-sac or pouch of Douglas, is an extension of peritoneum between the posterior wall of uterus and the rectum in females. It is the most dependent part of the peritoneal cavity and is analogous to the rectovesical pouch in males.

Applied Anatomy

- As it is the farthest point of the abdominopelvic cavity in women, it is a site where infection and fluids typically collect. The rectouterine pouch is used in the treatment of end-stage renal failure in patients who are treated by peritoneal dialysis. The tip of the dialysis catheter is placed into the deepest point of the pouch.

7. Write a short note on covering of the testis. (RUHS)

Answer

For answer, refer to Long Question no. 3(b), pg. no. 148

SHORT ANSWER QUESTIONS

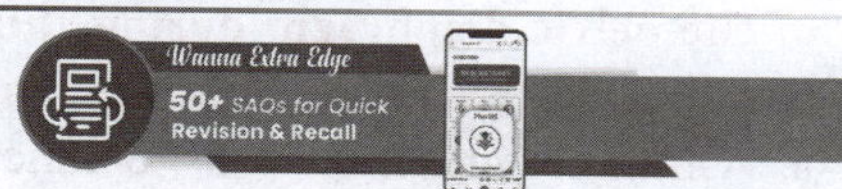

1. Enumerate parts of fallopian tube. (MGR)

Answer

Parts of Fallopian Tube

Infundibulum: The lateral end of the uterine tube is shaped like a funnel and is, therefore, called the infundibulum.
Ampulla: The part of the uterine tube medial to the infundibulum is called the ampulla.
Isthmus: It is narrow, rounded and cord like. It forms approximately the medial one-third.
Interstitial segment: The uterine or intramural or interstitial part of the tube is about 1 cm long and lies within the wall of the uterus.

2. Enumerate parts of spermatozoa. (MGR)

Answer

Parts of Spermatozoa

- Head
  - Egg-shaped
  - Has smooth surface
  - Contains the nucleus with 23 chromosomes
  - Contains a small secretory cap – acrosome
- Body
  - Contains mitochondria, which provide the energy to sperm to sustain its motion.
  - Centriole is present between the head and the body – it is involved in the production of mitotic apparatus—involved in separating chromosome during cell division.
- Tail
  - Thin elongated structure that makes up to 80% of the length of sperm.
  - Function—helps the sperm in movement in the vaginal cavity.

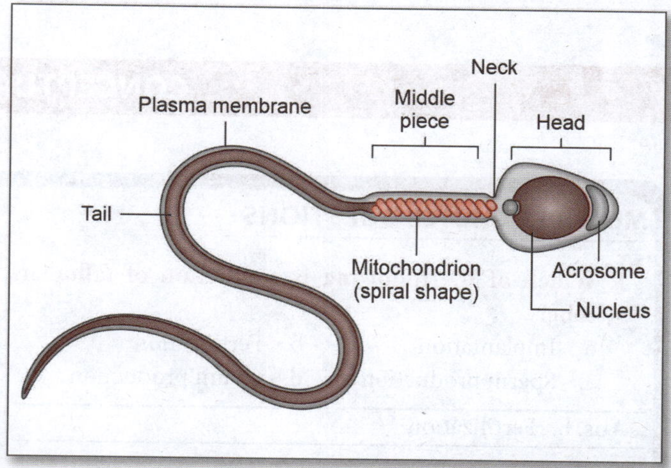

3. Classify the supports of uterus. (MGR)

Answer

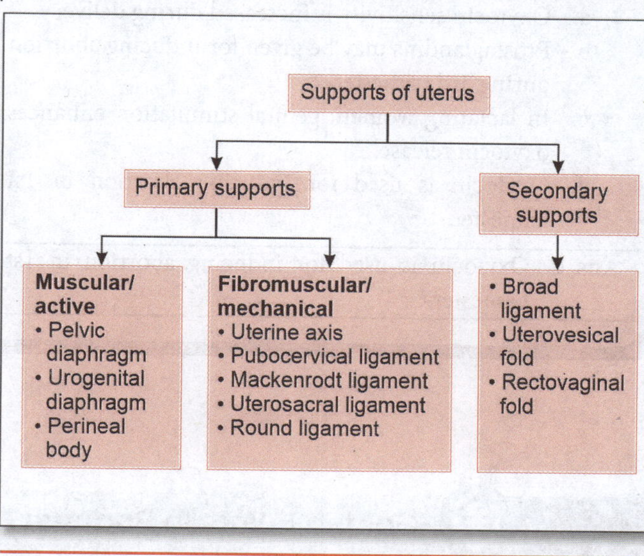

4. Write the functions of leydig's cells. (MGR)

Answer

Introduction

- Large rounded or polygonal in shape.
- Cytoplasm is eosinophilic and granular.
- Nucleus is absent.
- These cells are not affected by vasectomy as their secretion is poured directly into the blood.

Functions of Leydig's Cells

Secrete androgen, the male sex hormone which is responsible for the development and maintenance of male sex characteristics.

5. Write about lymphatic drainage of breast. (MGR)

Answer

Lymphatic Drainage of Breast

- **Dermal network:** Drain skin over the breast–except that from nipple and areola–pass radially lateral aspect: Drain into axillary lymph nodes
- **Superior aspect:** Supraclavicular nodes, few may reach nodes along cephalic vein in deltopectoral triangle
- **Medial aspect:** Drain into internal mammary nodes/ parasternal nodes
- **Inferior aspect:** Form a subperitoneal plexus and drain into subdiaphragmatic nodes. Cross midline and communicate with contralateral lymphatics
- Lymphatics from parenchyma of breast

CONCEPTUAL REVISION

MULTIPLE CHOICE QUESTIONS

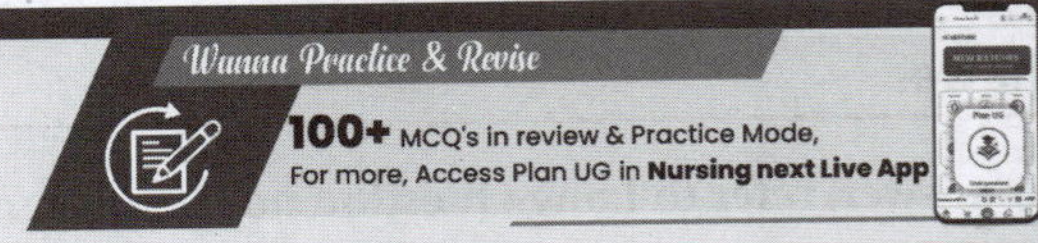

1. Which of the following is a function of fallopian tube?

a. Implantation b. Fertilization
c. Sperm production d. Ovum production

Ans. b. Fertilization

2. Normal pH of vagina:

a. 2–2.5 b. 3.5–4.5
c. 4.5–5.5 d. 5.0–6.5

Ans. c. 4.5–5.5

3. All of the following statements are true; except:

a. Oxytocin sensitivity is increased during delivery.
b. Prostaglandins may be given for inducing abortion during 3rd trimester.
c. In lactating women, genital stimulation enhances oxytocin release.
d. Oxytocin is used for inducing abortion in 1st trimester.

Ans. d. Oxytocin is used for inducing abortion in 1st trimester.

4. A 32-year-old lady is admitted to a hospital because the birth of her child is several days overdue. Tearing of the pelvic diaphragm during childbirth leads to paralysis of which of the following muscles?

a. Obturator internus b. Sphincter ani externus
c. Sphincter urethrae d. Levator ani

Ans. d. Levator ani

5. A young couple is having difficulty conceiving a child. Their physician at a reproduction and fertility clinic explains them that:

a. Erection of the penis is a sympathetic response.
b. Fertilization occurs in the infundibulum or ampulla of the uterine tube.
c. The glans clitoris is formed from the corpus spongiosum.
d. Ejaculation follows parasympathetic stimulation.

Ans. b. Fertilization occurs in the infundibulum or ampulla of the uterine tube.

CHAPTER 10

Nervous System

CONCEPTUAL THEORY

Terminology

Autonomic nervous system: Regulates involuntary activities of the body. Divided into sympathetic and parasympathetic components.
Blood-brain barrier: Formed by capillary endothelium, basement membrane of these cells, processes of astrocytes.
Central nervous system: Comprises brain and spinal cord.
Circle of Willis: Formed by branches of internal carotid artery and branches of basilar artery.
Edinger-Westphal nucleus: Part of III nerve complex contains parasympathetic motor fibers for the ciliary muscles and constrictor pupillae muscles
Erb's point: Meeting point of ventral rami of C5, C6, to form upper trunk which divides into anterior and posterior divisions and few branches. Klumpke's paralysis, which is paralysis of lower trunk of brachial plexus, leads to complete claw hand.
Meninges of brain: Dura mater (endosteal and meningeal layers), arachnoid mater and pia mater (from outside to inside).
Neuroglial cells: Astrocytes, oligodendrocytes and microglia.
Papez circuit: Its parts are hippocampus, fornix, mammillary body, anterior nucleus of thalamus, cingulate gyrus, parahippocampal gyrus. All of these are important for long-term permanent memory.
Parts of brain: Medulla oblongata, pons, midbrain, cerebellum, diencephalon and cerebral hemispheres
Peripheral nervous system: Comprises 31 pairs of spinal nerves and 12 pairs of cranial nerves.
Spinal nerves: Eight cervical, 12 thoracic, five lumbar, five sacral and one coccygeal.
Synapse: The point at which electrical signals move from one nerve cell to another.

PARTS OF NERVOUS SYSTEM

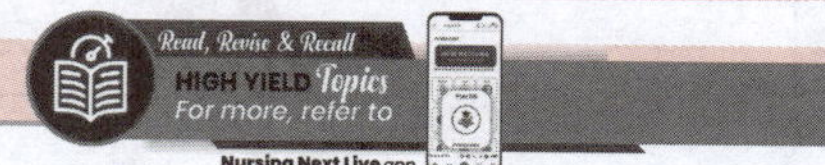

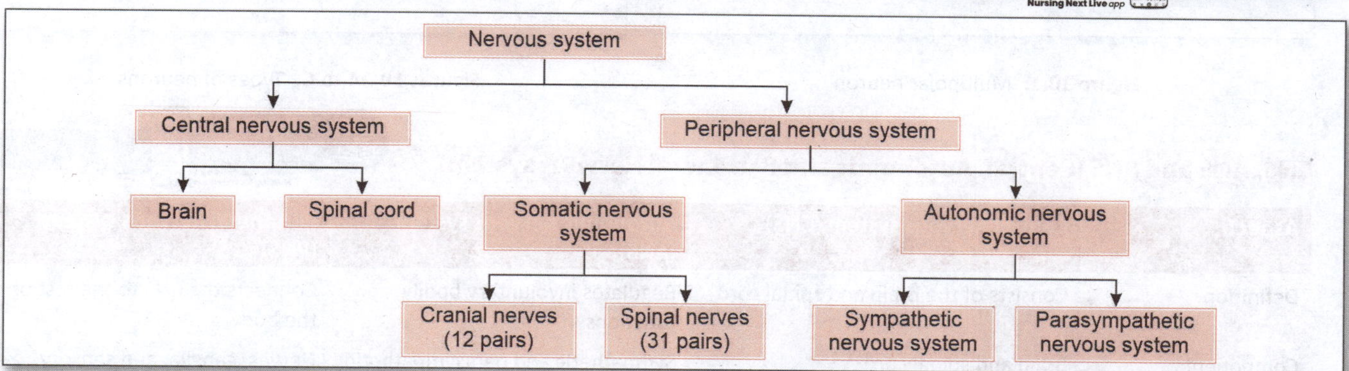

STRUCTURE OF NEURON

- **Cell Body (Soma):** The cell body is the main component of a neuron. It contains the nucleus, which houses the genetic material of the cell. The cell body also contains various organelles responsible for carrying out metabolic functions necessary for the neuron's survival.
- **Dendrites:** Dendrites are branch-like extensions that emanate from the cell body. They receive incoming signals from other neurons or sensory receptors and transmit those signals toward the cell body. Dendrites play a crucial role in integrating and processing incoming information.
- **Axon:** The axon is a long, slender projection extending from the cell body. It carries electrical impulses away from

the cell body and transmits them to other neurons or target cells. Axons can vary in length, with some extending over a meter in the human body.

- **Axon terminal:** At the end of the axon, there are small branches called axon terminals or terminal buttons. These specialized structures form synapses, which are junctions with other neurons or target cells. Axon terminals contain vesicles filled with neurotransmitters, which are chemical messengers that transmit signals across the synapse.
- **Myelin sheath:** In many neurons, the axon is covered by a fatty substance called the myelin sheath. The myelin sheath is formed by specialized cells called glial cells, specifically oligodendrocytes in the central nervous system and Schwann cells in the peripheral nervous system. It acts as an insulating layer, speeding up the conduction of electrical impulses along the axon.
- **Synapse:** Synapses are the points of communication between neurons or between neurons and target cells such as muscle fibers or glands. They consist of the presynaptic terminal of one neuron, the synaptic cleft (a tiny gap), and the postsynaptic membrane of the next neuron or target cell. Neurotransmitters released from the presynaptic terminal cross the synaptic cleft and bind to receptors on the postsynaptic membrane, transmitting the signal.
- **Nodes of Ranvier:** The myelin sheath is interrupted at regular intervals by small gaps called nodes of Ranvier. These nodes play a crucial role in facilitating the rapid transmission of electrical signals by allowing the signal to "jump" from node to node, a process known as saltatory conduction.

Figure 10.1: Multipolar neuron

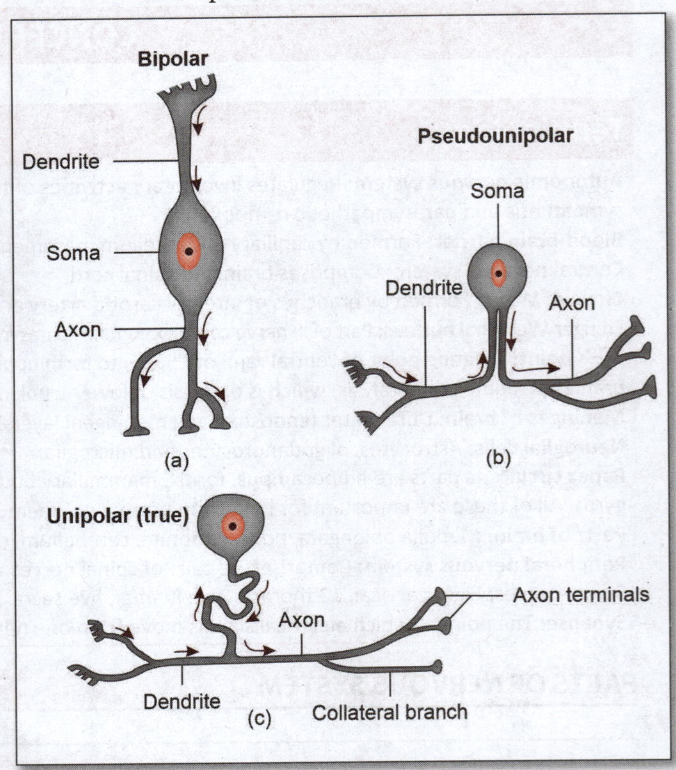

Figures 10.2A to C: Types of neurons

CNS, ANS and PNS (Central, Autonomic and Peripheral Nervous system)

Aspect	Central nervous system (CNS)	Autonomic nervous system (ANS)	Peripheral nervous system (PNS)
Definition	Consists of the brain and spinal cord	Regulates involuntary bodily functions	Connects the CNS to the rest of the body
Components	Brain and spinal cord	Sympathetic and parasympathetic divisions	Nerves, ganglia, and sensory receptors
Function	Integrates and processes information, coordinates responses	Regulates internal organs and involuntary processes	Transmits signals to and from the CNS
Protection	Protected by the skull and vertebral column	No specific protective structures	No specific protective structures

Contd...

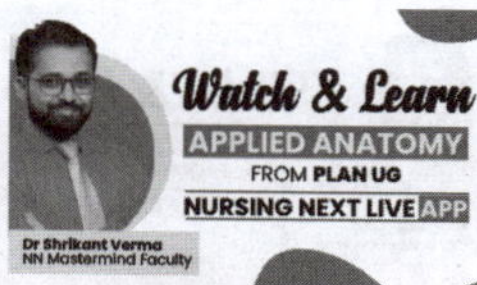

Aspect	Central nervous system (CNS)	Autonomic nervous system (ANS)	Peripheral nervous system (PNS)
Neural tissue	Composed of neurons and glial cells	Composed of neurons and glial cells	Composed of neurons and glial cells
Communication	Neurons transmit electrical signals	Neurons transmit electrical signals	Neurons transmit electrical signals
Brain	Consists of various regions and lobes	Controls and coordinates bodily functions	No direct involvement
Spinal Cord	Long bundle of nerve fibers in the vertebral column	Conducts sensory and motor signals	Connects the PNS to the brain
Sympathetic division	Regulates the "fight-or-flight" response	Activates during stressful situations	Connects to internal organs and glands
Parasympathetic Division	Controls the "rest and digest" response	Promotes relaxation and conserves energy	Connects to internal organs and glands
Cranial Nerves	12 pairs of nerves originating from the brain	Involved in regulating visceral functions	Connects to various head and neck structures
Spinal Nerves	31 pairs of nerves originating from the spinal cord	Transmit sensory and motor signals	Connects to the rest of the body
Sensory Receptors	Receive stimuli and transmit sensory information to the CNS	Monitor internal organ function and relay information	Detects stimuli and transmit sensory information
Motor Control	Initiates and coordinates voluntary movements	Controls involuntary muscle contractions	Initiates and controls voluntary movements
Reflexes	Involved in reflex actions and responses	Modulates reflex responses	Mediates reflex actions and responses

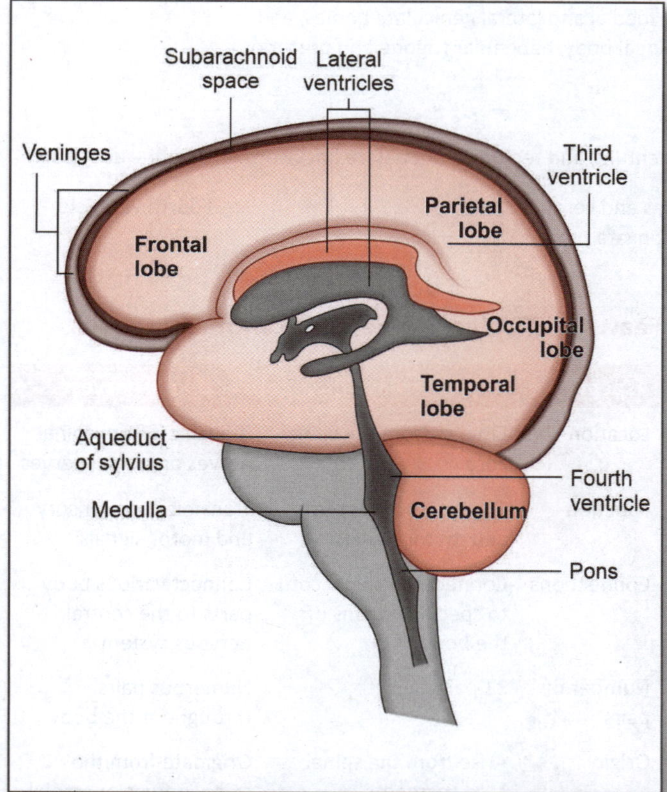

Figure 10.3: Structure of Brain

Structure of Brain, Spinal Cord, Cranial Nerves, Spinal Nerves, Peripheral Nerves, Functional Areas of Cerebral Cortex

- **Brain:** The brain is the central control center of the nervous system. It is protected by the skull and is divided into several main regions:
  - **Cerebrum:** The largest part of the brain responsible for conscious thought, memory, sensory processing, and voluntary muscle movement.
  - **Cerebellum:** Located at the back of the brain, it coordinates muscle movement, balance, and posture.
  - **Brainstem:** Connects the brain to the spinal cord and controls basic functions like breathing, heart rate, and digestion.
  - **Diencephalon:** Includes the thalamus and hypothalamus, involved in sensory processing, hormone regulation, and homeostasis.
- **Spinal cord:** The spinal cord is a long, cylindrical bundle of nerves that extends from the brainstem down the spinal column. It serves as a pathway for signals traveling to and from the brain. The spinal cord also integrates reflex actions without involving the brain.

- **Cranial nerves:** There are 12 pairs of cranial nerves that emerge directly from the brain. These nerves transmit sensory and motor signals between the brain and various parts of the head, neck, and organs.
- **Spinal nerves:** There are 31 pairs of spinal nerves that emerge from the spinal cord and extend to different parts of the body. They are responsible for relaying sensory information from the body to the spinal cord and transmitting motor signals from the spinal cord to muscles and glands.
- **Peripheral nerves:** Peripheral nerves are located outside the CNS and connect it to the limbs, organs, and other body parts. They consist of a network of nerves that branch off from the spinal nerves and cranial nerves. Peripheral nerves transmit sensory information from the body to the CNS and deliver motor commands from the CNS to the muscles and organs.
- **Functional areas of cerebral cortex:** The cerebral cortex is the outermost layer of the cerebrum and is highly folded to increase its surface area. It is responsible for higher cognitive functions, including perception, consciousness, memory, language, and problem-solving. The cerebral cortex is divided into different lobes, each associated with specific functions:
  - **Frontal lobe:** Involved in decision-making, reasoning, motor control, and speech production.
  - **Parietal lobe:** Processes sensory information, such as touch, temperature, and spatial awareness.
  - **Temporal lobe:** Plays a role in auditory processing, language comprehension, and memory.
  - **Occipital lobe:** Responsible for visual processing and interpretation.

Table 10.1: Parts of brain

Parts	Subdivisions	Cavity
1. Forebrain (prosencephalon)	• Telencephalon (cerebrum), made up of 2 cerebral hemispheres and the median part in front of the interventricular foramen	Lateral ventricle
	• Diencephalon (thalamencephalon), hidden by the cerebrum, consists of: ▪ Thalamus ▪ Hypothalamus ▪ Metathalamus, including the medial and lateral geniculate bodies, and ▪ Epithalamus, including the pineal body, habenular trigone and posterior commissure ▪ Subthalamus	Third ventricle
2. Midbrain (mesencephalon)	Crus cerebri, substantia nigra, tegmentum, and tectum, from before backward	Cerebral aqueduct
3. Hindbrain (rhombencephalon)	• Metencephalon, made up of pons and cerebellum • Myelencephalon or medulla oblongata	Fourth ventricle

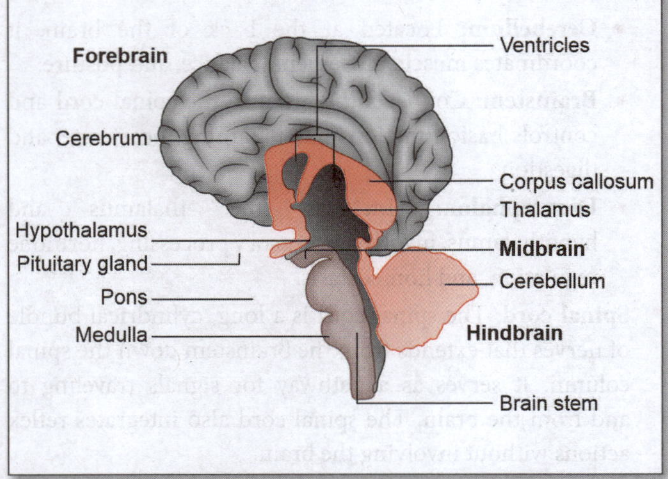

Figure 10.4: Transverse section of thoracic segment of spinal cord

Features of Spinal Nerves and Peripheral Nerves

Aspect	Spinal nerves	Peripheral nerves
Location	Emerge from the spinal cord	Branch off from spinal nerves or cranial nerves
Function	Transmit both sensory and motor signals	Transmit both sensory and motor signals
Connections	Connect the spinal cord to specific regions of the body	Connect various body parts to the central nervous system
Number of pairs	31 pairs	Numerous pairs throughout the body
Origin	Arise from the spinal cord segments	Originate from the spinal nerves or cranial nerves

Contd...

Aspect	Spinal nerves	Peripheral nerves
Distribution	Serve specific regions of the body based on their segment	Extend to peripheral organs, limbs, and other body regions
Structure	Consist of a dorsal (sensory) and ventral (motor) root	Comprise bundles of nerve fibers
Motor functions	Control voluntary muscle movement	Control voluntary muscle movement
Sensory functions	Transmit sensory information from the body to the CNS	Transmit sensory information from the body to the CNS
Reflex arcs	Participate in spinal reflexes	Participate in spinal reflexes
Examples	Cervical, thoracic, lumbar, sacral, and coccygeal nerves	Sciatic nerve, median nerve, ulnar nerve, facial nerve, etc.

Ventricular System – Formation, Circulation, and Drainage

- **Formation:** Formed during embryonic development
- **Components:** Consists of four interconnected ventricles:
  - Two lateral ventricles (one in each cerebral hemisphere)
  - Third ventricle (midline, between the two hemispheres)
  - Fourth ventricle (between the brainstem and cerebellum)
- **Cerebrospinal Fluid (CSF):** Produced by specialized cells called choroid plexus
  - **Production:** CSF is formed by filtration of blood plasma
  - **Circulation:**
    - CSF flows through the ventricles and into the subarachnoid space surrounding the brain and spinal cord
    - It circulates around the CNS, bathing and protecting it
  - **Functions:**
    - Provides cushioning and buoyancy to the brain
    - Transports nutrients, hormones, and waste products
    - Helps maintain a stable chemical environment in the CNS
    - Assists in the removal of metabolic waste from the brain
  - **Drainage:** CSF is absorbed by arachnoid granulations (or villi)
    - These structures protrude into the venous sinuses of the brain.
    - CSF is returned to the bloodstream for reabsorption.

CONCEPTUAL EXERCISES

LONG ANSWER QUESTIONS

1. Describe the gross anatomy of brain and spinal cord. (RUHS)

Answer

Brain

Part of CNS which lies within the cavity of the skull. The following are parts of brain:

- Forebrain
  - Cerebrum
  - Diencephalon
- Midbrain
  - Midbrain
- Hindbrain
  - Pons
  - Medulla oblongata
  - Cerebellum

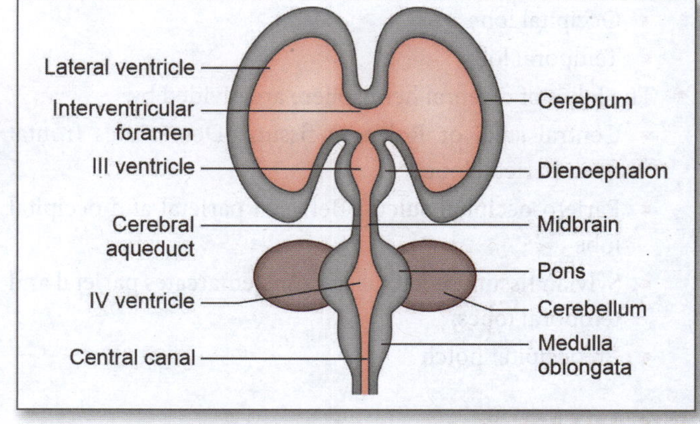

Figure 10.5: Parts of Brain

Cerebrum

- Largest part of brain.
- Consists of left and right cerebral hemispheres separated by fold of dura – falx cerebri.
- The median longitudinal fissure of the cerebrum intervenes between the medial surfaces of right and left surfaces.

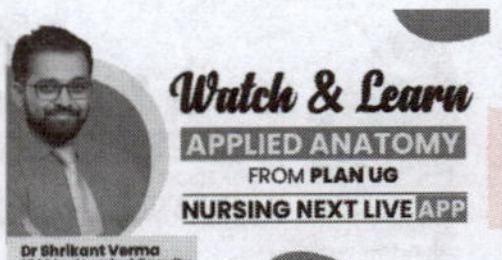

- Contents of longitudinal fissure are:
  - Falx cerebri
  - Arachnoid mater
  - Pia mater
  - Anterior cerebral vessels

External Features of Cerebrum

- Surface is not smooth. It has:
  - Sulci – grooves
  - Gyri – intervening surface between two sulci. These consist of central core of white matter covered by gray matter.
- Each cerebral cortex has three surfaces and three poles:
  - Pole – pointed ends
    - Anterior frontal pole
    - Posterior occipital pole
    - Temporal pole
  - Surfaces
    - Superolateral surface
    - Medial surface
    - Inferior surface: further divided into:
      - An anterior orbital surface
      - A posterior tentorial surface
- Lobes
  - Frontal lobe
  - Parietal lobe
  - Occipital lobe
  - Temporal lobe
- The lobes of cerebral hemisphere are divided by:
  - Central sulci or Rolandic fissure: Demarcates frontal from parietal lobes
  - Parieto-occipital sulcus: Between parietal and occipital lobe
  - Sylvian fissure or lateral sulcus: Demarcates parietal and temporal lobes.
  - Preoccipital notch

Internal Capsule

The internal capsule is a white matter structure situated in the inferomedial part of each cerebral **hemisphere** of the brain. It carries information past the basal ganglia, separating the caudate nucleus and the thalamus from the putamen and the globus pallidus.

Basal Ganglia

Region of the base of the brain that consists of three clusters of neurons responsible for involuntary movements and control of muscle tone.

Diencephalon

Hypothalamic sulcus divides the diencephalon into dorsal and ventral parts:

- Dorsal part of diencephalon
  - Thalamus
  - Metathalamus
    - Medial geniculate body – responsible for hearing
    - Lateral geniculate body – responsible for vision
  - Epithalamus
- Ventral part of diencephalon
  - Hypothalamus
  - Subthalamus

Brainstem

Connects the forebrain and spinal cord.

It consists of:

- Midbrain
- Pons
- Medulla oblongata

Hindbrain

Consists of pons, medulla oblongata and cerebellum.

Pons

- Lies between the midbrain and medulla oblongata.
- On each side, it is connected to the cerebellum by the middle cerebellar peduncle.
- Made up of gray and white matter.
- Role – center of respiration
- Nuclei of the cranial nerves – CN V, VII, VIII – are situated in the pons.
  - **External features**
    - Has a convex anterior surface marked by transversely running fibers.
    - Laterally these fibers collect to form a bundle known as middle cerebellar peduncle.
    - Trigeminal nerve originates here.
    - Posterior aspect of pons forms the upper part of the floor of the fourth ventricle.
  - **Functions**
    - Controlling sleep cycles.
    - Regulating the magnitude and frequency of the respiration.
    - Transfers information between the cerebellum and motor cortex.
    - Pons is also involved in sensations, such as the sense of taste, hearing and balance.

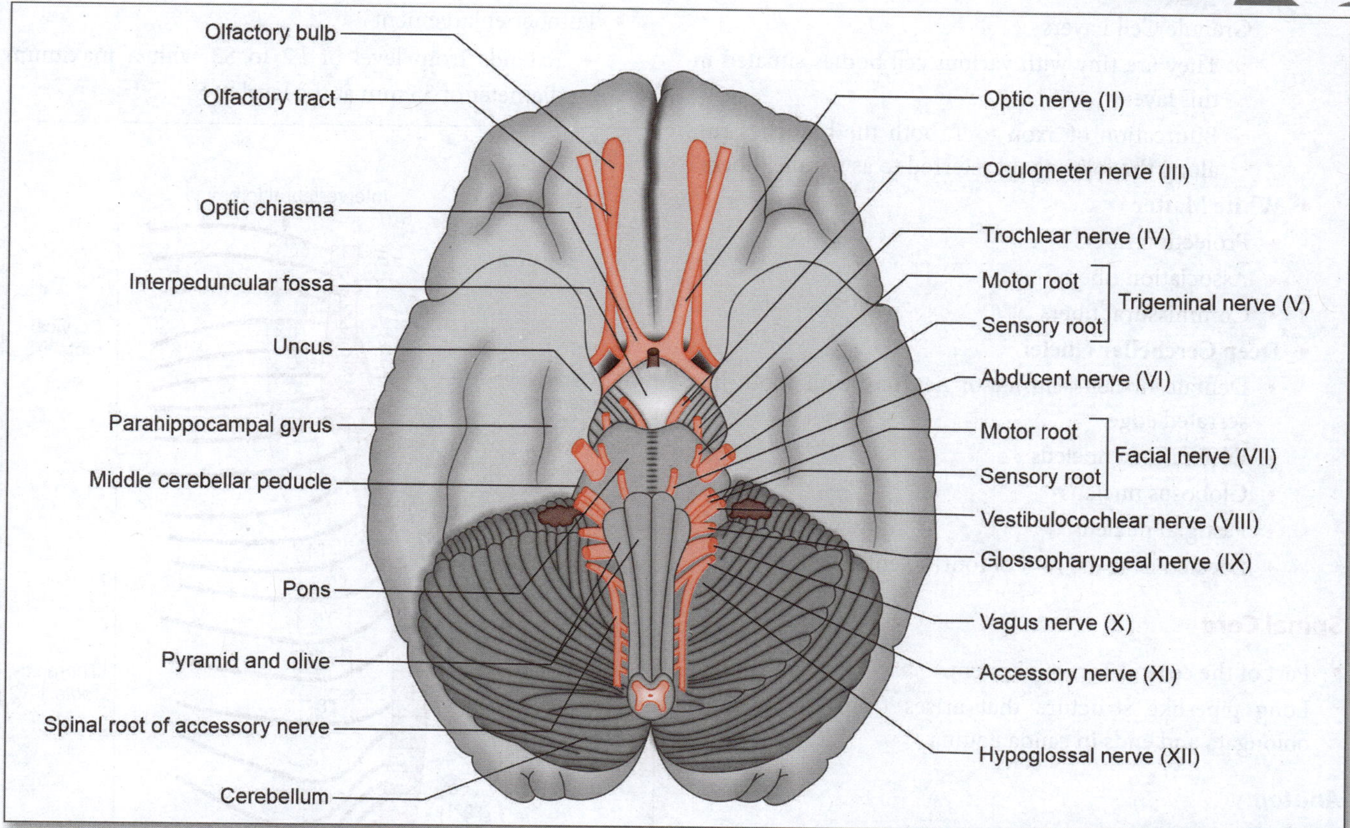

Figure 10.6: Brainstem

Medulla Oblongata

- Part of brainstem, about 3 cm in length.
- It is divided into:
  - Lower closed part – surrounds the canal
  - Upper open part – related to the fourth ventricle.

Important centers present in the medulla are:

- Respiratory center
- Cardiac center for the regulation of heart rate
- Reflex center for vomiting, coughing, sneezing, hiccuping and swallowing.
  - Helps in smooth performance

Cerebellum

- **Structure of Cerebellum**
  - **Cerebellar cortex**
    - Molecular layer
      - It further comprises nerve cells, viz. stellate cells and basket cells
      - Stellate cells are star-shaped; and superficially located basket cells are deeply located with sparse dendritic tree

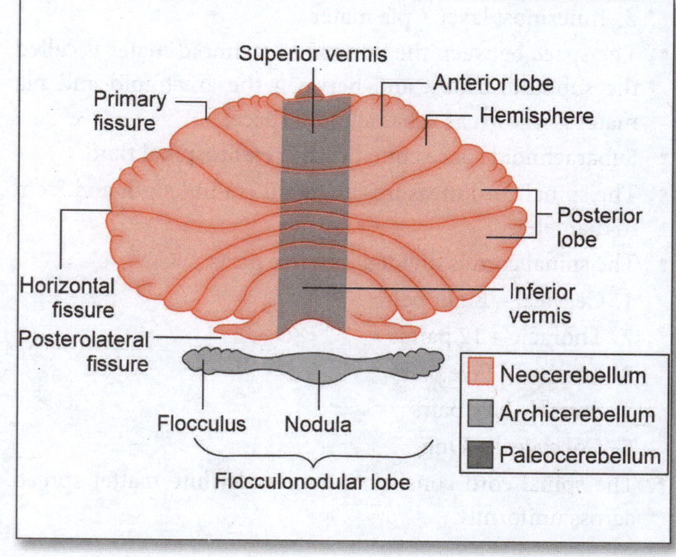

Figure 10.7: Structure of cerebellum

    - Purkinje cell layer
      - Flask-shaped Purkinje cells with extensive dendritic network with large surface area for axodendritic synapses

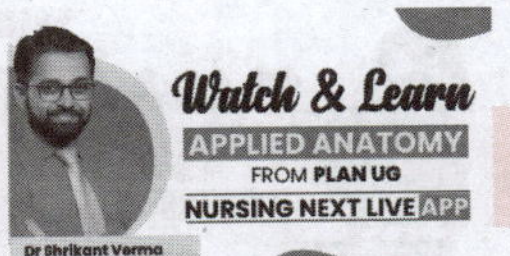

- Granule Cell Layers
  - They are tiny with various cell bodies situated in this layer
  - Bifurcation of axon to T, both the branches run along the folium and referred to as parallel fibers
- **White Matter**
  - Projection fibers
  - Association fibers
  - Commissural fibers
- **Deep Cerebellar Nuclei**
  - Dentate nucleus cluster of neurons with tooth-like serrated edge
  - Emboliform nucleus
  - Globosus nucleus
  - Fastigial nucleus
  - Located near the roof of fourth ventricle

Spinal Cord

- Part of the central nervous system.
- Long pipe-like structure that arises from the medulla oblongata and ends in cauda equina.

Anatomy

- The spinal cord is surrounded by three meninges.
  1. Outermost layer – dura mater
  2. Middle layer – arachnoid mater
  3. Innermost layer – pia mater
- The space between the dura and arachnoid mater is called the subdural space, and between the arachnoid and pia mater is known as subarachnoid space.
- Subarachnoid space contains the cerebrospinal fluid.
- The spinal cord measures about 40 cm in length and 2 cm in diameter.
- The spinal cord is divided into five parts:
  1. Cervical – Eight pairs
  2. Thoracic – 12 pairs
  3. Lumbar – Five pairs
  4. Sacral – Five pairs
  5. Coccygeal – One
- The spinal cord consists of gray and white matter spread across uniformly.

Enlargements

- Neurons at appropriate levels form enlargements to be able to supply the increased musculature. Presents as:
  - Cervical enlargement
    - Extends from C4 to T1 with a maximum diameter of 38 mm at the level of C6 segment.
    - For supply of upper limb muscles
  - Lumbar enlargement
    - Extends from level of L2 to S3 with a maximum diameter of 35 mm at the level of S1.

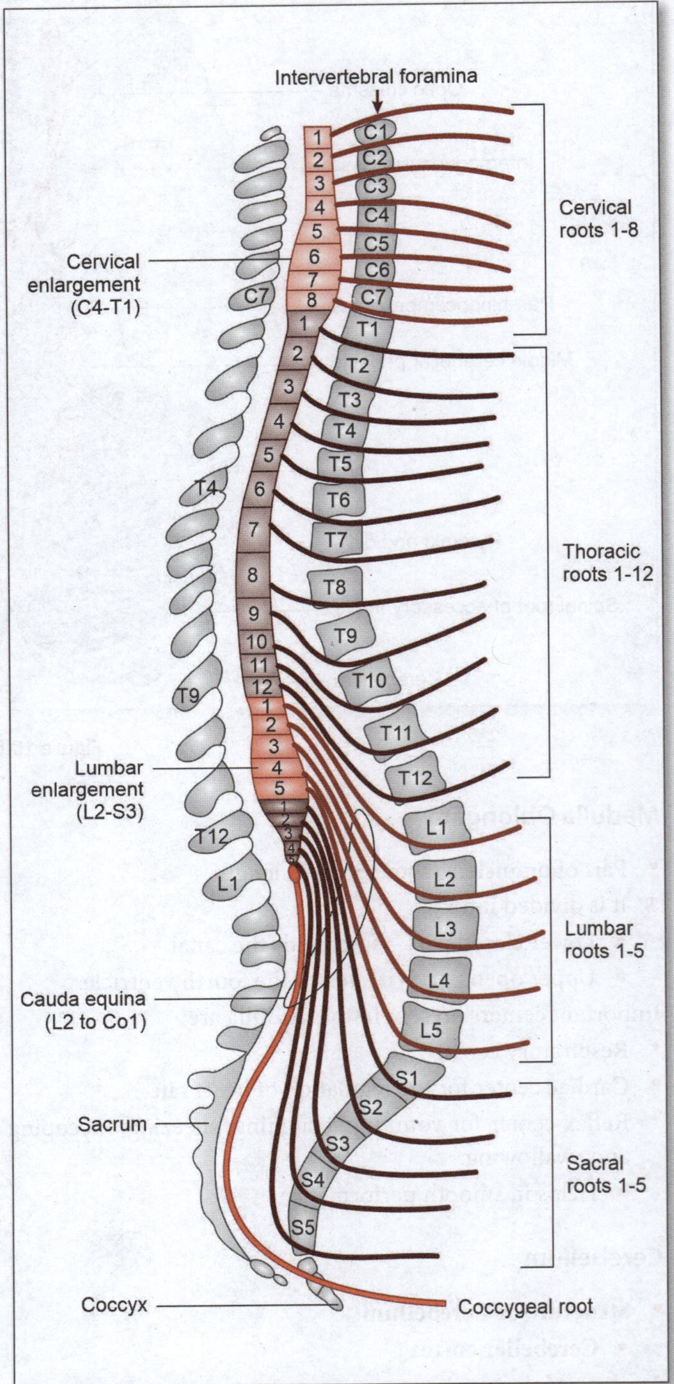

Cauda Equina

- Dorsal and ventral nerve roots of right and left sides of L2 to L5, S1 to S5 and Co1 nerves lie almost vertically around filum terminale. These are called cauda equina as these resemble the horse's tail.

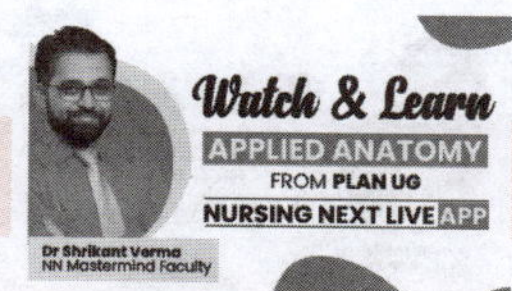

- The spinal cord extends in the lower part of the 1st lumbar vertebrae as conus medullaris. Below the level of the conus medullaris, only pia mater is continued as a thin fibrous cord, the filum terminale.

Internal Structure of Spinal Cord

- Spinal nerves arise from different regions of the vertebral column –
  - Eight – cervical
  - 12 – thoracic
  - Five – lumbar
  - Five – sacral
  - One – coccygeal
- Each spinal nerve arises by a series of six to eight dorsal and ventral nerve rootlets. These rootlets unite in or near the intervertebral foramen to form the spinal nerve.
- Cross-section of the spinal cord displays the gray matter shaped like a butterfly surrounded by the white matter.
  - Gray matter
    - Central canal
    - Filled with CSF
    - Consists of four projections and forms the core mainly containing the cells and neurons.
    - Forms two dorsal and two ventral horns.
  - White matter
    - Collection of axons permitting the communication between different layers of CNS.
    - Contains the tracts – ascending and descending tracts that send and transmit signals from the brain.

Blood Supply

- Anterior spinal artery – present in relation to the anterior median sulcus
- Two posterior spinal arteries – run along the posterolateral sulcus
- Both anterior and posterior spinal arteries are branches of vertebral arteries.

Functions of Spinal Cord

- Forms the connecting link between the brain and peripheral nervous system
- Provides the structural support and builds body posture
- Facilitates flexible movements
- Myelin present in the white matter acts as an electrical insulator
- Coordinates the reflexes.

2. Name the layers of cerebral cortex. Describe the main functional areas of the cerebral cortex. (DU)

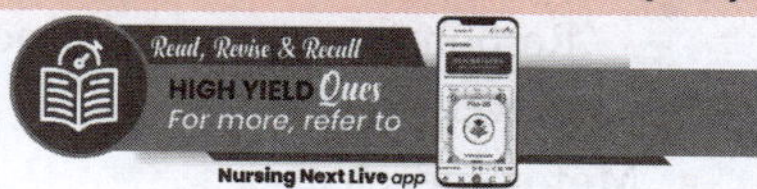

Answer

Layers of Cerebral Cortex

- The six layers of the cerebral cortex are:
  - Layer I – molecular layer
    - Lamina molecularis
    - Consists of only a few nerve cells (Cajal-Retzius cells)
  - Layer II – external granular layer
    - Lamina granularis externa
    - Consists of relatively thin layer of small, densely packed neurons
    - Contains stellate (granular) cells and pyramidal cells
  - Layer III – pyramidal layer/ external pyramidal layer
    - Lamina pyramidalis externa
    - Composed of medium sized pyramidal nerve cells
  - Layer IV – inner granular layer
    - Lamina granularis interna
    - Contains small irregularly shaped nerve cells (mainly pyramidal cells)
  - Layer V – ganglionic or inner pyramidal layer
    - Lamina pyramidalis interna
    - Includes large pyramidal cells and stellate cells
    - Narrowest layer
  - Layer VI – multiform layer
    - Lamina multiformis
    - Contains small polymorphic and fusiform cells and interneurons

Functional Areas of Cerebral Cortex

Functional areas of cerebral cortex can be described as lobewise:

- **Frontal lobe:** Consists of following areas:
  - **Primary motor area**
    - Extends throughout the precentral gyrus and adjoining lip of central sulcus.
    - Area 4 – located on the precentral gyrus of frontal lobe.
      - Acts as center of movement as it sends efferent fibers of primary motor area.
      - Activates the lower motor neurons in the spinal cord.
    - Main function is to control the voluntary movements in the opposite side of the body.
  - **Premotor area**
    - Contains the areas 6 and 8

- Lies anterior to the primary motor area in the precentral cortex.
- Responsible for acts producing orderly series of movements.

- **Motor speech area**
  - Situated in the inferior frontal gyrus
  - Present unilaterally in the dominant hemisphere.
  - Concerned with speech.
- **Prefrontal cortex**
  - Anterior part of frontal lobe (Areas 8 and 44)
  - Concerned with emotional reactions.
  - Forms the center for higher functions like emotions, learning, memory and social behavior.
  - Center for planned actions
  - Responsible for personality of the individuals.

- **Parietal lobe**
  - Contains the sensory areas of cerebral cortex
  - **First somatosensory area (S1)**
    - Corresponds to areas 3, 1 and 2 of Brodmann
    - Located in postcentral gyrus.
    - Sensory homunculus – the different sensory areas of body are represented in postcentral gyrus in an inverted manner as in the motor area.
  - **Second somatosensory area**
    - Situated in postcentral gyrus below the first somatosensory area.
    - Responsible for perception and integration of cutaneous sensations.
  - Area 1 – concerned with sensory perception
  - Area 2 – integration with senses
- **Temporal lobe**
  - **Contains:**
    - Primary auditory area
    - Auditopsychic area
    - Area for equilibrium
  - **Primary auditory area**
    - Includes areas 41, 42, Wernicke's area.
    - Concerned with perception of auditory impulses, analysis of pitch and determination of intensity and source of sound.
  - **Auditopsychic area**
    - Area 22
    - Occupies the superior temporal gyrus
    - Concerned with auditory sensation along the Wernicke's area.
  - **Area of equilibrium**
    - The area for equilibrium is located in the temporal lobe, near the hippocampus. It is responsible for processing information about balance and spatial orientation.
- **Occipital lobe**
  - Visual cortex.
  - Areas of occipital lobe – consists of three functional areas
    - Primary visual area - area 17
      - Concerned with visual impulses
    - Visual association area – area 18
      - Concerned with interpretation of visual impulses
    - Occipital eye field – area 19
      - Concerned with movement of eyes.

SHORT NOTES

1. Write a short note on corpus callosum. (RUHS)

Answer

Introduction

The corpus callosum forms the floor of the longitudinal **fissure** that separates the two cerebral hemispheres. It also forms a part of the roof of the **lateral** ventricles. The corpus callosum has four main parts; individual nerve tracts that connect different parts of the hemispheres.

Divisions

- The corpus callosum is divided into four parts: (i) rostrum, (ii) genu, (iii) body/trunk and (iv) splenium
- **The rostrum:** It is continuous with the lamina terminalis and connects the orbital surfaces of the frontal lobes.
- **The genu:** It is the bend of the anterior corpus callosum; and the forceps minor is a tract that projects fibers from the genu to connect the medial and lateral surfaces of the frontal lobes.
- **The body:** It forms the long central section and its fibers pass through the corona radiata to reach the surface of the hemispheres.
- **The splenium:** It tapers away at the posterior section, with the forceps major projecting fibers from the splenium to connect the two occipital lobes.

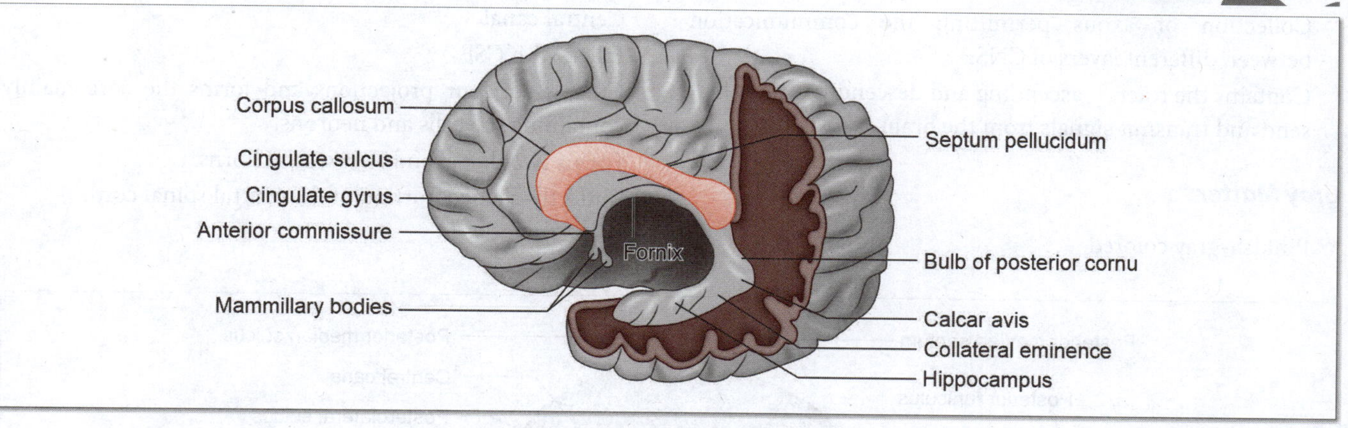

Figure 10.8: Relations of corpus callosum

Blood Supply

- The blood supply to the corpus callosum is rich and strengthened by anastomoses, that are rarely affected by infarcts.
- The anterior cerebral artery can be divided along its course as segment A1 between the internal carotid artery and the anterior communicating artery and as the pericallosal artery distal to the anterior communicating artery.
- A vast majority of the blood supply to the corpus callosum comes from callosal branches of the pericallosal artery, whose course follows the outer border of the corpus callosum, first in the subcallosal area, then in the callosal sulcus or in the cingulate sulcus.
- The posterior pericallosal (splenial) artery is mostly a branch of the posterior cerebral artery. It bifurcates into an inferior and a superior branch which supply the inferior and superior parts of the splenium respectively. The superior branch usually anastomoses with the pericallosal artery.
- The subcallosal artery supplies the hypothalamus in part, but also supplies the rostrum and genu of the corpus callosum.

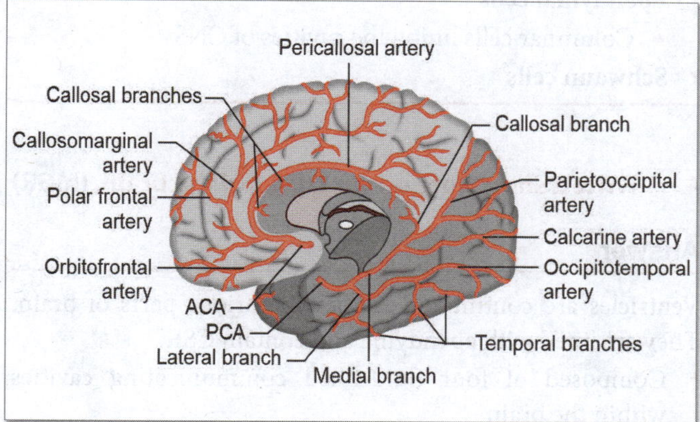

Figure 10.9: Blood supply

Applied Anatomy

- **Agenesis of the corpus callosum:** This is a rare congenital disorder, and is defined as the partial or complete absence of the corpus callosum. The disease usually occurs between the 3rd and 12th week of gestational life, the period when neurological development is at its peak.
- **Corpus callosum impingement syndrome:** Impingement of the corpus callosum fibers on the inferior free margin of the falx cerebri. It usually results from longstanding hydrocephalus. Ischemia results and finally causes atrophy.
- **Stereopsis/binocular vision:** This is the ability to perceive depth, and is dependent on corpus callosum, allowing us to interpret visual information from one eye in conjunction with the visual information from other eye.

2. Write a short note on gray matter and white matter of spinal cord, and spinal segments. (MGR)

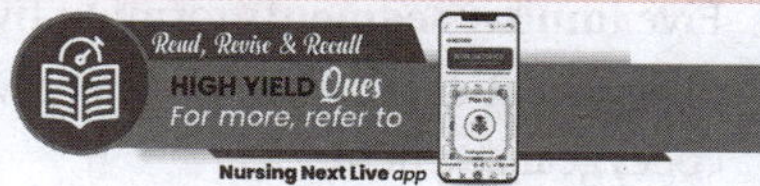

Answer

Spinal Cord

- Part of the central nervous system.
- Long pipe-like structure that arises from the medulla oblongata and ends in cauda equina.

White Matter

- The back portion of this butterfly shape is known as the posterior or dorsal gray horn.
- The front part, also known as ventral gray horn, sends descending nerve signals governing motor activities to the autonomic nerves.
- The white color is due to the presence of the myelin sheath, i.e., a mixture of proteins and lipids that helps in the conduction of the nerve signals and protection of axons.

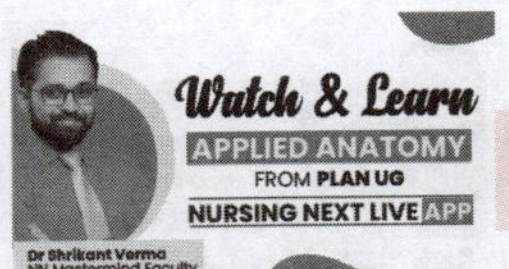

- Collection of axons permitting the communication between different layers of CNS.
- Contains the tracts – ascending and descending tracts that send and transmit signals from the brain.

Gray Matter

- Pinkish-gray colored
- Central canal
- Filled with CSF
- Consists of four projections and forms the core mainly containing the cells and neurons.
- Forms two dorsal and two ventral horns.
- Butterfly-shaped portion of the central spinal cord.

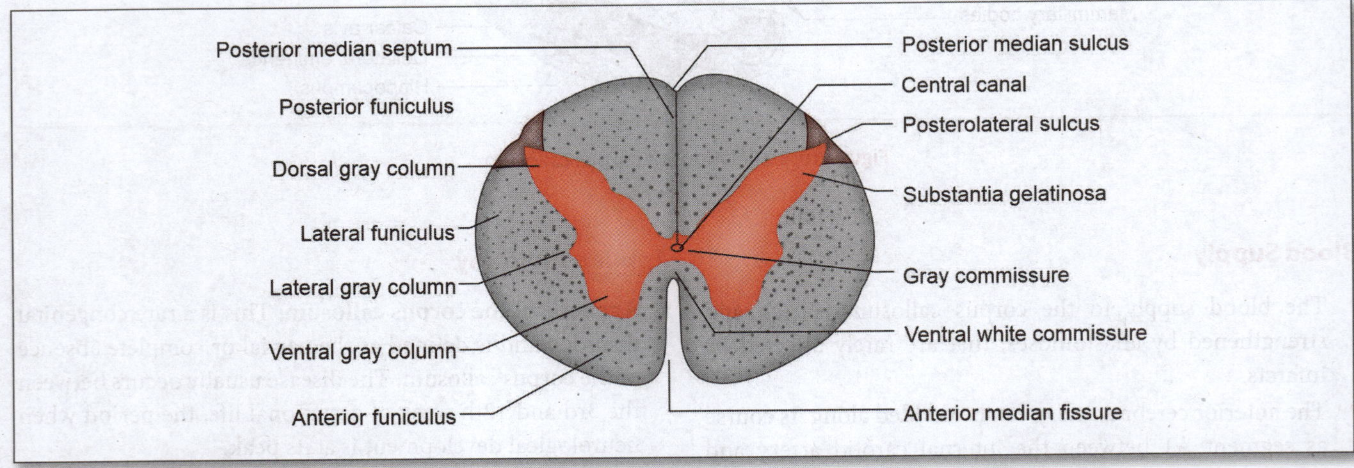

Figure 10.10: Microscopic structure of spinal cord

Spinal Segments

Part of spinal cord to which a pair of dorsal nerve roots (left and right) and a pair of ventral nerve roots are attached is called as spinal segment.

There are 31 spinal cord nerve segments in a human spinal cord:

- Eight **cervical segments** forming eight pairs of cervical nerves
- 12 **thoracic segments** forming 12 pairs of thoracic nerves
- Five **lumbar segments** forming five pairs of lumbar nerves
- Five **sacral segments** forming five pairs of sacral nerves coccygeal segment

3. Write a short note on neuroglial cells. (MGR)

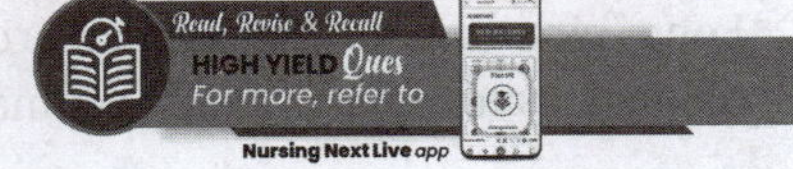

Answer

Neuroglial Cells

Various types of neuroglial cells are:

- **Astrocytes**
  - Star-shaped cells
  - Concerned with nutrition of the nervous tissue are star-shaped cells.
  - Form the blood-brain barrier.
  - Two types – protoplasmic and fibrous
  - These are absent in pineal gland and posterior pituitary.
- **Oligodendrocytes**
  - Counterparts of the Schwann cells. Schwann cells myelinate the peripheral nerves.
  - Function – myelination of cells.
- **Microglial cells**
  - Small elongated neuroglial cells that behave like macrophages of the CNS.
  - Nucleus is small, elongated and dark stained.
  - Cytoplasmic processes are short, thin and spinous.
  - Major function – phagocytosis
- **Ependymal cells**
  - Columnar cells lining the cavities of CNS
- **Schwann cells**

4. Write a short note on ventricles of the brain. (MGR)

Answer

Ventricles are continuous cavities in various parts of brain. They are lined with ependyma and contain CSF.

- Composed of four fluid-filled communicating cavities within the brain
- Consist of lateral ventricle in cerebrum, III ventricle in diencephalon and IV ventricle in pons and medulla.

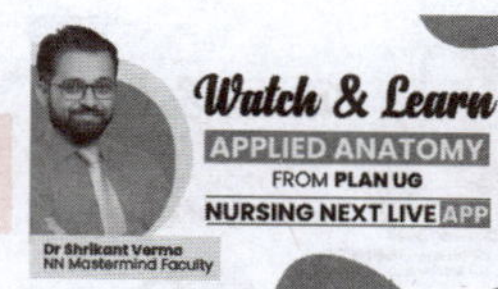

- Lateral ventricle:
  - Present within cerebral hemisphere.
  - Consists of central part and three horns
- Third ventricle:
  - Present between the two thalami and continues as aqueduct of brain
  - Communicates with lateral ventricle by interventricular foramen of Monro
  - Communicates with fourth ventricle by cerebral aqueduct of Sylvius
  - Contains choroid plexus in the roof
- Fourth ventricle:
  - It is the cavity of hindbrain (pons, medulla and cerebellum) and continues downward as central canal of spinal cord.

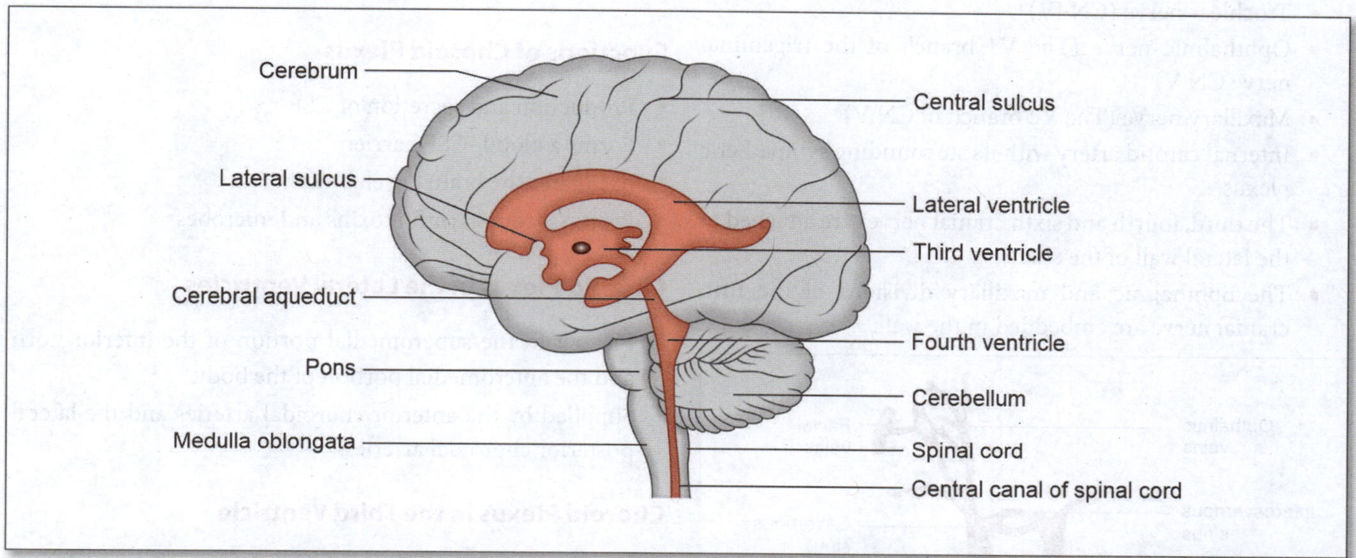

Figure 10.11: Ventricles of brain

5. Write a short note on fissure of Rolando (RUHS).

Answer

Introduction

- Also known as the central sulcus or groove
- Present in the cerebral cortex of the brain.
- Separates the parietal lobe and the frontal lobe, and primary motor cortex from the primary somatosensory cortex.
- Joins the Sylvian fissure in about 2% cases.

Characteristic Feature

- The Rolandic fissure curves posteriorly as it approaches the interhemispheric fissure and often terminates in the paracentral lobule, just anterior to the pars marginalis within the pars bracket.
- The invisible cortex sign is an accurate method of identifying the Rolandic fissure.

Nursing Implications

- Attention deficit hyperactivity disorder (ADHD)
  - Associated with sensorimotor deficits
  - Shape of the Rolandic fissure has been associated with ADHD.
- Focal cortical dysplasia is mainly located in the frontal region with a particular tropism for the central sulcus.

6. Write a short note on cavernous sinus (RUHS).

Answer

Cavernous Sinus

- The cavernous sinus is a large channel or cavity located in the skull, bordered by the sphenoid bone and the temporal bone. The cavernous sinus is an important structure because of its location and its contents which include the third cranial (oculomotor) nerve, the fourth cranial (trochlear) nerve, parts 1 (the ophthalmic nerve) and 2 (the maxillary nerve) of the fifth cranial (trigeminal) nerve, and the sixth cranial (abducens) nerve.

- The cavernous sinus is lined by a layer of endothelium, which separates the venous blood from the surrounding structures.
- Contents of the cavernous sinus include:
  - Oculomotor nerve (CN III)
  - Trochlear nerve (CN IV)
  - Ophthalmic nerve (The V1 branch of the trigeminal nerve CN V)
  - Maxillary nerve (The V2 branch of CN V)
  - Internal carotid artery with its surrounding sympathetic plexus
  - The third, fourth and sixth cranial nerves are attached to the lateral wall of the sinus
  - The ophthalmic and maxillary divisions of the fifth cranial nerve are embedded in the wall.

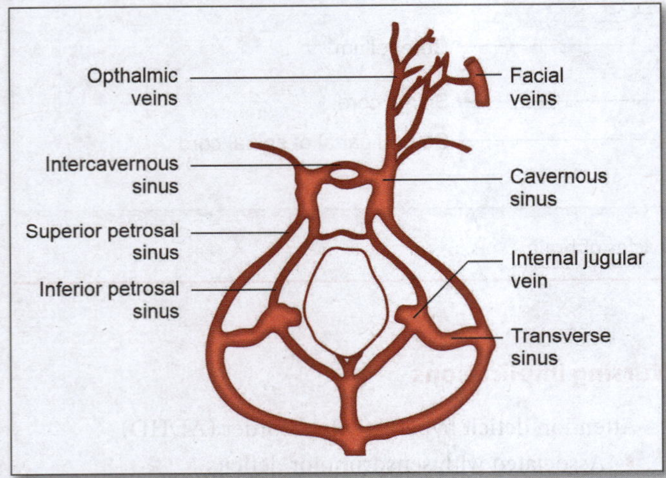

Figure 10.12: Lateral wall of cavernous sinus

7. Write a short note on choroid plexus (RUHS).

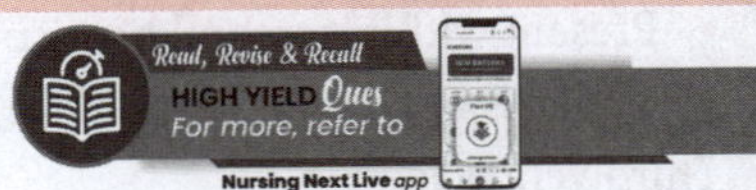

Answer

Introduction

Choroid plexus is the vascular plexus present at the floor of the lateral ventricles and the roof of the third and fourth ventricles.

Functions of Choroid Plexus

- Production and secretion of CSF
- Forms a blood–CSF barrier
- Facilitates the brain development
- Protects from harmful toxins and microbes

Choroid Plexus in the Lateral Ventricles

- Present in the superomedial portion of the inferior horn and the anteromedial portion of the body.
- Supplied by the anterior choroidal arteries and the lateral posterior choroidal arteries.

Choroid Plexus in the Third Ventricle

- The choroid plexus joins the roof of the third ventricle and projects into the superior part of the ventricle.
- It is supplied by the medial posterior choroidal arteries.

Choroid Plexus of the Fourth Ventricle

- The cerebral aqueduct is void of the choroid plexus.
- Located in the posterior medullary velum which partially forms the roof of the fourth ventricle.
- It is supplied by the posterior inferior cerebellar artery.

8. Write a short note on branches of facial nerve on face (RUHS).

Answer

The facial nerve originates in the brain and terminates by giving off five branches on the face, which are known as terminal branches.

The terminal branches of facial nerve are:

- Temporal branch
- Zygomatic branch
- Buccal branch
- Marginal mandibular branch
- Cervical branch

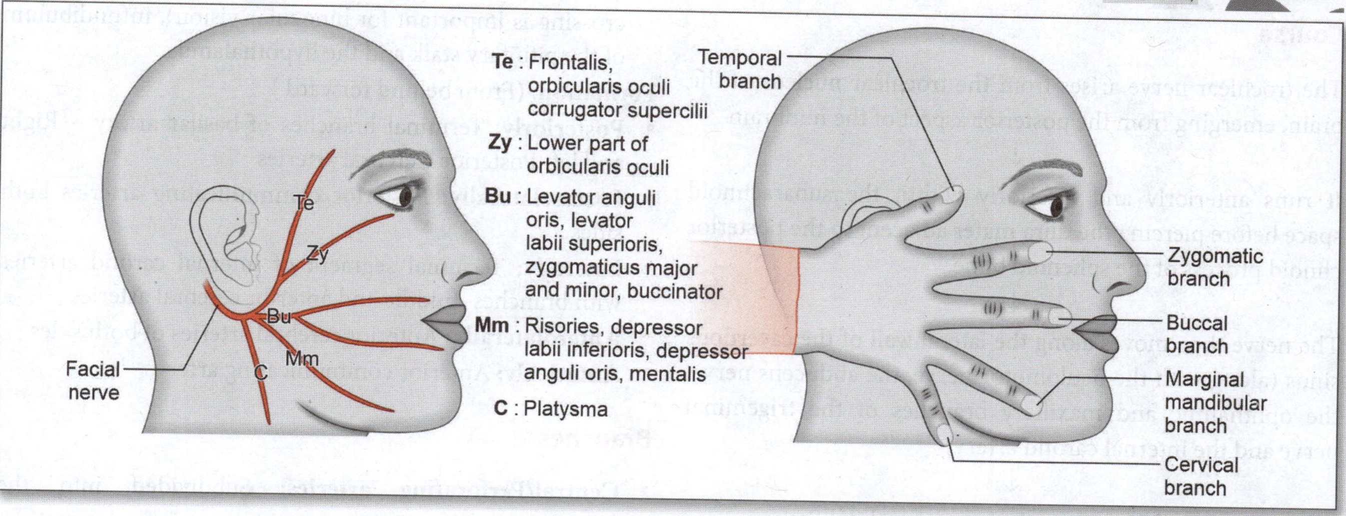

Figure 10.13: Terminal branches of facial nerve

9. Write a short note on fourth cranial nerve (RUHS).

Answer

Introduction

- Fourth cranial nerve or the trochlear nerve has several features that make it unique from the other cranial nerves.
- Trochlear nerve is the only nerve to exit from the dorsal surface of the brain.
- It is the only nerve in which all the lower motor neuron fibers decussate.
- It has the longest intracranial course.
- It has the smallest number of axons.
- The trochlear nerve, also called the fourth cranial nerve or CN IV, is a motor nerve (a somatic efferent nerve) that innervates only a single muscle: The superior oblique muscle of the eye, which operates through the pulley-like trochlea.

Nucleus

The nucleus of the trochlear nerve is located in the caudal mesencephalon beneath the cerebral aqueduct. The trochlear nucleus is unique in that its axons run dorsally and cross the midline before emerging from the brainstem posteriorly. Thus, a lesion of the trochlear nucleus affects the contralateral eye.

- The fibers of the trochlear nerve originate from the trochlear nucleus located in the tegmentum of the midbrain at the level of the inferior colliculus.
- The nucleus is located just ventral to the cerebral aqueduct. It is readily identifiable by its close association with the myelinated medial longitudinal fasciculus that allows communication between various brainstem nuclei.

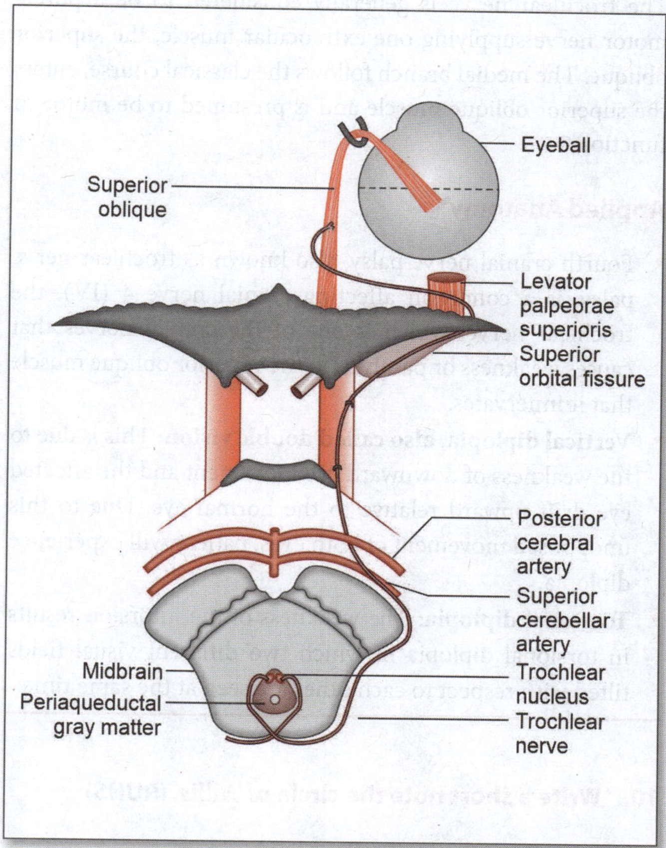

- Fibers leaving the trochlear nucleus travel dorsally to wrap around the cerebral aqueduct.
- All fibers of the two trochlear nerves decussate (i.e., cross) in the superior medullary velum and exit the dorsal surface of the brainstem just below the contralateral inferior colliculus.

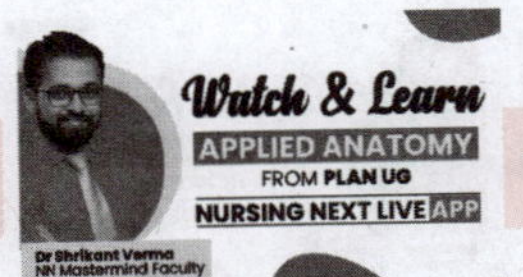

Course

The trochlear nerve arises from the trochlear nucleus of the brain, emerging from the posterior aspect of the midbrain

↓

It runs anteriorly and inferiorly within the subarachnoid space before piercing the dura mater adjacent to the posterior clinoid process of the sphenoid bone.

↓

The nerve then moves along the lateral wall of the cavernous sinus (along with the oculomotor nerve, the abducens nerve, the ophthalmic and maxillary branches of the trigeminal nerve and the internal carotid artery)

↓

Then the orbit of the eye via the superior orbital fissure.

Distribution

The trochlear nerve is generally considered to be a purely motor nerve supplying one extraocular muscle, the superior oblique. The medial branch follows the classical course, enters the superior oblique muscle and is presumed to be motor in function.

Applied Anatomy

- Fourth cranial nerve palsy, also known as trochlear nerve palsy, is a condition affecting cranial nerve 4 (IV), the trochlear nerve, which is one of the cranial nerves that causes weakness or paralysis to the superior oblique muscle that it innervates.
- **Vertical diplopia, also called double vision:** This is due to the weakness of downward eye movement and the affected eye drift upward relative to the normal eye. Due to this unopposed movement of both eyes, patient will experience diplopia.
- **Torsional diplopia:** The weakness of the intorsion results in torsional diplopia in which two different visual fields tilted with respect to each other are seen at the same time.

10. Write a short note the circle of Willis. (RUHS)

Answer

Introduction

- The circle of Willis is also known as the polygon of Willis.
- The circle of Willis is a ring of interconnecting arteries situated at the base of the brain around the optic chiasm or chiasma (partial crossing of the optic nerve - CNII; this crossing is important for binocular vision), infundibulum of the pituitary stalk and the hypothalamus.

Formation: (From behind forward)

- **Posteriorly:** Terminal branches of basilar artery – Right and left Posterior Cerebral arteries
- **Posterolaterally:** Posterior communicating arteries both sides
- **Laterally:** Terminal segment of internal carotid arteries with branches–middle and anterior cerebral arteries
- **Anterolaterally:** Anterior cerebral arteries of both sides
- **Anteriorly:** Anterior communicating artery.

Branches

- **Central/Perforating arteries:** Subdivided into the following groups:
  - **Anteromedial branches:** From anterior communicating artery and anterior cerebral arteries–pierce anterior perforated substance.
    - **Supply:** Optic chiasma, preoptic and supraoptic areas of hypothalamus, septum pellucidum, anterior columns of fornix, cingulate gyrus, rostrum of corpus callosum, anterior part of putamen and head of caudate nucleus.
  - **Anterolateral branches:** From proximal part of the middle cerebral arteries–also known as striate/ lateral striate/ lenticulostriate arteries. Pierce anterior perforated substance.
    - **Supply:** Posterior striatum, part of globus pallidus, anterior limb, genu, and posterior limb of internal capsule.
  - **Medial striate artery:** From middle or anterior cerebral arteries–supplies rostral part of caudate nucleus and putamen, anterior limb and genu of internal capsule.
  - **Posterolateral branches:** From distal part of posterior cerebral arteries
    - **Supply:** Cerebral peduncles, colliculi, pineal gland, and posterior thalamus and medial geniculate body (by thalamogeniculate branches)
  - **Posteromedial branches:** From proximal part of posterior cerebral arteries and posterior communicating arteries - pierce posterior perforated substance.
    - **Supply:** Parts of thalamus, hypothalamus, pituitary gland, mammillary bodies, subthalamus, globus pallidus.

Location of the Circle of Willis

This structure is a circle of interconnected arteries and it is located at the base of the brain. Its location is near to the pituitary stalk, optic chiasm and hypothalamus.

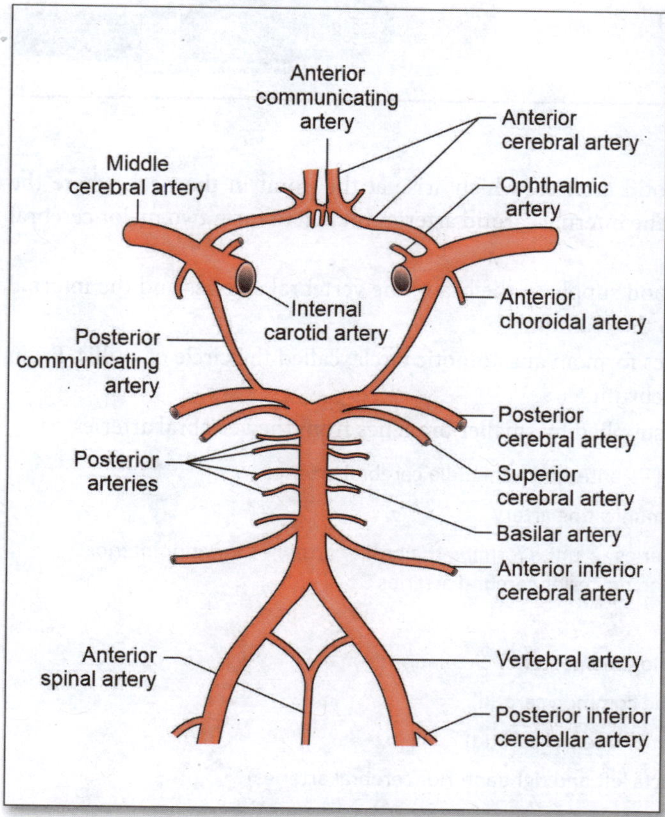

Figure 10.14: Circle of Willis

Clinical Importance

- Most important collateral arterial network to maintain cerebral blood flow.
- Obstruction in any one of the arterial systems (Internal carotid or Vertebral), the flow of blood from the unobstructed side replenishes the deficient supply.
- Berry aneurysm–rupture causes subarachnoid hemorrhage.
- Anterior choroidal artery–from internal carotid artery–artery of cerebral thrombosis.
- Charcot's artery–one of the lateral striate arteries is more susceptible to rupture–artery of cerebral hemorrhage.

11. Write a short note on the cranial nerves emerging from medulla oblongata. (MGR)

Answer

Medulla Oblongata

- Part of brainstem, about 3 cm in length.
- It is divided into:
  - Lower closed part – surrounds the canal
  - Upper open part – related to the fourth ventricle

Important centers present in medulla are:

- Respiratory center
- Cardiac center for the regulation of heart rate
- Reflex center for vomiting, coughing, sneezing, hiccuping and swallowing.

Nerves Emerging from the Medulla Oblongata

- Cranial nerve (CN IX) – glossopharyngeal nerve
- Cranial nerve (CN X) – vagus nerve
- Cranial nerve (CN XI) – hypoglossal nerve
- Cranial nerve (CN XII) – spinal accessory nerve

12. Write a short note on functions of cerebellum. (MGR)

Answer

Functions of Cerebellum

- Cerebellum is associated with cerebral cortex and basal ganglia for control of motor functions. It is a 'silent area' as it does not initiate movement but regulates it.
- **Equilibrium and body posture:** Cerebellum receives sensory information from the peripheral parts of the body and sequentially changes the movement by controlling muscle contraction.
- **Control of muscle reflexes and muscle tone:** Cerebellum receives information from the cerebellar motor cortex and peripheral sensory receptors; and is responsible for regulation of muscle tone and reflexes.
- **Control of voluntary movements:** Cerebellum sequences the motor movements and helps in corrective adjustment of those movements.
- **Comparator function to control voluntary movements:** Cerebellum functions in comparing the actual movement to the intended movement within a fraction of second and sends corrective signals to the motor area of cerebral cortex.
- **Damping of movement:** Cerebellum helps prevent overshooting of the intended movement.
- **Programming and timing of the movement:** Cerebellum helps in programming and timing of movement by comparing signals from the sensorimotor cortex and peripheral sensory receptors.
- **Control of rapid alternate movements:** Ballistic movements, lesion in cerebellum; thus, causes dysdiadochokinesia
- **Servomechanism:** Influence on sensorimotor cortex for correct execution of movement. If the actual movement is not according to the intended movement, it is corrected as per the intended movement from cerebral cortex.

13. Write a short note on the blood supply of brain. (MGR)

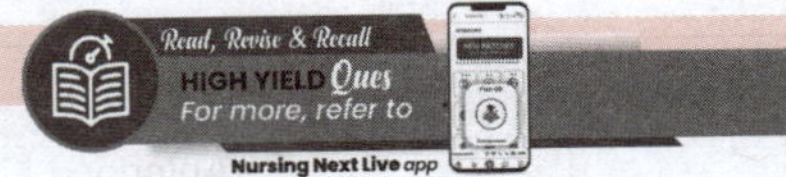

Answer

Introduction

- The brain receives blood from two sources: the internal carotid arteries, which arise at the point in the neck where the common carotid arteries bifurcate, and the vertebral arteries. The internal carotid arteries branch to form two major cerebral arteries, the anterior and middle cerebral arteries.
- There are two paired arteries which are responsible for the blood supply to the brain; the vertebral arteries and the internal carotid arteries. These arteries arise in the neck, and ascend to the cranium.
- Within the cranial vault, the terminal branches of these arteries form an anastomotic circle, called the circle of Willis. From this circle, branches arise which supply the majority of the cerebrum.
- Other parts of the CNS, such as the pons and spinal cord, are supplied by smaller branches from the vertebral arteries.

Anterior cerebral circulation	Common carotid → internal carotid → anterior and middle cerebral arteries
	ACA gives the branch anterior communicating artery
Posterior cerebral circulation	Subclavian arteries → vertebral arteries → unite forming the basilar artery → anterior inferior cerebellar (AICA), superior cerebellar, posterior cerebral arteries
Posterior cerebral gives the branch posterior communicating artery	
Circle of Willis	Polygonal anastomosis of the anterior and posterior circulation:
	Internal carotid artery (branch of the common carotid)
	Anterior cerebral artery (branch of the internal carotid)
Anterior communicating artery (branch of the anterior carotid, connects left and right anterior cerebral arteries)	
Posterior cerebral artery (branch of the basilar artery)	
Posterior communicating artery (branch of the posterior cerebral, connects the three cerebral arteries on the same side)	
Cerebellum	Superior cerebellar artery (branch of the basilar), anterior inferior cerebellar (branch of the basilar), posterior inferior cerebellar (branch of the vertebral artery)
Brainstem	Branches of the vertebral and basilar arteries: anterior spinal, posterior spinal, posterior inferior cerebellar, direct bulbar, paramedian, posterior cerebral, superior cerebellar, posterior communicating, anterior choroidal arteries
Spinal cord	Branches of the vertebral arteries: Anterior spinal, posterior spinal, posterior inferior cerebellar, direct bulbar arteries
Pons	Branches of the basilar artery: Paramedian, short and long circumferential branches
Midbrain	Branches of the basilar artery: Posterior cerebral, superior cerebellar, posterior communicating, anterior choroidal arteries
Cerebrum	Superolateral surface - mostly middle cerebral, but also anterior and posterior cerebral arteries
	Medial surface - mostly anterior cerebral, but also middle and posterior cerebral arteries
	Inferior surface - mostly posterior cerebral, but also anterior and middle cerebral arteries
	Deep structures - anterior communicating arteries, striate arteries, recurrent branches of the anterior cerebral artery
Clinical significance	Stroke, anterior, middle and posterior cerebral artery thrombosis, variations of the cerebral arterial circle, transient ischemic attack

14. Write a short note on the blood-brain barrier. (MGR)

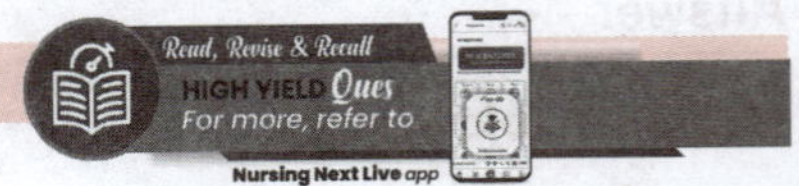

Answer

Definition

- The entry of numerous substances and pathogens is prohibited by a neuroprotective structure, viz. blood-brain barrier into the brain tissues from blood.

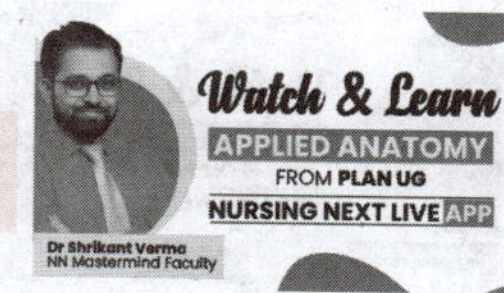

- Blood-brain barrier exhibits in the capillary membrane of all parts of the brain, except in some areas of hypothalamus.

Structure of Blood-Brain Barrier

- Blood-brain barrier functions due to the existence of tight junctions in the endothelial cells of brain capillaries.
- Since the fenestrae that allow transcytosis of substances through endothelium are absent in the brain capillaries unlike other organs due to fusion of the endothelial cells by tight junctions, there is formation of tight junctions between endothelial cells of the capillaries in childhood.
- Simultaneously, there is formation of astrocytes (neuroglial cells) around capillaries that reinforce the barrier and envelop the vasculature.
- Another significant component of blood-brain barrier, viz. pericytes help in the maintenance of tight junctions and structural stability.
- Pericytes work like macrophages in brain and function in defense.

Functions of Blood-Brain Barrier (BBB)

- BBB functions as mechanical barrier and plays a vital role in transport mechanisms.
- It prevents the entry of injurious chemical substances and allows metabolic and essential constituents into the brain tissues.
- A healthy environment persists for nerve cells of brain due to the prevention of harmful chemical substances.
- Numerous substances like oxygen, carbon dioxide, water, glucose, amino acids, electrolytes, drugs such as L-dopa, 5-hydroxytryptamine, sulfonamides, tetracycline and many lipid-soluble drugs, lipid-soluble anesthetic gases such as ether and nitrous oxide, other lipid-soluble substances pass through blood-brain barrier.
- Injurious chemical agents, pathogens such as bacteria, drugs such as penicillin and the catecholamines, dopamine cannot pass through blood-brain barrier.

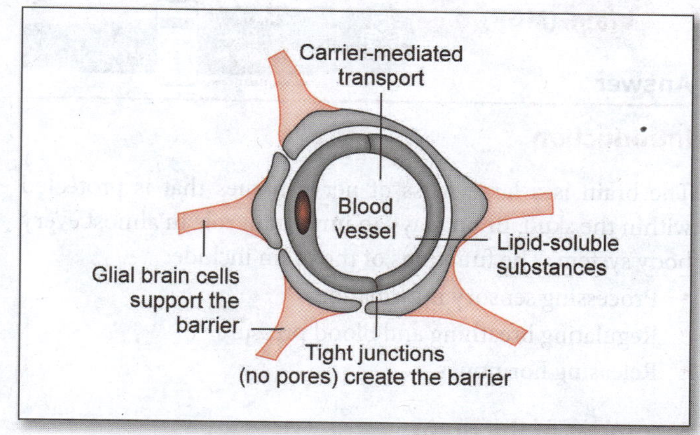

Figure 10.15: Blood-brain barrier

15. Write a short note on types of neurons. (MGR)

Answer

Types of Neurons

Type of neuron	Present in
According to the number of their processes	
Multipolar neurons	All motor and internuncial neurons
Bipolar neurons	Confined to the first neuron of the retina, ganglia of eighth cranial nerve, and the olfactory mucosa
Pseudounipolar neurons—actually unipolar to begin with but become bipolar functionally	Found in dorsal nerve root ganglia and sensory ganglia of the cranial nerves
Unipolar neurons—common in lower vertebrates	Mesencephalic nucleus of trigeminal nerve, and also occur during fetal life
Functional classification	
Sensory neurons • Primary or 1st order sensory neurons • Secondary or 2nd order sensory neurons • Tertiary or 3rd order sensory neurons	• In the dorsal root ganglion of spinal nerves • In the gray matter of spinal cord and in medulla • Seen in thalamus
Motor neurons • Upper motor neurons • Lower motor neurons	• In motor area of brain and synapse with cranial nerve nuclei and anterior horn of spinal cord • In cranial nerve nuclei and anterior horn of spinal cord

Contd...

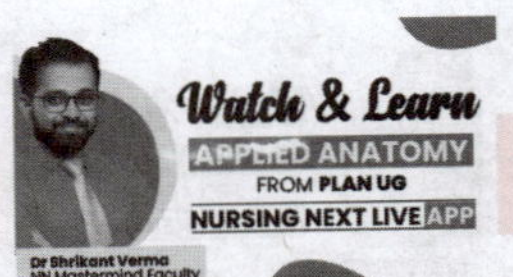

Type of neuron	Present in
Parasympathetic neurons—'craniosacral outflow'. • Preganglionic neurons • Postganglionic neurons	• Located in cranial nerves III, VII, IX and X, also in sacral 2–4 segments of the spinal cord • Located close to the wall or within the wall of the viscera
Sympathetic neurons—'thoracolumbar outflow'. • Preganglionic neurons • Postganglionic neurons	• Are located in the lateral horn of thoracic one to lumbar two segments of the spinal cord • Situated in the ganglia of the sympathetic trunk away from the viscera

16. Write a short note on name the coverings of the brain. (MGR)

Answer

Introduction

The brain is a large mass of nerve tissues that is protected within the skull. Brain plays an important role in almost every body system. The functions of the brain include:

- Processing sensory information
- Regulating breathing and blood pressure
- Releasing hormones

Meninges of the Brain

- Membranous coverings of the brain and spinal cord
- Separate the brain and spinal cord from the skull and the vertebral column.
- From superficial to deep
  - Dura mater
  - Arachnoid mater
  - Pia mater
- Spaces present between these layers
  - Epidural space
  - Subdural space
  - Subarachnoid space
- The major function of the meninges is the protection of the brain from the mechanical trauma.

Dura Mater

- Outermost meningeal layer
- Consists of dense irregular connective tissues
- Composed of two layers:
  - Superficial layer – periosteal cranial dura
    - Overlies the inner table of the cranial vault bones
  - Meningeal cranial dura
    - Lies superficial to the arachnoid mater
- The two dural membranes are mostly attached to each other – forming spaces between them – dural venous sinuses.
- Falx cerebri
  - Largest of the fibrous septa
  - Extends across the midline on the inner surface of the calvaria, from crista galli to internal occipital protuberance.
  - Separates the left and right cerebral hemispheres.
  - Contains the superior and inferior sagittal sinuses.
- Tentorium cerebelli
  - Separates the cerebrum from the cerebellum.
- Falx cerebelli
  - Separates the cerebral hemispheres.
  - Contains the occipital sinus.
- Diaphragma sellae
  - Flat membrane surrounding the pituitary stalk
  - Forms the roof of the hypophyseal fossa.
  - Houses the anterior and posterior intercavernous sinuses.

Arachnoid Mater

- Spiderweb-like meningeal layer
- Potential space present between
  - Arachnoid and dura – known as subdural space
  - Arachnoid and pia – known as subarachnoid space
- Subarachnoid space contains the cerebrospinal fluid (CSF).
- At the sites where the dura forms the venous sinuses, it forms mushroom-like protrusions called the arachnoid granulations.

Pia Mater

- Highly vascular membrane
- Separated from the membrane by a thin space called the subpial space.
- The subpial space is formed by the ends of astrocytes.
- Functions of pia mater
  - Separates the neural tissue from blood vessels in the subarachnoid space
  - Adds to the efficacy of blood-brain barrier.

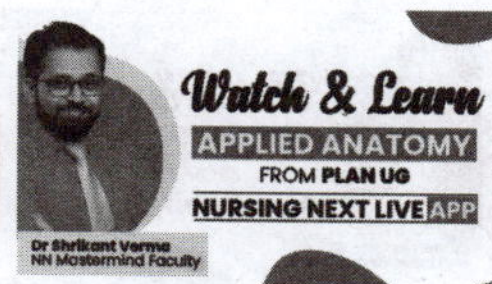

- Prevention of prolonged action of nerves by promoting degradation of neurotransmitters.

Meningeal Spaces

- Epidural space
  - Potential space between the dura mater and the skull.
  - Site for epidural anesthesia
- Subdural space
  - Potential space between the dura and arachnoid mater
  - Narrow space
  - Contains a thin film of fluid
- Subarachnoid space
  - Potential space between the arachnoid and the pia mater
  - Contains cerebrospinal fluid and major blood vessels
  - Provides extensions known as cisterns
  - The CSF is reabsorbed into the dural venous sinuses by diffusing into the subarachnoid granulations in the subarachnoid space.

17. Write a short note on Cerebrum. (KUHS)

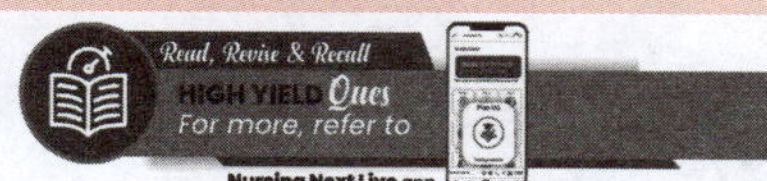

Answer

Cerebrum

- Largest part of brain.
- Consists of left and right cerebral hemispheres separated by fold of dura – falx cerebri.
- The median longitudinal fissure of the cerebrum intervenes between the medial surfaces of right and left surfaces.
- Contents of longitudinal fissure are:
  - Falx cerebri
  - Arachnoid mater
  - Pia mater
  - Anterior cerebral vessels.

External features of Cerebrum

- Surface is not smooth. It has:
  - Sulci – grooves
  - Gyri – intervening surface between two sulci. These consist of central core of white matter covered by gray matter.
- Each cerebral cortex has 3 surfaces and 3 poles:
  - **Pole** – pointed ends
    - Anterior frontal pole
    - Posterior occipital pole
    - Temporal pole
- **Surfaces**
  - Superolateral surface
  - Medial surface
  - Inferior surface: Further divided into:
    - An anterior orbital surface
    - A posterior tentorial surface
- **Lobes**
  - Frontal lobe
  - Parietal lobe
  - Occipital lobe
  - Temporal lobe
- The lobes of cerebral hemisphere are divided by:
  - Central sulci or Rolandic fissure: demarcates frontal from parietal lobes
  - Parieto-occipital sulcus: between parietal and occipital lobe
  - Sylvian fissure or lateral sulcus: demarcates parietal and temporal lobes.
  - Preoccipital notch

Borders

Each hemisphere has three borders:

1. Superomedial
2. Inferolateral
3. Inferomedial

These borders divide the surface into:

- Superolateral
- Medial
- Inferior: Further divided into anterior orbital and posterior tentorial part.
- Inferior border is divided into an anterior part – medial orbital border and posterior part – medial occipital border.
- Inferolateral border's orbital part is called the superciliary border.

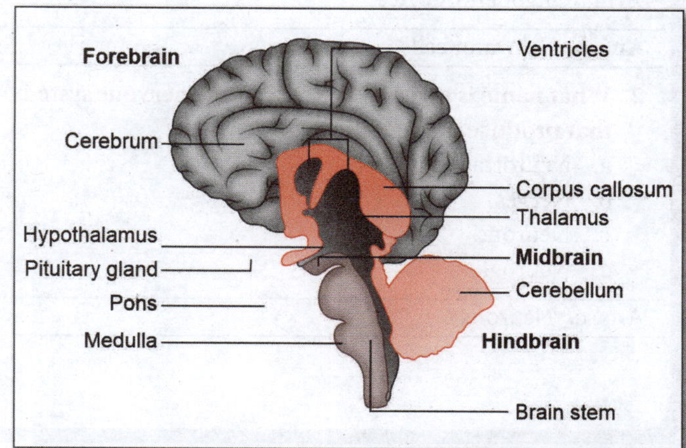

Figure 10.16: Cerebrum

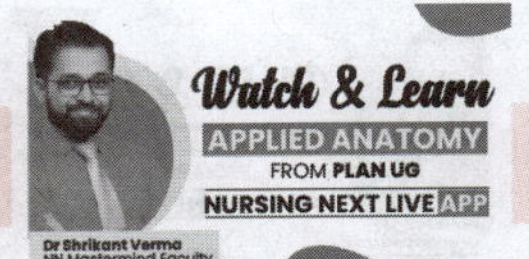

SHORT ANSWER QUESTIONS

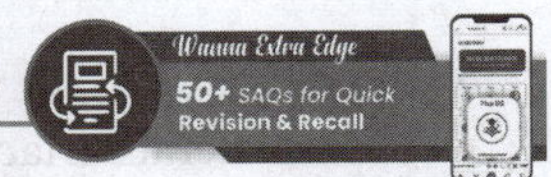

1. Name the arteries forming Circle of Willis. (MGR)

Answer

Anterior communicating artery, anterior cerebral arteries, internal carotid arteries, posterior communicating arteries, posterior cerebral arteries and basilar artery.

2. Mention any four functional areas of cerebrum. (MGR)

Answer

The cerebrum is the largest part of the brain and is responsible for a variety of functions, including sensation, perception, movement, thought, and consciousness.

3. Write the vertebral level for lumbar puncture and level of termination of spinal cord. (MGR)

Answer

A lumbar puncture is typically performed at a vertebral level between L3-L4 or L4-L5, which corresponds to the lower back and lies just below the spinal cord's terminus.

4. Define blood-brain barrier. (MGR)

Answer

The brain and spinal cord's blood arteries are lined with a specialized system called the blood-brain barrier (BBB), which is composed of densely packed cells. It creates a physical barrier that stops the majority of things from infiltrating the brain tissue from the bloodstream, including poisons, viruses, and big molecules.

5. Mention the upper and lower extent of the spinal cord in adult. (MGR)

Answer

In an adult, the spinal cord extends from the base of the brain, at the level of the foramen magnum, to the level of the first or second lumbar vertebra.

CONCEPTUAL REVISION

MULTIPLE CHOICE QUESTIONS

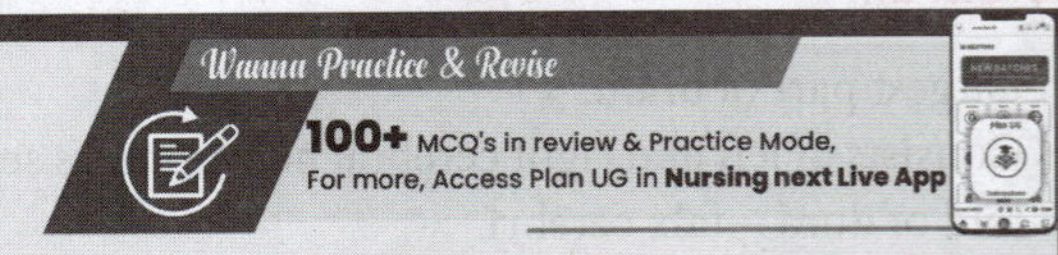

1. In the peripheral nervous system, which cells form the myelin sheath?

a. Ependymal cells
b. Schwann cells
c. Astrocytes
d. Oligodendrocytes

Ans. b. Schwann cells

2. What name is given to the cells in the nervous system that produce nerve impulses?

a. Neurotransmitters
b. Nerves
c. Neurons
d. Neuroglia

Ans. c. Neurons

3. When an action potential arrives at a synapse, what happens first?

a. A neurotransmitter is released into the synaptic cleft
b. Extracellular Na^+ crosses the post-synaptic membrane
c. Choline in the synaptic cleft enters the nerve cell and is converted to acetyl choline
d. Extracellular Ca^{++} enters the nerve cell

Ans. d. Extracellular Ca^{++} enters the nerve cell

4. Which of the following would conduct an action potential with the greatest speed?

a. Myelinated, large diameter fibers
b. Myelinated, small diameter fibers
c. Unmyelinated, large diameter fibers
d. Unmyelinated, small diameter fibers

Ans. a. Myelinated, large diameter fibers

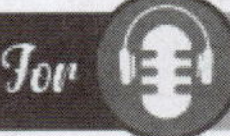

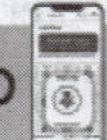

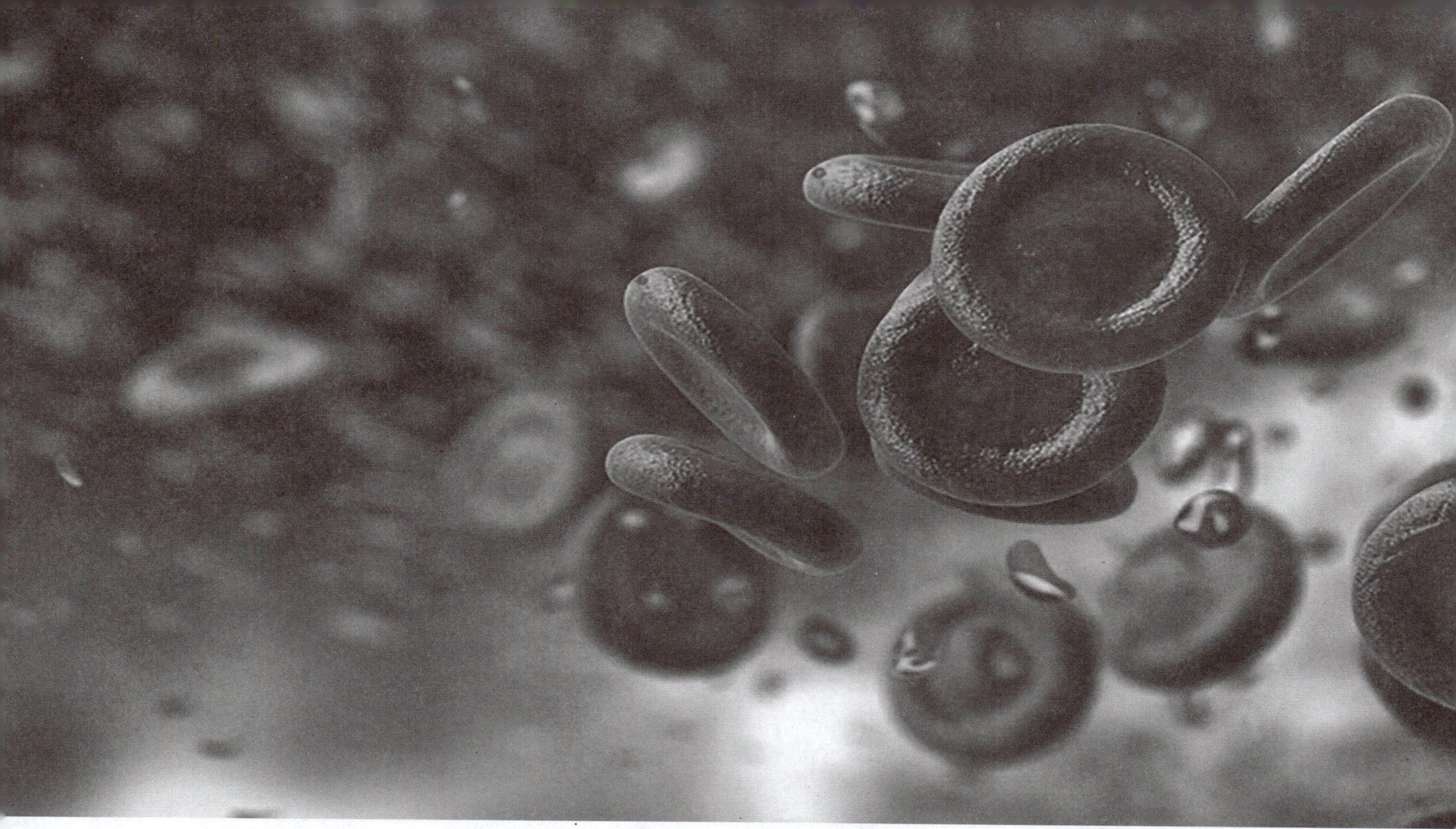

Applied Physiology

Unit Outline

CHAPTER 1

General Physiology—Basic Concepts

CONCEPTUAL THEORY

Terminology

Active transport: The transportation of molecules against their concentration ingredient is active transport.

Body fluid compartments: Intracellular compartment and extracellular compartment. Concentration of substances in the two compartments are constantly different, 55% of water is present in intracellular spaces.

Cell cycle: Comprises two phases: interphase and mitosis. Interphase consists of G1 (first gap phase); S phase (synthesis phase) and G2 second gap phase. Mitosis comprises prophase, metaphase, anaphase and telophase.

Cell: Small functional unit of the body. Cells group together to form tissues. Similar tissues join to form organs, which in turn form systems.

Electrolytes: Important electrolytes are Na^+, Ca^{++}, HPO_4^{2-} and Cl^-.

Homeostasis: It is dynamic equilibrium between extracellular fluid with Na^+, Cl^-, HCO_3^- and intracellular fluid with K^+, Mg, PO_4^{3-}. Most of the systems work to maintain homeostasis. In addition, there are negative and positive feedback mechanisms to maintain homeostasis.

Passive transport: The molecules move down the concentration gradient without involving energy.

Tissues: Cells of different types form tissues. Different tissues form organs. Organs serving similar functions form a system.

Transcellular fluid: Fluid separated from the other extracellular fluid by an epithelial membrane. Examples are CSF, synovial fluid, intraocular fluid, fluid in serous cavities, etc.

Water balance: Intake should be equal to the output to maintain the water balance. Acid base balance is maintained by lungs and kidneys.

CELL PHYSIOLOGY INCLUDING TRANSPORTATION ACROSS CELL MEMBRANE

- Cell physiology is the study of the functions and processes that occur within a cell.

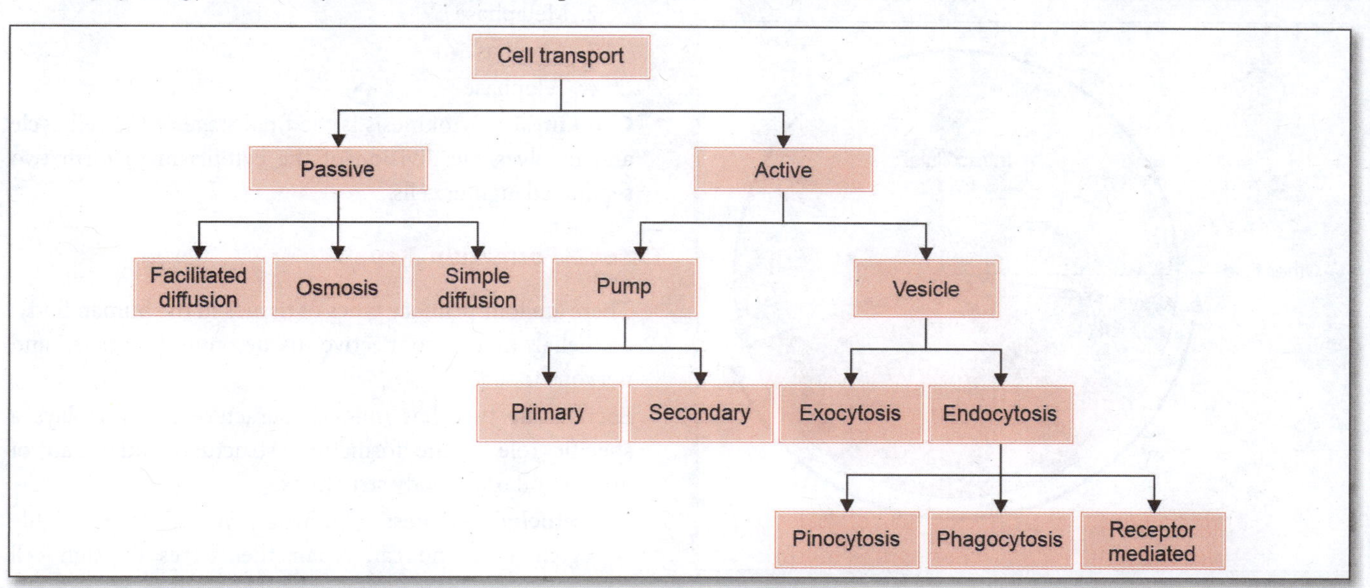

- One crucial aspect of cell physiology is the transportation of molecules across the cell membrane
- There are several mechanisms by which transportation occurs across the cell membrane:
  - **Passive diffusion:** This process occurs from an area of high concentration to an area of low concentration, following the concentration gradient.
  - **Facilitated diffusion:** Certain larger or charged molecules, such as glucose or ions, require the assistance of specific membrane proteins to cross the cell membrane. These proteins are called transporters or carrier proteins, and they facilitate the movement of molecules down their concentration gradient.
  - **Active transport:** Active transport is a process that moves molecules across the cell membrane against their concentration gradient. Active transport is carried out by specific membrane proteins called pumps. One well-known example is the sodium-potassium pump.
  - Endocytosis is the process by which cells engulf extracellular material by forming a vesicle around it. Example- Phagocytosis (engulfing solid particles) and pinocytosis (engulfing liquid droplets).
  - Exocytosis, on the other hand, involves the release of material from the cell by fusion of vesicles with the cell membrane.
  - Ion channels are specialized membrane proteins that allow the passage of specific ions across the cell membrane.

Body Water Content

Human body weight is primarily composed of water, which ranges from about 75% in infants to about 50–60% in adults and as little as 45% in the elderly.

Fluid Compartments

Interstitial fluid (IF), a subclass of extracellular fluid (ECF), is the liquid that exists between bodily cells. Extracellular fluid also includes the liquid found in blood vessels.

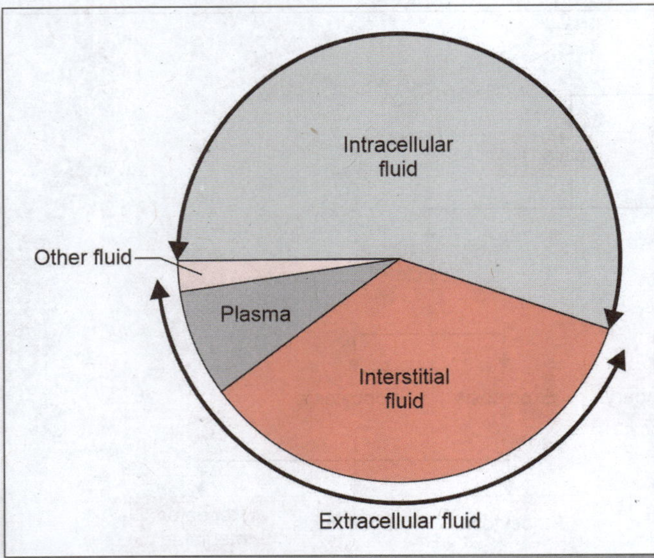

Intracellular fluid, or ICF, is the fluid that is present in the cytoplasm of every body cell.

The extracellular fluid (ECF) between the cells includes the interstitial fluid (IF). The second element of the ECF is blood plasma.

Maintenance of Homeostasis

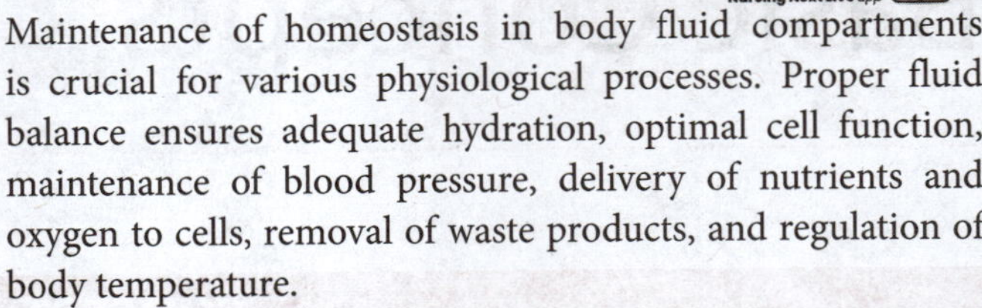

Maintenance of homeostasis in body fluid compartments is crucial for various physiological processes. Proper fluid balance ensures adequate hydration, optimal cell function, maintenance of blood pressure, delivery of nutrients and oxygen to cells, removal of waste products, and regulation of body temperature.

Cell Cycle

The cell cycle is the series of events that occur in a cell leading to its division and the production of two daughter cells.

It consists of several distinct phases, including interphase and mitosis.

- **Interphase:** Interphase is the longest phase of the cell cycle and can be further divided into three stages: G1 (Gap 1), S (Synthesis), and G2 (Gap 2).
  1. **G1 phase:** During G1 phase, the cell grows and carries out its normal functions.
  2. **S phase:** In the S phase, DNA replication occurs.
  3. **G2 phase:** During G2 phase, the cell continues to grow, synthesizes proteins, and prepares for mitosis.
- **Mitosis:**
  - Mitosis is the phase where the cell's nucleus divides into two identical daughter nuclei.
  - **It consists of four main stages:** Prophase, metaphase, anaphase, and telophase.
    1. Prophase
    2. Metaphase
    3. Anaphase
    4. Telophase
- **Cytokinesis:** Cytokinesis is the final stage of the cell cycle and involves the division of the cytoplasm to form two separate daughter cells.

Tissue—Formation, Repair

- There are four primary types of tissues in the human body: epithelial tissue, connective tissue, muscle tissue, and nervous tissue.
- Each tissue type has unique characteristics and plays a specific role in the formation, structure, and repair of organs and other body structures.
  - **Epithelial tissues:** Epithelial tissues are highly regenerative and can repair themselves through cell

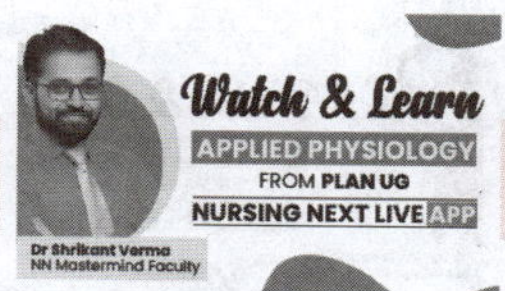

division, where new cells are produced to replace damaged or lost cells.

- **Connective tissues:** Connective tissues can repair through processes such as fibrosis, where damaged tissues are replaced with scar tissue, or regeneration, where new cells of the same type are generated to restore the original tissue structure.

- **Muscle tissues:**
  - **There are three types of muscle tissues:** Skeletal, cardiac, and smooth muscle.
  - In skeletal muscle, repair and regeneration occur through the activation of satellite cells, which differentiate and fuse with existing muscle fibers to repair or replace damaged muscle cells. Cardiac and smooth muscle have limited regenerative abilities, and repair often involves scar tissue formation.
- **Nervous tissues:** In the central nervous system (brain and spinal cord), damaged neurons have limited regenerative abilities, and repair often involves scar tissue formation. In the peripheral nervous system, certain neurons can regenerate over time, aided by specific growth factors and guidance from surrounding tissues.

Repair of tissues generally involves three overlapping processes:

1. **Inflammation:** In response to tissue injury or damage, inflammation occurs. It involves increased blood flow, recruitment of immune cells, and release of inflammatory mediators to remove damaged cells and initiate the repair process.
2. **Proliferation:** During the proliferation phase, new cells are generated to replace the damaged or lost cells. Cell division occurs, and specialized cells, such as fibroblasts in connective tissue or satellite cells in skeletal muscle, play a role in producing new cells to restore tissue integrity.
3. **Remodeling:** The remodeling phase involves the reorganization and maturation of newly-formed cells and tissues. The extracellular matrix is modified, and scar tissue may form to provide structural support. This phase can last for an extended period as the tissue gradually acquires its normal structure and function.

Membranes and Glands—Functions

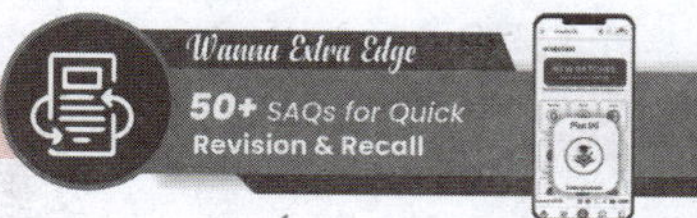

Membranes	Functions
Epithelial membranes	Provide a protective barrier against pathogens and physical damage
	Regulate the exchange of substances between body compartments and the external environment
	Secrete mucus, enzymes, and other substances for lubrication, absorption, or defense
	Absorb nutrients, gases, and water
	Participate in sensory reception and transmission
Mucous membranes	Line various body cavities and organs, including the respiratory, digestive, and reproductive tracts
	Produce mucus to lubricate and protect the underlying tissues
Serous membranes	Line the internal cavities of organs, such as the peritoneum, pleura, and pericardium
	Secrete serous fluid to reduce friction between organs during movement
Synovial membranes	Line the joint cavities and produce synovial fluid
	Lubricate the joints, reduce friction, and provide nourishment to the articular cartilage

Glands	Functions
Exocrine glands	Secrete substances, such as enzymes, hormones, mucus, or sweat, into ducts that lead to body surfaces or cavities
	Aid in digestion, cooling, lubrication, and protection
	Examples include salivary glands, sweat glands, mammary glands, and sebaceous glands
Endocrine glands	Secrete hormones directly into the bloodstream for distribution throughout the body
	Regulate various physiological processes, including metabolism, growth, reproduction, and homeostasis
	Examples include the pituitary gland, thyroid gland, adrenal glands, and pancreas
Mixed glands	Have both exocrine and endocrine functions
	Examples include the pancreas, which secretes digestive enzymes (exocrine) and hormones such as insulin (endocrine)

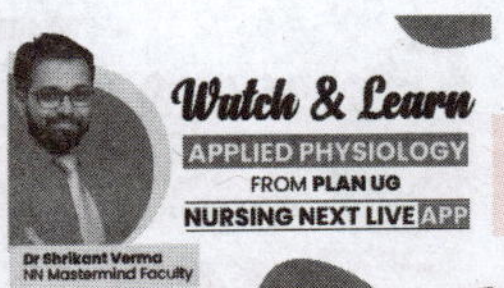

CONCEPTUAL EXERCISES

LONG ANSWER QUESTION

1. Explain the functional morphology of cell membrane and components of eukaryotic cell.

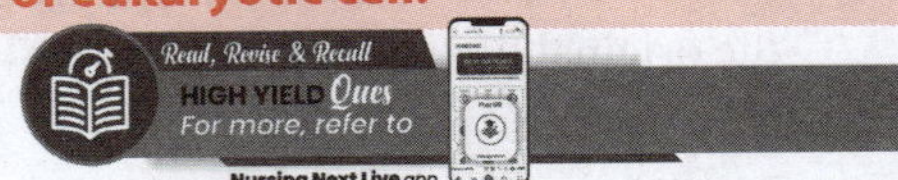

Answer

Introduction

Cell is the fundamental working unit of all the organisms. Cells in humans can be highly specialized in terms of both structure and function; conversely, cells from different organs might share traits and functions.

The cells in the various organs are highly specialized, and no cell can be called "typical" of all cells in the body. However, a few cell structures (organelles) are shared by all cells.

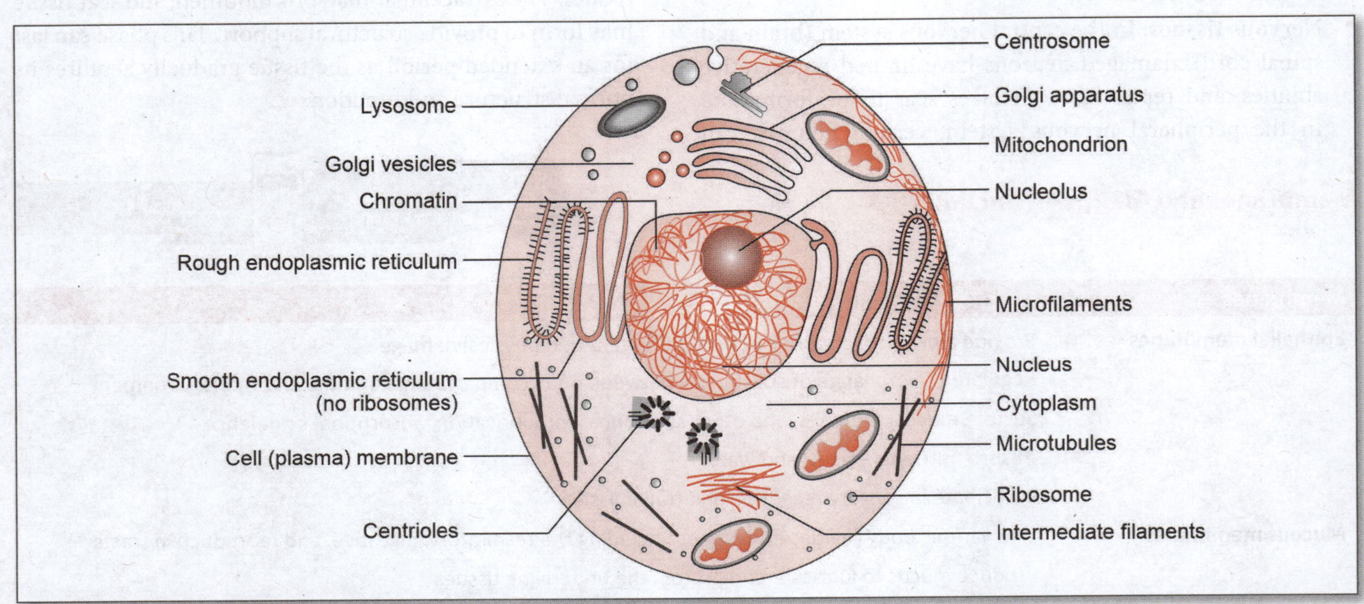

Figure 1.1: Simplified structure of a cell

Functional Morphology of Cell Membrane

- Membranes are composed of lipids and proteins, and they are semipermeable, allowing certain things to pass through while excluding others. Its permeability, however, can be altered since it contains several controlled ion channels and other transport proteins that can alter the quantity of items passing through it. It is commonly known as the plasma membrane.
- They are typically 7.5 nm (75 angstroms [Å]) thick. Phospholipids such as phosphatidylcholine, phosphatidylserine, and phosphatidylethanolamine are the most abundant lipids.
- The hydrophilic ends of the molecules are exposed to the aqueous environment that bathes the surface of the cells and the watery cytoplasm in the membrane, while the hydrophobic ends meet in the membrane's water-poor interior.
- The membrane contains several distinct proteins. Membrane proteins are divided into two types:
  1. Integral proteins (intrinsic membrane proteins)—embedded in one leaflet of the membrane
  2. Peripheral proteins (extrinsic membrane proteins)—associated with the inside or outside of the membrane
- Some proteins act as pumps, actively moving ions across the membrane. Other proteins act as transporters, facilitating the movement of molecules down electrochemical gradients. Others are ion channels, which, when activated, allow ions to enter or exit the cell.

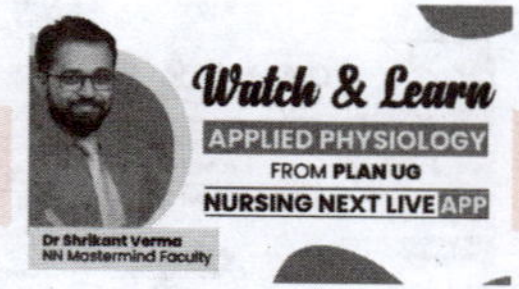

Various Cell Structures

Mitochondria

- Aerobic bacteria were engulfed by eukaryotic cells over a billion years ago and evolved into mitochondria, allowing eukaryotic cells to create the energy-rich chemical ATP via oxidative phosphorylation. It also plays role in regulation of apoptosis that is programed cell death.
- Hundreds to thousands of mitochondria can be found in each eukaryotic cell.
- It is an organelle in the shape of a sausage.
- Each has an outside membrane, an intermembrane space, a folded inner membrane (cristae), and a central matrix space.

Lysosomes

- Large, rather irregular structures are surrounded by membranes in the cell's cytoplasm.
- The core of these organelles, known as lysosomes, is more acidic than the rest of the cytoplasm, and they digest foreign material such as endocytosed bacteria and worn-out cell components.
- Over 40 different types of hydrolytic enzymes can be found in lysosomes.
- It is also known as a suicidal-bag because if the lysosomes rupture and expel their contents, the enzymes would be rendered ineffective.

Peroxisomes

- Peroxisomes are 0.5 m in diameter, covered by a membrane, and contain enzymes that can either create or degrade H_2O_2 (oxidases) (catalases).
- The peroxisome membrane contains a variety of peroxisome-specific proteins involved in the transport of chemicals into and out of the peroxisome matrix.
- More than 40 enzymes are found in the matrix, which work in tandem with enzymes found outside the peroxisome to catalyze a range of anabolic and catabolic events (e.g., breakdown of lipids).

Cytoskeleton

All cells have a cytoskeleton, which is a network of fibers that not only keeps the cell's structure but also allows it to change form and move. The cytoskeleton is primarily composed of microtubules, intermediate filaments, and microfilaments, as well as proteins that anchor and connect them.

Molecular Motors

- 100–500 kDa ATPases are the molecular motors that transport proteins, organelles, and other parts of cell throughout the cell.
- Molecular motors are classified into three superfamilies: kinesin, dynein, and myosin.

Centrosomes

- A centrosome is found in the cytoplasm of eukaryotic animal cells near the nucleus.
- The centrosome consists of two centrioles.
- When a cell splits, the centrosomes double and travel apart to the poles of the mitotic spindle, where they supervise the cell division process.

Nucleus and Related Structures

- The nucleus is made up of chromosomes, which are structures in the nucleus that carry a full blueprint for all heritable species and individual features of the animal.
- The DNA strand is around 2 m long, but it can fit in the nucleus because it is wrapped around a core of histone proteins at regular intervals to create a nucleosome.
- The beads represent nucleosomes, and the rope represents the linker DNA that connects them. Chromatin refers to the entire complex of DNA and proteins.
- The genes on the chromosomes are the ultimate units of inheritance.

Endoplasmic Reticulum

- The endoplasmic reticulum is a complicated sequence of tubules in the cell's cytoplasm with a folded inner limb of the membrane known as the cistern of endoplasmic reticulum.
- Membrane makes up the tubule walls. Ribosomes are connected to the cytoplasmic side of the membrane in rough (granular) endoplasmic reticulum, but not in smooth (agranular) endoplasmic reticulum.
- The rough endoplasmic reticulum is involved in protein synthesis and the first folding of polypeptide chains via disulfide bond formation.
- In steroid-secreting cells, the smooth endoplasmic reticulum is the site of steroid synthesis, while in other cells, it is the site of detoxifying processes.

Ribosomes

- Ribosomes in eukaryotes are roughly 22–32 nm in size. Each consists of a big and a small subunit known as the 60S and 40S subunits.
- They are protein synthesis sites.
- All transmembrane proteins, the majority of secreted proteins, and the majority of proteins stored in the Golgi apparatus, lysosomes, and endosomes are synthesized by ribosomes that get attached to the endoplasmic reticulum.

Golgi Apparatus

- The Golgi apparatus is a stack of membrane-enclosed sacs (cisternae) similar to a dinner plate.
- The Golgi apparatus is a polarized structure having cis and trans sides. The cis face is close to the endoplasmic reticulum, while the trans face is close to the plasma membrane.
- Membranous vesicles containing newly-generated proteins bud off from the rough endoplasmic reticulum and fuse with the Golgi apparatus's cistern on the cis side.
- The proteins are subsequently transported via additional vesicles to the middle cisterns and, eventually, to the trans side cistern, from which vesicles branch into the cytoplasm.

SHORT NOTES

1. Write a short note on active transport. (MGR)

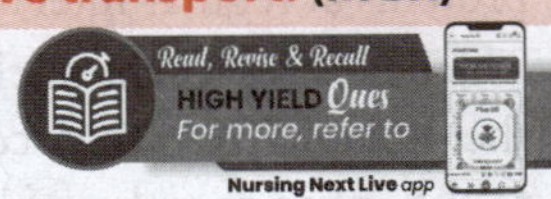

Answer

Active Transport

- Transport of substances occurs with the use of energy.
- **Two types:** Primary and secondary.

Primary Active Transport

- Active transport involves transport across cell membrane when energy is directly derived from ATP or some high-energy phosphate compound.
- **Examples:**
  - Na K ATPase pump
  - Potassium-hydrogen pump
  - Calcium pump.
- In active transport, carrier protein provides energy in the form of ATP for transport of substance against electrochemical gradient.
- Difference in ionic concentration across the membrane also provides energy to carrier proteins of secondary active transport.
- Primary active transport is responsible for causing electrical potential across cell membrane.
- The ions that are transported by primary active transport are: Na, K, Cl^-, H^+, etc.
- Pumps responsible for the primary active transport are present in almost all the cells of the body.
- Due to transport of the substances against the concentration gradient, primary active transport helps in maintaining cell volume. For example, proteins inside the cell are negatively charged and have the tendency to attract positive ions. Na^- K^+ ATPase pump helps in throwing three positively charged Na ions out and two positively charged K ions inside. This prevents loading of ions which prevents osmosis of water inside the cell. Thus, this prevents the bursting of the cell by osmosis.

Types of Primary Active Transport

- P Type transporters
  - The transporter protein is phosphorylated and dephosphorylated during the transport activity.
- V Type transporters
  - Present in the membrane of the lysosomes, the Golgi vesicles and the secretory vesicles, and are responsible for acidification of the interior of these vesicles.
- F Type transporters:
  - Present in mitochondria and are involved in ATP synthesis.

Secondary Active Transport

- Due to active transport of Na^+ by Na^+ K^+ ATPase pump across the cell membrane, there occurs an increased concentration of sodium outside the cell membrane and this excessive sodium outside the membrane has a tendency to diffuse inside the cell membrane from higher concentration to lower concentration.
- This causes diffusion energy which attracts other ions to diffuse across the cell membrane along with sodium.
- Also known as:
  - Ion gradient driven active transport
  - Free energy of the electrochemical gradient

Types of Secondary Active Transport

- Symporters or cotransporters, e.g., Na-Glucose cotransporters, Na-I symporters, transporters of amino acids.
- Countertransporters: Na–Ca2+ exchangers

Na-Glucose Cotransporter

- In this process, Na/K^+-ATPase located in the basolateral membrane pumps out the Na ions which in turn enter with glucose, i.e., the uptake of glucose and sodium is secondarily dependent on the Na gradient that is maintained primarily by Na/K-ATPase.
- Glucose enters intestinal epithelial cells by active transport using the electrogenic Na-glucose transporter-1 (SGLT1) in the apical membrane.
- This forms the principle of *oral rehydration therapy.*
  - Main ingredients of the oral rehydration solution (ORS) include glucose, NaCl or NaHCO, KCl and water.

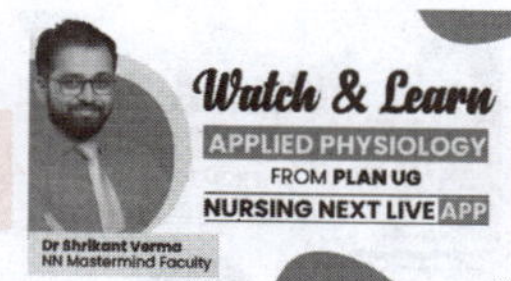

- On administration of ORS, glucose and Na' are reabsorbed by the sodium-glucose transporter-1 (SGLT1) in the apical membrane of enterocytes.
- This in turn increases the osmolarity, thereby favoring the absorption of water osmotically.
- Absorption of glucose accompanied by the obligatory increase in the absorption of NaCl and water helps to compensate for the diarrheal losses of water and solutes, which in turn treats dehydration.

2. Explain the functions of cell membrane. (MGR)

Answer

Cell membrane is a semipermeable membrane surrounding the cytoplasm of a cell. The functions of cell membrane are as follows:

- **Membrane transport:**
  - Cell membrane facilitates the transport of materials across it.
  - Selectively permeable to certain substances and helps in transport of substances needed for survival.
  - Two types:
    1. **Passive transport:** The molecules move down the concentration gradient without energy.
    2. **Active transport:** Transportation of molecules against their concentration gradient.
- **Protection of cell:** Surrounds the cytoplasm of cell and forms a physical barrier between intracellular and extracellular compartments.
- **Maintains structural integrity:** Anchors the cytoskeleton.
- The protein component of cell membrane acts as ligand receptors.
- The plasma membrane helps to take in food and also excretes waste products.
- Aids in cell recognition.
- Proteins in cell membrane act as enzymes and catalyze reactions.
- Modifications of plasma cell membrane
  - Brush border/microvilli in the absorptive cells of the small intestine
  - Flagella that form the tail of the spermatozoa
  - Ciliated cells of the respiratory tract
- Body fluid compartments, distribution of total body fluid, intracellular and extracellular compartments, major electrolytes and maintenance of homeostasis.

3. Differentiate between osmosis and diffusion. (KUHS)

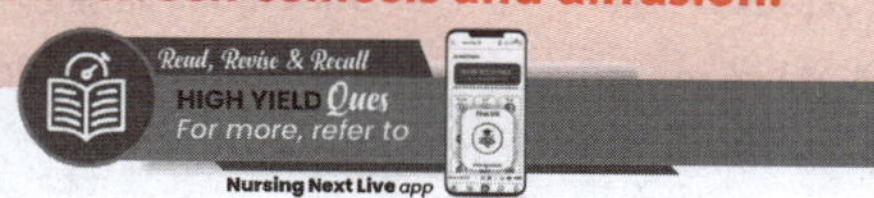

Answer

Table 1.1: Differences between osmosis and diffusion

Osmosis	Diffusion
Occurs in liquid medium	Occurs in liquid, gaseous and even solid medium
Depends on the concentration of solute in a solvent	Depends on the presence of other particles.
Requires a semipermeable membrane	Semipermeable membrane is not required.
Only the solvent diffuses	Both the solute and solvent can diffuse
Movement occurs in one direction only	Flow of particles occurs in all directions
Occurs between similar solutions	Occurs between similar as well as dissimilar solutions.
Does not require energy	Simple diffusion does not require energy, facilitated diffusion does.
Aids the body to get nutrients from food, removes waste from blood	Transport of water-soluble materials like sodium, calcium, exchange of gases

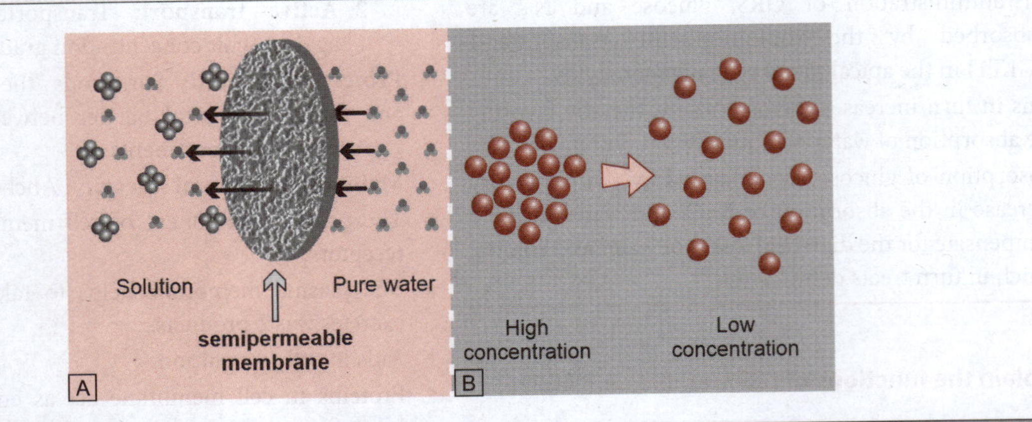

Figures 1.2A and B: A. Osmosis; B. Diffusion

4. Differentiate between mitosis and meiosis. (DU)

Answer

Table 1.2: Differences between mitosis and meiosis

	Mitosis	Meiosis
Definition	Cell division that produces identical daughter cells	Cell division that results in haploid daughter cells.
Nucleus	Undergoes single division	Undergoes two divisions
Mode of reproduction	Asexual reproduction	Sexual Reproduction
Occurrence	All the cells	Reproductive cells
Interphase	Chromosome replicates to form two genetically identical sister chromatids	Chromosomes are not yet visible but DNA has been duplicated
Prophase	Crossing over doesn't occur	Crossing-over and recombination take place
Metaphase	Chromosomes assemble at the metaphase plate.	Chromosomes adjust on the metaphase plate.
Anaphase	Centromeres split at anaphase	Centromeres do not split in anaphase I but occur in anaphase II
Function	General growth and repair, cell reproduction	Genetic diversity through sexual reproduction
Cytokinesis	Occurs in telophase	Occurs in telophase I and in telophase II

5. Differentiate between resting membrane potential and action potential. (KUHS)

Answer

Table 1.3: Differences between resting membrane potential and action potential

Features	Resting membrane potential	Action potential
Definition	Difference in the electrochemical potential across the outer and inner membrane at rest	Difference in the electrochemical potential across the neuron membrane when it is stimulated
Occurrence	At rest	When signals are transmitted along the neurons
Voltage	–70 mV	+40 mV
Ions	Na^+ is predominant outside and K^+ inside the cell membrane	Na^+ is present more inside; and less K^+ ions are present inside the cell

Contd...

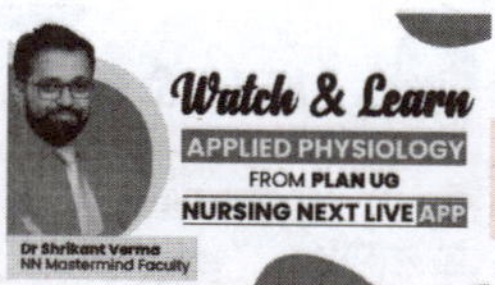

Features	Resting membrane potential	Action potential
Stability	Relatively static	Transient
Transmission of nerve impulse	Does not allow the transmission of nerve impulses	Allows the transmission of nerve impulses
Ion channels	Voltage-gated sodium and potassium ion channels are closed	Sodium ion channels are open; and voltage-gated potassium channels are closed.
Followed by	Action potential or graded potential	Hyperpolarization

6. Differentiate between extracellular fluid (ECF) and intracellular fluid (ICF). (KUHS)

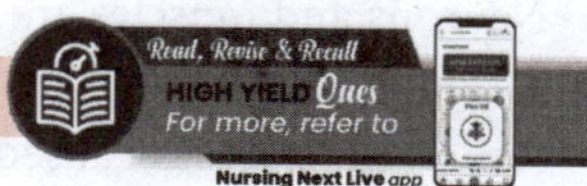

Answer

Table 1.4: Differences between extracellular fluid and intracellular fluid

Extracellular fluid	Intracellular fluid
Fluid present outside the cell aiding the functioning of tissue	Fluid present inside the cell, containing dissolved ions and components
Comprises the plasma, tissue fluid and transcellular fluid	Comprises the cytosol
Proteins and amino acids are present	Proteins and amino acids are absent
Major ions: Sodium (Na^+), chloride (Cl^-), bicarbonate (HCO_3^-), etc.	**Major ions:** Potassium (K^+), magnesium (Mg^{2+}), phosphate (PO_4^{3-}), etc.
The concentration of Na^+ ions > K^+ ions	Concentration of K^+ ions > Na^+ ions
Comprises about 45% of body water	Comprises about 55% of body water
Comprises 20% of total body weight	Comprises 40% of total body weight
Comprises 14 L of total body fluids	Comprises 25 L of total body fluids
Functions: Transports nutrients and oxygen to cells, removes waste products from cells, helps to maintain blood pressure	**Functions:** Maintains the structure of cells, provides a medium for chemical reactions, stores nutrients

7. Differentiate between active transport and facilitated diffusion. (KUHS)

Answer

The key difference between active transport and facilitated diffusion is that active transport occurs against the concentration gradient; hence, utilizes energy to transport molecules across the membrane; while facilitated diffusion occurs along the concentration gradient; hence, does not utilize energy to transport molecules across the membrane.

Table 1.5: Differences between active transport and facilitated diffusion

Features	Active transport	Facilitated diffusion
Definition	Transport of substances across the membrane with the use of energy	Transport of substances across the membrane without the use of energy
Process	Active	Passive
Concentration gradient	Occurs against the concentration gradient	Along the concentration gradient
Energy consumption	Uses energy either in form of ATP or electrochemical gradient	Does not use energy
Proteins involved	Sodium–potassium pump Sodium–glucose pump	Gated ion channels Transmembrane proteins
Termination	Doesn't stop even after the equilibrium is reached; Causes accumulation of substances inside the cell	Stops once the equilibrium is reached

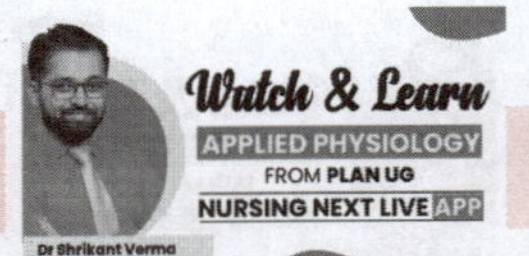

8. Describe briefly action potential. (DU)

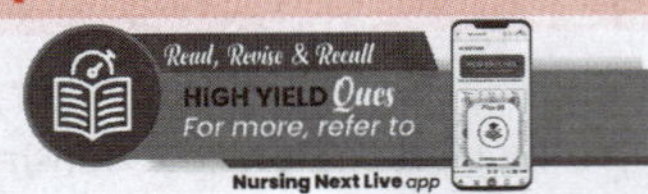

Answer

Action potential is sudden, fast, propagating change of the resting membrane potential.

- This property is known as excitability.
- Neurons and muscles are responsible for the generation of action potential.
- Action potential is caused by the temporary change in the membrane permeability.
- Changes in action potential cause the ion channels to open and the ions to diffuse through the membrane.
- Action potential has three phases:
  1. Depolarization
  2. Overshoot
  3. Repolarization
     - Hypopolarization—precedes depolarization
     - Hyperpolarization—follows repolarization

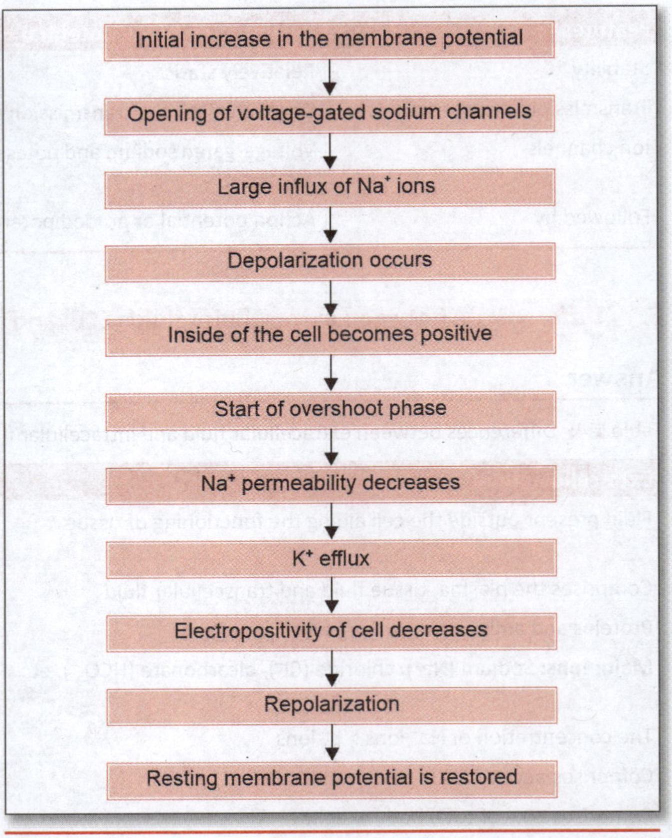

Refractoriness

Time lapse after an action potential during which the next action potential cannot be generated.

9. Write about meiosis. (RUHS)

Answer

Introduction

- Type of cell division that results in four daughter cells, each with half the number of chromosomes of the parent cell.
- A single cell divides twice to form four haploid daughter cells.
- Meiosis occurs in two stages:
  - During first division, the two DNA chains separate each serving as a template for synthesis of a new complementary chain. DNA polymerase catalyzes this reaction.
- Each stage is subdivided into several phases:
  1. Meiosis I:
     - Prophase I
     - Metaphase I
     - Anaphase I
     - Telophase I
     - Cytokinesis I
  2. Meiosis II:
     - Prophase II
     - Metaphase II
     - Anaphase II
     - Telophase II
     - Cytokinesis II

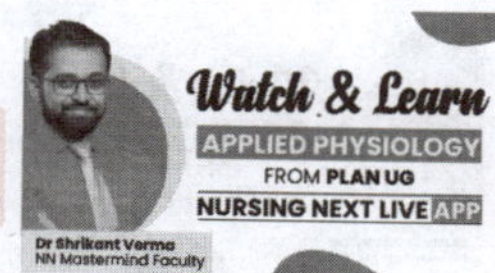

Stages of Meiosis

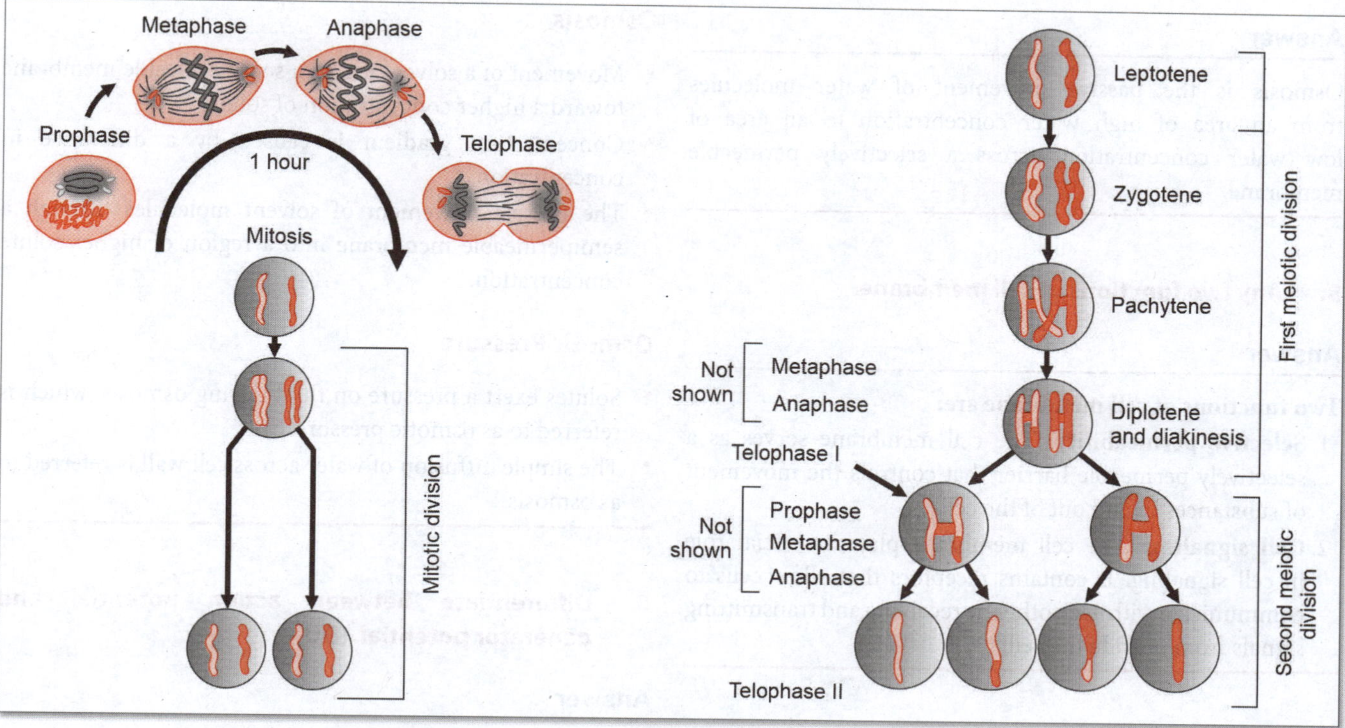

Figure 1.3: Meiosis

Meiosis cell division takes place in the following stages:

- **Meiosis I**
  - **Prophase I**
    - The nuclear envelope disintegrates.
    - Comprises
      - **Leptotene:** Chromosomes become visible, sister chromatids lie together.
      - **Zygotene:** Pairing of homologous chromosomes (tetrad chromosomes)
      - **Pachytene:** There is crossing over of chromatin material. The point of contact is chiasmata.
  - **Prometaphase II**
    - Spindle fibers attach to the chromosomes at the centromere.
  - **Metaphase I**
    - Chromosomes arrange on the spindle.
  - **Anaphase I**
    - Centromere does not split. Whole chromosome is pulled to opposite poles of the cell.
  - **Telophase I**
    - Spindle fibers disappear.
    - Nuclear envelope is reformed.
    - Daughter cells get half the number of chromosomes.
- **Meiosis II:** No duplication of chromatin material occurs.
  - **Prophase II**
    - The chromatin condenses into chromosomes.
    - Nuclear envelope disintegrates.
    - Centrosomes move to opposite poles.
    - Spindle fibers are visible.
  - **Metaphase II**
    - Chromosomes are arranged at the equatorial plate.
  - **Anaphase II**
    - Sister chromatids are pulled to the opposite poles.
  - **Telophase II**
    - Nuclear envelope reforms and the spindle fibers disappear.

SHORT ANSWER QUESTIONS

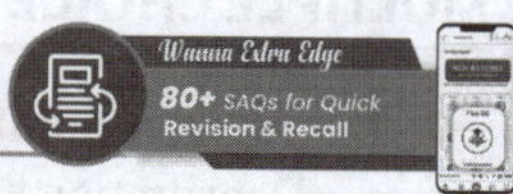

1. Active transport.

Answer

Active transport is a process in which cells use energy to move molecules or ions against their concentration gradient, from an area of lower concentration to an area of higher concentration.

2. Define osmosis.

Answer

Osmosis is the passive movement of water molecules from an area of high water concentration to an area of low water concentration across a selectively permeable membrane.

3. Any two functions of cell membrane.

Answer

Two functions of cell membrane are:

1. **Selective permeability:** The cell membrane serves as a selectively permeable barrier that controls the movement of substances in and out of the cell.
2. **Cell signaling:** The cell membrane plays a crucial role in cell signaling. It contains receptors that allow cells to communicate with each other by receiving and transmitting signals from outside the cell.

4. Name the plasma proteins.

Answer

Plasma proteins are also known as blood proteins or serum proteins found in blood plasma.

They help in controlling blood osmotic pressure and carrying substances like hormones and lipids.

It includes albumin, globulin, immunoglobulin, prothrombin, and fibrinogen

5. Write a short note on osmosis. (MGR)

Answer

Osmosis

- Movement of a solvent across a semipermeable membrane toward a higher concentration of solute.
- Concentration gradient is caused by a difference in concentration.
- The passive movement of solvent molecules through a semipermeable membrane into a region of higher solute concentration.

Osmotic Pressure

- Solutes exert a pressure on fluid during osmosis; which is referred to as osmotic pressure.
- The simple diffusion of water across cell wall is referred to as osmosis.

6. Differentiate between action potential and generator potential. (DU)

Answer

Table 1.6: Differences between action potential and generator potential

Action potential	Generator potential
Sudden, fast propagating change in the resting membrane potential	More gradual change
Requires an electrical stimulus of a certain threshold to occur	Occurs when a tonic receptor is stimulated
Follows all-or-none law	Doesn't follow all-or-none law
It is fixed and not proportional to the intensity of the stimulus	It is proportional to the intensity of the stimulus.

CONCEPTUAL REVISION

MULTIPLE CHOICE QUESTIONS

1. Decrease in colloidal osmotic pressure leads to:
   a. Dehydration
   b. No change in the body fluids
   c. Edema
   d. Acidosis

Ans. c. Edema

2. Na^+, K^+ gradient across the membrane is mainly maintained by:
   a. $Na^+ - Ca^+$ pump
   b. $Na^+ - K^+$ pump
   c. $H^+ - K^+$ pump
   d. Na^+ pumps

Ans. b. $Na^+ - K^+$ pump

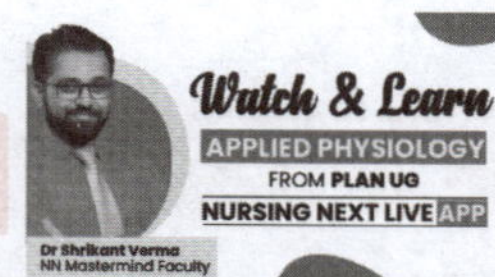

3. Normal ECF value of a 70 kg person:
a. 10 L
b. 14 L
c. 28 L
d. 2 L

Ans. b. 14 L

4. The major cation in extracellular fluid is:
a. Sodium
b. Potassium
c. Chloride
d. Bicarbonate

Ans. a. Sodium

5. Hypokalemia is:
a. Decrease in K concentration in the ECF
b. Increase in Na concentration in ECF
c. Increase in Na concentration in ICF
d. Decrease in Na concentration in ECF

Ans. a. Decrease in K concentration in the ECF

6. Which one is the major anion in Extracellular fluid?
a. Sodium
b. Chloride
c. Potassium
d. Phosphate

Ans. b. Chloride

7. The human body's ability to maintain a relatively constant internal temperature is an example of what?
a. Respiratory heat loss
b. Homeostasis
c. Vasodilation and evaporative heat loss
d. Positive feedback

Ans. b. Homeostasis

8. Which of the following would be a negative feedback response by the body to hyperthermia?
a. Shivering
b. Sweating
c. Vasoconstriction of blood vessels in the dermis
d. An increase in metabolic rate

Ans. b. Sweating

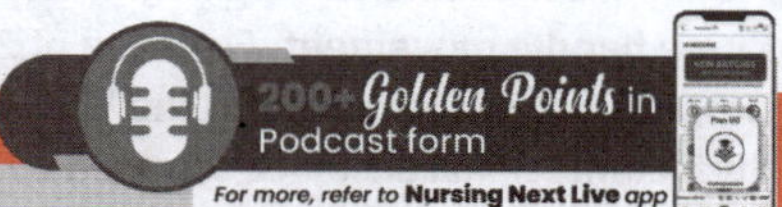

Golden Points

- Cell physiology is the study of individual activities of the cell to maintain homeostasis.
- **Electrolytes** are minerals in the human body that have an electric charge.
- Electrolytes are used to maintain voltages across their cell membranes and they also carry electrical impulses to other cells and across themselves.
- Endocrine glands discharge their secretion directly into the blood or lymphatic and are called ductless glands, e.g., thyroid.
- Exocrine glands discharge their secretions onto a surface directly or by means of ducts.
- Exocytosis is a process in which cells remove undigested or waste metabolites/products that were brought in the cell by endocytosis.
- Homeostasis is a state of dynamic equilibrium rather than constant, unchanging state.
- In pinocytosis process, fluid of smaller molecules can be engulfed and transported.
- Intracellular Fluid Compartment represents the sum of the fluid contents of all the cells of the body. This intracellular fluid contains about 30–40% of the body weight and holds about 55% of the whole-body water.
- Meiosis is a type of cell division that helps in production of egg and sperm cells.
- Mitosis is a process where a single cell divides into two identical daughter cells (cell division). Here the number of chromosomes remains constant through generations. Before mitosis, there is S phase where DNA duplicates itself.
- Mucous Membrane/Mucosa lines the alimentary tract, and the respiratory passage. It secretes mucus, which protects the cells from mechanical and chemical injuries.
- Physiology deals with learning and understanding the functions of the body.
- Systemic physiology is the study of the functioning of all the diverse systems of the body.
- The cell is the structural and functional unit of the living matter and is capable of carrying on the processes of life independently.
- The extracellular fluid compartment is a compartment containing heterogenous collections of fluids and not a continuous fluid phase.
- The most common cause of **electrolyte disturbances** is renal failure.
- Tissues are groups of cells that have a similar structure and act together to perform a specific function.

CHAPTER 2

Respiratory System

CONCEPTUAL THEORY

Terminology

150+ key terminologies for Quick Recall & Revision

Bucket handle movement: 7th–10th ribs get elevated to increase transverse diameter of the thorax.

Chemoreceptors: Aortic and carotid bodies act as chemoreceptors, i.e., respond to changes in pH, PO_2 and PCO_2.

Cyanosis: It is bluish discoloration of body tissues due to decreased levels of oxygen bound hemoglobin. If deoxy Hb levels increases more than 5 g/dL, it causes cyanosis.

Dyspnea: Difficulty in breathing

External respiration: Exchange of gases between the blood and the alveoli of the lungs.

Internal respiration: Interchange of gases in the tissues.

Piston-like movement: Diaphragm descends vertically like a piston to increase vertical diameter of thorax.

Pump handle movement: Elevation of 2nd–6th ribs with sternum increases anteroposterior diameter of the thorax.

Respiration: Taking oxygen in the body and expelling carbon dioxide from the body.

Surfactant: Lipid substance secreted by type II pneumocytes of alveoli is surfactant. It lowers the surface tension of alveoli and prevents them from collapsing.

Ventilation–perfusion ratio: It is the ratio of alveolar ventilation and the amount of blood that perfuses the alveoli.

FUNCTIONS OF RESPIRATORY ORGANS

The main functions of the respiratory organs include:

- Pulmonary ventilation
- Gas exchange
- Oxygen transport
- Acid-base balance
- Speech production
- Defense mechanism

PHYSIOLOGY OF RESPIRATION

Physiology of respiration can be divided into two main components: External respiration and internal respiration.

- **External respiration:** External respiration is completed in lung (alveoli) and blood from environment. It includes:
  - **Ventilation:** It starts with the process of ventilation, which includes the inhalation and exhalation of air.
  - **Gas exchange:** Once air reaches the lungs, the actual exchange of gases takes place across the respiratory membrane.
- **Internal respiration:** Internal respiration is completed in cells and tissues from the blood. It involves the following steps:
  - Oxygen delivery
  - Carbon dioxide removal
  - Gas exchange at tissues
  - Return to lungs

Pulmonary Circulation

Functional Features of Pulmonary Circulation

- Carries deoxygenated blood from the right ventricle of the heart to the lungs for oxygenation.
- Returns oxygenated blood from the lungs to the left atrium of the heart.
- Functions as a low-pressure system compared to the systemic circulation.
- Has shorter and wider blood vessels compared to the systemic circulation.
- Supplies the lungs with nutrients and removes waste products.
- Facilitates gas exchange between the alveoli (air sacs) and the pulmonary capillaries in the lungs.

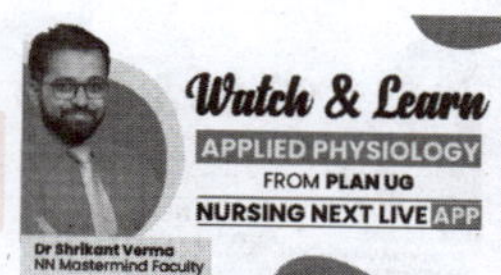

- Allows for the removal of carbon dioxide from the bloodstream and the intake of oxygen.
- Pulmonary arteries carry deoxygenated blood, while pulmonary veins carry oxygenated blood.
- The pressure in the pulmonary arteries is lower than in the systemic arteries.
- The pulmonary circulation is part of a closed circulatory system separate from the systemic circulation.
- Pulmonary circulation is essential for maintaining proper oxygenation of the blood and supporting overall respiratory function.

Pulmonary Ventilation, Exchange of Gases

Diffusion of Oxygen from the Alveoli to the Pulmonary Capillary Blood

- Curve shows the rapid rise in blood PO_2 as the blood passes through the capillary
- The blood PO_2 rises almost to that of the alveolar air by the time the blood has moved a third of the distance through the capillary, becoming almost 104 mm Hg.

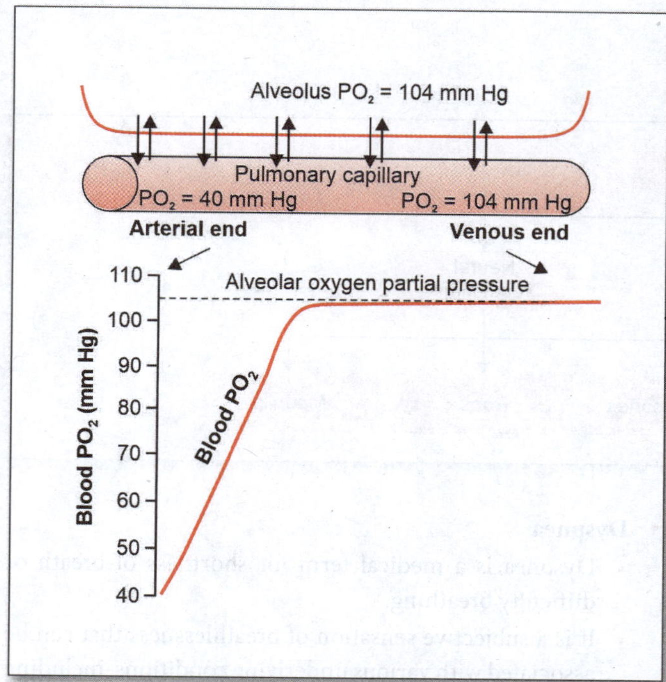

Diffusion of CO_2 from the Pulmonary Blood into the Alveolus

- PCO_2 at arterial end = 45 mm Hg
- PCO_2 of alveolar air = 40 mm Hg
- CO_2 diffusion with the difference of 5 mm Hg
- PCO_2 of the pulmonary capillary blood falls to almost exactly equal to the alveolar PCO_2 of 40 mm Hg

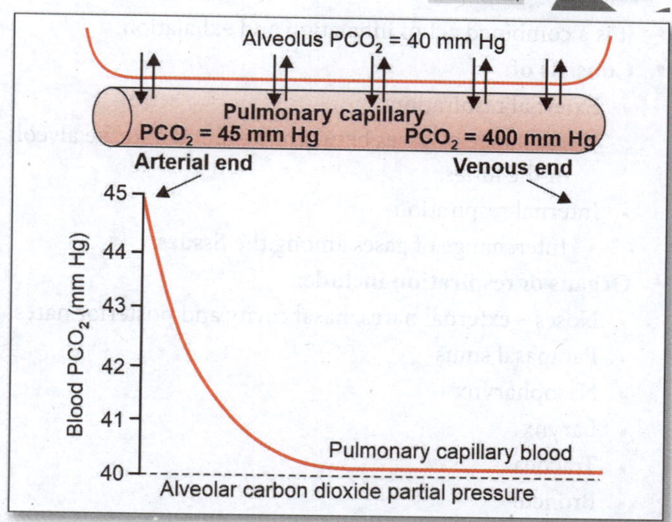

CARRIAGE OF OXYGEN AND CARBON DIOXIDE

Oxygen Transport

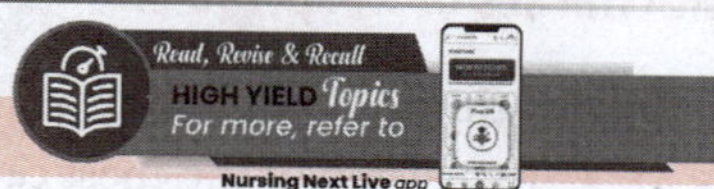

- Oxygen is transported from lungs to the tissues in two forms:
  1. Combination with hemoglobin (Hb) –98%
  2. Dissolved form –2%
     - Henry's law states the amount of gas that dissolves in a liquid at a given temperature is proportional to the partial pressure of the gas.
     - 0.3 mL of O_2 is transported in dissolved form in 100 mL of blood.
     - When 100% oxygen is inhaled in hyperbaric chamber, the dissolved oxygen is about 6 mL/dL of blood that accounts for supply of about 300 mL/min, which is adequate for tissue oxygenation

Transport of CO_2 in Blood

CO_2 is transported in blood in three forms:

1. Physically dissolved in the plasma (7%)
2. As bicarbonate ions in plasma and in red cells (70%)
3. As carbamino-Hb complexes (23%)
   - 70% of CO_2 is transported in the form of bicarbonate ions in the red cells
   - HCO_3^- can form in three ways:
     i. H_2CO_3 can dissociate into HCO_3^- and H^+
     ii. CO_2 can combine directly with OH^- to form HCO_3^-, the reaction catalyzed by carbonic anhydrase
     iii. HCO_3^- forms when carbonate combines with H^+

Exchange of Gases in Tissue

- Act of taking in oxygen into the lungs and tissues and expelling carbon dioxide outside.
- It involves exchange of gases.

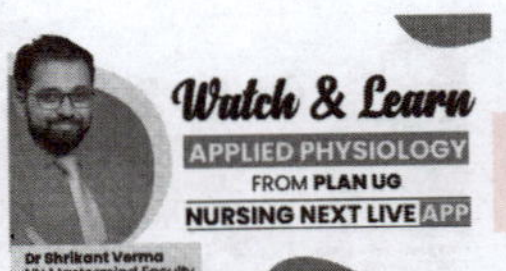

- It is a combined act of inhalation and exhalation.
- **Consists of:**
  - External respiration
    - Exchange of gases between the blood and the alveoli of the lungs.
  - Internal respiration
    - Interchange of gases among the tissues.
- **Organs of respiration include:**
  - Noses—external nares, nasal cavity and posterior nares.
  - Paranasal sinus
  - Nasopharynx
  - Larynx
  - Trachea
  - Bronchi
  - Lungs

Mechanics of Respiration

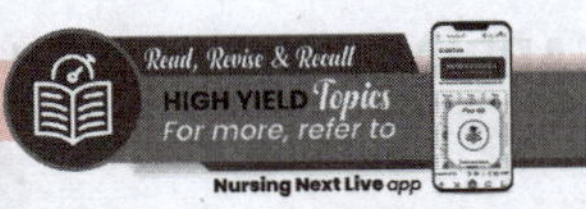

- **Inspiration:**
  - Expansion of the chest cavity leads to decrease in the intrathoracic pressure, causing the air to be pulled in—inhalation of air.
- **Expiration:**
  - Diaphragm is elevated leading to depression of chest, increasing the intrathoracic pressure, causing the air to flow out—exhalation of air.
- Intrapulmonary volume–volume within the lungs
- Intrapleural pressure–normal pressure within the pleural space.
- Nonrespiratory air movements–certain movements as a result of reflex, such as expiration.

Ventilation – Perfusion Ratio

- Ventilation – perfusion ratio is the ratio of alveolar ventilation and the amount of blood that perfuses the alveoli.
- In normal individuals at rest:
  - Alveolar ventilation (V) = 4 L/min and
  - Pulmonary blood flow (Q) = 5 L/min
  - Normal ventilation perfusion ratio V Q = 0.84

Regulation of Respiration

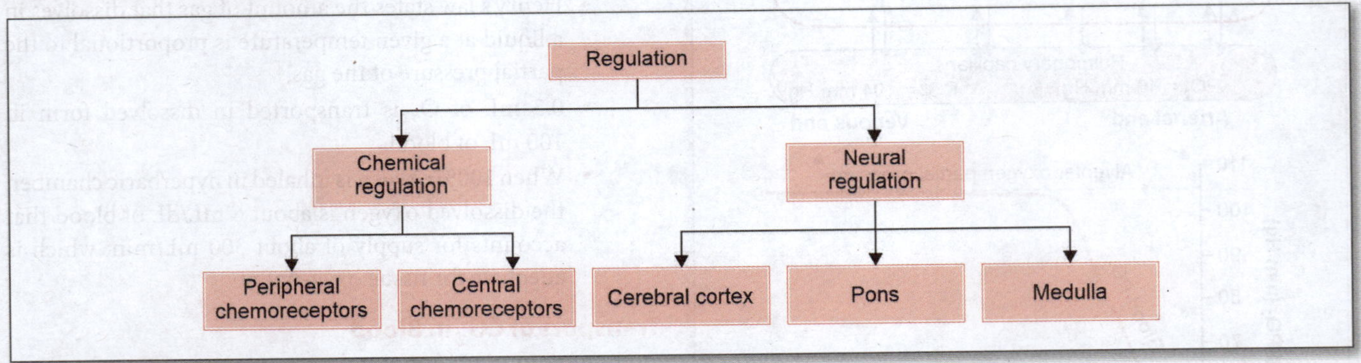

Hypoxia, Cyanosis, Dyspnea, Periodic Breathing

- **Hypoxia**
  - Hypoxia refers to a condition characterized by a deficiency of oxygen in the body's tissues.
  - It occurs when the oxygen supply to the tissues is insufficient, leading to inadequate oxygenation.
  - Hypoxia can result from various causes, such as respiratory diseases, heart conditions, high altitudes, carbon monoxide poisoning, or anemia.
- **Cyanosis**
  - Cyanosis is a bluish discoloration of the skin, lips, or nail beds, typically caused by a lack of oxygenated blood. It occurs when there is a significant reduction in the oxygen content of arterial blood.
- **Dyspnea**
  - Dyspnea is a medical term for shortness of breath or difficulty breathing.
  - It is a subjective sensation of breathlessness that can be associated with various underlying conditions, including respiratory disorders (e.g., asthma, chronic obstructive pulmonary disease), cardiac problems, anxiety, obesity, or physical exertion.
- **Periodic breathing**
  - Periodic breathing refers to a breathing pattern characterized by regular cycles of breaths followed by temporary pauses or cessation of breathing.
  - It is commonly seen in newborn infants, but it can also occur in adults during certain conditions.

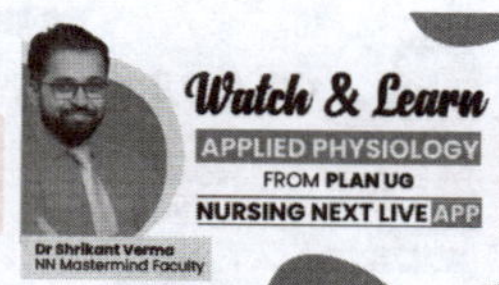

Respiratory Changes During Exercise

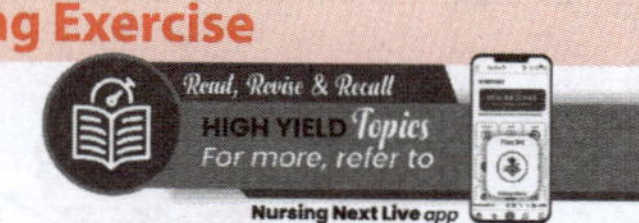

There are several changes occurring in the body during exercise. These changes are aimed at enhancing gas exchange, increasing oxygen delivery to the working muscles, and facilitating the removal of metabolic waste products. Few of these changes are:

- Increased respiratory rate
- Increased tidal volume
- Increased minute ventilation
- Enhanced gas exchange
- Activation of accessory respiratory muscles
- Maintenance of arterial blood gases

Application and Implication in Nursing

- **Assessment:** Nurses use their knowledge of respiratory physiology to perform a thorough respiratory assessment. This includes assessing respiratory rate, depth, and pattern, auscultating breath sounds, monitoring oxygen saturation levels, and evaluating cough and sputum production. These assessments aid in identifying abnormalities and changes in respiratory function.
- **Diagnosis:** A sound understanding of respiratory physiology assists nurses in interpreting assessment findings and identifying potential nursing diagnoses related to respiratory issues. For example, impaired gas exchange, ineffective airway clearance, or impaired breathing patterns may be diagnosed based on the patient's symptoms and physiological data.
- **Planning and intervention:** Nurses use respiratory physiology principles to develop and implement appropriate nursing care plans. This involves interventions aimed at improving oxygenation, promoting airway clearance, managing dyspnea, and facilitating effective breathing patterns.
- **Monitoring and evaluation:** Nurses continually monitor the patient's respiratory status and response to interventions, using their knowledge of respiratory physiology to interpret changes and make appropriate adjustments.
- **Patient education:** Nurses play a vital role in educating patients and their families about respiratory conditions, their underlying physiology, and self-management strategies.
- **Emergency response:** In emergency situations, nurses rely on their knowledge of respiratory physiology to recognize and respond promptly to respiratory distress or failure. This includes initiating appropriate interventions, such as administering oxygen, providing ventilatory support, and assisting with emergency procedures like cardiopulmonary resuscitation (CPR).

CONCEPTUAL EXERCISES

LONG ANSWER QUESTION

1. Write about regulation of respiration. (MGR, KUHS)

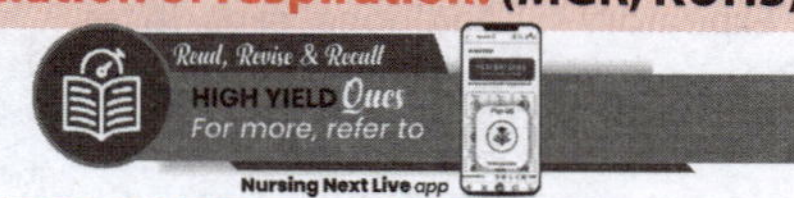

Answer

Introduction

- Body regulates the blood gas levels over a wide range of physiological and pathological conditions.
- Control of respiration is mainly involuntary. Voluntary control can be done in special cases such as speaking and singing but is overridden by involuntary mechanisms in case of hypercapnia.
- Respiratory center:
  - Present in medulla
  - Controls the rate and depth of respiration

Neural Regulation

- **Medullary center**
  - Dorsal group of inspiratory neurons: These neurons are present dorsally in the medulla and most of them are present in NTS (nucleus of tractus solitarius) which receives afferents from vagus and glossopharyngeal nerves from peripheral chemoreceptors, baroreceptors and lung receptors.
  - **Functions:**
    - Responsible for production of inspiratory neuronal action potential to generate respiratory ramp signals.
    - Ramp signal causes initiation of inspiration and causes inspiration which increases in ramp manner to provide nervous signal to inspiratory muscles and diaphragm. This inspiratory drive remains for two seconds and when it ceases, expiration occurs through relaxation of the diaphragm and elastic recoil of the lung and chest wall (normally 3 seconds).
    - Increase in inspiratory ramp causes increased filling of lungs.

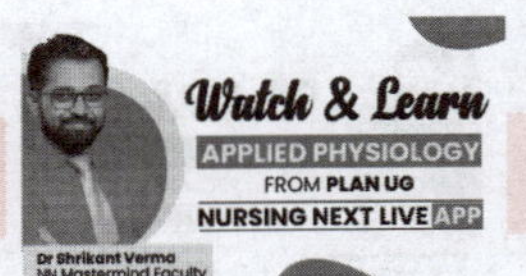

- Cessation of the ramp signal causes expiration. Thus shorter the duration of ramp, shorter is the duration of expiration.
- Ventral group of expiratory neurons in nucleus retro ambiguous caudally and nucleus ambiguous roastrally.
  - **Functions:**
    - These neurons are responsible for extra respiratory drive which results due to over spilling of basic oscillating neuronal signals from dorsal group of neurons to ventral group neurons during the period of high pulmonary ventilation (e.g., during heavy exercise).
    - Responsible for both inspiration and expiration during high levels of pulmonary ventilation. Reciprocal innervation of inspiratory and expiratory neurons occurs.
    - Vagus innervation of accessory muscles is controlled by its cranial division.
    - Respiratory drive to intercostal muscles is occurs by neurons of caudal division of **vagus**.
- **Pontine center**
  - Apneustic center in lower pons continuously stimulates dorsal group of inspiratory neurons.
  - Apneustic center is inhibited by vagus.
  - Pneumotaxic center in upper pons which is located in nucleus parabrachialis is responsible for 'switching off' of inspiratory ramp thus inhibits apneustic neurons.
  - Therefore, on strong stimulation of pneumotaxic center, duration of inspiration may decrease to as low as 0.5 seconds which also causes decreased duration of expiration causing increase in the rate of respiration (opposite happens on weak signal of pneumotaxic center).

Chemical Regulation

- The important sensory information arrives to the brainstem via chemoreceptors.
- Chemoreceptors play a vital role in regulation of respiration. **Types of chemoreceptors:**
  - **Central chemoreceptors:** Also referred to as medullary chemoreceptor. There is stimulation of central chemoreceptors by hydrogen ion that further stimulates inspiratory center and rate of respiration.
  - **Peripheral chemoreceptors:** Sensitive to reduction in partial pressure of oxygen, they get stimulated as the partial pressure of oxygen decreases and send impulses to inspiratory center.

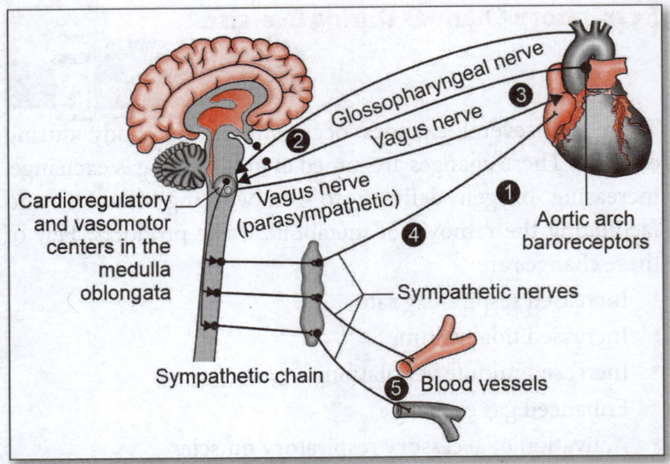

Figure 2.1: Regulation of respiration

SHORT NOTES

1. Write a short note on lung volumes and capacities. (MGR)

Answer

Lung Volumes

Tidal volume	Total amount of air that is exhaled or inhaled during each cycle of breathing.	About 500 mL at rest
Inspiratory reserve volume	Maximum volume of air, which a person can inhale from end inspiratory position.	2400–2600 mL
Expiratory reserve volume	Additional capacity of air that can be forcibly exhaled out after expiration.	1200–1500 mL
Residual volume	Volume of air present in lungs after maximal expiration.	1200–1500 mL
Dead space	Air present in respiratory tract that does not participate in diffusion.	150 mL
Alveolar ventilation	Volume of air that moves into and out of the alveoli per minute (tidal volume – anatomical dead space) × respiratory rate	5.25 L/min

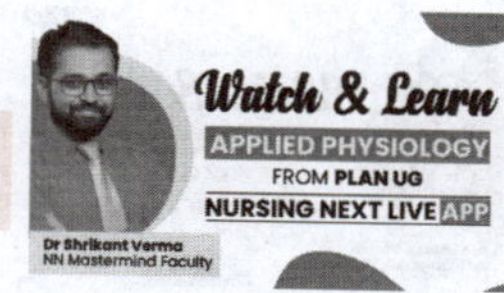

Lung Capacities

Inspiratory capacity	Total volume of air that can be inspired into the lungs	IC = TV + IRV 3600 mL
Functional residual capacity	Total volume of air that remains in lungs after normal exhalation	FRC = ERV + RV 2500 mL
Vital capacity	Maximum amount of air that can be exhaled after maximum inhalation.	IRV + TV + ERV 4200–4500 mL
Total lung capacity	Amount of air inspired to expand the lungs to its maximum extent.	TLC = TV + IRV + RV 6000 mL
Maximum breathing capacity	Maximum volume of air that can be breathed per minute. It is measured for 15 seconds and is expressed as liter/min	120–170 L/mm

2. Write a short note on Gas exchange in lungs. (MGR)

Answer

Gas Exchange

- Gas exchange in the lungs is the process by which oxygen and carbon dioxide are exchanged between the air in the lungs and the blood in the capillaries.
- It involves exchange of gases.
- It is a combined act of inhalation and exhalation.
- **Consists of:**
  - External respiration
    - Exchange of gases between the blood and the alveoli of the lungs.
  - Internal respiration
    - Interchange of gases among the tissues.

Mechanics of Respiration

- **Inspiration:**
  - Expansion of the chest cavity leads to decrease in the intrathoracic pressure, causing the air to be pulled in – inhalation of air.
- **Expiration:**
  - Diaphragm is elevated leading to depression of chest, increasing the intrathoracic pressure, causing the air to flow out – exhalation of air.

The process of gas exchange in the lungs is as follows:

- **Inhalation:** During inhalation, the diaphragm and other respiratory muscles contract, expanding the chest cavity and creating a negative pressure. This causes air to be drawn into the lungs through the airways.
- **Oxygen diffusion:** In the alveoli, oxygen from the inhaled air diffuses across the thin walls of the alveoli and into the surrounding capillaries. This diffusion occurs due to the difference in partial pressure of oxygen between the alveoli (higher) and the capillaries (lower).
- **Oxygen transport:** Oxygen binds to hemoglobin molecules within red blood cells, forming oxyhemoglobin. The oxygen-rich blood is then transported from the lungs to the body's tissues through the systemic circulation.
- **Carbon dioxide diffusion:** In the tissues, where cells are metabolizing oxygen and producing carbon dioxide as a waste product, the reverse process occurs. Carbon dioxide diffuses from the tissues into the capillaries, across the alveolar walls, and into the alveoli.
- **Exhalation:** During exhalation, the diaphragm and respiratory muscles relax, decreasing the size of the chest cavity. This creates a positive pressure, causing air with high levels of carbon dioxide to be expelled from the lungs through the airways.

Ventilation-Perfusion Ratio:

- The magnitude and distribution of ventilation perfusion play a vital role in determination of pulmonary gas exchange.
- Gas exchange abnormalities in major lung diseases is due to VA/Q inequality.
- Zones of Perfusion:
  - Zone 1 – No blood flow
  - Zone 2 – Intermittent blood flow
  - Zone 3 – Continuous blood flow

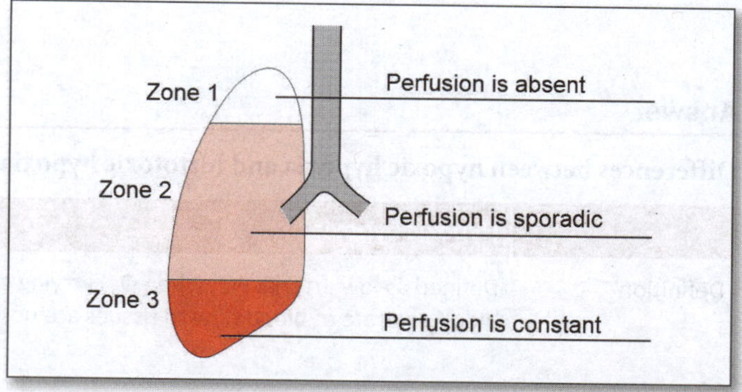

3. Write a short note on Hypoxia and its types. (KUHS)

Answer

Hypoxia

- Hypoxia is a condition in which body is deprived of adequate oxygen supply at the tissue level.

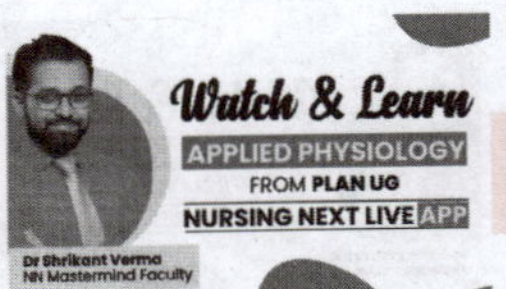

- Decreased supply of oxygen at the level of tissues, characterized by:
  - Cyanosis
  - Tachycardia
  - Tachypnea

Types of Hypoxia

Hypoxic Hypoxia

- Occurs when there is decreased partial pressure of oxygen.
- Causes:
  - It occurs due to low arterial PO_2 when the rate of blood flow to tissues and oxygen carrying capacity of blood is normal or elevated.
  - This occurs at high altitudes where there is low atmospheric oxygen.
  - Decrease in ventilation, e.g., bronchial asthma
  - Decreased diffusion across the alveoli, e.g., respiratory membrane disease
  - **Anatomical shunts:** Excessive blood from bronchial artery bypasses gas exchange and goes in pulmonary vein.
  - **Physiological shunts:** Venous admixture in pulmonary vein, e.g., pneumonia congenital heart diseases, e.g., Tetrology of Fallot
  - Characteristic features:
    - Low arterial oxygen content
    - Low arterial PO_2
    - Low arterial oxygen saturation of hemoglobin percentage
    - Low A-V PO_2 difference.
- **Histotoxic hypoxia**
  - In histotoxic hypoxia, there is decreased utilization of oxygen by tissues
  - O_2 carrying capacity of blood is normal
  - Causes include cyanide, sulphide poisoning
  - A-V PO_2 difference is nil
  - PO_2 arterial- 100, venous- 90
- **Anemic hypoxia**
  - Occurs due to reduced oxygen carrying capacity of the blood or reduced hemoglobin.
  - Arterial PO_2 is normal
  - Causes:
    - Severe anemia
    - Carbon monoxide poisoning
- **Stagnant anemia**
  - Occurs when the tissue blood flow is markedly reduced.
  - Causes include:
    - Shock
    - Heart failure
    - Local obstruction
  - PCO_2 and Hb concentration is normal.

Nursing Implications

Hypoxia causes increased levels of HIF-1 (hypoxia-induced factor-1) in tissues which binds with hypoxia response elements in the gene of erythropoietin which leads to transcription of mRNA to produce erythropoietin.

4. Differentiate between Hypoxic hypoxia and histotoxic hypoxia. (KUHS)

Answer

Differences between hypoxic hypoxia and histotoxic hypoxia

	Hypoxic hypoxia	Histotoxic hypoxia
Definition	Defined as low arterial PO_2 when O_2 carrying capacity of blood and rate of blood flow to tissues are normal.	Defined as normal delivery of O_2 to tissues but they cannot make use of O_2 supplied to them due to action of toxic agent.
Causes	Decreased PO_2, decreased pulmonary ventilation, defective V/P ratio	Cyanide poisoning
Arterial PO_2	Decreases	Normal
Arterial O_2 content	Decreases	Normal
Arterial %- O_2 saturation of hemoglobin	Decreases	Normal

Contd...

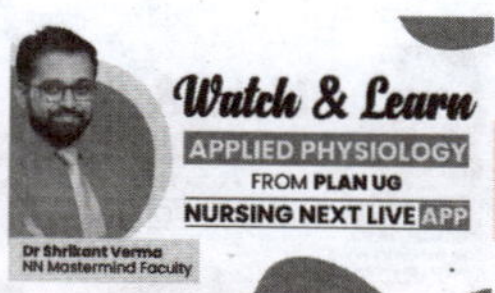

	Hypoxic hypoxia	Histotoxic hypoxia
A-V PO_2 difference	Decreases	Less than normal
Cyanosis	Present	Absent
Stimulation of peripheral chemoreceptors	Present due to decrease dissolved O_2 in plasma	Present because cyanide decrease O_2 utilization at tissue level.

SHORT ANSWER QUESTIONS

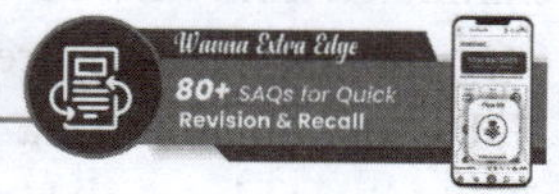

1. Dead space. (MGR)

Answer

Dead space refers to the portion of the respiratory system, such as the nose, mouth, trachea, and bronchi, where air moves in and out but doesn't participate in gas exchange with the blood.

2. Name the muscles for inspiration and expiration. (MGR)

Answer

Inspiration

- **Primary muscles:** Diaphragm, external intercostal muscles
- **Accessory muscles:** Sternocleidomastoid, scalene muscles, pectoralis minor

Expiration

- Internal Intercostal Muscles
- Abdominal Muscles

3. What is residual volume? Give the normal value. (MGR)

Answer

Residual volume (RV) refers to the amount of air that remains in the lungs after maximal expiration.

The normal value of residual volume in healthy adults ranges from 1.0 to 1.5 liters.

4. Define respiratory unit. (MGR)

Answer

A respiratory unit is a functional unit of the respiratory system that includes the respiratory bronchioles, alveolar ducts, and alveoli. This facilitates gas exchange between the lungs and the blood, allowing oxygen into the bloodstream and carbon dioxide removal.

5. What is vital capacity? Give the normal value (MGR)

Answer

Vital capacity refers to the maximum amount of air a person can exhale forcefully after taking a deep breath.

Normal vital capacity for a healthy adult can range between 4–5 liters.

6. What is surfactant? (MGR)

Answer

Surfactant is a mixture of phospholipids and proteins that is secreted by the type 2 alveolar cells in the lungs.

Surfactant reduces the surface tension of the alveolar fluid, preventing the collapse of the alveoli.

7. Write two functions of surfactant. (MGR)

Answer

Two functions of surfactant:

1. Surfactant reduces the surface tension and prevents the alveolar collapse during expiration and makes the alveoli more compliant.
2. Surfactant prevents intra-alveolar edema.

8. What are the neural centers for respiration? (MGR)

Answer

The respiratory nerve centers are found in the brainstem, specifically in the medulla oblongata and the pons.

Medulla generates the rhythm of respiration.

Pons regulates the timings of inspiration and expiration.

9. Enumerate four lung volumes (MGR)

Answer

1. **Tidal volume (TV):** The volume of air inhaled and expelled during regular breathing. The average tidal volume in healthy adults is 500 mL.
2. **Inspiratory reserve volume (IRV):** The additional volume of air that can be breathed forcefully after a normal inhalation. The typical IRV in healthy persons is around 3000 mL.
3. **Expiratory reserve volume (ERV):** The additional volume of air that can be exhaled forcibly after a regular exhalation. The average ERV in healthy adults is around 1000 mL.
4. **Residual volume:** The amount of air that remains in the lungs following a maximal exhale is referred to as the **residual volume** (RV). The average RV in healthy adults is around 1200 mL.

10. What is CO_2 transport. (MGR)

Answer

CO_2 is a waste product of cellular metabolism that must be eliminated from the body.

CO_2 is transported by three mechanisms:

1. Dissolution in plasma
2. Binding to hemoglobin
3. Conversion to bicarbonate ion.

CONCEPTUAL REVISION

MULTIPLE CHOICE QUESTIONS

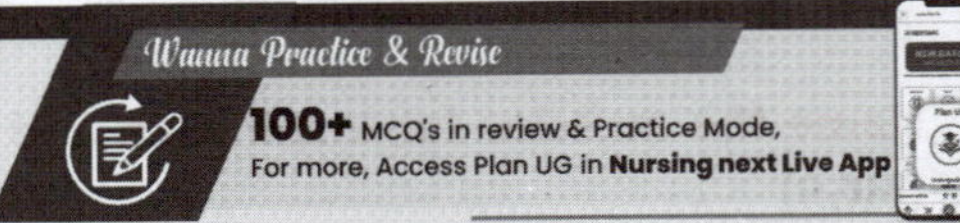

1. Which of the following could NOT be part of an acinus?

a. Alveolar sacs b. Alveolar ducts
c. Terminal bronchioles d. Respiratory bronchiole

Ans. c. Terminal bronchioles

2. In a healthy person, which of these lung volumes should be the largest?

a. Tidal volume b. Vital capacity
c. Expiratory reserve volume
d. Residual volume

Ans. b. Vital capacity

3. What ensures that the lungs expand as the chest wall expands?

a. Secreted surfactant
b. Negative pressure between the pleura
c. Serous liquid secreted by the pleura
d. The elastic recoil of the alveolar tissue

Ans. b. Negative pressure between the pleura

4. The wandering phagocytes found in the alveoli are called:

a. Alveolar macrophages b. Pulmonary cells
c. Goblet cells d. Chalice cells

Ans. a. Alveolar macrophages

5. A molecule that is important in maintaining normal lung structure is:

a. Immunoglobulin b. Hemoglobin
c. Peroxidase d. Surfactant

Ans. d. Surfactant

6. Normal expiration in a person at rest is due to:

a. Elastic tissues in the lung
b. Contraction of abdominal muscles
c. Contraction of the expiratory muscles
d. Diffusion

Ans. a. Elastic tissues in the lung

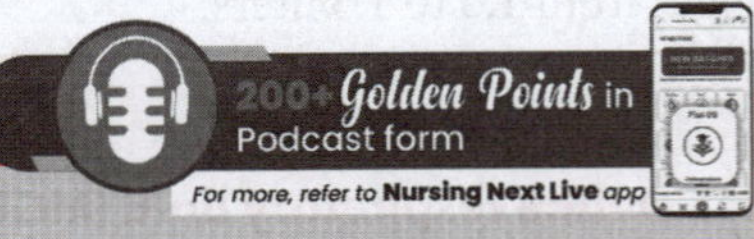

Golden Points

- External respiration occurs between the blood and the alveoli of the lungs.
- Functional residual capacity (FRC) is the amount of gas that remains in the lungs after normal expiration.
- Internal respiration is the interchange of gases in the tissues.
- Lung volume is the static volume of air breathed by an individual.

CHAPTER 3

Digestive System

CONCEPTUAL THEORY

Terminology

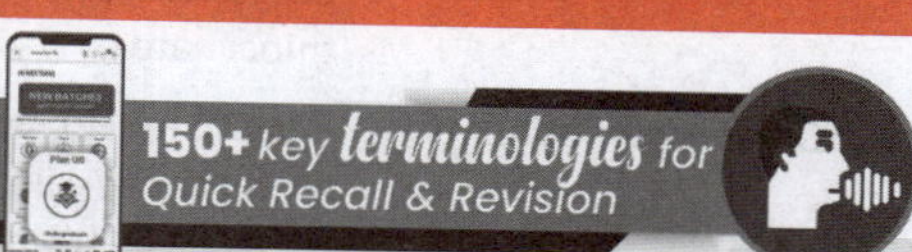

Absorption: Passage of products of digestion in blood and lymph capillaries.
Digestion: Mechanical and chemical breakdown of food.
Ejection: Expulsion of waste products through anus.
Ingestion: Taking in of the fluid/food.
Layers of GIT: Mucosa, submucosa, muscularis externa and serosa/adventitia.
Peristalsis: Pattern of smooth muscle contraction that propels foodstuffs distally through the esophagus and intestines.
Propulsion: Passage of fluid/food.

FUNCTIONS OF THE ORGANS OF DIGESTIVE TRACT

Read, Revise & Recall HIGH YIELD Topics For more, refer to Nursing Next Live app

- **Mouth:**
  - **Mechanical digestion:** Chewing breaks down food into smaller particles, increasing its surface area for chemical digestion.
  - **Chemical digestion:** Salivary glands secrete saliva containing enzymes (e.g., amylase) that initiate the breakdown of carbohydrates.
- **Esophagus:**
  - The esophagus transports chewed food (bolus) from the mouth to the stomach through rhythmic contractions called peristalsis.
- **Stomach:**
  - **Storage and mixing:** The stomach stores and mixes food with gastric secretions to form a semi-fluid mixture called chyme.
  - **Mechanical digestion:** The muscular walls of the stomach contract to mechanically break down food.
  - **Chemical digestion:** Gastric glands secrete gastric juice containing enzymes (e.g., pepsin) and hydrochloric acid, which aid in protein digestion.
- **Small intestine:**
  - The small intestine is the primary site for chemical digestion and nutrient absorption.
  - **Enzymatic digestion:** Pancreatic enzymes (e.g., amylase, lipase) and bile (from the liver) break down carbohydrates, fats, and proteins.
  - Nutrients, such as glucose, amino acids, fatty acids, vitamins, and minerals, are absorbed across the intestinal lining into the bloodstream.
- **Large intestine (colon):**
  - The colon absorbs water and electrolytes from undigested food, forming feces.
  - The colon stores feces and facilitates their elimination through defecation.
- **Rectum and anus:**
  - The rectum temporarily stores feces until it is voluntarily expelled through the anus during defecation.
- **Liver:**
  - The liver produces bile, which is stored in the gallbladder and released into the small intestine to aid in fat digestion and absorption.
- **Gallbladder:**
  - The gallbladder stores bile produced by the liver and releases it into the small intestine when needed.

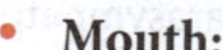

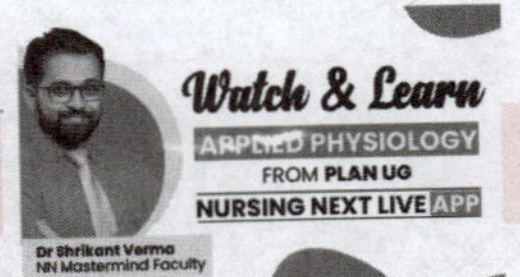

- **Pancreas:**
  - The pancreas secretes pancreatic enzymes into the small intestine to assist in the digestion of carbohydrates, proteins, and fats.

SALIVA

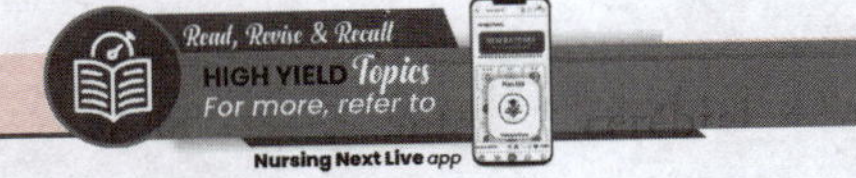

Saliva is produced by three pairs of salivary glands (the parotid, submandibular, and sublingual glands) that drain into the oral cavity.

Composition of Saliva

Water	99% (major component)
Inorganic components	Sodium, chloride, bicarbonate, potassium, phosphate, calcium, thiocynate
Organic components	Ptyalin, mucin, proline rich proteins, secretory IgA, lipase, lysozymes, peroxidase, histatins, statherin, kallikrein, lactoferrin

Functions of Saliva

- **Defense:**
  - Antibacterial
  - Antifungal
  - Immunological
- **Digestive function:**
  - Digestive enzymes—ptyalin, lipase
  - Formation of bolus
  - Taste
- **Protective function:**
  - Protective coating for hard tissues-teeth
  - Protective coating for soft tissues
- **Lubricative function:**
  - Keeps the oral cavity moist
  - Facilitates speech
  - Helps in mastication and swallowing
- **Buffering function**

Regulation of Salivary Secretion

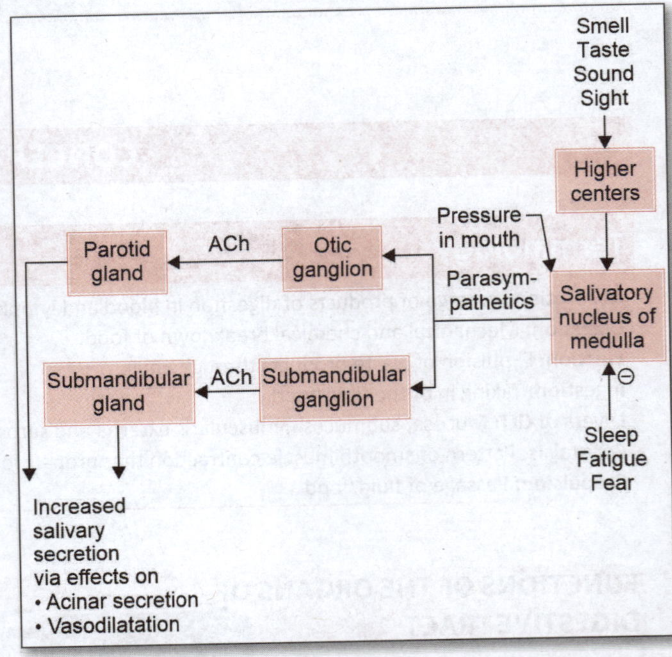

Figure 3.1: Regulation of salivary secretion by the parasympathetic nervous system. Saliva is also produced by the sublingual gland

Abbreviation: ACh, acetylcholine

GASTRIC JUICE

Composition, Function, Mechanism and Regulation of Gastric Secretion

Aspect	Gastric juice	Mechanism and regulation of gastric secretion
Composition	Hydrochloric acid (HCl)	Gastric secretion is primarily regulated by the vagus nerve, gastrin hormone, and local factors such as pH.
	Pepsinogen	Secreted by gastric chief cells
	Mucus	Secretion is by goblet cell and is regulated by autophagy and ER stress
	Intrinsic factor	Produced by parietal cell and is regulated by same biochemical parameters that are responsible for acid secretion
	Gastric lipase	
	Water	
Function	Acidifies gastric contents	Gastric secretion involves several functions that contribute to digestion and absorption:
	Activates pepsinogen to pepsin	• Hydrochloric acid (HCl) lowers the pH, creating an acidic environment necessary for pepsin activation and optimal digestion of proteins.

Contd...

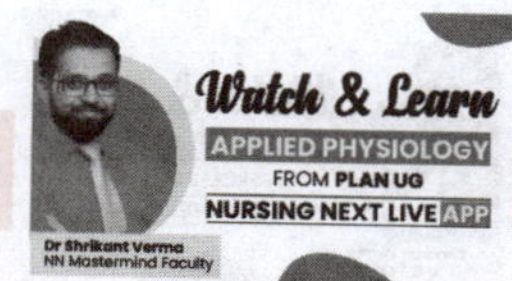

Aspect	Gastric juice	Mechanism and regulation of gastric secretion
	Begins protein digestion	• Pepsinogen, when converted to pepsin by the acidic pH, breaks down proteins into smaller peptides.
	Provides intrinsic factor	• Intrinsic factor is essential for the absorption of vitamin B12 in the small intestine.
	Lubricates and protects the stomach lining	• Mucus protects the stomach lining from the corrosive effects of gastric acid and enzymes.
	Partially digests dietary lipids	• Gastric lipase plays role in breaking down dietary fats.
		• Water helps facilitate the movement of food through the digestive tract.

Mechanism and Regulation

Gastric secretion is regulated by three main factors:

1. **Vagus nerve stimulation:** The parasympathetic vagus nerve stimulates gastric acid and enzyme secretion in response to the sight, smell, taste, or thought of food.
2. **Gastrin release:** Gastrin, a hormone produced by G-cells in the stomach, is released in response to the presence of food in the stomach. Gastrin stimulates gastric acid secretion.
3. **Local factors:** Local factors, such as low pH or partially digested proteins in the stomach, can stimulate gastric secretion through positive feedback loops.

Inhibition of gastric secretion can occur through negative feedback mechanisms, such as when the stomach becomes distended or the pH becomes too acidic.

PANCREATIC JUICE

Composition of Pancreatic Juice

- Water
- **Inorganic components:** Na^+, HCO_3^-, Cl^-
- **Organic components:**
  - **Proteolytic enzymes:** Trypsin, chymotrypsin and carboxypolypeptidase
  - **Amylolytic enzyme:** Pancreatic amylase
  - **Lipolytic:** Pancreatic lipase, cholesterol esterase, phospholipase
  - Trypsin inhibitors
  - Mucin

Functions of Pancreatic Juice

- **Carbohydrate digestion**
  - Amylase hydrolyzes starch into sugars
- **Fat digestion**
  - Lipase breaks down lipids into fatty acids, glycerol and monoglycerides. Emulsification of fat increases the surface area of fat droplets so that lipase can hydrolyze them.
  - 80% of fat digestion is due to pancreatic lipase.
  - Neutral fats break down into fatty acids and monoglycerides by pancreatic lipase.
  - Hydrolysis of cholesterol esters by cholesterol esterases.
  - Fatty acids break down to phospholipids by phospholipase.
- **Protein digestion**
  - Proteins break down into peptides by trypsin and chymotrypsin.
  - Peptides break down into amino acids by carboxypolypeptidase.
  - Trypsin inhibitor prevents digestion of pancreas.
- **Activation of pro-enzymes**
  - Trypsin acts on inactive precursors called chymotrypsinogen, procarboxypeptidase and proelastase to produce chymotrypsin, carboxypeptidase and elastase respectively.
- Mucin and bicarbonate secretion neutralizes acidic chyme from stomach.
- Presence of acidic chyme from stomach in duodenum stimulates the production of secretin and cholecystokinin (CCK) hormones from endocrine cells in the wall of duodenum. These hormones in turn stimulate the secretion of pancreatic juice.

LIVER

Functions of Liver

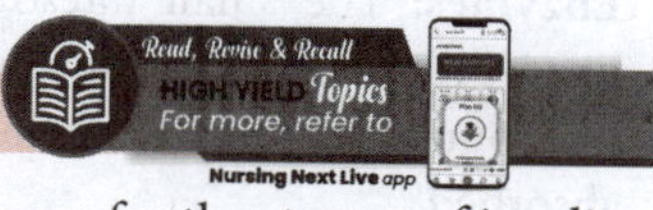

- Converts glucose into glycogen for the storage of insulin.
- **Carbohydrate metabolism:** Liver maintains the plasma glucose levels by converting glucose to glycogen and back with variations in blood glucose levels.
- **Protein metabolism:** Amino acids and nucleic acids are broken down to urea and uric acid in liver.
- **Fat metabolism:** Fat stored is metabolized to release energy.
- Liver secretes bile that contains the bile pigments, bile salts and cholesterol. Also stores iron and vitamins like B_{12}, A, D, E, K.
- Site for detoxification of toxic substances

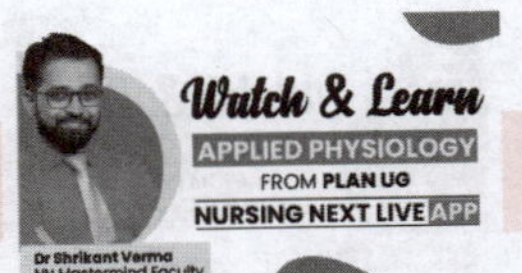

- Site for metabolism of thyroid hormones, alcohol and steroids.
- Site for protein synthesis.

Bile

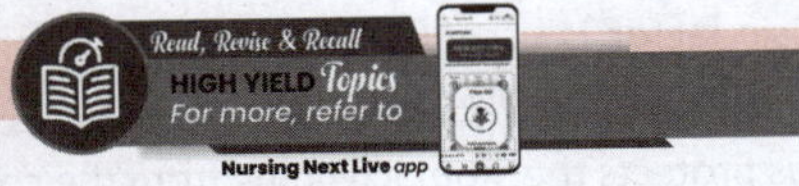

Composition of Bile

- Water (85%)
- Bile acids (Cholic acid and chenodeoxycholic acid)
- Bilirubin
- Phospholipids
- Cholesterol
- Xenobiotics
- Electrolytes (Sodium, calcium and bicarbonate)

Functions of Bile

- Emulsification of fats
- Acceleration of action of pancreatic lipase
- Micelle formation: Polymolecular aggregates formed by the interaction of monoglycerides, fatty acids, bile salts and electrolytes are referred to as micelles. Micelles help in the transport of lipids into intestinal cells
- Absorption of fat-soluble vitamins
- Formation of bile
- Intestinal motility

SMALL AND LARGE INTESTINE

Secretion of Small Intestine

The small intestine primarily secretes mucus, hormones, enzymes, and bile for digestion and absorption of nutrients. Here are some key secretions:

- **Mucus:** The small intestine produces mucus to protect its lining from the acidic chyme (partially digested food) coming from the stomach.
- **Enzymes:** The small intestine secretes various enzymes like—proteases, amylase and lipase to break down macronutrients into smaller molecules that can be absorbed.
- **Hormones:** The small intestine produces several hormones that regulate digestive processes. These include—cholecystokinin (CCK), secretin and gastric inhibitory peptide (GIP).
- **Bile:** Bile is produced by the liver and stored in the gallbladder. It is released into the small intestine to aid in the digestion and absorption of fats. Bile emulsifies fats, making them easier to digest by lipases.

Functions of Small Intestine

- **Digestion:** The small intestine receives partially digested food (chyme) from the stomach and continues the digestion process.
- **Absorption:** The small intestine has a large surface area due to the presence of villi and microvilli, which greatly enhance absorption.

Secretion of Large Intestine

The large intestine primarily secretes mucus and electrolytes (e.g., potassium, sodium) to facilitate the passage and elimination of waste materials.

Functions of Large Intestine

- Absorption of water and electrolytes
- Formation of feces
- Elimination of waste

MOVEMENTS OF ALIMENTARY TRACT

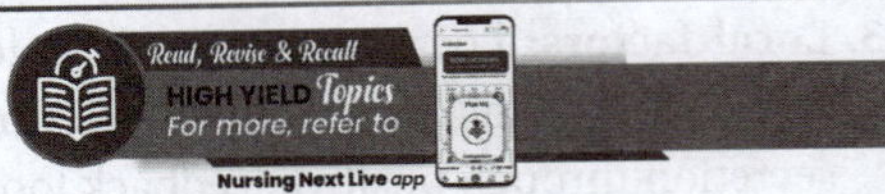

There are majorly four types of movement in GIT:

1. **Peristalsis:**
   - Peristalsis is a reflex response that occurs in all regions of the gastrointestinal tract, from the esophagus to the rectum, when the gut wall is stretched by lumen contents.
2. **Segmentation and mixing movements:**
   - When a meal is present, the enteric nervous system supports a motility pattern similar to peristalsis but designed to slow the passage of intestinal contents throughout the length of the intestinal tract to allow for digestion and absorption.
3. **Migrating motor complexes (MMC):**
   - The peristaltic wave that begins in the esophagus and moves through the entire gastrointestinal tract (migratory motor activity) during the interdigestive interval is known as the migrating motor complex (MMC).
4. **Retroperistalsis:**
   - Peristalsis is normally a forward movement. Yet, if the lumen becomes obstructed, reversal peristalsis occurs. This is known as retroperistalsis.
   - Vomiting is caused by retroperistalsis.

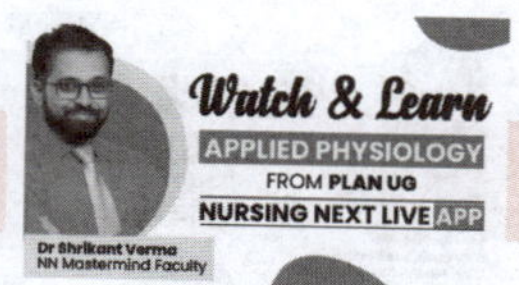

Digestion in Mouth, Stomach, Small intestine, Large intestine, Absorption of Food

Digestive process	Mouth	Stomach	Small intestine	Large intestine
Secretions	Saliva	Gastric juice (including HCl, enzymes)	Enzymes (proteases, lipases, amylase)	Mucus, electrolytes
Digestive enzymes	Amylase (breaks down carbohydrates)	Pepsin (breaks down proteins)	Proteases, amylase, lipases	None
Function	Mechanical breakdown, initial carbohydrate digestion	Mixing and churning, protein digestion	Final digestion, nutrient absorption	Water absorption, feces formation
Absorption	Limited absorption (some water, small lipids)	Limited absorption (some water, alcohol)	Main site of nutrient absorption	Water and electrolyte absorption
Key nutrient absorption	Not significant	Limited absorption of some nutrients	Carbohydrates, proteins, lipids, vitamins	Water, electrolytes
Key nutrients absorbed	Minimal	Limited (alcohol, some drugs)	Carbohydrates, proteins, lipids, vitamins	Water, electrolytes
Waste elimination	Swallowed for further digestion	Passage to small intestine for digestion	Passage from small intestine to large intestine for further digestion	Elimination of feces through rectum and anus

APPLICATION AND IMPLICATIONS IN NURSING

- **Assessment and monitoring:** Nurses need to assess and monitor patients' digestive system functioning to identify any abnormalities or changes. Understanding the normal physiological processes helps nurses identify potential issues and initiate appropriate interventions.
- **Nutrition and diet planning:** Knowledge of digestive system physiology enables nurses to consider factors such as digestive enzyme deficiencies, malabsorption conditions, and dietary restrictions to ensure patients receive adequate nutrients while managing their specific conditions.
- **Medication administration:** Understanding how medications interact with the digestive system helps nurses anticipate potential side effects or complications, educate patients about medication administration and possible gastrointestinal effects, and monitor for any adverse reactions.
- **Gastrointestinal procedures and preparations:** Knowledge of digestive system physiology helps nurses understand the purpose of procedures, like endoscopy, colonoscopy, tube feedings, etc. and prepare patients adequately, provide appropriate pre- and post-procedure care, and recognize and manage any complications that may arise.
- **Patient education:** Nurses educate patients and their families about various digestive system conditions, dietary modifications, medication management, and lifestyle changes.
- **Symptom management:** Nurses use their knowledge of digestive system physiology to implement interventions aimed at symptom management. This may include administering medications, recommending dietary modifications, promoting adequate fluid intake, and providing comfort measures.

CONCEPTUAL EXERCISES

LONG ANSWER QUESTIONS

1. Enumerate gastrointestinal hormones and describe movements of GIT. (RUHS)

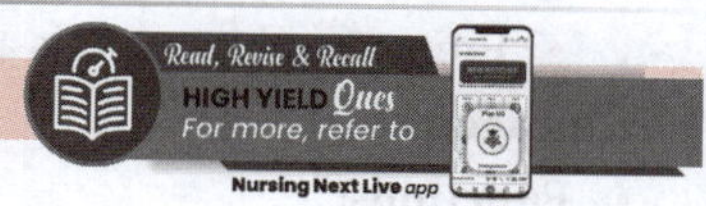

Answer

Gastrointestinal Hormones

- **Somatostatin**
  - **Functions:**
    - Decreases secretion of many other hormones, e.g., gastrin, bicarbonate, digestive enzymes.
    - Decreases nutrient absorption from gut by prolonging gastric emptying time.

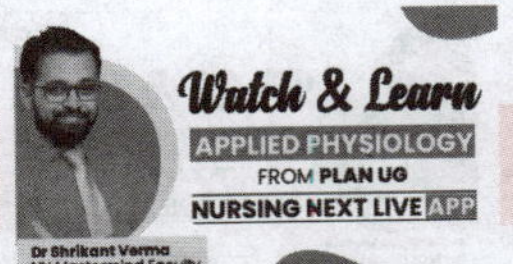

- Decreases pancreatic secretions
- Decreases visceral blood flow

- **Gastrin**
  - **Function:**
    - Induces gastric acid secretion
- **Motilin**
  - **Function:**
    - Stimulates gastric, pancreatic enzyme secretions.
- **Pancreatic peptide (PP)**
  - **Functions:**
    - Decreases gastric emptying
    - Decreases the motility of small intestine
    - Secreted by endocrine cells in pancreatic islets.
    - Vagal stimulation and hypoglycemia activate the pancreatic peptide.
- **Peptide Y**
  - **Functions:**
    - Inhibits gastric acid secretion
    - Decreases gastric and intestinal motility
    - Inhibits the pancreatic secretions
- **Secretin**
  - **Functions:**
    - Decreases acidity to improve pancreatic enzyme function
    - Increases the biliary bicarbonate, water and pancreatic secretions.
    - Plays a role in the regulation of pancreatic enzyme secretion.
    - Decreases the gastric emptying and gastric acid secretion.
- **Cholecystokinin (CCK)**
  - **Functions:**
    - Increases the contraction of gallbladder
    - Increases the enzymatic pancreatic secretion output.
    - Regulates the nutrient-stimulated enzyme secretion.
- **Insulin**
  - **Functions:**
    - Major anabolic hormone
    - Decreases blood glucose levels
    - Promotes glycogenesis and glycogen storage.
- **Glucagon**
  - **Functions:**
    - Action is opposite to that of insulin
    - Promotes glycogenolysis and increases the blood glucose concentration.
- **Incretins**
  - **Include:**
    - Glucagon like peptide I
    - Glucose-dependent insulinotropic peptide
  - **Functions:**
    - Stimulate the release of insulin from the pancreatic beta cells.
    - Increase levels of cAMP in the islet cells.
- **Gastric inhibitory peptide**
  - It is secreted by the duodenal mucosa.
- **Histamine**
  - It is secreted by the gastric mucosa.
  - Presence of food stimulates its secretion.
- **Serotonin**
  - **Function:**
    - Stimulates the contraction of muscle
- **Vasoactive intestinal peptide**
  - **Functions:**
    - Dilates intestinal capillaries
    - Increases secretions
    - Relaxes intestinal smooth muscle
    - It acts on small intestine, pancreas and stomach
- **Ghrelin**
  - Hunger stimulating hormone
- **Leptin**
  - Stimulates satiety
- **Enkephalins**
  - Causes smooth muscle constriction decreasing the fluid flow into the intestines

Movements of GIT

- The smooth muscles in the GI tract wall contract spontaneously to propel food forward, break it down into smaller particles, and mix it with GI secretions.
- This allows for optimal digestion and absorption. The enteric motor neurons also play a role in coordinating these movements.

Gastric Motility Initiation by Basal Electrical Rhythm

- The stomach has a single rhythmic contractile myogenic tone called the basic electrical rhythm (BER). The BER is a wave of smooth muscle cell depolarization that travels from the fundus of the stomach to the pyloric sphincter.
- Electrical slow waves are broad spontaneous rhythmic changes in membrane potential that range between –65 and –40 mV.

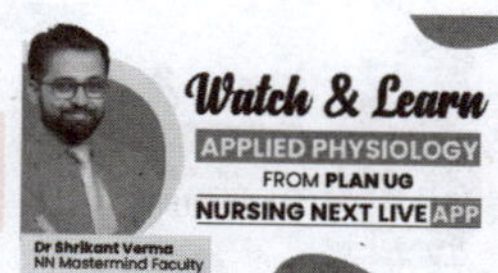

- Slow waves are produced by Cajal interstitial cells, which are found between the longitudinal and circular muscle layers.

Different Types of Gastric Motility

- Motility of empty stomach includes:
  - Migrating motor complex
  - Hunger contractions
- Gastric motility related to meal, includes:
  - Receptive relaxation
  - Mixing peristaltic waves
  - Gastric emptying.

Segment-specific Patterns of Motility in Mouth and Esophagus

1. **Mastication**
   - Mastication is the process of chewing food, which breaks down larger food particles into smaller ones.
   - It also increases salivary secretion, combines food and saliva, lubricates the contents of the oral cavity, and degrades starch.
2. **Swallowing (Deglutition)**
   - Swallowing is the process of moving food from the mouth to the esophagus. It is initiated voluntarily, but it is mostly involuntary.
   - The swallowing reflex is triggered when food is gathered in the mouth and forced backward into the throat.
   - The pharyngeal muscles then tighten involuntarily, pushing the food into the esophagus.
3. **Esophageal peristalsis**

In the esophagus, there are two types of peristalsis:

1. **Primary peristalsis:**
   - Primary peristalsis is a wave of contraction that begins in the esophagus and pushes food toward the stomach.
   - It is initiated by the deglutition reflex, which is the involuntary swallowing reflex.
   - Primary peristalsis occurs even when food is not present in the mouth, and it can also be activated by swallowing saliva.
2. **Secondary peristalsis:**
   - Secondary peristalsis begins when primary peristalsis fails to push the bolus from the body of the esophagus.

General Patterns of Motility in GI

- **Peristalsis:**
  - Peristalsis is a reflex response that occurs in all regions of the gastrointestinal tract, from the esophagus to the rectum, when the gut wall is stretched by lumen contents.
  - The stretch causes a circular contraction behind the stimulus and a relaxation zone in front of it.
  - The wave of contraction then travels from oral to caudal, forcing the lumen contents forward at rates ranging from 2 to 25 cm/s.
- **Segmentation and mixing movements:**
  - When a meal is present, the enteric nervous system supports a motility pattern similar to peristalsis but designed to slow the passage of intestinal contents throughout the length of the intestinal tract to allow for digestion and absorption.
  - This pattern of motility is known as segmentation, and it allows for adequate mixing of intestinal contents (known as chyme) with digestive juices.
  - A section of bowel contracts at both ends, followed by a second contraction in the center to force the chyme both backward and forward.
- **Migrating motor complexes (MMC)**
  - The peristaltic wave that begins in the esophagus and moves through the entire gastrointestinal tract (migratory motor activity) during the interdigestive interval is known as the migrating motor complex (MMC).
  - During the interdigestive interval, the MMCs eliminate any food that remains in the stomach.
  - During the interdigestive interval, the MMC wave travels at a constant velocity of 5 cm/min and occurs every 60–90 minutes.
  - Each cycle, or migrating motor complex (MMC), begins with a quiescent period (phase I), then moves on to a period of erratic electrical and mechanical activity (phase II), followed by a burst of regular activity (phase III) (phase III).
- **Retroperistalsis**
  - Peristalsis is normally a forward movement. Yet, if the lumen becomes obstructed, reversal peristalsis occurs. This is known as retroperistalsis.
  - Vomiting is caused by retroperistalsis.
  - Emotional circumstances or stimulation of medullary vomiting centers can also cause retroperistalsis.

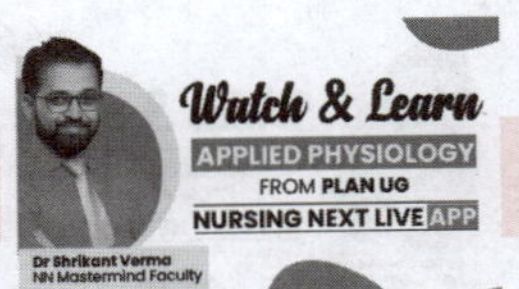

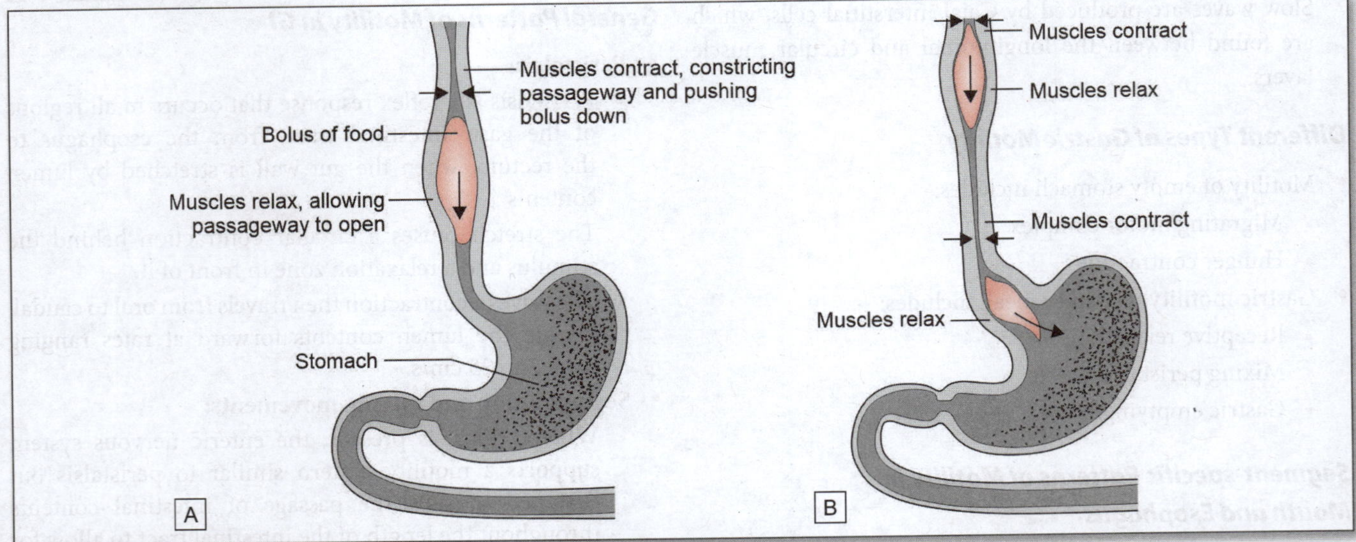

Figures 3.2A and B: Peristalsis in esophagus

2. Describe the composition, functions and regulation of gastric juice. (RUHS, DU)

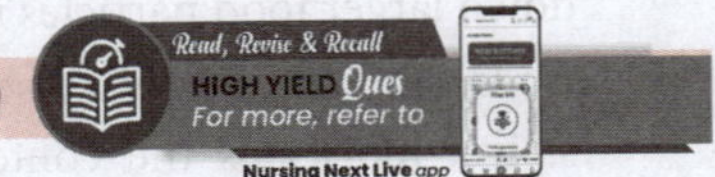

Answer

Introduction

- There are two types of glands in gastric mucosa which are responsible for the secretion of gastric juice.
  1. Oxyntic glands contain mucous (alkaline) secreting mucous neck cells, Pepsinogen secreting peptic/chief cells, HCl/ Intrinsic factor secreting parietal/oxyntic cells.
  2. Pyloric glands contain mucous neck cells, peptic cells and Gastrin hormone secreting G cells.

Composition of Gastric Juice

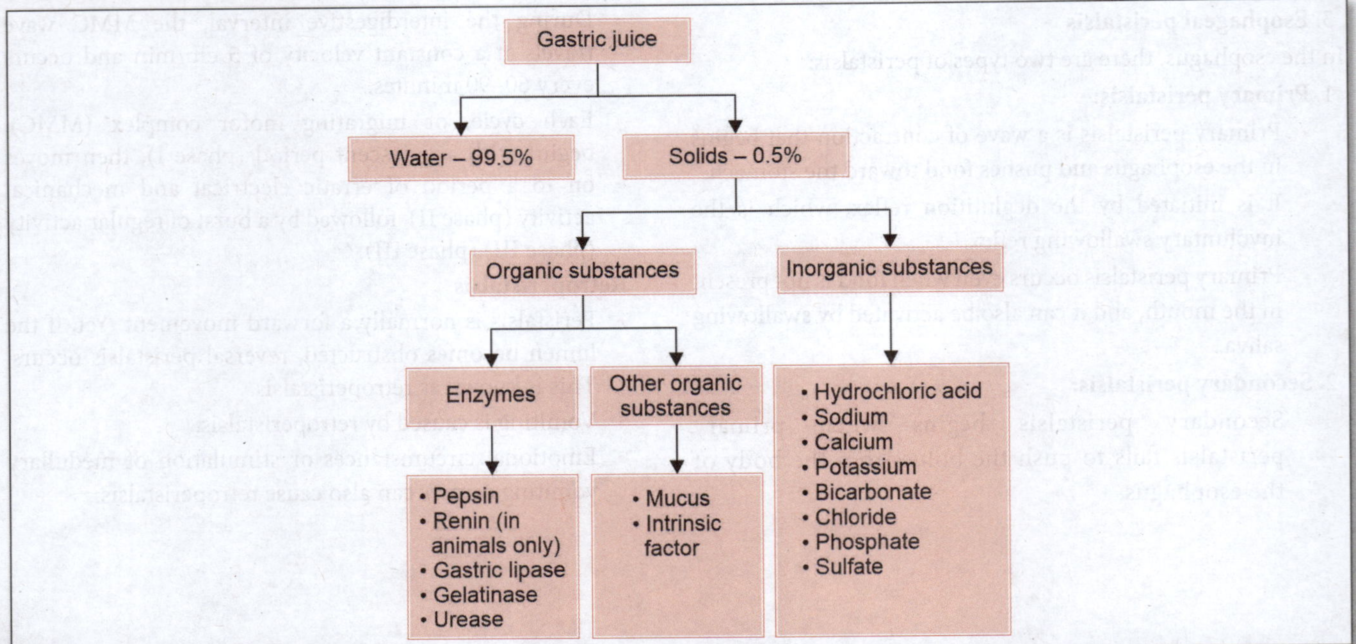

Figure 3.3: Composition of gastric juice

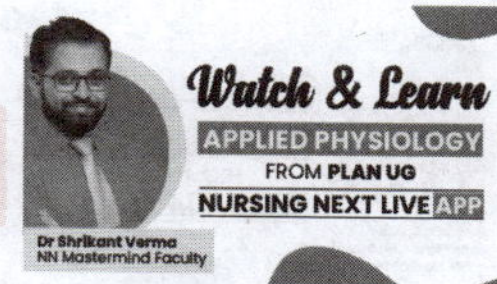

Regulation of Gastric Acid Secretion

- Gastrin stimulates gastric acid secretion by its action on CCK-B receptor which increases cytosolic calcium concentration.
- ACh increases gastric acid secretion by its action on M3 receptor which increases cytosolic calcium concentration.
- Histamine stimulates gastric acid secretion by adenyl cyclase and cAMP second messengers.
- Gastrin, Ach and histamine are physiologically highly synergistic in their function. This property of synergism helps to decrease acid secretion by H_2 antagonist drugs.
- Inhibition of gastric acid secretion occurs on increased acid content of the stomach and somatostatin.

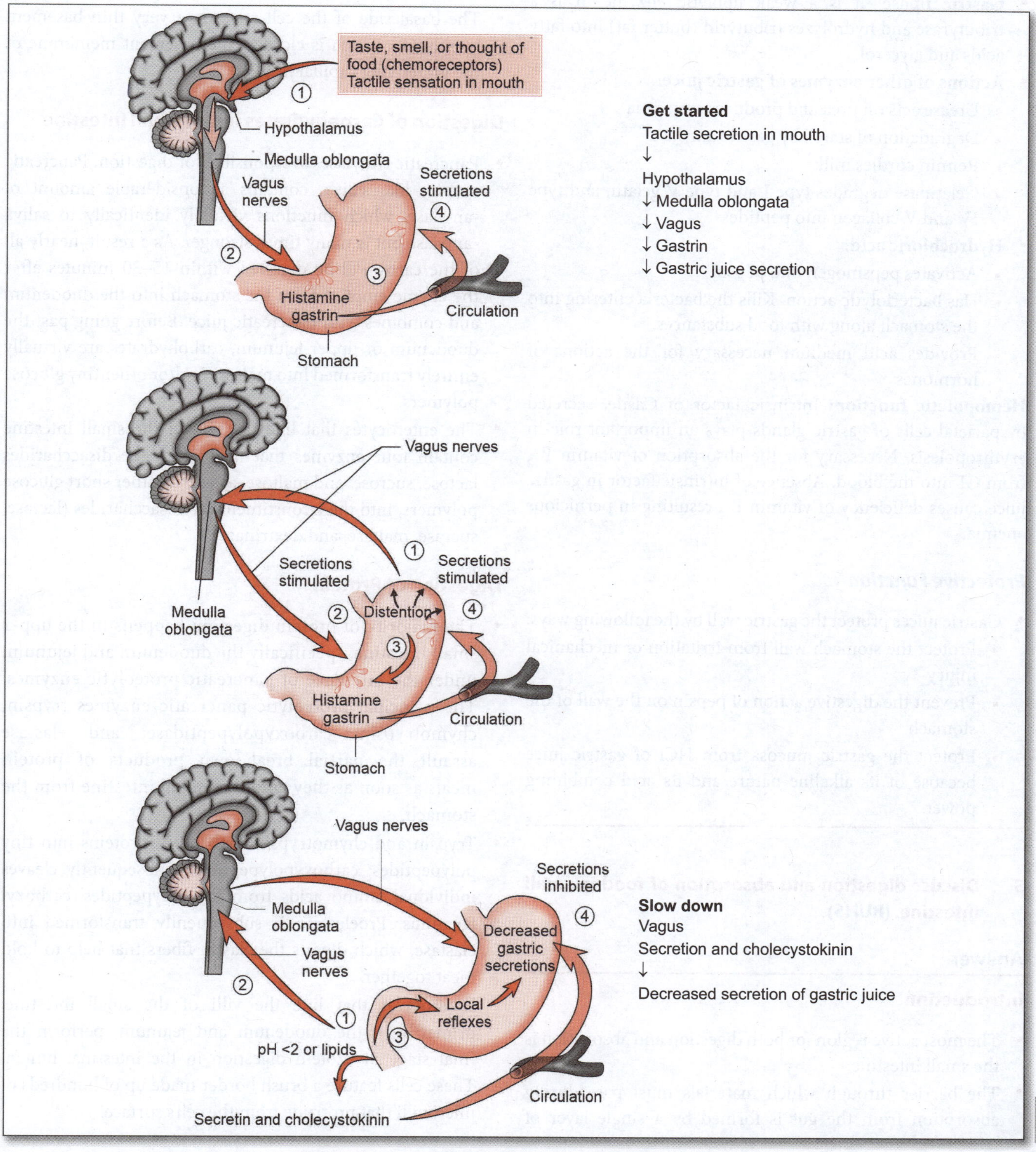

Figure 3.4: Mechanism and regulation of gastric secretion

Functions of Gastric Juices

Digestive function: The juices secreted are pepsin, gastric lipase and other enzymes. Gastric juice acts mainly on proteins.

- **Pepsin:** It converts proteins into proteases, peptones and polypeptides. It causes curdling and digestion of milk (casein)
- **Gastric lipase:** It is a weak lipolytic enzyme. It is a tributyrase and hydrolyzes tributyrin (butter fat) into fatty acids and glycerol.
- **Actions of other enzymes of gastric juice:**
  - Urease acts on urea and produces ammonia
  - Degradation of starch by gastric amylase
  - Rennin curdles milk
  - Gelatinase degrades type I and type V gelatin and type IV and V collagen into peptides
- **Hydrochloric acid:**
  - Activates pepsinogen into pepsin
  - Has bacteriolytic action. Kills the bacteria entering into the stomach along with food substances.
  - Provides acid medium necessary for the actions of hormones

Hemopoietic function: Intrinsic factor of Castle, secreted by parietal cells of gastric glands plays an important role in erythropoiesis. Necessary for the absorption of vitamin B_{12} from GI into the blood. Absence of intrinsic factor in gastric juice causes deficiency of vitamin B_{12} resulting in pernicious anemia.

Protective Function

- Gastric juices protect the gastric wall by the following ways:
  - Protect the stomach wall from irritation or mechanical injury
  - Prevent the digestive action of pepsin on the wall of the stomach
  - Protect the gastric mucosa from HCl of gastric juice because of its alkaline nature and its acid combining power.

3. Discuss digestion and absorption of food in small intestine. (RUHS)

Answer

Introduction

- The most active region for both digestion and absorption is the small intestine.
- The barrier through which materials must pass during absorption from the gut is formed by a single layer of epithelial cells on the surface of the villi, the finger-like projections.
- The area of the apical luminal surface of each epithelial cell is greatly increased by the presence of the brush-border.
- Below the villi in the mucosal membrane is a thick network of blood capillaries and small lymphatics.
- The basal side of the cell rests on a very thin basement membrane, which is close to the basement membrane of the underlying capillary.

Digestion of Carbohydrates in the Small Intestine

- Pancreatic Amylase is responsible for digestion. Pancreatic output, like saliva, contains a considerable amount of -amylase, which functions virtually identically to saliva -amylase but is many times stronger. As a result, nearly all of the carbs will be digested within 15–30 minutes after the chyme empties from the stomach into the duodenum and combines with pancreatic juice. Before going past the duodenum or upper jejunum, carbohydrates are virtually entirely transformed into maltose and/or other tiny glucose polymers.
- The enterocytes that line the villi of the small intestine contain four enzymes that may break the disaccharides lactose, sucrose, and maltose, as well as other short glucose polymers, into their constituent monosaccharides (lactase, sucrase, maltase, and dextrinase).

Digestion of Proteins

- The majority of protein digestion happens in the upper small intestine, specifically the duodenum and jejunum, under the influence of pancreatic proteolytic enzymes. The principal proteolytic pancreatic enzymes trypsin, chymotrypsin, carboxypolypeptidase, and elastase assault the partial breakdown products of protein meals as soon as they enter the small intestine from the stomach.
- Trypsin and chymotrypsin both break proteins into tiny polypeptides; carboxypolypeptidase subsequently cleaves individual amino acids from the polypeptides' carboxyl terminus. Proelastase is subsequently transformed into elastase, which digests the elastin fibers that help to hold meat together.
- Enterocytes that line the villi of the small intestine, primarily in the duodenum and jejunum, perform the final stage of protein digestion in the intestinal lumen. These cells feature a brush border made up of hundreds of microvilli that protrude from the cell's surface.

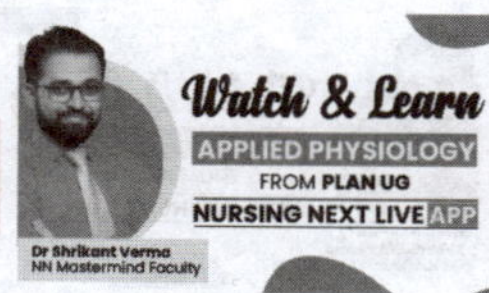

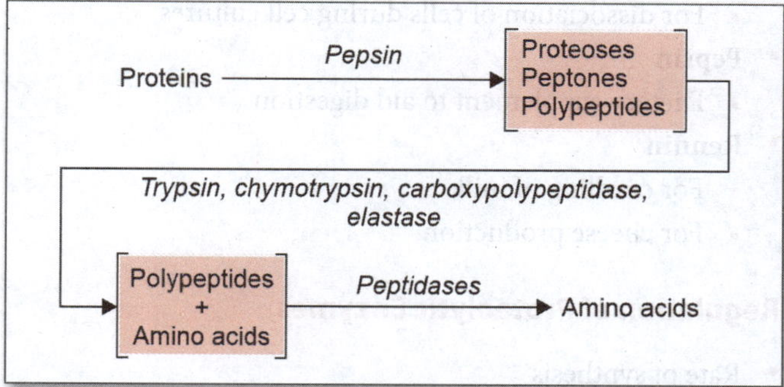

Figure 3.5: Digestion of proteins

Digestion of Fats

- Triglycerides are processed in the stomach by lingual lipase, which is released by lingual glands in the mouth and swallowed with saliva. This digesting amount is less than 10% and is often insignificant. Instead, almost all fat digestion takes place in the small intestine.
- The first step in fat digestion is emulsification by bile acids and lecithin.
- Triglycerides are digested by pancreatic lipase
- End products of fat digestion are free fatty acids.
- Bile salts form micelles that accelerate fat digestion
- Most cholesterol in the diet is in the form of cholesterol esters, which are combinations of free cholesterol and one molecule of fatty acid.

Absorption in the Small Intestine

Each day, several hundred grams of carbs, 100 or more grams of fat, 50–100 grams of amino acids, 50–100 grams of ions, and 7–8 L of water are absorbed from the small intestine.

Absorption of Carbohydrates

- Almost all carbohydrates in meals are absorbed as monosaccharides, with only a small fraction absorbed as disaccharides and essentially none absorbed as bigger carbohydrate molecules.
- Glucose is by far the most plentiful of the absorbed monosaccharides, accounting for more than 80% of the carbohydrate calories absorbed.

Absorption of Proteins as Dipeptides, Tripeptides, or Amino Acids

- After digestion, most proteins are absorbed as dipeptides, tripeptides, and a few free amino acids through the luminal membranes of intestinal epithelial cells.
- The majority of the energy for this movement is given through a sodium co-transport process, similar to how sodium co-transport of glucose happens. That is, most peptide or amino acid molecules attach to a specific transport protein in the cell's microvillus membrane, which requires sodium binding before transport can start.
- Following binding, the sodium ion proceeds down its electrochemical gradient to the cell's interior, dragging the amino acid or peptide along with it. This is known as co-transport (or secondary active transport) of amino acids and peptides.

Absorption of Fats

- When fats are digested to create monoglycerides and free fatty acids, both of these digestive end products initially dissolve in the bile micelle's core lipid part.
- The monoglycerides and free fatty acids are transferred to the surfaces of the microvilli of the brush border of the intestinal cell and subsequently enter into the recesses amid the moving, agitated microvilli.
- Because the lipids are also soluble in the epithelial cell membrane, the monoglycerides and fatty acids diffuse immediately out of the micelles and into the interior of the epithelial cells. In the presence of an abundance of bile micelles, about 97% of the fat is absorbed.

SHORT NOTES

1. Write in short about functions of stomach. (MGR)

Answer

Stomach performs the following functions:

- **Temporary storage organ**
  - Storage of ingested food till it reaches the small intestine.
- **Secretory functions**
  - Secretion of HCl and enzymes that aid in protein digestion.
  - Secretes pepsin
  - G cells of pyloric region secrete gastrin hormone
- **Digestive function**
  - This is because of pepsin enzyme that is proteolytic in nature.
- **Protective function**
  - This is due to high acidic medium provided by HCl. Due to high acidic medium, the microorganisms die and this protects the GI tract from the invading microorganisms.
- **Hematopoietic functions**
  - This is due to the presence of intrinsic factor.
  - It is secreted by the gastric glands of stomach.
  - Intrinsic factor is essential for the absorption of Vitamin B_{12} in the ileum region.

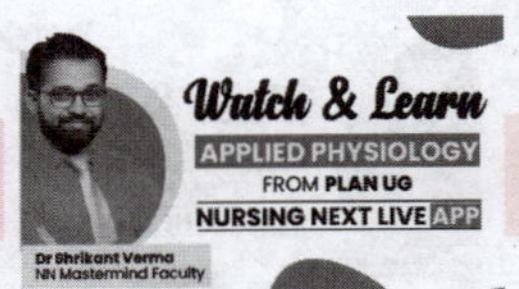

- **Absorptive function**
  - Small quantities of water and alcohol are absorbed directly from the stomach.
- **Motor function**
  - Peristaltic movements of stomach lead to pulverization of ingested food and mixing with the gastric secretions – this leads to the formation of chyme.
  - Chyme is emptied into the duodenum.
  - Enables the stomach to act as temporary reservoir of food.

2. Write in short about proteolytic enzymes in GIT. (RUHS)

Answer

Introduction

- Enzymes involved in the degradation of proteins
- Also known as proteases
- Secreted as zymogens – inactive enzymes
- Released by exocytosis
- Converted to active form by proteolysis

Activation of Proteolytic Enzymes

- **Chymotrypsinogen and trypsinogen**
  - By enzyme enterokinase in the duodenal lumen
  - Converted to chymotrypsin and trypsin
  - Also activated by its active form (autocatalytic)
- **Procarboxypeptidase**
  - Converted to carboxypeptidase
  - By enzyme trypsin
- **Proelastase**
  - Converted into elastase
  - Activated by trypsin
- **Pepsinogen**
  - Converted to pepsin
  - Activated by HCl and pepsin

Functions

- Proteolytic degradation is required for cellular maintenance
- Acts on the peptide linkages to break down proteins into small peptide chains and amino acids.
- **Trypsin**
  - In proteomics to break down proteins into peptides for spectrometry analysis
  - Baking enzyme
  - In the extraction of seasonings and flavorings
- **Papain**
  - Meat softener for cooking
  - For dissociation of cells during cell cultures
- **Pepsin**
  - Dietary supplement to aid digestion
- **Rennin**
  - For curdling of milk
  - For cheese production

Regulation of Proteolytic Enzymes

- Rate of synthesis
- Activation of proenzymes
- Rate of synthesis of inhibitors

3. Describe the composition and functions of the pancreatic juice. (RUHS)

Answer

Composition of Pancreatic Juice

- Water
- **Inorganic components:** Na^+, HCO_3^-, Cl^-
- **Organic components:**
  - **Proteolytic enzymes:** Trypsin, chymotrypsin and carboxypolypeptidase
  - **Amylolytic enzyme:** Pancreatic amylase
  - **Lipolytic:** Pancreatic lipase, cholesterol esterase, phospholipase
  - Trypsin inhibitors
  - Mucin

Functions of Pancreatic Juice

- **Carbohydrate digestion**
  - Amylase hydrolyzes starch into sugars
- **Fat digestion**
  - Lipase breaks down lipids into fatty acids, glycerol and monoglycerides. Emulsification of fat increases the surface area of fat droplets so that lipase can hydrolyze them.
  - 80% of fat digestion is due to pancreatic lipase.
  - Neutral fats break down into fatty acids and monoglycerides by pancreatic lipase
  - Hydrolysis of cholesterol esters by cholesterol esterases.
  - Fatty acids break down to phospholipids by phospholipase.
- **Protein digestion**
  - Proteins break down into peptides by trypsin and chymotrypsin
  - Peptides break down into amino acids by carboxypolypeptidase

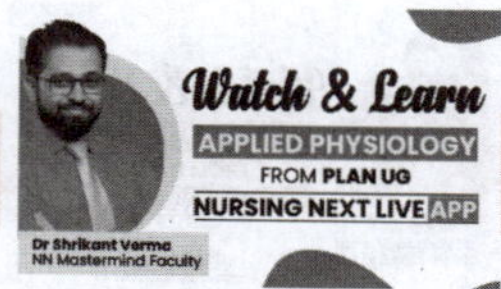

- Trypsin inhibitor prevents digestion of pancreas.
- **Activation of proenzymes**
  - Trypsin acts on inactive precursors called chymotrypsinogen, procarboxypeptidase and proelastase to produce chymotrypsin, carboxypeptidase and elastase respectively.
- Mucin and bicarbonate secretion neutralizes acidic chyme from stomach.
- Presence of acidic chyme from stomach in duodenum stimulates the production of secretin and cholecystokinin (CCK) hormones from endocrine cells in the wall of duodenum. These hormones, in turn, stimulate the secretion of pancreatic juice.

4. Write a short note on deglutition. (MGR)

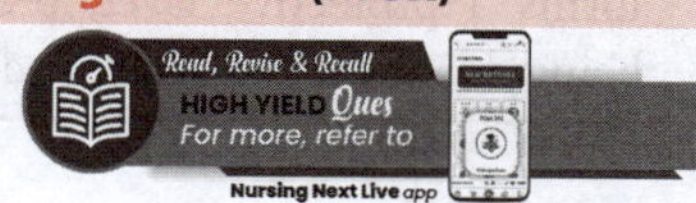

Answer

Introduction

Deglutition is also known as swallowing.

Stages of Deglutition

- Swallowing or deglutition consists of voluntary and involuntary stages (pharyngeal and esophageal).
- **Voluntary stage**
  - In this stage, the food present in the oral cavity is chewed and rolled into bolus with the help of tongue. The rolled out food is then pressed upward and backward against the soft palate with the help of tongue in such a way that it is pushed in the pharynx.
  - Chewed food is voluntarily rolled upward and backward against the palate by tongue.
- **Pharyngeal stage**
  - It is the transit of the food bolus through pharynx. It involves covering up of the nasopharynx by upward movement of soft palate.
  - Soft palate covers posterior nasopharynx as it is pulled upward
  - Formation of sagittal slit by pulling of palatopharyngeal folds sideways
  - Approximation of vocal cords
  - Epiglottis covers laryngeal opening as larynx is pulled anteriorly and upward
  - Opening of esophagus
  - Relaxation of upper esophageal sphincter
- **Esophageal stage**
  - Movement of food from esophagus to stomach
  - When the food bolus reaches the esophagus, the peristaltic wave pushes the food down the esophagus which causes receptive relaxation of the lower esophageal sphincter.
  - Primary peristalsis begins from posterior pharynx into esophagus
  - Secondary peristalsis in esophagus occurs due to distension by food bolus.
  - Receptive relaxation of the lower esophageal/gastroesophageal sphincter occurs.

5. Write in short about digestion in the stomach. (MGR)

Answer

- The stomach mucosa contains glands and cells, and secretes enzymes, hormones and acids that aid in digestion.
- Types of cells present in stomach are:
  - Parietal cells
  - Chief cells
  - G cells
  - Mucus cells
  - Endocrine cells

Role of Stomach in Digestion

- Digestion of carbohydrates
  - No carbohydrates are digested in stomach
  - Low gastric pH inactivates the salivary amylase
- Digestion of lipids
  - By Gastric Lipase—most effective for short and medium chain fatty acids
- Digestion of proteins
  - Protein digestion begins in stomach by:
  - Hydrochloric acid
    - pH of stomach is <2
    - This causes
      - Denaturation of proteins – makes proteins more susceptible to proteases
      - Killing of certain microorganisms
  - Pepsinogen—protease pro—enzyme
    - Converted to active pepsin by either autocatalysis or by gastric HCl.
    - Cleaves peptide bonds formed by amino groups of phenylalanine or tyrosine or leucine
    - Results in peptides and few amino acids which also act as stimulants for the release of the hormone cholecystokinin from duodenum.
  - Rennin
    - Also known as chymosin
    - Found in infants
    - Involved in curdling of milk.
    - Absent in adults.

6. Write a short note on the functions of saliva. (MGR)

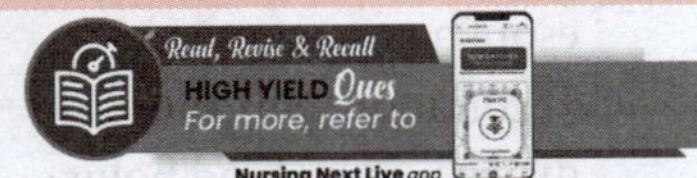

Answer

Functions of Saliva

- Lubrication and speech
  - Saliva helps moisten the food during mastication and helps in chewing.
  - Dissolves the food by forming bolus and facilitates swallowing.
  - Also helps in speech
  - Saliva keeps the oral cavity moist and maintains its health and integrity
- Taste
  - Foods dissolved in saliva stimulate the taste buds.
- Digestive functions
  - Enzymes like salivary amylase are present that help in the digestion of carbohydrates.
  - Lingual lipase also acts on fat digestion.
- Defense
  - It contains substances, like lysozyme, IgA, which can attach microorganisms, like bacteria and have defensive action.
- Excretory functions
  - Many substances such as mercury, potassium, iodide, lead and thiocyanate in saliva are excreted.
  - In certain conditions, excess urea or calcium may also be excreted.
- pH buffering action
  - Prevents sudden changes in pH
- Cleaning actions
  - Helps cleanse teeth
  - Washes away food debris and bacteria remaining in mouth.

SHORT ANSWER QUESTIONS

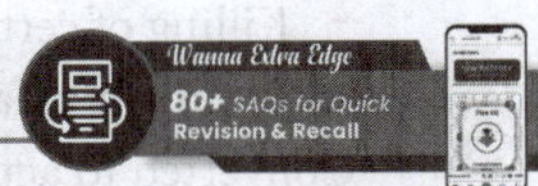

1. Mention two types of pancreatic secretions.

Answer

The two main types of pancreatic secretions are enzymes and bicarbonate.

Pancreatic enzymes, such as amylase, lipase, and protease, break down carbohydrates, fats, and proteins, respectively, into smaller molecules that can be absorbed by the small intestine.

2. Mention functions of stomach:

Answer

Functions of stomach are:

- **Storage:** The stomach can store food for several hours, allowing for a gradual release of partially digested food into the small intestine.
- **Mechanical digestion:** The stomach uses its muscular walls to mix food with digestive juices, breaking it down into smaller particles and creating a liquid mixture known as chyme.
- **Chemical digestion:** The stomach secretes hydrochloric acid and digestive enzymes, such as pepsin, to break down proteins into smaller molecules that can be absorbed by the small intestine.
- **Protection:** The stomach lining produces mucus that forms a protective layer, preventing the stomach from being damaged by the acidic digestive juices.

3. Name the two enzymes that help in the digestion of proteins.

Answer

Two enzymes that help in the protein digestion are:

1. Pepsin is a digestive enzyme produced by the stomach, which helps break down proteins into smaller peptides.
2. Trypsin is a digestive enzyme produced by the pancreas, which helps break down proteins into smaller peptides and amino acids.

4. List out functions of liver.

Answer

Functions of Liver

- Converts glucose into glycogen for the storage of insulin.
- **Carbohydrate metabolism:** Liver maintains the plasma glucose levels by converting glucose to glycogen and back with variations in blood glucose levels.
- **Protein metabolism:** Amino acids and nucleic acids are broken down to urea and uric acid in liver.
- **Fat metabolism:** Fat stored is metabolized to release energy.
- Liver secretes bile that contains the bile pigments, bile salts and cholesterol. Also stores iron and vitamins like B_{12}, A, D, E, K.
- Site for detoxification of toxic substances
- Site for metabolism of thyroid hormones, alcohol and steroids.
- Site for protein synthesis.

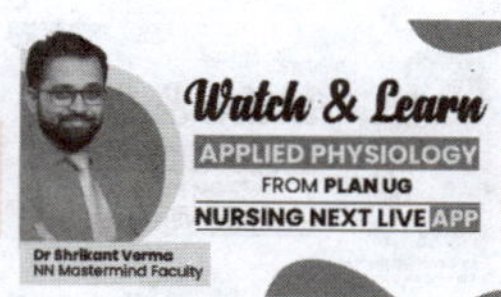

5. Mention functions of bile.

Answer

Functions of Bile

- Emulsification of fats
- Acceleration of action of pancreatic lipase
- **Micelle formation:** Polymolecular aggregates formed by the interaction of monoglycerides, fatty acids, bile salts and electrolytes are referred to as micelles. Micelles help in the transport of lipids into intestinal cells.
- Absorption of fat-soluble vitamins
- Formation of bile
- Intestinal motility

6. Mention the enzymes present in pancreatic juice.

Answer

- Amylase, protease, lipase and nuclease. These enzymes help break down carbohydrates into simpler sugars such as glucose.
- **Proteases:** The enzymes, including trypsin, chymotrypsin, and carboxypeptidase, break down proteins into smaller peptides and amino acids. Lipase breaks down fats or lipids into fatty acids and glycerol.

7. Name the bile salts.

Answer

The primary bile salts are cholic acid and chenodeoxycholic acid, which are conjugated with glycine or taurine and then stored in the gallbladder and released into the small intestine when needed.

8. Functions of hydrochloric acid. (MGR)

Answer

Functions of Hydrochloric Acid

- Acidification of the stomach
  - It maintains the pH of the stomach <2 by acidifying the stomach contents.
- Protective functions
  - Acts as a barrier against the foreign microorganisms and helps prevent infections.
- Role in digestion
  - Denaturation of proteins—makes proteins more susceptible to proteases
  - Activation of pro-enzymes such as pepsinogen into pepsin
  - Provides optimum pH for pepsin to act.
- Role in absorption
  - Helps in the absorption of iron and calcium in the stomach.
- Promotes secretion of pancreatic juice, bile and small intestine secretions.

9. Write two functions of gallbladder.

Answer

- The primary function of the gallbladder is to store and concentrate bile, a digestive fluid produced by the liver.
- The bile helps to emulsify the fats, making them easier to digest and absorb.

10. Name any two enzymes which help in digestion of carbohydrates.

Answer

Two enzymes that help in digestion of carbohydrates:

1. Amylase is an enzyme that breaks down starch and glycogen into smaller molecules, such as maltose and glucose, which can be easily absorbed by the body.
2. Lactase is an enzyme that breaks down lactose, a sugar found in milk and dairy products, into glucose and galactose.

11. List any two gastrointestinal hormones.

Answer

Two gastrointestinal hormones:

1. **Gastrin:** This hormone is produced by the G-cells of the stomach and stimulates the secretion of gastric acid, which helps to break down food in the stomach.
2. **Cholecystokinin (CCK):** This hormone is produced by the I-cells of the small intestine in response to the presence of fat and protein in the digestive tract.

12. Define peristalsis.

Answer

Peristalsis is a biological process that involves the rhythmic contraction and relaxation of smooth muscles in the digestive tract to propel food through it.

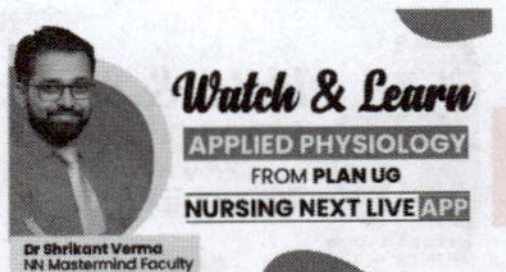

CONCEPTUAL REVISION

MULTIPLE CHOICE QUESTIONS

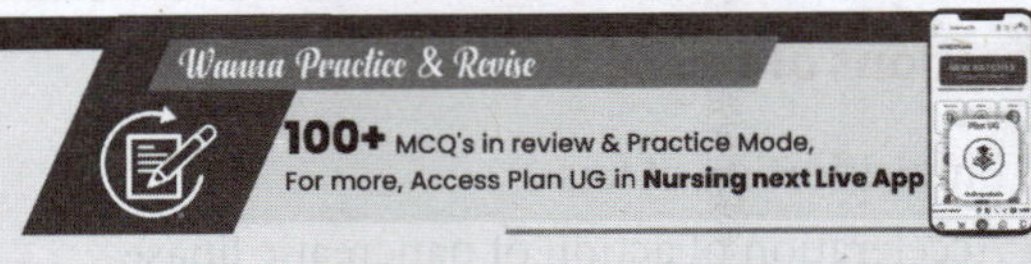

1. Which layer of the gastrointestinal tract is in contact with the contents of the gut?

a. Muscularis externa b. Mucosa
c. Serosa d. Submucosa

Ans. b. Mucosa

2. The pH of the stomach and the pH of the small intestine are BEST described (respectively) as:

a. Acidic and alkaline/basic
b. Strongly acidic and weakly alkaline/basic
c. Acidic and weakly alkaline/basic
d. Strongly acidic and strongly alkaline/basic

Ans. b. Strongly acidic and weakly alkaline/basic

3. What is the length of the rectum?

a. 5 cm b. 13 cm
c. 15 cm d. 20 cm

Ans. b. 13 cm

4. Which digestive enzyme in saliva breaks down starch?

a. Trypsin b. Lipase
c. Pepsin d. Amylase

Ans. d. Amylase

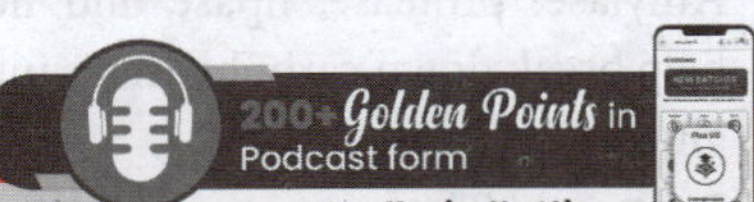

Golden Points

- 99.5% saliva is water and rest is made up of mucin, salts, proteins and amylase (ptyalin).
- About 1.5 L/day saliva is secreted by the three sets of salivary glands in the mouth. It lubricates and moistens the food.
- About 800 to 1000 mL bile is secreted daily.
- Absorption of about 90% of nutrients occurs in small intestine and the other 10% occurs in stomach and large intestine.
- **Amino acids** and **nucleic acids** are broken down to urea and uric acid in the liver.
- Bile acts as a medium for excretion of toxins and cholesterol.
- Bile salts are required for the emulsification of fats, i.e., reducing the size of globules, increasing their surface area and absorption.
- Carbohydrates are digested by amylase (salivary and pancreatic) to sugars.
- Cholecystokinin (CCK) hormone causes contraction of gallbladder and relaxation of sphincter of hepatopancreatic ampulla allowing the bile to flow into duodenum.

CHAPTER

4

Circulatory and Lymphatic System

CONCEPTUAL THEORY

Terminology

150+ key terminologies for Quick Recall & Revision

Atrial systole: Atria contract and pump the blood in ventricles.
Atrial diastole: Atria relax and receive the blood
Blood pressure: Lateral pressure exerted on the walls of arteries by column of blood is termed blood pressure.
Cardiac cycle: The sequence of events taking place in heart during each heart beat is known as cardiac cycle.
Cardiac output: Cardiac output is the quantity of blood pumped into the aorta each minute by the heart
His-Purkinje system: It carries the electrical signals throughout the ventricles to make them contract.
SA node (sinoatrial node): It is referred to as heart's natural pacemaker responsible for impulse generation
Stroke volume: It is indicator of width of the loop. After end diastolic volume (EDV), with next systole how much volume was ejected out.
Ventricular systole: Ventricular systole starts at the end of atrial systole because of AV nodal delay. Impulses reach the ventricles late.

FUNCTIONS OF HEART

- The primary duties of cardiovascular system include supplying nutrition and oxygen as well as removing metabolic waste.
- Each component of the system has a particular purpose. The purpose of the heart pump is to force blood through the arteries.
- To provide the lungs with oxygen, one ventricle pumps blood to the lungs. The other circulates blood throughout the body, carrying nutrition and oxygen.
- Blood vessels transport blood. They are hollow and are of different types depending on what they are used for.
- For instance, arteries have thick, muscular walls that allow them to squeeze blood under high pressure from the heart to the capillaries.
- Blood serves a variety of purposes. Hemoglobin in red blood cells draws oxygen.

CONDUCTION OR ELECTRICAL SYSTEM OF HEART

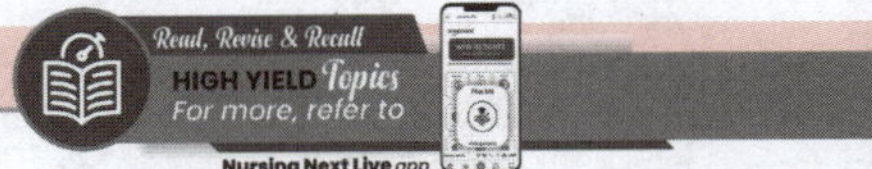

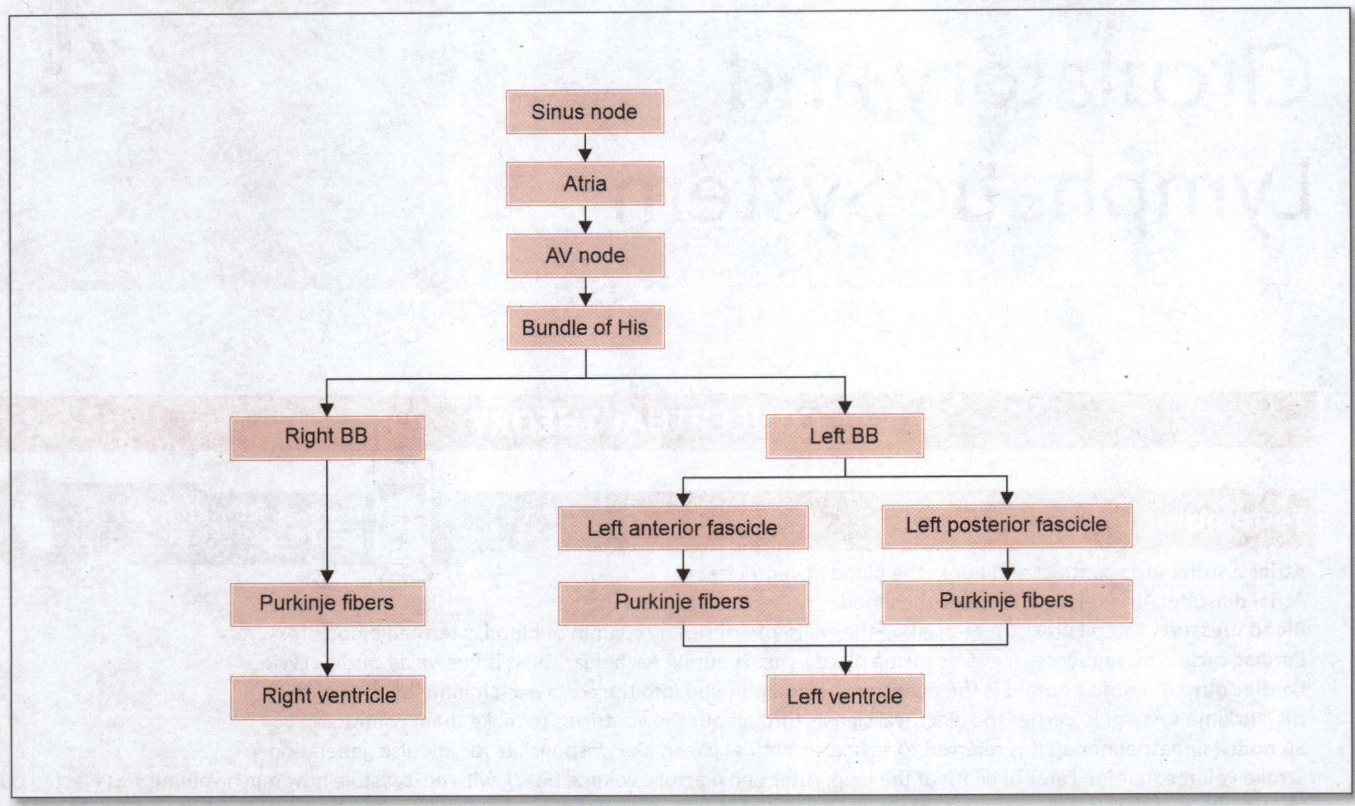

Figure 4.1: Conduction system of heart

SA Node (Sinoatrial Node)

- **SA node (sinoatrial node)** is referred to as heart's natural pacemaker. The SA node has special cells that create the electricity which makes your heart beat.
- It is pacemaker as it is responsible for impulse generation
- SA node contracts generating nerve impulses that travel throughout the heart wall and results in the contraction of both atria.

Functions

- SA node is part of the cardiac conduction system that ensures coordinated blood flow through various chambers of heart.
- Generates impulses for the contractions of the heart.
- Specialized conducting fibers between these different structures allow for quick transfer of impulses (four times faster than across normal myocardium).

AV Node (Atrioventricular Node)

- AV node is a small mass of cells situated in the right atrium in the posterior portion of interatrial septum.
- AV node is the bridge between the atria and ventricles. Electrical signals pass from the atria down to the ventricles through the AV node.

His-Purkinje System

His-purkinje system carries the electrical signals throughout the ventricles to make them contract. The components of His-Purkinje system include:

- His Bundle
- Right bundle branch
- Left bundle branch
- Purkinje fibers

CARDIAC CYCLE

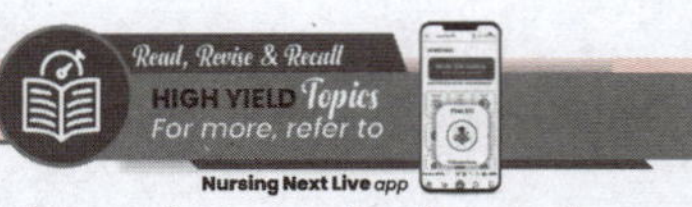

- The sequence of events taking place in the heart during each heart beat is defined as cardiac cycle.
- Total duration of cardiac cycle is 0.8 sec, if heart rate is 75 beats/min.
- Systole and diastole are the two major events.

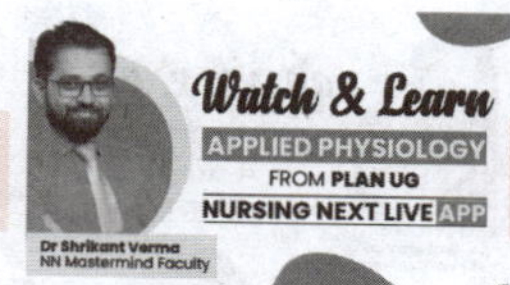

Cardiac cycle events		Duration (s)
Atrial	Systole	0.1
	Diastole	0.7
	Total	0.8
Ventricular	Systole	0.3
	Diastole	0.5
	Total	0.8

- **Atrial systole:** Atria contract and pump the blood in ventricles. It is referred to as meiotonic contraction in which the strength of contraction goes on decreasing as the contraction proceeds.
- **Atrial diastole:** Atria relax and receive the blood.
- **Ventricular systole:** Ventricular systole starts at the end of atrial systole because of AV nodal delay. Impulses reach the ventricles late.

  It includes isovolumetric contraction since all valves are closed and blood cannot go anywhere from the ventricles and the ventricles volume remains the same.
- **Ventricular diastole:** 70–80% of the ventricular filling is passive and last 20–30% of ventricular filling is active.

In first phase of diastole, sudden change in the direction of the blood is known as protodiastole and also includes isovolumetric relaxation phase.

After the first rapid filling, diastasis and last-rapid filling phases are also included.

Stroke Volume and Cardiac Output

- **Stroke volume:** It is indicator of width of the loop. After EDV (end diastolic volume), with next systole how much volume was ejected out. Usually stroke volume is 70 mL.

  Stroke volume = End diastolic volume – End systolic volume
- **Cardiac output:**
  - Cardiac output is the quantity of blood pumped into the aorta each minute by the heart.
  - Normal cardiac output in male is 5.6 L/min and in women is 4.9 L/min.
  - Measurement of cardiac output is done through direct Fick's method and thermodilution method.

$$CO = SV \times HR$$

cardiac output = store volume × heart rate
(mL/minute) (mL/beat) (beats/min)

BLOOD PRESSURE AND PULSE

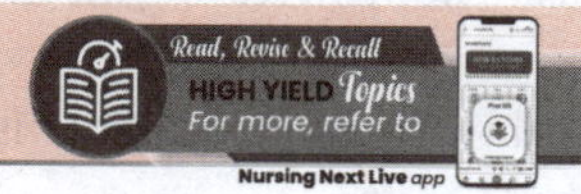

- Lateral pressure exerted on the walls of arteries by column of blood is defined as blood pressure.
- Blood pressure = Cardiac output. Total peripheral resistance
- It is expressed as mm Hg.
- It is usually referred to as systemic arterial blood pressure.
- Systolic blood pressure – maximum blood pressure exerted during the systolic phase of the cardiac cycle.
  - Normal values are 110–140 mm Hg
- Diastolic blood pressure – minimum blood pressure exerted during the diastolic phase of the cardiac cycle.
  - Normal values are 60–90 mm Hg
- So, the normal blood pressure – systolic/diastolic is 120/80 mm Hg.

Measurement of Blood Pressure

- Instrument used – Sphygmomanometer
- Principle – the pressure in the brachial artery is balanced with the pressure inside the BP cuff and is measured directly using the sphygmomanometer.
- Two methods
  1. Palpatory method
  2. Auscultatory method

Factors Influencing Blood Pressure

- **Blood pressure depends upon:**
  - Stroke volume (volume of blood ejected)
  - Heart Rate
    - It is affected by the Peripheral resistance and tone o arterioles. Also affected by the elasticity of arteriolar wall.

Blood Pressure= Cardiac output × Peripheral resistance

PRINCIPLES OF CIRCULATION

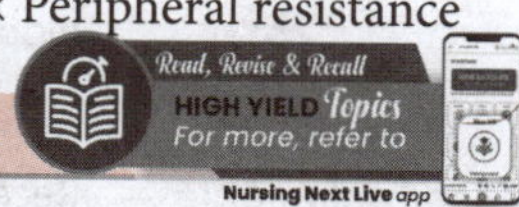

The principles of circulation refer to the fundamental concepts and mechanisms that govern the flow of blood throughout the circulatory system. These principles include:

- **Continuity:** The principle of continuity states that the volume of blood entering a given section of a blood vessel must equal the volume of blood leaving that section.
- **Pressure gradient:** Blood flow is driven by a pressure gradient. It flows from areas of higher pressure to areas of lower pressure. The heart acts as the central pump that creates the pressure gradient, pushing blood from the high-pressure arteries to the low-pressure veins.
- **Resistance:** Resistance refers to the impedance or opposition to blood flow within the blood vessels. It is primarily determined by the diameter of the blood vessels and their smooth muscle tone. The narrower the blood vessels, the higher the resistance, and the more difficult it is for blood to flow.

- **Compliance:** Compliance refers to the ability of blood vessels to stretch and accommodate changes in blood volume. Arteries have higher compliance, allowing them to expand and recoil, which helps maintain blood pressure and smooth out pulsatile flow.
- **Velocity of blood flow:** Blood flow velocity refers to the speed at which blood moves through the vessels. It is inversely proportional to the cross-sectional area of the vessel. Blood flow is slower in capillaries, allowing for exchange of gases and nutrients, while it is faster in larger arteries.
- **Filtration and reabsorption:** The capillaries play a crucial role in filtration and reabsorption of fluid. Blood pressure at the arterial end of the capillary bed forces fluid out of the capillaries, while osmotic pressure at the venous end helps reabsorb fluid back into the capillaries.
- **Autoregulation:** Autoregulation refers to the ability of tissues and organs to regulate their own blood flow based on their metabolic needs. It involves local vasodilation and vasoconstriction mechanisms to adjust blood flow in response to changes in oxygen and nutrient requirements.

Coronary, Pulmonary and Systemic Circulation

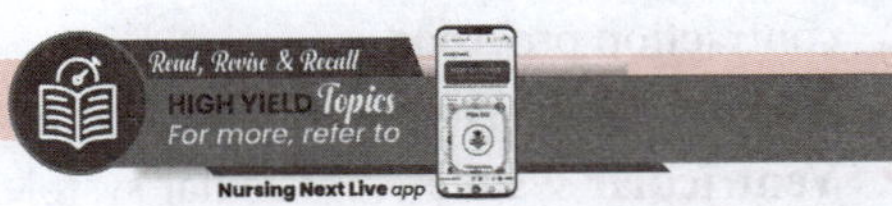

Circulation type	Coronary circulation	Pulmonary circulation	Systemic circulation
Function	Supplies blood to the heart muscle itself (myocardium)	Transports blood between the heart and the lungs	Transports blood between the heart and the rest of the body
Pathway	Begins at the aortic sinuses, which arise from the ascending aorta	Begins at the right ventricle, moves through the pulmonary artery, lungs, and returns to the left atrium	Begins at the left ventricle, moves through the aorta, arteries, arterioles, capillaries, venules, and veins, and returns to the right atrium
Oxygenation	Oxygenates the myocardium by supplying it with oxygen-rich blood	Oxygenates the blood by removing carbon dioxide and adding oxygen	Supplies oxygen and nutrients to body tissues while removing waste products, such as carbon dioxide
Deoxygenation	Removes waste products, such as carbon dioxide, from the myocardium	Collects deoxygenated blood from the body and returns it to the heart	Collects deoxygenated blood from the body and returns it to the heart
Blood pressure	Coronary arteries have the lowest blood pressure in the body	Pulmonary artery has lower blood pressure compared to systemic arteries	Systemic arteries have the highest blood pressure in the body
Blood volume	Receives about 4–5% of the total cardiac output	Receives the entire cardiac output from the right ventricle	Receives the entire cardiac output from the left ventricle
Blood composition	Contains oxygen, nutrients, and waste products	Contains deoxygenated blood, carbon dioxide, and waste products	Contains oxygenated blood, nutrients, and waste products

Heart Rate–Regulation of Heart Rate

- The rate of the heartbeat can be determined easily from an ECG because the heart rate is the reciprocal of the time interval between two successive heartbeats (the R-R interval).
- If the interval between two beats is determined from the time calibration lines is 1 second, the heart rate is 60 beats/min.
- The normal interval between two successive QRS complexes in an adult is about 0.83 second, which is a heart rate of 60/0.83 times/min, or 72 beats/min.
- Sympathetic stimulation markedly increases the activity of the heart, both increasing the heart rate and enhancing its strength and volume of pumping.
- Parasympathetic stimulation decreases heart rate and contractility. Circulatory effect is to control heart rate by way of parasympathetic nerve fibers to the heart in the vagus nerves.

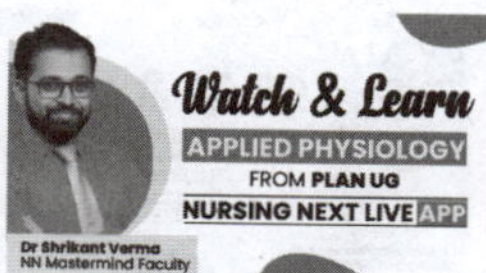

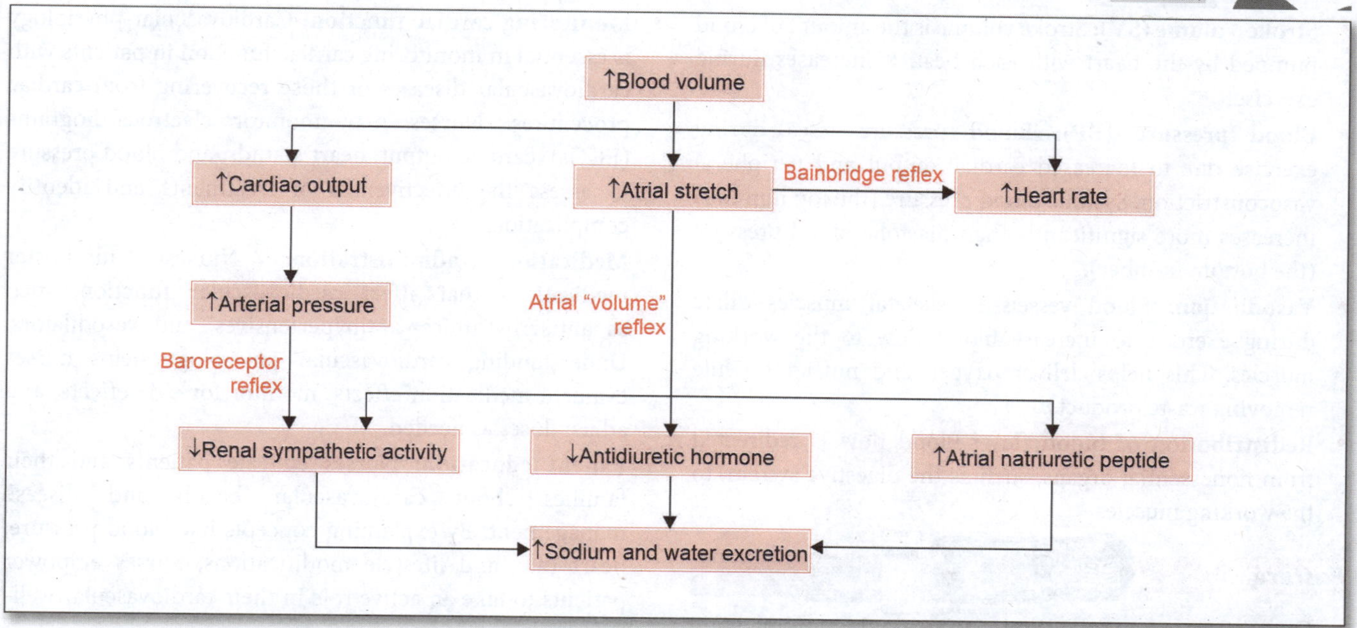

Figure 4.2: Reflex responses to increased blood volume which increases arterial pressure and atrial stretch

Normal Value and Variations

Parameter	Normal value/range	Variations
Heart rate	60–100 beats/min	Bradycardia - HR <60 bpm Tachycardia - HR >100 bpm
Blood pressure	Systolic: 90–120 mm Hg Diastolic: 60–90 mm hg	Elevated (at risk, or prehypertension): SBP 120–129 mm Hg; DBP <80 mm Hg. Hypertension stage 1: SBP 130–139 mm Hg; DBP 80–89 mm Hg Hypertension stage 2: SBP >140 mm Hg; DBP >90 mm Hg. Hypertensive Crisis: SBP >180 mm Hg; DBP >120 mm Hg.
Cardiac output	4–8 L/min	It increases during exercise and decreases during rest. Conditions such as heart failure can significantly affect cardiac output.
Stroke volume	60–100 mL per beat	It is affected by factors such as preload, afterload, and contractility of the heart.
Systemic vascular resistance	800–1200 dyn·s/cm^5	Conditions such as hypertension can increase resistance, while vasodilation can decrease it.
Central venous pressure	2–8 mm Hg	Central venous pressure can vary depending on factors such as blood volume, cardiac function, and intrathoracic pressure. It is influenced by factors like venous return, right heart function, and fluid balance.
Pulmonary artery pressure	Systolic: 15–30 mm Hg	Elevated pulmonary artery pressure may occur in conditions like pulmonary hypertension.
Oxygen saturation (SpO_2)	95–100%	It can vary based on factors like altitude, lung function, and cardiovascular health. Lower oxygen saturation levels may occur in respiratory or cardiovascular disorders.
Capillary refill time (CRT)	Less than 2 seconds	Prolonged capillary refill time may indicate decreased peripheral perfusion or circulatory impairment.

Cardiovascular Homeostasis in Exercise and Posture

Cardiovascular homeostasis refers to the maintenance of stable physiological conditions within the cardiovascular system.

This homeostasis is particularly important during exercise and changes in posture.

Exercise

- **Heart rate (HR) and cardiac output (CO):** During exercise, heart rate increases to meet the increased oxygen and nutrient demands of the muscles.

- **Stroke Volume (SV):** Stroke volume is the amount of blood pumped by the heart with each beat. It increases during exercise.
- **Blood pressure (BP):** Blood pressure rises during exercise due to increased cardiac output and peripheral vasoconstriction. Systolic blood pressure (the top number) increases more significantly than diastolic blood pressure (the bottom number).
- **Vasodilation:** Blood vessels in skeletal muscles dilate during exercise to increase blood flow to the working muscles. This helps deliver oxygen and nutrients while removing waste products.
- **Redistribution of blood flow:** Blood flow is redirected from nonessential organs, such as the digestive system, to the working muscles

Posture

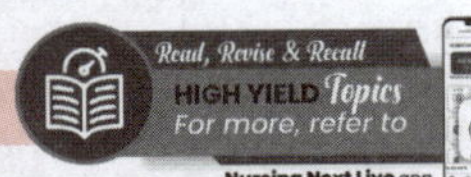

- **Orthostatic changes:** When transitioning from lying down to standing up, there is a temporary drop in blood pressure due to gravity pulling blood downward. This can lead to dizziness or lightheadedness. The body rapidly compensates through various mechanisms to maintain blood pressure.
- **Baroreceptor reflex:** Baroreceptors located in the carotid sinuses and aortic arch sense changes in blood pressure. When blood pressure drops upon standing, the baroreceptor reflex triggers vasoconstriction and an increase in heart rate to elevate blood pressure.
- **Venous return:** Maintaining venous return is crucial in upright posture. Skeletal muscle contractions during standing help facilitate blood return to the heart, aided by one-way valves in the veins preventing backflow.
- **Postural hypotension:** Some individuals may experience postural hypotension, where blood pressure drops significantly upon standing. This can occur due to factors such as dehydration, medication side effects, or autonomic nervous system dysfunction.

APPLICATION AND IMPLICATION IN NURSING

Cardiovascular physiology is highly relevant in the field of nursing as it provides the foundation for understanding and assessing the cardiovascular system. Here are some key applications and implications of cardiovascular physiology in nursing:

- **Patient assessment:** Nurses utilize cardiovascular physiology to assess patient's cardiovascular health. This includes measuring vital signs such as heart rate, blood pressure, and oxygen saturation levels. By understanding normal ranges and variations, nurses can identify abnormalities and provide appropriate interventions.
- **Monitoring cardiac function:** Cardiovascular physiology is essential in monitoring cardiac function in patients with cardiovascular diseases or those recovering from cardiac procedures. Nurses may monitor electrocardiograms (ECGs), cardiac output, heart sounds, and blood pressure to assess the effectiveness of treatments and identify complications.
- **Medication administration:** Nurses administer medications that affect cardiovascular function, such as antiarrhythmics, antihypertensives, and vasodilators. Understanding cardiovascular physiology helps nurses evaluate medication effects, monitor for side effects, and adjust doses as needed.
- **Patient education:** Nurses educate patients and their families about cardiovascular health and disease management. By explaining concepts like blood pressure, heart rate, and lifestyle modifications, nurses empower patients to take an active role in their cardiovascular well-being.
- **Cardiopulmonary resuscitation (CPR):** Nurses trained in CPR utilize their knowledge of cardiovascular physiology to provide immediate life-saving interventions during cardiac arrest. They perform chest compressions to maintain blood flow and deliver rescue breaths to oxygenate the patient.
- **Fluid balance management:** Nurses assess and manage fluid balance in patients, which directly impacts cardiovascular physiology. They monitor intake and output, administer intravenous fluids, and assess signs of fluid overload or dehydration to optimize cardiac function.
- **Pre- and postoperative care:** Before and after cardiovascular surgeries or procedures, nurses play a crucial role in preparing patients, monitoring hemodynamic stability, managing pain, preventing complications, and facilitating recovery.
- **Patient safety and risk assessment:** Nurses use cardiovascular physiology to identify patients at risk for cardiovascular events, such as those with hypertension, diabetes, or a family history of heart disease. By recognizing risk factors, nurses can implement preventive measures and advocate for appropriate interventions.
- **Health promotion:** Nurses promote cardiovascular health by educating patients about risk factors, promoting a healthy lifestyle, and supporting behavior changes such as smoking cessation, physical activity, and maintaining a balanced diet.
- **Collaboration with health care team:** Nurses collaborate with other health care professionals, such as physicians, cardiologists, and respiratory therapists, to provide comprehensive care to patients with cardiovascular conditions. A solid understanding of cardiovascular physiology allows nurses to effectively communicate and collaborate on patient care plans.

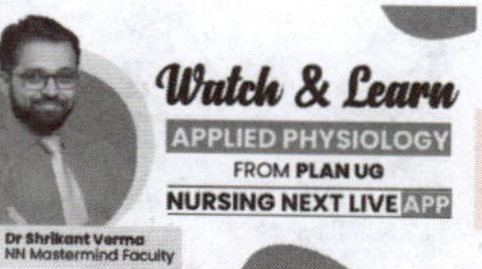

CONCEPTUAL EXERCISES

LONG ANSWER QUESTIONS

1. Define blood pressure. Write in detail about the factors controlling blood pressure. Add a note on hypertension. (KUHS, DU, MGR)

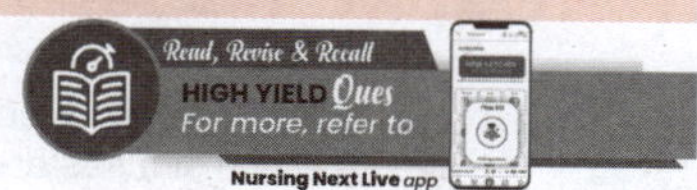

Answer

Blood Pressure

- Blood pressure is the force exerted by the blood against any unit area of the vessel wall. (Guyton and Hall)
- It is expressed as mm Hg.
- It is usually referred to as systemic arterial blood pressure.
- Systolic blood pressure—maximum blood pressure exerted during the systolic phase of the cardiac cycle.
  - Normal values are 110–140 mm Hg
- Diastolic blood pressure—minimum blood pressure exerted during the diastolic phase of the cardiac cycle.
  - Normal values are 60–90 mm Hg
- So, the normal blood pressure—systolic/diastolic is 120/80 mm Hg.

Factors Influencing Blood Pressure

- **Blood Pressure depends upon:**
  - Stroke volume (volume of blood ejected)
  - Heart rate
    - It is affected by the Peripheral resistance and tone o arterioles. Also affected by the elasticity of arteriolar wall.

Blood pressure = Cardiac output × Peripheral resistance

Other Factors Affecting Blood Pressure

- **Heredity:** Hypertension runs in families as people with parents and grandparents having hypertension are more likely to develop hypertension.
- **Gender:** Females are more likely to have lower blood pressure than males which can be attributed to higher estrogen levels in females. After menopause, there is no gender difference between males and females.
- **Age:** As the age advances, the rigidity of the arterial wall increases, this is called arteriosclerosis. Due to the above reason, arteries become less distensible and the blood pressure increases.
- **Built of the body:** Blood pressure recorded in obese individuals is apparently higher because of more subcutaneous tissues between the cuff and the artery.
- **Temperature:** On exposure to cold, there occurs vasoconstriction which causes an increase in blood pressure and on exposure to heat, there occurs vasodilation that causes a decrease in blood pressure
- **Diurnal variations:** Blood pressure is recorded higher in the evening and lower in the morning.
- **Sleep:** In NREM sleep, the blood pressure is relatively lower; whereas in REM sleep, it is usually higher because of increased muscle tone.
- **Meals:** Increase in systolic blood pressure is observed after meals due to release of epinephrine from adrenal medulla and due to distension of abdomen.
- **Effect of emotions:** Increased sympathetic activity occurs due to emotions like excitement and worry, this causes vasoconstriction bringing about an increase in systolic blood pressure.
- **Posture:** On standing, there occurs pooling of blood in the lower limbs, this causes decreased venous return to the right atrium which in turn decreases cardiac output and systolic blood pressure.
- **Exercise:** Due to sympathetic vasoconstriction during exercise, there occurs an increase in systolic blood pressure.
- **Gravity:** In upright position, there occurs pooling of blood in the lower limb. The gravity causes 0.77 mm Hg increase in pressure for every cm as we go down with mean blood pressure of 100 mm Hg at the level of heart.

Regulation of Blood Pressure

Blood pressure is regulated by two mechanisms:

1. **Short-term control:**
   - The short-term control of blood pressure is through nervous control by autonomic nervous system.
   - Mainly baroreceptor reflex and chemoreceptor reflex, higher centers and circulating hormones are involved.
   - Baroreceptors corrects up to 2/3 fall in BP.
   - Their physiological effect is to decrease the BP by decreased discharge from baroreceptors.
2. **Long-term control:**
   - Kidneys and renin – angiotensin - aldosterone system is involved in regulation of blood volume.

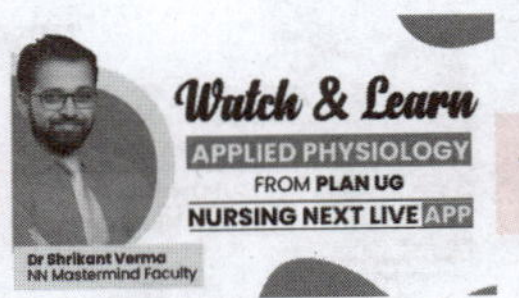

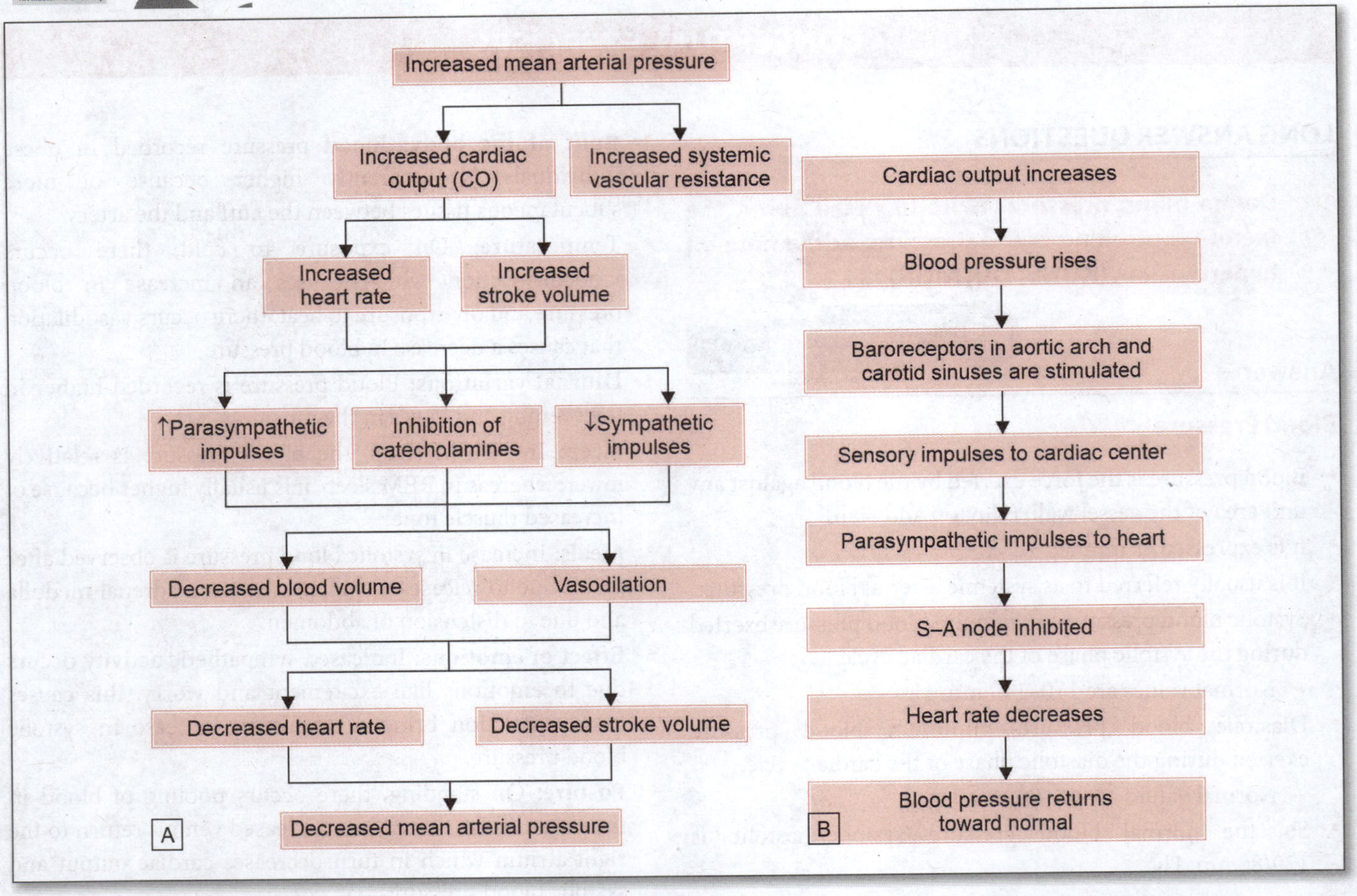

Figures 4.3A and B: Controlling mechanism of blood pressure. **A.** Long-term BP; **B.** Short-term regulation of BP

Hypertension

- Increase in systemic arterial blood pressure is known as hypertension.
- Systolic blood pressure >140 mm Hg, Diastolic blood pressure >90 mm Hg.
- Hypertension is characterized by increased cardiac output, sympathetic activity, Angiotensin II and aldosterone levels along with pressure natriuresis.

Table 4.1: Grades of hypertension

Category[a]	Systolic (mm Hg)		Diastolic (mm Hg)
Optimal	<120	and	<80
Normal	120–129	and/or	80–84
High normal	130–139	and/or	85–89
Grade 1 hypertension	140–159	and/or	90–99
Grade 2 hypertension	160–179	and/or	100–109
Grade 3 hypertension	≥180	and/or	≥110
Isolated systolic hypertension[b]	≥140	and	<90

Abbreviations: BP, blood pressure; SBP, systolic blood pressure.

[a]BP category is defined according to seated clinic BP and by the highest level of BP, whether systolic or diastolic.

[b]Isolated systolic hypertension is graded 1, 2 or 3 according to SBP values. The same classification is used for all ages from 16 years.

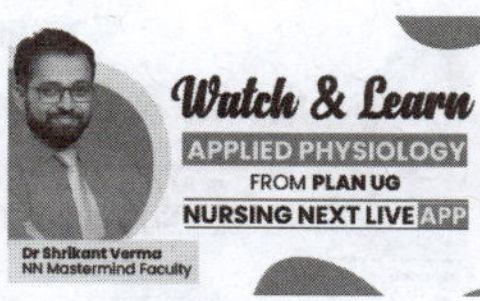

Classification of Hypertension

- **Essential or primary hypertension**
  - Hypertension of unknown origin
  - Risk factors include:
    - Obesity (increased waist hip ratio)
    - Family history
    - High salt intake
    - Sedentary lifestyle
    - Stress
    - Diabetes mellitus
- **Secondary hypertension**
  - Hypertension due to other causes such as:
    - Renal diseases
    - Adrenal gland disorders
      - Conn's syndrome
      - Cushing syndrome
      - Pheochromocytoma
    - Thyrotoxicosis
    - Certain medications

Complications of Hypertension

- Hemorrhagic stroke
- Acute renal failure
- Cardiac failure
- End—organ damage
- Cardiomyopathy
- Thrombosis—due to turbulent flow.

2. Briefly explain the conductive system of the heart. (MGR)

Answer

Conducting System of the Heart

Heart's electrical system includes:

SA Node (Sinoatrial Node)

- **SA node (sinoatrial node):** Referred to as heart's natural pacemaker, the SA node has special cells that create the electricity which makes your heart beat.
- It is pacemaker as it is responsible for impulse generation.
- SA node contracts generating nerve impulses that travel throughout the heart wall and results in the contraction of both atria.

Structure of SA Node

- Located in the posterolateral wall of the sinus of vena cava in the right atrium.
- Made of specialized cardiac muscle cells – cardiomyocytes, also known as the nodal or pacemaker cells.

Functions

- SA node is part of the cardiac conduction system that ensures coordinated blood flow through various chambers of heart.
- Generates impulses for the contractions of the heart.
- Specialized conducting fibers between these different structures allow for quick transfer of impulses (four times faster than across normal myocardium).

AV Node (Atrioventricular Node)

- AV node is a small mass of cells situated in the right atrium in the posterior portion of interatrial septum.
- AV node is the bridge between the atria and ventricles. Electrical signals pass from the atria down to the ventricles through the AV node.

His-Purkinje System

His-Purkinje system carries the electrical signals throughout the ventricles to make them contract. The components of His-Purkinje system include:

- His Bundle
- Left bundle branch
- Right bundle branch
- Purkinje fibers

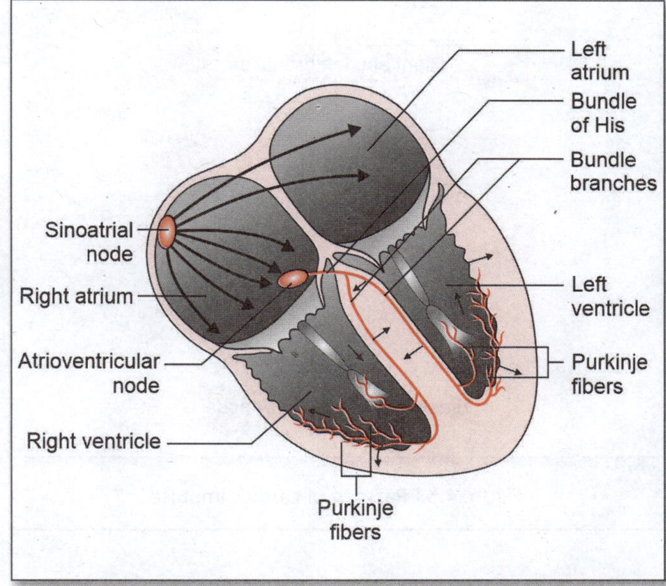

Figure 4.4: Conduction system of the heart and spread of impulse

Sequence of Cardiac Contraction

- **Pacemaker impulse generation**
  - SA node contracts generating nerve impulses that travel throughout the heart wall and results in the contraction of both atria.
- **AV node impulse conduction**
  - The AV node lies on the right side of the partition that divides the atria, near the bottom of the right atrium.

- When the impulses travel from SA node to AV node, they are delayed for about a tenth of a second allowing the atria to contract and empty their contents.
- **AV bundle impulse conduction**
  - The impulses are then sent to AV bundle. This bundle of fibers further divides into two bundles and the impulses travel down the center of the heart to the left and right ventricles.
- **Purkinje fibers impulse conduction**
  - At the base of the heart, the AV bundle starts to divide further into Purkinje fibers.
  - Ventricles contract due to muscle trigger as the impulses travel these fibers.

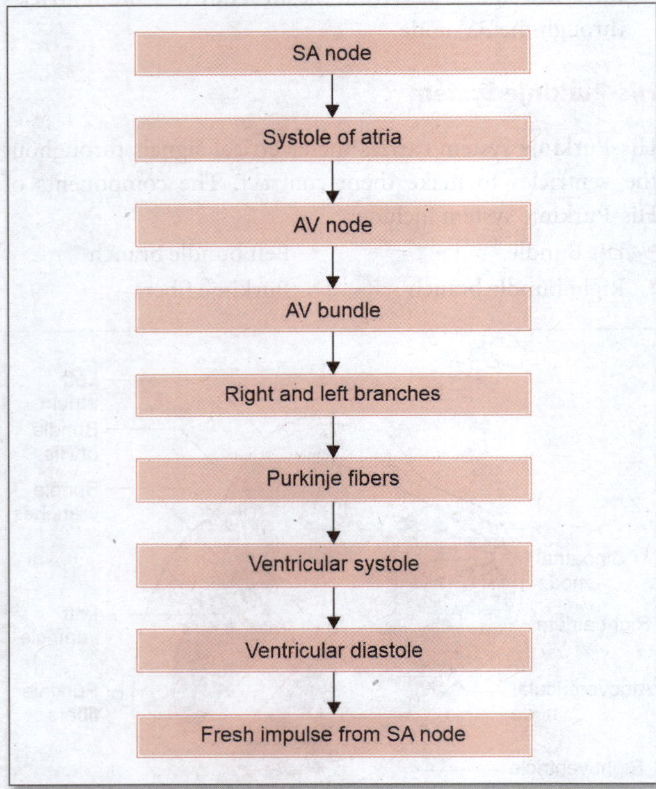

Figure 4.5: Passage of cardiac impulse

3. Define the cardiac cycle. What are the events in a cardiac cycle? Describe the ventricular events in detail. Add a note on heart sounds. (MGR)

Answer

Cardiac Cycle

- Cardiac cycle is the sequence of events that takes place between two successive heartbeats.
  - Atrial systole
  - Ventricular systole
  - Ventricular diastole
  - Atrial diastole

Duration

- If heart rate is 75/min, the duration of each cardiac cycle is 0.8 sec.
- All chambers of the heart are relaxed at the beginning of the cardiac cycle.
- The pressure in all the atria and ventricles is equal when the AV valves open.

Atrial Systole

- **Duration:** 0.1 seconds
- Occurs after generation of impulse from SA node
- Contraction of atrial muscles occurs
- Pressure increases in both right ventricle (4–6 mm Hg) and left ventricle (7–8 mm Hg)
- Atrial contraction propels 30 mL of blood into ventricles
- Resting ventricles usually have 100 mL of blood that is already present between them.

Atrial Diastole

- **Duration:** 0.7 seconds
- Atria relax and filling of atria occurs.
- AV valve opens.
- Coincides with the ventricular diastole; and diastasis phase causes an increase in the atrial pressure.

Ventricular Systole

- **Duration:** 0.3 seconds
- When the impulse reaches ventricle and at the beginning of QRS, complex ventricular depolarization causes ventricular contraction.
- **Two phases:** Isovolumetric/Isometric contraction of ventricles (0.05 seconds) and ventricular systole proper (0.25 seconds).
- **Isometric ventricular contraction**: Ventricles begin to contract, atria relax and AV valve closes.
- First heart sound (HS1) occurs. Ventricle contracts as closed chamber as myocardium presses on blood in ventricle. The pressure increases inside but no emptying occurs.

Ventricular systole proper: Pressure increases more than aorta in left ventricle and in right ventricle more than pulmonary artery causing opening of semilunar valves. There occurs rapid ejection phase: 0.1 sec, causing approximately 2/3 of stroke volume.

- Peak/Summit occurs till the aortic and pulmonary artery pressure exceeds the ventricular pressure. The momentum of the blood keeps it moving.
- **Slow ejection phase:** 0.15 seconds, pressure declines as contraction declines.

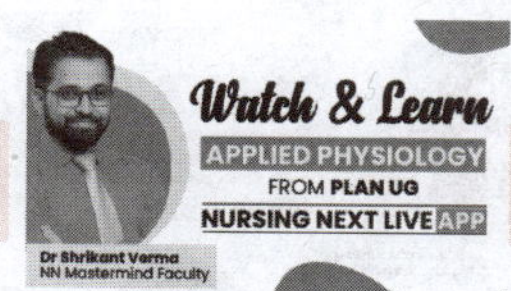

- Every stroke ejects 70–80 mL of blood from each ventricle.
- 65% of end-diastolic volume is ejected with every heartbeat which is ejection fraction.

Ventricular Diastole

- **Duration:** 0.5 sec
- **Protodiastole:** 0.04 sec, pressure drops, arterial pressure exceeds ventricular pressure, and causes the closure of semilunar valves. Second Heart Sound (HS2) occurs.
- **Isovolumetric ventricular relaxation:** Valves are closed, ventricle relaxes, pressure inside drops as a result AV valves open.
- **Ventricular diastole proper:** Responsible for 70% of filling. Rapid filling occurs for 0.1–0.12 seconds, slow filling/diastasis occurs for 0.18 to 0.20 seconds.
- **Last rapid filling phase:** Due to atrial systole, ventricles get completely filled. This ends the cardiac cycle.

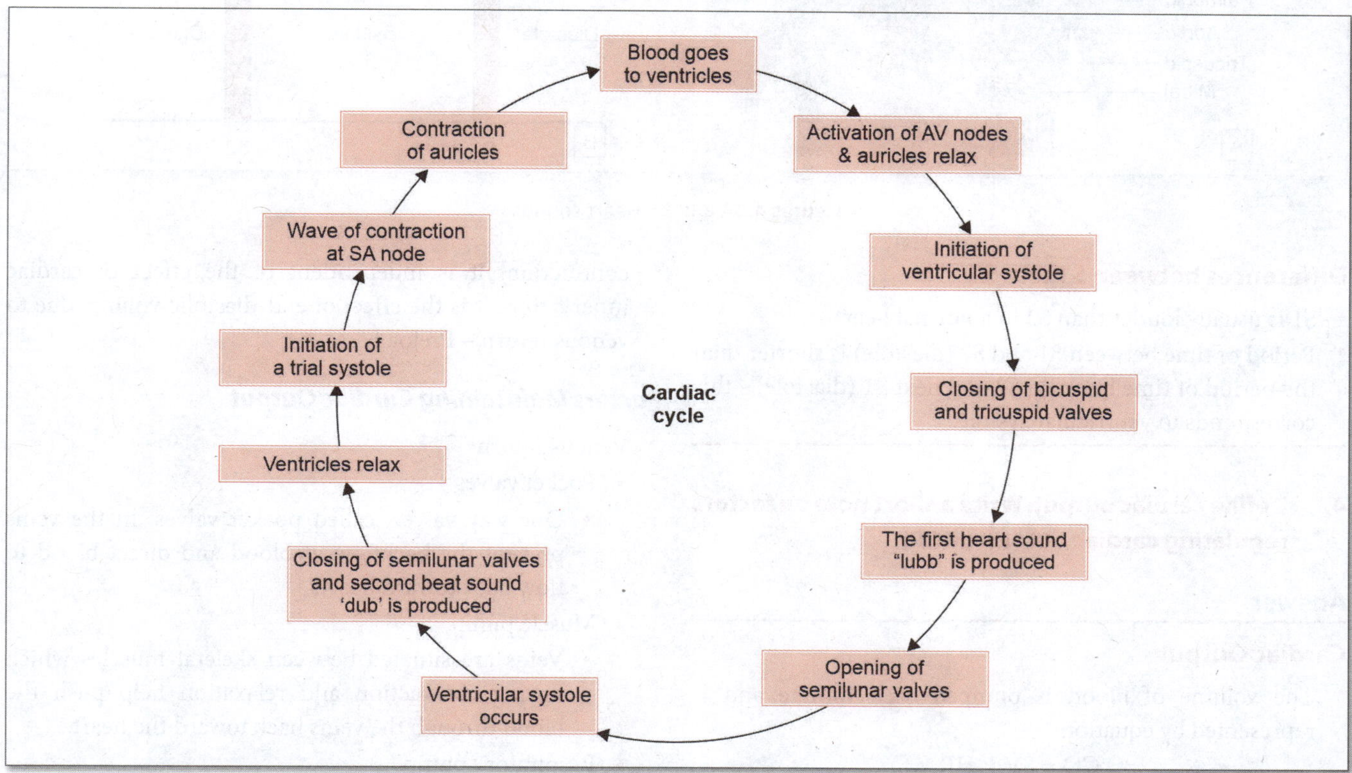

Figure 4.6: Cardiac cycle

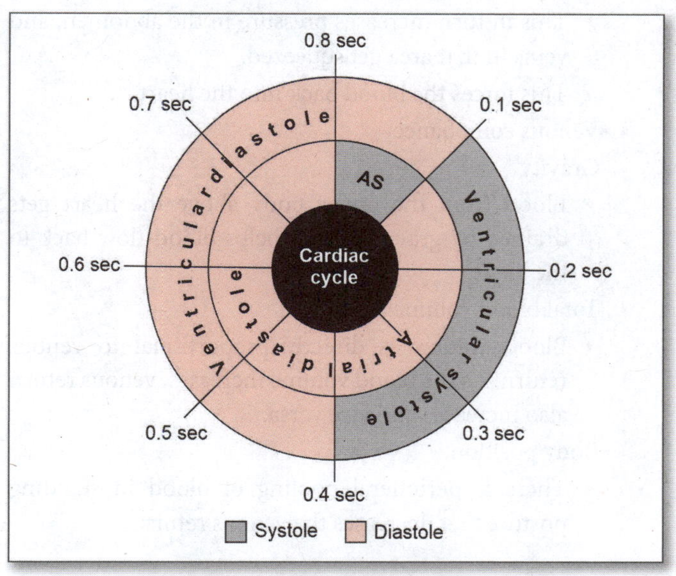

Figure 4.7: Cardiac cycle

Heart Sounds

- The sounds produced by the closure of heart valves during cardiac cycle are called heart sounds.
- Heart sounds can be heard by the examiner on auscultation by stethoscope.
- In a cardiac cycle, normally two heart sounds are heard, separated by a short nipple.
  - **First heart sound (S1):** It occurs due to the closure of both atrioventricular valves (mitral – M1 and tricuspid valves – T1). Sounds like LUB.
  - **Second heart sound (S2):** It occurs due to the closure of semilunar valves (aortic valve closure –A2, Pulmonary valve closure – P2). It sounds like DUB.
  - **Third heart sound:** It occurs due to turbulence of blood caused in rapid filling phase.
  - **Fourth heart sound:** It occurs during atrial systole.

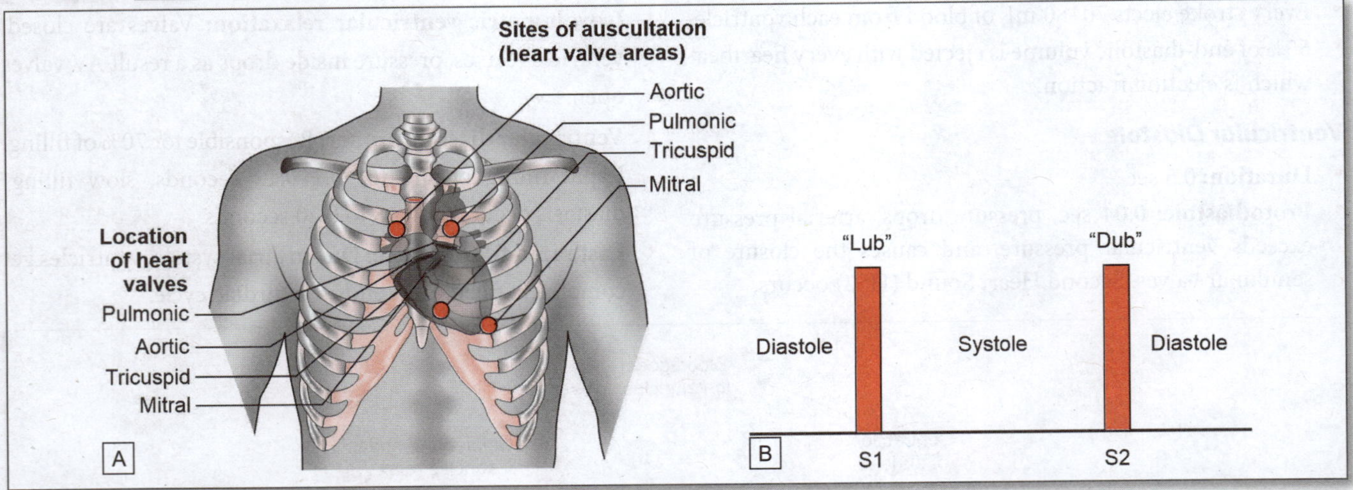

Figures 4.8A and B: Heart sounds

Differences between S1 and S2

- S1 is usually louder than S2 in a normal heart.
- Period of time between S1 and S2 (diastole) is shorter than the period of time between S2 and next S1 (diastole) - this corresponds to ventricular systole.

4. Define cardiac output. Write a short note on factors regulating cardiac output. (MGR)

Answer

Cardiac Output

- The volume of blood is pumped each minute and is represented by equation:

$$CO = SV \times HR$$

- Cardiac output is product of function of heart rate and stroke volume.
- Cardiac output = Heart Rate × Stroke volume.
- For example, if the HR = 72 and Stroke volume is 70 mL, then the Cardiac output is 72 × 70 = 5040 mL (5 L approx)
- It is expressed in liters per minute and normal value is 5 L/min.
- Regulation of cardiac output depends upon factors on which CO is calculated, i.e., HR and SV.
- Regulation of HR is primarily by cardiac innervation (sympathetic and parasympathetic) with effect from higher centers like cardiac vagal center and vasomotor center of medulla.
- Regulation of stroke volume depends upon heterometric and homometric regulation.
- Heterometric regulation is based on the Frank-Starling Law dependent length-tension relationship of cardiac muscle contraction. It is independent of the effect of cardiac innervation. It is the effect of end-diastolic volume due to venous return – Preload

Factors Maintaining Cardiac Output

- Venous return
  - Pocket valves
    - One-way valves, called pocket valves, in the veins prevent the backflow of blood and direct blood to flow back toward heart.
  - Muscle pump
    - Veins are situated between skeletal muscles which during contraction and relaxation help push the blood through the veins back toward the heart.
  - Respiratory pump
    - Pressure changes occur in the thorax and abdomen during exercise as breathing becomes faster.
    - This in turn increases pressure in the abdomen, and veins in that area get squeezed.
    - This forces the blood back into the heart.
  - Venous compliance
  - Gravity
    - Blood from the upper body above the heart gets drained by gravity, which helps blood flow back to the heart.
  - Total blood volume
    - Blood volume is directly proportional to venous return. As the blood volume increases, venous return also increases and vice versa.
  - Body position
    - There is peripheral pooling of blood in standing posture that decreases the venous return.

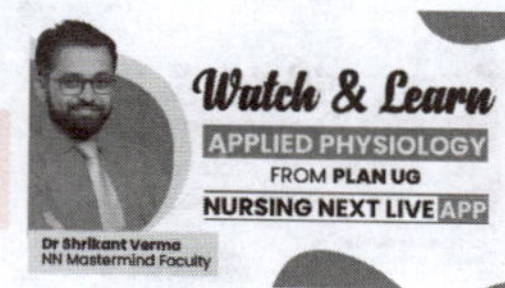

- Force of contraction
  - According to the Frank-Starling Law, before the onset of contraction, the force of contraction of heart is directly related to the initial length of muscle fibers.
  - Force of contraction depends upon preload and afterload.
- Heart rate
  - Heart rate is directly related to cardiac output provided all the other factors remain constant.
  - There is no alteration in cardiac output with moderate variation in heart rate.
  - Tremendous rise in heart rate increases cardiac output and vice versa.
- Peripheral resistance
  - It is a significant factor that maintains diastolic pressure.
  - Diastolic pressure is directly proportional to peripheral resistance.
  - Peripheral resistance is the resistance offered to the blood flow at the periphery.

Factors Affecting Contractility

- Sympathetic stimulation/catecholamines – increases
- Glucagon, digitalis, xanthine – increases
- Parasympathetic/vagal discharge – decreases
- Pathology MI, heart failure, hypoxia, acidosis, hyperkalemia and hypercapnia – decreases
- Anesthetics, barbiturates, quinidine and procainamide – decreases

Methods to Measure Cardiac Output

- Fick's principle

$$CO = \frac{VO_2}{O_2 \text{ art-} O_2 \text{ ven}}$$

Arterial O_2 = Hb × 1.34 × O_2 saturation
Venous O_2 = Mixed venous blood
VO_2 = Oxygen consumption

- Thermodilution

SHORT NOTES

1. Differences between central and peripheral cyanosis. (KUHS)

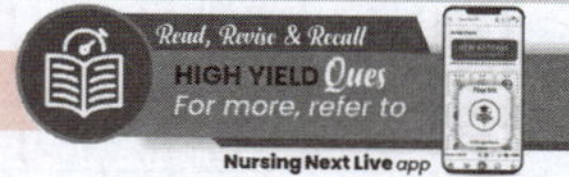

Answer

Central cyanosis	Peripheral cyanosis
It is due to diminished arterial oxygen saturation	Due to decreased blood flow to the local part
Usually present on skin and mucous membrane, like-tongue, lips, cheeks, etc.	Present on skin only
It is generalized	It is localized

2. Differences between systolic BP and diastolic BP. (KUHS)

Answer

Systolic BP	Diastolic BP
Maximum arterial pressure during the contraction of the left ventricle of the heart.	Minimum arterial pressure during the relaxation of the left ventricle of the heart.
Maximum blood pressure inside the arteries	Minimum blood pressure inside the arteries
Systolic pressure occurs when the left ventricle is contracted	Diastolic pressure occurs when the left ventricle is relaxed
Systolic pressure increases with the patient's age	Diastolic pressure decreases with age

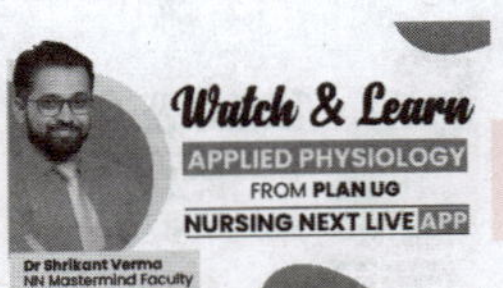

3. Differences between first and second heart sound. (KUHS)

Answer

First heart sound	Second heart sound
It is heard due to the closure of AV valves and marks the onset of ventricular systole	It is caused due to closure of semilunar valves and marks the onset of ventricular diastole
Character – Long, soft and low pitched, resembles the word LUBB	Character-short, sharp and high pitched resembles the word DUB
It is best heard over mitral and tricuspid areas It coincides with the peak of R wave in ECG	It is best heard over pulmonary and aortic area It coincides with peak of T wave in ECG

4. Normal ECG. (KUHS)

Answer

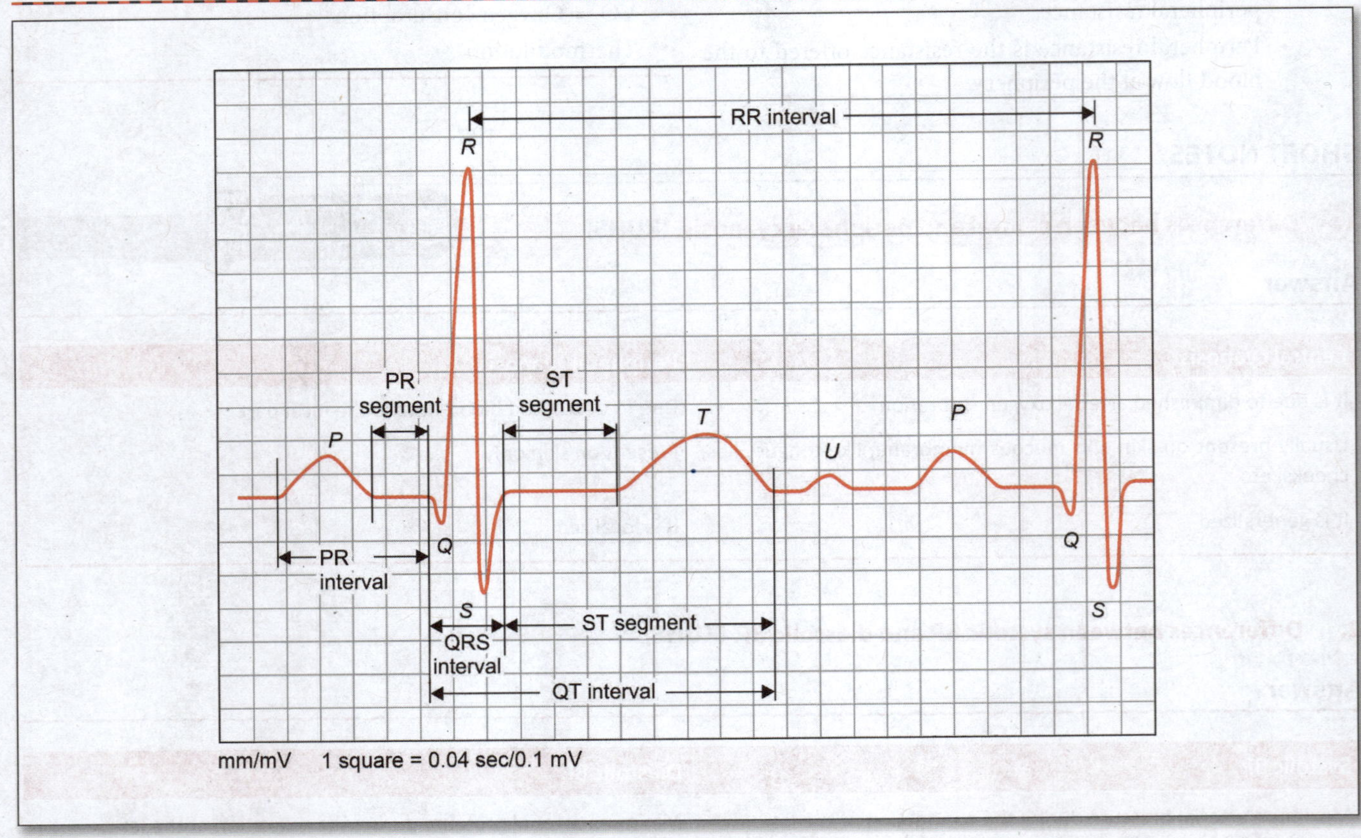

Figure 4.9: Normal ECG

- P wave – atrial depolarization, 0.5 mV, 0.1 sec
- QRS complex – ventricular depolarization, 0.08–0.12 sec
- T wave – ventricular repolarization, 0.5 mV, 0.27 sec
- U wave – repolarization of papillary muscle (slow/rare), 0.2 mV, 0.08 sec
- Q wave – depolarization of intraventricular septum, 0.2 mV, 0.04 sec
- R wave – depolarization of intraventricular septum and apex of both ventricles, 2.5 mV
- S wave – depolarization of base of ventricles

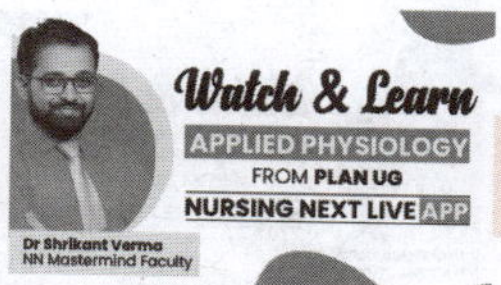

SHORT ANSWER QUESTIONS

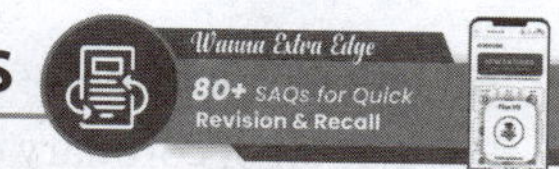

1. Name the leads of electrocardiogram. (MGR)

Answer

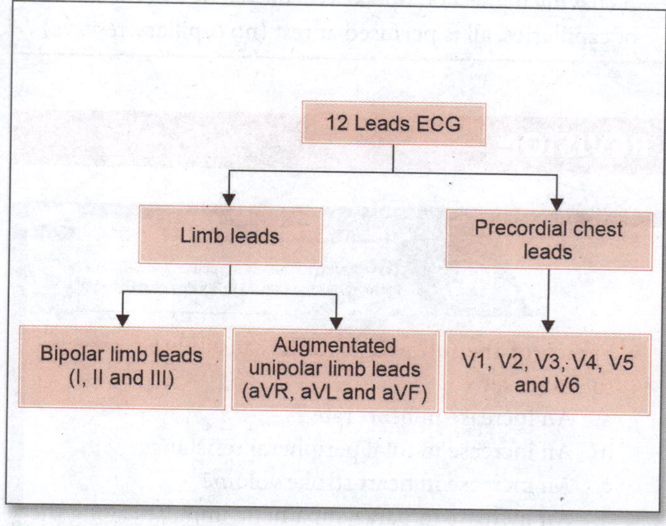

2. Name the pacemaker of heart. (MGR)

Answer

The pacemaker of the heart is a specialized group of cells called the sinoatrial node (SA node) that generates electrical impulses to initiate each heartbeat.

3. Define cardiac output. (MGR)

Answer

Cardiac output is defined as the amount of blood pumped by the heart per minute.

Cardiac output = Heart rate (HR) × Stroke volume (SV)

4. Mention two uses of ECG.

Answer

Two uses of ECG

1. Electrocardiogram (ECG) is a noninvasive diagnostic tool used to evaluate the electrical activity of the heart.
2. ECG is also used to monitor the cardiac function of patients with heart conditions.

5. Draw a diagram of conducting system of heart. (MGR)

Answer

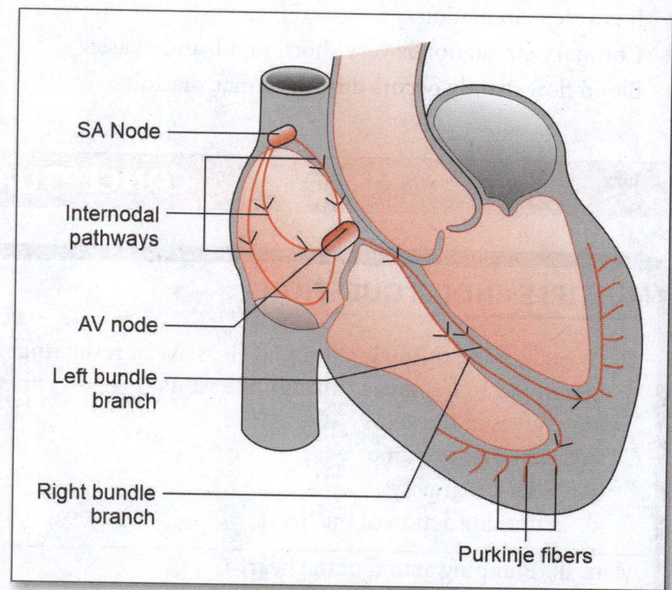

6 Define pulse. (MGR)

Answer

The cardiac pulse is the rhythmic contraction and relaxation of the heart muscles that create a wave of pressure in the arteries.

7. Define arterial blood pressure. (MGR)

Answer

Arterial blood pressure refers to the pressure exerted by the blood against the walls of the arteries as it circulates through the body.

Blood pressure = Systolic blood pressure
Diastolic blood pressure
= 120/80

8. Define cyanosis. (MGR)

Answer

Cyanosis is a medical disorder that causes bluish or purplish coloring of the skin and mucous membranes as a result of low oxygen saturation in the blood.

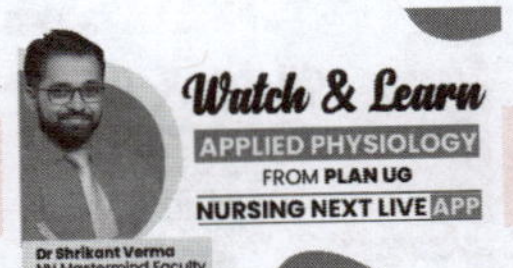

9. Special features of coronary circulation. (KUHS)

Answer

Special features of coronary circulation are:

- It is a rich circulation
- Coronary circulation is very short, rapid, and phasic.
- Blood flow mainly occurs during cardiac diastole.
- No efficient anastomoses between the coronary vessels.
- Regulation of coronary circulation is mainly by metabolites
- Capillary permeability is high (the cardiac lymph is rich in protein)
- Vessels are susceptible to degeneration and atherosclerosis.
- As having highest O_2 uptake is achieved by a dense network of capillaries, all is perfused at rest (no capillary reserve)

CONCEPTUAL REVISION

MULTIPLE CHOICE QUESTIONS

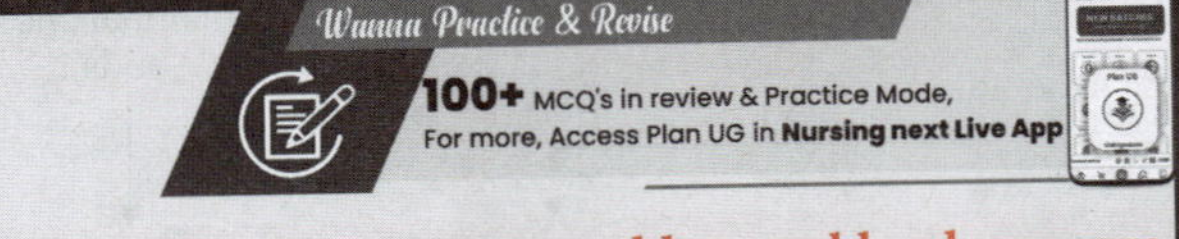

1. Which of the following does NOT assist in returning the blood to the heart through the veins?
a. Valves in the veins
b. Respiratory pump
c. Effect of gravity
d. Pumping action of the heart

Ans. d. Pumping action of the heart

2. What will cause the sinoatrial (SA) node to depolarize more frequently?
a. Acetylcholine
b. Norepinephrine
c. Parasympathetic stimulation
d. Vagus nerve

Ans. b. Norepinephrine

3. Which period of the heart cycle is completely occupied by the ventricles contracting?
a. Atrial systole
b. Atrial diastole
c. Ventricular systole
d. Ventricular diastole

Ans. c. Ventricular systole

4. Blood flow through the heart follows which of the sequences listed below?
a. From left atrium, then mitral valve, right ventricle, aorta, left ventricle
b. From right atrium, then mitral valve, right ventricle, pulmonary trunk, left ventricle.
c. From pulmonary trunk, then tricuspid valve, left atrium, aortic valve, aorta
d. From vena cava, then right ventricle, pulmonary trunk, left ventricle, aorta.

Ans. d. From vena cava, then right ventricle, pulmonary trunk, left ventricle, aorta

5. Which of the following would cause blood pressure to decrease?
a. An increase in heart rate
b. An increase in total peripheral resistance
c. An increase in heart stroke volume
d. An increase in parasympathetic impulses along the vagus nerve

Ans. d. An increase in parasympathetic impulses along the vagus nerve

6. The "systemic circulation" refers to which of the following?
a. The movement of blood from the pulmonary trunk, through capillaries into the pulmonary veins
b. The movement of blood into the coronary arteries, through capillaries into the coronary sinus
c. The flow of blood into the right atrium and eventually out of the left ventricle
d. The movement of blood from the aorta, through capillaries, then eventually into the vena cava

Ans. d. The movement of blood from the aorta, through capillaries, then eventually into the vena cava

7. If Sarah has a stroke volume of 70 mL and a cardiac output of 5950 mL/min, which of the following is her heart rate (in beats/min)?
a. 70
b. 75
c. 80
d. 85

Ans. d. 85

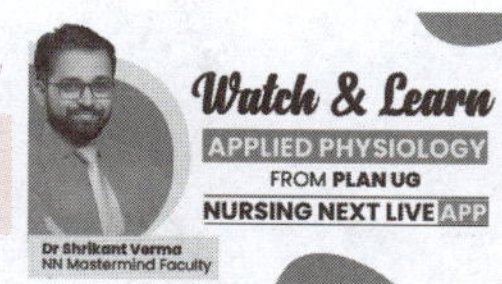

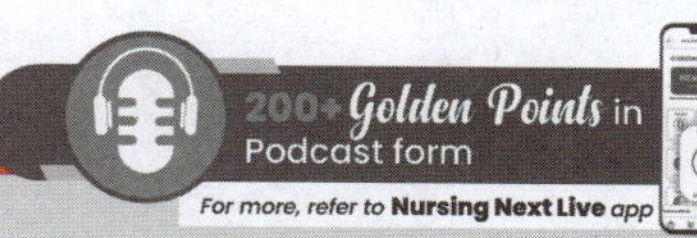

Golden Points

- Blood circulation between right ventricle and left atrium through lungs is known as **pulmonary circulation**.
  Blood pressure = Cardiac output × Peripheral resistance.
- Blood pressure is defined as the lateral pressure exerted by column of blood on the walls of blood vessels. Venous pressure is less than arterial pressure.
- Cardiovascular homeostasis refers to the maintenance of stable physiological conditions within the cardiovascular system. This homeostasis is particularly important during exercise and changes in posture.
- Circulation between left ventricle and right atrium through the tissues of upper limb, head, neck, brain and thorax, abdomen and lower limb is called systemic circulation.
- Circulatory system consists of heart, which acts as a pump and closed blood vessels.
- Contraction of the left ventricle during systole pushes blood into the arterial system. The pressure produced by this contraction is called the systolic blood pressure (SBP).
- During systole, the elastic artery expands to accommodate increased amount of blood. During diastole of the heart, there is elastic recoil of the artery, so there is continuous blood flow to the peripheral parts of the body.
- Heart rate is directly proportional to cardiac output.
- Long-term control of blood pressure is due to regulation of blood volume by kidneys, and renin-angiotensin-aldosterone system.
- Measurement of Blood Pressure is done by two methods - *Palpatory and Auscultatory*
- Pacemaker and the conducting system of the heart are formed of the sinoatrial node, the atrioventricular node, the bundle of His, and the Purkinje system.
- Pulse is felt by slightly compressing an artery against an underlying bone or flat muscle by the three middle digits.
- Pulse is usually felt in the radial, brachial, carotids, femoral and dorsalis pedis arteries.
- Sequence of events from one beat to the next is known as cardiac cycle. Its duration is 0.8 seconds.
- Short-term control of blood pressure is due to baroreceptor reflex and chemoreceptors, higher centers and circulating hormones.
- The blood pumped out by each ventricle in each systole is called stroke volume.
- The cardiovascular system's primary duties include supplying nutrition and oxygen as well as removing metabolic waste.
- The electrical changes in the heart can be easily recorded by electrodes placed on the body surface.

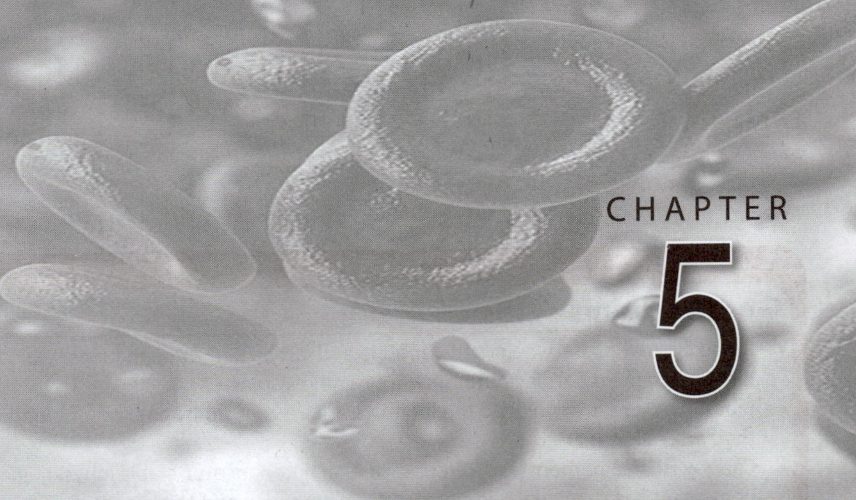

CHAPTER 5

Blood

CONCEPTUAL THEORY

Terminology

Blood bank: A bank where blood of different groups is stored.
Blood: Blood is described as a specialized connective tissue that transports oxygen and nutrients to the body cells and tissues and carries carbon dioxide and waste products from them.
Eryptosis: Process of removal of RBC after 120 days.
Erythropoiesis: Erythropoiesis is the process of red blood cell formation. It begins with the differentiation of hematopoietic stem cells into erythroid progenitor cells.
Erythropoietin: Hormone produced by kidney that is released during hypoxia.
Hematopoietic stem cells (HSC): All blood cells develop from the progenitor cells called HSC.
Leukopoiesis: Leukopoiesis is the process of white blood cell formation. It involves the differentiation of hematopoietic stem cells into myeloid or lymphoid progenitor cells.
Plasma: Blood minus the cellular components is plasma. (Made of water and solids)
Platelets: Thrombocytes they are small fragments that helps in clotting process.
RBC: Red blood cells
Red bone marrow: Cavities in the bones, like humerus, and femur where RBC, WBC and platelets are produced.
Thrombopoiesis: Thrombopoiesis is the process of platelet formation. It begins with the differentiation of hematopoietic stem cells into megakaryocytes in the bone marrow.
WBC: White blood cells
Yellow bone marrow: After puberty, red bone marrow in many bones is replaced by fat and is called yellow bone marrow. Red bone marrow only remains in the ends of long bones, sternum, iliac crest and skull bones.

BLOOD

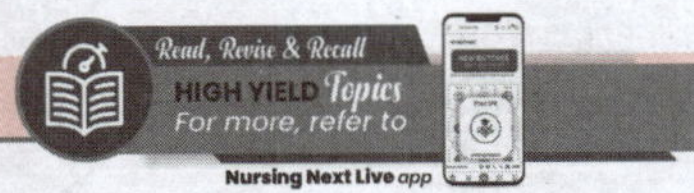

- Blood is described as a specialized connective tissue that transports oxygen and nutrients to the body cells and tissues and carries carbon dioxide and waste products from them.
- It consists of liquid intercellular substances known as plasma and formed elements, like red blood cells, white blood cells and platelets.

Functions of Blood

- Blood acts as a transportation system.
- Blood helps regulate several physiological processes.
- Blood regulates water balance and prevents excessive fluid loss or retention.
- Blood plays a crucial role in the immune response.
- Blood also contains antibodies and other immune components that help neutralize and eliminate foreign substances and toxins.

Physical characteristics	Descriptions
Composition	Cellular components: red blood cells (erythrocytes), white blood cells (leukocytes), platelets (thrombocytes)
	Fluid component: Plasma (water, electrolytes, proteins, hormones, nutrients, waste products)
Color	Oxygenated blood: bright red
	Deoxygenated blood: darker, bluish-red

Contd...

Physical characteristics	Descriptions
pH	Slightly alkaline, ranging from 7.35 to 7.45
Viscosity	Higher viscosity than water
Temperature	Slightly higher than body temperature (around 37°C or 98.6°F)
Volume	Varies based on factors such as age, gender, and body size
	Average adult blood volume: 4–6 L, approximately 7–8% of total body weight

Erythropoiesis

- The process of production of RBCs is referred to as erythropoiesis.
- It starts in 3rd week of IUL and continues as long as a person remains alive.

Functions of Red Blood Cells (RBCs)

- Oxygen transport
- Carbon dioxide transport
- Acid-base balance
- Oxygen release
- Flexible shape

Lifespan of red blood cells (RBCs): The lifespan of RBCs varies, but on average, it is around 120 days (approximately 3–4 months).

WBC—Types, Functions

White blood cell (WBC)	Function
Neutrophils	• Phagocytosis: Engulf and destroy pathogens and cellular debris
	• First line of defense against bacterial infections
Eosinophils	• Defense against parasites
	• Modulate allergic reactions
	• Phagocytosis of antigen-antibody complexes
Basophils	• Release histamine and other inflammatory mediators
	• Play a role in allergic reactions and hypersensitivity responses
Monocytes	• Phagocytosis: Engulf and destroy pathogens and cellular debris
	• Present antigens to T cells for immune response activation
Lymphocytes	• Adaptive immune response: Produce antibodies (B cells) or coordinate immune response (T cells)
	• Recognize and destroy infected or abnormal cells
	• Provide long-term immunity against specific pathogens

Platelets—Function and Production of Platelets

Platelets, also known as thrombocytes, are small, disc-shaped cell fragments that play a crucial role in blood clotting and hemostasis.

Function of Platelets

- Platelets are essential for the formation of blood clots, which help control bleeding and promote wound healing.
- Platelets contribute to the coagulation cascade, a complex process involving various proteins and enzymes.
- Platelets contain various growth factors, such as platelet-derived growth factor (PDGF) and transforming growth factor-beta (TGF-β). These growth factors play a role in tissue repair and regeneration by stimulating cell proliferation and promoting wound healing.

Clotting Mechanism

- The clotting mechanism of blood, also known as hemostasis, involves a series of complex interactions among various components in the blood to form a blood clot.
- There are three main stages in the clotting mechanism: vascular spasm, platelet plug formation, and coagulation cascade.

Clotting Time

- Clotting time refers to the time it takes for blood to form a clot after an injury.
- The normal clotting time is typically around 6 to 10 minutes.

Bleeding Time

- Bleeding time is a test that measures the time it takes for bleeding to stop after a standardized skin puncture.
- It evaluates the overall hemostatic function, including platelet function and the formation of a platelet plug.
- The normal bleeding time is typically around 2 to 7 minutes.

Partial Thromboplastin Time (PTT)

- PTT measures the time it takes for plasma to clot after the addition of an activator.
- It evaluates the function of various clotting factors involved in the intrinsic pathway.
- The normal range for PTT can vary depending on the laboratory, but it is typically around 25 to 35 seconds.

Coagulation Factors

Factor I – Fibrinogen
Factor II – Prothrombin
Factor III – Tissue thromboplastin
Factor IV – Calcium
Factor V – Proaccelerin

Factor VII – Proconvertin
Factor VIII – Antihemophilic factor
Factor IX – Plasma thromboplastin C
Factor X – Stuart-Prower factor
Factor XI – Plasma thromboplastin antecedent (PTA)
Factor XII – Hageman factor
Factor XIII – Fibrin stabilizing factor

Blood Groups

- Antigenic determinants present in human RBCs.
- The foremost vital blood groups determined before blood transfusions include:
  - Classical ABO blood groups
  - Rhesus (Rh) blood group
  - M and N Blood group ABO Blood Groups
- Landsteiner, a Nobel Prize laureate, discovered the ABO blood group system (1900–1901)
- Determined by ABO gene, located on chromosome 9
- ABO blood group system supported the presence or absence of substance A and substance B
- Blood groups are split into four types:
  1. 'A' group
  2. 'B' group
  3. 'AB' group
  4. 'O' group

Biochemical Basis of ABO Blood Group

- A and B antigens are carbohydrate groups bound to lipids.
- The specificity of antigen is based on the terminal sugar of carbohydrate.
- The one or two terminal sugar added to the substance determines the blood group.

Blood group	Antigens present in the RBC	Antibodies present in serum	Genotype
A	A antigen	Anti-B	AA or AO
B	B antigen	Anti-A	BB or BO
AB	A antigen and B antigen	None	AB
O	None	Anti-A and Anti-B	OO

Functions of Reticuloendothelial System, Immunity

- The reticuloendothelial system (RES), also known as the mononuclear phagocyte system (MPS), is a network of cells and tissues involved in various functions related to immunity and the clearance of foreign substances.
- The RES includes cells such as macrophages, monocytes, and dendritic cells, as well as tissues like the liver, spleen, bone marrow, and lymph nodes.
- Key functions of the reticuloendothelial system:
  - Phagocytosis
  - Immune surveillance
  - Clearance of old, damaged, or senescent red blood cells, as well as other cellular debris.
  - Plays a vital role in the metabolism and detoxification of various substances.

Immunity

The capability of the human body to resist all types of infections is immunity.

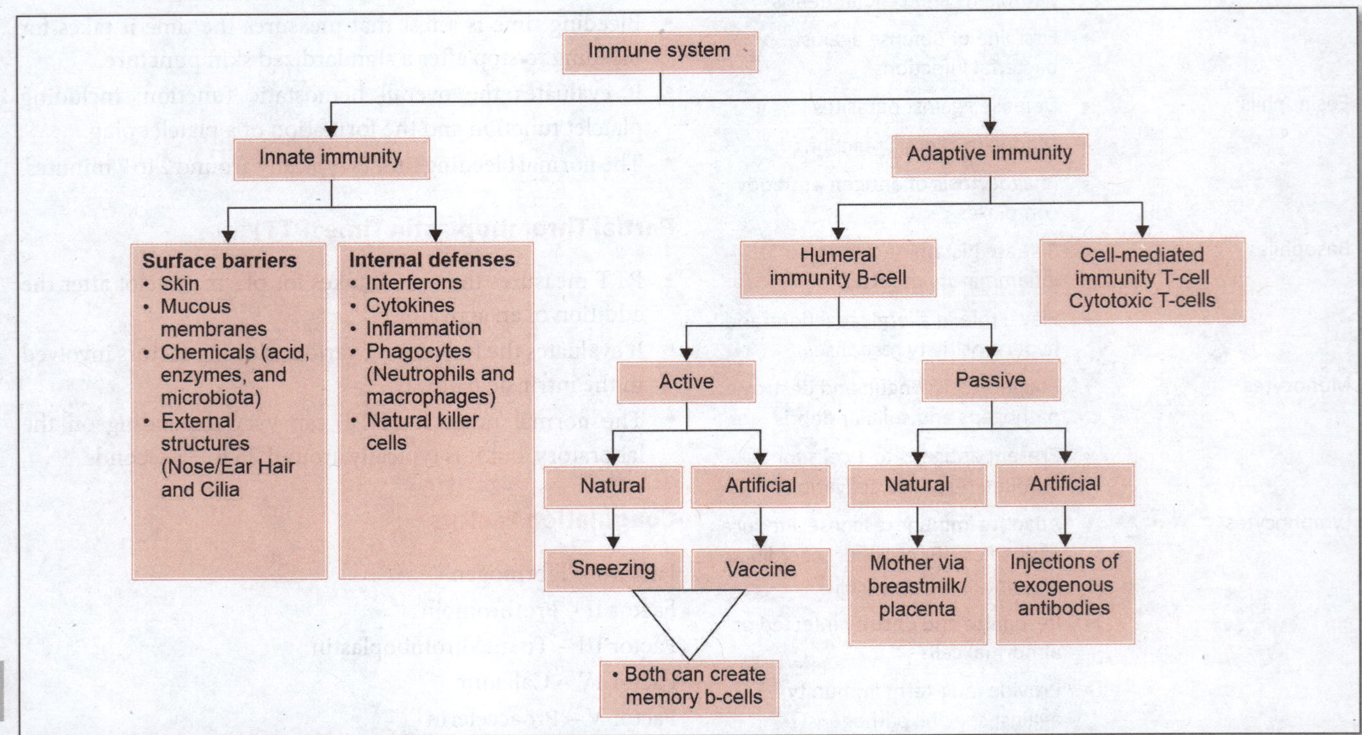

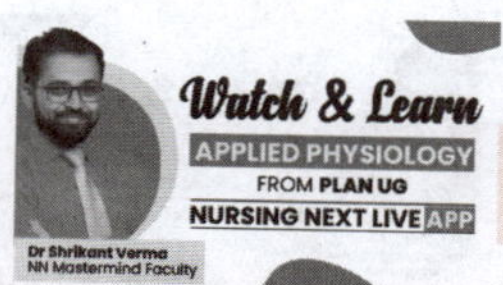

CONCEPTUAL EXERCISES

LONG ANSWER QUESTIONS

1. Write about various functions of blood. (MGR)

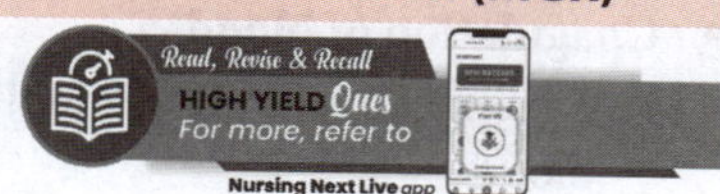

Answer

Blood

- Blood is described as a specialized connective tissue that transports oxygen and nutrients to the body cells and tissues, and carries carbon dioxide and waste products from them.
- It consists of liquid intercellular substances known as plasma and formed elements, like red blood cells, white blood cells and platelets.

Functions of Blood

Blood is a vital fluid. It performs the following functions:

Table 5.1: Functions of blood

Nutrition and hormones	It carries digested food material absorbed from the intestine to the tissue cells for utilization.
It acts as a vehicle	By its help, the hormones, the vitamins and other essential chemicals are brought to their places of activity.
Drainage of waste products	It carries the waste products of cellular activity.
Maintenance of water balance	Maintains 'Water balance' of the body.
Maintenance of acid-base equilibrium	It maintains acid-base equilibrium by its efficient buffering power (e.g., plasma proteins, reduced and oxidized hemoglobin, etc.) and with the help of kidney, skin and lungs.
Maintenance of ion balance	It maintains balance between the cells and the surrounding fluid.
Regulation of body temperature	The water content of blood possesses various qualities which make it very suitable for this purpose.
Defensive action	Blood acts as a great defensive mechanism.
Coagulation	By the property of coagulation it guards against hemorrhage.
Transportation	Carries oxygen from the lungs to the cells of the body and transports the carbon dioxide produced during cell metabolism from the cells back to lungs. Transports nutrients, hormones and waste products.
Regulation and maintenance	Maintenance of body temperature is done by: Plasma can absorb or give off heat. Speed at which the blood is flowing Expansion and constriction of the blood vessels affect the speed of blood flow, thereby affecting the heat loss.

Contd...

2. Describe the plasma proteins. (MGR)

Answer

Introduction

Plasma contains several types of proteins and these are serum albumin, serum globulin, fibrinogen, etc.

- Total concentration of plasma proteins–6–8 g/dL

Types of Plasma Proteins

- Albumin
- Globulin
- Fibrinogen
- Prothrombin

Serum Albumin

- Normal range – 3.4–5.5 g/dL (average 4.8 g/dL)
- Synthesized exclusively in liver
- Half-life – 20 days
- **Functions of albumin**
  - Osmotic function
    - Contributes to 75–80% of the total plasma osmotic pressure due to:
      - High concentration
      - Low molecular weight
      - Maintains blood volume and body fluid distribution
    - Decrease in plasma albumin results in
      - Fall in osmotic pressure
      - Fluid retention in fluid spaces
      - Edema
    - Transport function
      - Binds to several compounds such as free fatty acids, bilirubin, steroid hormones, calcium and copper; and aid in their transportation in the circulation
    - Nutritive function
      - Source of amino acids for tissue protein synthesis
    - Buffering action
      - Among the proteins, albumin has maximum buffering capacity

- **Clinical significance**
  - Binding of albumin to certain compounds prevents them from crossing the blood-brain barrier.
  - Hypoalbuminemia is seen in malnutrition; and nephrotic syndrome and cirrhosis are associated with edema.
  - Excretion of albumin in urine – albuminuria and microalbuminuria – helps in diagnosis and predicting the future risk of renal diseases.
  - Therapeutically useful for the treatment of burns and hemorrhage.

Globulins

- 2–3.5 g/dL
- Electrophoretically separated into:
  - α1 globulin
  - α2 globulin
  - β globulin
  - γ globulin

Alpha 1 Globulins

- Glycoproteins
- α1 antitrypsin – serine protease inhibitor
- α1 Lipoproteins – Transports cholesterol and phospholipids
- Retinol-binding proteins – transports vitamin A
- Thyroxine-binding globulin – transports thyroid hormones

Alpha 2 Globulin

- α2- macroglobulin – antitrypsin and antiplasmin activity
- Haptoglobins – bind with plasma free hemoglobin and prevent its excretion
- Prothrombin – participates in blood coagulation
- Ceruloplasmin – transport of copper

Beta Globulin

- Beta lipoproteins – transport triacylglycerols and cholesterol
- Transferrin – transports iron
- Hemopexin – transports heme
- Plasminogen – forms plasmin

γ Globulin

Immunoglobulins – Antibody functions

Fibrinogen

- Fibrinogen – 200–450 mg/dL
- Participates in blood coagulation

Prothrombin

- Normal range—40 mg/dL
- Participates in blood coagulation

Functions of Plasma Proteins

- **Coagulation of blood**
  - Fibrinogen and prothrombin help in the coagulation of blood.
- **Auxiliary transport**
  - Plasma proteins transport thyroxin.
  - Transport fatty acids, bilirubin, calcium and drugs.
  - Bind with plasma free hemoglobin and help in copper transport.
  - Help carbon dioxide carriage by forming carbamino proteins.
- **Protective function**
  - Globulin and antitrypsin combine with elastase, trypsin and thus, protect hydrolytic damage of tissues like lungs.
  - IgA and IgM globulins protect the body surface humoral immunity and act as first line of defense in humoral immunity and sensitivity.
- **Osmotic regulation**
  - Pressure exerted by proteins in blood plasma that usually pulls water into circulatory system and prevents edema.
  - Albumin has the smallest size and most symmetrical molecule, it exerts maximum osmotic pressure.
- **Maintains viscosity and blood pressure**
  - The plasma proteins, mainly globulins due to larger molecules and asymmetry of their structures, are responsible to some extent for the viscosity of blood. Viscosity is an important factor in maintaining blood pressure which is essential for efficient heart action.
- **Immunological function**
  - Complement activation – leading to lysis of microorganisms.
- **Buffering action**
  - Act in maintaining acid-base balance.

3. Define erythropoiesis. Describe in detail the stages of erythropoiesis. Add a note on maturation factors. (MGR)

Answer

Introduction

- The process of production of RBCs is referred to as erythropoiesis.
- It starts in 3rd week of IUL and continues as long as a person remains alive.

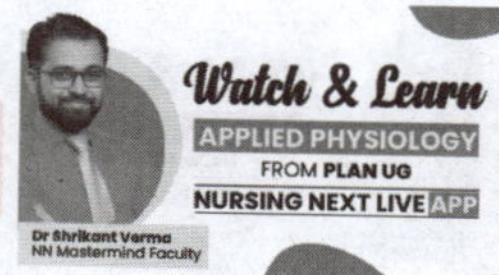

Stages of Erythropoiesis

- The various stages between stem cell and matured red blood cell are as follows:
  - Hemocytoblast
    - A big cell, 18–23 mm in diameter, with a large nucleus and a thin rim of deep basophilic cytoplasm.
  - Proerythroblast
    - 14–19 mm in diameter, basophilic cytoplasm, a large nucleus with distinct nucleoli and reticulum of fine chromatin threads.
    - Hemoglobin absent
    - Nuclear to cytoplasmic ratio high
    - Immature nuclear chromatin
    - 1–2 nucleoli
    - Basophilic cytoplasm
  - Early normoblast
    - Smaller in size
    - Nucleus is 11–17 mm
    - Chromatin is dense
    - Nucleoli are absent or rudimentary
    - Basophilic cytoplasm
  - Intermediate normoblast
    - Round nucleus with mature chromatin
    - Nucleoli absent
    - Cytoplasm is greyish in color due to hemoglobin synthesis occurring at this stage.
    - Cytoplasm is polychromatic
  - Late normoblast
    - Large 7–10 mm
    - Nucleus is very dense and pyknotic
    - Hemoglobin increases
  - Reticulocyte
    - Late erythroblasts extrude nuclei to become reticulocytes when stained with vital stain, these cells show a net-like structure in the cytoplasm.
  - Matured erythrocyte
    - Matured RBC is small, round and biconcave disk and appears like dumbbell.

Proerythroblast: High nuclear to cytoplasmic ratio, immature nuclear chromatin, 1–2 nucleoli, basophilic cytoplasm.

Early normoblast: High nuclear to cytoplasmic ratio, chromatin condenses, no nucleoli, basophilic cytoplasm.

Intermediate normoblast: Round nucleus with mature (clumped chromatin), no nucleoli, cytoplasm is greyish in color due to hemoglobin synthesis occurring at this stage. Cell division ceases at this stage.

Late normoblast: Pyknotic nucleus with well hemoglobinized cytoplasm (reddish).

Reticulocyte: Late erythroblast extrudes nuclei to become reticulocyte. Intermediate position between nucleated RBCs and and mature red blood cells. Has bluish tinge due to RNSs.

Mature RBCs: Size of a mature lymphocyte nucleus. Lack nucleus. Has central pallor 1/3rd the diameter of the cell.

Figure 5.1: Stages of Erythropoiesis

Factors Influencing Erythropoiesis

- **Erythropoietin**
  - Glycoprotein hormone is secreted by the kidneys and liver
  - Stimulates CFU-E to proliferate and differentiate to form pronormoblast
  - Deficiency results in the decreased RBC formation
- **Hemopoietic growth factors**
  - Include cytokines, interleukins, GM-CSF, etc.
  - Help in the differentiation of blood cells
- **Maturation factors**
  - Include vitamins, proteins, minerals and trace metals.
- **Hormones**
  - Androgens such as testosterone, thyroid hormones, catecholamines and growth hormone stimulate erythropoietin and thus, RBC proliferation.
- **Factors necessary for hemoglobin formation**
  - Various materials are essential for the formation of hemoglobin in the RBCs. Deficiency of these substances decreases the production of hemoglobin leading to anemia.
- **Maturation factors**
  - Vitamin B_{12} and folic acid are essential for the synthesis of DNA in the RBCs—hence, the maturation of the blast cells.
- In the absence or deficiency of vitamin B_{12} and folic acid, the blast cells are unable to divide and mature. The cellular content increases without the differentiation of the cells giving rise to megaloblasts (proerythroblast). This type of anemia is known as megaloblastic anemia.
- Also in deficiency of vitamin B_{12} and folic acid, the synthesis of DNA decreases leading to failure of maturation.
- Vitamin C is required for the absorption of iron from the gut.

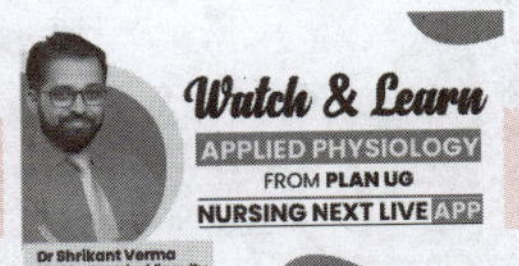

- Other vitamins required are:
  - Vitamin B_6
  - Thiamine
  - Nicotinic acid
- Proteins are required for the synthesis of globin and stroma of RBC.
- Minerals like iron, copper, cobalt, nickel, manganese and zinc, etc. are also required for erythropoiesis.
- Intrinsic factor of Castle
  - It is produced in the gastric mucosa of parietal cells of the gastric glands.
  - It is essential for the absorption of vitamin B_{12} from the intestine.
  - In the absence of intrinsic factor, vitamin B_{12} is not absorbed from the intestine.
  - This leads to pernicious anemia.
  - Deficiency of intrinsic factor occurs in severe gastritis, ulcer and gastrectomy.

4. Describe blood under the following heads: (KUHS)

a. **Composition of blood**
b. **Blood groups**
c. **Process of blood coagulation**
d. **Note on hemophilia**

Answer

Introduction

- Blood is described as a specialized connective tissue that transports oxygen and nutrients to the body cells and tissues and carries carbon dioxide and waste products from them.
- It consists of liquid intercellular substances known as plasma and formed elements, like red blood cells, white blood cells and platelets.

Composition of Blood

Blood is a connective tissue—so cells suspended in extracellular matrix—is the general composition of the blood like any other connective tissue of the body.

Extracellular matrix in blood is formed by the plasma; and the cells present in blood are red and white blood cells and platelets. Blood is made up of about 55% blood plasma and about 45% consists of different types of blood cells.

- **Cellular component**
  - Red blood corpuscles or erythrocytes
    - Disc-shaped cells.
    - Anucleate
    - Red color is due to the red pigment known as hemoglobin
    - Hemoglobin binds to oxygen and carries it to different body cells.
    - Also have a role in maintaining the pH of the blood-buffering action
    - Lifespan—120 days
  - White blood corpuscles or leukocytes
    - Nucleated cells
    - Don't contain hemoglobin
    - Types of WBCs include:
      - Granulocytes—contain granules
        - Monocytes
        - Lymphocytes
      - Agranulocytes—don't contain granules
    - Role and function:
      - Play a role in immunity
      - Role in allergic reactions
    - Lifespan is from a few hours to several days.
  - Platelets or thrombocytes
    - Don't contain nucleus
    - Important role in blood clotting and formation of platelet plug.
    - Lifespan – 5–9 days
- Extracellular matrix or Plasma
  - Obtained from blood after centrifugation/or addition of anticoagulant—cells settle down
  - Water—91–92% and solids—8–9%
  - Inorganic constituents (0.1%):
    - These constitute 0.9% sodium, potassium, calcium, magnesium, phosphorus, iron and copper, etc.
  - Organic constituents (8%):
    - **Proteins (7%):** Serum albumin, serum globulin, fibrinogen and prothrombin, etc.
    - Nonprotein nitrogenous (NPN) substances (1%): Urea, uric acid, xanthine, hypoxanthine, creatine, creatinine, ammonia and amino acids, etc.
    - **Carbohydrate:** Glucose, etc.
    - **Fats:** Neutral fats, phospholipid, cholesterol and cholesterides, etc.
    - **Other substances:** Internal secretions, antibodies and various enzymes.

b. **Blood groups**

Answer

Blood Groups

- Antigenic determinants present in human RBCs.
- The foremost vital blood groups determined before blood transfusions include:
  - Classical ABO blood groups
  - Rhesus (Rh) blood group
  - M and N Blood group ABO Blood Groups

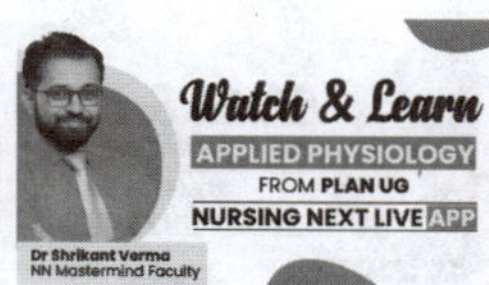

- Landsteiner, a Nobel Prize laureate, discovered the ABO blood group system (1900–1901)
- Determined by ABO gene, located on chromosome 9
- ABO blood group system supported the presence or absence of substance A and substance B
- Blood groups are split into four types:
  - 'A' group
  - 'B' group
  - 'AB' group
  - 'O' group

Biochemical Basis of ABO Blood Group

- A and B antigens are carbohydrate groups bound to lipids.
- The specificity of antigen is based on the terminal sugar of carbohydrate.
- The one or two terminal sugar added to the substance determines the blood group.

Blood group	Antigens present in the RBC	Antibodies present in serum	Genotype
A	A antigen	Anti-B	AA or AO
B	B antigen	Anti-A	BB or BO
AB	A antigen and B antigen	None	AB
O	None	Anti-A and Anti-B	OO

c. Process of blood coagulation

Answer

Coagulation

- Coagulation of blood or clotting of blood is a part of Hemostasis.
- Hemostasis consists of two terms: "hemo" meaning "blood" and "stasis" meaning "standing still". Thus, hemostasis is a term for how the body stops bleeding. The process of hemostasis consists of primary hemostasis and secondary hemostasis.
- Primary hemostasis means the formation of temporary platelet plug which temporarily seals the bleeding site.
- Secondary hemostasis consists of coagulation of blood and the formation of a permanent clot that seals the bleeding site.

Process of Secondary Hemostasis/Blood Coagulation

- The procoagulants present in the blood get activated when there is an injury or trauma to the blood vessels. This occurs in three steps:
  - Formation of prothrombin activator
  - Conversion of prothrombin into thrombin
  - Conversion of fibrinogen into fibrin fibers

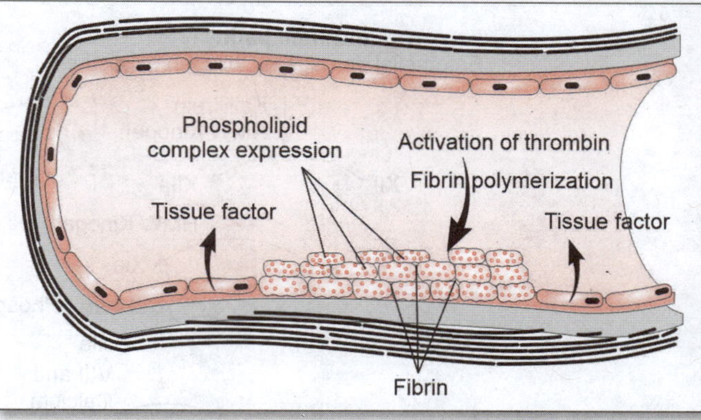

Figure 5.2: Secondary hemostasis

Steps

- **Step 1:** Formation of prothrombin activator
  - This is where the initiation of coagulation occurs. Here, the activation of procoagulants occurs due to injury to blood vessels or tissue trauma by intrinsic or extrinsic mechanisms.
  - Prothrombin activator is responsible for the conversion of prothrombin into thrombin.
  - Formation of prothrombin activator is by two mechanisms—intrinsic and extrinsic.
  - **Intrinsic mechanism:** This occurs due to exposure of collagen due to capillary endothelium. This causes activation of Hageman factor (XII) along with HMWK (high molecular weight kininogen) and Prekallikrein.
  - **Extrinsic mechanism:** This is initiated when there is tissue trauma due to which tissue thromboplastin or tissue factor (III) is released which causes activation of stable factor or Proconvertin (VII).
  - Activated factor X (Stuart-Prower factor) and activated factor V (labile factor) along with calcium together form prothrombin activator which converts prothrombin into thrombin. This is a common step of both intrinsic and extrinsic pathways.
- **Step 2:** Conversion of prothrombin into thrombin
- **Step 3:** Conversion of fibrinogen into fiber
  - Thrombin, which is proteolytic, converts fibrinogen into fibrin monomer
  - This fibrin monomer forms fibrin fibers which are stabilized by fibrin stabilizing factor (XIII), thrombin and calcium.
- **Step 4:** Clot retraction
  - This begins in two hours and is completed within 24 hours
  - This is the reason why an injured blood vessel does not remain clogged for a long time.
  - This occurs due to fibrin stabilizing factor, calcium and contraction of platelets.
  - The process of clotting ends with clot retraction.

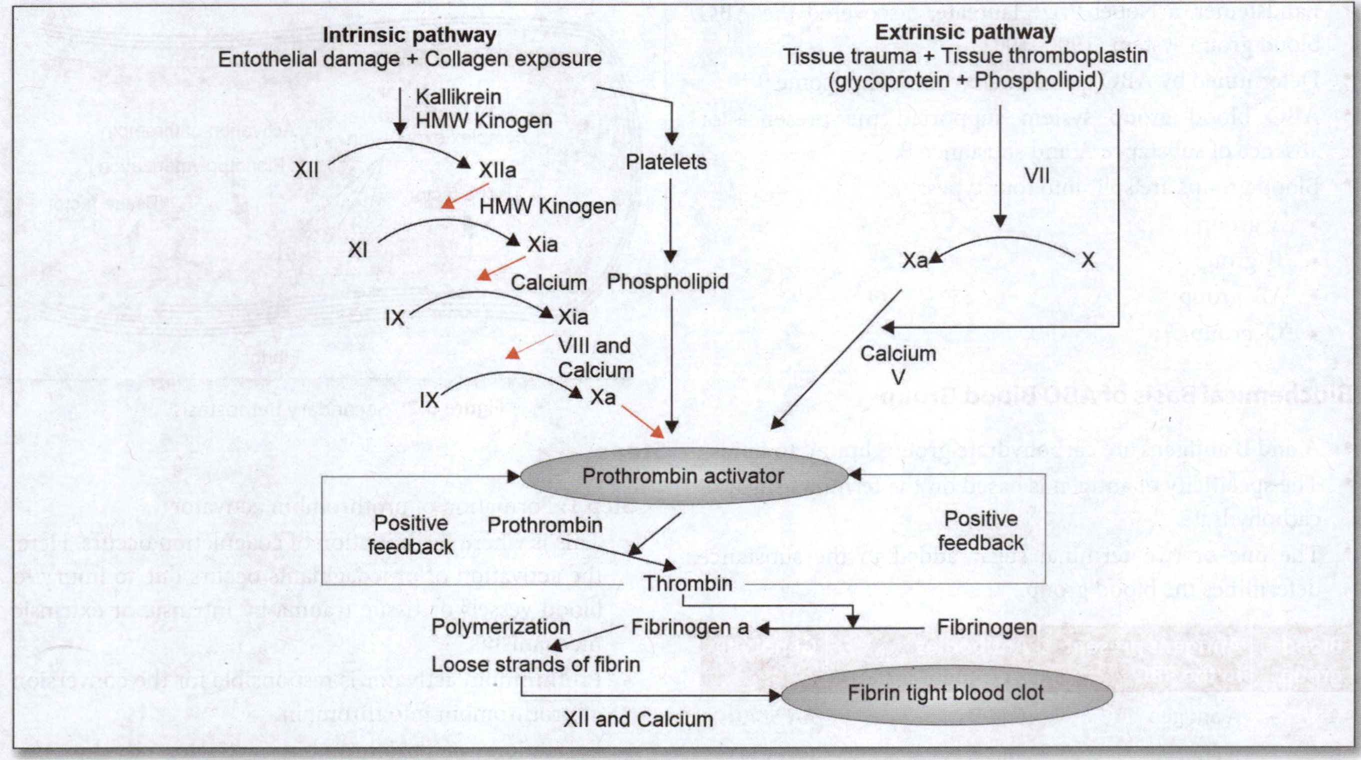

Figure 5.3 Coagulation cascade

d. **Note on hemophilia**

Answer

Hemophilia

- Hemophilia is the hereditary deficiency of coagulation factors. Due to the deficiency of coagulation factors in hemophilia, clotting time increases, whereas the bleeding time remains normal.
- **Types**
  - Hemophilia A or classical hemophilia due to factor VIII deficiency.
  - Hemophilia B due to deficiency of Factor IX or Christmas factor also known as Christmas disease.
  - Hemophilia C due to deficiency of Factor XI.
- **Inheritance**
  - Hemophilia A and B are X-linked recessive.
  - Hemophilia has Mendelian dominant inheritance.
- **Clinical features**
  - Excessive bleeding after trivial trauma. There can be episodes of spontaneous bleeds.
  - Bleeding in soft tissues, GIT, upper respiratory tract, urinary tract and joints
  - Joint damage due to recurrent hemorrhages
- **Treatment**
  - Fresh frozen plasma rich in factors VIII, IX or XI.
  - Cryoprecipitate of factor VIII.

5. Define Landsteiner's Law. Explain ABO blood grouping system. Add to a note on erythroblastosis fetalis. (MGR)

Answer

Landsteiner's Law

The presence of agglutinogen in the human RBCs corresponds to the absence of agglutinin in the plasma.

The absence of agglutinogen in the human RBCs corresponds to the presence of agglutinin in the plasma.

Landsteiner, a Nobel Prize laureate, discovered the ABO blood group system (1900–1901).

Determined by ABO gene, located on chromosome 9.

Requisites for Blood Typing

Blood group determination requires suspension of RBC and testing antisera. Suspension of RBC is formulated by mingling blood drops with isotonic saline (0.9%). Test sera are: 1. Antiserum A, containing anti-A or α-antibody. 2. Antiserum B, containing anti-B or β-antibody.

Inheritance of ABO Blood Groups

The four classical ABO blood groups depend on three genes, viz. A, B and O. An individual's blood group is determined by two genes obtained from either of the parents.

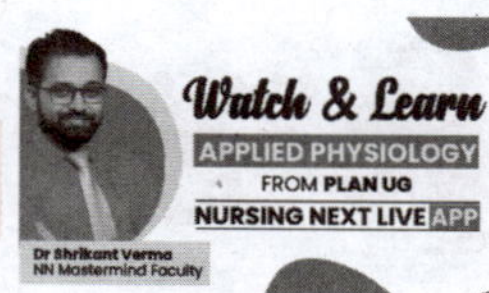

Blood Groups

- Antigenic determinants present in human RBCs.
- The foremost vital blood groups determined before blood transfusions include:
  - Classical ABO blood groups
  - Rhesus (Rh) blood group
  - M and N Blood group ABO Blood Groups
- ABO blood group system supported the presence or absence of substance A and substance B
- Blood groups are split into four types:
  1. 'A' group
  2. 'B' group
  3. 'AB' group
  4. 'O' group

Antibodies against ABO Antigens

The immune system forms antibodies against whichever ABO blood group antigens are present. For example, a person with blood group A will have B antibodies as shown in diagram.

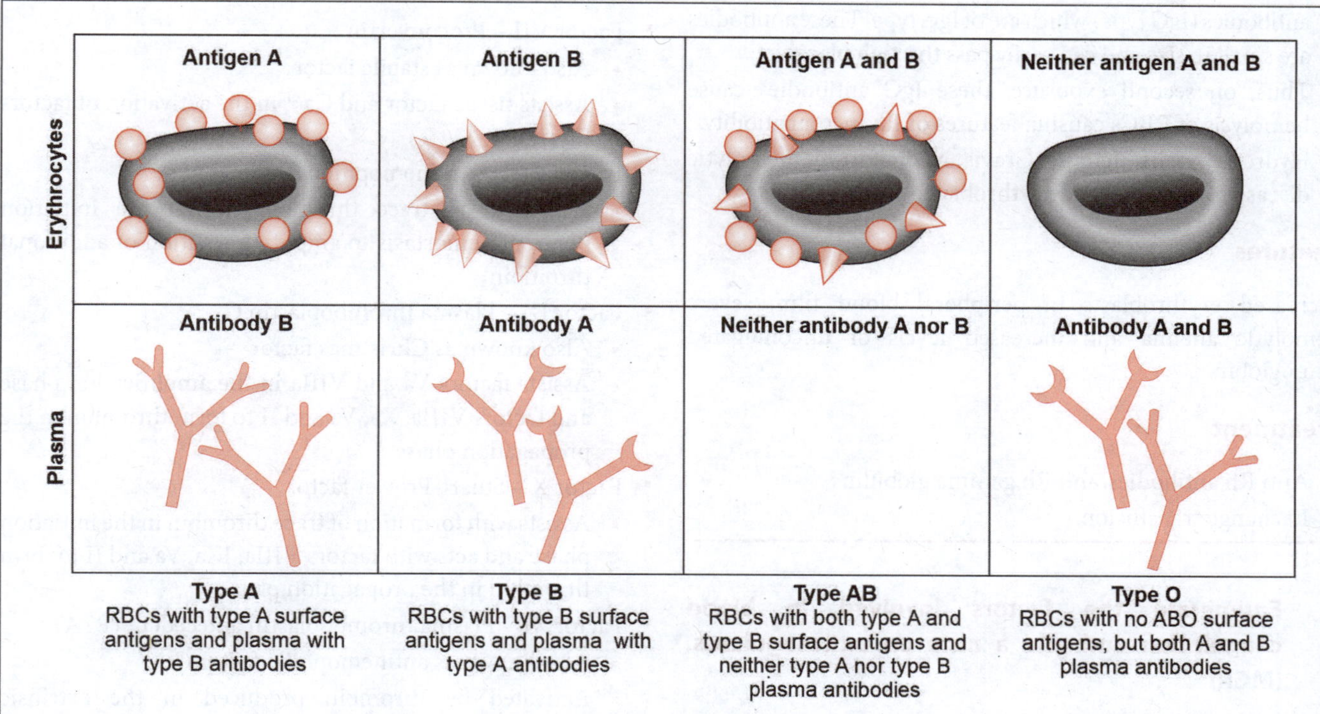

Biochemical Basis of ABO Blood Group

- A and B antigens are carbohydrate groups bound to lipids.
- The specificity of antigen is based on terminal sugar of carbohydrate.
- The one or two terminal sugar added to the substance determines the blood group.

Blood group	Antigen(s) present on the red blood cells	Antibodies present in the serum	Genotype(s)
A	A antigen	Anti-B	AA or AO
B	B antigen	Anti-A	BB or BO
AB	A antigen and B antigen	None	AB
O	None	Anti-A and Anti-B	OO

Universal Donor and Recipient

Universal Donor

- A person who can donate blood to any recipient of any blood group.
- People with O—(negative) blood type are the true universal donors.
- Biochemical basis of universal donor
  - Absence of any antigen on erythrocytes, i.e., their red blood cells do not carry antigens.
- So, they can donate blood to any other blood group.
- Positive blood group cannot be given to an Rh-negative individual.

Universal Recipient

- Can accept blood from anyone
- AB positive blood group
- Biochemical basis
  - Has all the antigens in its red blood cells.

Erythroblastosis Fetalis

- This occurs due to in utero Rh incompatibility
- The mother having Rh negative blood group is exposed to fetus having Rh positive blood group.
- On first exposure, there occurs development of anti Rh antibodies (IgG type) which are of IgG type. These antibodies are small in size and can easily pass through placenta.
- Thus, on second exposure, these IgG antibodies cause hemolysis of RBCs causing features of Rh incompatibility.
- Hydrops fetalis, Icterus Gravis Neonatorum, hemolytic disease of newborn and erythroblastosis fetalis.

Features

Increased erythroblasts in peripheral blood film, severe hemolytic anemia and increased levels of unconjugated hemoglobin.

Treatment

- Anti Rh antibodies/anti Rh gamma globulins
- Exchange transfusion.

---

6. Enumerate the factors involved in blood coagulation and add a note on anticoagulants. (MGR)

Answer

Blood Coagulation

Blood coagulation is a process that changes circulating substances within the blood into an insoluble gel and the insoluble gel plugs leaks in blood vessels and stops the loss of blood.

The process of coagulation requires coagulation factors, calcium and phospholipids.

Coagulation Factors

- Factor I – Fibrinogen
  - Globulin in nature with a molecular weight of 330000.
  - Assists in the formation of fibrin clot
- Factor II – Prothrombin
  - Assists factor Xa in formation of trace thrombin in the initiation phase and assists factors VIIIa, IXa, Xa and Va to form thrombin in the propagation phase of hemostasis.
  - Vitamin K is essential for its formation.
- Factor III – Tissue thromboplastin
  - Assists factor VII and Ca^{2+} in the activation of factors IX and X during the initiation phase of hemostasis
- Factor IV – Calcium
  - Acts as a cofactor
  - Essential for activation of multiple clotting factors
- Factor V – Proaccelerin
  - Also known as labile factor
  - Assists factors VIIIa, IXa, Xa, and II in the formation of thrombin during the amplification and propagation phases of hemostasis
- Factor VII – Proconvertin
  - Also known as stabile factor
  - Assists tissue factor and Ca^{2+} in the activation of factors IX and X
- Factor VIII – Antihemophilic factor
  - Activated by trace thrombin during the initiation phase of hemostasis to amplify formation of additional thrombin
- Factor IX – Plasma thromboplastin C
  - Also known as Christmas factor
  - Assists factors Va and VIIIa in the amplification phase and factors VIIIa, Xa, Va and II to form thrombin in the propagation phase
- Factor X – Stuart-Prower factor
  - Assists with formation of trace thrombin in the initiation phase and acts with factors VIIIa, IXa, Va and II to form thrombin in the propagation phase
- Factor XI – Plasma thromboplastin antecedent (PTA)
  - Also known as antihemophilic factor C
  - Activated by thrombin produced in the extrinsic pathway to enhance production of additional thrombin inside the fibrin clot via the intrinsic pathway; this factor also participates in slowing down the process of fibrinolysis.
- Factor XII – Hageman factor
  - Contact activator of the kinin system (e.g., prekallikrein, and high-molecular-weight kininogen)
  - Inactive form is activated on surface contact.
- Factor XIII – Fibrin stabilizing factor
  - Activated by thrombin and assists in formation of bonds between fibrin strands to complete secondary hemostasis
- Von Willebrand factor
  - Assists in platelet adhesion and thrombus formation

Anticoagulants

Substances that prevent coagulation to occur, i.e., inhibit the blood coagulation cascade.

Classification of Anticoagulants

- **In vivo**
  - Parenteral
    - Heparin, low molecular weight heparin, heparinoids
  - Oral
    - Coumarin derivatives
    - Indandione derivatives
- **In vitro**
  - Heparin
  - Calcium complexing agents
  - Sodium citrate, sodium oxalate, sodium edetate

Natural Anticoagulants

- Antithrombin III – inhibits factor X and thrombin
- Heparin
  - Secreted from the basophils and mast cells
  - Potentiates the effects of antithrombin III
  - Inhibits IX, X, XI, XII and thrombin
- Antithromboplastin
  - Inhibits tissue factors – tissue thromboplastins
- Protein C and S
  - Activated by thrombin
  - Degrades factors Va and VIIIa

SHORT NOTES

1. Types and functions of leukocytes. (MGR)

Answer

Types of Leukocytes

White blood cells or leukocytes play an important role in defense and immunity in human body.

- Agranulocytes
  - Lymphocytes
  - Monocytes
- Granulocytes
  - Neutrophils
  - Eosinophils
  - Basophils

Functions of Leukocytes

Table 5.2: Types and functions of white blood cells

Differential leukocytes	Percentage of white blood cells	Morphology	Life span	Function
Granulocytes				
Neutrophils (Cytoplasm; Granules; Multipartite nucleus)	50–70%	10–14 mm in diameter, multilobed nucleus (2–6 lobes) purple in color, cytoplasm is blue in color and fine sand like red brown colored granules are present	2–4 days	Phagocytosis—engulf and destroy bacterial pathogens and also act as mediators of pyrexia response
Eosinophils (Membrane; Secretion gland; Nucleus; Cytoplasm)	1–4%	10–14 mm in diameter, nucleus purple in color and has bilobed nuclei; eosinophilic pink colored cytoplasm with large, coarse brick red colored granules	8–12 days	Play a role in limiting allergic reactions. Mild phagocytic action and provides local mucosal immunity

Contd...

Differential leukocytes	Percentage of white blood cells	Morphology	Life span	Function
Basophils	<1%	10–14 mm in diameter, purple-colored bilobed nuclei, basophilic blue-colored cytoplasm, coarse, large purplish blue granules overlying the nucleus	12–15 days	Function as mediators of inflammation, mild phagocytic action and contains heparin which is an anti-coagulant
Agranulocytes				
Lymphocytes	20–40%	**Small lymphocyte:** 7–10 mm in diameter, Large Lymphocyte: 10–14 mm in diameter, Dense, purple staining, oval or round nucleus; little cytoplasm	More than a day to 2 or 3 days	The most important cells of the immune system; effective in fighting infectious organisms; act against a specific foreign molecule (antigen)
Monocytes (Cytoplasm, Nucleus, Lysosome, Chromatin)	2–8%	10–18 mm in diameter indented kidney-shaped nucleus, pale in color, cytoplasm abundant pale blue in color and cell is agranular	Mostly undergo apoptosis after about 24 hours	Transform into macrophages; phagocytic cells and detoxifies, killing tumor cells

2. Functions of platelets. (MGR)

Answer

Introduction

- Platelets are:
  - Smallest - Average size 2.5 mm
  - Colorless
  - Non-nucleated
  - Round or oval and flattened
  - Biconvex discs
  - Covered by unit membrane.
- Also known as thrombocytes
- Average life span – 8–9 days
- Normal range – 1.5–4 lakhs/mm^3 in blood.

Functions of Platelets

- **Responsible for primary hemostasis:** Injury to blood vessel causes release of vasoconstrictor substances from dense bodies, like adenine, serotonin, prostaglandins and activation of platelets and forms temporary platelet plug.
- **Platelet activation:** On exposure to collagen, the platelets develop pseudopodial extensions and become irregular in shape.
- Fibronectin present in alpha granules helps in binding platelet to trauma site.
- **Platelet adhesion and aggregation:** They attach themselves to the collagen through Von Willebrand factor and secrete large amount of ADP and Thromboxane A2 that helps platelet to aggregate and form platelet plug.
- Thrombospodin from alpha granules of platelet stabilizes the platelet plug. Platelets promote coagulation by platelet factor 4 as procoagulant.
- Platelets promote wound healing and fibrosis by releasing platelet derived growth factor.
- Lysosomes contain acid hydrolases.
- Catalases is present in micro peroxisomes of platelets.

SHORT ANSWER QUESTIONS

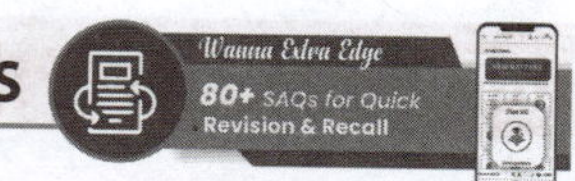

1. Any two important functions of platelets. (MGR)

Answer

Important Functions of Platelets

- Platelets prevent bleeding by forming plugs at the site of injury (temporary hemostatic plug).
- Platelets contribute to blood coagulation by releasing platelet factor 4, and synthesizing Clotting factors V and XI

2. Mention any two functions of blood. (MGR)

Answer

Two Functions of Blood

- Blood transports oxygen from lungs to tissues, and carbon dioxide from tissues to the lungs.
- Blood acts as the transport medium for various hormones, chemical substances, nutrients, vitamins, etc.

3. Functions of leukocytes. (MGR)

Answer

Functions of Leukocytes

Leukocytes help to identify and destroy harmful microorganisms such as bacteria, viruses, and fungi that can cause infections. They help in initiating and coordinating the body's immune response.

4. Functions of red blood cells. (MGR)

Answer

- The primary job of red blood cells is to transport oxygen from the lungs to the tissues. This is because red blood cells contain haemoglobin.
- Hemoglobins are also involved in the transport of carbon dioxide from tissues to the lungs and the maintenance of acid-base balance.

5. Name the first two clotting factors. (MGR)

Answer

The first two clotting factors in the coagulation cascade are:

1. Factor I (Fibrinogen) – deficiency leads to afibrinogenemia
2. Factor II (Prothrombin) – deficiency leads to Hypoprothrombinemia (hemorrhagic tendency in liver disease).

6. Classify WBC. (MGR)

Answer

Types of WBC's and their distribution

Table 5.3: Types of leukocytes and their distribution in peripheral blood as DLC and absolute count

Leukocytes	Percentage (DLC)	Absolute count (per cu mm)
A. Granulocytes		
1. Neutrophils	50–70	2000–2750
2. Eosinophils	1–4	40–440
3. Basophils	0–1	20–80
B. Agranulocytes		
1. Monocytes	2–8	1500–4000
2. Lymphocytes	20–40	500–800

7. What are the Vitamin K dependent clotting factors? (MGR)

Answer

The clotting factors that depend on vitamin K include:

Factor II (prothrombin)

Factor VII (proconvertin)

Factor IX (Christmas factor)

Factor X (Stuart-Prower factor)

8. Mention any two tests for anemia. (MGR)

Answer

- **Peripheral blood smear:** Microscopic evaluation of red blood cell morphology.
- **Serum ferritin test:** It helps to determine the total iron storage capacity of the body. Also helps to diagnose iron deficiency or iron overload.

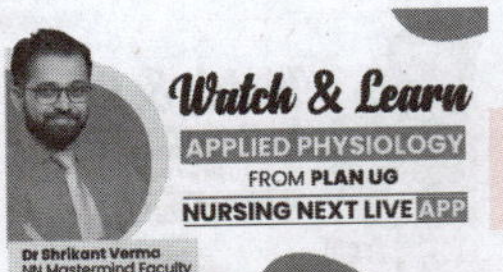

CONCEPTUAL REVISION

MULTIPLE CHOICE QUESTIONS

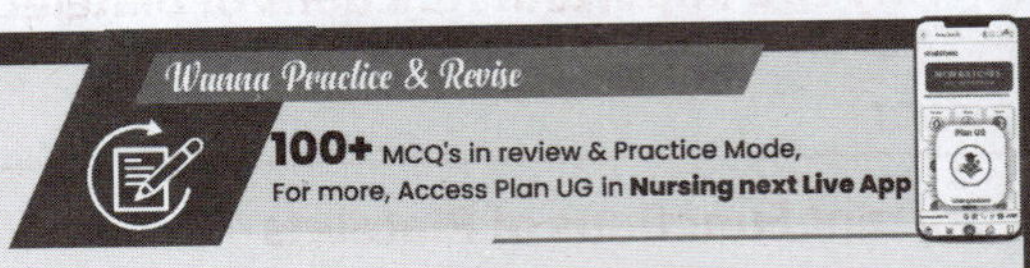

1. What is the term "formed elements" used to mean in a description of blood?

a. White blood cells, red blood cells and platelets
b. Blood plasma
c. Blood serum
d. The clotting factors in blood

Ans. a. White blood cells, red blood cells and platelets

2. What is the function of the plasma proteins in blood?

a. To transport oxygen
b. To regulate electrolyte balance
c. To exert osmotic pressure and so help maintain blood volume
d. To function as a non-specific body defense mechanism

Ans. c. To exert osmotic pressure and so help maintain blood volume

3. Which blood cells are involved in protecting the body from pathogens and foreign cells?

a. Erythrocytes
b. Leukocytes
c. Platelets
d. Hemoglobin

Ans. b. Leukocytes

4. Which cell in the list below is the MOST common white blood cell?

a. Basophils
b. Lymphocytes
c. Monocytes
d. Neutrophils

Ans. d. Neutrophils

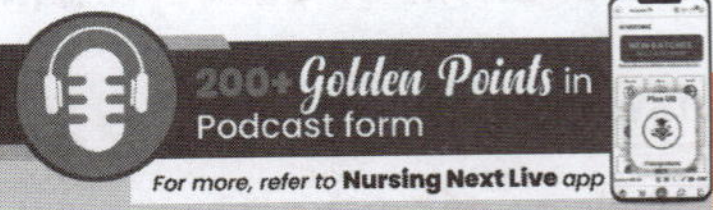

Golden Points

- Blood is described as a specialized connective tissue that transports oxygen and nutrients to the body cells and tissues and carries carbon dioxide and waste products from them.
- Disseminated intravascular coagulation is due to large areas of necrotic tissue and septicemia.
- Each molecule of hemoglobin when fully saturated with oxygen carries four molecules of oxygen.
- Erythropoiesis is a process in which human erythrocytes are produced.
- Functions of WBC are Phagocytosis, Antibody formation, Synthesis, Manufacture of trephines which exert great influence on the nutrition, growth and repair of tissues, Secretion of heparin and Antihistamine function.
- Hematopoiesis involves five processes: erythropoiesis, lymphopoiesis, granulopoiesis, monopoiesis and thrombopoiesis.
- Hemoglobin acts as an important buffer in the blood for maintaining pH.
- Hemoglobin has very important role as oxygen carrier in the blood and it also carries carbon dioxide in the blood.
- Hemoglobin is composed of heme or iron and protein globin.
- Hemoglobin plays a role in transport of nitric oxide (NO) from lungs to tissues where it causes vasodilation.
- Hemophilia is a hemorrhagic disease that results from deficiency of factor VIII.
- Leukopoiesis is defined as a process of development and maturation of the white blood cells. It takes a period of 12 days for the development of leukocytes.

CHAPTER 6

Endocrine System

CONCEPTUAL THEORY

Terminology

150+ key terminologies for Quick Recall & Revision

Acromegaly: Excessive secretion of growth hormone from acidophils of anterior pituitary after puberty. The look gets coarse, hands and feet become large. Person shows thick lips, macroglossia.

Addison's disease: Called adrenal insufficiency and is a chronic condition in which adrenal gland do not produce enough cortical hormones.

Cushing's syndrome: Obesity, hirsutism, diabetes and hypogonadism. This occurs due to excessive secretion of adrenal cortical hormones.

Diabetes mellitus: Hyperglycemia due to lack of insulin. Most common is type II/adult type of diabetes.

Gigantism: Excessive secretion of growth hormone from acidophils of anterior pituitary before puberty. Person becomes very tall looking like a 'giant'.

Hyperparathyroidism: Hypercalcemia, hypercalciuria and repeated renal calculi/stones, and repeated fracture of bones.

Hypoglycemia: Lack of glucose. It is very serious and may cause coma and death.

Tetany: Due to low levels of parathormone, hand goes into carpal spasm.

FUNCTIONS AND HORMONES OF PINEAL GLAND

- The main functions and hormones of the pineal gland are as follows:
  - The pineal gland is primarily responsible for the production and secretion of the hormone melatonin.
  - The pineal gland and its hormone melatonin play a crucial role in regulating the body's circadian rhythm.
  - The pineal gland and melatonin production have been found to influence reproductive function. Melatonin has been shown to regulate the release of reproductive hormones, such as luteinizing hormone (LH) and follicle-stimulating hormone (FSH), from the pituitary gland.
  - Melatonin, produced by the pineal gland, has potent antioxidant and anti-inflammatory properties. It scavenges free radicals and helps protect cells from oxidative stress, which can lead to cellular damage and aging.
  - There is evidence suggesting that melatonin, secreted by the pineal gland, may play a role in modulating immune function.

FUNCTIONS AND HORMONES OF PITUITARY GLAND

Anterior Pituitary

- Various hormones secreted by the anterior pituitary are:
  - **Growth hormone:**
    - Important for growth and development in the body.
    - Promotes linear growth of bones and skeletal muscles.
    - Promotes growth and maturation of genital organs and secondary sexual characteristics.
  - **Thyroid stimulating hormone:**
    - Stimulation and regulation of thyroid gland activity.
    - Secretion of T3 and T4 hormones.
  - **Adrenocorticotrophic hormone (ACTH)**
    - Regulates the secretion of steroid hormones
  - **Prolactin**
    - Stimulates lactation
  - **Gonadotrophins**
    - Follicle stimulating hormone (FSH) in both males and females stimulates the gamete production.
    - Luteinizing hormone (LH) along with FSH in females stimulates estrogen and progesterone secretion during the menstrual cycle.

- LH in males [also known as interstitial cell stimulating hormone (ICSH)] stimulates the interstitial cells of testes to produce testosterone.

Posterior Pituitary

Hormones secreted by posterior pituitary are:

- Oxytocin
  - Acts on the smooth muscles of the uterus and lactating breast
  - During labor, it stimulates uterine contractions and causes the expulsion of fetus.
  - Aids in the ejection of milk
- Anti-diuretic hormone (ADH)
  - Increases the permeability of the distal convoluted tubules and collecting tubules.
  - Increases reabsorption in kidney, which decreases the urine output.
  - Responsible for maintenance of acid-base balance.

THYROID GLAND

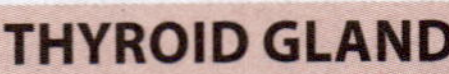
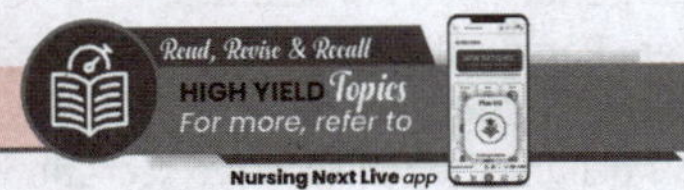

- Highly vascular gland situated in front of larynx and trachea at the level of 5th, 6th and 7th cervical and 1st thoracic vertebra.

Hormones of Thyroid Gland

- Thyroxine
- Triiodothyronine
- Calcitonin

Functions of Thyroid Gland

- Increases oxygen consumption
- Increases mitochondrial activity
- Increases utilization of vitamins
- Increases basal metabolic rate
- Increase in carbohydrate uptake, glycolysis, gluconeogenesis, increases plasma glucose levels, as a result increase in insulin secretion.
- Increase in T3 causes diarrhea, and decrease in T3 causes constipation.
- Increase in respiratory rate due to increased metabolic waste (CO_2).
- Increase in GFR
- Weakness in muscles (thyrotoxic myopathy). Fine tremors occur due to increased neuronal synaptic reactivity.
- **Reproductive:** Decreased levels of thyroid hormone cause menorrhagia and polymenorrhea, amenorrhea and loss of libido. Increased levels cause oligomenorrhea, rarely amenorrhea.

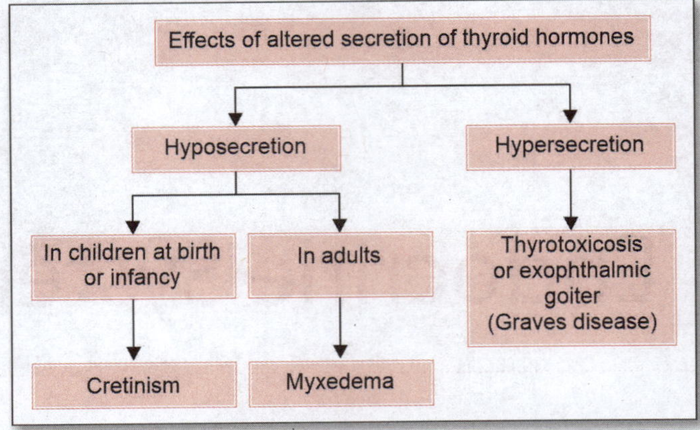

Figure 6.1: Effects of thyroid hormones

OTHER GLANDS

Hormones of Parathyroid Gland

- Parathyroid gland secretes parathormone. Its secretion is regulated by low plasma Ca 2+ concentration.
  - Primarily involved in increasing plasma Ca 2+ levels.
  - Action of PTH on bone
    - Increased osteoclastic activity, leading to demineralization of bones
  - Action on kidney and intestine:
    - PTH increases the synthesis of calcitriol, thus decreasing the excretion and increasing the absorption of calcium and phosphorus.

Thymus Gland

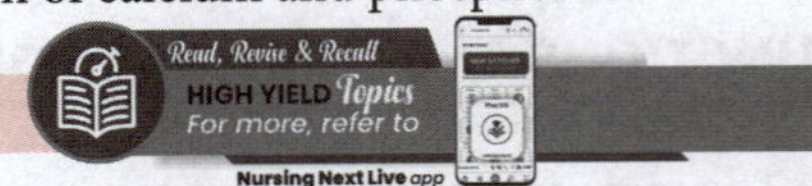

- **Thymopoietin:** Helps in the production of T-cells
- **Thymosin and thymulin:** Development of specialized types of T-cells.
- **Thymic humoral factor**

Pancreas

- Pancreas is 'J' shaped and secretes the digestive pancreatic juice; and the endocrine part secretes hormones, e.g., insulin.
- Contains both exocrine secretion for digestion of carbohydrates, fats and proteins; and endocrine secretion from islets of Langerhans, which acts in the carbohydrate metabolism.

Cell type	Secretion
A cells/Alpha cells	Glucagon
B cells/Beta cells	Insulin, Amylin, C peptide
D cells/Delta cells	Somatostatin
F cells	Pancreatic Polypeptide
Epsilon cells	Ghrelin

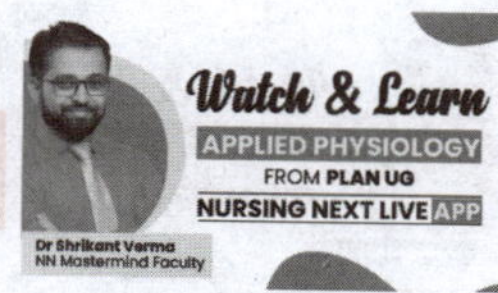

Adrenal Glands

- The adrenal glands (also known as suprarenal glands) are endocrine glands that produce a variety of hormones including adrenaline and the steroids aldosterone and cortisol.
- **Hormones produced by the adrenal cortex are:**
  - **Glucocorticoids:**
    - Regulation of carbohydrate metabolism
    - Sodium and water reabsorption from renal tubules
  - **Mineralocorticoids**
    - Stimulates reabsorption of the water and sodium
    - Role in renin-angiotensin system
  - **Androgens**
    - Deposition of proteins in muscles
    - Retention of nitrogen

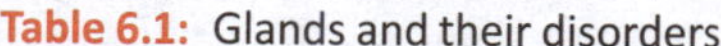

Alterations in Disease

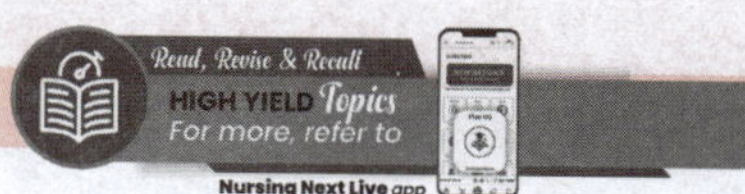

Table 6.1: Glands and their disorders

Gland	Hormones produced	Disorders
Hypothalamus	• Thyrotropin-releasing hormone (TRH) • Corticotrophin-releasing hormone (CRH) • Growth hormone-releasing hormone (GHRH) • Arginine vasopressin (AVP)	• Central diabetes insipidus • Depression • Anxiety
Pituitary gland (anterior)	• Thyroid-stimulating hormone (TSH) • Adrenocorticotropic hormone (ACTH) • Follicle-stimulating hormone (FSH) • Luteinizing hormone (LH) • Growth hormone (GH) • Prolactin	• Acromegaly • Dwarfism • Multiple endocrine neoplasia type 1 (MEN 1) • Pituitary tumors
(Posterior)	• Oxytocin • Antidiuretic hormone (ADH)	• SIADH
Thyroid	• Triiodothyronine (T3) • Thyroxine (T4) • Calcitonin	• Grave's disease • Hyperthyroidism • Thyroiditis • Nodules and cancers • Hypothyroidism • MEN 2A and 2B
Parathyroid	• Parathyroid hormone (PTH)	• Hypoparathyroidism • MEN 1, 2A and 2B
Pancreas	• Glucagon • Insulin	• Type 1 diabetes mellitus • Type 2 diabetes mellitus • Gestational diabetes • MEN 1
Adrenal	• Androgens • Glucocorticoids • Androgens • Adrenaline • Noradrenaline	• Addison's disease • Cushing's syndrome • MEN 2A and 2B
Ovary	• Estrogens • Progesterone	• Polycystic ovarian syndrome • Turner syndrome
Testes	• Testosterone	• Kallmann's syndrome • Hemochromatosis

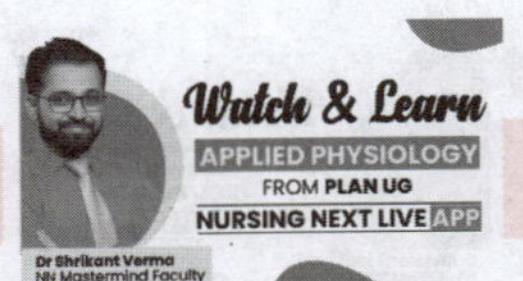

APPLICATION AND IMPLICATION IN NURSING

Assessment and Diagnosis

Medication administration: Endocrine disorders often require medication management. Nurses must understand the mechanism of action, side effects, and potential interactions of various endocrine medications.

Patient education: Nurses play a vital role in educating patients with endocrine disorders about their condition, treatment options, and self-management strategies.

Monitoring and management: Nurses closely monitor patients with endocrine disorders, including assessing blood glucose levels in diabetes, monitoring hormone replacement therapy, or evaluating thyroid function tests.

CONCEPTUAL EXERCISES

LONG ANSWER QUESTIONS

1. Explain the functions of pituitary gland in detail with a suitable diagram. (RUHS)

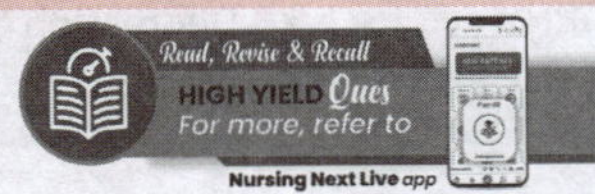

Answer

Introduction

- Pituitary gland – small ovoid structure attached to the base of brain.
- Lies in the hypophyseal fossa located on the superior surface of the body of sphenoid bone.
- Also known as hypophysis cerebri
- Divided into three parts:
  1. Anterior pituitary
  2. Posterior pituitary
  3. Pars media

Anterior Pituitary

- Constitutes a major part of the pituitary
- Linked to the hypothalamus by the hypothalamo-hypophyseal portal vessels.
- Various hormones secreted by the anterior pituitary are:
  - Growth hormone:
    - Important for growth and development in the body.
    - Active of GH is somatomedin
    - Promotes linear growth of bones and skeletal muscles.
    - Promotes growth and maturation of genital organs and secondary sexual characters.
    - Plays an important role in protein, fat and carbohydrate metabolism.
  - Thyroid stimulating hormone:
    - Stimulation and regulation of thyroid gland activity.
    - Secretion of T3 and T4 hormones.
  - Adrenocorticotrophic hormone (ACTH)
    - Regulates the secretion of steroid hormones
  - Prolactin
    - Stimulates lactation
  - Gonadotrophins
    - Follicle stimulating hormone (FSH) in both males and females stimulates the gamete production.
    - Luteinizing hormone (LH) along with FSH in females stimulates estrogen and progesterone secretion during the menstrual cycle.
    - LH in males [also known as interstitial cell stimulating hormone (ICSH)] stimulates the interstitial cells of testes to produce testosterone.

Posterior Pituitary

- Constitutes about 20% of the pituitary gland.
- Consists of nervous tissues and blood vessels.
- Linked with neural hypothalamohypophyseal tract.
- ADH and oxytocin are synthesized in the hypothalamus and transported by the neural tracts to the posterior pituitary and are released from there.
  - Oxytocin
    - Acts on the smooth muscles of the uterus and lactating breast
    - During labor, it stimulates uterine contractions and causes the expulsion of fetus.
    - Aids in the ejection of milk
  - Anti-diuretic hormone (ADH)
    - Increases the permeability of the distal convoluted tubules and collecting tubules.
    - Increases reabsorption in kidney, which decreases the urine output.
    - Responsible for maintenance of acid-base balance.

Intermediate Lobe

- Thin strip of tissue between anterior and posterior lobes.
- Produces melanocyte-stimulating hormone
- Stimulates melanocyte cells in deeper layers of epidermis to synthesize melanin.

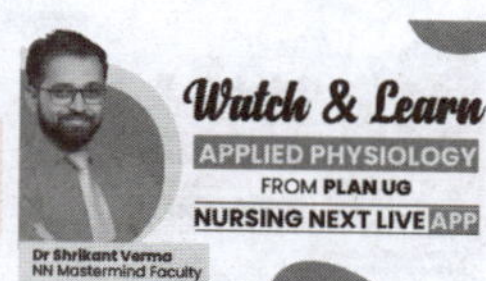

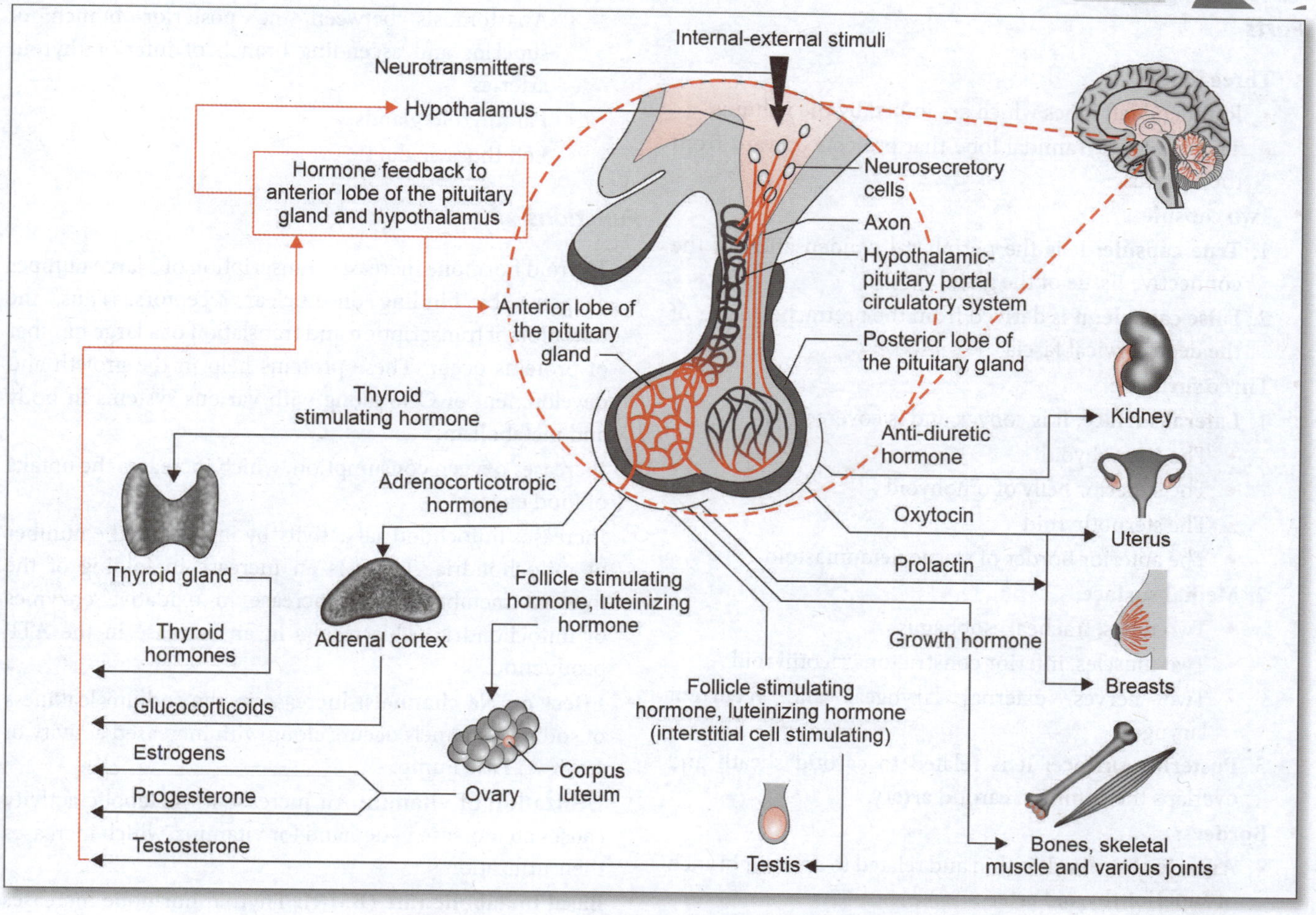

Figure 6.2: Hormones of the posterior and anterior pituitary

2. Enlist the various endocrine glands. Describe the structure and functions of thyroid gland in detail. (RUHS)

Answer

Endocrine Glands

The endocrine glands of the body control various activities by releasing hormones in the blood. The major endocrine glands are:

- Pituitary gland
- Thyroid gland
- Parathyroid gland
- Adrenal or suprarenal gland

Groups of endocrine cells may be present in organs that perform other functions. These include:

- Islets of Langerhans
- Interstitial cells of testes
- Follicle and corpus luteum of ovary
- Placenta

Thyroid Gland

Highly vascular gland situated in front of larynx and trachea at the level of 5th, 6th and 7th cervical and 1st thoracic vertebra.

Structure of Gland

- Weight of gland – 25 g
- The thyroid gland is located in the anterior neck, situated between the C5 and T1 vertebrae.
- It is an endocrine gland, divided into two lobes which are connected by an isthmus.
- Butterfly in shape, it consists of two lobes, one on either side of the thyroid cartilage and upper cartilaginous rings of the trachea.
- The lobes are joined by a narrow isthmus, lying in front of the trachea.
- The lobes are roughly cone-shaped and are about 5 cm long and 3 cm wide.

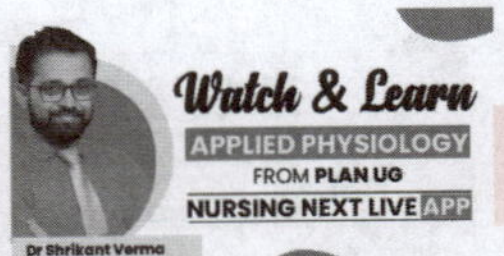

Parts

- **Three lobes:**
  - Right and left lobes which are joined by the isthmus.
  - The third is pyramidal lobe that projects upward from the isthmus.
- **Two capsules:**
  1. **True capsule:** It is the peripheral condensation of the connective tissue of the gland
  2. **False capsule:** It is derived from the pretracheal layer of the deep cervical fascia.
- **Three surfaces:**
  1. **Lateral surface:** It is convex and is covered by:
     - The sternohyoid
     - The superior belly of omohyoid
     - The sternothyroid
     - The anterior border of sternocleidomastoid
  2. **Medial surface:**
     - Two tubes, trachea, esophagus
     - Two muscles, inferior constrictor, cricothyroid
     - Two nerves, external laryngeal and recurrent laryngeal
  3. **Posterior surface:** It is related to carotid sheath and overlaps the common carotid artery.
- **Borders:**
  - **Anterior border:** It is thin and related to anterior branch of superior thyroid artery.
  - **Posterior border:** It is thick and round and separates medial and posterior surfaces. It is related to:
    - Inferior thyroid artery
    - Anastomosis between the posterior branch of superior and ascending branch of inferior thyroid arteries.
    - Parathyroid glands
    - Left thoracic duct

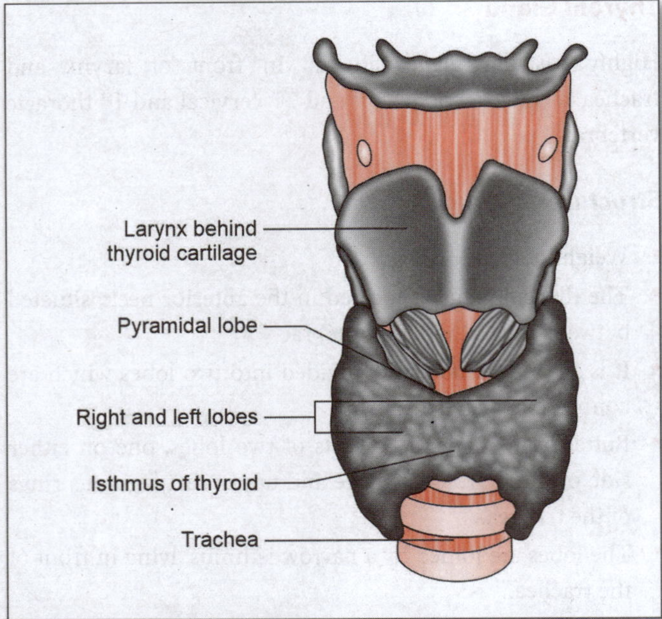

Figure 6.3: Thyroid gland

Functions

- Thyroid hormone increases transcription of a large number of genes by binding on nuclear receptors. Thus, the initiation of transcription and translation of a large number of proteins occur. These proteins help in the growth and development of CNS along with various systems in body and metabolism.
- Increases oxygen consumption, which increases the uptake of food energy.
- Increases mitochondrial activity by increasing the number of mitochondria. There is an increase in folding of the internal membrane and increase in oxidative enzymes of mitochondria. This results in an increase in the ATP production.
- **Effect on Na channels:** Increase in the sodium leakiness of sodium channels occurs along with increased activity of Na-K ATPase Pump.
- **Utilization of vitamin:** An increase in metabolic activity causes an increase in demand for vitamins, which increases their utilization.
- **Basal metabolic rate (BMR):** Thyroid hormone increases cellular metabolic processes by increasing mitochondrial activity, ATP production and accelerating other intracellular processes, which increases BMR. (Calorigenic action of T3 and T4)
- **Effect on carbohydrate metabolism:** Increase in carbohydrate uptake, glycolysis, gluconeogenesis, increase in plasma glucose levels and as a result increase in insulin secretion.
- **Effect on LDL, cholesterol and phospholipids:** Increased Lipoprotein receptors on hepatocytes cause increased uptake of LDL, cholesterol and phospholipids in hepatocytes thus decreasing their plasma levels.
- **CVS:** Due to an increase in tissue oxygenation, there occurs increased production of waste K^+ and H^+ ion causing vasodilation, which increases blood flow, cardiac output and heart rate. Due to increased secretion, systolic blood pressure increases and diastolic decreases, while mean arterial BP remains normal.
- **GIT:** Increase in T3 causes diarrhea, and decrease in T3 causes constipation.
- **Respiratory system:** Increase in metabolic activity causes an increase in metabolic waste (CO_2) which causes an increase in the respiratory rate.

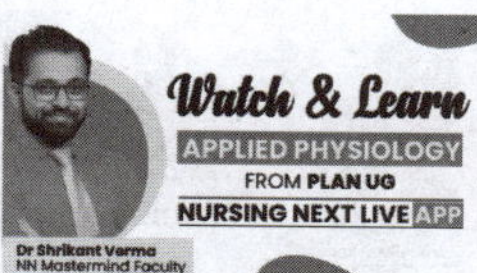

- **Kidney:** Increase in GFR
- **Musculoskeletal system:** Brisk reflexes, increased levels of T3/T4 cause muscle protein catabolism, which leads to weakness in muscles (thyrotoxic myopathy). Fine tremors occur due to increased neuronal synaptic reactivity.
- **Sleep:** Increase in level results in insomnia and somnolence on decrease on hormone level
- **Reproductive:** Decreased levels of thyroid hormone cause menorrhagia and polymenorrhea, amenorrhea and loss of libido. Increased levels cause oligomenorrhea, rarely amenorrhea.

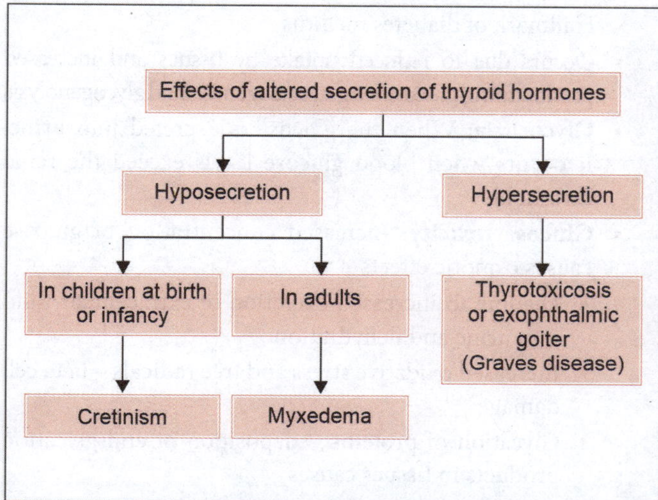

Figure 6.4: Effects of thyroid hormones

Calcitonin

- Secreted by parafollicular or C cells in the thyroid gland.
- Calcitonin lowers blood calcium levels. It does this by acting on:
  - Bone cells, promoting their storage of calcium
  - Kidney tubules, inhibiting the reabsorption of calcium

3. What is calcium homeostasis? Explain the role of parathyroid hormone in calcium homeostasis. Add a note on tetany. (MGR)

Answer

Introduction

- Calcium homeostasis refers to the maintenance of a stable and balanced level of calcium in the body.
- Calcium is the most abundant mineral in body.
- Normal serum value – 9–11 mg/dL

Factors regulating serum calcium levels are:

- Parathyroid hormone
- Calcitriol
- Calcitonin

Parathyroid Hormone

- Secreted by parathyroid gland
- Secretion is regulated by low plasma Ca^{2+} concentrations
- Primarily involved in increasing plasma Ca^{2+} levels.
- **Action of PTH on bone:**
  - Increased osteoclastic activity and reduced osteoblastic activity
- **Action on kidney and intestine:**
  - PTH increases the synthesis of calcitriol, thus decreasing the excretion and increasing the absorption of calcium and phosphorus.

Calcitriol

- **Action of calcitriol on the intestine:**
  - Increases the intestinal absorption of calcium and phosphate.
- **Action of calcitriol on the bone:**
  - Calcium uptake for deposition as calcium phosphate is stimulated.
  - Increased mobilization of calcium.
- **Action of calcitriol on the kidney:**
  - Reduces excretion of calcium and phosphate by kidney
  - Increases reabsorption

Calcitonin

- Secreted by parafollicular cells of thyroid gland
- Action is antagonist to that of PTH
- **Decreases serum calcium levels by:**
  - Promoting calcification by increasing activity of osteoblasts
  - Decreases bone reabsorption
  - Increases excretion of calcium into urine

Tetany

- Disorder of enhanced neuronal excitability associated with sensory disturbance
- Could be a clinical manifestation of hypoparathyroidism
- Plasma calcium level drops below 6 mg/dL (normal value of 9.4 mg/dL).
- Increased excitability of nerves is due to:
  - Hypocalcemia (low serum Calcium)
  - Alkalosis (proportion of serum calcium in iodized form is decreased)
- Hypomagnesemia

Pathophysiology

- Hypocalcemia results in hyperexcitability of muscles and nerve membranes, characterized by ischemia.
- There is increased permeability to sodium due to decrease in ionized calcium thus producing numbness, tingling, stiffness, extremity cramps owing to skeletal muscle spasm.

Signs and Symptoms

- Carpopedal spasm
- Muscle cramps
- Hyper-reflexia
- Paresthesia of hand and feet
- Circumoral numbness
- Flexion of wrist with hyperextensibility of fingers
- Severity of disorder may lead to laryngospasm, laryngeal stridor, seizures, arrhythmias and myocardial dysfunction.

Investigations

Tests to Unmask Latent Tetany

- **Trousseau sign:** Ionized calcium level drops to 1.75–2.25 mmol/L. A characteristic hand posture with the inflation of sphygmomanometer cuff above systolic pressure in 3 minutes leading to flexion of metacarpophalangeal joints.
- **Chvostek sign:** Jerk of the facial muscles, by a gentle tap over the facial nerve in pre-auricular region. It is due to the hyperirritability of facial nerve.
- **ERB sign:** Hyperexcitability of skeletal muscles in response to a mild stimulus is referred to as Erb sign. Also known as Erb-Westphal sign.

Latent Tetany

- Also referred to as subclinical Tetany
- Neuromuscular hyperexcitability that develops before the onset of tetany due to hypocalcemia
- Signs and symptoms include generalized weakness and cramps in arms and feet.

SHORT NOTES

1. Explain the metabolic changes in diabetes mellitus. (RUHS)

Answer

Diabetes Mellitus

- A chronic disorder in which the body cannot produce its own insulin which normally is produced in the pancreas.
- Diabetes occurs due to either an absolute (type 1) or a relative (type 2) deficiency of insulin.

Types

- Type 1 Diabetes (absolute insulin deficiency, autoimmune disease)
- Type 2 Diabetes (relative, progressive insulin deficiency; nonautoimmune etiology)
- Gestational (during pregnancy)
- Impaired glucose homeostasis.

Metabolic Changes in Diabetes

- **Hyperglycemia:**
  - Elevation of blood glucose level.
  - Hallmark of diabetes mellitus
  - Occurs due to reduced uptake by tissues and increased production of glucose via gluconeogenesis and glycogenolysis
  - **Glycosuria:** When the glucose is excreted into urine. It occurs when blood glucose levels exceed the renal threshold.
  - **Glucose toxicity:** Increased concentration of glucose causes osmotic effects
    - Leading to increased excretion of extracellular fluid into urine and dehydration
    - Increased oxidative stress and free radicals – beta cell damage
    - Glycation of proteins – deposition of end glycation products in tissues causes:
      - Diabetic nephropathy
      - Diabetic neuropathy
      - Diabetic retinopathy
- **Ketoacidosis:** Increased mobilization of fatty acids results in overproduction of ketone bodies.
- **Hypertriglyceridemia:** Conversion of fatty acids into triacylglycerols and the secretion of VLDL and chylomicrons are comparatively higher and activity of the enzyme lipoprotein lipase is low. Consequently, the plasma levels of VLDL, chylomicrons and triacylglycerols are increased.
- **Hypercholesterolemia:** An increase in the level of cholesterol is also frequently seen in diabetics.

2. Action of insulin. (RUHS)

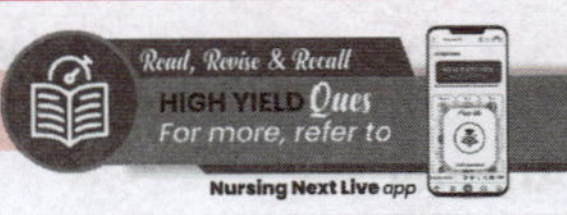

Answer

Introduction

- Secreted by the beta cells of pancreas.
- Insulin is a polypeptide hormone containing two amino acid chains (A and B) linked by disulfide bonds.
  - Chain A – contains 21 amino acids
  - Chain B – contains 30 amino acids
- Half-life of insulin is 5–6 minutes.

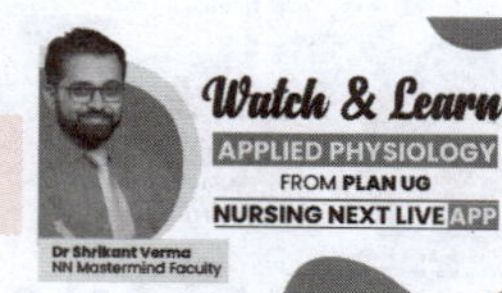

Actions of Insulin

- Major action is anabolic and causes storage of carbohydrates, proteins and fats.
- Target organs are liver, muscle, adipocytes
- Effects on carbohydrate metabolism
  - Insulin causes rapid uptake, storage and utilization of glucose by almost all tissues of our body, especially muscles, liver and adipocytes.
  - In liver
    - Stimulates glycogenesis
    - Inhibits gluconeogenesis
  - In muscles
    - Increases transport of glucose to the cells.
- Effect on fat metabolism
  - Helps in fat storage
    - Promotes fatty acid synthesis in the liver from excess glucose.
    - Insulin inhibits lipolysis.
- Effect on protein metabolism
  - Promotes protein synthesis and storage.
  - Stimulates transport of amino acids to the cells where they are used for synthesis of proteins
  - Inhibits catabolism of proteins

3. Enumerate the functions of hypothalamus. (RUHS)

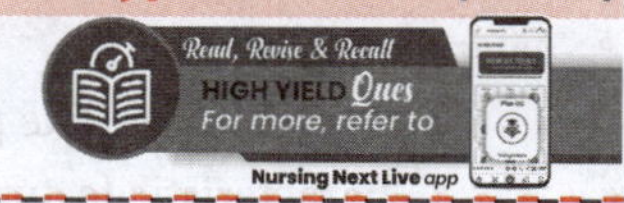

Answer

Functions of Hypothalamus

- **Endocrinal function:** Secretion of releasing and inhibitory hormones like:
  - Gonadotropin releasing hormone (GnRH)
  - Prolactin releasing hormone (PRH)
  - Growth hormone-releasing hormone (GHRH)
  - Thyrotropin releasing hormone (TRH)
  - Corticotropin releasing hormone (CRH)
  - Prolactin inhibiting hormone (PIH)
  - Growth hormone inhibiting hormone (somatostatin)
- **Autonomic function:** Anterior hypothalamus has parasympathetic function and posterior hypothalamus has sympathetic function.
- **Sleep:** Sleep facilitation centers are present in anterior hypothalamus and waking centers are present in posterior hypothalamus responsible for arousal.
  - Circadian Rhythm is maintained by hypothalamus through the tract formed by retinohypothalamic fibers and lateral geniculate nuclei. It is internally driven and is also known as 'Biological clock' of the body. Circadian rhythm is known to control following biological processes in our body.
    - Rhythmic secretion of hormones, e.g., adrenocorticotropic hormone (ACTH), growth hormone, melatonin and Gonadotropin releasing hormone (GnRH)
    - Sleep-wake cycle
    - Body temperature rhythm
- Feeding regulation is done by feeding center in lateral hypothalamic nucleus and satiety is regulated by ventromedial nucleus. Satiety center inhibits feeding center. Lesion in the ventromedial nucleus may cause hyperphagia.
- Reproductive function, maintenance of female estrous cycle and ovulation through tuberal region.
- Instinctual and emotional behavior is regulated by hypothalamus along with limbic system.
- Reward center along with medial forebrain bundle in lateral and ventromedial nucleus and punishment center in periventricular zone of medial hypothalamus.
- **Body temperature regulation:** Anterior hypothalamus is involved in heat loss and posterior hypothalamus is involved in heat gain.
- Thirst stimulated by lateral nucleus of hypothalamus and osmoreceptors in supraoptic nucleus secrete ADH.

4. Write a short note on cretinism. (MGR)

Answer

Cretinism

- Cretinism is a condition of hypothyroidism in children. Due to lack of thyroid hormone during fetal life, there is lack of myelination, growth and branching of neurons. Failure of the development of nervous system occurs due to which mental retardation occurs.
- Typical appearance of a cretin child is as follows:
  - Mentally retarded with stalky appearance
  - Protruding tongue because of normal growth of soft tissue as compared to retarded skeletal growth.
  - Short stature, decreased bone growth
  - Guttural breathing

Types of Cretinism

- **Congenital cretinism**
  - Due to genetic defect in the thyroid hormone synthesis
- **Endemic cretinism**
  - Occurs due to iodine deficiency
  - Also exposure to radioactive iodine during pregnancy may cause it.

- **Neurological cretinism:** Characterized by:
  - Retarded growth
  - Motor spasticity
  - Severe mental retardation
  - Squint
- **Myxedematous cretinism:** Characterized by:
  - Retarded growth
  - Incomplete maturation of facial expression
  - Thickened and dry skin
  - Delayed sexual maturation
  - Mental retardation

5. Write a note on dwarfism.

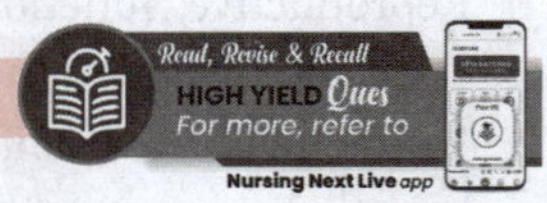

Answer

Medical or genetic condition that leads to someone being considerably shorter than an average-sized man or woman.

Classification of Dwarfs

- Familial
  - Constitutional growth delay
  - Genetic predisposition
  - Family history of stunted growth
- Endocrine
  - Pituitary dwarf
    - Occurs due to deficiency of growth hormone, viz. growth hormone-releasing hormone (GHRH)
    - Characteristic features
      - Plumpness
      - Immature facies
      - Small genitalia
      - Body proportion is in accordance with chronological age
  - Thyroid dwarf
    - Occurs due to deficiency of thyroid hormone
    - Characteristic features
      - Mental retardation
      - Body proportion remains infantile.
  - Cushing syndrome
    - Occurs due to overactivity of adrenal glands with consequent hypersecretion of glucocorticoids – hypercortisolism.
    - Characteristic features
      - Euphoria
      - Buffalo hump
      - Thinning of skin
      - Moon face
      - Bruising
      - Cataracts
      - Increased abdominal fat
      - Osteoporosis
      - Muscle weakness
- Nutritional
  - Marasmus
    - Characterized by protein energy malnutrition, energy deficiency
    - Characteristic features
      - Growth retardation
      - Muscle wasting
      - Loss of subcutaneous fat
      - Wrinkled skin
      - Vitamin deficiencies
      - Irritability
      - Diarrhea
      - Dehydration
  - Rickets
    - Caused due to deficiency of vitamin D in children
    - Characteristic features
      - Short stature
      - Frontal bossing
      - Thickening of wrists
      - Knock knees
      - Widening of epiphyseal plate
      - Bowing of legs
- Miscellaneous
  - Systemic diseases, like prolonged anemia
    - Characteristic features
      - Pallor
      - Tachycardia
      - Weight loss
      - Weakness
      - Clubbing
  - Chromosomal abnormalities, like Turner's syndrome
    - Dwarfism
    - Primary amenorrhea
    - Decreased sexual development
  - Achondroplasia
    - Abnormal dominant skeletal disorder
    - Characteristic features
      - Dwarfism
      - Large head
      - Short limbs
  - Emotional deprivation, like Kaspar Hauser Syndrome
    - Characteristic features
      - Immature behavior, intellect, facial appearance
      - Retarded bone age

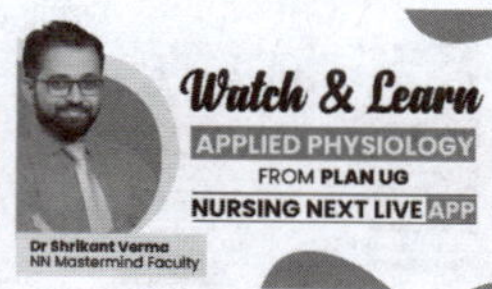

SHORT ANSWER QUESTIONS

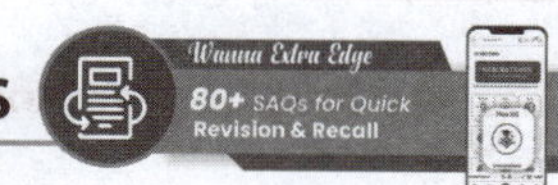

1. Name any four female sex hormones. (MGR)

Answer

Four female sex hormones are:

1. Estrogen
2. Progesterone
3. Follicle-stimulating hormone (FSH)
4. Luteinizing hormone (LH)

2. Define glands. (MGR)

Answer

Glands are biological organs or structures that generate and secrete substances, like hormones, enzymes, and other specialized products. These compounds are commonly discharged into the circulation, lymphatic system, or other body cavities.

3. Enlist hormones of anterior pituitary gland. (MGR)

Answer

The anterior pituitary gland produces and releases several hormones:

- Growth hormone (GH)
- Thyroid-stimulating hormone (TSH)
- Adrenocorticotropic hormone (ACTH)
- Follicle-stimulating hormone (FSH)
- Luteinizing hormone (LH)
- Prolactin (PRL)
- Melanocyte-stimulating hormone (MSH)

4. Define cretinism. (MGR)

Answer

Cretinism is a type of hypothyroidism that affects youngsters. Those that acquire hypothyroidism after or before birth are referred to as cretins. Patients are intellectually retarded and dwarf.

Symptoms:

- Stunted growth and mental retardation.
- Short stature (dwarfism).
- Mild neurological impairment with reduced muscle tone and coordination.
- Hearing and speech defects, etc.

5. Name the layers and secretions of adrenal cortex. (MGR)

Answer

There are three main layers of the adrenal cortex:

1. Zona glomerulosa—mineralocorticoids, particularly aldosterone
2. Zona fasciculata—glucocorticoids, particularly cortisol
3. Zona reticularis—androgens, particularly testosterone and DHEA

6. Write any two functions of thyroid hormone. (MGR)

Answer

Functions of Thyroid Hormone

- Thyroid hormones play a key role in regulating the body's metabolism.
- Thyroid hormones are important for normal growth and development, particularly in children.

7. Name two hormones of adrenal medulla.

Answer

Two hormones of adrenal medulla are:

1. Epinephrine (also known as adrenaline)
2. Norepinephrine (also known as noradrenaline)

Both Epinephrine and Norepinephrine rise the BMR, also increase the rate and force of cardiac contraction.

Epinephrine increases the blood glucose and norepinephrine produces vasoconstriction.

8. Define placental hormones. (MGR)

Answer

Placental hormones are produced by the placenta during pregnancy. They include:

- Human chorionic gonadotropin (hCG)
- Human placental lactogen (hPL)
- Progesterone
- Estrogen
- Relaxin
- Corticotropin-releasing hormone (CRH)
- Inhibin and activin
- Placental growth hormone (PGH)
- Prolactin
- Thyroid-stimulating hormone (TSH)

9. Enlist functions of calcium and its effect on serum calcium level. (MGR)

Answer

Calcium is a mineral that helps the body grow and maintain strong bones and teeth, as well as muscular function, nerve transmission, and blood coagulation.

When serum calcium levels are excessively high, the thyroid gland releases calcitonin, which stimulates the bones to take up calcium and decreases calcium reabsorption in the kidneys, so lowering serum calcium levels.

10. Define Gigantism. (MGR)

Answer

Gigantism is caused by GH hypersecretion prior to epiphysis union. Gigantism is caused by a pituitary tumor (of somatotroph) during childhood, which results in enhanced GH secretion.

11. Actions of glucocorticoid hormones. (RUHS)

Answer

Main Glucocorticoids

- Cortisone
- Cortisol
- Corticosterone

Actions of Glucocorticoids

- Regulation of carbohydrate metabolism
- Promote formation and storage of glycogen
- Promote sodium and water reabsorption from the renal tubules
- Gluconeogenesis, raising the blood glucose level
- Increase secretion of Glucocorticoid in response to stress, like surgery or infection.

CONCEPTUAL REVISION

MULTIPLE CHOICE QUESTIONS

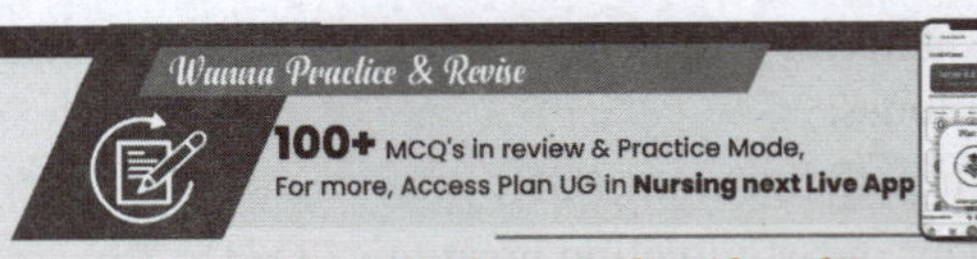

1. The thyroid gland:

a. Is located inferior to the larynx
b. Produces antidiuretic hormone
c. Secretes small amounts of insulin
d. Helps initiate milk production

Ans. a. Is located inferior to the larynx

2. What hormone(s) does the adrenal medulla produce?

a. Aldosterone
b. Epinephrine and norepinephrine
c. Corticosteroids
d. Glucocorticoids

Ans. b. Epinephrine and norepinephrine

3. Glucagon is produced in the pancreas by which cells?

a. Alpha cells
b. Beta cells
c. Delta cells
d. F cells

Ans. a. Alpha cells

4. A patient is admitted to the hospital with a diagnosis of primary hyperparathyroidism. A nurse checking the patient's lab results would expect which of the following changes in laboratory findings?

a. Low urine calcium
b. Elevated serum calcium
c. Elevated serum vitamin D
d. Low serum parathyroid hormone (PTH)

Ans. b. Elevated serum calcium

5. Hypoglycemia is seen in:

a. Acromegaly
b. Cushing's syndrome
c. Hyperthyroidism
d. Hypopituitarism

Ans. d. Hypopituitarism

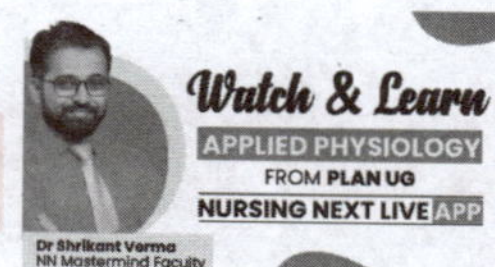

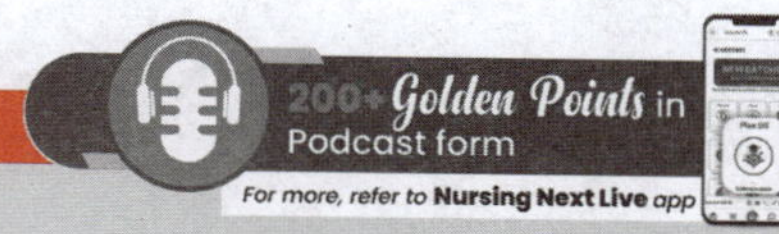

Golden Points

- Adrenal glands (also known as suprarenal glands) are responsible for the production of Glucocorticoids, Mineralocorticoids and androgens.
- Contains both exocrine secretion for digestion of carbohydrates, fats and proteins; and endocrine secretion from islets of Langerhans, which act in the carbohydrate metabolism.
- Hormone secretion is regulated by signals from nervous system, chemical changes in the blood or by other hormones.
- Hypothalamus regulates secretion of thyrotropin (TSH) corticotropin (ACTH), somatotropin (STH), prolactin, luteinizing hormone (LH), follicle stimulating hormone (FSH) and melanocyte stimulating hormone
- Hypothalamus serves as a major integrating link between nervous and endocrine systems.
- It is 'J' shaped and secretes the digestive pancreatic juice; and the endocrine part secretes hormones, e.g., insulin.
- Melatonin helps in coordination of circadian and diurnal rhythms of many tissues and it inhibits growth and development of sex organs till puberty.
- Parathyroid gland secretes parathormone. Its secretion is regulated by low plasma Ca++ concentration.
- Production of sperms and maintenance of male secondary sex characteristics is maintained by testosterone.
- Secretion of hormones and production of ova are governed by the follicle stimulating hormone (FSH) and the luteinizing hormone (LH) of the anterior pituitary
- The endocrine glands are devoid of ducts and the secretions are poured directly into the blood through the capillaries and numerous sinusoids draining and irrigating the gland.
- Thymus controls lymphopoiesis and maintains the lymphocytic population in various lymphoid organs.
- Thyroid gland regulates the basal metabolic rate and stimulates somatic and psychic growth, as well as plays an important role in calcium metabolism.

CHAPTER 7

Sensory Organs

CONCEPTUAL THEORY

Terminology

Accommodation: The process by which the curvature of the lens is increased is called accommodation.
Astigmatism: Leads to the image being focused on multiple places.
Hypermetropia: Common eye condition in which nearby objects appear blurred and far off ones are clear. Also known as long sightedness.
Myopia: When the shape of the eye causes the bending of light rays incorrectly, this causes the focusing of images in front of the retina instead of on the retina. Also known as nearsightedness.
Olfactory pathway: From the olfactory bulb, the signals are relayed to various regions of the brain, including the olfactory cortex, amygdala, and hippocampus. These regions are involved in the perception, recognition, and emotional response to odors.
Pupillary light reflexes: The pupillary light reflex is an autonomic reflex that constricts the pupil in response to light, thereby adjusting the amount of light that reaches the retina.

FUNCTIONS OF SKIN

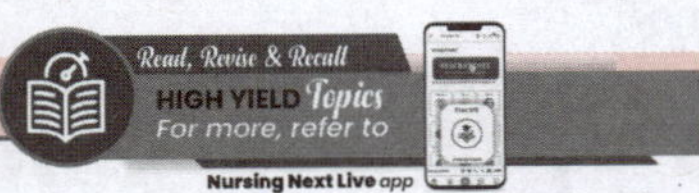

Five layers of epidermis are easily appreciable in thick skin as compared to thin skin. Going from superficial to deep, the layers are:

- **Stratum corneum:** Cornified layer
  - Main function is the protection of deeper layers.
- **Stratum lucidum:** Clear layer
  - Reduce friction between the other layers
- **Stratum granulosum:** Granular layer
  - This layer contributes to the selective permeability of skin, making it relatively waterproof.
- **Stratum spinosum:** Prickle cell layer
  - Helps to make the skin flexible and strong
- **Stratum basale/germinativum:** Basal layer
  - Stem cells continuously undergoing mitosis to regenerate the other layers

VISION

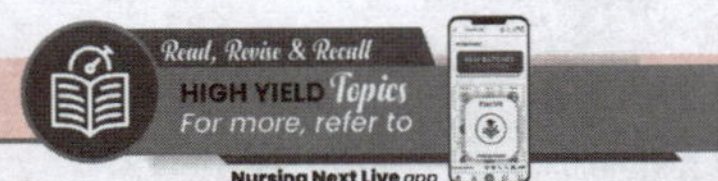

Accommodation

The process by which the curvature of the lens is increased is called accommodation.

Near Point of Vision

The nearest point to the eye at which an object can be brought into clear focus by accommodation is called the near point of vision.

Pupillary Light Reflexes

The pupillary light reflex is an autonomic reflex that constricts the pupil in response to light, thereby adjusting the amount of light that reaches the retina.

It includes direct light reflex and consensual light reflex. Optic nerve are the sensory fibers which initiates the reflex. Edinger-Westphal nuclei is main part in the reflex pathway.

Photoreceptors

Rod cells	Cone cells
Rods are responsible for vision in dim light.	The cones are responsible for color vision and works best in bright light.
The pigment present in the rods is rhodopsin, formed of a protein scotopsin and retinal (an aldeyde of vitamin A).	The pigment present in the cones is photopsin, formed of opsin protein and retinal.

Contd...

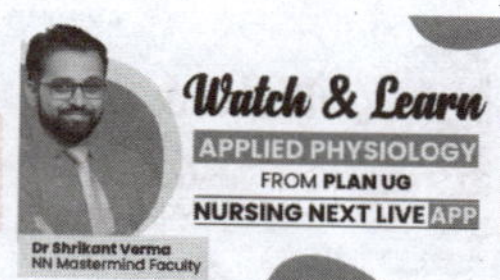

Rod cells	Cone cells
There are about 120 million rod cells.	There may be 6–7 million cone cells.
Rods are predominant in the extra fovea region.	Cones are concentrated in the fovea region.

Visual Pathway

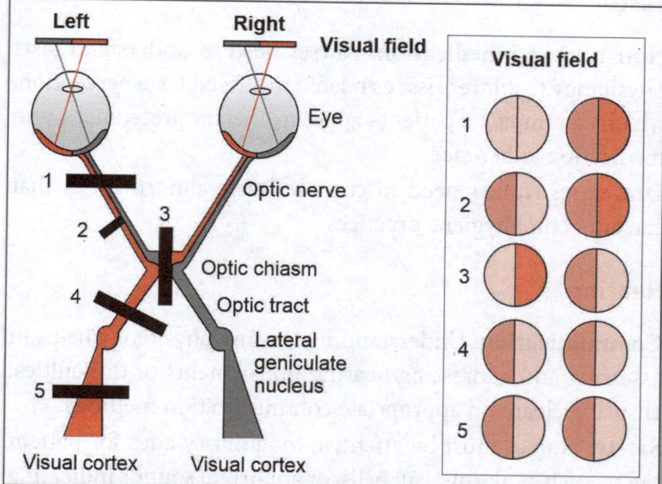

HEARING

Function of the Ear

The main divisions of the auditory system and their functions are as follows:

- **Outer ear:**
  - **Pinna (auricle):** Collects sound waves from the environment and funnels them into the ear canal.
  - **Ear canal:** Directs sound waves toward the middle ear.
- **Middle ear:**
  - **Tympanic Membrane (eardrum):** Vibrates in response to sound waves and transmits the vibrations to the ossicles.
  - **Ossicles (malleus, incus, and stapes):** Three small bones that amplify and transmit sound vibrations from the eardrum to the inner ear.
- **Inner ear:**
  - **Cochlea:** Spiral-shaped structure responsible for converting sound vibrations into electrical signals that can be interpreted by the brain.
  - **Vestibular saystem:** Consists of the semicircular canals and otolith organs, which contribute to the sense of balance and spatial orientation.
- **Auditory nerve:**
  - **Vestibulocochlear nerve (also known as the eighth cranial nerve):** Transmits electrical signals from the cochlea to the brainstem, where auditory processing begins.
- **Brainstem:**
  - **Cochlear nucleus:** First stage of auditory processing in the brainstem, where the auditory nerve fibers synapse.
  - **Superior olivary complex:** Involved in sound localization and processing binaural (two-eared) auditory information.
  - **Inferior colliculus:** Coordinates auditory information and relays it to higher-level auditory processing centers in the brain.
  - **Medial geniculate nucleus (MGN):** Located in the thalamus, relays auditory information to the auditory cortex.
- **Auditory cortex:**
  - **Primary auditory cortex (A1):** Located in the temporal lobe, responsible for basic sound processing and initial interpretation of auditory information.
  - **Auditory association areas:** Higher-level regions involved in complex sound analysis, speech perception, and sound recognition.

TASTE

Types of Taste

- There are five tastes perceived by the humans:

1. **Sweet:** Mainly on the tip of the tongue.
2. **Salty:** Mainly situated on the dorsum–anteriorly.
3. **Sour:** Detected on the edges of tongue.
4. **Bitter:** Detected on the back of the tongue.
5. **Umami:** Detected by the G receptors.

SMELL

Olfactory Epithelium

The olfactory process begins in the olfactory epithelium, which is a specialized tissue located high in the nasal cavity.

Olfactory Receptor Neurons

Olfactory receptor neurons have cilia, which are hair-like extensions that contain receptor proteins. These receptor proteins bind to odor molecules, initiating a chemical reaction that generates electrical signals in the ORNs.

Olfactory Bulb

The electrical signals generated by the ORNs travel along the olfactory nerve and reach the olfactory bulb, which is a structure located at the base of the brain. The olfactory bulb receives inputs from different ORNs and processes the signals.

Olfactory Pathway

From the olfactory bulb, the signals are relayed to various regions of the brain, including the olfactory cortex, amygdala, and hippocampus. These regions are involved in the perception, recognition, and emotional response to odors.

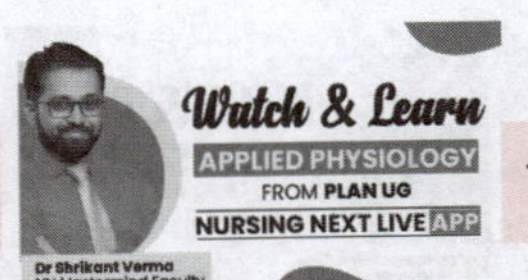

ERRORS OF REFRACTION

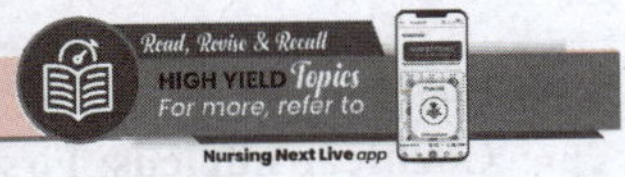

Myopia

- Also known as nearsightedness.
- **Cause:**
  - When the shape of the eye causes the bending of light rays incorrectly, this causes the focusing of images in front of the retina instead of on the retina.
- Far point of the vision decreases, is at <6 meters from the eye.
- **Management**
  - The defect is corrected by using concave lens as it diverges light rays and focuses them on the retina.

Hypermetropia

- Long sightedness
- Common eye condition in which nearby objects appear blurred and far off ones are clear.
- Management
  - The defect can be corrected by using convex lens which converges the rays and focuses them on the retina.

Astigmatism

- Common error and treatable.
- Leads to the image being focused on multiple places
- Common symptom is blurry vision.
- Management
  - The problem is corrected by using cylindrical lenses.

APPLICATION AND IMPLICATIONS IN NURSING

Smell

Assessment: Nurses can detect abnormal odors, such as foul-smelling wounds or infections, which can indicate an underlying issue.

Safety: Nurses need to be aware of potential hazards identified by smell, such as gas leaks or chemical spills, to ensure the safety of patients and themselves.

Nutrition: Nurses can assess changes in a patient's sense of smell that may affect their desire to eat, leading to potential nutritional issues.

Taste

Nutrition and medication: Nurses need to understand taste physiology to address issues related to altered taste perception, which can impact a patient's appetite, dietary preferences, and medication adherence.

Oral care: Nurses need to consider taste abnormalities that can affect oral hygiene practices.

Hearing

Communication: Understanding hearing physiology helps in assessing and addressing hearing impairments or difficulties, ensuring clear and appropriate communication methods.

Safety: Nurses must be attentive to auditory cues for patient safety, such as alarms, call bells, or abnormal sounds indicating potential risks or emergencies.

Vision

Assessment: Nurses need a basic understanding of visual physiology to assess visual acuity, peripheral vision, and color vision, which are important for patient safety and overall well-being.

Medication administration: Visual acuity and color vision are crucial when administering medications, especially when distinguishing between similar-looking medications or verifying dosages.

CONCEPTUAL EXERCISES

LONG ANSWER QUESTION

1. Describe the functions of skin. How body temperature is regulated? (RUHS)

Answer

Introduction

- The skin is the largest organ of the body, with a total area of about 20 square feet.
- The epidermis, the outermost layer of skin, provides a waterproof barrier and creates our skin tone. The dermis, beneath the epidermis, contains tough connective tissues, hair follicles and sweat glands.

Functions of Skin

- **Protection:** Skin protects the body's internal organs from the changes in the external environment.
  - **Physical barrier:** Due to stratum corneum, skin acts as a barrier against bacterial infections, heat and cold, acid or alkali.
  - **Defense and immunity:** Protects and acts as a barrier against microorganisms, viruses and bacteria present

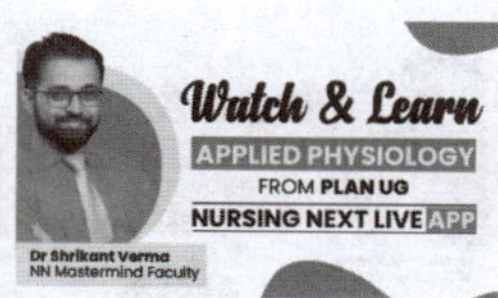

outside the body. The presence of Langerhans cells in skin is for phagocytosis.

- **Reflex action:** Sensory nerve endings start reflex action against painful stimuli and prevent it from damage.

- **Temperature regulation:** Regulation of body temperature occurs through skin, through vasodilation and vasoconstriction of the blood vessels supplying the skin and subcutaneous tissues. Heat is lost through convection, conduction and radiation through the skin itself.
- **Excretion:** Skin contains sweat glands which help in the excretion of urea and potassium. Excess water and salts are also excreted through sweat.
- **Vitamin D synthesis:** Exposure to ultraviolet rays of sun on the skin causes synthesis of cholecalciferol in the skin which forms 1,25 dihydroxycholecalciferol which is an active form of vitamin D.
- **Sensory:** Skin is sensory to touch, pain and temperature.
- **Absorption:** Oily substances are freely absorbed by the skin.
- **Regulation of pH:** Excretion of acid occurs through the skin which helps regulate pH.

Thermoregulation

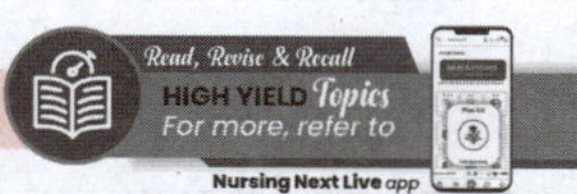

- Thermoregulation is the ability of an organism to maintain its body temperature within normal limits.
- The internal body temperature is maintained in a normal range by hemostatic mechanisms despite wide fluctuations in environmental temperature.
- Body temperature is least at 5 AM and is highest in the afternoon.
- Core temperature:
  - Temperature of the body structures that lie deep into the skin and subcutaneous layer.
- Shell temperature:
  - Temperature near body surface in the skin and the subcutaneous layer.
- If the core temperature declines, mechanisms that conserve heat and increase heat production to raise body temperature to normal become active *via* several negative feedback mechanisms. This is a major part of maintaining hemostasis.
- One of the major functions of the skin is thermoregulation. It does this by reacting differently to hot and cold conditions so that the internal body temperature is maintained within normal limits.

Hyperthermia

- Occurs when the body temperature rises above normal.
- The hypothalamic control center sends nerve impulses which stimulate heat losing center and inhibit heat promoting centers.
- Mechanisms of heat loss include:
  - Vasodilatation of the skin vessels: This leads to the loss of excess heat to the environment *via* radiation and conduction as an increased volume of blood flows from warmer core of body into cooler skin.
  - Decrease in metabolic rate.
  - Increased perspiration also results in heat loss.
  - Anorexia – loss of appetite results in reduced metabolism, which causes a reduction in heat production.
  - Decrease in muscular activity.
- Hyperthermia results in heatstroke. Clinical features include:
  - Cramps
  - Headache
  - Circulatory loss
  - Death occurs, if temperature rises above 44–46°C

Hypothermia

- Occurs when the core temperature is below 35°C.
- Compensatory mechanisms are:
  - Shivering
  - Vasoconstriction
  - Exercise increases the metabolic rate of the body, may increase up to 20 times the BMR due to contraction of the skeletal muscles.
  - **Nervous system:** Stimulation of the sympathetic division of the autonomic nervous system releases norepinephrine and epinephrine, both of which increase the metabolic rate.
  - Thyroid hormones regulate the BMR
  - Ingestion of food
  - Metabolic rate is also affected by gender. Higher in men than women except during pregnancy.
- Compensatory mechanisms fail below 32°C. Clinical features include:
  - Muscle rigidity
  - Cramps
  - Lowered body temperature
  - Low pulse and respiratory rate
  - Mental confusion
  - Disorientation
  - Death, if temperature falls below 25°C

Skin-based Thermoregulation

- Skin is the largest organ and serves as a barrier between the internal and external environment.

- Owing to its location and large surface area, it plays a very important role in thermoregulation.
- Skin plays a role in thermoregulation by the following means:
  - Temperature receptors in skin and hypothalamus send nerve impulses to control centers in hypothalamus, which in turn sends impulses to heat promoting center.
  - These impulses also cause the release of thyroid-stimulating hormone. These impulses help to raise the core temperature by:
    - **Constriction of blood vessels of the skin:** Decreases heat loss through skin by decreasing the flow of blood to skin. Piloerection, i.e., contraction of arrector pili muscles, which causes skin hair to stand up. These form an insulating layer to conserve heat.
    - **Increased release of hormones by adrenal medulla:** These hormones bring about an increase in cellular metabolism, which increases heat production.
    - Increased TSH releases; increased secretion of thyroid hormones from the thyroid gland, which in turn increases metabolic rate.
    - Impulses from the brain cause shivering (skeletal muscles contract in a repetitive cycle, (increasing the metabolic rate).
  - All the above mechanisms result in an increase in body temperature.
  - Decrease in body temperature occurs by:
    - If the body needs to cool down, vasodilatation occurs. The enlarged peripheral vessels of the skin allow for greater amounts of blood to flow near the surface of the skin, allowing thermal radiation through the skin, i.e., transferring the heat to environment.
    - Body also loses heat by convection and conduction through skin.
      - **Conduction:** It is the exchange of heat that occurs between molecules of two materials that are in direct contact with each other.
      - **Convection:** It is the transfer of heat by movement of gas/liquid between areas of different temperatures. Contact of air/water with human body results in heat transfer by both conduction and convection.
  - Perspiration or sweating is also a means of heat loss through skin. Sweating begins when the body temperature rises above 37°C.

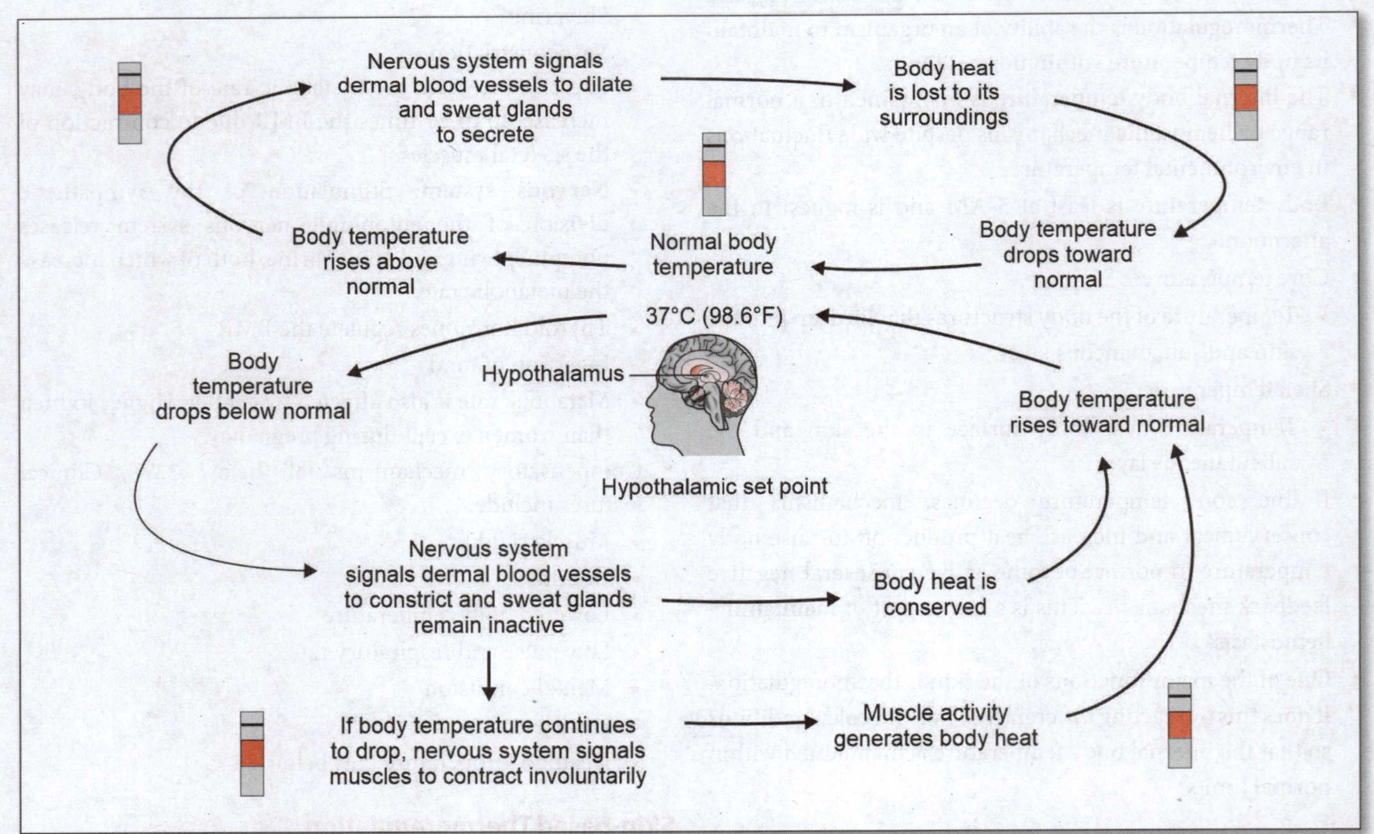

Figure 7.1: Regulation of body temperature

SHORT NOTES

1. Write in short about different types of taste. (MGR)

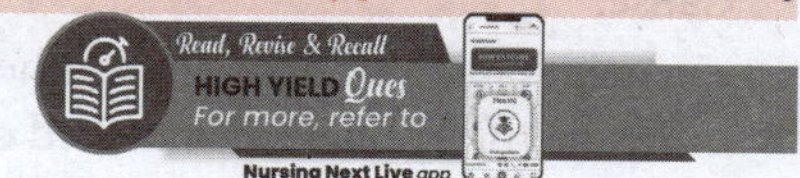

Answer

Types of Taste

- There are five tastes perceived by the humans:
  1. **Sweet**
     - Involves the detection of glucose and monosaccharides.
     - Mainly on the tip of the tongue.
  2. **Salty**
     - Detection of the presence of sodium ions in the saliva which directly diffuse into the gustatory sensory epithelial cells causing them to depolarize and release neurotransmitters.
     - Mainly situated on the dorsum–anteriorly.
  3. **Sour**
     - Detection of the presence of a high concentration of hydrogen ions will cause the depolarization of gustatory cells.
     - Detected on the edges of tongue.
  4. **Bitter**
     - Detection of long chain organic compounds such as alkaloids that contain basic nitrogen ions.
     - Detected by the G coupled receptors.
     - Detected on the back of the tongue.
  5. **Umami**
     - Detected by the G receptors.

Taste Buds

- Microscopic sensory organs containing peripheral chemoreceptors present throughout the mouth, maximum on the tongue.
- **Number of taste buds:** 500–5000
- **Number of cells in one taste bud:** Up to 150
- **Average turnover time of gustatory cells:** 8–12 days.

Nursing Implications

- Taste dysfunction
- May be due to viral/bacterial infections or neurological disorders.
  - Ageusia – total absence of taste sensation
  - Hypogeusia – decreased sense of taste
  - Hypergeusia – increased sense of taste

2. Write a short note on cataract. (RUHS)

Answer

Introduction

- It is the clouding of the lens of an eye.
- It affects the lens of the eye.
- It leads to shadiness or obscuring of the lens, keeping light from separating back to the retina.
- It is linked with the clumping together of proteins of lens.
- It shows early symptoms.
- It progresses slowly.

Types of Cataract

- Nuclear cataract
- Cortical cataract
- Congenital cataract
- Posterior capsular cataract

Symptoms

- Distressed or yellowing colors
- Blurred vision
- Needing updated prescription glasses more often.
- Glare or halos around lights, particularly at night
- Poor night vision
- Double vision

Management

- Regular eye examination
- Quit smoking
- Management of underlying systemic conditions
- Can be treated surgically.

3. Write a note on refractive errors of the eye. (RUHS)

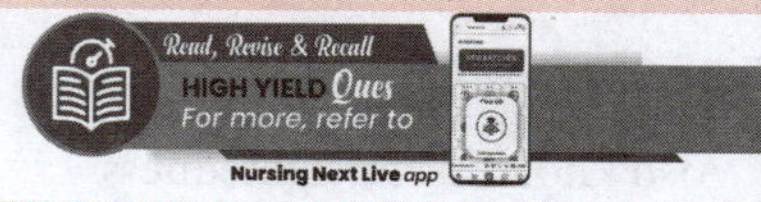

Answer

Introduction

- In normal eyes, emmetropic, parallel rays from distant objects converge to focus on retina, provided that the ciliary muscles are completely relaxed.
- If this does not occur, it leads to an error in refraction.

Signs/Symptoms

- Blurry vision
- Double vision
- Difficulty in focusing
- Headache
- Squinting

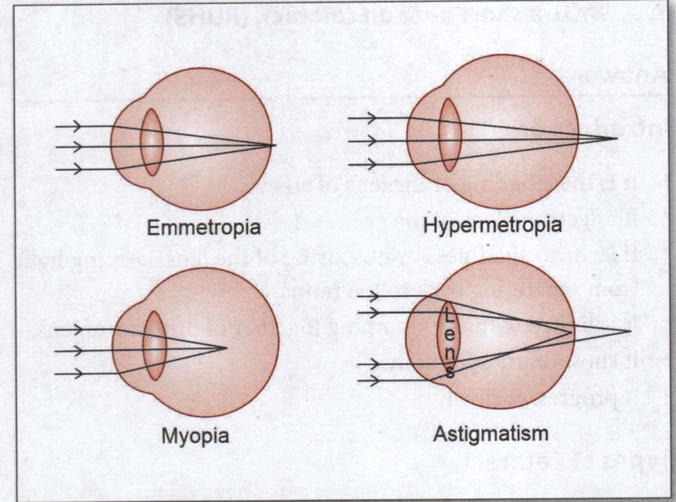

Types of Refractive Errors

- Myopia
- Hypermetropia
- Astigmatism

Myopia

- Also known as nearsightedness.
- Person is able to see the near objects clearly, but the farther ones are blurry.
- Cause:
  - When the shape of the eye causes the bending of light rays incorrectly, this causes the focusing of images in front of the retina instead of on the retina.
- Far point of the vision decreases, is at <6 meters from the eye.
- Management
  - The defect is corrected by using concave lens as it diverges light rays and focuses them on the retina.

Hypermetropia

- Also known as farsightedness
- Common eye condition in which nearby objects appear blurred and far off ones are clear.
- It occurs when the eyeball is too short or the cornea has insufficient curvature, causing light to focus behind the retina instead of directly on it.
- Management
  - The defect can be corrected by using convex lens which converges the rays and focuses them on the retina.

Astigmatism

- The front surface of the eye or the lens inside the eye is curved differently in one direction than the other.
- Common error and treatable.
- Leads to the image being focused on multiple places
- Cause:
  - Astigmatism occurs when either the cornea or the lens inside the eye has mismatched curves.
- Common symptom is blurry vision.
- Management
  - The problem is corrected by using cylindrical lenses.

4. Write a note on color blindness. (MGR)

Read, Revise & Recall HIGH YIELD Ques For more, refer to Nursing Next Live app

Answer

Introduction

- Decreased ability to see different colors or recognize the differences in color.
- More common in males than females.

Causes of Color Blindness

- Genetic reasons
- Variation in the function of cone cells
- Damage to the optic nerve

Diagnosis

By Ishihara color test

Types of Color Blindness

- Red green color blindness
  - Most common
- Blue yellow color blindness
- Total color blindness
  - Least common
- Based on the severity, color blindness can be classified as:
  - Monochromatic
    - No ability to see colors
    - Also known as total color blindness or cerebral achromatopsia.
    - Primarily of two types:
      1. Rod monochromacy
         - When the retina contains no cone cells
         - Vision in lights of normal intensity is difficult
      2. Cone monochromacy
         - Having single type of cones
  - Dichromacy
    - Can distinguish only between two primary colors.
    - Can be protanopia, deuteranopia and tritanopia.

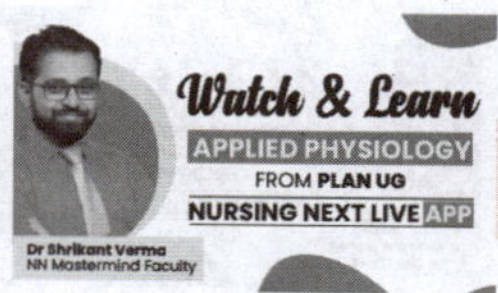

5. What is myopia? Name the corrective lens used for myopia. (MGR)

Answer

Myopia

- Also referred to as nearsightedness.
- Occurs due to either too long eyeball or too much refractive power in the lens of eye.
- Parallel rays of light from distant object get focused in front of the retina.
- Far point of vision decreases, is at ≤6 meters from the eye.

Cause of Myopia

When the shape of the eye causes the bending of light rays incorrectly, this causes the focusing of images in front of the retina instead of on the retina.

Management

Correction is done by concave lens.

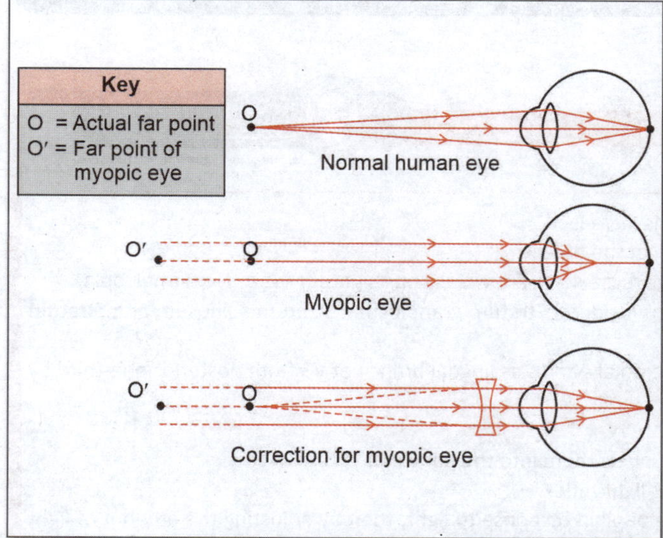

SHORT ANSWER QUESTIONS

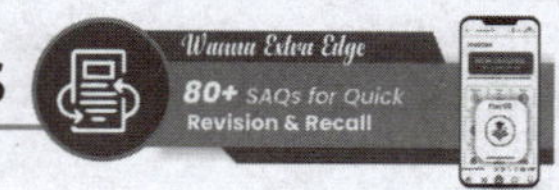

1. Enumerate different types of taste.

Answer

The five different types of tastes are:

1. Salt
2. Sweet
3. Bitter
4. Sour
5. Umami

2. Mention any two functions of skin.

Answer

The two most important functions of skin:

1. It provides protection and acts as a barrier from harmful external factors.
2. It plays role in providing sensation as it contains a network of sensory receptors.

3. Name the three compartments of cochlea.

Answer

Cochlea is the coiled part of the inner ear. Three compartments of cochlea are:

1. **Scala vestibuli:** Filled with perilymph and opens at the oval window.
2. **Scala media:** Filled with the endolymph and contains organ of Corti.
3. **Scala tympani:** Filled with perilymph and opens into the middle ear through the round window.

4. Enumerate different refractory errors of the eye.

Answer

- Myopia
- Hypermetropia/Hyperopia
- Presbyopia
- Astigmatism

5. Define Hypermetropia/Hyperopia

Answer

Hyperopia, also known as "farsightedness," is usually due to either an eyeball that is too short or, occasionally, to a lens system that is too weak.

The person can clearly see distant objects, while close-up objects are hazy. This happens when the cornea is not sufficiently curved or the eyeball is too short, leading light to focus behind the retina rather than on it.

CONCEPTUAL REVISION

MULTIPLE CHOICE QUESTIONS

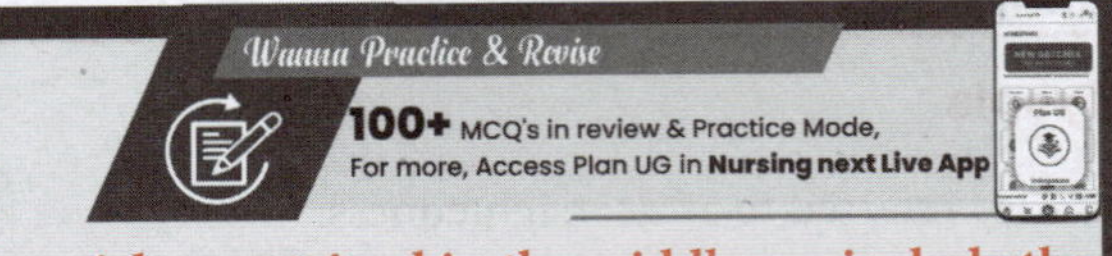

1. Which of the following is false about cones?

a. Dark adaptation later
b. Sensitive to high-intensity light
c. Higher visual acuity
d. Color vision

Ans. a. Dark adaptation later

2. The optic nerves from each eyeball cross at the:

a. Optic chiasma
b. Vitreous humor
c. Optic disc
d. Visual cortex

Ans. a. Optic chiasma

3. The ossicles contained in the middle ear include the malleus, the incus and the:

a. Pars tensa
b. Pars flaccida
c. Umbo
d. Stapes

Ans. d. Stapes

4. Otosclerosis is a common cause of conductive hearing loss. What is true for such partial hearing loss?

a. Air conduction is more effective than bone conduction
b. Stapedectomy is the procedure of choice
c. The patient is usually unable to hear bass tones
d. Hearing aids usually restore some hearing

Ans. d. Hearing aids usually restore some hearing

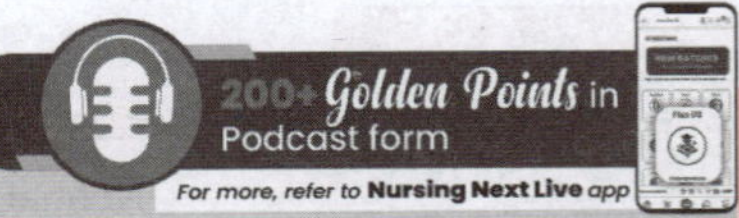

Golden Points

- Accommodation is the process by which the curvature of the lens is increased.
- Binocular vision is important to perceive the depth and proportion of the object.
- Condition in which nearby objects appear blurred and far off ones are clear are known as Long sightedness or Hypermetropia.
- From superficial to deep, the layers are Stratum corneum, Stratum lucidum, Stratum granulosum, Stratum spinosum and Stratum basale/germinativum.
- General sensation from anterior two-third of tongue is carried by cranial nerves as lingual branch of V3 from posterior one-third by IX; from posterior most part by X.
- In astigmatism, image is focused on multiple places.
- Pinna (auricle): Collects sound waves from the environment and funnels them into the ear canal.
- The constriction of pupils upon which light is shown is called direct light reflex.
- The pupillary light reflex is an autonomic reflex that constricts the pupil in response to light, thereby adjusting the amount of light that reaches the retina.
- The sensation of taste is carried by cranial nerve branch of VII (facial) from most of the anterior two-thirds; by branch of IX (glossopharyngeal) from vallate papillae and posterior one-third of tongue; by branch of X (vagus) from posterior most part of tongue.
- Three small bones that amplify and transmit sound vibrations from the eardrum to the inner ear known as ossicles (malleus, incus, and stapes).
- Vestibular System: Consists of the semicircular canals and otolith organs, which contribute to the sense of balance and spatial orientation.
- When the shape of the eye causes the bending of light rays incorrectly, this causes the focusing of images in front of the retina instead of on the retina known as nearsightedness or myopia.

CHAPTER 8

Musculoskeletal System

CONCEPTUAL THEORY

Terminology

150+ key terminologies for Quick Recall & Revision

Abduction: Moving a bone away from the midline of the body.
According to action, skeletal muscles are classified as: Prime movers—chief muscles, Synergist—assisting chief muscles, Antagonist—opposing chief muscles
Adduction: The movement of a bone toward the midline of the body.
Change of length/tension in the muscle: Isotonic—Length of muscle may decrease or increase but tension is constant.
Concentric: Muscle shortens with increased tension.
Disc prolapse: Nucleus pulposus (soft mass) of intervertebral disc may herniate posterolaterally to press on the spinal nerves
Fixators: Fix the proximal joints so that distal parts, i.e., hand can do the movements.
Intracartilaginous ossification: Process of ossification from cartilaginous cells and is seen in the spine and long bones.
Intramembranous ossification: Development of bone directly from sheets of mesenchymal (undifferentiated) connective tissue.
Isometric: Tension increases, but length remains same, e.g., holding glass of water in air.
Osteophytes: Bony spicules in relation to intervertebral foramina, which may press on the emerging spinal nerve roots/nerves.
Pronation: The action of rotating the forearm so that the palm of the hand is turned down or back.
Supination: The action of rotating the forearm so that the palm of the hand is turned up or forward.

BONE

Functions of Bone

- Forms framework of the body.
- Attaches muscle and tendon.
- Permits the movements in body parts.
- Protects organs.
- Plays role in hematopoiesis
- Is a reservoir of minerals and fats.

Division of skeleton	Bone movements
Axial skeleton	**Skull:** Minimal movement, jaw opening, lateral and forward movements of the mandible, rotation (temporomandibular joint)
	Vertebral column: Flexion, extension, lateral flexion, rotation
	Ribs and Sternum: Expansion and contraction of the chest during breathing
	Hyoid bone: No direct bone movements, but serves as a site for muscle attachments involved in swallowing and speech
Appendicular skeleton	**Upper limb:** Flexion, extension, abduction, adduction, medial and lateral rotation, circumduction
	Lower limb: Flexion, extension, abduction, adduction, medial and lateral rotation, circumduction
	Pelvis: Anterior tilt, posterior tilt, side-to-side tilting, rotation
	Joints: Various movements including flexion, extension, rotation, abduction, adduction, and circumduction in specific joints such as shoulder, elbow, hip, knee, and ankle

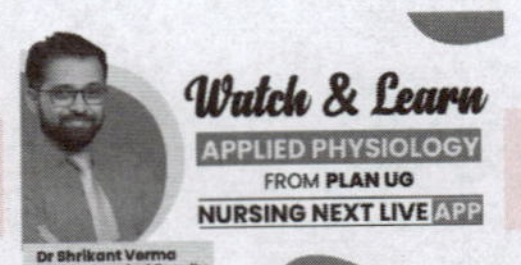

Process of Bone Healing

- **Stage 1:** From 1–3 days after the injury. Hematoma formation
- **Stage 2:** Within 3 days to 3 weeks. Formation of fibrocartilage
- **Stage 3:** Within 3 to 6 weeks after the injury. Formation of fibrocartilaginous callus
- **Stage 4:** Between 3 to 8 weeks. Initiation of Endochondral ossification
- **Stage 5:** Remodeling and consolidation

Joints and Joint Movements

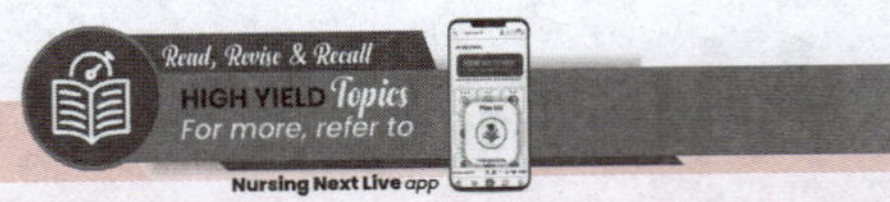

Joint Type	Joint Movement	Example
Ball and socket	Allows for movement in all directions: Flexion, extension, abduction, adduction, rotation	Shoulder joint
Hinge	Allows for flexion and extension in one plane	Elbow joint, knee joint
Pivot	Allows for rotational movement around a central axis	Atlantoaxial joint (between C1 and C2 vertebrae)
Saddle	Allows for flexion, extension, abduction, adduction, and circumduction	Carpometacarpal joint of the thumb
Condyloid	Allows for flexion, extension, abduction, adduction, and circumduction	Wrist joint
Gliding	Allows for sliding or gliding movements between flat surfaces	Intercarpal joints (between carpal bones)
Fixed/immovable	No movement	Sutures of the skull

Alteration of Joint Disease

- **Osteoarthritis:** Osteoarthritis is a degenerative joint disease that primarily affects the articular cartilage, which is the smooth and protective covering of the joint surfaces.
- **Rheumatoid arthritis:** Rheumatoid arthritis is an autoimmune disease that primarily affects the synovial membrane, the lining of the joint.
- **Gout:** Gout is a type of arthritis caused by the deposition of uric acid crystals in the joints.

MUSCLES

Skeletal Muscles

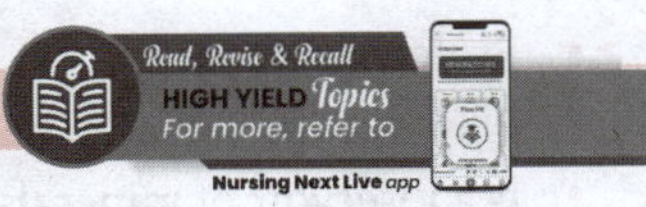

Skeletal muscles are a type of striated muscle that are attached to bones and enable voluntary movements of the body. They have several key properties and functions:

Properties of Skeletal Muscles

- Skeletal muscles can respond to stimuli, such as nerve signals, by initiating muscle contraction.
- Skeletal muscles have the ability to contract or shorten in length, generating force to produce movement.
- Skeletal muscles can be stretched or extended without damage, allowing for a range of motion at joints.
- After being stretched, skeletal muscles have the ability to return to their original length due to their elastic properties.

Functions of Skeletal Muscles

- The primary function of skeletal muscles is to produce voluntary movements of the body.
- Skeletal muscles help maintain proper body posture and provide stability to the skeletal system.
- Skeletal muscles provide support and stability to joints, preventing excessive movement or dislocation. They act as dynamic stabilizers during movement and static stabilizers to maintain joint integrity.
- Skeletal muscle contractions generate heat as a byproduct of energy metabolism.

MECHANISM OF MUSCLE CONTRACTION

- Skeletal muscle contraction is initiated by a nerve impulse (action potential) that travels from the central nervous system to the muscle fibers via motor neurons.
- The nerve impulse stimulates the release of calcium ions from the sarcoplasmic reticulum (a specialized structure within the muscle fiber).
- Conformational change in the myosin head resulting in muscle contraction

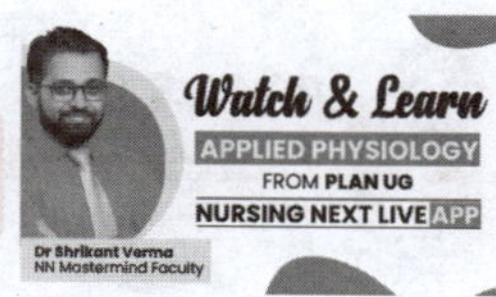

Cardiac Muscles and Smooth Muscles

Property	Cardiac muscles	Smooth muscles
Location	Found exclusively in the heart	Found in the walls of various organs and structures (e.g., blood vessels, digestive tract)
Appearance	Striated (striped) appearance	Nonstriated (smooth) appearance
Nuclei	Typically one or two centrally located nuclei	Single, centrally located nucleus
Intercalated Discs	Present, allowing for electrical and mechanical coupling between adjacent cells	Not present
Contraction	Involuntary and rhythmic	Involuntary and slow, sustained or rhythmic
Regulation of Contraction	Controlled by the electrical conduction system of the heart and autonomic nervous system	Controlled by hormones, local factors, and the autonomic nervous system
Fatigue Resistance	Highly fatigue-resistant due to a rich supply of mitochondria and myoglobin	Moderately fatigue-resistant
Force of Contraction	Strong and forceful contraction	Relatively weaker contraction
Speed of Contraction	Rapid and synchronized contraction	Slower and more prolonged contraction
Cell-to-Cell Communication	Gap junctions allow for rapid electrical coupling between cells	Gap junctions present, allowing for slow electrical coupling between cells
Regeneration Potential	Limited regenerative capacity	Limited regenerative capacity

APPLICATION AND IMPLICATION IN NURSING

- **Assessment and diagnosis:** Nurses need to perform comprehensive assessments and accurately diagnose musculoskeletal conditions. This includes assessing range of motion, muscle strength, joint stability, and gait patterns to identify abnormalities or potential issues.
- **Patient education:** They provide information on proper body mechanics, posture, and ergonomics to prevent musculoskeletal injuries and promote healthy movement patterns.
- **Safe patient handling:** Musculoskeletal injuries are a significant concern for health care providers, especially when it comes to lifting, transferring, and repositioning patients.
- **Pain Management:** Many musculoskeletal conditions, such as fractures, sprains, or arthritis, can cause significant pain. This may include administering medications, applying therapeutic modalities, or assisting with non-pharmacological pain relief techniques like positioning and relaxation techniques.
- **Rehabilitation and mobility:** Nurses often play a role in assisting patients with their rehabilitation and mobility.

CONCEPTUAL EXERCISES

LONG ANSWER QUESTION

1. Describe in detail with help of a diagram the mechanism of skeletal muscle contraction. (MGR)

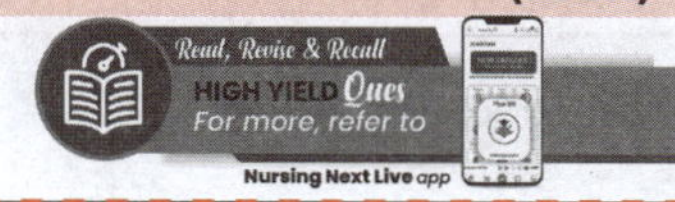

Answer

Skeletal Muscle

- Each muscle is made up of numerous subunits or bundles called fascicles that are surrounded by connective tissue called the permysium.
- Each fascicle is composed of numerous muscle fibers.
- Muscle cells are enclosed by endomysium and is made up of myofibrils.
- These myofibrils are composed of long protein molecules called myofilaments.

Mechanism of Skeletal Muscle Contraction

- Proposed by Jean Hanson and HE Huxley (1954)
- The excitation-contraction coupling is the process that occurs in between the excitation and contraction of the muscle. This process involves a series of events which are responsible for the contraction of the excited muscle.
- Calcium ions act as coupler.

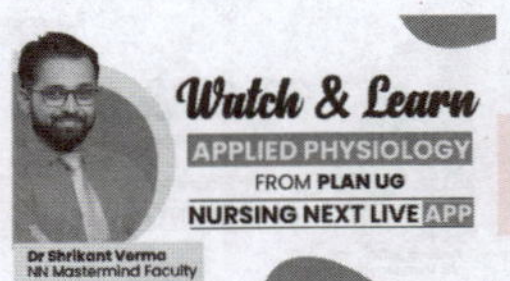

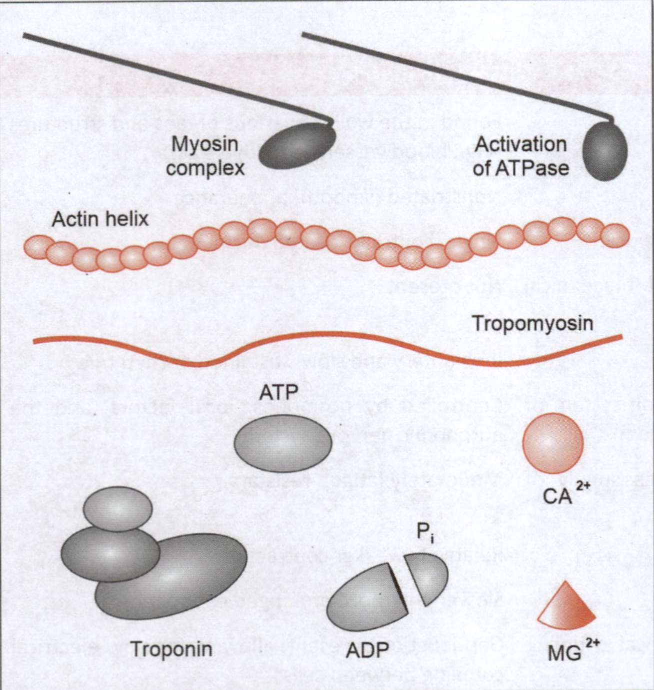

Figure 8.1: Components of muscle contraction

- **Sequence of events:**
  - Muscle shortening occurs due to the movement of actin filament over the myosin filament
  - There is reduction in the distance between Z lines of the sarcomere
  - Nerve impulses are sent to neuromuscular junction
  - Acetylcholine diffuses in and causes calcium ions to be released in the sarcoplasmic reticulum
  - Calcium ions bind with troponin
  - Removal of tropomyosin from actin
  - Actin and myosin join together and myosin pulls actin inward
  - ATP enables quick detachment of actin and myosin in preparation for power stroke
  - ATP breaks down
  - Sarcomere and distance between Z disc shortens
  - This process continues at a high rate in the presence of calcium ions
  - Once the impulse stops; calcium ions are sent back to sarcoplasmic reticulum
  - Tropomyosin rejoins actin, sarcomere and Z disc distance increases causing the relaxation of muscle.

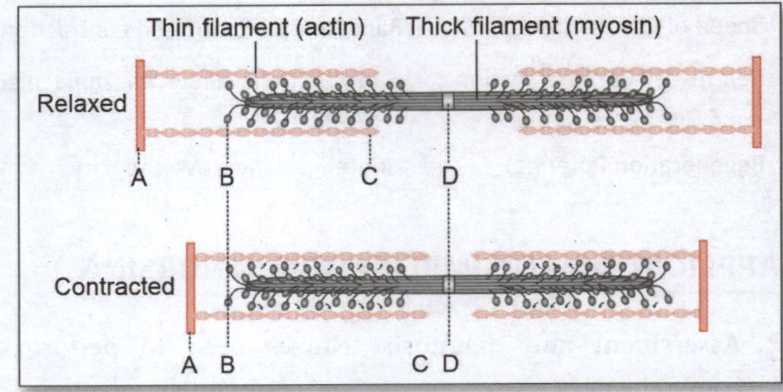

Figure 8.2: Sliding filament theory relaxation and contraction

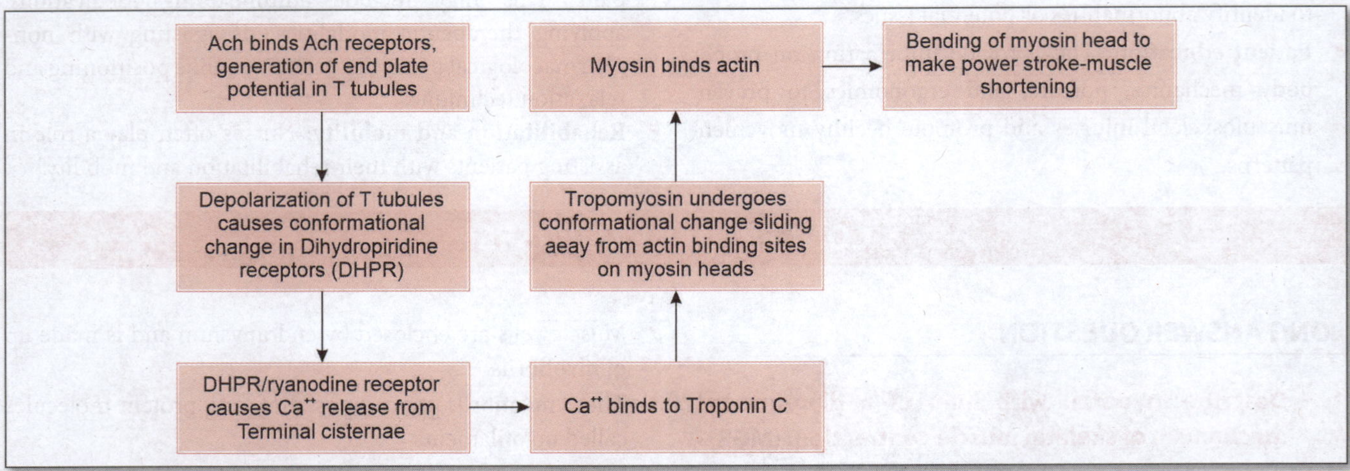

Figure 8.3: Steps in excitation contraction coupling

- **Role of calcium ions in muscle contraction**
  - The attachment of myosin cross bridges to actin and requires calcium ions.
  - The action potential causes the sarcoplasmic reticulum to release stored calcium ions into the sarcoplasm.
  - When the action potential ends, calcium ions are immediately reabsorbed into the sarcoplasmic reticulum storage areas and the muscle cell relaxes and settles back to its original length.

SHORT NOTES

1. Write a short note on synapse. (MGR)

Answer

Introduction

- Synapse is also known as neuronal junction.
- It is the site present between two nerve cells or between a neuron and a gland or between neuron and a muscle cell for transmission of electric nerve impulses.

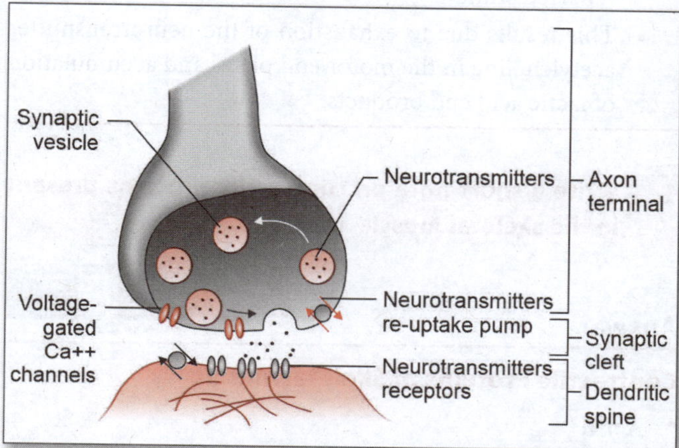

Figure 8.4: Synapse

Properties of Synapse

- **One way conduction – Bell-Magendie law:** This law states the transmission of impulses in one direction from presynaptic to postsynaptic neurons.
  - Direction of an impulse can be elicited at one way gate synapse as axons transmit impulses in either direction easily.
- **Convergence and divergence:** Numerous presynaptic neurons terminate on a single postsynaptic neuron, this is referred to as convergence, e.g., spinal motor neuron.
  - One presynaptic neuron terminates on many postsynaptic neurons, this is referred to as divergence.
- **Synaptic delay:** During impulse conduction, there is a delay of 0.5 msec before a reaction is elicited in the postsynaptic neuron.
  - It occurs as a consequence of time required for release of neurotransmitter and movement of neurotransmitter from axon terminal to postsynaptic membrane.
  - Synaptic delay helps in determination of reflex pathway whether it is monosynaptic or polysynaptic.
- **Summation:** Multiple excitatory postsynaptic potentials (EPSPs) can summate to reach the threshold required to fire an action potential in the postsynaptic neuron.
- **Fatigue:**
  - Fatigue is observed at synapse due to exhaustion of neurotransmitter acetylcholine
- **Occlusion:** With stronger stimuli, the effect of stimulating two nerve fibers may turn out to be less than the sum of stimulating either of them separately
- **Subliminal fringe:** Subliminal fringe is referred to as below threshold border.
  - If postsynaptic neurons are not discharged by the activity of presynaptic neurons instead possess their increased excitability, they obey property of subliminal fringe
- **Synaptic plasticity habituation:** If a stimulus gets repeated over and over again, the response to stimulus disappears.
- **Sensitization:** If a stimulus gets accompanied by unpleasant sensation, response increases.
- **Post-tetanic potentiation:** Increased production of post synaptic potentials due to excitation that lasts for minutes to hours.
- **Long-term potentiation:** Persistent prolongation of post-tetanic potentiation lasting for days is referred to as long-term-potentiation.
  - Occurs as a result of increase in intracellular calcium in postsynaptic neuron

2. Write a short note on Neuromuscular junction. (RUHS)

Answer

Neuromuscular Junction

- The junction between a motor nerve and a skeletal muscle fiber
- Also known as the myoneural junction
- When the nerve axons come close to the muscle fibers, they lose their myelin sheath exposing the axis cylinder.
- The terminal portion of the axis cylinder is expanded like a bulb—terminal buttons or end feet.
- The axon terminal contains mitochondria and synaptic vesicles.
- The synaptic vesicles contain the neurotransmitter substance, acetylcholine (Ach). It is synthesized in the mitochondria and stored in the vesicles located in the axon terminal.
- The end feet invaginates inside the muscle fiber and forms a depression. The membrane of the muscle fiber below the end feet is thickened and is called the postsynaptic membrane or the motor end plate.
- The membrane of the nerve ending is called the presynaptic membrane. The space between these two is known as synaptic cleft, it contains the enzyme acetylcholinesterase.

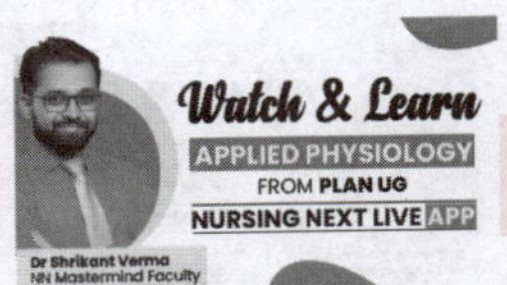

- Postsynaptic membrane – membrane of the muscle fiber. It is thrown into numerous folds called subneural clefts.
- The postsynaptic membrane contains the receptors called nicotinic acetylcholine receptors.

Resting Membrane Potential

When the muscle is in resting condition, the electrical potential is called resting membrane potential. It is –90 mV.

Action Potential

When the muscle is stimulated, electrical changes occur – action potential.

Neuromuscular Transmission

- Neuromuscular transmission is defined as the transfer of information from motor nerve endings to the muscle fiber through neurovascular junction.
- It is the mechanism that initiates muscle contraction.

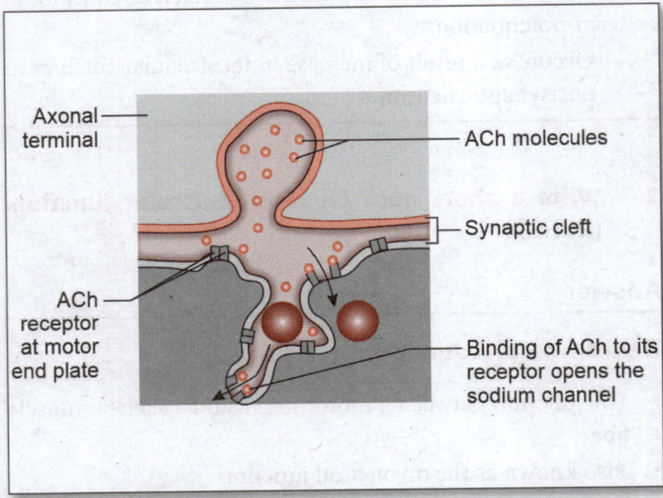

Figure 8.5: Neuromuscular junction

3. List the properties of skeletal muscle. (MGR)

Answer

Skeletal Muscle

- Each muscle is made up of numerous subunits or bundles called fascicles that are surrounded by connective tissue called the perimysium.
- Each fascicle is composed of numerous muscle fibers.
- Muscle cells are enclosed by endomysium and is made up of myofibrils.
- These myofibrils are composed of long protein molecules called myofilaments.

Properties of Skeletal Muscle

- **Excitability**
  - Reaction or response of a tissue to irritation or stimulation.
- **Contractility**
  - Response to a stimulus by change in length of the muscle fibers
- **Muscle tone**
  - Plays an important role in maintenance of posture.
  - Allows movement of the joints and the body as a whole.
- **Muscle fatigue**
  - Decrease in muscular activity due to prolonged or repeated stimuli.
  - This results due to exhaustion of the neurotransmitter acetylcholine in the motor end plates and accumulation of lactic acid end products.

4. Write a short note on contractile proteins present in the skeletal muscle. (MGR)

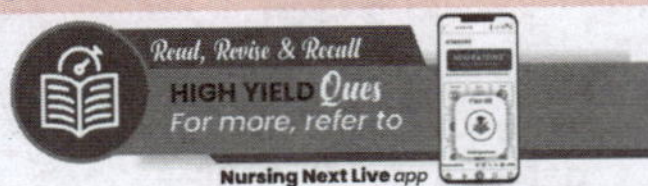

Answer

Contractile Proteins of Skeletal Muscle

- **Actin**
  - Most abundant protein in nonmuscle cells 1–5%
  - Functions
    - Role in maintaining the shape of the cell
    - Polarization
    - Locomotion
    - Division of the cell
- **Myosin**
  - Part of the large family of myosin related proteins
  - Contains one or two heavy chains and several light chains
  - Heavy chain contains:
    - Large globular head
      - Contains actin binding regions
      - Contains the ATPase regions
    - Alpha helical neck region
      - Binds the light chain
    - Tail
      - For oligomerization or cargo binding.
  - Light chain contains
    - Calmodulin – calcium binding protein
    - Has a role in regulation of myosin activity
- **Accessory contractile proteins are:**
  - **Titin**
    - Large elastic protein that anchors the Z lines and thick filaments
    - Prevents excessive stretching of the myofibril

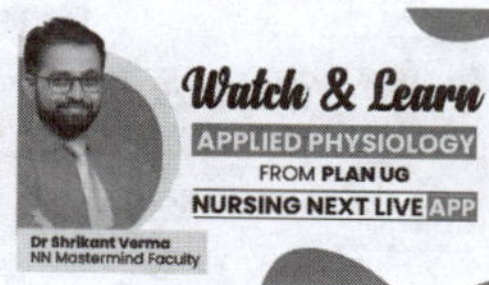

- **Tropomodulin**
  - Attached to the free end of an actin filament
  - Maintains the length of the actin filament
- **Myomesin**
  - Anchors the thick filaments to M line
- **Desmin**
  - Intermediate filament
  - Attaches the Z line to subsarcolemmal cytoskeleton and the plasma membrane
- **Alpha actinin**
  - Short rod-shaped protein that arranges thin filaments into parallel bundles
  - Anchors the thin filaments to Z line
- **Nebulin**
  - Thin elongated protein running parallel to thin filaments
  - Assists alpha actinin in function.

5. Write a short note on myasthenia gravis. (MGR)

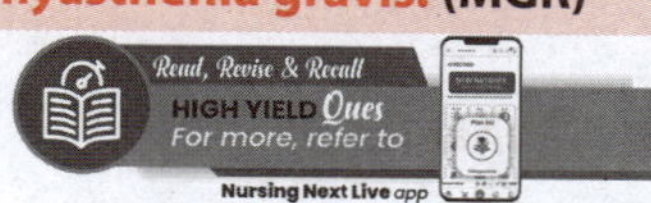

Answer

Myasthenia Gravis

- Myasthenia gravis is an autoimmune disorder that affects acetylcholine receptor (AChR) of muscle fibers resulting in abnormal progressive fatigability of skeletal muscle.
- Females 2:1; any age; often begins with small muscle of head and neck
- Caused by autoimmune condition. Antibodies are formed against acetyl choline receptors at the NMJ.
- Characterized by increased muscle weakness and fatigue
- Eventually death from respiratory failure
- Neuromuscular junction is severely affected due to depletion of acetylcholine

Mechanism

- Caused by autoantibody against acetylcholine receptor
- Reduction in the size of end plate potential results in difficulty to depolarize muscle membrane to threshold and thus generation of action potential.

Signs and Symptoms

- Characterized by increased muscle weakness and fatigue
- Lids and Extraocular Muscles
  - Drooping eyelids is an early and prominent sign.
  - Diplopia and Ptosis
- Facial muscles
  - "Worried or surprised look "snarling appearance"
- Masticatory Muscle Weakness
  - Weakness while chewing
- Speech
  - Myasthenic speech
  - Dysarthria – Mushy quality
- Dysphagia
  - Nasal regurgitation
  - Aspiration of liquids or foods
  - Eventually death from respiratory failure

Diagnosis

- Weakness and Fatigability
- No loss of reflexes
- No impairment of sensations
- Edrophonium
  - Rapid onset–30 s
  - Short duration–5 minutes
  - Initial dose–2 mg IV
  - Additional dose–8 mg IV
- Neostigmine: 15 mg orally
- Electrodiagnostic testing: Electric shock: 2–3 per sec
- Ice pack test

Treatment

- Neostigmine acts by decelerating the breakdown of acetylcholine
- Therefore, unavailability of acetylcholine prevents its attachment to the muscle receptor resulting in the strengthening of muscles
- Responds dramatically to AchE inhibitors such as Neostigmine
- Oral Pyridostigmine is started within 15–30 minutes lasting for 3–4 hours. Moderate dose, 60 mg 3–5 times/ day, Maximum dosage – 120 mg every 3 hours/day

SHORT ANSWER QUESTIONS

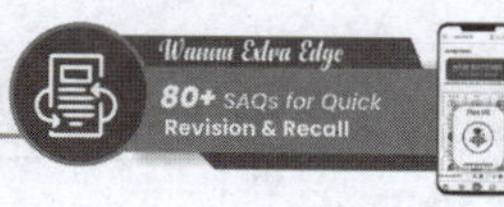

1. Define sarcomere.

Answer

Sarcomere is the structural and functional unit of myofibril.

In each myofibril, thick and thin filaments are arranged in a repeating pattern in the form of sarcomere between two successive Z lines.

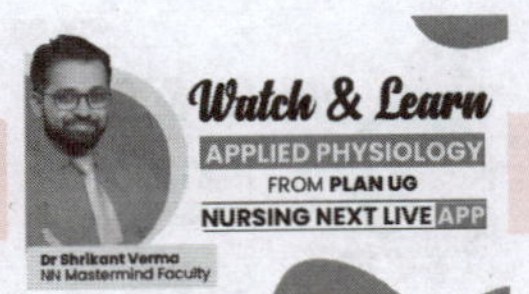

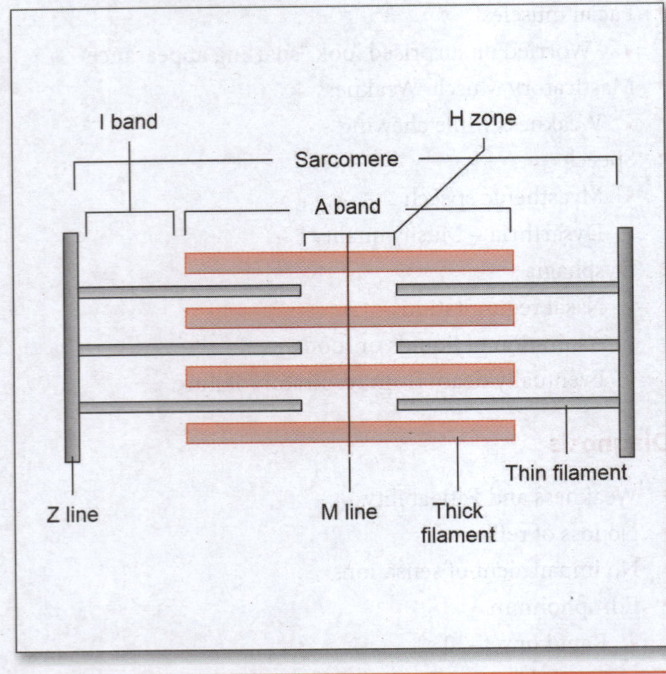

2. Define rigor mortis.

Answer

Rigor mortis refers to the stiffening of the muscle after death. Rigor mortis develops 3 to 6 hours after death as a result of a drop in ATP levels in all types of cells, including muscle cells.

3. Name any two contractile proteins.

Answer

Two contractile proteins found in muscle cells are:

1. Actin is a thin filamentous protein that is involved in muscle contraction.
2. Myosin is a thick filamentous protein that is also involved in muscle contraction.

4. List any two physiological properties of skeletal muscle.

Answer

Two physiological properties of skeletal muscle.

1. **Excitability:** Refers to the ability of skeletal muscle cells to respond to signals from CNS for muscle contraction
2. **Contractility:** Refers to the ability of skeletal muscle cells to generate force and shorten in response to a stimulus.

5. What is tetany?

Answer

Tetany is a medical condition characterized by involuntary contractions of skeletal muscles that occur as a result of low levels of calcium in the blood. Chvostek's sign and Trousseau's sign are two key features.

CONCEPTUAL REVISION

MULTIPLE CHOICE QUESTIONS

1. Bones contain yellow marrow that is composed mainly of:

a. Fat
b. Protein
c. Cartilage
d. Carbohydrates

Ans. a. Fat

2. Which type of bone cell is responsible for the formation of bone?

a. Osteocyte
b. Osteoclast
c. Osteoblast
d. Sarcomere

Ans. c. Osteoblast

3. Bones in synovial joints are joined together by:

a. Cartilage
b. Ligaments
c. Tendons
d. Periosteal tissue

Ans. b. Ligaments

4. Articulation between the head of the femur and the acetabulum is in the:

a. Knee joint
b. Tibial joint
c. Ankle joint
d. Hip joint

Ans. d. Hip joint

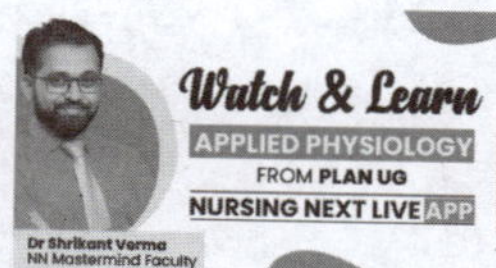

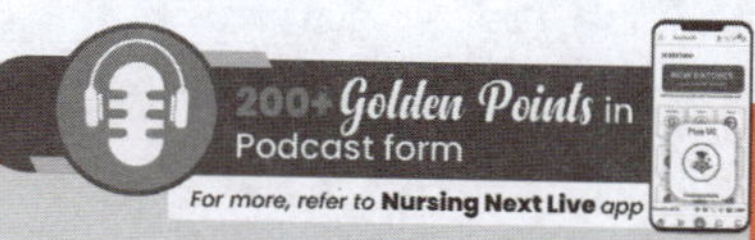

Golden Points

- All bones develop from the mesenchymal tissue of the embryo.
- Ball and socket joint allows for movement in all directions.
- Bone is able to regenerate.
- Bone is made up of 2/3rd inorganic matter, i.e., $Ca_{10}(PO_4)_6OH_2$ and 1/3rd organic matter is made up of collagen fibers.
- Cardiac muscles are striated muscles found exclusively in heart with involuntary and rhythmic contraction controlled by the electrical conduction system of the heart and autonomic nervous system.
- Five main properties of the muscular system are – Contractibility, Elasticity, Excitability, Extensibility and Adaptability.
- Hinge joint allows for flexion and extension in one plane
- Osteoarthritis is a degenerative joint disease that primarily affects the articular cartilage.
- Pivot joint allows for rotational movement around a central axis
- Rheumatoid arthritis is an autoimmune disease that primarily affects the synovial membrane.
- Skeletal muscle contraction is initiated by a nerve impulse (action potential) that travels from the central nervous system to the muscle fibers via motor neurons.
- Skeletal muscles help maintain proper body posture and provide stability to the skeletal system.
- Smooth muscle cells can divide and multiply
- The primary function of skeletal muscles is to produce voluntary movements of the body.
- The process of bone healing consists of five stages- Hematoma formation, formation of fibrocartilage, formation of fibrocartilaginous callus, initiation of endochondral ossification and remodeling and consolidation.
- The smooth muscle is small fusiform and non-striated cells with a single nucleus.
- There are two types of bone tissues: Cortical which is compact and cancellous which is trabecular and spongy.

CHAPTER 9

Renal System

CONCEPTUAL THEORY

Terminology

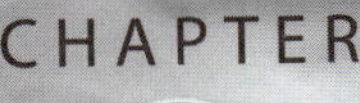

Filtration: The first step in renal function is filtration, which occurs in the glomerulus of the nephron.
Glomerular filtration rate: (GFR) is the amount of plasma ultrafiltrate formed each minute. Normal adult GFR - 125mL/min
Homeostasis: Self-regulating process by which biological systems tend to maintain stability while adjusting to conditions that are optimal for survival.
Micturition: Process by which urinary bladder empties when it is filled.
Reabsorption: After filtration, reabsorption takes place in the renal tubules.
Secretion: In addition to reabsorption, the renal tubules also participate in secretion, where certain substances are actively transported from the blood into the tubules.

FUNCTIONS OF KIDNEY

Major functions of kidney are the regulation of:
- Water homeostasis
- Electrolyte composition
- Acid-base homeostasis
- Regulation of the extracellular volume (blood pressure)

As nephrons are the functional unit of kidney it consists of renal corpuscle, PCT, Loop of Henle, DCT and collecting duct system.

Role of Kidney in Maintaining Homeostasis

- Regulates blood pressure and blood volume
- Regulates plasma ion concentration
- Helps in stabilization of blood pH
- Helps conservation of valuable nutrients
- Helps liver in detoxification of poison

GFR

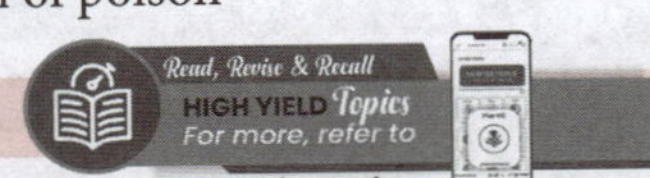

Glomerular filtration rate (GFR) is the amount of plasma ultrafiltrate formed each minute. Normal adult GFR – 125mL/min.

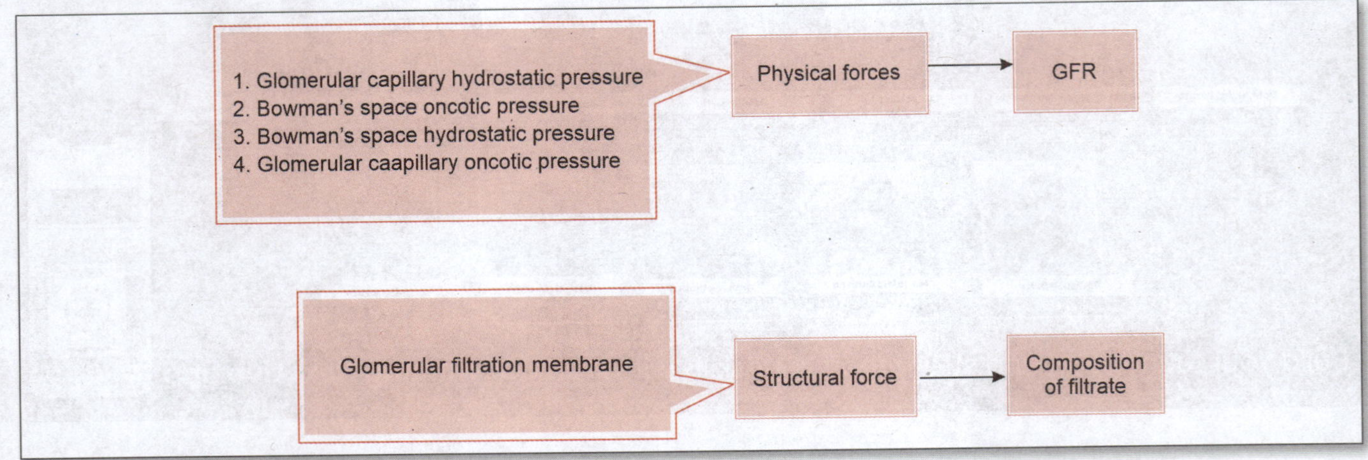

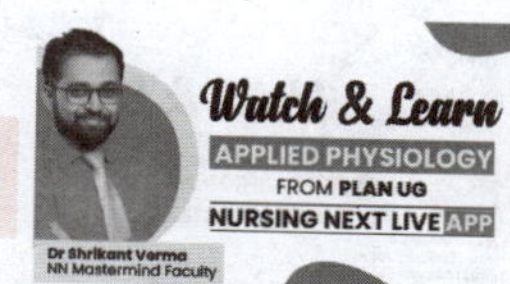

i Net driving force (P_{UF}):
[(PGC – PBS) – (πGC- πBS)]

ii GFR= Kf × Net filtration pressure,
where Kf is glomerular capillary filtration coefficient.

Factors Affecting the Glomerular Filtration

- **Renal Blood Flow:** Glomerular filtration rate (GFR) is directly proportional to renal blood flow.
  - **Age:** GFR is inversely proportional to age, as the age increases GFR decreases.
- **Changes in hydrostatic pressure in the glomerular capillaries (PCap)**
  - Glomerular filtration rate increases with increase in glomerular capillary pressure.
  - Capillary pressure is dependent on renal blood flow and arterial blood pressure.
  - PCap is directly proportional to systemic blood pressure.
- **Changes in hydrostatic pressure in Bowman's capsule (PBow)**
  - GFR is inversely proportional to PBow
  - Certain conditions like urethral obstruction and edema of kidney increases PBow decreases GFR.
- **Changes in the Concentration of Plasma Proteins**
  - GFR is inversely proportional to plasma oncotic pressure
  - During hypoproteinemia colloidal osmotic pressure in capillaries (COP)cap decreases, thus GFR increases
  - Dehydration increases COPcap decreases GFR
- **Constriction of Afferent and Efferent Arteriole**
  - Blood flow to glomerular capillaries reduces due to afferent arteriole constriction reducing GFR
  - Initially there is increase in GFR due to constriction of efferent arteriole

FUNCTIONS OF URETERS, BLADDER AND URETHRA

Ureter

- The ureters are muscular tubes that connect the kidneys to the bladder.
- The primary function of the ureters is to transport urine from the kidneys to the bladder.
- The ureters accomplish this by using peristaltic contractions, which are wave-like muscular movements, to propel urine down into the bladder.
- The ureters also have valves called ureterovesical valves at their junction with the bladder, which prevent the backflow of urine.

Bladder

- The bladder is a hollow, muscular organ located in the lower abdomen.
- It serves as a reservoir for urine storage until it can be voluntarily released from the body.
- The main function of the bladder is to store urine and stretch to accommodate increasing volumes of urine without a significant increase in internal pressure.
- The bladder wall is made of smooth muscle, which contracts during urination to expel urine through the urethra.
- The bladder also has a triangular area called the trigone, which acts as a sensory region that signals the brain when the bladder is full.

Urethra

- The urethra is a tube that connects the bladder to the external urethral orifice, allowing urine to exit the body.
- In males, the urethra serves a dual function by also being a part of the reproductive system, as it transports semen during ejaculation.
- The length of the urethra is different in males and females, with males generally having a longer urethra.
- The external urethral sphincter, a ring of muscles at the opening of the urethra, helps control the voluntary release of urine.

MICTURITION

- Process by which urinary bladder empties when it is filled.
- Involves two steps:
  - First the bladder fills progressively till the tension in its walls rises above a threshold level.
  - Secondly, the nervous reflex sets in that is the micturition reflex that empties the bladder.

Higher Centers that Control Micturition

- Pontine micturition center
  - Present in the Barrington's nucleus of pons
  - Facilitates micturition
- Posterior hypothalamus – facilitates micturition
- Midbrain – inhibits micturition
- Paracentral lobule
- It is concerned with regulation of physiological function such as defecation and micturition
- It is supplied by anterior cerebral artery
- Lesion in this area causes urinary incontinence

REGULATION OF RENAL FUNCTION

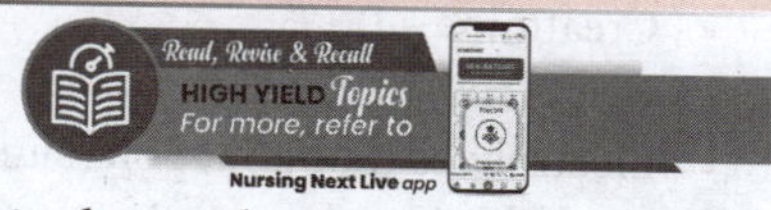

Main processes involved in the regulation of renal function:

- **Filtration:** The first step in renal function is filtration, which occurs in the glomerulus of the nephron.
- **Reabsorption:** After filtration, reabsorption takes place in the renal tubules.

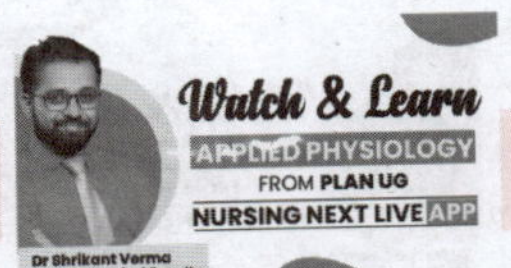

- **Secretion:** In addition to reabsorption, the renal tubules also participate in secretion, where certain substances are actively transported from the blood into the tubules.
- **Renin-Angiotensin-Aldosterone system (RAAS):** The RAAS is a hormonal system that regulates blood pressure and fluid balance. When blood pressure drops or there is a decrease in sodium levels, the kidneys release an enzyme called renin.
- **Antidiuretic hormone (ADH):** ADH, also known as vasopressin, is released by the pituitary gland in response to changes in blood osmolality or volume. ADH acts on the collecting ducts of the nephron, increasing their permeability to water.
- **Autoregulation:** The kidneys have intrinsic mechanisms to regulate their own blood flow and glomerular filtration rate (GFR). Autoregulation helps maintain a relatively constant blood flow and filtration despite changes in systemic blood pressure. The two main mechanisms of autoregulation are the myogenic mechanism and the tubuloglomerular feedback mechanism.

APPLICATION AND IMPLICATION IN NURSING

Renal physiology plays a crucial role in nursing practice, as it directly affects the overall health and well-being of patients. Here are some applications and implications of renal physiology in nursing:

- **Assessment of renal function:** Nurses are responsible for assessing and monitoring the renal function of patients. This includes evaluating urine output, measuring laboratory values such as blood urea nitrogen (BUN) and creatinine levels, and assessing fluid and electrolyte balance.
- **Administration and monitoring of medications:** Many medications are excreted by the kidneys, and renal dysfunction can significantly impact their pharmacokinetics.
- **Fluid and electrolyte management:** Maintaining fluid and electrolyte balance is crucial for patients with renal dysfunction or undergoing renal replacement therapy (such as hemodialysis or peritoneal dialysis).
- **Prevention and management of acute kidney injury (AKI):** AKI is a common condition in hospitalized patients and can have serious implications.
- **Patient education and support:** Nurses are responsible for educating patients about kidney health, managing chronic kidney disease (CKD), and promoting self-care strategies.
- **Collaboration with the interdisciplinary team:** Nursing professionals collaborate with other healthcare providers, such as nephrologists, dietitians, and pharmacists, to provide comprehensive care to patients with renal conditions.

CONCEPTUAL EXERCISES

LONG ANSWER QUESTION

1. Describe the composition of Urine. Discuss the mechanism of urine formation. (RUHS, MGR, DU)

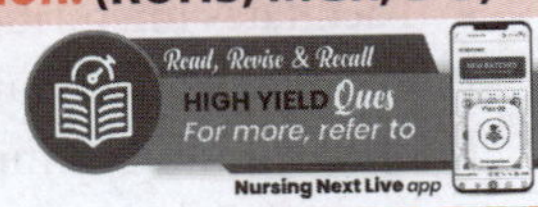

Answer

Composition of Urine:

- Composition of urine depends on the amount of substances secreted and absorption of water and electrolytes.
- Composition:
  - Water – 95%
  - Urea – 2%
  - Creatinine – 0.1%
  - Uric Acid – 0.03%
  - Electrolytes (Sodium, potassium, chloride, bicarbonate)
- Normal physical characteristics of urine are:
  - Color: Amber
  - Specific gravity: 1.010–1.030
  - Odor: mild
  - Volume: 1,500–2000 mL/day
  - Turbidity: Transparent when freshly passed
  - pH: 5–8
  - Water content –97%
  - Solids: Less than 3%

Mechanism of Urine Formation

Urine is formed by the collective action of the following three processes:

1. Glomerular filtration.
2. Tubular reabsorption of the substance from the tubular fluid into the blood.
3. Tubular secretion of the substance from the blood into the tubular fluid.

Glomerular Filtration

- First step in the formation of urine.
- Renal blood flow is about 1200 mL/min.
- As the glomerular capillaries are narrower than the glomerular arterioles, hydrostatic pressure is exerted.

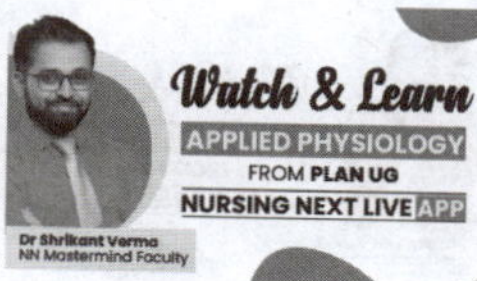

- Due to this pressure, the blood is filtered through the pores of podocytes. This filtrate is known as glomerular filtrate and the process is known as ultrafiltration.
- This filtrate consists of water, electrolytes, glucose, amino acids and waste products of metabolism.
- The volume of filtrate formed by both kidneys each minute is called glomerular filtration rate (GFR) which is about 125 mL/min.
- Factors affecting the glomerular filtration are:
  - Glomerular blood hydrostatic pressure
  - Opposing forces: plasma colloid osmotic pressure and capsular hydrostatic pressure.
- Glomerular filtration is regulated by:
  - Myogenic mechanism: Increase in blood pressure increases the pressure in afferent arterioles that results in increased blood flow to the glomerulus.

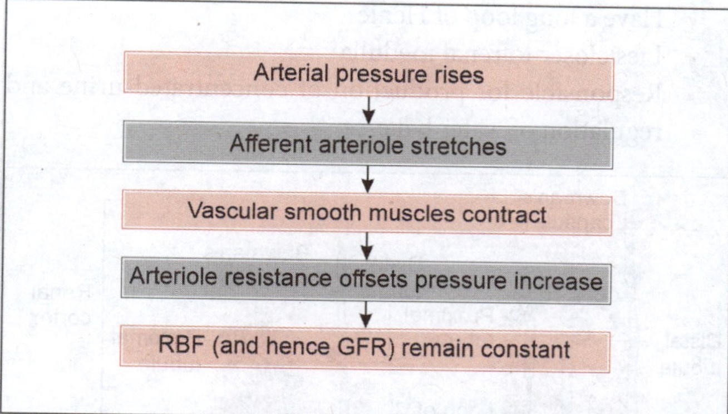

Figure 9.1: Myogenic Mechanism

- Juxtaglomerular mechanism: Secretes an enzyme renin, which controls the blood pressure and the GFR – renin-angiotensin mechanism.

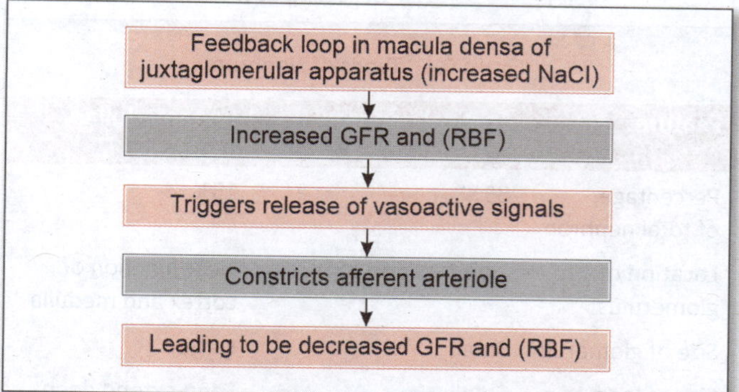

Figure 9.2: Tubuloglomerular feedback mechanism

- Neural control:
  - Autoregulation prevails when the sympathetic nervous system is at rest.
  - Under stress and effect of epinephrine, afferent arterioles constrict and filtration is inhibited.

Tubular Reabsorption

- **Proximal convoluted tubule**
  - As the filtrate passes through the PCT, 70% of the water and electrolytes and 100% of the glucose and amino acids are reabsorbed.
  - Reabsorption of vitamins, hormones, chlorides and sodium also occurs.
  - Thus, filtrate is isotonic to plasma.
- **Loop of Henle**
  - Continuation of the proximal convoluted tubule.
  - Consists of ascending and descending parts.
  - Water is reabsorbed in the descending limb and not the solutes; thus, filtrate is hypertonic to blood plasma.
  - In the ascending limb, solutes are reabsorbed, making the filtrate hypotonic.
- **Distal convoluted tubule (DCT)**
  - Under the influence of aldosterone, sodium ions are reabsorbed.
  - Under the influence of ADH, water is reabsorbed.
- **Collecting duct**
  - More water is reabsorbed, thereby making the filtrate hypertonic.
  - This concentrated filtrate is known as urine.

Hormones Regulating Tubular Reabsorption

Parathormone - ↑ reabsorption of Ca^{2+}, Mg
Calcitonin - ↓ Ca^{2+} reabsorption
Aldosterone - ↑ Na^{+} reabsorption
Angiotensin II - ↑ Na reabsorption
Antidiuretic hormone - ↑ water reabsorption

Tubular Secretion

- Till the time the filtrate reaches the end of the proximal tubule, it has already reabsorbed:
  - 60–70% of water and sodium
  - About 100% of glucose and amino acids.
  - 90% of K^{+}, bicarbonate, Ca^{2+}, uric acid.
- Distal convoluted tubules and collecting ducts:
  - Dependent on ADH
  - Secretion of harmful toxic materials like ammonia, creatinine, urea, hippuric acid, etc.
  - ADH is also responsible for facultative water reabsorption.
  - Parathyroid hormone increases Ca^{2+} reabsorption.
  - Many electrolytes, e.g., H^{+}, Cl^{-}, K^{+} etc. are secreted from blood into the tubular fluid.
- This takes place by:
  - **Passive diffusion:** Movement occurs from the peritubular capillaries to the interstitial fluid within the nephron.

- **Active transport:**
  - Movement occurs with the use of ATPase pumps.
  - ATPase pumps transport substances across the renal epithelium into the lumen of nephron.

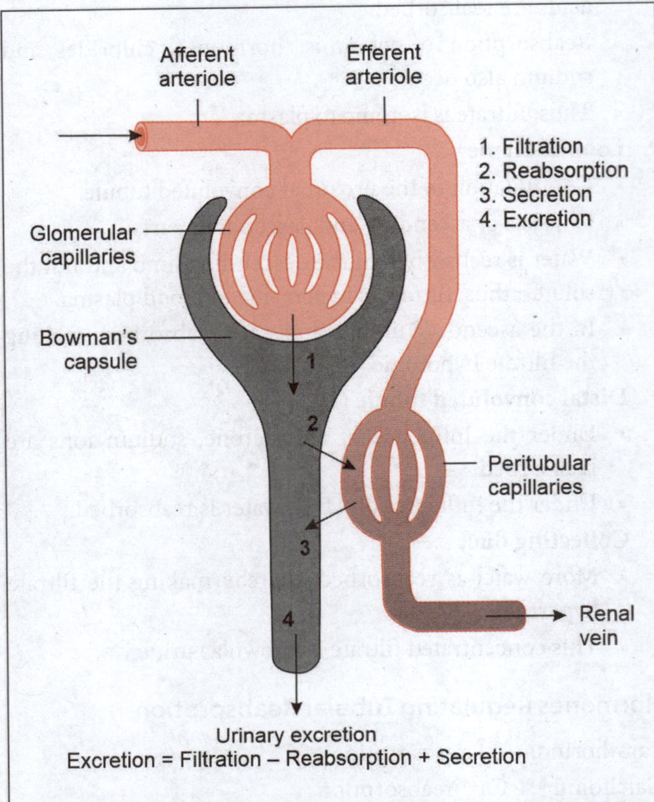

Figure 9.3: Tubular secretion—steps involved in urine formation.

Countercurrent Mechanism

- A countercurrent system is a system of 'U'-shaped tubes in which the flow of fluid is in opposite direction in two limbs of the 'U'-shaped tubules.
- In kidney, countercurrent system is seen in the loop of Henle and vasa recta in renal medulla. This concentrates urine. Urine formed in the kidneys comes down to the urinary bladder through ureters and then is expelled out of the body. This expulsion is called micturition.

Significance of Urine Formation

- Removing wastes such as creatinine and urea.
- Regulating the extracellular fluid volume by removal of extra fluid.
- Regulating blood pH.
- Maintaining the electrolyte-water balance by concentrating or diluting the urine.

SHORT NOTES

1. Describe types of nephron and its functions. (MGR)

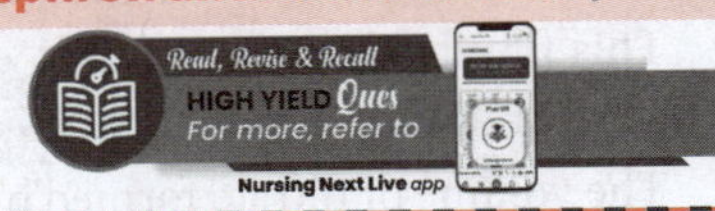

Answer

Nephron

- Structural and functional unit of the kidneys.
- Consists of malpighian body and renal tubules.

Types of Nephron

- **Cortical nephron**
  - Short nephrons
  - Lie in the cortical region of the kidney.
  - Regulates electrolytes, blood pH and overall fluid balance
- **Juxtamedullary nephron**
  - Have a long loop of Henle
  - Lies closer to renal medulla
  - Responsible for production of concentrated urine and regulation of water balance

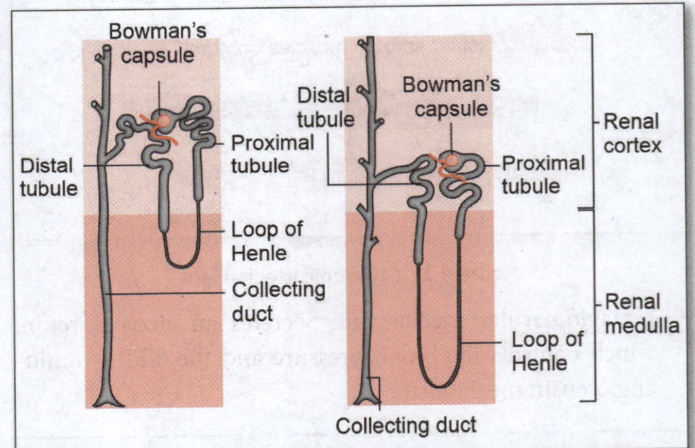

Figure 9.4: Types of Nephron

Feature	Cortical nephron	Juxtamedullary nephron
Percentage of total nephron	85%	15%
Location of glomerulus	Upper region of cortex	Near junction of cortex and medulla
Size of glomeruli	Small	Large
Size of loop of Henle	Small	Long-extend deep into medulla
Capillaries	Surrounded by peritubular capillaries	Surrounded by Vasa recta
Major unction	Excretion of waste products in urine	Concentration of urine by the counter current system

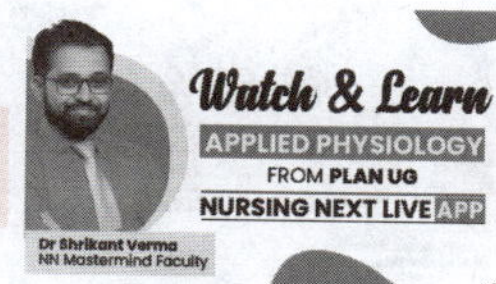

Both the cortical and juxtamedullary nephron work together to filter blood, removal of waste products and maintenance of fluid and electrolyte balance in the body.

2. Factors affecting glomerular filtration rate. (MGR)

Answer

Factors affecting the glomerular filtration rate

- **Renal Blood Flow:** Glomerular filtration rate (GFR) is directly proportional to renal blood flow.
- **Age:** GFR is inversely proportional to age, as the age increases GFR decreases.
- **Changes in hydrostatic pressure in the glomerular capillaries (PCap)**
  - Glomerular filtration rate increases with increase in glomerular capillary pressure.
  - Capillary pressure is dependent on renal blood flow and arterial blood pressure.
  - PCap is directly proportional to systemic blood pressure.
- **Changes in hydrostatic pressure in Bowman's capsule (PBow) w**
  - GFR is inversely proportional to PBow
  - Certain conditions like urethral obstruction and edema of kidney increases PBow decreases GFR.
- **Changes in the Concentration of Plasma Proteins**
  - GFR is inversely proportional to plasma oncotic pressure.
  - During hypoproteinemia colloidal osmotic pressure in capillaries (COP) cap decreases, thus GFR increases.
  - Dehydration increases COPcap decreases GFR
- **Constriction of Afferent and Efferent Arteriole**
  - Blood flow to glomerular capillaries reduces due to afferent arteriole constriction reducing GFR
  - Initially there is increase in GFR due to constriction of efferent arteriole.

3. Write a short note on micturition. (MGR)

Answer

Micturition

- Process by which urinary bladder empties when it is filled.
- Involves two steps:
  - First the bladder fills progressively till the tension in its walls rises above a threshold level.
  - Secondly, the nervous reflex sets in that is the micturition reflex that empties the bladder.

Micturition Reflex

- It is a self-regenerative reflex.
- It occurs due to stimulation of the sensory stretch fibers carrying signal through pelvic nerves to sacral segment and brings the signal back to bladder through parasympathetic nerve fibers.
- Its initiation occurs by rapid and progressive increase in pressure. Initially the sensation to void the urine starts with 200 mL.
- Pressure equals basal tone of bladder, when the pressure increases it stimulates sensory fibers of stretch receptors. The afferent are carried through pelvic nerve
- Initiation of micturition reflex causes stimulation of postganglionic neuron in intramural ganglion in urinary bladder which causes contraction of the detrusor muscle.
- Relaxation of the external sphincter by its inhibition through pudendal nerve.
- Voiding of bladder occurs when micturition reflex gets powerful enough (urine >500 mL).

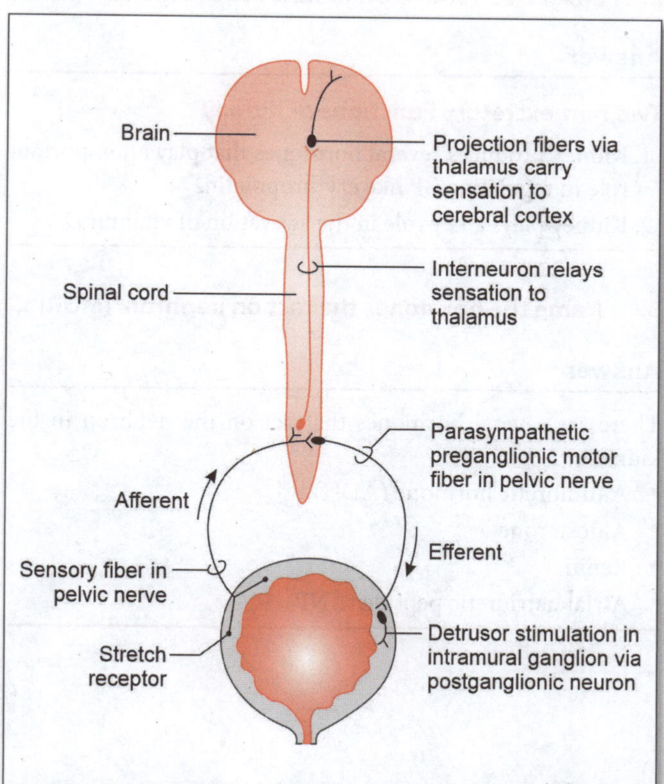

Figure 9.5: Micturition reflex

Higher Centers that Control Micturition

- Pontine micturition center
  - Present in the Barrington's nucleus of pons
  - Facilitates micturition

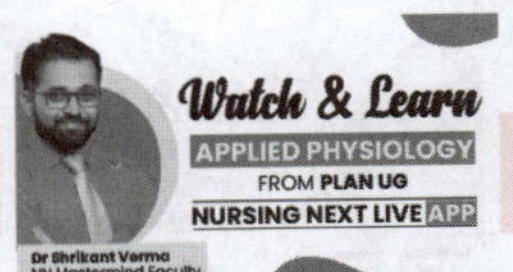

- Posterior hypothalamus facilitates micturition
- Midbrain inhibits micturition
- Paracentral lobule
- It is concerned with regulation of physiological function such as defecation and micturition.
- It is supplied by anterior cerebral artery.
- Lesion in this area causes urinary incontinence.

SHORT ANSWER QUESTIONS

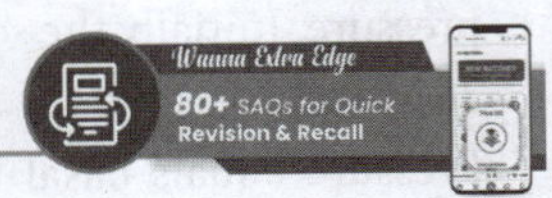

1. What is renal failure? (MGR)

Answer

A medical illness known as renal failure, or as kidney failure, occurs when the kidneys are unable to adequately filter waste materials from the blood. It result in accumulation of harmful compounds in the body like urea and creatinine.

2. Enlist two nonexcretory functions of kidney. (MGR)

Answer

Two non-excretory Functions of Kidney

1. Kidney produces several hormones that play an important role in regulating BP like erythropoietin.
2. Kidney plays a key role in the activation of vitamin D.

3. Name the hormones that act on nephron. (MGR)

Answer

There are several hormones that act on the nephron in the kidneys:

- Antidiuretic hormone (ADH)
- Aldosterone
- Renin
- Atrial natriuretic peptide (ANP)

4. Define glomerular filtration rate. (MGR)

Answer

Glomerular filtration rate (GFR) is the amount of filtrate produced by the glomerular filtering membrane of both kidneys in a unit of time. In the normal range, it is 125 mL/min (7.5 L/hr or 180 L/day).

5. Write two functions of kidneys. (MGR)

Answer

Two Functions of Kidneys

1. The primary function of kidneys is to excrete waste products of metabolisms from the body such as urea, creatinine, uric acid, etc. dissolved in urine.
2. Kidneys contribute mainly to long-term regulation of arterial volume and pressure.

6. Name two important waste products excreted by the kidneys. (MGR)

Answer

The two important waste products excreted by the kidneys are:

1. Urea is a waste product that is produced when the body breaks down proteins.
2. Creatinine is a waste product that is produced by the muscles when they use energy.

7. Define juxtaglomerular apparatus. (MGR)

Answer

A unique kidney structure called the juxtaglomerular apparatus (JGA) is situated next to the glomerulus, which is where blood is filtered. The macula densa, juxtaglomerular cells, and extraglomerular mesangial cells are the three primary parts of the JGA.

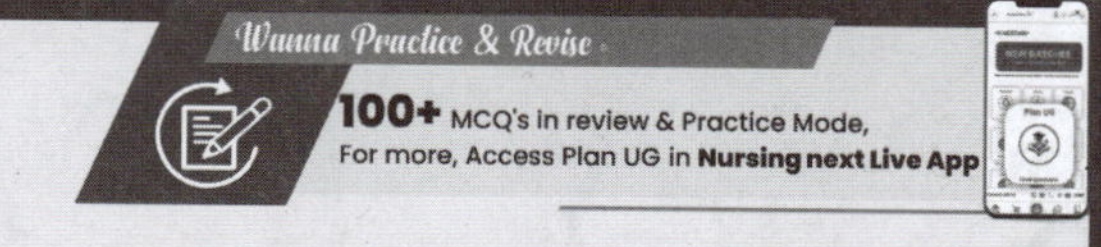

CONCEPTUAL REVISION

MULTIPLE CHOICE QUESTIONS

1. **Which of the following structures is not a part of the nephron?**
   a. The calyx
   b. The distal convoluted tubule
   c. The ascending loop of Henle
   d. The collecting duct

Ans. a. The calyx

2. **The kidneys produce all of the following EXCEPT one. Which one?**
   a. Erythropoietin
   b. Angiotensinogen
   c. Hydronium ions
   d. Bicarbonate ions

Ans. b. Angiotensinogen

3. **Approximately what volume of filtrate enters the glomerular capsule space each day?**
   a. 80 L
   b. 130 L
   c. 180 L
   d. 230 L

Ans. c. 180 L

4. **Which of the following acts as the filtration apparatus of the kidneys?**
   a. The descending loop of Henle
   b. The glomerular capsule
   c. The collecting duct
   d. The renal pelvis

Ans. b. The glomerular capsule

Golden Points

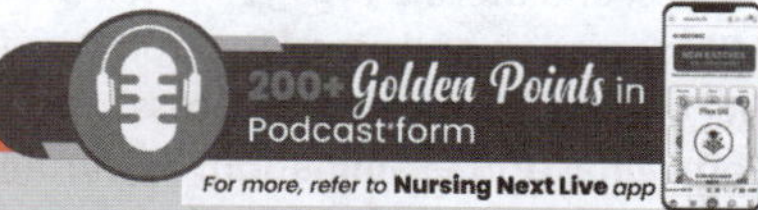

- Glomerular filtration rate (GFR) is the amount of plasma ultrafiltrate formed each minute. Normal adult GFR - 125 mL/min.
- In males, the urethra serves a dual function by also being a part of the reproductive system, as it transports semen during ejaculation.
- Major functions of kidney are water homeostasis, electrolyte composition, acid-base homeostasis and regulation of the extracellular volume.
- Micturition is a process by which urinary bladder empties when it is filled.
- Nephrons are the functional unit of kidney.
- The main function of bladder is to store urine and stretch to accommodate increasing volumes of urine without a significant increase in internal pressure.
- The ureter is the muscular tube that connect the kidneys to the bladder and its primary function is to transport urine from the kidneys to the bladder.
- The urethra is a tube that connects the bladder to the external urethral orifice, allowing urine to exit the body.
- Urine is formed and regulated by the collective action of three processes- Glomerular filtration, Tubular secretion and Tubular reabsorption.

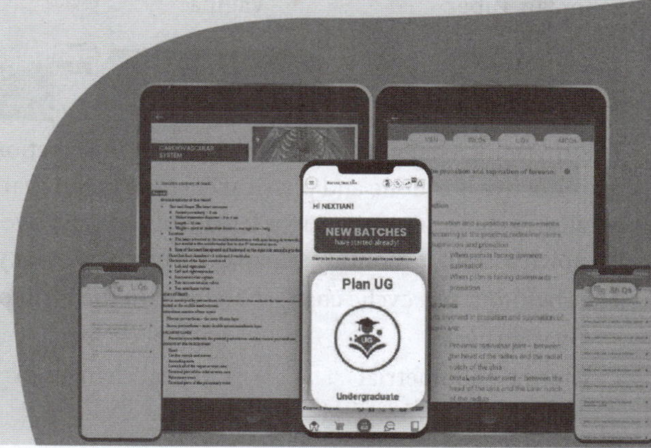

CHAPTER

10

Reproductive System

CONCEPTUAL THEORY

Terminology

Fertilization: Fertilization is the process by which male and female gametes are fused together and initiate the development of a new organism.
Implantation: Implantation is burrowing of an embryo deep into the lining of the uterus, where it can then begin to grow.
Menstrual cycle: The rhythmic changes that occur monthly in secretion of reproductive hormone and physical changes in the ovarian, cervical and uterine organs in a female of reproductive age is known as female monthly sexual cycle or menstrual cycle.
Milk secretion and ejection: Prolactin, with estrogen, and progesterone cause milk secretion. Oxytocin helps in milk ejection.
Oogenesis: It is a growth process in which the primary egg cell (or ovum) becomes a mature ovum.
Pervaginal (PV) examination: By introducing gloved index and middle fingers into vagina, one can palpate vagina, cervix, uterus, ovaries, pulsation of uterine arteries during pregnancy.
Puberty: Puberty in females is marked by first episode of menstrual flow at about 12–14 years.
Spermatogenesis: Spermatogenesis is the process by which male primary sperm cells undergo meiosis and produce a number of cells called spermatogonia, from which the primary spermatocytes are derived.

FEMALE REPRODUCTIVE SYSTEM

The female reproductive system is a complex system of organs that are responsible for producing and nurturing eggs (ova), facilitating fertilization, supporting embryo development, and giving birth to offspring. It also plays a role in hormone production and regulation.

The primary organs of the female reproductive system include:

- Ovaries
- Fallopian Tubes
- Uterus
- Cervix
- Vagina

Menstrual Cycle

- The rhythmic changes that occur monthly in secretion of reproductive hormone and physical changes in the ovarian, cervical and uterine organs in a female of reproductive age is known as female monthly sexual cycle or menstrual cycle.
- The rhythmic and cyclic changes are seen in the form of:
  - Ovarian cycle
  - Uterine endometrial cycle
  - Uterine cervix cycle
  - Vaginal cycle
  - Cyclical changes in breast

Function and Hormones of Ovary

Functions	Hormones
Production of gametes	• Oocytes (immature egg cells)
	• Follicle-stimulating hormone (FSH)
	• Estrogen
	• Inhibin
Regulation of menstrual cycle and ovulation	• Estrogen
	• Progesterone
	• Luteinizing hormone (LH)
	• Follicle-stimulating hormone (FSH)
Maintenance of reproductive tissues	• Estrogen
	• Progesterone
	• Inhibin
Endocrine functions	• Estrogen
	• Progesterone
	• Inhibin

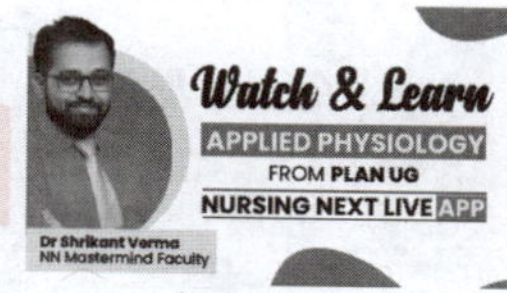

Oogenesis

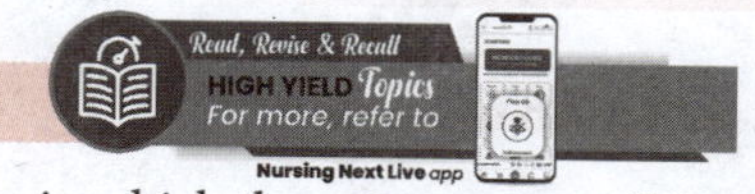

Oogenesis is growth process in which the primary egg cell (or ovum) becomes a mature ovum.

Fertilization

- Fertilization is the process by which male and female *gametes* are fused together and initiate the development of a new organism.
- The male gamete or *'sperm'*, and the female gamete, *'egg'* or *'ovum'* are specialized sex cells, which fuse together to begin the formation of a *zygote*.

Implantation

Implantation is the burrowing of an embryo deep into the lining of the uterus, where it can then begin to grow. Implantation occurs after fertilization when sperm meets egg.

Functions of Breast

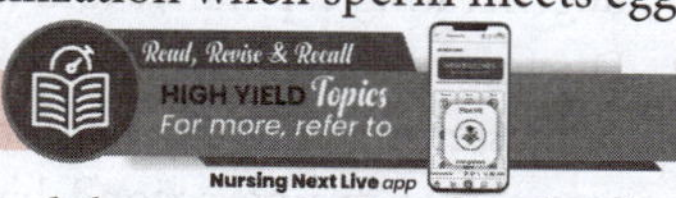

The breast is a specialized glandular organ in females that has several important functions, primarily related to reproduction and lactation. The key functions of the breast:

- Lactation of newborn
- The breast also has the function of ejecting or releasing milk during breastfeeding.
- The breast tissue produces hormones, including estrogen and progesterone, which play a crucial role in the development and maintenance of the breast structure.
- The breast also plays a role in body image and self-identity for many individuals

MALE REPRODUCTIVE SYSTEM

The system consists of:

- **Testes:** The testes, or testicles, are the primary male reproductive organs.
- **Epididymis:** The epididymis is a coiled tube located on the back of each testicle. It serves as a storage and maturation site for sperm.
- **Vas deferens:** The vas deferens is a muscular tube that transports mature sperm from the epididymis to the ejaculatory ducts.
- **Seminal vesicles:** The seminal vesicles are glands located near the base of the bladder.
- **Prostate gland:** The prostate gland is a walnut-sized gland located just below the bladder.
- **Bulbourethral glands:** The bulbourethral glands, also known as Cowper's glands, are located on either side of the urethra
- **Urethra:** The urethra is a tube that runs through the penis and carries both urine from the urinary bladder and semen from the reproductive system.
- **Penis:** The penis is the external organ of the male reproductive system.

Spermatogenesis: Spermatogenesis is the process by which male primary sperm cells undergo meiosis and produce a number of called calls spermatogonia, from which the primary spermatocytes are derived.

Male Hormones and their Functions

Hormone	Source	Function
Testosterone	Testes	• Development of male reproductive organs
		• Development of secondary sexual characteristics
		• Sperm production
		• Regulation of sex drive (libido)
		• Maintenance of muscle mass and strength
		• Maintenance of bone density
Luteinizing hormone	Pituitary gland	• Stimulation of testosterone production in the testes
Follicle-stimulating hormone	Pituitary gland	• Stimulation of sperm production in the testes
Prolactin	Pituitary gland	• Regulation of reproductive function
		• Stimulation of milk production in mammary glands (in some cases)

Semen Composition

Color: White, opalescent	
Specific gravity: 1.028	
pH: 7.35–7.50	
Sperm count: Average about 100 million/mL, with <20% abnormal forms	
Other components: Fructose (1.5–6.5 mg/mL) Phosphorylcholine Ergothioneine Ascorbic acid Flavins Prostaglandins	From seminal vesicles (contributes 60% of total volume)

Contd...

Spermine Citric acid Cholesterol, phospholipids Fibrinolysin, fibrinogenase Zinc Acid phosphatase	From prostate (contributes 20% of total volume)
Phosphate Bicarbonate	Buffers
Hyaluronidase	From the acrosome of the sperm cells after it has reached the oocyte

Function of Semen

- The primary function of semen is to transport sperm from the male reproductive system into the female reproductive tract during sexual intercourse.
- The components of semen, including seminal fluid and sperm, work together to enhance sperm motility, provide nutrition and protection to sperm, and create an optimal environment for fertilization and the journey of sperm to reach the female egg.

CONCEPTUAL EXERCISES

LONG ANSWER QUESTION

1. Describe physiological changes occurring in different phases of menstrual cycle. Add a note on female contraceptive devices. (MGR, KUHS)

Answer

Menstrual Cycle

- The rhythmic changes that occur monthly in secretion of reproductive hormone and physical changes in the ovarian, cervical and uterine organs in a female of reproductive age is known as female monthly sexual cycle or menstrual cycle.
- The rhythmic monthly changes that occur in the ovaries is known as ovarian cycle.
- The result of ovarian cycle each month is the release of single ovum (for fertilization).
- FSH and LH are the hormones responsible for the initiation of the ovarian cycle.
- On birth of the female child, the ovaries have Primordial follicles (ovum that are covered by granulosa cell sheath and suspended in prophase stage of meiotic division).
- On menarche, the release of FSH and LH causes these primordial follicles to enlarge, increasing the granulosa cell layers and enlargement of ovum.
- Hormones secreted during the cycle are regulated by negative feedback mechanisms.

Physiological Changes Occurring in Different Phases of Menstrual Cycle

Menstrual Phase

- When the ovum is not fertilized, the corpus luteum starts to degenerate.
- Progesterone and estrogen levels fall, and the functional layer of endometrium, which is dependent on high levels of these ovarian hormones, is shed in menstruation.
- The menstrual fluid consists of the secretions from endometrial glands, endometrial cells, blood from the degenerating capillaries and the unfertilized ovum.
- During the menstrual phase, levels, of estrogen and progesterone are very low because corpus luteum, which was active during second half of the previous cycle, has degenerated. This means that the hypothalamus and anterior pituitary can resume their cyclical activity, and levels of FSH begin to rise, initiating a new cycle.

Proliferative Phase

- Each month FSH causes accelerated growth of primary follicle, increased thickness of granulosa cell layer around ovum. Outside the granulosa layer there occurs formation of theca layer that divides into theca interna and theca externa.
- Theca interna secretes estrogens and progesterone while theca externa becomes highly vascular.
- Granulosa cells secrete follicular fluid that accumulates around ovum which is rich in estrogen. This results in formation of antrum around ovum.
- Estrogen causes accelerated growth of granulosa cells, causes upregulation of FSH receptors and increased follicular secretion.
- 3–4 times increase in the size of the ovum occurs
- Increase in FSH is followed by increase in estrogen and LH from anterior pituitary.
- Out of 5–11 enlarging follicles, only 1 follicle outgrows to form mature ovum. Others undergo atresia.
- Selection of the dominant follicle occurs on day 5–7. It depends on:
  - The intrinsic capacity of the follicle to synthesize estrogen
  - Highest ratio in the follicular fluid.
- As the follicle matures, the follicle with the highest number of FSH receptors will continue to thrive.

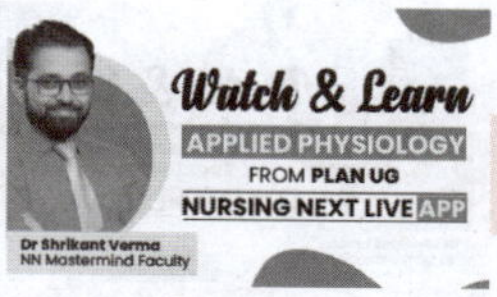

Ovulation

- On 14th day, swelling of the outer wall of the follicle occurs. This occurs as a result of increase in LH (6 to 10 times), also known as LH surge.
- LH causes granulosa cells to secrete progesterone, decrease estrogen secretion, thus increasing the rapid growth of blood vessels in follicle wall along with release of prostaglandins.
- The ovum may survive in a fertilizable form for nearly 8 hours.
- A small nipple-like stigma protrudes from the center of the follicle due to proteolytic enzyme secreted from theca externa. From this stigma, oozing of the fluid proceeds the rupture of the follicle and release of the ovum along with viscous fluid and granulosa cells (in the form of corona radiata) around it.

Secretory Phase/Luteal Phase

- This phase begins after the ovum is released.
- After ovulation, LH from the anterior pituitary stimulates development of the corpus luteum from the ruptured follicle, which produces progesterone, estrogen and inhibin.
- Under the influence of progesterone, the endometrium becomes edematous and the secretory glands produce increased amounts of watery mucus. This assists the motile spermatozoa through the uterus to the uterine tubes, where the ovum is usually fertilized.
- In this phase under the effect of LH, luteinization occurs. Here the follicle cells enlarge and are filled with lipid inclusions and the lipid laden mass of cells is known as Corpus Luteum.
- At this time, granulosa cells secretions consist of higher levels of progesterone and lower levels of estrogen.
- Theca cells secrete androstenedione and testosterone which is later converted to estrogen by aromatase enzyme.
- Estrogen released in this phase causes feedback inhibition of FSH and LH produced from pituitary.
- This causes involution (degeneration) of the corpus luteum around 26th day of the menstrual cycle.
- During this time, the placenta develops and produces estrogen, progesterone and gonadotrophins.

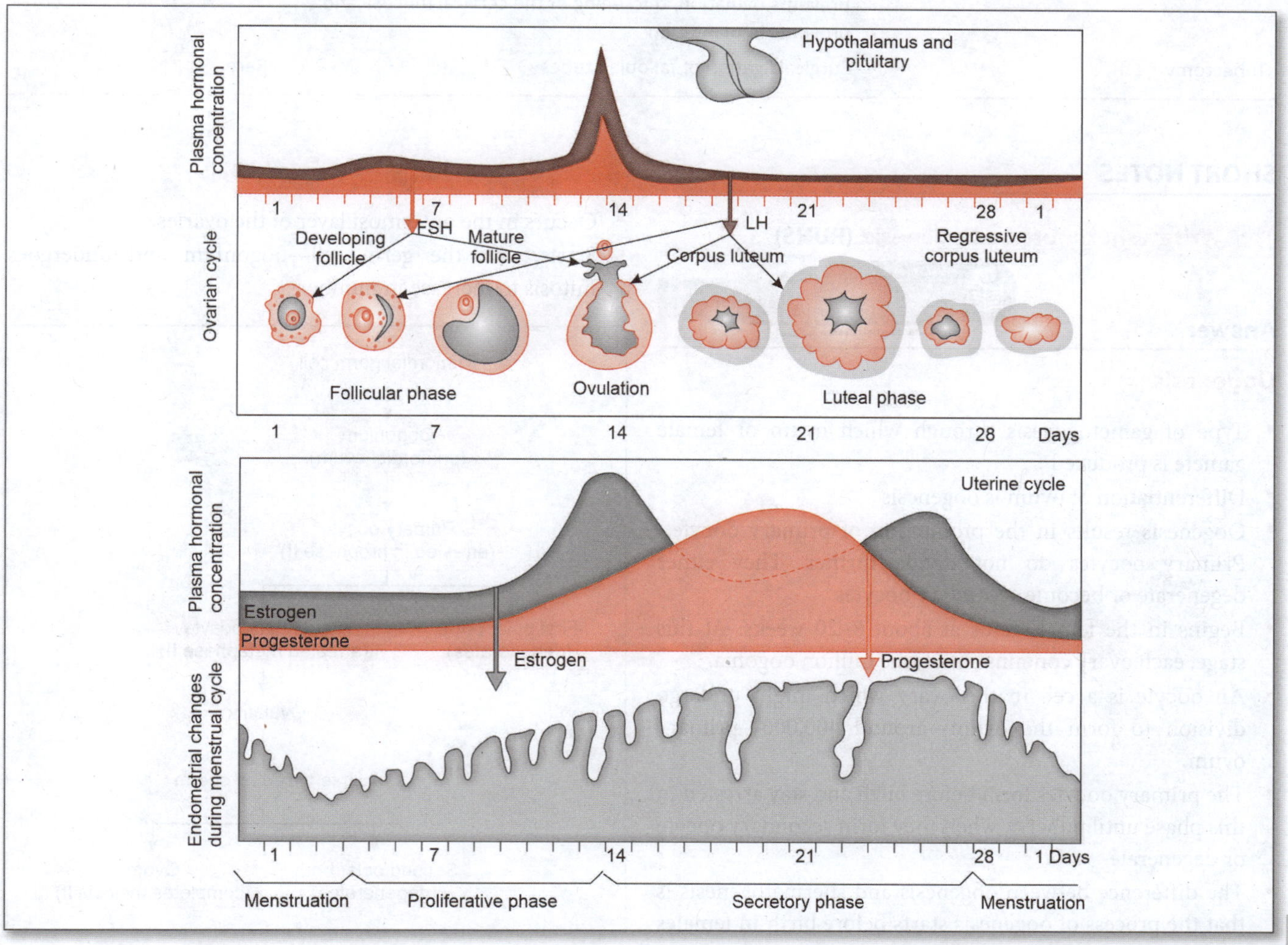

Figure 10.1: Effects of hormones leading to ovarian cycle including phases of endometrium in menstrual cycle

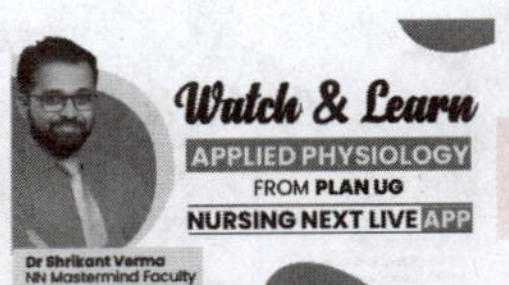

Female Contraceptive Devices

Read, Revise & Recall HIGH YIELD Topics For more, refer to Nursing Next Live app

Contraceptive methods are often classified as either:

Modern: Barrier methods such as male and female condoms, diaphragm, cervical cap and sponge; hormonal contraceptives that include oral, injectable, transdermal, vaginal ring, and implants; intrauterine device (IUD).

Or

Traditional: Rhythm method (periodic abstinence), withdrawal (coitus interruptus), fertility awareness-based methods, the lactational amenorrhoea method and folk methods.

Method	Mechanism of action	Failure rate
Calender method/natural family planning	Abstinence during fertile period	Highest failure rate
Condom	Barrier method	Moderate failure rate
Cervical diaphragm/cervical cap	Barrier method	Failure is more if used incorrectly
Intrauterine devices	Copper T, progestin containing device causes thickening of the cervical mucus and makes uterine wall unfavorable for implantation.	Low failure rate
Contraceptive pills • Mini pill (progesterone only) • Contraceptive injections	Prevents implantation and ovum release. Thickening of cervical mucosa.	Very low
Contraceptive injections	Progesterone injection given once every 12–13 weeks prevents ovulation, thickening of the cervical mucosa and prevents implantation	Very low
Tubectomy	Surgical ligation of fallopian tubes	Rare

SHORT NOTES

1. Write a short note on Oogenesis. (RUHS)

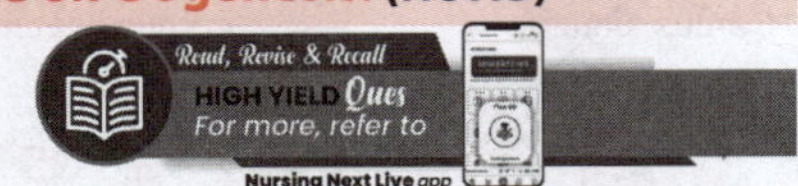

Answer

Oogenesis

- Type of gametogenesis through which ovum or female gamete is produced.
- Differentiation of ovum is oogenesis
- Oogenesis results in the production of primary oocytes. Primary oocytes do not divide further. They either degenerate or become secondary oocytes.
- Begins in the female fetus at about 8–20 weeks. At this stage, each ovary contains about one million oogonia.
- An oocyte is a cell in the ovary which might undergo division to form the ovum—around 400,000—primary ovum.
- The primary oocytes form before birth and stay arrested in this phase until puberty, when they form secondary oocyte or degenerate.
- The difference between oogenesis and spermatogenesis is that the process of oogenesis starts before birth in females whereas spermatogenesis begins at puberty in males.

Stages of Oogenesis

- Occurs in the outermost layer of the ovaries.
- Starts with the germ cell—oogonium and undergoes mitosis to increase in number.

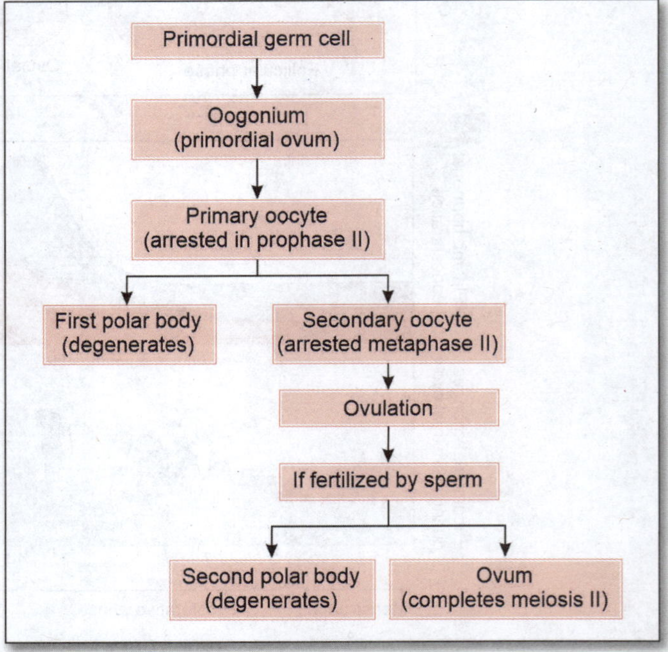

Figure 10.2: Oogenesis

- Stages of oogenesis are:
  - Prenatal
  - Antral
  - Preovulatory

2. Ovarian changes and capacities. (RHUS)

Answer

Ovarian Changes in Menstrual Cycle

- The rhythmic changes that occur monthly in secretion of reproductive hormone and physical changes in the ovarian, cervical and uterine organs in a female of reproductive age is known as female monthly sexual cycle or menstrual cycle.
- The rhythmic monthly changes that occur in the ovaries is known as ovarian cycle.

Proliferative Phase

- It follows the menstrual phase during which part of the endometrium is shed off. This phase lasts from 5th to 14th days of the cycle.

Ovarian Changes

- Many secondary follicles grow in the beginning of the cycle. Approximately on day 6, one follicle grows faster and matures into a Graafian follicle.
- The cells of the follicle secrete estrogen.
- Amount of estrogen secreted by the follicle rises and is responsible for the proliferative changes in the uterine endometrium.

Secretory Phase

Ovarian Changes

- Corpus luteum (CL) grows and secretes progesterone and estrogen.
- Corpus luteum continues as CL of pregnancy if it ensues. If no pregnancy occurs, CL retrogresses' after 20th day and is known as CL of menstruation
- Levels of progesterone and estrogen rise and then decline if no pregnancy occurs but remain high in case of pregnancy.

Menstrual Phase

Ovarian Changes

- CL retrogresses and is called corpus albicans.
- Levels of estrogen, progesterone, FSH and LH are very low. After the menstruation, FSH begins to rise and causes growth of the primordial follicles.

Ovarian Capacities

- Size and volume of ovary is usually determined with an ultrasound.
- The volume is calculated for the formula for an ellipsoid where D1 D2 and D3 are the three axial measurements
- $D1 \times D2 \times D3 \times 0.52$
- The normal adult, non pregnant mean ovary volume is 6–7 mL.
- Above 20 mL is considered abnormal
- Variation in volume of ovary
  - Varies with age
    - 14–15 mL <30 years
    - 13 mL – >30 years
    - 11 mL – 40s
    - 5–6 mL – 50s
    - Less than 5 – >60
  - Body weight
  - Fertility
    - Increases to about 24 mL in fertile years.

3. Spermatogenesis. (RUHS)

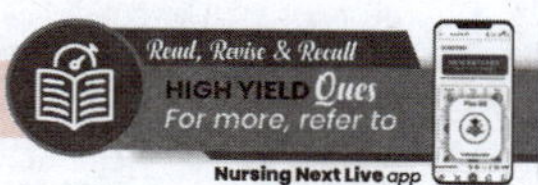

Answer

Definition

The sequence of events by which spermatogonia gets transformed into mature sperms is referred to as spermatogenesis.

Sequence of Events

- During Spermatogenesis
  - Spermatogonia remain dormant in the seminiferous tubules till the fetal period and the process begins during puberty.
  - Sertoli cells nurture the germ cells and play a pivotal role in regulation of spermatogenesis.
  - Spermatogonia get transformed into primary spermatocytes, the largest germ cells by mitotic division.
  - Each primary spermatocyte undergoes meiosis (1st meiotic division) to form two haploid secondary spermatocytes, approximately half the size of primary spermatocyte.
  - With the second meiotic division of secondary spermatocytes, four haploid spermatids are formed.
  - Spermeiogenesis further involves gradual transformation of spermatids to four mature sperms.
  - The duration of the entire process of spermatogenesis takes approximately 74 days.

- After the completion of spermeiogenesis, sperms enter the lumen of seminiferous tubules.
- There is passive transport of sperm to epididymis, a coiled duct in continuation with vas deferens that transports the sperms to urethra.
- Mature sperms are free –swimming actively motile cells consisting of a head and tail.

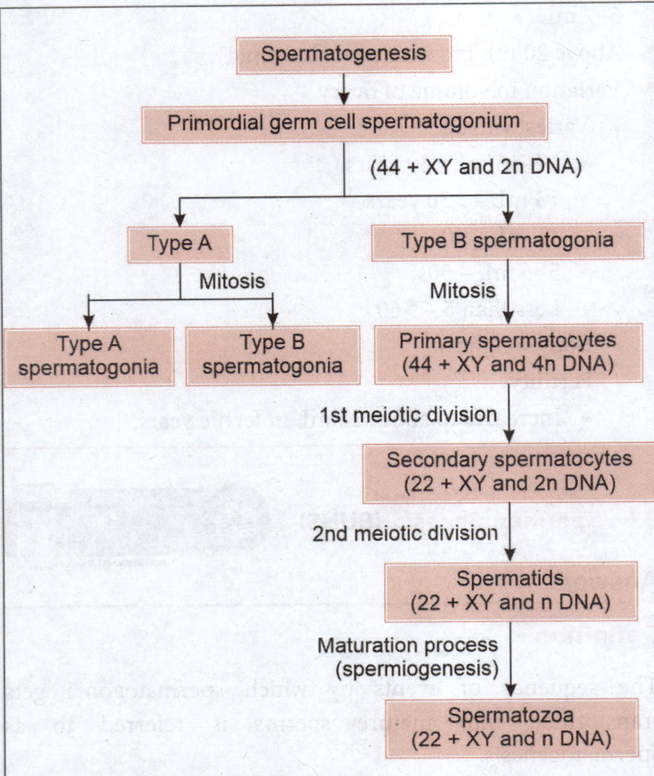

Figure 10.3: Spermatogenesis

4. Write about contents of spermatic cord. (RUHS)

Answer

Introduction

The spermatic cord is the cord-like structure in males formed by the vas deferens (ductus deferens) and surrounding tissue that runs from the deep inguinal ring down to each testicle.

Contents of Spermatic Cord

The spermatic cord consists of vessels, nerves and ducts that run to and from the testes. They are surrounded by fascia, which forms a cord-like structure.

- Via the Deep Inguinal Ring
    - Vas
    - Artery to vas (inferior vesicle)
    - Testicular artery (aorta)
    - Cremasteric artery (inferior epigastric)
    - Cremasteric vein (inferior epigastric)
    - Testicular vein (IVC/left renal)
    - Obliterated processus vaginalis
    - Lymphatics
    - Sympathetics
    - Genital branch of genitofemoral nerve (L2)
- In Canal
    - Internal spermatic fascia
    - Cremasteric fascia
    - Cremasteric muscle
    - Ilio- inguinal nerve
- Outside Superficial Ring
    - External spermatic fascia

Arteries of the Spermatic Cord

- Testicular artery–branch of the aorta that arises just inferiorly to the renal arteries.
- Cremasteric artery and vein–supply the cremasteric fascia and muscle.
- Artery to the vas deferens–branch of the inferior vesicle artery, which arises from the internal iliac.
- Pampiniform plexus of testicular veins–drains venous blood from the testes into the testicular vein.

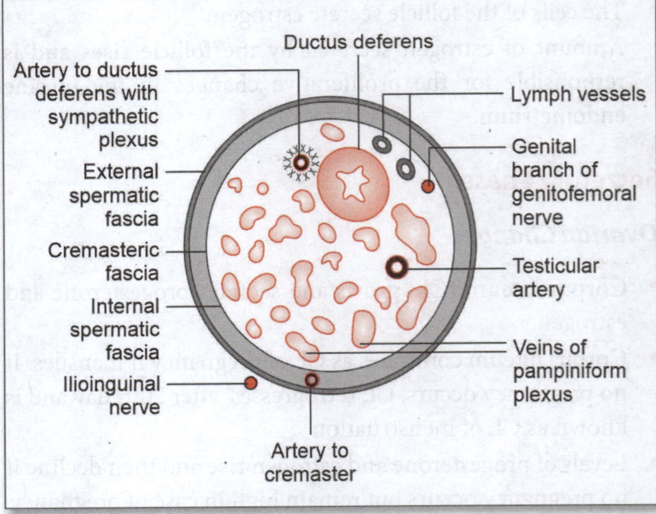

Figure 10.4: Transverse section through the spermatic cord

Coverings of Spermatic cord (From within outwards)

- Internal spermatic fascia
- Cremasteric fascia
- External cremasteric fascia

5. Contraceptive methods in male and female. (RUHS)

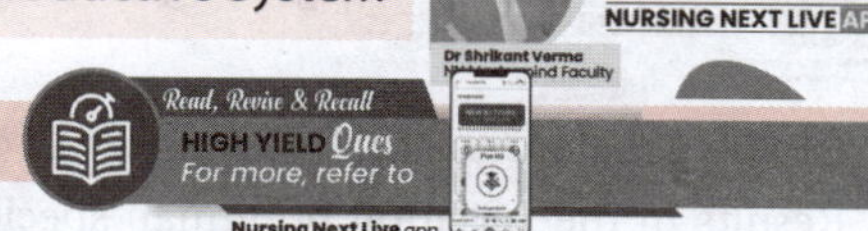

Answer

Contraceptive Methods

- Birth control measures – contraceptive measures – any method, device or medicine that is used to prevent pregnancy.
- There are different types of contraceptive measures for both females and males, both permanent and temporary.
- The choice depends mainly on the individual.

Contraceptive Methods in Male and Female

Method	Advantage		Disadvantage
Conventional			
Condoms	Male and female	Protection against STD	Effective only if used consistently
Diaphragm	Female		Requires training Local infection if left in vagina
Coitus interruptus	Male		Minor time error or drop of semen may lead to pregnancy
Douches	Female		Burning sensation
Modern			
Intrauterine Devices • Non medicated • Copper IUD • Hormone releasing	Female		Periodical replacement at duration of 2-4 years
Sterilization	Male & Female		
Subdermal Implants	Female		
Oral Contraceptives • Classical • Sequential • Mini	Female	100% success in prevention of pregnancy	Increase incidence of carcinoma of endometrium Precipitate thromboembolism Increase risk of diabetes
Emergency Pills		Female	
Injectables		Female	
Vasectomy	Male	Safe and convenient	50% develops antibodies against sperms
Tubectomy	Female		Safe Permanent measure preventing pregnancy

6. Write a short note on fertilization. (RUHS)

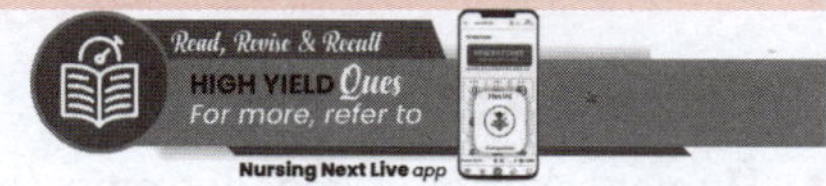

Answer

Fertilization

- Fertilization is the fusion of haploid gametes, egg and sperm, to form the diploid zygote. Note: Through there can be subtle differences in the fertilization process which occurs naturally within the body or through reproductive technologies outside the body, the overall product in both cases is a diploid zygote.
- The result of fertilization is a cell (zygote) capable of undergoing cell division to form a new individual. The fusion of two gametes initiates several reactions in the egg.

Result of Fertilization

- Stimulates the secondary oocyte to complete meiosis.

- Restores the normal diploid number of chromosomes (46).
- Results in the variation of human species as maternal and paternal chromosomes intermingle.
- The embryo contains only maternal mitochondria because the sperm mitochondria are dispersed into the egg cytoplasm and discarded.
- Determines the sex of the embryo.
- The sex chromosomes (Y or X) carried by the sperm determines embryonic sex.
- The sperm can only survive 48 hours within the female genital tract.

7. Name any four female sex hormones and their functions. (MGR)

Answer

Female Sex Hormones: Hormones secreted by the females include :

- Estrogen
- Progesterone
- Follicle-stimulating hormone (FSH)
- Human chorionic gonadotropin

Estrogen

Estrogens are compounds consisting of steroid hormones with cholesterol as its main precursor.

- Estrogen plays a vital role in pubertal changes in vagina, fallopian tubes and uterus.
  - In vagina, it helps in cornification and thickening of vaginal epithelium.
  - During preovulation, it helps in proliferation of endometrium.
  - In cervix, it causes rhythmic contractions of uterus and fallopian tubes resulting in increased cervical mucus and alkaline watery secretion that facilitates sperm penetration.
- **Mammary glands:**
  - Plays a vital role in FSH/LH feedback mechanism.
  - Estrogen is also responsible for development of secondary sexual characteristics in females viz breast development, pigmentation of nipples, fat accumulation in body and feminine type hair pattern and voice.
- **Bone:**
  - Estrogen helps in the maintenance of bone mass by reducing bone resorption.
  - Estrogen defends against parathormone mediated resorption of bone.
  - It reduces the activity of osteoclasts by modification of regulatory cytokines from osteoblasts.
  - In estrogen—deficient conditions, such as that after menopause, the unabated effect of PTH on bone contributes to the development of osteoporosis.
- **Brain:**
  - It maintains body temperature, delays memory loss and helps in regulation of organs of brain that prepares body for sexual and reproductive development.
- **Heart and liver:**
  - Plays a significant role in regulation of production of cholesterol thus prevents buildup of plaque in arteries.

Progesterone

Progesterone is the active principle of corpus luteum. It is secreted by corpus luteum, placenta and adrenal cortex.

Functions of Progesterone

- Progesterone is essential for the maintenance of pregnancy and various other changes associated with it. It also takes part in menstruation.
- Responsible for premenstrual changes of uterine mucosa and takes an essential part in pregnancy.
- Development of breasts during pregnancy, due to proliferation of glandular elements.
- Inhibits menstrual cycle and ovulation and during pregnancy, maturation of follicles, and ovulation, menstrual cycle are also inhibited. The production of pituitary luteinizing hormone (LH) is inhibited by large doses of progesterone.
- **Causes enlargement of birth canal:** At full term, birth canal enlarges due to growth of vagina and relaxation of pelvic ligaments
- Antagonizes the action of estrogen
- Protein catabolic activity
- Causes water and salt retention.
- **Stimulates respiration:** Alveolar pCO_2 is higher in females in luteal phase.
- Inhibits ovulation as it inhibits gonadotrophin releasing hormones from hypothalamus.
- Increases body temperature due to formation of eticholanolone and pregnanediol.

Human Chorionic Gonadotropin

- Human chorionic gonadotropin (hCG) is a glycoprotein secreted by placenta
- It has luteinizing and luteotrophic properties
- It maintains the secretory activity of corpus luteum that secretes estrogen and progesterone leading to termination of ovulation
- It is found in serum 10 days after ovulation

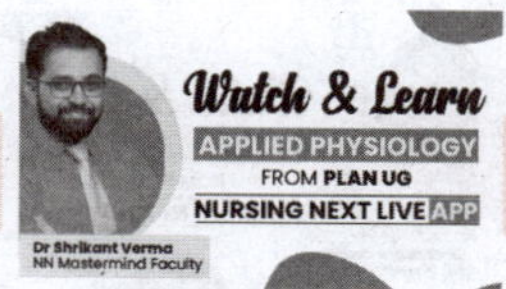

- The concentration of hCG upsurges in serum and urine and reaches a peak at 50–60 days after last menstrual cycle and falls to 0 before labor
- Not an absolute measure of pregnancy
- hCG acts on fetal testes to stimulate the interstitial cells of Leydig that secretes testosterone and helps in development of sex organs in male fetus.

Follicle-stimulating hormone (FSH):

- Although FSH is not exclusive to females, it plays a crucial role in female reproduction.
- FSH is responsible for stimulating the growth and development of ovarian follicles, which contain immature eggs.

8. Functions of placenta. (MGR)

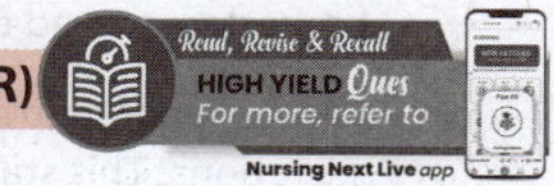

Answer

Functions of Placenta

Nutritive Function

Placenta plays a vital role in the exchange of nutrients and electrolytes, viz-amino acids, fatty acids, carbohydrates and vitamins.

Excretory Function

Excretion of metabolic waste products from fetus into the mother's blood occurs via placenta.

Transmission of Maternal Antibodies

- Transportation of IgG immunoglobulin from mother to fetus occurs at approximately 14 weeks of pregnancy.
- This helps in acquiring passive immunity to fetus against numerous infections.

Exchange of Gases

- Exchange of gases like oxygen, carbon dioxide and carbon monoxide occurs via diffusion.
- Fetus achieves its oxygen requirement from maternal circulation extracting 20–30 mL of oxygen per minute.

Endocrine Function

Placenta secretes numerous hormones like estrogen, progesterone, human chorionic gonadotropin (hCG), human chorionic thyrotropin (HCT), human chorionic somatomammotropin (hCS).

Human Chorionic Gonadotropin

- Human chorionic gonadotropin (hCG) is a glycoprotein secreted by placenta
- It has luteinizing and luteotrophic properties
- It maintains the secretory activity of corpus luteum that secretes estrogen and progesterone leading to termination of ovulation
- It is found in serum ten days after ovulation

- The concentration of hCG upsurges in serum and urine and reaches a peak at 50–60 days after last menstrual cycle and falls to 0 before labor
- Not an absolute measure of pregnancy
- hCG acts on fetal testes to stimulate the interstitial cells of Leydig that secretes testosterone and helps in development of sex organs in male fetus.

9. Hormonal regulation of menstrual cycle. (MGR)

Answer

Hormonal Control of Menstrual Cycle

- Menstrual cycle is under the impact of Hypothalamo-pituitary-ovarian axis
- Menstrual cycle is controlled by hypothalamus, however, this can be influenced by stress or anxiety
- Hypothalamus releases gonadotropin releasing hormone in pulsatile manner which further stimulates anterior pituitary to release LH and FSH
- Follicular stimulating hormone (FSH)—stimulation of follicular maturation during follicular phase
- Stimulates steroid hormone secretion—estrogen (by the granulosa cells of mature ovarian follicle)
- Luteinizing Hormone (LH)—glycoprotein stimulates steroid hormone secretion estrogen
- Ovulation- mid cycle surge of LH
- Progesterone production by corpus luteum
- Negative feedback mechanism control cycle.

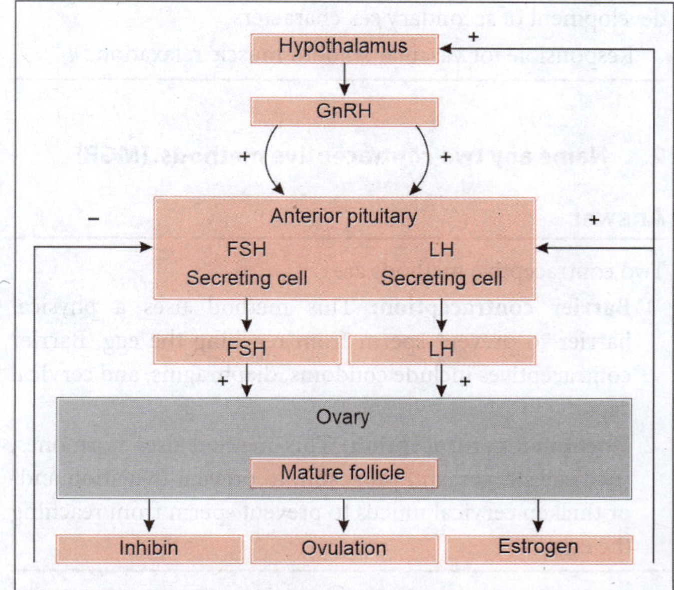

Hormonal Changes during Menstrual Cycle

Steps	Stimulus	Target location	Result
1	Gonadotropin releasing hormone (GnRH) is released by hypothalamus	Anterior pituitary gland	Stimulates the release of follicle stimulating hormone (FSH). This starts the follicular phase
2	FSH is released from anterior pituitary gland into blood	Ovary	Stimulates follicle development in the ovaries. As follicles mature, there is release of estrogen and inhibin into blood
3	Increase in estrogen concentrations in blood Inhibin concentrations increase in blood	Hypothalamus Uterus Anterior pituitary gland	Causes increase in GnRH production. Causes endometrium to develop and regenerate Inhibits further release of FSH
4	Increased GnRh production	Anterior pituitary gland	Stimulates the use of luteinizing hormone (LH) in blood
5	Sudden increase of LH in blood	Ovaries	Promotes formation of corpus luteum. Produces progesterone and estrogen
6	Progesterone and estrogen concentrations in blood increases	Uterus Hypothalamus	Causes endometrium to thicken further and produce secretions. This starts the secretory phase Decreases production of GnRH
7	Decreased GnRH production	Anterior pituitary gland	Decreases the release of LH
8	Decrease of LH in blood	Ovaries	Corpus luteum begins to degenerate- progesterone and estrogen decreases
9	Progesterone and estrogen concentrations in blood decreases	Hypothalamus Uterus	Begins production of GnRH. Starts the cycle all over again Endometrium is shed. This starts menstruation.

SHORT ANSWER QUESTIONS

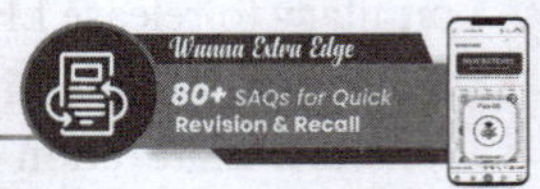

1. Functions of testosterone. (MGR)

Answer

Functions of Testosterone

Testosterone is an anabolic hormone and it is the principal androgen hormone of the testes.

It promotes growth of male reproductive system and causes development of secondary sex characters.

Responsible for vascular smooth muscle relaxation

2. Name any two contraceptive methods. (MGR)

Answer

Two contraceptive methods are :

1. **Barrier contraception:** This method uses a physical barrier to prevent sperm from reaching the egg. Barrier contraceptives include condoms, diaphragms, and cervical caps.
2. **Hormonal contraception:** This method uses hormones, such as estrogen and progestin, to prevent ovulation and/or thicken cervical mucus to prevent sperm from reaching the egg.

3. Name any two hormones produced by the ovary. (MGR)

Answer

The ovaries produce several hormones, but here are two important ones:

1. **Estrogen:** Responsible for the development of female sexual characteristics and the regulation of the menstrual cycle.
2. **Progesterone:** Plays an important role in preparing the uterus for pregnancy by thickening the uterine lining.

4. List out the methods of contraception in females. (MGR)

Answer

Hormonal contraception

Barrier contraception

Intrauterine device (IUD)

Sterilization

Natural family planning

Contraceptive pills

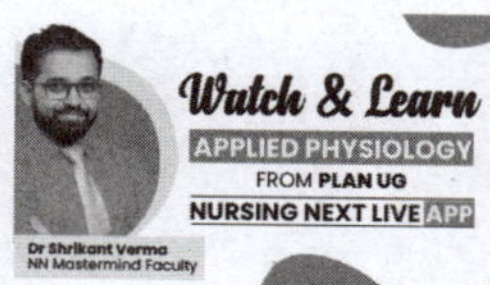

5. Define spermatogenesis. (MGR)

Answer

The process of development of male germ cells into spermatozoa is known as spermatogenesis. The primordial germ cells migrate into the gonad during embryogenesis.

CONCEPTUAL REVISION

MULTIPLE CHOICE QUESTIONS

1. A fertilized ovum is called:

a. A blastocyst
b. A secondary oocyte
c. A diploid cell
d. A zygote

Ans. d. A zygote

2. The female external genitalia are called:

a. Pubic symphysis
b. Vagina
c. Vulva
d. Clitoris

Ans. c. The vulva

3. Maximum number of mucosa folds are found in which part of fallopian tube?

a. Intramural
b. Isthmus
c. Ampulla
d. Infundibulum

Ans. c. Ampulla

4. Which structure of the female breast carries milk from the alveoli to the lactiferous sinuses?

a. Ducts
b. Areola
c. Nipple
d. Adipose tissue

Ans. a. Ducts

5. What are the phases of the ovarian cycle?

a. Menarche, menstrual cycle, menopause
b. Luteal phase, menses and proliferative phase
c. Follicular phase and the luteal phase
d. Menses, proliferative phase and secretory phase

Ans. c. Follicular phase and the luteal phase

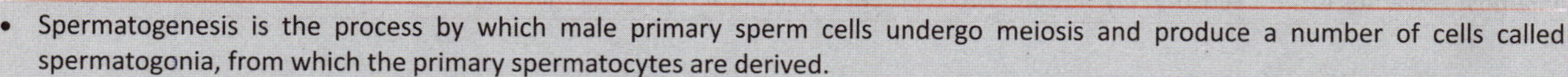

Golden Points

- Spermatogenesis is the process by which male primary sperm cells undergo meiosis and produce a number of cells called spermatogonia, from which the primary spermatocytes are derived.
- The female reproductive system is a complex system of organs that are responsible for producing and nurturing eggs (ova), facilitating fertilization, supporting embryo development, and giving birth to offspring. It also plays a role in hormone production and regulation.

CHAPTER

11

Nervous System

CONCEPTUAL THEORY

Terminology

Anosmia: Loss of sense of smell with aging.

Autonomic nervous system: Regulates involuntary activities of the body. Divided into sympathetic and parasympathetic components.

Cerebellum: Primarily responsible for coordinating voluntary muscle movements, balance, posture, and motor learning.

CSF Rhinorrhea: Leakage of CSF through nose in injury to the anterior cranial fossa of skull.

Limbic system: It is collection of neural structures involved in emotion, olfaction, behavior modulation, long-term memory and ANS function.

Motor nervous system: Transmits motor signals from the central nervous system to muscles and glands.

Nerve impulse: A nerve impulse, also known as an action potential, is an electrical signal that travels along a nerve fiber. It is the means by which information is transmitted within the nervous system.

Neuron: It is the functional unit of CNS and its number is 10^{11}.

Papez circuit: Its parts are hippocampus, fornix, mammillary body, anterior nucleus of thalamus cingulate gyrus, parahippocampal gyrus. All these are important for long-term permanent memory.

Peripheral nervous system: The peripheral nervous system (PNS) is one of the two main parts of the nervous system and the other part is the central nervous system (CNS).

Reflex: Fast involuntary action for muscular contraction/glandular secretion.

Sensory nervous system: Transmits sensory information from sensory receptors (such as eyes, ears, skin, etc.) to the central nervous system (brain and spinal cord).

Thalamus: Thalamus is the " Sensory rely station" which processes all the sensory information (except olfaction) that reaches the cortex.

OVERVIEW OF NERVOUS SYSTEM

- Nervous system
  - Central nervous system (CNS)
    - Brain and spinal cord
  - Peripheral nervous system (PNS)
    - All nerves and sensory structures outside of the brain and spinal cord
      - Somatic
        - Voluntary control of skeletal muscle
      - Autonomic
        - Involuntary control of glands and smooth muscle
          - Sympathetic → "Fight or flight"
          - Parasympathetic → "Rest and digest"

NEURONS

Types, Structure and Functions of Neurons

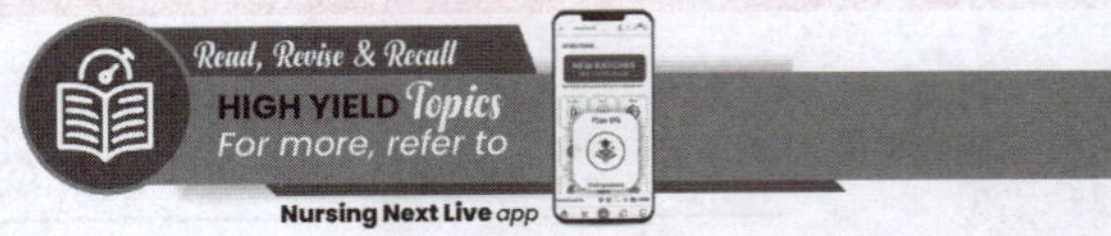

- Neuron is the functional unit of CNS and its number is 10^{11}.
- Parts of neuron include:

a. **Cell body:** Contain nucleus and is metabolic center.

b. **Dendrites:** It receives information and has dendritic spines which are small projections.

c. **Axon hillock:** It is the thickened area of cell body.

d. **Axon:** Part of neuron that transmits impulses to the nerve endings.

e. **Initial segment:** It is the site for the generation of the action potential.

f. **Nerve endings:** It is the site in neuron for storage and release of neurotransmitters.

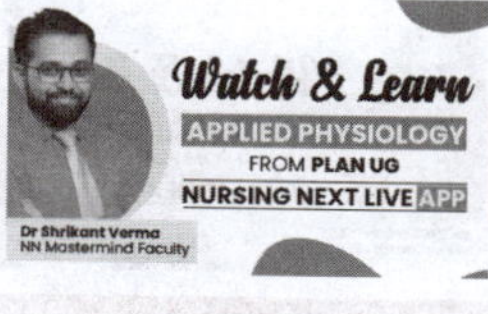

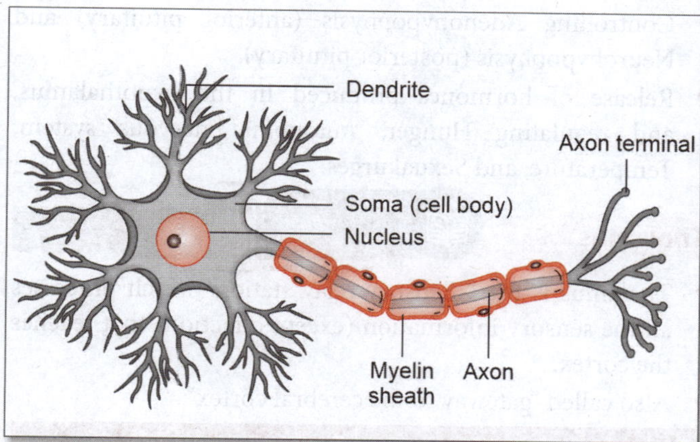

Figure 11.1: Structure of Neuron

Classification of Neurons

Neuron type	Characteristics	Example
Unipolar	Single process originating from cell body	Invertebrate neurons
Bipolar	Two functionally specialized types of processes that are dendrite and axon	Olfactory neuron, Bipolar retinal neurons
Pseudo unipolar	It is variant of bipolar cells in which one end goes to peripheral skin and other goes to spinal cord	Dorsal root ganglion cell
Multipolar	Most common type of neuron in CNS which has 1 axon and multiple dendrites	Sympathetic ganglia, spinal motor neuron

Nerve Impulse

- A nerve impulse, also known as an action potential, is an electrical signal that travels along a nerve fiber. It is the means by which information is transmitted within the nervous system.
- Nerve impulses are generated and propagated through a series of events involving the movement of ions across the cell membrane of nerve cells, also called neurons.

FUNCTIONS OF BRAIN-MEDULLA, PONS, CEREBRUM, CEREBELLUM

Brainstem

Medulla

- The medulla oblongata is located at the base of the brainstem and connects the spinal cord to the rest of the brain.
- It plays a vital role in controlling several automatic functions of the body, including regulating heart rate, blood pressure, breathing, swallowing, and digestion.

Pons

- The pons is situated above the medulla and acts as a bridge between different parts of the brain.
- It serves as a relay center, transmitting signals between the cerebrum, cerebellum, and other areas of the brain.
- The pons also plays a role in controlling certain aspects of breathing, sleep, and facial expressions.

Cerebrum

- The cerebrum is the largest and most highly developed part of the brain.
- It is divided into two hemispheres (left and right) and is responsible for various higher-level functions, including conscious thought, reasoning, sensory perception, voluntary muscle movement, language processing, and memory formation.
- The cerebrum is further divided into lobes (frontal, parietal, temporal, and occipital), each with its own specific functions.

Cerebellum

- The cerebellum is located at the back of the brain, beneath the cerebrum.
- Although it is smaller in size compared to the cerebrum, it contains a significant number of neurons. The cerebellum is primarily responsible for coordinating voluntary muscle movements, balance, posture, and motor learning.
- It receives input from various sensory systems and helps fine-tune movements to ensure smooth coordination and precision.
  - Vestibulocerebellum

Sensory and Motor Nervous System

Sensory nervous system	Motor nervous system
Transmits sensory information from sensory receptors (such as eyes, ears, skin, etc.) to the central nervous system (brain and spinal cord)	Transmits motor signals from the central nervous system to muscles and glands
Detects and processes sensory stimuli (e.g., touch, temperature, pain, vision, hearing, taste, smell)	Initiates and controls voluntary muscle movements
Comprises sensory neurons that carry information from the body to the brain and spinal cord	Comprises motor neurons that carry signals from the brain and spinal cord to the muscles and glands

Contd...

Sensory nervous system	Motor nervous system
Involves specialized receptors, such as photoreceptors in the eyes, mechanoreceptors in the skin, etc.	Utilizes effectors, including muscles and glands, to produce appropriate responses
Allows us to perceive and interpret the environment around us	Enables us to perform physical actions and respond to stimuli
Involves ascending pathways (afferent pathways) that carry sensory signal towards the brain	Involves descending pathways (efferent pathways) that transmit motor signals from the brain to the muscles
Examples include detecting pain from a burn, feeling the touch of an object, hearing a sound, or tasting food	Examples include voluntary movements like walking, talking, writing, and blinking

Peripheral Nervous System

- The peripheral nervous system (PNS) is one of the two main parts of the nervous system and the other part is the central nervous system (CNS).
- The PNS consists of the nerves and ganglia outside of the brain and spinal cord.
- **Functional Component:**
  - Autonomic nervous system (ANS): Involuntary and connect CNS to the visceral organs such as the heart, stomach, intestines, and glands.
  - Somatic nervous system (SNS): Voluntary and responsible for conscious activities.
- **Anatomical Component:**
  - Spinal nerves
  - Cranial nerves
  - Autonomic nerves
  - Ganglia

Autonomic Nervous System

- The autonomic nervous system (ANS) is comprised of:
  - Sympathetic nervous system
  - Parasympathetic nervous system
  - Enteric nervous system.
- Also known as involuntary nervous system because it carries out its functions.
- It shows various physiological process *via* its innervation of cardiac muscle, pacemaker cells, smooth muscle, exocrine and endocrine glands, liver cells, adipose tissue and lymphatic tissue.

Hypothalamus

- Maintains homeostasis by regulating thirst and water balance
- Controlling Adenohypophysis (anterior pituitary) and Neurohypophysis (posterior pituitary).
- Release of hormones produced in the hypothalamus, and regulating Hunger, Autonomic nervous system, Temperature, and Sexual urges.

Thalamus

Read, Revise & Recall HIGH YIELD Topics For more, refer to Nursing Next Live app

- Thalamus is the " Sensory relay station" which processes all the sensory information (except olfaction) that reaches the cortex.
- Also called "gateway to the cerebral cortex"

Thalamic nuclei	Function
Lateral geniculate bodies	Related to vision
Medial geniculate bodies	Related to hearing
Anterior nuclei	Part of papez circuit and related to learning and memory
Ventral anterior and ventral lateral nuclei	Related to motor functions Input from basal ganglia and cerebellum
Ventral posterior lateral and ventral posteromedial nuclei	Transmission of somatosensory information to sensory cortex
Dorsomedial thalamic nucleus	Related to olfaction

Limbic System

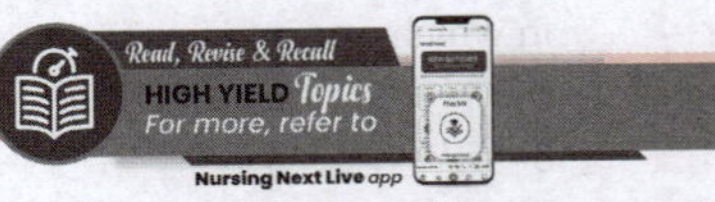

- Limbic system is collection of neural structures involved in emotion, olfaction, behavior modulation, long-term memory and ANS function.
- It consists of rim of cortical tissues that is around the hilum of cerebral hemisphere.
- Main concerned functions are emotions, sexual behavior, rage, motivation, fear.
- The most important role played by limbic system is in papez circuit.

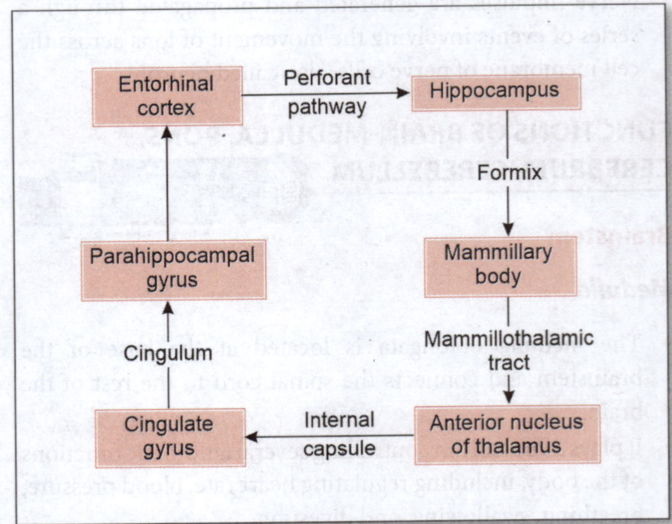

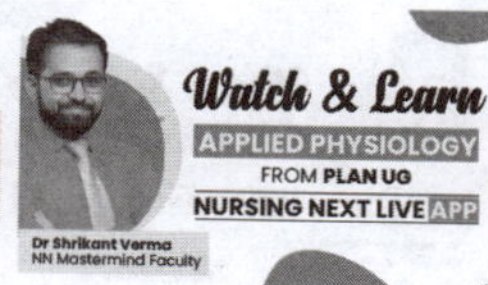

Vestibular System

- The vestibular system can be divided into:
  - Vestibular apparatus - detects head motion and position and transduces this information to a neural signal
  - Central vestibular nuclei - maintains the position of the head in space
- The cerebellum, reticular formation, and spinal cord all receive information from the descending vestibular nucleus, which also receives input from the otolith.
- Controlling eye movements are the ascending connections to the cranial nerve nuclei, and the ascending projections of the vestibular nuclei to the thalamocortical neurons.

Autonomic Functions

The autonomic functions controlled by the ANS include:

- Regulation of heart rate and blood pressure
- Control of respiratory rate and depth
- Digestion and absorption of nutrients
- Regulation of body temperature
- Control of bladder and bowel function
- Modulation of sexual arousal and function
- Regulation of pupil size and accommodation of the lens in the eye
- Control of sweat production
- Modulation of salivation and tear production

Physiology of Pain-Somatic, Visceral and Referred

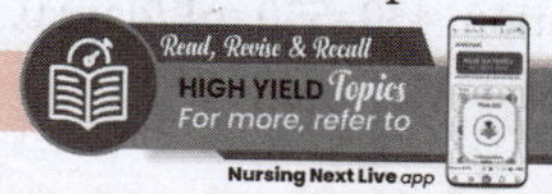

Aspect	Somatic pain	Visceral pain	Referred pain
Location	Arises from the skin, muscles, joints, bones, and ligaments	Originates from internal organs and tissues	Felt in a different area from the actual source of the pain
Sensory receptors	Nociceptors (pain receptors) in the skin and deep tissues	Nociceptors within organs and tissues	Nociceptors in one area, refer pain to another area
Character of pain	Well-localized, sharp, or throbbing pain	Diffuse, dull, deep, and aching pain	Dull, aching, or sharp pain experienced away from the source
Awareness of pain	Easily localized and identified by the individual	Vague and difficult to precisely localize	Felt in a different area, often with less precision
Description by patient	Patient can point to the exact area of pain	Patient may describe pain as "cramping" or "aching"	Patient may describe pain as being "radiated" or "referred"
Neural pathways	Pain signals travel *via* somatic sensory nerves to the brain	Pain signals travel *via* visceral sensory nerves to the brain	Pain signals from internal organs misinterpreted as somatic pain
Associated symptoms	Swelling, redness, heat, or visible signs of injury	Nausea, vomiting, and autonomic responses (sweating, etc.)	No visible signs of injury or inflammation in the referred area
Examples	Cut, burn, fracture, sprain	Appendicitis, kidney stone, intestinal obstruction	Pain from a heart attack felt in the left arm or jaw

CONCEPTUAL EXERCISES

LONG ANSWER QUESTIONS

1. Explain the composition, circulation and functions of CSF. (MGR)

Answer

Introduction

Cerebrospinal fluid (CSF)

- Modified tissue fluid contained in the ventricular system of the brain and in the subarachnoid space around the brain and the spinal cord.
- It acts as a water cushion – protects the brain from injury.

Composition of CSF

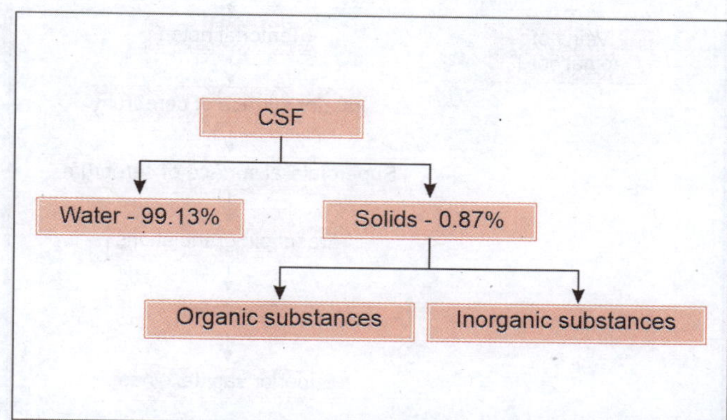

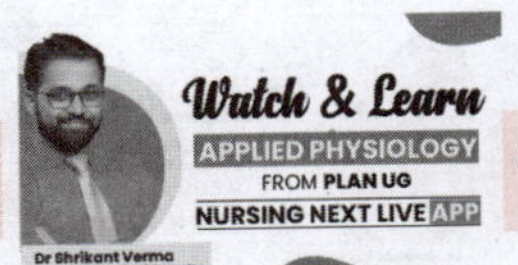

Table 11.1: Composition of CSF

Composition of normal CSF	
Protein	15–14 mg/dL
Glucose	50–80 mg/dL
Urea	6.0–16 mg/dL
Uric acid	0.5–3.0 mg/dL
Creatinine	0.6–1.2 mg/dL
Cholesterol	0.2–0.6 mg/dL
Ammonia	10–35 µg/dL

Characteristics of CSF

- Total volume: 130–150 mL
- Rate of formation: 430–530 mL/day.; 0.3–0.4 mL/min
- CSF pressure: 60–100 mm H_2O

Formation of CSF

- Site of formation–choroid plexus of lateral ventricles.
- CSF is an ultrafiltrate of the plasma
- Circulation of CSF

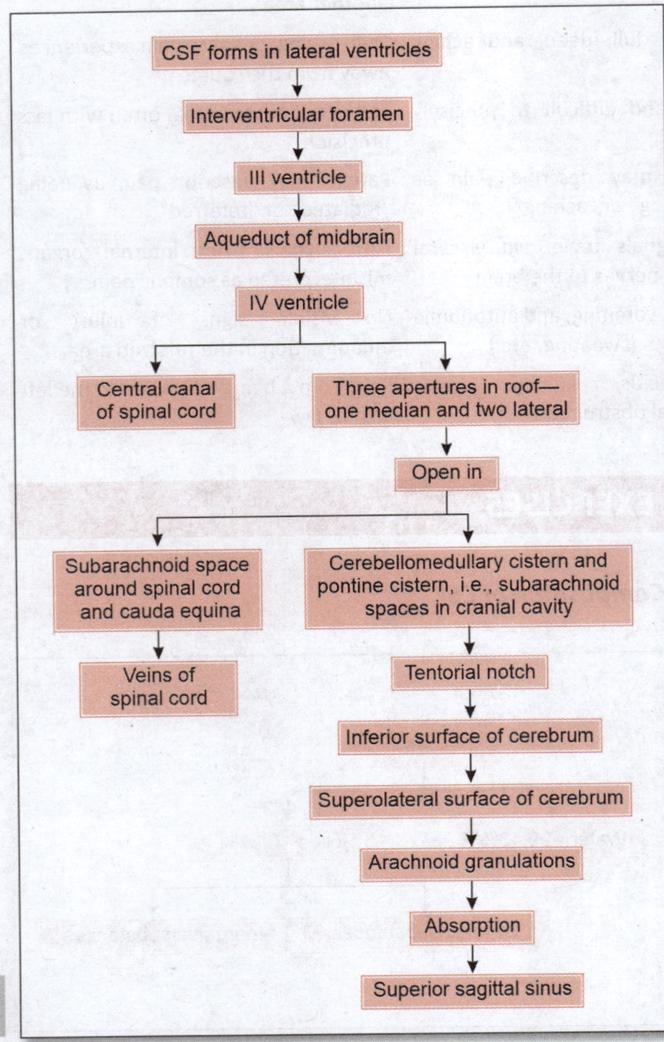

Circulation of cerebrospinal fluid

Absorption of CSF

Absorption of CSF occurs into the dural venous sinuses:

- Drained into the superior sagittal sinus and into the arachnoid villi.
- Arachnoid villi
  - Project into dural venous sinuses, especially superior sagittal sinus.
  - Covered by endothelium of the venous sinus
  - Tend to be grouped together to form elevations known as arachnoid granulations.
- CSF pressure >> Sinus pressure
- Thus, rate of absorption of CSF through the arachnoid villi controls the CSF pressure.
- Small amount fluid is absorbed into the cervical lymphatic system through the sheaths over the cranial nerves.

Functions of CSF

- CSF acts as fluid buffer thus, providing optimal atmosphere to neurons and protects the brain from shock.
- Brain floats in the CSF due to similar specific gravity of brain and CSF and thus, braces the brain in cranial vault.
- CSF maintains the volume of cranial content. Blood volume of brain is inversely proportional to CSF, i.e., if blood volume decreases, CSF is retained and *vice versa*.
- The nutritive substances and waste materials gets exchanged between blood and brain tissues through CSF.
- Brain capillaries are selectively permeable thus, protects the brain from fluctuations in neurotransmitter.

Nursing Implications

- Hydrocephalus: Excess CSF in the ventricles of brain causing ventricles to widen that puts pressure on the tissues of brain.
- Raised intracranial pressure: It is an emergency condition that arises due to rise in pressure around your brain. It may be due to an increase in the amount of fluid surrounding your brain.

2. Functions of cranial nerves.

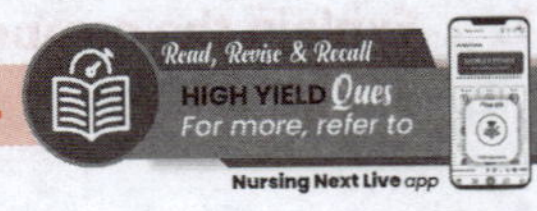

Answer

- **Introduction** Nerves that originate from the brain and brain stem are known as cranial nerves.
- These are paired nerves mainly responsible for vision, smell, hearing and muscle movements.
- Cranial nerves are 12 in number, numbered I to XII depending on their origin.

These may be motor, sensory or mixed cranial nerves and their functions.

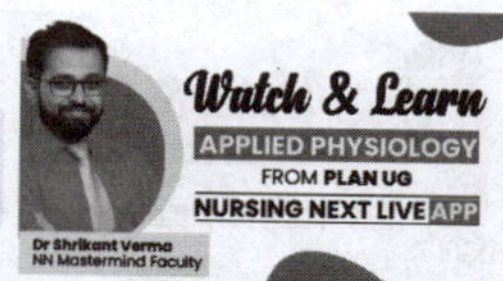

Cranial nerve	Sensory, motor or both	Function	Symptoms after injury
(I) Olfactory	Pure sensory	Smell	Loss of smell (Anosmia)
(II) Optic	Sensory	Vision	Loss of vision (Anopsia)
(III) Oculomotor	Mainly motor	Supplies levator palpebrae superioris, inferior oblique, superior, medial and inferior rectus along with pupillary sphincter and muscles of ciliary body	Strabismus
(IV) Trochlear (thinnest and smallest cranial nerve in terms of axons it carries and has greatest intracranial length)	Motor	Innervates superior oblique muscle	Upward drifting of the eye resulting in double vision or diplopia
(V) Trigeminal-(largest and thickest of the 12 cranial nerves)	Both sensory and motor	Innervation of muscles of mastication, taste sensation from anterior 2/3rd of tongue, hard and soft palate	Bilateral damage–Drooping of jaw, atrophy, asymmetric chewing, inability to bite firmly (injury to mandibular branch), loss of corneal reflex, (trigeminal neuralgia- severe, shooting pain like an electric shock, triggering factors–touching, brushing, speaking, chewing, etc. Usually affect one side of the face and pain last for few seconds to several minutes, mainly involves the lower face and jaw with less frequent involvement of area around the nose and above the eye
(VI) Abducens	Mainly motor	Innervation of lateral rectus eye muscle	Medial deviation of eye-Strabismus, double vision
(VII) Facial	Both sensory and motor	Motor supply to muscles of facial expressions, posterior belly of digastric, stylohyoid and stapedius muscle. Secretomotor innervation to salivary gland and lacrimal gland. Special taste sensation from anterior 2/3rd of tongue.	Facial paralysis, drooping eyelids, loss of taste sensation on the affected side,↓ed salivation and tear secretion, drooping of the corner of the mouth (Bell's palsy)
(VIII) Vestibulocochlear	Usually sensory	Mainly balance and hearing (vestibular branch – impulses for equilibrium and cochlear branch provide impulses for hearing	Deafness, Nystagmus
(IX) Glossopharyngeal	Both sensory and motor	Receives taste sensation from posterior 1/3rd of tongue Secretomotor innervation to parotid gland Motor supply to stylopharyngeus Also involved with vagus nerve in gag reflex	Difficulty in swallowing, choking
(X) Vagus – (As name suggest it means "wandering". It is the longest cranial nerve as it runs all the way from brainstem to the part of colon)	Both sensory and motor	Branchiomotor innervation to pharyngeal and laryngeal muscles, except stylopharyngeus Parasympathetic innervation to thoracic and abdominal viscera Receives special taste sensation from epiglottis. Controls muscles and soft palate for voice and resonance	Inspiratory dyspnea, hoarseness of voice, impaired gag reflex

Contd...

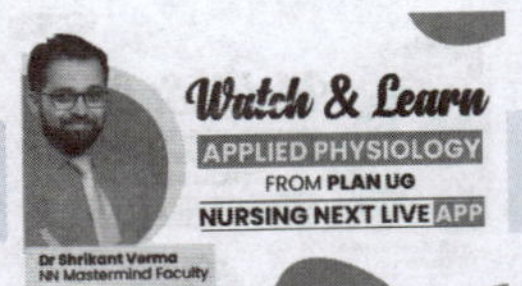

Cranial nerve	Sensory, motor or both	Function	Symptoms after injury
(XI) Spinal accessory	Mainly motor	Supplies trapezius and sternocleidomastoid. Few fibers overlaps with vagus nerve function and supplies to viscera	Difficulty in turning neck, shrug shoulders
(XII) Hypoglossal	Mainly motor	Innervates extrinsic and intrinsic muscles of tongue, except palatoglossus	Deviation of tongue toward affected side (injury)

SHORT NOTES

1. Classification of reflexes. (RUHS)

Answer

Introduction

- Reflex is an involuntary and instantaneous movement in response to a stimulus.
- It is automatic response to a stimulus that does not require to reach the brain.
- Reflex arc acts on an impulse before it reaches the brain.

Classification of Reflexes

- **Based on function:**
  - Based on the movement of the organs or parts of body that move due to reflex.
  - Reflexes that involve skeletal muscles are extensor, flexor, locomotor and statokinetic
  - Reflexes that involve the function of internal organs are cardiovascular, digestive, secretory and excretory.
- **Based on the degree of complexity:**
  - Monosynaptic or monosegmental
  - Polysynaptic or intersegmental
- **Based on the development:**
  - Innate reflexes or genetically predetermined
  - Acquired reflexes or learned reflexes
- **Based on the response:**
  - Somatic
  - Visceral or autonomic
- **Based on depth:**
  - Superficial reflexes
    - Plantar response, abdominal reflex, cremasteric reflex, corneal reflex
  - Deep reflexes
    - Biceps, brachioradialis, triceps, ankle jerk, knee jerk

Importance of Reflexes

- Protection from danger: These are involuntary responses of effectors to the stimulus
- Reduce the reaction time

Examples of Reflexes

- Myotatic reflexes
  - Also known as the muscle stretch reflex or deep tendon reflex
- Tendon reflexes
  - Contraction of muscle in reaction to the striking of its tendon
- Cough and accommodation reflexes

2. Write in short about Vasovagal shock. (RUHS)

Answer

Introduction

- Sudden loss of consciousness due to temporary decrease in the blood flow.
- Usually caused by certain triggers.

Prodromal Symptoms

- Most patients experience prodromal symptoms before a vasovagal shock. These include:
  - Dizziness
  - Pallor
  - Nausea
  - Sweating
  - Palpitations

Etiopathogenesis

- Occurs due to activation of parasympathetic nervous system in response to certain emotional or environmental triggers.
- These cause bradycardia, followed by vasodilatation of the peripheral blood vessels.
- Hypotension occurs, that leads to the reduction of the oxygen supply of the brain – finally resulting in cerebral hypoperfusion and loss of consciousness.
- One common cause of vasovagal shock is orthostatic hypotension, i.e., sudden drop in blood pressure due to abrupt change in position of the person – occurs as a result of delay in venoconstriction upon standing – leading to pooling of blood in the legs, reduced cardiac output and blood pressure.

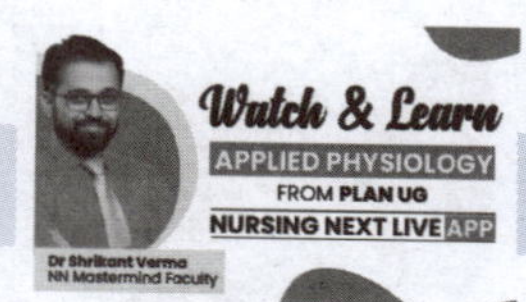

3. Write in short about postural reflexes. (MGR)

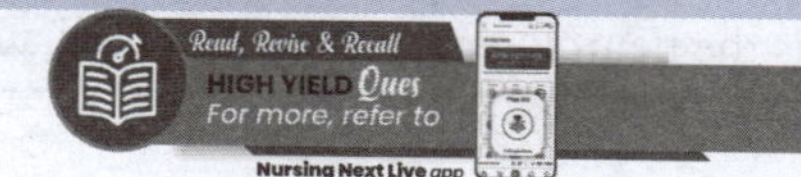

Answer

Introduction

Postural reflexes resist displacement of the body caused by gravity or acceleratory forces.

Functions of the Postural Reflexes

- Maintenance of the upright posture of the body
- Restoration of the body posture, if disturbed
- Provides a suitable postural background for performance of voluntary movements.

Types of Postural Reflexes

- Segmental reflexes—center lies in the spinal cord
  - Stretch reflex
  - Crossed extensor
  - Positive support reaction
  - Negative support reaction
- Tonic reflexes—center lies in medulla
  - Tonic neck
  - Tonic labyrinthine
- Righting
  - Neck righting
  - Labyrinthine righting
  - Body righting
  - Limb righting
  - Optical righting

SHORT ANSWER QUESTIONS

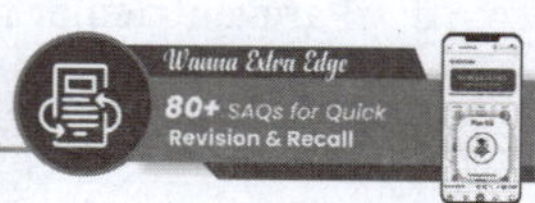

1. Define Myasthenia gravis.

Answer

It is an autoimmune neuromuscular illness that is characterized by skeletal muscle weakness and fatigability that gradually gets worse as the muscles are used. It results from a decrease in the number of AChR lead to formation of autoantibodies.

2. Functions of cerebellum. (MGR)

Answer

Cerebellum, also known as "little brain," is located at the back of the brain, underlying the occipital and temporal lobes of the cerebral cortex.

It plays an important role in motor learning and higher mental functions

It has three parts:

1. Spinocerebellum- for motor coordination
2. Neocerebellum- responsible for motor planning
3. Vestibulocerebellum-for balance and eye movements

3. Define muscle tone. (MGR)

Answer

Muscle tone is the degree of resistance or tension that a muscle exhibits while at rest and is controlled by the neurological system. The body can maintain posture, stability, and balance, thanks to the constant and passive partial contraction of its muscles.

4. List the name of any two neuroglial cells. (MGR)

Answer

1. Astrocytes: These are star-shaped cells that play a critical role in maintaining the structural and functional integrity of the nervous system.
2. Oligodendrocytes: These are cells that produce myelin in CNS.

5. Enlist types of neurons. (MGR)

Answer

They are of three types:

1. Sensory neurons (afferent neurons): The sensory neurons convert signals from the external environment into corresponding internal stimuli. They are pseudounipolar in structure
2. Motor neurons (efferent neurons): Transmission of information from the brain to the muscles of the body. Most common type of neuron.
3. Interneurons: Help in passing signals between two neurons. They are multipolar in structure.

6. Mention two functions of neuroglia. (MGR)

Answer

1. Neuroglia plays a crucial role in providing structural support to neurons and the nervous system.

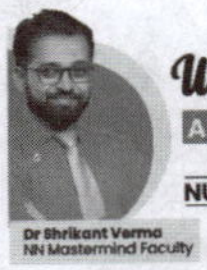

2. Neuroglia provides protection to neurons and the nervous system by removing cellular debris and dead cells, preventing the spread of infection and inflammation.

7. Define reflex action. (MGR)

Answer

A reflex action is a quick, unconscious response that is automatic and involuntary to a stimuli. The reflex arc, which consists of sensory neurons, interneurons, and motor neurons, is the neurological system that mediates a reflex action.

8. Functions of thalamus. (MGR)

Answer

a. It is the major relay station for sensory inputs in humans and higher order of animals, whereas in lower order of animals, it acts as the center for sensory integration.

b. Participate in the arousal mechanism.

CONCEPTUAL REVISION

MULTIPLE CHOICE QUESTIONS

1. Based upon the typical distribution of ions across a cell membrane, which of the following values best represents the appropriate resting membrane potential?

a. +70 mV b. −70 mV
c. 0 mV d. +30 mV

Ans. b. −70 mV

2. The hyperpolarization of a neuron is governed by the action of which of the following ions?

a. Potassium and sodium b. Sodium only
c. Chloride and potassium d. Sodium and calcium

Ans. c. Chloride and potassium

3. Identify the lumbar vertebrae in the following image:

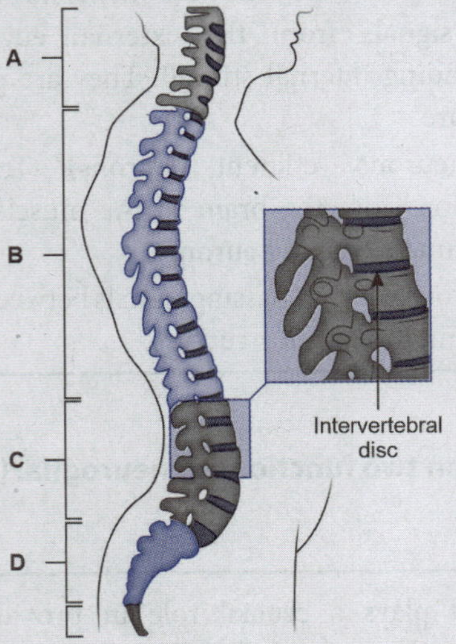

a. A b. B
c. C d. D

Ans. c. C

4. A 17-year-old boy is admitted to the hospital with a traumatic brain injury, sustained when he fell off his motorcycle. He develops a fever of 102.2°F (39°C), which is unrelated to an infection or inflammation. The fever is most likely due to a lesion of which of the following?

a. Lateral hypothalamus
b. Posterior nucleus
c. Anterior hypothalamus
d. Paraventricular nucleus

Ans. c. Anterior hypothalamus

5. Speech in words and not in sentence occurs due to the lesion of:

a. Wernicke's sensory speech area
b. Broca's motor speech area
c. Arcuate fasciculus
d. Primary auditory area

Ans. b. Broca's motor speech area

6. Basal ganglia consists of all of the following; except:

a. Caudate nucleus b. Putamen
c. Thalamus d. Globus pallidus

Ans. c. Thalamus

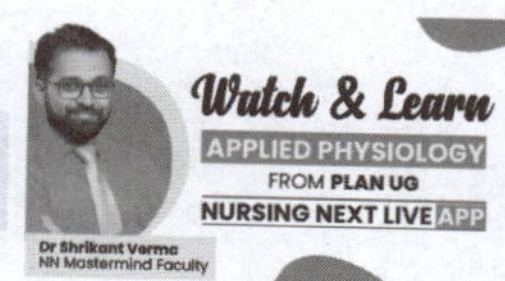

Golden Points

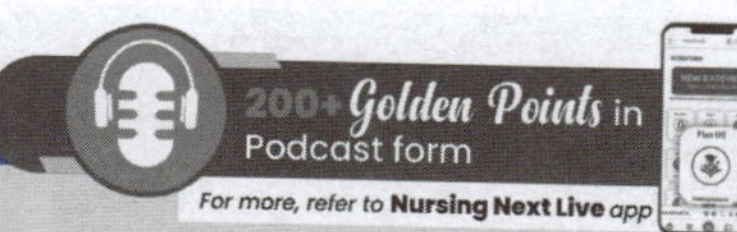

- A nerve impulse, also known as an action potential, is an electrical signal that travels along a nerve fiber. It is the means by which information is transmitted within the nervous system.
- A small gap exists at the membrane-to-membrane junction point called synapse.
- Axons receive signals from other neurons and transmit flow of the messages to the adjacent connected neurons and to glands.
- Central nervous system (CNS) comprises brain and spinal cord and is responsible for integrating, coordinating the sensory information and ordering appropriate motor actions.
- Gray matter is the part of nervous tissue containing the cell body (soma), neuroglial cells and abundance of blood vessels.
- In brain, white matter lies deep to cortex of brain.
- Myelin sheath insulates the axon and increases the speed of the flow of signals through the axon.
- Neuron is the functional unit of CNS and there number is 10^{11}.
- Neurons convert the chemical signals into electrical impulses and further carry electrical impulses toward the next part of the neuron, the cell body.
- Neurotransmitters are the biochemical messengers, or carriers of information between cells.
- Peripheral nervous system (PNS) includes 12 pairs of cranial nerves and 31 pairs of spinal nerves.
- Synapse contains molecular structures that control energy by allowing electrical or chemical signals to be rapidly transmitted through biochemical neurotransmitters.
- The autonomic motor division is divided into two complementary subsystems: the sympathetic and the parasympathetic system.
- The autonomic nervous system primarily regulates involuntary or unconscious activities of body such as heart rate, breathing and pupil dilation.
- The spinal cord receives sensory information from the skin, joints, and muscles of the trunk, limbs, and contains the motor neurons responsible for both voluntary and reflex movements.
- White matter comprises only the fibers, i.e., axons, dendrites, neuroglial cells and fewer blood vessels.

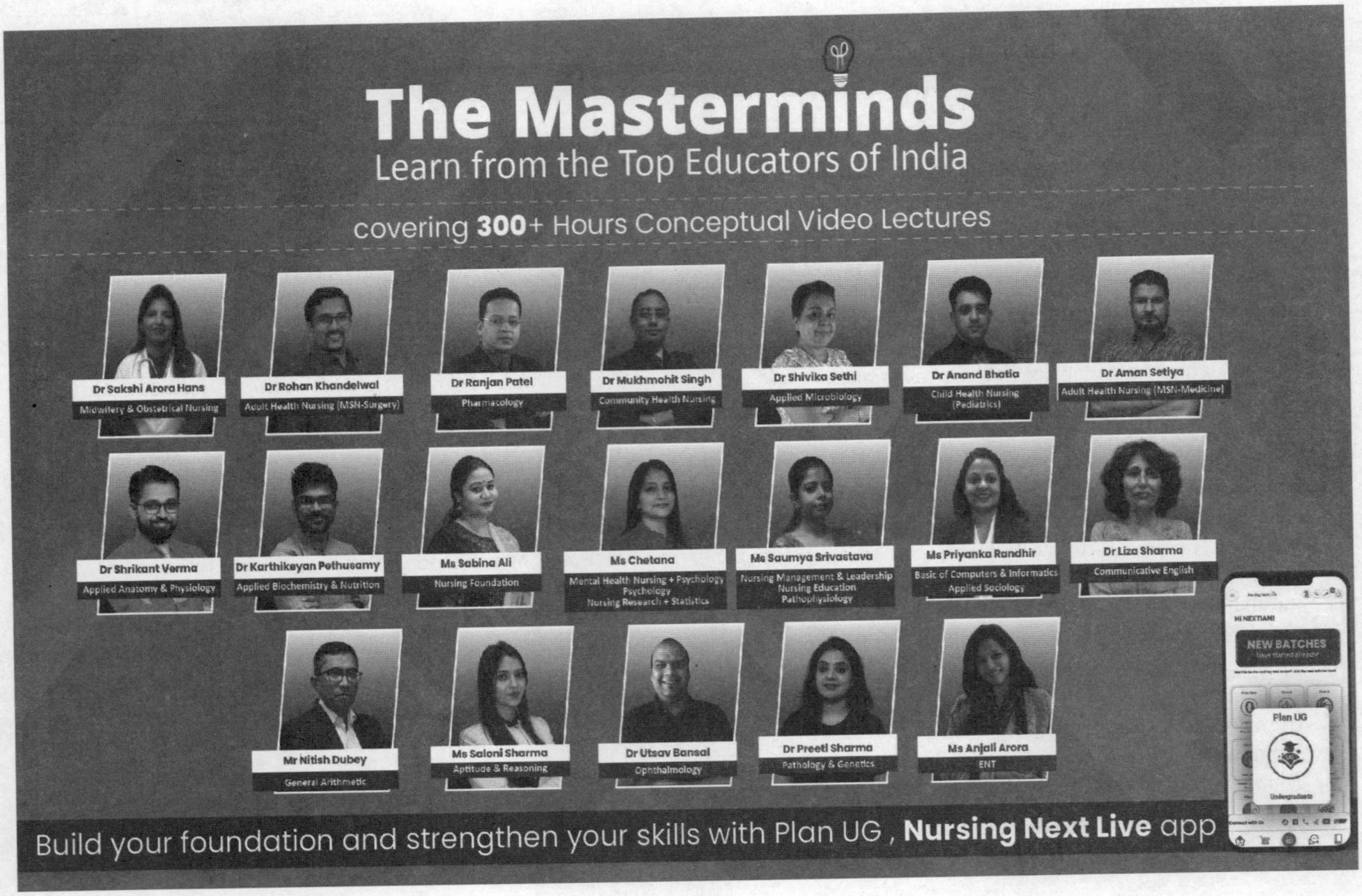

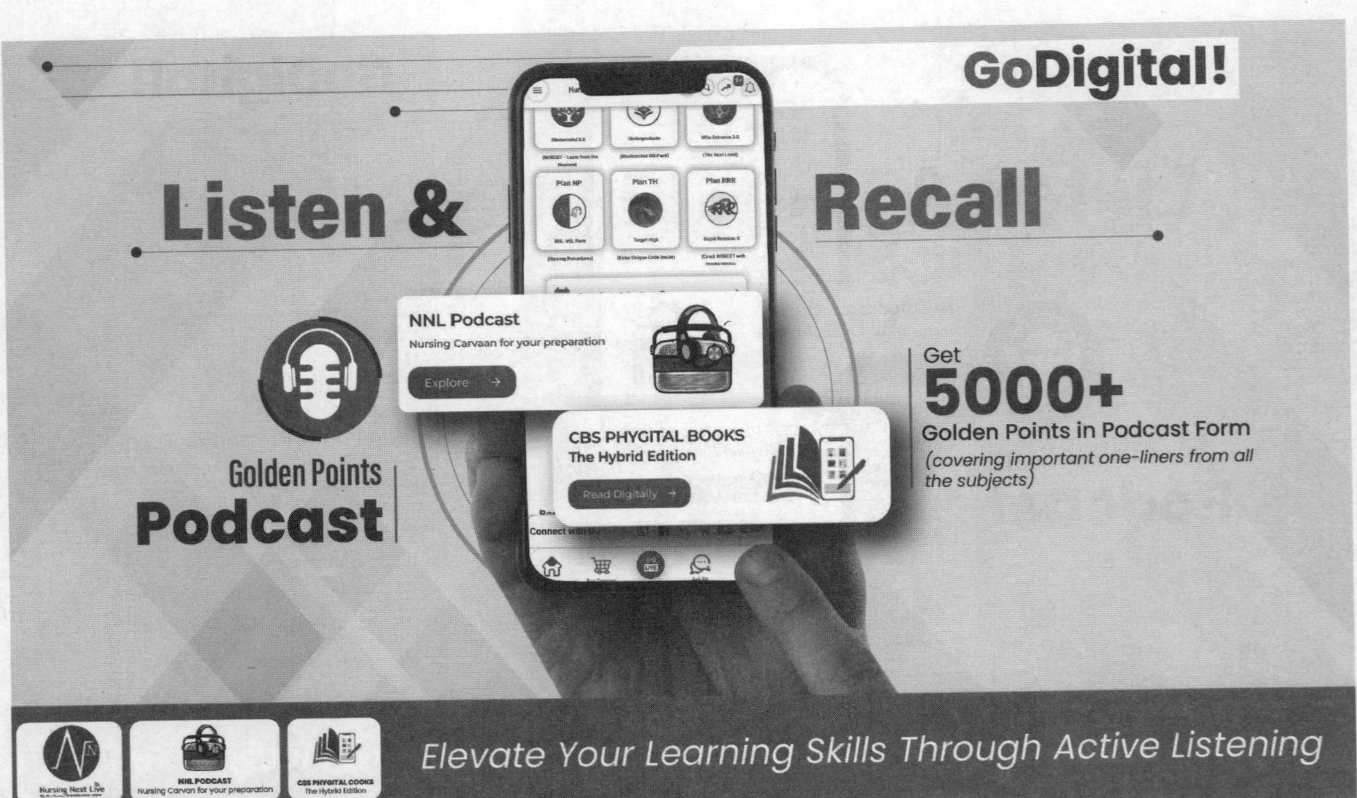

GoDigital!
Listen &
Recall
Plan NP
Plan TH
Plan RRR
NNL Podcast
Nursing Carvaan for your preparation
Explore
CBS PHYGITAL BOOKS
The Hybrid Edition
Read Digitally
Golden Points
Podcast
Get
5000+
Golden Points in Podcast Form
(covering important one-liners from all the subjects)
Nursing Next Live
NNL PODCAST
Nursing Carvan for your preparation
CBS PHYGITAL BOOKS
The Hybrid Edition
Elevate Your Learning Skills Through Active Listening

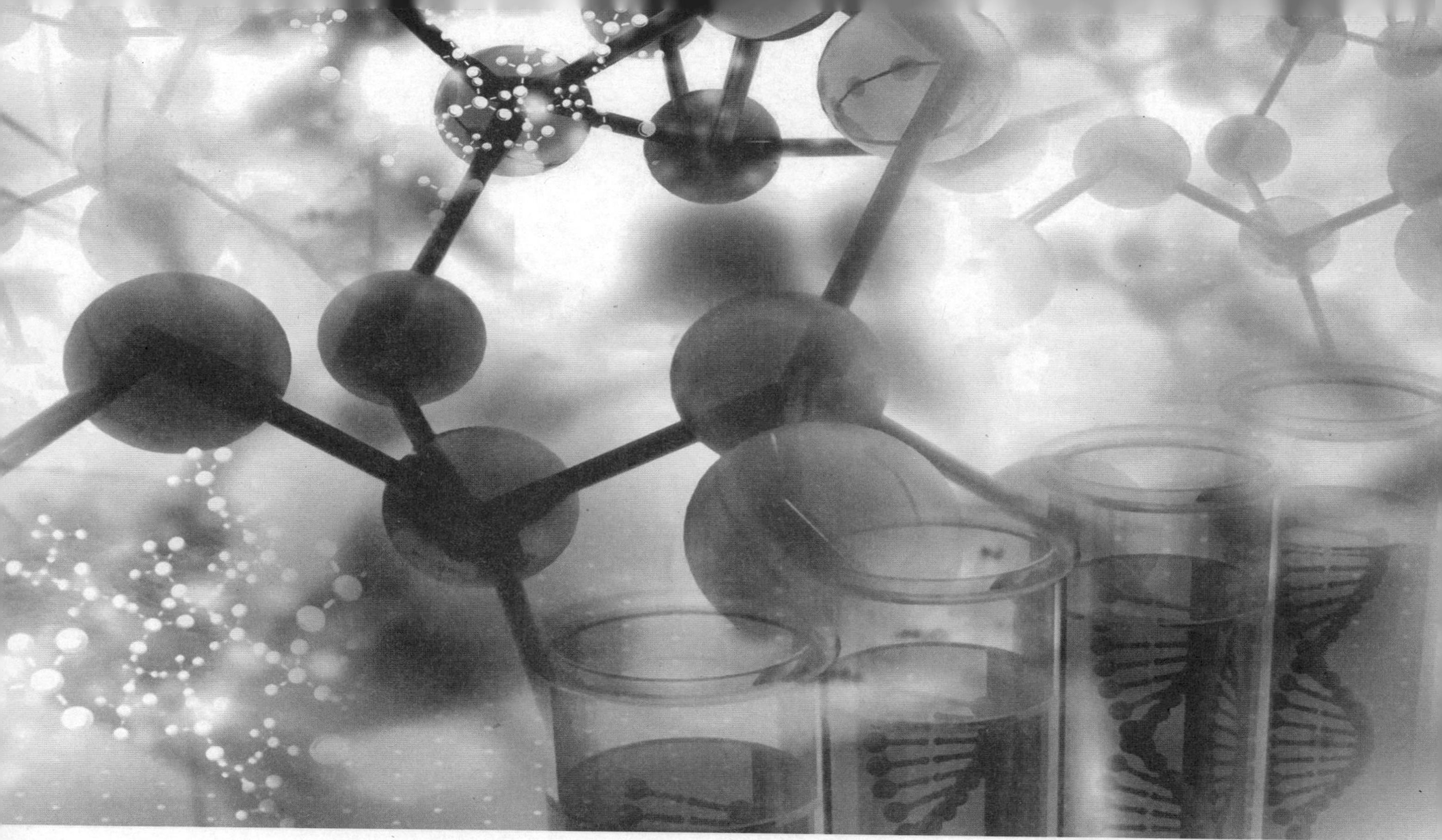

Applied Biochemistry

Unit Outline

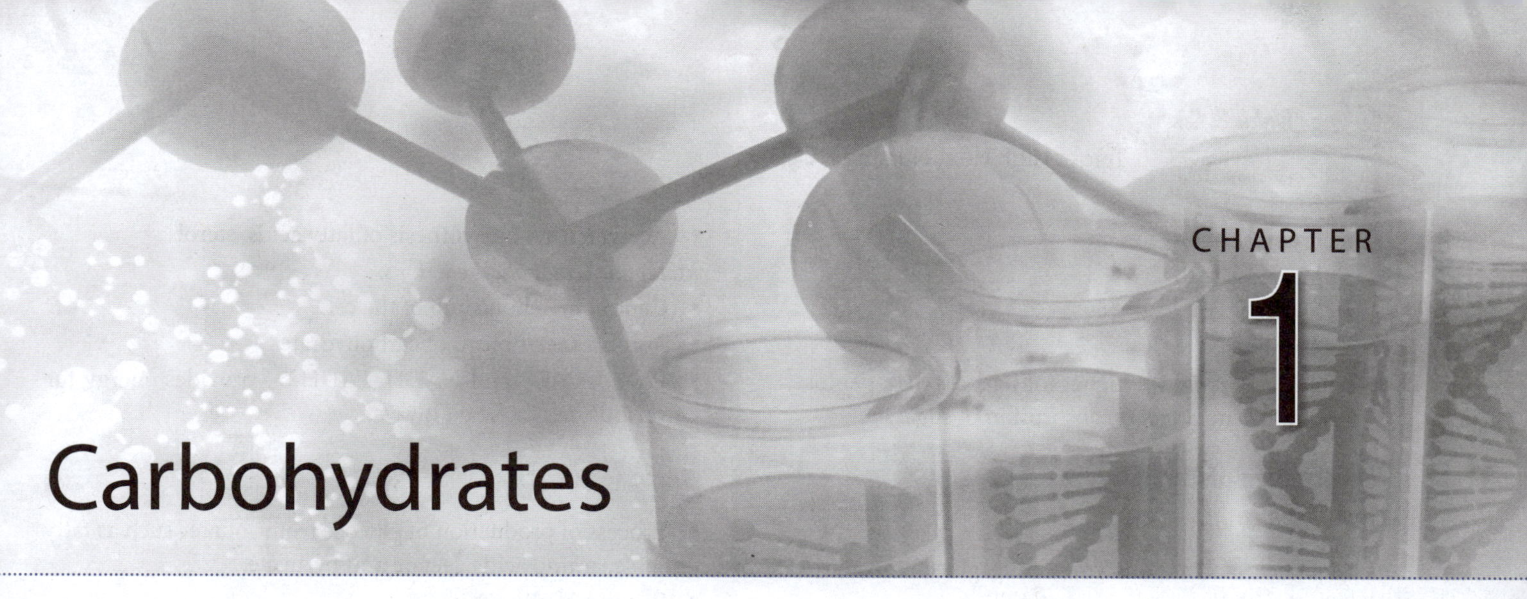

Carbohydrates

CONCEPTUAL THEORY

Terminology

150+ key terminologies for Quick Recall & Revision

Aldose: The sugar is an aldose when it has an aldehyde (-CHO) group on carbon -1

Carbohydrates: Carbohydrates are defined as the aldehyde or ketone derivatives of higher polyhydroxy alcohols or their anhydrides.

Gluconeogenesis: Gluconeogenesis (neoglucogenesis) is the process of the formation of glucose from various non-carbohydrate sources.

Glycogenolysis: Glycogenolysis is the process of conversion of glycogen to either glucose-6-phosphate in muscle or free glucose in liver and kidney

Glycolysis: Glycolysis is also called Embden-Meyerhof-Parnas pathway or the Embden-Meyerhof Pathway.

Glycosides = Sugar + alcohol (such as methanol), e.g., methylglycoside. These are found in glycosaminoglycans.

Hypoglycemia: Hypoglycemia refers to a condition when plasma glucose concentration is below 40 mg/dL.

Ketoses: The sugar is a ketose when it has a ketone (-CO) group at carbon-2

Lactose: Lactose is a reducing disaccharide, made up of beta-D glucose and beta-D galactose. It is also known as milk sugar, as it is found in milk.

Oligosachharides: Oligosachharides consist of more than two (usually 3–10) monosaccharide units by O glycosidic bonds, e.g., maltotriose, raffinose.

Polysaccharides: Polysaccharides, also called glycans, are polymers of a large number (>10) of monosaccharides linked by glycosidic bonds.

Sucrose: Sucrose consists of alpha-D glucose and beta-D fructose. It is a nonreducing sugar due to the absence of a free carbonyl carbon.

DIGESTION, ABSORPTION AND METABOLISM OF CARBOHYDRATES AND RELATED DISORDERS

Digestion of Carbohydrates

- Digestion of carbohydrate begins in the mouth.
- Salivary amylase in the mouth hydrolyzes starch into smaller polysaccharides and maltose.
- *In the stomach:*
  - No carbohydrates are digested in stomach
  - Low gastric pH inactivates the salivary amylase
- The digestion of carbohydrates is then continued in the small intestine by the:
  - Pancreatic amylase, which converts the partially hydrolyzed dextrins/oligosaccharides into dextrins, maltose and isomaltose
  - Alpha dextrinases convert the alpha limit dextrins into maltotriose and glucose
  - Disaccharidases such as sucrase, lactase, maltase break down disaccharides such as sucrose, lactose, maltose into monosaccharides

Absorption of Carbohydrates

- Site of absorption – duodenum and upper jejunum
- Monosaccharides are produced by digestion of carbohydrates, i.e., glucose, fructose and galactose
- Of these, glucose accounts for 80% of the total
- *The relative rates of absorption of important monosaccharides are (in reference to Glucose):*
  - Glucose – 100
  - Galactose – 110

- Fructose – 43
- Mannose – 20
- Xylose – 15
- Arabinose – 9
- Rate of absorption is higher for hexoses than pentoses
- Insulin has no effect on absorption of sugars

Metabolism of Carbohydrates

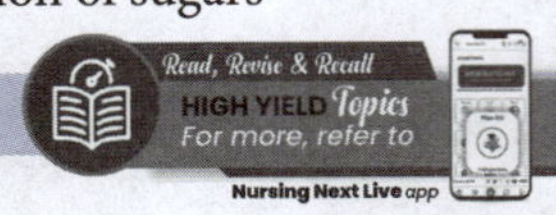

Glycolysis

- Sequence of reactions converting glucose to pyruvate or lactate with the production of ATP.
- Also known as Embden- Meyerhof- Parnas (EMP) pathway.
- Takes place in the cytoplasm of the cells.
- In *aerobic conditions* – pyruvate is the end product.
- In *anaerobic conditions* – lactate is the end product.
- Major pathway for ATP synthesis in tissues lacking mitochondria, e.g., RBCs, cornea, lens, etc.

Steps in Glycolysis

Three phases:

1. Energy investment phase or preparatory phase
2. Splitting phase
3. Energy generation phase

Overall Reaction

Glucose (6C) + 2 NAD^+ + 2 ADP + 2 inorganic phosphates (Pi) $\Rightarrow$ 2 pyruvate (3C) + 2 $NADH^+$ + 2 H^+ + 2 H_2O

Citric Acid Cycle

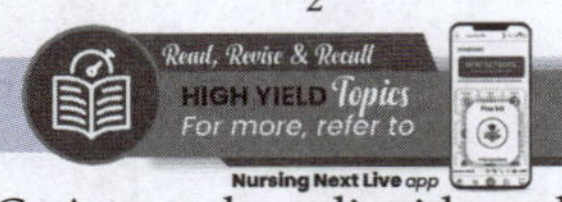

- Involves the oxidation of acetyl CoA to carbon dioxide and water
- Utilizes about 2/3rds of the oxygen consumed by the body
- Connecting link between most metabolic pathways
- Location: Mitochondrial Matrix
- Cyclic process – open cycle – many compounds enter the cycle and leave.
- *Also known as:*
  - Tricarboxylic acid cycle
  - Krebs cycle

Amphibolic Nature of TCA

TCA is known as amphibolic because of both synthetic and metabolic reactions. These are:

Synthetic (anabolic) reactions :

- Oxaloacetate and α – ketoglutarate – serve as precursor for synthesis of asparate and glutamate, used in the synthesis of non-essential amino acids, purine and pyrimidines.
- Succinyl CoA – synthesis of porphyrins and heme
- Acetyl CoA – biosynthesis of fatty acids, sterols

Metabolic (catabolic) reactions:

- Central metabolic hub of the cell.
- Aerobic metabolism of carbohydrates
- Provides ATP and NADH, FADH2 – provides energy for various metabolic pathways.

Gluconeogenesis

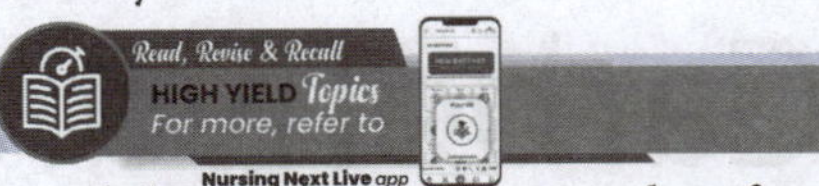

- Process of production of glucose from sources such as fatty acids, amino acids, lactate and pyruvate.
- Reverse of glycolysis.
- Main site is liver – mitochondria and cytoplasm.
- Provides energy during fasting and starvation.

Metabolic Disorders Associated with Carbohydrate Digestion and Metabolism

- Hereditary metabolic disorder
- Usually X-linked
- Disorders associated with carbohydrate digestion
  - Lactose intolerance
    - Due to deficiency of lactase
    - Lactose accumulates in the large intestine and draws water by osmosis causing diarrhea
  - Congenital Sucrase-Isomaltase deficiency
    - Deficiency of enzyme sucrose and isomaltase
    - Leads to non-utilization of lactose
  - Disacchariduria
    - Deficiency of enzyme disaccharidases
    - Leads to excretion of large amounts of disaccharides in urine.
- Disorders associated with carbohydrate metabolism
  - Galactosemia
    - Most common form is due to the deficiency of enzyme galactose 1 phosphate uridyl transferase.
  - Glycogen storage disease
    - Occurs due to the deficiency of enzymes related to glycogen metabolism.
    - This leads to an abnormal type or quantity of glycogen deposition in different tissues.
  - Hereditary fructose intolerance
    - Occurs due to deficiency of enzyme aldose B
  - Pyruvate metabolism disorder
    - Occurs due to the deficiency of enzymes pyruvate dehydrogenase and pyruvate carboxylase

REGULATION OF BLOOD GLUCOSE

- *Fasting blood glucose levels less than 100 mg/dL are considered*

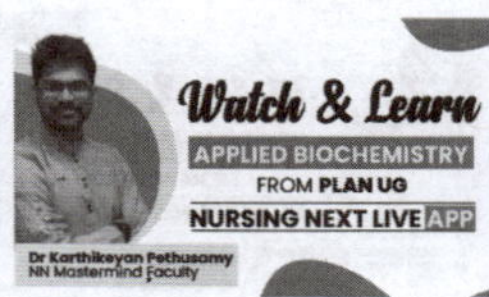

- *Normal Blood glucose levels are maintained mainly by:*
  - Liver
  - Kidney
  - Reciprocal regulation of blood glucose occurs by glycolysis and gluconeogenesis
- **Key element** in this reciprocal pathway is a bifunctional allosteric enzyme that contains two different regulatory domains:
  i. Phosphofructokinase – 2 (PFK-2)
  ii Fructose bisphosphatase -2 (FBP-2)
  - *This bifunctional enzyme exists in two states:*

  1. *Unphosphorylated state*
     - PFK-2 is active
     - FBP-2 is inhibited
     - PFK-2 converts fructose – 6- phosphate to fructose 2, 6 bisphosphate
  2. *Phosphorylated State*
     - PFK-2 is inhibited
     - FBP-2 is active
     - FBP-2 causes dephosphorylation of fructose 2, 6 bisphosphate to fructose–6–phosphate

Effects of Hormones

- Insulin and glucagon affect the rate of gene transcription
- Insulin stimulates:
  - Phosphofructokinases
  - Pyruvate kinase
  - Glucose transporter (GLUT – 4)
  - Glucagon inhibits the above enzymes

DIABETES MELLITUS – TYPE I AND TYPE II, SYMPTOMS, COMPLICATIONS AND MANAGEMENT

Diabetes Mellitus

- Metabolic disorder of fuel metabolism
- Characterized by hyperglycemia

Types of Diabetes Mellitus

- Insulin dependent DM (IDDM)
  - Also known as type I diabetes or juvenile onset diabetes,
  - Age of onset—12–15 years age
  - Less common, accounts for about 10–20% of the known diabetics.
  - Etiology - Almost total deficiency of insulin due to destruction of B-cells of pancreas
- Non-insulin dependent DM (NIDDM)
  - Also called type II diabetes or adult-onset diabetes
  - Most common, accounting for 80–90%
  - Age of onset - above 35 years
  - Less severe than IDDM.
  - Etiology - due to genetic and environmental factors and obesity

Metabolic Changes in Diabetes

- *Hyperglycemia*
  - Elevation of blood glucose level
- *Glycosuria*
  - When the glucose is excreted into urine
- *Ketoacidosis*
  - Increased mobilization of fatty acids results in overproduction of ketone bodies
- *Hypertriglyceridemia*
  - Conversion of fatty acids to triacylglycerols and the secretion of VLDL and chylomicrons are comparatively higher and activity of the enzyme lipoprotein lipase is low. Consequently, the plasma levels of VLDL, chylomicrons and triacylglycerols are increased.
- *Hypercholesterolemia*
  - An increase in level of cholesterol is also frequently seen in diabetics.

Acute Complications of Type I and II Diabetes

- *Diabetic ketoacidosis*
  - Acute and dangerous complication
  - Low insulin levels cause the liver to turn fatty acid to ketone for fuel (i.e., ketosis)
  - Elevated levels of ketone bodies in the blood decrease the blood's pH, leading to DKA.
  - More common in type I diabetes than type II.
- *Hyperglycemia hyperosmolar state*
  - With blood glucose levels above 300 mg/dL (16 mmol/L)), water is osmotically drawn out of cells into the blood
  - This results in loss of water and an increase in blood osmolarity.
  - More common in type II diabetes than type I.
- *Hypoglycemia*
  - Abnormally low blood glucose
  - Acute complication of diabetes treatment
- *Diabetic coma*
  - Severe diabetic hypoglycemia
  - Diabetic ketoacidosis
  - Hyperosmolar nonketotic coma

Investigation of Diabetes Mellitus

Oral Glucose Tolerance Test

- Diagnosis of diabetes is made on the basis of individual's response to oral glucose load – Glucose tolerance test (GTT)
  - Used for diagnosis of Diabetes in doubtful cases:
    - Gestational diabetes
    - Prediabetes
    - Insulin resistance

Preparation of Subject

- Carbohydrate rich diet for at least 3 days prior to test
- Fasting for 10 hours before test

Procedure for GTT

- Conducted preferably in morning
- Fasting sample is taken
- Subject is given 75 g of glucose dissolved in 300 mL of water – to be drunk in 5 minutes
- Blood and urine samples are taken at 30 minutes intervals for the next 2 hours
- Blood samples – glucose elimination
- Urine samples – quantitative glucose estimation

Interpretation

People Without Diabetes	• Fasting value (before test): Under 6 mmol/L • At 2 hours: Under 7.8 mmol/L
People with Impaired Glucose Tolerance (IGT)	• **Fasting value (before test):** 6.0 to 7.0 mmol/L • **At 2 hours:** 7.9 to 11.0 mmol/L
Diabetic Levels	• **Fasting value (before test):** Over 7.0 mmol/L • **At 2 hours:** Over 11.0 mmol/L

Mini GTT

- Also known as modern glucose tolerance test
- In this, only two blood samples are collected:
  i. At zero hour or fasting
  ii. 2 hours post glucose
- Urine samples are also collected at the same time.

Interpretation

	Zero hour	After 2 hours
Normal person	<110 mg/dL	<140 mg/dL
Increased glucose tolerance	110–126 mg/dL	140–199 mg/dL

Extended GTT

- Also known as extended glucose tolerance test
- It is a diagnostic test to measure:
  - Blood Glucose
  - Insulin
  - C – peptide

Technique

For **extended GTT**, blood samples are to be collected at **30, 60, 120 and 180 minutes** for glucose, insulin and c-peptide.

Glucose Challenge Test

- Measures body's response to glucose
- Done during pregnancy to screen for gestational diabetes

Procedure

- Done in two steps at any time of day, not on an empty stomach
  1. First step
     - Drink 50 g of glucose
  2. Second step
     - One hour later – blood sugar levels are measured

Intravenous GTT

- Glucose is intravenously injected
- Blood glucose levels are measured within 5 minutes of administration of glucose

Advantages

- Accurate assessment of first phase of insulin release
- Abnormal results can be detected even prior to the onset of diabetes.
- Since the glucose does not pass through the GI tract, as is the case in OGTT, IV GTT allows for greater sensitivity.

Disadvantages

- Use of intravenous line – difficult to start and maintain throughout the procedure
- Risk of hyperglycemia is more
- Risk of beta cell damage is there
- Needs proper equipment
- It bypasses the response of incretin hormone stimulated by oral glucose ingestion.

HbA1c

- Glycated or glycosylated hemoglobin – glucose derived products of normal adult hemoglobin HbA
- Glycation – post-translational, nonenzymatic addition of sugar residue to amino acids

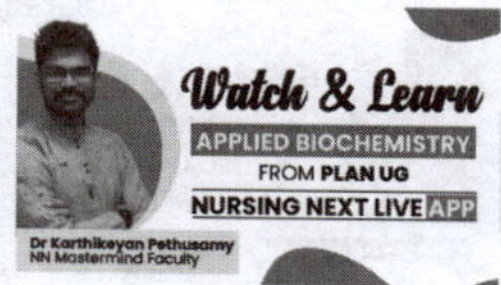

- HbA1c – most abundant glycated hemoglobin – produced by condensation of glucose with N-terminal valine of each β-chain of HbA

Normal Range

- In healthy nondiabetic – 4–5.6%
- Prediabetic – 5.7%–6.4%
- Diabetic – 6.5% or higher

HYPOGLYCEMIA

- Blood glucose levels fall below 45 mg/dL
- Leads to the glucose deprivation to the central nervous system (particularly brain)

Symptoms

- Headache
- Anxiety
- Confusion
- Sweating
- Slurred speech
- Seizures
- Coma

Conditions Associated with Hypoglycemia

- Deficiency of growth hormone, pituitary hormone
- Maple syrup urine disease
- Glycogen storage diseases type I and II
- Insulin-induced hypoglycemia
- Addison's disease

CONCEPTUAL EXERCISES

LONG ANSWER QUESTIONS

1. Describe the process of glycolysis. Explain how many ATP molecules are formed in anaerobic and aerobic glycolysis. (MGR)

Answer

Introduction

- Sequence of reactions converting glucose to pyruvate or lactate with the production of ATP.
- Also known as Embden- Meyerhof- Parnas (EMP) pathway.
- Takes place in the cytoplasm of the cells.
- In *aerobic conditions* – pyruvate is the end product.
- In *anaerobic conditions* – lactate is the end product.
- Major pathway for ATP synthesis in tissues lacking mitochondria, e.g., RBCs, cornea, lens, etc.

Steps in Glycolysis

Three phases:

1. Energy investment phase or preparatory phase
2. Splitting phase
3. Energy generation phase

Energy Investment Phase

- Phosphorylation of glucose to glucose 6-phosphate
  - Enzyme – hexokinase or glucokinase
    - Dependent on Mg^{2+} and ATP
  - Hexokinase – present in all tissues
  - Glucokinase – present in liver
- Isomerization of glucose 6-phosphate to fructose 6-phosphate in presence of enzyme phosphohexose isomerase and Mg^{2+}
- Phosphorylation of Fructose 6-phosphate to fructose 1, 6-bisphosphate
  - Enzyme – phosphofructokinase
  - Irreversible step
  - Regulatory step in glycolysis

Splitting Phase

- Breakdown of the fructose 1, 6-bisphosphate (6C) to glyceraldehyde 3-phosphate (3C) and dihydroxyacetone phosphate (3C)
  - Enzyme – aldolase
- Glyceraldehyde 3-phosphate and dihydroxyacetone phosphate are reversibly interconvertible
  - Enzyme – Phosphotriose isomerase

Energy Generation Phase

- Conversion of glyceraldehyde 3-phosphate to 1, 3-bisphosphoglycerate
  - Enzyme – glyceraldehyde 3-phosphate dehydrogenase
  - $NADH + H^+$ is formed.
- 3-phosphoglycerate is formed from 1,3-bisphosphoglycerate in the presence of enzyme phosphoglycerate kinase
  - ATP is formed (***Substrate Level phosphorylation I***)
  - Reversible step
- Isomerization of 3-phosphoglycerate to 2-phosphoglycerate
  - Enzyme – phosphoglycerate mutase
- 2-phosphoglycerate is converted to phosphoenol pyruvate
  - Enzyme – enolase
    - Dependent on Mg^{2+} or Mn^{2+}
    - Inhibited by fluoride

- Transfer of high energy phosphate from phosphoenol pyruvate to ADP
  - ATP is formed
  - Enzyme – pyruvate kinase
  - Product formed is pyruvate
  - Irreversible step

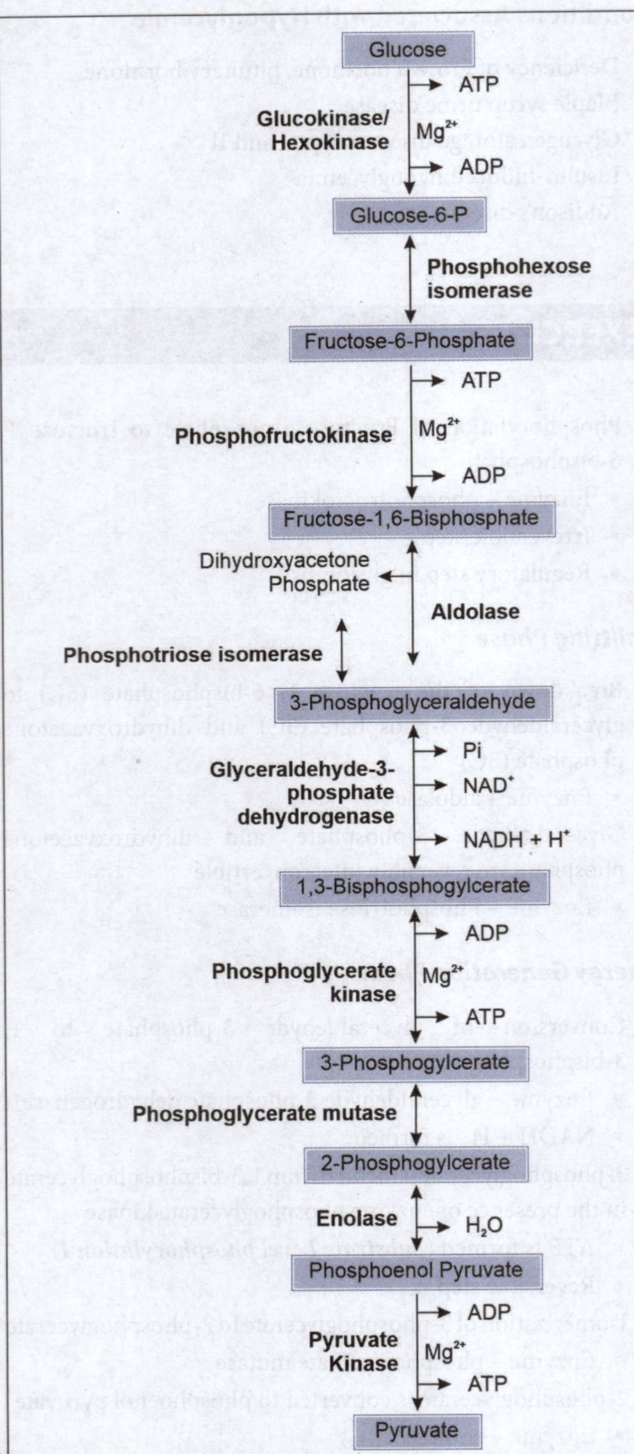

Figure 1.1: Metabolism of glucose via aerobic glycolysis

Energetics of Glycolysis – Aerobic Conditions

Overall Reaction

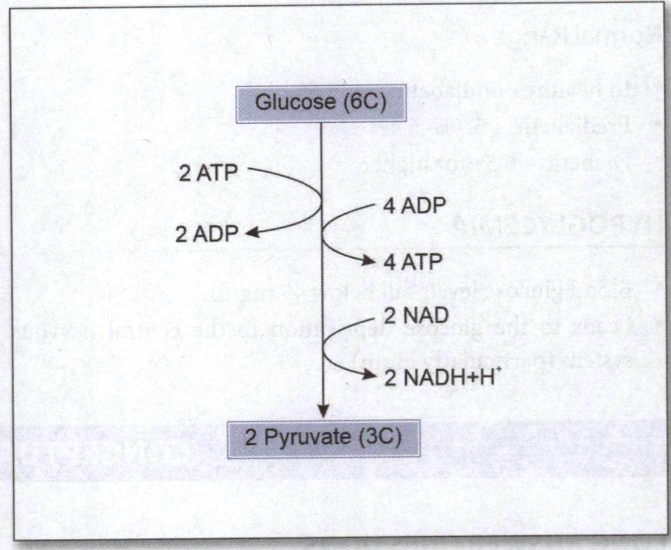

Glycolysis – Aerobic Conditions

Glucose (6C) + 2 NAD^+ + 2 ADP + 2 inorganic phosphates (Pi) $\Rightarrow$ 2 pyruvate (3C) + 2 $NADH^+$ + 2 H^+ + 2 H_2O

- ATP consumed per glucose – 2
- ATP produced per glucose – 4
- NADH produced = 2
- 2 NADH yields 6 ATP

Net ATP: 8 per glucose

Energetics of Glycolysis–Anaerobic Conditions

- ATP consumed per glucose – 2
- ATP produced per glucose – 4
- NAD^+ produced during the pathway is used for the conversion of pyruvate to lactate.

So, Net ATP = 2 ATP per glucose.

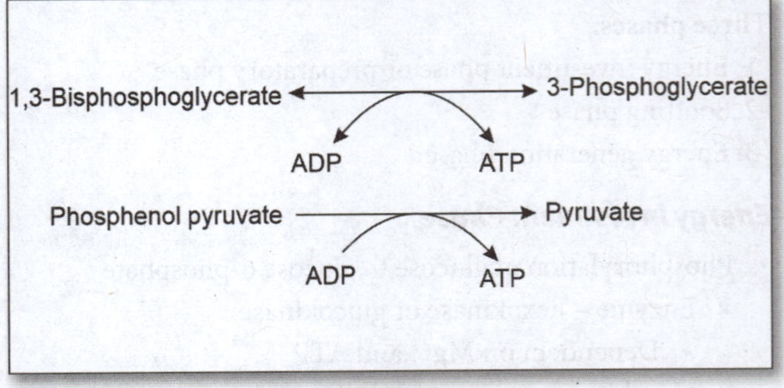

Figure 1.2: Energy-yielding steps in glycolysis

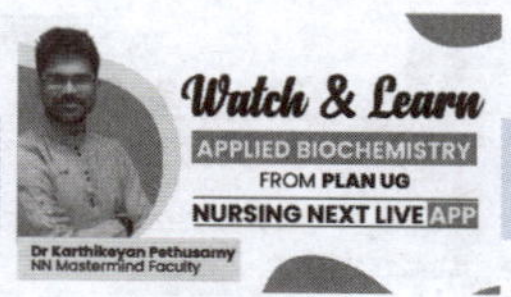

2. Write the gluconeogenesis process in detail and explain the action of key enzymes on it. (MGR, DU)

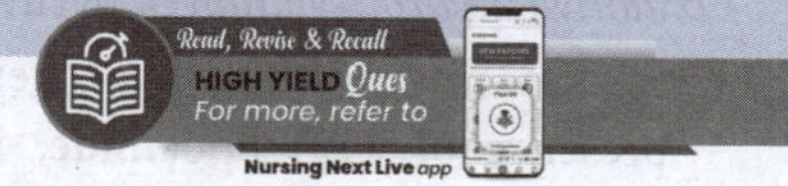

Answer

Gluconeogenesis

- Process of production of glucose from sources such as fatty acids, amino acids, lactate and pyruvate.
- Reverse of glycolysis.
- Main site is liver – mitochondria and cytoplasm.
- Provides energy during fasting and starvation.

Significance of Gluconeogenesis

- Maintenance of blood sugar levels
- Major source of D-glucose
- Large amounts of lactate produced during anaerobic glycolysis at the time of exercise or starvation are utilized during gluconeogenesis.
- Protein can also act as substrate for gluconeogenesis.

Steps of Gluconeogenesis

Three irreversible reactions of glycolysis that are bypassed in gluconeogenesis are:

1. **Conversion of pyruvate to phosphoenol pyruvate:**
   - Two steps
     i. Pyruvate is converted to oxaloacetate in mitochondria by pyruvate carboxylase
     ii. Oxaloacetate is transported to the cytosol by malate shuttle where it converts to phosphoenol pyruvate in the presence of enzyme phosphoenolpyruvate carboxykinase
2. **Conversion of fructose 1,6 bisphosphate to fructose-6-phosphate:**
   - Enzyme – fructose 1,6 bisphosphatase – requires Mg^{2+} ions
   - Absent in smooth muscle and heart muscle
   - *Regulatory enzyme in gluconeogenesis*
3. **Conversion of glucose 6-phosphate to glucose:**
   - Enzyme – glucose 6-phosphatase
   - Present in liver and kidney
   - Absent in muscle, brain and adipose tissue

Glucose-alanine Cycle

- There is a continuous transport of amino acids from muscle to liver, mostly during starvation.
- Alanine is the most common amino acid transported.
- Pyruvate in skeletal muscle undergoes transamination to produce alanine.
- Alanine is transported to liver and used for Gluconeogenesis and the process is called glucose-alanine cycle.

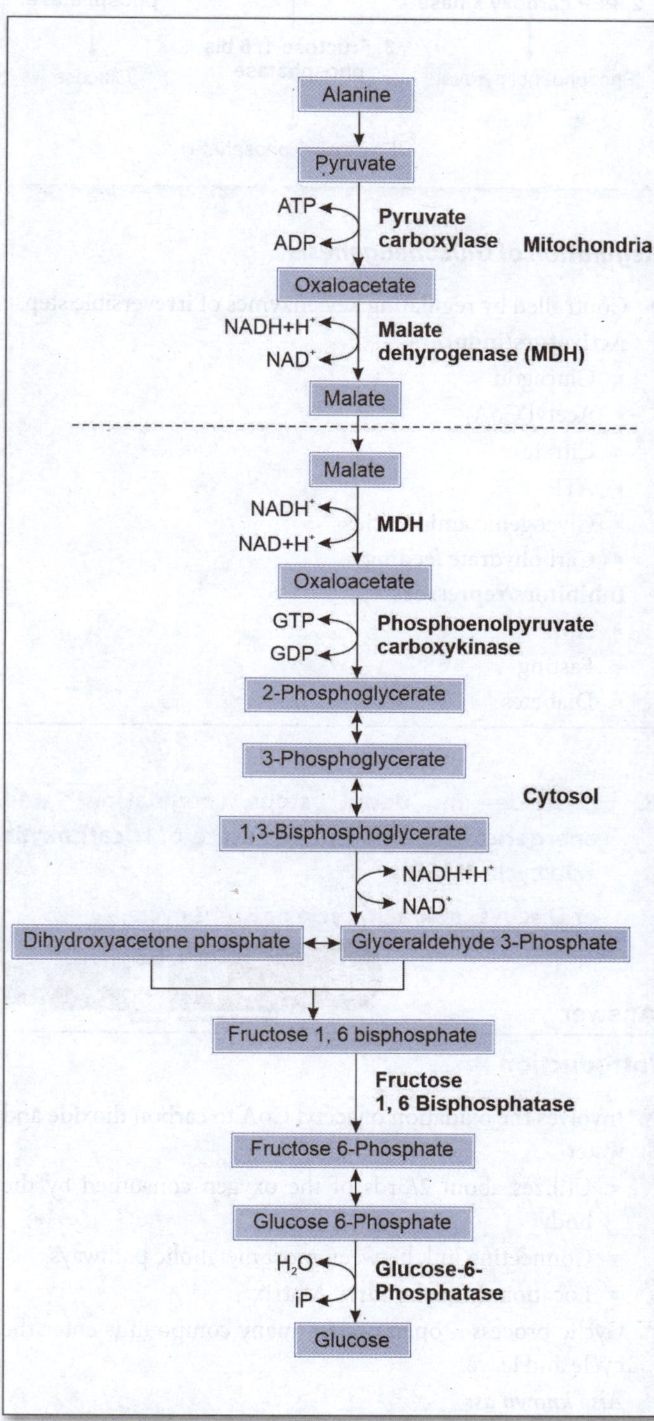

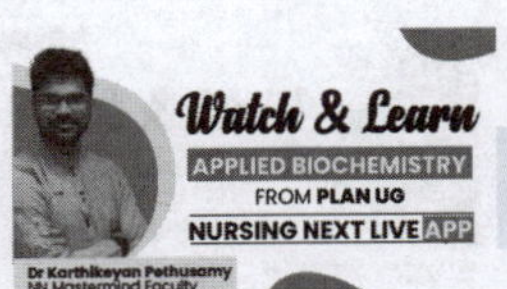

Key Enzymes in Gluconeogenesis

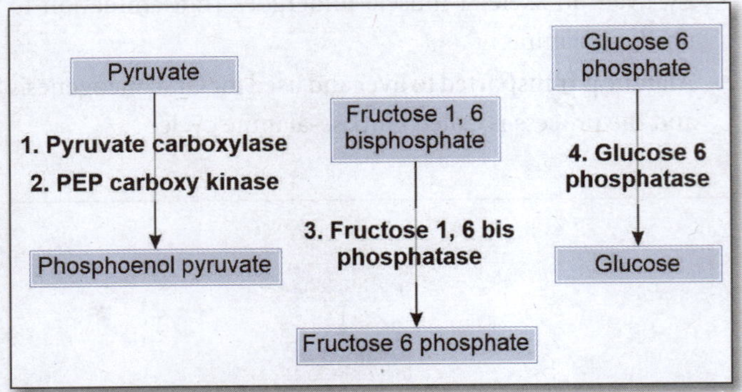

Regulation of Gluconeogenesis

- Controlled by regulating key enzymes of irreversible steps
- **Activators/inducers**
  - Glucagon
  - Acetyl CoA
  - Citrate
  - ATP
  - Glycogenic amino acids
  - Carbohydrate feeding
- **Inhibitors/repressors**
  - AMP
  - Fasting
  - Diabetes

3. Describe in detail steps, regulation, and energetics and amphibolic nature of tricarboxylic acid cycle. (MGR)

or Discuss citric acid cycle or Krebs cycle.

Answer

Introduction

- Involves the oxidation of acetyl CoA to carbon dioxide and water
  - Utilizes about 2/3rds of the oxygen consumed by the body
  - Connecting link between most metabolic pathways
  - Location: Mitochondrial Matrix
- Cyclic process – open cycle – many compounds enter the cycle and leave.
- *Also known as:*
  - Tricarboxylic acid cycle
  - Krebs cycle
  - Citric acid cycle

Citric Acid Cycle

- *Oxidative decarboxylation* of pyruvate to citric acid cycle
  - Enzyme pyruvate dehydrogenase complex, in the presence of TPP, lipoamide, FAD, coenzyme A and NAD^+.
  - Connecting link between glycolysis and Krebs cycle.
- **Step 1:** Formation of Citrate
  - Acetyl CoA (2C) combines with oxaloacetate (4C) to give (S)-citryl CoA (6C).
  - Enzyme - citrate synthase.
  - (S)-citryl CoA is hydrolyzed to citrate by citrate synthase to produce CoA-SH and citrate.
- **Step 2:** Formation of Isocitrate
  - Citrate, isomerized to isocitrate
  - Enzyme-aconitase.
- **Step 3: Oxidation of Isocitrate**
  - Involves oxidation-reduction and decarboxylation.
  - Enzyme - isocitrate dehydrogenase is complex
    - Isocitrate is oxidized to oxalosuccinate by NAD^+, releasing 2 hydrogen atoms and NADH is formed
    - The oxalosuccinate further undergoes decarboxylation, to form α-ketoglutarate (5C), CO_2 and NADH.
- **Step 4:** Oxidation of α-ketoglutarate
  - α-ketoglutarate undergoes both redox reaction and decarboxylation in the presence of NAD^+, CoA-SH, to produce CO_2, NADH and succinyl CoA (4C)
  - Enzymes - α-ketoglutarate dehydrogenase complex.
- **Step 5:** Thioester bond cleavage in Succinyl CoA and Phosphorylation of GDP
  - Succinyl CoA is converted to succinate to produce GTP
  - Enzyme - succinyl CoA synthetase
- **Step 6:** Oxidation of Succinate
  - Succinate is dehydrogenated by FAD catalyzed by succinate dehydrogenase to produce fumarate, and FADH2.
- **Step 7:** Hydration of Fumarate
  - The enzyme fumarase catalyzes the addition of water to produce L-malate.
- **Step 8:** Oxidation of L-Malate to Regenerate Oxaloacetate
  - Malate undergoes oxidation to regenerate oxaloacetate in the presence of NAD^+
  - NADH + H^+ is released
  - Enzyme - malate dehydrogenase.
  - Oxaloacetate combines with Acetyl CoA to enter the cycle again.

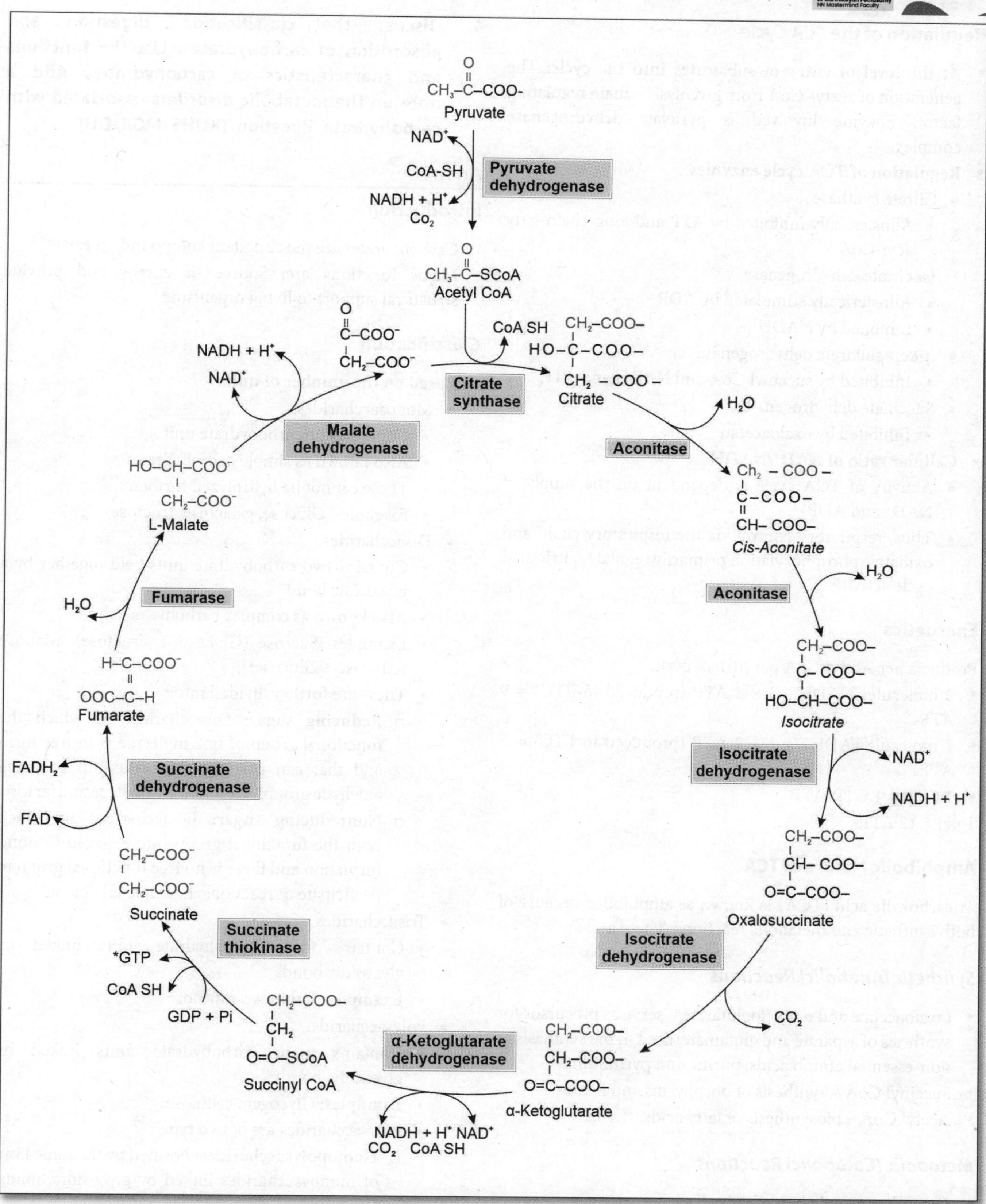
CH3–C(=O)–COO-
Pyruvate
NAD+
CoA-SH
NADH + H+
CO2
Pyruvate dehydrogenase
CH3–C(=O)–SCoA
Acetyl CoA
CoA SH
Citrate synthase
CH2–COO–
HO–C–COO–
CH2 COO –
Citrate
H2O
Aconitase
Ch2 – COO –
C–COO–
CH– COO–
Cis-Aconitate
H2O
Aconitase
CH2–COO–
C– COO–
HO–CH–COO–
Isocitrate
Isocitrate dehydrogenase
NAD+
NADH + H+
CH2–COO–
CH– COO–
O=C–COO–
Oxalosuccinate
Isocitrate dehydrogenase
CO2
CH2–COO
CH2–COO–
O=C–COO–
α-Ketoglutarate
α-Ketoglutarate dehydrogenase
NADH + H+ NAD+
CO2 CoA SH
CH2–COO–
CH2
O=C–SCoA
Succinyl CoA
GDP + Pi
*GTP
CoA SH
Succinate thiokinase
CH2–COO-
CH2–COO-
Succinate
FAD
FADH2
Succinate dehydrogenase
H–C–COO-
-OOC–C–H
Fumarate
H2O
Fumarase
HO–CH–COO-
CH2–COO-
L-Malate
Malate dehydrogenase
NADH + H+
NAD+
C(=O)–COO-
CH2–COO-

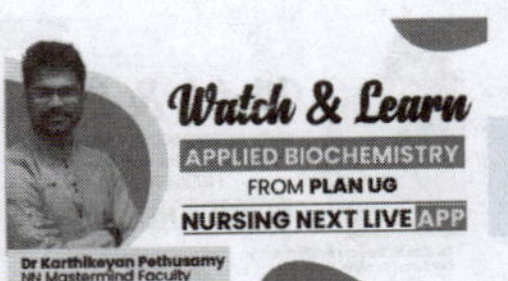

Regulation of the TCA Cycle

- **At the level of entry of substrates into the cycle:** The generation of acetyl-CoA from glycolysis – main regulating factor. Enzyme involved is pyruvate dehydrogenase complex.
- **Regulation of TCA cycle enzymes**
  - Citrate synthase
    - Allosterically inhibited by ATP and long-chain fatty acyl-CoA.
  - Isocitrate dehydrogenase
    - Allosterically stimulated by ADP,
    - Inhibited by NADH
  - α-ketoglutarate dehydrogenase
    - Inhibited by succinyl CoA and NADH and ATP.
  - Succinate dehydrogenase
    - Inhibited by oxaloacetate
- **Cellular ratio of NAD^+/NADH**
  - Activity of TCA cycle is dependent on the supply of NAD^+ and ADP
  - Thus, respiratory control via the respiratory chain and oxidative phosphorylation primarily regulates citric acid cycle activity.

Energetics

Products per Acetyl CoA per turn of cycle

- 3 molecules NADH - 3 × 3 ATP (produced in ETC) = 9 ATPs
- 1 molecule FADH2 – 1 × 2 ATP (produced in ETC) = 2 ATPs
- 1 GTP = 1 GTP/ATP

Total = 12 ATPs

Amphibolic Nature of TCA

Tricarboxylic acid (TCA) is known as amphibolic because of both synthetic and metabolic reactions. These are:

Synthetic (Anabolic) Reactions

- Oxaloacetate and α – ketoglutarate – serve as precursor for synthesis of asparate and glutamate, used in the synthesis of non-essential amino acids, purine and pyrimidines.
- Succinyl CoA – synthesis of porphyrins and heme
- Acetyl CoA – biosynthesis of fatty acids, sterols

Metabolic (Catabolic) Reactions

- Central metabolic hub of the cell.
  - Aerobic metabolism of carbohydrates
- Provides ATP and NADH, FADH2 – provides energy for various metabolic pathways.

4. Discuss the classification, digestion and absorption of carbohydrates. List the functions and characteristics of carbohydrates. Add a note on the metabolic disorders associated with carbohydrate digestion. (KUHS, MGR, DU)

Answer

Introduction

- Carbohydrates are the abundant compound on earth.
- Major functions are: Source of energy and provide structural support to living organisms.

Classification

- **Based on the number of units**
  - Monosaccharides:
    - Contains one carbohydrate unit
    - Also known as simple carbohydrates
    - These cannot be hydrolyzed further.
    - Examples: Glucose, galactose, fructose
  - Disaccharides
    - Contains two carbohydrate units held together by a glycosidic bond.
    - Also known as complex carbohydrates
    - Examples: Sucrose (Glucose + Fructose), Maltose (Glucose + Glucose)
    - These are further divided into:
      - **Reducing sugar:** Disaccharides in which the functional group of one molecule is in free form and that can participate in reactions reducing aldehyde groups. Example are maltose and lactose.
      - **Nonreducing sugar:** Disaccharides in which both the functional groups are engaged in bond formation and there is no free functional group to participate in reactions. Example is sucrose.
  - Trisaccharides
    - Contains three carbohydrate units linked by glycosidic bonds.
    - **Examples:** Rabinose, raffinose
  - Polysaccharides
    - Contains many carbohydrate units linked by glycosidic bonds.
    - **Examples:** Glycogen, cellulose
    - Polysaccharides are of two types:
      - **Homopolysaccharides:** Formed by the same kind of monosaccharides linked by glycosidic bonds. Examples are glycogen, starch, cellulose
      - **Heteropolysaccharides:** Formed by two or more types of monosaccharides joined together by glycosidic linkages.

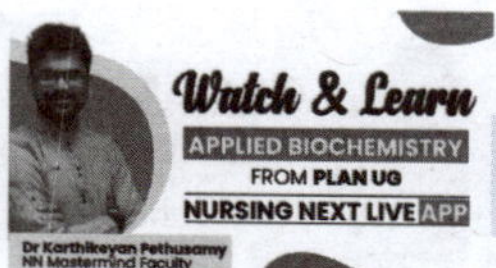

- Mucopolysaccharides
  - Heteropolysaccharides in which there is a mixture of sugar units.
  - **Examples:** Hyaluronic acid, chondroitin sulfate, heparin
- **Based on position of carbonyl position**
  - Carbonyl at C1 is aldehyde – Aldose
  - Carbonyl at any other carbon – Ketone
- **Based on number of carbon**
  - Three carbons – triose
  - Four carbons – tetrose
  - Five carbons – pentose
  - Six carbons – hexose
  - Seven carbons – heptose
- **Stereochemistry**
  - Dextro or levo rotatory depending on the stereochemistry of chiral carbon.

Dietary Carbohydrates Mainly Include

- Polysaccharides – starch, glycogen
- Disaccharides – lactose, sucrose
- Monosaccharides – glucose, fructose – to a minor extent.

Digestion of Carbohydrates

- The polysaccharides get hydrated during heating which is essential for the efficient digestion.
- Glycosidases bring about the hydrolysis of glycosidic bonds of carbohydrates.
- **In the oral cavity:**
  - Salivary alpha amylase (ptyalin) acts on starch and breaks down into alpha dextrins, maltotriose and maltose by cleaving the 1,4 glycosidic bonds.
- **In the stomach:**
  - No carbohydrates are digested in stomach
  - Low gastric pH inactivates the salivary amylase
- **In the small intestine:**
  - Pancreatic alpha amylase breaks down starch into disaccharides and oligosaccharides by acting on alpha 1,4 glycosidic bonds
  - In the upper jejunum, oligosaccharidases and disaccharidases act on the disachaarides and oligosaccharides to form monosaccharides
  - The enzyme sucrase hydrolyzes sucrose, and lactase acts on lactose.

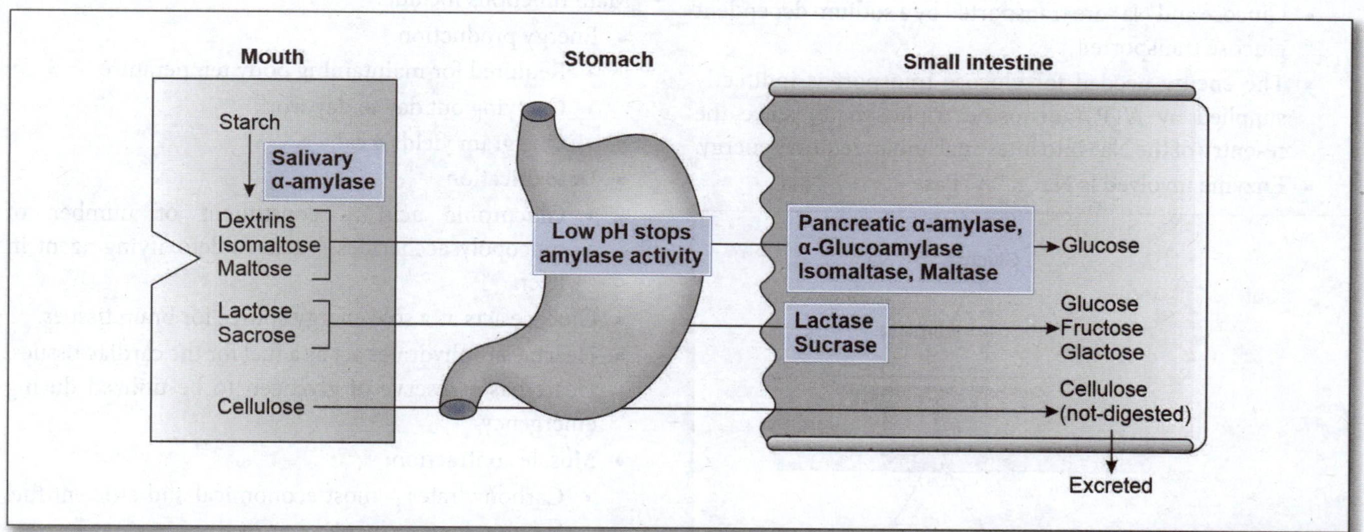

Enzyme	Site of action	Catalytic action
Salivary amylase	Mouth	Starch/Glycogen→ Partially hydrolyzed dextrins, oligosaccharides, isomaltose and maltose
Pancreatic amylase	Small intestine	Partially hydrolyzed dextrins/oligosaccharides→Dextrins, maltose, isomaltose, maltotriose
α–Dextrinase	Small intestine	α–Limit dextrins →Maltotriose, glucose
Disaccharidases	Small intestine	
Sucrase		Sucrose → Glucose and fructose
Lactase		Lactose → Glucose and galactose
Maltase		Maltose/Maltotriose → Glucose
Isomaltase		Isomaltose → Glucose

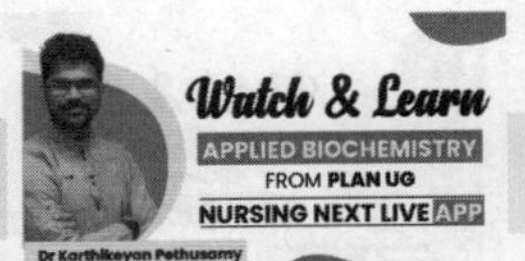

Absorption of Monosaccharides

- Site of absorption – duodenum and upper jejunum
- Monosaccharides are produced by digestion of carbohydrates, i.e., glucose, fructose and galactose
- Of these, glucose accounts for 8% of the total
- **The relative rates of absorption of important monosaccharides with reference to Glucose are:**
  - Glucose – 100
  - Galactose – 110
  - Fructose – 43
  - Mannose – 20
  - Xylose – 15
  - Arabinose – 9
- Rate of absorption is higher for hexoses than pentoses
- Insulin has no effect on absorption of sugars

Mechanism of Absorption

- Different sugars possess different mechanisms for their absorption
- **Glucose**
  - Transported into the intestinal mucosal cells by a carrier-mediated process that requires energy
  - Glucose and Na^+ are transported by a sodium dependent glucose transporter
  - The energy needed for glucose transport is indirectly supplied by ATP (adenosine triphosphate) since the re-entry of the Na^+ into intestinal luman requires energy.
  - Enzyme involved is Na^+ K^+ ATPase

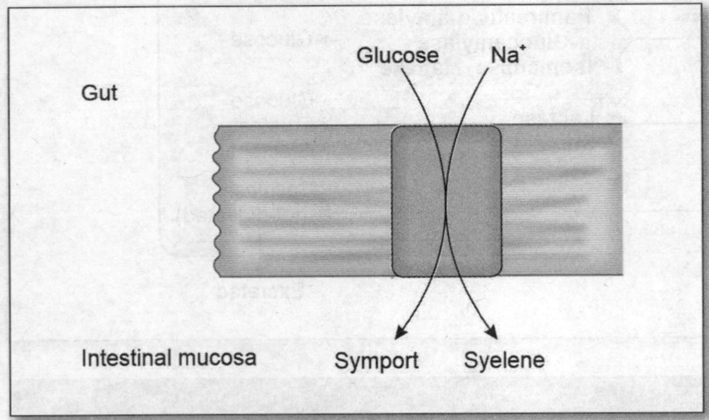

- **Fructose**
  - Not energy dependent
  - Independent of Na^+ transport
  - Transported by facilitated diffusion mediated by a carrier
  - Fructose is converted to glucose inside the epithelial cells.
- **Pentoses**
  - Absorbed by simple diffusion
- **Nondigestible carbohydrates**
  - Complex carbohydrates such as cellulose, hemicellulose, pectins, etc. are not digested by humans.
  - These act as fibers in the diet

Rate of Absorption

Absorption mainly occurs in jejunum.

Rate is regulated by:

- Rate of entry
- Mobility in stomach
- Tone of pyloric sphincter
- Vitamin B
- Endocrine glands - Thyroid and pituitary hormones.
- Insulin has no effect in absorption.

Characteristics and Functions of Carbohydrates

- Carbohydrates in diet mainly constitute of monosaccharides, oligosaccharides and polysaccharides.
- Repeating units of monosaccharides held together by glycosidic bonds form polysaccharides
- May be linear or branched
- Two major functions – structural and storage of energy
- Main functions include:
  - Energy production
    - Required for maintaining body temperature
    - Carrying out day to day work
    - One gram yields 4 cal.
  - Detoxification
    - Glucuronic acid – constituent of number of mucopolysaccharides – acts as detoxifying agent in liver.
  - Glucose acts as a sole energy source for brain tissues.
  - Heart: Carbohydrates act as a fuel for the cardiac tissues. Heart has a reserve of glycogen to be utilized during emergency.
  - Muscle contraction:
    - Carbohydrates – most economical and efficient fuel for muscle movement.
    - Glycogen – storage form of carbohydrate.
  - Protein sparing effect:
    - Proteins are spared for growth and repair when fats and carbohydrates are sufficiently able to meet the energy demands.
  - Required for the complete oxidation of fats. In their absence, fats are broken down rapidly leading to formation of ketones, resulting in a condition known as ketosis.
  - Lactose:
    - Required for growth of gut bacteria

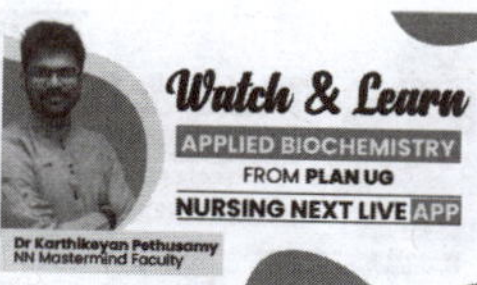

- Aids in absorption of minerals, calcium and phosphorus.
- Dietary fibers:
  - Prevent constipation
  - Lower cholesterol
- Provide carbon skeletal for the synthesis of certain nonessential amino acids.
- Heparin, a mucopolysaccharide, is an anticoagulant.

Metabolic Disorders Associated with Carbohydrate Digestion

- Metabolic disorders associated with carbohydrate digestion and metabolism:
  - Lactose intolerance: Inability to digest lactose due to a deficiency of the enzyme lactase.
  - Galactosemia: Genetic disorder resulting in the inability to metabolize galactose due to enzyme deficiencies.
  - Fructose malabsorption: Impaired absorption of fructose leading to digestive symptoms after consuming fructose-rich foods.
  - Diabetes mellitus: Chronic condition characterized by high blood sugar levels due to inadequate insulin production or insulin resistance.
  - Glycogen storage diseases: Inherited disorders affecting glycogen metabolism, leading to abnormal storage or release of glycogen.
  - Hyperinsulinism: Excessive insulin secretion causing low blood sugar levels.
  - Disorders of glucose transport: Impaired transport of glucose across cell membranes, affecting glucose utilization and metabolism.
  - Reactive hypoglycemia: Low blood sugar levels occurring after a meal due to an exaggerated insulin response.
- Hereditary fructose intolerance: Genetic disorder resulting in the inability to metabolize fructose due to enzyme deficiencies.

SHORT NOTES

1. Classification of carbohydrates. (MGR)

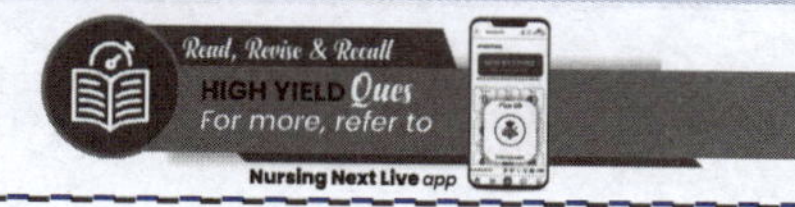

Answer

Introduction

- Most abundant compound on earth.
- Major functions are: Source of energy and provide structural support to living organisms.

Classification

I. Based on the Number of Units

- Monosaccharides:
  - Contains one carbohydrate unit
  - Also known as simple carbohydrates
  - These cannot be hydrolyzed further.
  - Examples: Glucose, galactose, fructose
- Disaccharides:
  - Contains two carbohydrate units held together by a glycosidic bond.
  - Also known as complex carbohydrates
  - Examples: Sucrose, maltose
  - These are further divided into:
    - Reducing sugar: Disaccharides in which the functional group of one molecule is in free form and that can participate in reactions reducing aldehyde groups. Examples are maltose and lactose.
    - Nonreducing sugar: Disaccharides in which both the functional groups are engaged in bond formation and there is no free functional group to participate in reactions. Example is sucrose.
- Trisaccharides:
  - Contains three carbohydrate units linked by glycosidic bonds.
  - Examples: Rabinose, raffinose
- Polysaccharides:
  - Contains many carbohydrate units linked by glycosidic bonds.
  - Examples: Glycogen, cellulose
  - Polysaccharides are of two types:
    - Homopolysaccharides: Formed by the same kind of monosaccharides linked by glycosidic bonds. Examples are glycogen, starch, cellulose.
    - Heteropolysaccharides: Formed by two or more types of monosaccharides joined together by glycosidic linkages.
- Mucopolysaccharides:
  - Heteropolysacharides in which there is a mixture of sugar units.
  - Examples: Hyaluronic acid, chondroitin sulfate, heparin

II. Based on Position of Carbonyl Position

- Carbonyl at C1 is aldehyde – Aldose
- Carbonyl at any other carbon – Ketone

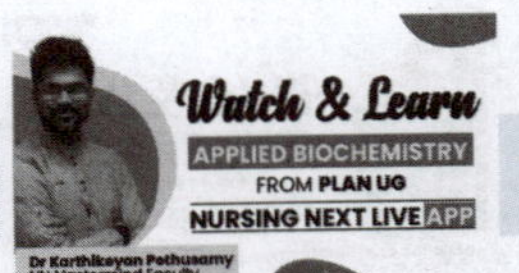

III. Based on Number of Carbon

- Three carbons – triose
- Four carbons – tetrose
- Five carbons – pentose
- Six carbons – hexose
- Seven carbons – heptose

IV. Stereochemistry

Dextro or levo rotatory depending on the stereochemistry of chiral carbon.

2. Glycogen storage disease. (MGR)

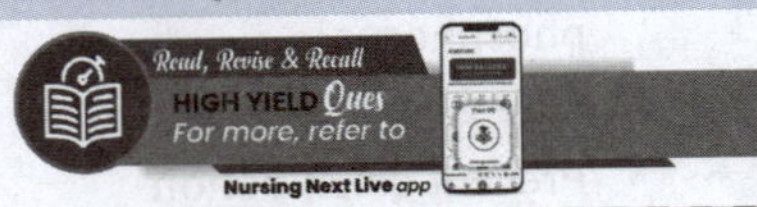

Answer

Introduction

- Metabolic defects concerned with glycogen synthesis and degradation
- Characterized by deposition of normal or abnormal glycogen in one or more tissues.
- Incidence – 1:40,000 births

Type of Glycogen Storage Diseases/Glycogenosis

Type	Name	Defective enzyme	Involved organs	Characteristic features
0	GSD 0	Glycogen synthase	Liver	• Hypoglycemia • Ketonemia • Extra glycogen is not stored in liver • Early death
I	Von Gierke's disease	Glucose 6-phosphatase	Liver, kidney, intestine	• Glycogen accumulation in hepatocytes and renal cells • Enlarged liver and kidney • Fasting hypoglycemia • Lactic acidemia • Gouty arthritis • Ketosis
II	Pompe's disease	Lysosomal α-1,4 glucosidase	All organs	• Accumulation of glycogen in lysosomes • Enlarged liver and heart • Affects nervous system • Early death due to heart failure
III	Cori's disease (Forbe's disease)	Amylo α-1,4 glucosidase (debranching enzyme)	Liver, muscle, leukocytes, heart	• Accumulation of branched chain glycogen • S/S similar to Von Gierke's disease
IV	Anderson's disease (amylopectinosis)	Glucosyl 4-6 transferase (branching enzyme)	Most tissues	• Rare • Liver cirrhosis • Impaired liver function
V	McArdle's disease	Muscle glycogen phosphorylase	Skeletal muscle	• Increased glycogen storage in muscle – not available during exercise • Inadequate energy supply to muscles
VI	Her's disease	Liver glycogen phosphorylase	Liver	• Enlarged liver • Hypoglycemia • Ketosis
VII	Tarui's disease	Phosphofructokinase	Skeletal muscle, erythrocytes	• Muscle cramps • Elevated blood lactate • Hemolysis

3. Write a short note on Cori cycle. (MGR)

Answer

Introduction

Gluconeogenesis from lactate – Cori cycle

Cori Cycle

- The cycle of lactate produced in the muscles being transported to the liver, converted back to glucose, and released back to the muscles is known as the Cori cycle.
  - Lactate in muscle cannot be converted to glucose due to the absence of enzymes glucose-6-phosphatase and fructose 1,6 bisphosphatase.
- The accumulation of lactate in the muscle cells can lead to a decrease in pH, contributing to muscle fatigue. To prevent this, lactate produced in the muscles is transported to the liver via the bloodstream.
  - Lactate is converted to pyruvate in liver, which is converted to glucose by gluconeogenesis.
- Glucose is subsequently released into the bloodstream and can be transported back to the muscles to serve as an energy source.
- The Cori cycle plays an essential role in maintaining blood glucose levels during periods of high energy demand, such as intense exercise.

Significance of Cori Cycle

Regenerates NADH so that glycolysis can occur continuously in skeletal muscles.

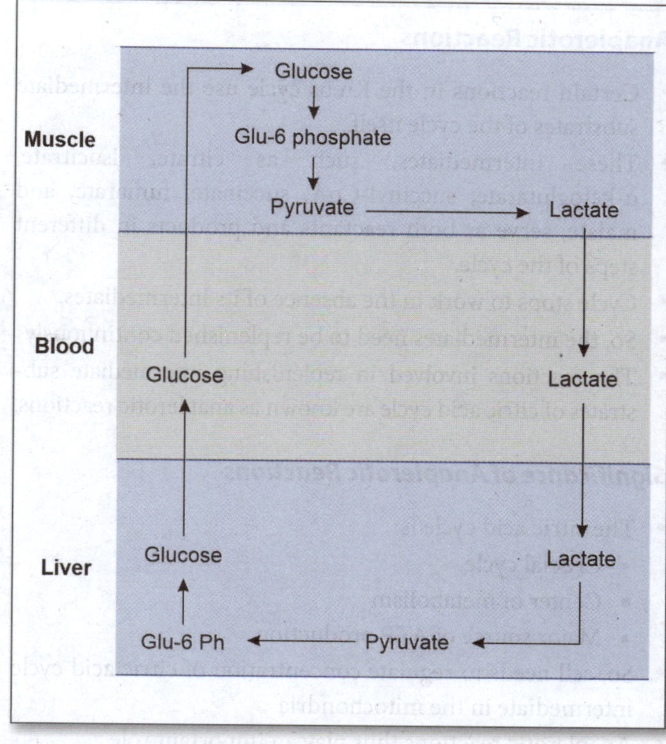

4. Differentiate between amylose and amylopectin. (DU)

Answer

Differences between Amylose and Amylopectin

	Amylose	Amylopectin
Structure	Straight chain polymer of D-glucose units	Branched chain polymer of D glucose units
Linkage	Linked by alpha 1,4 glycosidic bonds	Linked by alpha 1,4 and alpha 1,6 glycosidic bonds
% component	Constitutes about 20% of starch	Constitutes about 80% of starch
Water solubility	Soluble	Insoluble
Reaction with iodine	Stains blue black	Stains reddish brown
Hydrolysis	Hydrolyzed by enzymes such as alpha and beta amylase	Hydrolyzed by alpha and beta amylases, but alpha 1, 6 glycosidic linkages cannot be hydrolyzed.
Reaction with hot water	Doesn't form a gel	Forms a gel

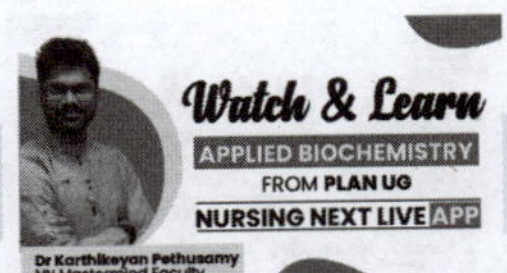

5. What are anaplerotic reactions? What are the three fates of pyruvate? (DU)

Answer

Anaplerotic Reactions

- Certain reactions in the Krebs cycle use the intermediate substrates of the cycle itself.
- These intermediates, such as citrate, isocitrate, α-ketoglutarate, succinyl-CoA, succinate, fumarate, and malate, serve as both reactants and products in different steps of the cycle.
- Cycle stops to work in the absence of its intermediates.
- So, the intermediates need to be replenished continuously
- The reactions involved in replenishing intermediate substrates of citric acid cycle are known as anaplerotic reactions.

Significance of Anaplerotic Reactions

- The citric acid cycle is:
  - Crucial cycle
  - Center of metabolism
  - Major source of ATP production
- So, cell needs to regulate concentration of citric acid cycle intermediate in the mitochondria
- Anaplerotic reactions thus play an important role
- Anaplerotic flux balances cataplerotic flux in order to retain homeostasis of cellular metabolism.

Metabolic Fate of Pyruvate

The metabolic fate of pyruvate depends on a number of factors, including the availability of oxygen, the energy needs of the cell, and the presence of other metabolic intermediates. Three fates of Pyruvate include:

1. **Acetyl-CoA production:**
   - This is the most common fate of pyruvate in aerobic conditions.
   - Pyruvate is converted to acetyl-CoA by the enzyme pyruvate dehydrogenase complex (PDC).
   - Acetyl-CoA is then used in the Krebs cycle to generate ATP and NADH.
2. **Lactate production:**
   - This occurs in anaerobic conditions, when there is not enough oxygen available for pyruvate to be converted to acetyl-CoA.
   - Pyruvate is converted to lactate by the enzyme lactate dehydrogenase. Lactate can be used by the liver to produce glucose in a process called gluconeogenesis.
3. **Ethanol fermentation:**
   - Occurs in yeast
   - Pyruvate is converted to acetaldehyde by enzyme pyruvate decarboxylase, which gets reduced to ethanol by NADH in the presence of enzyme alcohol dehydrogenase.
   - This regenerates NAD^+.

6. Differentiate between starch and glycogen. (KUHS)

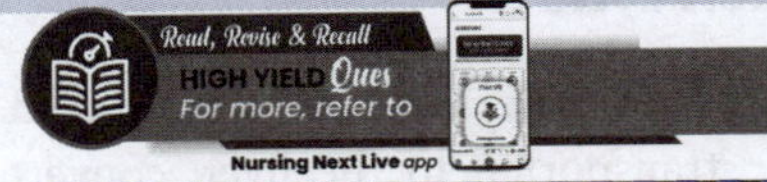

Answer

Differences between Starch and Glycogen

Starch	Glycogen
Plant reserve food. It is mostly stored in the form of seeds/grains.	Glycogen is animal reserve food. It is mainly stored in the liver and muscle.
Less branched. Branching occurs after 20–30 glucose units	Highly branched. Branching occurs after nearly 10–12 glucose units.
Consists of amylose and amylopectin	No such structures are present
It is sparingly soluble in cold water and forms a paste in hot water	Soluble in water. It forms an opalescent solution in water
It gives violet color with iodine	It gives brown to red color with iodine.

7. Write a note on polysaccharides.

Answer

Introduction

- Contains many carbohydrate units linked by glycosidic bonds.
- Examples: Glycogen, cellulose
- Polysaccharides are of two types:
  1. Homopolysaccharides: Formed by the same kind of monosaccharides linked by glycosidic bonds. Examples are glycogen, starch, cellulose
  2. Heteropolysaccharides: Formed by two or more types of monosaccharides joined together by glycosidic linkages.

Homopolysaccharides

- *Starch*
  - Carbohydrate reserve of plants
  - Dietary component of higher animals including man
  - Homopolysaccharides of D-glucose units held together by α-glycosidic bonds.
  - Consists of two polysaccharide components

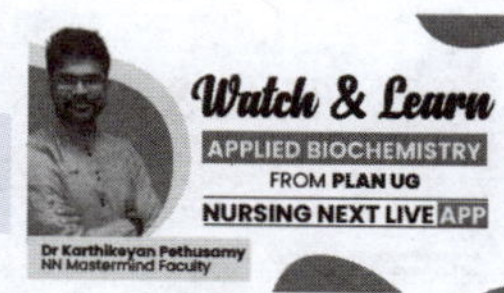

- Amylose
  - Water soluble
  - Unbranched chain of D glucose units held by α (1,4)-glycosidic bonds
- Amylopectin
  - Water insoluble
  - Branched with α (1-6)-glycosidic bonds at branching points.
- Hydrolyzed by amylase to liberate dextrins, and finally maltose and glucose.

- *Inulin*
  - Polymer of fructose
  - Water soluble
  - Present in dahlia bulbs, onion, garlic
  - Used for measurement of glomerular filtration rate.
- *Glycogen*
  - Carbohydrate reserve in animals
  - Also known as Animal starch
  - Highly concentrated in liver and muscles
  - Structurally similar to amylopectin with more branching
- *Cellulose*
  - Present exclusively in plants
  - Composed of β-D glucose units linked by β-(1-4) glycosidic bonds
  - Hydrolysis yield cellobiose followed by β-D-glucose
  - Cannot be digested by humans
  - Major constituent of fiber – nondigestible carbohydrate
  - Functions:
    - Decreasing absorption of glucose and cholesterol from intestine
    - Increasing bulk of feces.

Heteropolysaccharides

- Heteropolysaccharides – when polysaccharides are composed of different types of sugars and their derivatives.
- These include:
  - Mucopolysachharides
  - Glycoproteins
  - Agar
  - Blood group substances
  - Pectins

8. Write a short note on oxidative phosphorylation. (MGR)

Answer

Introduction

- It is the process of synthesizing ATP from ADP and inorganic phosphate coupled with the electron transport chain.
- ATP generation during the transport of electrons through the electron transport chain
- Site - complex V of the inner mitochondrial membrane
- Inhibitors of oxidative phosphorylation
  - Uncouplers: Substances altering the permeability of inner mitochondrial membrane
  - Ionophores: Lipophilic substances that promote the transport of ions across biological membranes

Theories Proposed for Oxidative Phosphorylation

- Chemiosmotic theory
- Boyer's binding change mechanism
- Chemical coupling hypothesis

Chemiosmotic Theory

- Most widely accepted theory of electron transport chain
- Proposed by Peter Mitchell
- Explains the mechanism of ATP production by the transport of electrons in the respiratory chain
- According to this theory, ATP synthesis in the respiratory chain is linked to the H^+ electrochemical gradient

Boyer's Binding Change Mechanism

- Binding change mechanism proposed originally by Paul Boyer and it is the most widely accepted mechanism of ATP synthesis
- According to this theory, conformational changes in the protein play a crucial role in the binding change mechanism. The energy from the proton gradient doesn't directly drive ATP synthesis. Instead, the energy is utilized to release tightly bound ATP from the enzyme's active site.

Chemical Coupling Hypothesis

- This theory suggests that during the oxidation of a component in the electron transport chain, the released energy is captured by forming a bond (~) with a molecule outside the chain.
- Examples of this theory include the oxidation of glyceraldehyde-3-P to 3-phosphoglycerate and the oxidation of succinyl CoA to succinate, where ATP is generated through the transfer of phosphate or the formation of a reactive intermediate, respectively.

9. Write about significance of HMP shunt. (MGR)

Answer

Introduction

- Alternative Glucose oxidation pathway.

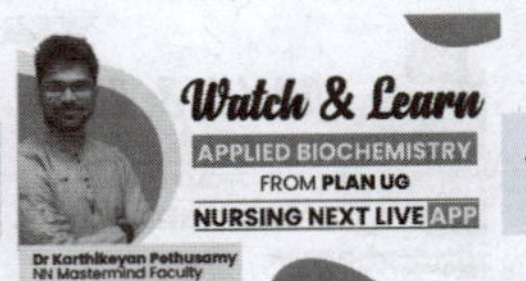

- Results in production of NADPH from NADP.
- **HMP pathway is also known as**
  - Hexose monophosphate shunt
  - Pentose phosphate pathway

Importance of HMP Shunt

- HMP pathway – major source of NADPH in body
  - Required for the biosynthesis of fatty acids, steroids and amino acids
  - Cytochrome P450 is NADPH dependent. Cyt P450 is responsible for the detoxification of various drugs
  - NADPH oxidase plays a crucial role in host defense by neutrophils and macrophages.
  - **Role in RBCs**
    - Regulates the concentration of glutathione
    - Prevents the integrity of RBC membrane
    - Maintains the ferrous of hemoglobin in ferrous state, preventing the formation of methemoglobin in RBC
- **Provides Ribose-5-Phosphate:**
  - Required for Purine biosynthesis.
  - The enzyme Glucose-6-Phosphate dehydrogenase in HMP shunt optimizes the concentration of Ribose-5-Phosphate.
- **Producing Glycolytic Intermediate:**
  - Glycolytic intermediates- Glyceraldehyde-3-Phosphate and Fructose-6-Phosphate are produced during HMP pathway.

10. Why is sucrose a nonreducing sugar? (MGR)

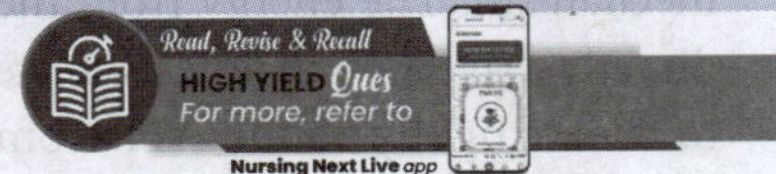

Answer

Sucrose

- Sucrose is a saccharide which is made up of glucose and fructose molecules.

Nonreducing Sugar

- Reducing sugars have a free aldehyde group. Reducing sugars are capable of reducing other substances by donating electrons, which leads to the oxidation of the sugar itself. Examples of reducing sugars include glucose, fructose, and lactose.
- Nonreducing sugars are the sugars that don't have a free ketone or aldehyde group.
- Instead of hemiacetal, these sugars have acetal that consists of two O-R groups, one –R and –H group all attached to the same carbon atom.
- Sucrose consists of one molecule each of α-D glucopyranose and β-D fructofuranose which are linked by β-1,2-glycosidic linkage.
- Since the carbonyl groups of both the monosaccharides, i.e., carbon-1 of glucose and carbon-2 of fructose participate in the formation of the glycosidic bond and that as such there is no free carbonyl carbon on any of its monosaccharides, hence, sucrose is nonreducing sugar.
- Anomeric carbons of both the monosaccharides are involved in glycoside or acetal formation. So, it does not have a free -CHO group.

11. Write a note on anomers. (MGR)

Answer

Anomers

- When a monosaccharide cyclizes, its carbonyl carbon atom, called the anomeric carbon also becomes asymmetric and exhibits two configurations, which are referred to as the alpha form and beta form.
- Such stereoisomers that differ in configuration at the anomeric carbon, i.e., at carbon 1 in an aldose or carbon 2 in a ketose are called anomers. Both the anomers have different physical and chemical properties, including optical rotation.

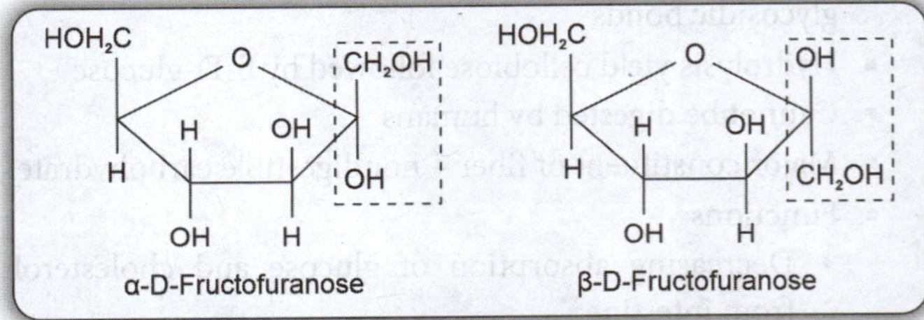

Figure 1.3: α and β anomers of fructose.

Anomerization

- Process of conversion of one anomer to the other.
- In case of reducing sugars, it is referred to as mutarotation.
- This process occurs readily and leads to an anomeric mixture in which the alpha and beta anomers are in equilibrium.
- The ratio of two anomers is specific for the specific sugar.
- Two anomers of glucose are freely interconvertible in an aqueous solution. At equilibrium, D glucose is a mixture of beta-anomer and alpha-anomer which are found in a ratio of approximately 2:1.
- Example:
  - A solution containing D-glucose will gradually move toward a mixture of approximately 64% beta-D glucopyranoside and 36% of alpha-D-glucopyranose.
  - As the ratio changes, the optical rotation of the mixture changes and this is known as mutarotation.

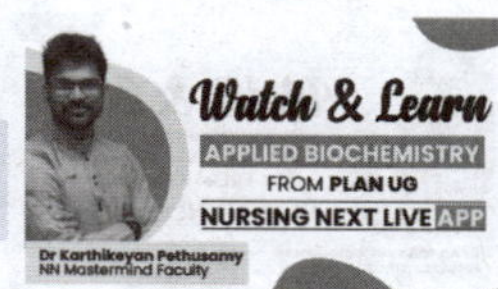

Physical Properties

- Anomers differ in structure, so have different stabilizing and destabilizing effects.
- Usually beta anomer of D-glucopyranoside is more stable in water.
- These differ in polarity and specific rotation.

12. Write in short about Inhibitors of electron transport chain. (DU)

Answer

Inhibitors of ETC

- The inhibitors of electron transport chain bind to one or more components of ETC and block the transport of electrons.
- Lead to accumulation of reduced components before the inhibitor blockade step and oxidized components after that step.
- ATP synthesis is dependent on ETC.
- Hence all inhibitors of ETC also inhibit ATP synthesis.

Three Possible Sites of Action for ETC Inhibition

1. **NADH and coenzyme Q**
   - Inhibited by:
     - Fish poison – rotenone
     - Barbiturate drug – amytal
     - Antibiotic – piercidin A
2. **Between cytochrome b and c1**
   - Inhibited by:
     - Antibiotic – antimycin A
     - British anti-Lewisite (BAL)
3. **Inhibitors of cytochrome oxidase**
   - Inhibited by:
     - Carbon monoxide
     - Cyanide
     - Hydrogen sulphide
     - Azide

13. Write about functions of glycogen in the body. (KUHS)

Answer

Introduction

- Glycogen – highly branched polymer and storage form of glucose.
- Mainly found in muscles and liver
- Involved in the maintenance of blood glucose homeostasis.
- Exists as granules in the cytosol.
- Glycogenesis – synthesis of glycogen from glucose.
- Glycogenolysis – breakdown of glycogen.

Functions of Glycogen in the Body

- Liver cells
  - Make up 6 – 10% of the liver weight
  - Glycogen is synthesized in the presence of high glucose levels and sufficient insulin levels.
  - Insulin activates the enzyme glycogen synthase that promotes glycogenesis
  - When the blood glucose levels decline, glycogen breaks down to glucose to maintain the blood glucose levels.
  - Act as energy reservoir.
- Muscle cells
  - Account for 1 – 2% of the muscle weight
  - Muscle glycogen does not compensate for the decreased blood glucose levels in contrast to the liver glycogen.
  - This is due to the absence of the enzyme glucose 6-phosphatase in the muscles.
  - Thus muscle glycogen is only available for energy generation during muscle contraction.
- Other tissues
  - Glycogen is present in smaller amounts in red and white blood cells, kidney cells and glial cells.
  - Also provides for the energy needs of the embryo in the uterus
- Other organisms
  - Glycogen also provides for energy storage form in lower organisms such as fungi and bacteria.

14. Write a short note on lactose intolerance. (KUHS)

Answer

Introduction

- Lactose is a common dairy sugar.
- Lactose intolerance is a common condition characterized by a decreased ability to digest lactose.
- This occurs due to lack of enzyme lactase in the small intestines, that breaks lactose to glucose and galactose.

Pathophysiology

- Lactose, a disaccharide molecule, is commonly found in milk and dairy products.
- It cannot be absorbed directly into the body, so in the absence of lactase, it is passed on unabsorbed.
- Bacteria in the colon metabolize lactose, and the resulting fermentation produces copious amounts of gas, that causes the various abdominal symptoms.

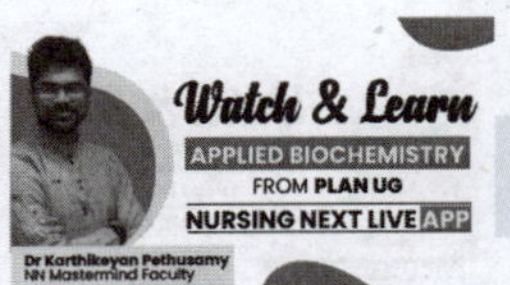

Clinical Manifestations

- Patients present with:
  - Abdominal pain
  - Bloating
  - Diarrhea
  - Flatulence
  - Nausea

Types of Lactose Intolerance

- Primary
  - Occurs as amount of enzyme lactase declines with age
- Secondary
  - Occurs due to injury to the small intestines
- Developmental
  - Usually occurs in premature babies
  - May improve with age
- Congenital
  - Rare genetic disorder
    - Primary hypolactasia

Diagnosis

- Differential diagnosis includes:
  - Irritable bowel syndrome
  - Celiac disease
  - Inflammatory bowel disease
- Definite diagnosis can be made by:
  - Hydrogen breath test
  - Stool acidity test

15. Differentiate between diabetic ketoacidosis and starvation ketoacidosis. (KUHS)

Answer

Differences between Diabetic ketoacidosis and Starvation ketoacidosis

	Diabetic ketoacidosis	Starvation ketoacidosis
Definition	Ketoacidosis that occurs due to lack of insulin	Ketoacidosis that occurs due to prolonged fasting
Causes	• Uncontrolled diabetes • Compliance with insulin therapy • Physical or emotional trauma • Pregnancy • Certain medications	• Eating disorders • Reduced intake due to socioeconomic reasons • Issues with swallowing or absorption
Clinical Manifestation	• Polydipsia, polyphagia, polyuria • Shortness of breath • Fruity scented breath • Increased blood glucose levels • Increased blood ketone bodies	• Lower body mass • Lower muscle mass • Hypotension • Hypothermia • Dry skin • Dehydration • Kussmaul breathing
Diagnosis	• Blood glucose levels • Blood insulin levels • Blood ketone bodies • Urine analysis • ECG	• Physical examination • Blood tests • Urine analysis
Management	• Fluid and electrolyte replacement • Insulin therapy	• Fluid and electrolyte replacement • Dextrose

16. Biochemical derangements in Diabetes mellitus. (KUHS)

Answer

Metabolic Changes in Diabetes

- **Hyperglycemia:** Elevation of blood glucose level.
- **Glycosuria:** When the glucose is excreted into urine.
- **Ketoacidosis:** Increased mobilization of fatty acids results in overproduction of ketone bodies.
- **Hypertriglyceridemia:** Conversion of fatty acids to triacylglycerols and the secretion of VLDL and chylomicrons are comparatively higher and activity of the enzyme

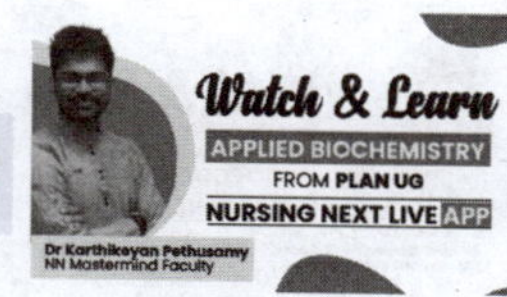

lipoprotein lipase is low. Consequently, the plasma levels of VLDL, chylomicrons and triacylglycerols are increased.

- **Hypercholesterolemia:** An increase in level of cholesterol is also frequently seen in diabetics.

Acute Complications of Type I and II Diabetes

- **Diabetic ketoacidosis**
  - Acute and dangerous complication
  - Low insulin levels cause the liver to turn fatty acid to ketone for fuel (i.e., ketosis)
  - Elevated levels of ketone bodies in the blood decrease the blood's pH, leading to DKA.
  - More common in type I diabetes than type II.
- **Hyperglycemia hyperosmolar state**
  - With blood glucose levels above 300 mg/dL (16 mmol/L), water is osmotically drawn out of cells into the blood
  - This results in loss of water and an increase in blood osmolarity.
  - More common in type II diabetes than type I.
- **Hypoglycemia**
  - Abnormally low blood glucose
  - Acute complication of diabetes treatment.
- **Diabetic coma**
  - Severe diabetic hypoglycemia
  - Diabetic ketoacidosis
  - Hyperosmolar nonketotic coma

17. Write a short note on Van den Bergh test. (KUHS)

Answer

Introduction

- Specific test for identification of increased serum bilirubin levels
- Normal serum gives a negative Van den Bergh reaction

Mechanism of Reaction

- Van den Bergh reagent – mixture of equal volume of sulfanilic acid and sodium nitrite
- ***Principle*** – diazotized sulfanilic acid reacts with bilirubin to form a purple colored azobilirubin
- *Direct and indirect reactions*
  - Bilirubin is insoluble in water
  - Conjugated bilirubin is soluble
  - Van den Bergh reagent reacts with conjugated bilirubin and gives a purple color within 30 seconds – *Direct positive test*
  - Addition of methanol dissolves the unconjugated bilirubin and gives Van den Bergh reaction positive within 30 minutes – *Indirect positive*

Significance

- *Van den Bergh Reaction and Jaundice*
  - Indirect positive – Hemolytic jaundice
  - Direct positive – Obstructive jaundice
  - Biphasic – Hepatic jaundice

18. Write a short note on glycosuria. (MGR)

Answer

Glycosuria

- Defined as the presence of reducing sugars in urine
- Monosaccharides seen in urine are:
  - Glucose
  - Lactose
  - Fructose
- Glucosuria – presence of glucose in the urine
- This happens when the glomerular filtrate contains more glucose than the proximal convoluting tubules can reabsorb.
- The term glucosuria is used when the glucose levels in urine exceed 25 mg/dL.

Conditions Associated with Glycosuria

- Elevated plasma glucose levels as seen in diabetes mellitus
- Impairment with the reabsorption by the PCT as seen in
  - Fanconi syndrome
  - Familial renal glucosuria

Pathophysiology

↑ Plasma glucose

↓

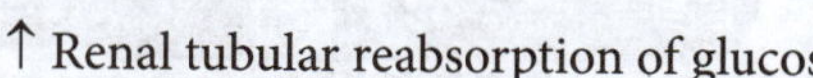

↑ Renal tubular reabsorption of glucose

- Renal threshold for glucose
  - Capacity of proximal tubule to reabsorb glucose to prevent its excretion in urine.
- Membrane proteins present in the PCT responsible for reabsorption of glucose from the glomerular filtrate are the
  - SGLT 1 and 2
  - GLUT 2
- Defects in these transporters can also lead to the presence of glucose in urine.

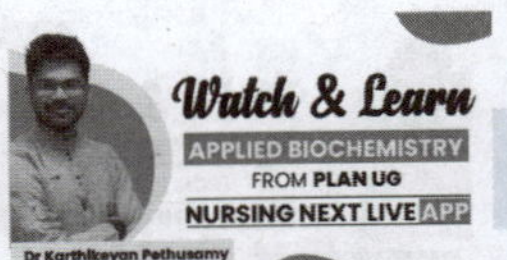

19. Write about Benedict's test.

Answer

Introduction

- Test for simple carbohydrates
- Identifies reducing sugars – monosaccharides and some disaccharides – which have free ketone or aldehyde functional groups
- Used to test the presence of glucose in urine

Composition of Benedict's Solution

- Anhydrous sodium carbonate
- Sodium citrate
- Copper sulfate pentahydrate

Principle

- When benedict's solution and simple carbohydrates are heated, the cupric ions (copper II) are reduced to cuprous ions (Copper I), which form a brick-red precipitate.
- Copper (I) oxide is red in color, insoluble in water and precipitates.
- As the reducing sugar increases, the darker the red.

Results

If color changes to

- Blue/no change – no sugar
- Green – 0.1–0.5% sugar
- Yellow – 0.5–1% sugar
- Orange – 1–1.5% sugar
- Red – 1.5–2.0% sugar
- Brick red - >2% sugar

20. Write a short note on Glucose Tolerance Test. (MGR, KUHS)

Answer

Glucose Tolerance Test (GTT)

Administration of glucose to determine how quickly glucose is absorbed and cleared from the blood and homeostasis is achieved.

Indications

- To establish presence of diabetes in patients who show normal fasting and postprandial blood sugar levels.
- To establish gestational diabetes
- To investigate glycosuria
- Diagnostic evaluation in obese person.

Preparation

- Preferably have a carbohydrate rich diet for atleast 3 days prior to test.
- Overnight fasting on the day of test.
- Discontinuation of any medication that may interfere with test results.
- Avoid smoking/alcohol prior to test
- Avoid strenuous exercise prior to test

Procedure

- Preferably done in early hours.
- Fasting sample is taken.
- 75 g glucose in 300 mL of water is given orally
- Blood samples taken every 30 minutes for 2 hours.
- Urine samples are also collected simultaneously.
- Each blood sample is analyzed and a graph is plotted.

Interpretation

	Fasting	2 hour	Implications
No diabetes	≤6.0	<7.8	No excess micro- nor macro-vascular risk
Prediabetes	6.1–6.9	7.8–11.0	Excess macro- but not micro-vascular risk
Diabetes	≥7.0	≥11.1	Excess macro- and micro-vascular risk

21. Differentiate between hypoglycemia and hyperglycemia. (KUHS)

Answer

Table 1.1: Differences between Hypoglycemia and Hyperglycemia

	Hypoglycemia	Hyperglycemia
Definition	Deficiency of glucose in blood	Excessive glucose in the blood
Range	Blood glucose level <70 mg/dL	Blood glucose level > 130 mg/dL
Causes	• Reduced dietary intake • Excessive use of insulin/oral hypoglycemic drugs • Excessive exercise	• Increased/excessive intake of dietary sugars • Missed insulin/oral drugs • Infections
Complication	Most common complication is neuroglycopenia which leads to neurological damage.	Most common complication is hyperosmolar hyperglycemic non ketotic syndrome

Contd...

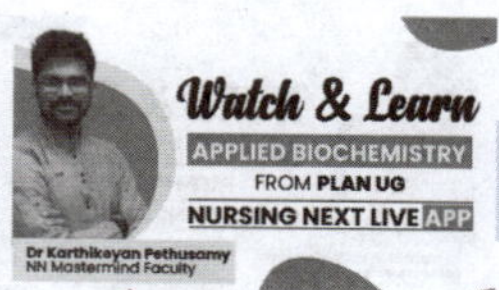

	Hypoglycemia	Hyperglycemia
Clinical Presentation	• Pale, clammy skin • Rapid pulse • Hypertension • Normal or shallow breathing • Irritable, confused behavior • Dizziness • Loss of consciousness	• Hot flushed dry skin • Weak rapid pulse • Hypotension • Labored breathing • Nausea and vomiting • Polydipsia, polyphagia and polyuria • Restlessness • Unconsciousness

SHORT ANSWER QUESTIONS

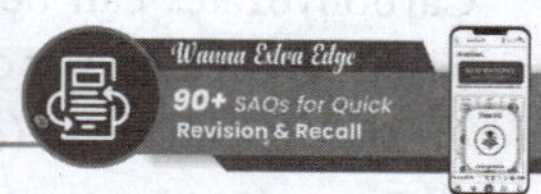

1. Examples for monosaccharide. (MGR)

Answer

Glucose, fructose, galactose, ribose, deoxyribose and mannose are few examples of monosaccharide.

2. What are hetero-polysaccharides? Give example. (MGR)

Answer

Hetero-polysaccharides are complex carbohydrates made up of repeating units of two or more different types of monosaccharides.

For example: 1. Heparin (glucosamine and uronic acid). 2. Chondroitin sulfate (N-acetylgalactosamine and glucuronic acid).

3. Significance of HMP shunt. (MGR)

Answer

Significance of HMP shunt is

- HMP pathway – major source of NADPH in body
- *Provides Ribose-5-Phosphate* required for purine biosynthesis.
- Glycolytic intermediates such as Glyceraldehyde-3-Phosphate and Fructose-6-Phosphate are produced during HMP pathway.

4. Define glycolysis. (MGR)

Answer

- Glucose is broken down into two pyruvate molecules during the metabolic process known as glycolysis, which takes place in the cytoplasm of cells. Also known as Embden- Meyerhof- Parnas (EMP) pathway.

5. Examples for disaccharides. (MGR)

Answer

Some examples of disaccharides are:

- Sucrose (composed of Glucose and Fructose)
- Lactose (composed of Glucose and Galactose)
- Maltose (composed of Glucose and Glucose)

6. Sucrose is nonreducing sugar, why? (MGR)

Answer

- Sucrose is a nonreducing sugar because it does not have a free aldehyde or ketone group that can be oxidized. When a reducing sugar, such as glucose or fructose, is mixed with Benedict's reagent and heated, it reduces the copper ions in the reagent to form a red precipitate of copper oxide.
- Sucrose is formed by a condensation reaction between glucose and fructose, resulting in the formation of a glycosidic bond between the two monosaccharides. This bond blocks the free aldehyde or ketone group on both glucose and fructose, making sucrose a nonreducing sugar.

7. Oxidative phosphorylation. (MGR)

Answer

It is a metabolic process that takes place in the mitochondria of eukaryotic cells and produces ATP by oxidizing NADH and FADH2 molecules.

8. What are homopolysaccharides? Give example. (MGR)

Answer

Homopolysaccharides are polysaccharides composed of a single type of monosaccharide subunit. Examples are Cellulose and starch.

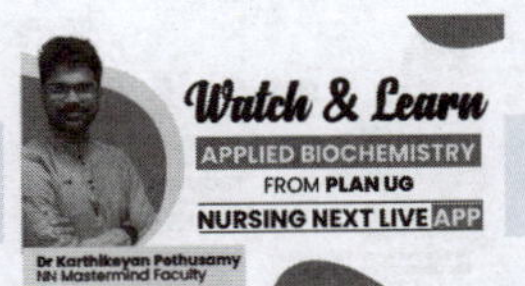

9. Name two reducing disaccharides. (MGR)

Answer

Maltose and lactose are two reducing disaccharides.
- Maltose (composed of Glucose and Glucose)
- Lactose (composed of Glucose and Galactose)

10. Name the two conditions in which blood sugar level is raised. (MGR)

Answer

- Diabetes mellitus: A chronic metabolic disorder characterized by high levels of glucose in the blood, which is caused by a lack of insulin or the body's inability to use insulin effectively.
- Hyperglycemia: A condition characterized by abnormally high levels of glucose in the blood. It can be caused by a variety of factors, including diabetes.

11. Gluconeogenesis. (KUHS)

Answer

A metabolic mechanism called gluconeogenesis produces glucose largely in the liver and kidneys from non-carbohydrate precursors like amino acids, lactate, and glycerol.

12. Epimerism. (KUHS)

Answer

Stereoisomerism known as epimerism occurs when two molecules only differ in the location of one chiral center.

13. Galactosemia. (KUHS)

Answer

Galactosemia is a rare genetic condition in which Galactose, a sugar present in milk and other dairy products, cannot be metabolized properly by the body.

14. Hyperglycemia. (KUHS)

Answer

Hyperglycemia is a medical condition characterized by high levels of glucose (sugar) in the blood. More specifically, Hyperglycemia is blood glucose greater than 125 mg/dL while fasting and greater than 180 mg/dL 2 hours postprandial.

15. Carbohydrates. (KUHS)

Answer

- A macronutrient known as carbohydrates which gives the body energy, can be found in a variety of foods, such as grains, fruits, vegetables, and dairy products. They are organic molecules made up of carbon, hydrogen, and oxygen atoms. Carbohydrates provide approximately 4 calories of energy per gram.
- Carbohydrates can be divided into three main categories based on the number of sugar units they contain:
  1. Monosaccharides (one sugar unit), e.g., Glucose
  2. Disaccharides (two sugar units), e.g., Sucrose
  3. Polysaccharides (many sugar units), e.g., Starch

16. Mini GTT. (KUHS)

Answer

Mini glucose tolerance test is a diagnostic test for gestational diabetes, a form of the disease that develops during pregnancy. It is a simplified version of the standard glucose tolerance test, which is used to assess how well the body is able to regulate blood sugar levels. The test involves consuming a high-carbohydrate drink and measuring blood sugar levels at specific intervals.

17. Lactose intolerance. (KUHS)

Answer

A digestive illness known as lactose intolerance is characterized by an inability to completely digest lactose, a sugar present in milk and other dairy products.

18. Diabetes mellitus. (KUHS)

Answer

It is a chronic metabolic disorder characterized by high levels of glucose (sugar) in the blood due to lack or ineffective use of insulin.

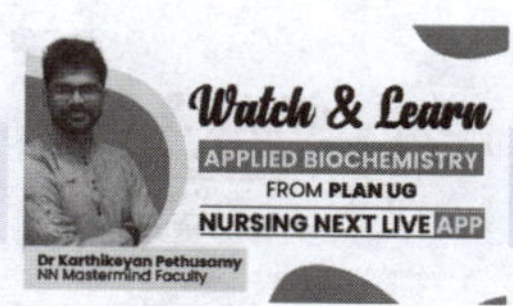

19. Functions of glycogen in the body. (KUHS)

Answer

A complex carbohydrate called glycogen is stored in the muscles and liver of both humans and animals. It provides the body with an easily accessible source of energy.

20. GTT. (MGR)

Answer

GTT stands for Glucose Tolerance Test, which is a medical test used to diagnose diabetes or other disorders related to glucose metabolism. The GTT involves fasting for a period of time (overnight), drinking a glucose solution, and having blood samples taken at regular intervals over several hours to evaluate how the body processes glucose.

21. Name the ketone bodies. (MGR)

Answer

The three ketone bodies are:
- Acetoacetate
- β-hydroxybutyrate
- Acetone

CONCEPTUAL REVISION

MULTIPLE CHOICE QUESTIONS

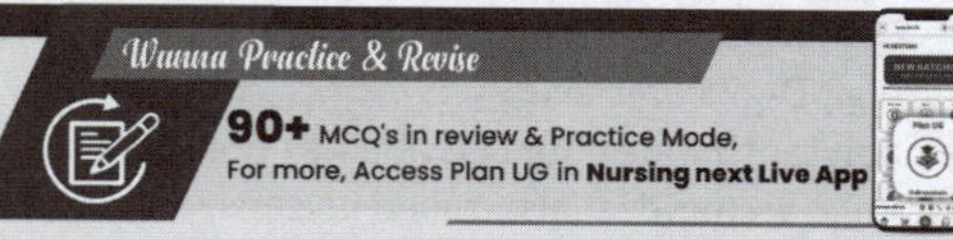

1. Which of the following is an aldose sugar?
a. Fructose b. Erythrulose
c. Glucose d. None

Ans. c. Glucose

2. A 30-year-old presents with intractable vomiting and inability to eat or drink for the past 3 days. His blood glucose level is normal. Which of the following is the most important source of blood glucose?
a. Liver b. Heat
c. Skeletal muscle d. Lysosome

Ans. a. Liver

3. Aldose sugar is converted to ketose sugar by:
a. Oxidoreductase b. Aldose
c. Decarboxylase d. Isomerase

Ans. d. Isomerase

4. Which one of the following metabolites is used by all cells for glycolysis, glycogen synthesis and the hexose monophosphate shunt pathway?
a. Glucose-1-phosphate
b. Fructose-6-phosphate
c. Glucose-6-phosphate
d. Phosphoenolpyruvate

Ans. c. Glucose-6-phosphate

5. Anaerobic glycolysis occurs in all places, except:
a. Muscles b. RBCs
c. Brain d. Kidney

Ans. c. Brain

6. The end product of one stage fermentation is:
a. Formic acid b. Pyruvate
c. Lactate d. Ethanol

Ans. c. Lactate

7. Pyruvate can be converted directly into all the following, except:
a. Phosphoenol pyruvate b. Acetyl CoA
c. Alanine d. Lactate

Ans. a. Phosphoenol pyruvate

8. Normal Fasting Blood sugar value:
a. < 60 mg/dL b. 80 to 140 mg/dL
c. < 140 mg/dL d. 70 to 110 mg/dL

Ans. d. 70 to 110 mg/dL

9. The client is taking rosiglitazone for control of his diabetes. Which laboratory result should be reported to the physician?
a. Blood glucose level of 110 mg/dL
b. Blood urea nitrogen level of 10 mg/dL
c. Creatinine level of 3.0 mg/dL
d. White blood cell count of 8,000

Ans. c. Creatinine level of 3.0 mg/dL

10. Fluoride, used in the collection of blood samples for glucose estimation, inhibits the enzyme:
a. Glucokinase b. Hexokinase
c. Enolase d. Glucose-6-phosphatase

Ans. c. Enolase

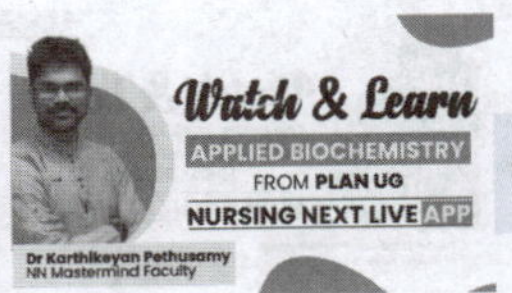

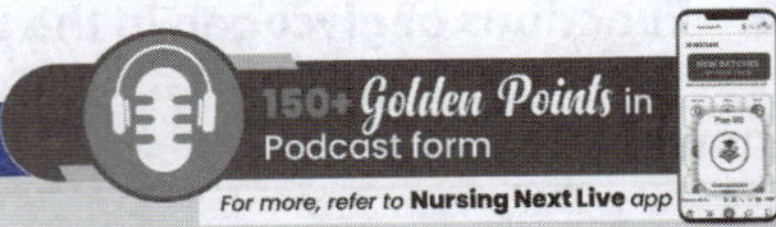

Golden Points

- Biochemistry is the study of chemical processes within the living organism.
- Biologically important disaccharides are maltose, lactose and sucrose.
- Carbohydrates may be classified into monosaccharides, disaccharides, oligosaccharides or polysaccharides depending on the number of the monomer units.
- Common homosaccharides of biological significance are starch, glycogen and cellulose and inulin.
- Derived sugars are derivatives of monosaccharides such as acids, alcohols, amino acid derivatives.
- Disaccharides consist of two similar or dissimilar monosaccharides linked together by a glycosidic bond.
- Heteropolysaccharides contain repeating disaccharide units, which bear negatively charged groups.
- Homopolysaccharides are polymers of the identical monosaccharide units.
- Lactose is a reducing disaccharide, made up of beta –D-glucose and beta-D galactose. It is also known as milk sugar, as it is found in milk.
- Maltose consists of two alpha-D-glucose units linked together by alpha 1,4-glycosidic linkage. It is hydrolyzed by the enzyme maltase in the intestinal lumen.
- Monosaccharides are divided according to the chemical nature of their carbonyl group into aldoses and ketoses.
- Most important glycosaminoglycans are hyaluronic acid, chondroitin sulfates, heparin, etc.
- Oligosachharides consist of more than two (usually 3 to 10) monosaccharide units by O glycosidic bonds, e.g., maltotriose, raffinose.
- Oxidation of carbon 1 of an aldose converts its aldehyde group to its carboxyl group and forms an acid which is called aldonic acid, e.g., D-gluconic acid.
- Polysaccharides are classified as homopolysaccharides and heterosaccharides.
- Polysaccharides, also called glycans, are polymers of a large number (more than 10) monosaccharides linked by glycosidic bonds.
- Sucrose consists of alpha –D glucose and beta-D Fructose. It is a non reducing sugar due to the absence of a free carbonyl carbon.
- Sucrose is also as invert sugar, table sugar and cane sugar.

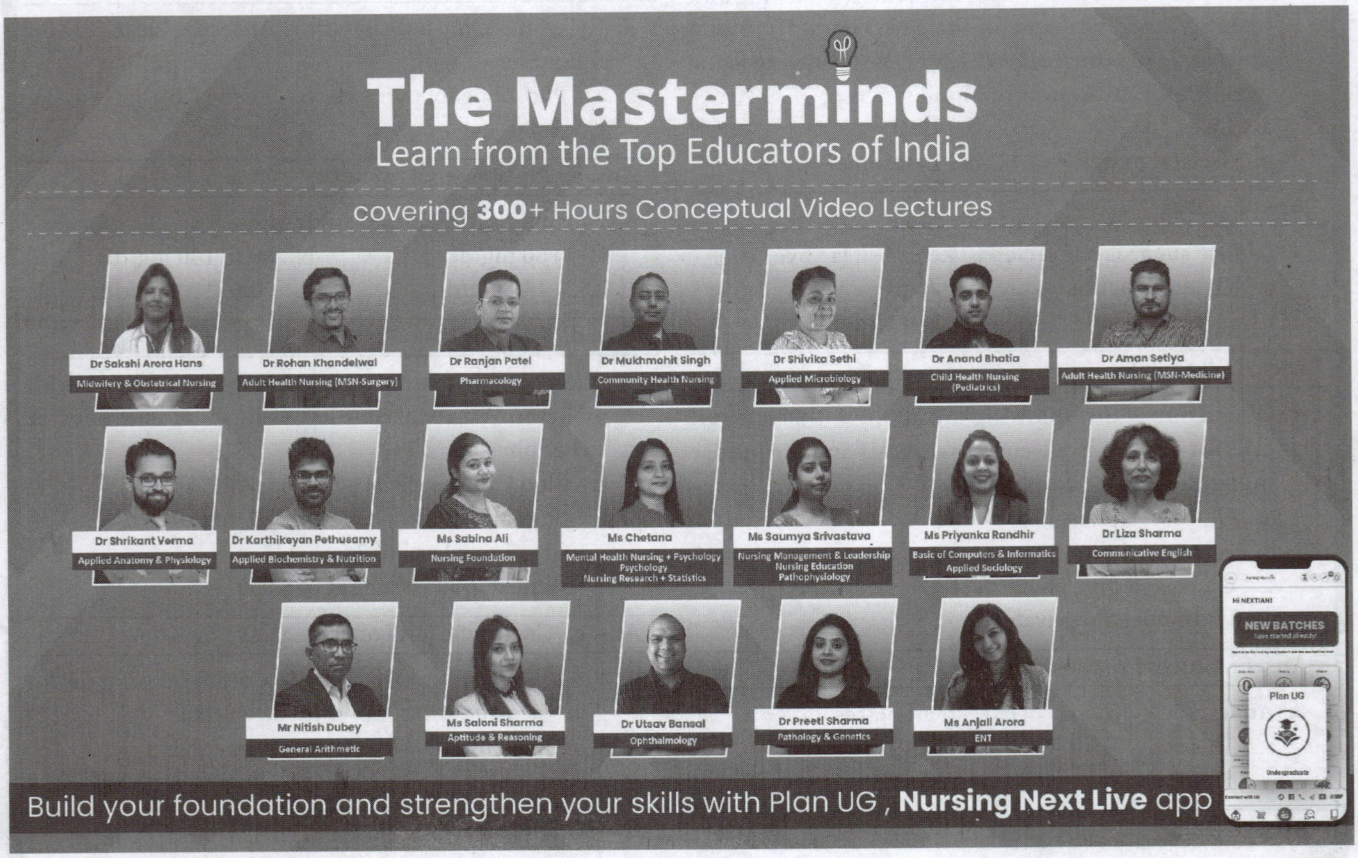

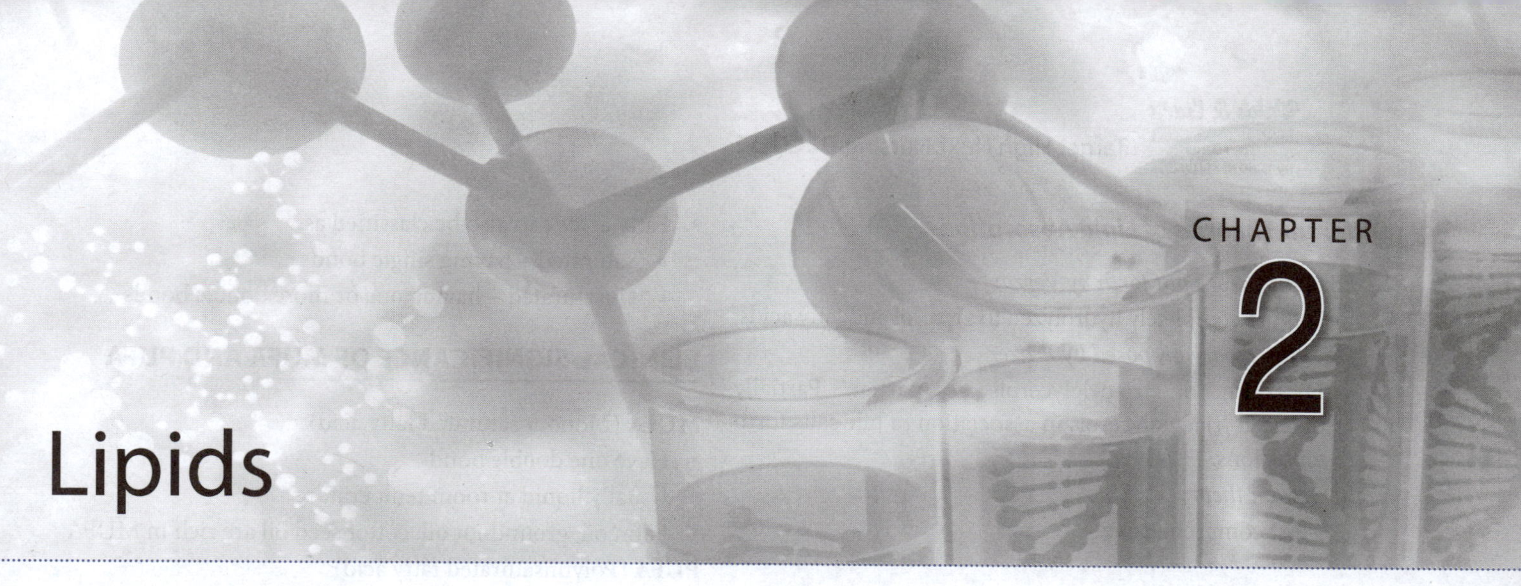

Lipids

CONCEPTUAL THEORY

Terminology

150+ key terminologies for Quick Recall & Revision

Atherosclerosis: Atherosclerosis (arteriosclerosis) is a disease of arterial wall. It is characterized by the accumulation of cholesterol and its esters in cells, which are derived from monocyte-macrophage line smooth muscle cells. This in turn results in the formation of atherosclerotic plaque, which narrows the blood vessels and serves as the site of thrombus formation.

Fatty acids: Fatty acids are the carboxylic acids with a long hydrocarbon side chain which may be saturated or unsaturated with one or more double bonds.

Lipid: Lipid is a heterogeneous group of hydrophobic organic molecules found in cells. Sparingly soluble in water but is soluble in organic solvents.

Lipid profile: Lipid profile refers to the estimation of total cholesterol, LDL-cholesterol, HDL-cholesterol and triglycerides in serum. Serum lipids and lipoproteins should be measured after a 10-hour fast because chylomicrons normally are present in plasma up to 10 hours after a meal.

Phospholipids: Phospholipids are predominant lipids of a cell membrane, component of lung surfactants, Essential components of the bile and help in regulation of serum cholesterol.

PUFAs: PUFAs are essential components of cell membranes. While Ω-6 PUFAs are predominant in all cells, the nerve tissue has high levels of long chain Ω-3 PUFA.

Trans fatty acids: Trans fatty acids are isomers of the normal cis (cis) fatty acids, produced when PUFAs are hydrogenated, such as in the production of margarine and vegetable shortening.

LIPIDS—DEFINITION

Lipids are a diverse group of organic compounds that are insoluble in water but soluble in organic solvents such as alcohol, ether, and chloroform.

LIPIDS—DIGESTION, ABSORPTION AND METABOLISM

Digestion of Lipids

- *Digestion in mouth*
  - Triglyceride degradation: by lipases to form free fatty acids and glycerol
- *Digestion in stomach*
  - By gastric lipase- most effective for short and medium chain fatty acids
- *Digestion in small intestine*
  - Major site of fat digestion
  - Effective digestion due to the presence of pancreatic lipase and bile salts.

Absorption of Lipids

- Direct absorption from the intestinal lumen—Glycerol, short and medium chain fatty acids
- Long chain fatty acids, free cholesterol and β- acyl glycerol together with bile salts form mixed micelles.
- *Micelles*
  - Disk-shaped clusters of amphipathic lipids
  - Soluble in water
  - Absorption may be facilitated by specific transport proteins.

Different Theories of Lipid Absorption

- *Lipolytic theory put forth by Verzar*
  - Fats are completely hydrolyzed to glycerol and fatty acids.
- *Partition theory proposed by Frazer*
  - Digestion of triacylglycerols is partial. Partially digested triacylglycerols in association of bile salts form emulsions.
- *Bergstrom theory*
  - Most comprehensive

Metabolism of Lipids

β-Oxidation Proper

- Enzymes for fatty acid oxidation – collectively known as fatty acid oxidase system – present in mitochondria
- **Four steps**
  1. **Oxidation**
     - Acyl CoA undergoes dehydrogenation to form trans enoyl CoA
     - Enzyme – FAD-dependent acyl CoA dehydrogenase
  2. **Hydration**
     - Enoyl CoA forms **β**-hydroxyacyl CoA
     - Enzyme – enoyl CoA hydratase
  3. **Oxidation**
     - **β**-hydroxyacyl CoA forms **β**-ketoacyl CoA under the effect of **β**-hydroxyacyl CoA dehydrogenase
  4. **Cleavage**
     - Liberation of acetyl CoA from acyl CoA
     - Thiolytic cleavage
     - Enzyme – **β**-ketoacyl CoA thiolase
- The newly formed acyl CoA (with 2 carbon less) enters the **β**-oxidation cycle again till the complete fatty acid oxidation takes place.
- *The summary of beta-oxidation of palmitic acid (16C) is as follows:*

Palmitoyl CoA + 7 CoASH + 7 FAD + 7 NAD$^+$ + 7 H_2O ---→ 8 Acetyl CoA + 7 $FADH_2$ + 7 NADH + 7 H^+

FATTY ACIDS—DEFINITION AND CLASSIFICATION

Read, Revise & Recall HIGH YIELD Topics For more, refer to Nursing Next Live app

Fatty Acids

- Carboxylic acids (-COOH) having hydrocarbon side chains.
- Naturally occurring ones are even chain fatty acids.
- Fatty acids are classified as:
  - Short chain fatty acids – contain 4–8 carbons
  - Medium chain fatty acids – contain 10–14 carbons
  - Long chain fatty acids – contain 16 or more carbons
- Fatty acids can also be classified as:
  - Saturated – having single bonds
  - Unsaturated – having one or more double bonds

CLINICAL SIGNIFICANCE OF MUFA AND PUFA

MUFA (Monounsaturated fatty acid)

- Have one double bond
- Usually liquid at room temperature
- Palm oil, groundnut oil, cottonseed oil are rich in MUFA

PUFA (Polyunsaturated fatty acid)

Two families–omega represents the position of first double bond

- Omega 3
- Omega 6

Advantages of PUFA

- **Component of essential fatty acids:** Linoleic acid, linolenic acid, arachidonic acid–cannot be synthesized in body
- **Component of membrane structure:** Responsible for the flexibility of membrane
- Improves circulation and oxygen uptake by RBCs
- Required for cholesterol formation, transport and function
- **Essential for the synthesis of eicosanoids:** Inhibits inflammatory process and blood coagulation
- Reduces platelet aggregation
- Prevents fatty liver and coronary heart disease.
- Supports CVS, reproductive, immune and nervous systems.

ESSENTIAL FATTY ACIDS, TRANS FATTY ACIDS

Essential Fatty Acids

- They cannot be synthesized by the body; so, they have to be supplied in the diet.
- Polyunsaturated fatty acids
- ***Essential fatty acids include:***
  - Linoleic acid (18:2; 9, 12)
  - Linolenic acid (18:3; 9, 12, 15)
  - Arachidonic acid (20:4; 5, 8, 11, 14)
    - Essential only in the deficiency of linolenic acid

Trans Fatty Acids

- Trans fat is **formed from the chemical process called hydrogenation.**
- Have no nutritional value.
- Eating **foods rich in trans fat increases the amount of bad cholesterol** (LDL-cholesterol) in the blood and **reduces the amount of good cholesterol** (HDL-cholesterol).
- Trans fats create inflammation, which is linked to heart disease, stroke, diabetes and other chronic conditions.

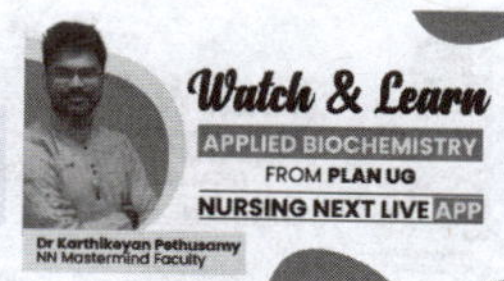

KETONE BODIES (NAME, TYPE AND SIGNIFICANCE)

Introduction

- Acetone, acetoacetate, β-hydroxyl butyrate
- Ketone bodies are water soluble
- Energy yielding

Ketogenesis

- Ketogenesis is the metabolic process by which ketone bodies are produced in the liver.
- Enzymes are present in mitochondrial matrix
- Acetyl CoA – precursor of ketone bodies
- β-oxidation of fatty acids yields acetyl CoA

Significance of Ketone Bodies

In Starvation

- State of metabolic stress
- Due to scarcity of food
- Imposes certain metabolic compulsions on the organism
- Biochemical changes occur to maintain adequate supply of energy to the various tissues

During Prolonged Starvation

- **Ketone bodies:** Fuel source for brain–meets 50–70% of its energy needs.
- Rest of the demands is met by glucose.
- Glucose during starvation is provided by gluconeogenesis in liver.
- **Ketone bodies:** More important during periods of starvation and diabetes mellitus
  - Ketone bodies – beta-hydroxybutyrate – serve as fuel source for peripheral tissues
    - After 3-day fast – serves 1/3rd of brain's demand
    - After 40 days – 70% of energy demands

LIPOPROTEINS (TYPES AND FUNCTIONS)

Introduction

Lipoproteins:

- Lipoproteins consist of lipids (such as cholesterol and triglycerides) and proteins.
- Transport lipids in plasma

Types of Lipoproteins

Four major types—differentiated based on specific proteins attached to the phospholipid outer layer, called the apolipoprotein

- Chylomicron
  - Chylos – juice; micron - small
  - Transports exogenous/dietary triacylglycerols to various tissues.
  - Consists of triglycerides, phospholipids, cholesterol, proteins (mainly apoprotein B48)
  - Least in density in lipoproteins
  - Largest size
  - Stabilizes the lipid droplets.
  - Increases the solubility of lipids.
- VLDL
  - Consists of protein, fats and cholesterol synthesized in the liver.
  - Associated with five different apoproteins - B-100, C-I, C-II, C-III and E
  - Converted to IDL and LDL by removal of the apoproteins
  - Second only to chylomicrons in the percentage triglyceride content.
- LDL
  - Bad-cholesterol.
  - Transports cholesterol from liver to peripheral tissues.
  - LDL contains only one lipoprotein Apo B-100.
  - LDL particles are derived from VLDL.
  - Small part is directly released from liver.
  - Binding of LDL to receptor is by apo-B-100.
- HDL
  - HDL is a good cholesterol.
  - Transports cholesterol from peripheral tissues to liver.
  - Synthesized in liver.
  - Major apoproteins in HDL are Apo A1, with some Apo A2, Apo C and Apo E.
  - HDL is a plasma reservoir of Apo C and Apo E, which can be transferred to VLDL and chylomicrons

LIPID PROFILE

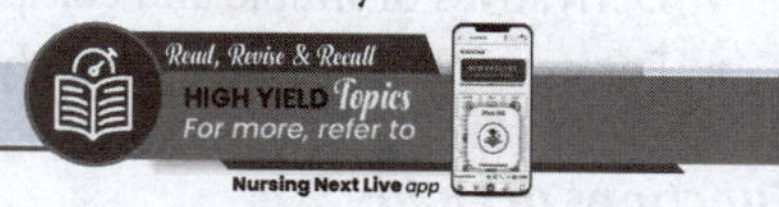

- **Lipid profile** refers to the estimation of total cholesterol, LDL-cholesterol, HDL- cholesterol and triglycerides in serum.
- Should be measured after a 10-hour fast
- For differentiation of disorders of lipoproteins, triglycerides and total cholesterol are routinely measured.
- Most of the cholesterol present in plasma is found in LDL.
- The fasting lipid profile, i.e., the concentration of total cholesterol, LDL cholesterol, HDL cholesterol and triglycerides, provides information about the main lipid markers of cardiovascular risk.

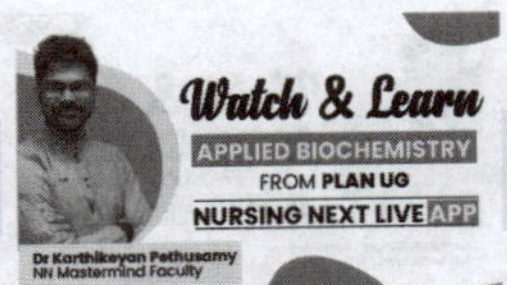

ATHEROSCLEROSIS

Atherosclerosis

- Atherosclerosis – complex disease characterized by thickening or hardening of arteries due to the accumulation of lipids in the inner arterial wall.

Causes

- Directly related to:
  - Plasma cholesterol
  - LDL levels
  - High blood pressure
- Indirectly related to plasma HDL levels

CONCEPTUAL EXERCISES

LONG ANSWER QUESTIONS

1. Classify lipids. Write in detail about the functions of phospholipids. (MGR)

Answer

Lipids

- Organic molecules that are insoluble in water and soluble in organic solvents.
- Hydrophobic in nature.
- Naturally occurring molecules include fats, waxes, sterols and fat-soluble vitamins.

Classification of Lipids

- **Simple lipids:**
  - Esters of fatty acids with alcohol.
  - For example: Oil, fats, waxes
- **Complex lipids:**
  - Esters of fatty acids with alcohol-containing amphipathic groups.
  - Also known as compound lipids.
  - Example: Phospholipids
- **Derived lipids:**
  - Derivatives of simple and complex lipids.
  - For example: Fatty acids and glycerol

Functions of Lipids

- Source of energy
- Form an important component of the cell membrane
- Source of fat-soluble vitamins
- Fat provides insulation and protection from cold.

Phospholipids

- Compound lipids containing phosphoric acid along with nitrogenous base and alcohol.
- Major component of cell membrane.
- Amphiphilic in nature as they are made up of hydrophilic heads and hydrophobic tails joined together by glycerol molecule.

Classification of Phospholipids

- Two types:
  1. Glycerophospholipids
  2. Sphingophospholipids

Functions of Phospholipids

- Phospholipids are a class of lipids that play vital roles in biological systems. The functions of phospholipids are as follows:
- **Formation of cell membranes:** Phospholipids are fundamental building blocks of cell membranes.
- **Membrane fluidity and flexibility:** Phospholipids contribute to the fluidity and flexibility of cell membranes.
- **Signal transduction:** Certain phospholipids serve as important signaling molecules in cellular communication.
- **Cell adhesion:** Phospholipids can interact with other molecules, such as proteins and carbohydrates, to help cells stick together.
- **Energy storage:** Some phospholipids, such as phosphatidylcholine, can store energy in the form of fatty acids.
- **Biosynthesis:** Phospholipids are involved in the synthesis of other molecules, such as cholesterol and triglycerides.
- **Protective coating:** Phospholipids provide a protective coating in certain tissues and organs. For instance, in the lungs, a specialized phospholipid mixture called pulmonary surfactant lines the air sacs (alveoli) and reduces surface tension.
- **Protein anchoring:** Phospholipids anchor proteins to cell membranes.
- **Emulsification and absorption of fats:** In the digestive system, phospholipids aid in the emulsification and absorption of dietary fats.
- **Intracellular membranes and organelles:** Phospholipids are also present in intracellular membranes and organelles.

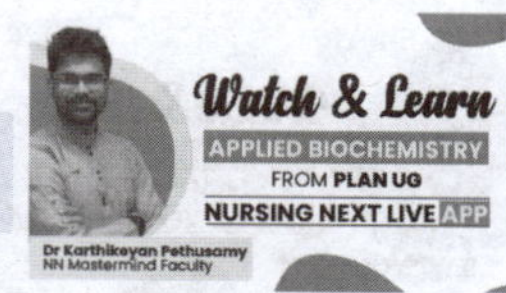

2. Discuss the biological importance of saturated and unsaturated fatty acids. (DU)

Answer

Biological Importance of Saturated Fatty Acids

- Saturated fatty acids are fatty acids that contain single bonds. They are simplest form of fats. Fatty acids derived from animal sources are usually saturated fatty acids with even number carbon atoms.
- **Biological imporance includes:**
  - **Energy storage:** Saturated fatty acids are a concentrated source of energy in the body. When consumed in the diet or released from adipose tissue, they can be broken down through beta-oxidation to produce ATP, the energy currency of cells.
  - **Structural role:** Saturated fatty acids contribute to the structural integrity of cell membranes. Their straight and rigid structure allows them to tightly pack together, resulting in a more stable and less permeable membrane. This is important for maintaining cellular compartments and protecting cells from the external environment.
  - **Hormone production:** Saturated fatty acids serve as precursors for the synthesis of various hormones and signaling molecules in the body. Saturated fatty acids are involved in the production of steroid hormones such as cortisol, estrogen, and testosterone.
  - **Absorption of fat-soluble vitamins:** Saturated fatty acids play a role in the absorption of fat-soluble vitamins (A, D, E, and K) in the digestive system. They form micelles with bile salts, helping to solubilize and transport these vitamins for absorption into the body.

Biological Importance of Unsaturated Fatty Acids

- Unsaturated fatty acids are fatty acids with one or more double bonds. They are complex fatty acids. Types of unsaturated fatty acids includes monounsaturated fatty acids, Diunsaturated fatty acids and Polyunsaturated fatty acids.
- **Biological importance includes:**
  - **Cell membrane fluidity:** Unsaturated fatty acids introduce kinks in their structure due to double bonds, which prevent them from tightly packing together. This increases the fluidity and flexibility of cell membranes.
  - **Essential fatty acids:** Certain unsaturated fatty acids, such as omega-3 and omega-6 fatty acids, are essential for human health. They cannot be synthesized by the body and must be obtained through the diet. These essential fatty acids play critical roles in cell signaling, inflammation regulation, and maintaining the integrity of cell membranes.
  - **Cardiovascular health:** Unsaturated fatty acids, particularly monounsaturated and polyunsaturated fats, have been associated with improved cardiovascular health. They help lower levels of LDL cholesterol (bad cholesterol) in the blood, reducing the risk of heart disease. Omega-3 fatty acids, in particular, have anti-inflammatory properties and are beneficial for heart health.
  - **Brain function and development:** Unsaturated fatty acids, particularly omega-3 fatty acids like docosahexaenoic acid (DHA), are crucial for brain development and function. DHA is a major component of neuronal membranes and plays a role in neurogenesis, synaptic function, and cognitive performance.
  - **Inflammation and immune response:** Certain unsaturated fatty acids, such as omega-3 fatty acids, have anti-inflammatory properties and can modulate immune responses. They can help reduce chronic inflammation and contribute to the resolution of inflammatory processes.

3. Describe the β-oxidation of fatty acids. Mention the energetics and its deficiency. (MGR)

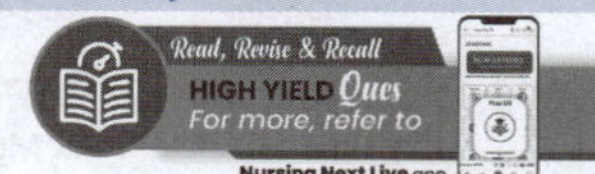

Answer

Introduction

- Fatty acid breakdown takes place in body mainly by β-oxidation
- β-oxidation is the oxidation of fatty acids on the β-carbon
- Resulting in sequential removal of 2 carbon atoms

Fatty Acid Oxidation

- *It involves three stages:*
  1. Activation of fatty acids—in cytosol.
  2. Transport of fatty acids to mitochondria.
  3. β-oxidation proper—in mitochondria.

Fatty Acid Activation

- Activated by thiokinase or acyl CoA synthase to acyl CoA
- Requires two high energy phosphates
- Irreversible reaction

Transport of Acyl CoA into Mitochondria

- The inner mitochondrial membrane is impermeable to fatty acids.
- It is transported through carnitine carrier system or carnitine shuttle.

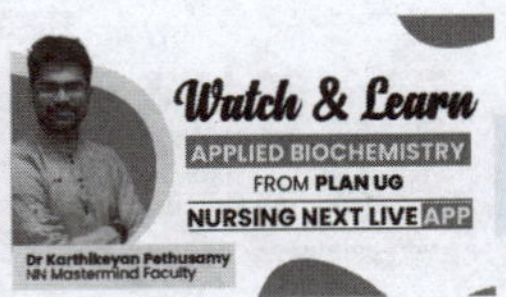

β-Oxidation Proper

- Enzymes for fatty acid oxidation – collectively known as fatty acid oxidase system – present in mitochondria
- **Four steps:**
  - **Oxidation**
    - Acyl CoA undergoes dehydrogenation to form trans enoyl CoA
    - Enzyme – FAD dependent acyl CoA dehydrogenase
  - **Hydration**
    - Enoyl CoA forms β-hydroxyacyl CoA
    - Enzyme – enoyl CoA hydratase
  - **Oxidation**
    - β-hydroxyacyl CoA forms β-ketoacyl CoA under the effect of β-hydroxyacyl CoA dehydrogenase
  - **Cleavage**
    - Liberation of acetyl CoA from acyl CoA
    - Thiolytic cleavage
    - Enzyme – β-ketoacyl CoA thiolase
- The newly formed acyl CoA (with 2 carbon less) enters the β-oxidation cycle again till the complete fatty acid oxidation takes place.

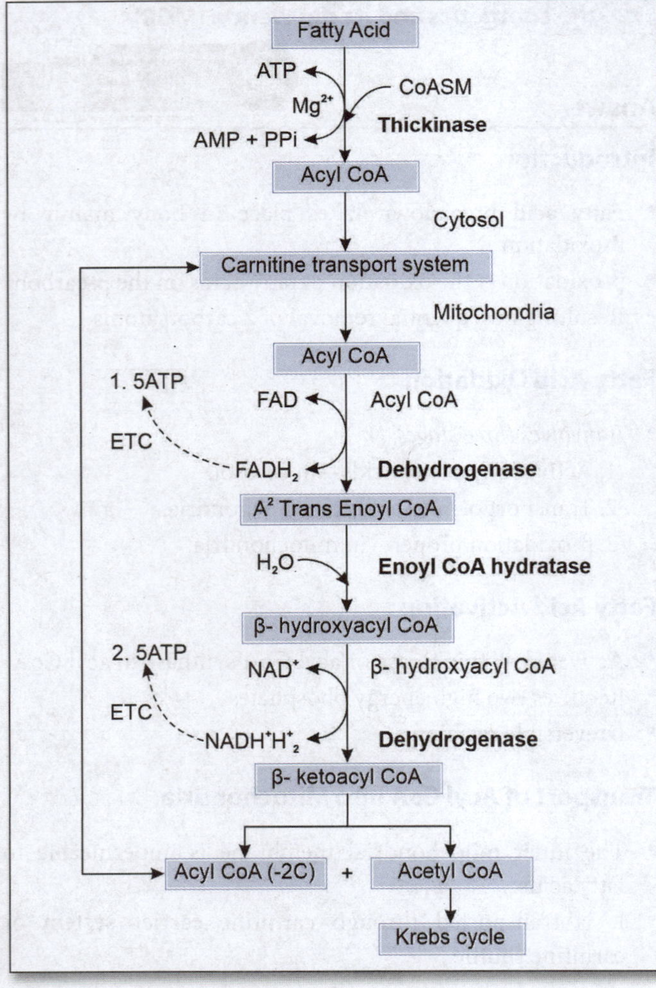

Energetics

The summary of beta-oxidation of palmitic acid (16C) is as follows:

Palmitoyl CoA + 7 CoASH + 7 FAD + 7 NAD^+ + 7 H_2O ---→ 8 Acetyl CoA + 7 $FADH_2$ + 7 NADH + 7 H^+

Palmitic acid undergoes 7 cycles of beta-oxidation to yield 8 acetyl CoA which enters citric acid cycle and undergoes oxidation to CO_2 and H_2O.

Net yield for one molecule of palmitic acid – 106 ATP

Deficiency

Medium chain fatty acyl CoA dehydrogenase deficiency leads to an autosomal recessive disorder called Sudden Infant Death Syndrome (SIDS).

4. Classify lipoproteins. Describe the metabolism of very low density lipoprotein. Add a note on atherosclerosis. (KUHS)

Answer

Introduction

- Lipoproteins are complex particles composed of both proteins and lipids.
- They play a crucial role in the transport and metabolism of lipids in the body.

Types of Lipoproteins

Four major types - differentiated based on specific proteins attached to the phospholipid outer layer, called the apolipoprotein.

The major classes of lipoproteins include chylomicron, very low-density lipoprotein (VLDL), low-density lipoprotein (LDL), and high-density lipoprotein (HDL).

- **Chylomicron**
  - Chylos – juice; micron – small
  - Transports exogenous/dietary triacylglycerols to various tissues.
  - Consists of:
    - Triglycerides: 85–92%
    - Phospholipids: 6–12%
    - Cholesterol: 1–3%
    - Proteins: 1–2% (mainly apoprotein B48)
  - Least in density in lipoproteins
  - Largest size
  - Stabilizes the lipid droplets.
  - Increases the solubility of lipids.

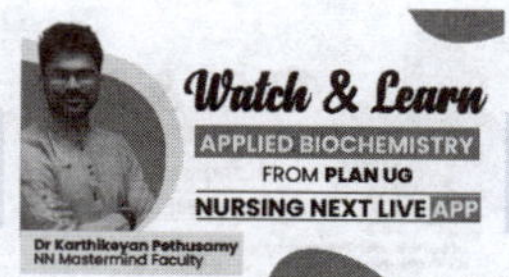

- VLDL
  - Consists of protein, fats and cholesterol—synthesized in the liver.
  - Associated with five different apoproteins:
    - B-100
    - C-I
    - C-II
    - C-III
    - E
  - Converted to IDL and LDL by removal of the apoproteins
  - Second only to chylomicrons in the percentage triglyceride content.
- LDL
  - Bad-cholesterol.
  - Transports cholesterol from liver to peripheral tissues.
  - LDL contains only one lipoprotein Apo B-100.
  - LDL particles are derived from VLDL.
  - Small part is directly released from liver.
  - Binding of LDL to receptor is by apo B-100.
  - Half-life is 2 days.
- HDL
  - HDL is a good cholesterol.
  - Transports cholesterol from peripheral tissues to liver.
  - Synthesized in liver.
  - Major apoproteins in HDL are Apo A1, with some Apo A2, Apo C and Apo E.
  - HDL is a plasma reservoir of Apo C and Apo E, which can be transferred to VLDL and chylomicrons.

Metabolism of Very Low Density Lipoprotein

- Very low density lipoproteins are also called pre-beta-lipoproteins.
- Composed of triacylglycerols like chylomicrons.
- The major function is to transport lipids from liver to peripheral tissues.
- VLDL is released from the liver as nascent VLDL, similar to the release of nascent chylomicrons from the intestinal mucosa.
- Nascent VLDL particles contain apo B-100 and apo A-1. Subsequently, they acquire apo C-II and apo E from circulating HDL.
- During the circulation, lipoprotein lipase hydrolyzes triacylglycerols and releases free fatty acids, which are taken up by the peripheral tissues.
- Apo C and apo E are transferred to HDL.
- In addition, cholesteryl esters which are synthesized in the plasma, as a result of the action of lecithin cholesterol acyltransferase (LCAT), are transferred from HDL to VLDL and IDL via the cholesteryl ester transfer protein (CETP).
- As a result of it, the particle size is reduced and density is increased.
- VLDL particles are hence converted into VLDL remnants.
- These are also known as intermediate density lipoproteins (IDLs)
- IDL particles are removed by the liver or converted into LDL.

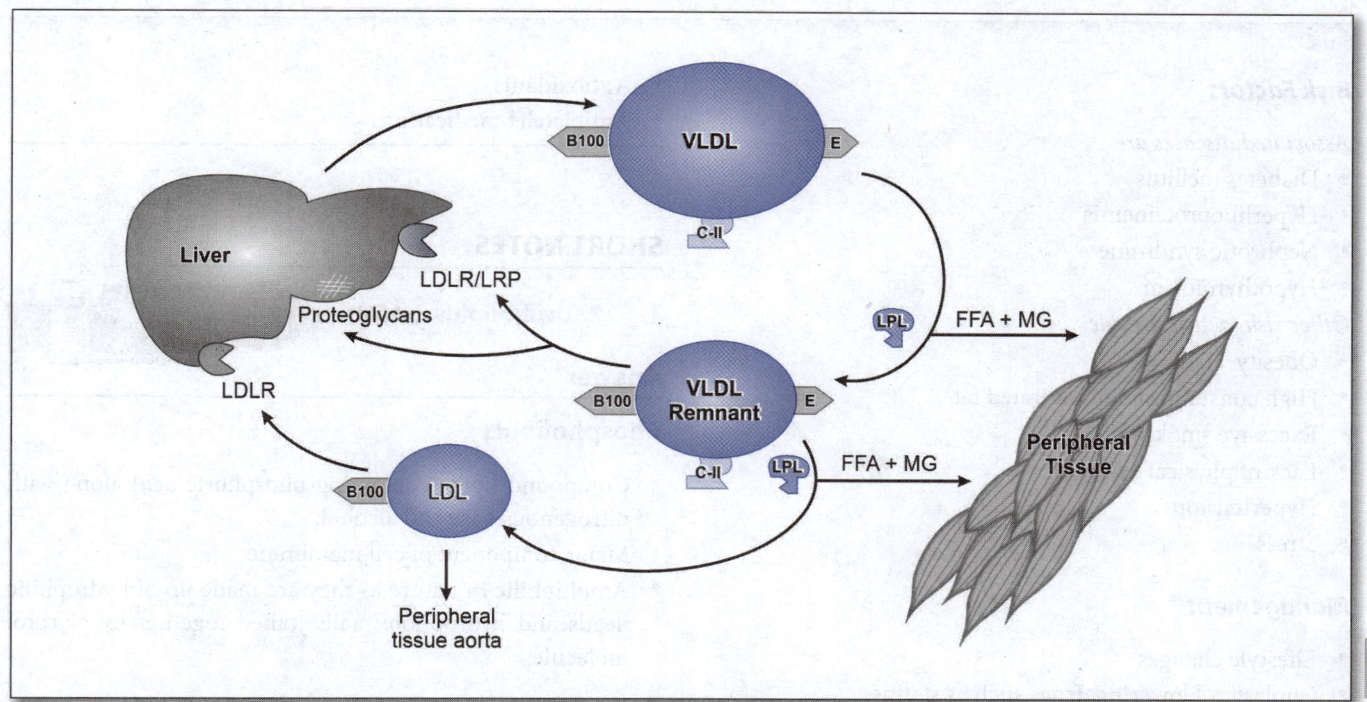

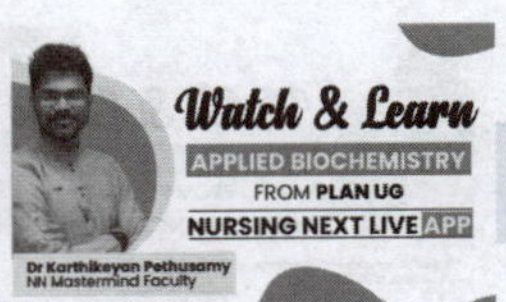

Atherosclerosis

Atherosclerosis – complex disease characterized by thickening of hardening of arteries due to the accumulation of lipids in the inner arterial wall.

Causes

- Directly related to:
  - Elevated serum cholesterol and triglycerides.
  - Elevated LDL levels
  - High blood pressure
- Indirectly related to decreased plasma HDL levels

Pathophysiology

- Develops as a chronic inflammatory response to endothelial injury of the arterial wall.
- Endothelial injury causes increased permeability, leukocyte adhesion and thrombosis.

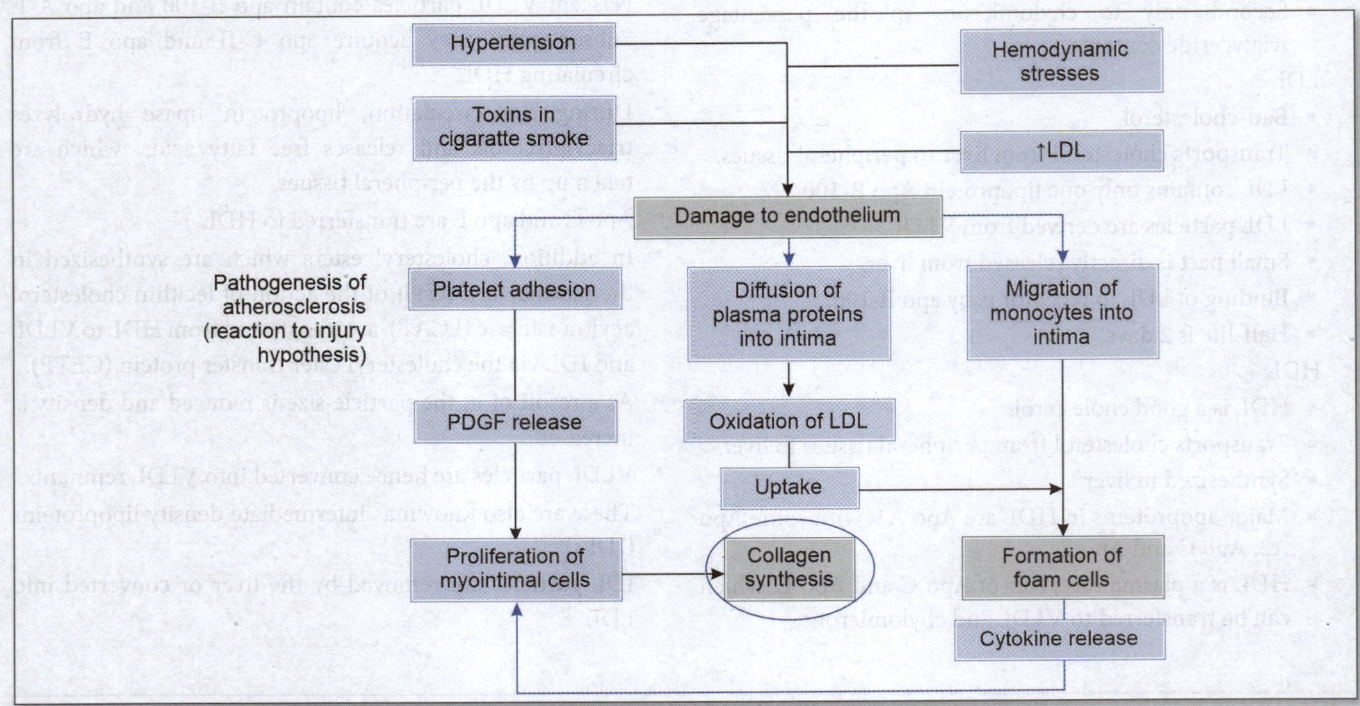

Risk Factors

Associated diseases are:

- Diabetes mellitus
- Hyperlipoproteinemia
- Nephrotic syndrome
- Hypothyroidism

Other risk factors include:

- Obesity
- High consumption of saturated fat
- Excessive smoking
- Lack of physical exercise
- Hypertension
- Stress

Management

- Lifestyle changes
- Cholesterol lowering drugs such as statins
- Antioxidants
- Antiplatelet medications

SHORT NOTES

1. Phospholipids. (MGR)

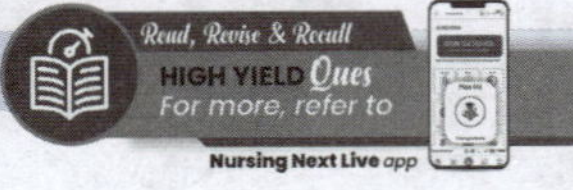

Answer

Phospholipids

- Compound lipids containing phosphoric acid along with nitrogenous base and alcohol.
- Major component of cell membrane.
- Amphiphilic in nature as they are made up of hydrophilic heads and hydrophobic tails joined together by glycerol molecule.

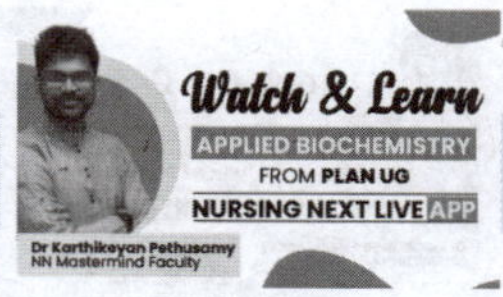

Functions

- Structural components of cell membrane and regulate membrane permeability
- Component of lung surfactant
- Act as lipotropic factors
- Essential component of bile.
- Mitochondrial phospholipids maintain the conformation of ETC and thus cellular respiration
- Role in absorption of fats from intestine
- Synthesis and transport of certain lipids
- Role in reverse cholesterol transport.

Classification of Phospholipids

- Two types:
  1. Glycerophospholipids
  2. Sphingophospholipids

Glycerophospholipids:

- Also known as phosphoglycerides.
- Contain glycerol as the alcohol.
- Synthesized from phosphatidic acid.
- Major lipids in cell membrane
- Important ones are:
  - Phosphatidic acid – simplest phospholipid
  - Lecithins (phosphatidylcholine)
    - Phosphatidic acid + choline as base
    - Contain choline at carbon 3
    - Present in brain, nerve cells, sperm and egg yolk.
    - Help in emulsification of fats.
    - Most abundant in cell membrane
  - Cephalins – phosphatidylethanolamine
    - Present in RBC membrane, brain and many other tissues.
    - Ethanolamine is the nitrogenous base
  - Phosphatidylinositol
    - Phosphatidic acid + myo-inositol
    - Mainly found in brain.
  - Cardiolipins
    - Carbon 1 is linked with unsaturated fatty acids.
    - Present in cardiac and skeletal muscles.

Sphingophospholipids:

- Sphingosine is the amino alcohol group - Important constituent of myelin sheath
- Ceramide – acts as second messenger
- Important sphingophospholipids are:
  - Sphingomyelins
    - Contain phosphocholine or phosphoethanolamine.
    - Myelin sheath is rich in sphingomyelins
  - Cerebrosides
    - Contain ceramide
  - Gangliosides
    - Consist of oligosaccharides.
    - Present in ganglion cells of nervous system.

2. Differentiate between saturated fatty acids and unsaturated fatty acids. (KUHS)

Answer

Differences between Saturated and Unsaturated Fatty Acids

	Saturated fatty acids	Unsaturated fatty acids
Definition	Unbranched linear chain of CH_2 groups linked by carbon-carbon single bonds with a terminal carboxylic acid	Bent and branched hydrocarbon chains linked by carbon-carbon double bonds with a terminal carboxylic acid group
No. of bonds	Single bond	Double bond
Saturation of hydrogen atoms	Maximum	Less than maximum
Hydrogenation	Not possible	Possible as the double bonds can be converted to single bonds
Source	Abundant in fats of animal origin like butter, meat, whole milk	Abundant in fats of plant origin like vegetable oil, sunflower oil, mustard oil.
Configuration	Trans and cis configuration are not possible	Exist in cis and trans configuration
Melting point	High	Low
State at room temperature	Exist in solid state	Exist in liquid state
Rancidity	Low rancidity	High

Contd...

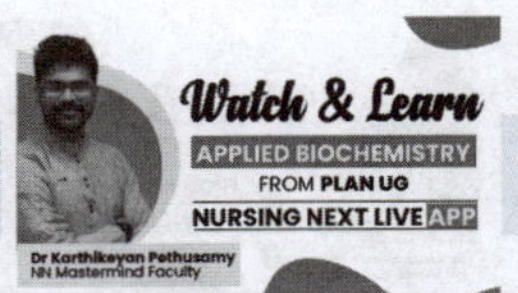

	Saturated fatty acids	Unsaturated fatty acids
Shelf life	Higher shelf life	Lesser shelf life
Low density lipoprotein (LDL) levels	Saturated fatty acids increase LDL levels	Unsaturated fatty acids decrease LDL levels
Calorie	Provide for 10% of the total calories	Provide for 30% of the total calories
Solubility in vitamins	Soluble	Insoluble
Storage	Stored in liver and adipose tissue	Stored in seeds and fruits of plants
Excessive consumption leads to	Heart disease	Reduction in cholesterol levels
Examples	Stearic acid, palmitic acid, capric acid	Linoleic acid, linolenic acid, oleic acid

3. Name the lipotropic factors. (MGR)

Answer

Lipotropic Factors

- Substances that prevent accumulation of fats in liver.
- *Important lipotropic factors are:*
  - Choline–present in egg yolks, organ meats and fish
  - Betaine
  - Methionine
  - Inositol – beans, brown rice, meats
  - Folic acid, vitamin B_{12}, glycine and serine – to some extent

Action of Lipotropic Factors

- Choline and inositol – components of phospholipids – required for their synthesis
- Also concerned with transmethylation reactions
- Other lipotropic factors are used for synthesis of choline.

Deficiency of Lipotropic Factors

- Decreased phospholipid synthesis
- Impaired formation of lipoprotein membrane
- Reduced synthesis of carnitine due to insufficient supply of methyl groups
- Impairment in fatty acid oxidation

4. Define fatty acids. (MGR)

Answer

Fatty Acids

- Carboxylic acids (-COOH) having hydrocarbon side chains.
- Naturally occurring ones are even chain fatty acids.
- Fatty acids are classified as:
  - Short chain fatty acids: contain 4–8 carbons
  - Medium chain fatty acids: contain 10–14 carbons
  - Long chain fatty acids: contain 16 or more carbons.
- Fatty acids can also be classified as:
  - Saturated: having single bonds
  - Unsaturated: having one or more double bonds

5. Digestion of fat. (MGR)

Answer

Introduction

- Typical diet consists of 25–160 g of lipids
- Mainly triglycerides
- *Enzymes required for lipid digestion*
  - Lipases
  - Lingual
  - Gastric
  - Pancreatic – synthesized in pancreas and works in duodenum
- Maximum lipid digestion occurs in duodenum.

Emulsification of Lipids in Small Intestine

- Breakdown of lipids into smaller droplets
- Reduces surface tension and increases surface area
- Essential for effective digestion
- *Occurs by three mechanisms*

1. *Detergent action of bile salts:*
   - Interact with lipid particles and the aqueous duodenal contents and convert them into smaller ones
   - Stabilize the smaller lipid particles from coalescing back.
2. *Surfactant action of degraded lipids*
   - Initial lipid products acted by lipases, free fatty acids and monoglycerols promote emulsification
3. *Mechanical mixing due to peristalsis*

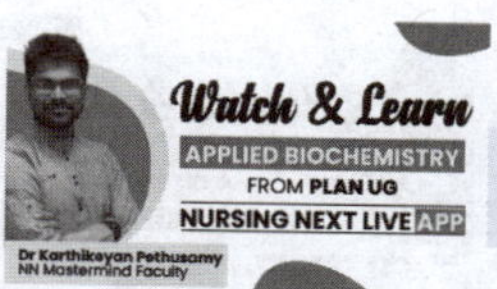

Digestion of Lipids

- *Digestion in mouth*
  - Triglyceride degradation: by lipases to form free fatty acids and glycerol
- *Digestion in stomach*
  - By gastric lipase—most effective for short and medium chain fatty acids
- *Digestion in small intestine*
  - Major site of fat digestion
  - Effective digestion due to the presence of pancreatic lipase and bile salts.
  - Secretion of pancreatic juice is stimulated by:
    - Passage of acidic gastric contents into the duodenum
    - Secretion of Secretin, Cholecystokinin and Pancreozymin, the gastrointestinal hormones
    - Triacylglycerol degradation by pancreatic lipase
    - Digestion of triglycerides proceeds by the removal of a terminal fatty acid to produce an α, β diglyceride.
    - The other terminal fatty acid is then removed to produce β monoglyceride.
    - The last fatty acid is linked by secondary ester group; hence, cannot be hydrolyzed by pancreatic lipase.
    - β-monoacylglycerol can be converted to α-monoacylglycerol by isomerase enzyme and then hydrolyzed by pancreatic lipase.

Absorption of Lipids

- Direct absorption from the intestinal lumen—Glycerol, short and medium chain fatty acids
- Long chain fatty acids, free cholesterol and β-acyl glycerol together with bile salts form mixed micelles.
- *Micelles*
  - Disk-shaped clusters of amphipathic lipids
  - Soluble in water
  - Absorption may be facilitated by specific transport proteins.

Different Theories of Lipid Absorption

- *Lipolytic theory put forth by Verzar*
  - Fats are completely hydrolyzed to glycerol and fatty acids.
- *Partition theory proposed by Frazer*
  - Digestion of triacylglycerols is partial. Partially digested triacylglycerols in association with bile salts form emulsions.
- *Bergstrom theory*
  - Most comprehensive

6. Write a short note on essential fatty acids. (MGR)

Answer

Introduction

- Essential fatty acids cannot be synthesized by the body; so, they have to be supplied in the diet.
- Polyunsaturated fatty acids
- ***Essential fatty acids include:***
  - Linoleic acid (18:2; 9, 12)
  - Linolenic acid (18:3; 9, 12, 15)
  - Arachidonic acid (20:4; 5, 8, 11, 14)
    - Essential only in the deficiency of linolenic acid

Conditionally Essential Fatty Acids

- Fatty acids that become essential under certain developmental or diseased conditions
- Examples:
  - *Docosahexaenoic acid (DHA; omega-3 fatty acid 22:6)*
    - DHA is synthesized from linoleic acid
    - In preterm infants, this capacity is limited; so, supplementation is required
    - Source – fish oils

Biomedical Importance of Essential Fatty Acids

- Essential fatty acids are the structural components of biological membrane.
- They participate in the transport and utilization of cholesterol.
- They prevent fat accumulation in the liver.
- They are required for the synthesis of prostaglandins.
- They maintain proper growth and reproduction of organisms.
- They are required for healthy skin and hair.
- They regulate blood clotting.

Deficiency of Essential Fatty Acids

- Leads to phrynoderma.
- Symptoms include dry, scaly skin, poor wound healing, loss of hair and growth failure.

7. Write functions of lipids. (MGR)

Answer

Introduction

- Typical diet consists of 25–160 g of lipids
- Mainly triglycerides

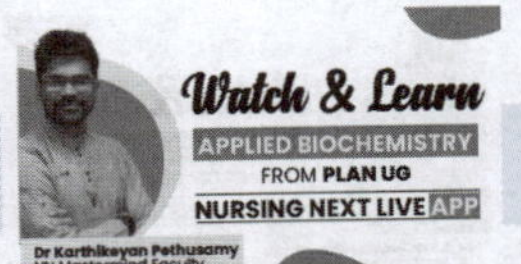

- *Problems associated with lipid digestion and absorption:*
  - Insoluble or sparingly soluble in water
  - Lipophilic and hydrophilic
  - Form fat droplets
  - Digestive enzymes work in aqueous medium

Functions of Lipids

- Source of energy
- Form an important component of the cell membrane
- Source of fat soluble vitamins
- Provide insulation and protection from cold
- Participate in the transport and utilization of cholesterol
- Prevent fat accumulation in the liver
- Required for the synthesis of prostaglandins.
- Maintain proper growth and reproduction of the organisms.

8. Write a short note on chylomicrons. (MGR)

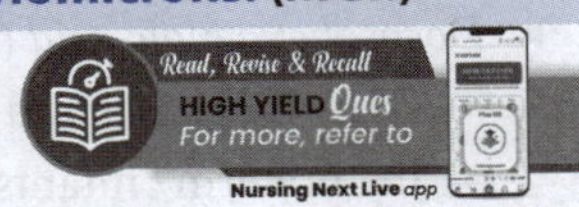

Answer

Chylomicrons

- "Chylos" means juice and "micron" means small particle.
- Transport exogenous/dietary triacylglycerols to various tissues.
- Consist of lipids (99%) and protein (1%)
- Least in density among lipoproteins
- Largest size.
- Stabilize the lipid droplets
- Increase the solubility of lipids.

Composition of Chylomicrons

- **Lipids are resynthesized in intestinal cells:** hydrophobic in nature
- **Lipid droplets are surrounded by a thin layer consisting of mostly apoproteins.**
- Chylomicrons consist of:
  - **Triglycerides:** 85–92%
  - **Phospholipids:** 6–12%
  - **Cholesterol:** 1–3%
  - **Proteins:** 1–2% (mainly apoprotein B48)
    - Apo B48 –apoprotein contains 48% of protein coded by apo B gene.

Metabolism of Chylomicrons

- Three stages of chylomicron life cycle:
  i. Nascent chylomicron
  ii. Mature chylomicron
  iii. Chylomicron remnant
- **Nascent chylomicron**
  - Emulsification of triglycerides by bile.
  - Lipoprotein lipase hydrolyzes triacylglycerols present in chylomicrons to form fatty acids and monoglycerides; these pass through intestinal lumen into enterocytes
  - Re-esterification occurs to form triglycerides
  - Triglycerides combine with phospholipids and apo B48–form nascent chylomicron
  - Released into lymph to enter systemic circulation
- **Mature chylomicron**
  - In blood, nascent chylomicrons take up apo C-II and apolipoproteins from HDL to form mature chylomicron.
  - Lipoprotein lipase hydrolyzes triacylglycerols present in chylomicrons
  - Liberates free fatty acids
  - Lipoprotein lipase is activated by apo C-II
- **Chylomicron remnant**
  - After the degradation, chylomicrons lose apo C-II which is returned to HDL
  - Chylomicron remnants attach to the receptors present on hepatocytes.

9. Name the bile salts and explain their role in digestion. (MGR)

Answer

Bile Salts

- Bile salts are biological detergents
- Synthesized from cholesterol in liver
- Secreted with bile into duodenum

The Bile salts include:

- Primary bile salts are:
  - Cholic acid
  - Chenodeoxycholic acid
- Secondary bile salts are:
  - Deoxycholic acid (formed from cholic acid)
  - Lithocholic acid (formed from chenodeoxycholic acid)
- Conjugated bile salts are:
  - Glycocholic acid
  - Taurocholic acid
  - Glycochenodeoxycholic acid
  - Taurochenodeoxycholic acid

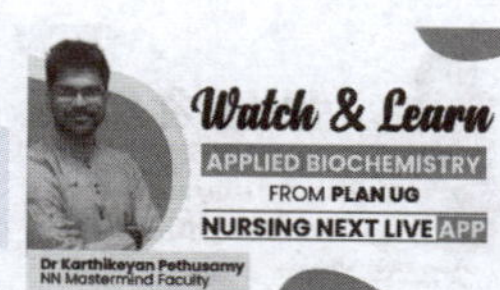

Functions

Role of bile salts in digestion:

- **Emulsification of fats:** Bile salts play a crucial role in the digestion and absorption of dietary fats. They act as natural detergents by emulsifying large fat globules into smaller droplets. This process increases the surface area of fats, allowing pancreatic enzymes called lipases to break them down into smaller molecules.
- **Micelle formation:** Bile salts form micelles in the small intestine. Micelles are tiny structures composed of bile salts, fatty acids, cholesterol, and fat-soluble vitamins. Within the micelles, fats are solubilized and transported to the surface of the intestinal lining for absorption.
- **Fat absorption:** Bile salts facilitate the absorption of fatty acids, cholesterol, and fat-soluble vitamins across the intestinal lining.
- **Recycling and enterohepatic circulation:** After aiding in fat digestion and absorption, bile salts are reabsorbed in the terminal ileum and transported back to the liver through a process called enterohepatic circulation. The liver then re-secretes these recycled bile salts into the bile, promoting their continuous reuse in digestion.

10. Write a short note on hypercholesterolemia. (MGR)

Answer

Hypercholesterolemia

- Hypercholesterolemia is defined as increase in plasma concentration of cholesterol above 200 mg/dL.
- Elevated levels of LDL cholesterol, VLDL cholesterol
- **Associated with:**
  - Atherosclerosis
  - Coronary heart disease
  - Peripheral vascular diseases
  - Stroke
- Usually seen in diabetes mellitus, hypothyroidism, obstructive jaundice, nephrotic syndrome, etc.
- **Risk factors:**
  - Diet
  - Obesity
  - Genetic diseases such as LDL receptor mutations
  - Presence of other diseases
  - Smoking
  - Having high BP
- **Diagnosis**

In mg/dL	Desirable	Borderline	High
Total cholesterol	<200	200–239	>240
LDL cholesterol	<100	100–129	>130
HDL cholesterol	>60	41–59	<40

Management

- Lifestyle modifications
- Medications
  - **Statins**
    - Cholesterol reducing drugs
      - E.g., lovastatin, atorvastatin, simvastatin, fluvastatin
      - **Competitive inhibitors of enzyme HMG CoA reductase**
  - **Cholestyramine:** Cholesterol lowering drug
    - Bile acid sequestrant

11. Describe good and bad cholesterol in blood. Explain their role. (DU)

Answer

Good Cholesterol

- HDL (High density lipoprotein) is a good cholesterol.
- Transports cholesterol from peripheral tissues to liver.
- Synthesized in liver.
- Major apoproteins in HDL are Apo A1, with some Apo A2, Apo C and Apo E.
- HDL is a plasma reservoir of Apo C and Apo E, which can be transferred to VLDL and chylomicrons.

Antiatherogenic Role of HDL

Attributed to:

- Reverse cholesterol transport
- Antioxidant role – due to the presence of enzyme paraoxonase – protects low density lipoproteins from getting oxidized.

Bad Cholesterol

- LDL (low density lipoprotein) is known as bad cholesterol
- Transports cholesterol from liver to peripheral tissues.
- LDL contains only one lipoprotein Apo B-100.
- LDL particles are derived from VLDL.
- A small part is directly released from liver.
- Binding of LDL to receptor is by apo-B-100.
- Half-life is 2 days.

Clinical Significance

- LDL concentration increases in cardiovascular diseases.
- A small fraction of cholesterol is taken up by macrophages.
- Increased levels of LDL or modified LDL or oxidized LDL increase the fraction of cholesterol taken by macrophages.
- There is an LDL infiltration through arterial walls and taken up by macrophages or scavenger cells.
- This is the starting event of atherosclerosis, leading to myocardial infarction (MI).
- Cells become engorged with cholesterol, foam cells are formed and deposited in subendothelial space triggering the formation of atheromatous plaque.
- Leads to thrombosis and coronary artery disease.
- Defect in LDL receptor synthesis leads to familial hypercholesterolemia.

12. Write a short note on compounds synthesized from cholesterol. (MGR)

Answer

Compounds Synthesized from Cholesterol

Steroid Hormones

- **Adrenal gland hormones**
  - Glucocorticoids
    - Blood sugar regulation
    - Anti-inflammatory
    - Immunosuppressive action
  - Mineralocorticoids
    - Electrolyte balance and fluid balance
- **Sex hormones**
  - Progesterone
    - Regulates endometrial lining of the uterus
  - Estrogens
    - Role in the growth and development of female secondary sex organs
  - Testosterone
    - Key role in the development of male reproductive tissues – testes and prostate, and the secondary sexual characteristics.
- **Bile acids**
  - Essential for digestion and absorption of fats and fat-soluble vitamins
- **Vitamin D**
  - Essential for calcium absorption
  - Essential for bone growth and development

13. Write a short note on ketone bodies and its significance. (MGR)

Answer

Introduction

- Ketone bodies are acetone, acetoacetate, β-hydroxyl butyrate
- Ketone bodies are water soluble and energy yielding
- Ketone bodies are produced in liver cells by the breakdown of fatty acids. They are released into the blood after glycogen stores in the liver have been depleted.

Ketogenesis

- Ketogenesis is the metabolic process by which the liver produces ketone bodies from fatty acids.
- Ketone bodies are readily transported into tissues outside the liver, where they are converted into acetyl-CoA—which then enters the citric acid cycle and is oxidized for energy.
- Ketogenesis is triggered by a lack of carbohydrates in the diet. When there are not enough carbohydrates available for energy, the body breaks down fatty acids for fuel. This process produces ketone bodies, which are then released into the bloodstream.
- Ketone bodies can be used by the brain and other tissues as an alternative source of energy. However, they are not as efficient as carbohydrates for providing energy.

Regulation of Ketogenesis

- **Hormonal regulation**
  - Glucagon stimulates ketogenesis
  - Insulin inhibits ketogenesis
- **Regulation mainly takes places in three stages:**
  1. Mobilization of free fatty acids from adipose tissue
  2. Carnitine palmitoyltransferase–1 activity is low in fed state and increases in starvation, which results in elevated fatty acid oxidation
  3. Low oxaloacetate concentration impairs Krebs cycle leading to accumulation of acetyl CoA.

Utilization of Ketone Bodies

- Easily transported to various tissues from liver as they are water soluble
- **Source of energy for peripheral tissues such as skeletal muscle**
- During prolonged starvation
  - Fuel source for brain – meets 50–70% of its energy needs.
- More important during periods of starvation and diabetes mellitus

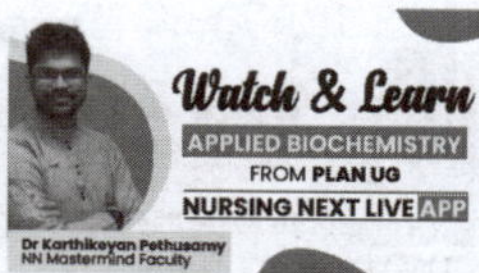

Significance of Ketone Bodies

Role of Ketone Bodies in Starvation

In Starvation

- State of metabolic stress
- Due to scarcity of food
- Imposes certain metabolic compulsions on the organism
- Biochemical changes occur to maintain adequate supply of energy to various tissues.

During Prolonged Starvation

- **Ketone bodies:** Fuel source for brain–meets 50–70% of its energy needs
- Rest of the demands are met by glucose
- During starvation, glucose is provided by gluconeogenesis in liver
- **Ketone bodies:** More important during periods of starvation and diabetes mellitus
  - Ketone bodies – beta-hydroxybutyrate – serve as fuel source for peripheral tissues
    - After 3-day fast – serves 1/3rd of brain's demand
    - After 40 days – 70% of energy demands

14. Write a short note on Rothera's test.

Answer

Rothera's Test

- Test for detection of ketone bodies in urine
- Principle
  - Acetoacetic acid and acetone react with sodium nitroprusside (alkaline solution) to form a purple color complex.
- Significance
  - Can detect acetone above 10–20 mg/dL
  - Can detect acetoacetic acid above 1–5 mg/dL
  - Cannot detect beta-hydroxyacetate.
- Procedure
  - Add 5 mL of urine to test tube
  - Add Rothera's reagent to it and mix well
  - Add 1–2 mL of concentrated ammonium hydroxide
  - Observe the results at the interface
- Observations and results
  - Presence of purple permanganate colored ring at the interface – Result positive, i.e., ketone bodies are present.
  - Absence of any purple permanganate colored ring at the interface – Result negative, i.e., ketone bodies are absent.

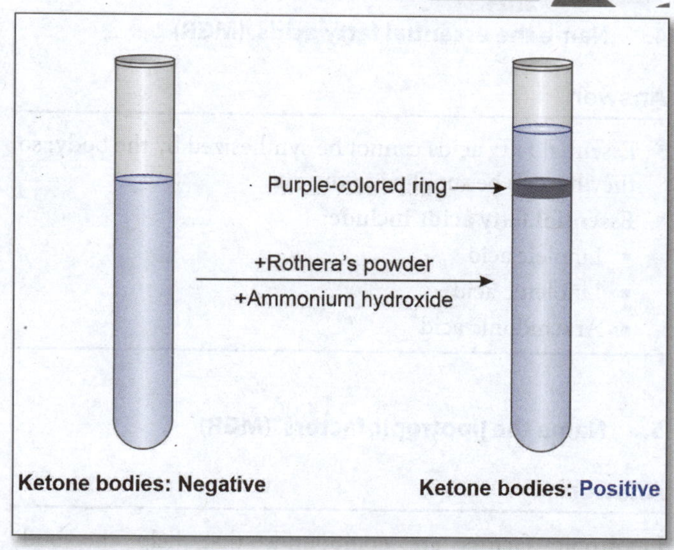

SHORT ANSWER QUESTIONS

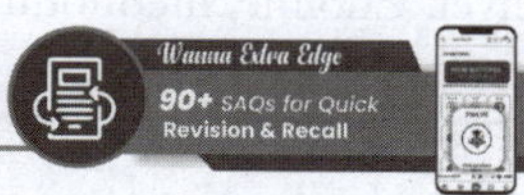

1. What are phospholipids? (MGR)

Answer

Phospholipids are a heterogeneous group of compounds, which contain one or more phosphoric acid residues and a polar group that may be a nitrogenous base, an amino acid or a polyhydroxy alcohol.

2. What saturated fatty acids refer to? (MGR)

Answer

When the carbon atoms in a fatty acid are totally saturated with hydrogen atoms, there are no double bonds between the carbon atoms. This form of fatty acid is referred to as saturated fatty acids, e.g., stearic acid.

3. What are lipids? Write any two functions of lipids. (KUHS, MGR)

Answer

- Lipids are a heterogeneous group of molecules, which are soluble in organic solvents but are sparingly soluble in water.
- Important functions of lipids are:
  - They act as storage form of energy.
  - They make structural components of biomembranes.

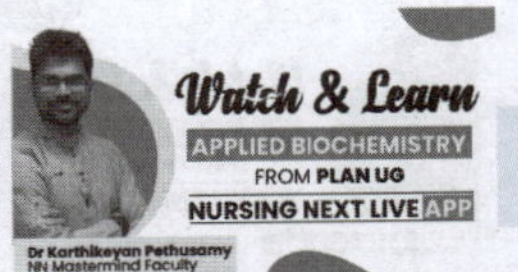

4. Name the essential fatty acids. (MGR)

Answer

- Essential fatty acids cannot be synthesized by the body; so, they have to be supplied in the diet
- **Essential fatty acids include:**
  - Linoleic acid
  - Linolenic acid
  - Arachidonic acid

5. Name the lipotropic factors. (MGR)

Answer

Lipotropic factors are compounds that help the body metabolize fats and prevent the buildup of excess fat in the liver. Choline, methionine, inositol and betaine are lipotropic factors.

6. Name four lipoproteins. (MGR)

Answer

Chylomicron, very-low-density lipoprotein (VLDL), low-density lipoprotein (LDL) and high-density lipoprotein (HDL) are lipoproteins.

7. What is micelle? (KUHS)

Answer

A micelle is a small spherical structure composed of hydrophilic head and hydrophobic tail. In an aqueous environment, such as the digestive tract, micelles are commonly formed by the aggregation of bile salts, fatty acids, monoglycerides, and cholesterol.

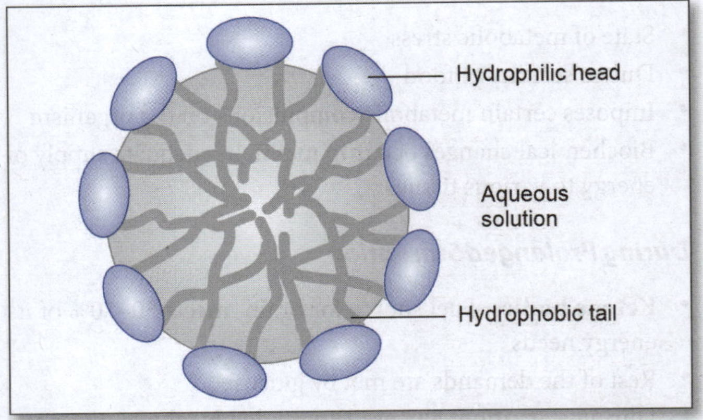

8. Polyunsaturated fatty acids. (KUHS)

Answer

Polyunsaturated fatty acids (PUFAs) have more than one double bond in the molecule and are liquid at room temperature. They are an essential component of cell membranes.

9. Normal serum values of HDL cholesterol and LDL cholesterol. (KUHS)

Answer

Lipoprotein	Normal serum values
HDL cholesterol	>40 mg/dL for men, > 50 mg/dL for women
LDL cholesterol	<130 mg/dL (or <100 mg/dL for individuals at high risk for cardiovascular disease)

CONCEPTUAL REVISION

MULTIPLE CHOICE QUESTIONS

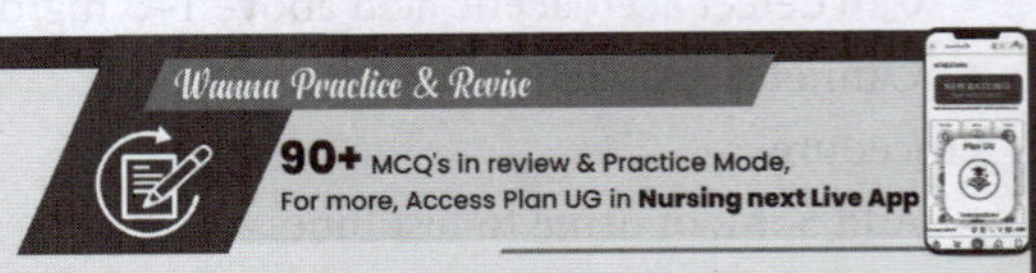

1. Which fatty acid is not synthesized by man?

a. Linoleic acid
b. Stearic acid
c. Palmitic acid
d. Oleic acid

Ans. a. Linoleic acid

2. Which of the following is a cardioprotective fatty acid?

a. Palmitic acid
b. Stearic acid
c. Oleic acid
d. Omega-3-fatty acid

Ans. d. Omega-3-fatty acid

3. The normal concentration of serum bilirubin ranges from:

a. 1.2–1.7 mg/dL
b. 0.5–1.0 mg/200 mL
c. 1.5–2.0 mg/dL
d. 0.2–1.2 mg/dL

Ans. d. 0.2–1.2 mg/dL

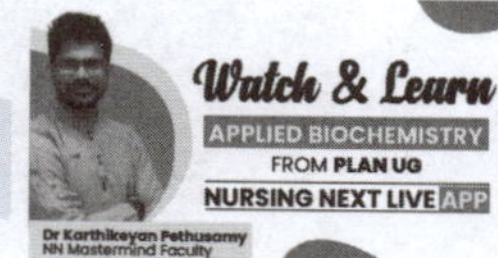

Golden Points

- Acetoacetate, β-hydroxybutyrate and acetone are collectively referred to as ketone bodies (acetone bodies).
- Atherosclerosis (arteriosclerosis) is a disease of arterial wall. It is characterized by the accumulation of cholesterol and its esters in cells, which are derived from monocyte-macrophage line smooth muscle cells. This in turn results in the formation of atherosclerotic plaque, which narrows the blood vessels and serves as the site of thrombus formation.
- Cholesterol content in normal human blood varies from 130 mg to 220 mg/100 mL
- Elevated levels of HDL in plasma protect the body against atherosclerosis.
- Esters of long chain fatty acids with high molecular weight like monohydroxy aliphatic alcohols are called waxes. They are used in the manufacturing of wax-polish.
- Fatty acids are the carboxylic acids with a long hydrocarbon side chain which may be saturated or unsaturated with one or more double bonds.
- HDL serves as a circulating reservoir of apo C-II.
- Lipid is a heterogeneous group of hydrophobic organic molecules found in cells. Sparingly soluble in water but are soluble in organic solvents.
- Lipid profile refers to the estimation of total cholesterol, LDL-cholesterol, HDL-cholesterol and triglycerides in serum. Serum lipids and lipoproteins should be measured after a 10 hours fast because chylomicrons normally are present in plasma up to 10 hours after a meal.
- Lipids are classified into three groups as simple lipids, compound lipids and derived lipids.
- Liver is the primary tissue for de novo synthesis of fatty acids.
- Most fat absorption takes place in the duodenum or jejunum of the small intestine.
- **Omega-3 fatty acids:** α-Linolenic acid is referred to as ω-3 fatty acid.
- Omega-6 fatty acid: Linoleic acid is referred to as ω-6 fatty acid.
- Phospholipids are amphipathic in nature, i.e., they contain both, a hydrophilic head and a long hydrophobic tail.
- Primary function of LDL is to transport cholesterol from liver to the extrahepatic tissues.
- Saturated fatty acids end in word "-anoic", e.g., octadecanoic acid (stearic acid), a fatty acid with 18 carbon atoms. Saturated fatty acids are commonly found in animal fat, e.g., butter.
- Simple lipids are esters of fatty acids with alcohol. These include neutral fats, oils and waxes.
- The oxidation of fatty acids derived from adipose tissue is the major source of energy in hepatic tissue, during prolonged fasting.
- The process of the formation of ketone bodies is called ketogenesis.
- The process of β-oxidation occurs in the mitochondrial matrix.
- Trans (trans) fatty acids are isomers of the normal cis (cis) fatty acids, produced when PUFAs are hydrogenated, such as in the production of margarine and vegetable shortening.
- Unsaturated fatty acids end with word "-enoic", e.g., octadecenoic acid (oleic acid), a fatty acid having 18 carbon atoms and one double bond. Unsaturated fatty acids have one or more double bonds.

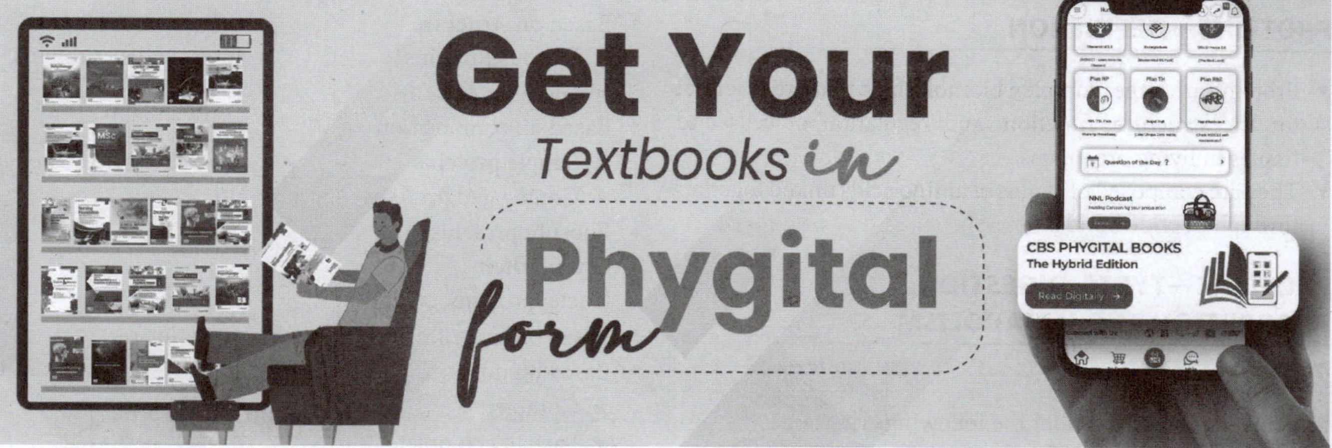

CHAPTER

3

Amino Acids and Proteins

CONCEPTUAL THEORY

Terminology

150+ key terminologies for Quick Recall & Revision

Coenzyme: A coenzyme is a dialyzable, thermostable, low-molecular weight, organic substance.

Cystinuria: It involves the carrier for sulfur-containing amino acid, cystine and the basic amino acids, i.e., lysine and arginine.

Enzymes: Enzymes are organic molecules that increase the rate of a biochemical reaction without being utilized in the overall process. They are non-dialyzable, colloidal particles which are thermolabile proteins with highly specific catalytic activity. An enzyme increases rate of a chemical reaction by lowering its free energy barrier that separates a substrate (reactant) from the product.

Hartnup disease: The inability to reabsorb amino acids by the kidney manifests in the excretion of neutral amino acids including tryptophan and other indole derivatives in the urine, resulting in neutral aminoaciduria.

Hydrolases: Hydrolases bring about hydrolysis of a substrate with the addition of a molecule of water.

Isomerases: Isomerases are involved in the conversion of one isomeric form of the substrate into another.

Ligases: Ligases are involved in the synthesis of a product by linking two substrates together.

Lyases: Lyases catalyze splitting of a substrate into two products without the addition of water.

Oxidoreductases: Oxidoreductases are involved in oxidation and/or reduction of the substrate.

Primary structure: Primary structure of a protein refers to the order and sequence of amino acids in a protein chain.

Protein: Protein is a class of natural products, which contain nitrogen.

Secondary structure: Secondary structure of a protein refers to folding and twisting pattern of a polypeptide chain, i.e., the spatial arrangement of a polypeptide. Secondary structures include α-helix and β-sheets.

Tertiary structure: Tertiary structure involves intramolecular folding of the polypeptide chain thereby forming a compact three dimensional structure which has a specific shape.

Transamination: Transamination is a process of transfer of the α-amino group from an amino acid to a keto acid.

Transferases: Transferases catalyze transfer of a particular group from one substrate to another.

Urea cycle: Urea cycle is the process by which ammonia, i.e., is a highly toxic substance, is converted to urea, which is a less toxic, water soluble, excretory waste product, in the liver.

PROTEINS—DEFINITION

- Proteins are large, complex biomolecules that are essential for the structure, function, and regulation of cells and tissues in living organisms.
- They are composed of chains of amino acids linked together through peptide bonds.

PROTEINS—TYPES, DIGESTION, ABSORPTION AND METABOLISM

Types

Proteins are classified under the following criteria:

- Based on structure
  - Fibrous Proteins
  - Globular proteins
  - Intermediate proteins
- Based on composition
  - Simple proteins
  - Conjugated proteins
- Phosphoproteins
- Glycoproteins
- Nucleoproteins, etc.
- Based on function (Functional classification)
- Based on quality
  - Complete
  - Partially complete
  - Incomplete

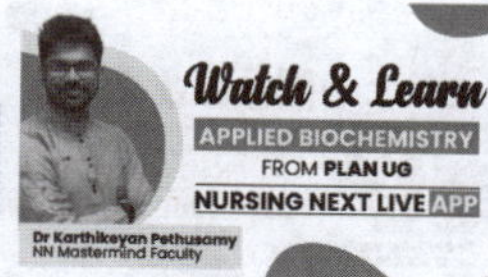

Sources of Protein

- Dietary
- Endogenous

Note: Dietary proteins are denatured on cooking and therefore, easily digested.

- *Enzymes responsible for degradation of protein*
  - Endopeptidases (proteases)
    - Break the internal peptide bonds
    - Examples – pepsin, trypsin
  - Exopeptidases
    - Act on the peptide bonds of terminal amino acids.
    - Two types
      - Carboxypeptidases – act on C terminal amino acid
      - Aminopeptidases – act on N-terminal amino acid

Digestion of Proteins by Gastric Secretion

- Protein digestion in the stomach begins with the secretion of hydrochloric acid (HCl).
- Pepsinogen, an inactive proenzyme, is then activated by HCl to form the active enzyme pepsin, which breaks down proteins into smaller fragments.
- In infants and children, rennin (chymosin) is present in gastric juice and aids in the digestion of milk proteins.

Digestion of Proteins by Pancreatic Proteases

- Pancreatic proteases are secreted as inactive zymogens.
- The zymogens are activated by two polypeptide hormones: **cholecystokinin (CCK)** and **secretin.**
- CCK activates trypsinogen, which then activates the other zymogens.
- The activated proteases are trypsin, chymotrypsin, and elastase.
- Trypsin cleaves the peptide bond (-CO-) carbonyl groups contributed by lysine or arginine.
- Chymotrypsin cleaves the peptide bond after hydrophobic amino acids, such as phenylalanine, leucine, and isoleucine.
- The pancreatic proteases are active at neutral pH. The gastric pH is neutralized by pancreatic $NaHCO_3$.
- The digestion of proteins by pancreatic proteases results in the formation of small peptides and free amino acids.

Digestion of Proteins by Small Intestinal Enzymes

- Small intestine enzymes: Aminopeptidases and dipeptidases.
- Produce small peptides (usually dipeptides) and free amino acids.

Absorption of amino acids and dipeptides

- Absorbed by intestinal epithelial cells
- *Two mechanisms*
  - Absorbed by Na^+ dependent active process
  - γ- glutamyl cycle or Meister cycle
    - Involves glutathione

AMINO ACIDS

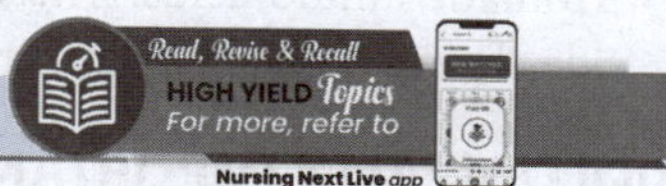

- Amino acids – building blocks of proteins.
- Alpha amino substituted carboxylic acid.

Classification of Amino Acids

- Amino acids are classified into two main groups:
  - Essential amino acids
  - Nonessential amino acids.

Essential Amino Acids

Essential amino acids are those that the human body cannot synthesize and must be obtained from the diet.

- There are nine essential amino acids:
  1. Histidine
  2. Isoleucine
  3. Leucine
  4. Lysine
  5. Methionine
  6. Phenylalanine
  7. Threonine
  8. Tryptophan
  9. Valine

Nonessential Amino Acids

Nonessential amino acids are those that the body can synthesize from other compounds.

- They are:
  - Alanine
  - Asparagine
  - Aspartic Acid
  - Cysteine
  - Glutamic Acid
  - Glutamine
  - Glycine
  - Proline
  - Serine
  - Tyrosine

Amino Acids can also be Classified According to their Side Chain

- Nonpolar amino acids: These amino acids have nonpolar side chains. E.g., alanine, valine, etc.
- Polar amino acids: These amino acids have polar side chains. E.g., serine, threonine, etc.

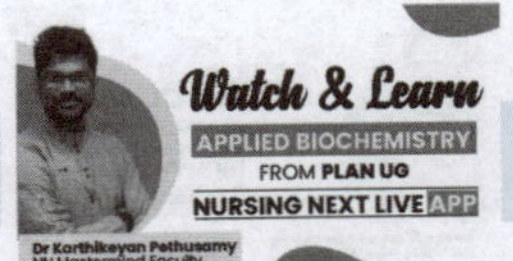

- Charged amino acids: These amino acids have charged side chains. E.g., lysine, arginine
- Aromatic amino acids: These amino acids have aromatic side chains. E.g., phenylalanine, tyrosine

BIOLOGICALLY IMPORTANT COMPOUNDS SYNTHESIZED FROM VARIOUS AMINO ACIDS

- There are many biologically important compounds that are synthesized from various amino acids. Following are some examples:
  - Hormones. E.g., adrenaline, noradrenaline
  - Coenzymes. E.g., NAD^+, $NADP^+$
  - Neurotransmitter. E.g., dopamine, serotonin
  - Pigments. E.g., melanin, bilirubin
  - Nitrogenous bases (building blocks of DNA)
  - Immunoglobulin.

INBORN ERRORS OF AMINO ACID METABOLISM

Table 3.1: Inborn errors of aromatic amino acids metabolism

Metabolic disorder	Deficient enzyme
Phenylketonuria	Phenylalanine hydroxylase
Tyrosinemia type I	Fumarylacetoacetate hydrolase
Tyrosinemia type II	Tyrosine transaminase
Alkaptonuria	Homogentisic acid oxidase
Albinism	Tyrosinase

PLASMA PROTEIN – TYPES, FUNCTION AND NORMAL VALUES

- Total concentration of plasma proteins–6-8 g/dL
- *Types of plasma proteins*
  - Albumin
  - Globulins
  - Fibrinogen

Albumin

- Albumin – major constituent of plasma proteins
- Normal concentration – 3.5–5.0 g/dL
- **Functions of Albumin**
  - *Osmotic function*
    - Maintains blood volume and body fluid distribution
  - *Transport function*
    - Binds to several compounds such as free fatty acids, bilirubin, steroid hormones, calcium, copper and aids in their transportation in the circulation
  - *Nutritive function*
    - Source of amino acids for tissue protein synthesis
  - *Buffering action*

Globulins

- Normal plasma range of Globulin: 2.3 to 3.5 g/dL
- Electrophorectically separated into:
  - α1 globulin
  - α2 globulin
  - β globulin
  - γ globulin

Alpha 1 globulins

- Glycoproteins
- α1 antitrypsin – serine protease inhibitor
- α1 Lipoproteins – transport cholesterol and phospholipids
- Retinol binding proteins – transport vitamin A
- Thyroxine binding globulin – transports thyroid hormones

Alpha 2 globulin

- α2- macroglobulin – antitrypsin and antiplasmin activity
- Haptoglobulins – bind with plasma free hemoglobulin and prevent its excretion
- Prothrombin – participates in blood coagulation
- Ceruloplasmin – transport of copper

Beta globulin

- Beta lipoproteins – transport triacylglycerols and cholesterol
- Transferrin – transports iron
- Hemopexin – transports heme
- Plasminogen – forms plasmin

γ globulin

- Immunoglobulins – antibody functions

Fibrinogen

Participates in blood coagulation

CAUSES OF PROTEINURIA, HYPOPROTEINEMIA, HYPERGAMMAGLOBULINEMIA

Causes of Proteinuria

- Prerenal causes:
  - Heavy exercise
  - Fever
  - Hypertension
  - Multiple myeloma
  - Eclampsia
- Renal causes:
  - Acute and chronic Glomerulonephritis
  - Renal Tubular dysfunction
  - Polycystic kidney
  - Nephrotic syndrome

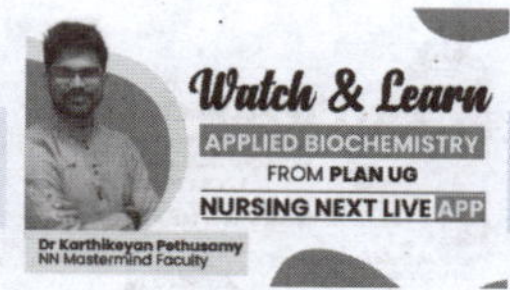

- Post renal causes:
  - Acute and chronic cystitis
  - Tuberculosis cystitis

Causes of Hypoproteinemia

- Overhydration
- Excessive loss through kidney such as in nephrotic syndrome, and from the skin after burns or loss through the intestine such as in protein losing enteropathy
- Decreased synthesis such as in a severe liver disease
- Reduced intake either due to severe dietary protein deficiencies like kwashiorkor or severe malabsorption.

Causes of Hypergammaglobulinemia

- Increase in globins occurs most commonly in advanced liver disease (e.g., cirrhosis)
- Chronic infectious diseases
- Multiple myeloma

PRINCIPLE OF ELECTROPHORESIS

- The movement of charged molecules in an electric field toward the oppositely charged electrode
- Negatively charged particles move toward the cathode, while positively charged particles move toward anode.
- Electrophoresis is a technique used to separate molecules based on their size and charge.
- It is a common laboratory method used to separate serum proteins, lipoproteins and immunoglobulins.
- Electrophoresis is used to analyze DNA, and RNA.
- The concentration of these components can be determined by densitometric scanning.
- Factors affecting electrophoresis are:
  - pH of the medium
  - Net charge on the particles
  - Temperature
  - Molecular weight
  - Shape of molecule
  - Solvation of ions
  - Viscosity of solution
  - Extent of current
- *Different types of electrophoresis include:*
  - Zone electrophoresis
    - Paper
    - Gel
  - Isoelectric focusing
  - Immunoelectrophoresis

CONCEPTUAL EXERCISES

LONG ANSWER QUESTIONS

1. Describe urea cycle and how it is regulated? What is the normal blood urea level? (MGR)

Answer

Introduction

- Ammonia is released during amino acid metabolism.
- Urea cycle is a metabolic pathway that converts ammonia to urea
- Exists as NH_4^+ ions (ammonium ions)
- Reference range for serum urea – 10–40 mg/dL

Detoxification Process

- Known as urea cycle/Krebs-Henseleit cycle
- Urea is the end product of protein metabolism
- Ammonia is converted to urea
- Ammonia is toxic, while urea is nontoxic
- Urea is excreted in urine.
- Takes place partly in mitochondria and partly in cytosol

Regulation of Urea Cycle

- Key regulating enzyme of urea cycle is carbamoyl phosphate synthase.
- This enzyme is stimulated by:
  - N-acetylglutamate
  - High protein diet
  - Starvation

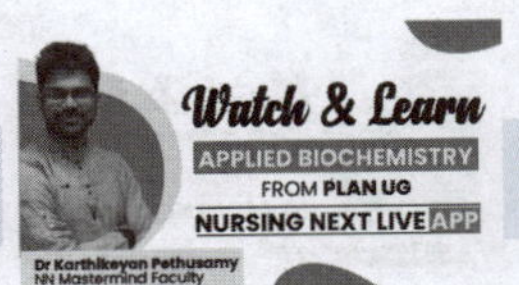

Target High Next Nursing **DECODE**

Urea Cycle

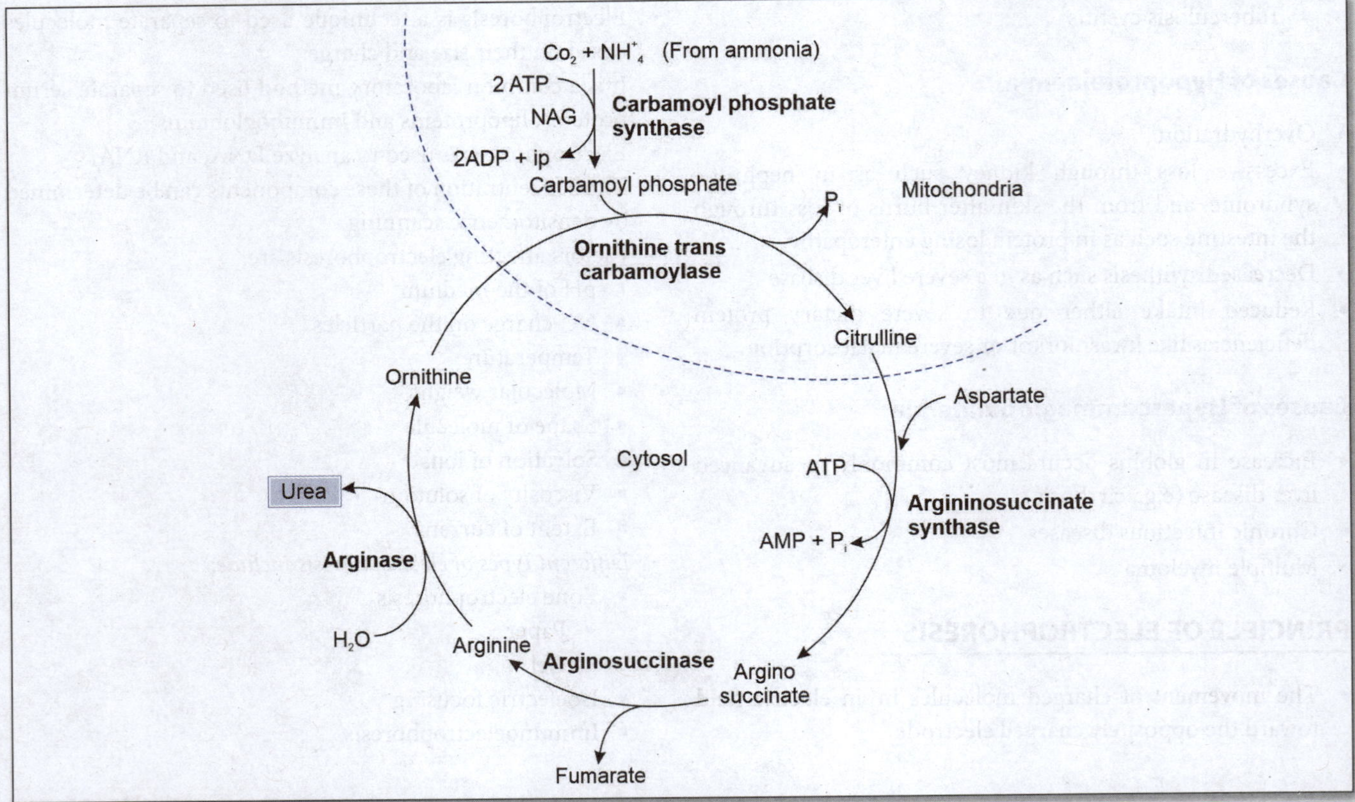

Step 1: Formation of Carbamoyl Phosphate

Carbamoyl phosphate synthase I

- Catalyzes the condensation of **NH ions** with CO_2 to form carbamoyl phosphate
- Present in mitochondria
- Consumes 2 ATPs and N-acetyl glutamate
- Irreversible step

Step 2: Formation of Citrulline

Citrulline is synthesized from:

- Carbamoyl phosphate synthase I
- Ornithine by ornithine transcarbamoylase

Step 3: Formation of Arginosuccinate

- Arginosuccinate is produced from citrulline in the presence of enzyme arginosuccinate synthase.
- **The second amino group of urea is involved here.**
- ATP is broken down to AMP.

Step 4: Formation of Arginine

- Arginosuccinate is broken down to arginine and fumarate
- Catalyzed by arginosuccinase

Step 5: Formation of Urea

- Enzyme – Arginase
- Arginine is broken down to urea and ornithine
- Ornithine enters mitochondria and is reused in urea cycle.

Overall Reaction

NH_4^+ *(from ammonia)* + CO_2 + Aspartate + 3 ATP Urea

2. Describe the biologically important compounds derived from phenylalanine. Mention the inborn errors associated with phenylalanine. (KUHS)

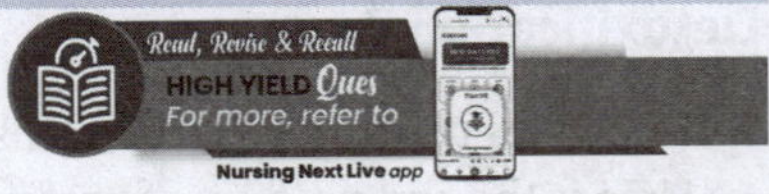

Answer

Introduction

- Phenylalanine is classified as an aromatic amino acid due to its chemical structure containing a phenyl group.
- Phenylalanine is an essential amino acid that serves as a precursor for the synthesis of various biologically important compounds.

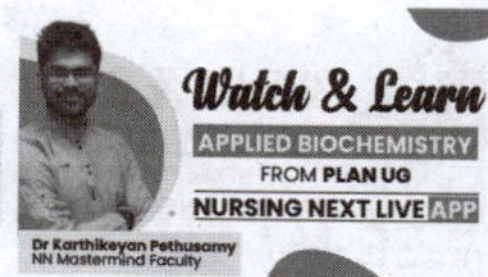

- **Following are the biologically important compounds derived from phenylalanine:**
  - Thyrosine: Phenylalanine is converted to tyrosine through hydroxylation. Tyrosine involved as precursor in the synthesis of:
    - Epinephrine
    - Norepinephrine
    - Dopamine (catecholamines)
    - Thyroid hormones
    - Melanin
    - Precursors for glycolysis and lipogenesis

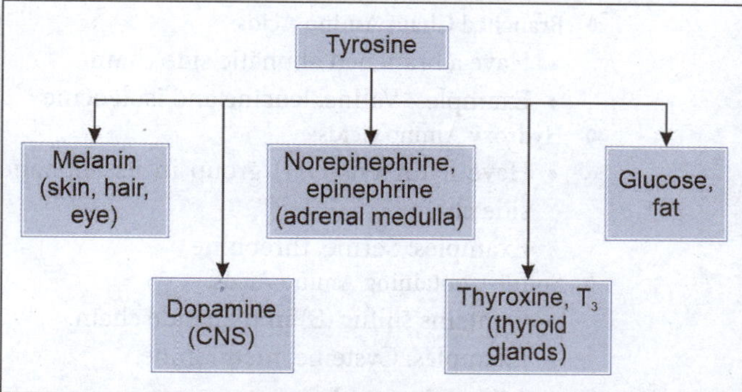

Biochemical Significance

- *Synthesis of melanin:*
  - Pigment of skin, hair, eyes
  - Synthesized from tyrosine
  - Enzyme involved – tyrosinase
- *Synthesis of thyroid hormones:*
  - Thyroid hormones are:
    - Thyroxine (tetraiodothyronine)
    - Triiodothyronine
  - Produced from tyrosine residues of thyroglobulin
  - Tyrosine ring is iodized to mono-, di-, tri and tetra iodothyronine.
- *Synthesis of catecholamines:*
  - Tyrosine acts as precursor for the synthesis of epinephrine, norepinephrine, dopamine
  - Occurs in CNS and adrenal medulla
  - Enzyme – tyrosine hydroxylase

Inborn Errors Associated with Phenyalanine Metabolism

1. **Phenylketonuria**
   - Deficiency of enzyme - phenylalanine hydroxylase
   - Autosomal recessive disorder
   - Characterized by:
     - Mental retardation
     - Hypopigmentation
2. **Tyrosinemia Type I**
   - Deficient enzyme – maleylacetoacetate isomerase
   - Characteristics:
     - Liver failure
     - Renal dysfunction
     - Polyneuropathy
3. **Tyrosinemia Type II**
   - Enzyme defective – tyrosine transaminase
   - Characterized by:
     - Dermatitis
     - Eye lesion
     - Mental retardation
4. **Alkaptonuria**
   - Defective enzyme – homogentisate oxidase
   - Accumulation of homogentisate occurs - undergoes oxidation - produces alkapton – causes ochronosis
   - Characteristics:
     - Black colored urine
     - Arthritis
5. **Albinism**
   - Deficient melanin synthesis
   - Autosomal recessive disorder
   - Due to:
     - Deficiency of enzyme tyrosinase
   - Characteristics
     - Sensitivity to sunlight
     - Susceptibility to skin cancer
     - Photophobia

SHORT NOTES

1. Classification of amino acids. (MGR)

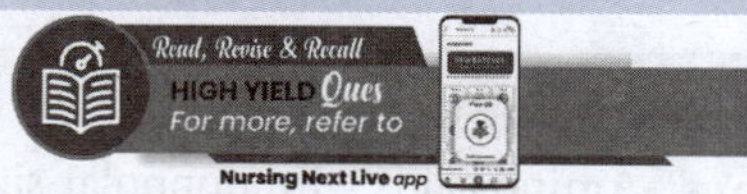

Answer

Classification of Amino Acids

- ***According to their dietary requirement***
  - Essential amino acids:
    - Amino acids that are not synthesized by the human body.
    - Need to be supplied through diet.
    - They include:
      - Leucine
      - Isoleucine
      - Histidine
      - Lysine
      - Tryptophan
      - Phenylalanine

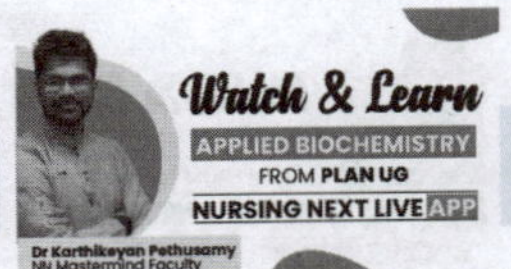

- Methionine
- Threonine
- Valine

- Semiessential amino acids
  - Amino acids that are synthesized by the body from the essential amino acids.
  - So, these must be provided through diet to prevent the deficiency of essential amino acids.
  - They include:
    - Arginine
    - Tyrosine
    - Cysteine
    - Glycine
    - Serine
- Nonessential amino acids
  - Amino acids that can be synthesized by the human body.
  - They include:
    - Glutamic acid
    - Aspartic acid
    - Alanine
    - Proline
    - Hydroxyproline

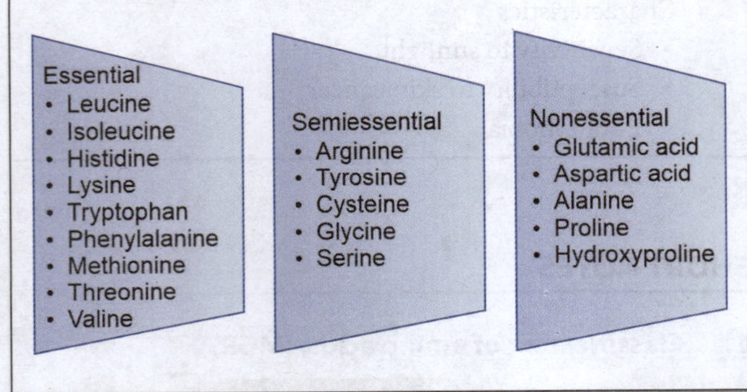

- **According to polarity**
  - Amino acids with nonpolar side chains
    - **Examples:** Glycine, alanine, valine, leucine, isoleucine, methionine, phenylalanine, tryptophan and proline.
  - Amino acids with polar side chains
    - Have uncharged polar side chains with zero net charge at neutral pH
      - **Examples:** Serine, threonine and tyrosine
    - Have charged polar side chains as they contain an additional amide group
      - **Examples:** Asparagine and glutamine.
- **According to their structure**
  - Neutral amino acid
    - These amino acids are neutral in reaction.
    - Have one amino acid group ($-NH_2$) and one carboxyl group (-COOH).
    - Also referred to as mono amino monocarboxylic acids.
    - According to the presence of the R group, these amino acids are further subdivided into:
      - **Aliphatic amino acids:**
        - Simple Amino Acids:
          - Have either hydrogen or a methyl group in the aliphatic side chain.
          - Glycine has hydrogen (H), whereas alanine has a methyl group ($-CH_3$) as a side chain
        - Branched Chain Amino Acids:
          - Have a branched aliphatic side chain
          - Examples: Valine, leucine and isoleucine
        - Hydroxy Amino Acids:
          - Have hydroxyl(-OH) group in its aliphatic side chain.
          - Examples: Serine, threonine
        - Sulfur-Containing Amino Acids:
          - Contains sulfur (S) in their side chain.
          - Examples: Cysteine, methionine.
      - **Aromatic amino acids**
        - Have an aromatic ring in their side chains.
        - Examples - Phenylalanine (alanine attached to a phenyl group), tyrosine (4-hydroxyphenylalanine) and tryptophan (alanine attached to an indole ring)
      - **Acidic amino acids**
        - Have more than one, generally two, **carboxyl groups**.
        - Also referred to as monoamino dicarboxylic acids. These are **aspartic acid** and **glutamic acid**
        - Amide of aspartic acid - **asparagine**
        - Amide of glutamine acid - **glutamine**
      - **Basic amino acids**
        - Basic amino acids have **one carboxyl group** with either **more than one amino group** in its aliphatic side chain **or a heterocyclic ring,** which is basic in reaction.
        - Examples: Lysine, arginine and histidine.
- **Imino Acid**
  - In addition to the above amino acids that are found in most of the proteins, some proteins, e.g., collagen, are rich in proline.
  - Proline does not contain a primary alpha-amino group (-NH) in its side chain but has a secondary imino group (-NH-), which forms a part of the heterocyclic ring. Hence, proline is not an amino acid but imino acid.
    - However, for uniformity, proline is included in the list of alpha –amino acid. Proline can be converted to its 4-hydroxyl derivative, called **Hydroxyproline,** in the body.

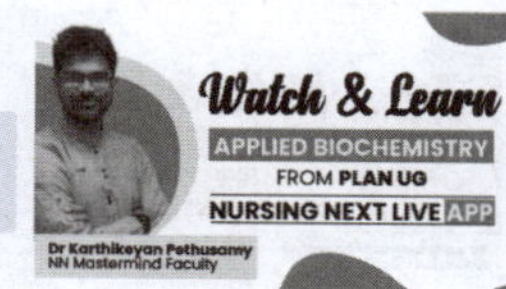

2. Essential amino acids.

Or

Differentiate between semiessential amino acids and essential amino acids. (KUHS)

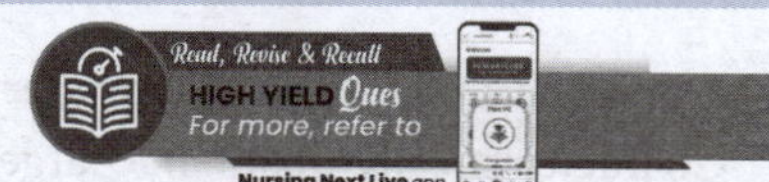

Answer

Introduction

- 24 amino acids are required for protein synthesis and other biological activities
- All of these are not synthesized by body.
- Those that cannot be synthesized by the body – essential
- Those amino acids that can be synthesized by the body – nonessential

Essential or Indispensable Amino Acids

- Cannot be synthesized by the body
- Need to be supplemented in the diet
- Required for growth and maintenance of the human body
- Nine essential amino acids are:
  - Valine
  - Histidine
  - Isoleucine
  - Leucine
  - Lysine
  - Methionine
  - Phenylalanine
  - Threonine
  - Tryptophan

Semiessential Amino acids

- Those amino acids that can be synthesized by adults and not by children
- Include:
  - Arginine
  - Histidine

Conditionally Essential Amino Acids

- Those amino acids that can be synthesized by the body to a limited extent.
- But in certain conditions, either their synthesis is limited or their requirement surpasses the body's capacity to synthesize them.
- Need to be supplemented in diet during certain pathophysiological conditions
- These are:
  - Arginine
  - Cysteine
  - Glycine
  - Glutamine
  - Proline
  - Tyrosine

3. Write a note on classification of proteins. (MGR)

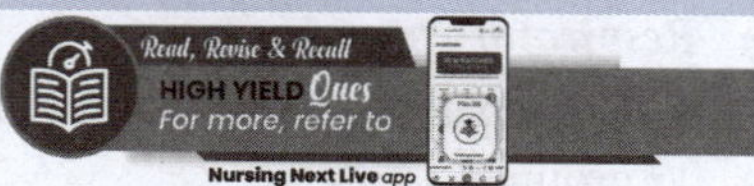

Answer

Classification Based on Structure

- ***Fibrous proteins***
  - Linear in shape
  - Function
    - Perform the structural functions in cells
  - Examples – collagen, Myosin, Silk, Keratin
- ***Globular proteins***
  - Spherical or globular in shape
  - Functions
    - Antibodies
    - Certain hormones
    - Enzymes
  - Examples – insulin, hemoglobin, RNA and DNA polymerases
- ***Intermediate proteins***
  - Function
    - Blood clotting
  - Example – fibrinogen

Classification Based on Composition

- **Simple proteins**
  - Composed of only amino acids
  - Example – albumin in egg white
- **Conjugated or complex proteins**
  - Protein + Nonprotein molecule
  - Examples – lipoprotein, nucleoprotein, hemoprotein
- **Derived proteins**
  - Obtained as a result of heat or chemical action on simple or complex proteins.
  - Example – polypeptides

Functional Classification of Proteins

- ***Structural proteins***
  - Part of the connective tissue, cartilage, tendons, bone
  - Mainly fibrous proteins
  - Insoluble in water
  - Examples – collagen, elastin, keratin
- ***Enzymes***
  - Biological catalysts
  - Reduces the activation energy of reactants
  - Mostly globular conjugated proteins
  - Examples – DNA polymerase, Lipase

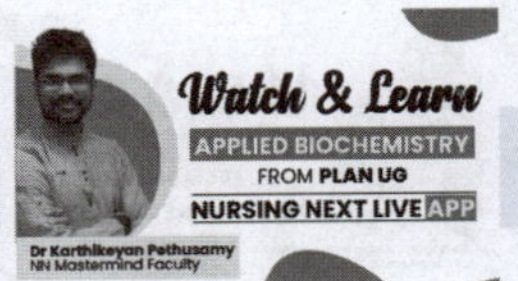

- ***Hormones***
  - Proteinaceous hormones
  - Examples – insulin, ACH, Glucagon
- ***Respiratory proteins***
  - Conjugated Proteins containing chrome as prosthetic group
  - Examples – hemoglobin, myoglobin
- ***Transport proteins***
  - Transport materials in cells
  - Form channels in plasma membrane
  - Examples – transferrin, albumin
- ***Contractile proteins***
  - Part of the muscle
  - Examples – actin, Myosin
- ***Storage proteins***
  - Act as storage form of metal ions and amino acids
  - Examples – ferritin, casein, gluten
- ***Toxins***
  - Toxic in nature
  - Example – snake venom

Classification Based on Quality

- ***Complete proteins***
  - Contain all essential amino acids in sufficient quantities.
- ***Partially complete proteins***
  - Do not contain all essential amino acids
  - Are used to sustain life but do not promote growth.
- ***Incomplete proteins***
  - Deficient in essential amino acids.
  - Do not promote growth and repair.

4. Give one example of each transport protein and fibrous protein. (DU)

Answer

Transport Proteins

- Also known as transmembrane pump
- Types of transport proteins include carrier proteins and membrane transport protein.
- These are involved in the movement of ions and molecules across the cell membrane.
- Also assist in the movement of molecules by facilitated diffusion.
- Form channels in plasma membrane
- Examples
  - Transferrin
  - Albumin

Fibrous Proteins

- Exhibit certain mechanical properties.
- Characteristically contain large amounts of regular secondary structures and have long rod-like shapes.
- Have low solubility in water
- Functions
  - Protective
  - Connective
  - Supportive
  - Component of skin and cornea
- Examples
  - Collagen
  - Keratin
  - Tropomyosin

5. Differentiate between integral proteins and transmembrane proteins. (KUHS)

Answer

Integral proteins and transmembrane proteins are both types of proteins that are embedded in the cell membrane.

Integral Proteins

Peripheral integral proteins: Peripheral integral proteins are only partially embedded in the membrane.

Integral membrane proteins: Integral membrane proteins are completely embedded in the membrane.

Transmembrane Proteins

Transmembrane proteins are a type of integral protein that spans the cell membrane. They have a hydrophobic region that runs through the middle of the membrane, and they have hydrophilic regions on either side of the membrane.

There are some key differences between the two types of proteins.

- All integral proteins are not transmembrane proteins, but all transmembrane proteins are integral proteins.
- Integral proteins are also related to processes other than facilitated diffusion.
- Both types of proteins play a variety of important roles in cells, including transport, signal transduction, and cell adhesion.

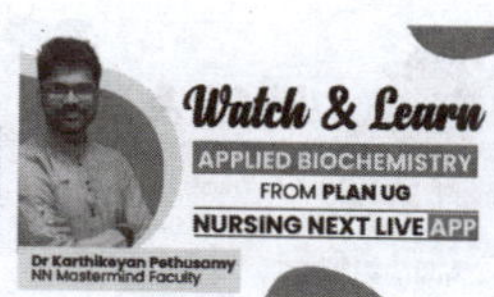

6. Differentiate between essential amino acids and nonessential amino acids. (KUHS)

Answer

Differences between the essential and nonessential amino acids

Features	Essential amino acids	Nonessential amino acids
Definition	Amino acids that cannot be synthesized by the body	Amino acids that can be synthesized by the body
Source	Foods such as soya, egg, chicken etc are important sources of essential amino acids	These are produced in the body
Biological role	Growth and repair of body tissues Formation of neurotransmitters	Synthesis of RBC and WBC Removal of toxins Promotion of brain function
Deficiency	Probability of deficiency is high if dietary intake is inadequate	Probability of deficiency is rare
Examples	**Essential amino acids:** Histidine, Isoleucine, Leucine, Lysine, Methionine, Phenylalanine, Threonine, Tryptophan, Valine	**Nonessential amino acids:** Alanine, asparagine, aspartic acid, cysteine, glutamic acid, glutamine, glycine, proline, serine, tyrosine

7. Conjugated protein. (KUHS)

Answer

Conjugated or Complex Proteins

- Protein that functions in combination with nonprotein molecule attached by a covalent bond.
- Protein + Nonprotein molecule
- The nonprotein part of the conjugated protein is known as prosthetic group.
- Most prosthetic groups are vitamin in nature.
- Conjugated are classified on the basis of chemical nature of their prosthetic groups.
- Examples:
  - Lipoprotein – lipids + proteins
  - Nucleoprotein – nucleic acid + proteins
  - Hemoprotein – heme + proteins
  - Glycoprotein – Carbohydrate + proteins

Lipoproteins

- Lipids + proteins
- Most lipids are phospholipids
- Primary component of cell membrane

Nucleoprotein

- Nucleic acid + proteins
- Present mainly in the chromosomes
- These include ribosomes, nucleosomes, viral nucleocapsid proteins

Chromoproteins

- Pigmented prosthetic part + proteins
- It can act as phytochrome and phototropin
- Examples include:
  - Hemoglobin – iron containing heme
  - Rhodopsin – carotenoid pigment
  - Cytochrome – heme
  - Flavoproteins – riboflavin
  - Hemocyanin – copper

Phosphoproteins

- Phosphoric acid + protein
- Water insoluble
- Milk protein and egg yolk are its examples

Glycoproteins

- Carbohydrate + protein
- Present on the surface of lipid bilayer of cell membranes

Metalloproteins

- Metal + proteins
- Integral part of the structure

8. Write short note on transamination. (MGR)

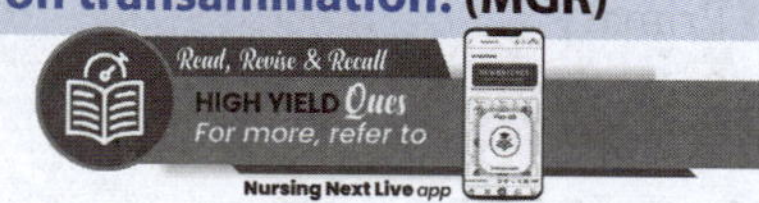

Answer

Transamination

- Transfer of amino group from amino acid to keto acid

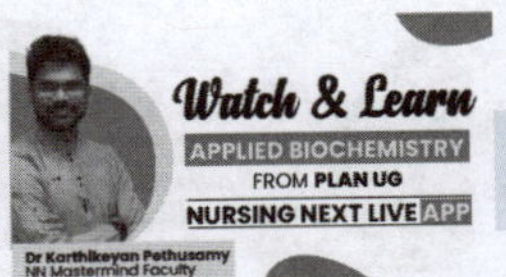

- Initiating point for amino acid metabolism
- Involves interconversion of amino acids and keto acids
- Enzymes involved are transaminases.

Salient Features of Transamination

- Enzyme transaminases require pyridoxal phosphate as coenzyme
- No free amino group or ammonia is released, only transfer of groups
- Reversible reaction
- Essential for the synthesis of nonessential amino acids
- It diverts excess amino acids for energy production
- Amino acids undergo transamination to finally concentrate nitrogen in glutamate.
- All amino acids except *lysine, threonine, proline and hydroxyproline participate* in transamination
- Transaminases have diagnostic and prognostic importance.

Mechanism of Transamination

Occurs in two stages:

- Transfer of amino group from the amino acid to the pyridoxal phosphate to form pyridoxamine phosphate.
- Transfer of amino group from pyridoxamine phosphate to the keto acid.

Clinical Significance

- Aspartate amino transferase (AST) – elevated in myocardial infarction
- Alanine amino transferase (ALT) – elevated in liver disorders.

9. Write a note on gout disease. (MGR)

Answer

Gout

- Metabolic disorder associated with excessive production of uric acid.
- Blood uric acid levels >7 mg/dL in males and >6 mg/dL in females lead to uric acid crystal deposition in urinary tract.

Types

- Primary
- Secondary

Primary Gout

- Inborn error of metabolism due to overproduction of uric acid
- Related to increased synthesis of purine nucleotides
- *Metabolic defects in primary gout*
  - *PRPP synthase*
    - Normally it is under feedback control by purine nucleotides
    - Variant forms not subjected to feedback control – lead to increased production of purines
  - *PRPP glutamylamidotransferase*
    - Lack of feedback control leads to increased purine synthesis
  - *HGPRT deficiency*
    - Leads to defect in purine salvage pathway
    - Decreased utilization of purines
    - Decreased levels of IMP and GMP
  - *Glucose-6-phosphatase deficiency*
    - Increased utilization of glucose-6-phosphate for HMP shunt
      - Increased production of ribose 5 phosphate and PRPP
      - Increased purine production
  - *Increased glutathione reductase*
    - Increased NADPH+
    - Increased HMP shunt – increased ribose – 5 phosphate
    - Thus, increased purine synthesis

Secondary Gout

- Due to various diseases causing increased synthesis or decreased excretion of uric acid
- *Causes of secondary gout*
  - *Increased uric acid synthesis*
  - Increased degradation of nucleic acids
- Seen in:
  - Leukemias
  - Polycythemia
  - Lymphoma
  - Psoriasis
- Increased tissue breakdown
  - Seen in:
    - Trauma
    - Starvation
- *Decreased uric acid excretion*
- Impaired renal function

Signs and Symptoms

- Painful joints
- Gouty arthritis (big toe)
- Urolithiasis and renal damage in chronic gout.

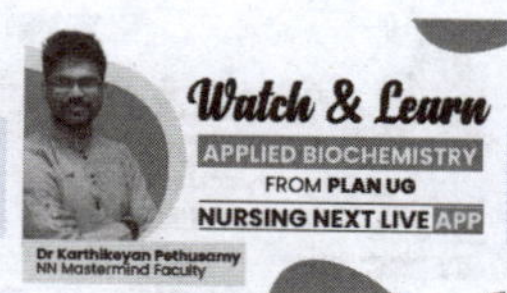

Management of Gout

- Drug of choice – Allopurinol
  - Acts as competitive inhibitor of xanthine oxidase, thereby inhibiting the conversion of hypoxanthine and xanthine to uric acid
  - Allopurinol oxidizes to form alloxanthine – more potent inhibitor
- Uricosuric agents
  - Prevent renal reabsorption of uric acid; thus, more uric acid is excreted in urine
  - Dietary restriction of purines and alcohol

10. Write a note on digestion and absorption of proteins. (MGR)

Answer

Introduction

- Dietary proteins are denatured on cooking and therefore easily digested.
- *Enzymes responsible for degradation of protein*
  - Endopeptidases (proteases)
    - Break the internal peptide bonds
    - Examples – pepsin, trypsin
  - Exopeptidases
    - Act on the peptide bonds of terminal amino acids.
    - Two types:
      - Carboxypeptidases – act on C terminal amino acid
      - Aminopeptidases – act on N-terminal amino acid

Digestion of Proteins by Gastric Secretion

- Protein digestion begins in stomach by
  - Hydrochloric acid
    - pH of stomach is <2
    - This causes:
      - Denaturation of proteins – makes proteins more susceptible to proteases
      - Killing of certain microorganisms
  - Pepsinogen – protease proenzyme
    - Converted to active pepsin by either autocatalysis or by gastric HCl.
    - Cleaves peptide bonds formed by amino groups of phenylalanine or tyrosine or leucine
    - Results in peptides and few amino acids which also act as stimulants for the release of the hormone cholecystokinin from duodenum.
  - Rennin
    - Also known as chymosin
    - Found in infants and children
    - Involved in curdling of milk
    - Absent in adults

Digestion of Proteins by Pancreatic Proteases

- Secreted as zymogens
  - Activated by two polypeptide hormones
    - Cholecystokinin
    - Secretin
- Pancreatic proteases
  - Trypsin
    - Cleaves the peptide bond (-CO-) carbonyl groups contributed by lysine or arginine
  - Chymotrypsin
    - Elastase
    - Active at neutral pH
    - Gastric pH is neutralized by pancreatic $NaHCO_3$
    - Results in the formation of small peptides and free amino acids.

Digestion of Proteins by Small Intestinal Enzymes

- Aminopeptidases and dipeptidases
- Produce small peptides (usually dipeptides) and free amino acids.

Absorption of Amino Acids and Dipeptides

- Absorbed by intestinal epithelial cells
- *Two mechanisms*
  - Absorbed by Na^+ dependent active process
  - γ- glutamyl cycle or Meister cycle
    - Involves glutathione

11. Write a short note on deamination. (DU)

Answer

Deamination

- Process of removal of the alpha – amino group from amino acids is referred to as deamination.
- It may take place either by oxidative or nonoxidative process.

Sites of Deamination

- Liver
- Kidney

Oxidative Deamination

- Liver and kidney contain several enzymes which catalyze deamination of amino acids such as amino acid oxidases, glutamate dehydrogenase, etc.
- Amino acid oxidases:
  - L-amino acid oxidase is linked to FMN group and catalyzes the oxidation of an L-amino acid producing alpha-keto acid, ammonia and water, as the final products.
  - Some of these tissues also contain FAD linked D amino acid oxidases which catalyze the oxidation of glycine and the D amino acids.
- Glutamate dehydrogenase
  - Glutamate is produced from alpha ketoglutarate by the enzyme glutamate dehydrogenase (GDH).
  - This enzyme plays a role in the release of ammonia from glutamate during glutamate degradation and used for gluconeogenesis
  - Coenzymes used:
    - During synthetic reaction – NADPH
    - During catabolic reaction – NAD^+
  - GDH catalyzes reversible set of reactions.

Nonoxidative Deamination

- Dehydratase, sulfhydrase and histidase catalyze deamination of serine, cysteine and histidine, respectively.
- They catalyze dehydration followed by nonoxidative deamination of the amino acids.
- This occurs spontaneously.

12. Write about denaturation of proteins.

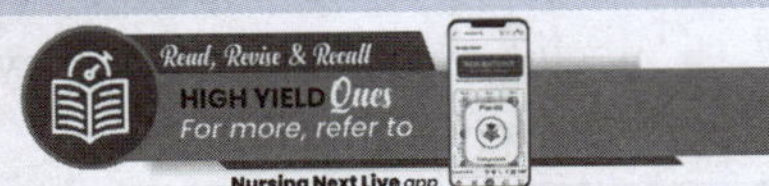

Answer

Introduction

- Loss of original protein structure due to disruption of weak bonds and interactions is known as denaturation
- Results in change in physical, chemical and biological properties.
- Loss of secondary, tertiary and quaternary protein structure
- No change is seen in the primary structure

Denaturation Reactions

- Due to change in pH
  - Changes the charges on many of the side chains.
  - Disrupts electrostatic attractions and hydrogen bonds.
- Due to reagents such as urea and guanidine hydrochloride
  - Leads to formation of stronger hydrogen bonds to the protein groups than the hydrogen bonds formed between the groups.
- Due to detergents such as sodium dodecyl sulfate
  - Interfere with the normal hydrophobic interactions by associating with the nonpolar groups of protein
- Due to organic solvents such as acetone alcohols
  - Disrupt hydrophobic interactions.
- Due to heat
  - Increase molecular motion that can disrupt the attractive forces.

Agents of Denaturation

Physical

- Heat
- Trauma – violent shaking
- Radiations – X-rays, UV rays

Chemical

- Change in pH
  - Acids
  - Alkalis
- Salts of heavy metals
- Organic solvents

Characteristics of Denaturation

- Loss of helical structure
- Loss of biological activity
- Change in solubility of the denatured proteins
- Increase in viscosity
- Decreased surface tension
- Increase in ionizable and sulfhydryl groups of proteins
- Easily digestible
- Usually irreversible, in some cases, it is reversible – known as renaturation
- Denatured proteins cannot be crystallized.

13. What are the sources of ammonia? How ammonia is detoxified. (KUHS)

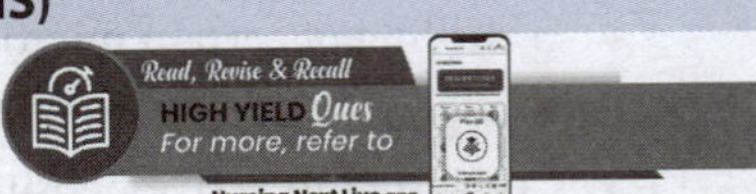

Answer

Sources of Ammonia

- From amino acids by the process of
  - Transamination
    - Transamination of amino acids with alpha ketoglutarate to form glutamate

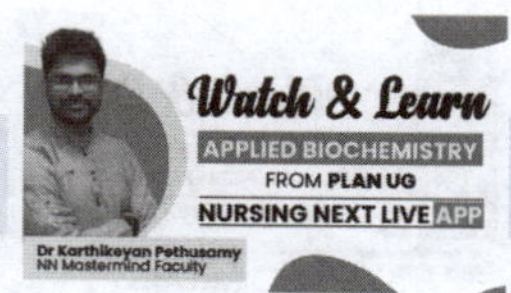

- Deamination
  - Both oxidative and nonoxidative deamination
- Transsulfuration
- Degradation of amino sugars
- Monoamine oxidase
- Pyrimidine and purine catabolism
- By action of intestinal bacteria on the unabsorbed dietary amino acids

Ammonia Toxicity

- Normal plasma levels of ammonia – 15–45 µg/dL
- Above 45 µg/dL – Hyperammonemia
- **Slight elevation of ammonia levels – leads to toxicity**

Detoxification Process

- Ammonia is a waste product that is generated during the metabolism of proteins, and it is toxic to the body
- The detoxification process of ammonia primarily occurs in the liver through a series of biochemical reactions called the urea cycle/ Krebs-Henseleit cycle or ornithine cycle.
- The process of detoxification is as follows:
  - **Conversion to glutamate:** Ammonia is initially converted to glutamate through an enzyme called glutamate dehydrogenase.
  - **Formation of glutamine:** Glutamate is then combined with ammonia by an enzyme called glutamine synthetase to produce glutamine.
  - **Transportation to liver:** Glutamine, along with other amino acids, is transported to the liver through the bloodstream.
  - **Urea cycle:** In the liver, the ammonia from glutamine is released through the urea cycle. The urea cycle consists of a series of enzymatic reactions that convert ammonia into urea.
    a. **Carbamoyl phosphate synthesis:** Ammonia is converted into carbamoyl phosphate by the enzyme carbamoyl phosphate synthetase.
    b. **Citrulline formation:** Carbamoyl phosphate combines with ornithine, an amino acid, to form citrulline. This reaction is catalyzed by the enzyme ornithine transcarbamylase (OTC).
    c. **Argininosuccinate formation:** Citrulline is converted into arginine by the enzyme argininosuccinate synthetase.
    d. **Arginine formation:** Argininosuccinate is cleaved by the enzyme argininosuccinase to yield arginine and fumarate.
    e. **Urea formation:** Finally, arginine is converted into urea and fumarate by the enzyme arginase
    f. Urea is a water-soluble compound that can be easily excreted by the kidneys. Fumerate is nontoxic that can be used for energy production.

14. Write a note on alkaptonuria.

Answer

Alkaptonuria

- Alkaptonuria is an inborn error tyrosine metabolism.
- It is a rare inherited disorder that prevents the breaking down of two amino acids called tyrosine and phenylalanine.
- Autosomal recessive disorder
- Prevalence is 1 in 25,000
- Occurs due to the presence of defective enzyme – homogentisate oxidase

Biochemical Manifestations

- Due to the presence of defective enzyme in tyrosine metabolism, homogentisate accumulates in tissues and blood and is excreted in urine
- Homogentisate is oxidized to benzoquinone acetate, which polymerizes to give black or brown colored pigment known as **alkapton**
- Thus, urine of alkaptonuric patients turns black on standing
- Alkapton deposition occurs in connective tissues, bones and various organs
- This is known as **ochronosis**
- Deposition of alkapton in joints can lead to arthritis

15. Write a note on Hartnup disease. (KUHS)

Answer

Introduction

- Also known as neutral amino aciduria
- Neutral amino acids include - tryptophan, alanine, serine, threonine, valine
- Caused by a mutation of the gene that controls the processes of amino acid absorption and reabsorption
- Due to the inability of intestinal and renal epithelial cells to absorb neutral amino acids
- Impaired conversion of tryptophan to NAD^+ and $NADP^+$, the coenzymes of niacin – this results in typical symptoms of pellagra.

Symptoms

- Sensitivity to light

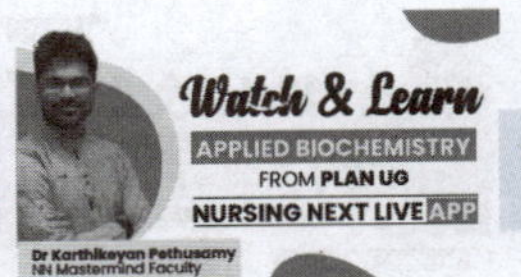

- Anxiety
- Rapid mood swings
- Hallucinations
- Delusions
- Intention tremor
- Speech difficulties
- Abnormalities in muscle tone: more tight (hypertonia) or exhibit decreased muscle tone (hypotonia).

Treatment

- Dietary modification, avoidance of sunlight, and sulfonamide drugs
- Niacin, rich foods provide symptomatic relief.

16. Give a brief account of glutathione. (MGR)

Answer

Introduction

- Tripeptide is composed of three amino acids – Glutamine, Cysteine, Glycine
- Chemically, glutathione is γ-glutamyl-cysteinyl-glycine.
- Exists in reduced or oxidized states in a ratio of 100:1 = reduced:oxidized.

$$2G{-}SH \rightleftharpoons G{-}S{-}S{-}G$$

Reduced Oxidized

Functions of Glutathione

Biological function is due to reversible oxidation – reduction capability of glutathione

- Serves as a coenzyme for certain enzymes such as prostaglandin synthase, glyoxylase
- Prevents oxidation of sulfhydryl (-SH) groups to disulfide (-S-S-) groups
  - Essential for protein/enzyme function
- Has a role in formation of correct disulfide bonds in several proteins
- In RBCs
  - Reduced glutathione plays a role in maintenance of structure and integrity of RBC membrane
  - Protects hemoglobin from oxidation by peroxidases
- Involved in the transport of amino acids *via* the γ-glutamyl cycle or Meister cycle
- Plays a role in detoxification
- Glutathione peroxidase – acts as free radical scavenger.

17. Name the specialized products formed from glycine. (MGR)

Answer

Important Products Derived from Glycine

- Purine ring
  - Glycine contributes to the formation of positions 4 and 5 of carbon and position 7 of nitrogen of purines
  - Purines are an essential component of
    - DNA and RNA (adenine and guanine)
    - Energy storing molecules ATP, GTP
    - Cyclic AMP, NADH and coenzyme A
  - Function as neurotransmitters
- Glutathione
  - Tripeptide, requires glycine for its formation
  - Prevents oxidation of sulfhydryl (-SH) groups to disulfide (-S-S-) groups
    - Essential for protein/enzyme function
  - Has a role in formation of correct disulfide bonds in several proteins
  - In RBCs
    - Reduced glutathione plays a role in maintenance of structure and integrity of RBC membrane
    - Protects hemoglobin from oxidation by peroxidases
  - Involved in the transport of amino acids *via* the γ glutamyl cycle or Meister cycle
  - Plays a role in detoxification
  - Glutathione peroxidase – acts as free radical scavenger.
- Heme
  - Glycine combines with succinyl CoA to form δ-amino levulinate that serves as a precursor for heme synthesis
  - Iron containing substance
  - Part of several proteins/enzymes
  - Important part of hemoglobin, myoglobin, cytochromes, peroxidases, etc.
- Creatine
  - Present in muscle, brain, blood, etc.
  - Exists in any of the following forms:
    - Free creatine
    - Phosphocreatine – high energy compound
    - Serum creatine – 0.2–0.6 mg/dL
  - Glycine, arginine and methionine are required for creatine synthesis
  - Arginine transfers guanidine group to glycine to form guanidoacetate (glycocyamine) under the effect of enzyme arginine-glycine transamidinase
  - Active methionine donates its methyl group to glycocyamine to form creatine

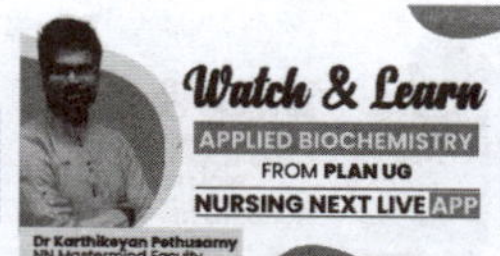

- Creatinine is an anhydride of creatine.
- Serum creatinine and serum creatine are diagnostic tests for assessing the renal function.

18. Write about collagen. (MGR)

Answer

Introduction

- *Collagen*
  - Most abundant insoluble fibrous connective tissue protein
  - 25% - 35% of whole body protein
  - 19 different types of collagen are present in body
- *Structure*
  - Triple helix
  - Left handed helix
  - Each alpha chain has glycine at every position
  - Other A are proline and hydroxyproline
  - Stabilized by hydrogen bonds, covalent cross linking, hydrophobic and van der Waals forces

Types of Collagen

- Superfamily of proteins – includes 27 distinct types.
- Based on their functions and locations in the body, collagens are organized into three groups:
  - Fibril forming collagen
    - Includes type I, type II, type III
  - Network forming collagen
    - Form three-dimensional mesh
    - Includes type IV and VII collagen
  - Fibril associated collagens
    - Type IX collagens are found in cartilage, whereas type XII collagen occurs in tendons and ligaments.
- *Biosynthesis of collagen*

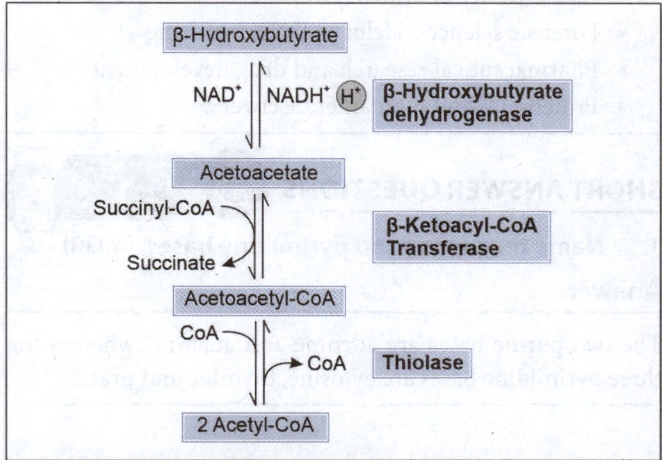

19. Add a note on phenylketonuria. (MGR)

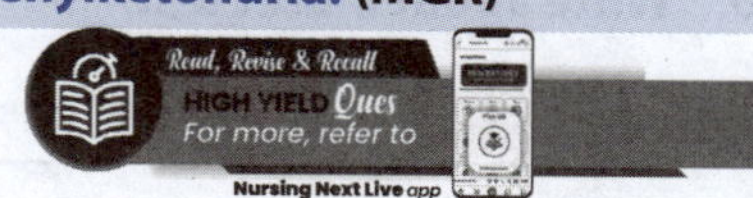

Answer

Introduction

- Most common amino acid metabolic disorder
- Occurs due to deficiency of enzyme - phenylalanine hydroxylase
- Autosomal recessive disorder
- Phenylalanine is not converted to tyrosine, leading to accumulation of phenylalanine in tissues

Phenylalanine Metabolism in Phenylketonuria

- Increased excretion in urine
- Excessive production of phenylpyruvate, phenylacetate and phenyl lactate
- These metabolites are excreted in urine
- Phenylacetate imparts urine of PKU patients a mousey odor.

Clinical/Biochemical Manifestations of PKU

- Effect on central nervous system
  - Characterized by:
    - Mental retardation
    - Seizures
    - Failure to walk and talk
  - This is due to:
    - Accumulation of phenylalanine in brain impairing the metabolism and transport of other amino acids.
    - Deficiency of serotonin
    - Defective myelin formation
- Hypopigmentation – defective melanin synthesis

Diagnosis

- Increased plasma phenylalanine levels in newborns to about 20–65 mg/dL
- Normal values – 1–2 mg/dL
- Guthrie test – bioassay for the detection of phenyalanine in newborns
- Ferric chloride test – detection of phenylpyruvate in urine
- Prenatal diagnosis – using cultured amniotic cells

Treatment

- Decreased intake of food rich in phenylalanine.
- Increased intake of tyrosine-rich foods.
- Drug sapropterin, in certain cases, increases tolerance to phenylalanine.

20. Write about Biuret test.

Answer

Introduction

- Chemical test used to detect the presence of peptide bonds/ proteins.
- Biuret – compound formed by heating urea to 180°C.

Biuret Agent

Sodium hydroxide, hydrated copper (II) sulfate and potassium sodium tartrate.

Principle of Biuret Test

When biuret is treated with dilute copper sulfate in alkaline medium, a purple color is obtained.

Significance

- Used for identification of proteins and peptides.
- Given by compounds containing two or more CO-NH groups, i.e., peptide bonds.
- Proteins containing at least two peptide linkages, i.e., tripeptides give positive biuret test.
- 5–160 mg/mL can be determined.

21. Define electrophoresis. Mention the factors affecting, types and uses of electrophoresis.

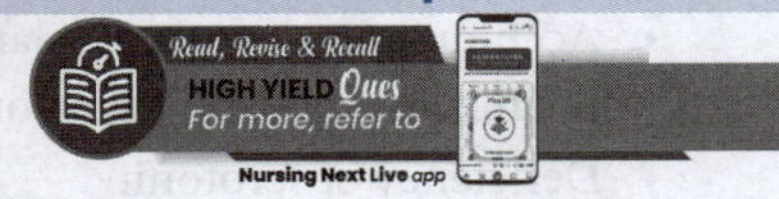

Answer

Definition

Electrophoresis is defined as the motion of dispersed particles relative to a fluid under the influence of a spatially uniform electric field.

Principle of Electrophoresis

- The movement of charged molecules in an electric field toward the oppositely charged electrode
- Negatively charged particles move toward the cathode, while positively charged particles move toward anode.
- Separates biological molecules such as serum proteins, lipoproteins and immunoglobulins.
- The concentration of these components can be determined by densitometric scanning.
- Factors affecting electrophoresis are:
  - pH of the medium
  - Net charge on the particles
  - Temperature
  - Molecular weight
  - Shape of molecule
  - Solvation of ions
  - Viscosity of solution
  - Extent of current

Different Types of Electrophoresis

- Zone Electrophoresis: It involves the separation of charged molecules based on their migration rates through a supporting medium. It includes:
  - Paper Electrophoresis: A filter paper strip acts as the supporting medium.
  - Gel Electrophoresis: It employs a gel matrix, typically agarose or polyacrylamide, as the supporting medium
- Isoelectric Focusing (IEF): It is a technique used to separate molecules based on their isoelectric point (pI). It uses pH gradient across a gel matrix.
- Immunoelectrophoresis: It is a combination of electrophoresis and immunodiffusion techniques based on electrophoretic mobility of proteins and their reaction with antibodies.

Uses of Electrophoresis

- Electrophoresis has a wide range of applications across various scientific fields. It is useful in:
  - Nucleic acid analysis: Used in DNA sequencing, genotyping, genetic finger printing, etc.
  - Testing vaccines: Used for the creation and production of vaccines.
  - Protein analysis: Used to identify protein and determine their structure.
  - Clinical diagnosis, e.g., cystic fibrosis, sickle cell anemia, and HIV.
  - Quality Control in Biotechnology and Pharmaceuticals: Assess purity of protein samples.
  - Forensic sciences: Helps in DNA matching
  - Pharmaceutical research and drug development
  - Proteomics and biomarker discovery.

SHORT ANSWER QUESTIONS

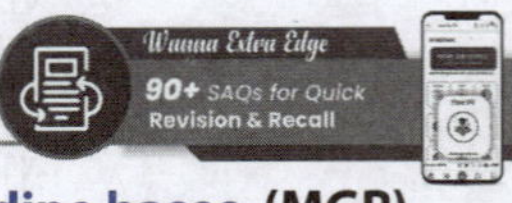

1. Name the purine and pyrimidine bases. (MGR)

Answer

The two purine bases are adenine and guanine, whereas the three pyrimidine bases are cytosine, thymine and uracil.

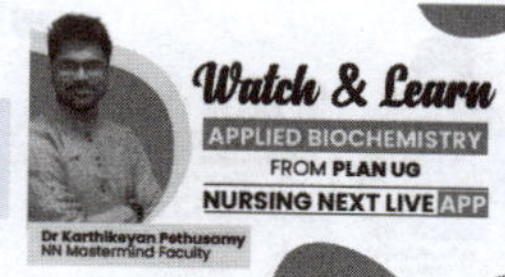

2. Essential amino acids. (MGR)

Answer

The body cannot synthesize essential amino acids; hence, they must be consumed through diet. There are nine essential amino acids.

- Phenylalanine
- Methionine
- Tryptophan
- Threonine
- Histidine
- Isoleucine
- Leucine
- Lysine
- Valine

3. Differences between DNA and RNA (any two). (MGR)

Answer

DNA	RNA
Double stranded molecule carries the genetic material in eukaryotes	Single stranded molecule mainly involved in protein synthesis
DNA content is constant in all the cells except during cell division	RNA varies from cell to cell

4. Serum proteins and their normal values. (MGR)

Answer

Serum protein	Normal range (g/L)
Albumin	35–50 g/L
Globulin	20–35 g/L
Total protein	60–80 g/L

5. What is semiessential amino acid? (MGR)

Answer

Amino acids that are considered semiessential can occasionally become conditionally necessary, even though they are typically nonessential and can be produced by the body on its own. E.g., Arginine and Histidine.

6. Define ribosome. (MGR)

Answer

Ribosomes are small, complex molecular machines found in cells that are responsible for synthesizing proteins. They are composed of two subunits, each of which is made up of ribosomal RNA (rRNA) and proteins. All living cells, including prokaryotic and eukaryotic cells, use ribosomes as their primary means of protein synthesis.

7. Define elastin. (MGR)

Answer

A fibrous protein is a complex network of proteins and other molecules. It provides elasticity to many tissues like skin, lungs and ligaments.

8. Define cytoskeleton. (MGR)

Answer

The cytoskeleton is a complex network of protein filaments that gives cells their shape, mechanical strength, and ability to move. They are composed of microfilaments, intermediate filaments, and microtubules.

9. Define collagen. (MGR)

Answer

Collagen is most abundant and a structural protein which forms the framework for connective tissues like skin, tendons, ligaments, cartilage, and bones.

10. Name the specialized products formed from glycine. (MGR)

Answer

Glycine can be modified to form specialized products, such as collagen, creatine, glutathione and porphyrins.

11. Purine catabolism and its normal value. (MGR)

Answer

Purines are nitrogen-containing chemicals that can be found in many meals. Purine catabolism is the process by which purines are broken down into simpler compounds and removed from the body in the form of uric acid. Value lies between 3.4 and 7.2 mg/dL for men, and between 2.4 and 6.0 mg/dL for women.

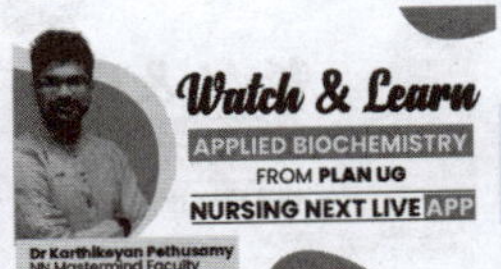

12. Lipoproteins. (MGR)

Answer

Lipoproteins are complex compounds that carry lipids through the bloodstream. They are made up of proteins, lipids (fats), and other chemicals. E.g., Chylomicrons, VLDL, LDL and HDL.

13. Mention any two functions of proteins. (MGR)

Answer

1. Structural function: Proteins are an essential component of cells and tissues and provide structural support to various organs and structures in the body.
2. Enzymatic function: Proteins can also function as enzymes, which are molecules that catalyze chemical reactions in the body.

14. Name two clinically significant transaminases measured in the laboratory. (MGR)

Answer

Alanine transaminase (ALT) and Aspartate transaminase (AST) are two clinically significant transaminases measured in the laboratory.

15. Name two special products from tyrosine and their functions. (MGR)

Answer

Two special products from tyrosine are dopamine (helps in regulating mood and movement) and thyroid hormone (regulating metabolism and growth).

16. What is the end product of purine catabolism? What is its normal level? (MGR)

Answer

- The end product of purine catabolism is uric acid.
- The normal range of serum uric acid is between 3.4 and 7.2 mg/dL for men and between 2.4 and 6.0 mg/dL for women.

17. What are the different bases found in DNA? How are they paired? (MGR)

Answer

These bases pair with each other in a specific way. Adenine (A) always pairs with thymine (T), forming an A-T base pair. Guanine (G) always pairs with cytosine (C), forming a G-C base pair. This base pairing is known as complementary base pairing.

18. Deamination. (DU)

Answer

Deamination is a chemical process that involves removal of the α-amino group from amino acids. The main organs involved in the process are liver and kidney.

19. Hypoproteinemia. (KUHS)

Answer

A medical disease known as hypoproteinemia is characterized by unusually low quantities of protein in the blood. It can be brought on by autoimmune diseases, liver illness, kidney disease, or malnutrition.

CONCEPTUAL REVISION

MULTIPLE CHOICE QUESTIONS

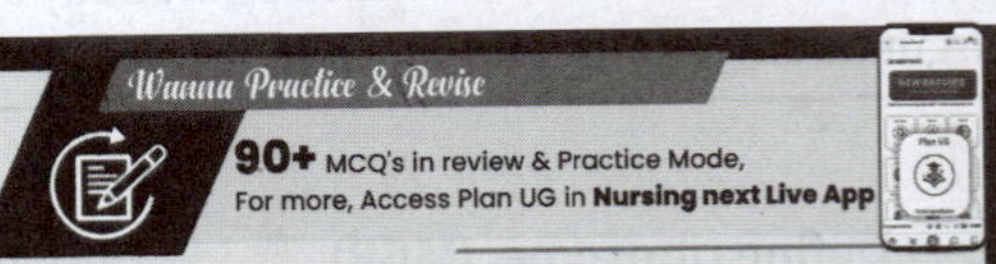

1. Primary structure of protein is represented by which of the following?

a. Linear structure of protein joined by peptide bonds
b. 3-dimensional structure of protein
c. Helical structure of proteins
d. Subunit structure of protein

Ans. a. Linear structure of protein joined by peptide bonds

2. Which type of collagen is maximum in skin?

a. Type-I
b. Type-II
c. Type-III
d. Type-IV

Ans. a. Type-I

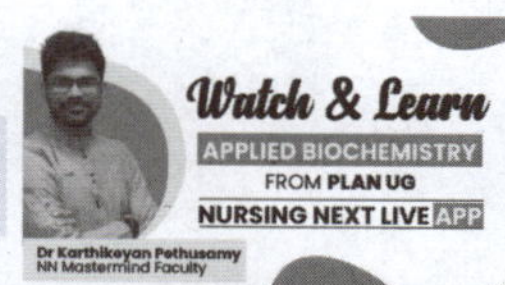

3. Blood urea level is markedly increased in:
a. Liver disease
b. Renal disease
c. Cardiac disease
d. Protein intake

Ans. b. Renal disease

4. Urea is formed from which substrate?
a. Arginine
b. Ornithine
c. Citrulline
d. Alanine

Ans. a. Arginine

5. Which of the following is not an aromatic amino acid?
a. Phenylalanine
b. Tyrosine
c. Tryptophan
d. Valine

Ans. d. Valine

6. Under normal conditions in blood, which of the following amino acid residues of albumin is neutral?
a. Glutamate
b. Aspartate
c. Histidine
d. Glutamine

Ans. d. Glutamine

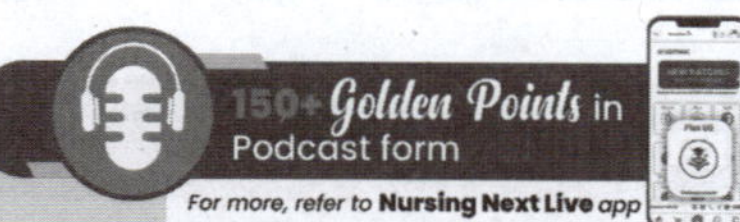

Golden Points

- A/G ratio refers to plasma albumin: globulin ratio. The normal plasma A/G ratio is 1.2 – 2.0:1.
- Absorption of amino acids may be affected in specific transport disorders or other diseases involving the small intestine or the immune system, such as Hartnup's disease and cystinuria.
- Albumin, globulins and fibrinogen are the major plasma proteins, all of which are synthesized in the liver (except γ-globulins).
- Glucogenic amino acids serve as precursors of gluconeogenesis, for glucose formation, include glycine, alanine, serine, aspartic acid, asparagine, glutamic acid, glutamine, proline, valine, methionine, cysteine, histidine and arginine.
- Glucogenic amino acids, e.g., alanine, serve as a source of energy.
- Glycine is a precursor of creatine, glutathione, heme, bile acids and purines.
- Main function of albumin is maintenance of plasma colloidal osmotic pressure and hence the regulation of blood volume.
- Molecules with equal number of ionizable groups, i.e., when the number of cations is equal to the number of anions, are called zwitterions.
- Plasma proteins are separated by paper electrophoresis.
- Primary structure of a protein refers to the order and sequence of amino acids in a protein chain.
- Protein is the class of natural products, which contain nitrogen.

CHAPTER 4

Enzymes and Clinical Enzymology

CONCEPTUAL THEORY

Terminology

150+ key terminologies for Quick Recall & Revision

Apoenzyme: Apoenzyme is the catalytically-inactive, protein component of the enzyme.
Catalysts: Catalysts are those substances which alter the rate of reaction by changing the path of reaction.
Coenzyme: A coenzyme is a dialyzable, thermostable, low-molecular weight, organic substance required for proper functioning of enzyme.
Cofactors: These are inorganic molecules required for proper functioning of enzyme. Example- ions of copper, Iron, magnesium, etc.
Enzyme: An enzyme is a type of protein that acts as a biological catalyst, facilitating chemical reactions within living organisms.
Holoenzyme: Catalytically-active form of the enzyme, consisting of the apoenzyme and the cofactor.

ENZYMES—DEFINITION

- An enzyme is a type of protein that acts as a biological catalyst, facilitating chemical reactions within living organisms.
- Enzymes play an important role in various biological processes by increasing the rate of specific biochemical reactions without being consumed or altered in the process.

CLASSIFICATION

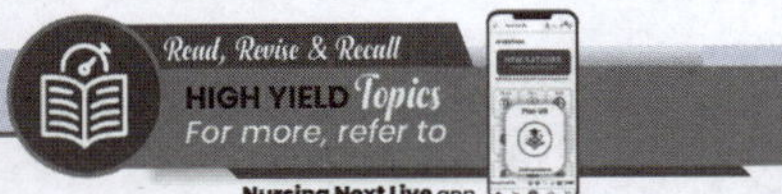

Enzymes are classified based on the type of reaction they catalyze.

- **Oxidoreductases:** catalyze oxidation-reduction reactions, in which electrons are transferred from one molecule to another.
- **Transferases:** catalyze the transfer of a functional group, such as a methyl or phosphate group, from one molecule to another.
- **Hydrolases:** catalyze the hydrolysis of bonds, which is the splitting of a molecule by the addition of water.
- **Lyases:** catalyze the breaking of bonds without the addition of water.
- **Isomerases:** catalyze the rearrangement of atoms within a molecule.
- **Ligases:** catalyze the joining of two molecules by the formation of a new bond.

ISOENZYMES—DEFINITION AND PROPERTIES

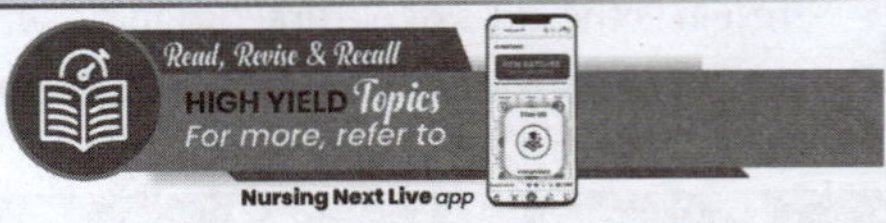

- Multiple forms of a single enzyme catalyzing the same reaction are isoenzymes.
- Isoenzymes have similar enzyme activity.
- They differ in their physical and chemical properties such as:
  - Amino acid sequence
  - Quaternary structure
  - Electrophoretic and immunological properties
  - Km and Vmax values
  - pH optimum
  - Relative susceptibility to inhibitors and
  - Degree of denaturation.
- Usually synthesized from different genes.

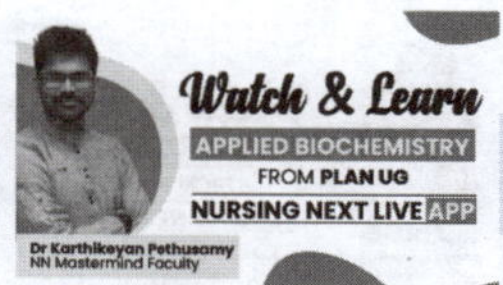

ENZYMES OF DIAGNOSTIC IMPORTANCE—LIVER DISEASE, MI, MUSCLE DISEASE, BONE DISEASE, PROSTATE CANCER

Table 4.1: Some enzymes of diagnostic importance

Enzyme	Principal source	Clinical situation in which altered
Acid phosphatase	Prostate and RBC	**Increases** in carcinoma of prostate
Alkaline phosphatase	Liver, bone, placenta and kidney	**Increases** in obstructive jaundice, rickets, Paget's disease and hyperparathyroidism
Aldolase	Skeletal muscle and heart	**Increases** in muscular dystrophies and acute liver diseases
Amylase	Salivary glands, pancreas and ovaries	**Increases** in acute pancreatitis, intestinal obstruction and acute parotitis. **Decreases** in acute liver diseases
Ceruloplasmin	Liver	**Increases** in cirrhosis. **Decreases** in Wilson's disease
Cholinesterase	Liver	**Increases** in nephrotic syndrome and organophosphorus poisoning. **Decreases** in acute liver diseases
Creatine phosphokinase	Skeletal muscle, brain and heart	**Increases** in myocardial infarction and muscular dystrophies
Glutamate oxaloacetate transaminase (GPT)	Liver, skeletal muscle, heart, kidney and RBCs	**Increases** in myocardial infarction, toxic liver cell necrosis, acute liver diseases, and muscle diseases
γ-glutamyl transferase	Liver and kidney	**Increases** in alcoholism and hepatobiliary diseases
Lactate dehydrogenase	Heart, liver, skeletal muscle, RBCs and platelets	**Increases** in acute myocardial infarction, acute hepatitis, and muscle disorders
Lipase	Pancreas	**Increases** in acute pancreatitis and pancreatic carcinoma. **Decreases** in liver diseases and diabetes mellitus
5′-nucleotidase	Hepatobiliary tract	**Increases** in liver diseases, obstructive jaundice and hepatic carcinoma
Trypsin	Pancreas	**Increases** in acute pancreatic diseases

CONCEPTUAL EXERCISES

LONG ANSWER QUESTIONS

1. Clinical applications of enzymes with normal ranges. (MGR)

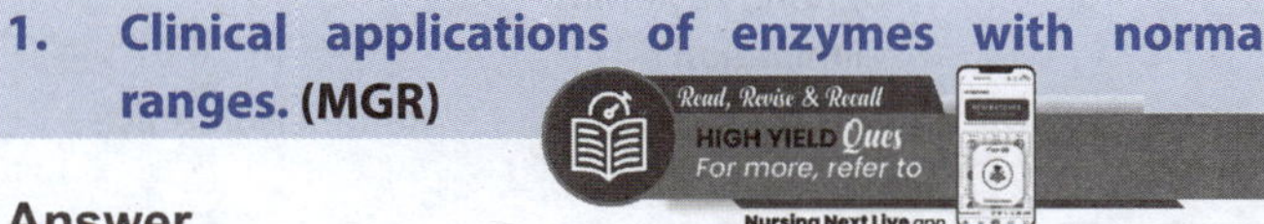

Answer

Introduction

- Plasma level of an enzyme is an estimation of the balance between the synthesis and release of the enzyme during normal metabolism.
- *Change in the level of enzymes is usually indicative of:*
  - Cellular damage
  - Increased rate of proliferation of cells
  - Change in cell turnover
  - Altered synthesis of enzymes, etc.
- Thus, indicative of disease diagnosis – **biomarker**

Examples of Certain Enzymes as a Diagnostic Tool

Alkaline Phosphatase Enzyme

- Mainly derived from the bone and cells lining the bile canaliculi
- Normal serum ALP value 50–100 U/L
- Elevated ALP levels are seen in:
  - Obstructive/posthepatic jaundice
  - Hepatic tumors
  - Cirrhosis of liver
  - Rickets
  - Hyperparathyroidism
  - Carcinoma of bone
- **Significance of isoenzymes**
  - α2 – heat labile ALP- suggests hepatitis
  - Pre β ALP suggests bone diseases

Lactate Dehydrogenase

- Important in the diagnosis of heart and liver disorders
- LDH_2 >>> LDH_1 – healthy individuals
- LDH_1 >>> LDH_2 – myocardial infarction (within 12–24 hours after infarction)
- Increased activity of LDH_5 – indicator of liver disease
- LDH activity in RBC >> LDH activity in serum (80–100 times)
- So, for estimation of LDH – serum should be hemolysis free

Creatine Phosphokinase (CK)

- First enzyme to be released into circulation
- Within 6–12 hours after infarction
- Reaches a peak within 24–30 hours
- Returns to normal by 2nd or 3rd day
- Earliest marker of myocardial infarction (MI)

Aspartate transaminase (AST or SGOT)

- Rises after CK
- Reaches a peak after 2nd day of infarction
- Returns to normal in 4–5 days

Alanine Aminotransferase (ALT)

- Normal Range: 10–40 U/L
- Clinical Applications: Elevated levels can indicate liver damage or disease, such as hepatitis or liver cirrhosis.

Gamma-Glutamyl Transferase (GGT)

- Normal Range: Up to 45 U/L in males and 30 U/L in females.
- Clinical Applications: Elevated levels can indicate liver disease, alcohol abuse, or certain drug reactions.

Troponin

- Normal Range:
  - Troponin T-Below 0.04 ng/mL; Troponin I-Below 0.03 ng/mL
- Clinical Applications: Elevated levels can indicate acute myocardial injury or other cardiac conditions.

Prostate-Specific Antigen (PSA)

- Normal Range: typically below 4 ng/mL
- Clinical Applications: Elevated levels may indicate prostate cancer or benign prostatic hyperplasia (BPH).

Amylase

- **Normal levels:** 30–150 U/L
- Elevated levels are seen in:
  - Acute pancreatitis
  - Acute parotitis

2. Classify enzymes. Explain the properties of enzymes and influence of various factors on enzyme activity. (MGR)

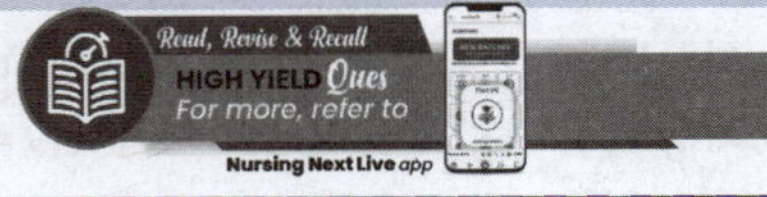

Answer

Introduction

- Enzymes are defined as biological catalysts that catalyze biochemical reactions.
- Mainly protein in nature.
- Colloidal and thermolabile.
- Highly specific.

Classification of Enzymes

Enzymes are classified into six major groups according to the type of reaction they catalyze:

Enzyme class	Catalyzes	Examples
Oxidoreductases	Enzymes involved in oxidation-reduction reactions	Alcohol dehydrogenase
Transferases	Catalyze transfer of functional groups	Hexokinase
Hydrolases	Cause hydrolysis of various compounds by addition of water	Lipase
Lyases	Cause cleavage of bonds by atom elimination	Aldolase
Isomerases	Involved in isomerization reactions	Retinol isomerase
Ligases	Cause joining of two molecules – synthetic reaction	Succinate thiokinase

Each class is further divided into subclasses which are further divided into sub-subclasses.

A four-digit Enzyme Commission (EC) number is assigned to each enzyme representing:

1. **First digit:** Class
2. **Second digit:** Subclass
3. **Third digit:** Sub-subclass
4. **Fourth digit:** Individual enzyme

Properties of Enzymes

- Act as biocatalyst

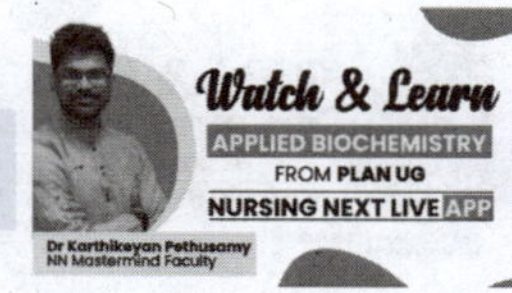

- Physical properties
  - Act as colloids
  - Enzymes are inactivated typically below the boiling point of water.
  - Most active at 25°–45°C
  - Activity is pH dependent.
- Chemical properties
  - Protein in composition
  - Enzyme Specificity
    - Catalyze a specific reaction

Enzyme Specificity

- Enzymes are highly specific, interacting with only one or a few substrates and catalyzing one type of a chemical reaction only.
- Various types of enzyme specificities are:
  - Stereo specificity
  - Reaction specificity

Stereo Specificity

- Only one specific isomer of the compound acts as the substrate for a particular enzyme.
- This is known as stereo specificity.
- Examples:
  - L-amino acid oxidase will act only on L-amino acids.
  - Succinate dehydrogenase will act only on succinate and not on malate.

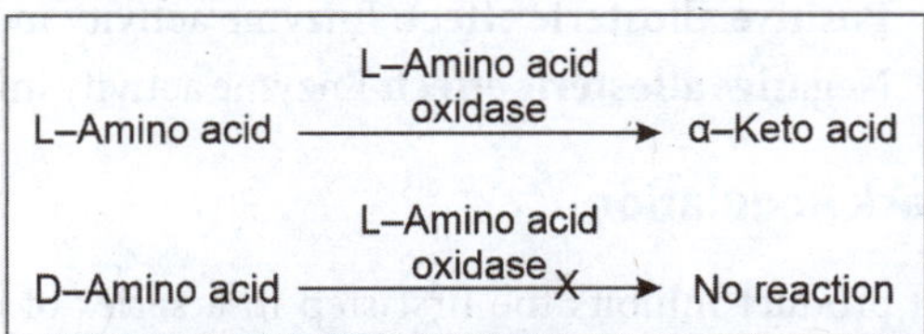

Figure 4.1: Stereo-specificity.

Reaction Specificity

- Though a substrate can be used in several reactions, but a particular enzyme will catalyze only one of these reactions.
- This is known as reaction specificity.
- Example:
  - Oxaloacetate can be converted to aspartate as well as to malate but the two reactions are catalyzed by two separate enzymes and not by the same enzyme.

Factors Affecting Enzyme Activity

Contact between the enzyme and substrate is a prerequisite for enzyme action.

Important factors that influence the velocity of enzyme are:

- **Enzyme concentration**
  - As the enzyme concentration increases, the velocity of reaction increases proportionately.
  - This property is used for determining the activities of serum enzymes during the diagnosis of diseases.

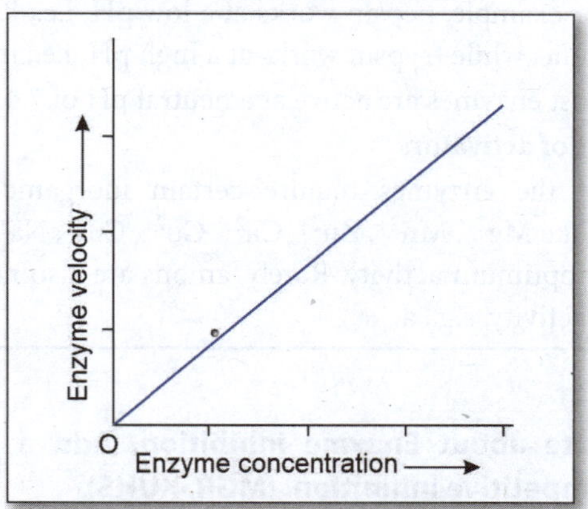

- **Substrate concentration**
  - Substrate concentration is directly proportional to the velocity of enzyme reaction within a limited range.
  - Rectangular hyperbola is formed.
- **Effects of temperature**
  - Enzymes are sensitive to minor thermal changes due to their protein nature.
  - Active only within a narrow range of temperature; optimal temperature range is 37°–40°C.

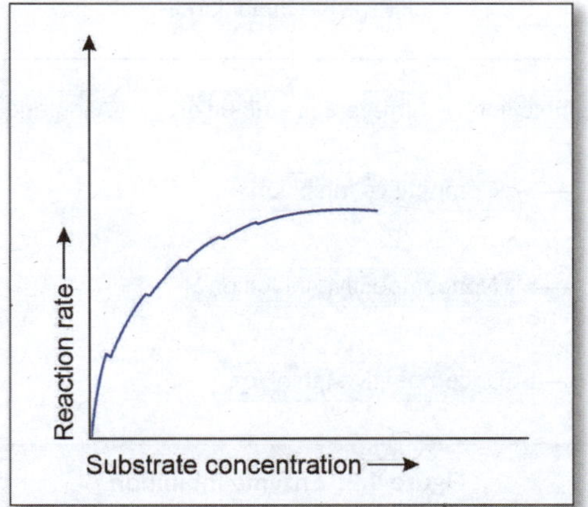

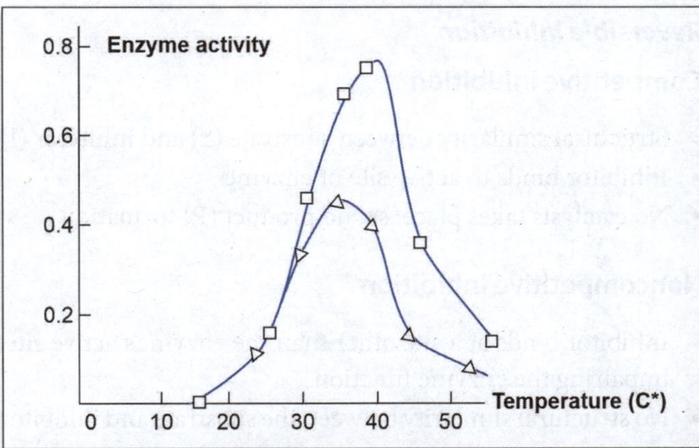

- **Effects of pH**
  - pH at which enzyme activity is at maximum efficiency is called optimal pH.
  - Change in pH decreases the enzyme activity.
  - For example, pepsin works at a low pH, i.e., it is highly acidic, while trypsin works at a high pH, i.e., it is basic.
  - Most enzymes are active at a neutral pH of 7.4.
- **Effect of activators**

Some of the enzymes require certain inorganic metallic cations, like Mg^{2+}, Mn^{2+}, Zn^{2+}, Ca^{2+}, Co^{2+}, Cu^{2+}, Na^{+}, K^{+}, etc., for their optimum activity. Rarely, anions are also needed for enzyme activity, e.g., a.

3. Write about Enzyme inhibition. Add a note on competitive inhibition. (MGR, KUHS)

Answer

Introduction

- Enzyme inhibition – decrease in the catalytic activity of an enzyme
- Enzyme inhibitor – substance that causes enzyme inhibition

Types of Enzyme Inhibition

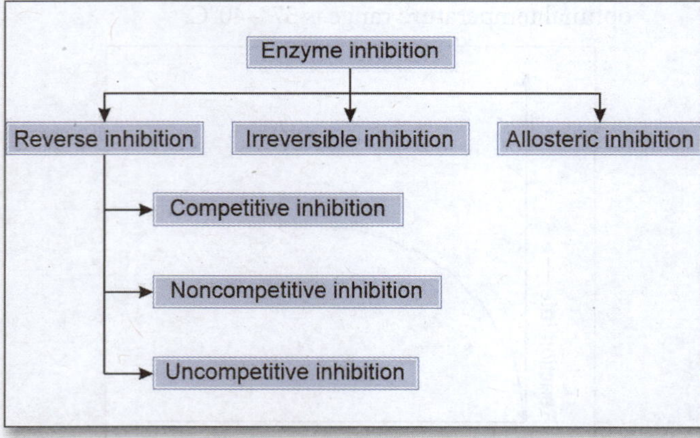

Figure 4.2: Enzyme Inhibition

Reversible Inhibition

Competitive Inhibition

- Structural similarity between substrate (S) and inhibitor (I)
- Inhibitor binds to active site of enzyme
- No catalysis takes place; so, no product (P) formation

Noncompetitive Inhibition

- Inhibitor binds at a site other than the enzyme's active site, impairing the enzyme function
- No structural similarity between the substrate and inhibitor
- Binding of inhibitor causes distortion in enzyme conformation
- K_m value is unchanged, while V_{max} is lowered

Uncompetitive Inhibition

- The inhibitor will only bind to an enzyme-substrate complex; therefore, it does not compete with the substrate for the binding site.
- Both K_m and V_{max} values decrease.

Irreversible Inhibition

- Inhibitors bind covalently with enzymes and inactivate them irreversibly
- Usually toxic or poisonous substances
- Example: Cyanide inhibits cytochrome oxidase of electron transport chain.
- Suicide inhibition: Specialized form of irreversible inhibition. In this, the structural analogue or the competitive inhibitor is converted to more potent form of the same enzyme that needs to be inhibited

Allosteric Regulation/Inhibition of Enzyme Activity

- Allo=other
- Steric=site
- Allosteric=other site in addition to active site
- *Allosteric effectors/modulators*
  - Regulate the enzyme activity by binding at allosteric site.
    - **Positive allosteric effect:** Enzyme activity increases
    - **Negative allosteric effect:** Enzyme activity inhibition

Feedback Regulation

- Final product inhibits the first step in a series of enzyme regulated reactions of a pathway.
- Helps to control the concentration of final product in the system.
- Specialized type of allosteric inhibition.

Competitive Inhibition

- Structural similarity between substrate (S) and inhibitor (I)
- Inhibitor binds to active site of enzyme
- Thus, substrate is not able to attach to the enzyme (E)
- No catalysis takes place; so, no product (P) formation
- *To summarize:*

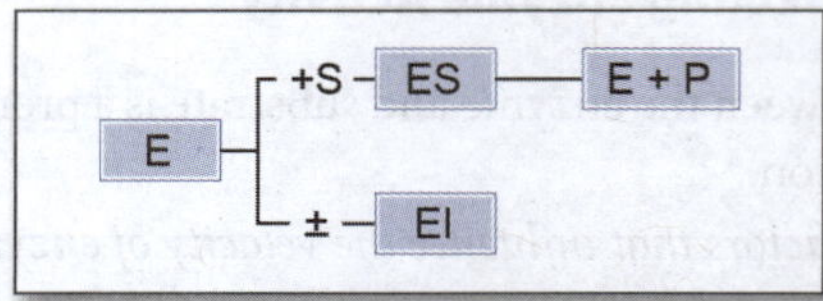

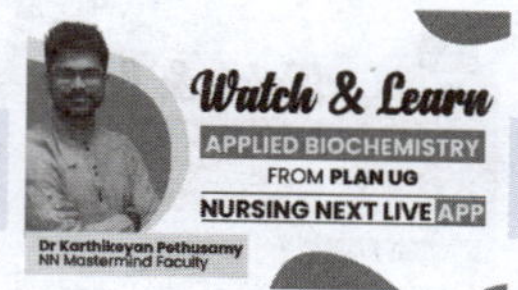

Factors Affecting Competitive Inhibition

- Relative concentration of the substrate and inhibitor
- Affinity of inhibitor with the enzyme
- Can be overcome by increasing the substrate concentration.

In competitive inhibition, the value of K_m increases, whereas that of V_{max} remains unchanged.

Examples

1. Enzyme xanthine oxidase
   - Competitive inhibitor - Allopurinol
   - Substrate – Hypoxanthine xanthine
   - Product – Uric acid
   - Allopurinol has structural similarity to hypoxanthine xanthine, which forms the basis of treatment of gout.
2. Glutaric acid and malonic acid are structural analogs of succinic acid, actively compete with it for binding at the active site of succinate dehydrogenase.

SHORT NOTES

1. Write a short note on coenzyme. (MGR)

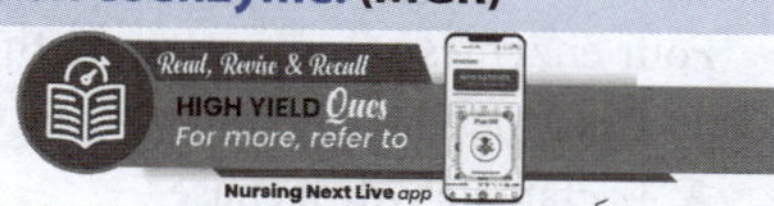

Answer

Introduction

- A coenzyme is an organic nonprotein compound that binds with an enzyme to catalyze a reaction.
- Coenzymes are often called cofactors, but they are chemically different.
- Also referred to as second substrates as they have enzyme affinity comparable to that of substrates.
- A coenzyme cannot function alone, but can be reused several times when paired with an enzyme.
- They undergo alterations during enzymatic reactions and are later regenerated.

Some Examples of Coenzyme

- NAD^+ (Nicotinamide adenine dinucleotide): NAD is a coenzyme that is involved in many reactions, including the oxidation of glucose in the cellular respiration pathway.
- $NADP^+$ (Nicotinamide adenine dinucleotide phosphate): Similar to NAD^+, $NADP^+$ functions as a coenzyme in redox reactions, particularly in anabolic processes such as fatty acid and nucleotide synthesis.
- FAD (Flavin adenine dinucleotide): FAD is a coenzyme that is involved in many reactions, including the oxidation of fatty acids.
- Coenzyme A (CoA): CoA is a coenzyme involved in numerous metabolic pathways including citric acid cycle, fatty acid metabolism, and amino acid metabolism.
- TPP (Thiamine pyrophosphate): TPP is a coenzyme derived from vitamin B1 (thiamine). It plays a crucial role in the citric acid cycle and glucose metabolism.
- PLP (Pyridoxal phosphate): PLP is derived from vitamin B_6 (pyridoxine) and serves as a coenzyme in various enzymatic reactions, particularly in amino acid metabolism and the synthesis of neurotransmitters.

Functions of Coenzymes

- Participate in a variety of reactions such as transfer of atoms or groups.
- Essential for biological activity of enzymes
- Coenzymes help to stabilize enzymes and prevent them from denaturing
- Coenzymes help to transport molecules across membranes
- Coenzymes regulate enzyme activity by binding to the enzyme and changing its shape.

2. Define K_m value. What is its significance?

Answer

K_m – Michaelis-Menten Constant

- Defined as the substrate concentration (mol/L) to produce half-maximum velocity in enzyme catalyzed reaction.
- Reflection of the affinity of enzyme for its substrate
- Characteristic of a particular enzyme-substrate system.
  - The smaller the value of K_m, the more strongly the enzyme binds the substrate.
  - Kinetic values of enzyme catalyzed reactions are usually measured under steady state conditions and described by a simple expression called Henri-Michaelis-Menten equation.

Significance of Michaelis-Menten Constant

- By knowing the K_m value of a particular enzyme-substrate system, one can predict whether the cell needs more enzymes or more substrate to speed up the enzymatic reaction.

3. Write about enzymes of diagnostic importance in liver disease.

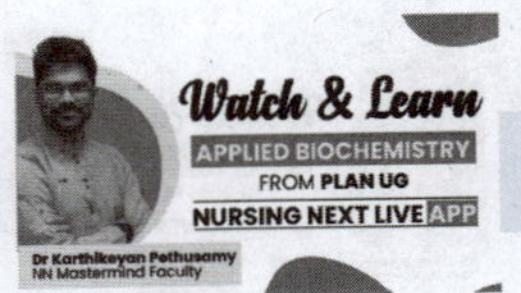

Answer

Introduction

- *Enzymes used in the diagnosis of various liver diseases are:*
  - Viral hepatitis, jaundice, toxic hepatitis, cirrhosis and hepatic necrosis
    - Alanine transaminase
    - Aspartate transaminase
    - Lactate dehydrogenase
  - Intrahepatic and extrahepatic cholestasis:
    - Alkaline phosphatase
    - 5'-nucleotidase
  - Alcoholic liver disease
    - Serum gamma-glutamyl transpeptidase

Plasma enzymes	Hemolytic jaundice	Obstructive jaundice	Hepatic jaundice
Aspartate aminotransferase (AST) or serum glutamic oxaloacetic transaminase (SGOT)	No change	Marginally increased	Increased
Alanine aminotransferase (ALT) or serum glutamic pyruvic transaminase (SGPT)	No change	Marginally increased	Considerably increased
Alkaline phosphatase (ALP)		Considerably increased	Marginally increased

Alanine Transaminase

- **Normal serum levels:** 10–45 IU/L
- *Increased in:*
  - Acute hepatitis
  - Jaundice
  - Cirrhosis of liver

Alkaline Phosphatase Enzyme

- Mainly derived from the bone and cells lining the bile canaliculi
- **Normal serum ALP value:** 50–100 U/L
- **Elevated ALP levels are seen in:**
  - Obstructive/posthepatic jaundice
  - Hepatic tumors
  - Cirrhosis of liver
- **Significance of isoenzymes**
  - α_2 – heat labile ALP- suggests hepatitis
  - Pre β ALP suggests bone diseases

Lactate Dehydrogenase

- Important in the diagnosis of heart and liver disorders
- LDH_2 >>> LDH_1 – healthy individuals
- LDH_1 >>> LDH_2 – myocardial infarction (within 12–24 hours after infarction)
- Increased activity of LDH_5 – indicator of liver disease
- LDH activity in RBC >> LDH activity in serum (80–100 times)
- So, for estimation of LDH – serum should be hemolysis free

γ- Glutamyl Transpeptidase

- Sensitive diagnostic marker for the detection of alcoholism
- Increased in:
  - Infective hepatitis
  - Obstructive jaundice

4. Write about enzymes related to cardiac diseases.

Answer

Enzymes in Myocardial Infarction (MI)

- Four enzymes are important in the diagnosis of MI:
  1. Creatine Phosphokinase-MB (CPK-MB)
  2. Lactate dehydrogenase
  3. Aspartate transaminase
  4. Troponin T and Troponin I

Creatine Phosphokinase-MB (CPK-MB)

- First enzyme to be released into circulation
- Within 6–12 hours after infarction
- Reaches a peak within 24–30 hours
- Returns to normal by 2nd or 3rd day
- Earliest marker of MI

Aspartate Transaminase (AST or SGOT)

- Rises after CK
- Reaches a peak after 2nd day of infarction.
- Returns to normal in 4–5 days.

Lactate Dehydrogenase (LDH_1)

- Rises 2nd day after MI
- Peaks at 3rd or 4th day
- Returns to normal in 10–15 days
- Last enzyme to rise and last enzyme to return to normal.

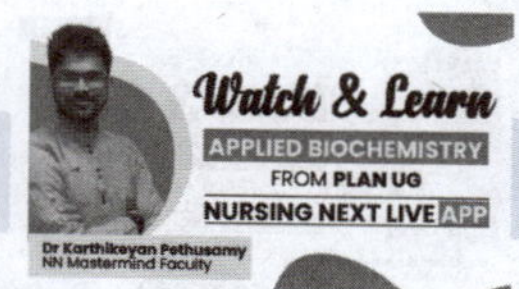

Troponin

- Normal Range:
  - Troponin T-Below 0.04 ng/mL; Troponin I-Below 0.03 ng/mL
- Clinical Applications: Elevated levels can indicate acute myocardial injury or other cardiac conditions.

SHORT ANSWER QUESTIONS

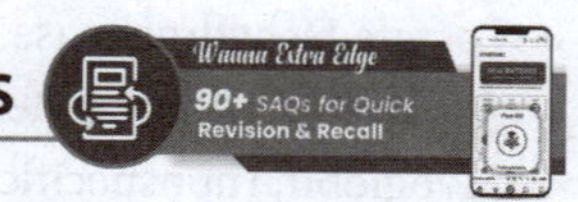

1. What are Holoenzymes and APOenzymes? (MGR)

Answer

- A holoenzyme is complete and active form of an enzyme. It consists of both the protein component, called the apoenzyme, and a non-protein component known as a cofactor or a coenzyme.
- An apoenzyme, also known as an inactive enzyme is the protein component of an enzyme that lacks the necessary cofactor for its activity.

2. What is a suicide bag? (MGR)

Answer

Lysosomes are known as the "suicide bags" of the cell because they can cause autodigestion and cell death when they release their hydrolytic enzymes into the cytoplasm during cellular damage.

3. Power house of the cell (MGR)

Answer

Mitochondria are known as the powerhouse of the cell because they generate most of the cell's supply of ATP (adenosine triphosphate), which is the molecule that provides energy to drive most cellular processes.

4. Define coenzyme. (MGR)

Answer

A coenzyme is an organic nonprotein molecule that interacts with an enzyme to support the enzyme's activity. Some examples of coenzymes include NAD^+ (nicotinamide adenine dinucleotide), Biotin, ATP (adenosine triphosphate), FAD (flavin adenine dinucleotide).

5. Induced fit model of enzyme activity. (MGR)

Answer

An explanation of the interactions between enzymes and substrates during enzymatic processes is provided by the induced fit model of enzyme activity caused by the conformational change in the enzyme.

6. Write any two functions of antioxidants. (MGR)

Answer

1. Protecting against oxidative stress: Protection of cells and tissues from the damaging effects of free radicals by neutralizing them.
2. Maintenance of cellular health and function: By preventing or reducing oxidative damage to important cellular components such as membranes, organelles, and DNA and supporting the immune system.

7. Functions of lysosomes. (MGR)

Answer

The intracellular digestion of large molecules such as proteins, nucleic acids, carbohydrates, and lipids is carried out by lysosomes, which also participate in the autophagy process.

8. Two examples for isoenzymes. (MGR)

Answer

- Examples of isoenzymes include:
  - Lactate dehydrogenase (LDH) - LDH 1, LDH 2, LDH 3, LDH 4, and LDH 5 are isoenzymes.
  - Creatine Kinase (CK) - CK-MB, CK-MM, CK-BB are isoenzymes.

9. Name four clinically important enzymes. (MGR)

Answer

Clinically important enzymes include:

- Alanine aminotransferase (ALT): Elevated in Liver disease.
- Alkaline phosphatase (ALP): Elevated in Liver disease.
- Creatine kinase: Elevated in myocardial infarction.
- Amylase: Elevated in pancreatitis, salivary gland infection.

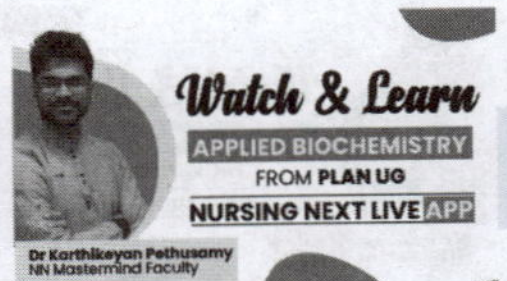

10. What are the coenzymes of pyridoxine? Mention a reaction where it is used? (MGR)

Answer

Pyridoxal phosphate (PLP) and pyridoxamine phosphate (PMP) are two coenzymes of pyridoxine. They are involved in the metabolism of amino acids.

11. What is enzyme inhibition? Classify. (MGR)

Answer

When a molecule (the inhibitor) attaches to an enzyme, it decreases or stops the activity of the enzyme. This process is known as enzyme inhibition. It is classified into reversible, irreversible and allosteric inhibitors.

12. Give four examples for detoxification by conjugation. (MGR)

Answer

Glucuronidation, Sulfation, Methylation and Acetylation are four examples for detoxification by conjugation.

13. Classify the enzymes. (MGR)

Answer

Enzymes can be broadly classified as:

- Oxidoreductases
- Transferases
- Hydrolases
- Lyases
- Isomerases
- Ligases

14. Enzymes elevated in myocardial infarction. (KUHS)

Answer

Some of the enzymes that are elevated in myocardial infarction are:

- Troponin
- Creatine kinase (CK)
- Lactate Dehydrogenase (LDH)
- Aspartate aminotransferase (AST)
- Myoglobin (nonspecific)

15. One enzyme indicating hepatocellular damage. (KUHS)

Answer

Hepatocytes, which are the cells of the liver, contain a large amount of the enzyme alanine aminotransferase (ALT). ALT is a sensitive indicator of hepatocellular injury because it is released into the bloodstream when liver cells are injured or destroyed.

16. Competitive inhibition. (KUHS)

Answer

When a substance with a structure identical to the substrate attaches to the enzyme's active site, it prevents the substrate from binding and lowers the enzyme's activity. This is referred to as competitive inhibition.

CONCEPTUAL REVISION

MULTIPLE CHOICE QUESTIONS

1. In the human body, enzyme activity is most efficient at:

a. 0°C b. 37°C
c. 42°C d. 60°C

Ans. b. 37°C

2. Definition of ribozyme:

a. t-RNA
b. RNA molecule that acts catalytically to change itself or another RNA molecule
c. Ribonucleoprotein
d. Ribosome

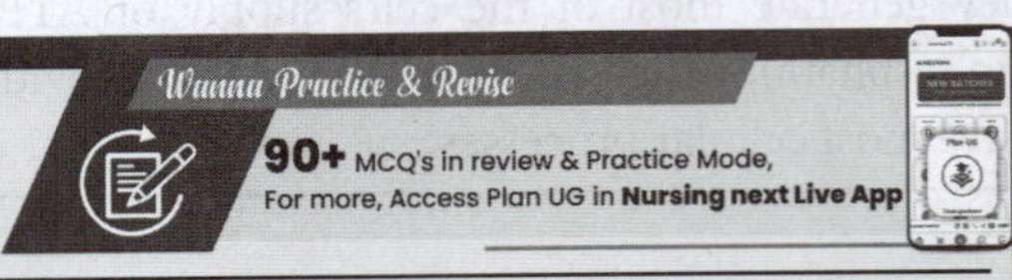

Ans. b. RNA molecule that acts catalytically to change itself or another RNA molecule

3. Which of these is not used by the body for energy?

a. Fat b. Carbohydrate
c. Protein d. Water

Ans. d. Water

4. Enzyme which splits C-C bond?

a. Lyase b. Ligase
c. Isomerase d. Transferase

Ans. a. Lyase

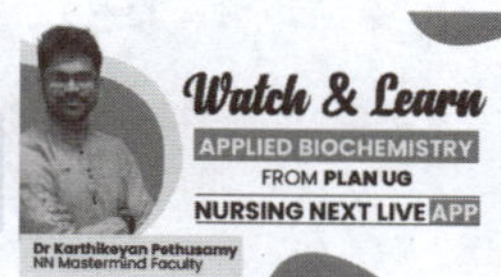

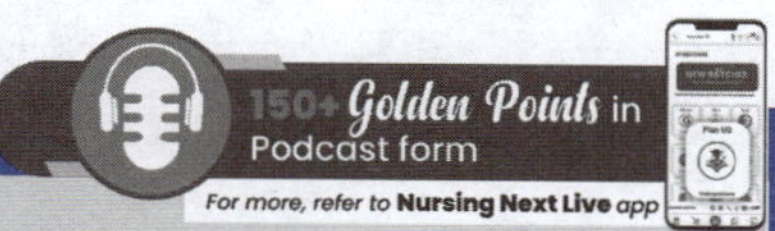

Golden Points

- A coenzyme is a dialyzable, thermostable, low-molecular weight, organic substance.
- A competitive inhibitor competes with the substrate for binding at the active sites of the enzyme.
- A metal ion may be either tightly bound to the enzyme (metalloenzymes) or loosely associated with it (metal-associated enzymes).
- A noncompetitive inhibitor may also bind at a site other than the substrate-binding site. a reversible noncompetitive inhibitor thus decreases V_{max} but does not change the K_m.
- According to IUBMB, each enzyme is assigned a four-digit systematic code, commonly known as Enzyme Commission number (E.C. number).
- According to the enzyme commission, enzymes are classified into six classes.
- All enzymes are proteinaceous in nature and have large molecular weights. Some RNA molecules called ribozymes, also have catalytic activity.
- Enzyme activity is expressed in terms of international units (IU).
- Enzymes are organic molecules that increase the rate of a biochemical reaction without being utilized in the overall process. They are non-dialyzable, colloidal particles which are thermolabile proteins with highly specific catalytic activity. An enzyme increases rate of a chemical reaction by lowering its free energy barrier that separates a substrate (reactant) from the product.
- High levels of ALP may indicate liver inflammation, blockage of the bile duct or a bone disease.
- Measurement of CK-MB, in serum, is used in the diagnosis of acute MI, where initial rise occurs within 4 – 6 hours.
- Most of the intracellular enzymes are secreted in their active form called zymase inactive form called proenzyme or zymogen
- Multienzyme complexes are single polypeptide chains with several catalytic sites.
- Oligomeric enzymes, having two or more subunits, have two different sites, which are called the catalytic site or regulatory site (also known as the allosteric site) and the substrate-binding site. Such enzymes are called allosteric enzymes or regulatory enzymes. Proenzyme (protein) + prosthetic group (non-protein component) = Holoenzyme
- Several enzymes require certain metal ions called cofactors for their activity, e.g., Mg^{2+}, Zn^{2+} or Cl^-, etc.
- The enzymes that occur in a number of different forms and differ from each other chemically, immunologically and electrophoretically are called isoenzymes or isozymes.
- These enzymes are referred to as holoenzymes (conjugated proteins). The protein part of such an enzyme is called apoenzyme (apo-protein) while the nonprotein component is called prosthetic group.

CHAPTER 5

Acid-Base Maintenance

CONCEPTUAL THEORY

Terminology

150+ key terminologies for Quick Recall & Revision

Acid: Acid is a substance whose dissociation in water releases hydrogen ions (H^+). Addition of an acid to a solution thus, increases the concentration of free H^+ ions in the solution.

Acidosis: Acidosis refers to a decrease in pH of the blood. It includes respiratory acidosis and metabolic acidosis.

Alkalosis: Alkalosis refers to an increase in pH of the blood. It includes respiratory alkalosis and metabolic alkalosis.

Amphoteric substances: Amphoteric Substances are substances, such as amino acids and proteins, that can act as acid as well as base, e.g., glycine.

Anion gap: Anion gap is a difference between the sum of Na^+ and K^+ (cations) from the sum of Cl^- and HCO_3^- (anions).

Buffer: A buffer is a solution, which resists change in pH.

Compensation: Compensation is the body's attempt to correct the imbalance, i.e., it is the system in the body, which it is trying to compensate for an abnormality in another system.

pH: pH is defined as the negative logarithm to the base 10 of the molar concentration of the hydrogen ions (H^+) in a solution.

ACID-BASE BALANCE

- Acid-base balance refers to the regulation and maintenance of the pH level in the body fluids, particularly the blood.

Normal Arterial Blood Gas (ABG) values:

Parameter	Normal range
pH	7.35–7.45
$PaCO_2$	35–45 mm Hg
PaO_2	80–100 mm Hg
HCO_3	22–26 mEq/L
SaO_2	95–100%

ACID-BASE DISORDER

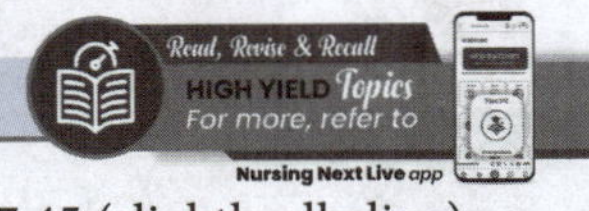

- Normal pH of blood – 7.35–7.45 (slightly alkaline)
- pH of erythrocytes – 7.2
- Acid-base disorders refers to a change in the normal value of extracellular pH
- Results when
  - Renal/respiratory function is abnormal
  - An acid or base load overwhelms excretory capacity
- Clinical disturbances of acid-base metabolism classically are defined in terms of the HCO_3^-/CO_2 buffer system.
- Acidosis –decrease in the blood pH below normal range
  - Process that increases $[H^+]$ by increasing pCO_2 or by reducing $[HCO_3^-]$
- Alkalosis – Elevation in blood pH above the normal range
  - Process that reduces $[H^+]$ by reducing pCO_2 or by increasing $[HCO_3^-]$

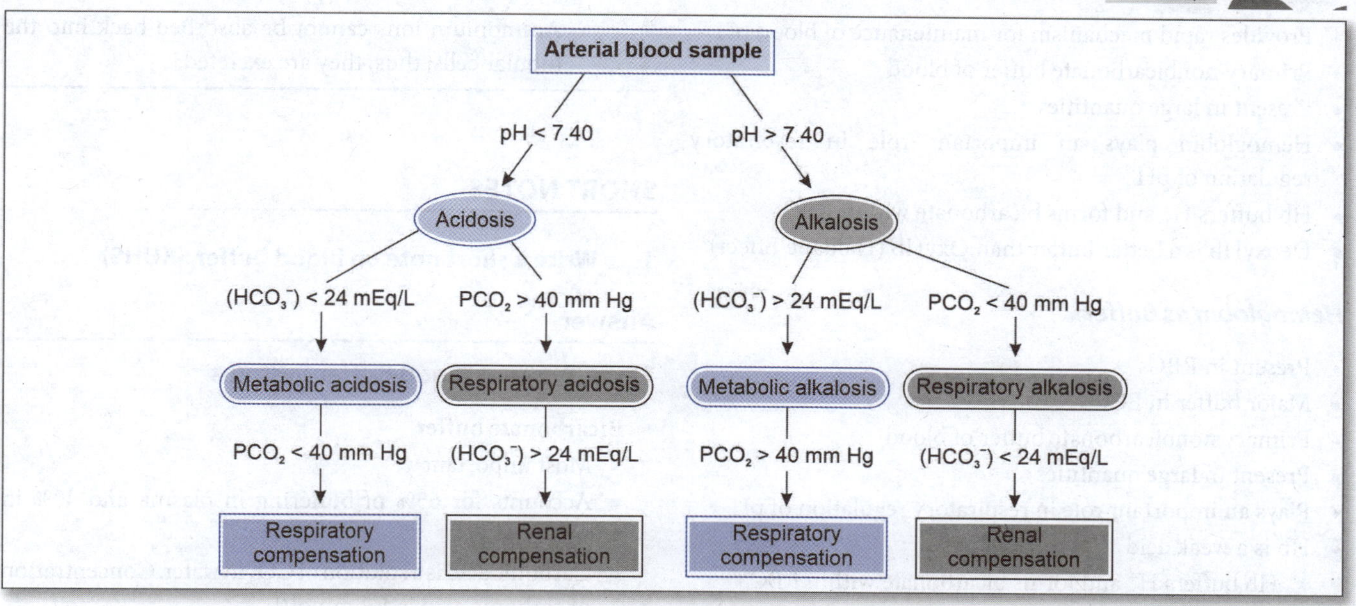

CONCEPTUAL EXERCISES

LONG ANSWER QUESTION

1. Explain the mechanisms that maintain pH of blood.

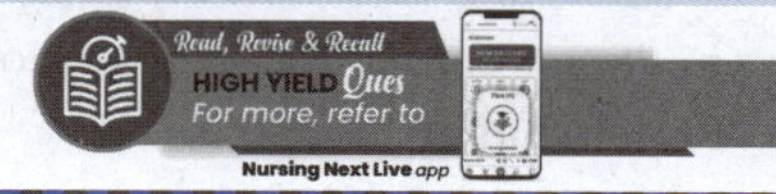

Answer

Introduction

- **Buffers:** Maintain pH
- **Blood buffers:** Maintain and regulate blood pH
- Defined as solution of weak acid and its salt with strong base
- **Function:** Maintains the blood pH at 7.4

Three lines of defense for regulation of blood pH

- Blood buffers
- Respiratory buffers
- Renal mechanism

Three types of blood buffer systems:

- **Bicarbonate buffer**
  - Most important
  - Accounts for 65% of buffering in plasma and 40% in whole body
  - Carbonic acid is a solution of CO_2 in water. Concentration of carbonic acid is 1.2 mmol/L
  - At blood pH, ratio of bicarbonate to carbonic acid is 20:1
  - Higher bicarbonate concentration – *alkali reserve* – buffering of hydrogen ions
- **Phosphate buffer**
  - Intracellular buffer
  - Sodium dihydrogen phosphate and disodium hydrogen phosphate constitute the phosphate buffer
  - Plasma concentration is very low
- **Protein buffer**
  - **Protein buffer:** Plasma proteins + hemoglobin
  - Dependent on pK of ionizable group of amino acid.

Respiratory Mechanism

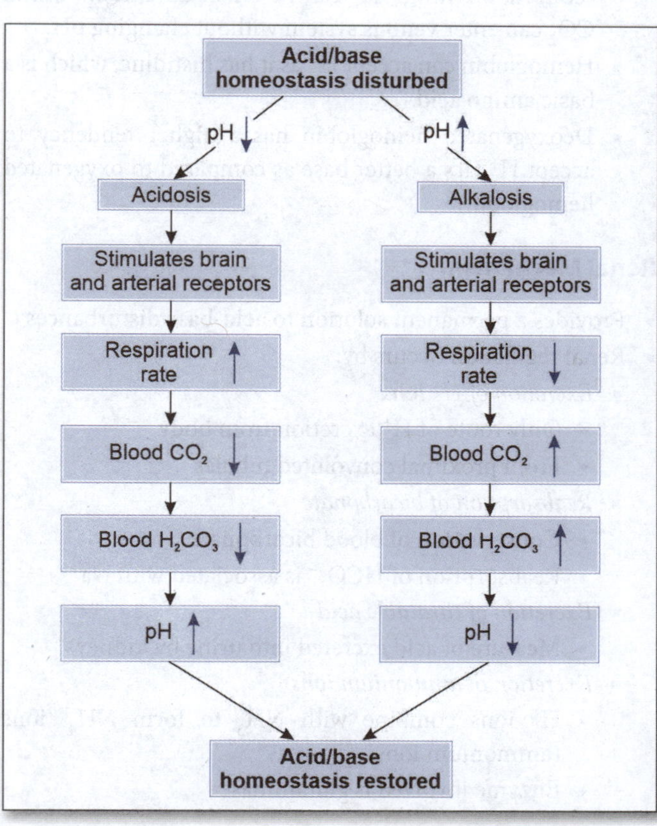

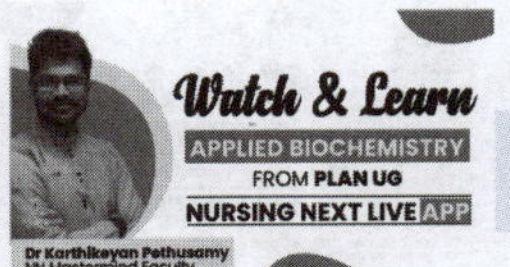

- Provides rapid mechanism for maintenance of blood pH
- Primary nonbicarbonate buffer of blood
- Present in large quantities
- Hemoglobin plays an important role in respiratory regulation of pH
- Hb buffers H^+ and forms bicarbonate within RBC
- DeoxyHb is a better buffer than OxyHb (Haldane Effect)

Hemoglobin as Buffer

- Present in RBCs
- Major buffer in ECF
- Primary nonbicarbonate buffer of blood
- Present in large quantities
- Plays an important role in respiratory regulation of pH
- Hb is a weak acid
  - Hb buffers H^+ and forms bicarbonate within RBC
  - Intracellular HCO_3 - increases, leading to diffusion down the concentration gradient out of the cell
  - The presence of an acid in the ECF leads to the maintenance of the concentration gradient and the continued movement of HCO_3 - from within the RBC
  - This contributes to 30% of the Haldane effect
- DeoxyHb is a better buffer than OxyHb (Haldane Effect)
  - DeoxyHb (pKa 8.2) dissociates more than OxyHb (pKa 6.6)
  - Isohydric buffering – for each mmol oxyHb that is reduced, 0.7 mmol H^+ can be taken up and 0.7 mmol CO_2 can enter venous system without changing pH.
  - Hemoglobin can accept H^+ as it has histidine, which is a basic amino acid.
  - Deoxygenated hemoglobin has a higher tendency to accept H^+ (It's a better base as compared to oxygenated hemoglobin)

Renal Mechanism

- Provides a permanent solution to acid-base disturbances
- Renal regulation occurs by:
  - *Excretion of H^+ ions*
    - Only route of H^+ excretion from body
    - From proximal convoluted tubules
  - *Reabsorption of bicarbonate*
    - Conservation of blood bicarbonate
    - Reabsorption of HCO_3^- is associated with Na^+
  - *Excretion of titratable acid*
    - Measure of acid excreted into urine by kidneys
  - *Excretion of ammonium ions*
    - H^+ ions combine with NH_3 to form NH_4^+ ions (ammonium ions)
    - Enzyme involved is glutaminase
    - Ammonium ions cannot be absorbed back into the tubular cells; thus, they are excreted.

SHORT NOTES

1. Write a short note on blood buffer. (KUHS)

Answer

Three Types of Blood Buffer Systems

- **Bicarbonate buffer**
  - Most important
  - Accounts for 65% of buffering in plasma and 40% in whole body
  - Carbonic acid is a solution of CO_2 in water. Concentration of carbonic acid is 1.2 mmol/L
  - At blood pH, ratio of bicarbonate to carbonic acid is 20:1
  - Higher bicarbonate concentration – *alkali reserve* – buffering of hydrogen ions
- **Phosphate buffer**
  - Intracellular buffer
  - Sodium dihydrogen phosphate and disodium hydrogen phosphate constitute the phosphate buffer
  - Plasma concentration is very low
- **Protein buffer**
  - **Protein buffer:** plasma proteins + hemoglobin
  - Dependent on pK of ionizable group of amino acid.

Hemoglobin as Buffer

- Present in RBCs
- Major buffer in ECF
- Primary nonbicarbonate buffer of blood
- Present in large quantities
- Plays an important role in respiratory regulation of pH

2. Add a note on role of kidney in acid-base balance. (MGR)

Answer

Introduction

- Renal response to an acid-base disturbance is slow but more accurate.
- The kidney regulates acid-base balance by controlling bicarbonate reabsorption and secreting acid.
- Both of these processes depend upon the formation of H^+ and HCO_3^- from CO_2 and H_2O within the tubule cells.

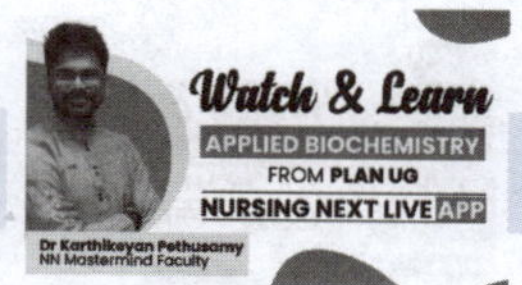

Secretion of H^+

Normally H^+ formed in the reaction is actively secreted into the tubular fluid, in exchange for Na^+. Within the tubule cell, Na^+ as well as HCO_3^- is pumped out of the cell into the interstitial fluid. Sodium uptake by the tubular cell is partly passive, flowing down the electrochemical gradient and partly active via $Na^+ - H^+$ antiport system.

Renal Mechanism

- Tries to provide a permanent solution to acid-base disturbances
- Maintains the alkali reserve and excretion of acidic substances
- Carbonic anhydrase enzyme – central importance in the renal regulation of blood pH
- Urine pH
  - Lower than blood pH
  - Usually acidic – pH 6.0, this is because H^+ ions are excreted mainly by urine
- **Renal regulation occurs by:**
  - *Excretion of H^+ ions*
    - Only route of H^+ excretion from body
    - From proximal convoluted tubules along with regeneration of bicarbonate
    - Carbonic anhydrase catalyzes the reaction between carbon dioxide and water to form carbonic acid (H_2CO_3)
    - Carbonic acid then breaks down to H^+ ions and HCO_3^-
    - H^+ is further secreted into the PCT in exchange for Na^+ ions
    - This effectively eliminates acids (H^+) from the body and regenerates bicarbonate
    - Builds up alkali reserve of the body
- **Reabsorption of bicarbonate**
  - Conservation of blood bicarbonate
  - Reabsorption of HCO_3^- is associated with the excretion of H^+ ions
  - Bicarbonate freely diffuses into the tubular cell lumen.
- **Excretion of titratable acid**
  - Measure of acid excreted into urine by kidneys
  - Estimated by titration of urine to blood pH
  - Occurs by phosphate buffer mechanism
- **Excretion of ammonium ions**
  - H^+ ions combine with NH_3 to form NH_4^+ ions (ammonium ions)
  - Enzyme involved is glutaminase
  - Ammonium ions cannot be absorbed back into the tubular cells, thus they are excreted.
  - NH_4^+ major urine acid

3. Differentiate between metabolic acidosis and metabolic alkalosis. (DU)

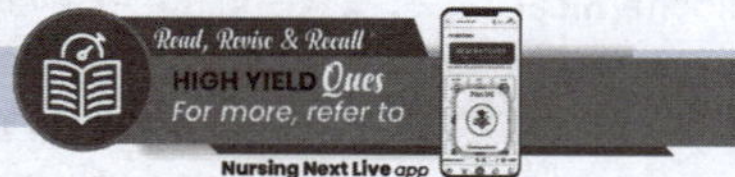

Answer

Differences between Metabolic Acidosis and Metabolic Alkalosis

	Metabolic acidosis	Metabolic alkalosis
Definition	Occurs as a result of excessive production of organic acids which combine with $NaHCO_3^-$ and deplete the alkali reserve.	Occurs as a result of decreased hydrogen ion concentration leading to an increase in bicarbonate concentration.
Effect on pH	Condition in which pH is decreased (below pH 7.35)	Condition in which pH is increased (above pH 7.45)
Causes	• Uncontrolled diabetes mellitus • Lactic acidosis • Ketoacidosis • Liver failure • Cardiac failure • Ethylene glycol • Renal tubular acidosis • Diarrhea – results in hypokalemia	• Excessive vomiting • Gastric lavage • Diuretic therapies • Prolonged diarrhea • Cystic fibrosis

Contd...

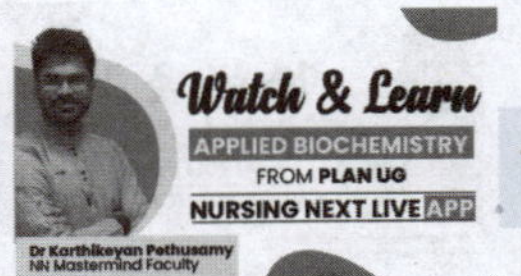

	Metabolic acidosis	Metabolic alkalosis
Clinical Manifestations	• Healthy individuals - 15 mEq/L (range – 8-18 mEq/L) • Acid-base disorders – associated with alteration in anion gap • Increased accumulation of organic acids – increased anion gap – in metabolic acidosis • Seen in diabetic ketoacidosis.	• Abnormal sensations • Neuromuscular irritability • Tetany • Abnormal heart rhythms • Electrolyte abnormalities ▪ Low potassium levels • Neurological symptoms such as coma and seizures • Temporary waxing and waning state of confusion
Compensatory mechanism	• Respiratory buffers – hyperventilation of lungs which causes increased carbon dioxide elimination – short lived • Renal mechanism – sets in 3–4 days and more long lasting	• Respiratory mechanism ▪ Hypoventilation causing retention of CO_2. • Renal compensation • Increased excretion of bicarbonate

4. Differentiate between respiratory acidosis and respiratory alkalosis. (DU)

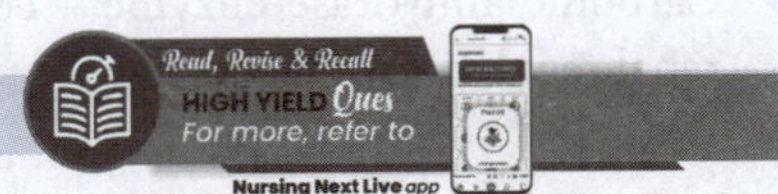

Answer

Differences between Respiratory Acidosis and Respiratory Alkalosis

	Respiratory acidosis	Respiratory alkalosis
Definition	• Due to increase in $PaCO_2$. • The level of $PaCO_2$ is determined by the rate of carbon dioxide production (VCO_2) and the rate of alveolar ventilation (VA), as follows: $PaCO_2 = K \times VCO_2/VA$, where K is a constant.	• Primary decrease in the partial pressure of carbon dioxide. • This may occur with or without compensatory decrease in bicarbonate • Occurs as a result of hyperventilation.
Biochemical assessment	• Acute –Elevated $PaCO_2$ is elevated and accompanying acidemia (pH <7.36). • Chronic – Elevated $PaCO_2$ is elevated with a normal blood pH secondary to renal compensation and an elevated serum bicarbonate	• Fall in arterial pCO_2. • pH may be high or normal

Causes	• Three possible mechanisms:
	  ▪ Presence of excess CO_2 in the inspired gas
	  ▪ Decreased alveolar ventilation
	  ▪ Increased production of CO_2 by the body: The increase in $PaCO_2$, in turn, decreases the bicarbonate (HCO_3^-)/$PaCO_2$ ratio, thereby decreasing the pH.
		• Anxiety
		• Central nervous system injury involving the respiratory center
		• Salicylate poisoning
		• Fever
		• High altitude, due to decrease in total atmospheric pressure, alveolar pCO_2 falls and there is chronic respiratory alkalosis.

Clinical manifestations	• Hyperpnea • Lightheadedness	• Hyperpnea • Lightheadedness • Confusion • Paresthesia • Carpopedal cramps • Syncope

Contd...

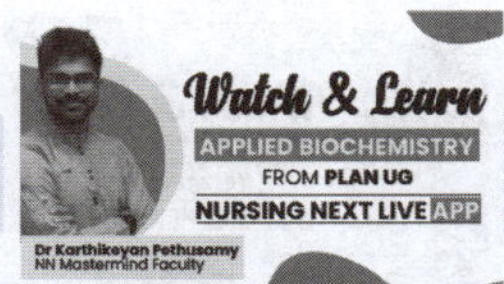

	Respiratory acidosis	Respiratory alkalosis
Compensatory mechanism	• Respiratory buffers – hyperventilation of lungs which causes increased carbon dioxide elimination – short lived • Renal mechanism – sets in 3–4 days and more long lasting	• Excretion of HCO_3^- in the urine • Low CO_2 leads to decreased H^+ secretion by the tubular epithelium • This, in turn, results in reduced reabsorption of the filtered bicarbonate and increases its excretion in the urine. • This loss of bicarbonate in the urine results in further decrease in plasma bicarbonate and brings plasma pH toward normal.

5. Normal values of serum electrolytes. (MGR)

Answer

Electrolytes Present in Serum

Electrolytes Present in Water

Electrolytes	
• Sodium	135–145 mEq/L
• Potassium	3.5–5.3 mEq/L
• Chloride	100–106 mEq/L
• Bicarbonate	• Normal arterial concentration – 22–26 mEq/L • Normal venous concentration – 24–30 mEq/L
• Calcium	4–5 mEq/L
• Magnesium	1.5–2.4 mEq/L
• Phosphate	2.5–4.5 mEq/L

- Sodium
  - Major cation in ECF
  - Normal concentration – 135–145 mEq/L
  - Maintains balance of extracellular fluid
  - Transmission of nerve impulses, neuromuscular and myocardial impulses
- Potassium
  - Major cation in ICF
  - Normal concentration – 3.5–5.3 mEq/L
  - Regulates neuromuscular excitability and muscle contraction
  - Regulates acid-base balance
- Chloride
  - Major anion in ECF
  - Normal concentration – 100–106 mEq/L
  - Maintains the electrical neutrality
- Bicarbonate
  - Normal arterial concentration – 22–26 mEq/L
  - Normal venous concentration – 24–30 mEq/L
  - Major chemical buffer
  - Essential component of carbonic acid – bicarbonate buffer
- Calcium
  - Most abundant element in the body
  - Normal concentration – 4–5 mEq/L
  - Regulated by:
    - Thyroid gland
    - Parathyroid gland
  - Maintains cell membrane integrity and structure
  - Conducts nerve impulses in skeletal muscle
  - Plays a role in blood coagulation, muscle relaxation and formation of bones
- Magnesium
  - Normal concentration – 1.5–2.4 mEq/L
  - Functions include:
    - Enzyme activity
    - Neurochemical activity
    - Muscular excitability
- Phosphate
  - Major anion in ICF
  - Normal concentration – 2.5–4.5 mEq/L
  - Has role in:
    - Development and maintenance of bones and teeth
    - Neuromuscular action
    - Acid-base regulation

6. Write a short note on metabolic acidosis. (MGR)

Answer

Metabolic Acidosis

- Result of excessive production of organic acids which combine with $NaHCO^-{}_3$ and deplete the alkali reserve.
- Increased anion gap

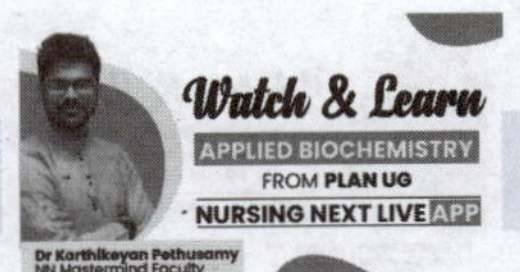

Causes

- Uncontrolled diabetes mellitus
- Lactic acidosis
- Ketoacidosis
- Liver failure
- Cardiac failure
- Ethylene glycol
- Renal tubular acidosis
- *Diarrhea – results in hypokalemia*

Anion Gap

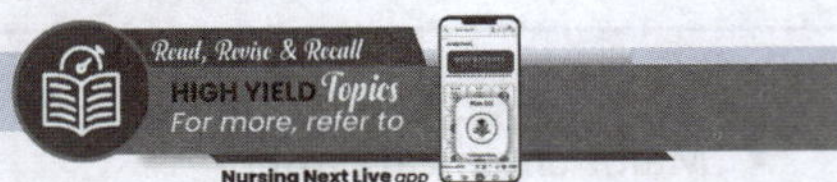

- Represented as A^-
- Defined as the difference between the total concentration of measured cations and anions
- Represents the unmeasured anions in plasma

Calculation of Anion Gap

- Measured in mEq/L
  $Na^+ + K^+ = Cl^- + HCO_3^- + A^-$
  $136 + 4 = 100 + 25 + A^-$
  $A^- = 15$ mEq/L

Significance of Metabolic Acidosis

- Healthy individuals: 15 mEq/L (range – 8–18 mEq/L)
- Acid-base disorders are associated with alteration in anion gap
- Increased accumulation of organic acids – increased anion gap – in metabolic acidosis
- Seen in diabetic ketoacidosis.

Compensatory Mechanism of Metabolic acidosis

- Respiratory buffers – hyperventilation of lungs which causes increased carbon dioxide elimination – short lived
- Renal mechanism – sets in 3–4 days and more long lasting

7. Write a short note on metabolic alkalosis. (MGR)

Answer

Metabolic Alkalosis

- Condition in which pH is increased
- Occurs as a result of decreased hydrogen ion concentration leading to an increase in bicarbonate concentration.
- Characterized by:
  - Intake of excess alkali, i.e., by the gain of strong base or HCO_3^-
  - Abnormal loss of acid

Clinical Manifestations

- Abnormal sensations
- Neuromuscular irritability
- Tetany
- Abnormal heart rhythms
- Electrolyte abnormalities
  - Low potassium levels
- Neurological symptoms such as coma and seizures
- Temporary waxing and waning – a state of confusion

Causes

- Excessive vomiting
- Gastric lavage
- Diuretic therapies
- Prolonged diarrhea
- Cystic fibrosis

Biochemical Assessment

- Increase in plasma bicarbonate concentration
- Rise in pH
- Compensatory increase in pCO_2

Compensatory Mechanism

- Respiratory mechanism
  - Hypoventilation causing retention of CO_2
- Renal compensation
  - Increased excretion of bicarbonate

SHORT ANSWER QUESTIONS

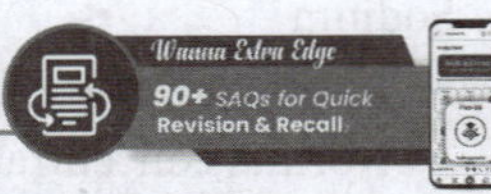

1. Write any two functions of calcium. (MGR)

Answer

- A vital component of bone tissue, calcium gives bones their strength and shape.
- Muscle contraction, which enables movement and functional performance, involves calcium.

2. Name of the hormones regulating blood calcium level. (MGR)

Answer

1. **Parathyroid hormone:** It is produced by the parathyroid glands. It increases blood calcium levels by stimulating the release of calcium from bones, promoting the reabsorption of calcium in the kidneys, and increasing the absorption of calcium from the intestines.

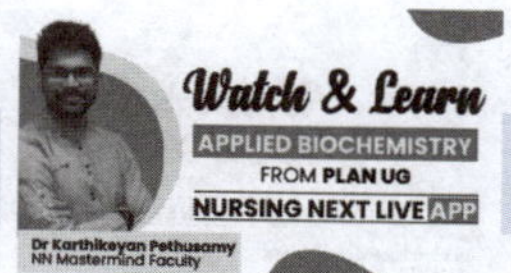

2. **Calcitonin:** It is produced by the thyroid gland. It acts on the bones to decrease blood calcium levels by inhibiting the release of calcium from bones.

3. Optimum pH. (MGR)

Answer

The pH range where a specific enzyme or chemical reaction operates most effectively is referred to as the optimal pH. The optimum pH level of human blood is from 7.35 to 7.45.

4. Define metabolic acidosis. (MGR)

Answer

In metabolic acidosis, the pH of the blood drops below the normal range of 7.35 to 7.45. Metabolic acidosis is a medical condition in which the body produces too much acid due to metabolic causes, or cannot effectively remove acid from the body. It may be due to accumulation of lactic acid due to anaerobic metabolism, the accumulation of ketones due to uncontrolled diabetes, or loss of bicarbonates.

5. Define acidosis. (MGR)

Answer

A fall in blood pH below 7.35 as a result of the medical condition is known as acidosis. It is characterized by an excess of acid in the blood and bodily tissues.

6. Define metabolic alkalosis. (MGR)

Answer

Metabolic alkalosis occurs when the body's tissues and blood have an excessive amount of the base bicarbonate and insufficient amounts of acid. In metabolic alkalosis, the pH of the blood rises above the normal range of 7.35 to 7.45. It can result from various causes such as excessive vomiting, the use of diuretics, or the excessive intake of alkali substances such as antacids.

7. Bicarbonate buffer. (DU)

Answer

The pH balance of the blood and other biological fluids is maintained by the bicarbonate buffer system. The bicarbonate buffer system is a physiological mechanism that helps to regulate the pH of the blood and other body fluids. It works by using bicarbonate ions (HCO_3^-) and carbonic acid (H_2CO_3) to maintain the pH within a narrow range of 7.35 to 7.45.

8. What are blood buffers. (DU)

Answer

- Blood buffers are chemical systems in the blood that help to maintain the pH of the blood and other body fluids within a narrow range of 7.35 to 7.45. They work by absorbing or releasing hydrogen ions (H^+) in response to changes in acid-base balance.
- The three main blood buffer systems include:
  - Bicarbonate Buffer system
  - Phosphate buffer system
  - Protein buffer system

9. Define anion gap. (KUHS)

Answer

Anion gap is a measure of the difference between the concentration of cations (positively charged ions) and anions (negatively charged ions) in the blood. Anion gap is an important diagnostic tool that can help identify the underlying cause of an acid-base disorder, such as metabolic acidosis.

Anion Gap = $([Na^+] + [K^+]) - ([Cl^-] + [HCO_3^-])$

10. Define respiratory alkalosis. (KUHS)

Answer

Respiratory alkalosis is a medical disorder in which an excessive quantity of breathing causes the blood pH to become overly alkaline (above the 7.45), increasing the amount of carbon dioxide expelled from the lungs.

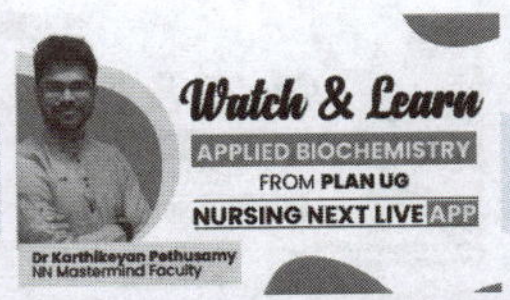

CONCEPTUAL REVISION

MULTIPLE CHOICE QUESTIONS

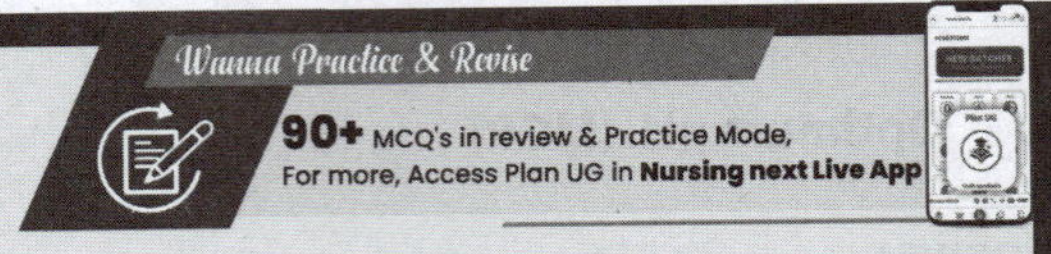

1. A pH of 7.1 is considered:

a. Neutral b. Weakly acidic
c. Weakly alkaline d. Strongly acidic

Ans. c. Weakly alkaline

2. At the time of measuring the oxygen saturation of a COVID client, the nurse Reena noted down 65 mm Hg. The client asks the nurse what should be the normal laboratory value of arterial PO_2?

a. 60–100 mm Hg b. 75–100 mm Hg
c. 40–80 mm Hg d. 33–44 mm Hg

Ans. b. 75–100 mm Hg

3. A 32-year-old client comes to the to emergency department with muscle twitching, severe vomiting and confusion due to excess intake of alcohol. The physician diagnosed that the client has metabolic alkalosis. Which of the following ABG values of the client suggests metabolic alkalosis?

a. pH <7.35, HCO_3^- = 20 mEq/L
b. pH <7.2, HCO_3^- = 28 mEq/L
c. pH >7.5, HCO_3^- = 32 mEq/L
d. pH = 7.4, PCO_2 = 40 mm Hg

Ans. c. pH > 7.5, HCO_3^- = 32 mEq/L

4. A client with diabetes mellitus has a carbon dioxide level of 46 mEq/L. The nurse would expect to see which symptom in the client with a carbon dioxide level of 46 mEq/L?

a. Absence of audible respirations
b. Eupnea
c. Kussmaul breathing
d. Slow respirations

Ans. c. Kussmaul breathing

5. A patient has the following arterial blood gases (ABGs): pH 7.38, HCO_3 24 and PCO_2 38. How do you interpret these results?

a. Metabolic acidosis b. Respiratory acidosis
c. Metabolic alkalosis d. Normal

Ans. d. Normal

6. A patient with AKI has a serum potassium level of 6.7 mEq/L (6.7 mmol/L) and the following arterial blood gas results: pH 7.28, $PaCO_2$ 30 mm Hg, PaO_2 86 mm Hg, HCO_3^- 18 mEq/L (18 mmol/L). The nurse recognizes that treatment of the acid-base problem with sodium bicarbonate would cause a decrease in which value?

a. pH b. Potassium level
c. Bicarbonate level d. Carbon dioxide level

Ans. b. Potassium level

7. Blood pH is 7.2, PCO_2 is 30 mm Hg and HCO_3^- is 10 mEq/L. It is a picture of which partially compensated disorder?

a. Metabolic acidosis b. Metabolic alkalosis
c. Respiratory acidosis d. Respiratory alkalosis

Ans. a. Metabolic acidosis

8. An unconscious patient presented with tachypnea. His blood sugar was 350 mg/dL and pH was 7.2. He has:

a. Metabolic acidosis b. Metabolic alkalosis
c. Respiratory acidosis d. Respiratory alkalosis

Ans. a. Metabolic acidosis

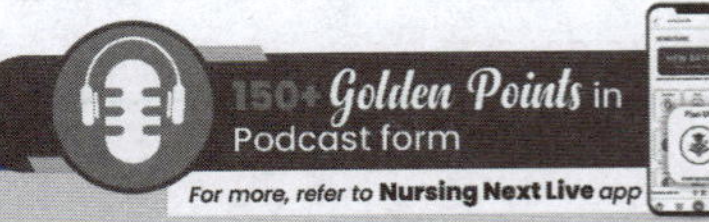

Golden Points

- Amphoteric Substances are substances such as amino acids and proteins that can act as acid as well as base, e.g., glycine.
- Metabolic acidosis is characterized by the accumulation of nonvolatile acids (gain of fixed acids other than H_2CO_3) and loss of HCO_3
- Metabolic alkalosis is characterized by the intake of excess alkali, i.e., by the gain of strong base or HCO_3^-, or abnormal loss of acid other than H_2CO_3.

CHAPTER 6

Heme, Porphyria and Jaundice

CONCEPTUAL THEORY

Terminology

150+ key terminologies for Quick Recall & Revision

Bilirubin: Bilirubin is an orange-yellow pigment, derived from the breakdown of red blood cells in the liver, spleen and bone marrow.

Direct bilirubin: Direct bilirubin refers to the bilirubin which undergoes chemical change (conjugation) in the liver.

Hemoglobin: Hemoglobin is a globular protein, which is present in high concentration in red blood cells. A molecule of hemoglobin consists of four heme groups along with the four polypeptide chains.

Indirect bilirubin: Indirect bilirubin refers to the bilirubin formed by the breakdown of red blood cells which travels from the blood to the liver.

Jaundice: Jaundice is a physical sign characterized by yellow appearance of the patient and is the most characteristic clinical manifestation of hyperbilirubinemia.

Unconjugated bilirubin: Unconjugated bilirubin is hydrophobic and, therefore, cannot be excreted in urine. Conversely, conjugated bilirubin is hydrophilic and, thus, can be excreted in the urine.

Van den Bergh: Van den Bergh test is a chemical reaction used to measure bilirubin levels in blood.

HEME DEGRADATION PATHWAY

- Life span of erythrocytes is 120 days.
- Erythrocytes are degraded by the macrophages of reticulo endothelial system in spleen.
- Hemoglobin breaks down into heme and protein.
- The globin protein is either reutilized for hemoglobin synthesis or broken down to individual amino acids.

Fate of Heme

- **Sources of heme:** Erythrocytes (80%) and immature RBCs, myoglobin, cytochromes (20%)
- **Heme oxygenase:** With the help of this enzyme, heme breaks down into biliverdin (green pigment), Fe^{3+} iron and carbon dioxide in the presence of NADPH and oxygen
- Biliverdin is excreted in birds and amphibians, while in mammals it is degraded to form bilirubin (yellow pigment) by biliverdin reductase.
- **Bilirubin**
  - Bilirubin and its derivatives – bile pigments
  - Lipophilic – insoluble in aqueous medium
- **In liver**
  - The albumin-bilirubin complex dissociates and bilirubin is taken up by sinusoidal surface of the hepatocytes by a carrier mediated active transport.
  - Bilirubin conjugates with glucuronate in the presence of bilirubin glucuronyltransferase to form water soluble bilirubin diglucuronide
  - Bilirubin diglucuronide is excreted in bile by an active energy dependent process.
- Bilirubin diglucuronide is hydrolyzed in the intestine by special enzymes – diglucuronidases – to liberate bilirubin which is converted to urobilinogen (colorless), a part of which is reabsorbed in circulation.
- Urobilinogen is converted to urobilin (yellow pigment) in kidney and excreted in urine (*urobilin imparts the yellow color to urine*)
- Major part of urobilinogen is converted to stercobilin, which is excreted along with feces (*stercobilin imparts the brown color to feces*).

Disorders Associated with Bilirubin Metabolism

Jaundice

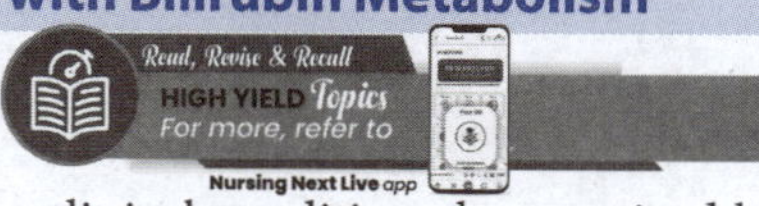

- Jaundice or icterus is a clinical condition characterized by yellow discoloration of skin and sclera.

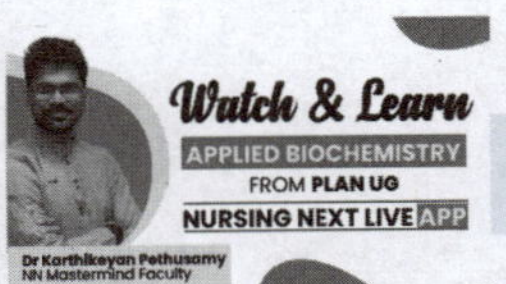

- Results from the increased serum bilirubin concentration leading to bilirubin deposition.
- Divided into three types:

1. Hemolytic 2. Hepatic 3. Obstructive

Van den Bergh Test for Bilirubin

- Specific test for identification of increased serum bilirubin levels
- Normal serum gives a negative Van den Bergh reaction

Mechanism of Reaction

- **Van den Bergh reagent:** Mixture of equal volume of sulfanilic acid and sodium nitrite
- **Principle:** Diazotized sulfanilic acid reacts with bilirubin to form a purple colored azobilirubin
- **Direct and indirect reactions**
  - Bilirubin is insoluble in water
  - Conjugated bilirubin is soluble
  - Van den Bergh reagent reacts with conjugated bilirubin and gives a purple color within 30 seconds – *Direct positive test*
  - Addition of methanol dissolves the unconjugated bilirubin and gives Van den Bergh reaction positive within 30 minutes – *Indirect positive*

Significance

- **Van den Bergh reaction and jaundice**
  - Indirect positive – Hemolytic jaundice
  - Direct positive – Obstructive jaundice
  - Biphasic – Hepatic Jaundice

CONCEPTUAL EXERCISES

LONG ANSWER QUESTION

1. Write in detail about the synthesis and break down of heme and the disorders associated with bilirubin metabolism. (MGR)

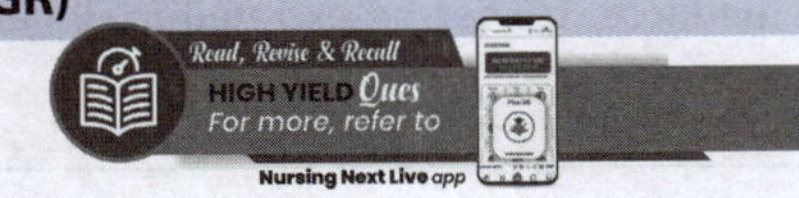

Answer

Biosynthesis of Heme

- Occurs mainly in liver and erythroid cells
- Absent in mature RBCs lacking mitochondria.
- **Occurs in the following steps:**
  - Formation of δ aminolevulinate (ALA) by the fusion of glycine and succinyl CoA in the presence of enzyme δ aminolevulinate synthase in the mitochondria. – rate limiting step

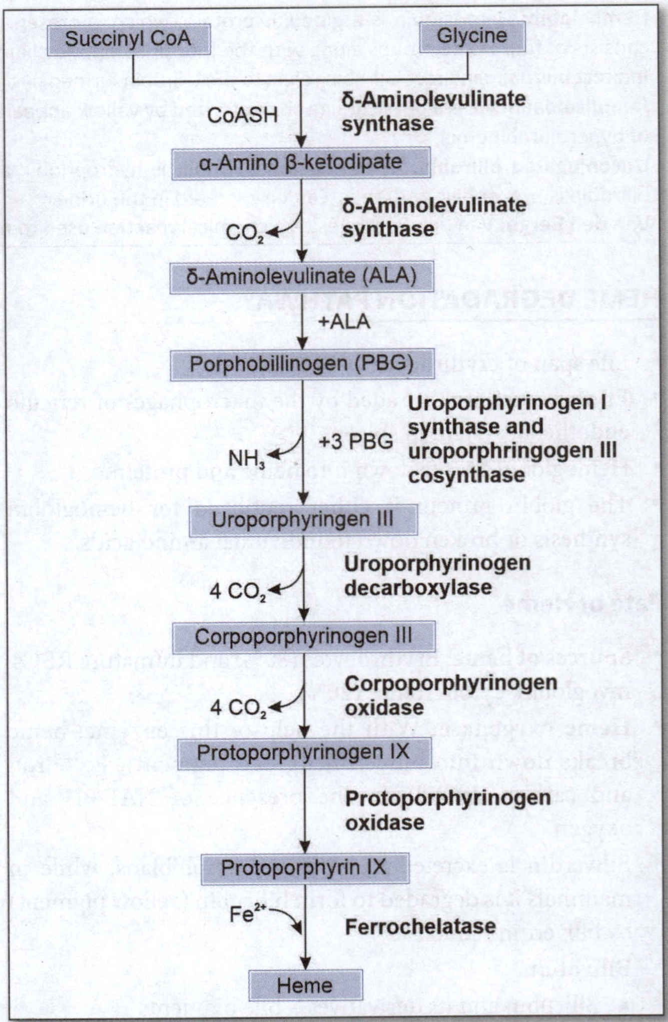

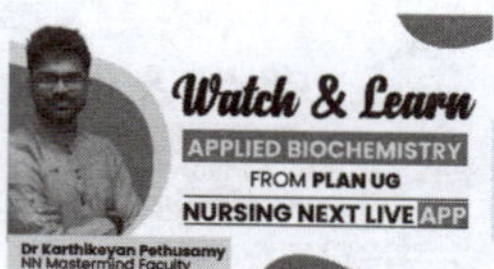

- 2 molecules of ALA condense to form porphobilinogen in the presence of ALA dehydrase
- 4 molecules of porphobilinogen condense to porphyrin.
- Pyrrole rings are interconnected by methylene bridges from alpha carbon of glycine.
- Uroporphyrinogen I synthase and uroporphyrinogen III cosynthase causes condensation of porphobilinogen followed by ring closure to form uroporphyrinogen III
- Uroporphyrinogen III undergoes a series of reactions to form protoporphyrin IX.
- Ferrochelatase incorporates a ferrous ion into the protoporphyrin IX leading to the formation of heme. This enzyme is inhibited by lead.

Two Mechanisms of Regulation Exist

- In liver
- In erythroid cells

Mechanism in Liver

- First step in heme biosynthesis in the presence of δ amino levulinate (ALA) synthase is regulated by heme or its oxidized product hemin by:
  - Feedback inhibition
  - Repression of ALA synthase
  - Inhibition of transport of ALA synthase from cytosol to mitochondria (site of action)
- **Effects of drugs on ALA synthase activity**
  - Activity is increased by drugs such as phenobarbital, insecticides, carcinogens
  - These lead to depletion of cellular levels of heme due to its increased corporation into cyctochrome P450.

Mechanism in Erythroid Cells

- Uroporphyrinogen synthase and ferrochelatase regulate heme formation in erythroid cells
- Cellular uptake of iron also affects the heme synthesis Heme stimulates globin synthesis

Degradation of Heme

- **Heme oxygenase:** With the help of this enzyme, heme breaks down into biliverdin (green pigment), Fe^{3+} iron and carbon dioxide in the presence of NADPH and oxygen
- **Bilirubin**
  - Bilirubin and its derivatives – bile pigments
  - One gram of hemoglobin on degradation yields 35 mg of bilirubin
  - Lipophilic – insoluble in aqueous medium
  - Transported to liver by binding to plasma albumin (25 mg – tightly bound, 10 mg – loosely bound)
- **In liver**
  - The albumin-bilirubin complex dissociates, and bilirubin is taken up by sinusoidal surface of the hepatocytes by a carrier mediated active transport.
  - Bilirubin conjugates with glucuronate in the presence of bilirubin glucuronyl transferase to form water soluble bilirubin diglucuronide
  - Bilirubin diglucuronide is excreted in bile by an active energy dependent process.
- Bilirubin diglucuronide is hydrolyzed in the intestine by special enzymes – diglucuronidases – to liberate bilirubin which is converted to urobilinogen (colorless), a part of which is reabsorbed in circulation.

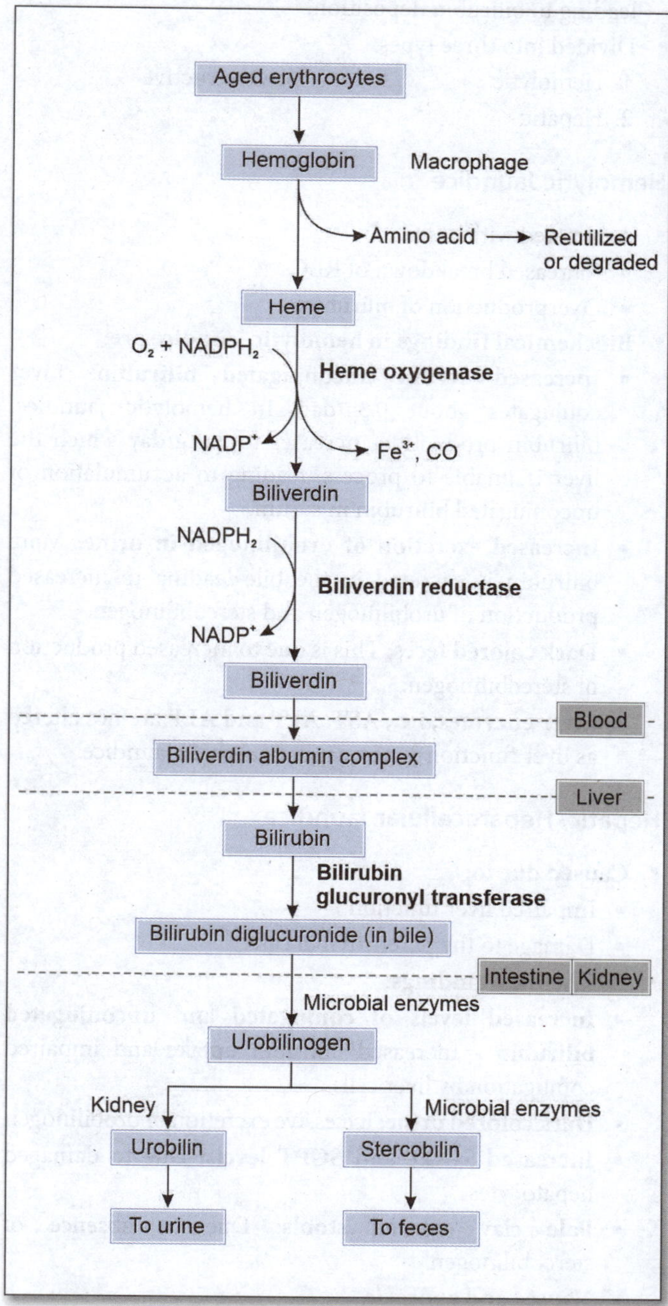

- Urobilinogen is converted to urobilin (yellow pigment) in kidney and excreted in urine (*urobilin imparts the yellow color to urine*)
- Major part of urobilinogen is converted to stercobilin, which is excreted along with feces (*stercobilin imparts the brown color to feces*)

Disorders Associated with Bilirubin Metabolism

Jaundice

- Jaundice or icterus is a clinical condition characterized by yellow discoloration of skin and sclera.
- Results from the increased serum bilirubin concentration leading to bilirubin deposition.
- Divided into three types:
  1. Hemolytic
  2. Hepatic
  3. Obstructive

Hemolytic Jaundice

- Associated with:
  - Increased breakdown of RBCs
  - Overproduction of bilirubin.
- **Biochemical findings in hemolytic jaundice are:**
  - **Increased serum unconjugated bilirubin:** Liver conjugates about 0.3g/day. In hemolytic jaundice, bilirubin production increases to 3.0 g/day which the liver is unable to process, leading to accumulation of unconjugated bilirubin in serum.
  - **Increased excretion of urobilinogen in urine:** More bilirubin is excreted in the bile leading to increased production of urobilinogen and stercobilinogen.
  - **Dark colored feces:** This is due to increased production of stercobilinogen.
  - **Liver enzymes, i.e., AST, ALT and ALP** are not altered as liver function is normal in hemolytic jaundice.

Hepatic/ Hepatocellular Jaundice

- **Caused due to:**
  - Impaired liver function
  - Damage to the parenchymal cells
- **Biochemical findings:**
  - **Increased levels of conjugated and unconjugated bilirubin** - Increased bilirubin uptake and impaired conjugation by liver cells
  - **Dark colored urine:** Excessive excretion of urobilinogen
  - **Increased SGOT and SGPT levels:** Due to damaged hepatocytes
  - **Pale clay colored stools:** Due to absence of stercobilinogen
  - **Nausea and anorexia**

Obstructive Jaundice

- Due to obstruction in the bile duct
- Obstructs the passage of bile to intestine
- Obstruction may be due to:
  - Gallstones
  - Tumors
- **Biochemical/Laboratory findings:**
  - **Increased serum conjugated bilirubin (>1 mg/dL):** Due to bile duct blockage, conjugated bilirubin enters blood circulation
  - **Increased serum alkaline phosphatase (>147 U/L):** Released from damaged bile duct cells
  - **Dark colored urine:** Due to increased excretion of bilirubin
  - **Clay colored stools:** Absence of stercobilinogen
  - **Nausea and GI pain**

SHORT NOTES

1. What is methemoglobin? What is its significance? (MGR)

Answer

Introduction

- Hemoglobin combines with different ligands and forms hemoglobin derivatives.
- **Hemoglobin derivatives include:**
  - Oxyhemoglobin
  - Deoxyhemoglobin
  - Methemoglobin
  - Carboxyhemoglobin

Methemoglobin

- Biological function of hemoglobin – carrying oxygen – occurs when iron is in ferrous state (Fe^{2+})
- When hemoglobin (Fe^{2+}) is oxidized, it forms methemoglobin (Fe^{3+})
- Normally, molecular oxygen does not oxidize Hb, it only loosely binds to form oxyhemoglobin

Causes

The oxidation of hemoglobin to methemoglobin is caused by:

- H_2O_2
- Free radicals
- Drugs

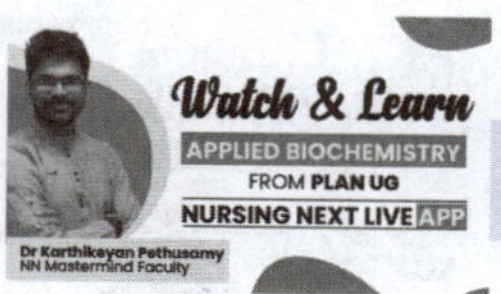

Clinical Significance

- Fe^{3+} is unable to bind oxygen as its site is occupied by water.
- This is corrected by enzyme methemoglobin reductase in normal cases.

2. Write about types of jaundice and laboratory findings in a case of obstructive jaundice. (MGR)

Answer

Types of Jaundice

- Jaundice or icterus is a clinical condition characterized by yellow discoloration of skin and sclera.
- Results from the increased serum bilirubin concentration leading to bilirubin deposition.
- Divided into three types:
  - Hemolytic
    - Associated with:
      - ❒ Increased breakdown of RBCs
      - ❒ Overproduction of bilirubin
  - Hepatic
    - Caused due to:
      - ❒ Impaired liver function
      - ❒ Damage to the parenchymal cells
  - Obstructive
    - Due to obstruction in the bile duct
    - Obstructs the passage of bile to intestine
    - Obstruction may be due to:
      - ❒ Gallstones
      - ❒ Tumors

Laboratory Findings

- **Increased serum conjugated bilirubin:** Due to bile duct blockage, conjugated bilirubin enters blood circulation
- **Increased serum alkaline phosphatase:** Released from damaged bile duct cells
- **Dark-colored urine:** Due to increased excretion of bilirubin
- **Clay-colored stools:** Absence of stercobilinogen
- **Nausea and GI pain**

3. Differentiate between the prehepatic jaundice and obstructive jaundice. (KUHS)

Answer

Differences between Prehepatic Jaundice and Obstructive Jaundice

Features	Prehepatic (Hemolytic jaundice)	Posthepatic (Obstructive jaundice)
Cause	Excessive breakdown of RBC producing ↑ed bilirubin that cannot be conjugated by normal liver	Obstruction of bile ducts (head of pancreas mostly). Conjugated bilirubin cannot be excreted
Types of excessive bilirubin in plasma	Unconjugated	Conjugated
Van den Bergh test	Indirect positive	Direct positive
Plasma protein profile:		
Albumin	Normal	May reduce in later stage
Globulin	Normal	Normal
A:G ratio	Normal	Usually normal
Serum enzymes level		
ALP/GGT	Normal	↑↑ed
SGOP/AST	Normal	↑ed/normal
SGPT/ALT	Normal	↑ed/normal
Urine bilirubin	Absent (acholuric jaundice)	Present (choleric jaundice)
Urobilinogen	↑	Absent in complete obstruction
Fecal stercobilinogen	↑↑	Absent, if complete obstruction
Fat	Normal	↑↑
Thymol turbidity	Nil	Usually slight

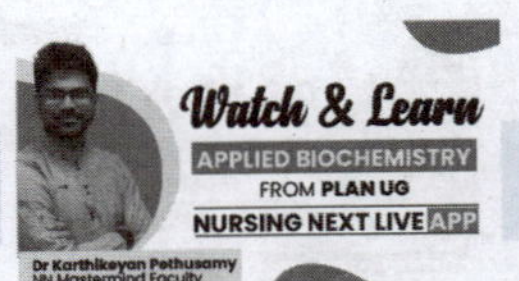

SHORT ANSWER QUESTIONS

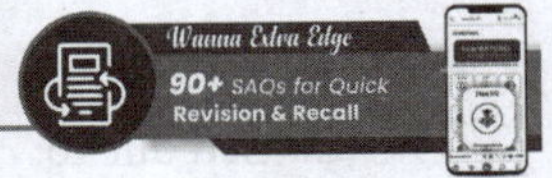

1. Types of jaundice. (MGR)

Answer

There are various types of jaundice:

- **Prehepatic:** Usually due to excessive breakdown of blood cells (excessive bilirubin)
- **Hepatic:** Due to liver problems
- **Posthepatic jaundice (obstructive jaundice):** Due to blockage of bile ducts
- **Physiological jaundice:** Due to breakdown of fetal red blood cells in newborns
- **Drug-induced jaundice:** As a side effect of certain drugs

2. Laboratory findings in case of obstructive jaundice. (MGR)

Answer

- Elevated bilirubin levels (conjugated or direct bilirubin) (>1 mg/dL)
- Elevated alkaline phosphatase (ALP) levels (>147 U/L)
- Elevated transaminase levels (>36 U/L) and
- Abnormal liver function tests are the findings in case of obstructive jaundice.

3. Name the primary and secondary bile acids. (MGR)

Answer

- Primary bile acids are cholic acid and chenodeoxycholic acid.
- Secondary bile acids are deoxycholic acid and lithocholic acid.

4. What is methemoglobin? What is its significance? (MGR)

Answer

- Hemoglobin can be oxidized to generate methemoglobin, which changes iron from the ferrous (Fe^{2+}) state to ferric (Fe^{3+}) state.
- Methemoglobinemia is a condition characterized by elevated levels of methemoglobin which can lead to hypoxia.

5. What is the normal total serum bilirubin level? Mention the name of the test for it. (MGR)

Answer

- The normal total serum bilirubin level is usually <1.2 mg/dL.
- The Van den Bergh test, also known as the bilirubin test or diazo reaction, is a laboratory test used to measure the levels of bilirubin in the blood.

6. Van den Bergh test. (MGR)

Answer

A chemical method called the Van den Bergh reaction is used to assess blood bilirubin levels. The Van den Bergh test is commonly used to distinguish between unconjugated (indirect) and conjugated (direct) bilirubin in the blood. This examination aids in determining the type of jaundice.

7. Jaundice. (KUHS)

Answer

Jaundice is a medical condition that results in yellowing of the skin, sclera (white of the eyes), and mucous membranes, caused by an excess of bilirubin in the blood.

8. Urinary findings in obstructive jaundice. (KUHS)

Answer

In obstructive jaundice, dark urine (brownish-yellow or even dark brown in color), elevated bilirubin level and proteinuria are observed in urine.

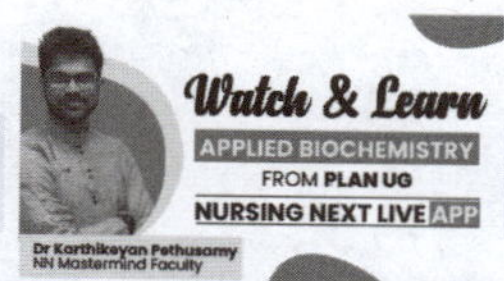

CONCEPTUAL REVISION

MULTIPLE CHOICE QUESTIONS

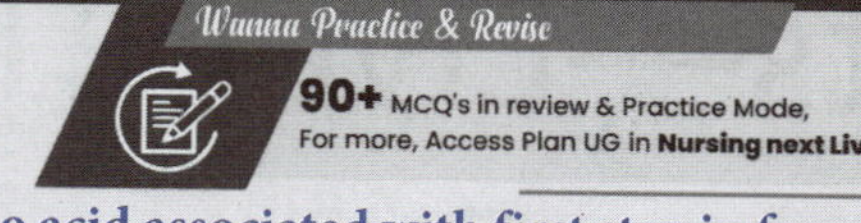

1. **Heme is which porphyrin?**
   a. Type I b. Type II
   c. Type III d. Type IV

Ans. c. Type III

2. **A patient seen in the ER has ingested antifreeze in a suicide attempt. Other than bicarbonate, which one of the following is the major buffer of acids to help maintain the pH in the blood within the range compatible with life?**
   a. Hemoglobin b. Acetoacetate
   c. Phosphate d. Collagen

Ans. a. Hemoglobin

3. **Amino acid associated with first step in formation of Heme is:**
   a. Histidine b. Glycine
   c. Alanine d. Lysine

Ans. b. Glycine

4. **Which one of the following is the amino acid in hemoglobin that accepts H^+ and allows hemoglobin to act as a buffer to acids?**
   a. Alanine b. Histidine
   c. Serine d. Aspartate

Ans. b. Histidine

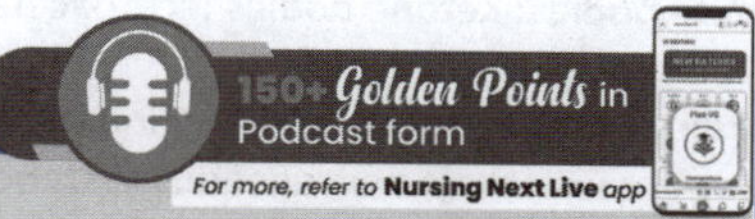

Golden Points

- β-thalassemias also exhibit different degrees of severity and can be caused by a variety of defects or deletions.
- Bilirubin fractionation is also helpful in differential diagnosis of jaundice.
- Bilirubin is an orange-yellow pigment, derived from the breakdown of red blood cells in the liver, spleen and bone marrow.
- Biliverdin is reduced to bilirubin by the enzyme biliverdin reductase.
- Degradation of heme occurs mainly in the liver.
- Hemoglobin is a globular protein, which is present in high concentration in red blood cells. A molecule of hemoglobin consists of four heme groups along with the four polypeptide chains.
- Jaundice is a physical sign characterized by yellow appearance of the patient and is the most characteristic clinical manifestation of hyperbilirubinemia.
- Normally, almost all the bilirubin in plasma is unconjugated.
- One gram of hemoglobin yields about 35 mg of bilirubin.
- Red blood cells have limited lifespan of approximately 100–120 days.

Organ Function Tests—Liver, Thyroid, Kidney, Pancreas

CHAPTER 7

CONCEPTUAL THEORY

Terminology

150+ key terminologies for Quick Recall & Revision

Bile pigments: Bile pigments are the degradation products of hemoglobin.
Bile salts: Bile salts are the sodium and potassium salts of glycocholic and taurocholic acids.
Bilirubin: Bilirubin is an orange-yellow pigment, derived from the breakdown of red blood cells in the liver, spleen and bone marrow.
Clearance: Clearance is defined as the volume of plasma that has cleared-off a particular substance by the two kidneys in one minute.
Ketone bodies: Ketone bodies (acetoacetate, β-hydroxybutyrate and acetone) are formed in considerable amounts when fat is metabolized.
Proteinuria: Proteinuria or albuminuria may be physiological (benign albuminuria) or pathological (renal albuminuria).
Urea: Urea is a major nitrogenous metabolic product of protein catabolism in man, accounting for more than 75% of the nonprotein nitrogen which is eventually excreted. Urea is a principal end product of protein catabolism in mammals. An adult man excretes 25–30 g of urea under normal conditions, in 24 hours.

RENAL FUNCTION TEST (RFT)

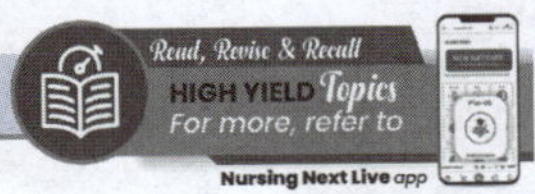

- To assess the renal function
- 2/3rds of the renal tissue needs to be damaged to show any abnormality in tests.
- **Four groups of tests:**
  1. **Glomerular function tests**
     - Measure the glomerular filtration rate
     - Creatinine clearance **test normal value 8.9-186.3 L/day (6.2-129.4 mL/min)**
     - Urea clearance tests normal value- **428.4 to 714 mmol/day**
  2. **Tubular function tests**
     - Measure the specific gravity of urine
     - Urine concentration measurement
     - **Normal – 1.020 in early morning sample**
  3. **Analysis of blood/serum**
     - To assess overall kidney function
     - Serum urea measurement—The normal range of urea nitrogen in blood or serum is **5 to 20 mg/dL, or 1.8 to 7.1 mmol urea per liter.**
     - Serum creatinine measurement – **0.7 to 1.3 mg/dL for adult males. 0.5 to 1.1 mg/dL for adult females.** Also assess GFR
     - Cystatin C **0.67–6.15 mg/L**– biomarker of kidney function
  4. **Urine examination**
     - Volume 800 to 2,000 milliliters per day
     - pH normal values. 4.6 to 8.0
     - Specific gravity 1.005 to 1.030
     - Osmolality - 50 to 1200 mOsm/kg

LIVER FUNCTION TEST

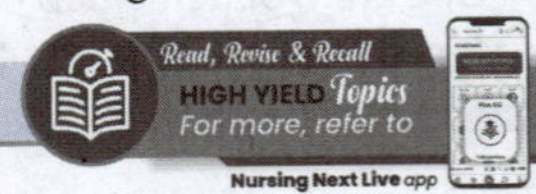

Classification of Liver Function Test (LFT)

- Based on excretory function
  - Measurement of bile pigments, bile salts and bromosulphthalein
- Based on serum enzymes derived from liver
  - Measurement of transaminases (4–36 U/L),
  - Alkaline phosphatase (44 and 147 U/L), etc.
- Based on metabolic activity
  - Galactose tolerance: The plasma galactose should be <5.4 mmoVL at 45 min, <2.3 mmoVL at 60 min and undetectable at 75 and 120 min.
  - Antipyrine clearance: Antipyrine-clearance values in normal subjects is 58.7 +/– 4,8 mL/min

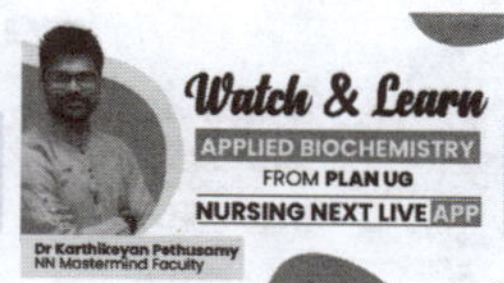

- Based on synthetic functions
  - Prothrombin time: The normal range for PT is 10–13 seconds.
  - Serum albumin: A normal albumin range is 3.4–5.4 g/dL
- Based on detoxification
  - Serum Ammonia: The normal range is 15–45 µ/dL (11–32 µmol/L)

THYROID FUNCTION TEST

- Initially **basal metabolic rate (BMR)** and serum **protein bound iodine** (PBI) estimation
- Hypothyroidism - PBI score of less than 3 µg/100 mL.
- **Assessment of thyroid hormones**
  - Two principle hormones **thyroxine** (T4) and **tri iodothyronine** (T3)
  - Secretion is under the influence of **thyroid-stimulating hormone** (TSH) by pituitary.
  - **Thyroid-binding globulin** (TRG) - binds most of the thyroid hormones T3 and T4, only the free T3/T4 is active. Free T3 and T4, and TSH are measured by Radioimmunoasay or ELISA.
- **Normal serum concentration** of free hormone is:
  - Free T3 – 80–220 ng/dL
  - Free T4 – 0.8–2.4 ng/dL
  - TSH – <10 µg/mL

CONCEPTUAL EXERCISES

SHORT NOTES

1. Name the clearance test used to assess the renal function. (MGR)

Answer

Creatinine Clearance

Volume (in mL) of plasma that would be completely cleared of creatinine per minute.

Procedure

Traditional Method

- Creatinine concentration of 24 hours urine and plasma concentration is estimated.
- Creatinine clearance in mg/dL or mmol/dL (C) = Urine concentration of creatinine (U) × Urine output in mL/min (V)/Plasma concentration of creatinine (P)
- C = U × V/P

Modified Procedure

- Instead of 24-hour urine collection, 1-hour urine sample is collected.
- Creatinine clearance is calculated by the same formula.

Referred Values

- Normal range of creatinine clearance – 120–145 mL/min
- Lower in females
- Can be expressed in terms of body surface area.

Diagnostic Importance

- Decrease in creatinine clearance - <75% normal – indicator of a decreased GFR, renal damage
- Useful for early detection of impaired kidney function.
- Creatinine is freely filtered across the glomerulus and is neither reabsorbed nor metabolized by the kidney.
- Only marginally secreted by tubule
- Hence, creatinine clearance is close to GFR
- Sensitive measurement to assess GFR

2. Write a note on renal function test. (MGR)

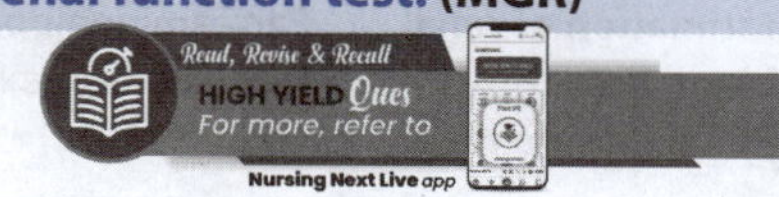

Answer

Introduction

- To assess the renal function
- 2/3rd of the renal tissue needs to be damaged to show any abnormality in tests.
- **Four groups of tests:**
  1. **Glomerular function tests**
     - Measure the glomerular filtration rate
     - Creatinine clearance test normal value 8.9-186.3 L/day (6.2–129.4 mL/min)
     - Urea clearance tests 428.4 to 714 mmol/day
  2. **Tubular function tests**
     - Measure the specific gravity of urine
     - Urine concentration measurement
     - Normal – 1.020 in early morning sample
  3. **Analysis of blood/serum**
     - To assess overall kidney function

- Serum urea measurement: The normal range of urea nitrogen in blood or serum is 5–20 mg/dL, or 1.8–7.1 mmol urea per liter.
- Serum creatinine measurement – **0.7–1.3 mg/dL for adult males. 0.5–1.1 mg/dL for adult females.** Also assess GFR
- Cystatin C **0.67–6.15 mg/L**– biomarker of kidney function

4. **Urine examination**
   - Volume 800–2,000 mL/day
   - pH normal values. 4.6–8.0
   - Specific gravity 1.005–1.030
   - Osmolality - 50–1200 mOsm/kg

Choice of Renal Function Tests

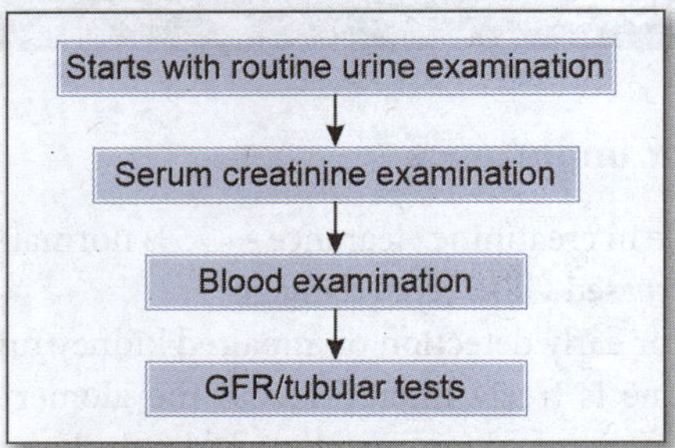

Estimation of glomerular function	Creatinine clearance test Inulin clearance test (used to assess glomerular filtration rate)
Estimation of tubular function	Water deprivation test (used to assess distal tubular function)
Estimation of renal blood flow **Renal plasma flow**	Para-aminohippurate (PAH) clearance (used to assess renal plasma flow – RPF)

3. Write a short note on liver function tests. (MGR)

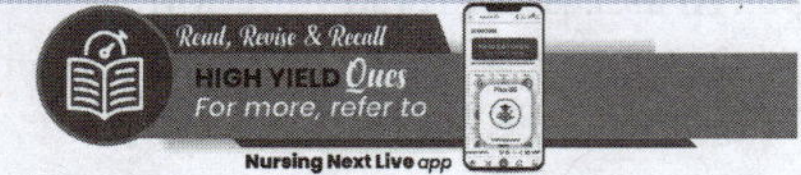

Answer

Introduction

Liver function tests (LFT) are biochemical investigations to assess the capacity of liver to carry out its functions and detect abnormalities.

Diagnostic Significance

- Differential diagnosis of jaundice
- Ascertaining the presence of liver disease
- Evaluating the prognosis of liver disease
- Evaluating the response to therapy in a case of known liver disease.

Classification of Liver Function Tests

• Based on excretory function	• Measurement of bile pigments, bile salts and bromosulphthalein
• Based on serum enzymes derived from liver	• Measurement of transaminases, alkaline phosphatase, etc.
• Based on metabolic activity	• Participates in carbohydrates, lipid, protein, mineral and vitamin metabolism ▪ Galactose tolerance ▪ Antipyrine clearance
• Based on synthetic functions	• Participates in formation of blood • Produces clotting factors like factor V, VII • Synthesis of plasma proteins and destruction of erythrocytes. ▪ Prothrombin time ▪ Serum albumin
• Based on detoxification	• Ammonia is detoxified to urea • Kupffer cells of liver perform phagocytosis • Metabolism of xenobiotics • Hippuric acid synthesis

4. What is the normal total serum bilirubin level? Mention the name of the test for it.

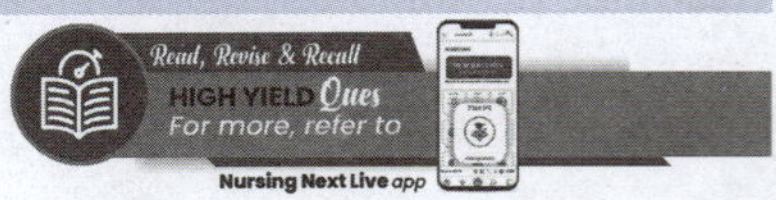

Answer

- Bilirubin is a tetrapyrrole and a breakdown product of heme catabolism.
- Most bilirubin (70–90%) is derived from hemoglobin degradation and, to a lesser extent, from other heme proteins. In the serum, bilirubin is usually measured as both direct bilirubin and total value bilirubin.
- **Normal findings:**
  - **Adult/elderly/child:**
    - **Total bilirubin:** 0.3–1.0 mg/dL or 5.1–17 µmol/L (SI units)
    - **Indirect bilirubin:** 0.2–0.8 mg/dL or 3.4–12.0 µmol/L (SI units)
    - **Direct bilirubin:** 0.1–12.0 mg/dL or 1.7–5.1 µmol/L (SI units)
  - **Newborn:**
    - **Total bilirubin:** 1.0 – 12.0 mg/dL or 17.1–205 µmol/L (SI units)
- **Possible critical values: Total bilirubin:**
  - **Adult:** >12 mg/dL
  - **Newborn:** >15 mg/dL

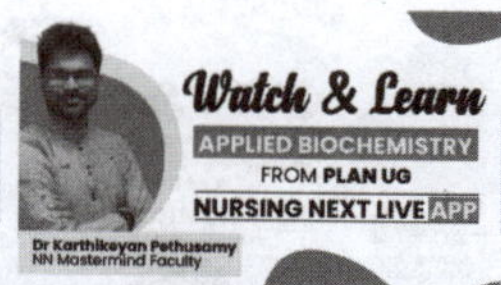

Test for Bilirubin

Van den Bergh Test for Bilirubin

- Specific test for identification of increased serum bilirubin levels
- Normal serum gives a negative Van den Bergh reaction

Mechanism of Reaction

- Van den Bergh reagent – mixture of equal volume of sulfanilic acid and sodium nitrite
- **Principle:** Diazotized sulfanilic acid reacts with bilirubin to form a purple-colored azobilirubin
- **Direct and indirect reactions**
  - Bilirubin is insoluble in water
  - Conjugated bilirubin is soluble
  - Van den Bergh reagent reacts with conjugated bilirubin and gives a purple color within 30 seconds – *Direct positive test*
  - Addition of methanol dissolves the unconjugated bilirubin and gives Van den Bergh reaction positive within 30 minutes – *Indirect positive*

Significance

- **Van den Bergh Reaction and Jaundice**
  - **Indirect positive:** Hemolytic jaundice
  - **Direct positive:** Obstructive jaundice
  - **Biphasic:** Hepatic jaundice

SHORT ANSWER QUESTIONS

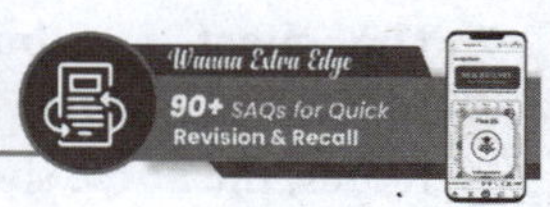

1. Glycosuria. (MGR)

Answer

Glycosuria is a medical condition characterized by the presence of glucose in the urine. The most common method for measuring glucose in urine is through a dipstick test. Urine glucose test is also used.

2. Normal values of serum electrolytes. (MGR)

Answer

Electrolyte	Normal range
Sodium (Na^+)	135-145 mEq/L
Potassium (K^+)	3.5-5.0 mEq/L
Chloride (Cl^-)	95-105 mmol/L
Bicarbonate (HCO_3^-)	22-28 mmol/L
Calcium (Ca^{2+})	8.5-10.5 mg/dL or 2.2-2.6 mmol/L
Magnesium (Mg^{2+})	1.5-2.5 mg/dL or 0.6-1.0 mmol/L
Phosphate (PO_4^{3-})	2.5-4.5 mg/dL or 0.81-1.45 mmol/L

3. Write the normal value of serum urea and serum creatinine. (MGR)

Answer

Test	Normal range
Serum Urea	7–20 mg/dL or 2.5–7.1 mmol/L
Serum Creatinine	0.7–1.3 mg/dL or 62–115 µmol/L

4. Name any two liver function tests. (MGR)

Answer

The two main liver functions tests are as follows:

1. Alanine aminotransferase (ALT) (normal range: 10–40 U/L)
2. Aspartate aminotransferase (AST) (normal range: 10–34 U/L)

5. Define Hypercholesterolemia. (MGR)

Answer

Hypercholesterolemia is defined as having high levels of total cholesterol in the blood, typically greater than 200 mg/dL.

6. Renal function test. (MGR)

Answer

Test used to evaluate proper functioning of the kidney and few function tests involved are blood urea nitrogen, serum creatinine, urinalysis and GFR.

Test name	Normal range
Blood Urea Nitrogen	7–20 mg/dL
Creatinine	0.6–1.3 mg/dL (adult males)
	0.5–1.1 mg/dL (adult females)
Glomerular Filtration Rate (GFR)	90–120 mL/min
Albumin	3.4–5.4 g/dL
Total Protein	6.4–8.3 g/dL
Urine Creatinine	20–370 mg/dL
Urine Protein	Negative or trace
Urine Glucose	Negative or trace
Urine Ketones	Negative or trace

7. Define clearance. How is it calculated? (MGR)

Answer

Clearance is a measure of how efficiently the kidneys are able to remove a substance from the blood and excrete it in the urine.

$$\text{Renal Clearance} = \frac{\text{(Urine Concentration of substance} \times \text{urine volume per unit time)}}{\text{Plasma Concentration of Substance}}$$

CONCEPTUAL REVISION

MULTIPLE CHOICE QUESTIONS

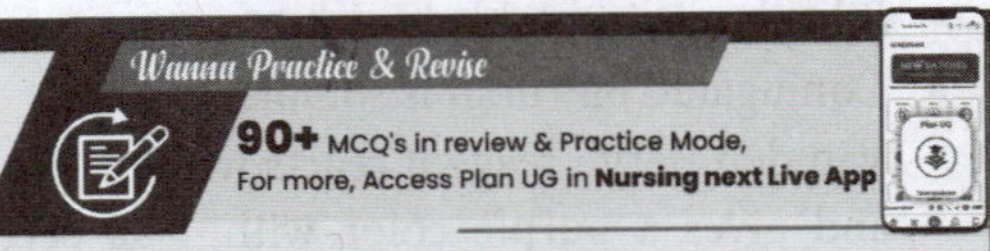

1. Exceeding which of the following serum cholesterol levels significantly increases the risk of coronary artery disease?

a. 100 mg/dL
b. 150 mg/dL
c. 175 mg/dL
d. 200 mg/dL

Ans. d. 200 mg/dL

2. The nurse Priyanka is going through the lab report of client, who has been admitted in the Emergency ward. In which condition the nurse Priyanka gives a call to nephrologist?

a. The client's serum creatinine is 0.8 mg/dL
b. The client's serum creatinine is 1 mg/dL
c. The client's serum creatinine is 7 mg/dL
d. The client's serum creatinine is 0.6 mg/dL

Ans. c. The client's serum creatinine is 7 mg/dL

3. Best timing of routine sample collection:

a. 12 hours after the last ingestion of food
b. 15 hours after the last ingestion of food
c. 6 hours after the last ingestion of food
d. 24 hours after the last ingestion of food

Ans. a. 12 hours after the last ingestion of food

4. Which of the following laboratory result indicates hypoparathyroidism?

a. Serum magnesium level of 1.7 mg/dL
b. Serum phosphorus level of 5.7 mg/dL
c. Serum calcium level of 4.3 mEq/L
d. Serum potassium of 3.6 mEq/L

Ans. b. Serum phosphorus level of 5.7 mg/dL

5. What is the normal amount of White Blood Cells in a Complete Blood Count?

a. 4,500–11,000
b. 11,000–15,000
c. 1,000–2,000
d. 30,000–35,000

Ans. a. 4,500–11,000

6. Normal amount of NEUTROPHILS in Complete Blood Count:

a. 1–2%
b. 5–8%
c. 10–15%
d. 50–70%

Ans. d. 50–70%

7. The client is admitted with a sodium level of 100 mEq/L. After checking the other laboratory values, the nurse should:

a. Chart the finding
b. Contact the doctor
c. Teach the client about low-sodium meal options
d. Check the client's deep tendon reflexes for hyperreflexia

Ans. b. Contact the doctor

8. An adult male client has a hemoglobin count of 12.5 g/dL. Based on the result, the client is most likely having this due to which of the following noted in the client's record?

a. Client living at a high altitude
b. Emphysema
c. Dehydration
d. History of splenomegaly

Ans. a. Client living at a high altitude

CHAPTER

8

Immunochemistry

CONCEPTUAL THEORY

Terminology

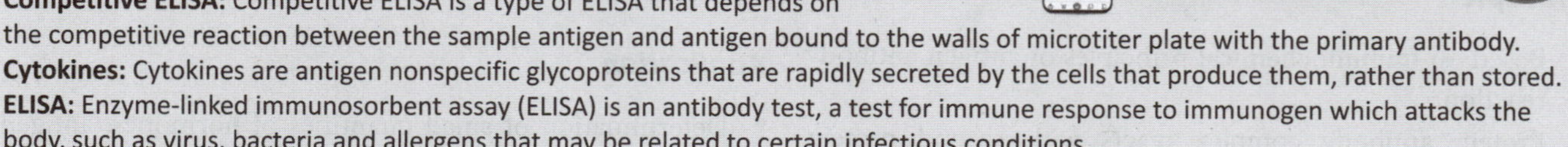

Competitive ELISA: Competitive ELISA is a type of ELISA that depends on the competitive reaction between the sample antigen and antigen bound to the walls of microtiter plate with the primary antibody.
Cytokines: Cytokines are antigen nonspecific glycoproteins that are rapidly secreted by the cells that produce them, rather than stored.
ELISA: Enzyme-linked immunosorbent assay (ELISA) is an antibody test, a test for immune response to immunogen which attacks the body, such as virus, bacteria and allergens that may be related to certain infectious conditions.
Hypervariable sequences: Hypervariable sequences (the antigen-binding sites) are complementary to the topology of the antigen and are designated as complementary-determining regions.
Immunochemistry: Immunochemistry is the study of biochemical and molecular aspects of immunology, especially the nature of antibodies (immunoglobulins), antigens, their interactions, and determination of immune materials by immunochemical techniques such as enzyme-linked immunosorbent assay (ELISA), immunoblotting, and precipitation and agglutination reactions.
Immunogen: Any substance that is capable of stimulating an immune response is referred to as immunogen.
Microplate ELISA: Microplate ELISA reader, also known as microplate readers or microplate photometers, are instruments which are used to detect biological, chemical or physical events of samples in microtiter plates.

STRUCTURE OF IMMUNOGLOBULIN

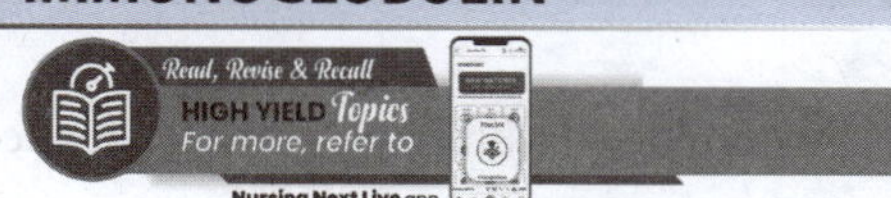

- Consists of two identical heavy (H) and light (L) chains held together by disulfide linkages and non-covalent interactions.
- Each chain has constant (C_H and C_L) and variable regions (V_H and V_L)
- Y-shaped tetramer (H_2L_2)
- Types of light chains – differ C_L regions
  - Kappa κ
  - Lambda λ
- Types of heavy chains
  - γ – IgG
  - α – IgA
  - δ – IgD
  - μ – IgM
  - ε – IgE

Five types based on the heavy chain present in it.

1. **Immunoglobulin G (IgG)**
   - Most abundant (75 – 80%)
   - Composed of single Y-shaped unit
   - Functions
     - Causes foreign cell destruction
     - Mediated by complement
     - Can cross the placenta – transfers mother's immunity to fetus
2. **Immunoglobulin A (IgA)**
   - Found in body secretions – saliva, sweat, tears
   - Composed of a monomer or dimer held by J chain
   - Most predominant in colostrum
   - Function
     - Prevents the entry of foreign substances
3. **Immunoglobulin M (IgM)**
   - Largest Ig
   - Composed of 5 Y-shaped units held by J polypeptide chain
   - Functions
     - Cannot traverse blood vessels, hence restricted to blood stream
     - Most effective against antigens
     - First antibody to be produced

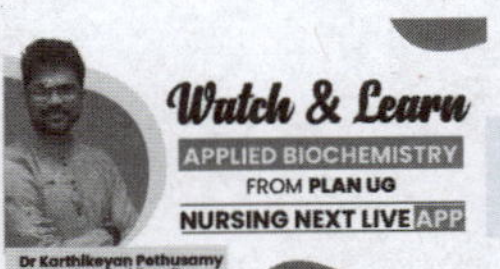

4. **Immunoglobulin D (IgD)**
   - Composed of single Y-shaped unit
   - Present on surface of B cell
   - Functions as B cell receptor
5. **Immunoglobulin E (IgE)**
   - Single Y-shaped monomer
   - Associated with allergic reactions
   - Functions
     - Associate with mast cells
     - Release histamine

ELISA

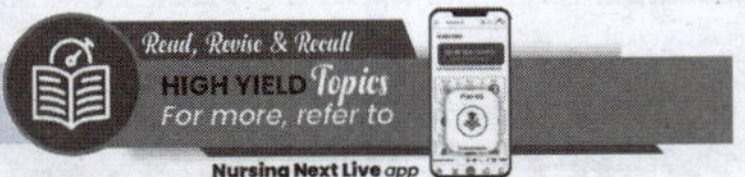

- Enzyme-linked immunosorbent assay – ELISA
- Non-isotopic assay
- Sensitive test

Principle

- Based on immunochemical principles of antigen antibody reaction
- Protein antibody complex reacts with second protein specific antibody to which enzyme is covalently linked

Procedure

- The antibody against the concerned protein is coated onto the plate
- Antibody coated surface is conjugated with the sample containing the protein to be determined
- The protein antibody complex is then reacted with a second protein specific antibody to which an enzyme is covalently linked.
- Chromophores are added
- Unbound antibody linked enzyme is washed, and enzyme bound to second antibody complex is assayed.

Types of ELISA

- Solid phase immunoassay
- Enzyme label
  - Competitive assay
  - Noncompetitive assay
    - Sandwich assay
    - Direct ELISA
    - Indirect ELISA

Application

- Determination of small quantities of hormones, antigens and antibodies
- Pregnancy test based on urine hCG is based on ELISA
- Diagnosis of AIDS

CONCEPTUAL EXERCISES

SHORT NOTES

1. Write a short note on acquired immunity. (DU)

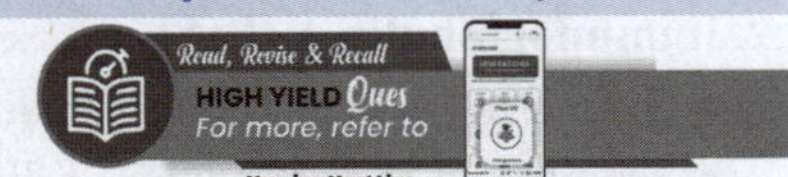

Answer

Immunity

Ability of an organism to resist foreign substances or infections from entering the body.

Acquired Immunity

- Immunity is divided into natural immunity and acquired immunity.
- Acquired immunity is further divided into active and passive immunity:
  - Active immunity
    - Active or adaptive immunity results from the development of the immune response when an individual is stimulated by an antigen, such as those associated with invading microorganisms.
    - Response is specific to a particular antigen.
  - Passive immunity
    - Results when a non-immune individual receives immunity from an immune person.
    - Example: injection of horse antitoxin for tetanus.

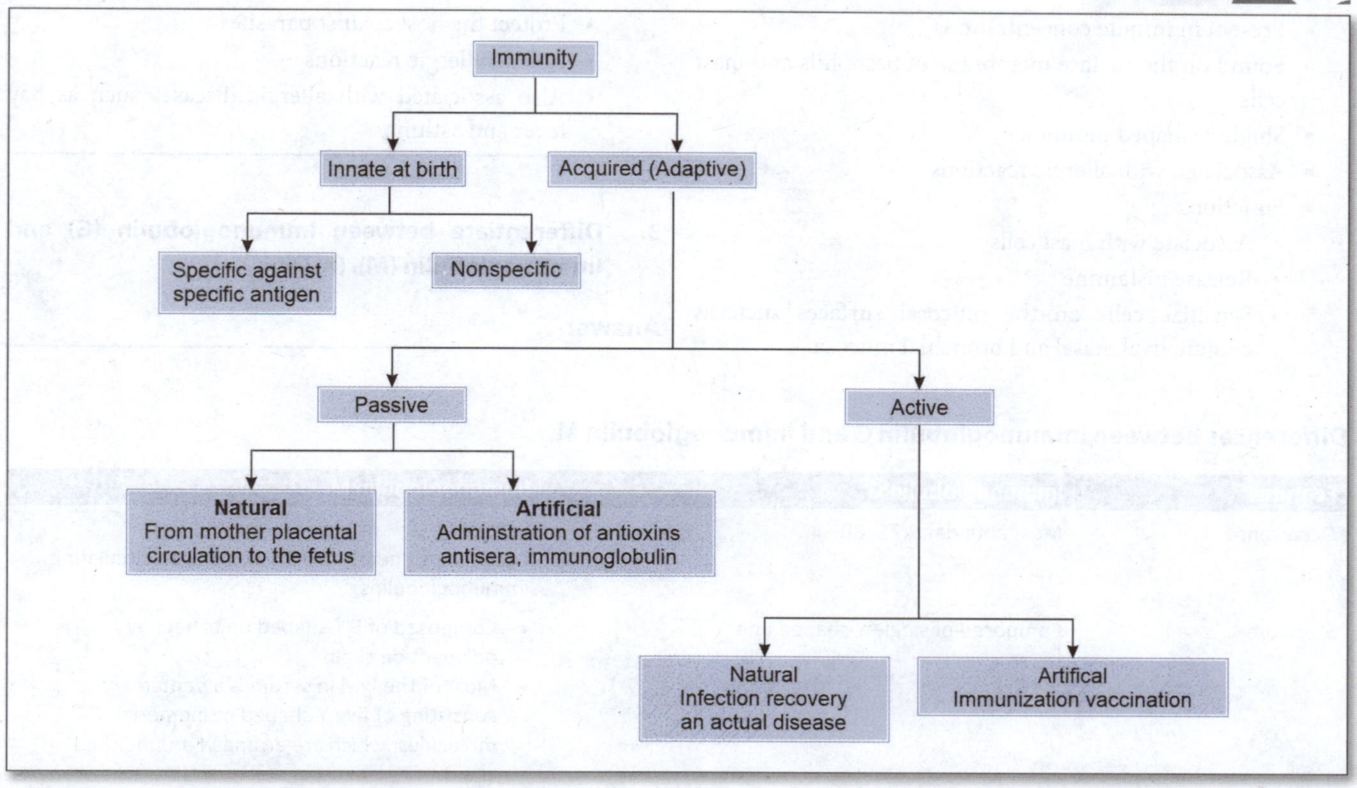

2. Name the types of Immunoglobulins and their functions. (DU)

Answer

Introduction

- Classes of immunoglobulins called IgG, IgA, IgM, IgD and IgE.
- Each one differs from the other with respect to the type of its H chain.

Functions of Immunoglobulins

- **Immunoglobulin G (IgG)**
  - Most abundant (75–80%)
  - Produced in response to most bacteria and viruses.
  - These antibodies bind to macrophages and neutrophils, and promote phagocytosis.
  - **Functions**
    - Causes foreign cell destruction
    - Mediated by complement
    - Can cross the placenta – transfers mother's immunity to fetus
- **Immunoglobulin A (IgA)**
  - Accounts for 15–20% of the total serum immunoglobulins
  - In human beings, 80% of IgA occurs as a monomer.
  - Found in body secretions – saliva, sweat, tears
  - **Function:** Prevents the entry of foreign substance
- **Immunoglobulin M (IgM)**
  - Largest immunoglobulin
  - Composed of 5 Y-shaped units held by J polypeptide chain
  - Functions
    - Cannot traverse blood vessels, hence, restricted to blood stream
    - Most effective against antigens
    - First immunoglobulin to be synthesized by the cell – first line of defense
    - Only immunoglobulin that a neonate can synthesize.
    - Predominant in primary immune response
    - Largely confined to the intravascular pool and is frequently associated with the immune response to antigenically complex blood borne infectious organism
- **Immunoglobulin D (IgD)**
  - Accounts for <1% of the total
  - Present on surface of B cell
  - Function
    - Plays a role in the antigen triggered lymphocyte differentiation
- **Immunoglobulin E (IgE)**

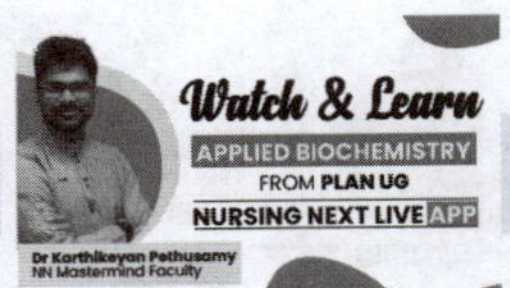

- Present in minute concentrations
- Found on the surface membrane of basophils and mast cells
- Single Y-shaped monomer
- Associated with allergic reactions
- Functions
    - Associate with mast cells
    - Release histamine
    - Sensitize cells on the mucosal surfaces such as conjunctival, nasal and bronchial mucosa.
    - Protect the host against parasites
    - Role in allergic reactions
    - Also associated with allergic diseases such as hay fever and asthma.

3. Differentiate between Immunoglobulin (G) and Immunoglobulin (M). (KUHS)

Answer

Differences between Immunoglobulin G and Immunoglobulin M

Features	Immunoglobulin G	Immunoglobulin M
Occurrence	Most abundant (75–80%)	Largest Ig Accounts for nearly 5–10% of the total circulating immunoglobulins.
Structure	Composed of single Y-shaped unit	• Composed of 5 Y-shaped units held by J polypeptide chain • Most of the IgM in serum is a pentamer consisting of five Y-shaped monomeric molecules, which are arranged around the J chain.
Features	Occurs in secondary immune response and is distributed evenly between the intravascular and extra vascular pools	• Abundance of oligosaccharide units • Associated with μ chain • Presence of an additional peptide chain – joining chain (J chain) – assist the process of polymerization prior to its secretion.
Effector stimuli	Produced in response to most bacteria and viruses.	
Effector mechanism	• These antibodies bind to macrophages and neutrophils, and promote phagocytosis • The major effector mechanism of the human IgG1 and IgG3 subclasses is the activation of the classical pathway of a complement.	• Predominant in primary immune response
Functions	Causes foreign cell destruction Mediated by complement Can cross the placenta – transfers mother's immunity to fetus	Cannot traverse blood vessels, hence, restricted to blood stream Most effective against antigens First immunoglobulin to be synthesized by the cell – first line of defense Only immunoglobulin that a neonate can synthesize. Largely confined to the intravascular pool and is frequently associated with the immune response to antigenically complex blood borne infectious organism
Subclasses	Four classes – IgG1 – IgG4 These subclasses differ, primarily in the hinge region.	–

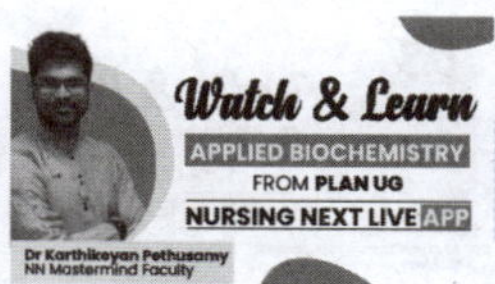

4. Differentiate between IgM and IgA. (KUHS)

Answer

Differences between Immunoglobulin M and Immunoglobulin A

Features	Immunoglobulin M	Immunoglobulin A
Occurrence	• Largest Ig • Accounts for nearly 5–10% of the total circulating immunoglobulins.	• Accounts for 15–20% of the total serum immunoglobulins • In human beings, 80% of IgA occurs as a monomer
Structure	• Composed of 5 Y-shaped units held by J polypeptide chain • Most of the IgM in serum is a pentamer consisting of five Y-shaped monomeric molecules, which are arranged around the J chain.	• Found in body secretions – saliva, sweat, tears • **Secretory IgA** ▪ Most important form of IgA ▪ Predominant immunoglobulin in seromucous secretions such as saliva, colostrum, milk and tracheobronchial and genitourinary secretions. • Structure ▪ Occurs in dimeric form ▪ Occurs in association with another protein that is known as a secretory component
Features	• Abundance of oligosaccharide units • Associated with u chain • Presence of an additional peptide chain – joining chain (J chain) – assist the process of polymerization prior to its secretion.	• Predominant in all secretions
Effector mechanism	• Predominant in primary immune response	• Secretory IgA gets assembled during the active transport process, as the locally produced IgA passes across the mucosal epithelium.
Functions	• Cannot traverse blood vessels, hence, restricted to blood stream • Most effective against antigens • First immunoglobulin to be synthesized by the cell – first line of defense • Only immunoglobulin that a neonate can synthesize. Largely confined to the intravascular pool and is frequently associated with the immune response to antigenically complex blood borne infectious organism	• IgA_1 ▪ Predominant subclass ▪ Accounts for 75–90% ▪ Present in many secretions such as nasal secretions, tear, saliva and milk • IgA_2 ▪ Predominant in colon ▪ Composed of a monomer or dimer held by J chain ▪ Most predominant in colostrum ▪ Functions ◆ Prevents the entry of foreign substance
Subclasses	–	• Subclasses of IgA • Two subclasses – IgA_1 and IgA_2

5. Write a short note on structure of immunoglobulin. (KUHS)

Answer

Structure of Immunoglobulin

- Consists of two identical heavy (H) and light (L) chains held together by disulfide linkages and non-covalent interactions.
- Each chain has constant (C_H and C_L) and variable regions (V_H and V_L)
- Y-shaped tetramer (H2L2)
- Types of light chains – differ C_L regions
  - Kappa κ
  - Lambda λ
- Types of heavy chains
  - γ – IgG
  - α – IgA
  - δ – IgD
  - μ – IgM
  - ε – IgE

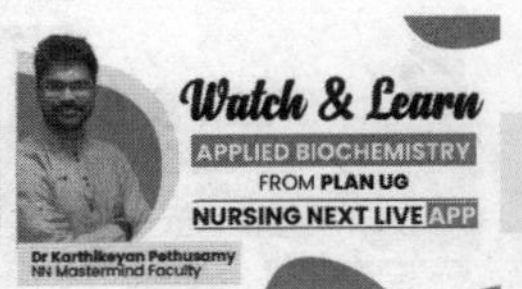

- Heavy chains of immunoglobulins are attached to carbohydrates – hence, glycoproteins
- The amino acid sequence of variable regions of light and heavy chains is responsible for specific binding of immunoglobulin with antigen

Immunoglobulin Four Polypeptide Chains

- Has a basic unit compromising of four polypeptide chains.
  - Two identical small polypeptides – L chains
  - Two identical large polypeptides – H chains
- They occur in light-heavy-heavy-light arrangement.

Light Chains

- Smaller polypeptides (about 25 kD each)
- Each L chain has approximately 220 amino acids.
- Two types
  - Kappa
  - Lambda
- Kappa chains are more prevalent than lambda chains.

Heavy Chains

- Larger subunits that are found in the immunoglobulins
- Five different types of H chains, each containing 440–450 amino acids, are found in immunoglobulins
- Molecular mass of an H chain may vary from 50 to 75 kD
- The type of immunoglobulin is based on the type of H chains.

Each Polypeptide—Two Regions

- Each chain has two regions called constant region and variable region.
- **Variable regions:**
  - Amino acid sequences that are found in the NH_2 terminal half of the L chain and one fourth of the H chains are highly variable between the different immunoglobulin molecules.
  - Thus NH_2 terminal regions are called variable regions (V regions).
- The V regions of the L chains and H chains are designated as the V_L regions and the V_H region, respectively.
- **Constant regions:**
  - Half of the L chain toward the COOH- terminal end and three fourths of the H chains are designated as V_L and V_H regions, respectively.
  - CH region is further subdivided into three parts, each comprising of about 110 amino acids.
  - Each of these segments contains an intra chain disulphide bond.
  - The μ type and € type of H chains have four CH regions instead of three found in others.
- **Hypervariable regions:** V regions of immunoglobulin is involved in recognition and binding of the antigen with the antibody. This ability of the antibody resides in several short sequences which are located in small loops within the V region.
  - Only 5–10 amino acids in each of the hypervariable sequence contribute to the antigen binding site.
  - Amino acid segments separating different hypervariable sequences from each other are referred to as framework regions.

Proteolytic Cleavage of Ig

An immunoglobulin is split by enzyme papain to form two identical antigen binding fragments (Fab) and one crystallizable fragment (Fc) at a site between CH1 and CH2 regions – that is referred to as hinge region.

- **Fab Fragment**
  - Entire L chain and half of H chain (comprising of the VH and the CH1 regions). Each of the Fab fragments can bind to an antigen with the affinity similar to that of the intact antibody.
- **Fc Fragment**
  - The Fc fragment consists of the C terminal halves of the two H chains, i.e., the CH2 and CH3 regions, which are joined together by disulfide bridges.
  - All antibodies are bifunctional, i.e., in addition to the antigen binding, they also exhibit one or more effector function, such as complement activation and cell binding.
- **Hinge region**
  - Two fab factors of the immunoglobulin are connected to the Fc fragment by a flexible region, referred to as the hinge region.
  - Present between the CH1 and CH2 regions and confers flexibility to the molecules.

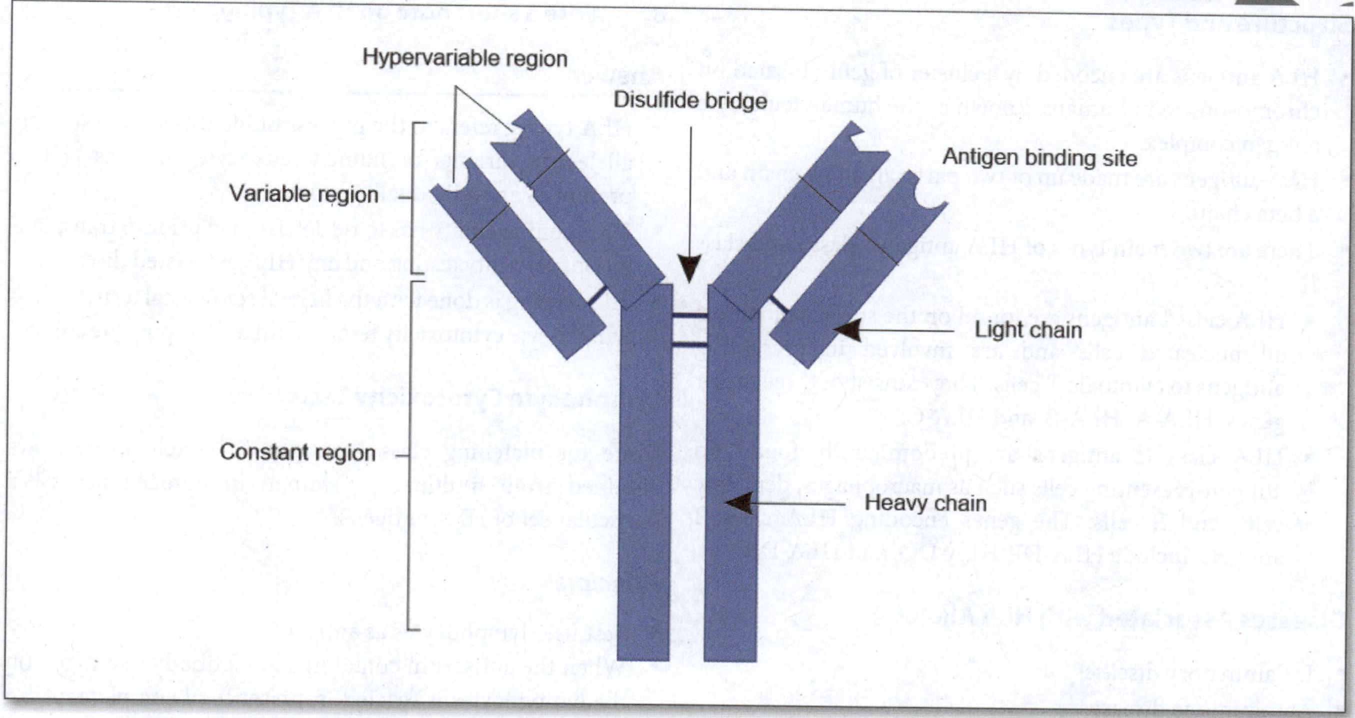

Figure 8.1: Structure of immunoglobulin molecule

6. Write about mechanism of antibody production. (MGR)

Answer

Introduction

The production of antibodies, also known as immunoglobulins, involves a complex process that begins with the activation of B lymphocytes (B cells) in response to an antigen.

Mechanism of Antibody Production

The mechanism of antibody production is as follows:

- **Antigen recognition:** B cells have surface receptors called B cell receptors (BCRs) that are specific to particular antigens. When an antigen (foreign protein or pathogen) enters the body, it is recognized by BCRs on B cells that have a complementary shape to the antigen. This binding triggers the activation of the B cell.
- **B cell activation:** Once activated, the B cell undergoes a series of changes called gene rearrangement to initiate antibody production. The B cell internalizes the antigen through endocytosis and processes it into small peptide fragments.
- **Antigen presentation:** The B cell then presents these antigen fragments on its surface in association with a protein called major histocompatibility complex class II (MHC II). This complex acts as a signal to activate helper T cells, which play a crucial role in the immune response.
- **Helper T cell activation:** Activated helper T cells recognize the antigen on B cells and release cytokines. These cytokines stimulate the B cells to make more antibodies and turn into plasma cells.
- **Antibodies production:** Plasma cells are responsible for the production and secretion of large amounts of antibodies. Antibodies are Y-shaped proteins composed of two heavy chains and two light chains. Each chain has a variable region that determines the specificity of the antibody for a particular antigen and a constant region that mediates other immune functions.

7. Write a short note on HLA antigens. (MGR)

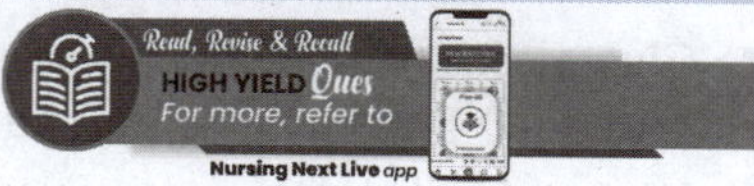

Answer

Introduction

- HLA antigens, also known as Human Leukocyte Antigens, are proteins that are found on the surface of all nucleated cells in the body.
- It regulates immune system in humans
- Located on short arm of chromosome 6
- Inherited as haplotypes one from each parent
- Codominantly expressed

Structure and Types

- HLA antigens are encoded by a cluster of genes located on chromosome 6 in humans, known as the human leukocyte antigen complex.
- HLA antigens are made up of two parts: an alpha chain and a beta chain.
- There are two main types of HLA antigens: class I and class II.
  - HLA class I antigens are found on the surface of almost all nucleated cells and are involved in presenting antigens to cytotoxic T cells. They consist of three major genes: HLA-A, HLA-B, and HLA-C.
  - HLA class II antigens are predominantly found on antigen-presenting cells such as macrophages, dendritic cells, and B cells. The genes encoding HLA class II antigens include HLA-DP, HLA-DQ, and HLA-DR.

Diseases Associated with HLA Alleles

- Inflammatory diseases
- Autoimmune diseases

Inflammatory Diseases

- HLA is known to be associated with Ankylosing Spondylitis (AS), Psoriasis, and Inflammatory Bowel Disease (IBD)

Autoimmune Diseases

HLA types are inherited, and some HLA disease associations

- **HLA-B27:** Ankylosing Spondylitis, Postgonococcal arthritis, Acute anterior uveitis
- **HLA-DR4:** Rheumatoid arthritis
- **HLA-DR3:** Autoimmune hepatitis, Primary Sjogren syndrome, Type 1 diabetes mellitus
- HLA typing is used as diagnostic tool in autoimmunity example in celiac disease

In Cancer

- Gluten-sensitive enteropathy - associated with enteropathy-associated T-cell lymphoma, and DR3-DQ2 homozygotes.
- HLA molecules play a protective role by targeting abnormal cells for apoptosis.

HLA Typing

- HLA compatability has to be determined prior to transplantation, paternity testing and any HLA associated diseases.
- Done with the help of serological tests, such as lymphocyte cytotoxicity tests and mixed lymphocyte culture.

8. Write a short note on HLA Typing.

Answer

- HLA typing refers to the process of identifying the specific alleles or variants of human leukocyte antigens (HLA) present in an individual's genome.
- HLA compatability has to be determined prior to transplantation, paternity testing and any HLA associated diseases.
- HLA typing is done with the help of serological tests, such as lymphocyte cytotoxicity tests and mixed lymphocyte culture.

Lymphocyte Cytotoxicity Tests

Done for matching class I antigen in which antisera are obtained from multiparous women immunized against a particular set of HLA antigens.

Principle

- Test uses lymphocytes as antigens.
- When the antiserum containing an antibody to antigen on the lymphocytes is reacted in presence of complement, an antigen antibody reaction takes place with the binding of the complement.
- This induces cell lysis.
- Stain eosin is introduced. The stain is taken up by the nonviable or dead cells.
- The extent of lymphocytotoxicity is estimated and the lymphocyte antigens are identified by using different groups of antisera.
- Newer techniques use monoclonal antibodies and polymerase chain reaction.

Mixed Lymphocyte Culture

Identifies class II antigens by using pure B lymphocyte population that is homozygous for the particular HLA-D allele.

Principles

- Culturing of the lymphocytes in the presence of antigens.
- Stimulation of the cells to divide resulting in blast formation
- Blast cells are metabolically very active, in which the DNA synthesis is enhanced.
- The rate of DNA synthesis can be estimated by tritiated thymidine (3H- thymidine).
- The donor lymphocytes are treated with mitomycin C to prevent their division, in response to recipient's lymphocytes.

9. Write a short note on Antioxidant. (MGR)

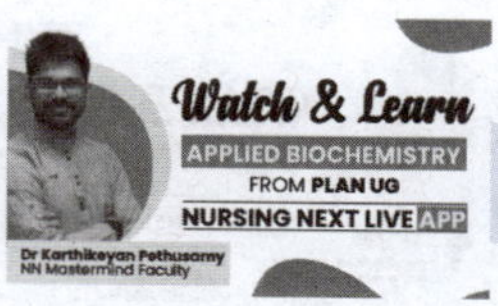

Answer

Introduction

- Mitigate harmful effects of free radicals
- Substance that significantly delays or inhibits oxidation of a substrate
- Scavenger of free radicals
- Present in low concentration as compared to an oxidizable substrate

Classification of Antioxidants

- **According to location**
  - **Plasma antioxidants:** E.g., beta carotene, ascorbic acid, bilirubin
  - **Cell membrane antioxidants:** E.g., alpha-tocopherol
  - **Intracellular antioxidants:** E.g., superoxide dismutase, catalase, glutathione peroxidase
- **According to nature and action**
  - **Enzymatic antioxidants:** E.g., superoxide dismutase, catalase, glutathione peroxidase, glutathione reductase
  - **Non-enzymatic antioxidants**
    - **Nutrient:** E.g., carotenoids, alpha tocopherol, vitamin C, selenium
    - **Metabolic:** E.g., glutathione, ceruloplasmin, albumin, bilirubin, transferrin, ferritin, uric acid

Antioxidant Enzyme System

- **Superoxide dismutase** converts superoxide to hydrogen peroxide and oxygen. First line of defense against superoxide
- **Catalase** metabolizes hydrogen peroxide
- **Glutathione peroxidase** detoxifies hydrogen peroxidase

Nutrient Antioxidants

- **Tocopherols** present in all cellular membranes. Prevents against lipid peroxidation
- **Vitamin C** scavenges free radicals and prevents lipid peroxidation
- **Carotenoids** like beta carotene, lycopene, lutein and zeaxanthin – act as antioxidant under low partial pressure of oxygen.
- **Selenium** in association with Vitamin E is a significant antioxidant. Also required for function of glutathione peroxidase

Metabolic Antioxidants

- **Uric acid** – scavenger of singlet oxygen and OH^- radicals
- **Ceruloplasmin** inhibits iron and copper dependent lipid peroxidation
- **Transferrin** binds iron and prevents iron catalyzed free radical formation

10. Write a short note on Free radicals. (DU, MGR)

Answer

Introduction

- Uncharged highly reactive molecule
- Capable of independent existence
- Short lived
- Generate new radicals by chain reaction
- Causes damage to cell, tissue
- Oxygen derivatives O_2–
  - H_2O_2
  - OH–
  - Singlet oxygen
  - Hydroperoxy radical
  - Lipid peroxide radical
  - Nitric oxide
  - Peroxynitrite

Source of Free Radicals

- Due to metabolic activity of cells—few examples are:
  - Leakage of electrons from ETC
  - Lipid peroxidation reaction
  - Production of peroxide and oxides by oxidase enzymes
  - During phagocytosis
- Environmental sources
  - Drug metabolism
  - Ionizing radiation damage
  - Cigarette smoke
  - Alcohol
  - Photo excitation and photolysis of oxygen molecules in tissue

Harmful Effects of Free Radicals

- Causes oxidation of sulfhydryl groups of proteins, causes fragmentation and cross-linking of amino acids – loss of protein function
- Causes lipid peroxidation – PUFA – most susceptible to free radical damage
- Cause DNA breakage, fragmentation of bases.
- Associated with various diseases such as cardiovascular diseases, cancer, diabetes mellitus, etc.

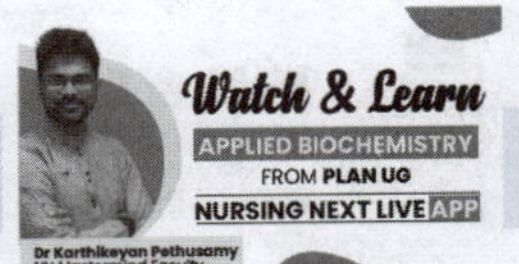

SHORT ANSWER QUESTIONS

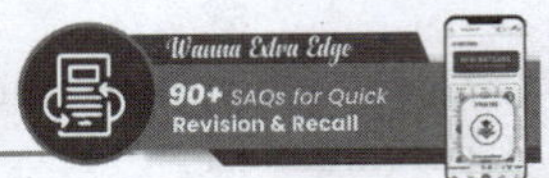

1. ELISA. (MGR)

Answer

Enzyme-Linked Immunosorbent Assay, or ELISA, is a frequently employed scientific technique for identifying and quantifying a particular protein or molecule in a sample, such as blood or urine.

2. Mention the types of immunoglobulins. (MGR)

Answer

The main five types of immunoglobulins includes:

1. IgG
2. IgA
3. IgM
4. IgD and
5. IgE

3. Functions of Immunoglobulin. (DU)

Answer

Some of the main functions of immunoglobulins are:

- **Opsonization:** Immunoglobulins can also tag antigens for destruction by immune cells, a process known as opsonization.
- **Neutralization of antigens:** Immunoglobulins can bind to and neutralize antigens by preventing them from entering or damaging cells.
- **Complement activation:** Immunoglobulins can activate the complement system, a group of proteins that work together to destroy pathogens by causing cell lysis.

4. Acquired immunity. (DU)

Answer

It is a form of immunity that develops gradually over time as a result of exposure to diverse diseases or foreign substances over time, e.g., immunity to chicken pox post exposure.

5. Immunoglobulin E. (KUHS)

Answer

IgE is a monomeric molecule which is minutely found in the blood and is commonly associated with allergic diseases.

6. Immunoglobulin G. (KUHS)

Answer

IgG is the most abundant immunoglobulin produced by plasma cells. These antibodies promote phagocytosis by binding to macrophages and neutrophils.

7. Immunoglobulin M. (KUHS)

Answer

IgM is a large pentameric antibody, which means that it is made up of five monomers (single protein molecules) that have been bonded together. B cells create an antibody called immunoglobulin M (IgM) in response to a recent infection.

CONCEPTUAL REVISION

MULTIPLE CHOICE QUESTIONS

Wanna Practice & Revise
90+ MCQ's in review & Practice Mode, For more, Access Plan UG in **Nursing next Live App**

1. IgE antibody is secreted by:

a. Plasma cells
b. Macrophages
c. Mast cells
d. Eosinophils

Ans. a. Plasma cells

2. Major subclass of IgG immunoglobulin is:

a. IgG1
b. IgG2
c. IgG3
d. IgG4

Ans. a. IgG1

3. The secretory component of IgA is formed by:

a. Plasma cell
b. Epithelial cells of lining mucosa
c. Both (a) and (b)
d. MALT

Ans. b. Epithelial cells of lining mucosa

4. Which of the following antibody participates in specific immunity to respiratory viral disease?

a. IgA
b. IgD
c. IgG
d. IgM

Ans. a. IgA

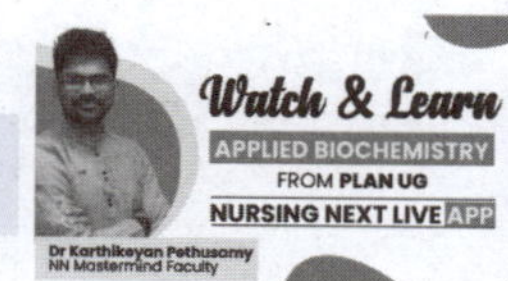

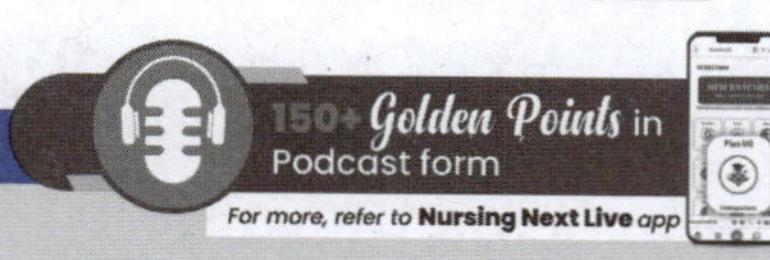

Golden Points

- A molecule of immunoglobulin has Y-shaped structure with two arms and a stem.
- Antibodies are highly specific for the three-dimensional conformation of the epitope.
- Any substance that is capable of stimulating an immune response is referred to as immunogen.
- Cytokines are antigen nonspecific glycoproteins that are rapidly secreted by the cells that produce them, rather than stored.
- Cytotoxic T cells (Tc cells) are involved in killing foreign cells. They recognize foreign antigens, imbedded in MHC class I molecules.
- Enzyme-linked immunosorbent assay (ELISA) is an antibody test, a test for immune response to immunogen which attack the body, such as virus, bacteria and allergens that may be related to certain infectious conditions.
- Five different types of the H chains, each containing 440 - 450 amino acids, are found in immunoglobulins, in human beings.
- Helper T cells (Th cells) are required for the production of normal levels of antibody by B cells and aid in development of cell-mediated immunity.
- IgE is commonly associated with the allergic diseases, such as hay fever and asthma.
- Immunochemistry is the study of biochemical and molecular aspects of immunology, especially the nature of antibodies (immunoglobulins), antigens, their interactions, and determination of immune materials by immunochemical techniques such as enzyme-linked immunosorbent assay (ELISA), immunoblotting, and precipitation and agglutination reactions.
- Immunoglobulin G (IgG) is a major immunoglobulin produced by the plasma cells.
- Inflammation is the localized tissue reaction to injury, caused by physical and chemical agents. Components C3a to C5a contribute to acute inflammation.
- Macrophages function as antigen presenting cells (APC).
- Opsonization is the promotion of phagocytosis by specific antibody in conjunction with complement.
- Proteolytic cleavage by pepsin: Action of pepsin on an immunoglobulin molecule results in a fragment that has 2 Fab regions only, i.e., $F(ab)_2$ while the Fc fraction is hydrolyzed to oligopeptides and amino acids.
- Rocket immunoelectrophoresis is used to quantify antigen.
- Secretory IgA (sIgA) is the most important form of IgA.

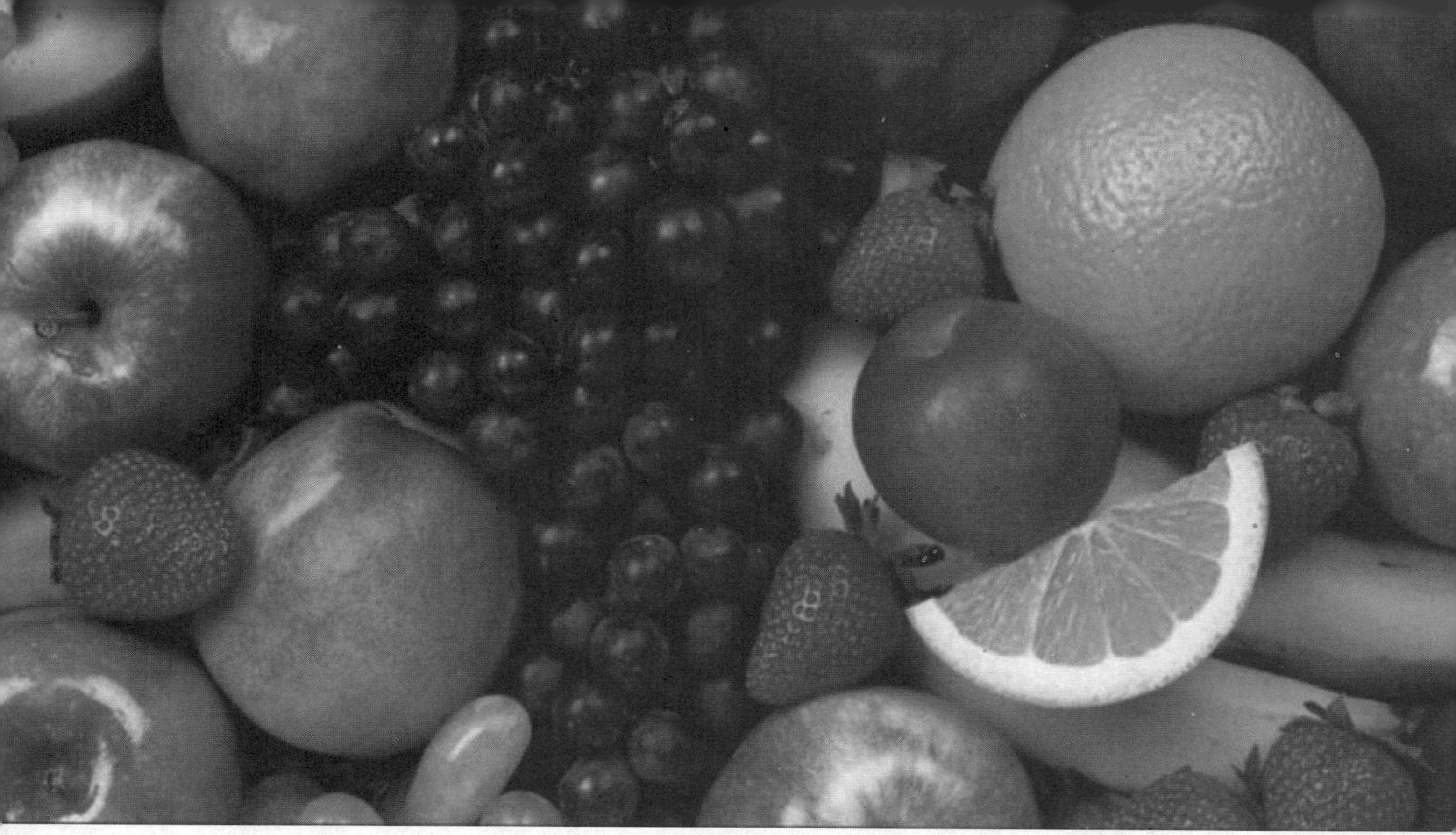

Applied Nutrition and Dietetics

Unit Outline

CHAPTER

1

Introduction to Nutrition

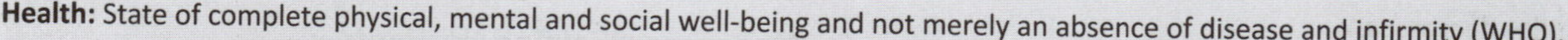

CONCEPTUAL THEORY

Terminology

150+ key terminologies for Quick Recall & Revision

Food taboos: Religion-based food habits like vegetarianism in Hindu society and prohibition of pork in Muslim society.
Health: State of complete physical, mental and social well-being and not merely an absence of disease and infirmity (WHO).
Macronutrients: Required in large quantity and from the bulk of our food, e.g., proteins, fats and carbohydrates.
Micronutrients: Required in small amounts but play an important role in the regulation of metabolic activities, e.g., vitamins and minerals.
Nutrient: A substance essential for the growth, maintenance, function and reproduction of a cell or of an organism.

DEFINITIONS OF NUTRITION AND HEALTH

Nutrition

- Nutrition is defined as the science of food and its relationship with health.
- It is also defined as the science of food, nutrients and other substances with their actions, interaction, balance and relationship with health and illness.

Health

According to WHO, health is defined as the 'state of complete physical, mental and social well-being and not merely the absence of disease or infirmity.'

MALNUTRITION—UNDER NUTRITION AND OVER NUTRITION

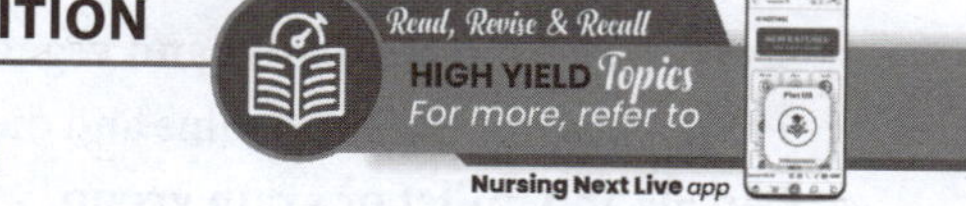

Malnutrition

- Malnutrition is the condition resulting from dietary nutrient deficiency, excess or imbalance of nutrients.
- It may be related to proteins, fats, vitamins and minerals.
- **Two types**
  1. **Under nutrition:** Refers to deficiency of calories/ nutrients
  2. **Over nutrition:** Refers to excess of nutrients, usually calories

ROLE OF NUTRITION IN MAINTAINING HEALTH

- **Growth and development:** Food helps in the formation of new protoplasm or repairing the worn out cells and tissues.
- **Provide resistance:** Proper nutrition helps to reduce the risks of infection and build up resistance against diseases.
- **Mortality and morbidity:** Malnutrition contributes a lot to general death rates, infant mortality rates, stillbirths and premature deliveries or over nutrition responsible for obesity, diabetes, hypertension and cardiovascular diseases.
- **Regulating metabolic process:** Energy is required for performing various life processes such as ingestion, digestion and absorption. Energy required for these processes is released by oxidation of food.
- Many organic substances such as hormones and enzymes are required by living beings.
- Malnutrition is directly responsible for certain specific nutritional diseases, e.g., PEM, malnutrition, goiter and anemia. So, a balanced amount of nutrition is very important to prevent deficiencies.

FACTORS AFFECTING FOOD AND NUTRITION

Socioeconomic Factors

- Fundamental need of life is nourishment through food. Depends upon family resources for adequate and nutritive food.

- Economic status of the family also makes a difference in the choice of food.

Cultural Factors

- Every culture has its own customs and beliefs regarding nutritional practice.
- Religious beliefs affect the food choices and health of the individual directly or indirectly.

Traditional Factors

Traditional taboos are certain beliefs regarding the food intake and its effects.

System of Distribution

- Adequate availability of food is an important factor in determining the adequate intake of food and nutrition.
- Market imperfections and government restrictions affect the free movement of the food grains across the borders. Due to these reasons, cost of food grains increase and availability decreases.

Lifestyle and Food Habit Factors

- During the growth period, basal metabolism is higher so food and nutrition requirement is higher.
- Body mass index affects the food and nutritional requirements.
- Larger body has a greater amount of muscles and glandular tissues requiring higher energy requirement.
- Presence of physical activity increases the energy expenditure above the basal energy need.
- Excessive amount of stress can lead to risk of strokes, heart attacks, depression, etc.

NUTRIENTS

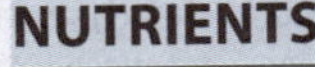

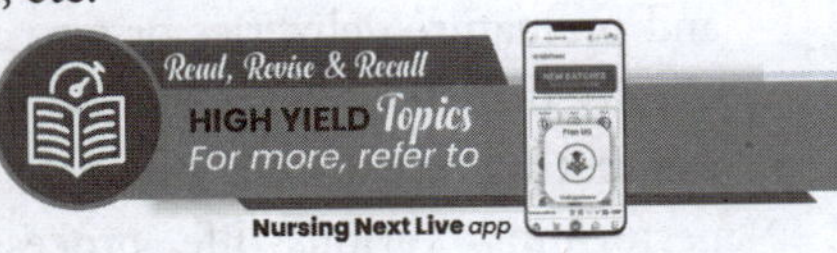

Classification

Macronutrients

- They are required in a large amount in our body; they form the bulk of food:
  - Carbohydrates
  - Fats
  - Proteins

Micronutrients

- Essential dietary elements that are needed only in very small quantities
- Also known as trace elements.
- This includes vitamins and minerals.

Organic and Inorganic

- The presence or absence of carbon is what differentiates organic nutrients from inorganic nutrients.
- Carbohydrates, lipids, proteins and vitamins have carbon in their structure, thus are classified as organic, whereas water and minerals do not have carbon, so these are termed inorganic.

Energy Yielding Nutrients

- These include the energy rich foods, i.e., carbohydrates, fats and proteins.
- These are usually known as macronutrients.
- These are needed in large quantities and provide most of the energy requirements of the body.
- The amount of energy provided by these nutrients is measured in calories.

Nonenergy Yielding Nutrients

- These include micronutrients, like vitamins and minerals.
- These are needed in small quantities and do not provide energy to the body directly.

Food

Classification—Food Groups

- Foods are classified into five groups according to their functions in the human body. These are:
  1. **Protein food group**
     - Includes milk, pulses, nuts, legumes, eggs, meat, fish and poultry
  2. **Primary protective vegetables and fruit group**
     - Includes two subgroups
       - Foods rich in beta carotene and green leafy vegetables—spinach, fenugreek, papaya, apricots, mango, carrot
       - Food rich in vitamin C—pineapple, tomato, strawberries, citrus fruits.
  3. **Secondary protective food and vegetable groups**
     - Supplies minerals, vitamins and dietary fiber
  4. **Cereals and millet or grain group**
     - Supplies half of the daily requirement of proteins and calories.
     - Includes jawar, bajra, maize, wheat, rice.
     - Contains no cholesterol.

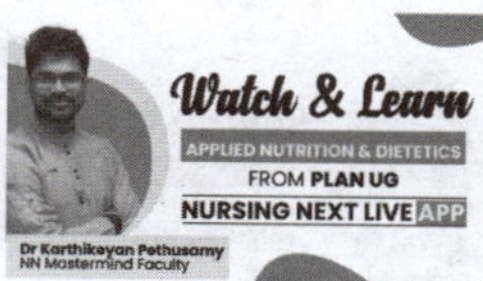

5. **Oil, fat and sugar group**
   - Also known as fuel group
   - Sugars – sweeten the food
   - Fats and oil – increase the palatability of foods.
   - Source of fat soluble vitamins such as vitamin A, D, E and K

Origin

- Based on the origin of food, the food is classified into:
  - Animal origin
  - Plant origin

CONCEPTUAL EXERCISES

LONG ANSWER QUESTION

1. **What do you mean by nutrition and health? Explain.**

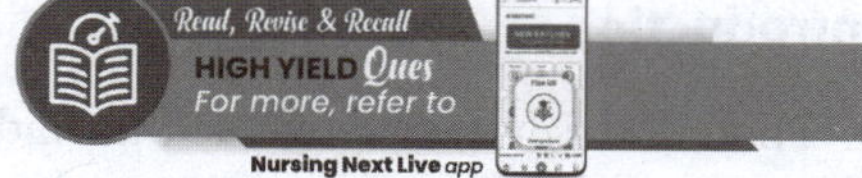

Answer

Nutrition

- Nutrition is defined as the science of food and its relationship with health. It plays an important role in growth, development and maintenance of the body system. It is also defined as the science of food, nutrients and other substances with their actions, interaction, balance and relationship with health and illness. It includes the ingestion, digestion, absorption and utilization of food, and disposal of their end products.
- It is the science of food, the nutrients and the substances, their action, interaction and balance in relation to health and disease, the process by which the organism ingests, digests, absorbs, transport, utilizes and excretes food substances.

Elements of Nutrition

Macronutrients	Micronutrients
They are required in a large amount in our body; they form the bulk of food	They are required in a small amount that may vary fraction of 1 mg to several grams
• Carbohydrates • Fats • Proteins	• Vitamins • Minerals

Health

- According to WHO, health is defined as the 'state of complete physical, mental and social well-being and not merely the absence of disease or infirmity.'
- Earlier, the concept of health revolved around healing the sick and helping them to maintain their health by educating those regarding foods that can strengthen the body.

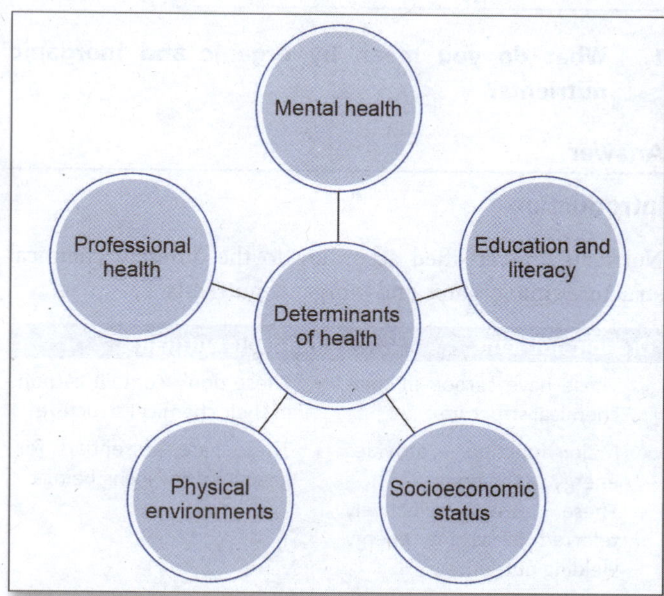

Relationship between Health and Nutrition

Growth and development	Body cells multiply regularly. They increase in size as well. For all these processes, the new protoplasm is required. Food helps in the formation of new protoplasm or repairing the worn out cells and tissues.
Provide resistance	Proper nutrition helps to reduce the risks of infection and build up resistance against diseases. If a person takes an adequate amount of nutrients, then his/her body remains free from all the infections.
Mortality and morbidity	Malnutrition contributes a lot to general death rates, infant mortality rates, stillbirths and premature deliveries or over nutrition responsible for obesity, diabetes, hypertension and cardiovascular diseases.
Regulating metabolic process	Adequate nutrition is required for regulating and maintaining and repairing various parts, the food provides basic raw materials
Release of energy	Energy is required for performing various life processes such as ingestion, digestion and absorption. Energy required for these processes is released by oxidation of food.

Contd...

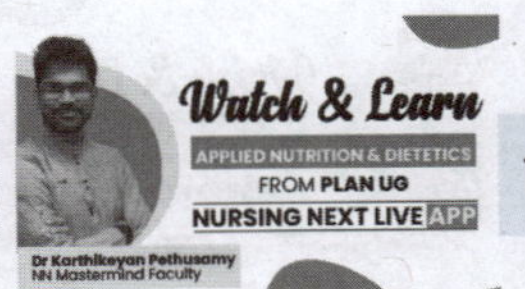

Formation of organic substances	Many organic substances such as hormones and enzymes are required by living beings.
Specific deficiency diseases	Malnutrition is directly responsible for certain specific nutritional diseases, e.g., PEM, malnutrition, goiter and anemia. So, a balanced amount of nutrition is very important to prevent deficiencies.

SHORT NOTES

1. What do you mean by organic and inorganic nutrients?

Answer

Introduction

Nutrients are classified according to the different chemical structures into organic and inorganic nutrients.

Organic nutrients	Inorganic nutrients
• These have carbon in their chemical structure	• These don't contain carbon in their chemical structure
• Major function – provides energy to the body. • These are collectively referred to as the energy yielding nutrients	• These are essential for growth of the living beings
• Includes carbohydrates, proteins, lipids and vitamins	• Includes minerals and water.

2. Give classification of food according to its origin.

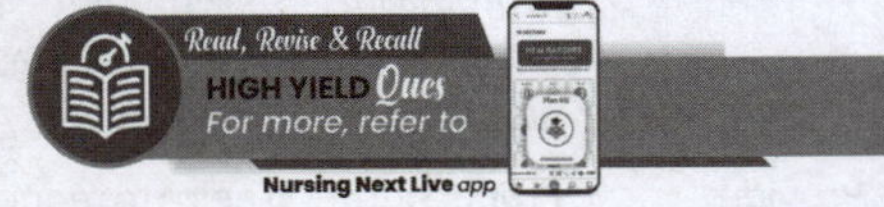

Answer

Introduction

Food is any substance consumed to provide nutritional support for the body.

Classification of Food

Based on the origin of food, the food is classified into:
- Animal origin
- Plant origin
- **Fruits and vegetables:** Apples, bananas, carrots, broccoli, etc.
- **Grains and cereals:** Rice, wheat, oats, barley, etc.
- **Meat and poultry:** Beef, chicken, pork, lamb, etc.
- **Seafood:** Fish, shrimp, lobster, crab, etc.
- **Dairy products:** Milk, cheese, yogurt, butter, etc.
- **Legumes:** Lentils, beans, chickpeas, etc.
- **Fats and oils:** Olive oil, butter, coconut oil, etc.
- **Sweets and desserts:** Chocolate, cakes, ice cream, etc.

Animal origin	Plant origin
Those derived from animals	Those derived from vegetable/plants
Example—meat, fish, eggs, etc.	Example—pulses, cereals, fruits

3. How lifestyle and habits affect nutritional status of an individual?

Answer

Introduction

- Food is a term used to refer to the solid or liquid substances that are ingested.
- It is the source of nutrition to the body for the growth and maintenance of the body and its processes.

Lifestyle and Food Habit Factors Affecting Nutritional Status of an Individual

Age	During the growth period, basal metabolism is higher so food and nutrition requirement is higher. During adolescence, calorie requirement is higher.
Weight	Associated with range of adverse health consequences such as cardiovascular diseases, diabetes and some cancers.
Body size	Body mass index affects the food and nutritional requirements. Larger body has a greater amount of muscles and glandular tissues requiring higher energy requirement.
Physical activity	Presence of physical activity increases the energy expenditure above the basal energy need. Regular physical activity have lower risk of many chronic diseases.
Altered physiological states	Certain conditions such as pregnancy and lactation, energy requirements of the individual are increased due to elevated BMR. The need of extra energy is associated with deposition of tissues during pregnancy and secretion of milk during lactation.
Psychological stress	Excessive amount of stress can lead to risk of strokes, heart attacks, depression, etc.

- **Food habits:** Healthy food habits impart healthy growth and improves cognitive development.
- It provides longer term health benefits such as reducing the risk of becoming overweight or obese and developing noncommunicable diseases, like-diabetes, stroke, etc. later in life.

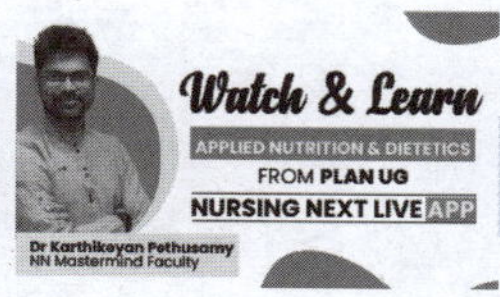

SHORT ANSWER QUESTIONS

1. Classification of food. (MGR)

Answer

According to their origin, the food is classified into two groups:

- Plant origin—seeds, fruits and vegetables
- Animal origin—meat, milk and eggs

Classified based on chemical constituents:

- Macronutrients:
  - Carbohydrate
  - Protein
  - Lipids (Fat)
- Micronutrients:
  - Vitamins
  - Minerals

2. Define health. (MGR)

Answer

According to WHO health is defined as "a state of complete physical, mental and social well-being and not merely the absence of disease".

3. Define nutrition. (MGR)

Answer

Nutrition is well defined as the science of food and its association with the health.

4. What is active transport? (MGR)

Answer

The process of moving substances across a biological membrane against their concentration gradient, or from regions of lower concentration to regions of greater concentration, is known as active transport.

CONCEPTUAL REVISION

MULTIPLE CHOICE QUESTIONS

1. Who is considered the Father of modern nutrition?
   a. Hippocrates b. Louis Pasteur
   c. Antoine Lavoisier d. Antoine Parmentier

Ans. c. Antoine Lavoisier

2. Which of the following historical figures is credited with discovering the importance of Vitamin C in preventing scurvy?
   a. James Cook b. Christopher Columbus
   c. Marco Polo d. Vasco da Gama

Ans. a. James Cook

3. Which of the following was the first nutrient to be discovered?
   a. Carbohydrates b. Proteins
   c. Fats d. Vitamins

Ans. b. Proteins

4. The first national nutrition survey in India was conducted in which year?
   a. 1947 b. 1958
   c. 1975 d. 1998

Ans. b. 1958

Golden Points

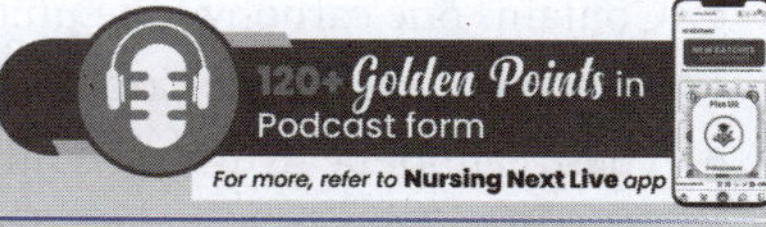

- A social or religious custom prohibiting or restricting a particular practice is known as Taboos.
- Basal metabolic rate (BMR) is the rate of metabolism when an individual is at complete rest in a warm environment and is in postabsorptive state (12 hours after taking a meal).

CHAPTER

2

Carbohydrates

CONCEPTUAL THEORY

Terminology

150+ key terminologies for Quick Recall & Revision

Basal metabolism: The energy metabolism of a subject at complete physical and mental rest, and having normal body temperature and in the post absorptive state (i.e., 12 hours after the intake of last meal) is known as basal metabolism.

BMR: The basal metabolic rate (BMR) is the measurement of an organism's energy expenditure when at rest. Amount of minimum energy required to carry on the basic involuntary work of the body is known as BMR.

Body mass index (BMI): Body mass index is a value derived from the weight and height of an individual. The BMI is defined as a body mass divided by square of the body height. It is expressed in the unit of kg/m^2.

Brush border enzymes: Enzymes responsible for the final digestion of carbohydrates in the villi of intestine are called brush border enzymes, like maltase, sucrase and lactase.

Calorie (kcal or C): The amount of heat required to raise the temperature of 1 kg of water by 1°C (from 15°C to 16°C).

Carbohydrates: The organic compounds, sugar, starches and dietary fiber that occur in plant foods and provide energy to body.

Empty calories: Term used for foods that provide only energy without any other nutrient, e.g., white sugar and alcohol.

Glycogenesis: The conversion of glucose to glycogen for storage in the liver.

Glycogenolysis: The splitting up of glycogen in the liver, yielding glucose.

Glycolysis: A metabolic process that occurs nearly in all living cells in which glucose is converted in a series of steps to pyruvic acid and during which energy is released in the form of adenosine triphosphate (ATP).

Hydrolysis: Chemical decomposition in which a compound is split into other compounds by reacting with water.

Ketosis: Ketosis is a metabolic process that occurs when the body does not have enough glucose for energy. Stored fats are broken down for energy, resulting in a build-up of acids called ketones within the body.

Lactose intolerance: Disorders resulting from improper digestion of milk sugar called lactose, due to lack of enzyme, lactose in the intestinal mucosa.

CARBOHYDRATES

- Carbohydrates are hydrates of carbon. The presence of carbon, hydrogen and oxygen in carbohydrates is in the ratio of 1:2:1.
- Monosaccharides:
  - Contains one carbohydrate unit
  - Also known as simple carbohydrates
  - These cannot be hydrolysed further.
  - Example: Glucose, galactose, fructose
- Disaccharides:
  - Contains two carbohydrate units held together by a glycosidic bond.
  - Also known as complex carbohydrates
  - Example: Sucrose, maltose
  - These are further divided into:
    - **Reducing sugar:** Disaccharides in which the functional group of one molecule is in free form and that can participate in reactions reducing aldehyde groups. Example: maltose and lactose.
    - **Nonreducing sugar:** Disaccharides in which both the functional groups are engaged in bond formation and there is no free functional group to participate in reactions. Example: sucrose.
- Trisaccharides
  - Contains three carbohydrate units linked by glycosidic bonds.
  - Examples: Rabinose, raffinose

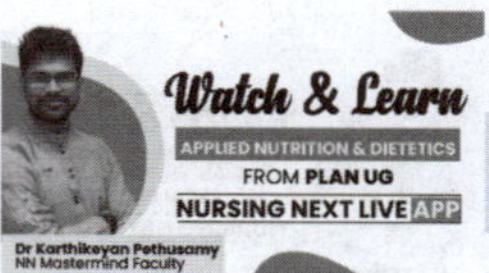

- Polysaccharides
  - Contains many carbohydrate units linked by glycosidic bonds.
  - Example: Glycogen, cellulose
  - Polysaccharides are of two types:
    1. **Homopolysaccharides:** Formed by the same kind of monosaccharides linked by glycosidic bonds. Example: glycogen, starch, cellulose
    2. **Heteropolysaccharides:** Formed by two or more types of monosaccharides joined together by glycosidic linkages.
- Mucopolysaccharides
  - Heteropolysacharides in which there is a mixture of sugar units.
  - Example: Hyaluronic acid, chondroitin sulphate, heparin.

RECOMMENDED DAILY ALLOWANCE

- Amount of nutrient and calorie intake per day is considered necessary for maintenance of good health.
- Amount of nutrient is calculated for males and females of various ages and recommended by the Food and Nutrition Board of National research council.
- Total energy requirement of an individual is mainly made up of three components.
- Its requirement during work can be calculated by adding together the energy requirement for:
  - Basal metabolism
  - Additional energy requirement for work
  - Specific dynamic action of food.

Energy Requirement (RDA)

- Adult man doing sedentary work—2400 kcal
- Adult women doing sedentary work—1900 kcal

The WHO suggests that carbohydrates should constitute 55% to 75% of the total daily energy intake to meet the body's energy needs.

DIETARY SOURCES

Main dietary sources of carbohydrates include grains, vegetables and fruits. Complex carbohydrates are present in whole grains (such as cereals and rice), bran, beans, bread and pasta.

Milk and milk products provide lactose, while beverages, jams, jellies and candies provide refined sugar, such as glucose and fructose.

Foods which are rich in carbohydrate include:

- **Dairy:** Milk, yogurt and ice cream
- **Fruits:** Whole fruits and fruit juice
- **Grains:** Cereal grains, bread and rice
- **Legumes:** Beans and pulses
- **Starchy vegetables:** Potatoes and corn
- **Sugary sweets:** Soda, candy, cookies and other deserts.

Functions

Carbohydrates are necessary for good health and give a variety of benefits:

- **Brain health:** Carbohydrates are important for brain functions. They are a quick source of energy and have influence on mood and memory.
- **Weight loss:** Although, carbohydrates are often blamed for weight gain, the right kind of carbohydrate can actually help to maintain a healthy weight. This can happen due to the consumption of many good carbohydrates, especially, whole grains and vegetables with skin, which contain fiber.
- **Good sources of nutrients:** Whole, unprocessed fruits and vegetables are well known for their nutrient contents. Due to the same reason, some of the food stuffs are even considered as super foods, such as the green leafy vegetables, sweet potatoes, berries, citruses and apples. Whole grains also have significantly higher amounts of fiber, energy and polyunsaturated fats, as well as all micronutrients (except vitamin B_{12} and sodium). Further, whole grains have also been shown to contain antioxidants.
- **Heart health:** Fiber also helps to lower cholesterol. This is due to the reason that the digestive process requires bile acids, which are made, partly, from cholesterol. As the digestion improves, liver pulls cholesterol from blood, to form more bile acid, thereby, reducing the amount of LDL (the bad cholesterol).

ENERGY

- Capacity to do work is known as energy.
- It is required for each activity.
- It is derived from the metabolism of carbohydrates, fats and proteins.

Unit of Energy

- Kilocalorie – most commonly used
- Joule – SI unit. It is defined as the energy required to move 1 kg mass by 1 meter by a force of 1 newton acting on it.

Energy Value of Food

- 1 g of carbohydrate – 4 kcal
- 1 g of protein – 4 kcal
- 1 g of fat – 9 kcal

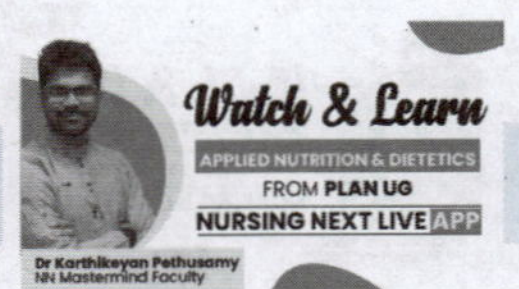

Basal Metabolic Rate (BMR)

- Minimum amount of energy per unit time required by the body to maintain function at the rest.
- Affected by body surface area

FACTORS AFFECTING BMR

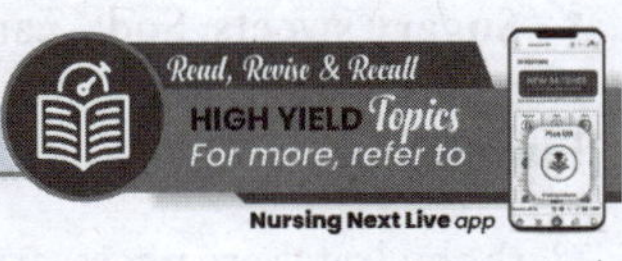

Surface area:

Sex: Males > Females

Age:

Physical work:

Hormones:

Climatic conditions:

Racial variations:

Disease states:

Diet:

Muscle mass:

CONCEPTUAL EXERCISES

LONG ANSWER QUESTION

1. Define basal metabolism. Explain factors affecting basal metabolic rate and write the determination of basal metabolism. (MGR, KUHS)

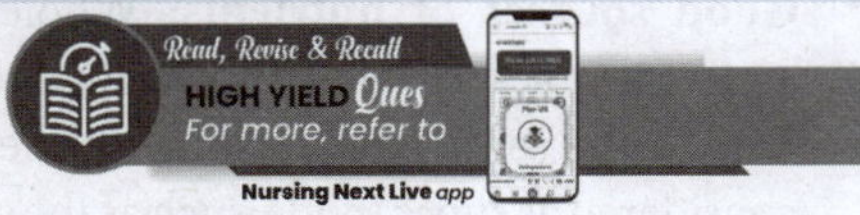

Answer

Introduction

- Minimum amount of energy per unit time required by the body to maintain function at the rest.
- Affected by body surface area
- **Body functions contributing to BMR**
  - Cardiac activities
  - Organ functions
  - Nerve impulse conduction
  - GI motility
  - Reabsorption by renal tubules
  - Ion transport across membranes
  - NA^+- K^+ pump utilized 50% of basal energy

Units of BMR

- Calories consumed per square meter per hour by body
- Cal/sq.m/h

Normal Values

- Adult man – 35–38 Cal/sq.m/hr or 1600 Cal/day
- Adult woman – 32–35 Cal/sq.m/hr or 1400 Cal/day

Factors Affecting BMR

- **Surface area:** BMR is directly proportional to surface area, i.e., weight and height of individual.
- **Sex:** Males > Females. Because of the presence of more lean muscle mass in males.
- **Age:** More in infants and growing children than adults. BMR decreases 2% per 10 years in adults.
- **Physical work:** BMR increases with increase in regular physical activity.
- **Hormones:** Thyroid hormones (T3 and T4) have stimulatory effect on body metabolism, i.e., BMR. So BMR increases in hyperthyroidism and decreases in hypothyroidism.
- **Climatic conditions:** Hot climate <Cold climate areas
- **Racial variations:** Higher in eskimos
- **Disease states:** BMR increases with increase in body temperature, in presence of infections, leukemias, hypertension, cardiac failure and polycythemia.
- **Diet:** Vegetarians have 11% less BMR than meat eaters. BMR falls after prolonged starvation.
- **Muscle mass:** Higher muscle mass means higher BMR.

Determination of Basal Metabolism

- Usually determined by using the Benedict's and Roth apparatus.
- Benedict and Roth apparatus is a closed circuit system in which the subject breathes in oxygen from a metal cylinder of about 6L capacity and carbon dioxide produced is absorbed by soda-lime present in the tower.
- The oxygen cylinder floats on water present in an outer rank.
- The subject wears a nose clip and breathes through a mouthpiece.
- Duration of the process is 6 minutes.
- The volume of oxygen used is recorded on a graph paper attached to a revolving drum by a pen attached to it.
- Since the subject is in the post-absorptive state, calorific value of one liter of oxygen consumed is taken as 4.8 kcal.

Example

- Adult male, 50 kg body weight consumes oxygen in 6 min = 1.1
- Heat produced in 6 minutes = 48 × 1.1 = 5.28 kcal
- Heat produced in 24 hours = 5.28 × 10 × 24 = 1267

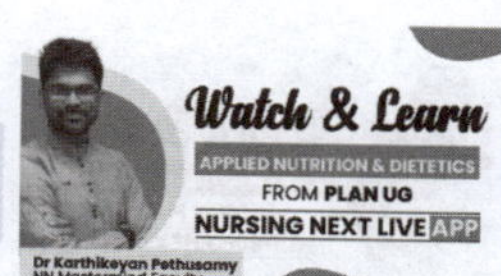

Factors Affecting the Determination of Basal Metabolism

- Test is done in post-absorptive state, i.e., 10–12 hours after the last meal.
- Subject should be resting position but awake.
- Both body temperature and surrounding temperature should be maintained at normal.
- Subject should have a normal pulse rate and free from stress or fear.

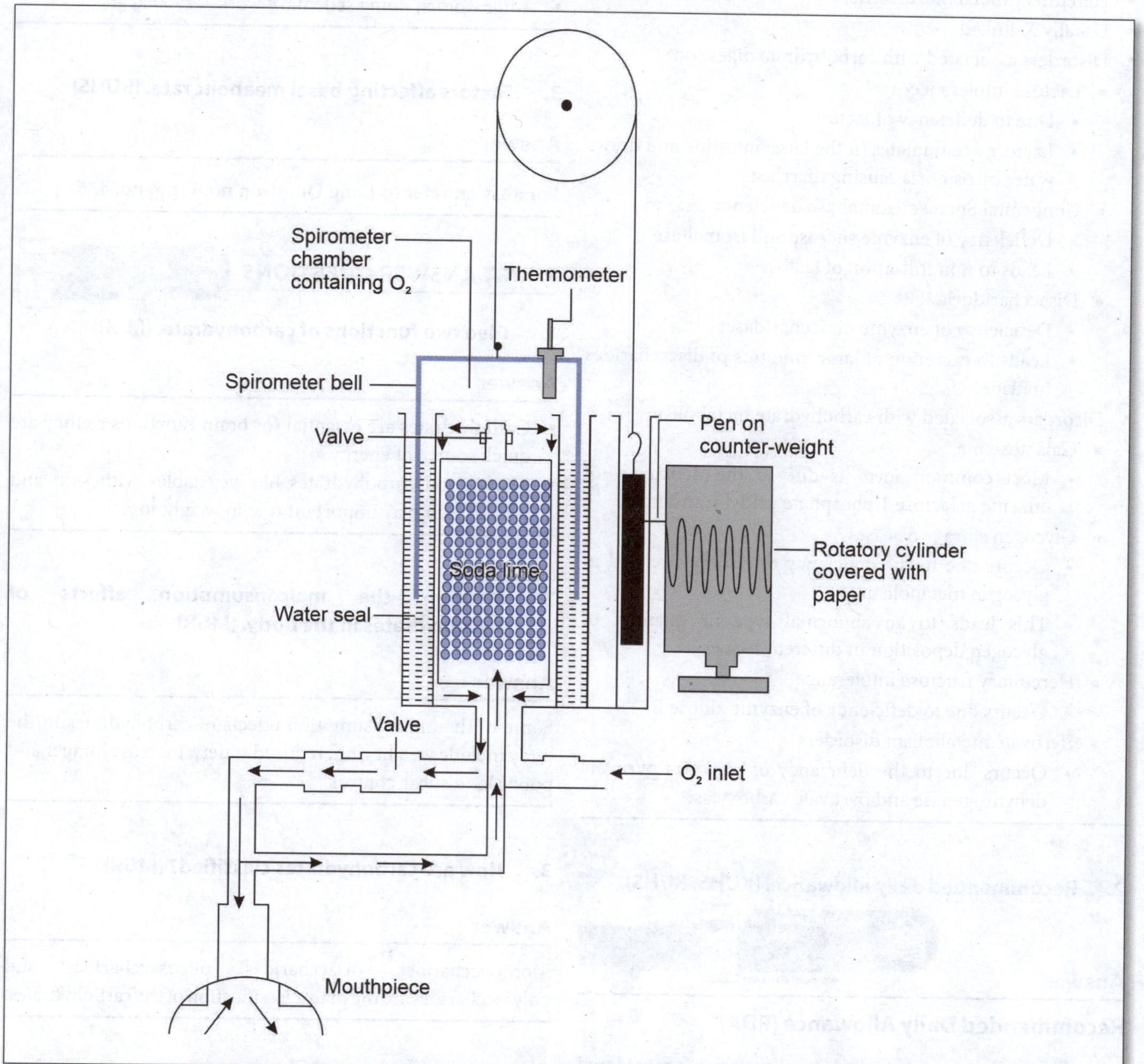

Figure 2.1: Apparatus of Benedict and Roth (spirometer) used for determination of BMR

SHORT NOTES

1. Write a note on the metabolic disorders associated with carbohydrate digestion. (KUHS)

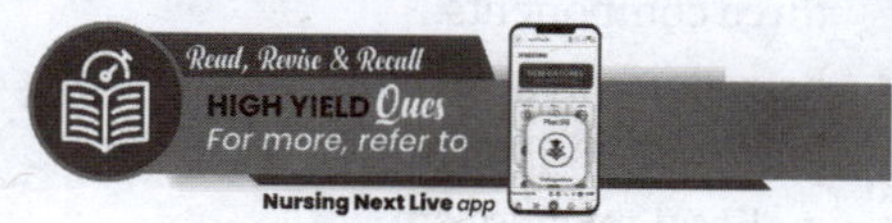

Answer

Metabolic Disorders Associated with Carbohydrate Digestion

- Hereditary metabolic disorder
- Usually X-linked
- Disorders associated with carbohydrate digestion
  - Lactose intolerance
    - Due to deficiency of lactase
    - Lactose accumulates in the large intestine and draws water by osmosis causing diarrhea
  - Congenital Sucrase-Isomaltase deficiency
    - Deficiency of enzyme sucrose and isomaltase
    - Leads to nonutilization of lactose
  - Disacchariduria
    - Deficiency of enzyme disaccharidases
    - Leads to excretion of large amounts of disaccharides in urine.
- Disorders associated with carbohydrate metabolism
  - Galactosemia
    - Most common form is due to the deficiency of enzyme galactose 1 phosphate uridyl transferase.
  - Glycogen storage diseases
    - Occurs due to the deficiency of enzymes related to glycogen metabolism.
    - This leads to an abnormal type or quantity of glycogen deposition in different tissues.
  - Hereditary fructose intolerance
    - Occurs due to deficiency of enzyme aldose B
  - Pyruvate metabolism disorders
    - Occurs due to the deficiency of enzymes pyruvate dehydrogenase and pyruvate carboxylase

2. Recommended daily allowance. (KUHS, RUHS)

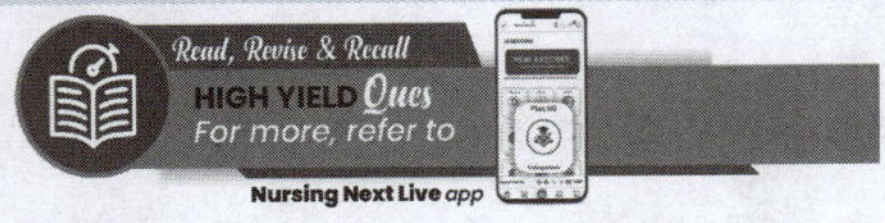

Answer

Recommended Daily Allowance (RDA)

- Amount of nutrient and calorie intake per day is considered necessary for maintenance of good health.
- Amount of nutrient is calculated for males and females of various ages and recommended by the Food and Nutrition Board of National research council.
- Total energy requirement of an individual is mainly up of three components.
- Its requirement during work can be calculated by adding together the energy requirement for:
  - Basal metabolism
  - Additional energy requirement for work
  - Specific dynamic action of food.

Energy Requirement (RDA)

- Adult man doing sedentary work – 2400 kcal
- Adult women doing sedentary work – 1900 kcal

3. Factors affecting basal meabolic rate. (RUHS)

Answer

For answer, refer to Long Question no. 1, pg. no. 436

SHORT ANSWER QUESTIONS

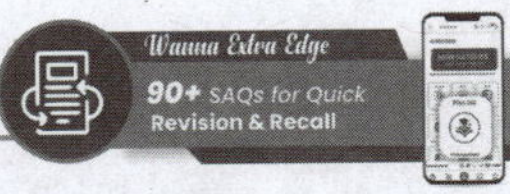

1. Give two functions of carbohydrate. (MGR)

Answer

- Carbohydrates are essential for brain functions as they are quick source of energy.
- Many good carbohydrates like vegetables with skin and whole grain play important role in weight loss.

2. Mention the malconsumption effects of carbohydrates in the body. (MGR)

Answer

Some of the malconsumption effects of carbohydrates in the body include weight gain, reduced satiety, increase hunger and poor blood sugar control.

3. How are carbohydrates classified? (MGR)

Answer

Monosaccharides, disaccharides, oligosaccharides and polysaccharides are the main classification of the carbohydrates.

4. List out four foods avoided by a diabetic patient. (MGR)

Answer

Diabetic patients avoid foods that are heavy in refined carbohydrates, sugary drinks, high-fat foods, and foods with a lot of added sugar.

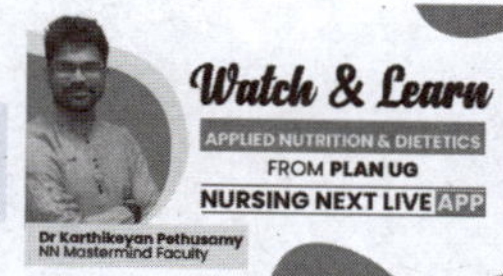

5. Write the energy value of a diet prescribed with 150 g of carbohydrate. (DU)

Answer

Carbohydrates provide 4 calories per gram. Thus, energy value of a diet with 150 grams of carbohydrates would be:

Energy value = 150 grams × 4 calories/gram = 600 calories

6. Name the glucose tolerance factor. (DU)

Answer

Chromium is considered to be the primary component of GTF and is often referred to as "glucose tolerance factor chromium" (GTFCr).

CONCEPTUAL REVISION

MULTIPLE CHOICE QUESTIONS

1. Desirable intake of dietary fiber per 2000 kcal energy intake is:

a. 20 g b. 40 g
c. 60 g d. 100 g

Ans. b. 40 g

2. Energy (kcal/g) obtained from fiber:

a. 2 b. 4
c. 7 d. 9

Ans. a. 2

3. Energy (kcal/g) obtained from alcohol:

a. 2 b. 4
c. 7 d. 9

Ans. c. 7

4. Rich source of fiber is:

a. Spinach b. Ragi
c. Green Gram d. Wheat

Ans. b. Ragi

5. Fiber content is highest in:

a. Maize b. Oat
c. Rice d. Wheat

Ans. a. Maize

6. True about dietary fibers:

i. Decrease post prandial glucose
ii. Decrease bile salt reabsorption
iii. Decrease LDL cholesterol
iv. Increases bulk of stool

a. If i, ii, iii are correct
b. If i and iii are correct
c. If ii and iv are correct
d. If all four (i, ii, iii and iv) are correct

Ans. d. If all four (i, ii, iii and iv) are correct

7. Food with low glycemic index is:

a. Sucrose b. Potato
c. Wheat bread d. Rice

Ans. d. Rice

8. Glycemic index is defined as ability of the food item to:

a. Stimulate the release of glucagon
b. Raise blood sugar
c. Stimulate Insulin release
d. Others

Ans. b. Raise blood sugar

Golden Points

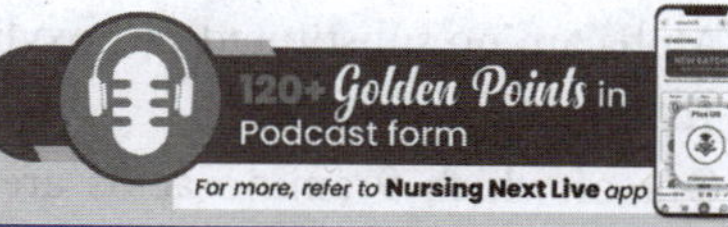

- Carbohydrates have a protein sparing action. It prevents the breakdown of proteins for energy.
- Digestion of carbohydrates particularly starch begins in the mouth with the action of salivary amylase.
- Glycogen is also called animal starch. It is the reserve form of carbohydrates found in liver and muscle of animals and man.
- Glycogen stored in liver is used to maintain blood sugar levels and energy levels throughout the day.

CHAPTER 3

Proteins

CONCEPTUAL THEORY

Terminology

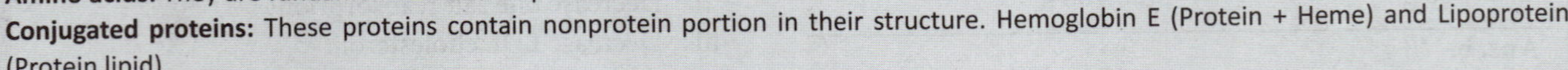

Amino acids: They are fundamental blocks of proteins.

Conjugated proteins: These proteins contain nonprotein portion in their structure. Hemoglobin E (Protein + Heme) and Lipoprotein (Protein lipid).

Derived proteins: These are produced by the action of acids, alkaline, heat and enzymes on native proteins, polypeptides, proteases, etc.

Enzyme: Biological catalysts which enhance the role of chemical reactions in the body.

Lactoferrin: Minor protein of milk containing iron.

Protein: A macromolecule composed of one or more polypeptide chains, each with a characteristic sequence of amino acids linked by peptide bonds and is essential for muscle mass.

Transport or carrier proteins: Certain proteins are involved in the transportation of many essential biological factors to various parts of organisms. These are known as carrier or transport proteins.

COMPOSITION

Proteins

- Protein is defined as a macromolecule composed of one or more polypeptide chains, each with a characteristic sequence of amino acids linked by peptide bonds and is essential for muscle mass.
- It accounts for about 16% of body weight.
- It contains carbon, hydrogen, and oxygen and also nitrogen.
- The basic units of proteins are called amino acids that are linked through peptide bonds.

Amino Acids

- Amino acids – building blocks of proteins.
- Alpha amino substituted carboxylic acid.
- Total – 21 amino acids
- Out of which 9 amino acids are not synthesized by the human body, so are essential.

EIGHT ESSENTIAL AMINO ACIDS

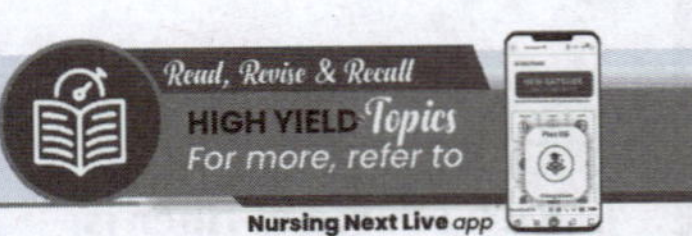

Essential or Indispensable Amino Acids

- Cannot be synthesized by the body
- Need to be supplemented in the diet
- Required for growth and maintenance of the human body
- The ten essential amino acids are:
  1. Arginine
  2. Valine
  3. Histidine
  4. Isoleucine
  5. Leucine
  6. Lysine
  7. Methionine
  8. Phenylalanine
  9. Threonine
  10. Tryptophan

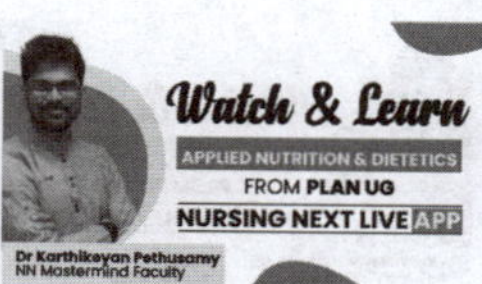

FUNCTIONS

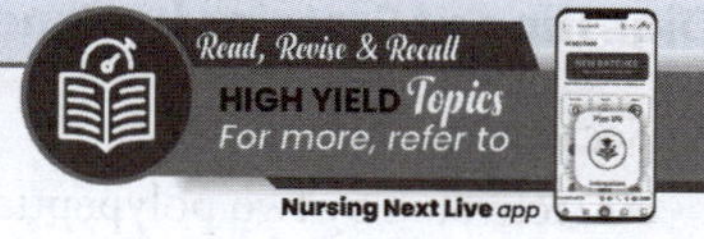

Functions of Proteins

- **Structural proteins**
  - Part of the connective tissue, cartilage, tendons, bone
  - Mainly fibrous proteins
  - Example – Collagen, elastin, keratin
- **Enzymes**
  - Biological catalysts
  - Reduce the activation energy of reactants
  - Mostly globular conjugated proteins
  - Example – DNA polymerase, Lipase
- **Hormones**
  - Proteinaceous hormones
  - Example – Insulin, ACH, Glucagon
- **Respiratory proteins**
  - Conjugated Proteins containing chrome as prosthetic group
  - Example – Hemoglobin, myoglobin
- **Transport proteins**
  - Transport materials in cells
  - Form channels in plasma membrane
  - Example – transferrin, albumin
- **Contractile proteins**
  - Part of the muscle
  - Example – Actin, Myosin
- **Storage proteins**
  - Act as storage form of metal ions and amino acids
  - Example – ferritin, casein, gluten
- **Toxins**
  - Toxic in nature
  - Example – snake venom

DIETARY SOURCES

Dietary Sources of Proteins

- Animal Sources
  - Animal products are rich sources of proteins. It has a balanced combination of all the amino acids, hence known as complete protein.
  - Important sources include:
    - Meat
    - Egg
    - Milk
    - Cheese
    - Fish
  - Egg protein is the best protein – due to its high biological value and digestibility.
- Vegetable sources
  - Plant protein is incomplete except soybean proteins.
  - Incomplete protein is deficient in one for more of the essential amino acids.
  - Important sources include:
    - Pulses
    - Beans

PROTEIN REQUIREMENTS – RDA

Daily Requirement of Protein

The recommended daily allowances for proteins are as follows:

- Average man – 60 g/day
- Average women – 55 g/day
- Lactating women – additional 25 g/day
- Children – 22–40 g/day
- Adolescent boy – 70 g/day
- Adolescent girl – 65 g/day

CONCEPTUAL EXERCISES

LONG ANSWER QUESTIONS

1. Explain the classification, digestion and deficiency manifestations of protein. (KUHS)

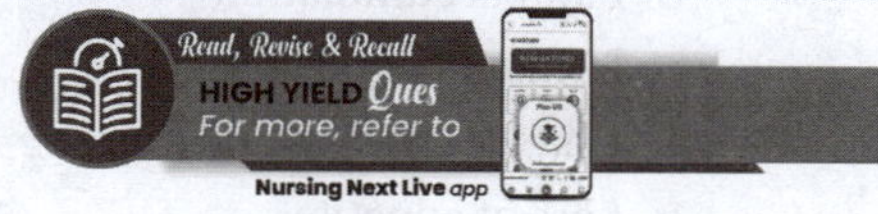

Answer

Protein

- Protein is defined as a macromolecule composed of one or more polypeptide chains, each with a characteristic sequence of amino acids linked by peptide bonds and is essential for muscle mass.
- It accounts for about 16% of body weight.
- It contains carbon, hydrogen, and oxygen and also nitrogen.
- The basic units of proteins are called amino acids that are linked through peptide bonds.

Classification

- Proteins are classified under three criteria

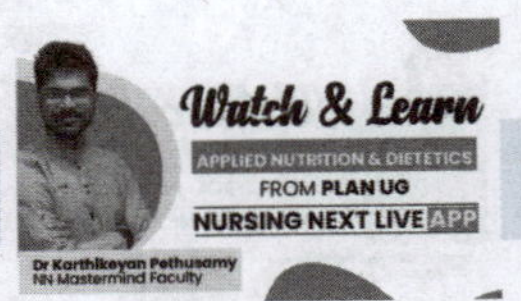

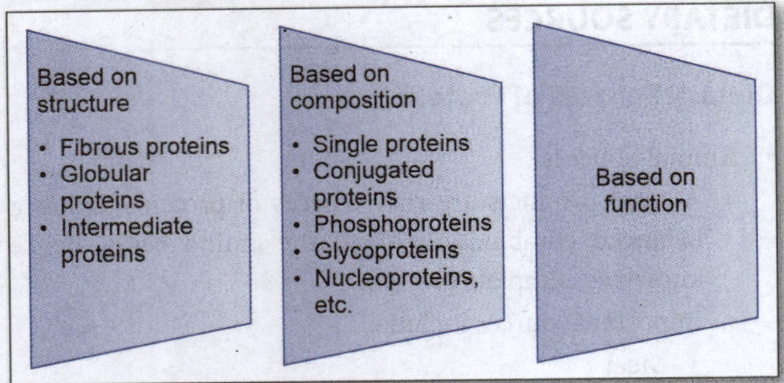

Digestion and Absorption

- **Source of protein**
  - Dietary
  - Endogenous
- Dietary proteins are denatured on cooking and therefore, easily digested.
- **Enzymes responsible for degradation of protein**
  - Endopeptidases (proteases)
    - Break the internal peptide bonds
    - Example – pepsin, trypsin
  - Exopeptidases
    - Act on the peptide bonds of terminal amino acids.
    - Two types:
      - Carboxypeptidases – act on C terminal amino acid
      - Aminopeptidases – act on N-terminal amino acid

Digestion of Proteins by Gastric Secretion

- Protein digestion begins in stomach by
  - Hydrochloric acid
    - pH of stomach is <2
    - This causes
      - Denaturation of proteins – makes proteins more susceptible to proteases
      - Killing of certain micro-organisms
  - Pepsinogen – protease proenzyme
    - Converted to active pepsin by either autocatalysis or by gastric HCl.
    - Cleaves peptide bonds formed by amino groups of phenylalanine or tyrosine or leucine
    - Results in peptides and few amino acids which also act as stimulants for the release of the hormone cholecystokinin from duodenum.
  - Rennin
    - Also known as chymosin
    - Found in infants and children
    - Involved in curdling of milk.
    - Absent in adults.

Digestion of Proteins by Pancreatic Proteases

- Secreted as zymogens
  - Activated by two polypeptide hormones
    - Cholecystokinin
    - Secretin
- Pancreatic proteases
  - Trypsin
    - Cleaves the peptide bond (-CO-) carbonyl groups contributed by lysine or arginine
  - Chymotrypsin
    - Elastase
    - Active at neutral pH
    - Gastric pH is neutralized by pancreatic $NaHCO_3$
    - Results in the formation of small peptides and free amino acids.

Digestion of Proteins by Small Intestinal Enzymes

- Aminopeptidases and dipeptidases
- Produce small peptides (usually dipeptides) and free amino acids.

Deficiency of Proteins

- Deficiency of proteins for longer periods may lead to weight loss, anemia, nutritional edema, low resistance to infection and poor healing of wounds.
- As there is continuous protein building as well as degradation in human body for its normal functions, their regular optimal intake is very essential for keeping good health.
- Protein deficiency diseases occur in developing countries due to poverty as well as lack of knowledge about nutritional needs.
  - Protein energy malnutrition
    - Clinical disorders resulting from deficiency of proteins and energy.
    - Primarily occurs in young children
    - Two types – Kwashiorkor and marasmus
    - Clinical symptoms
      - Reduced growth, thinning, wasting of muscles
      - Fluid accumulation
      - Irritability and apathy
      - Changes in skin and hair
      - Loss of appetite
      - Liver enlargement
      - Anemia
      - Increased susceptibility to infections

Differences between Kwashiorkor and Marasmus

Aspect	Kwashiorkor	Marasmus
Definition	A severe form of malnutrition resulting from inadequate protein intake despite sufficient caloric intake	A severe form of malnutrition resulting from overall energy deficiency, including inadequate protein and calorie intake
Etiology	Inadequate protein intake, infections, or diseases causing malabsorption	Severe and prolonged calorie deficiency
Age of onset	1–3-year-old	6–18-month-old
Appearance	Edema (swelling) of the feet, legs, and abdomen; skin changes (rash, peeling, discoloration)	Severe wasting of muscle and fat; skin appears dry, loose, and wrinkled
Hair and nails	Hair changes color and texture, easily pulled out; brittle, ridged nails	Normal hair color and texture; thin, brittle, and easily plucked hair; thin and fragile nails
Appetite	Often has a poor appetite	Anorexia (lack of appetite)
Mental status	Normal or irritable	Apathy and lack of emotional expression
Body weight	Normal or slightly below normal for age and size	Significantly below normal for age and size
Growth retardation	Less likely to experience stunted growth	Likely to experience stunted growth
Treatment	Protein-rich diet; gradual introduction of food; correction of underlying infections or diseases	Gradual reintroduction of calories and protein to avoid refeeding syndrome; correction of underlying infections or diseases; fluid and electrolyte replacement

SHORT NOTES

1. High biological value proteins. (DU)

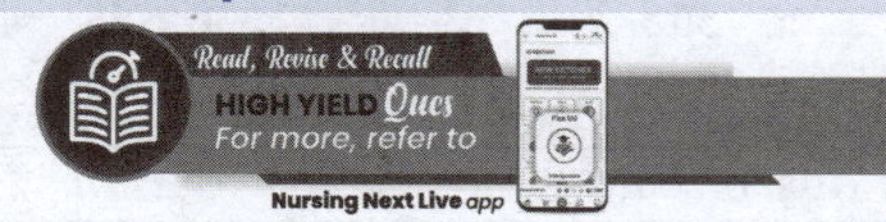

Answer

Biological Value Proteins

- Quality of proteins based on the content of the essential amino acids.
- Index to measure the quality of proteins
- Proteins rich in essential amino acids are known as **high biological value proteins.**
- Also known as complete protein, i.e., have essential amino acids in adequate quantities to meet the minimum requirement of the body.

Essential amino acids include phenylalanine, lysine, leucine, isoleucine, valine, threonine, tryptophan, methionine.

Sources of High Biological Value Proteins

- Animal origin proteins such as eggs, cow meat, chicken meat, fish, cow milk.
- Vegetable origin proteins such as legumes, whole grains.

Examples of Low Biological Value Proteins

Bread, cereals, pulses

2. Write a note on functions of protein.

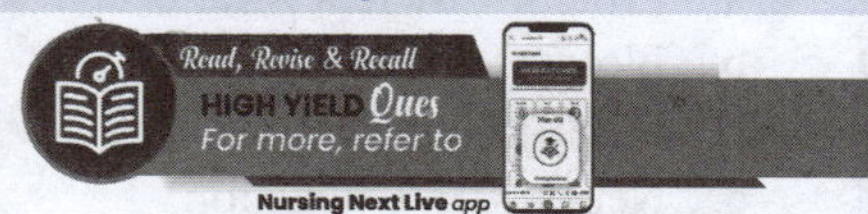

Answer

- Protein is defined as a macromolecule composed of one or more polypeptide chains, each with a characteristic sequence of amino acids linked by peptide bonds and is essential for muscle mass.
- It accounts for about 16% of body weight.
- It contains carbon, hydrogen, and oxygen and also nitrogen.
- These are responsible for the body's growth, maintenance and repair.

Functions of Proteins

Structural proteins	• Part of the connective tissue, cartilage, tendons, bone • Mainly fibrous proteins • Insoluble in water • Example – Collagen, elastin, keratin
Enzymes	• Biological catalysts • Reduces the activation energy of reactants • Mostly globular conjugated proteins • Example – DNA polymerase, Lipase
Hormones	• Proteinaceous hormones • Example – Insulin, ACH, Glucagon

Contd...

Respiratory proteins	• Conjugated proteins containing chrome as prosthetic group • Example – Hemoglobin, myoglobin
Transport proteins	• Transport materials in cells • Form channels in plasma membrane • Example – transferrin, albumin
Contractile proteins	• Part of the muscle • Example – Actin, Myosin
Storage proteins	• Act as storage form of metal ions and amino acids • Example – ferritin, casein, gluten
Toxins	• Toxic in nature • Example – snake venom

Contd...

CONCEPTUAL REVISION

MULTIPLE CHOICE QUESTIONS

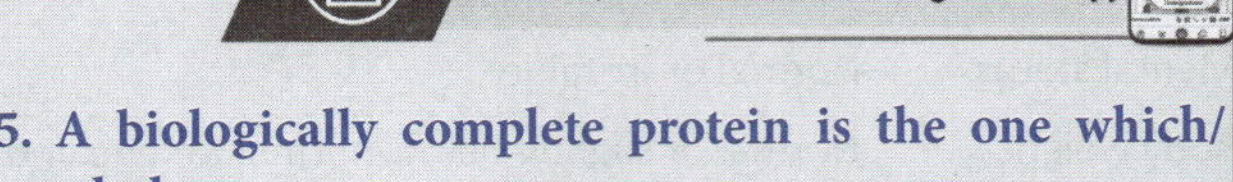

1. **Proteins with highest biological value are found in:**
   a. Legumes
   b. Cereals
   c. Protein of animal source
   d. Milk

Ans. c. Protein of animal source

2. **Which one of the following is the best indicator of protein quality for recommending the dietary protein requirement?**
   a. Protein-Efficiency Ratio
   b. Biological Value
   c. Digestibility Coefficient
   d. Net Protein Utilization

Ans. d. Net Protein Utilization

3. **Net Protein Utilization is given by the formula:**
   a. Weight gained/Amount of protein consumed × 100
   b. Nitrogen retained by body/Nitrogen intake × 100
   c. Nitrogen retained/Nitrogen absorbed × 100
   d. Biological value/Digestibility coefficient

Ans. b. Nitrogen retained by body/Nitrogen intake × 100

4. **Protein constitute % of body weight in adults:**
   a. 10 b. 20
   c. 25 d. 30

Ans. b. 20

5. **A biologically complete protein is the one which/whole:**
   a. Net protein utilization is 100
   b. Amino acid score is 100
   c. Contains all amino acids
   d. Contains all essential amino acids

Ans. d. Contains all essential amino acids

6. **ICMR recommends 1.0 g of protein/kg body weight for an Indian adult, assuming a NPU for dietary proteins:**
   a. 55 b. 65
   c. 85 d. 100

Ans. b. 65

7. **Energy (kcal/g) released from protein:**
   a. 2 b. 4
   c. 7 d. 9

Ans. b. 4

8. **The average daily nutrient intake level estimated to meet the requirement of half of the healthy individuals in a particular life stage and gender group is called:**
   a. Adequate intake
   b. Estimated average requirement
   c. Tolerable upper intake level
   d. Recommended dietary allowance

Ans. b. Estimated average requirement

Golden Points

120+ Golden Points in Podcast form
For more, refer to Nursing Next Live app

- Amino acids are fundamental blocks of proteins.
- Arginine and histidine are called semi essential amino acids as they are required in the diet of children, pregnant women and lactating women.

CHAPTER

4

Fats

CONCEPTUAL THEORY

Terminology

150+ key terminologies for Quick Recall & Revision

Atherosclerosis: Atherosclerosis is a build-up of plaque in the wall of the arteries causing narrowing and loss of elasticity. Plaque contains deposits of fats, cholesterol and cell waste products.
Chylomicrons: These are lipoproteins; serve to transport dietary lipids from the intestines to other locations in the body.
Chyme: Chyme is a liquid substance found in stomach before entering into small intestine. Contains partly digested food, water, hydrogen chloride and digestive enzymes.
Fatty acids: These are long chain of lipid carboxylic acid molecules found in fats and oils. It is an important component of cell membrane as phospholipids and glycolipids.
Glycolipid: A lipid containing a carbohydrate group.
Hydrogenation: It is the process in which liquid vegetable oils convert into solid and semi-solid fats. It occurs in presence of catalyst.
Lipases: These are enzymes which help in hydrolysis of fats.
Lipid: A small water insoluble biomolecule generally containing fatty acids, sterols or isoprenoid compounds.
Lipogenesis: Apart from lipoproteins, cholesterol and phospholipids are also synthesized in the liver. This is called lipogenesis.
Lipolysis: The blood transports lipids to the rest of the body and cells absorb them and utilize for energy. This breakdown of fats to yield energy is called lipolysis.
Lipoprotein: A lipid protein aggregate that serves to carry water insoluble lipids in the blood.
Phospholipids: A lipid containing one or more phosphate group.
Prostaglandins: Physiologically active substance participates in body functions like contraction and relaxation of smooth muscle, dilatation of blood vessels, etc.
Rancidity of fat: This process is also known as rancidification. It means complete or incomplete oxidation or hydrolysis of fats and oils when exposed to light, air or moisture or by bacterial action resulting in disagreeable smell, texture or appearance.
Saturated fatty acids: Fatty acids without double bond are known as saturated fatty acids.
Sterol: Sterol is an important class of organic molecules. They are also known as steroid alcohols and subgroup of the steroids. They are usually found in plants, animals and fungi and can be produced by some bacteria.
Triacylglycerol: An ester derived from glycerol and omega 3 fatty acids.
Unsaturated fatty acids: Fatty acids which have carbon-carbon double bond are known as unsaturated fatty acids.
Visible fats: Fats and oils that can be used directly or in cooking.

CLASSIFICATION

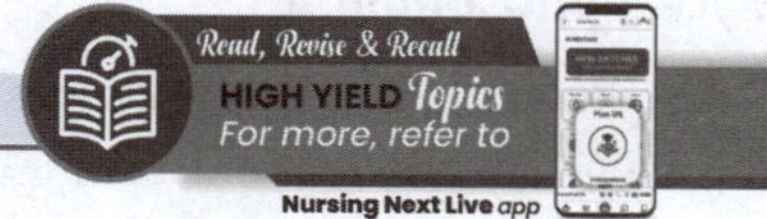

Saturated and Unsaturated Fatty Acids

Saturated Fatty Acids

- Saturated fatty acids are fatty acids that contain single bonds.
- These are simplest form of fats.
- These are defined as unbranched linear chains of CH_2 groups linked together by C-C bonds with a terminal carboxylic acid.
- General formula is $C_nH_{2n+1}COOH$
- Fatty acids derived from animal sources are usually saturated fatty acids with even number of carbon atoms
- Examples of saturated short fatty acids include butyric acid (C_4) and caproic acid (C_6).

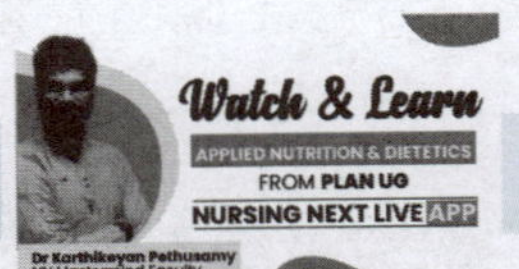

Unsaturated Fatty Acids

- Unsaturated fatty acids are fatty acids with one or more double bonds.
- These are complex fatty acids
- Contain a bent hydrocarbon chain linked together by C=C or C=C bonds with a terminal carboxylic acid group.
- These don't have enough hydrogen atoms bound to carbon atoms.

Fatty acids are divided into:

- **Monounsaturated:** Containing one double bond, e.g., monoethenoid
- **Polyunsaturated:** Containing two or more double bonds.
- **Eicosanoids:** Containing 20-carbon PUFA, e.g., prostaglandins

Caloric Value

- One kilocalorie (1 kcal or 1000 calories) is the amount of heat (energy) needed to raise the temperature of one kg of water by one degree Celsius (°C).
- The SI standard unit for energy is Joule (J).

Calorific value of various nutrients is:

- 1 g of Carbohydrates gives 4 kcal
- 1 g of Fats gives 9 kcal
- 1 g of Proteins gives 4.5 kcal

FUNCTIONS

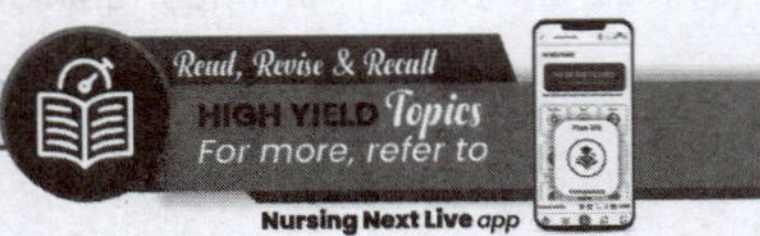

- Source of energy
  - Along with carbohydrates, fats also source of energy.
  - Provides almost double the calories per gram as compared to carbohydrates.
  - Act as reserved fuel of body.
- Form an important component of the cell membrane
- Source of fat soluble vitamins
- Fat provides insulation and protection from cold.
  - They help in maintaining the body temperature due to the presence of thin layer of fats located under the skin.
  - Also protects the inner core of body from extreme temperature changes.
- Participate in the transport and utilization of cholesterol
- Prevent fat accumulation in the liver
- Required for the synthesis of prostaglandins
- Maintain proper growth and reproduction of the organisms.
  - These include:
    - Coconut oil
    - Butter
    - Animal fats
    - Chocolate
    - Fish oil
    - Cream
    - Nuts
    - Cheese
    - Meat
- Foods rich in unsaturated fats
  - Also known as good fats
  - Control cholesterol levels
  - These include:
    - Avocado
    - Peanut butter
    - Walnuts
    - Vegetable oils
    - Peas
    - Beans

FAT REQUIREMENTS—RDA

The ICMR recommended dietary allowances for fat for Indians as per 100 g:

- Energy – 300 kcal
- Fat – 24.3 g of which
  - Saturates – 4.97 g
  - Mono unsaturates – 11.21 g
  - Polyunsaturates – 7 g

CONCEPTUAL EXERCISES

SHORT NOTES

1. Write a note on Phospholipids. (DU)

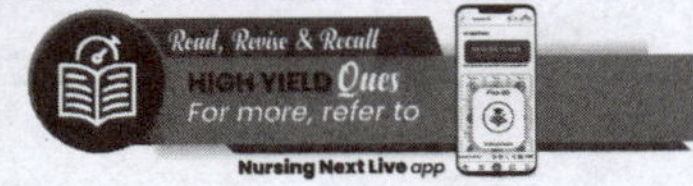

Answer

Phospholipids

- Compound lipids containing phosphoric acid along with nitrogenous base and alcohol.
- Major component of cell membrane.
- Amphiphilic in nature as they are made up of hydrophilic heads and hydrophobic tails joined together by glycerol molecule.

Types of Phospholipids

- Two types
  1. Glycerophospholipids
  2. Sphingophospholipids

Glycerophospholipids

- Also known as phosphoglycerides
- Contain glycerol as the alcohol
- Major lipids in cell membranes
- Important ones are:
  - Phosphatidic acid – simplest phospholipid
  - Lecithins (phosphatidylcholine)

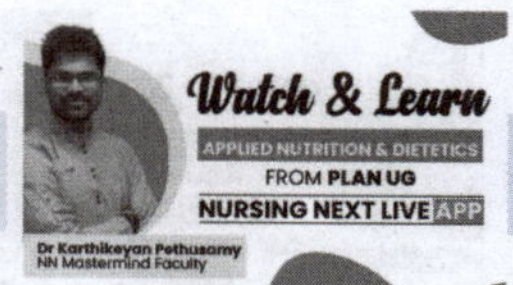

- Phosphatidic acid + choline as base
  - Most abundant in cell membrane
- Cephalins – phosphatidylethanolamine
- Ethanolamine is the nitrogenase base
- Phosphatidylinositol – phosphatidic acid + myo-inositol

Sphingomyelins

- Also known as sphinophospholipids
- Sphingosine is the amino alcohol group - Important constituent of myelin sheath
- Ceramide – acts as second messenger

Functions of Phospholipids

- Structural components of cell membrane and regulate membrane permeability
- Mitochondrial phospholipids maintain the conformation of ETC and thus, cellular respiration
- Role in absorption of fats from intestine
- Synthesis and transport of certain lipids
- Role in reverse cholesterol transport.

2. Write a note on sources and digestion of fat. (DU, KUHS)

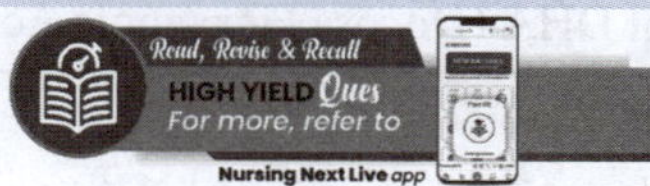

Answer

Sources of Fat

Foods rich in saturated fats	Foods rich in unsaturated fats
• Derived from mainly animal sources. • These include: ▪ Coconut oil ▪ Butter ▪ Animal fats ▪ Chocolate ▪ Fish oil ▪ Cream ▪ Nuts ▪ Cheese ▪ Meat	• Also known as good fats • Control cholesterol levels • These include: ▪ Avocado ▪ Peanut butter ▪ Walnuts ▪ Vegetable oils ▪ Peas ▪ Beans

Digestion of Fat

- Typical diet consists of 25–160 g of lipids
- Mainly triglycerides
- Enzymes required for lipid digestion
  - Lipases
  - Lingual
  - Gastric
  - Pancreatic – synthesized in pancreas and works in duodenum
  - Maximum lipid digestion occurs in duodenum

Emulsification of Lipids in Small Intestine

- Breakdown of lipids into smaller droplets
- Reduce surface tension and increase surface area
- Essential for effective digestion
- **Occurs by three mechanisms**
  1. **Detergent action of bile salts:**
     - Interact with lipid particles and the aqueous duodenal contents and convert them into smaller ones
     - Stabilize the smaller lipid particles from coalescing back.
  2. **Surfactant action of degraded lipids**
     - Initial lipid products acted by lipases, free fatty acids and monoglycerols promote emulsification
  3. **Mechanical mixing due to peristalsis**

Digestion of Lipids

- **Digestion in mouth**
  - Triglyceride degradation: By lipases to form free fatty acids and glycerol
- **Digestion in stomach**
  - By Gastric Lipase- most effective for short and medium chain fatty acids
- **Digestion in small intestine**
  - Major site of fat digestion
  - Effective digestion due to the presence of pancreatic lipase and bile salts.
  - Secretion of pancreatic juice is stimulated by
    - Passage of acid gastric contents in to the duodenum
    - By secretion of Secretin, Cholecystokinin and Pancreozymin, the gastro intestinal hormones
    - Gastro Intestinal hormones
    - Triacyl glycerol degradation by pancreatic lipase
    - Digestion of Triglycerides proceeds by removal of a terminal fatty acid to produce an α, β diglyceride.
    - The other terminal fatty acid is then removed to produce β mono glyceride.
    - The last fatty acid is linked by secondary ester group, hence cannot be hydrolyzed by pancreatic lipase.
    - β-Mono acyl glycerol can be converted to α- Mono acyl glycerol by isomerase enzyme and then hydrolyzed by Pancreatic lipase.

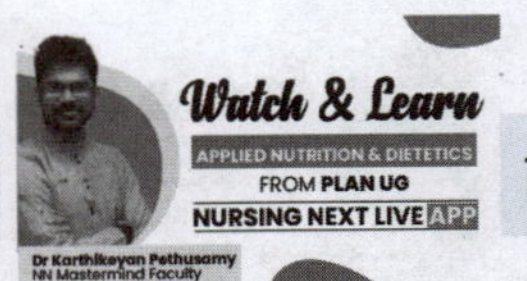

SHORT ANSWER QUESTIONS

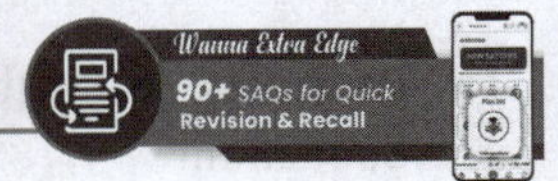

1. Two functions of fat. (MGR)

Answer

- Fats serve as a very rich source of energy.
- It also promotes absorption of vitamin -A, D, E and K these are fat soluble vitamins.

2. What is trans fat? (MGR)

Answer

Trans fats are more hazardous type of fat and are formed by hydrogenation and are usually not metabolized by the body.

3. Define fatty acids. (MGR)

Answer

Fatty acids are the long chains or building blocks of the fat in our bodies which is commonly divided as saturated and unsaturated fatty acids.

4. Write types of lipoprotein. (MGR)

Answer

Main types of lipoproteins include Low-Density Lipoprotein, High-Density Lipoprotein, Very Low-Density Lipoprotein and Chylomicrons.

5. Write two functions of lipids. (MGR)

Answer

- Lipids play a crucial role in the structure and function of cell membranes.
- Lipids are a major source of energy in the body.

6. Write two properties of lipids. (MGR)

Answer

Hydrophobic or water-repelling nature and Lipid Solubility are the two major properties of lipids.

7. List out the essential fatty acids. (MGR)

Answer

Linoleic acid and Linolenic acid are referred to as essential fatty acids.

8. Sources of DHA (Docosa Hexaenoic Acid). (DU)

Answer

Fish Oil Supplements, Fatty Fish and Fortified Foods such as certain dairy products, eggs, and breakfast cereals are sources of DHA (Docosa Hexaenoic Acid)

9. Energy value of 2 tea-spoon of vegetable oil. (DU)

Answer

A teaspoon of vegetable oil typically has between 40 and 45 calories. Consequently, 2 teaspoons of vegetable oil would have 80–90 calories.

10. Write two source of Omega-3 fatty acids. (DU)

Answer

Fish and Fish oils are biologically more active form of omega 3 fatty acids.

CONCEPTUAL REVISION

MULTIPLE CHOICE QUESTIONS

1. Highest quantity of PUFA and EFA are present in:

a. Coconut oil b. Sunflower oil
c. Safflower oil d. Soybean oil

Ans. c. Safflower oil

2. 1 kg of adipose tissue is equal to kcal energy:

a. 4400 b. 5500
c. 6600 d. 7700

Ans. d. 7700

3. Not true regarding hydrogenation of fats is:

a. Unsaturated fatty acids are converted into saturated fatty acids
b. EFA content is drastically reduced
c. Partial hydrogenation of PUFA creates trans fatty acids
d. Trans fatty acids are not atherogenic

Ans. d. Trans fatty acids are not atherogenic

4. Linoleic acid is maximum/highest in:

a. Groundnut oil b. Mustard oil
c. Safflower oil d. Coconut oil

Ans. c. Safflower oil

5. Most important essential fatty acid is:

a. Linoleic acid
b. Linolenic acid
c. Arachidonic acid
d. Eicosapentaenoic acid

Ans. a. Linoleic acid

6. Fortification of Vanaspati ghee is done with:

a. Iron b. Iodine
c. Vitamin A d. Calcium

Ans. c. Vitamin A

7. More than 50% PUFA is seen in multiple correct options:

i. Soyabean oil ii. Safflower oil
iii. Corn oil iv. Mustard oil

a. If i, ii, iii are correct
b. If i and iii are correct
c. If ii and iv are correct
d. If all four (i, ii, iii and iv) are correct

Ans. a. If i, ii, iii are correct

8. Which of the following is a cardio protective fatty acid?

a. Palmitic acid b. Stearic acid
c. Oleic acid d. Omega-3-fatty acid

Ans. d. Omega-3-fatty acid

9. Fatty acid metabolism gives:

a. Acetyl CoA b. Malonyl CoA
c. Ketone bodies d. Cholesterol

Ans. a. Acetyl CoA

10. Which cholesterol is designated as "Good Cholesterol"?

a. VLDL b. LDL
c. HDL d. IDL

Ans. c. HDL

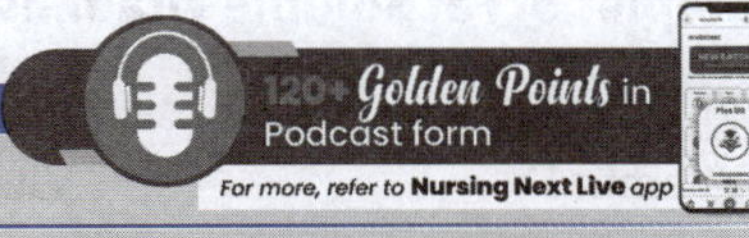

Golden Points

- Chylomicrons are lipoproteins; serve to transport dietary lipids from the intestines to other locations in the body.
- Essential fatty acids that are required by the human body but cannot be made in sufficient quantity from other substrates and must be obtained from food are called essential fatty acids, e.g., linolenic acid, linoleic acid.
- Fat is a group of components that are generally soluble in organic solvents and largely insoluble in water.
- Fats are made up of glycerol and fatty acids. Each glycerol is attached to three fatty acids.
- Fatty acids are obtained from the hydrolysis of oils and fats. They have methyl group ($-CH_3$) at the one end and a carboxyl group ($-COOH$) at the other end with the chain of carbon and hydrogen atom in the middle.
- Nonessential fatty acids are those fatty acids that can be synthesized by the body and need not be supplied through the diet, e.g., palmitic acid, oleic acid, etc.
- Phospholipids are lipids containing one or more phosphate group.

CHAPTER

5

Vitamins

CONCEPTUAL THEORY

Terminology

Lathyrism: Paralyzing disease of human and animals by consuming "KHESARI DAL" *(Lathyrus sativus)*

Ophthalmoplegia: Refers to weakness, paralysis of one or more extraocular muscles which is responsible for eye movements.

Stomatitis: Inflammation of mouth and lips.

Syndrome: It is a set of signs and symptoms which are correlated with each other.

Vitamin: Vitamin is the term used for a group of potent organic compounds other than proteins, carbohydrates and fats which occur in minute quantities in food and which are essential for some specific body functions, such as regulation, maintenance, growth and protection. There are two types of vitamins—water soluble and fat soluble.

CLASSIFICATION—FAT SOLUBLE AND WATER SOLUBLE VITAMINS

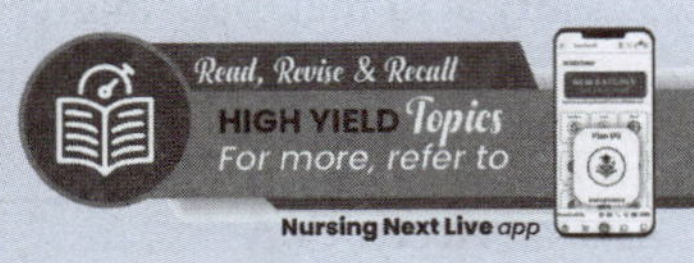

Fat Soluble Vitamins

- These are absorbed in the lumen, in the presence of fat and are emsulfied with bile.
- Precursors of fat soluble vitamins are known as provitamins.
- Stored in liver.

Examples of Fat Soluble Vitamins

- Vitamin A
- Vitamin D
- Vitamin E
- Vitamin K

Water Soluble Vitamins

- These vitamins are soluble in water and thus excreted in urine.
- Most function as coenzyme for various important biochemical reactions.
- Hypervitaminosis is rare.
- These include:
  - Vitamin B_1 (Thiamine)
  - Vitamin B_2 (Riboflavin)
  - Niacin
  - Vitamin B_6 (Pyridoxine)
  - Vitamin B_{12}
  - Folic acid
  - Vitamin C

CONCEPTUAL EXERCISES

LONG ANSWER QUESTIONS

1. Describe the sources, RDA, biochemistry, functions and deficiency manifestations of vitamin D. (DU)

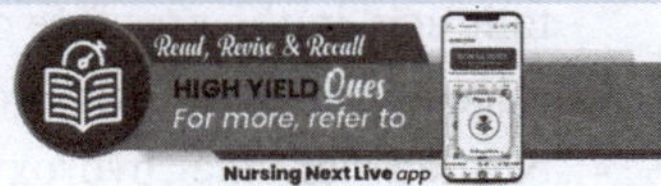

Answer

Introduction

- Vitamin D – fat soluble vitamin
- Functions like hormone
- Derived from ergocalciferol and cholecalciferol
- Biosynthesized from cholesterol on exposure to sunlight – sunshine vitamin
- Antirachitic vitamin

Food Sources

- Salmon
- Egg yolk
- Fortified milk
- Fortified cereal
- Cod liver oil

Recommended Daily Allowance

- Adults – 2.5 mcg
- Pregnant and lactating women – 10 mcg

Role of Vitamin D in Mineral Metabolism

- Calcitriol (1, 25-DHCC) — biologically active form.
  - Regulates the plasma calcium and phosphate levels.
  - Acts at intestine, kidney and bone in response to low plasma Ca levels
- **Action of calcitriol on the intestine:**
  - Increases the intestinal absorption calcium and phosphate.

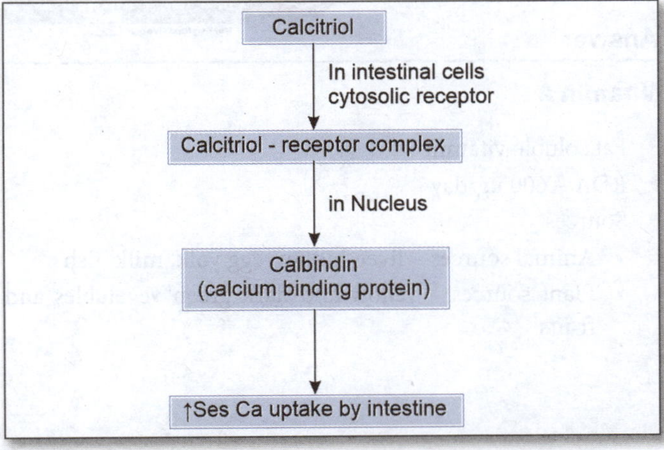

- **Action of calcitriol on the bone:**
  - Essential for bone formation
  - Calcium uptake for deposition as calcium phosphate is stimulated.
  - Increased mobilization of calcium.
- **Action of calcitriol on the kidney:**
  - Reduces excretion of calcium and phosphate by kidney
  - Increases reabsorption
- Dihydroxycholecalciferol (24, 25-DHCC)—another metabolite of vitamin D.
  - Synthesized in the kidney by 24-hydroxylase.
- When calcitriol concentration increases, 24-hydroxylase leads to synthesis 24, 25-DHCC, maintaining calcium homeostasis.

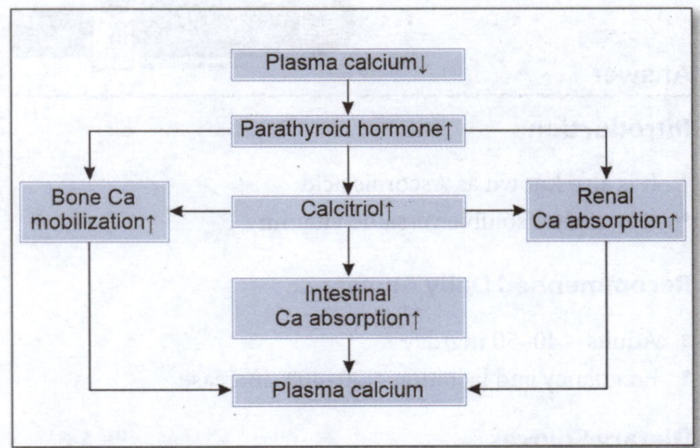

Deficiency Symptoms

- Rare since biosynthesis is possible.
- Seen in
  - Due to insufficient exposure to sunlight
  - Strict vegetarians
  - Chronic alcoholics
  - Individual with liver and kidney diseases
  - Fat malabsorption syndromes
  - People following purdah

Symptoms

Rickets in the Children

- Bone deformities
- Due to incomplete mineralization
- Delayed tooth eruption
- Bow legs
- Elevated alkaline phosphatase activity

Osteomalacia in Adults

- Demineralization of bones
- Increased susceptibility to fracture

Diagnosis of Vitamin D Deficiency

Plasma levels <30–40 ng/mL of 25-hydroxycholecalciferol

Renal Rickets (Renal Osteodystrophy)

- Chronic renal failure patients.
- Due to decreased synthesis of calcitriol in kidney.
- Treatment – intake of calcitriol

2. Describe the sources, biochemical functions, and requirement and deficiency manifestations of vitamin C. (DU)

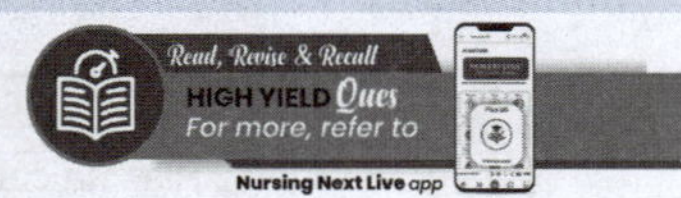

Answer

Introduction

- It is also known as Ascorbic acid
- It is a water soluble versatile vitamin

Recommended Daily Allowance

- Adults – 40–50 mg/day
- Pregnancy and lactation – 20–40% increase

Dietary Sources

- Citrus fruits
- Gooseberry (Amla)
- Guava, green vegetables, tomatoes
- Adrenal glands, gonads
- Milk – poor source

Biochemical Functions

Mainly due to its property to undergo reversible oxidation – reduction, i.e., interconversion of ascorbic acid and dehydroascorbic acid

- **Collagen formation**
  - Acts as a coenzyme in the hydroxylation of proline and lysine – post- translational modifications
- Required for bone formation
- Enhances iron absorption – reduces iron to ferrous state
  - Helps in storage of iron in ferritin state
- Essential for synthesis of serotonin
- **Tyrosine metabolism**
  - Required for the oxidation of p-hydroxyphenylpyruvate to homogentistic acid
  - Essential for dopamine beta-hydroxylase for the synthesis of epinephrine and norepinephrine.
- **Folic acid metabolism**
  - Required for the formation of tetrahydrofolate from folic acid in the presence of folic acid reductase
- **Corticosteroid synthesis**
  - Needed for the hydroxylation reaction during the corticosteroid synthesis.
- Strong antioxidant – prevents other vitamins from oxidation
- Essential for the synthesis of immunoglobulins

Deficiency Symptoms

- **Scurvy**
  - Characteristics
    - Sore gums
    - Loose teeth
    - Anemia
    - Swollen joints
    - Fragile blood vessels
    - Decreased immunocompetence
    - Delayed wound healing
    - Osteoporosis
  - Occurs due to:
    - Defective collagen synthesis
    - Impairment in the antioxidant property of vitamin C
- Infantile scurvy – Barlow's disease
  - Occurs in infants aged 6–12 months

3. Describe the sources, biochemistry, functions, requirement and deficiency manifestations of vitamin A. (DU, KUHS, MGR)

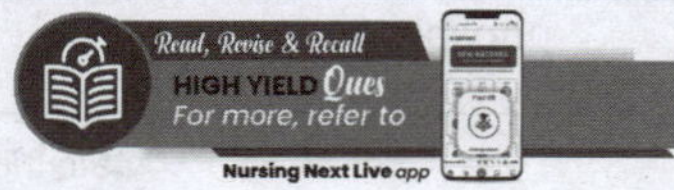

Answer

Vitamin A

- Fat soluble vitamin
- RDA – 600 ug/day
- Sources
  - Animal sources – liver, kidney, egg yolk, milk, fish
  - Plant sources – yellow and dark green vegetables and fruits

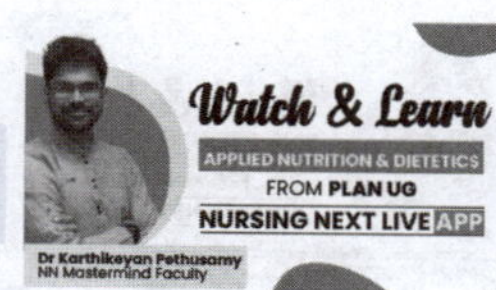

Fat soluble vitamins	Water soluble vitamins
• Precursors - provitamins • Stored in liver. • These include: ▪ Vitamin A ▪ Vitamin D ▪ Vitamin E ▪ Vitamin K	• These vitamins are soluble in water and thus excreted in urine. • Most function as coenzyme for various important biochemical reactions. • Hypervitaminosis is rare. • These include: ▪ Vitamin B_1 (Thiamine) ▪ Vitamin B_2 (Riboflavin) ▪ Niacin ▪ Vitamin B_6 (Pyridoxine) ▪ Vitamin B_{12} ▪ Folic acid ▪ Vitamin C

Chemistry

- Exists as retinol, retinal, retinoic acid and beta carotene (provitamin)
  - Retinol – vitamin A alcohol
    - Primary alcohol containing beta-ionone ring
  - Retinal – vitamin A aldehyde
    - Obtained by oxidation of retinol
  - Retinoic acid – vitamin A acid
    - Obtained by oxidation of retinal
  - Beta carotene – provitamin A
    - Found in plants

Biochemical Functions

- Retinoic acid – functions as steroid hormones
  - Regulates gene expression
- Plays important role in:
  - Vision
    - Helps to maintain the cornea
    - Conversion of light energy into nerve impulses at the retina
    - Rhodopsin is a light-sensitive pigment of the retina that contains a protein called opsin.
  - Cell growth and differentiation
    - Important for cellular differentiation, embryo development and gene expression
    - Important for development and function of epithelial cells
  - Maintenance of epithelial tissue
  - Preventing keratin synthesis
  - Synthesis of glycoproteins and mucopolysaccharides
  - Reproduction
    - Important for
      - Sperm development
      - Fetal development
      - Growth in children
      - Bone remodeling
  - Maintenance of proper immune system
    - Cholesterol synthesis
    - Carotenoids – antioxidant role

Causes of Vitamin A Deficiency

- Inadequate intake
- Impaired absorption
- Impaired storage
- Impaired transport
- Excessive excretion
- Chronic alcoholism

Deficiency Manifestations

- Ocular changes in vitamin A deficiency
  - Night blindness (Nyctalopia)
    - Dark adaptation time is increased
    - Difficulty to see in dim light
    - Irreversible damage occurs to visual cells in case of prolonged deficiency
  - Xerophthalmia
    - Characterized by:
      - Dryness in conjunctiva and cornea
      - Keratinization of epithelial cells
      - Bitot's spots – white triangular plaques in conjunctiva
      - Keratomalacia – corneal destruction
    - Prolonged xerophthalmia leads to:
      - Corneal ulceration
      - Corneal degeneration
      - Can cause total blindness
- Growth retardation – impaired skeletal formation
- Effect on reproduction – degeneration of germinal epithelium – sterility in males
- Keratinization of epithelial cells
- Formation of urinary stones

4. Briefly explain about water soluble vitamins. (MGR, KUHS)

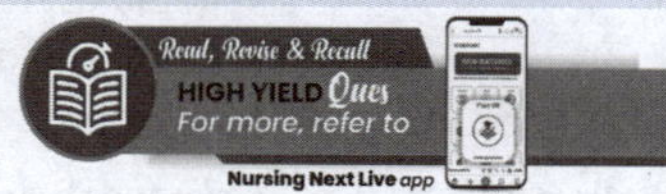

Answer

Water Soluble Vitamins

- These vitamins are soluble in water and thus excreted in urine.
- Most vitamins function as coenzyme for various important biochemical reactions.
- Hypervitaminosis is rare.
- These include:
  - Vitamin B1 (Thiamine)
  - Vitamin B2 (Riboflavin)

- Niacin
- Vitamin B_6 (Pyridoxine)
- Vitamin B_{12}
- Folic acid
- Vitamin C

Table 5.1: Water soluble vitamins

Water soluble vitamin	Dietary source	RDA	Functions	Deficiency symptoms
Vitamin B_1 (thiamine)	• Pork • Liver • Kidney • Yeast • Whole cereals • Milk	1.2–1.8 mg	Acts as pyrophosphate, is coenzyme in decarboxylation reaction	• Korsakoff syndrome • Wernicke syndrome • Dry and wet beri beri
Vitamin B_2 (riboflavin)	All food	11.2 mg	• Cofactors for many enzymes in intermediary metabolism • Converted to coenzymes flavin mononucleotide and flavin adenine dinucleotide	• Seborrheic dermatitis • Dermatitis • Stomatitis • Cheilosis • Moeller's glossitis • Ariboflavinosis • Corneal vascularization
Niacin	• Liver • Yeast • Whole grains • Cereals • Beans • Peanuts	12–20 mg	• Involved in a variety of redox reactions • Incorporated into nicotinamide adenine dinucleotide and NAD phosphate	• Diarrhea • Dementia • Dermatitis • Pellagra
Vitamin B_6 (pyridoxine)	• Fish • Beef • Liver • Starchy vegetables • Fruits	2 mg	• Coenzymes in many intermediary reactions	• Dermatitis • Glossitis • Cheilosis • Peripheral neuropathy
Vitamin B_{12}	Foods of animal origin, synthesized by intestinal bacteria	1–3 mg	• Maintenance of myelination of spinal cord tracts • Required for normal folate metabolism and DNA synthesis	• Combined system disease (megaloblastic pernicious anemia and degeneration of posterolateral spinal cord tracts)
Vitamin C	• Citrus fruits • Gooseberry (Amla) • Guava, green vegetables, tomatoes • Adrenal glands, gonads • Milk – poor source	• Adults – 40–50 mg/day • Pregnancy and lactation – 20–40% increase	• Hydroxylation of collagen • Serves in many oxidation reduction reactions • Enhances iron absorption – reduces iron to ferrous state	Scurvy
Folic acid	• Green leafy vegetables • Whole grains, • Cereal • Liver, kidney, yeast and egg.	• 10–20 microgram • Pregnant women – 400 microgram • Lactating mothers – 300 microgram	• Prevents neural cord defects in fetus • Required for DNA synthesis, cell growth, RBC formation • Synthesis of thiamine	• Megaloblastic anemia • Folate deficiency during pregnancy leads to neural tube defects and spina bifida.
Biotin (Vitamin B_7)	• Liver • Kidney • Egg yolk • Milk • Tomatoes • Grains	20–30 ug	• Involved in carbohydrate and lipid metabolism • Binds to histones – plays a role in DNA replication and transcription	• Dermatitis • Lack of appetite • Nausea • Mental depression • Anemia

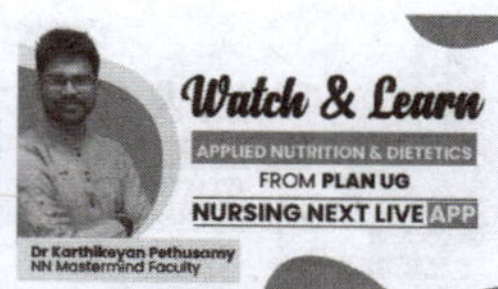

5. Classify the vitamins. Explain about the functions, sources and deficiencies of fat soluble vitamins. (MGR, RUHS)

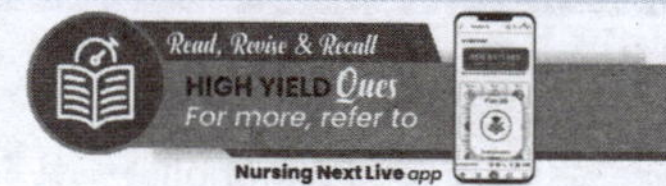

Answer

Vitamins

- Vitamins are classified as a micro-nutrient.
- They are required for the proper growth and functioning of the body.
- Based on the solubility of the vitamins, these are classified as:

	Fat soluble vitamins	Water soluble vitamins
	• These are absorbed in the lumen, in the presence of fat and are emulsified with bile. • Precursors of fat soluble vitamins are known as provitamins • Stored in liver.	• These vitamins are soluble in water and thus excreted in urine. • Most function as coenzyme for various important biochemical reactions. • Hypervitaminosis is rare.
Includes	• Vitamin A • Vitamin D • Vitamin E • Vitamin K	• Vitamin B_1 (Thiamine) • Vitamin B_2 (Riboflavin) • Niacin • Vitamin B_6 (Pyridoxine) • Vitamin B_{12} • Folic acid • Vitamin C

Fat Soluble Vitamins

Vitamins	Sources	RDA	Functions	Deficiency symptoms
Vitamin A	• Animal sources – liver, kidney, egg yolk, milk, fish • Plant sources – yellow and dark green vegetables and fruits	600 µg/day	Retinoic acid – functions as steroid hormones • Regulates gene expression • Plays important role in vision, helps to maintain the cornea • Important for cellular differentiation, embryo development and gene expression • Maintenance of epithelial tissue • Preventing keratin synthesis • Synthesis of glycoproteins and mucopolysaccharides Reproduction • Maintenance of proper immune system • Cholesterol synthesis • Carotenoids – antioxidant role	• Ocular changes in vitamin A deficiency ▪ Night blindness (Nyctalopia) ▪ Xerophthalmia • Growth retardation – impaired skeletal formation • Effect on reproduction – degeneration of germinal epithelium – sterility in males • Keratinization of epithelial cells • Formation of urinary stones
Vitamin D	• Salmon • Egg yolk • Fortified milk • Fortified cereal • Cod liver oil	• Adults – 2.5 mcg • Pregnant and lactating women – 10 mcg	Calcitriol (1,25-DHCC)—biologically active form. • Regulates the plasma calcium and phosphate levels. • Acts at intestine, kidney and bone in response to low plasma Ca levels *Action of calcitriol on the intestine*: • Increases the intestinal absorption calcium and phosphate. *Action of calcitriol on the bone*: • Essential for bone formation • Calcium uptake for deposition as calcium phosphate is stimulated. • Increased mobilization of calcium. *Action of calcitriol on the kidney:* • Reduces excretion of calcium and phosphate by kidney • Increases reabsorption Dihydroxycholecalciferol (24, 25-DHCC)—another metabolite of vitamin D. • Synthesized in the kidney by 24-hydroxylase.	Rickets in the children • Bone deformities • Due to incomplete mineralization • Delayed tooth eruption • Bow legs • Elevated alkaline phosphatase activity Osteomalacia in adults. • Demineralization of bones • Increased susceptibility to fracture

Contd...

Vitamins	Sources	RDA	Functions	Deficiency symptoms
Vitamin E	• Wheat germ oil • Cotton seed oil • Peanut oil • Meat • Milk • Eggs	• Man – 10 mg • Woman – 8 mg	• Antioxidant property – acts synergistically with selenium • Essential for the structure and integrity of cell membrane • Prevents peroxidation of PUFA. • Protects RBCs from hemolysis • Involved in the maintenance of germinal epithelium in the gonads – anti sterility vitamin	• Sterility • Degenerative changes in muscle • Megaloblastic anemia • Increased fragility of RBCs
Vitamin K	Synthesized by gut bacteria	70–100 µg/day	• ***Formation of γ-carboxyglutamate (Gla):*** Vitamin K is required in the hepatic synthesis of prothrombin and blood clotting factors II, VII, IX, and X.	• Lack of active prothrombin • Defective blood coagulation • Blood clotting time is increased

SHORT NOTES

1. Write a note on vitamin deficiencies. (MGR)

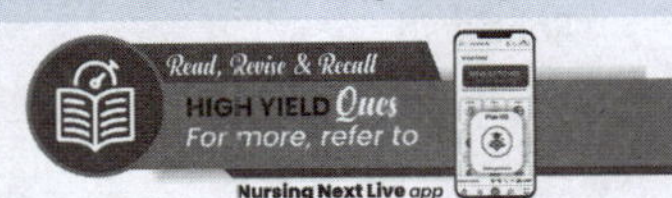

Answer

Vitamins	Deficiency symptoms
Vitamin A	• Ocular changes in vitamin A deficiency ▪ Night blindness (Nyctalopia) ▪ Xerophthalmia • Growth retardation – impaired skeletal formation • Effect on reproduction – degeneration of germinal epithelium – sterility in males • Keratinization of epithelial cells • Formation of urinary stones
Vitamin D	• Rickets in the children ▪ Bone deformities ▪ Due to incomplete mineralization ▪ Delayed tooth eruption ▪ Bow legs ▪ Elevated alkaline phosphatase activity • Osteomalacia in adults. ▪ Demineralization of bones ▪ Increased susceptibility to fracture
Vitamin E	• Sterility • Degenerative changes in muscle • Megaloblastic anemia • Increased fragility of RBCs
Vitamin K	• Lack of active prothrombin • Defective blood coagulation • Blood clotting time is increased
Vitamin B_1 (thiamine)	• Korsakoff syndrome • Wernicke syndrome • Dry and wet beri beri
Vitamin B_2 (riboflavin)	• Seborrheic dermatitis • Dermatitis • Stomatitis • Cheilosis • Moeller's glossitis • Ariboflavinosis • Corneal vascularization
Niacin	• Diarrhea • Dementia • Dermatitis • Pellagra
Vitamin B_6 (pyridoxine)	• Dermatitis • Glossitis • Cheilosis • Peripheral neuropathy
Vitamin B_{12}	• Combined system disease (megaloblastic pernicious anemia and degeneration of posterolateral spinal cord tracts)
Vitamin C	• Scurvy
Folic acid	• Megaloblastic anemia • Folate deficiency during pregnancy leads to neural tube defects and spina bifida.
Biotin (Vitamin B_7)	• Dermatitis • Lack of appetite • Nausea • Mental depression • Anemia

Contd...

2. Write a short note on Vitamin C. (MGR)

Answer

For answer, refer to Long Question no. 2, pg. no. 452

3. Write a note on hypervitaminosis. (MGR)

Answer

Hypervitaminosis

The result of toxic levels of all vitamins on the system. Mostly the water soluble vitamins are excreted through urine, so chances of toxicity of these vitamins is rare. Mostly the toxicity of fat soluble vitamins such as vitamin A, D, E and K are seen.

Hypervitaminosis A

- Occurs due to overdose of vitamin A such as ingestion of polar bear liver
- Types of hypervitaminosis A

	Acute hypervitaminosis A	Chronic hypervitaminosis A
	Occurs due to excessive dietary intake of vitamin A	Occurs due to excessive intake of 50,000 IU/day for at least 3 months
Signs and symptoms	• Headache • Abdominal pain and discomfort • Nausea and vomiting • Visual changes • Increased intracranial pressure leading to bulging fontanelles in kids, papilledema, diplopia • Anemia • Thrombocytopenia	• Teratogenic – birth defects • Skin irritation • Pain in bones and increased tendency to fracture • Pseudotumor cerebri • Liver cirrhosis • Bone mineral loss • Raised intracranial pressure

Hypervitaminosis D

- Rare
- Occurs in patients who intake excessive amounts of Vitamin D supplements
- Leads to hypercalcemia
- Increased calcitriol production
- **Signs/symptoms**
  - Nausea
  - Weight loss
  - Hypertension
  - Reduced appetite
  - Polyuria, polydipsia
  - Tetany, seizures
  - Headache
  - Weakness
  - Blurred vision

Hypervitaminosis E

- Signs and symptoms
  - Nausea and vomiting
  - Fatigue

Hypervitaminosis K

- Causes excess clotting of blood
- Leads to thrombosis
- Death may occur due to blood or heart clots

Hypervitaminosis B$_1$

- Rare
- Signs/Symptoms
  - Blocks nerve transmission
  - Restlessness
  - Convulsion
  - Respiratory paralysis
  - Cardiac failure
  - Death

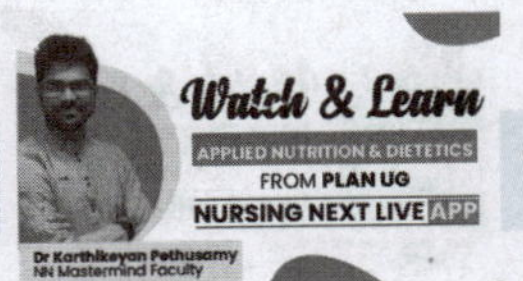

Hypervitaminosis B_2

- Signs/symptoms
  - Bright yellow urine
  - Itching
  - Burning or pricking sensations
  - Numbness
  - Photosensitivity

4. Write about vitamin B_2. (MGR)

Answer

Vitamin B_2

- Also known as riboflavin
- Present in high quantities in milk
- Coenzyme associated with riboflavin are flavin nucleotides – flavin mononucleotide (FMN) flavin adenine dinucleotide (FAD)

Recommended Daily Allowances

- For adult men – 1.1–1.3 mg/day
- For adult women – 0.9–1.1 mg/day
- Pregnant – 1.4 mg/day
- Lactation – 1.6 mg/day

Dietary Sources

- Beef
- Chicken
- Salmon
- Cheese
- Avocado
- Peanuts
- Almonds
- Mushrooms
- Eggs
- Beans

Functions

- Riboflavin (Vitamin B_2) gives rise to flavin coenzymes
- Flavin mononucleotide (FMN) and Flavin adenine dinucleotide (FAD)
- Acts as prosthetic groups for enzymes
- Critically important electron carriers.
- FMN (Flavin mononucleotide)
  - Contains a molecule of riboflavin and phosphoric acid
- FAD (flavin adenine dinucleotide)
  - Dinucleotide of FMN and AMP
- The coenzyme forms an integral part of the flavoprotein containing enzymes and participates in several oxidative reduction reaction.

Deficiency – Ariboflavinosis

- Usually rare, but can be seen with:
  - Alcoholics
  - Vegetarian athletes
  - Certain conditions such as hypothyroidism, adrenal insufficiency, etc.
- Signs and symptoms include:
  - Angular stomatitis
  - Sore throat
  - Painful red tongue – Glossitis
  - Cheilosis
  - Seborrheic dermatitis
  - Anemia
  - Hair loss
  - Peripheral nerve dysfunction
  - Increased risk for preeclampsia
  - Increased risk of fetal birth defects

Hypervitaminosis B_2

- Signs/symptoms
  - Bright yellow urine
  - Itching
  - Burning or pricking sensations
  - Numbness
  - Photosensitivity

5. Write in short the role of vitamin A in vision. (MGR)

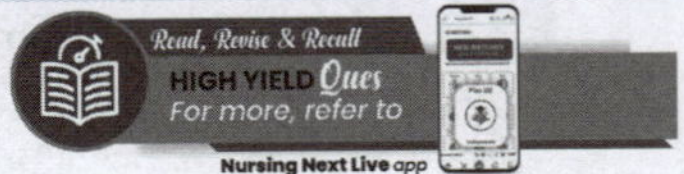

Answer

Role of Vitamin A

Vitamin A plays a vital role in vision. It is essential for the

- **Retinal formation:** Vitamin A is a precursor for the formation of a pigment called retinal, which is a component of the light-sensitive cells in the retina called rods and cones.
- **Rhodopsin production:** Rhodopsin, the visual pigment found in the rods of the retina, consists of a protein called opsin and a molecule of retinal.
- **Phototransduction:** This process converts light energy into electrical signals that can be transmitted to the brain for visual processing. Vitamin A is vital for this phototransduction process to occur effectively.
- **Maintenance of the cornea:** Vitamin A is also involved in maintaining the health and integrity of the cornea. It helps in the production of the mucous-like substance that covers the cornea, called the tear film.
- **Antioxidant properties:** Vitamin A acts as an antioxidant, helping to protect the cells of the retina and other ocular tissues from oxidative stress and damage caused by free radicals.

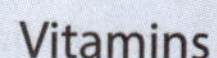

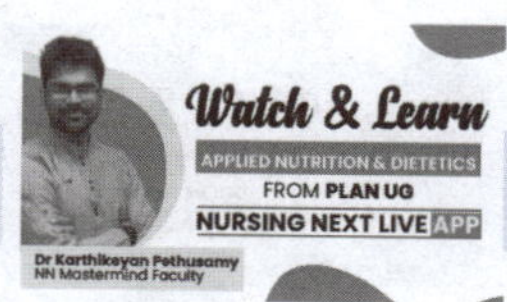

Ocular Changes in Vitamin A Deficiency

Night blindness (Nyctalopia)	• First symptom of vitamin A deficiency • Dark adaptation time is increased • Difficulty to see in dim light • Irreversible damage occurs to visual cells in case of prolonged deficiency • Since retinal is essential for the synthesis of rhodopsin (by rods) and vitamin A deficiency interferes with the production of rhodopsin, thus vitamin A impairs the rod functions and results in night blindness. • Night blindness responds to vitamin A therapy.
Xerophthalmia	• Dryness in conjunctiva and cornea • Keratinization of epithelial cells • Bitot's spots – white triangular plaques in conjunctiva • Keratomalacia – corneal destruction • Prolonged xerophthalmia leads to ▪ Corneal ulceration ▪ Corneal degeneration ▪ Can cause total blindness
Bitot's spots	• Accumulation of foamy-cheesy material on the conjunctiva, often in association with other signs of xerophthalmia, such as conjunctival xerosis. • Spots may differ in size, location or shape.
Corneal xerosis and ulceration	• Cornea becomes dry • If left untreated, it can progress to corneal ulceration.
Keratomalacia	• Melting or wasting of cornea • Indicates destruction of a part or complete corneal stroma, which in turn results in permanent structural alterations.
Corneal scar	• Leads to perforation of cornea • At this stage a corneal scar is formed which remains forever.

6. What are the coenzymes of pyridoxine? Mention a reaction where it is used. (MGR)

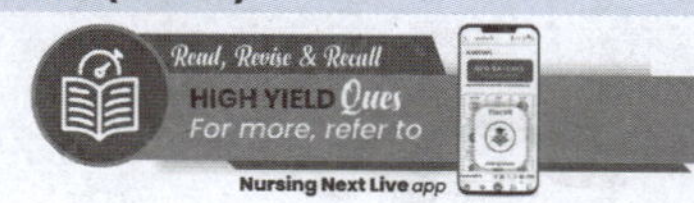

Answre

Pyridoxal Coenzymes

- Active form of vitamin B6 – coenzyme pyridoxal phosphate (PLP)
- Pyridoxal (the aldehyde form) converts to its phosphate – pyridoxal phosphate (PLP) by the loss of ATP
- The so formed PLP acts as a coenzyme for many reactions such as:
  - **Transamination**
    - *AST and ALT – transaminases require PLP as coenzyme for its actions*
  - **Decarboxylation**

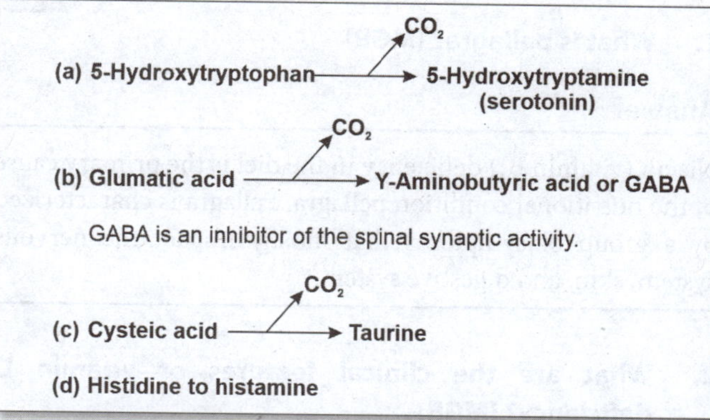

  - **Oxidative deamination**
    - Coenzyme for diamine oxidase which catalyzes the oxidative deamination of diamines like cadaverine and putrescine
    - These enzymes are involved in catabolism of histamine

7. Add a note on antioxidant vitamins. (MGR)

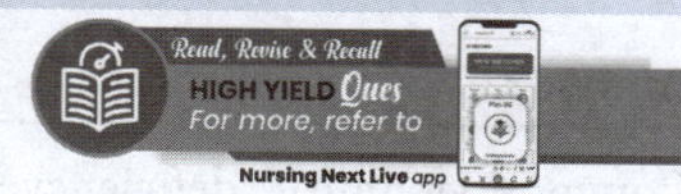

Answer

Antioxidant

- Any substance that delays or inhibits oxidation of another substance.
- Oxidation leads to the formation of free radicals that are harmful to the biological tissues.
- So to prevent the free radical damage, antioxidants are required.
- These are scavengers of free radicals

Antioxidant Vitamins

Vitamin E	Tocopherol – alpha – tocopherol Protection against lipid peroxidation Directly acts on oxyradicals and serves as important chain breaking antioxidant
Vitamin C	Efficiently scavenges free radicals Inhibits lipid peroxidation
Carotenoids	*Beta – carotene – most important* Acts as antioxidant under low partial pressure Acts in association with vitamin C and vitamin E
Alpha- lipoic acid	Vitamin like compound Plays a role in recycling other antioxidants such as ascorbic acid, alpha – tocopherol and glutathione

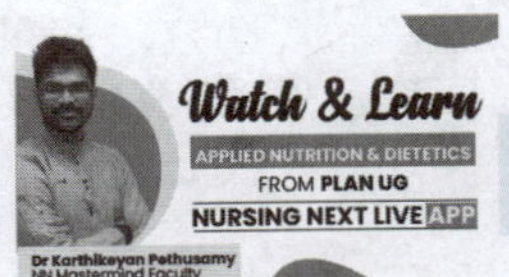

SHORT ANSWER QUESTIONS

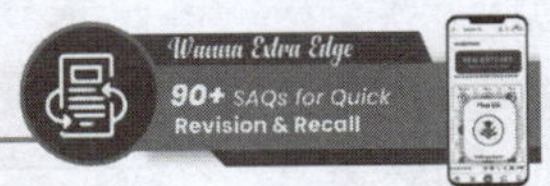

1. **What is pellagra? (MGR)**

Answer

Niacin (vitamin B_3) deficiency in the diet is the primary cause of the nutritional condition pellagra. Pellagra is characterized by a group of symptoms that mostly impact the nervous system, skin, and digestive system.

2. **What are the clinical features of vitamin D deficiency? (MGR)**

Answer

The few clinical signs of vitamin D insufficiency include rickets, delayed growth, and decreased bone formation, weakening bones, increased risk of fractures, fatigue, and weakness.

3. **What are the deficiency manifestations of vitamin K? (MGR)**

Answer

Common vitamin K deficiency symptoms include decreased blood clotting, which increased bleeding and hemorrhage. The likelihood of bleeding diseases like hemophilia is increased, weaker bones and sluggish wound healing.

4. **Functions of vitamin 'C'. (MGR)**

Answer

Antioxidant property of vitamin C commonly known as ascorbic acid and increased absorption of nonheme iron are most important functions of vitamin C

5. **List four sources of vitamin E. (MGR)**

Answer

Wheat germ oil, safflower oil, cottonseed oil, sunflower oil, nuts, seeds, green leafy vegetables and avocado are good sources of vitamin E.

6. **List down the sources of ascorbic acid. (MGR)**

Answer

Amla, tomatoes, spinach, citrus fruits, guava, potatoes and other green leafy vegetables are good sources of ascorbic acid.

7. **List two deficiency diseases of vitamin A. (MGR)**

Answer

Night blindness and Xerophthalmia are the two most common deficiency diseases of vitamin-A.

8. **Write the revised RDA of vitamin A for a lactating mother. (DU)**

Answer

The RDA for vitamin A in breastfeeding females is 950 μg/day.

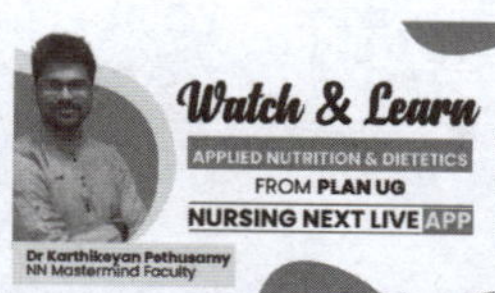

CONCEPTUAL REVISION

MULTIPLE CHOICE QUESTIONS

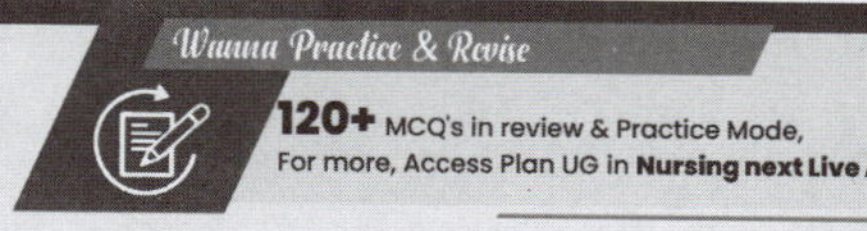

1. Green leafy vegetables are rich source of:

a. Vitamin A b. Vitamin B
c. Vitamin C d. Vitamin D

Ans. a. Vitamin-A

2. Which one of the following vitamin helps in wound healing?

a. Vitamin A b. Vitamin B
c. Vitamin C d. Vitamin D

Ans. c. Vitamin C

3. Which of the following deficiency disease is caused by the deficiency of Thiamine (vit-B1):

a. Angular Stomatitis b. Pellagra
c. Glosittis d. Beri-Beri

Ans. d. Beri-Beri

4. Pernicious anemia occurs due to deficiency of:

a. Vitamin A b. Vitamin B_{12}
c. Vitamin D d. Vitamin K

Ans. b. Vitamin B_{12}

5. Anti Beri-Beri factor is called:

a. Vitamin B_2 b. Vitamin B_5
c. Vitamin B_1 d. Vitamin B_6

Ans. c. Vitamin-B1

6. Vitamin B_3 is called as:

a. Riboflavin b. Pantothenic acid
c. Pyridoxin d. Niacin

Ans. d. Niacin

7. Deficiency of vitamin D in children may cause:

a. Osteomalacia b. Rickets
c. Pellagra d. Beri-Beri

Ans. b. Rickets

8. One of the fat soluble vitamin involved in coagulation is:

a. Vitamin K b. Vitamin E
c. Vitamin D d. Vitamin A

Ans. a. Vitamin K

120+ Golden Points in Podcast form
For more, refer to Nursing Next Live app

Golden Points

- A deficiency of niacin is known as pellagra which means rough skin (from the Italian word "pelle" for skin and "agra" for rough).
- A dietary deficiency of riboflavin leads to ariboflavinosis, a deficiency syndrome marked by stomatitis (inflammation of mouth and lips) including painful red tongue with sore throat and chapped lips.
- Deficiency of thiamine can cause beriberi and Wernicke's Korsakoff syndrome (comprising Wernicke's encephalopathy and Korsakoff psychosis).
- Eating excess amounts of egg whites may also cause biotin deficiency because egg whites contain avidin, a substance that binds biotin.
- Folic acid is found mostly in dark green vegetables like broccoli, spinach, legumes such as beans, peas and enriched grains.
- Megaloblastic anemia is characterized by large, abnormally nucleated erythrocytes.
- Prolonged deficiency of vitamin C results in scurvy.
- Scurvy in adults: The disease is characterized by general weakness, spongy bleeding gums, loose teeth with swollen tender joints and hemorrhages under the skin.
- The deficiency of vitamin D in children can lead to rickets and osteomalacia.
- The four fat-soluble vitamins are vitamin A, vitamin D, vitamin E and vitamin K.
- Vitamin A plays an important role to protect the digestive tract by boosting immune system.
- Vitamin B_{12} is also known as cobalamin.
- Vitamin D is an important regulator of calcium metabolism.
- Vitamin D is derived from both sunlight and food.
- Vitamin D is synthesized in the body by the action of ultraviolet rays of sunlight on 7 dehydrocholesterol stored in the skin.
- Vitamin E acts as antioxidant. It itself gets oxidized and protects cell membranes from oxidative damage.
- Vitamins are natural substances found in plants and animals and are known as essential nutrients for human beings.
- Water-soluble vitamins are absorbed in our intestine, pass directly to the blood and are carried to the tissue in which they will be utilized.

CHAPTER 6

Minerals

CONCEPTUAL THEORY

Terminology

150+ key terminologies for Quick Recall & Revision

Flavonoids: Pigments widely distributed in nature in flowers, fruits and vegetables.

Minerals: Inorganic compounds that occur naturally in the earth's crust, have diverse functions within the body and are required in the diet in very small amounts.

Myoglobin: An iron-containing protein that carries oxygen and carbon dioxide in muscle tissue.

Osteoporosis: A condition which bones become porous and fragile due to loss of minerals.

pH: A term used to express a substances acidity or alkalinity as measured on a scale from 0 (extreme acid) to 14 (extreme base).

Phytochemicals: General name of chemicals present in plants.

Ration: The ration or food basket usually consists of variety of basic food items like cereals, oils and pulses. Additional food known as complementary foods consist of meat, fish, vegetables and fruits, condiments that enhance nutritional adequacy and palatability.

Trace minerals: Needed in smaller amounts, occur in the body in minute quantities, <100 mg/day.

CLASSIFICATION—MAJOR MINERALS (CALCIUM, PHOSPHORUS, SODIUM, POTASSIUM AND MAGNESIUM) AND TRACE ELEMENTS

Minerals

Minerals – inorganic elements essential for the normal functioning of the body

Classification of Minerals

Macrominerals

- Also known as principal elements
- Constitute 60–80% of the body's inorganic elements
- **Includes**
  - Calcium
  - Phosphorus
  - Magnesium
  - Sodium
  - Potassium
  - Chloride
  - Sulfur

Microminerals

- Require in <100 mg/day
- **Subdivided into three categories:**
  1. Essential trace elements
  2. Possibly essential trace elements
  3. Non-essential trace elements

FUNCTIONS

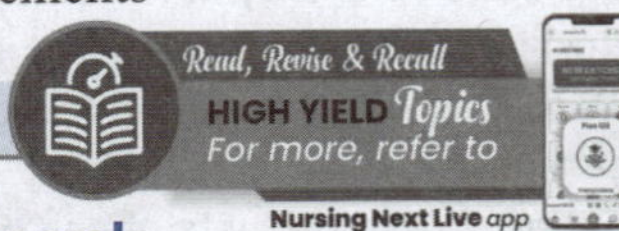

General Functions of Minerals

- Plays a role in the maintenance of osmotic pressure, and thus, regulate the exchange of water and solutes within the human body.
- Essential constituents of skeletal structures such as bones and teeth.
- Serve as structural constituents of soft tissues.
- Essential for the transmission of nerve impulses and muscles contraction.
- Plays a vital role in the acid-base equilibrium of the body, and thus, regulate the pH of the blood and other body fluids.
- Essential components of many enzymes, vitamins, hormones and respiratory pigments.

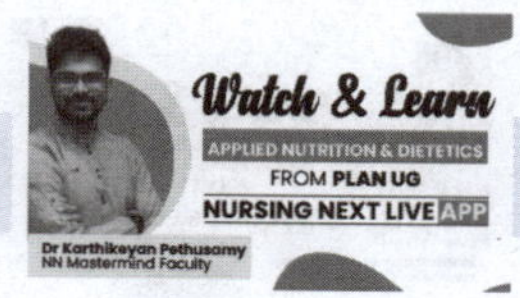

DIETARY SOURCES

Sources of Calcium

Milk and milk products, canned fish with bones, fortified tofu and fortified soy milk, green broccoli, mustard greens, legumes.

Sources of Iron

- Liver (richest), heart, kidney, leafy vegetables, pulses, cereals, fish, apples, dried fruits, molasses, jaggery
- Poor sources—milk, wheat, polished rice.

Sources of Potassium

Meats, milk, fresh fruits, vegetables, whole grains, legumes

Sources of Iodine

Seafood, drinking water, vegetables, fruits

Sources of Zinc

Meat, Fish, Eggs, Milk, Beans

CONCEPTUAL EXERCISES

LONG ANSWER QUESTIONS

1. Classify minerals. Discuss the functions, absorption and metabolism of calcium. (MGR, KUHS)

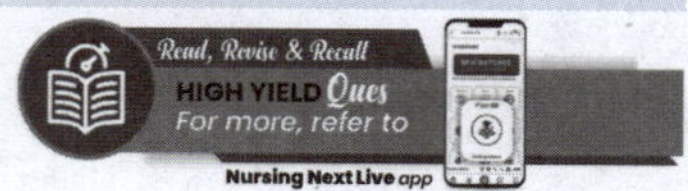

Answer

Minerals

Introduction

Minerals – inorganic elements essential for the normal functioning of the body.

Macrominerals	Microminerals
• Also known as principal elements • Constitute 60–80% of the body's inorganic elements • Includes ▪ Calcium ▪ Phosphorus ▪ Magnesium ▪ Sodium ▪ Potassium ▪ Chloride • Sulfur	• Require in less than 100 mg/day • Subdivided into three categories • Essential trace elements • Possibly essential trace elements • Non essential trace elements

Calcium

- Most abundant mineral in the body.
- Major constituent of the bones and teeth in the form of hydroxyapatite.
- Provides support to the skeletal structure and function.

Recommended daily allowance (rda)	• Adult – 800 mg • Pregnant and lactating women – 1.5 g • Children – 0.8–1.2 g
Dietary sources	Milk and milk products, canned fish with bones, fortified tofu and fortified soy milk, green broccoli, mustard greens, legumes.
Serum calcium levels	**9–11 mg/dL**

Contd...

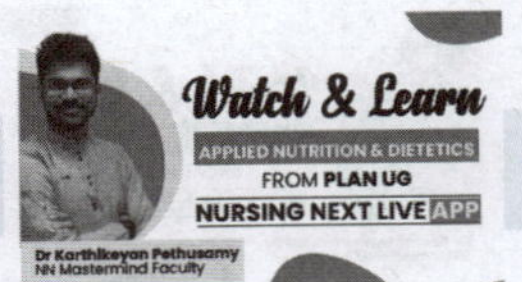

Biochemical functions	• **Development of bones and teeth:** Along with phosphate, it forms hydroxyapatite – basic structure of bones and teeth • **Muscle contraction:** ▪ Causes contraction of muscle by activating troponin C ▪ Activates ATPase – increases actin – myosin interaction • Role in **blood coagulation** – factor IV of clotting cascade is dependent on calcium • Necessary for **nerve impulse transmission** • Plays an important role in maintaining **membrane integrity and permeability** • **Enzyme activation:** ▪ Enzymes such as ATPase, lipase, etc., require calcium for activation ▪ Enzymes such as protein kinases, phospholipase C, glycogen synthase are activated by Ca – calmodulin complex. • Acts as a **second messenger** for hormones such as epinephrine in liver glycogenolysis, as a **third messenger** for hormones such as ADH. • Facilitates **release of certain hormones** such as insulin, PTH, calcitonin from the endocrine glands. • Regulates microfilament and microtubule mediated processes such as endocytosis, exocytosis and cell motility • Action on heart: Acts on myocardium and **prolongs systole**.
Absorption and metabolism of calcium	• Occurs mostly in duodenum • **Factors promoting absorption of calcium** ▪ Calcitriol ▪ Parathyroid hormone ▪ Acidity or low pH ▪ Lactose promotes calcium uptake by cells ▪ Lysine and arginine
	• **Factors inhibiting calcium absorption** ▪ Phytates and oxalates as they form insoluble salts ▪ High dietary content of phosphates ▪ Alkaline conditions ▪ High dietary fiber
Deficiency of calcium	Deficiency of calcium leads to hypocalcemia that can result in rickets in children and osteomalacia in adults • Rickets ▪ Results in delayed closure of fontanelles, ▪ Incomplete mineralization of bone leads to the formation of soft and pliable bones ▪ Delayed teeth formation ▪ Weight bearing bones are bent to form bow legs ▪ **Biochemical features** ◆ Increased activity of alkaline phosphatase ◆ Occurs due to increased cellular activity of bone. ▪ **Management** ◆ Vitamin D supplementation ◆ Calcium supplementation • **Adult rickets (Osteomalacia)** ▪ Results due to vitamin D deficiency in adults ▪ Defective mineralization of bones occurs ▪ Bones become softer and more prone to fracture

2. Write the following, sources and deficiency disorders of Iodine. (DU)

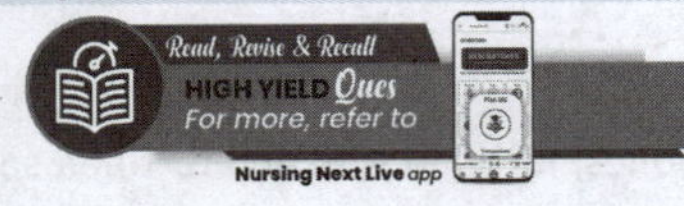

Answer

Introduction

- Total body content of iodine – 20 mg
- Tissue distribution of iodine
  - Thyroid gland – 80%
  - Muscle
  - Salivary glands
  - Ovaries

Recommended Daily Allowance

- Adults – 100–150 ug
- Pregnant women – 200 ug

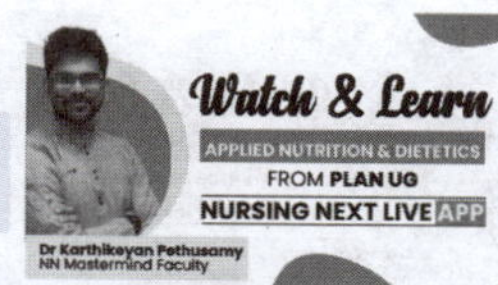

Sources

- Seafood
- Drinking water
- Vegetables
- Fruits

Biochemical Functions

- Required for the synthesis of thyroid hormones – thyroxine (T4) and triiodothyronine (T3)
- Thyroid hormones are involved in several biochemical functions
- T3 is more active than T4.

Deficiency of Iodine – Results in goiter

Definition	Enlarged thyroid gland
Types	• Simple goiter ▪ When thyroid gland does not make enough hormones • Endemic goiter ▪ Occurs due to iodine deficiency • Sporadic goiter ▪ Occurs due to certain drugs
Biochemical basis	• When TSH increases, thyroid gland uses iodine to make T3 and T4 • When iodine is deficient, thyroid hormones decrease • To compensate this, the thyroid gland activity increases to maximize the iodine uptake • This leads to hypertrophy of thyroid gland leading to goiter

Contd...

Definition	Enlarged thyroid gland
Clinical Manifestations	• Swelling in the neck • Hoarseness • Feeling of tightness in neck • Difficulty in swallowing • Cough
Diagnosis	• Thyroid function tests • Anti – TPO • MRI • Thyroid scan
Management	• Thyroid hormone replacement drugs • Antithyroid drugs • Radioactive iodine treatment • Surgical options
Prevention	• Including iodine rich diet such as: ▪ Seafood ▪ Foods grown in iodine rich soil ▪ Iodized salt ▪ Bread and dairy products

SHORT NOTES

1. Write a short note on function, sources and deficiency of calcium. (MGR, DU, KUHS)

Answer

For answer, refer to Long Question no. 1, pg. no. 463

2. Write a short note on Fluorosis. Add a note on causes and prevention of fluorosis. (MGR, DU, KUHS)

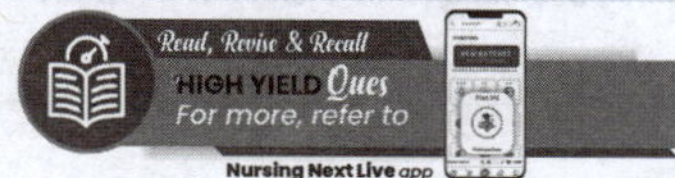

Answer

Fluorosis

Caused by excessive intake of fluorine

Types of Fluorosis

	Dental fluorosis	Skeletal fluorosis	Non skeletal fluorosis
Etiology	Caused by intake above 2 ppm in children	Caused by intake above 20 ppm	
Characteristics	• Mottling of teeth • Discolored teeth • Teeth become weak and rough with brown or yellow patches on the surface	• Hypercalcification of bones • Increased density of spine, pelvis and limbs • Calcification of spine ligaments and bone collagen • Neurological disturbances • Crippling of bone	• Calcification of muscles, actin and myosin filaments • Mitochondria lose their structural integrity • Erythrocyte membrane loses its calcium content • Infertility due to oligospermia and azoospermia

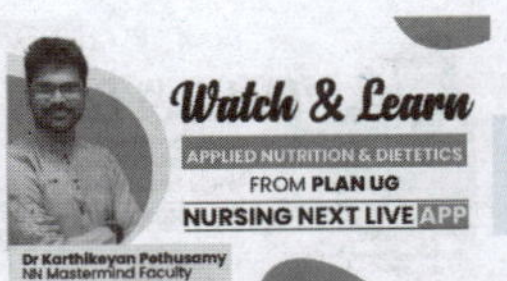

Target High Next Nursing **DECODE**

Fluorosis: Causes and Prevention

Causes	Most common cause - Intake of fluorine rich water
Types	• Two types – Skeletal and nonskeletal • Hypercalcification of bones, muscles, spinal ligaments • Increased risk of fractures • Teeth discoloration and mottling • Neurological disturbance
Management	• Palliative management • Cosmetic treatments for dental fluorosis
Preventive measures	• Identification of fluorine rich areas and defluoridation of the water supply

3. Write a short note on functions of water, distribution in body and its daily requirement. (MGR, KUHS)

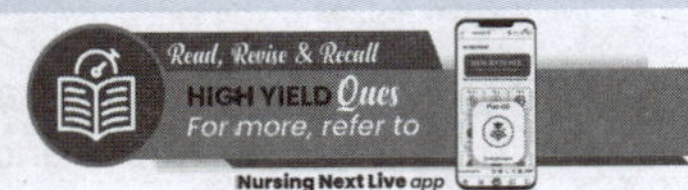

Answer

Introduction

- Special type of nutrient
- Most abundant substance present in the body.
- 45–75% of human body is formed of water – Total Body Water
- Intracellular fluid – 70% TBW
- Extracellular fluid – 30% TBW
  - Interstitial fluid
  - Plasma volume
  - Transcellular fluid

Physiological Functions of Water

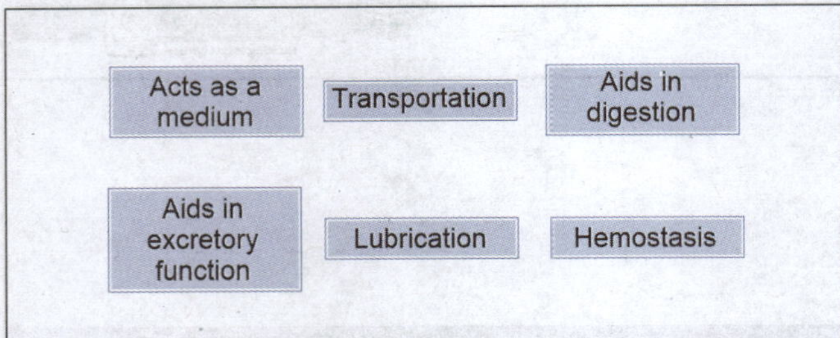

Distribution of Water

- Human body contains about 70% water
  - Men – 55–70%
  - Women – 45–60%
- Women and obese individuals – lesser percentage of water
- Normally, a 70 kg man contains
  - Total – 42 L of water
    - Intracellular fluid – 28 L
    - Extracellular fluid – 14 L
      - Interstitial fluid – 10.5 L
      - Plasma – 3.5 L

Water intake – 2500 mL/day	Water output – 2500 mL/day

• Two sources
• Exogenous sources
  ▪ Ingested water and beverages
  ▪ Water content of solid foods
  ▪ Highly variable
  ▪ Range from 0.5–5 L
• **Endogenous sources**
  ▪ Metabolic water produced within the body
  ▪ Derived from oxidation of foodstuffs
  ▪ Vary from 300–350 mL/day
	• **Four routes of excretion**
	  ▪ Urine – 1500 mL
	  ▪ Skin – 500 mL
	  ▪ Lungs – 300 mL
	  ▪ Feces – 200 mL
	• Urine
	  ▪ Major route for water loss
	  ▪ Medium for elimination of waste products from the body

4. Classify minerals. Explain the dietary sources, absorption and metabolism, daily requirements and deficiency of iron. (MGR)

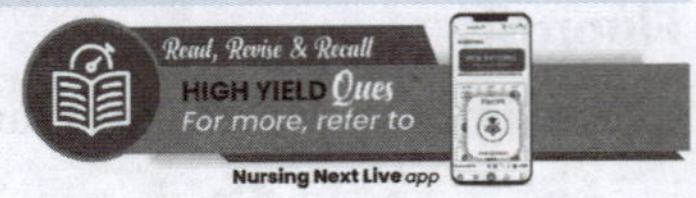

Answer

Classification of Minerals

Macro minerals	Microminerals
Also known as principal elements Constitute 60–80% of the body's inorganic elements Includes: • Calcium • Phosphorus • Magnesium • Sodium • Potassium • Chloride • Sulfur	Require in less than 100 mg/day Subdivided into three categories: • Essential trace elements • Possible essential trace elements • Nonessesntial trace elements

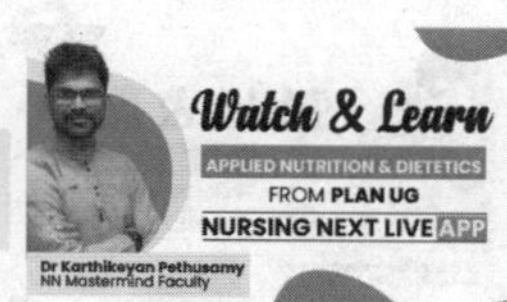

Iron

- Total body content of iron – 3–5 g.
  - ≈ 70% - present in RBCs – as hemoglobin.
  - ≈ 5% – myoglobin of muscle.
  - Remaining as
    - Heme - iron-containing substance. Part of several proteins/enzymes myoglobin, cytochromes, peroxidase, etc.
    - Nonheme iron, e.g., transferrin
    - Hemoproteins-hemoglobin ferritin, hemosiderin.

Biochemical functions	• Transport of O_2 and CO_2 by hemoglobin and myoglobin • Oxidation and phosphorylation reactions – cytochrome, nonheme proteins • Electron transport chains – cytochromes • Has a role in phagocytosis and immunity
RDA	• Adults – 10 mg • Menstruating woman – 18 mg • Pregnant and lactating woman – 40 mg
Dietary sources	• Liver (richest) • Heart, • Kidney • Leafy vegetables • Pulses • Cereals, • Fish, • Apples, • Dried fruits, • Molasses, • Jaggery • Poor sources – Milk, wheat, polished rice.
Absorption and metabolism	• Site of absorption – stomach, duodenum and upper jejunum. • Only 10% of dietary iron is absorbed • Increased in high body demands like anemia • Usually present as ferric state, binds to proteins or organic acids. • Iron is released as Ferric form in the presence of acid in stomach • Ferric form is converted to ferrous state by reducing substances such as vitamin C and cysteine • Ferrous form is soluble and readily absorbed. • In mucosal cells, ferrous is converted back to ferric form by enzyme ferroxidase. • Ferric combines with protein apoferritin to form ferritin (temporary storage form) • When required, iron enters the blood stream from mucosal cells.
Functions of iron	• Exerts its function through the compounds in which it is present. • Transport of O_2 and CO_2 by hemoglobin and myoglobin • Oxidation and phosphorylation reactions – cytochrome, nonheme proteins • Electron transport chains and oxidative phosphorylation – cytochromes • Peroxidase – lysosomal enzyme, required for phagocytosis and killing of bacteria by neutrophils • Associated with effective immunocompetence of the body
Deficiency of iron	• Iron deficiency anemia • Microcytic anemia • *Symptoms/Signs* ▪ Fatigue ▪ Pallor ▪ Dizziness ▪ Irritability ▪ Plummer vinson syndrome • Causes ▪ Blood loss ▪ Inadequate dietary intake ▪ Drugs interfering with iron absorption ▪ Malabsorption syndromes ▪ Increased demands

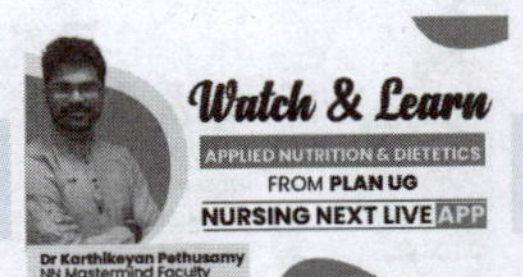

5. Write about water balance and its regulation (KUHS)

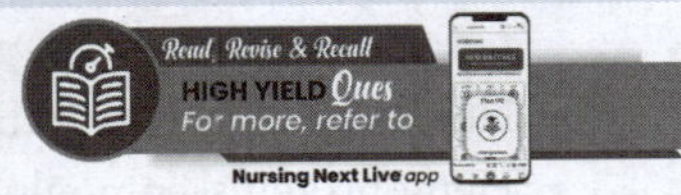

Answer

Introduction

- Human body contains about 70% water
  - Men – 55–70%
  - Women – 45–60%
- Women and obese individuals – lesser percentage of water
- Normally, a 70 kg man contains
  - Total – 42 L of water
    - Intracellular fluid – 28 L
    - Extracellular fluid – 14 L
      - Interstitial fluid – 10.5 L
      - Plasma – 3.5 liters

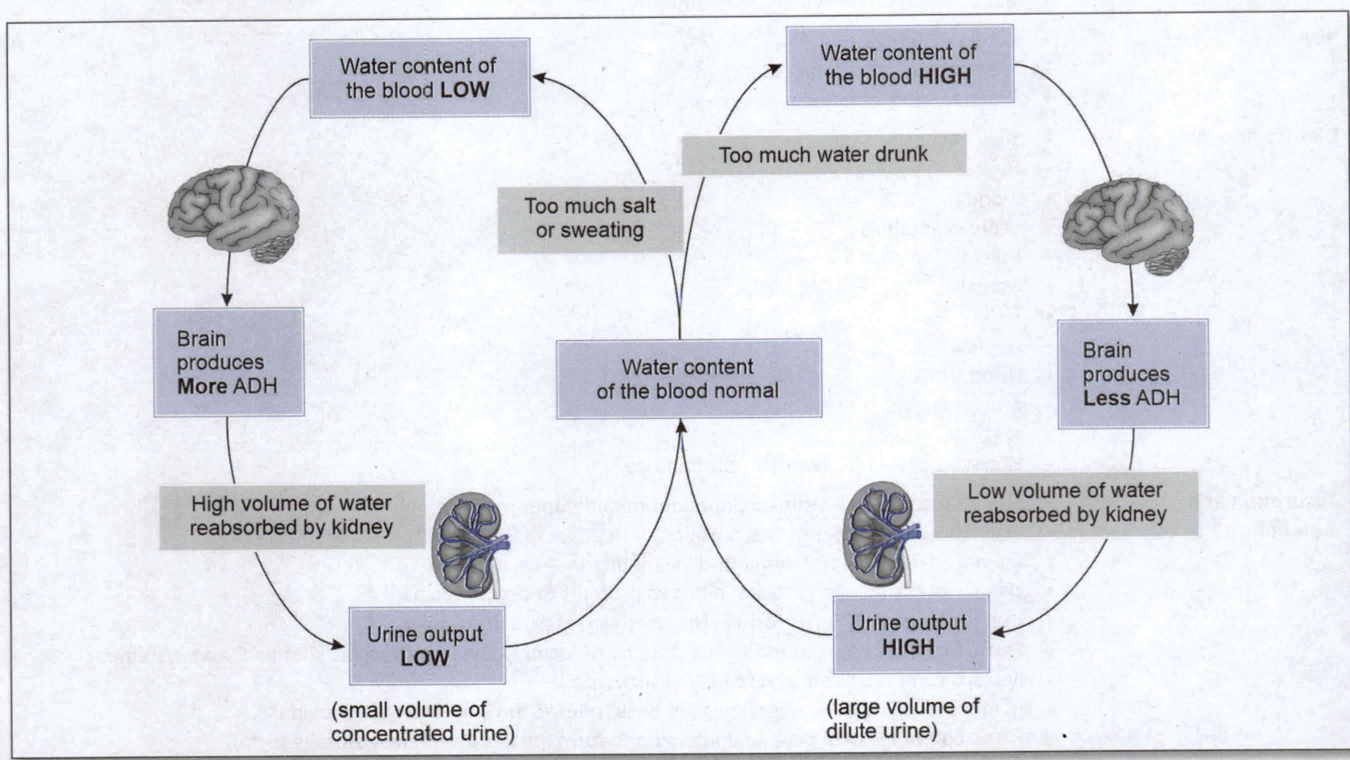

Figure 6.1: Regulation of water balance

- **Water loss**
  - Depends on atmospheric temperature and humidity
  - Increased loss occurs in
    - Hot climate
    - Fever
- Water intake
  - Controlled by thirst center located in the hypothalamus
  - Increase in the osmolality of plasma – stimulates thirst center – leads to increased water intake.
    - Thirst center is stimulated by
    - Angiotensin II
    - Antidiuretic hormone
    - Osmocenters
    - Controls salivation
- Water output
  - Urine production is regulated by
    - Sodium reabsorption
    - Water follows sodium reabsorption
    - Antidiuretic hormone (ADH)
    - Secreted by the posterior pituitary gland
    - Regulated by the osmotic pressure of plasma
    - Increased osmolality promotes ADH secretion
    - Dependent on sodium concentration

Role of Vasopressin (ADH)

- Sensory impulses travel through osmotic receptors to the hypothalamus
- Stimulation of supraoptic nucleus in the hypothalamus to secrete vasopressin *via* hypothalamic hypophyseal tract.
- Vasopressin released acts on vasopressin receptors in the collecting duct.
- Insertion of aquaporin channels
- Increased water reabsorption
- Maintenance of osmolarity

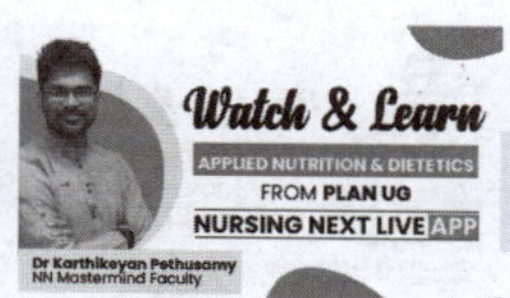

6. Explain how the body maintains electrolyte balance. (MGR, KUHS)

Answer

In body, electrolyte balance is maintained through various mechanisms:

- **Kidney:** selective reabsorption or excretion of electrolytes such as sodium, potassium, calcium, etc. is carried out by kidneys and process is regulated by hormones like-aldosterone and ADH
- **Hormones:** Aldosterone from adrenal gland regulate the electrolyte balance. It increases the reabsorption of sodium and excretion of potassium in the kidneys maintaining the proper level of electrolytes in the body.
- **Nervous system**: It regulate the electrolyte balance through various feedback mechanism and signals.
- **Intestine:** Absorption and excretion of electrolytes in the intestine is regulated to maintain balance. For example, if sodium levels are too high, intestine may decrease its absorption.
- **Sweating:** Sweating is a process in which electrolytes esp. sodium and chloride are lost. In order to maintain balance, sweat glands in the skin selectively reabsorb sodium and maintain appropriate electrolyte balance.
- **Diet:** Consumption of food rich in electrolytes help in maintaining electrolyte balance. Foods like banana, nuts, dairy products provide essential electrolytes required for the proper functioning of the body.

7. Write a short note on hyperkalemia. (MGR)

Answer

Definition	• Elevated levels of potassium (K^+) in blood • Normal serum potassium levels – 3.5 – 5.0 mmol/L • Above 5.5 mmol/L – hyperkalemia
Types	• Mild – 5.5–5.9 mmol/L • Moderate – 6.0–6.4 mmol/L • Severe – >6.6 mmol/L
Symptoms – ***non specific***	• Palpitations • Hyperventilation – compensatory mechanism to metabolic acidosis
Causes	• Renal failure • Hypoaldosteronism • Rhabdomyolysis • Medications such as • NSAIDs • Spironolactone • Angiotensin converting enzyme inhibitors

Contd...

Diagnosis	• ECG changes • Pseudokalemia – due to cell breakdown in blood sample
Treatment	• Low potassium diet

SHORT ANSWER QUESTIONS

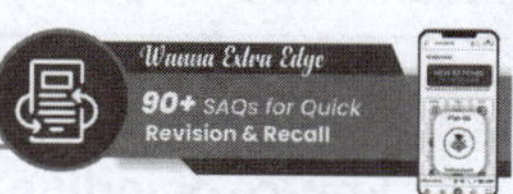

1. Give four rich sources of calcium. (MGR)

Answer

Calcium-rich foods include milk, yoghurt, cheese, leafy green vegetables like broccoli and cabbage, tofu, breakfast cereals, and plant-based milk substitutes like almond, soy, and oat milk. They also include canned salmon and sardines.

2. Dietary sources of zinc. (MGR)

Answer

Zinc rich foods include colostrum, wholegrain cereals, milk, egg, cheese, nuts and pulses.

3. Sources of iron. (MGR)

Answer

Food cooked in iron cookware, red meat, poultry like chicken and turkey, seafood, legumes, tofu nuts, seeds and fortified cereals are rich source of iron.

4. Write the role of water and electrolytes in the body. (MGR)

Answer

Electrolytes are important in maintaining adequate fluid balance, regulating nerve activity, and supporting muscular function. Water is vital for maintaining proper hydration levels in the body.

5. Define lathyrism and fluorosis. (MGR)

Answer

The ingestion of the bean Lathyrus sativus, also referred to as grass pea, results in lathyrism, a persistent neurotoxic illness.

Fluorosis is a disorder brought on by an excessive intake of fluoride, which is typically obtained by drinking water, food, or dental products.

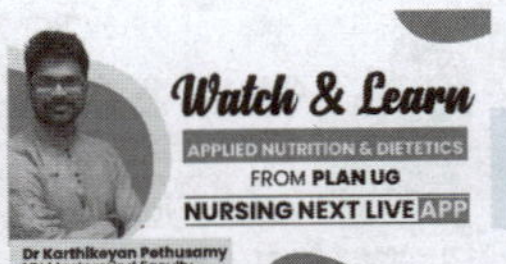

6. Define positive nitrogen balance. (MGR)

Answer

A physiological condition known as positive nitrogen balance occurs when the body retains more nitrogen than it excretes.

7. Source of iodine. (MGR)

Answer

Seafoods, vegetables, fruits, cereals and meat are good sources of Iodine.

8. Sources of potassium. (MGR)

Answer

Potassium rich foods are fruits, dairy products, vegetables and fresh meats.

CONCEPTUAL REVISION

MULTIPLE CHOICE QUESTIONS

1. All of the following are a result of Zinc deficiency; except:

a. Sexual infantilism
b. Impaired immunity
c. Skeletal abnormalities
d. Increased appetite

Ans. d. Increased appetite

2. Acrodermatitis enteropathica is:

a. Inherited disorder of excessive excretion of zinc from body
b. Inherited disorder of impaired uptake of zinc from body
c. Inherited disorder of excessive excretion of copper
d. Inherited disorder of impaired uptake of copper

Ans. b. Inherited disorder of impaired uptake of zinc from body

3. RDA of calcium in normal adult male is:

a. 800 mg
b. 600 mg
c. 400 mg
d. 100 mg

Ans. b. 600 mg

4. Daily elemental calcium requirement for an elderly women is:

a. 1200 mg
b. 300 mg
c. 2000 mg
d. 2500 mg

Ans. a. 1200 mg

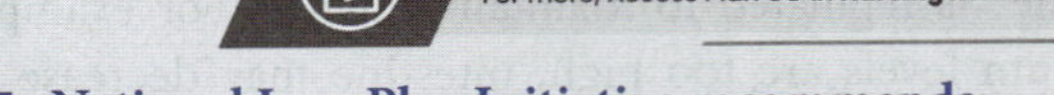

5. National Iron Plus Initiative recommends:

a. Biweekly IFA to pregnant and lactating mothers
b. Biweekly IFA to children 6-60 months
c. Biweekly IFA to adolescent girls
d. None of the above

Ans. b. Biweekly IFA to children 6–60 months

6. True about Anemia Mukt Bharat scheme for Lactating females:

a. 60 mg iron + 500 mcg folic acid tablet daily for 6 months
b. 100 mg iron + 500 mcg folic acid tablet daily for 6 months
c. 60 mg iron 400 mcg folic acid tablet biweekly for 6 months
d. 100 mg iron + 400 mcg folic acid tablet for 100 days at delivery

Ans. a. 60 mg iron + 500 mcg folic acid tablet daily for 6 months

7. False statement regarding folic acid supplementation:

a. Fortified in all wheat products in India like as in USA
b. Preconceptionally given for prevention of neural defects
c. It is present in leafy vegetables, spinach, and paneer
d. Requirement per day in pregnancy is 500 mcg

Ans. a. Fortified in all wheat products in India like as in USA

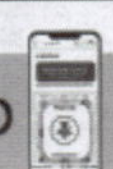

CHAPTER

7

Balanced Diet

CONCEPTUAL THEORY

Terminology

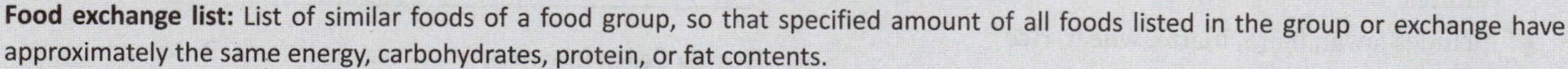

Balanced diet: It is defined as a diet which provides all nutrients in proper proportion, obtained from various food groups to maintain the body functions in working order.

Food exchange list: List of similar foods of a food group, so that specified amount of all foods listed in the group or exchange have approximately the same energy, carbohydrates, protein, or fat contents.

Food groups: Grouping of food in different groups depending upon their major nutrients, e.g., cereals and grains, pulses and legumes, etc.

Food guides: Guidelines stating the amount and kind of nutrients are called food guides.

Meal planning: Meal planning is defined as a simple process which involves application of knowledge of food, nutrients, food habits and likes and dislikes to plan wholesome and attractive meals.

Recommended dietary allowance (RDA): Food and Nutrition Board defines the RDA as the level of intake of essential nutrients considered in the judgment of the committee on Dietary Allowance of the Food and Nutrition Board, on the basis of available scientific knowledge, to be adequate to meet the nutritional needs of practically healthy persons.

Weaning: It is the process of gradually introducing food other than breast milk in the child's feeding schedule.

NUTRITION ACROSS LIFE CYCLE

- Meal planning/Menu planning—definition, principles, steps
- Infant and Young Child Feeding (IYCF) guidelines—breast feeding, infant foods
- Changes in Adolescence
- Diet in pregnancy—nutritional requirements and balanced diet plan
- Anemia in pregnancy—diagnosis, diet for anemic pregnant women, iron and folic acid supplementation and counseling
- Nutrition in lactation—nutritional requirements, diet for lactating mothers, complementary feeding/weaning.

DEFINITION, PRINCIPLES, STEPS

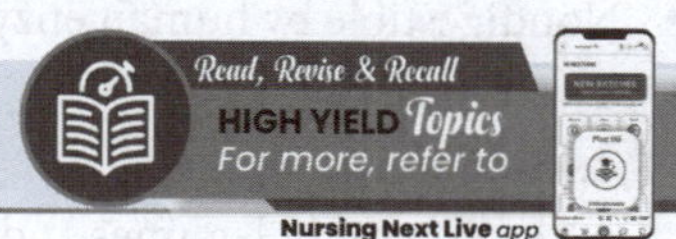

Balanced Diet

- Also known as prudent diet.
- Defined as diet containing different types of foods possessing the various nutrients in required amount and proper proportions to meet the body requirements.
- **Various nutrients include**
  - Carbohydrates
  - Fats
  - Proteins
  - Vitamins and minerals
  - Fiber
  - Water

Principles of Balanced Diet

Balanced Diet Should Provide

- 50–60% calories from carbohydrates
- 10–15% calories from proteins
- 20–30% calories from fats

FOOD GUIDES—BASIC FOUR FOOD GROUPS

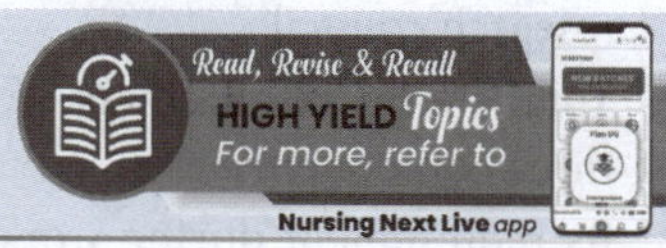

Food Groups

Food is classified into five groups according to their functions in the human body. These are:

1. **Protein food group**

- Includes Milk, Pulses, Nuts, Legumes, Eggs, Meat, Fish and poultry
- Provides
  - Proteins for growth and maintenance
  - Vitamin B complex
  - Iron and calcium
- Each serving of this group supplies 4–6 g of protein

2. **Primary protective vegetables and Fruit Group**
   - Includes two subgroups:
     - Foods rich in beta carotene and green leafy vegetables – spinach, fenugreek, papaya, apricots, mango, carrot
     - Food rich in vitamin C – pineapple, tomato, strawberries, citrus fruits.
   - Serving size – 50–75 g
3. **Secondary protective food and vegetable groups**
   - Supplies minerals, vitamins and dietary fiber
   - Serving size – 50–70 g
4. **Cereals and millet or grain group**
   - Supplies half of the daily requirement of proteins and calories.
   - Includes jawar, bajra, maize, wheat, rice
   - Contains no cholesterol
   - Good source of iron and vitamin B
   - Serving size – 25 g
5. **Oil, fat and sugar group**
   - Also known as fuel group
   - Provides energy
   - Sugars – sweeten the food
   - Fats and oil – increase the palatability of foods.
   - Source of fat soluble vitamins such as vitamin A, D, E and K
   - Serving size – 25 g

RDA—DEFINITION, LIMITATIONS, USES

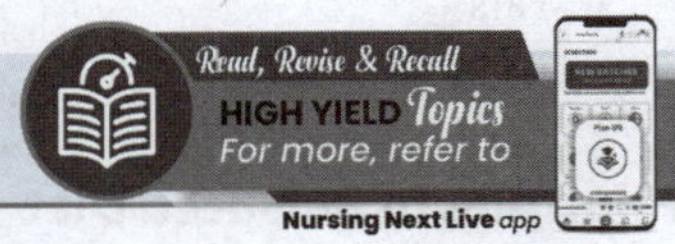

RDA

- Amount of nutrient and calorie intake per day considered necessary for maintenance of good health.
- Calculated for males and females of various ages and recommended by the Food and Nutrition Board of National research council.
- Total energy requirement of an individual is mainly up of three components.
- Its requirement during work can be calculated by adding together the energy requirement for:
  - Basal metabolism
  - Additional energy requirement for work
  - Specific dynamic action of food.

Energy Requirement (RDA)

- Adult man doing sedentary work – 2400 kcal
- Adult women doing sedentary work – 1900 kcal

FOOD EXCHANGE SYSTEM

Food Exchange System

Food exchange system allows one to choose a variety of food with adequate nutrient. The food exchange system is important in planning a nutritious diet. It can be used to select a food in familiar measures that are adequate in nutrient content and safety the requirements of a given individual. Foods commonly used are divided into seven main groups on the basis of similarities in nutrient composition. Food items falling under similar groups have approximately equal carbohydrates, proteins, fats, vitamins and minerals contents. (Fruits and vegetables being exception)

CALCULATION OF NUTRITIVE VALUE OF FOODS

Bomb Caloriemeter

- Constant volume calorimeter
- For determination of energy changes during a reaction
- Measures the heat of reaction at a fixed volume – change in internal energy
- Measures the combustion heat of oxygen burnable samples
- Determines the calorific values of solid and liquid fuels.
- Bomb calorimeter gets its name from the strong steel shell known as a bomb.

Uses of Bomb Calorimeter

- Determines the heat emitted from a given quantity of biomass sample combustion and calculate the HHV of that fuel.
- The calorific value of food can be measured by heating a pre measured mass of food and igniting it in an oxygen atmosphere.

DIETARY FIBER

Read, Revise & Recall
HIGH YIELD Topics
For more, refer to
Nursing Next Live app

Dietary Fiber

- Complex carbohydrates
- Nondigestible by human enzymes
- **Two types:**
  1. **Soluble:**
     - Present in legumes and fruits
     - Water soluble
     - Results in gel formation
     - E.g., pectins

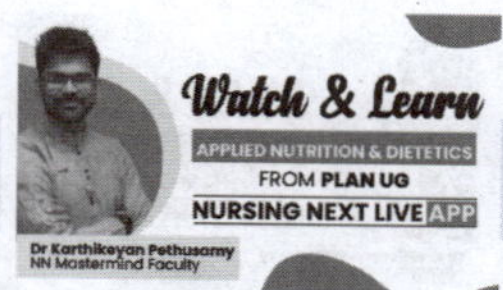

2. **Insoluble:**
   - Found in vegetables and grains
   - Adsorb water
   - E.g., cellulose and hemicellulose
- Intestinal bacteria can digest certain fibers, e.g., Pectins

Beneficial Effects of Fiber

- Prevents constipation
- Eliminates bacterial toxins
- Decreases risk of GIT cancer
- Improves glucose tolerance
- Reduces serum cholesterol levels

NUTRITION ACROSS LIFE CYCLE MEAL PLANNING/MENU PLANNING—DEFINITION, PRINCIPLES

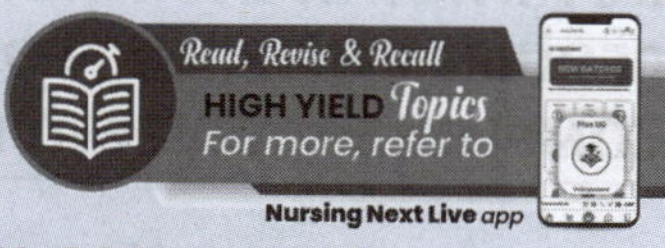

Menu Planning

Defined as a simple process which involves application of knowledge of food, nutrients, food habits and likes and dislikes to plan wholesome and attractive meals.

Importance of Menu Planning

- Early recovery of patient
- Provide variety
- Save money, time and energy
- Financial concerns of patient
- Improve quality of food
- Improve appetite

Principles of Meal Planning

- According to need of the patient
- According to the composition of family
- Should be nourishing, appealing and tasty
- Should include variety
- Should be colorful and pleasing
- Have contrast of texture, flavor and methods of preparation.
- Storage/shelf life options should be considered.
- Availability of raw materials

INFANT AND YOUNG CHILD FEEDING (IYCF) GUIDELINES—BREASTFEEDING, INFANT FOODS

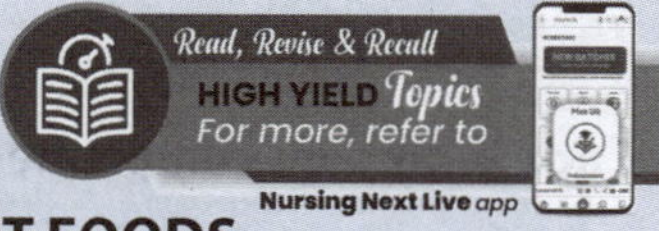

According to WHO UNICEF Recommendation

- Initiate breastfeeding as early as possible within 1 hour of birth
- For first six month of life exclusive breastfeeding should be done
- At 6 months of age introduce nutritionally adequate and safe complementary (solid) food up to 2 years of age.
- However, many of the infants and children are not able to receive optional feeding. Recommendation are also refined to address the needs of HIV-infected infants. Anteretroviral drugs allows these infants to have exclusively breastfeeding for at least 12 months of age.

Breastfeeding Guidelines

- There should be skin to skin contact between mother and baby immediately after birth and breastfeeding should be initiated within the first hour of life.
- Breast feed the infant as often as it needs.
- Allow the mothers and infants to remain together for 24 hours a day.

Complimentary Feeding Guidelines

- Complimentary feed should be started after 6 month of age on demand and breastfeed until 2 years of age.
- Feed the child slowly and patiently and encourage him to eat food by making eye to eye contact and do not force the child to eat.

CHANGES IN ADOLESCENCE

- Adolescent period
  - Also known as teenage.
  - Age group: 12–18 years
- Process of physical development from child to adult is called puberty.

DIET IN PREGNANCY—NUTRITIONAL REQUIREMENTS AND BALANCED DIET PLAN

- **Guidelines for meal planning during pregnancy**
  - Fulfil all requirements of calories and other nutrients
  - Nonvegetarians have good choice of meat to fulfil protein requirement but vegetarians should add legumes and grains.
  - Milk and milk products according to the requirement.
  - Use variety of whole grains and cereals, rice and other grains in menu.
  - Use fruits and vegetables in the form of salads.
  - Should include fiber, folic acid, iron, vitamin B6 and zinc.
  - Use iodized salt.
- **Energy required to have gestational weight gain**
  - Additional 850 calories
  - 1st trimester – 0.5 g
  - 2nd trimester – 6.9 g
  - 3rd trimester – 22.7 g

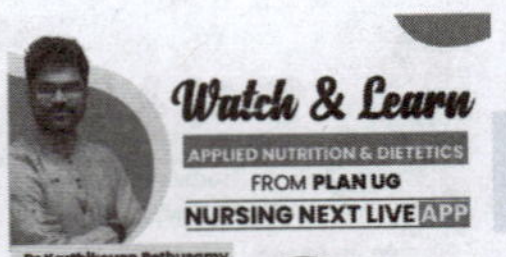

According to ICMR-NIN, nutritional requirements in pregnancy are as follows:

- Preferable weight gain during pregnancy – 10–12 kg
- Additional energy requirements during pregnancy is 350 kcal.
- Also the diet should contain additional 23 g of protein during the third trimester of pregnancy.
- Some micronutrients (vitamins and minerals) are also required in extra amount.
  - Additional RDA during pregnancy for:
    - Vitamin B_{12} – 1.2 µg/day
    - Thiamine – 0.2 mg
    - Riboflavin – 0.3 mg
    - Niacin – 2 mg
    - Pyridoxine – 2.5 mg
    - Vitamin C – 60 mg
    - Vitamin A – 800 mg

ANEMIA IN PREGNANCY—DIAGNOSIS, DIET FOR ANEMIC PREGNANT WOMEN, IRON AND FOLIC ACID SUPPLEMENTATION AND COUNSELING

Anemia in Pregnancy

- Anemia is one of the most frequent complications related to pregnancy.
- Normal physiologic changes in pregnancy affect the hemoglobin concentration.
- Anemia increases the risk of:
  - Preterm delivery
  - Low birth weight
  - Postpartum maternal infections
- Clinical manifestations of anemia in pregnancy:
  - Fatigue
  - Light headedness
  - Mild dyspnea during exertion
  - Pallor
  - Tachycardia
  - Hypotension

Menu Plan for Pregnant Women Who is Anemic

Breakfast	½ cup oats and 2 egg whites or 1 banana and 1 cup yogurt or ½ cup muesli
Lunch	Wholegrain chapatti and beet root yogurt and iron rich vegetable or Vegetable sandwich and beetroot salad
Dinner	Broccoli soup and oven baked chicken or Baked potatoes and cucumber/lettuce salads with wholegrain chapatti
Snacks	Fruit salads/nuts/collagen protein shake/eggs/ banana.

NUTRITION IN LACTATION—NUTRITIONAL REQUIREMENTS, DIET FOR LACTATING MOTHERS, COMPLEMENTARY FEEDING/WEANING

Guidelines for Meal Planning of Nursing/Lactating Mothers

- Proteins – 70 g/day
- Fluids – water, milk, fruit juices and soups should be added.
- Calories – increased by 400 to 600 calories/day
- DHA – important for baby's visual and mental development.
- Iron – Add iron rich foods such as legumes, pulses, egg, red meat, etc.
- Vitamin D and calcium rich foods such as tuna, salmon, milk and milk products should be included.
- Lactating mothers should eat at least three nutritious meals a day
- Avoid sugar and fat rich foods, alcohol and smoking.

Weaning

- Process of gradually introducing food other than breast milk in the child's feeding schedule.
- Fully weaned – when the baby is no longer fed with breast milk.
- Concentrated, energy dense complementary foods are essential for maintenance of adequate velocity of growth.

CONCEPTUAL EXERCISES

LONG ANSWER QUESTIONS

1. Write the nutritional requirements during infancy and add a note on complementary foods and discuss the feeding problems of infants. (DU)

Answer

- Infant and young child feeding is a key area to improve child survival and promote healthy growth and development.

- According to WHO and UNICEF, under nutrition is estimated to be associated with approximately 45% of all child deaths.

Nutritional Requirements During Infancy

Nutrient	Per kg body weight/day
Energy	92 kcal
Protein	1.16 g
Iron	46 ug
Niacin	710 ug
Thiamine	0.2 mg/day
Riboflavin	0.3 mg/day
Pyridoxine	0.1 mg/day
Magnesium	30 mg/day

- These requirements can be met from breast milk and thus, it is essential to promote exclusive breast feeding for 6 months and if possible, up to 2 years.
  - Breast milk contains all the nutrients, which are essentially required for infants.
  - Colostrum, the milk secreted during the first 3–4 days after child birth, is rich in proteins, minerals, vitamins and antibodies.

Complementary Feeding

- Feed provided to the infants in addition to breastfeed, when it is not sufficient to provide for the infant's nutrition, especially in infants above 6 months of age.
- Complementary foods must be:
  - Timely introduced
  - Provide sufficient protein, energy and micronutrients to meet the child's nutritional needs.
  - Hygienically stored and prepared.
  - Properly fed to the child

Feeding Problems of the Infants

Feeding problems	Causes	Prevention/management
Regurgitation	Occurs due to backward flowing of feed from stomach along with swallowed air.	Frequent burping
Vomiting	Occurs due to overfeeding, excessive swallowing of air, prolonged burping or pathological causes such as gastroenteritis, congenital pyloric stenosis, and intestinal obstruction.	Correct the incorrect feeding technique. Treat the cause.
Suckling and swallowing difficulty	Prolonged suckling problem may be due to congenital malformations. Like cleft palate, cleft lip, large tongue, etc. Preterm babies have more chances.	Assess the cause and specific management is required.
Dehydration and fever	Refusal of feed, lethargy, fever and drowsiness are common in neonates in first 3–4 days. Inadequate feeding or infections may be the cause.	Antibiotics are required in case of infections. Mothers should be educated about personal hygiene.
Excessive crying	This may be related to hunger, wet napkins, abdominal colic, etc.	Mothers should be educated about technique and adequacy of breastfeeding.
Underfeeding	Low breast milk production, economic problems or ignorance. Infants fail to gain weight.	Teach the mother proper breastfeeding technique.
Overfeeding	Forcing the babies to overfeed may lead to infantile obesity. Fatty diarrhea, excessive crying, emotional problems.	Education of the mother is very important.

2. (a) Describe the changes in adolescence. (b) What dietary advice would you give for an adolescent girl suffering from severe anemia? (DU)

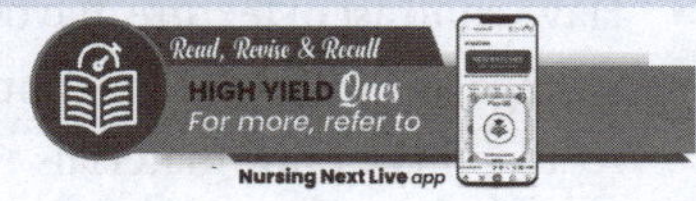

Answer

Changes in Adolescence

- Adolescent period
  - Also known as teenage.
  - Age group 12–18 years
- Process of physical development from child to adult is called puberty.
- In females, its peak is at the age of 12 and is completed by age 15. In males, its peak is at 14 and it is completed by age of 19.
- Growth spurt is seen.
- Changes during adolescence:
  - Weight gain is about 50%.
  - Physical growth is seen

- Sexual growth occurs due to several endocrine hormones.
- As a result of development of bones, and physical and sexual growth, body's requirement for almost all the nutrients (both macronutrients as well as micronutrients) is significantly increased.
- Increased basal metabolic rate (BMR), body requires extra calories which met by increasing the dietary intake of carbohydrates and fat.
- Before puberty the proportion of fat and muscles is similar but now at this stage, males put on twice as muscle as females and females gain more fat.
- Change in body composition of boys and girls also leads to a difference in their nutritional requirements. Males now need more calories, proteins, iron and zinc for muscle and bone development whereas females require more iron due to the onset of menstruation.

- Growth also increases the demands of protein. Bone growth also needs extra vitamin D, calcium, phosphorus and magnesium.
- Increased BMR and the extra consumption of carbohydrates and proteins require additional amount of vitamins, particularly, B vitamins (such as thiamine or vitamin B_1, vitamin B_{12}, vitamin C and protein. Thus, it is essential to plan their diet accordingly.

Dietary Advice for an Adolescent Girl Suffering from Severe Anemia

- Iron requirement increases in the adolescent girls due to the onset of mensturation. Increased demands are also present due to pubertal growth spurts. Thus, anemia is very common in this age group, if proper diet is not given.

Table 7.1: Guidelines for menu planning for adolescents (13–18 years)

Food groups	Quantity	
	Boys	Girls
Cereals and millets	420	300
Pulses	60	60
Milk (mL)	500	500
Roots and tubers	200	100
Green leafy vegetables	100	100
Other vegetables	100	100
Fruits	100	100
Sugar	35	30
Fats/oils (visible)	25	25

- Foods that are rich in iron should be included:
  - Liver (richest)
  - Heart,
  - Kidney
  - Leafy vegetables
  - Pulses
  - Cereals,
  - Fish,
  - Apples,
  - Dried fruits,
  - Molasses,
  - Jaggery
- Poor sources—Milk, wheat, polished rice.

3. What is balanced diet? Narrate a day's menu for a normal pregnant woman in second trimester. List down the principles of meal planning. Describe the importance of Menu planning. (KUHS, RUHS)

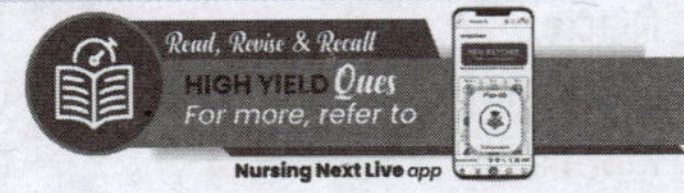

Answer

Balanced Diet

- Also known as prudent diet.
- Defined as diet containing different types of foods possessing the various nutrients in required amount and proper proportions to meet the body requirements.
- **Various nutrients include**
  - Carbohydrates
  - Fats
  - Proteins
  - Vitamins and minerals
  - Fiber
  - Water

Balanced Diet Should Provide

- 50–60% calories from carbohydrates
- 10–15% calories from proteins
- 20–30% calories from fats

Menu Planning

Defined as a simple process which involves application of knowledge of food, nutrients, food habits and likes and dislikes to plan wholesome and attractive meals.

Principles of Meal Planning

- Meal should meet the caloric needs of the patient.
- Meal should consists a balanced diet
- According to need of the patient
- According to the composition of family
- Should be nourishing, appealing and tasty
- Should include variety
- Should be colorful and pleasing
- Have contrast of texture, flavor and methods of preparation.
- Storage/shelf life options should be considered.
- Availability of raw materials

Importance of Menu Planning

- Early recovery of patient
- Provide variety
- Save money, time and energy

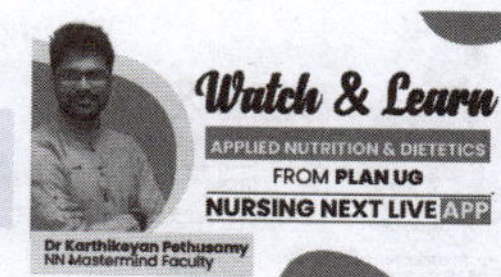

- Financial concerns of patient
- Improve quality of food
- Improve appetite

Menu for a Pregnant Women in Second Trimester

- **Guidelines for meal planning during pregnancy**
  - Fulfil all requirements of calories and other nutrients
  - Nonvegetarians have good choice of meat to fulfil protein requirement but vegetarians should add legumes and grains
  - Milk and milk products according to the requirement.
  - Use variety of whole grains and cereals, rice and other grains in menu.
  - Use fruits and vegetables in the form of salads.
  - Should include fiber, folic acid, iron, vitamin B6 and zinc.
  - Use iodized salt.
- **Energy required to have gestational weight gain**
  - Additional 850 calories
  - 2nd trimester – 6.9 g
- **One day menu plan for pregnant women**

Meal	Food stuffs
Breakfast	Besan parantha -2 Curd – one katori or Omelette – 2 eggs Bread – 4 slices
Mid day morning	Fresh juice or 1 cup tea with roasted chanas
Lunch	Vegetables – one katori Rice – one plate Raita – one katori Green salad – one plate Chapatti – one or two
Evening tea	Milk – 1 cup Biscuits – 4–6
Dinner	Chapatti – 2–3 Dal/meat – one katoori Kheer/ice cream/fruit custard

4. Define balanced diet. What are the factors to be considered in preparing a menu? (MGR)

Answer

Balanced Diet

- Also known as prudent diet.
- Defined as diet containing different types of foods possessing the various nutrients in required amount and proper proportions to meet the body requirements.
- **Various nutrients include:**
  - Carbohydrates
  - Fats
  - Proteins
  - Fiber
  - Vitamins and minerals
  - Water

Balanced Diet Should Provide

- 50–60% calories from carbohydrates
- 10–15% calories from proteins
- 20–30% calories from fats

Menu Planning

- Simple process which involves application of knowledge of food, nutrients and personal preferences to plan a nutritive and wholesale meals.
- **Aims of menu planning**
  - Provide variety of food in single menu
  - To help in easy recovery of patient
  - To save money, time and energy by planning before cooking a meal for family
  - To plan menu according to the financial condition of family
  - Improvement of food quality
  - Improvement in appetite of the person.
- **Factors to be considered in preparing a menu**
  - Type of consumer
  - Food availability
  - Geographical location
  - Weather
  - Economic factors
  - Time availability
  - According to the need of the client
    - Diabetic diet
    - Liquid diet
  - Family factors like:
    - Age
    - Occupation
    - Sex
  - Planned meals should be nourishing, fulfiling and appetizing.
  - Should be serving variety of food
  - Strive for contrast of texture, flavor and methods of preparation.

5. Write the RDA for a pregnant woman and plan a day's menu for a pregnant woman who is suffering from anemia. (MGR)

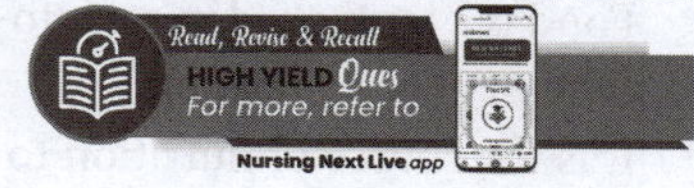

Answer

Introduction

A good nutrition level in women minimizes the risk of childbirth and ensures a healthy baby.

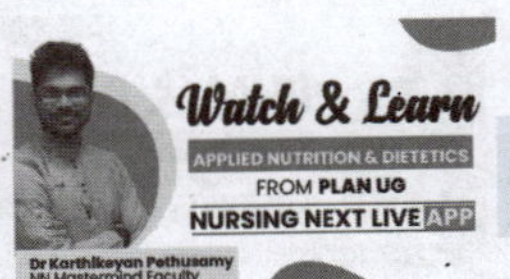

Weight gain during pregnancy is about 11–12 kg, of which 40% is due to child's placenta and amniotic fluids.

Anemia in Pregnancy

- Anemia is one of the most frequent complications related to pregnancy.
- Normal physiologic changes in pregnancy affect the hemoglobin concentration.
- Anemia increases the risk of:
  - Preterm delivery
  - Low birth weight
  - Postpartum maternal infections
- Clinical manifestations of anemia in pregnancy
  - Fatigue
  - Light headedness
  - Mild dyspnea during exertion
  - Pallor
  - Tachycardia
  - Hypotension

Menu Plan for Pregnant Women Who is Anemic

Breakfast	½ cup oats and 2 egg whites or 1 banana and 1 cup yogurt or ½ cup muesli
Lunch	Wholegrain chapatti and beetroot yogurt and iron rich vegetable or Vegetable sandwich and beetroot salad
Dinner	broccoli soup and oven baked chicken or Baked potatoes and cucumber/lettuce salads with wholegrain chapatti
Snacks	Fruit salads/nuts/collagen protein shake/eggs/banana.

6. Describe the role of nutrition in maintaining health. Explain the factors affecting food and nutrition. (RUHS)

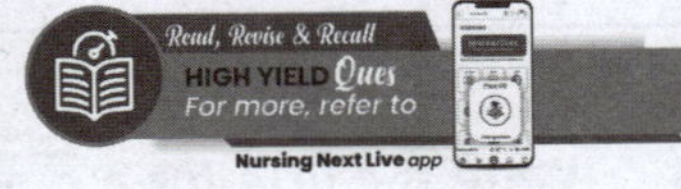

Answer

Introduction

- Food is a term used to refer to the solid or liquid substances that are ingested.
- It is the source of nutrition to the body for the growth and maintenance of the body and its processes.

Objectives of Nutrition

- To apply the principle of nutrients and dietetics in health and sickness.
- To make nutrition an important part of daily nursing practices.
- To recognize the values of nutrition in maintaining personal and patient health.
- To plan and prepare normal and therapeutic diet for different types of patients.

Elements of Nutrition

Macronutrients	Micronutrients
They are required in a large amount in our body; they form the bulk of food.	They are required in a small amount that may vary from 1 mg to several grams.
• Carbohydrates • Fats • Proteins	• Vitamins • Minerals

Relationship with Health and Nutrition

Growth and development	Body cells multiply regularly. They increase in size as well. For all these processes, the new protoplasm is required. Food helps in the formation of new protoplasm or repairing the worn out cells and tissues.
Provide resistance	Proper nutrition helps to reduce the risks of infection and build up resistance against diseases. If a person takes an adequate amount of nutrients, then his/her body remains free from all the infections.
Mortality and morbidity	Malnutrition contributes a lot to general death rates, infant mortality rates, stillbirths and premature deliveries or over nutrition responsible for obesity, diabetes, hypertension and cardiovascular diseases.
Regulating metabolic processes	Adequate nutrition is required for regulating, maintaining and repairing various parts: the food provides basic raw materials.
Release of energy	Energy is required for performing various life processes such as ingestion, digestion and absorption. Energy required for these processes is released by oxidation of food.
Formation of organic substances	Many organic substances such as hormones and enzymes are required by living beings.
Specific deficiency diseases	Malnutrition is directly responsible for certain specific nutritional diseases, e.g. PEM, malnutrition, goiter and anemia. So, a balanced amount of nutrition is very important to prevent deficiencies.

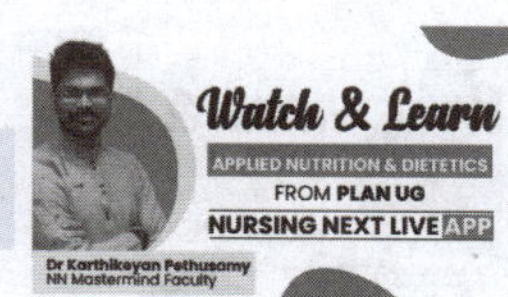

Factors Affecting Food and Nutrition Intake

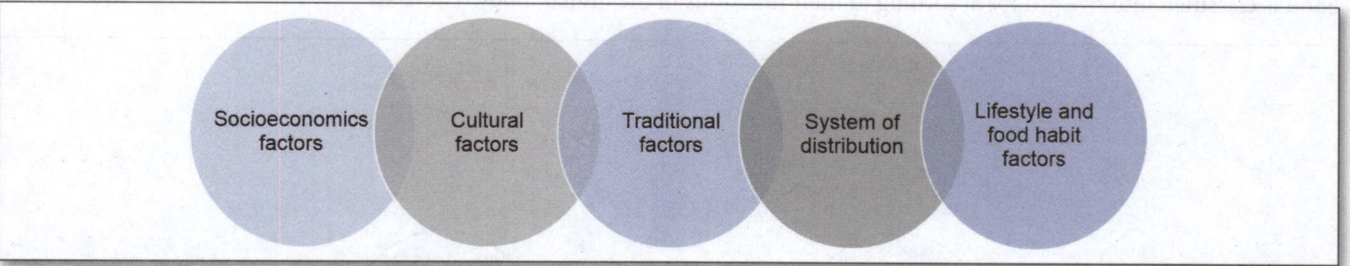

Socioeconomic Factors

- Fundamental need of life is nourishment through food. Depends upon family resources for adequate and nutritive food.
- Economic status of the family also makes a difference in the choice of food.

Cultural Factors

- Every culture has its own customs and beliefs regarding nutritional practice.
- Religious beliefs affect the food choices and health of the individuals directly or indirectly.

Traditional Factors

- Traditional taboos are certain beliefs regarding the food intake and its effects.
- For example:
  - Consumption of garlic by lactating mother increases milk production.
  - Consumption of certain foods may lead to the development of boils (hot foods) and some may be lead to cold, sore throat (cold foods).

System of Distribution

- Adequate availability of food is an important factor in determining the adequate intake of food and nutrition.
- Market imperfections and government restrictions affect the free movement of the food grains across the borders. Due to these reasons, cost of food grains increase and availability decreases.

Lifestyle and Food Habit Factors

Age	During the growth period, basal metabolism is higher so food and nutrition requirement is higher. During adolescence, calorie requirement is higher
Weight	Associated with a range of adverse health consequences such as cardiovascular diseases, diabetes and some cancers.
Body size	Body mass index affects the food and nutritional requirements. Larger body has a greater amount of muscles and glandular tissues requiring higher energy requirement.
Physical activity	Presence of physical activity increases the energy expenditure above the basal energy need. Regular physical activity have lower risk of many chronic diseases.
Altered physiological states	Certain conditions such as pregnancy and lactation, energy requirements of the individual are increased due to elevated BMR. The need of extra energy is associated with deposition of tissues during pregnancy and secretion of milk during lactation.
Psychological stress	Excessive amounts of stress can lead to risk of strokes, heart attacks, depression, etc.
Food habits	Healthy food habits impart healthy growth and improves cognitive development. It provides longer term health benefits such as reducing the risk of becoming overweight or obese and developing non-communicable diseases, like-diabetes, stroke, etc. later in life.

Contd...

SHORT NOTES

1. Write a short note on basic five food groups. (MGR, DU)

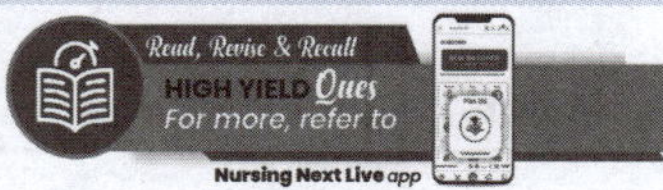

Answer

Introduction

Food is an edible substance ingested by an individual for nutritional support. Food contains nutrients as carbohydrates, fats, proteins, vitamins or minerals.

Food Groups

Food is classified into five groups according to their functions in the human body. These are:

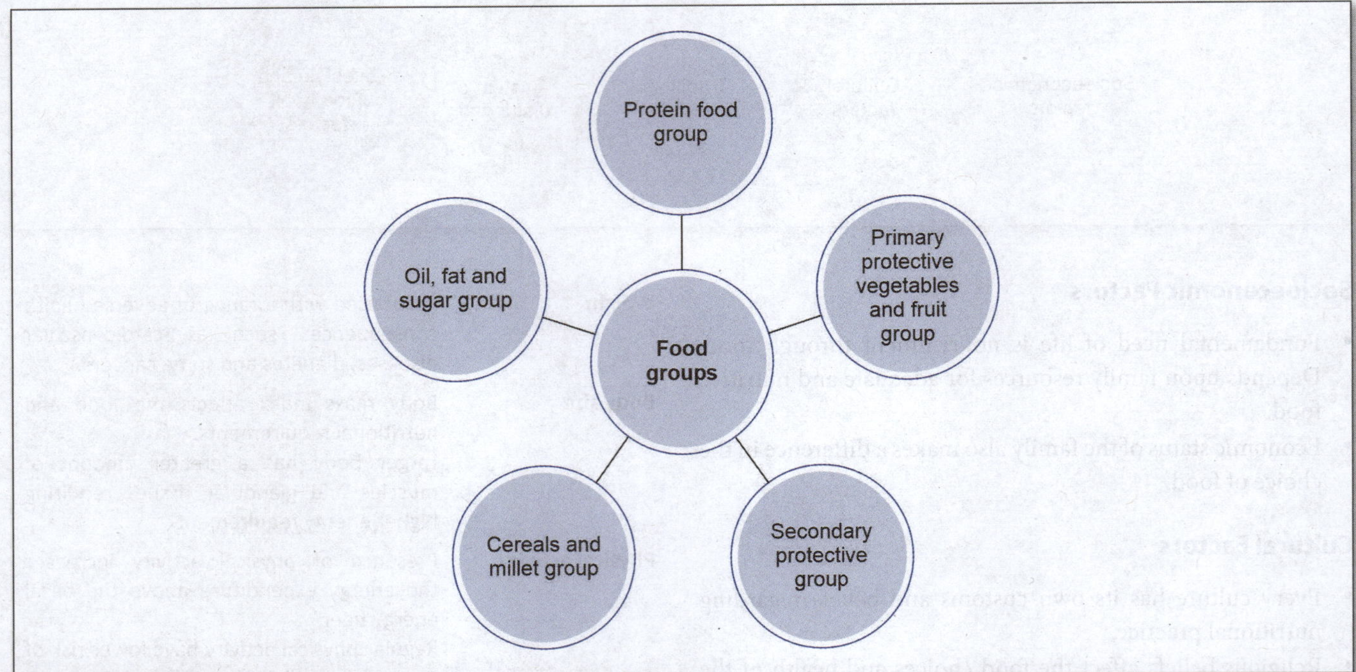

Protein food group	Primary protective vegetables and fruit group	Secondary protective food and vegetable groups	Cereals and millet or grain group	Oil, fat and sugar group
Includes • Milk • Pulses • Nuts • Legumes • Eggs • Meat • Fish and poultry Provides • Proteins for growth and maintenance • Vitamin B complex • Iron and calcium Each serving of this group supplies 4–6 g of protein	Includes two subgroups 1. Foods rich in beta carotene and green leafy vegetables – spinach, fenugreek, papaya, apricots, mango, carrot 2. Food rich in vitamin C – pineapple, tomato, strawberries, citrus fruits. Serving size – 50–75 g	Supplies minerals, vitamins and dietary fiber Serving size – 50–70 g	Supplies half of the daily requirement of proteins and calories. Includes jawar, bajra, maize, wheat, rice Contains no cholesterol Good source of iron and vitamin B Serving size – 25g	Also known as fuel group Provides energy Sugars – sweeten the food Fats and oil – increase the palatability of foods. Source of fat soluble vitamins such as vitamin A, D, E and K Serving size – 25g

2. Discuss the factors influencing meal planning. (DU, KUHS)

Answer

Menu Planning

- Simple process which involves application of knowledge of food, nutrients and personal preferences to plan a nutritive and wholesale meals.
- **Factors to be considered in preparing a menu**

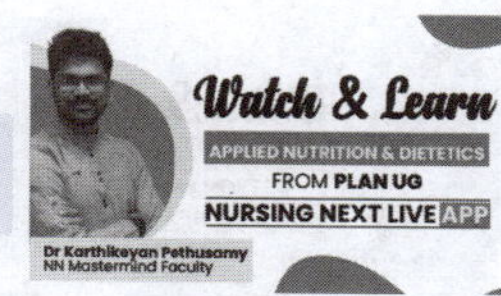

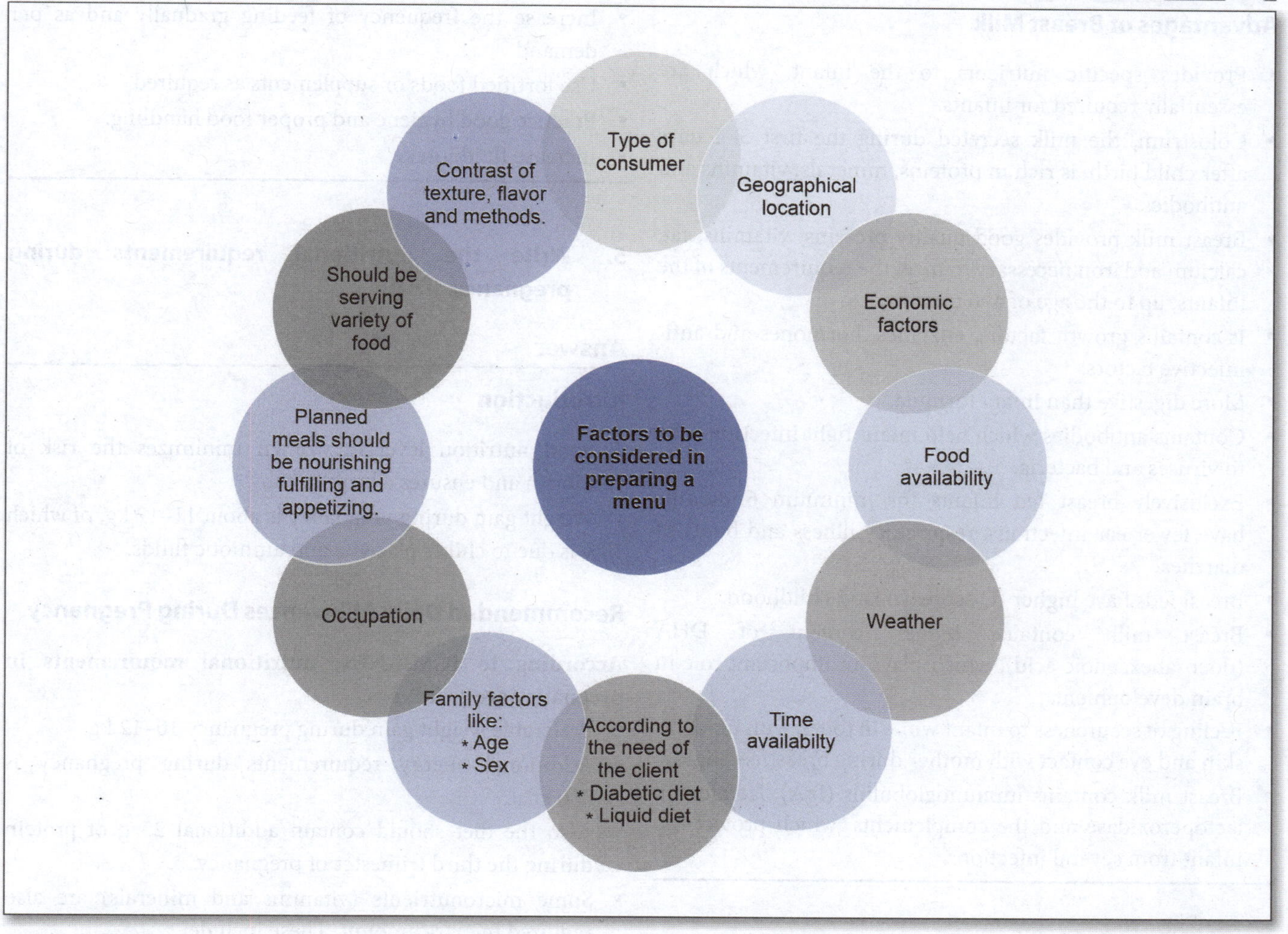

Factors to be considered in preparing a menu

Type of consumer

Geographical location

Economic factors

Food availability

Weather

Time availabilty

According to the need of the client
* Diabetic diet
* Liquid diet

Family factors like:
* Age
* Sex

Occupation

Planned meals should be nourishing fulfilling and appetizing.

Should be serving variety of food

Contrast of texture, flavor and methods.

Importance of Menu Planning

- Early recovery of patient
- Provide variety
- Save money, time and energy
- Financial concerns of patient
- Improve quality of food
- Improve appetite

3. Justify "Breast milk is the Best milk" for infants. (DU)

Answer

Breastfeeding

It is recommended that the infants should be exclusively breastfed up to 6 months of age.

Composition of Breast Milk

Nutrient	Content/100 mL
Calories	67 kcal
Fat	3.5 g
Proteins	1.1 g
Sodium	0.9 mEq
Lactose	7.0 g
Potassium	1.4 mEq
Iron	30 – 50 ug
Zinc	120 ug
Calcium	35 mg
Vitamin C	5.2 mg
Vitamin A	60 ug

Advantages of Breast Milk

- Provides specific nutrients to the infant, which are essentially required for infants.
- Colostrum, the milk secreted during the first 3–4 days after child birth, is rich in proteins, minerals, vitamins and antibodies.
- Breast milk provides good quality proteins, vitamins, fat, calcium and iron necessary to meet the requirements of the infants, up to the age of 4–6 months.
- It contains growth factors, enzymes, hormones and anti-infective factors.
- More digestive than infant formula.
- Contains antibodies which help infant fight infections due to viruses and bacteria.
- Exclusively breast fed infants for minimum 6 months have fewer ear infections, respiratory illness and bouts of diarrhea.
- Breast feds have higher IQ scores in later childhood.
- Breast milk contains higher content of DHA (docosahexaenoic acid), which plays an important role in brain development.
- Feeling of secureness to infant while in touch with mother's skin and eye contact with mother during breastfeeding.
- Breast milk contains immunoglobulins (IgA), lactoferrin, lactoperoxidase and the complements, which protect the infant from several infections.

4. Write in short about complementary foods for infants. (DU)

Answer

Complementary Feeding

- Feed provided to the infants in addition to breastfeed, when it is not sufficient to provide for the infant's nutrition, especially in infants above 6 months of age.
- Complementary foods must be:
  - Timely introduced
  - Provide sufficient protein, energy and micronutrients to meet the child's nutritional needs.
  - Hygienically stored and prepared.
  - Properly fed to the child

Principles of Complementary Feeding

- Continue frequent, on demand breastfeeding until 2 years of age
- Increase the consistency and variety of food gradually
- Increase the frequency of feeding gradually and as per demand.
- Use fortified foods or supplements as required
- Practice good hygiene and proper food handling.
- Increase fluid intake

5. Write the nutritional requirements during pregnancy. (DU)

Answer

Introduction

A good nutrition level in women minimizes the risk of childbirth and ensures a healthy baby.

Weight gain during pregnancy is about 11–12 kg, of which 40% is due to child's placenta and amniotic fluids.

Recommended Daily Allowances During Pregnancy

According to ICMR-NIN, nutritional requirements in pregnancy are as follows:

- Preferable weight gain during pregnancy 10–12 kg
- Additional energy requirements during pregnancy is 350 kcal.
- Also the diet should contain additional 23 g of protein during the third trimester of pregnancy.
- Some micronutrients (vitamins and minerals) are also required in extra amount. These include:
  - Extra iron is also required by the mother as well as the growing fetus, to meet the increased demand of erythropoiesis, i.e., the formation of RBCs. RDA for iron has been suggested to be 35 mg during pregnancy.
  - Calcium, which is essential for proper formation of bones and to prevent osteoporosis in the mother. RDA of calcium has been suggested to be 1200 mg during pregnancy.
  - Folic acid which should be taken throughout the pregnancy, to reduce the risk of congenital malformations and increase the birth weight. RDA for dietary folate has been suggested to be 500 µg during pregnancy.
  - Additional RDA during pregnancy for:
    - Vitamin B_{12} – 1.2 µg/day
    - Thiamine – 0.2 mg
    - Riboflavin – 0.3 mg
    - Niacin – 2 mg
    - Pyridoxine – 2.5 mg
    - Vitamin C – 60 mg
    - Vitamin A – 800 mg

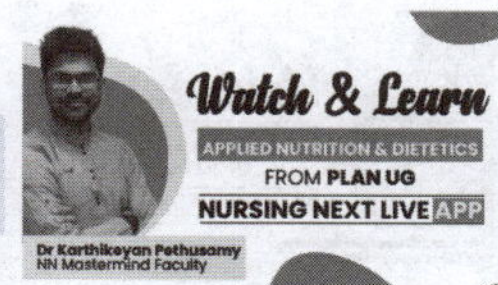

6. Write a note on nutritional classification of food. (MGR, KUHS)

Answer

Classification of Food Based on Functions

Food class	Food group	Functions
Energy rich foods	• Carbohydrates and fats • Whole grains, cereals, millets, nuts • Vegetable oils, ghee, butter • Sugars	• Source of energy to the body and brain • Supplies half the daily requirement for proteins and calories • Sweetens the food, increases the palatability • Also act as source of vitamin A
Body building foods	• Proteins • Pulses, nuts and oilseeds • Milk and milk products • Meat, fish and poultry	• Provides proteins for growth and maintenance • Provides vitamin B complex such as thiamine, niacin and riboflavin • Also a source of calcium
Protective foods	• Vitamins and minerals • Green leafy vegetables • Other vegetables and fruits • Eggs, milk, milk products and flesh foods.	• Serve as a source of antioxidants, fibres and carotenoids • Are sweet and provide sweetness to food • Act as source of proteins.

7. What is balanced diet and bland diet ? Write a note on elements of balanced diet. (MGR, RUHS, KUHS)

Answer

Balanced Diet

- Also known as prudent diet
- Defined as diet containing different types of foods possessing the various nutrients in required amount and proper proportions to meet the body requirements.
- **Various nutrients include:**
  - Carbohydrates
  - Fats
  - Proteins
  - Vitamins and minerals
  - Fiber
  - Water

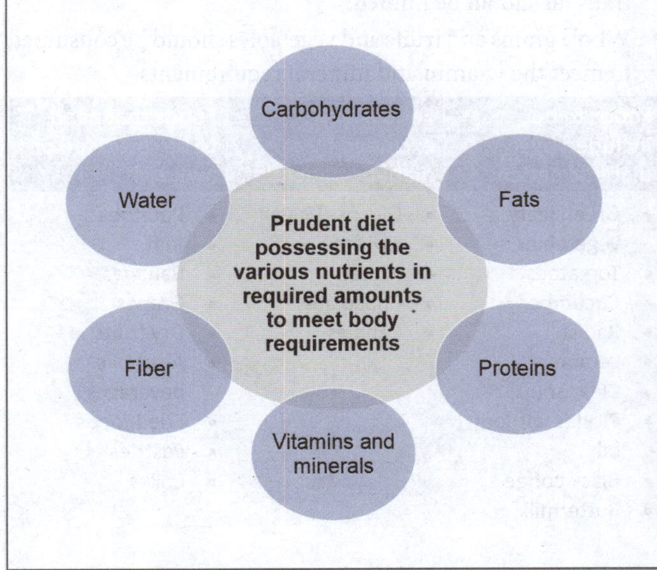

Balanced Diet Should Provide

- 50–60% calories from carbohydrates
- 10–15% calories from proteins
- 20–30% calories from fats

Bland Diet

- Consists of easily digested foods that do not irritate the gastrointestinal tract.
- It is useful for patients with gastric problems such as peptic ulcers.
- Bland diet doesn't include the following foods:
  - Fried foods
  - Highly seasoned food
  - Coarse food
  - Alcohol
  - Tea, coffee
  - Carbonated drinks

Elements of Balanced Diet

Six major elements form the basis of all nutritional requirements.

Carbohydrates	Major source of energy. Derived from whole grains, fruits and vegetables. Should provide 45–60% of energy needs.
Fats	Helps in insulation of the body and maintenance of body temperature. Mainly of two types – saturated and unsaturated. Provides 15–30% of the body's energy needs.

Contd...

Proteins	Responsible for growth and repair of the body. Important role in maintaining water, pH balance and immune system. Provides 10–15% of the body's energy needs.
Vitamins	Required for various important metabolic reactions. Two types – fat and water soluble.
Minerals	Responsible for growth and development of the body. Maintenance of water and electrolyte balance. Two types – macro and micro minerals.
Water	Major nutritional element Acts as solvent and regulates body temperature, provides lubrication to joints.

8. Write a note on daily requirement and functions of fiber/roughage. (KUHS)

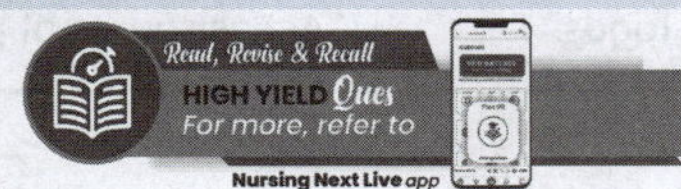

Answer

Introduction

- Complex carbohydrates
- Nondigestible by human enzymes

Sources and Classification of Dietary Fibers

Classification	Description	Sources
Soluble fibers	• Fermentable fiber/ prebiotic fiber • Dissolves in water • Generally viscous • Delays gastric emptying	• Beta glucans – oats, barley mushrooms • Psyllium • Inulin
Insoluble fibers	• Does not dissolve in water • Inert to digestive enzymes • Provides bulk to the food.	• Wheat bran • Cellulose • Lignin

Daily Requirement of Fiber (g/day)

Age	Males	Females
<2 years	19	19
2–8 years	25	25
9–15 years	31	31
16–50 years	38	25
>50 years	30	21

Role of Fiber

- Dietary fiber comprises carbohydrates (pectin, cellulose, hemicellulose) and noncarbohydrates (lignin) in plant food resistant to endogenous digestive enzymes of human gastrointestinal tract.
- It increases volume and softens consistency of stool (low fiber diet leads to constipation).
- It decreases the glycemic response (rise in postprandial glucose) to an oral carbohydrate meal.
- It lowers atherosclerosis (decreasing total serum cholesterol and LDL and increasing HDL) and CHD.
- It has a protective role against cancer, especially cancer colon, stomach, breast, prostate.
- It has a role in weight reduction.
- It has a role in management of irritable bowel syndrome and recurrent diverticulis.

9. Write a menu plan for a sedentary diabetic patient. (KUHS)

Answer

Introduction

Diabetes mellitus is characterized by the decreased ability or complete inability of tissues to utilize carbohydrates, accompanied by changes in the metabolism of fat, proteins, electrolytes and water. It arises due to deficiency of insulin, a hormone secreted by pancreas.

Essential Consideration in Diabetic Patient Diet

- Reduce the intake of calories, helps to reduce weight.
- Limit refined carbohydrates like wheat bread, pasta, rice, soda, packed foods.
- Add high fiber complex carbohydrates.
- Proteins from plant sources should be included.
- Intake of fried foods and other foods high in saturated and trans fat should be limited.
- Whole grains and fruits and vegetables should be consumed to meet the vitamin and mineral requirements.

Foods to be included by a diabetic patient	Foods to be excluded by a diabetic patient	Foods that need to be restricted or avoided
• Green leafy vegetables • Tomatoes • Cucumber • Radish • Lemon • Clear soup • Pickles without oil • Black coffee • Buttermilk	• Glucose/Sugar • Sweets • Honey • Chocolates • Candies	• Potatoes • Jam • Bananas • Grapes • Dry fruits • Alcoholic beverages • Fried foods • Pastries • Cakes

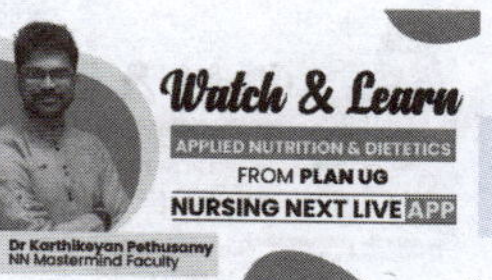

One Day Menu Plan for Diabetic Patient

Table 7.2: One-day menu plan for diabetic patient

Meal	Foodstuff	Quantity in sedentary worker	Quantity in moderate worker	Quantity in heavy worker
Early morning	Lemon water	1 cup	1 cup	1 cup
	Lemon tea	1 cup	1 cup	1 cup
	Toned milk	1 cup	1 cup	2 cup
Breakfast	Bread slices	2 slices	2	2 slices
	Missi roti	1	1	1
	Curd (200 g)	1 katori	1 katori	1 katori
	Butter	—	—	10 g
	Fruit citrus	1	1	1
Mid–morning	Sprouted dals	30 g	30 g	30 g
	Black gram	30 g	30 g	30 g
	Roasted channa	30 g	30 g	30 g
Lunch/Dinner	Salad	1 plate	1 plate	1 plate
	Diabetic chapati	1	2	3
	Green leafy vegetables	1 katori	1 katori	1 katori
	Dal or chicken	1 katori	1 katori	1 katori
	Tea	1 cup	1 cup	1 cup
Evening Tea	Bran biscuits or	2	2	4
	Paneer	30 g	30 g	30 g

Daily Nutrient Requirement of Sedentary Diabetic Patient

Nutrients	
Calories	1300 kcal
Protein	60 g
Carbohydrates	170 g
Fat	33 g

10. Prescribe a balanced diet for a preschool child. (KUHS)

Answer

Balanced Diet for a Preschool Child

- Preschool/Toddlers: 1–3 years of age
- Points to be kept in mind for preparing a meal for toddlers are:
  - Avoid mixing of food
  - Let child identify what they are eating
  - Add color and variety to food
  - Like nutritious food in all food groups
  - Vegetables can be served raw and cut as finger foods

Table 7.3: Menu plan of a day for child 3–5-year-old

Time	Food	Amount
8–9 am	Cooked cereal-dal preparation	2–3 spoons
	Or	
	Idli	1–2 idlis
	Bread with butter	1–2 slices
	Or	
	Puffed whole ragi with milk	Small amount
	Soft boiled, poached or scrambled	1 egg
	Or	
	Boiled dals	
10:30 am	Boiled milk (cow, buffalo)	1 spoon
	Fruit juice	1½ tumbler
	Or	1½ tumbler
12:30–1 pm	Fresh seasonal fruit	
	Cooked rice	One serving
	Or	2–4 spoons
	Wheat or ragi chapati	
	Boiled potato, sweet potato or tapioca (occasionally)	1–2 chapatis
	Curd or milk	Small portion
	Cooked green leafy or green vegetable	½ tumbler
	Or	½ spoon
3–4 pm	Raw vegetable salad three times a week in place of cooked vegetable	1½-2 spoons ½ tumbler
7–8 pm	Boiled milk (cow, buffalo)	1 teaspoon
	Fish liver oil	2–3 spoons
	Cooked cereal like suji, broken wheat or ragi porridge	2 spoons
	Boiled dal, fish or meat preparation	
	Boiled milk (at bed time)	½ tumbler

11. RDA for a lactating women doing moderate work. (KUHS)

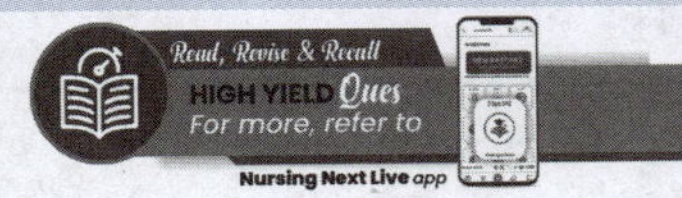

Answer

Guidelines for Meal Planning of Nursing/ Lactating Mothers

- Proteins – 70 g/day
- Fluids – water, milk, fruit juices and soups should be added.
- Calories – increased by 400–600 calories/day
- DHA – important for baby's visual and mental development.
- Iron – Add iron rich foods such as legumes, pulses, egg, red meat, etc.
- Vitamin D and calcium rich foods such as tuna, salmon, milk and milk products should be included.
- Lactating mothers should eat at least three nutritious meals a day
- Avoid sugar and fat rich foods, alcohol and smoking.

Table 7.4: Vegetarian diet for Nursing Mother doing moderate work

Food group	Quantity in (g)
Cereals and millets	330
Milk	500
Green leafy vegetables	150
Root and tubers	100
Other vegetables	100
Pulses	90
Fruits	200
Fats and oils	30
Sugar	20

For nonvegetarians, substitute 30 g of pulse with 50 g of meat/ fish/chicken/eggs.

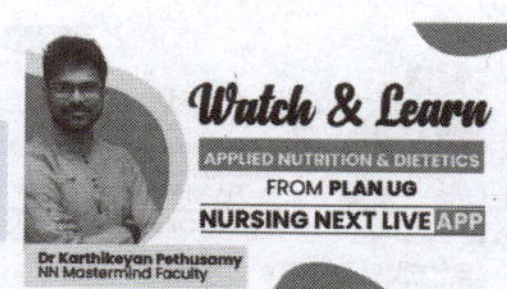

12. Write a note on nutritional problems during adolescence. (KUHS)

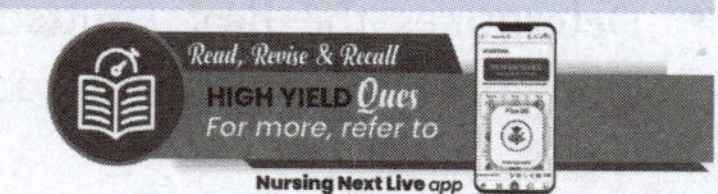

Answer

Factors Effecting Adolescent Food Choices

- Nutrition education
- Perceived body image
- Time constraints
- Social and cultural differences
- Lack of family guidance
- Mass media
- Peer pressure

Nutritional Problems During Adolescence

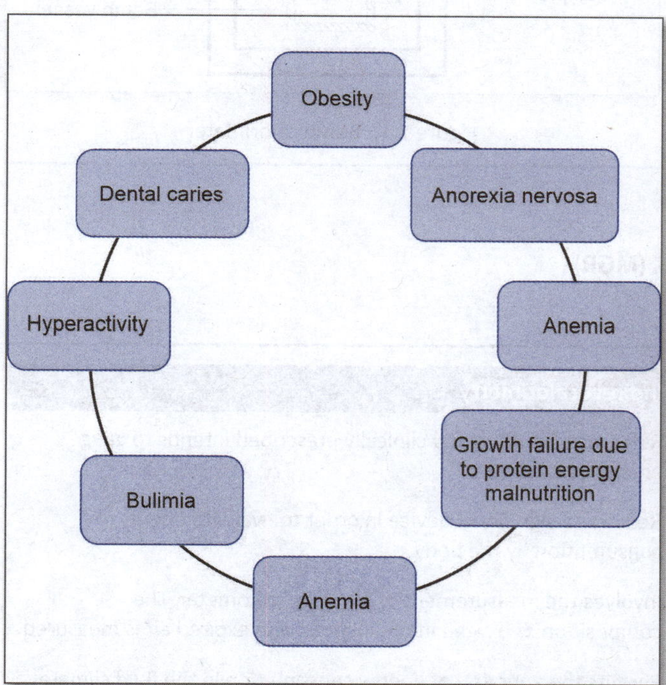

Obesity	Calorie rich foods are consumed in greater quantities and more frequently.
Underweight	Detected by height and weight. More emphasizes is given to slimness More susceptibility to infections.
Anorexia nervosa	Physiological disorder seen in adolescent females. Leads to self-starving Characterized by extreme weight loss. Symptoms include amenorrhea, constipation, hypotension, bradycardia.
Bulimia	Characterized by episodes of bulk eating followed by self-induced vomiting.
Anemia	Common in children who consume less green leafy vegetables. Supplementary iron therapy is effective
Dental Caries	Develops due to deficiency of protein, calcium, fluorides, etc. and poor oral hygiene.
Hyperactivity	Seen in adolescence. Diet free of additives, artificial flavoring is beneficial.

13. Write a short note on weaning. (MGR, KUHS)

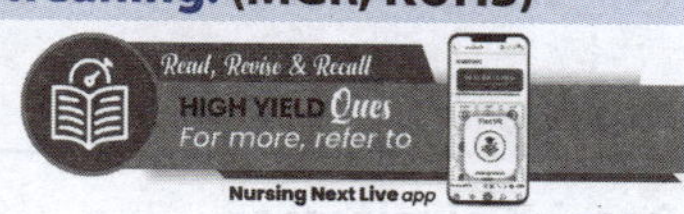

Answer

Weaning

- Process of gradually introducing food other than breast milk in the child's feeding schedule.
- Fully weaned – when the baby is no longer fed with breast milk.
- Concentrated, dense energy complementary foods are essential for maintenance of adequate velocity of growth.

Table 7.5: Progress of weaning from 6 months to 1 year of infant's life

6 months → 1 year		
Smooth/pureed	Mashed	Chopped
First food	Add more taste and texture	Add 3 meals + snacks
Baby rice + breast milk Mashed banana, cooked apple and pear Mashed and cooked carrots and sweet potato Sticks of soft/ cooked fruit or cooked vegetable	Milk mixed with wheat cereals + breast milk Cooked pasta/rice/ noodles Hard boiled eggs Mashed beans, peas Yogurt/cheese Soft ripe fruit and vegetables Bread or chapatti	Porridge and chopped banana Finger toast with cheese Full fat yogurt Rice pudding Cottage pie and green beans

Principles of Weaning

- Start weaning at the age of 6 months
- Introduce one food item at a time
- At proper time, introduce feeding with a cup
- Avoid highly allergic foods

Recommendations on Weaning: WHO and UNICEF

- Start with liquids, then gradually shift to semi-solid and then to solid foods.

Contd...

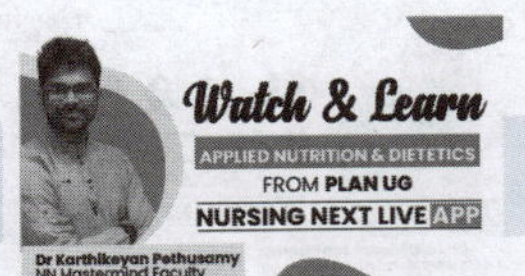

- Foods rich in iron should be added.
- Increase the zinc intake by adding zinc containing foods such as dairy products, wheat and rice.
- Start with smaller portions and gradually increase according to need and requirement of child.
- Food should not be fried or spicy.
- Add variety to child's diet.
- If child dislikes a particular food, remove that item from the diet and reintroduce sometime later.

14. Write a note on Bomb calorimeter. (MGR)

Answer

Bomb Calorimeter

- Constant volume calorimeter
- For determination of energy changes during a reaction
- Measures the heat of reaction at a fixed volume – change in internal energy
- Determines the calorific values of solid and liquid fuels.
- Bomb calorimeter gets its name from the strong steel shell known as a bomb.

Uses of Bomb Calorimeter

- Determines the heat emitted from a given quantity of biomass sample combustion and calculate the HHV of that fuel.
- The calorific value of food can be measured by heating a pre measured mass of food and igniting it in an oxygen atmosphere.

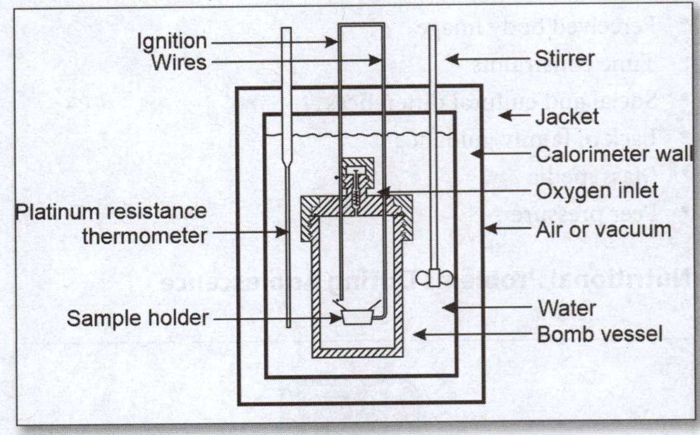

Figure 7.1: Bomb calorimeter

15. Differentiate between Direct and indirect calorimetry. (MGR)

Answer

Direct calorimetry	Indirect calorimetry
Direct measure of the heat produced by the body.	Reference standard and clinically prescribed intends to gauge energy consumption.
Requires proper equipment to determine it.	Requires a significant device in order to evaluate energy consumption by the body.
Involves placing the individual inside an insulated chamber and directly measuring the temperature rise of known mass of water.	Involves the measurement of air using spirometer. The composition of oxygen in the inspired and expired air is measured.
Most precise technique to evaluate the metabolic rate.	Permits the appraisal of energy consumption in the field climate.
Its major disadvantage is the requirement of complex designing and requirement of proper spaces.	Its major disadvantage is that it can't quantify energy creation by anaerobic cycles.
It is expensive.	It is less expensive as compared to direct calorimetry.

16. Write a note on energy nutrients. (MGR)

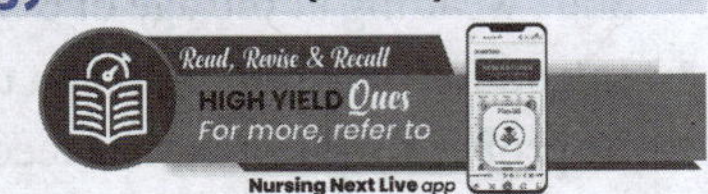

Answer

Energy Nutrients

- These include the energy rich foods, i.e., carbohydrates and fats and proteins.
- These are usually known as macronutrients
- These are needed in large quantities and provide most of the energy requirements of the body.
- The amount of energy provided by these nutrients is measured in calories.

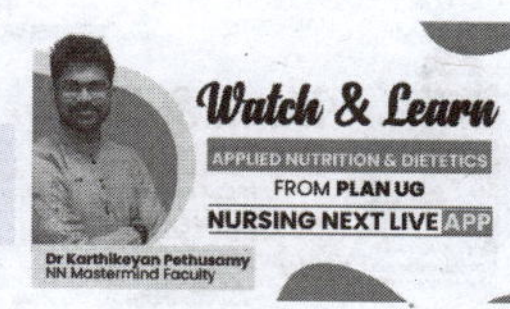

Table 7.6: Types of energy nutrients

	Carbohydrates	Fats	Proteins
Definition	Major source of energy	Also known as lipids	Building blocks of body tissues
Types	Monosaccharides Oligosaccharides Polysaccharides	Saturated fats Unsaturated fats	Essential amino acids Nonessential amino acids
Calorific value of carbohydrates	4 calories	9 calories	4 calories
Recommended daily allowance	130 g Provides for 45–65% of the body's daily energy needs.	About 60 g	50 g
Sources	Cereals, millets, roots, tubers, pulses, sugar, jaggery	Ghee, oil	Meat, egg, cheese, fish, pulses, beans, cereals.

17. Discuss the dietary modifications in elderly. (MGR)

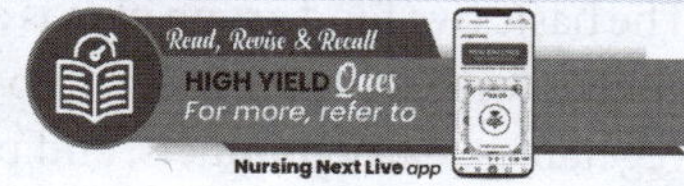

Answer

Introduction

- Old age – period that starts at a point when active contribution by a person is no longer possible.
- More vulnerable to malnutrition.
- Irreversible biological change.

Changes in Elderly Persons that Lead to Nutritional Insufficiency

- Different body organs lose their capacity to work efficiently.
- Loss of senses.
- Decline in neuromuscular communication.
- Anorexia or loss of appetite.
- Slowly down of digestion.
- Decline in lean body mass that leads to reduced metabolic rate.
- Financial constraints.

Dietary modifications in elderly

Energy requirements	Decline with age Is about 2100–2330 kcal/day in 60 + males and 1800–1900 kcal/day in 60 + females.
Proteins	Slightly lower in elderly men - 53.3 g/day as compared to 55.5 g/day Increases in women after 50 years of age to 46 g/day as compared to 45 g/day
Vitamin D	Due to reduced exposure to sunlight, chances of deficiency are increased. Add vitamin D rich foods in their diet.
Calcium	Age related bone loss can be decreased with the help of sufficient calcium in diet. Recommended intake of calcium per day is 700 mg in adults over 50-year-old.
Vitamin C	RDA of vitamin C is same as in young individuals
Iron	Requirement of iron in females is less. Iron absorption decreases from the stomach.
Fiber	Increase fiber content to aid in digestion.
Salt and fats	Elderly have many underlying medical conditions, so preferably reduce salt and fats in diet.
Fluids	Drink plenty of fluids. Avoid alcohol

Contd...

18. Menu plan for school going child. (MGR)

Answer

Meal Planning for School Going Children

- More variety is required.
- Good snacking options are required.
- Choking is an important concern, particularly in younger ones.
- All children up to the age of 10 years need to eat every 4–6 hours which helps to keep the blood sugar level at desirable level.
- Meals and snacks should be good source of calcium, iron and zinc.

Table 7.7: Menu plan of a day for school going child

Food groups	Quantity (g)		
	7–9 years	10–12 years	
		Boys	Girls
Cereals and millets	270	330	270
Pulses	60	60	60
Milk (mL)	500	500	500
Roots and tubers	100	100	100
Green leafy vegetables	100	100	100
Other vegetables	100	100	100
Fruits	100	100	100
Sugar	30	35	30
Fats/oils (visible)	25	25	25

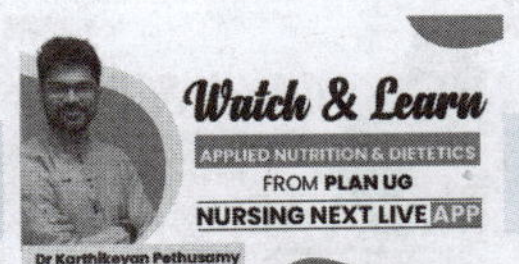

19. Write a note on RDA. (RUHS)

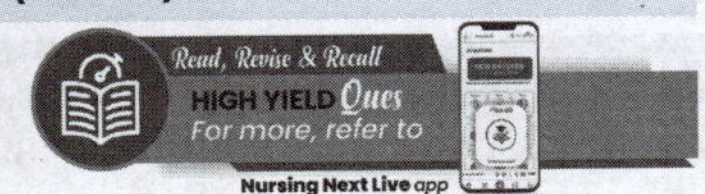

Answer

RDA (Recommended Dietary Allowance)

- Amount of nutrient and calorie intake per day considered necessary for maintenance of good health.
- Calculated for males and females of various ages and recommended by the Food and Nutrition Board of National research council.

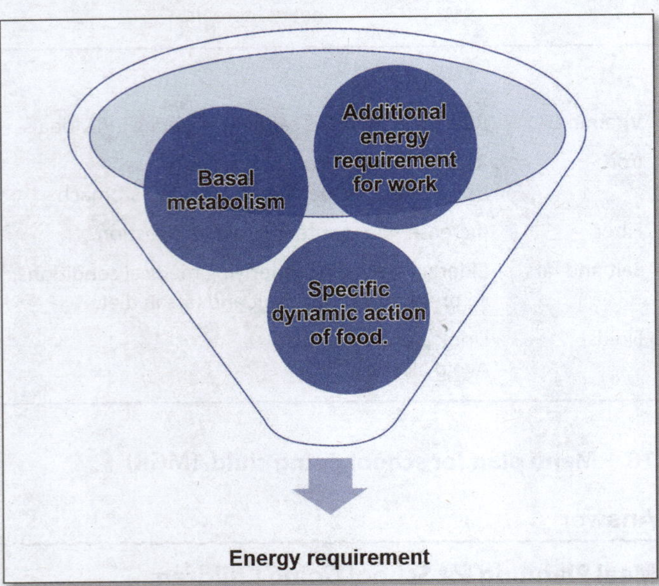

- Total energy requirement of an individual is mainly up of three components.
- Its requirement during work can be calculated by adding together the energy requirement for:
  - Basal metabolism
  - Additional energy requirement for work
  - Specific dynamic action of food.

Energy Requirement (RDA)

- Adult man doing sedentary work – 2400 kcal.
- Adult women doing sedentary work – 1900 kcal.

SHORT ANSWER QUESTIONS

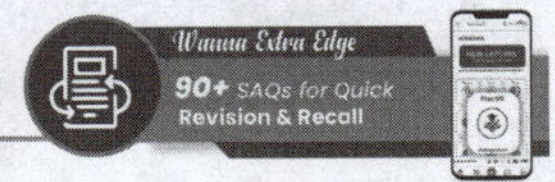

1. Define balanced diet with example. (MGR)

Answer

A balanced diet is one that has all the food items required in appropriate proportions to meet the body's nutritional needs. Example of protein food includes, meat, eggs, fish, beans, nuts, and legumes.

2. Define nutritional status.

Answer

Nutritional status has been defined as an individual's health condition as it is influenced by the intake and utilization of nutrients (Todhunter, 1970).

The optimal nutritional status should be attained by consuming sufficient, but not excessive, sources of energy, essential nutrients, and other food components (such as dietary fiber) not containing toxins or contaminants.

3. List out the basic five food group plan. (MGR)

Answer

The basic five food group plan is a straightforward and popular system for classifying foods into several groups. grains, fruits, vegetables, dairy products, and proteins.

4. Sources and classification of dietary fibres. (MGR)

Answer

There are two types of dietary fibers that is soluble (oats, apple, orange, carrot, broccoli and nuts) and insoluble (whole grains, brans and edible seeds).

5. Enlist the sources of fat soluble vitamins.

Answer

Sources of fat soluble vitamins are -Eggs, shrimp, fish, fortified milk, sweet potatoes, carrots, pumpkins, spinach, mangoes, beef, liver, fortified milk and cereals.

6. Write the classification of food.

Answer

Food is classified into five groups according to their functions in the human body.

These are:

1. **Protein food group:** Includes Milk, Pulses, Nuts, Legumes, Eggs, Meat, Fish and poultry
2. **Primary protective vegetables and fruit group:** Foods rich in beta carotene, vitamin C and green leafy vegetables
3. **Secondary protective food and vegetable groups:** Provide minerals, vitamins and dietary fiber
4. **Cereals and millet or grain group:** Supplies half of the daily requirement of proteins and calories.
5. **Oil, fat and sugar group:** Provide energy and increases the palatability of the food.

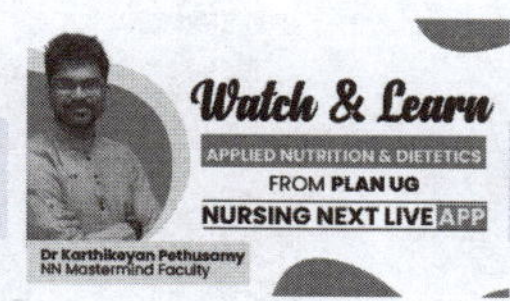

7. What is the energy requirement (RDA) for an adult man and adult women doing sedentary work?

Answer

- Adult man doing sedentary work – 2400 kcal
- Adult women doing sedentary work – 1900 kcal

8. Define dietary fibre. Enumerate sources and classification of dietary fibers.

Answer

Dietary Fibers

Dietary fiber are nutrients in the diet that are not digested by gastrointestinal enzymes but still plays an important role.

Sources and classification of dietary fibers

Classification	Sources
Soluble fibers	• Beta glucans – oats, barley mushrooms • Psyllium • Inulin
Insoluble fibers	• Wheat bran • Cellulose • Lignin

CONCEPTUAL REVISION

MULTIPLE CHOICE QUESTIONS

1. Which of the following food groups should be included in a balanced diet?

a. Carbohydrates b. Proteins
c. Fats d. All of these

Ans. d. All of these

2. Which of the following is an example of a good source of carbohydrates?

a. White bread b. Brown rice
c. Fried potatoes d. Sugary drinks

Ans. b. Brown rice

3. Which of the following nutrients is essential for the growth and repair of tissues in the body?

a. Carbohydrates b. Proteins
c. Fats d. Vitamins

Ans. b. Proteins

4. Which of the following is an example of a good source of healthy fats?

a. Fried chicken b. Butter
c. Avocado d. Bacon

Ans. c. Avocado

5. Which of the following vitamins is essential for the absorption of calcium in the body?

a. Vitamin A b. Vitamin B_{12}
c. Vitamin C d. Vitamin D

Ans. d. Vitamin D

6. Which of the following minerals is important for the proper functioning of the thyroid gland?

a. Iron b. Zinc
c. Iodine d. Calcium

Ans. c. Iodine

7. Which of the following is a good source of vitamin C?

a. Oranges b. Milk
c. Eggs d. Fish

Ans. a. Oranges

8. Which of the following is a good source of iron?

a. Spinach b. White bread
c. Cheese d. Soft drinks

Ans. a. Spinach

CHAPTER

8

Nutritional Deficiency Disorder

CONCEPTUAL THEORY

Terminology

150+ key terminologies for Quick Recall & Revision

Kwashiorkor: It is a form of severe Protein energy malnutrition (PEM). The main symptoms of Kwashiorkor are pitting edema, irritability, anorexia, distended and enlarged liver with fatty infiltrates.

Marasmic kwashiorkor: Children suffering from the disease show the signs of both kwashiorkor and marasmus. They are severely underweight but also have edema.

Marasmus: Marasmus results from severe deficiency of proteins and calories in the diet. It is due to continuous restriction of every intake. The important features are growth retardation and severe wasting of muscles and loss of subcutaneous fat.

Obesity: The generalized accumulation of excess adipose tissue in the body.

Protein energy malnutrition (PEM): A wasting condition resulting from a diet inadequate in either protein or energy or both.

PROTEIN ENERGY MALNUTRITION

Malnutrition

Malnutrition is the condition resulting from dietary nutrient deficiency, excess or imbalance of nutrients.

Two Types

Under nutrition: Refers to deficiency of calories/nutrients

Over nutrition: Refers to excess of nutrients, usually calories

Marasmus and Kwashiorkor – Protein Energy Malnutrition

- Nutritional disorder
- Seen in developing countries
- Mostly seen in young children and infants

SEVERE ACUTE MALNUTRITION

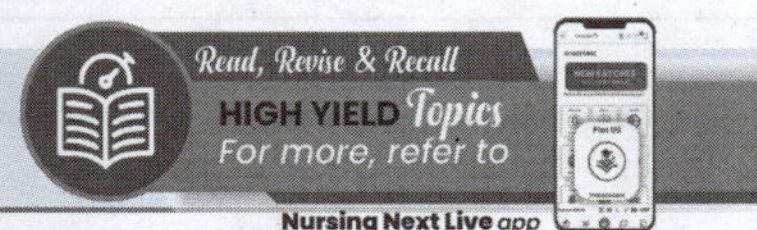

Severe acute malnutrition (SAM) is defined by a very low weight for height (below – 3 z scores of the median WHO Growth Standards), by visible severe wasting, or by the presence of nutritional edema characterized by swollen feet, face and limbs. It is the most extreme and visible form of undernutrition. About two–thirds of these children live in Asia and almost one third live in Africa. It is a life–threatening condition requiring urgent treatment.

CHILDHOOD OBESITY

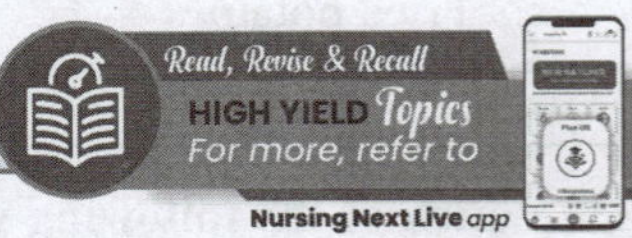

- State of being overweight in children and adolescents.
- Due to excessive body fat.
- Obese children are above the normal weight for their age and height.
- More likely to be obese in adulthood as well.
- Females > Males

Causes of Obesity

- Excess consumption of calories
- Lack of physical activity
- Viral infection (adenovirus–36)
- Hereditary reasons (gene responsible is ob gene expressed in white adipose tissue)
- Leptin defects – body weight regulatory hormone

Obesity and Adipose Tissue

- Increase in both size and number of adipocytes in adipose tissue

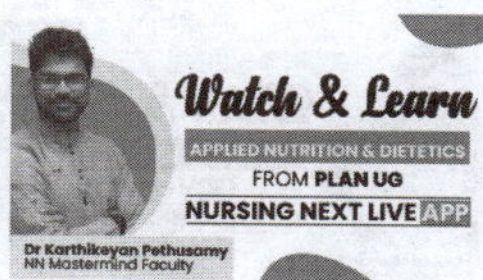

- Two types of adipose tissue:
  1. **Brown:**
     - Less fat
     - More metabolically active
     - More mitochondria
     - More diet induced thermogenesis
     - Present in hibernating animals and newborns
     - Absent in obese individuals
  2. **White:**
     - More fat
     - Less metabolically active

Obesity Indicators

Clinical obesity is measured by
- Body mass index (BMI)
- BMI (kg/m^2) is calculated as weight in kgs divided by (height in meters)^2
  - Reference Range for BMI
    - 18.5–24.9 kg/m^2 - healthy
  - 25–30 – grade I obese
    - >30 – grade II obese or clinical obesity
    - >40 – grade III obese or morbid obesity
- Waist hip ratio – more effective
  - Ratio between waist size and hip size
  - <0.9 – men
  - <0.85 – women
- Lower the waist hip ratio – lower the risk of heart diseases

VITAMIN DEFICIENCY DISORDERS

Vitamins	Deficiency disorders
Vitamin A	Xerophthalmia, bitot's spots
Vitamin B1 (Thiamine)	Beriberi
Vitamin B2 (Riboflavin)	Dermatitis, angular stomatitis
Vitamin B3 (Niacin)	Pellagra
Vitamin B12	Pernicious anemia, irreversible nerve damage
Vitamin C	Scurvy
Folic acid	Macrocytic anemia
Vitamin D	Rickets, Osteomalacia

MINERAL DEFICIENCY DISEASES

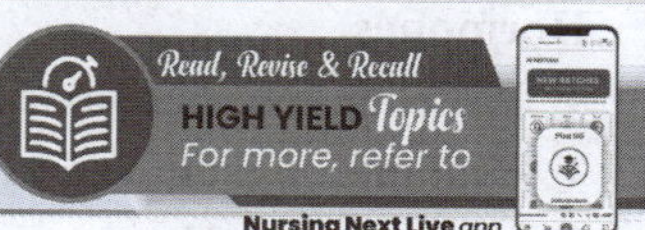

Mineral	Deficiency disorders
Calcium	Decreased bone mineralization, rickets, osteomalcia
Iodine	Goiter, iodine deficiency disorders, birth defects
Zinc	Genetic disorders, impaired growth, decreased resistance to infectious diseases
Fluoride	Increased dental decay
Selenium	Cardiomyopathy, increased risk of cardiovascular diseases
Chromium	Impaired glucose tolerance, peripheral neuropathy
Iron	Anemia, decreased alertness
Magnesium	Increased cholesterolemia, decreased clotting factors

CONCEPTUAL EXERCISES

LONG ANSWER QUESTION

1. Classification, function, dietary sources and deficiency disorder of proteins. (RUHS)

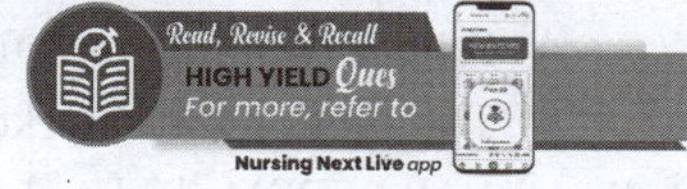

Answer

Introduction

- Protein is defined as a macromolecule composed of one or more polypeptide chains, each with a characteristic sequence of amino acids linked by peptide bonds and is essential for muscle mass.
- It accounts for about 16% of body weight.
- It contains carbon, hydrogen, oxygen and nitrogen as well.
- These are responsible for the body's growth, maintenance and repair.
- **Classification of Proteins:** Structural classification:
  - **Fibrous proteins:** These proteins have a long, elongated shape and provide structural support. Examples include collagen and keratin.
  - **Globular proteins:** These proteins have a compact, spherical shape and are involved in various biological functions. Examples include enzymes, antibodies, and hormones.
  - **Derived proteins:** These are proteins that have been modified by chemical or enzymatic processes. They are often more soluble than their parent proteins and have different properties. Examples of derived proteins include denatured proteins, peptides, and glycoproteins.

Functions of Proteins

- **Structural proteins**
  - Part of the connective tissue, cartilage, tendons and bones.
  - Mainly fibrous proteins.
  - Insoluble in water.
  - Example – Collagen, Elastin, Keratin.
- **Enzymes**
  - Biological catalysts.
  - Reduces the activation energy of reactants.
  - Mostly globular conjugated proteins.
  - Example – DNA polymerase, Lipase.
- **Hormones**
  - Proteinaceous hormones.
  - Example – Insulin, ACH, Glucagon.
- **Respiratory proteins**
  - Conjugated Proteins containing chrome as prosthetic group.
  - Example – Hemoglobin, Myoglobin.
- **Transport proteins**
  - Transport materials in cells.
  - Form channels in plasma membrane.
  - Example – Transferrin, Albumin.
- **Contractile proteins**
  - Part of the muscle.
  - Example – Actin, Myosin.
- **Storage proteins**
  - Act as storage form of metal ions and amino acids.
  - Example – Ferritin, Casein, Gluten.
- **Toxins**
  - Toxic in nature.
  - Example – Snake Venom.

Dietary Sources of Proteins

- Animal sources
  - Animal products are rich sources of proteins. It has a balanced combination of all the amino acids, hence known as complete protein.
  - Important sources include:
    - Meat
    - Egg
    - Milk
    - Cheese
    - Fish
  - Egg protein is the best protein due to its high biological value and digestibility.
- Vegetable sources
  - Plant protein is incomplete except soybean proteins.
  - Incomplete protein is deficient in one or more of the essential amino acids.
  - Important sources include:
    - Pulses
    - Beans
    - Cereals
    - Nuts
    - Oilseeds

Daily Requirement of Protein

The recommended daily allowances for proteins are as follows:

- Average men – 60 g/day
- Average women – 55 g/day
- Lactating women – additional 25 g/day
- Children – 22–40 g/day
- Adolescent boy – 70 g/day
- Adolescent girl – 65 g/day

Deficiency of Proteins

- Deficiency of proteins for longer periods may lead to weight loss, anemia, nutritional edema, low resistance to infection and poor healing of wounds.
- As there is continuous protein building as well as degradation in human body for its normal functions, their regular optimal intake is very essential for keeping good health.
- Protein deficiency diseases occur in developing countries due to poverty as well as lack of knowledge about nutritional needs.
  - Protein energy malnutrition:
    - Clinical disorders resulting from deficiency of proteins and energy.
    - Primarily occurs in young children.
    - Two types – kwashiorkor and marasmus.

1. **Kwashiorkor:** PEM that is characterized by a deficiency of protein.
2. **Marasmus:** PEM that is characterized by a deficiency of both protein and energy.

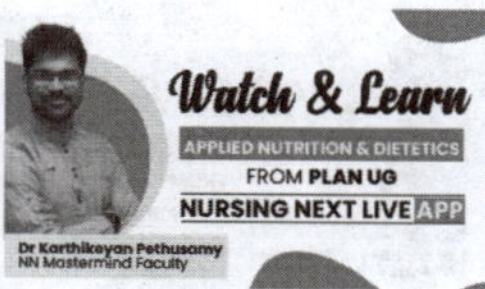

Discuss about Protein Energy Malnutrition

	Marasmus	Kwashiokor
Introduction	Marasumus – meaning to waste	Protein calorie malnutrition
Etiology	Deficiency of calories, insufficient intake of proteins, fats and carbohydrates due to failed breastfeeding, feeding inadequate infant formula or suffering from some disease like diarrhea	Insufficient intake of proteins, due to weaned from mother's milk to a diet low in protein
Symptoms	Large belly sticking out, diarrhea, change in skin pigment, muscle wasting, diarrhea, growth retardation, fatigue, hair changes, etc.	Peeling and alternately pigmented skin, hair loss, edema or swelling, skin folds are formed, etc.
Age of onset	Generally, children under age of 1	Generally, children of age 1– 5 years
Muscle wastage	Yes	No
Bloating of abdomen	No	Yes
Biochemical findings	Serum albumin 2–3 mg/dL Increased serum cortisol	Serum albumin less than 2 mg/dL Decreased serum cortisol
Treatment	Providing a nutritious, well-balanced diet with lots of fresh fruits and vegetables, grains, and protein. Especially adding vitamin B to the diet.	Providing carbohydrates followed by high protein foods. Dried milk specially

SHORT NOTES

1. Write a note on pellagra. (MGR, RUHS)

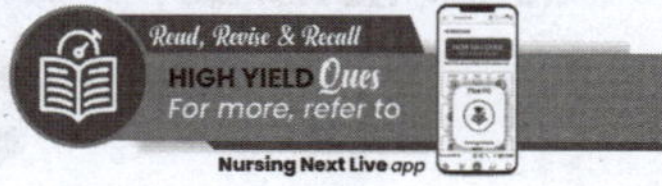

Answer

Pellagra

- Also known as rough skin.
- Involves skin, gastrointestinal tract and central nervous system
- **Symptoms include 3 Ds**
  - Dermatitis
    - Inflammation of skin
    - Occurs in sun exposed areas
  - Diarrhea
    - Loose stools often with blood and mucus
  - Dementia
    - Degeneration of nervous tissues
    - Symptoms include
      - Anxiety
      - Irritability
      - Memory loss
      - Insomnia
  - Death (4th D)

Causes

- Seen in people whose staple diet is corn or maize.
- Mainly due to deficiency of niacin and tryptophan
- Other factors include:
  - Deficiency of riboflavin or pyridoxine
- Seen in Women > Men due to inhibition of tryptophan metabolism by estrogen metabolism

Management

- Consumption of food rich in niacin such as:
  - Liver
  - Yeast
  - Whole grains
  - Cereals
  - Beans
  - Peanuts

2. Describe the deficiency manifestation of thiamine. (MGR, KUHS)

Answer

Thiamine is a water soluble vitamin. It is also known as vitamin B1 or Anti beriberi vitamin or Antineuritic vitamin.

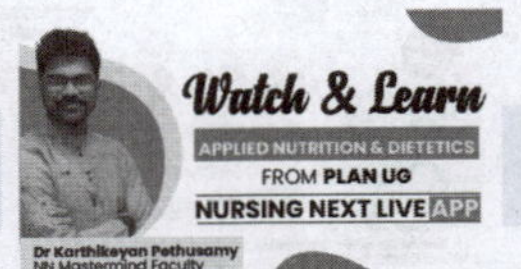

Recommended Daily Allowance

- Adults – 1-1.5 mg/day
- Children – 0.7 – 1.2 mg/day
- Pregnancy and lactation, old age, alcoholism – 2 mg/day

Deficiency Symptoms

Beriberi

- Seen in exclusively polished rice consumers
- **Types**
  - Wet beriberi – affects the heart and circulatory system.
  - Dry beriberi – affects the nerves and muscles
- **Symptoms**
  - Loss of appetite
  - Weakness
  - Constipation
  - Nausea
  - Decreased muscle function
  - Mental depression
  - Peripheral neuropathy
  - Numbness in legs
- **Biochemical changes in B1 deficiency**
  - Impaired carbohydrate metabolism. Pyruvate accumulates in tissues and is excreted in urine.
  - Blood brain barrier is altered and pyruvate is able to cross the BBB. Pyruvate accumulation in brain results in polyneuritis.
  - Due to lack of TPP, nerve impulse transmission is impaired.
  - Decreased activity of transketolase in RBCs is seen.

Wernicke-Korsakoff Syndrome

- Also known as cerebral beriberi
- Seen in chronic alcoholism
- Due to increased demands in alcoholism
- **Characteristics**
  - Loss of memory
  - Apathy
  - Rhythmical to and fro motion of eye balls

3. Write a short note on Scurvy. (MGR, RUHS, DU, KUHS)

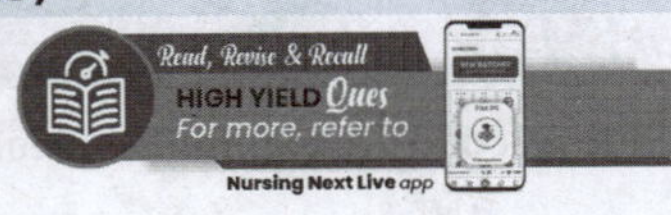

Answer

Definition	• Occurs due to deficiency of a water-soluble vitamin – vitamin C • Also known as ascorbic acid
Clinical characteristics	• Sore gums • Loose teeth • Anemia • Swollen joints • Fragile blood vessels • Decreased immunocompetence • Delayed wound healing • Osteoporosis
Etiology	• Defective collagen synthesis • Impairment in the antioxidant property of vitamin C
Management	• Including vitamin C rich foods such as: • Citrus fruits • Gooseberry (Amla) • Guava, green vegetables, tomatoes • Adrenal glands, gonads • Milk – poor source
Infantile scurvy – Barlow's disease	Occurs in infants aged 6–12 months

4. Discuss about Protein Energy Malnutrition. (MGR, KUHS, DU)

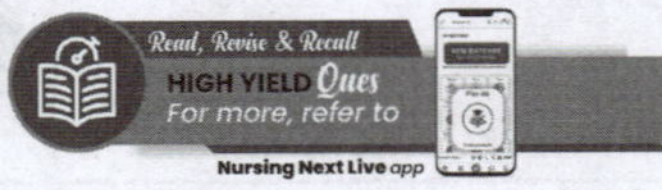

Answer

Introduction

Protein-energy malnutrition (PEM) is a condition that occurs when the body does not get enough protein or energy (calories) to meet its needs.

This can lead to a number of health problems, including growth retardation, weight loss, impaired immunity, and increased risk of death.

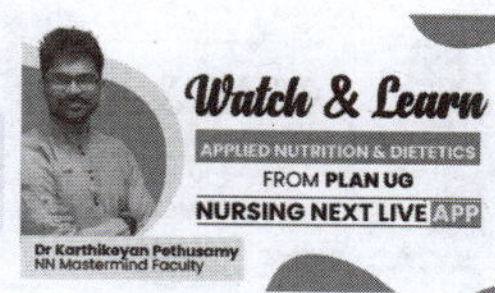

Mostly seen in young children and infants PEM can be classified into two main types:

1. **Kwashiorkar:** PEM that is characterized by a deficiency of protein.
2. **Marasmus:** PEM that is characterized by a deficiency of both protein and energy.

	Marasmus	Kwashiokor
Introduction	Marasumus – meaning to waste	Protein calorie malnutrition
Etiology	Deficiency of calories, insufficient intake of proteins, fats and carbohydrates due to failed breastfeeding, feeding inadequate infant formula or suffering from some disease like diarrhea	Insufficient intake of proteins, due to weaned from mother's milk to a diet low in protein
Symptoms	Large belly sticking out, diarrhea, change in skin pigment, muscle wasting, diarrhea, growth retardation, fatigue, hair changes, etc.	Peeling and alternately pigmented skin, hair loss, edema or swelling, skin folds are formed, etc.
Age of onset	Generally, children under age of 1	Generally, children of age 1 – 5 years
Muscle wastage	Yes	No
Bloating of abdomen	No	Yes
Biochemical findings	Serum albumin 2–3 mg/dL Increased serum cortisol	Serum albumin less than 2 mg/dL Decreased serum cortisol
Treatment	Providing a nutritious, well-balanced diet with lots of fresh fruits and vegetables, grains, and protein. Especially adding vitamin B to the diet.	Providing carbohydrates followed by high protein foods. Dried milk specially

5. Distinguish between overweight and obesity. (MGR, KUHS)

Answer

Differences between overweight and obesity

	Overweight	Obesity
Definition	Condition where a person weighs more than normal for his particular age, height and sex	Disease marked by excessive fat deposition
BMI	Between 25 and 29.9	Over 30
Associated risks	Depression, hypertension	Cardiovascular diseases, diabetes
Causes	Excess intake of calories than required, reduced or no physical activity	Excessive intake of calories through junk foods, etc, stress, hormonal imbalance, sedentary lifestyle
Occurrence	About a billion	>300 million
Management	Lifestyle modifications, reduced intake of food	Reduce calories, exercise, surgical options

6. Write a short note on Obesity. (MGR, KUHS)

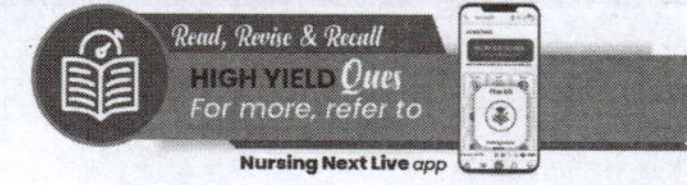

Answer

Obesity

- State of being overweight is termed obesity.
- Result due to excessive body fat.
- Associated with number of diseases
    - Type II diabetes
    - Cardiovascular disease
    - Hypertension
    - Arthritis
    - Stroke

Causes of Obesity

- Excess consumption of calories
- Lack of physical activity
- Viral infection (adenovirus–36)

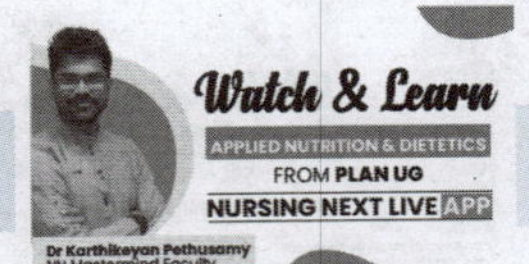

- Hereditary reasons (gene responsible is of gene expressed in white adipose tissue)
- Leptin defects – body weight regulatory hormone

Obesity and Adipose Tissue

- Increase in both size and number of adipocytes in adipose tissue
- Two types of adipose tissue:
  1. Brown:
     - Less fat
     - More metabolically active
     - More mitochondria
     - More diet induced thermogenesis
     - Present in hibernating animals and newborns
     - Absent in obese individuals
  2. White:
     - More fat
     - Less metabolically active

Obesity Indicators

Clinical obesity is measured by

- Body mass index (BMI)
- BMI (kg/m^2) is calculated as weight in kgs divided by (height in meters)^2
  - Reference Range for BMI
    - 18.5-24.9 kg/m^2 - healthy
    - 25–30 – grade I obese
    - >30 – grade II obese or clinical obesity
    - >40 – grade III obese or morbid obesity
- **Waist hip ratio – more effective**
  - Ratio between waist size and hip size
  - <0.9 – men
  - <0.85 – women
  - Lower the waist hip ratio – lower the risk of heart diseases

Treatment of Obesity

- Diet control
- Exercise
- Pharmacological interventions
- Synthetic lipids like Olestra and Orlistat

7. What measures can be taken for prevention of Iron deficiency anemia among adolescent girls? (KUHS)

Answer

Dietary Advice for an Adolescent girl for Prevention of Anemia

- Iron requirement increases in the adolescent girls due to the onset of menstruation. Increased demands are also present due to pubertal growth spurts. Thus, anemia is very common in this age group, if proper diet is not given.
- Foods that are rich in iron should be included:
  - Liver (richest)
  - Heart
  - Kidney
  - Leafy vegetables
  - Pulses
  - Cereals
  - Fish
  - Apples
  - Dried fruits
  - Molasses
  - Jaggery
- Poor sources—milk, wheat, polished rice.

Prophylactic dose and regime for iron folic acid supplementation

Weekly provide 1 tablet of iron and folic acid. Each tablet contains 60 mg elemental iron + 500 mcg folic acid.

Anemia Management Protocol for Adolescents

Table 8.1: Anemia management protocol for adolescents

Target group	All school-going adolescents 10–19 years in government/government-aided schools
Who will screen and place of screening	In school premises by RSBK team
Periodicity	Annually
Mild and moderate anemia	
First level of treatment (at all levels of care)	Two IFA tablets (each with 60 mg elemental iron and 500 mcg folic acid), once daily, for 3 months, orally after meals.

Contd...

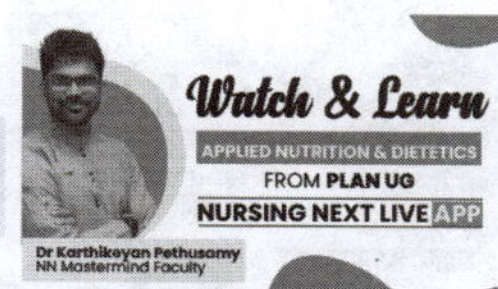

Target group	All school-going adolescents 10–19 years in government/government-aided schools
Follow-up	• Line listing of all anemic cases to be maintained in the school register for Iron Folic Acid supplementation and given to the ANM/LHV/MPHW of designated area • Follow-up by ANM/LHV/MPHW of designated area, as feasible for the state • Parents to ensure follow-up of adolescent after 45–90 days at the nearest sub-center/ health facility • If hemoglobin levels have improved to normal level, discontinue the treatment, but continue with the prophylactic IFA dose
If no improvement after first level of treatment	If no improvement after three months of treatment (i.e., still in mild/moderate category), ANM/MO of nearest facility to refer adolescent to First Referral Unit (FRU)/District Hospital (DH)
If Hemoglobin is <8 g/dL (severe anemia)	
First dose of treatment	Management of severe anemia in adolescents 10–19 years is to be done by the medical officer at FRU/DH based on investigation and subsequent diagnosis

8. Write a note on beriberi. (MGR)

Answer

Introduction	• Caused by a vitamin B_1 (thiamine) deficiency • Seen in persons consuming exclusively polished rice
Types	• Wet beriberi affects the heart and circulatory system. • Dry beriberi – affects the nerves and muscles
Symptoms	• Loss of appetite • Weakness • Constipation • Nausea • Decreased muscle function • Mental depression • Peripheral neuropathy • Numbness in legs
Etiology	• Female gender • Increasing age • Family history • White or Asian ethnicity • Small stature • Early menopause • Excess alcohol intake • Cigarette smoking
Management	• Diet Therapy • Weight bearing exercises • Decrease risk factors

9. What are the deficiency manifestations of vitamin K and clinical features of Vitamin-D deficiency? (MGR)

Answer

Vitamin K

- Fat soluble vitamin
- Specific coenzyme function
- Required for production of blood clotting factors
- Essential for coagulation

Deficiency of Vitamin K

- Uncommon
- Causes
  - Faulty absorption
  - Diarrheal diseases

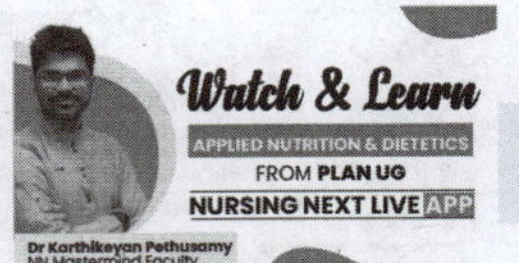

    - Over administration of antibiotics
- Leads to
    - Lack of active prothrombin
    - Defective blood coagulation
    - Blood clotting time is increased
- Newborns have sterile intestines and so initially lack the bacteria that synthesize vitamin K.
- Because human milk provides only about one fifth of the daily requirement for vitamin K, it is recommended that all newborns receive a single intramuscular dose of vitamin K as prophylaxis against hemorrhagic disease.

Vitamin D

- Vitamin D – fat soluble vitamin
- Functions like hormone
- Derived from ergocalciferol and cholecalciferol
- Biosynthesized from cholesterol on exposure to sunlight – sunshine vitamin
- Antirachitic vitamin

Clinical Features of Vitamin D Deficiency

Rickets in the children	Osteomalacia in adults
• Bone deformities • Due to incomplete mineralization • Delayed tooth eruption • Bow legs • Elevated alkaline phosphatase activity	• Demineralization of bones • Increased susceptibility to fracture

10. Differentiate between osteomalacia and osteoporosis. (MGR)

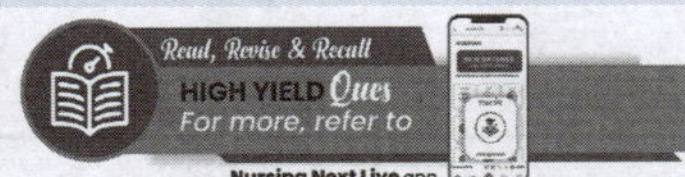

Answer

Differentiating Features between Osteomalacia and Osteoporosis

	Osteomalacia	Osteoporosis
Definition	• Bone disease characterized by defective mineralization of bone and impaired bone metabolism. • Occurs due to deficiency of phosphate, calcium and vitamin D.	• Systemic skeletal disorder • More common in elderly. • Chronic pain • More common in elderly and post menopausal women.
Clinical characteristics	• Generalized bone condition in which there is inadequate mineralization of bone. • Patients usually present with: ▪ Diffuse joint and bone pain – symmetrical and non-radiating pain ▪ Muscle weakness ▪ Hypocalcemia ▪ Pelvic flattening ▪ Tendency to fracture	• Low bone mass • Deterioration of bone tissue • Increased bone fragility • Increased risk of fractures
Causes	• Insufficient calcium absorption ▪ This may be due to: ◆ Inadequate dietary calcium intake ◆ Inadequate calcium absorption due to deficiency of vitamin D or any celiac disease • Deficiency of phosphate ▪ This may be due to increased renal excretion	• Main reason for the imbalance between the bone resorption and the bone formation. • In a normal bone, a balance between the bone formation and resorption occurs which leads to matrix remodeling of the bone. • Mechanisms leading to osteoporosis are: ▪ Excessive bone resorption ▪ Inadequate formation of new bone ▪ Inadequate mineralization • Hormones such as parathyroid hormone and calcitonin play a role in the pathogenesis of calcium metabolism and vitamin D. • Deficiency of calcium and vitamin D levels leads to impaired bone deposition. • Parathormone increases bone resorption leading to increased calcium levels in blood. • Calcitonin increases bone deposition. • Balance between parathormone and calcitonin maintains the calcium metabolism and bone health.
Management	Vitamin D_3 supplementation and calcium supplementation	Exercise and lifestyle modifications

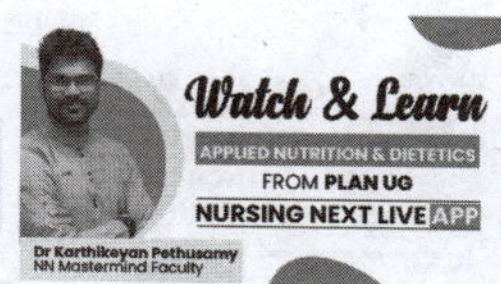

11. Mention the clinical symptoms of hypokalemia and hyponatremia. (MGR)

Answer

Clinical Symptoms of Hypokalemia and Hyponatremia

Hypokalemia	Hyponatremia
• Decreased serum potassium concentration • Potassium concentration is below <3.5 mEq/L	• Serum sodium levels falls below normal. • Serum sodium concentration of <135 mEq/L
Manifestations • Nausea • Vomiting • Chest pain • Respiratory distress/weakness • Decreased strength/cardiac contractility • ECG changes (prolonged PR, wide QRS) • Reflexes (hyper or areflexia)	**Manifestations** • Hypotension • Circulatory failure • Seizures • Lethargy • Altered mental status • Muscle cramps

12. Discuss the management of moderate acute malnutrition (MAM). (DU)

Answer

Moderate Acute Malnutrition (MAM)

- Defined as the weight for height Z score between –2 and –3
- Mid upper arm circumference (MUAC) between 115 and 125 millimeters
- Results in the loss of body mass relative to height.

Management of MAM

- This can be broadly categorized into prevention and treatment strategies.

Prevention strategies	Treatment strategies
• Promotion of breastfeeding and complementary feeding practices • Improving equitable access to health services • Improved access to quality food • Improved sanitation and hygiene practices • Use of supplements to augment the home diet.	• Early detection and recognition of malnutrition • Use of highly fortified ready to use foods at home (RUTFs) • Diagnosis of underlying systemic illness or infections. • Counselling to the caregivers and decision making framework for selecting appropriate supplementary feeding.

13. Describe functions, sources and deficiency problems of vitamin B_6. (DU)

Answer

Vitamin B_6

- Vitamin B_6, also known as pyridoxine, is a water-soluble vitamin
- Available in three forms:
  1. Pyridoxine
  2. Pyridoxal
  3. Pyridoxamine

- **Functions:**
  - Important for the metabolism of fat, carbohydrates and proteins.
  - Promote red blood cell production.
  - Maintenance of normal nerve function.
  - Production of antibodies to fight against many diseases.
  - Deficiency of vitamin B6 can cause anemia because it helps in the production of hemoglobin and hemoglobin carries oxygen in the red blood cells to the tissues.
- **Sources:**
  - Fish

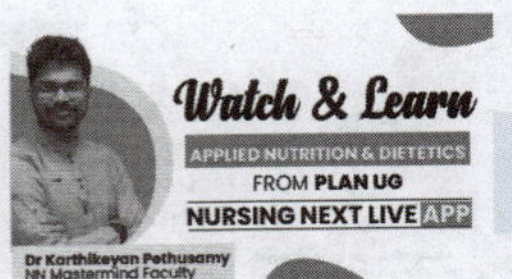

- Beef, liver and other organ meats
- Whole cereals
- Legumes, oil seeds, nuts
- Eggs, milk, green leafy vegetables
- **Deficiency Manifestations:**
  - Muscle weakness
  - Depression
  - Irritability
  - Short-term memory loss
  - Nervousness
  - Difficulty in concentration
  - Risk of heart disease
  - Peripheral neuritis
  - Convulsive seizures in children

SHORT ANSWER QUESTIONS

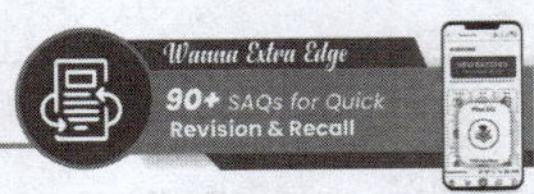

1. Distinguish between osteoporosis and osteomalacia. (MGR)

Answer

Osteoporosis is condition characterized by low bone mass, deterioration of bone tissue, and increased risk of fractures where as **Osteomalacia** a condition characterized by softening of bones due to inadequate mineralization, usually caused by vitamin D deficiency.

2. Mention the clinical symptoms of hypokalemia and hyponatremia. (MGR)

Answer

Clinical symptoms of hypokalemia: Weakness, fatigue, and muscle cramps, abnormal heart rhythms (arrhythmias), constipation, abdominal cramping or bloating.

Clinical symptoms of hyponatremia: Nausea, vomiting, and loss of appetite, headache and confusion, weakness, lethargy, and fatigue, seizures or convulsions, restlessness, irritability, and mood changes, swelling or edema, usually in extremities

3. Scurvy. (MGR)

Answer

Scurvy is a disorder caused by a significant ascorbic acid (vitamin C) deficit in the diet.

4. Define water intoxication. (MGR)

Answer

Hyponatremia, also known as water intoxication, is a disorder that develops when there is an excessive intake of water or a problem with the body's ability to expel water, which causes a dilution of sodium levels in the blood.

5. Give the clinical symptoms of iron deficiency. (MGR)

Answer

Fatigue, pale skin, brittle nails and hairs, shortness of breath, increased heart rate and pica are some of the common symptoms of iron deficiency.

6. Protein energy malnutrition. (MGR)

Answer

Protein-energy malnutrition (PEM) is a medical condition that develops when the diet contains insufficient amounts of protein and energy (calories), impairing physical and cognitive growth.

7. Write the symptoms of osteomalacia. (MGR)

Answer

Muscle weakness, bone pain, bone tenderness and deformities, risk of fracture, disturbance of gait, fatigue and weakness are common symptoms of osteomalacia.

8. Describe Bitot's spots. (MGR)

Answer

Bitot's spots are small, raised, foamy, white or grayish plaques that appear on the conjunctiva of the eyes.

9. Dental fluorosis (MGR)

Answer

Dental fluorosis is a condition that alters how teeth look because it results from consuming too much fluoride while teeth are developing, usually in childhood.

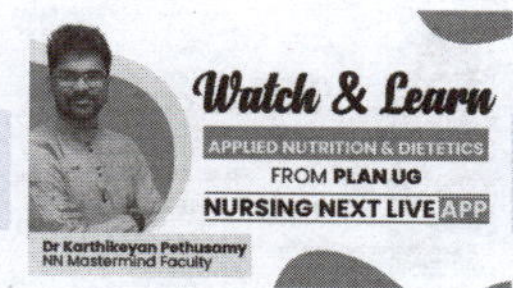

10. What is rickets? (MGR)

Answer

Rickets is a condition characterized by weak or soft bones in children, usually caused by a deficiency of vitamin D, calcium, or phosphorus.

11. Define dehydration. (MGR)

Answer

An imbalance of fluid levels occurs in the body when there is not enough water present, which is the hallmark of dehydration.

12. What is osteomalacia? (MGR)

Answer

Due to the impairment of calcium and phosphorus deposition, osteomalacia is a disorder that affects bone mineralization and causes the bones to soften and weaken.

13. What is nutritional anemia? (MGR)

Answer

Micronutrient deficits either due to inadequate intake or absorption, such as those in iron, vitamin B12, folate (vitamin B9), and vitamin C, can result in nutritional anemia.

14. Define malnutrition. (MGR)

Answer

Malnutrition is a condition when a person's nutritional status is out of balance, either as a result of insufficient intake or excessive intake of vital nutrients. That is in the form of undernutrition, overnutrition, or a combination of both.

15. Name two signs and two symptoms of PEM. (MGR)

Muscle wasting and edema are the signs of PEM and Fatigue and growth retardation are the symptoms of PEM.

16. Write two signs and two symptoms of rickets. (MGR)

Answer

Various skeletal deformities, such as bowing of the legs or knock-knees and delayed tooth eruption are the two signs and muscle weakness and pain and poor height gain are the two symptoms of rickets.

CONCEPTUAL REVISION

MULTIPLE CHOICE QUESTIONS

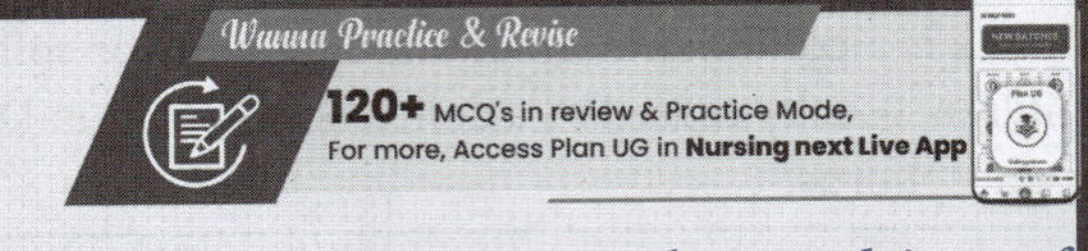

1. Marasmus disease is caused due to the deficiency of:
a. Proteins and calorie b. Proteins
c. Calorie d. None of these

Ans. a. Proteins and calorie

2. Best indicator for nutritional status for a child is:
a. Chest circumference
b. Mild arm circumference
c. Rate of increase of height and weight
d. Head circumference

Ans. c. Rate of increase of height and weight

3. What is the cut off value of mild arm circumference below which severe malnutrition is diagnosed in children up to 5 years of age?
a. 11 cm
b. 11.5 cm
c. 12 cm
d. 12.5 cm

Ans. b 11.5 cm

4. All are seen in rickets; except:
a. Cupping of metaphysis
b. Defective mineralization
c. Soft bone
d. Epiphyseal dysgenesis

Asn. d. Epiphyseal dysgenesis

5. A 5-year-old boy presents with complaints of prolonged fever for 7 days with palpable neck nodes. He also has bilateral watery eye discharge. Peelings of skin over palms are seen for the past 1 day along with macular rash over the trunk. What is the diagnosis?
a. Dengue fever b. Rubella
c. Scarlet fever d. Kawasaki disease

Ans. d. Kawasaki disease

6. Nutritional Supplementation of preterms include all; except:
a. Vitamin A at 1000 IU/day
b. Iron at 1 mg/kg
c. Calcium to phosphate ratio is 2:1
d. Vitamin E at 15 IU/day

Ans. b. Iron at 1 mg/kg

7. Chronic malnutrition is measures by:
a. Weight/age b. Weight/Height
c. Mid arm circumference d. Height/age

Ans. d. Height/age

8. In children, which disease occur due to protein deficiency.
a. Marasmus b. Kwashiorkor
c. Beriberi d. Scurvy

Ans. b. Kwashiorkor

Golden Points

- Childhood obesity is when child ideal weight for height is over then it signifies obesity.
- Children suffering from the disease marasmic kwashiorkor show the signs of both kwashiorkor and marasmus.
- Kwashiorkor is a form of severe PEM. The main symptoms of Kwashiorkor are pitting edema, irritability, anorexia, distended and enlarged liver with fatty infiltrates.
- Nurse can discuss with the parents of child early signs of childhood obesity and measures to control it at initial phase of life through activities and diet and by guiding them for healthy food items available at home in day-to-day meal planning.
- Protein deficiency diseases occur in developing countries due to poverty as well as lack of knowledge about their nutritional requirements.
- Protein energy malnutrition is a term used to describe clinical disorders, resulting from deficiency of protein and energy.
- The first indicator of PEM is underweight for age. Maintaining of growth chart (road to health) is the most practical method to detect PEM.
- The most extreme forms of malnutrition or PEM are kwashiorkor and marasmus.

CHAPTER

9

Therapeutic Diet

CONCEPTUAL THEORY

Terminology

Bland diet: A bland diet is made of foods that are soft, not very spicy and low in fiber. Mostly prescribed in patient with gastric and duodenal ulcers gastritis or ulcerative colitis.

Diarrhea: Diarrhea may be defined as the frequent passage of loose stool, watery stool and unformed stool which may also contain blood or mucus. When there is presence of mucus or blood, then the condition is known as dysentery.

Enteral nutrition: Enteral feeding is a method to provide nutrients in the gastrointestinal tract with the help of tube when oral intake is inadequate to maintain optimal nutritional status in body.

Food Allergy: Food allergy means any adverse reaction to any food. The food intolerance is an adverse, nonimmunological reaction related to chemical composition of food.

Obesity: Obesity is an abnormal growth of the adipose tissues due to an enlargement of fat cell size or an increase in fat cell number or in combination of both conditions.

Parenteral feeding: Parenteral nutrition is defined as the provision of nutrients directly into the bloodstream in the patient who cannot feed through enteral route.

Peripheral access: The feed can be infused through a peripheral intravenous catheter placed in a vein, i.e., peripheral parenteral nutrition (PPN).

Semi-liquid: The semi-liquid diet includes egg yolk, milk powder, honey, horlicks, complan, milk fruit shake and cornflakes.

Soft diet: This type of diet provides soft whole food that is likely seasoned and almost similar to the regular diet.

Total parenteral nutrition (TPN): With septic technique, catheters are inserted into the subclavian vein and continued until the catheter tip reaches the superior vena cava. TPN is also known as central access.

THERAPEUTIC DIET

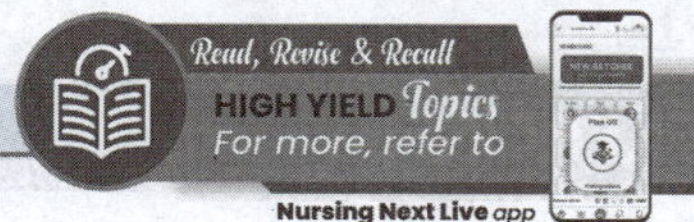

Therapeutic Diet

- Meal plan that helps to control and plan the intake of certain nutrients and food.
- It is a modification of the normal diet of the patient prescribed by a physician and planned by the dietician to supplement the medical therapy.

Objectives of Therapeutic Diet

- Correction of nutritional deficiencies caused by a disease or restoration of optimum nutritional status.
- Maintenance of good nutritional status
- Affording rest to whole body or specific affected organ in diseased condition like gastritis
- Increase/decrease or maintain weight
- Adjustment of tolerance of food intake in certain cases.
- Adjustment of mechanical difficulties in elderly or special patients.
- Alteration in diet to aid in treatment of certain diseases.

Principles of Therapeutic Diet

- To maintain good nutritional status
- To correct deficiency diseases
- To provide rest to body or specific organ
- To help metabolize the nutrients
- To make changes in body weight when necessary

Attributes in Therapeutic Diets

- Adequacy
- Accuracy
- Economy
- Palatability

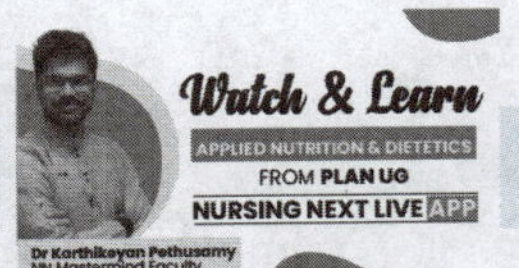

MODIFICATIONS – CONSISTENCY, NUTRIENTS

Modifications in Therapeutic Diets

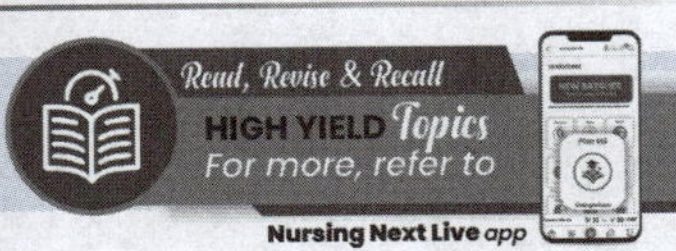

- Therapeutic diets are modified for consistency or texture to fit the nutritional needs of clients on their medical condition.
- According to nature of diet
  - Qualitative diets
    - Restriction of nutrient
    - Excess of nutrient
  - Quantitative diets
    - Change in consistency
    - Rearrangement of meals
    - Deletion/omission of nutrient
- According to consistency
  - Full clear
    - Diet consisting of clear liquids
    - Nonstimulating, nonirritating and nongas forming
    - Nutritionally inadequate
    - Can be given for short period of time (24 – 48 hours)
  - Liquid diet
    - Diet that includes all foods that are liquid or can be liquefied
    - Free from cellulose and irritating spices
    - Average composition is 1200 kcal and 35 g protein.
  - Soft and mechanical diet
    - Transitional diet between full fluid and normal diet
    - It is of soft consistency, easy to chew.
    - Contains limited fiber
    - Average composition provides 1800 kcal and 50g protein
    - Can be given in certain conditions such as elderly, edentulous
  - Balanced diet
- According to taste
  - Bland diet
    - Diet made up of soft foods, non-spicy and low fiber
    - Nonirritating to GI tract
    - Prescribed in patients with gastric or peptic ulcers
- According to modification in nutrients
  - Modifications are made in diet to treat deficiencies or treat diseases
- According to modification in meal frequency
  - Small and frequent meals.
  - Modified meal frequency is useful in GERD patients.

FEEDING TECHNIQUES

Different techniques used in hospitals for different diseases, include:

- **Tube Feeding**
  - Tube feedings (nutrition support) are used for people, who cannot take adequate food or fluid by mouth.
  - The tube may be passed through the nose into the stomach (nasogastric), duodenum (nasoduodenal) or jejunum (nasojejunal). When there is an obstruction in the esophagus, enteral feeding is done by passing a tube surgically through an incision in the abdominal wall into the stomach (gastrostomy), duodenum (duodenostomy) or jejunum (jejunostomy).
- **Total Parenteral Nutrition (TPN)**
  - The delivery of nutrients directly into the circulation through the peripheral or central vein is termed parenteral nutrition. This technique is used for long term purpose. In this method, a cannula is inserted in large veins to reach superior vena cava in the heart.

CONCEPTUAL EXERCISES

LONG ANSWER QUESTIONS

1. a. Enumerate the etiology of hypertension.
b. Discuss the dietary management.
c. Write the foods to be included and avoided in hypertension. (KUHS, MGR)

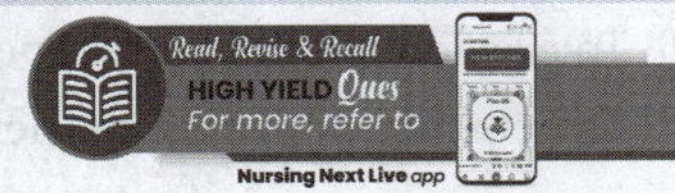

Answer

Hypertension

- Increase in systemic arterial blood pressure is known as hypertension.
- Systolic blood pressure >140 mm Hg, Diastolic blood pressure >90 mm Hg.

Etiology of Hypertension:

Genetic Factors:

- **Lifestyle factors** diet, physical activity, obesity,
- Increased age
- Secondary to medical conditions: E.g. Kidney disease, cardiovascular conditions, endocrine disorders.
- Stress

b. Dietary management of hypertensive patient

Answer

Energy requirement – 1600 kcal

Fat – 40 g

Protein – 65 g

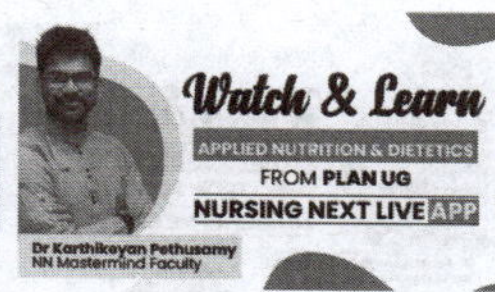

Table 9.1: One-day menu plan for CV diseases

Meal	Food stuff	Quantity
Early morning (Breakfast)		
	Lemon water	1 glass
	Milk (skimmed)	1 cup 200 mL
	Sugar	1 tsp
	Missi roti or stuffed roti	1
	Curd	½ katori
	Boiled egg (white)	1–2
Mid-morning	Bread	1–2 slices
	Fresh fruits	1
Lunch		
	Salad	150 g
	Chapati	2–3 (30 g each)
	Rice	60 g (raw)
	Vegetable	250 g
	Curd	1 katori (200 g)
Evening tea		
	Tea	1 cup
	Sugar	1 tsp
	Biscuits	3–4
Dinner	Vegetable soup	1 cup
	Chapati	2 (30 g each)
	Vegetables	250 g
	Dal sabot	1 katori
	Paneer	50 g
	Chicken or fish	100 g
	Whole day's cooking oil	20 g

c. **Write the foods to be included and avoided in hypertension. (KUHS, MGR)**

Answer

Foods to be included and Avoided in Hypertension

Foods recommended in hypertension	Foods avoided in hypertension
• Skimmed milk, paneer from skimmed milk • Cereals and pulses • Whole grains • Vegetables and all fruits • High fiber diet • Egg white and fish • Vegetable oil, sugar and jaggery	• Cholesterol rich food • Fat containing food, e.g., cheese, butter and cream, etc. • Indian sweet meals • Egg yolk, fish • Organ meat such as liver • Alcohol • Fried food

2. What is therapeutic diet? Write briefly on modifications in therapeutic diet (MGR)

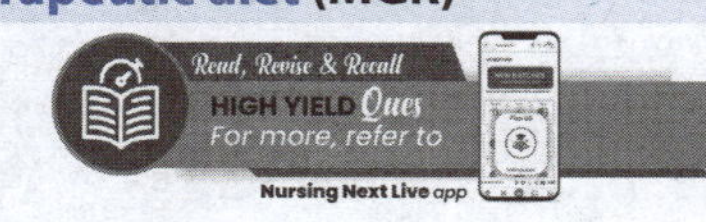

Answer

Therapeutic Diet

- Meal plan that helps to control and plan the intake of certain nutrients and food.
- It is a modification of the normal diet of the patient prescribed by a physician and planned by the dietician to supplement the medical therapy.

Objectives of therapeutic diet

- Correction of nutritional deficiencies caused by a disease or restoration of optimum nutritional status.
- Maintenance of good nutritional status
- Affording rest to whole body or specific affected organ in diseased condition like gastritis
- Increase/decrease or maintain weight
- Adjustment of tolerance of food intake in certain cases.
- Adjustment of mechanical difficulties in elderly or special patients.
- Alteration in diet to aid in treatment of certain diseases.

Modifications in Therapeutic Diets

- Therapeutic diets are modified for consistency or texture to fit the nutritional needs of clients on their medical condition.
- **According to nature of diet**

Qualitative diets	Quantitative
• Restriction of nutrient • Excess of nutrient	• Change in consistency • Rearrangement of meals • Deletion/omission of nutrient

- **According to consistency**
  - Full clear
    - Diet consisting of clear liquids
    - Nonstimulating, nonirritating and nongas forming
    - Nutritionally inadequate
    - Can be given for short period of time (24 – 48 hours)
  - Liquid diet
    - Diet that includes all foods that are liquid or can be liquefied
    - Free from cellulose and irritating spices
    - Average composition is 1200 kcal and 35 g protein.
  - Soft and mechanical diet
    - Transitional diet between full fluid and normal diet
    - It is of soft consistency, easy to chew.
    - Contains limited fiber
    - Average composition provides 1800 kcal and 50g protein
    - Can be given in certain conditions such as elderly, edentulous
  - Balanced diet
- **According to taste**
  - Bland diet
    - Diet made up of soft foods, non-spicy and low fiber
    - Non irritating to GI tract

- Prescribed in patients with gastric or peptic ulcers
- **According to modification in nutrients**
  - Modifications are made in diet to treat deficiencies or treat diseases
- **According to modification in meal frequency**
  - Small and frequent meals.
  - Modified meal frequency is useful in GERD patients.

3. Discuss the etiology and dietary management would you suggest for a patient suffering from tuberculosis. (KUHS)

Answer

Introduction

- Tuberculosis is a debilitating disease. Patients are usually malnourished and thus prone to more infections.
- Tuberculosis is caused by Mycobacterium tuberculosis.
- It usually affects the lungs, but can affect other organs as well.
- It spreads from one person to other due to air droplets.
- The common symptoms of TB include chronic cough, fever, night sweats, blood stained sputum, weight loss, etc.

Dietary Management of Tuberculosis Patient

- Nutrition status is an important determinant of the clinical outcome in tuberculosis.
- Good nutrition is necessary to boost the patient's immunity.
- Addition of ginger and garlic in the patient's diet has been found to be very beneficial.
- It is a vicious cycle – active Tb can lead to malnutrition, and poor nutrition can debilitate a TB patient and make him more prone to infections.

Dietary Modifications for a Patient Suffering from Tuberculosis

- Additional good quality protein to boost the immune system. These include dairy and dairy products, meat, eggs, legumes.
- Dietary fiber – to keep the gut healthy. These are provided by whole grains, cereals, sprouted legumes.
- Energy dense foods – to meet the increasing calorie demands for healing – examples include banana, cereal, peanuts, ragi, etc.
- Variety of fruits and vegetables to meet the demands of vitamins such as vitamin C, A, D, E and minerals like selenium, iron and zinc.
- These also provide antioxidants for the body.

Foods to be limited	Foods to be included
Oily and fried foods Trans fatty acids Refined carbohydrates Caffeine and alcohol	Protein rich diet Micronutrient intake should be increased such as vitamin A, E, C and B complex, zinc and selenium Antioxidant rich foods

SHORT NOTES

1. Write about the medicinal value of ginger and garlic.

Answer

Medical Value of Ginger and Garlic

Nutrient	Ginger	Garlic
Selenium	0.7 µg	14.2 µg
Calcium	16 mg	181 mg
Vitamin B_6	0.16 mg	1.235 mg
Manganese	0.229 mg	1.672 mg
Vitamin C	5 mg	31.2 mg
Phosphorus	34 mg	153 mg
Zinc	0.34 mg	1.16 mg
Iron	0.6 mg	1.7 mg
Magnesium	43 mg	25 mg

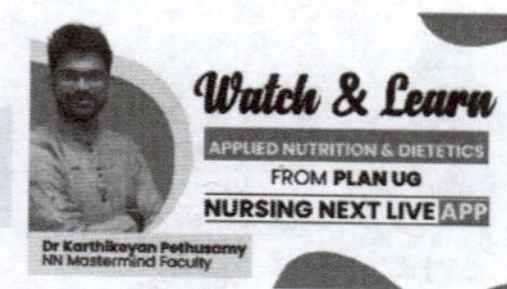

Benefits of Garlic and Ginger

Benefits of garlic	Benefits of ginger
• Provides relief from acne and asthma • Helps in digestion • Helps cure hypertension • Aids in ear aches and infections • Reduces cholesterol levels • Relieves cold and cough	• Improves blood flow • Promotes respiratory health • Improves immunity • Minimizes motion sickness and morning sickness • Aids in digestion • Decreases the risk of colon and ovarian cancer

2. Write about preoperative and postoperative diet. (DU)

Answer

Preoperative Diet	Postoperative Diet
• In case of elective surgeries, body nutrient stores can be accumulated by use of fortified diet according to the type of surgery and patient's requirements. • This helps in better wound healing and speedy recovery. • Increase the intake of proteins, energy and vitamins and minerals.	• Adequate nutritional support aids recovery from surgery • Aids in healing. • Optimal protein and energy to aid in building and healing tissues. • Sufficient fluid intake is required to prevent dehydration • Vitamin C helps in wound healing. Other important vitamins and minerals are B complex vitamins, iron, phosphorus and zinc.

3. General characteristics and nutritional importance of clear fluid, full fluid and soft diet. (DU)

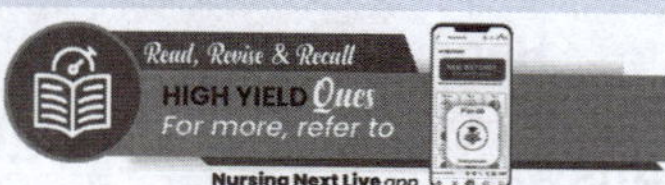

Answer

Full clear	Liquid diet	Soft and mechanical diet
• Diet consisting of clear liquids • Non stimulating, nonirritating and nongas forming • Nutritionally inadequate • Can be given for short period of time (24–48 hours)	• Diet that includes all foods that are liquid or can be liquefied • Free from cellulose and irritating spices • Average composition is 1200 kcal and 35 g protein.	• Transitional diet between full fluid and normal diet • It is of soft consistency, easy to chew. • Contains limited fiber • Average composition provides 1800 kcal and 50 g protein • Can be given in certain conditions such as elderly, edentulous

4. Write a note on food fortification. (DU, RUHS)

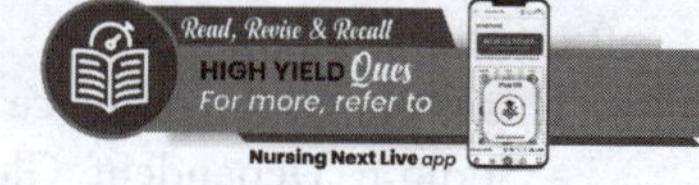

Answer

Food Fortification

Means deliberate addition of essential micronutrients in the food to increase its nutritional quality.

Advantages of Food Fortification

- Socially acceptable—as people don't need to alter their eating methods
- Doesn't affect the existing properties of the food
- Can be done on community level.

Examples

- Fluoridation of drinking water in endemic areas to prevent dental caries
- Iodization of salt
- Vitamin A fortification for preventing ocular diseases

5. Discuss the dietary management of Type 2 Diabetes mellitus. (DU, MGR, KUHS)

Answer

Essential Consideration in Diabetic Patient Diet

- Reduce the intake of calories, helps to reduce weight
- Limit refined carbohydrates like wheat bread, pasta, rice, soda, packed foods.

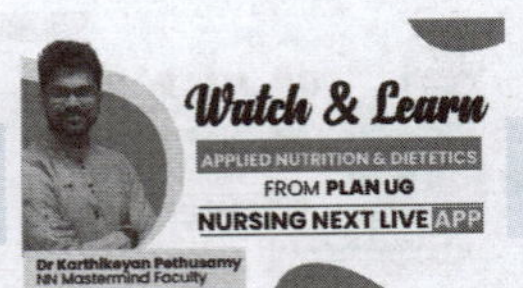

- Add high fiber complex carbohydrates
- Proteins from plant sources should be included.
- Intake of fried foods and other foods high in saturated and trans fat should be limited.
- Whole grains and fruits and vegetables should be consumed to meet the vitamin and mineral requirements.

Foods to be included by a diabetic patient	Foods to be excluded by a diabetic patient	Foods that need to be restricted or avoided
• Green leafy vegetables • Tomatoes • Cucumber • Radish • Lemon • Clear soup • Pickles without oil • Black coffee • Buttermilk	• Glucose/Sugar • Sweets • Honey • Chocolates • Candies	• Potatoes • Jam • Bananas • Grapes • Dry fruits • Alcoholic beverages • Fried foods • Pastries • Cakes

6. List the foods to be included and avoided in Hepatitis. (DU, RUHS)

Answer

Dietary Considerations in Hepatitis

- Patients with a liver disease should be given small but more frequent meals.
- Frequent feeding also improves nitrogen balance and prevents hypoglycaemia.
- Increased lipid and protein intake.
- Vitamin and mineral supplementation is required.
- Zinc, magnesium, calcium supplementation is required.

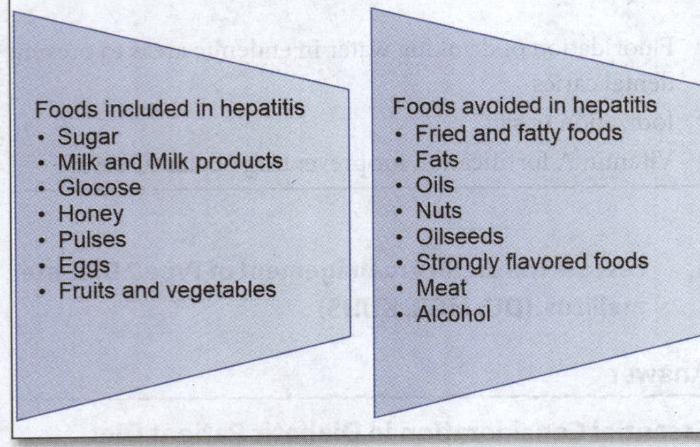

7. Discuss the dietary modification in constipation. (DU) or Foods to manage constipation (DU)

Answer

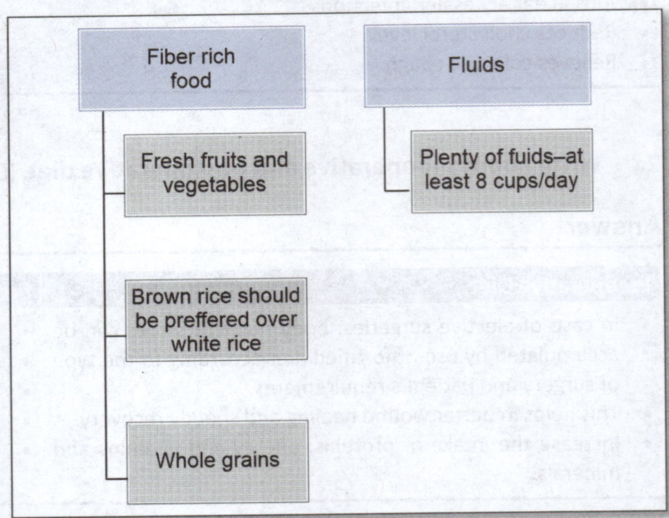

8. Oral rehydration therapy (MGR)

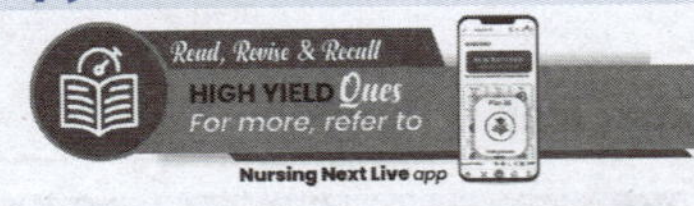

Answer

Oral Rehydration Therapy

- Given orally
- Cheap, simple, effective and noninvasive
- Involves drinking water with salts and glucose
- Fluid replacement therapy
- Does not treat diarrhea
- Replenishes fluid and electrolyte balance
- Glucose in ORT enables intestine to absorb sodium efficiently
  - This is due to the presence of Glucose and Na^+ symport – Sodium Dependent Glucose Transporter – in the intestinal mucosal cells
  - Should be taken every time the stool is passed
- Main ingredients of the oral rehydration solution (ORS) include glucose, NaCl or NaHCO, KCl and water.
- On administration of ORS, glucose and Na' are reabsorbed by the sodium-glucose transporter-1 (SGLT1) in the apical membrane of enterocytes.
- This in turn increases the osmolarity thereby favoring the absorption of water, osmotically.
- Absorption of glucose accompanied by the obligatory increase in the absorption of NaCl and water helps to compensate for the diarrheal losses of water and solutes and in turn treat dehydration.

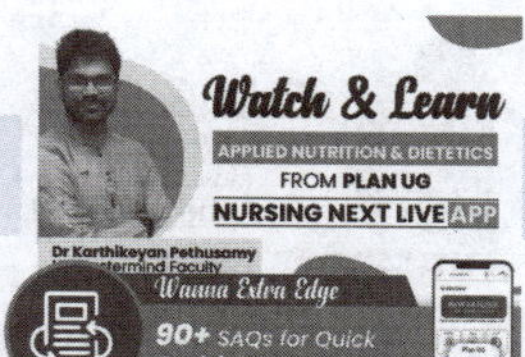

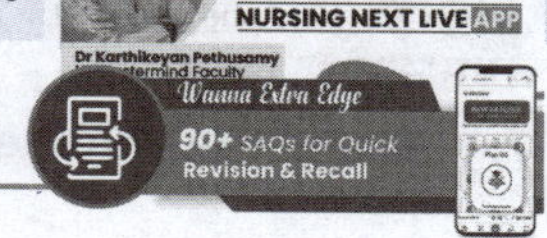

9. Write a note on fluid diet. (MGR)

Answer

Description	• Diet that consists of foods that are liquid at room temperature • These are made from fluids and foods that are normally liquid and foods that turn to liquid at room temperature. • Diet consisting of clear liquids • Nonstimulating, nonirritating and nongas forming • Nutritionally inadequate • Can be given for short period of time (24–48 hours) • Provides more calories than the clear diet.
Examples of fluid diet	• Tea • Juice • Clear soups • Pudding
Beneficial for patients with	• After surgery • Acute infections or digestive problems • In patients with vomiting, diarrhea
Disadvantages	• Nutritionally inadequate • Can be used for shorter duration

10. Planning a diet for a client who is suffering from renal disorders (RUHS)

Answer

Dietary Management in Chronic Renal Failure

When planning a diet for a client with renal disorders, it is essential to consider individualized dietary restrictions or recommendations provided by their healthcare provider.

Dietary guidelines for patient with renal disorders:

- Maintain balanced diet
- Limit Sodium Intake
- Limit potassium in diet
- Choose lean protein, e.g., chicken, fish, beans, and lentils.
- Control fluid intake—depends on the severity of renal disease.

Table 9.2: Daily nutrient requirement for chronic renal disease patient

Nutrients	Sedentary worker	Moderate worker	Heavy worker
Proteins	20 g	30 g	40 g
Calories	2,040	2,197	2,363
Sodium	180 mg	215 mg	255 mg
Potassium	1,226 mg	1,382 mg	1,982 mg
Phosphorus	441 mg	586 mg	717 mg

SHORT ANSWER QUESTIONS

1. Two types of weaning foods. (MGR)

Answer

Mashed foods and finger foods are two preferred weaning foods.

2. Give two examples of supplementary foods. (MGR)

Answer

- Vitamin and mineral supplements - vitamin D supplements, and calcium supplements
- Protein supplements - whey protein, soy protein, and pea protein supplements

3. Discuss any four factors you will consider while planning a menu. (MGR)

Answer

Four factors that should be considered while planning a menu are nutritional requirement, food preferences, seasonal availability and resources.

4. What are therapeutic diets? (MGR)

Answer

Therapeutic diets are tailored to meet the unique nutritional needs of individuals with certain health conditions, and are designed to help improve their health outcomes.

5. Name few full fluid diet. (DU)

Answer

Full fluid diets are also called clear fluid diets which include clear broth, fruit juices, clear soups, plain gelatin, ice chips and honey syrups.

6. Sources of high residual food. (DU)

Answer

High residual food sources are whole grain, legumes, fruits and vegetables as they fulfil individuals dietary needs.

7. Name the glucose tolerance factor. (KUHS)

Answer

Glucose Tolerance Factor

- Biologically active form of chromium
- Combination of trivalent chromium, amino acids and vitamins
- Has a role in regulating carbohydrate metabolism.
- Essential dietary agent that potentiates the action of insulin by:
  - Promotes strong bonding between insulin and insulin receptor
  - Stimulates the biological activity of insulin.
  - Improves the sensitivity of insulin receptors.

CONCEPTUAL REVISION

MULTIPLE CHOICE QUESTIONS

1. You are taking care of a patient with severe COPD. What type of diet would best suit this patient's needs?

a. Cut apples, fresh broccoli, and grilled chicken
b. Pureed sweet potatoes, ground turkey and gravy with mash potatoes
c. Green beans, boiled carrots, and steamed fish
d. Fried chicken, French fries, and pudding

Ans. b. Pureed sweet potatoes, ground turkey and gravy with mash potatoes

2. A patient who has a colostomy is complaining about having excess gas. You ask the patient to tell you what he has eaten in the past 48 hours. What food would you suspect is causing the patient excessive gas?

a. Cherries, radish, and watermelon
b. Caraway seeds, tomato soup, and eggs
c. Chicken, grapes, and raspberries
d. Squash, spinach, and pickles

Ans. a. Cherries, radish, and watermelon

3. A patient is diagnosed with Congestive Heart Failure and must follow a specific diet. Which spices are okay for the patient to use daily?

a. Onion salt and garlic powder
b. Ginger and bay leaves
c. Sea salt and pepper
d. Garlic sodium and nutmeg

Ans. b. Ginger and bay leaves

4. A patient with gout should follow what type of diet?

a. High-calcium diet
b. Potassium-modified diet
c. Low-purine diet
d. Renal diet

Ans. c. Low-purine diet

5. The patient is on a low potassium diet that includes food such as applesauce, green beans, cabbage, lettuce, grapes, and raspberries. What type of patient would you expect to be on this type of diet?

a. A patient with heart disease
b. A patient with osteoporosis
c. A patient with Addison's disease
d. A patient who recently had gastric bypass surgery

Ans. c. A patient with Addison's disease

6. A patient with anemia would benefit from which diet?

a. Legumes, organ meat, and dark green leafy vegetables
b. Nuts and seeds, fruits, and soy products
c. Vegetables, fish, and pasta
d. Grains, berries, and organic vegetables

Ans. a. Legumes, organ meat, and dark green leafy vegetables

7. A patient is on a lacto-ovo vegetarian diet. What type of foods can the patient eat?

a. Fish, milk, and poached eggs
b. Chicken, cheese, and grilled eggplant
c. Boiled eggs and chocolate milk
d. Oysters, yogurt, and turkey

Ans. c. Boiled eggs and chocolate milk

8. A patient is suffering from a broken jaw. Which foods would be most beneficial for this patient?

a. Carrots, fried chicken, and cereal
b. Soup, pudding, and ice cream
c. Rice, watermelon, and smoked fish
d. Tacos, peanuts, and fresh broccoli

Ans. b. Soup, pudding, and ice cream

CHAPTER

10

Cookery Rules and Preservation of Nutrients

CONCEPTUAL THEORY

Terminology

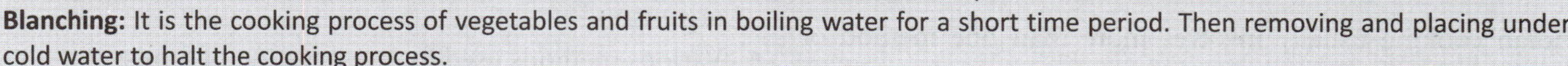

Adulteration: Inferior substances added with food or drink that are unfit for consumption.
Blanching: It is the cooking process of vegetables and fruits in boiling water for a short time period. Then removing and placing under cold water to halt the cooking process.
Carbonated water: Water into which CO_2 gas is dissolved under pressure.
Oxidation: It is effect of oxygen present in the air on food items. It changes the color and taste of food.
Pasteurization: Method of sterilization of food products such as milk, fruit juices by heating, at a specific temperature for a specific time period followed by immediate cooling and packing into an airtight container using aseptic techniques.
Preservatives: These are the substances that are added to food products to prevent growth of microorganisms.
Processed food: Transformation of raw food into other form that can be easily prepared by the consumers.
Saute: It is the method of tossing the food in a pan or cooking food in small amount of oil over high heat.
Toxins: These are the substances capable of producing harmful effects if consumed in a large amount.

COOKING—PRINCIPLES, METHODS, ADVANTAGES AND DISADVANTAGES

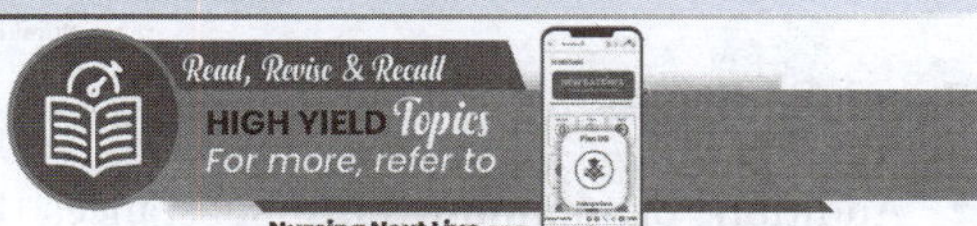

- Conversion of raw ingredients to deem it fit for consumption.
- Cooking is essential to make the food:
  - Pleasing in appearance
  - Easy to digest
  - Appealing in taste, texture
  - Enhances flavor
  - Destroys pathogenic organisms
  - Increases the nutritional value

Principles of Cooking

- Heat causes chemical, physical and biological changes in the food ingredients. In cooking, there is transfer of energy from a heat source to food.
- Transfer of energy occurs by three methods:
  - Conduction
    - Transfer of heat by direct contact.
    - Cooking pans are made up of copper and aluminum that conduct heat very efficiently.
  - Convention
    - Transfer of heat occurs through fluid.
    - The fluid may be in liquid or gaseous form.
    - This is seen in convention oven.
    - Responsible for baking, pizza, cakes, etc.
  - Radiation
    - Transfer of heat occurs through electromagnetic radiations.
    - This is seen in microwave oven that uses strong radio waves.
    - It works by spinning water, fat, sugars and oils inside the food. It causes friction which then heats the food and cooks it from inside.

Methods of Cooking

- **Moist heat method**
- In this method, the heat is conducted to the food product by water or steam.
- **Types of Moist heat method:**
  - Boiling

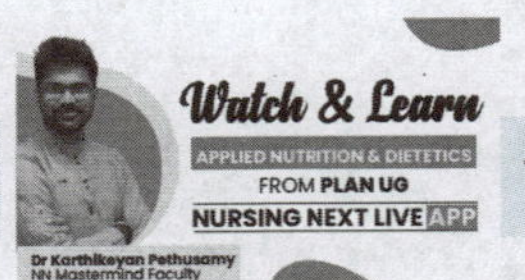

- Simmering
- Stewing
- Poaching
- Blanching
- Steaming
- Cooking by pressure cookers

Dry Heat Method

- In this method, the heat is conducted without moisture, i.e., by hot air, hot metal radiation or hot fat.
- **Types of dry heat method:**
  - Roasting and Baking
  - Broiling
  - Grilling
  - Saute
  - Frying

Combined Method

Indian cooking usually involves more than one method of cooking.

Methods of Cooking

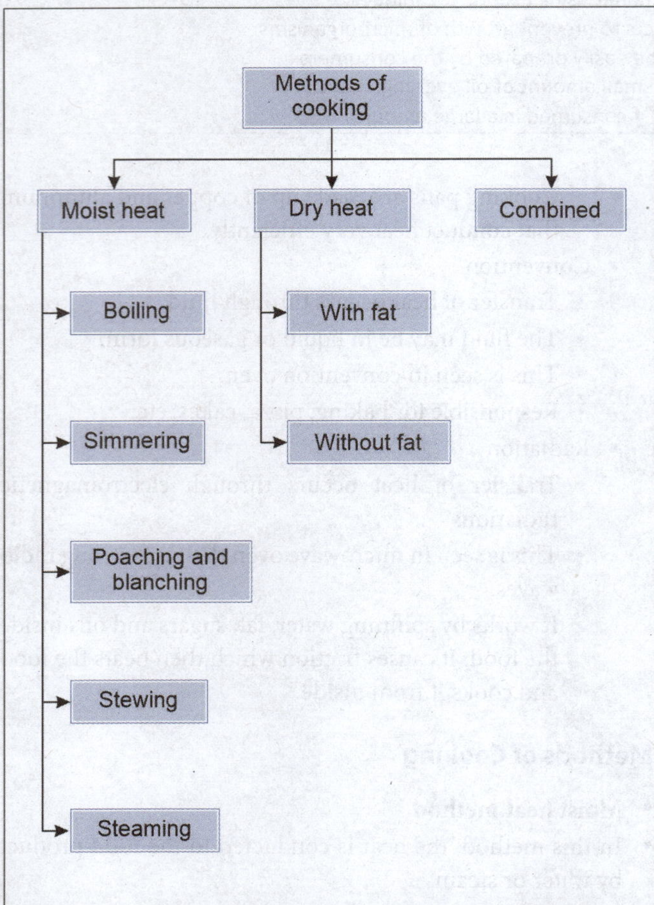

SAFE FOOD HANDLING AND STORAGE OF FOODS

Food Hygiene

- Collection of practices and guidelines to protect against the risks of foodborne illnesses caused by microbial contamination.
- Concerned with food handling, proper storage and processing of materials.
- Basic principles of good food hygiene:
  - Avoid bacterial contamination.
  - Prevent multiplication of bacteria in case it has gain access to food.

FOOD PRESERVATION

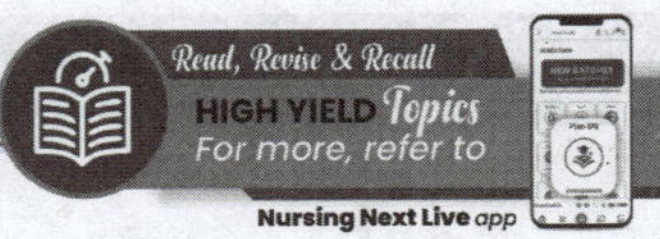

Food preservation

- Technique used to prevent food from spoiling.
- Prevents the growth of bacteria, fungi or other micro-organisms.
- Various methods used for preservation of foods:
  - Canning
  - Pickling
  - Drying
  - Freezing
  - Pasteurization
  - Smoking
  - Addition of chemicals

FOOD ADDITIVES AND FOOD ADULTERATION

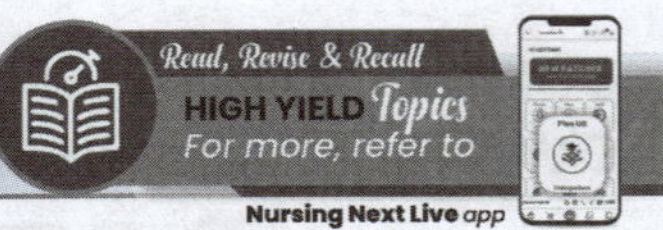

Food Additives

- Addition of nonnutritious substances that are added intentionally to food in smaller quantity to improve its appearance, texture or storage properties.
- Substances added to food to enhance or preserve its flavor, color and taste.

Food Adulteration

- Defined as a process of degrading the quality of food being sold by the addition or use of inferior quality substances or by extracting some valuable components of a food article. It is a common fraudulent practice adopted by the sellers to earn profit.
- Adulteration usually refers to mixing of any inferior or harmful quality matter with food and drink becomes unfit for human consumption.
- Prevention of food adulteration act was given in the year 1954.

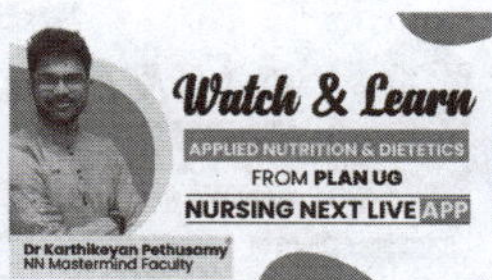

FOOD STANDARDS

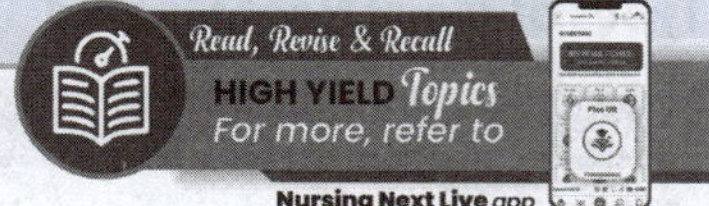

Food standards

- Set of standards laid down to regulate the manufacture, storage, sale and distribution of the food.
- Also ensures the availability of safe food for the consumption by humans.
- Controlled by the Food Safety and Standards Authority of India (FSSAI) and Food Safety and Standards Act, 2006.

CONCEPTUAL EXERCISES

LONG ANSWER QUESTIONS

1. Discuss the methods of cooking in detail. (MGR) (KUHS, RUHS)

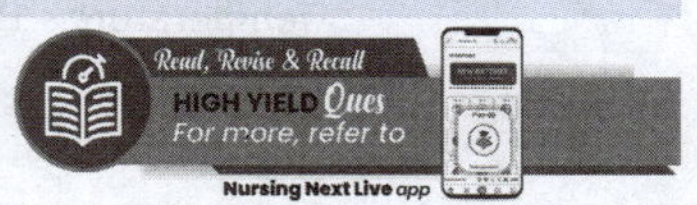

Answer

Cooking

- Conversion of raw ingredients to deem it fit for consumption.
- Cooking is essential to make the food:

Methods of Cooking

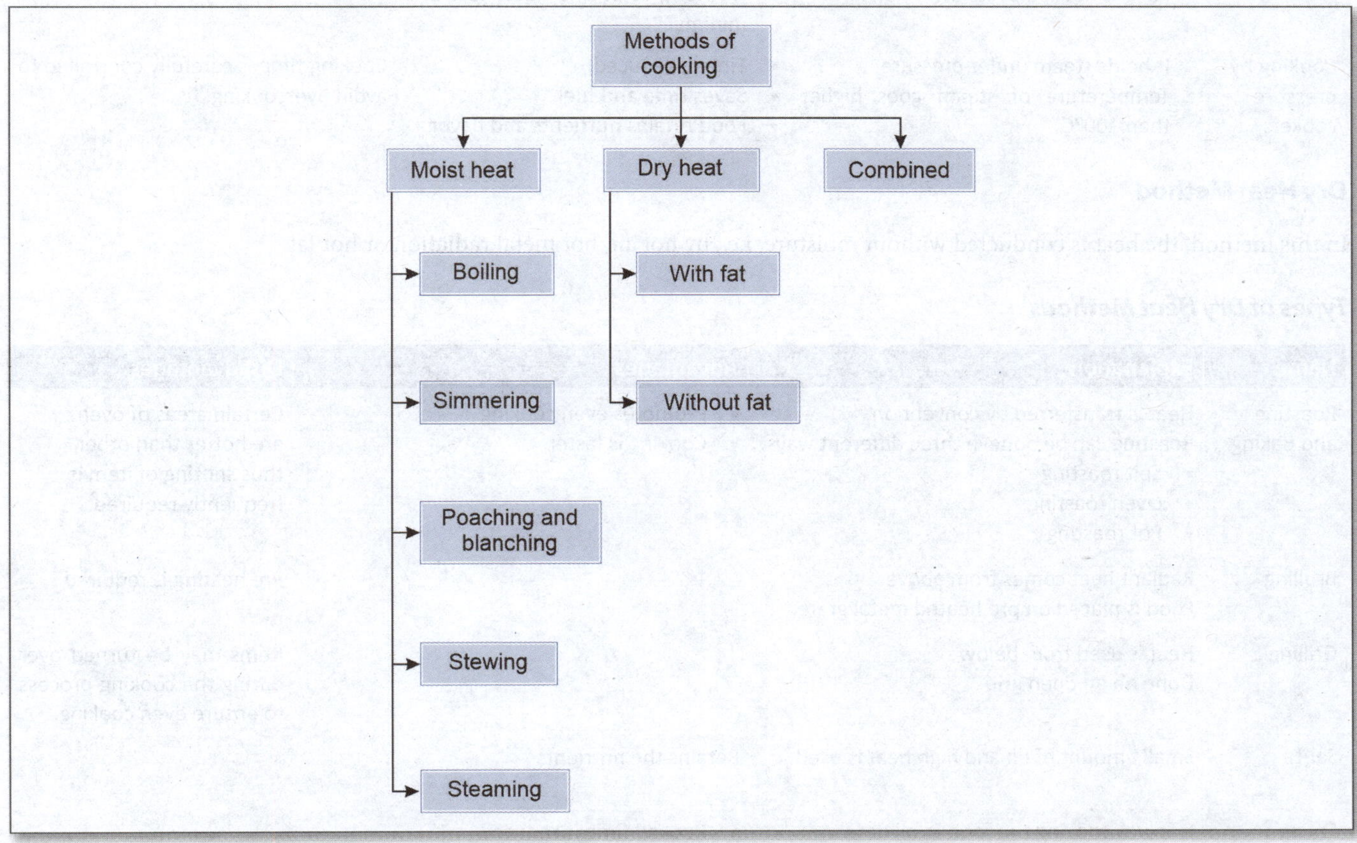

Moist Heat method

- In this method, the heat is conducted to the food product by water or steam.

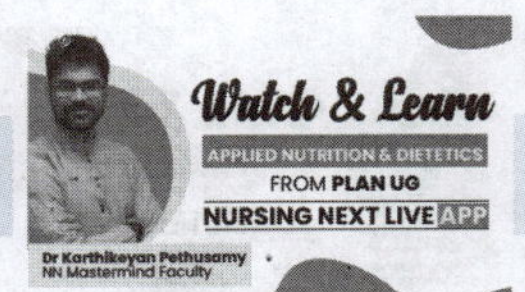

Types of Moist Heat Method

Name	Explanation	Advantages	Disadvantages
Boiling	Cooking in a boiling liquid. High temperature causes the proteins to toughen and rapid bubbling breaks up the delicate products.	• Easy • Time and fuel efficient • Cooked food is easily digestible.	• High temperature causes protein foods to toughen • Affects the flavor, color and appearance of food. • Some nutrients may be lost
Simmering	Cooked in small amounts of liquid that is bubbling very gently. Temperature - 85 – 96°C.	• Cooking at longer periods makes the food tender and digestible. • Enhances taste and flavor of the food.	• Slow process • Vitamin C is destroyed by slow process of cooking.
Stewing	Similar to stewing. Solid food is cooked in liquid and served with the resultant gravy. Temperature - 180°C	• Nourishing since it is cooked in covered pan. • Almost all nutrients are retained as gravy which is also served.	
Poaching	Cooking in a small amount of hot liquid. Temperature - 80 – 82°C	• Undesired odors and flavors are eliminated. • Softens the food.	Partial cooking occurs
Blanching	Food items are plunged into the boiling water for short periods and then removed and placed under cold water.	• Maintains the nutritive value of food. • Maintains the color of the food.	Partial cooking occurs
Steaming	Cooking occurs by direct exposure to steam. Food is cooked by its own moisture.	• Food is cooked rapidly and without agitation. • Nutrient, color and flavor loss are minimal.	
Cooking by pressure cookers	It holds steam under pressure. Temperature of steam goes higher than 100°C	• Time is reduced • Saves time and fuel • Food retains nutrients and flavor	Cooking time is carefully controlled to avoid overcooking.

Dry Heat Method

In this method, the heat is conducted without moisture, i.e., by hot air, hot metal radiation or hot fat.

Types of Dry Heat Methods

Name	Explanation	Advantages	Disadvantages
Roasting and Baking	Heat is transferred by convention. Roasting can be done in three different ways: • Spit roasting • Oven roasting • Pot roasting	• Promotes even cooking • Cooking is faster	Certain areas of oven are hotter than other, thus shifting of item is frequently required.
Broiling	Radiant heat comes from above Food is placed on pre heated metal grate.		Pre heating is required
Grilling	Heat is used from below Done on an open grid		Items may be turned over during the cooking process to ensure even cooking.
Saute	Small amount of oil and high heat is used	Retains the nutrients	
Frying	Involves cooking the food in oil or fats	• Cooked time is reduced • Impacts the crispiness, color and flavor.	

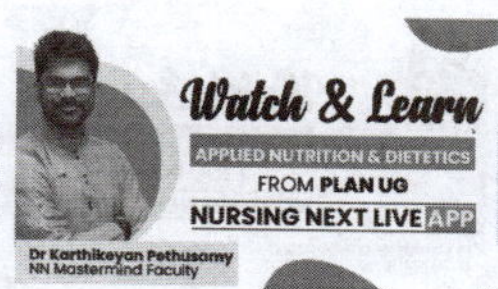

Combined Method

Indian cooking usually involves more than one method of cooking.

- Braising
- Combination of dry and moist method of cooking.
- First the item is cooked by dry heat to ensure proper caramelization.
- Then liquid is added, simmer it until it becomes soft and tender.

2. a. What is food hygiene? (MGR)

b. Explain the process involved in maintaining milk and meat hygiene. (MGR)

c. List the essential hygienic requirements of food handlers. (MGR)

Read, Revise & Recall HIGH YIELD Ques For more, refer to Nursing Next Live app

Answer

Food Hygiene

- Collection of practices and guidelines to protect against the risks of foodborne illnesses caused by microbial contamination.
- Concerned with food handling, proper storage and processing of materials.

Aims of Food Hygiene

- To protect the food spoilage, mainly due to biological contamination.
- To educate and motivate people about safe food handling and sanitary practices.
- To extend the shelf life of food.
- To detect the unsafe food and prevention of foodborne illnesses.

b. Explain the process involved in maintaining the milk hygiene

Answer

- Clean surroundings
- Clean hands while milking
- Free from communicable diseases
- Immediate cooling of milk <10°C
- Milking machines

Pasteurization of Milk

- Various milk pasteurization methods are:
  - Holder method
  - UHT method
  - HTST method
- Tests of pasteurized milk
  - Phosphatase test
  - Coliform count
  - Standard plate count

Meat Hygiene

- **The characteristics of good meat are:**
  - Neither deep purple nor pink
  - Should not contain excess fluids
  - Should not have an offensive odor
  - Should be acidic in reaction
- **Common infections in the meat are:**
  - Tapeworm infestations – *Taenia solium, T. saginata, Trichinella spiralis, Fasciola hepatica*
  - Bacterial infections–anthrax, actinomycosis, tuberculosis, food poisoning
- **Prevention**
  - Meat inspection – ante mortem and post mortem
  - Important factors for proper hygienic slaughter houses:
    - Location and structure of the slaughter house
    - Proper ventilation and disposal of waste
    - Water supply
    - Transportation of meat
    - Inspection of animals and storage of meat

c. List the essential hygienic requirements of food handlers

Answer

- Proper hand-washing
- Proper grooming
- Keep fingernails trimmed, filed and maintained
- Protective gears
- Clean uniforms
- Change apron when it becomes soiled
- Health status of personnel

3. Comment on "Prevention of Food Adulteration Act (PFA)". (RUHS)

Read, Revise & Recall HIGH YIELD Ques For more, refer to Nursing Next Live app

Answer

Prevention of Food Adulteration

- Prevention of Food Adulteration Act came into effect in the year 1954.
- This act covers the following:
  - Protection against food adulteration
  - Maintain food standards
  - General procedures for sampling
  - Analyzing food
  - Power of authorized officers
  - Enrichment and fortification of food.

- Nature of penalties
- Other parameters related to food.
- Regulates the use of chemicals, pesticides, flavors and other additives in food preparation.
- Dumping of substandards foods

Objectives

- To protect the public from poisonous and harmful food.
- To protect the sale of substandard foods.
- To protect the interest of the consumer by eliminating fraudulent practice.

Concept of Adulteration

- An article of food shall be deemed to be adulterated if the food contains any other substance which affects the quality of food. If the article has been prepared, packed or kept under unsanitary conditions whereby it has become injurious to health.
- If the article is obtained from rotten, decomposed or diseased animal.
- If the article contains any poisonous ingredient.
- If the article contains any prohibited preservative or permitted preservative in excess of the prescribed limit.
- If the amount of prescribed coloring matter is not within the prescribed limits.

Sale is Prohibited in Case of

- A cream which has not been prepared from the milk or contains less than 25% of milk fat.
- Milk which contains added water
- Mixture of two or more edible oils.
- Food which contains any artificial sweetener beyond the prescribed limit.
- Curd not made out of milk.
- Turmeric containing any other foreign substance.

Procedure for Sampling and Analysis

A food inspector can inspect anywhere an article

Preventive Measures on Food Adulteration

Common methods that are used to avoid food adulteration:

- Check for the food inspection regularity and report.
- Check whether the premises are pest free and clean
- Check the panel for the production date, expiry date and their ingredients
- Check the packaging

4. What is preservation? Explain methods of preservation. Add a note on canning. (MGR)

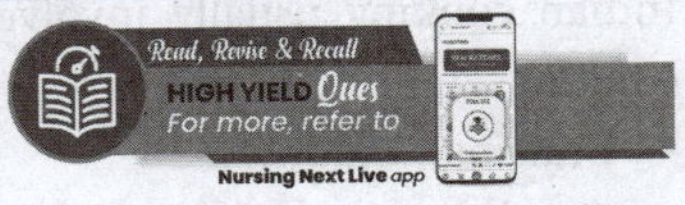

Answer

Food Preservation

- Technique used to prevent food from spoiling
- Prevents the growth of bacteria, fungi or other micro-organisms.

Importance of Food Preservation

- Increases the shelf life of food item
- Decreases the wastage of food by processing and preserving food products
- Maintains texture, flavor and nutritive value of food.
- Food is easy to store and can distributed from one place to another
- It can be made available beyond their natural season of production
- This can increase income in agriculture sector.

Methods of Food Preservation

- Long period preservation
- Short period preservation

Long Period Preservation

Dehydration	• Simple method • Process of removal of moisture under controlled conditions of temperature and humidity • Inhibits growth of microorganisms • Apparatus - dehydrator
Sun drying	• Oldest method • Process of reducing the water content to prevent or delay the bacterial growth. • Drying in sun enhances color and flavor of the food items • Used for fish, fruits, nuts, raisins, dates and vegetables
Cooling	• Slows down the growth and reproduction of the microorganisms • Slows the action of enzymes • Apparatus – Refrigerator • Used for fresh fruits, vegetables and dairy products
Freezing	• Convenient and easy method • Preserves the food quality, texture and nutritional values • Control enzymes activation • Used for fruits, vegetables, meat, sea foods and prepared foods

Contd...

Boiling	• Kills harmful bacteria • Used for liquids such as milk and water
Salting	• Draws moisture from food items through the process of osmosis • High salt concentration prevents bacterial growth due to hypertonic nature of the salt. • Pickling, fermenting and curing technique • Used for vegetables, fish and meat
Sugaring	• Used for preservation of fruits such as apple, pears and plums. • Cooked in sugar to the point of crystallization and the resultant product is then stored dry. • Used in jams and jellies
Pickling	• Method of preserving food in a vinegar sauce or salty water • Pickling agent includes vinegar, alcohol, vegetable oil, brine (high in salt). • Mechanism involved is anaerobic fermentation.
Canning	Process of preserving food in sealed airtight containers and heating them to temperature that kills microorganisms
Smoking	Meat or fish is exposed to smoke generated by burning wood fire.

Short Period Preservation

Washing	• Thoroughly washing of food item is done to remove dirt and microorganisms
Safe handling	• Proper selection of food items take place. Any damaged item must be discarded.
Packaging	• After washing and selection of food item, packing is done to reduce microbial growth to a great extent. • Three methods are used: ▪ Use of low temperature ▪ Use of high temperature ▪ Vacuum packing

Canning

- Process of preserving food in airtight containers.
- Involves placing foods in vacuum containers and heating them to a temperature that kills microorganisms. Then the containers are sealed and cooled down.

Two types of canning methods:

1. Water bath canning
2. Pressure canning

Two Types of Canning Methods

Water bath canning	Pressure canning
• Used for high acid foods such as tomatoes, fruits, jams, jellies and pickles. • In this method, containers are immersed in boiling water and cooked for a specified period of time.	• Used for low acid foods such as meat, poultry, sea food and vegetables. • Containers are placed in two to three inches of water in a pressure cooker which is heated to temperature of at least 240°C.

SHORT ANSWER QUESTIONS

1. Safe methods of handling food. (DU)

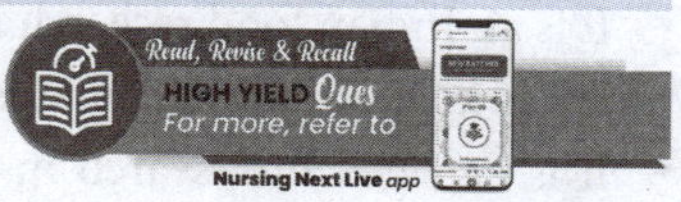

Answer

Safe Handling of Food

- Required to be taken for safe food handling, to avoid the risk of food-borne illnesses.
- Include general precautions and specific steps at different stages such as during shopping, storage in the house, freeze or refrigerator, before, during and after cooking and storage of leftover food.

General precautions for safe food handling	• Use of fresh ingredients. • Use of rotten or unwashed vegetables should be forbidden. • Personal hygiene should be maintained. • Packed foods may be considered safer than that kept in open.
Safe food handling during shopping	• Purchase from reliable sources having high turnover rate to ensure freshness. • Purchase foods with certification marks. • Always look for date of packaging, best before or date of expiry while purchasing packaged food. • Food grains should be infestation free and free of foreign matter. • Artificially colored food should be avoided. • Fats/oils should not be purchased loose.
Safe food handling while storing	• Always refrigerate perishable foods within 2 hours. • Cook or freeze poultry, fish and meat within 2 days. • Always store eggs in refrigerator. • High acid canned foods can be stored on shelf for 12 – 18 months. • Discard dented, leaking, bulging or rusted cans.
Safe food handling while cooking	• Handwashing before cooking. • Do not cross contaminate the foods, raw foods should be kept away from cooked food.

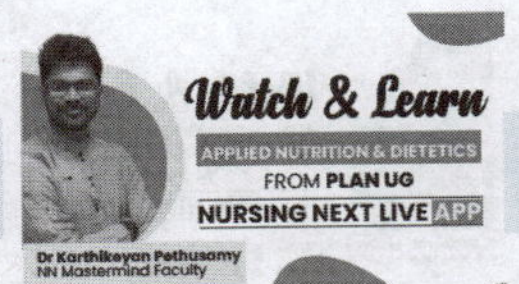

2. Write a short note on Prevention of Food Adulteration (PFA). (PFA) (DU)

Answer

For answer, refer to Long Question no. 3, pg. no. 517

3. Write a short note on CFTRI. (DU)

Answer

CFTRI

- The full form of CFTRI is Central Food Technological Research Institute.
- It is an Indian food research institute and laboratory.
- It has its headquarters in Mysore.
- It is engaged in research in the production and handling of grains, pulses, oilseeds, fruits, vegetables, meat, poultry and fish.

4. Principles of cooking and serving. (KUHS)

Answer

Principles of Cooking

- Heat causes chemical, physical and biological changes in the food ingredients. In cooking, there is transfer of energy from a heat source to food.
- Transfer of energy occurs by three methods:

Conduction	Convention	Radiation
• Transfer of heat by direct contact. • Cooking pans are made up of copper and aluminum that conduct heat very efficiently.	• Transfer of heat occurs through fluid. • The fluid may be in liquid or gaseous form. • This is seen in convention oven. • Responsible for baking, pizza, cakes, etc.	• Transfer of heat occurs through electromagnetic radiations. • This is seen in microwave oven that uses strong radio waves. • It works by spinning water, fat, sugars and oils inside the food. It causes friction which then heats the food and cooks it from inside.

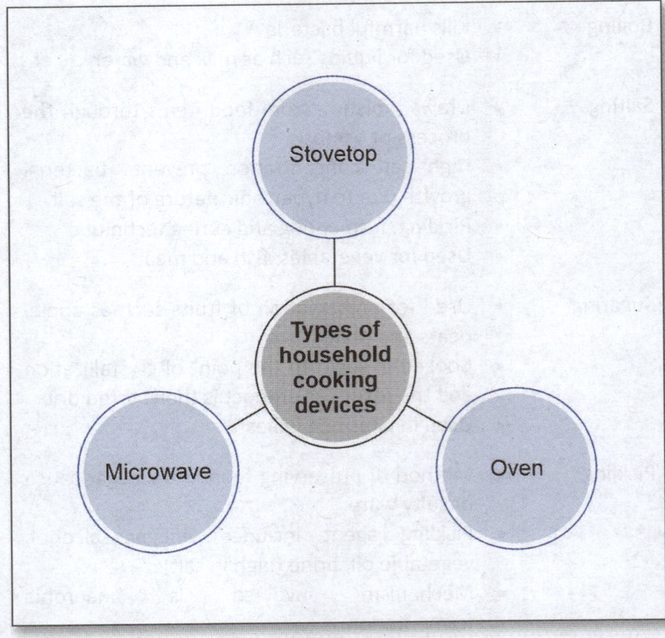

5. Write a note on food preservation by drying and canning. (MGR, KUHS)

Answer

Drying

Long-term preservation method.
This can be of two types—dehydration or sun drying.

Dehydration	• Simple method • Process of removal of moisture under controlled conditions of temperature and humidity • Inhibits growth of microorganisms • Apparatus - dehydrator
Sun drying	• Oldest method • Process of reducing the water content to prevent or delay the bacterial growth. • Drying in sun enhances color and flavor of the food items. • Used for fish, fruits, nuts, raisins, dates and vegetables.

Canning

- Process of preserving food in airtight containers.
- Involves placing foods in vacuum containers and heating them to a temperature that kills microorganisms. Then the containers are sealed and cooled down.

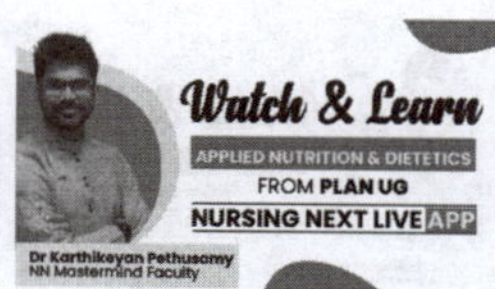

Two Types of Canning Methods

Water bath canning	Pressure canning
• Used for high acid foods such as tomatoes, fruits, jams, jellies and pickles. • In this method, containers are immersed in boiling water and cooked for a specified period of time.	• Used for low acid foods such as meat, poultry, sea food and vegetables. • In this method, containers are placed in two to three inches of water in a pressure cooker which is heated to a temperature of at least 240°C.

6. Write a note on household methods and principles of food preservation. (MGR, KUHS)

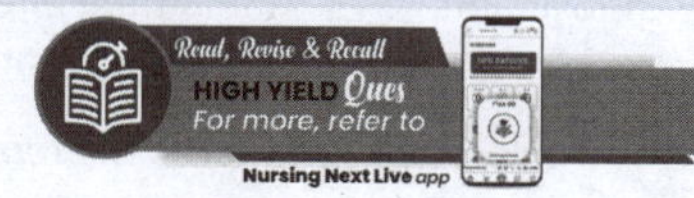

Answer

Food Preservation

- Technique used to prevent food from spoiling.
- Prevents the growth of bacteria, fungi or other micro-organisms.

Household Methods of Food Preservation

Sun drying	• Oldest method • Process of reducing the water content to prevent or delay the bacterial growth. • Drying in sun enhances color and flavor of the food items • Used for fish, fruits, nuts, raisins, dates and vegetables
Cooling	• Slows down the growth and reproduction of the microorganisms • Slows the action of enzymes • Apparatus – Refrigerator • Used for fresh fruits, vegetables and dairy products
Freezing	• Convenient and easy method • Preserves the food quality, texture and nutritional values • Controls enzyme activation • Used for fruits, vegetables, meat, sea foods and prepared foods
Boiling	• Kills harmful bacteria • Used for liquids such as milk and water
Salting	• Draws moisture from food items through the process of osmosis. • High salt concentration prevents bacterial growth due to hypertonic nature of the salt. • Pickling, fermenting and curing technique. • Used for vegetables, fish and meat.
Sugaring	• Used for preservation of fruits such as apple, pears and plums. • Cooked in sugar to the point of crystallization and the resultant product is then stored dry. • Used in jams and jellies.
Pickling	• Method of preserving food in a vinegar sauce or salty water. • Pickling agent includes vinegar, alcohol, vegetable oil, brine (high in salt). • Mechanism involved is anaerobic fermentation.
Smoking	Meat or fish is exposed to smoke generated by burning wood fire.
Washing	Thoroughly washing of food item is done to remove dirt and microorganisms.
Safe handling	Proper selection of food items take place. Any damaged item must be discarded.

Principles of Food Preservation

Principles

Preservation of food by any method is based on the following principles:

- Asepsis for prevention or delay of microbial decomposition
  - By canning
  - Packaging of food
  - Pasteurization of milk
- By removal of microorganisms
  - Filtration allows for the complete removal of the microorganisms.
- By impeding the growth and activity of microorganisms
  - This may be done by:
    - Low temperature
    - Anaerobic conditions
    - Drying of foods
- By killing the microorganisms using heat or radiation
  - Use of gamma rays or high speed electrons
- Prevention or delay of self-decomposition of food: Done by:
  - Destruction or inactivation of food enzymes by blanching.

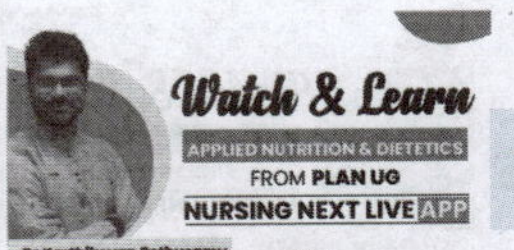

7. Write a note on Food standards. (MGR, KUHS)

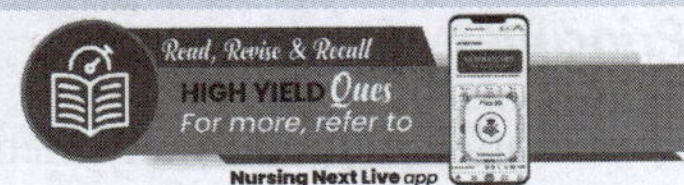

Answer

Food Standards

- Set of standards laid down to regulate the manufacture, storage, sale and distribution of the food.
- Also ensures the availability of safe food for the consumption by humans.
- Controlled by the Food Safety and Standards Authority of India (FSSAI) and Food Safety and Standards Act, 2006.

Key Features of Food Safety and Standard Act

- Packaging and labeling
  - There should be declaration on package, either in Hindi or English.
  - Pre-packaged food on the label shall not be presented or described on any label.
  - Label should not be separated from the container.
  - Contents should be clear, prominent, indelible and readily legible by consumers.
  - If the container is covered by a wrapper, the necessary information or the label on the container should not be obscured by the wrapper.
- **Licensing registration and health and sanitary permits:** Food business operators are instructed to be registered or licensed. The conditions with regard to sanity safety and hygienic requirements have to be met at all times.
- **Signage and customer notice:** No person shall engage himself in any unfair trade practice for the purpose of sale, supply, use and consumption of articles or adopt any deceptive practice of making any statement whether orally or in writing which gives public any guarantee of the efficacy that is not based on an adequate or scientific justification.

8. Write a short note on food additives. (KUHS)

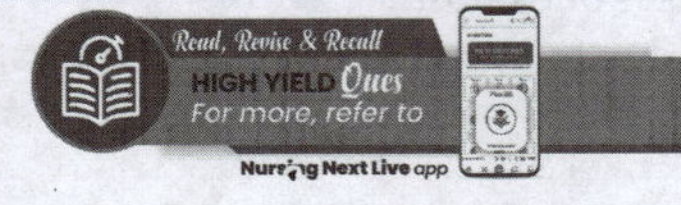

Answer

Food Additives

Addition of nonnutritious substances that are added intentionally to food in smaller quantity to improve its appearance, texture or storage properties.

Use of Additives

- To improve the taste of food item.
- To improve flavor.
- To enhance its texture and color.
- To improve its storage properties.
- To increase the shelf life of food.

Types of Food Additives

Natural	Nature Identical	Artificial
Those found naturally such as beetroot (for colors)	Synthesized copies of natural substances	Synthetic substances such as vanillin or ethyl maltol.

Classification of Food Additives

Acids	• Act as preservatives and antioxidants. • Example: Vinegar, citric acid and lactic acid.
Antioxidants	• Inhibit the effect of oxygen on food • Example: Vitamin C
Food colors	• Makes the food more attractive
Antifoaming agent	• Reduce foaming in food
Bulking agent	• Increase the bulk of the food without affected the taste • Example: Arrowroot or starch
Flavor	• Enhance the taste and flavor of the food items. • May be naturally or artificially derived.
Preservatives	• Prevent the spoilage of food from micro-organisms.
Stabilizers	• They give firmer texture to jams and jellies.
Sweeteners	• Sweeteners are added to keep the food calories low, mostly they are used by diabetic patients.
Glazing agents	• Give shiny appearance to foods.
As emulsifiers	• Improve texture, volume and body of baked products and maintain an even distribution of ingredients. • Example: Lecithin

Importance of Food Additives in Food Processing

Food additives in food processing are used for:

- Safe and sure food products.
- Isolation of the specific compounds and exploit biological potential of constituents.
- Improving safety and freshness of products.
- Increase the storage life of food products.
- Develop the traditional and innovative food products.
- Improving or maintaining the nutritional values.

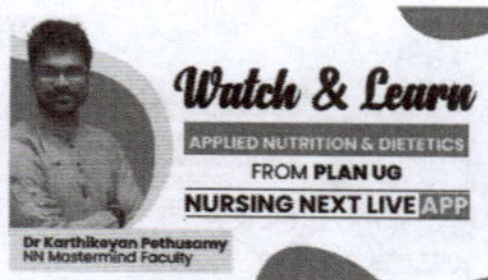

9. Write a note on steaming and grilling. (MGR)

Answer

Steaming

Definition	• Cooking occurs by direct exposure to steam. • Food is cooked by its own moisture. • Steaming is done with a lid on the utensil.
Advantages	• Food is cooked rapidly and without agitation • Nutrient, color and flavor loss are minimal in this method. • Flavors can be added in the form of vapors. • Little monitoring is required.

Grilling

Definition	• Dry heat method of cooking. • Food is cooked by radiant heat from below. • An open grid is used for this type of cooking.
Types of grilling	• Direct ▪ Similar to broiling ▪ Food is cooked directly over heat source. • Indirect ▪ Similar to roasting ▪ Food is cooked evenly on all sides.
Advantages	Charred or smokey flavor is produced in the food being grilled.
Disadvantages	Items need to be turned over during cooking process to ensure even cooking.
Foods suitable for grilling	• Chicken • Fish • Steaks • Bacon • Sausages • Vegetables • Fruits

10. Write about food toxicity. (RUHS)

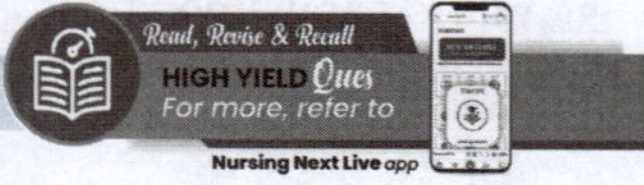

Answer

Food Toxicity

Food contains harmful toxicants including nutrients. Toxins are poisonous substances capable of causing diseases when consumed in large amount.

Types of Toxins

Food toxins	
Mercury	Some species of fish for example Shark, Broadbill, Marlin and Swordfish. Mercury exposure produces harmful effects on CNS, digestive system, immune system, lungs and kidneys. Symptoms of mercury poisoning include insomnia, memory loss and headache, cognitive and motor dysfunction.
Furocoumarin toxins	Natural toxin produced by the plants to protect themselves from being damaged by insects and mammals. Symptoms include stomach ache, skin reactions.
Lecitins	Toxins found in grains and kidney beans. Symptoms are severe stomach ache, vomiting and diarrhea.

Contd...

Food toxins	
Sodium nitrate and arsenic	Potatoes contain these toxins. They have hazardous effect on the health if consumed in large quantities. Consuming a large variety of foods minimizes the amount of toxic substances.
Protein gluten	It is the toxin present in wheat and other cereal grains. It can damage the intestines and causes conditions like obesity and diabetes.
Soya products	Soya contains trypsin inhibitors that inhibit protein digestion. It contains phytic acid which reduces the absorption of minerals like calcium, iron and zinc.
Green tea	Green tea can also lead to disturbing effects like impaired vision, impaired hearing, breathing problems, and other symptoms if consumed in high amount.
Lathyrus poisons	This is commonly observed in India and Mediterranean countries. The disease is caused due to the ingestion of legume *Lathyrus sativus*. It causes a neurologic and a crippling disease. Symptoms include weakness of leg muscle, dragging of feet, and loss of sensation of heat, pain and spinal cord lesion.
Fungal Toxins Mycotoxins	Natural death cap mushroom is a poisonous fungus that is responsible for 80% of all deaths. Symptoms of toxicity are severe stomach ache, nausea, vomiting, diarrhea and liver damage.
Ergot	Associated with eating rye infected by a fungus *Claviceps purpura*. Symptoms include nausea, vomiting, giddiness and drowsiness.
Aflatoxins	Produced by the mould *Aspergillus flavus*. These are powerful hepatocarcinogens. This affects the liver and causes cancer in many animals.

Other important toxins are:

- Artificial toxins include:
  - Pesticides and industrial chemicals
  - Growth hormones given to mulching animals
  - Flavored drinks
  - Artificial colors
- Bacterial Food Toxins
  - Staphylococcus aureus
  - Salmonella
  - Clostridium botulinum
  - Bacillus cereus
  - Vibrio parahemolyticus

SHORT ANSWER QUESTIONS

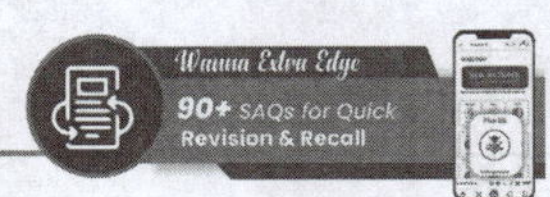

1. What is adulteration? (MGR)

Answer

Adulteration is a legal offence. When the food fails to meet the legal standards set by the government, it is said to have been adulterated.

Food is considered adulterated when it doesn't adhere to the government's legal standards, which is considered a criminal violation. When purposely or accidentally adding ingredients that lower food quality, food adulteration occurs. Therefore, the contamination or adulteration of food or food products by the addition of dangerous chemicals can be described as food adulteration.

2. List out two dry heat methods of cooking. (MGR)

Answer

Two dry methods of cooking are roasting, and baking.

3. Define food adulteration. (MGR)

Answer

Food Adulteration can be defined as the practice of adulterating food or contamination of food materials by adding a few substances, which are collectively called adulterants.

4. List the food preservation methods. (MGR)

Answer

- Always refrigerate perishable food within 2 hours.
- Perishable foods such as meat and poultry, should be wrapped securely.
- Canned the food items like fish, meat, and poultry and store it for 2–5 years.

5. Objectives of cooking. (MGR)

Answer

1. Food is kept fresher longer when it is cooked.
2. The bacteria found in raw food items are eliminated during cooking.

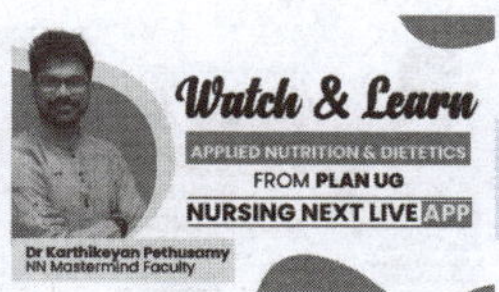

3. Cooking stimulates the digestive system, which increases appetite by pleasing the sight, palate, and digestive fluids.
4. The menu can be varied by cooking a single item in a number of different ways.
5. Cooking keeps the nutrients and flavors of the ingredients.
6. Boost the flavor.
7. The food is simple to masticate.
8. It aids in food digestion.

6. Write three chemical preservatives. (MGR)

Answer

- Benzoic acid, sodium benzoate, benzoates: jams, salad dressing, juices, pickles, fizzy drinks, soy sauce.
- Sorbic acid, sodium sorbate, and sorbates: cheese, wine, baked goods.
- Sulphur dioxide, sulfites: fruits, wines.

7. List out the two types of cooking methods. (MGR)

Answer

Boiling, grilling and frying are various methods of cooking.

8. Food fortification. (DU)

Answer

Adding vitamins and minerals to frequently consumed foods during processing to improve their nutritional value is known as food fortification. It is a tried-and-true, risk-free, and economical method for enhancing diets and preventing and controlling micronutrient deficiencies.

9. Reference fortification. (DU)

Answer

Micronutrient deficits can be prevented, reduced, and controlled with the use of fortification, an evidence-based strategy. It can be used to treat a proven micronutrient deficiency in the whole population (mass or large-scale fortification) or in particular demographic groups (targeted fortification), such as kids, pregnant women, and those who get benefits from social protection programs. Point-of-use fortification is the practice of adding vitamins and minerals to food immediately before it is consumed at home, in a classroom, or in a nursery.

10. Phytochemicals. (DU)

Answer

- Phytochemicals are compounds that are produced by plants, phytochemicals protect cells from damage.
- Phytochemicals such as polyphenols, flavones, also afford protection against oxidative damage.

CONCEPTUAL REVISION

MULTIPLE CHOICE QUESTIONS

1. The movement of molecules through air or liquid:

a. Convection b. Roasting
c. Conduction d. Radiation

Ans. a. Convection

2. A liquid has reached its highest temperature in normal conditions:

a. Baking b. Braising
c. Broiling d. Boiling

Ans. d. Boiling

3. ………. creates high pressured atmosphere by trapping steam in an airtight chamber:

a. Moist heat cooking b. Pan-broiling
c. Dry heat cooking d. Pressure cooking

Ans. d. Pressure cooking

4. Cooking food surrounded by heat in an oven - Meat and poultry is:

a. Baking b. Poaching
c. Broiling d. Roasting

Ans. d. Roasting

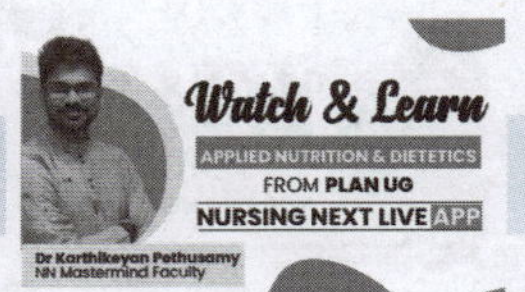

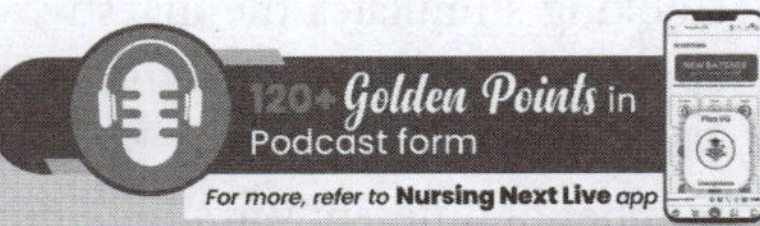

Golden Points

- Box cooker is the easiest and most popular device to build and use. It has a lid on a cardboard box and sunlight is reflected into pots kept under glass. Box cooker works slow and provides even cooking of large quantities of food.
- Canning is the process of preserving food in sealed airtight containers.
- Carbonated water is water into which CO2 gas is dissolved under pressure.
- Cooking is the skill of preparing food fit for consumption by combining.
- Food adulteration can be defined as a process of degrading the quality of food being sold by the addition or use of inferior quality substances or by extracting some valuable components of a food article. It is a common fraudulent practice adopted by the sellers to earn profit.
- Food processing includes some methods and techniques which are used to transform raw ingredients into food or other forms of food items for consumption.
- Frying is a dry heat cooking method as water is not used in this method. It involves cooking of food item in oil or other edible fats such as vegetable oil, olive oil, coconut oil, ghee, etc.
- Green beans, broccoli, fruits and other green vegetables are cooked by blanching.
- In conduction method, heat is transferred through direct contact. When cooking on the stovetop, the heat from the flame or electric grill is applied directly to the fry pan to cook food but it requires flip and toss around the food to cook it properly.
- In convection method, heat transfers through the fluid. The fluid can be liquid or gas and even in case of convection oven it may be air. An oven is a confined area that because hot by flames or electric coils.
- In electronic heat transfer, specially-designed microwave ovens or electronic ranges are used for cooking food. Microwave ovens have magnetron fitted in it which converts electric currents to microwaves that are similar to light or radio waves. This energy is focused toward the food to be cooked.
- In microwave cooking method, the high frequency electromagnetic waves, also called microwaves are used for cooking. The microwaves are emitted when food is cooked in the microwave oven.
- In radiation, heat is transferred using electromagnetic radiations. A microwave oven uses strong radio waves which are very weak and not hot. Microwave ovens work by spinning water, fat, sugars and oils inside the food. This causes friction, which then heats the food and cooks it from inside.
- Low acid foods such as meat, poultry, sea food and vegetables are best preserved by pressure canning.
- Pasteurization Method of sterilization of food products such as milk, fruit juices by heating, at a specific temperature for a specific time period followed by immediate cooling and packing into an airtight container using aseptic techniques.
- Pickling is an act of preserving food in a vinegar sauce or salty water.
- Poaching means to cook in a small amount of hot liquid that is not actually boiling.
- Simmering means to cook in a small amount of liquid that is bubbling very gently. Temperature is generally 185 – 205°F (85 – 96°C).
- The Food Safety and Standards Authority of India (FSSAI) has been established under Food Safety and Standards Act, 2006 which consolidates various acts and orders that have hitherto handled food.

CHAPTER 11

Nutritional Assessment and Nutrition Education

CONCEPTUAL THEORY

Terminology

150+ key terminologies for Quick Recall & Revision

Anthropometry: Anthropometric measurements include height, weight, skin fold thickness and circumference, etc. These changes of body composition is used to assess the nutritional status.

Food frequency questionnaires (FFQ) method: It is a type of dietary assessment instrument that attempts to capture the amount of food consumed and its frequency of consumption with the help of predefined food list.

Mid upper arm circumference (MUAC): It involves measuring the circumference of the mid-point on upper arm using a tape measure. This is a surrogate measure of both fat mass and fat free mass. It is a useful measure when a person cannot, be weighed or if the weight is not likely to be a true reflection of the person's actual weight.

Nutrition education: It is the process of teaching the science of nutrition to population by health professionals in different settings like community clinic, etc. With the help of this education, health professionals enable individuals to incorporate changes in eating patterns and behavior into their lives.

Nutritional assessment: It is a process of collecting and interpreting information related to health issues and to make decisions related to these health issues.

OBJECTIVES OF NUTRITIONAL ASSESSMENT

Nutritional Assessment

- It is defined as the process of collecting and interpreting information related to health issues and to make decisions related to these health issues.

Objectives of Nutritional Assessment

- To find out the severity and distribution of malnutrition in community.
- To find out high risk groups which may fall under malnourished category in near future.
- To find out ecological factors responsible for malnourishment
- To suggest corrective measures or develop appropriate health care programs.
- To alert concerned authorities or policy makers to make them realize the extent of the problems.
- To find out the result of existing nutritional programs in community.

Methods of Nutritional Assessments

- Clinical/physical examination
- Laboratory and biochemical assessment
- Anthropometric measurement
- Functional assessment
- Dietary assessment
- Vital and health statistics
- Assessment of Socioeconomic Status
- Food Frequency Questionnaires method

NUTRITION EDUCATION – PURPOSES, PRINCIPLES AND METHODS

Nutrition Education

- Process of teaching the science of nutrition to a population or individual by health professionals in health care center, community or clinic.
- It enables the individuals to incorporate changes in behavior related to nutrition and health in their day to day life.

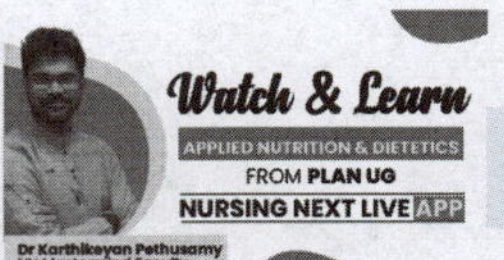

Principle of Nutrition Education

- Imaprt right knowledge in right direction
- Educate people for correct and healthy choices of food
- Education of correct and appropriate eating habits.
- Tells about appropriate eating habits.
- After health education, health status of whole family could be improved and problems related to nutrition in coming future may be reduced.

Purposes of Nutritional Education

- Improvement in nutritional level of community
- Initiation of supplementary nutrition programs,if required
- Development of Nutrition education programs and nutrition advisory services.

Methods of Nutrition Education

The various important methods of nutrition education are as follows:

- Workshops
- Film and slide shows
- Posters, charts and exhibition
- Books, bulletins, pamphlets and newspaper
- Radio and television
- Lectures and demonstrations

CONCEPTUAL EXERCISES

LONG ANSWER QUESTIONS

1. Define nutritional assessment. Write methods of nutritional assessment and role of nurse in nutritional care. (MGR, KUHS, RUHS)

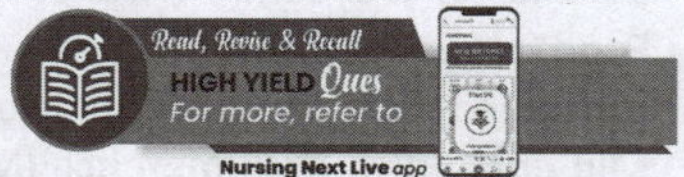

Answer

Nutritional Assessment

It is defined as the process of collecting and interpreting information related to health issues and to make decisions related to these health issues.

Methods of Nutritional Assessments

Clinical/physical examination	• The examination is done from head to foot. Quantification of malnutrition may be done in the scores of 1, 2 and 3.0 stands for no deficiency and 1, 2, 3 stand for mild, moderate and severe degrees of deficiency, respectively. • General malnutrition may be due to deficient dietary intake or inadequate absorption of nutrients.
Laboratory and biochemical assessment	• Identifies specific nutrition related abnormalities such as anemia, iron deficiency or protein. • Biochemical tests provide the first indication of nutritional abnormality before clinical or anthropometric changes occur. These tests are specific for the particular nutrient being investigated.
Anthropometric measurement	• Anthropometric measurement such as height, weight, skinfold thickness and arm circumference are valuable indicators of nutritional status. In young children, additional measurements such as head and chest circumference are made.
Functional assessment	• Functional indices of nutritional status are emerging as an important class of diagnostic tool, for example, sperm count, heart rate, nerve conduction, EEG, etc.
Dietary assessment	• Description of dietary intake may help to explain any observed clinical or biochemical abnormalities and may suggest proper remedial steps. 24 hour recall is one of the most common methods of dietary assessment. In this, the individual is asked to recall all food and beverages consumed over the preceding 24 hours and sometimes the physical activity level during the period. • Subjective method and not fully reliable.
Vital and health statistics	• Vital statistics involve mortality and morbidity data showing which group is at higher risk. Include rates used for vital statistics are low birth weight babies, infant mortality rate, second year mortality rate and life expectancy. They all are influenced by nutritional status of a particular group.
Assessment of socioeconomic status	• Low food availability, increased family size, unsanitary living conditions, inadequate knowledge of nutritional needs, and inadequate weaning practices are powerful, social, cultural and economic factors which influence nutritional status.
Food Frequency Questionnaires method	• It is a type of dietary assessment instrument that attempts to capture the amount of food consumed and its frequency of consumption with the help of predefined food list.

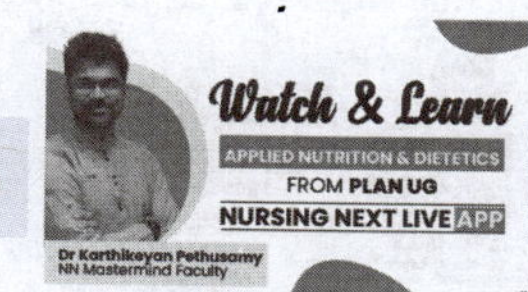

Role of Nurse in Nutritional Care

- Acts as a connecting link between the physician and dietician regarding the patient's response to the prescribed diet.
- Provides information about the patient's diet, his response to the prescribed diet to physician or dietician.
- Conducts nutrition screening.
- Performs assessment and intervention.
- Assist the patient during their meal times by providing pleasant environment favorable to eating.
- Gives full information to patient regarding the reasons for prescribing particular diet and its importance and expected outcomes and clarifying doubt about the diet.
- Focuses on nutritional needs of every patient during every shift.
- Keep records and reports of patient's response to dietician and physician.
- Counsels for home diet for family members and the patient.
- In community setting, nurse can provide nutrition education to breastfeeding and weaning mothers, old age persons and to whole family regarding importance of nutritional diet and deficiency disorders related to imbalanced diet.

2. Write about nutrition education in detail. (MGR)

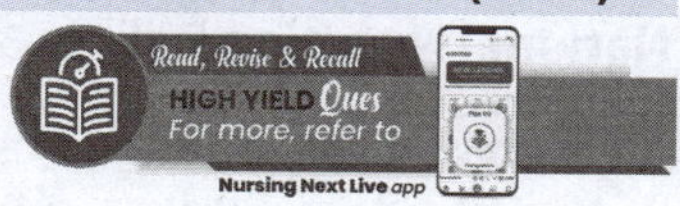

Answer

Nutrition Education

- Process of teaching the science of nutrition to a population or individual by health professionals in health care center, community or clinic.
- It enables the individuals to incorporate changes in behavior related to nutrition and health in their day-to-day life.
- According to Society for Nutrition Education and behavior which "Nutrition education is a combination of educational strategies, accompanied by environment support, is designed to facilitate voluntary adaptation of food choices and other food and nutrition related behavior conducive to health and well-being. It requires participation at individual, community and policy levels."

Principle of Nutrition Education

- Gives knowledge in right direction and corrects faulty practices.
- Educates people to make best use of their limited resources
- Educates people to make wise food choices for health and well-being of family members.
- Tells about appropriate eating habits.
- After health education, health status of whole family could be improved and problems related to nutrition in coming future may be reduced.

Purposes of Nutritional Education

- To improving the nutritional levels of community by available means.
- To develop supplementary nutrition program where and whenever needed.
- To develop nutrition advisory services and nutrition education programs.

Methods of Nutrition Education

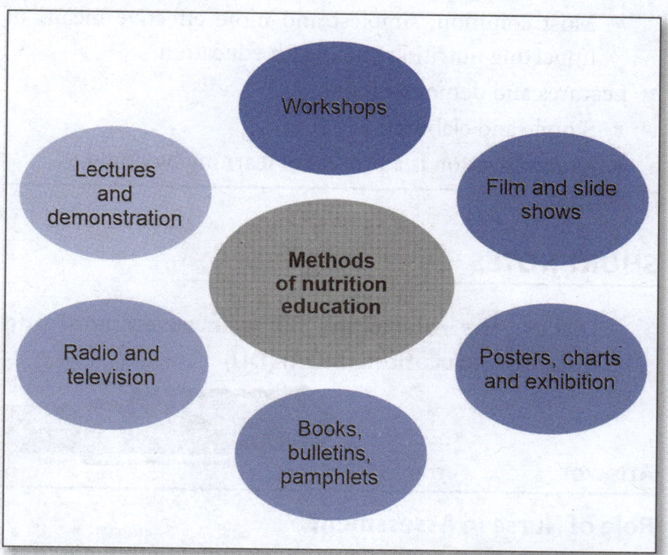

The various important methods of nutrition education are as follows

- Workshops:
  - Includes current topics related to nutrition and its deficiencies.
- Film and slide shows:
  - Most effective method of education.
  - Practical, illustrative and time effective.
  - Needs to be supplemented with literature, posters, demonstration and discussion.
  - Slideshows/Slide are single picture usually in color. Slides are used in a cardboard frame.
- Posters, charts and exhibition:
  - Posters and charts should be simple, attractive and should be written in regional language.
  - Exhibition is a systematic display of models, specimens, charts, photograph, pictures, posters, etc. in a sequence around a theme to create awareness and interest in community.

- Books, bulletins, pamphlets and newspaper:
  - Printed material
  - Used singly or in combination
  - Reach number of people quickly
  - Provide accurate, motivating, credible and distortion free information
  - Used as source of future reference.
- Radio and television
  - Electronic medium
  - One way communication
  - Radio – audio medium
  - Television – audio – visual medium
  - Reach a large number of audience within no time.
  - Most common, simplest and more effective means of imparting nutrition and health education.
- Lectures and demonstrations
  - Simple and elaborate
  - Demonstration is a process of learning by doing.

SHORT NOTES

1. Discuss the role of the nurse in assessment and nutrition education. (MGR) (DU)

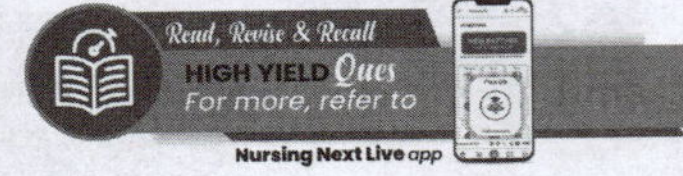

Answer

Role of Nurse in Assessment

Nurses assess the health by interviewing, inspecting and observing the patients in a variety of heath setups. These assessments help the nurse:

- In gathering information about the patient's condition.
- Conducting primary physical information and collection of relevant information.
- To identify families at risk and investigate problems in families.
- To obtain prenatal and family history
- Forming a nursing care plan
- Continuous health assessment helps to assess whether the desired effect is achieved or not in the patient.
- To evaluate the patient's health status in order to recommend discharge.
- To impart discharge teaching to the patient.

Role of Nurse in Nutritional Care

- Acts as a connecting link between the physician and dietician regarding the patient's response to the prescribed diet.
- Provides information about the patient's diet, his response to the prescribed diet to physician or dietician.
- Conducts nutrition screening.
- Performs assessment and intervention.
- Assist the patient during their meal times by providing pleasant environment favorable to eating.
- Gives full information to patient regarding the reasons for prescribing particular diet and its importance and expected outcomes and clarifying doubt about the diet.
- Focuses on nutritional needs of every patient during every shift.
- Keep records and reports of patient's response to dietician and physician.
- Counseling for home diet for family members and the patient.
- In community setting, nurse can provide nutrition education to breastfeeding and weaning mothers, old age persons and to whole family regarding importance of nutritional diet and deficiency disorders related to imbalanced diet.

2. Write about goals of national nutritional policy. (MGR, DU, KUHS)

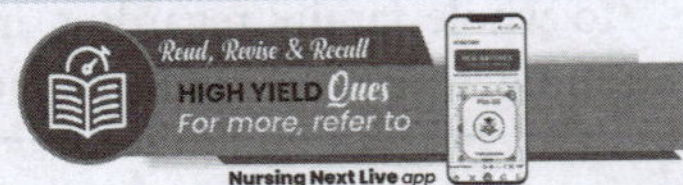

Answer

National Nutrition Policy

Advocates a multisectoral strategy for eradication of malnutrition across the country.

Aims/Goals of National Nutritional Policy

- To improve nutrient intake
- To advocate intersectoral coordination
- To observe nutrition as an outcome of the sectoral activities
- To reduce the incidence of malnutrition across the country
- To improve access and food availability
- To establish various strategies to achieve the nutritional goals
- To prevent and reduce food and vector borne diseases
- To improve mother and child care
- To strengthen the nutritional capacity within all levels and sectors of GoI

3. Discuss methods of assessing nutritional status. (DU, RUHS)

Answer

Nutritional

For answer, refer to Long Question no. 1, pg. no. 528

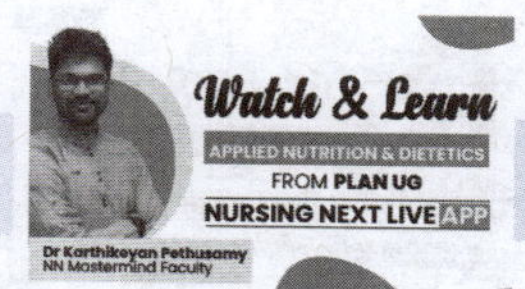

4. Dietary recall method. (DU)

Answer

Dietary Recall Method

- Structured interview to capture the food and beverages consumed by the individual in the past 24 hours.
- Person is asked to recall the detailed information about the food consumed.
- Open-ended response structure
- Comprehensive and detailed report of all foods and beverages consumed.
- Takes about 20–60 minutes
- Advantages
  - Easy and quick method
- Disadvantages
  - Need of an experienced interviewer
  - Dependent on the patient's memory

5. Write a note on Anthropometric measurement. (MGR, KUHS)

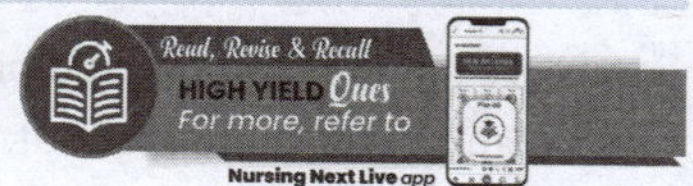

Answer

Anthropometry

- Refers to the measurement of the human body.
- Helps in understanding the physical variations of the human body.
- This involves the systematic measurement of the physical properties such as height, weight, skinfold thickness and arm circumference are valuable indicators of nutritional status.
- For purpose of anthropometric assessment, a representative sample of the population may be drawn.

Measurement	Equation/method	Interpretation of results
Weight and % weight change	% weight change = (current weight – previous weight/current weight) x 100	A patient is indicated for nutrition support if he has: • Unintentional weight loss of >10% in the previous 3–6 months • BMI <20 kg/m^2 and unintentional weight loss – 5% in the previous 3–6 months
Body mass index	BMI (kg/m^2) = weight (kg)/height^2 (m^2)	• If BMI is >18.5 kg/m^2, patient is underweight • If BMI is 18.5 – 25 kg/m^2, patient is in normal BMI range. • If BMI >25 – patient is overweight
Height	• Taken in a standing position without footwear, and is recorded to the nearest.	• Height is a stable measurement of growth as opposed to body weight. Whereas weight reflects only the present health status of the child, height indicates the events in past also.
Mid upper arm circumference (MUAC)	• Involves measuring the circumference of the mid-point on upper arm using a tape measure. This is a surrogate measure of both fat mass and fat free mass.	• If MUAC is >23.5 cm—at low risk of malnutrition. • If MUAC is <23.5 cm—the patient is at risk of malnutrition.
Skin fold thickness	• Taken at different site, suprailiac subscapular, biceps, triceps. • Measurement should be repeated 3 times and the mean result is recorded.	• Centile tables can be used to interpret skin fold thickness measurement.
Mid arm muscle circumference (MAMC)	MAMC is a surrogate measure of fat free mass and is calculated by using MUAC and TSF	• Centile tables allow assessment of changes in total body muscle mass.
Head circumference	Measurement of head circumference is a standard procedure to detect pathological condition in children. Head circumference is related mainly to assess brain size.	• At birth, the circumference of head is greater than that of the chest.

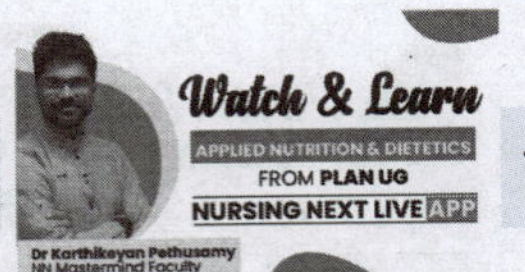

SHORT ANSWER QUESTIONS

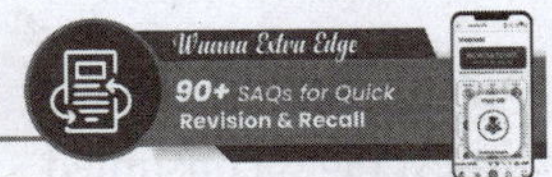

1. Define BMR. (MGR)

Answer

The energy required by an individual during the period of rest, either physical, emotional or digestive rest.

2. Give medicinal value of any two foods. (MGR)

Answer

Foods are having many medicinal values like:

- Rice and banana are given at the time of diarrhea.
- Corn is recommended for intestinal disorders, like irritable bowel syndrome, it also reduces the cholesterol because of presence of bran in it.
- Oats provide vitamin B_1, fatty acid, glucose and phosphoros, it helps in neuron functioning.

3. What is the energy requirement (RDA) for an adult man and adult women doing sedentary work? (MGR)

Answer

RDA (energy requirement) for an adult man and adult women doing sedentary work is 2350 kcal/day and 1900 kcal/day.

4. Distinguish between overweight and obesity. (MGR)

Answer

For adults, WHO defines overweight and obesity in the following manner:

- Overweight is a BMI greater than or equal to 25; and
- Obesity is a BMI greater than or equal to 30.

5. List down the methods of nutrition education. (MGR)

Answer

1. General lectures and discussion.
2. Slide shows
3. Nukkar natak

6. What is edema? (MGR)

Answer

Edema is swelling or puffiness of parts of the body. Edema can occur in ankle, feet, around eyes (Periorbital edema), hands, face and legs.

7. Define kilo calorie. (MGR)

Answer

Kilocalorie is defined as the energy required for raising the temperature of 1 kg water by 1°C. It is a unit of energy.

8. Anthropometric measurement. (MGR)

Answer

The Center for Disease Control and Prevention (CDC) claim that anthropometry is a useful tool for determining both children's and adults' nutritional status. It is a non-invasive quantitative measurements of the body.

9. BMI (Body Mass Index) (DU)

Answer

BMI (Body Mass Index) is computed by dividing the weight in kilograms by the square of the height in meters.

The ideal range of BMI is:

Normal= 18.5 – 25

Overweight = equal to or >25

Obese = 30 or more

10. Write the revised additional RDA of energy for a lactating mother. (DU)

Answer

An additional 330–400 kcal/day is recommended for well-nourished breastfeeding mothers.

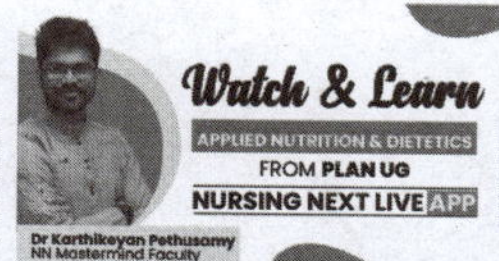

CONCEPTUAL REVISION

MULTIPLE CHOICE QUESTIONS

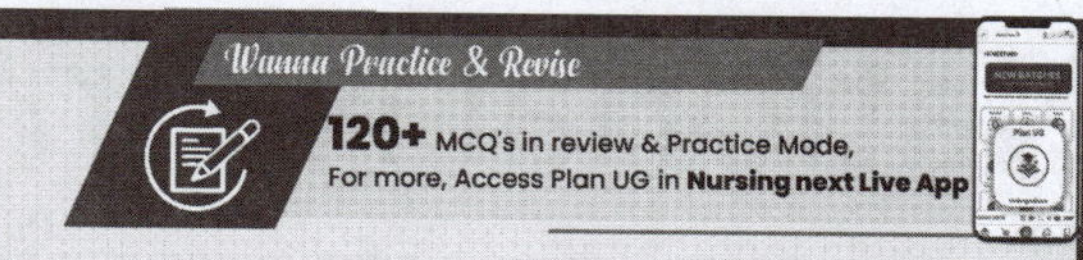

1. Which of the following is NOT a component of a nutritional assessment?

a. Anthropometric measurements
b. Biochemical assessments
c. Psychological evaluation
d. Dietary assessment

Ans. c. Psychological evaluation

2. What is the purpose of a dietary assessment?

a. To determine the adequacy of nutrient intake
b. To identify specific foods to avoid
c. To diagnose food allergies
d. To assess body composition

Ans. a. To determine the adequacy of nutrient intake

3. Which of the following is an example of a subjective assessment tool for evaluating dietary intake?

a. Food frequency questionnaire
b. 24-hour dietary recall
c. Weighed food record
d. Dual-energy X-ray absorptiometry (DXA) scan

Ans. a. Food frequency questionnaire

4. Which of the following is NOT a component of a comprehensive nutritional assessment?

a. Anthropometric measurements
b. Dietary intake assessment
c. Blood pressure measurement
d. Biochemical tests

Ans. c. Blood pressure measurement

5. Which of the following is an example of a nutrition screening tool?

a. 24-hour dietary recall
b. Food frequency questionnaire
c. Malnutrition Universal Screening Tool (MUST)
d. Bioelectrical Impedance Analysis (BIA)

Ans. c. Malnutrition Universal Screening Tool (MUST)

6. Which of the following is the best approach for assessing a patient's dietary intake?

a. 24-hour dietary recall
b. Food frequency questionnaire
c. Diet history
d. All of the above

Ans. a. 24-hour dietary recall

7. What is the most reliable indicator of fluid status?

a. Body weight
b. Serum electrolyte levels
c. Urine output
d. Skin turgor

Ans. a. Body weight

8. Which of the following is an important consideration when providing nutrition education to a patient?

a. The patient's health literacy
b. The patient's cultural background
c. The patient's personal preferences
d. All of the above

Ans. d. All of the above

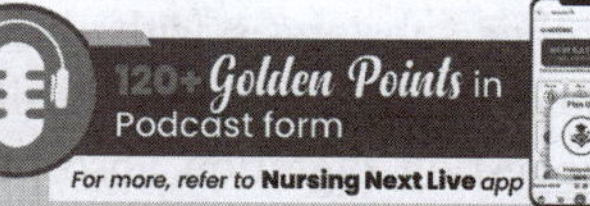

Golden Points

- Anthropometric measurements include height, weight, skin fold thickness and circumference, etc. These changes of body composition is used to assess the nutritional status.
- In community setting, nurse can provide nutrition education to breastfeeding and weaning mothers, pregnant and lactating mothers, old age persons and to whole family regarding importance if nutritional diet and deficiency disorders related to imbalanced diet.
- Nurse acts as a liason between physician and dietician regarding the patient's response to the prescribed diet to physician or dietician.
- Nutritional status of an individual is influenced by the adequacy of food intake both in terms of quantity and quality and also by the physical health of an individual.

CHAPTER

12

National Nutritional Program and Role of Nurse

CONCEPTUAL THEORY

Terminology

150+ key terminologies for Quick Recall & Revision

CARE: Cooperative for Assistance and Relief Everywhere.
CFTRI: Central Food Technology and Research Institute, Mysore.
FAO: Food and Agriculture Organization.
FDTRC: Food and Drug Toxicology Research Center.
FFS: Farmer Field School.
IAAH: International Alliance Against Hunger.
ICDS: Integrated Child Development Scheme.
IDD: Iodine Deficiency Disorder.
NIN: National Institute of Nutrition.
NIPCCD: National Institute of Public Cooperation and Child Development.
NNMB: National Nutrition Monitoring Bureau.

NUTRITIONAL PROBLEMS IN INDIA

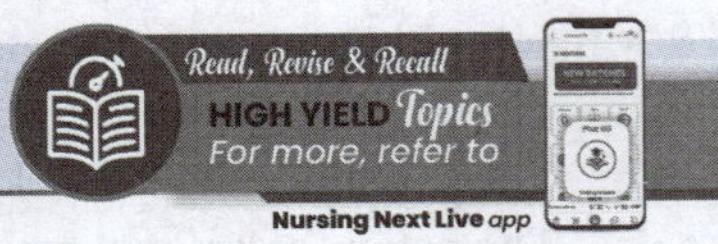

Nutrition

- Nutrition is defined as the science of food and its relationship with health. It plays an important role in growth, development and maintenance of the body system. It is also defined as the science of food, nutrients and other substances with their actions, interaction, balance and relationship with health and illness. It includes the ingestion, digestion, absorption and utilization of food, and disposal of their end products.

People who are at Risk of Nutritional Problems

- Low socioeconomic status
- Elderly
- Pregnant women
- Nursing mothers
- Infants/Low birth weight infants
- Preschool children and adolescents

Nutritional Problems in India

- Kwashiorkor
- Marasmus
- Micronutrient deficiencies
- Lathyrism
- Fluorosis

NATIONAL NUTRITION POLICY

National Nutrition Policy

- Advocates a multisectoral strategy for eradication of malnutrition across the country.
- In order to handle the nutritional problems, various developmental policy instruments have been developed that include:
- Direct short-term intervention
- Indirect policy instruments

Various Nutritional Program in India

- Vitamin A prophylaxis program
- Integrated child development services scheme (ICDS)
- National nutritional prophylaxis program
- Midday meal scheme
- Iodine deficiency disorder program

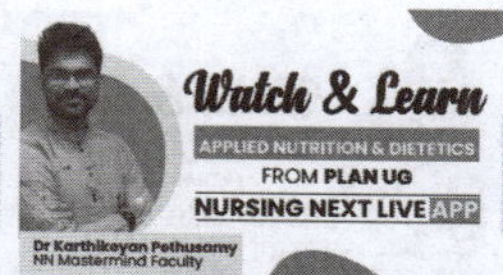

CONCEPTUAL EXERCISES

LONG ANSWER QUESTIONS

1. Discuss the nutritional programs in detail. (RUHS)

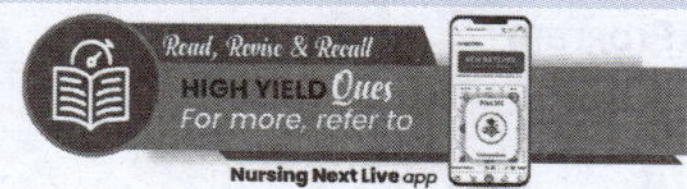

Answer

Various Nutritional Program in India

India has a number of national nutritional programs in place to improve the nutritional status of its population. These programs target different groups of people, including children, pregnant and lactating women, and the elderly.

These include:

- Vitamin A prophylaxis programs
- Integrated child development service (ICDS) scheme
- National nutritional Anemia prophylaxis program
- Midday meal scheme
- Iodine deficiency disorders control program

Suggestion

- The content can be presented Descriptively.
- One by one covering all these 6 points.
- It will be easy to follow.
- It will save pages too.

Nutritional program	Description	Modifications if any	Goals/Objectives	Beneficiaries	Services	Role of nurse
Vitamin A Prophylaxis Program	• To prevent blindness due to deficiency of vitamin A • Started in 1970	• In 1994, the National prophylaxis against National Blindness due to Vitamin A deficiency • First dose – 1 lakh IU 9 -12 month-old infant • Second dose – 2 lakh IU at the time of DPT and OPV booster • Afterward 2 lakh IU given at 6 monthly intervals till the age of 3 years.	• Administration of vitamin A solution to children • Promotion of exclusive breastfeeding for newborn in mothers	• Young children due to increased demands and low intake	2 lakh IU of oral vitamin A concentrate is given to children between 2 and 6 years at intervals of 6 months.	• To providing education to community regarding importance of vitamin A rich food and breastfeeding. • To promote exclusive breastfeeding for newborn • To ensure regular intake of vitamin A in children • To administer vitamin A to children • To identify the under five children of that area • To prepare a plan of action • To ensure supply of vitamin A solution • To supervise and monitor in the field. • To regular monitoring of services to watch the progress of the program • To submit of report to authorities from time to time.

Contd...

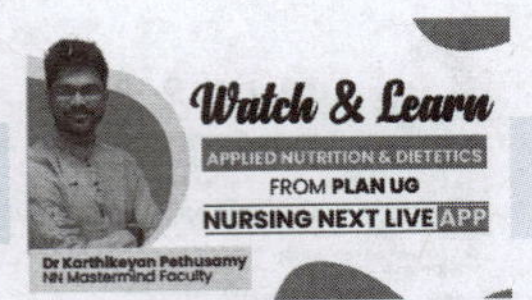

Nutritional program	Description	Modifications if any	Goals/Objectives	Beneficiaries	Services	Role of nurse
National Nutritional Anemia Prophylaxis Program	• Launched in 1970 during the fourth Five-year plan. • The program consists of distribution of iron and folic acid tablets to pregnant women and young children.		• Assessment of prevalence of anemia in mother and children. • Reduction of iron deficiency anemia in pregnant women • Providing anti-anemia treatment to women with Hb <10 g and preschool children with Hb <8 g. • Monitoring of quality, distribution and consumption of tablets. • Education of the mother	• Children in 1 – 5 years of age • Pregnant and nursing mothers • Female acceptors of terminal methods of family planning and IVDs	• Promotion of regular consumption of iron rich foods. • Providing iron and folate supplements. • Identification and treatment of severely anemic cases. • RDA • Children (1–5 yrs): 20 mg Fe + 0.1 mg FA for 100 days • School children (6 – 10 yrs): 30 mg Fe + 2.5 mg FA • Adults and adolescents: 100 mg Fe + 0.5 mg FA for 100 days. • Pregnant women: 100 mg elementary iron + 0.5 mg folic acid daily	• Firstly identify the antenatal, postnatal mothers and under five children of that particular area for further care. • Deworming in the area of heavy worm infestation • To ensure that there is adequate supply of iron and folic acid to the needy person. • It is also the responsibility of the nurse to supervise her junior nurses or health workers time to time for effective monitoring and providing care. • Checking of samples of iron and folic acid in the field • To refer the severe cases • Time to time organization of health education camps. • To submit report to higher authorities for further action. • Timely and regular follow-up
Midday meal Scheme	Provided to primary school children with 300 calories of energy and 8 – 12 g protein per day for minimum 200 days	• 2006– calories intake was increased to 450 and 12 g of protein • 2007 – covered the upper primary classes • 2008 – extended to Madrasas under Sarva Siksha Abhiyaan	• Provision of energy and protein rich foods to school children • Free supply of food grains	School children	Provision of central assistance for: • Cooking cost- ₹1/child/school day • Transport subsidy was raised from ₹50/ quintal to ₹100/quintal • Management, monitoring and evaluation cost at 2% of the cost of food grains, transport subsidy and cooking assistance.	• To act as a nutrition counselor in community • Assessment of the nutritional status of school children with the help of nutrition assessment tools. • To convey information related to nutrition and health to teachers, parents and children. • Plans the weekly menu • Evaluation of failure or success of the program • Referral of the severely malnourished • To organize of regular health education camps. School health nurse is responsible to maintain the health records of school children.

Contd...

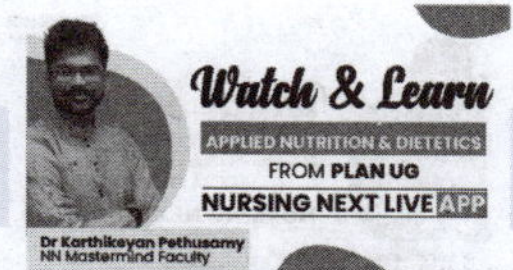

Nutritional program	Description	Modifications if any	Goals/Objectives	Beneficiaries	Services	Role of nurse
Iodine Deficiency Disorders Control Program	Later renamed as National IDD Control Program (NIDDCP) in 1992.		• To conduct surveys to assess the magnitude of IDD • To reduce the prevalence of IDD below 10% in the endemic districts of the country by 2012. • To supply iodized salt in place of normal salt • Health education and publicity • To conduct resurveys to assess the extent of IDD and impact of the iodized salt. • To laboratory monitor the iodized salt and urinary iodine excretion.	School children and adults suffering from iodine deficiency	• Technical guidance to the state/UTs • Intersectoral coordination at various levels • Undertaking various IDD surveys • Imparting training • Collection, compilation and analysis of relevant data • Monitoring the quality control of iodized salt • Monitoring the procurement and distribution of iodized salt • Managing the IFC activities at the apex level • Managing the financial and other physical aspects of state level IDD cells.	• Identification of children from school and community with goiter and other iodine deficiency disorders. • Nutritional or development assessment of community children (growth, muscle size, etc.) • Conduction of goiter examination of identified children and refer the cases • Salt and urine sample collection from identified children. • To create awareness among the community regarding the high risk group (infants, pregnant and lactating women) and importance of iodized salt for them. • To advise the people to eat iodized salt for household consumption. • To educate the public to understand the importance of proper storage of iodized salt • Training of paramedical staff a as nurse teacher • To evaluate of IDD program periodically through community survey.

Contd...

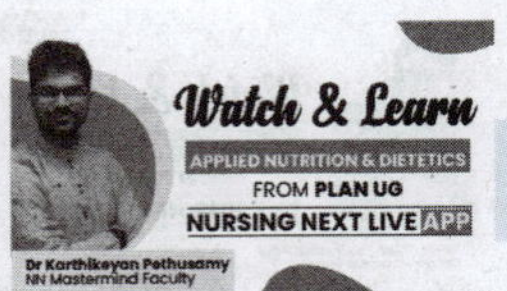

Nutritional program	Description	Modifications if any	Goals/Objectives	Beneficiaries	Services	Role of nurse
Integrated Child Development Service (ICDS)	ICDS was launched on October 2, 1975 by the Government of India under the Ministry of Social and Women Welfare in the pursuance of National Policy for Children. ICDS is one of the world's largest and most unique programs for early childhood care and development. Now, the goal is universalization of ICDS throughout the country.		• Improve the nutritional and health status of children below the age of 6 years. • Lay the foundation for proper psychological, physical and social development. • Reduce the incidence of mortality, morbidity, malnutrition and school droupouts. • Achieve effective coordination and implementation of policy among various departments. • Enhance the capacity of the mother to look after the normal health and nutrition needs through proper nutrition and health education.	• Children below 6 years • Pregnant and lactating women • Women in the age group of 15–44 years • Adolescent girls in selected girls • The ninth five year plan aims to universalize the ICDS.	• Health checkups • Growth promotion and supplementary feeding • Immunization • Referral services • Nutrition and health education to women • Early childhood care and preschool education. • Treatment of minor illnesses • Convergence of other supportive services like water supply, sanitation, etc. • Anganwadi center is the focal point of delivery of these projects. Anganwadi centers are managed by anganwadi workers, assisted by anganwadi helpers.	• Regular and timely health checkups of children and expecting mothers • Regular immunization of under 5 children • Referral in severe cases • Providing education regarding health and nutrition to expectant mothers • Organizing nonformal education for children of 3 – 6 years of age groups • Coordination of health checkups, immunization • Organization of supplementary nutrition free for under 6 children and expecting/lactating mothers • Carrying out surveys • Training of ICDS staff and supervision of staff activities • Periodic evaluation and comparing it with previous data.

2. Define nutrition. Explain in detail nutritional problems in India with preventive measures. (MGR)

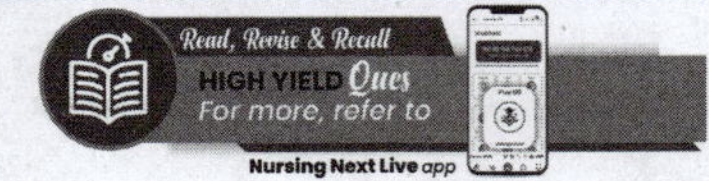

Answer

Nutrition

- Nutrition is defined as the science of food and its relationship with health. It plays an important role in growth, development and maintenance of the body system. It is also defined as the science of food, nutrients and other substances with their actions, interaction, balance and relationship with health and illness. It includes the ingestion, digestion, absorption and utilization of food, and disposal of their end products.
- It is the science of food, the nutrients and the substances, their actions, interaction and balance in relation to health and disease, the process by which the organism ingests, digests, absorbs, transports, utilizes and excretes food substances.

Nutritional Problems in India

Nutritional problems in India:

- Protein Energy malnutrition
  - Kwashiorkor
  - Marasmus
- Micronutrient deficiency
- Chronic diseases

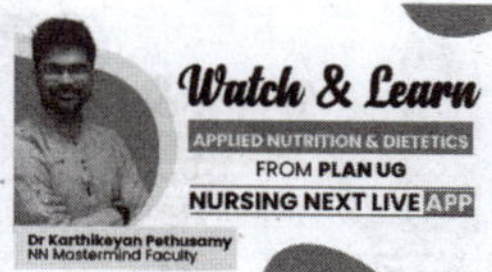

- Lathyrism
- Fluorosis
- Easting disorders

Nutritional problem	Causes	Clinical presentation	Management	Preventive measures
Kwashiorkor	Insufficient intake of proteins, due to weaning from mother's milk to a diet low in protein	• Seen in children of age 1–5 years • Peeling and alternately pigmented skin • Hair loss • Edema or swelling • Skin folds	Providing carbohydrates followed by high protein foods. Dried milk specially	• Encouraging breast feeding for at least 6 months • Improving the health of nursing mothers • Increased intake of protein rich diet.
Marasmus	Deficiency of calories, insufficient intake of proteins, fats and carbohydrates due to failed breastfeeding, feeding inadequate infant formula or suffering from some disease like diarrhea	• Seen in children under age of one year • Large belly sticking out • Diarrhea • Change in skin pigmentation • Muscle wasting • Diarrhea • Growth retardation • Fatigue • Hair changes	Providing a nutritious, well-balanced diet with lots of fresh fruits and vegetables, grains, and protein. Especially adding vitamin B to the diet.	Increasing awareness and availability of protein and calorie rich diet.
Micronutrient deficiencies	Vitamin and mineral deficiencies such as vitamin A, B_1, B_2, B_3, B_6, B_{12} and C; iodine, iron, zinc, calcium, selenium, fluorine	• A plethora of signs and symptoms occurs due to these deficiencies • Common ones are weakness, fatigue and failure to thrive. • Iodine deficiency leads to goiter; and vitamin A deficiency is a leading cause of blindness	• Supplementation through diet or medications • Managing the etiology, i.e., either reduced intake or insufficient absorption.	• Dietary supplementation • Use of iodized salt to prevent iodine deficiency • Vitamin A drops
Lathyrism	Consumption of certain legumes like 'khesari dal'	• Neurological disease • Spastic paralysis of lower limbs	Antispastic drugs and physiotherapy	Eating the chickling pea with grains having high concentration of sulfur based amino acids reduces the risk of lathyrism
Fluorosis	Most common cause - Intake of fluorine rich water	• Two types—Skeletal and nonskeletal • Hypercalcification of bones, muscles, spinal ligaments • Increased risk of fractures • Teeth discoloration and mottling • Neurological disturbance	• Palliative management • Cosmetic treatments for dental fluorosis	Identification of fluorine rich areas and defluoridation of the water supply

SHORT NOTES

1. Discuss the National Nutrition Policy. (MGR, DU)

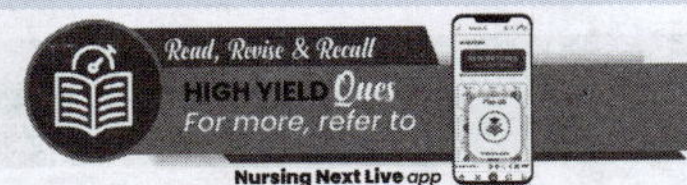

Answer

National Nutrition Policy

Advocates a multisectoral strategy for eradication of malnutrition across the country.

Aims/Goals of National Nutrition Policy

- To improve nutrient intake
- To advocate intersectoral coordination
- To observe nutrition as an outcome of the sectoral activities
- To reduce the incidence of malnutrition across the country
- To improve access and food availability
- To establish various strategies to achieve the nutritional goals
- To prevent and reduce food and vector-borne diseases
- To improve mother and child care
- To strengthen the nutritional capacity within all levels and sectors of GoI

Nutrition Policy Instruments

In order to handle the nutrition problems, various developmental policy instruments have been developed that include:

Direct short-term intervention	Indirect policy instruments
• Includes all vulnerable groups such as ▪ Children below 6 years ▪ Mothers of 0–3-year-old children ▪ Pregnant and lactating mothers ▪ Adolescent girls • This includes: ▪ Use of fortified foods ▪ Production of low cost nutritious foods ▪ Control of micronutrient deficiencies.	• Encouraging food security • Prevention of food adulteration • Improvement in dietary patterns • Policies for effective income transfer • Health and family welfare • Regular monitoring of nutrition programs • Improving educational and literacy levels of women.

Administration and Monitoring

- To analyze the nutritional relevance of sectoral proposals
- To incorporate of nutritional considerations
- To analyze, discuss and resolve the technical issues and nutrition aspects of all plans
- The council will be the national forum for policy coordination, review and direction at the national level.
- Monitoring of nutrition situation.

Role of State Governments

- Decentralization at provincial and district level.
- Prioritized targeting at rural, urban levels.
- Integrating nutrition interventions into all relevant sectors.
- Establishing coordination mechanisms for planning, implementation, management and M+E of the nutrition program
- To ensure that women and vulnerable groups play an active decision-making role in the planning and implementation of the strategies.
- To establish and strengthen participatory monitoring and evaluation systems.

Strength of the Policy

- Identified that nutrition is key to country's development
- Both direct and indirect interventions were identified.
- Identified that malnutrition has to be taken care through multisectoral approach.
- Identified a series of activities like production, distribution of food, women empowerment and nutrition surveillance.

2. Write about the iodine Deficiency Control (IDD) program. (MGR)

Answer

Iodine Deficiency Disorders Control Program

- Iodine deficiency disorders include mental and physical retardation, deaf, mutism, cretinism, still birth, abortion etc.
- Taken care by the Ministry of Health and Family Welfare
- **Objectives**
  - To conduct surveys to assess the magnitude of IDD
  - To laboratory monitor the iodized salt and urinary iodine excretion.
  - To supply iodized salt in place of normal salt
  - To conduct resurveys to assess the extent of IDD and impact of the iodized salt.
  - Health education and publicity
- **Goal**
  - To reduce the prevalence of IDD below 10% in the endemic districts of the country by 2012.
- **Activities**
  - Imparting training
  - Technical guidance to the state/UTs
  - Intersectoral coordination at various levels
  - Collection, compilation and analysis of relevant data
  - Monitoring the quality control of iodized salt
  - Undertaking various IDD surveys

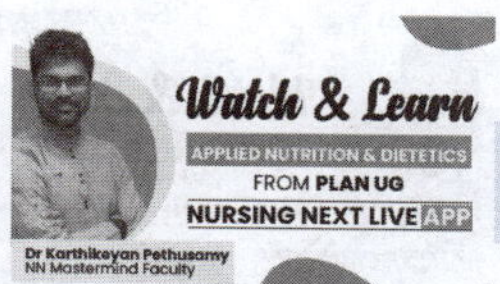

- **Role of nurse in IDDCP**
  - Identification of children from school and community with goiter and other iodine deficiency disorders.
  - Nutritional or development assessment of community children (growth, muscle size, etc.)
  - Conduction of goiter examination of identified children and refer the cases
  - Salt and urine sample collection from identified children.
  - Creating awareness among the community regarding the high risk group (infants, pregnant and lactating women) and importance of iodized salt for them.
  - Advise the people to eat iodized salt for household consumption.
  - Educate the public to understand the importance of proper storage of iodized salt
  - Training of paramedical staff as nurse teacher
  - Evaluation of IDD program periodically through community survey.

3. Write a note on midday meal program. (MGR, DU, KUHS)

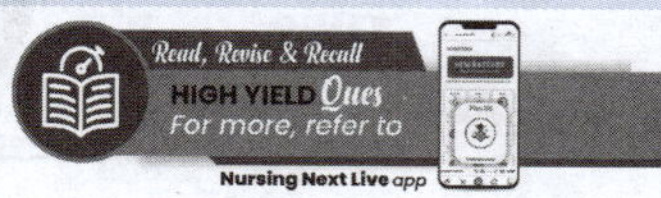

Answer

Midday Meal Scheme

- Midday meal is provided to primary school children with 300 calories of energy and 8–12 g protein per day for minimum 200 days.
- Modifications/Revisions
  - 2004 – free supply of food grains, cooking cost at Rs 1/ child/school day and transport subsidy
  - 2006 – calories intake was increased to 450 and 12 g of protein
  - 2007 – covered the upper primary classes
  - 2008 – extended to Madrasas under Sarva Siksha Abhiyaan

Role of Nurse

- Acts as a nutrition counselor in community
- Assesses the nutritional status of school children with the help of nutrition assessment tools.
- Conveys information related to nutrition and health to teachers, parents and children.
- Plans the weekly menu
- Evaluates failure or success of the program
- Refers the severely malnourished
- Organizes regular health education camps.
- School health nurse is responsible to maintain the health records of school children.

4. Write a note on integrated Child Development Scheme (ICDS program). (MGR, DU, KUHS)

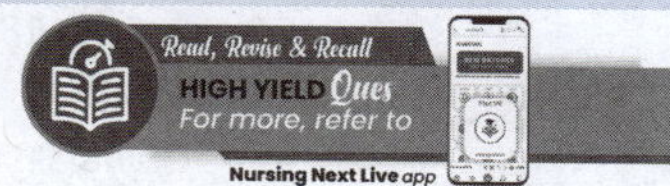

Answer

Integrated Child Development Scheme (ICDS)

- One of the world's largest and most unique programs for early childhood care and development
- The ninth five year plan aims to universalize the ICDS.

Objectives	• To improve the nutritional and health status of under 6 years children • To lay the foundation for proper psychological, physical and social development. • To reduce the incidence of mortality, morbidity, malnutrition and school dropouts. • To achieve effective coordination and implementation of policy • To educate the mother about proper nutrition and child development.
Beneficiaries	• Children under 6 years of age • Pregnant and lactating women • Women in the age group of 15 – 44 years • Adolescent girls
Services of ICDS	• Health checkups • Growth promotion and supplementary feeding • Immunization • Referral services • Nutrition and health education to women • Early childhood care and preschool education. • Treatment of minor illnesses • Convergence of other supportive services like water supply, sanitation, etc. • Anganwadi center - focal point of delivery of these projects.
Delivery of services	• Supplementary nutrition • Nonformal preschool education • Immunization • Health checkups: It includes ▪ Antenatal and postnatal care of expectant mothers ▪ Care of children under 6 years of age. ▪ Providing iron and folic acid tablet along with protein supplements to expectant mothers. • Nutrition and health education ▪ Giving health education to expectant and nursing mothers regarding nutrition and other health related topics by anganwadi workers during their home visit. Nutritional program for Adolescent Girls 2003 • Given to girls that weigh less than 35 kg and pregnant women <45 kg • Get ration of 6 kg/month free of cost in the form of wheat and rice

Contd...

	Scheme for adolescent girls (Kishori Shakti Yojana) • Educating the adolescent girls in the age group of 11–18 years (70%) about menarche, immunization, training for minor ailments, deworming ▪ General health checkups for anemia, goiter and vitamin deficiencies, etc. ▪ Referral to PHC, district hospital, if required
Role of nurse	• Regular and timely health checkups of children and expecting mothers • Regular immunization of under 5 children • Referral in severe cases • Providing education regarding health and nutrition to expectant mothers • Organizing nonformal education for children of 3–6 years of age groups • Coordination of health checkups, immunization • Organization of supplementary nutrition free for under 6 children and expecting/lactating mothers • Carrying out surveys • Training of ICDS staff and supervision of staff activities • Periodic evaluation and comparing it with previous data.

5. What are the objectives of Applied Nutrition Program. (MGR)

Answer

Applied Nutritional Programme

- First started in Andhra Pradesh and Orissa in 1959, later expanded to other states of India.
- Factors affects the nutritional status improvement:
  - Awareness and knowledge
  - Availability of food

Objectives of Applied Nutrition Program

- To combat malnutrition and improvement in nutritional status in affected groups, young children and mothers.
- To increase awareness about the nutritional needs.
- To provide supplementary nutrition through locally produced foods.
- To increase the production of nutritional food and their consumption.

Features

- Improves nutrition in the underprivileged groups
- Success is dependent on the political willingness.
- Community participation is an important aspect.
- Continuous monitoring and evaluation are required.
- Repeated incidence of food poisoning reported in mid-day meals causes serious threat to the existence of these programs.

6. Write a note on types of supplementary foods. (MGR)

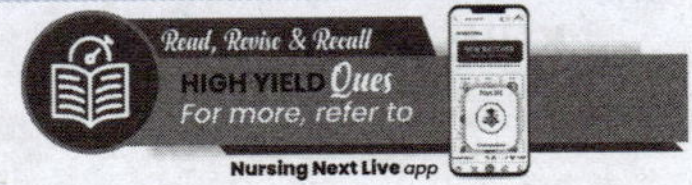

Answer

Supplementary Nutrition/foods

- Given to children after weaning from breast milk below 6 years of age.
- In this, 500 calories and 12–15 g of protein are given to children between 6–72 months of age.
- In case of severely malnourished, 800 calories and 20–25 g of proteins are given.

Types of Supplementary Foods

Liquid supplements	Solid supplements	Solid supplements unmashed
• Milk: By the 6th month, animal milk is introduced and breast milk is reduced. • Fresh fruit juice: Fruit juices such as sweet lime, oranges, grapes etc. are added to supplement the protective nutrients that are present in insufficient amounts in milk. • Soup: vegetable soup, initially strained and later unstrained provides for several vitamins and minerals.	• Mashed food: Started around 7th and 8th month. • Cereal and starchy food: This takes care of the increasing calorie demands • Vegetables: Cooked, mashed vegetables like potato, green leafy vegetables and carrots add variety of colors, tastes and vitamins. • Fruits: Stewed fruits are given to children below 1 year. Banana are given as mashed • Nonvegetarian: Small amounts of minced and cooked/boiled eggs/meat/fish should be given with gradual increase in quantity. • Pulses: Khidchi/pongal/porridge	• Slowly as the child grows teeth, chopped vegetables, cooked cereals, pulses and vegetables can be introduced. • Solids like idli, chapatti, rice can be added to diet as the child gets accommodated with semi solids.

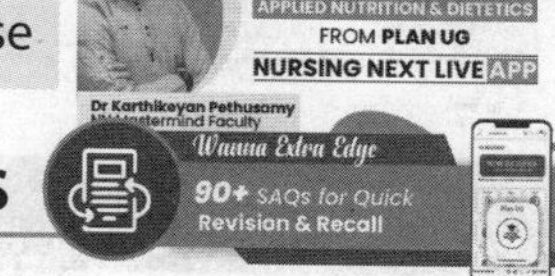

7. Explain the role of nurse in nutritional program with reference to vitamin A drops program. (MGR)

Answer

Vitamin A Drops/Prophylaxis Program:

- The program was started in 1970
- To prevent blindness due to deficiency of vitamin A
- Goals
  - Administration of vitamin A solution to children
  - Promotion of exclusive breastfeeding for newborn in mothers

Role of Nurse

- As an educator and counselor
  - Providing education to community regarding importance of vitamin A rich food and breastfeeding.
  - Promote exclusive breastfeeding for newborn
  - Ensure regular intake of vitamin A in children
- As a caregiver
  - Administer vitamin A to children
- As a manager
  - Identify the under five children of that area
  - Prepare a plan of action
  - Ensure supply of vitamin A solution
  - Supervise and monitor in the field.
  - Regular monitoring of services to watch the progress of the program
  - Submission of report to authorities from time to time.

SHORT ANSWER QUESTIONS

1. Objectives of applied nutrition program. (MGR)

Answer

Applied nutrition programme was introduced at Orissa in 1963 which extended to Tamil Nadu and Uttar Pradesh. The objectives are:

- Promoting production of protective food such as vegetables and fruits and
- Ensure their consumption by pregnant and nursing mothers and children.

2. Two national organizations associated with nutrition. (MGR)

Answer

- National Institute of Nutrition (ICMR)
- Food and Agriculture Organization
- Food and Nutrition Board, Ministry of Women and Child Development, Government of India
- Indian Dietetic Association

3. NIPCCD (National Institute of Public Cooperation and Child Development) (DU)

Answer

NIPCCD is a premier organization devoted to promotion of voluntary action research, training and documentation in the overall domain of women and child development.

The objectives of NIPCCD are to develop and promote programs in pursuance of the National Policy for Children and to work for child development.

CONCEPTUAL REVISION

MULTIPLE CHOICE QUESTIONS

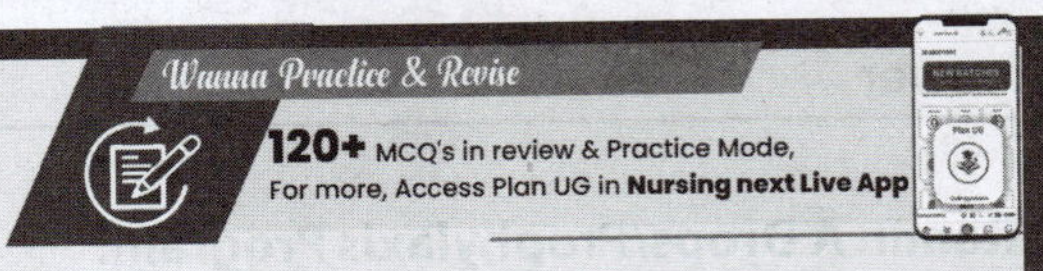

1. What is the primary objective of National Nutritional Programs?
- a. To promote healthy eating habits
- b. To reduce malnutrition among the population
- c. To increase the availability of nutritious foods
- d. To prevent the spread of food-borne illnesses

Ans. b. To reduce malnutrition among the population

2. What is the role of nurses in National Nutritional Programs?
- a. To provide nutrition education to patients and their families
- b. To conduct nutritional assessments of patients
- c. To provide referrals to nutritionists and dietitians
- d. All of the above

Ans. a. To provide nutrition education to patients and their families

3. Which of the following groups is most at risk for malnutrition?
- a. Children under the age of 5
- b. Elderly adults
- c. Pregnant women
- d. All of the above

Ans. d. All of the above

4. What are some common causes of malnutrition?
- a. Poverty and food insecurity
- b. Chronic illness and medication use
- c. Poor access to health care
- d. All of the above

Ans. d. All of the above

5. What are some key components of a healthy diet?
- a. Adequate protein and healthy fats
- b. A variety of fruits and vegetables
- c. Whole grains and fiber
- d. All of the above

Ans. a. Adequate protein and healthy fats

6. What is the role of micronutrients in the body?
- a. To provide energy for physical activity
- b. To support growth and development
- c. To regulate bodily processes
- d. All of the above

Ans. b. To support growth and development

7. How can nurses promote healthy eating habits in their patients?
- a. By providing nutrition education and resources
- b. By encouraging patients to track their food intake
- c. By making recommendations for healthier food choices
- d. All of the above

Ans. a. By providing nutrition education and resources

8. What is the WIC program?
- a. A federal program that provides food and nutrition assistance to low-income pregnant women, new mothers, and young children
- b. A state-level program that promotes healthy eating habits in schools
- c. A national initiative to reduce childhood obesity
- d. A program that provides funding for community gardens and urban agriculture projects

Ans. a. A federal program that provides food and nutrition assistance to low-income pregnant women, new mothers, and young children

9. What is the role of community health workers in National Nutritional Programs?
- a. To provide education and support to individuals and families in the community
- b. To conduct nutritional assessments and provide referrals to health care providers
- c. To advocate for policies and programs that promote healthy eating
- d. All of the above

Ans. a. To provide education and support to individuals and families in the community

10. Which government agency is responsible for implementing national nutritional programs in India?
- a. Ministry of Health and Family Welfare
- b. Ministry of Women and Child Development
- c. National Institute of Nutrition
- d. All of the above

Ans. d. All of the above

CHAPTER

13

Food Safety

CONCEPTUAL THEORY

Terminology

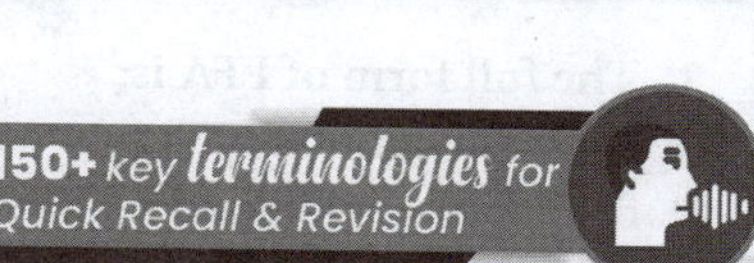

Food taboos: Religion-based food habits like vegetarianism in Hindu society and prohibition of pork in Muslim society.
Health: State of complete physical, mental and social well-being and not merely an absence of disease and infirmity (WHO).
Macronutrients: Required in large quantity and from the bulk of our food, e.g., proteins, fats and carbohydrates.
Micronutrients: Required in small amounts but play an important role in the regulation of metabolic activities, e.g., vitamins and minerals.
Nutrient: A substance essential for the growth, maintenance, function and reproduction of a cell or of an organism.

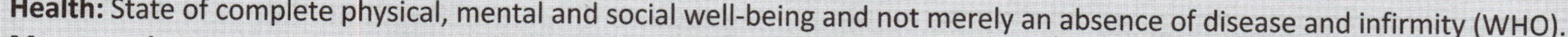

DEFINITION, FOOD SAFETY CONSIDERATIONS AND MEASURES

Food Safety Regulatory Measures in India

Food safety is used as a scientific method/discipline describing good food handling, preparation, supply and storage of food in a manner that will result in prevention of food-borne illness.

Five Keys to Safer Food:
1. Keep clean
2. Separate raw and cooked
3. Cook thoroughly
4. Keep food at safe temperature
5. Use safe water and raw material

CONCEPTUAL EXERCISES

SHORT NOTE

1. Write a note on five keys to safer food.

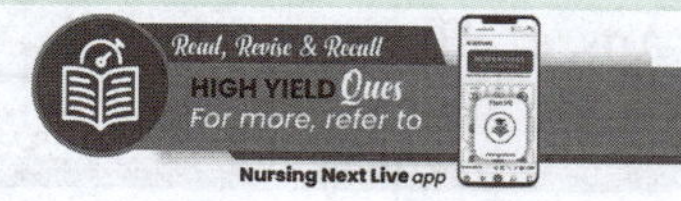

Answer

Five Keys to Safer Food

1. **Keep clean:**
   - Wash your hands before food handling and during preparation of food.
   - Wash hands after using toilet.
   - Wash and sanitize all the equipment used for preparing food.
   - Kitchen should be protected against insects, pests and animals.
2. **Separate raw and cooked:**
   - Allow separate the raw meat, poultry and seafood from other foods.
   - For handling raw food, always use separate equipment.
   - Always store raw food in container to avoid contact between raw food and prepared food.
3. **Cook thoroughly:**
   - Food should be cooked thoroughly especially raw food.
   - For preparing soups and stews, boiling temperature should reach up to 70°C.
   - For preparing raw food, make sure that meat is clean and is free from juices. The preparing temperature should be assumed by the use of thermometer.
   - Cooked food should be reheated thoroughly

4. **Keep food at safe temperature:**
   - Cooked food should not be left at room temperature for more than 2 hours.
   - Cooked and perishable food should be placed in refrigerator below 5°C.
   - Before serving food should be hotter than 60°C.
   - Even in refrigerator food should not be stored for long time.
   - Frozen food should always be thawed in the refrigerator.
5. **Use safe water and raw material:**
   - To make food safe, use safe water.
   - To prepare food always select fresh and whole some food.
   - Always wash fruits and vegetables especially when you eat raw food.
   - Always check expiry date before using food.

CONCEPTUAL REVISION

MULTIPLE CHOICE QUESTIONS

1. The full form of PFA is:
   a. Prevention of food act
   b. Protection of food act
   c. Prevention of food adulteration act
   d. None of the above

Ans. c. Prevention of food adulteration act

2. The preservation of food through 'Cold sterilization' involves
   a. Dehydration b. Lyophilization
   c. Refrigeration d. Radiation

Ans. d. Radiation

3. This method dehydrates microbial cells by plasmolysis thereby causing them to die
   a. Heating b. Smoking
   c. Pasteurization d. Sugaring

Ans. d. Sugaring

4. Under the PFA Act, when is the food said to be adulterated
   a. If any ingredient is injurious to health
   b. If it is obtained from a diseased animal
   c. If spices are sold without their essence
   d. All of the above

Ans. d. All of the above

5. This statement about Potassium Bromate is/are true
   1. Potassium Bromate is a category 2B carcinogen
   2. Potassium Bromate increases dough strength, leads to higher rising and uniform finish to baked products
   3. Food Safety and Standards Authority of India (FSSAI) allows them upto 50 parts per million

   a. 1, 2 b. 1, 3
   c. 2, 3 d. All of these

Ans. d. All of these

6. In cattle, this factor is critical that would lead to increased milk yield
   a. Provision of ideal environmental conditions to cattle
   b. Hygiene and stringent cleanliness
   c. Disease-resistant
   d. Selection of good breeds

Ans. d. Selection of good breeds

7. This is an adulterant:
   a. Pesticides b. Urea
   c. Iron filings in tea d. All of these

Ans. d. All of these

Golden Points

- Additives are substances added to food to improve flavor, color and texture or to preserve foods to help extend the self-life.
- Food safety is used as a scientific method/discipline describing good food handling, preparation, supply and storage of food in a manner that will result in prevention of food-borne illness.
- Nonperishable foods are all canned foods such as jams, jelly, pickles, whole pulses, cereals, legumes, sugar, jaggery and pure honey, pure ghee, tea, coffee, spices, condiments and food flavors, etc.
- Perishable foods are fish, meat, poultry, milk and milk products, bread and bread products, butter, cream, cheese, fruits and vegetables and cooked food.

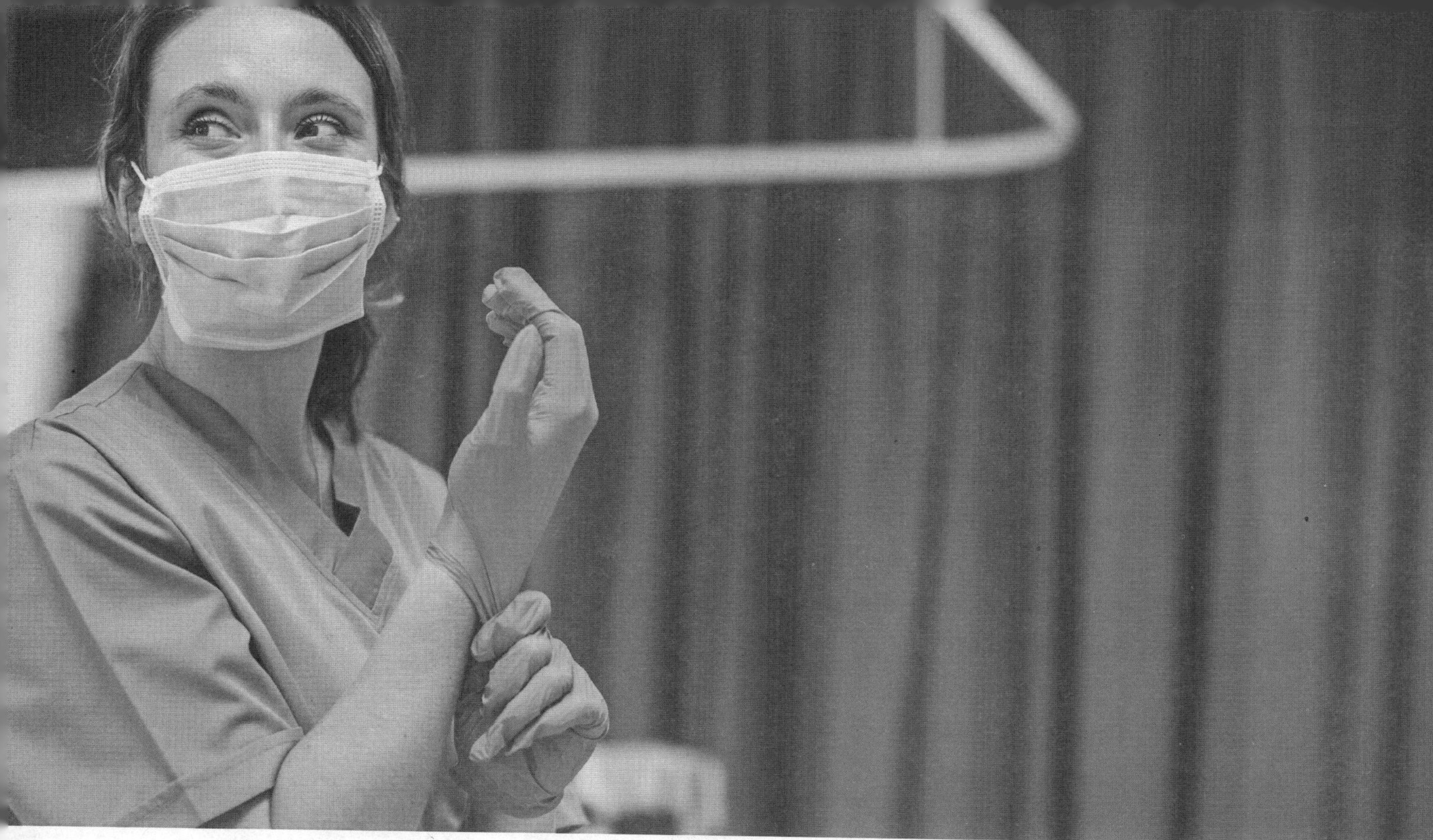

Nursing Foundation

Unit Outline

CHAPTER 1

Introduction to Health and Illness

CONCEPTUAL THEORY

Terminology

Acquired immunity: Immunity which is developed later in life after microbial infection or through vaccination in host is called acquired or developed immunity.
Health: It is a state of complete physical, mental and social well-being and not merely the absence of disease or infirmity.
Illness: A disease or period of sickness affecting the body or mind.
Illness behavior: It is any behavior undertaken by an individual who feels ill to relieve that experience or to better define the meaning of the illness experience.
Immunization: It is the process whereby a person is made immune or resistant to an infectious disease, typically by the administration of a vaccine. Vaccines stimulate the body's own immune system to protect the person against subsequent infection or disease.
Innate immunity: Immunity with which an individual is born is called innate or natural immunity.
The term immunity refers to the body's specific protective response to an invading foreign agent or organism. The human body has the ability to resist almost all types of organisms or toxins that tend to damage the tissues and organs. The capability is called immunity.
Wellness: It is a state of well-being.

HEALTH

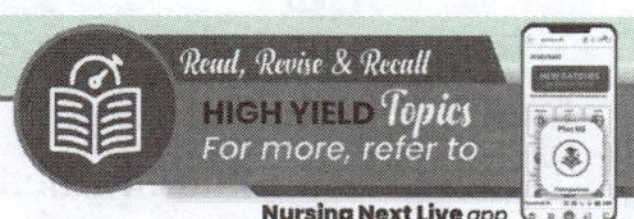

According to WHO, "Health is a state of complete physical, mental, social and spiritual well-being and not merely an absence of disease or infirmity."

Dimensions of Health

- Physical dimension
- Emotional dimension
- Sociocultural dimension
- Intellectual dimension
- Environmental dimension
- Spiritual dimension

Health-Illness Continuum

Composed of two arrows:

1. Movement towards right indicates increasing state of health
2. Movement towards left indicates deterioration in health

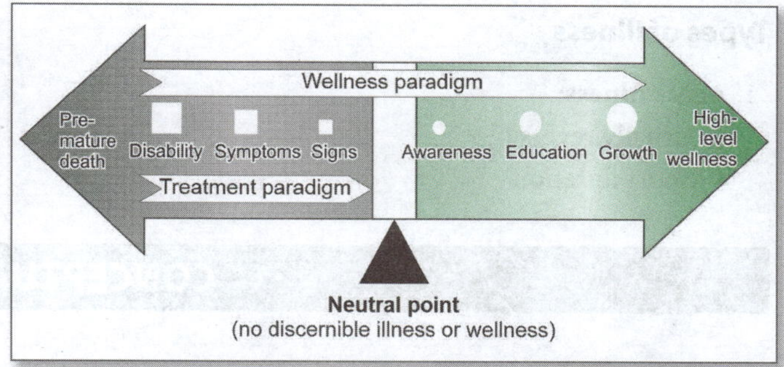

Figure 1.1: Health-illness continuum

Maslow's Hierarchy of Needs

According to Abraham Maslow, people are motivated to fulfill their basic needs. People need to satisfy their most important needs first, when they achieved this, they can move onto the next need.

- **The first stage of hierarchy:** Physiological stage
- **The second stage of hierarchy:** Safety stage
- **The third stage of hierarchy:** Love/Belonging stage
- **The fourth stage of hierarchy:** Esteem stage
- **The fifth stage of hierarchy:** Self-actualization stage

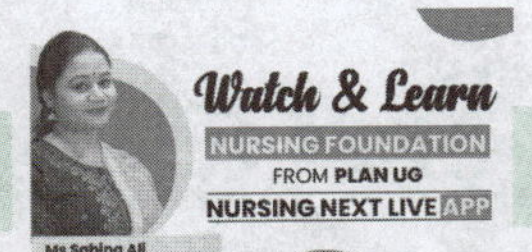

Factors Influencing Health

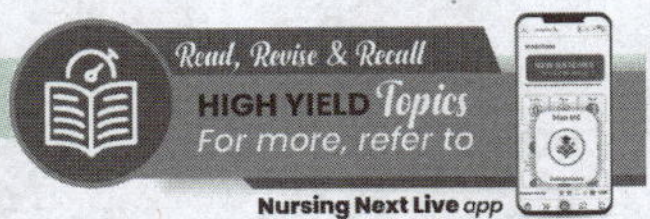

- The factors are multifactorial present within the individual and externally in the society.
- These factors are broadly classified into the following:
  1. **Genetic factors:**
     - The mental and physical traits of individuals are determined by genes to some extent.
     - Health depends on the genetic predisposition.
  2. **Environmental factors:**
     - It can be external or internal.
     - The internal environment pertains to body tissues, organs and organ system.
     - The external environment comprises three components:
       1. **Physical environment**—water, air, sunlight, climate, season, soil, housing-facilities, waste and excreta disposal, etc.
       2. **Biological environment**—all living things, plants, animals, insects and microorganisms.
       3. **Social environment**—people, customs, culture, society, income, occupation, religion, etc.

ILLNESS

It is the state in which a person's physical, emotional, intellectual, social, developmental, or spiritual functioning is diminished or impaired.

Types of Illness

1. **Acute illness:**
   - Usually reversible
   - Short duration
   - Intense
   - Short period illness
2. **Chronic illness:**
   - Persists longer than 6 months
   - Irreversible
   - May be life threatening

Illness Behavior

Illness behavior refers to the way individuals respond to and behave when they are experiencing symptoms or are faced with a health condition.

Stages of Illness Behavior

- **Stage 1:** Experiencing symptoms
- **Stage 2:** Assuming the sick role
- **Stage 3:** Medical care seeking
- **Stage 4:** Assuming the dependent role
- **Stage 5:** Achieving resources and rehabilitation

Impact of Illness on Patient

- Irrespective of type of illness, all patients exhibit certain illness behaviors
- These behaviors are unique in nature
- Illness behavior also depends upon age, sex, family, cultural and education level, etc.

Impact of Illness on Family

- Whenever any illness occurs, both the patient and the family get affected.
- The responses of family members to an illness are also unique.
- Some family members want to be with the patient all the time, while others might avoid visiting.

CONCEPTUAL EXERCISES

LONG ANSWER QUESTION

1. Write about Health-illness continuum. Explain the illness and illness behavior along with the impact of illness on patient and family. (MGR, KUHS, RUHS)

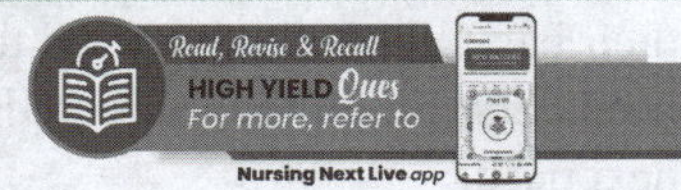

Answer

Health-illness Continuum

- Concept proposed by John W Travis in 1972.
- The health-illness continuum is a graphic illustration of a well-being,
- Composed of two arrows pointing in opposite direction and joined at a neutral point.
- Movement to the right to the arrows (toward the high level of wellness) indicates increase in level of health and well-being.
- Health and well-being can be achieved in three steps:
  1. Awareness
  2. Education
  3. Growth

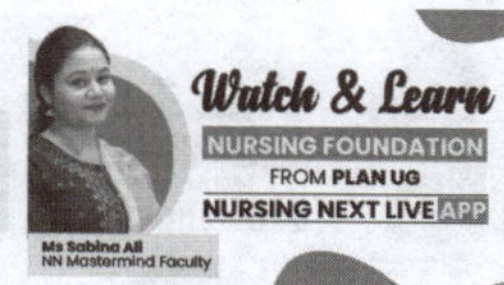

Movement to the left to the arrows (toward premature death) shows decreasing state of health.

This can be achieved in three steps:

1. Signs
2. Symptoms
3. Disability

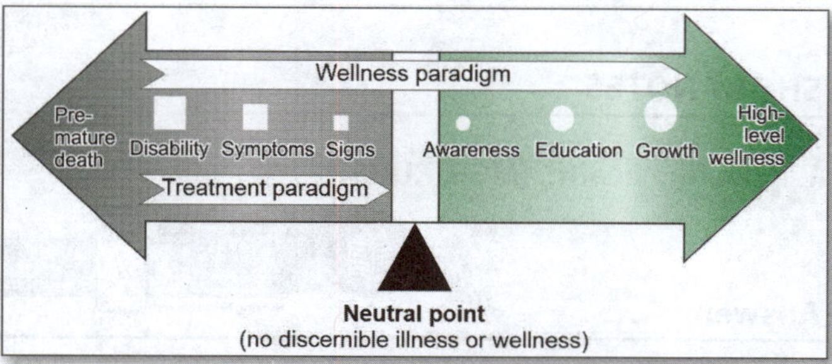

Figure 1.2: Health-illness continuum

Illness and Illness Behavior

Illness

It is the state in which a person's physical, emotional, intellectual, social, developmental, or spiritual functioning is diminished or impaired.

General Classification of Illness

1. **Acute illness:**
   - Usually reversible
   - Short duration
   - Often severe
   - Symptoms appear abruptly
   - Intense
   - Short period illness
2. **Chronic illness:**
   - Persists longer than 6 months
   - Irreversible
   - Affects one or more systems
   - May be life threatening

Illness Behavior

- How the people act when they are ill that the medical sociologists called it an illness behavior.
- How people react to illness.
- It involves explaining the symptoms, seek medical help, and use the health care-related resources.
- Illness behavior has two variables:
  1. **Internal variables**—patient perception of symptoms.
  2. **External variables**—economic condition, accessibility of health care system and social group.

Impact of Illness on Patient and Family

Impact of Illness on Patient

- Irrespective of type of illness, all patients exhibit certain illness behaviors.
- These behaviors are unique in nature.
- Illness behavior also depends upon age, sex, family, cultural and education level, etc.

Stage1: Experiencing Symptoms

- The ways how people cope with alterations in functions due to the presence of disease.
- Unique for each individual.
- If symptoms are of short duration, individual does not take any intervention.

Stage 2: Assuming the Sick Role

- If symptoms persist, person may choose not to take anything but also can buy over-the-counter drugs.
- May seek medical help.

Stage 3: Medical Care Seeking

In this stage, individuals decide whether to seek medical care or not. Factors like perceived severity of symptoms, perceived effectiveness of treatment, availability of healthcare, previous experiences, and social influences can influence the decision to seek medical help.

Stage 4: Assuming the Dependent Role

- Person may depend on others.
- May seek assistance in daily activities.
- If illness is serious, it may require hospitalization.

Stage 5: Achieving Resources and Rehabilitation

- Recovery and rehabilitation may start in hospital.
- Person gives up the dependency.
- Resume normal activities and responsibilities.

Impact of Illness on Family

- Family dynamics will be adversely affected due to illness in the family. It includes.
- Whenever any illness occurs, both the patient and the family get affected.
- The responses of family members to an illness are also unique.
- **Financial burden:** The cost of healthcare, loss of income due to caregiving responsibilities, and other related

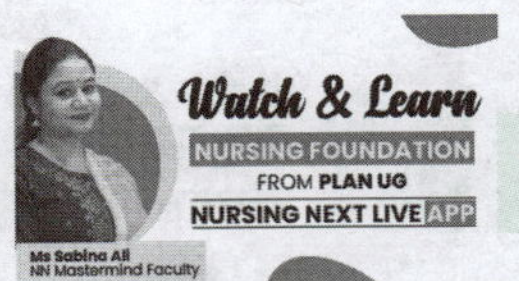

expenses can cause financial strain and impact the family's overall financial stability.

- **Disruption of daily life:** Family members may need to allocate time and resources to seek treatment. This disruption can impact the family's ability to maintain a balanced lifestyle and engage in social activities.
- **Social isolation:** Families dealing with illness may experience social isolation due to the need for specialized care, hospitalizations, or the stigma associated with certain illnesses. This isolation can lead to a lack of social support, feelings of loneliness, and difficulties in maintaining social connections.
- **Increased stress and burnout:** Caring for a family member with an illness can be physically and emotionally demanding. Family caregivers may experience increased stress levels, fatigue, and burnout due to the constant caregiving responsibilities.

Behavioral and Emotional Changes

- People react differently to illness.
- Individual behavioral and emotional reactions depend on the nature of the illness.
- Severe illness can lead to more emotional and behavioral changes.

Impact on Family Roles

When an illness occurs, the client and family often require specific counseling and guidance to assist them in coping due to role changes.

Impact on Body Changes

- Some illnesses results in changes in physical appearance.
- Client and family may show emotions such as shock, withdrawal, acknowledgment, acceptance and rehabilitation.

Impact on Self-concept

- Due to illness, patients may no longer meet the expectations of family.
- Tension and conflicts may also occur.

Impact on Family Dynamics

- Family makes decisions and supports the individual.
- Copes with everyday changes and challenges.
- Illness can disrupt the normal family dynamics and roles. Family members may need to take on new roles or responsibilities, such as caregiving, which can lead to changes in routines and power dynamics within the family. This can create stress and tension within family relationships.
- Emotional and Psychological Impact: Illness can create emotional distress and psychological challenges for both the individual and the family members. Family members may experience feelings of worry, anxiety, fear, and sadness. They may also feel overwhelmed by the responsibilities of care-giving and the uncertainty of the illness.

SHORT NOTES

1. Define health. (MGR, RUHS)

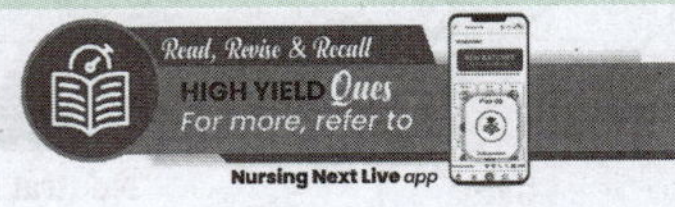

Answer

Health is defined as:

- A series of successful and continuous adaptations to a continuously changing environment.
- The condition of being sound in body, mind and spirit and especially free from physical disease or pain. —*Webster*
- Soundness of body or mind; that condition in which their functions are duly and efficiently performed. —*Oxford English Dictionary*
- A state of relative equilibrium of body's form and function, which results from its successful dynamic adjustment to forces tending to disturb it. It is not passive interplay between body substance and forces impinging upon it but active response of body forces working toward readjustment. —**Perkin**
- **World Health Organization (WHO)** states that "Health is a state of complete physical, mental, social and spiritual well-being and not merely an absence of disease or infirmity."

2. State the factors influencing health. (KUHS, MGR, DU)

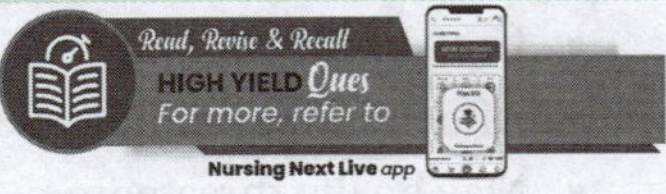

Answer

Factors Influencing Health

- The factors are multifactorial present within the individual and externally in the society.
- These factors are broadly classified into:
  1. **Genetic factors/Heredity/Human biology:**
     - The mental and physical traits of individuals are determined by genes to some extent.
     - Health depends on the genetic predisposition.
  2. **Environmental factors:**
     - Environment has a close relation to the health of an individual.

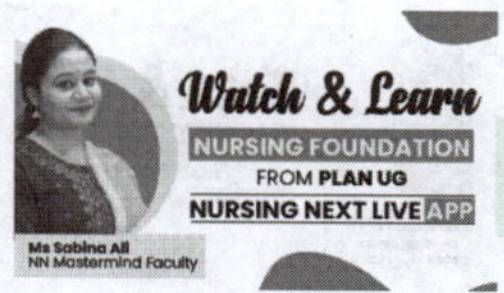

- It can be external or internal.
- The internal environment pertains to body tissues, organs and organ system.
- The external environment is all external conditions of physical and mental capacities he/she has inherited.
- External environment comprises three components:
  1. **Physical environment**—water, air, sunlight, climate, season, soil, housing-facilities, waste and excreta disposal, etc.
  2. **Biological environment**—all living things, plants, animals, insects and microorganisms.
  3. **Social environment**—people, customs, culture, society, income, occupation, religion, etc.

Lifestyle/Ways of Living

- The way people live
- Reflects social values, attitudes and activities.
- Lifestyle is based upon social interactions with parents, peer groups, friends, and siblings and through school and mass media.
- It is composed of cultural and behavioral patterns of life-long personal habits.
- Adoption of healthy lifestyle leads to promoting optimal health.

Resources

- Help in maintaining and determining health of an individual.
- Health status is determined by socioeconomic factors.

Economic Status

The socioeconomic factors have a major role in reducing morbidity, increasing life expectancy and improving quality of life.

Education

- Education is important factor that affects health.
- Lack of education closely coincides with ill health, high infant mortality rate, malnutrition, etc.
- Education compensates the effects of poverty on health.

Occupation

- Occupation promotes health.
- Unemployment deteriorates the socioeconomic status which can lead to deterioration in health status.

Political System

- Political system is responsible for implementation of health technologies.
- Political system is concerned with resource allocation, manpower policy, and the degree to which health services are made available and accessible to different segments of society.

Health Services

Health services are directed toward treatment of diseases, prevention of illness and promotion of health.

3. Mention the various dimensions of health. (MGR)

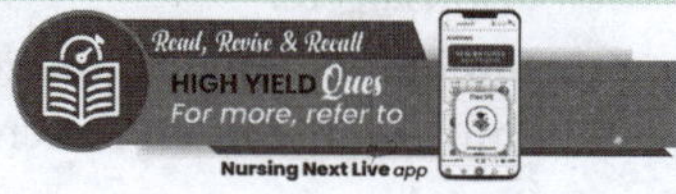

Answer

Dimensions of Health

- Physical dimension
- Emotional dimension
- Sociocultural dimension
- Intellectual dimension
- Environmental dimension
- Spiritual dimension

Physical Dimension

- All the organs of the body function normally.
- All special senses are intact.
- Physiological parameters are normal for the individual's age and sex.

Emotional Dimension

- People feel comfortable about themselves.
- They accept their shortcomings.
- They are internally adjusted.
- They are self-confident.
- They are free from internal conflicts.
- They have good self-control.
- They are not dominated by emotions.
- They have problem solving skills.

Sociocultural Dimension

- Capable of making friendships
- Responsible according to one's capabilities
- Satisfied in accomplishments of everyday tasks
- Live happily with others.

Intellectual Dimension

- Cognitive abilities, past experiences and emotional background.
- Plays an important role in health behavior.

Environmental Dimension

- Environment has a close relation to the health of an individual.
- It can be external or internal.
- The internal environment pertains to body tissues, organs and organ system.
- The external environment is all external conditions of physical and mental capacities he/she has inherited.
- External environment comprises three components:
  1. **Physical environment**—water, air, sunlight, climate, season, soil, housing-facilities, waste and excreta disposal, etc.
  2. **Biological environment**—all living things, plants, animals, insects and microorganisms.
  3. **Social environment**—people, customs, culture, society, income, occupation, religion, etc.

Spiritual Dimension

- Maintains faith in religion
- Believes in empathy
- Believes in goodness of all.

4. Discuss the concept of health. (DU)

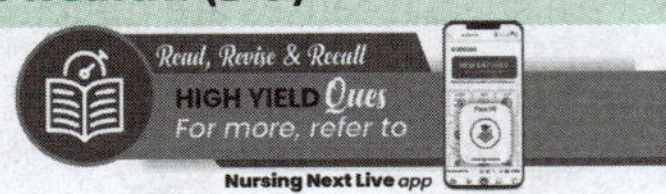

Answer

The concepts of health are discussed below:

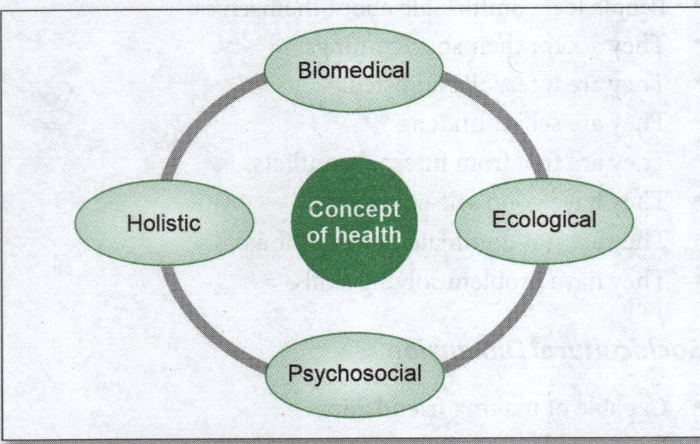

Figure 1.3: Concept of health

- An understanding of health is the basis of all the health care.
- Health is not perceived the same way by all the members of a community.

1. Biomedical Concept

- It is based on the "germ theory of the disease".
- This concept has minimized the role of the environment, social and cultural determinants of the health.

2. Ecological Concept

- Health as a dynamic equilibrium between man and his environment,
- Perceived disease as a maladjustment of the human organism to environment.

3. Psychosocial Concept

Health is also influenced by social, psychological, cultural, economic and political factors of the people.

4. Holistic Concept

- Recognizes the strength of social, economic, political and environmental factors of health.
- Multidimensional process involving the well-being of the person as a whole.
- Emphasis is on the promotion and protection of health.

5. Write short note on health-illness continuum.

Answer

For answer, refer to Long Question no. 1, pg. no. 550

6. Explain the determinants of health.

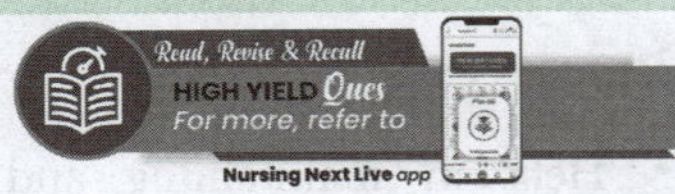

Answer

- The factors are multifactorial present within the individual and externally in the society.
- These factors are broadly classified into:
  1. **Genetic factors/Heredity/Human biology:**
     - The mental and physical traits of individuals are determined by genes to some extent.
     - Health depends on the genetic predisposition.
  2. **Environmental factors:**
     - Environment has a close relation to the health of an individual.
     - It can be external or internal.
     - The internal environment pertains to body tissues, organs and organ system.
     - The external environment is all external conditions of physical and mental capacities he/she has inherited.
     - External environment comprises three components:
       1. **Physical environment**—water, air, sunlight, climate, season, soil, housing-facilities, waste and excreta disposal, etc.
       2. **Biological environment**—all living things, plants, animals, insects and microorganisms.
       3. **Social environment**—people, customs, culture, society, income, occupation, religion, etc.

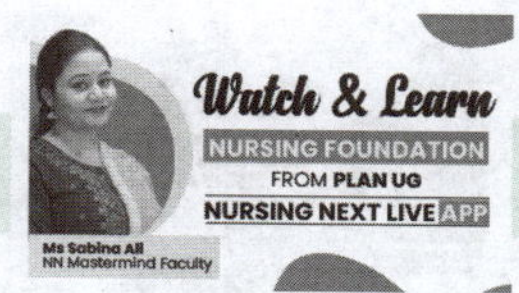

Lifestyle/Ways of Living

- The way people live
- Reflects social values, attitudes and activities.
- Lifestyle is based upon social interactions with parents, peer groups, friends, and siblings and through school and mass media.
- It is composed of cultural and behavioral patterns of life-long personal habits.
- Adoption of healthy lifestyle leads to promoting optimal health.

Resources

- Help in maintaining and determining health of an individual.
- Health status is determined by socioeconomic factors.

Economic Status

The socioeconomic factors have a major role in reducing morbidity, increasing life expectancy and improving quality of life.

Education

- Important factor that affects health.
- Lack of education closely coincides with ill health, high infant mortality rate, malnutrition, etc.
- Education compensates the effects of poverty on health.

Occupation

- Occupation promotes health.
- Unemployment deteriorates the socioeconomic status which can lead to deterioration in health status.

Political System

- Political system is responsible for implementation of health technologies.
- Political system is concerned with resource allocation, manpower policy, and the degree to which health services are made available and accessible to different segments of society.

Health Services

Health services are directed toward treatment of diseases, prevention of illness and promotion of health.

7. Explain the illness and illness behavior.

Answer

For answer, refer to Long Question no. 1, pg. no. 550

8. Explain the impact of illness on patient and family.

Answer

For answer, refer to Long Question no. 1, pg. no. 550

9. Write the stages of illness behavior.

Answer

For answer, refer to Long Question no. 1, pg. no. 550

10. Mention the Maslow's Hierarchy of needs.

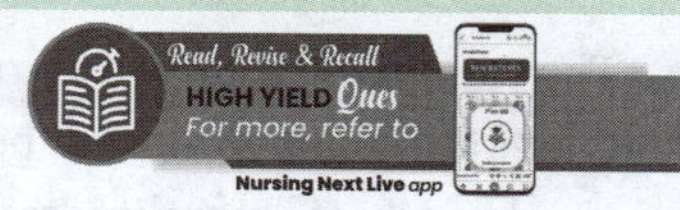

Answer

According to Abraham Maslow, people are motivated to fulfill their basic needs. People need to satisfy their most important needs first, when they achieved this, they can move onto the next need.

The First Stage of Hierarchy—Physiological Stage

It includes 'basic' needs of human life such as breathing, excretion and the desire for food, water, sex, sleep and homeostasis.

The Second Stage of Hierarchy—Safety Stage

Once physiological needs have been met, desire turns to safety and security such as living in a safer place, financial/job security and good health.

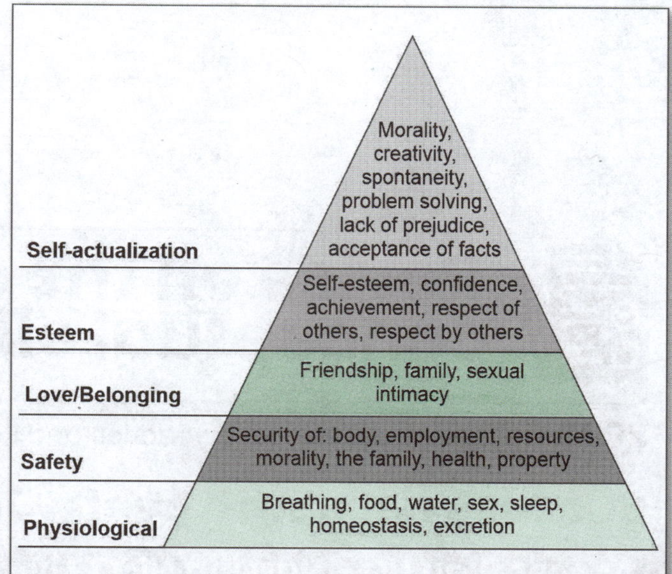

Figure 1.4: Maslow's hierarchy of needs

The Third Stage of Hierarchy—Love/Belonging Stage

- Also referred to as the 'social needs stage'.
- Needs such as family, friendship and sexual intimacy.

The Fourth Stage of Hierarchy—Esteem Stage

- Esteem needs can be external or internal.
- Internal esteem needs are related to self-esteem, such as the need to respect yourself and achieve.
- External esteem needs are those such as social status, reputation and recognition.

The Fifth Stage of Hierarchy—Self-Actualization Stage

- The summit of Maslow's hierarchy of needs.
- Quest of reaching your full potential.
- Needs such as: morality, creativity, problem-solving, and lack of prejudice, acceptance of facts, truth, justice, wisdom and meaning.
- These need can never be satisfied as the people grow, change and continue to challenge themselves.

SHORT ANSWER QUESTIONS

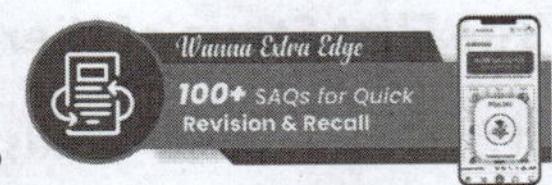

1. Define health. (MGR, RUHS)

Answer

World Health Organization (WHO) states that "Health is a state of complete physical, mental, social and spiritual well-being and not merely an absence of disease or infirmity."

2. Mention the various dimensions of health. (MGR)

Answer

Dimensions of Health

- Physical dimension
- Emotional dimension
- Sociocultural dimension
- Intellectual dimension
- Environmental dimension
- Spiritual dimension

3. Define illness and enumerate stages of illness behavior.

Answer

Definition

Illness: It is the state in which a person's physical, emotional, intellectual, social, developmental, or spiritual functioning is diminished or impaired.

Stages of Illness Behavior

- **Stage 1:** Experiencing symptoms
- **Stage 2:** Assuming the sick role
- **Stage 3:** Medical care seeking
- **Stage 4:** Assuming the dependent role
- **Stage 5:** Achieving resources and rehabilitation

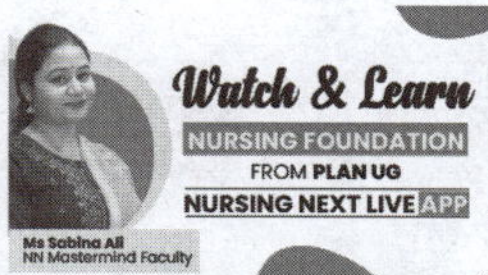

CONCEPTUAL REVISION

MULTIPLE CHOICE QUESTIONS

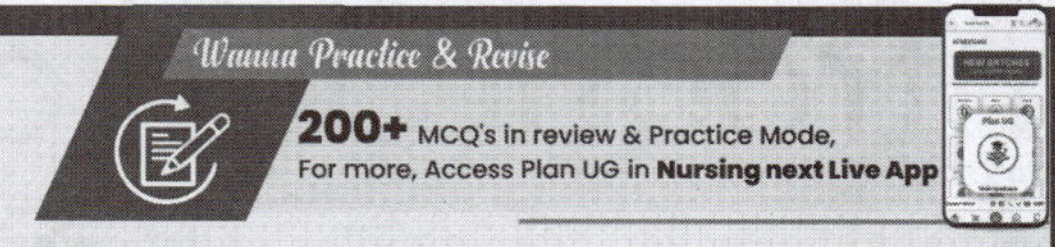

1. Managing frustration and anger is a part of which dimension?

a. Physical b. Emotional
c. Intellectual d. Social

Ans. b. Emotional

2. Interacting with people face to face, via email, Skype, texting or snap chat are examples of which wellness dimension?

a. Social b. Physical
c. Occupational d. Intellectual

Ans. a. Social

3. Who among the following has described the nursing as autonomous and collaborative care of individuals of all ages, families, groups and communities, sick or well and in all settings?

a. Indian Nursing Council
b. American Nurses Association
c. International Council of Nurses
d. Virginia Henderson

Ans. c. International Council of Nurses

4. Who gave the hierarchy of needs?

a. Abraham Maslow b. David McClelland
c. Frederick Herzberg d. Douglas McGregor

Ans. a. Abraham Maslow

5. How many levels are there in Needs Hierarchy theory of motivation?

a. 6 b. 5
c. 4 d. 3

Ans. b. 5

6. Which among the following is not a deficiency need that arises due to deprivation?

a. Physiological need b. Safety and security needs
c. Self-esteem needs d. Self-actualization needs

Ans. d. Self-actualization needs

7. In the Health Belief Model, the nurse recognizes that the focus is placed on the:

a. Relation of perceptions and compliance with therapy
b. Multidimensional nature of clients and their interaction with the environment
c. Functioning of the individual in all dimensions Basic human needs for survival

Ans. a. Relation of perceptions and compliance with therapy

8. Who was the original author of the Illness-Wellness Continuum?

a. Dr John W Travis in 1972
b. Florence Nightingale in 1875
c. Dr Benjamin Carson in 1997
d. Dr William S Travis in 1972

Ans. a. Dr John W Travis in 1972

9. The hospitals run for the dual purpose, i.e. teaching the medical, nursing and other health care students, as well providing care to people are called ....?

a. Long-term hospitals b. Short-term hospitals
c. Private Hospitals d. Teaching hospitals

Ans. d. Teaching hospitals

Golden Points

- Health is a state of complete physical, mental and social well-being and not merely the absence of disease or infirmity (WHO 1948).
- Illness can be defined as a state of poor health or disease in an individual. It refers to a deviation from the normal functioning of the body or mind, resulting in physical or mental discomfort, impairment, or dysfunction. Illness can be categorized into Acute illnesses and Chronic illnesses.
- Maslow's hierarchy of needs illustrates the five levels of human needs, from the most basic to the most complex. The five levels are: Physiological needs, Safety needs, Love and belonging needs, Self-esteem needs and Self-actualization needs.
- Various dimensions of heath are: Physical health, Mental health, Social health and Spiritual health.

CHAPTER 2

Introduction of Basic Concepts and Meanings

CONCEPTUAL THEORY

Terminology

150+ key terminologies for Quick Recall & Revision

Hospital: A hospital is an integral part of a social and medical organization, the function of which is to provide for the population, the complete care both curative and preventive and whose outpatient services reach out to the family and his home environment.

Health care team: The health care team consists of a group of people who coordinate their particular skills in order to assist a patient or his family. The health care team consists of Physicians, Nurses, Dietitians, Physiotherapists, Social Workers, etc.

Health promotion: It is the process of "enabling people to increase control over, and to improve, their health.

Primary prevention: Can be defined as action taken prior to the onset of disease.

Primordial prevention: It is the prevention of emergence of risk factors in populations, in which they have not yet appeared.

Secondary Prevention: The action which halts the progress of a disease at its incipient stage and prevents complications.

Tertiary prevention: All measures available to reduce or limit impairments and disabilities, minimize suffering caused by existing departures from good health and to promote the patient's adjustment to irremediable conditions.

LEVELS OF DISEASE PREVENTION

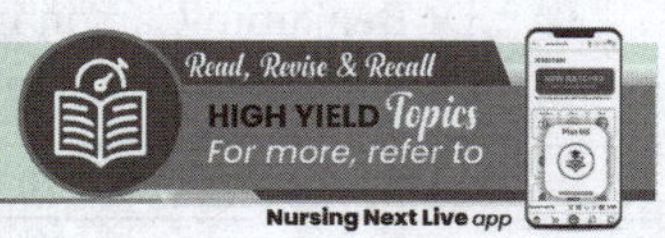

Primordial Prevention

Primordial prevention, a new concept, is receiving special attention in the prevention of chronic diseases. In primordial prevention, efforts are directed toward discouraging children from adopting harmful lifestyles.

Primary Prevention

Primary prevention can be defined as "action taken prior to the onset of disease".

Health Promotion

Health Promotion Behaviors
- Wearing seat belts, safety helmets, etc.
- Eating well-balanced diet
- Maintaining ideal body weight
- Refraining from using tobacco, etc.
- Obtaining immunization

Specific protection like immunization, chemoprophylaxis.

Secondary Prevention

It can be defined as "action which halts the progress of a disease at its incipient stage and prevents complications". The specific interventions are **early diagnosis and adequate treatment**.

Tertiary Prevention

Tertiary prevention can be defined as "all measures available to reduce or limit impairments and disabilities, minimize sufferings and maximizing potential years of quality life". It includes:
- Disability limitation
- Rehabilitation

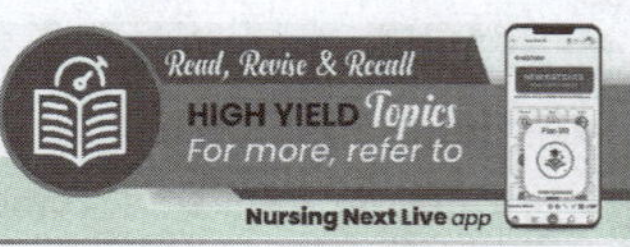

PRIMARY HEALTH CARE

Primary health care is essential health care made universally accessible to individuals and families in the community, by means acceptable to them, through their full participation and at a cost that community and country can afford.

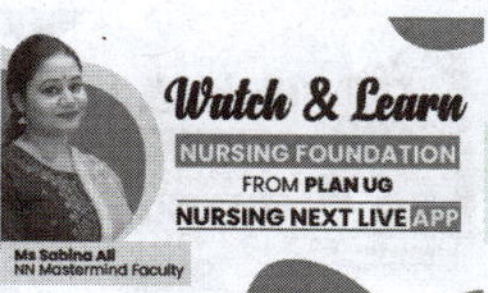

Elements of Primary Health Care

As per Alma-Ata declaration, primary health care includes:

- Education concerning prevailing health problems and methods of identifying, preventing and controlling them
- Promotion of food supply and proper nutrition
- An adequate supply of water and basic sanitation
- Maternal and child health care including family planning
- Immunization against the major infectious diseases
- Prevention and control of locally endemic diseases
- Appropriate treatment of common diseases and injuries
- Promotion of mental health
- Provision of essential drugs

Principles of Primary Health Care

- Equitable distribution
- Community participation
- Coverage and accessibility
- Intersectoral coordination
- Appropriate health technology
- Human resource
- Referral system
- Logistics of supply
- Physical facilities
- Control and evaluation

LEVELS OF CARE OR HEALTH SERVICES

Primary Health Promotion

This is the first level of contact between the individual and the health system where "essential health care" is provided.

Secondary Health Promotion

At this level, most complex problems are dealt with. The care comprises essentially curative services and is provided by the district hospitals and community health centers.

Tertiary Health Promotion

This level offers super-specialty care.

The major purpose of tertiary (rehabilitative) care is to restore an individual to the state of health.

Levels of Health Care

- **Primary care**
  - Prenatal care
  - Nutritional care
  - Well baby care
  - Family planning
- **Preventive care**
  - Body weight, BP and blood sugar monitoring
  - Risk assessment
  - Crisis prevention
  - Counseling services
- **Secondary care**
  - Acute care (medical and surgical)
  - Emergency care
  - Diagnostic services
- **Tertiary care**
  - ICU care
  - Subacute care
- **Restorative care**
  - Rehabilitation and home-based care
- **Continuing care**
  - Care to ill/disabled
  - Geriatric care

HEALTH CARE AGENCIES

- **Classification according to Length of stay**
  - Short stay hospital
  - Acute care
  - Long stay hospitals
- **Classification according to ownership**
  - Government or public hospitals
  - Voluntary hospitals
  - Private nursing homes/hospitals
  - Corporate hospitals
- **Classification according to objectives**
  - Teaching cum research hospitals
  - General hospitals
  - Specialized hospitals
  - Isolation hospitals
- **Classification according to size**
  - Teaching hospitals
  - District hospitals
  - Taluk hospitals
  - Community health centers
  - Primary health centres
- **Classification according to management**
  - Union government or government of India
  - State government
    - Local bodies
    - Autonomous bodies
    - Private
    - Voluntary agencies

- **Classification according to system**
  - Allopathic hospital
  - Ayurveda, Unani, Siddha and Homeopathy (AYUSH)

HEALTH CARE TEAM

Health care team, health professionals or health care providers are considered the team members who are directly or indirectly responsible for the improvement in the health of the clients. These personnel are from the different disciplines who coordinate with each other to assist the clients.

Health care team includes:

- Nurse
- Physician
- Dietitian/Nutritionist
- Physiotherapist
- Occupational therapist
- Dentist
- Paramedics
- Pharmacist
- Respiratory therapist
- Social worker
- Spiritual support personnel, etc.

CONCEPTUAL EXERCISES

LONG ANSWER QUESTION

1. What all are the levels of prevention?

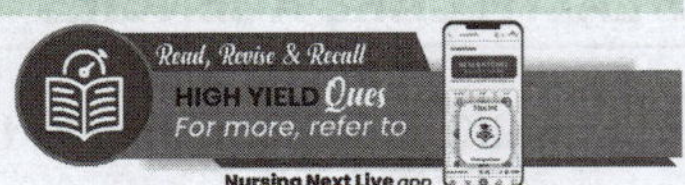

Answer

- In the field of public health, there are four commonly recognized levels of prevention: primordial prevention primary prevention, secondary prevention, and tertiary prevention.
- These levels aim to prevent disease and promote health at different stages. Here's an overview of each level:

Primordial Prevention

- It focuses on addressing the underlying social, economic, and environmental determinants of health to prevent the development of risk factors and disease conditions in the first place.
- It aims to create conditions that promote health and well-being at a population level.

Primary Prevention

This level focuses on preventing the onset of a disease or injury before it occurs. It aims to promote health and well-being in the general population.

Primary prevention strategies include:

- Health promotion campaigns
- Immunizations

Environmental interventions such as implementing measures to improve safety standards, clean water initiatives, prevention of accidents or exposure to harmful substances.

Secondary Prevention

- This level involves early detection and intervention to halt or slow the progression of a disease in its early stages.
- It focuses on individuals who are at higher risk or have already developed certain health conditions.

Secondary prevention strategies include:

- **Regular screenings and medical check-ups:** These aim to identify diseases or conditions at an early stage, such as mammograms for breast cancer or blood pressure screenings for hypertension.
- **Diagnostic tests:** Conducting tests to identify specific conditions or risk factors, such as cholesterol tests to detect cardiovascular disease risk.
- **Prompt treatment:** Providing timely medical interventions, medications, or therapies to prevent the disease from progressing or complications from developing.

Tertiary Prevention

- This level focuses on managing and improving the quality of life for individuals who have already experienced a disease or injury.
- Tertiary prevention aims to prevent complications, reduce disability, and improve overall functioning.

Strategies for tertiary prevention include:

- **Rehabilitation programs:** These focus on physical, occupational, or psychological therapies to help individuals recover and regain their functionality after an illness or injury.
- **Support groups and counseling:** Providing emotional support and counseling services to individuals and their families to cope with the challenges of living with a chronic condition or disability.
- **Disease management programs:** Offering comprehensive care and interventions to individuals with chronic conditions, such as diabetes or asthma, to prevent exacerbations and promote self-management.

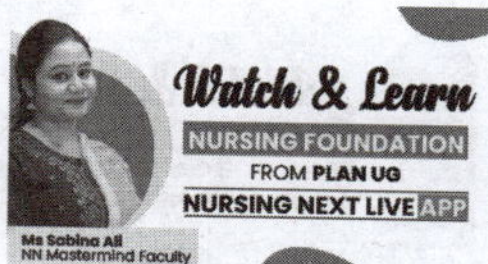

SHORT NOTES

1. Write a note on different levels of disease prevention. (MGR, DU)

Answer

For answer, refer to Long Question no. 1, pg. no. 560

2. Write about Health promotion model. (MGR)

Answer

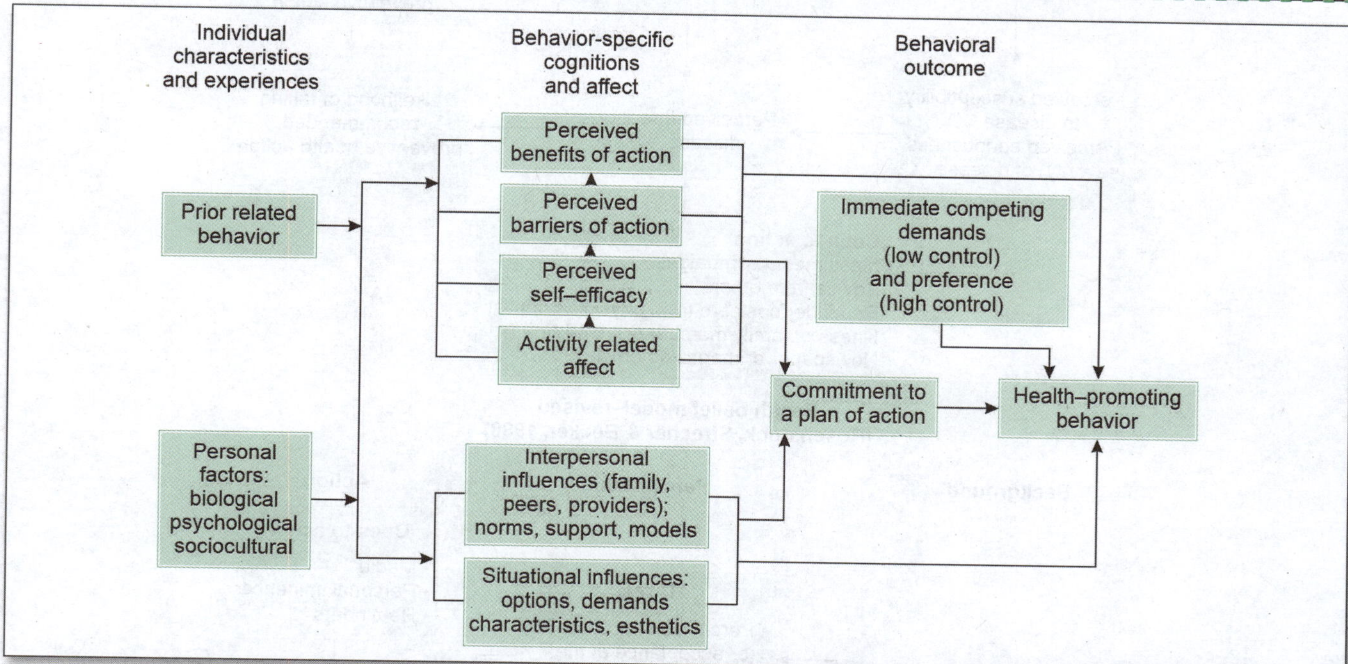

Adapted from: Revised Health Promotion Model. (From Current Nursing (2010) Health Promotion Model in italic form)

The Health Promotion Model is based upon on behavior and personal factors. It has Major various concepts and these are:

- Prior related behaviour
- Personal biological factors
- Personal psychological factors
- Personal sociocultural factors
- Perceived benefits of action
- Perceived barriers to action
- Perceived self-efficacy
- Activity-related affect
- Interpersonal influences
- Situational influences
- Commitment to a plan of action
- Immediate competing demands and preferences
- Health-promoting behaviour

The four global concepts are addressed in the Health Promotion Model in the figure:

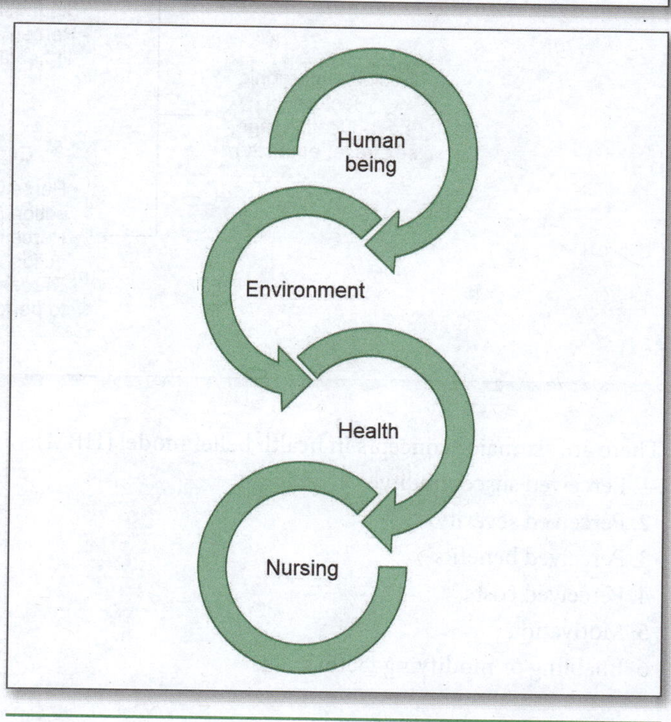

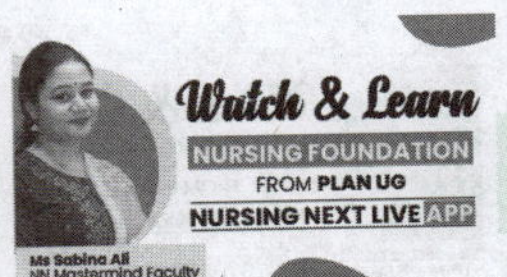

3. Write a note on health belief model. (DU)

Answer

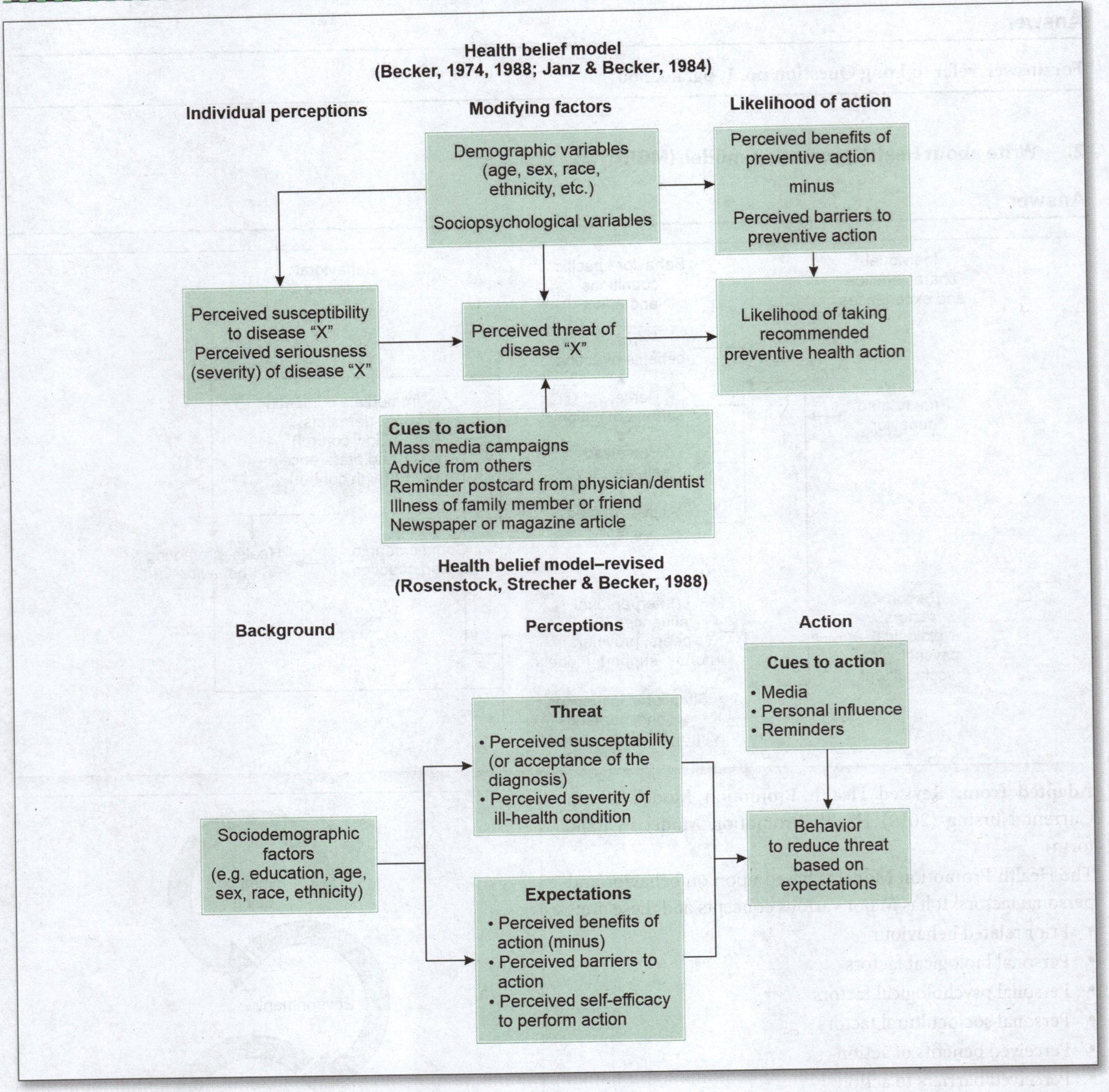

Health belief model
(Becker, 1974, 1988; Janz & Becker, 1984)

Individual perceptions | **Modifying factors** | **Likelihood of action**

Demographic variables (age, sex, race, ethnicity, etc.)
Sociopsychological variables

Perceived benefits of preventive action
minus
Perceived barriers to preventive action

Perceived susceptibility to disease "X"
Perceived seriousness (severity) of disease "X"

Perceived threat of disease "X"

Likelihood of taking recommended preventive health action

Cues to action
Mass media campaigns
Advice from others
Reminder postcard from physician/dentist
Illness of family member or friend
Newspaper or magazine article

Health belief model–revised
(Rosenstock, Strecher & Becker, 1988)

Background | **Perceptions** | **Action**

Sociodemographic factors (e.g. education, age, sex, race, ethnicity)

Threat
- Perceived susceptibility (or acceptance of the diagnosis)
- Perceived severity of ill-health condition

Expectations
- Perceived benefits of action (minus)
- Perceived barriers to action
- Perceived self-efficacy to perform action

Cues to action
- Media
- Personal influence
- Reminders

Behavior to reduce threat based on expectations

There are six major concepts in health belief model (HBM):

1. Perceived susceptibility
2. Perceived severity
3. Perceived benefits
4. Perceived costs
5. Motivation
6. Enabling or modifying factors

1. **Perceived susceptibility:** perception that health related issue is relevant.
2. **Perceived severity:** Even when one recognizes or perceives the severity to be high enough to have serious threat to the life.
3. **Perceived benefits:** Belief that a given treatment will cure the illness or help to prevent it.
4. **Perceived costs:** Refers to the duration and accessibility of the treatment

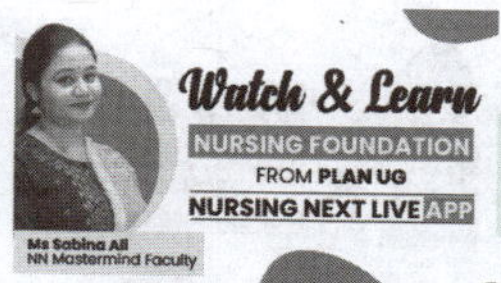

5. **Motivation:** Desire to comply with the treatment
6. **Modifying factors:** Such as personality variables, socio-demographic variables and patient satisfaction.

SHORT ANSWER QUESTIONS

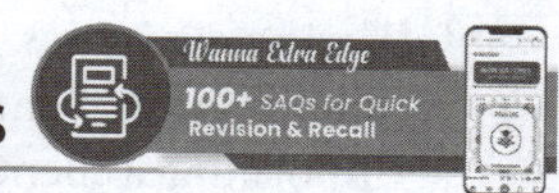

1. Enumerate different levels of disease prevention. (MGR, DU)

Answer

Different levels of disease prevention are:

- **Primordial prevention:** Individual and mass education for not adopting harmful lifestyles e.g., bad eating habits, exercise, smoking, etc.
- **Primary prevention:** It includes Health Promotion, Specific Protection like immunization
- **Secondary prevention:** It includes Early diagnosis and adequate treatment.
- **Tertiary prevention:** It includes Disability limitation and Rehabilitation.

2. Define Health promotion. (RUHS)

Answer

- Health promotion is not only an illness prevention. It means assisting individuals to improve the health.

Or

- **Pender (1987) describes** health promotion as being an activity that is concerned with sustaining or increasing one's level of well-being. Self-actualization and personal fulfillers.
- It is the process of enabling people to increase control over and to improve health.
- It include health measures such as health education, environmental sanitation, nutrition etc.

Examples are- wearing seat belts, eating balanced diet and obtaining immunization.

3. List the role of Nurses in health promotion. (RUHS)

Answer

Nurses play a vital role in improving health as well as health promotion, various role of nurses are discuss below:

- Health education
- Adequate food supply
- Promote environmental sanitation
- Encourage MCH and family planning services
- Promote immunization
- Prevention of communicable diseases
- Appropriate interventions for prevention of common diseases.
- Assessment of high risk population in a community.
- Provide support for life style changes
- Counsellor
- Educator
- Leader
- Motivator

CONCEPTUAL REVISION

MULTIPLE CHOICE QUESTIONS

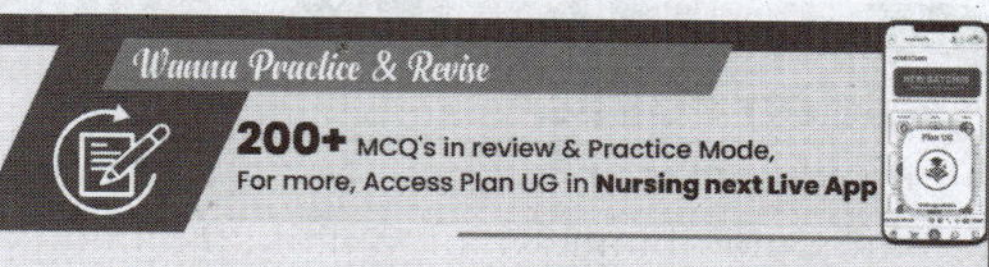

1. In the Health Belief Model, the nurse recognizes that the focus is placed on the:

a. Relation of perceptions and compliance with therapy
b. Multidimensional nature of clients and their interaction with the environment
c. Functioning of the individual in all dimensions
d. Basic human needs for survival

Ans. a. Relation of perceptions and compliance with therapy

2. There are different ways to look on health and illness. When formulating a definition of "health," a person should consider that health, within its current definition, is:

a. The ability to pursue activities of daily living
b. A function to the physiological state
c. A state of wellbeing involving whole person
d. The absence of disease

Ans. c. A state of wellbeing involving whole person

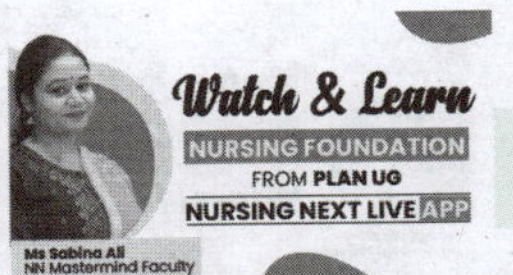

3. A nurse is using a holistic approach with a client. To incorporate all of the factors that may influence the client, the nurse should respond to the client as follows:

a. "Your physician has left orders for you to know."
b. "The laboratory tests reveal the need to reduce your daily percentage of fat grams."
c. "Adapting your diet and activity will lower your blood glucose levels."
d. "I would like you to perform this exercise once a day."

Ans. c. "Adapting your diet and activity will lower your blood glucose levels."

4. In the Health Belief Model, the nurse recognizes that the focus is placed on the:

a. Relation of perceptions and compliance with therapy
b. Multidimensional nature of clients and their interaction with the environment
c. Functioning of the individual in all dimensions
d. Basic human needs for survival

Ans. a. Relation of perceptions and compliance with therapy

5. The hospitals run for the dual purpose i.e. teaching the medical, nursing and other health care students, as well providing care to people are called ....:

a. Long term hospitals
b. Short term hospitals
c. Private Hospitals
d. Teaching hospitals

Ans. d. Teaching hospitals

6. The nurse incorporates the levels of prevention as a basis for the types of clients' needs that are evident and the nursing care that is provided. Which of the following activities of the nurse is an example of tertiary level preventive care giving?

a. Informing a client that immunizations for her infant are available through the health department
b. Providing a class on hygiene for an elementary school class
c. Arranging for a hospice nurse to visit with the family of a client with cancer
d. Teaching a client how to irrigate a new colostomy

Ans. c. Arranging for a hospice nurse to visit with the family of a client with cancer

7. The client is a paraplegic and is in the hospital for an electrolyte imbalance. Based on the levels of prevention, the client is receiving care at the:

a. Tertiary Prevention
b. Primary Prevention
c. Secondary Prevention
d. Health Promotion Level

Ans. c. Secondary Prevention

8. When assessing the external variables that influence a client's health beliefs and practices, the nurse must consider his:

a. Income status
b. Reaction to the heart disease
c. Educational background
d. Religious practices

Ans. a. Income status

Golden Points

- Health care team includes—Nurse, Physician, Dietician/Nutritionist, Physiotherapist, Occupational therapist, Dentist, Paramedics, Pharmacist, Respiratory therapist, Social worker, Spiritual support personnel, etc.
- Levels of health care are: Primary care, Preventive care, Secondary care, Tertiary care, Restorative care and Continuing care.
- Primary health care is essential health care made universally accessible to individuals and families in the community, by means acceptable to them, through their full participation and at a cost that community and country can afford.
- Primary prevention can be defined as "action taken prior to the onset of disease".
- Primordial prevention, a new concept, is receiving special attention in the prevention of chronic diseases. In primordial prevention, efforts are directed toward discouraging children from adopting harmful lifestyles.
- Secondary Prevention can be defined as "action which halts the progress of a disease at its incipient stage and prevents complications". The specific interventions are early diagnosis and adequate treatment.
- Tertiary prevention can be defined as "all measures available to reduce or limit impairments and disabilities, minimize sufferings and maximizing potential years of quality life. It includes: Disability limitation and Rehabilitation.

CHAPTER

3

History of Nursing and Nursing as a Profession

CONCEPTUAL THEORY

Terminology

150+ key terminologies for Quick Recall & Revision

Assault: It is the unjustifiable attempt to touch another person or the threat.
Autonomy: Independence; self-determination; self-reliance
Battery: An intentional act that is harmful or offensive without that person's consent.
Beneficence: Actively seeking benefits; promotion of good
Code of ethics: A **code of ethics** is a set of ethical principles, ideals and values shared by members of the group, and serves as a standard for their professional actions.
Defamation: Publication of a false statement about an individual made either verbally which damages his/her reputation.
Ethical principles: Refer to those general judgments that serve as a justification for particular ethical prescriptions and evaluations of human actions.
Ethics: It refers to the moral code of nursing and is based on obligation to service and respect for human life (Melanie and Evelyn)
False imprisonment: It is an intentional act which prevents an individual from moving about where s/he wants to be.
Fidelity: Faithfulness; striving to keep promises
Informed consent: All patients should be given the complete knowledge and understanding about any treatment/procedure and agrees to sign for treatment/procedure.
Intentional torts: Interfere in individual's privacy, mobility, property or personal interests. Intentional torts can be assault, battery, false imprisonment or defamation.
Justice: Fairness or equity
Legal issue: A legal issue is something that happens, that has legal implications and may need the help of a lawyer to sort out.
Malpractice: Professional misconduct; negligence performed in professional practice; any unreasonable lack of skill in professional duties.
Negligence: Lack of proper care and attention; carelessness; 'An act of carelessness'
Nonmaleficence: Actively seeking to do no harm.
Nursing: According to Florence Nightingale, Nursing is to bring healthy and those who are suffering from disease to a condition for nature to act for preserving health, preventing disease and injury and to restore health and cure disease.
Profession: A **profession** is defined as " an occupation or calling requiring advanced training and experience in some specific or specialized body of knowledge which provides service to society in that special field."
Trend: Trend means a change or movement in a particular direction. A trend in nursing profession is a change that is taking place in present days in any field of nursing, may it be in education or practice which affects the profession as a whole.
Values: Values are enduring beliefs or attitudes about the worth of a person, idea or actions. They are important because they influence decisions and actions, including nurses' ethical decision-making.
Vocation: It is the particular occupation for which you are trained. This possesses a particular combination of characteristics.

BACKROUND

The word Nurse is derived from a Latin word-nutrix which means to nourish. According to *Shakespeare* Nurse is one who looks after, fosters, or advises.

EDUCATIONAL PREPARATION OF A NURSE

In nursing, many changes took place after independence including establishment of Indian Nursing Council (INC) and Trained Nurses Association of India (TNAI) who brought various changes in nursing practice as well nursing education.

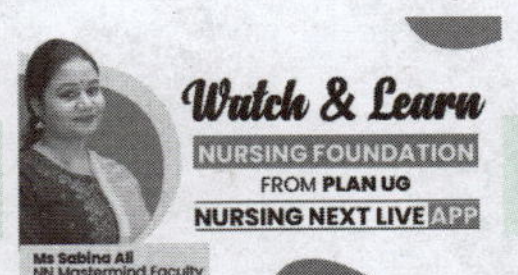

CATEGORIES OF NURSING EDUCATION

- General nursing and midwifery
- Auxiliary nursing midwifery
- Diploma in nursing education and administration
- Diploma courses in nursing specialties
- University-level programs
  - Basic BSc nursing
  - Post Basic BSc Nursing
  - Post Basic Nursing by distance education mode.
  - Postgraduate education—MSc nursing
  - M Phil
  - PhD in Nursing

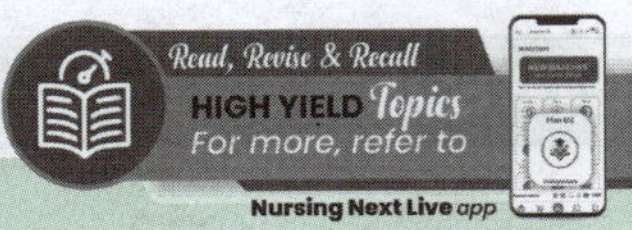

NURSING

The meaning of nursing is to nourish, to cherish, and to educate.

According to **Florence Nightingale**, "Nursing is to bring healthy and those who are suffering from disease to a condition for nature to act for preserving health, preventing disease and injury and to restore health and cure disease."

International Council of Nursing defines Nursing in the following manner. "Nursing encompasses autonomous and collaborative care of individuals of all ages, families, groups and communities, sick or well and in all settings. Nursing includes the promotion of health, prevention of illness, and the care of ill, disabled and dying people. Advocacy, promotion of a safe environment, research, participation in shaping health policy and in patient and health systems management, and education are also key nursing roles."

Scope of Nursing Practice

The scope of nursing practice is divided into extended roles as well as expanded roles of nursing. For the better upliftment of nursing career or for futuristic nursing, the roles of nursing practice has been increasing worldwide focusing on meeting patient needs as well as patient safety. Nurse provides care for Individual, Family and Community.

Nursing practice involves four areas:

1. Promotion of health and wellness
2. Prevention of illness
3. Restoration of health
4. Care for the dying or facilitating coping with disability and death

Nursing as a Profession

Nursing has been called the oldest of arts and the youngest of professions. Nursing is a profession due to the following characteristics:

- Has a theoretical body of knowledge and skills.
- Provides scientific service.
- Has autonomy in decision making and practice.
- Has a whole code of ethical practice.
- Requires an extended education.
- Has is strong service orientation
- His is ongoing research process
- Professional organization that sets standards.

Nursing as an Art

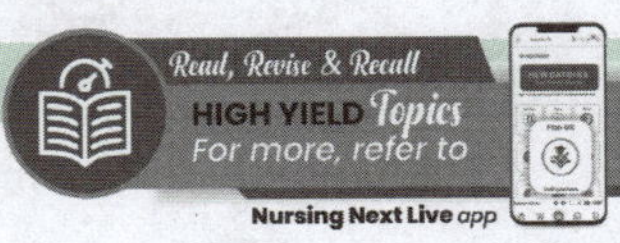

- Nursing was largely the care of the ill in the hospital and the care of the mothers and children in the community.
- Nursing was primarily the art of caring, based on intuition and skills training rather than on science.
- **Roles of a professional nurse**
  - Caregiver
  - Teacher
  - Communicator
  - Client advocate
  - Counselor
  - Change agent
  - Leader
  - Researcher
  - Collaborator
- **Expanded educational and career roles of nurses**
  - Clinical Nurse Specialist
  - Nurse-practitioner
  - Nurse-midwife
  - Nurse-educator
  - Nurse-administrator
  - Nurse-researcher
  - Nurse-entrepreneur

VALUES

Values are enduring beliefs or attitudes about the worth of a person, idea or actions. They are important because they influence decisions and actions, including nurses' ethical decision making. The professional values in nursing are:

- Altruism
- Autonomy
- Human dignity
- Integrity
- Social justice

ETHICS

Ethics refers to the moral code of nursing and is based on obligation to service and respect for human life (Melanie and Evelyn).

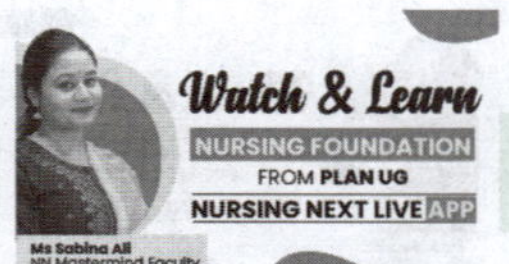

Values and ethics are inherent in all nursing acts. Values influence decisions and actions, such as nurses' ethical decision making.

Professional Ethics

A code of ethics is a set of ethical principles, ideals and values shared by members of the group, and serves as a standard for their professional actions.

Nursing Code of Ethics in India

- The Nurse respects the uniqueness of an individual in provision of care.
- Nurse respects the rights of individuals as partners in care and help in making informed choices.
- Nurse respects the individual right to privacy, maintains confidentiality and shares information judiciously.
- Nurse maintains competence in order to render quality nursing care.
- Nurse is obliged to practice within the framework of ethical, professional and legal boundaries.
- Nurse is obliged to work harmoniously with members of health care team.
- Nurse commits to reciprocate the trust invested in nursing profession by society.

Ethical Principles in Nursing

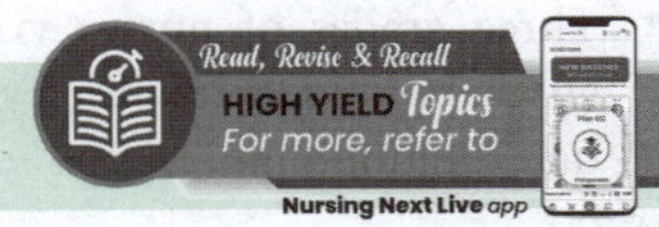

Ethical principles refers to those general judgments that serve as a justification for particular ethical prescriptions and evaluations of human actions.

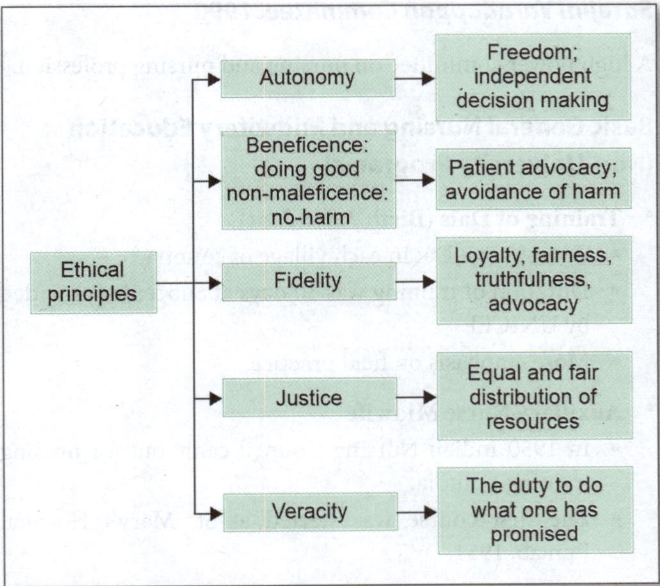

Figure 3.1: Institutional review board

LEGAL ISSUES IN NURSING

A ***legal issue*** is something that happens that has legal implications and may need the help of a lawyer to sort out.
—**Solicitors Regulation Authority**

- **1st nursing law:** Nursing registration- 1903
- **Indian Nursing Council Act:** Enacted in 1947
- Amended in 1957
- **Malpractice:** Professional misconduct; negligence performed in professional practice; any unreasonable lack of skill in professional duties.
- **Negligence:** Lack of proper care and attention; carelessness; 'An act of carelessness'
- **Informed consent:** All patients should be given the complete knowledge and understanding about any treatment/procedure and agrees to sign for treatment/procedure.
- **Intentional torts:** Interfere in individual's privacy, mobility, property or personal interests. Intentional torts can be assault, battery, false imprisonment or defamation.
  - **Assault:** It is the unjustifiable attempt to touch another person or the threat.
  - **Battery:** An intentional act that is harmful or offensive without that person's consent.
  - **False imprisonment:** It is an intentional act which prevents an individual from moving about where s/he wants to be.
  - **Defamation:** Publication of a false statement about an individual made either verbally which damages his/her reputation.

CONCEPTUAL EXERCISES

LONG ANSWER QUESTIONS

1. Write in detail about history of Florence Nightingale.

Answer

Florence Nightingale—the Pioneer of Modern Nursing

- She was born in Italy on May 12, 1820.
- Founder of modern nursing profession
- She was of british nationality.
- Died in London on August 13, 1910.

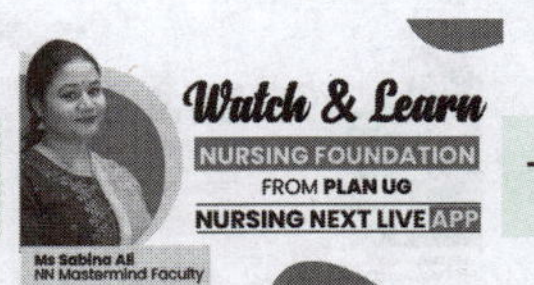

Education

- Home schooled by her father.
- Parents did not want her to become a nurse.
- She was 30-year-old when went to Germany and Paris to study nursing.
- She studied medicine books herself for years.
- Florence Studied at the Institute for Protestant Deaconesses at Kaiserswerth, Germany.
- Trained in nursing at the Institute of Saint Vincent De Paul in Alexandria, Egypt.

Ambition in Life

- Interest in politics
- More attraction toward various charitable institution and social conditions.
- Driven by attraction to nursing — A 'calling' to fulfill a 'Mission of mercy.'
- Visited several convents, hospitals, schools, orphanages.
- Went to Kaiserswerth for 3 months training in Nursing.
- Formulated organized training for nurses.
- Became Superintendent of an 'Establishment for gentle women during illness.'
- Organizer and an administrator.

During **Crimean War**, she scrubbed the floors, cleaned the wards/units and washed the linen and clothes as well. In the night she carried a lamp hence called "The Lady with the Lamp".

- After her dedicated care, all the soldiers were recovered well and after that the whole World appreciated the power of Nursing.
- After two years she returned from Crimea.
- Nightingale was also chosen as the first female member in Royal Statistical Society.

Honours

- She became a Fellow of the Royal Statistical Society and American Statistical Association.
- She changed the hospitals all over the world.

Nursing Contributions

- Founded the Nightingale School and Home for Nurses at Saint Thomas' Hospital in London
- Wrote Notes on Nursing, the first textbook for nurses
- As a pioneer in statistics, she visualized her analysis so that the conclusions and practical information can be derived easily.
- She was famous for using polar area diagrams (Nightingale rose diagrams)

2. Describe history of nursing education in India. (DU)

Answer

On 15th August 1947 India became independent and self-governing country. The INC was constituted to establish a uniform standard of education for nurses, midwives, health visitors and auxiliary nurse midwives in 1949.

Recommendations of Various Committees Pertaining to Nursing Education

Health survey and Development Committee (Bhore Committee, 1946)

- Establishment of nursing college.
- Creation of an all India Nursing Council.

Shetty Committee, 1954

- Improvement in conditions of training of nurses.
- Minimum requirement for admission to be in accordance with regulation of the INC.

Health Survey and Planning Committee (Mudaliar Committee 1959–61)

- Three grades of nurses viz. the basic nurses (4 years), auxiliary nurse midwife (2 years) and nurses with a degree qualification.

Mukherjee Committee, 1966

Training of nurses and ANM'S required for family planning.

Sarojini Varadappan Committee, 1990

A high power committee on nursing and nursing profession.

Basic General Nursing and Midwifery Education (Non-University Programs)

- **Training of Dais (Birth Attendant)**
  - To train one Dai in each village of country
  - Duration of training was 30 days at Subcenter provided by UNICEF.
  - More emphasis on field practice.
- **Auxiliary Nurse Midwife**
  - In 1950 Indian Nursing Council came out for nursing training in India.
  - The first course was started at St. Mary's Hospital Punjab, 1951.

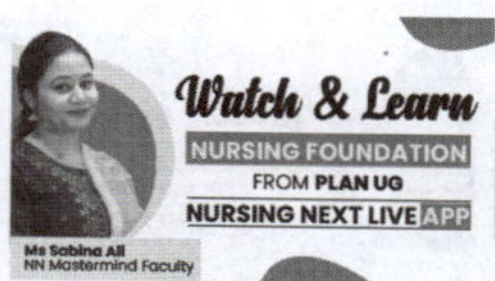

- In 1977, multipurpose health worker were prepared and vocationalization of higher secondary education was established.

- **Lady Health Visitor (CHV) Course**
  - Training of LHV course continued postindependence.
  - The duration was two and a half years which reduced to 2 years.
- **General Nursing and Midwifery Course**
  - In 1951, syllabus was prescribed by INC. In 1954 a special provision was made for male nurse and public health was integrated into basic nursing course.
  - In 1964–65 Psychiatric nursing was included.
  - The duration of course was reduced from 4 years to 3.5 years and further reduced to 3 years in 1982.
- **Post-Basic/Post Certificate Short-term Courses and Diploma Programs**
  - In 1951 a one year course in public health was started at college of nursing.
  - During 1953–54, first organized course at All India Institute of Mental Health.
  - In 1962 diploma in pediatric nursing was established at J.J.Group of Hospitals, Bombay.

University-Level Programs

- **Basic BSc Nursing**
  - First university program started just before independence in 1946 at university of Delhi and CMC Vellore.
  - At present the BSc Nursing program which is recommended by the INC is of four years.
- **Post Basic BSc Nursing**
  - The need was stressed by the Mudaliar Committee in1962.
  - Two years post basic certificate BSc(N) program was started in December 1962 for nurses with diploma in general and midwifery
- **Post Basic Nursing by Distance Education Mode**
  - In1985 Indira Gandhi National Open University was established
- **Post- Graduate Education-MSc Nursing**
  - First two years course in masters of nursing was started at RAK College of Nursing in 1959 and in 1969 in CMC Vellore.
  - At present there are many colleges imparting MSc Nursing degree course in different specialties.
- **M Phil**
  - In 1986 one year full time and two years part time program was started in RAK College of nursing Delhi.
- **PhD in Nursing**
  - From1992 PhD in nursing is also available in India.

Current Educational Patterns in Nursing

Non University Program

- **Basic**—ANM and GNM
- **Advance**—Post-Certificate diploma

University Program

- **Basic**—BSc(N), Post-Basic BSc (Regular) and Post Basic BSc(N), IGNOU
- **Advance**—MSc (Nursing), M Phil and PhD

SHORT NOTES

1. Write short notes on educational preparation of a nurse. (DU)

Answer

For answer, refer to Long Questions no. 2, pg. no. 568

2. Define nursing. Write about the roles of a professional nurse. (KUHS)

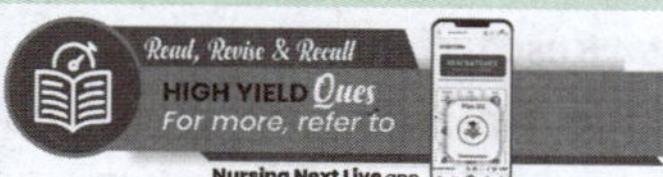

Answer

According to **Florence Nightingale,** Nursing is to bring healthy and those who are suffering from disease to a condition for nature to act for preserving health, preventing disease and injury and to restore health and cure disease.

International Council of Nursing, defines Nursing as Nursing encompasses autonomous and collaborative care of individuals of all ages, families, groups and communities, sick or well and in all settings. Nursing includes the promotion of health, prevention of illness, and the care of ill, disabled and dying people. Advocacy, promotion of a safe environment, research, participation in shaping health policy and in patient and health systems management, and education are also key nursing roles.

Roles of a Professional Nurse

Roles of the Nurse

- **Caregiver**
  - To provide complete care for the completely dependent client.
  - To provide partial care for the partially dependent client.
  - To provide supportive and educative care to assist clients in attaining health and wellness.

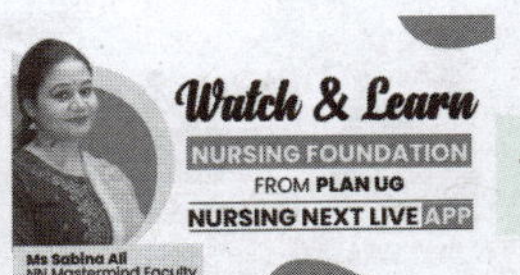

- **Teacher**
  - To restore or maintain their health.
  - To assesses the client's learning needs and readiness to learn.
  - To utilizes various teaching strategies.
  - To evaluates learning.
- **Communicator**
  - Nurses identify client's problems.
  - Communicate these needs/problems verbally or in writing to other members of the health team.
  - Communication must be clear and accurate to meet client's health care.
- **Client advocate**
  - To protect the client.
- **Counsellor**
  - To recognize and cope with psychological or social problems
  - To develop interpersonal relationship
  - To helps in developing new attitudes, behaviors
- **Change agent**
  - To make modifications in their behaviors.
- **Leader**
  - To work together to accomplish a specific goal.
- **Researcher**
  - By participating or conducting research to improve patient care based on evidence-based practice.
- **Collaborator**
  - To facilitate the functions of all members of the health care team.

Expanded Educational and Career Roles of Nurses

Clinical Nurse Specialist

An expert in a specialized area of nursing.

Nurse-practitioner

- Completes a course in anesthesia,
- Carried out preoperative assessments, administers and monitor anesthesia during surgery and evaluates postoperative state of patients.

Nurse-midwife

- Provides prenatal and postnatal care
- Delivers with uncomplicated pregnancies.

Nurse-educator

- Teaches theoretical knowledge
- Teaches clinical skills along with conducting research.

Nurse-administrator

- Functions at various levels of management in health care settings
- Responsible for the management and administration

Nurse-researcher

Conducts research for enhancement of nursing practice and education.

Nurse-entrepreneur

Consultant to institutions, political agencies.

3. Explain, How nursing is an art? (MGR)

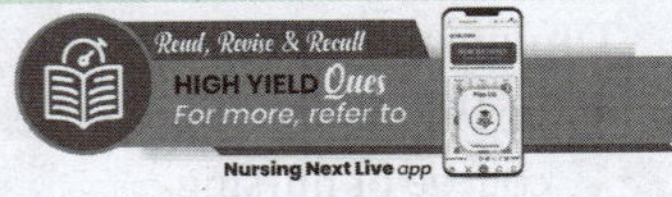

Answer

Nursing as an Art

- Nursing is an art because it has creativity, empathy, and intuition. It also parts emphasis on soft skills for nurses such as compassion, concern, and communication. These soft skills are also an art aspect of nursing.
- Effective nurses deliver the care from sickness to health which is artful in any sense of the word.
- Florence Nightingale has indicated that the nursing profession is more than the administration of medications but actually an art of providing comprehensive care to each patient.
- The art of nursing also refers to compassion, concern, commitment, and communication among nontechnical skills.

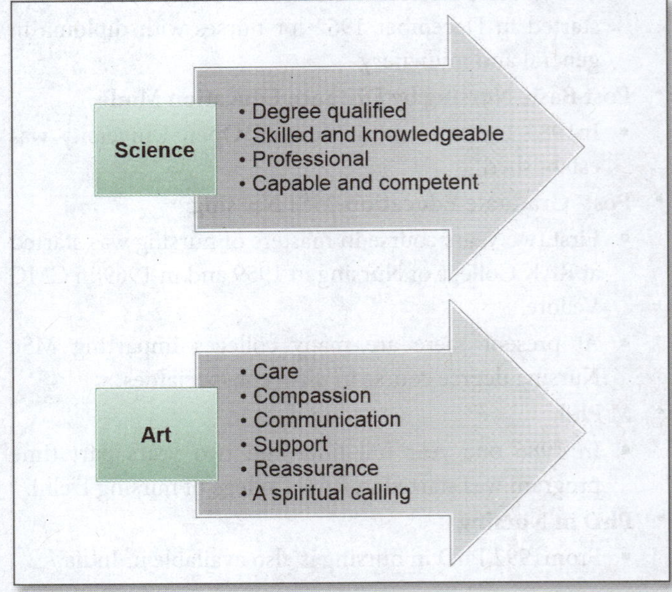

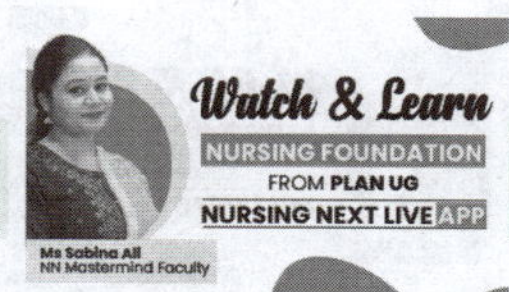

- Nursing model known as the Circle of Caring seeks to build the "artistic" aspects of nursing. It includes a holistic nursing assessment which should include comprehensive understanding to the overall social determinants of health.
- All these statements allow to practice the artful aspects in nursing profession such as empathy, patient communication, and advocacy.
- Nursing was largely the care of the ill in the hospital and the care of the mothers and children in the community.
- Nursing was primarily the art of caring, based on intuition and skills training rather than on science.

4. Define vocation.

Answer

It is the particular occupation for which you are trained. This possesses a particular combination of characteristics.

Characteristics

- On job training
- Length of training varies
- Largely manual work
- Guided decision-making
- Values, beliefs and ethics not part of preparation
- Commitment may vary
- Supervision may include
- Often change jobs
- Motivated by reward
- Employer is primarily accountable

5. Define nursing. (DU, MGR)

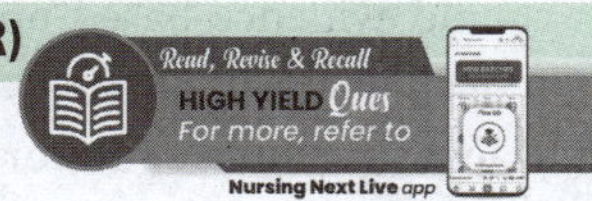

Answer

The meaning of nursing is to nourish, to cherish, and to educate.

According to **Florence Nightingale**, Nursing is to bring healthy and those who are suffering from disease to a condition for nature to act for preserving health, preventing disease and injury and to restore health and cure disease.

International Council of Nursing, defines Nursing as: Nursing encompasses autonomous and collaborative care of individuals of all ages, families, groups and communities, sick or well and in all settings. Nursing includes the promotion of health, prevention of illness, and the care of ill, disabled and dying people. Advocacy, promotion of a safe environment, research, participation in shaping health policy and in patient and health systems management, and education are also key nursing roles.

6. Discuss scope of nursing practice.

Answer

Nursing is a profession that ensures quality care for all. The scope of nursing practice is divided into extended roles as well as expanded roles of nursing. For the better upliftment of nursing career or for futuristic nursing, the roles of nursing practice has been increasing worldwide focusing on meeting patient needs as well as patient safety.

The Nursing Scope of Practice describes the "who," "what," "where," "when," "why," and "how" of nursing practice:

- **Who:** Registered Nurses (RN) should be educated and maintain nursing standards and follow legal and ethical norms to practice in nursing profession.
- **What:** Nursing is the way of health promotion and illness prevention; alleviation of suffering through the early diagnosis and appropriate treatment of individuals, families, groups, communities, and populations.
- **Where:** A patient in need of care.
- **When:** A need for nursing knowledge, compassion, and expertise/competency.
- **Why:** To achieve the most positive patient and health outcomes.

Nurse provides care for three types:

1. Individual care
2. Family care
3. Community care.

Nursing Practice for Individual

- Nurses promote health promotion and wellness in patients who are both healthy and ill. They are also play an important role in enhancing healthy lifestyles such as proper nutrition and prevention of drug and alcohol abuse, restrict smoking, etc.
- Nurses also provide direct care to the ill person and also help in performing diagnostic procedures.

Nursing Practice for Family and the Community

- Nurses identify and assess the family health-related issues.
- She also provides the nursing services to the family of a community.
- In the community, nurses encourage the whole community to utilize the resources provided by the government.

- Nurses also play a vital role in implementation of various national policies and health programs.

Nursing practice involves four areas:

1. Promotion of health and wellness
2. Prevention of illness
3. Restoration of health
4. Care for the dying or facilitating coping with disability and death.

Patient and family education: Nurses teach self-care techniques, promote health literacy, explain treatment plans, and offer guidance on managing chronic conditions and lifestyle modifications.

Health assessment and diagnostic skills: Nurses are trained in conducting comprehensive health assessments, which involve collecting and analyzing patient data, conducting physical examinations, and interpreting diagnostic tests.

Advocacy and patient rights: Nurses serve as advocates for their patients, ensuring their rights and preferences are respected. They actively participate in care decisions, safeguard patient privacy and confidentiality, and raise concerns about patient safety or quality of care.

Leadership and Management: Nurses often take on leadership and management roles within healthcare settings. They may supervise and delegate tasks to other members of the healthcare team, contribute to quality improvement initiatives, and participate in policy development and implementation.

Research and evidence-based practice: Nurses contribute to the advancement of nursing knowledge and practice through research. They participate in evidence-based practice, applying the latest research findings to improve patient outcomes and enhance nursing care.

7. "Nursing is a profession", justify the statement.

Answer

A **profession** is defined as "an occupation or calling requiring advanced training and experience in some specific or specialized body of knowledge which provides service to society in that special field."

Criteria of Profession

- To provide a service needed in the society.
- To enhance knowledge in the field.
- To protect its members
- To practice effectively.

Bixler and Bixler Criteria for Profession

A profession is a form of employment, especially one that is respected in society as honourable and is possible only for an educated person and after training in some special branch of knowledge.

Nursing has been called the oldest of arts and the youngest of professions.

Nursing is a profession due to the following characteristics:

- **Specialized knowledge and expertise:** Nursing requires specialized knowledge and expertise acquired through formal education and training. Nurses undergo rigorous education programs that encompass a wide range of subjects, including anatomy, physiology, pharmacology, nursing theory, and clinical skills. This specialized knowledge equips nurses with the necessary competence to provide comprehensive care to individuals, families, and communities.
- Nurses deliver care based on evidence-based practice.
- **Autonomy and responsibility:** Nurses exercise a significant level of autonomy and responsibility in their practice. They make independent judgments, assessments, and decisions related to patient care, treatment plans, and health promotion strategies. Nurses collaborate with other healthcare professionals while assuming accountability for their actions and the outcomes of patient care.
- **Ethical standards and codes of conduct:** Nursing is guided by ethical standards and codes of conduct that emphasize the importance of patient-centered care, confidentiality, respect for autonomy, and the promotion of the well-being and dignity of patients. These ethical principles and professional guidelines help shape nurses' behavior and decision-making in providing safe and compassionate care.
- It requires an extended education.
- It strong service orientation
- Ongoing research in nursing aims to address gaps in knowledge, evaluate interventions and strategies, and guide evidence-based practice to enhance the quality and effectiveness of nursing care.
- **Licensing and regulatory bodies:** Nursing is regulated by licensing boards and regulatory bodies in most countries. These bodies establish and enforce standards of practice, educational requirements, and professional conduct. Nurses must meet specific qualifications, pass licensing exams, and maintain their licensure through continuing education and adherence to professional standards.Nursing has a regulatory body which sets standards of education and practice.
- **Continuing professional development:** Nursing recognizes the importance of lifelong learning and professional development. Nurses engage in continuing education, attend conferences, participate in research, and stay updated with advancements in healthcare practices and technology. This commitment to ongoing learning ensures that nurses provide evidence-based and quality care to their patients.

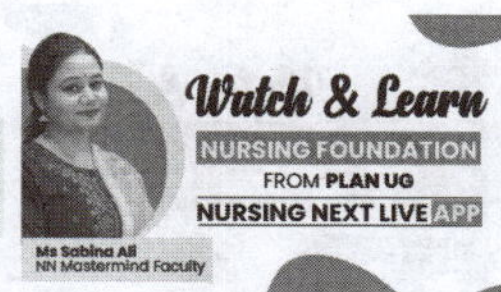

- **Professional associations and advocacy:** Nursing is supported by professional associations and organizations at local, national, and international levels. These associations advocate for the nursing profession, promote standards of practice, provide resources for professional development, and facilitate networking and collaboration among nurses.
- All these aspects justify that nursing is a profession.

8. List down the qualities of a nurse.

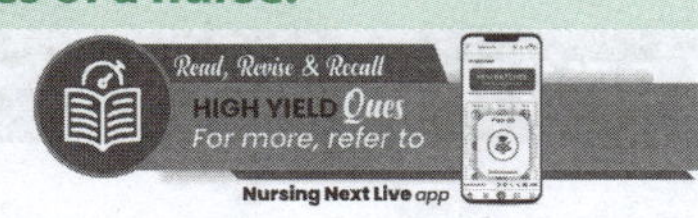

Answer

The word **Nurse is derived** from a Latin word-**nutrix** which means to nourish.

Nurse is defined as a person who has completed a programmed of basic nursing education and is qualified and authorized in her/ his country to practice nursing.

Quality of the Nurses Include

- **Communication skills:** Nurses must be able to communicate effectively with patients, families, and other healthcare professionals.
- **Emotional stability:** Nurses must be able to remain calm and collected under pressure, even when dealing with difficult patients or situations.
- **Empathy:** Nurses must be able to understand and relate to the feelings of their patients.
- **Flexibility:** Nurses must be able to adapt to changing situations and priorities.
- **Attention to detail:** Nurses must be able to pay close attention to detail in order to provide safe and effective care.

Figure 3.2: Qualities of the professional nurse

- **Interpersonal skills:** Nurses must be able to build rapport with patients and their families.
- **Physical endurance:** Nurses must be able to work long hours and be physically active.
- **Problem solving skills:** Nurses must be able to identify and solve problems quickly and effectively.
- **Quick response:** Nurses must be able to respond to emergencies quickly and efficiently.
- **Respect:** Nurses must treat all patients with respect, regardless of their background or circumstances.

SHORT ANSWER QUESTIONS

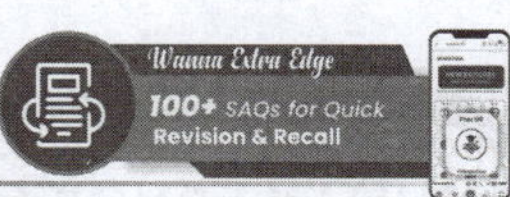

1. Define Vocation.

Answer

Profession is defined as "a vocation requiring advanced training and usually involving mental rather than manual work, as teaching, engineering, especially medicine, law."

2. What are the characteristics of a profession?

Answer

- It has a theoretical body of knowledge and skills.
- It provides scientific service.
- It has autonomy in decision making and practice.
- It has a whole code of ethical practice.
- It requires an extended education.
- It has strong service orientation.
- Ongoing research.
- It is a professional organization that sets standards.

3. Write about the criteria of a profession.

Answer

According to Bixler, criteria of profession are as follows:
- **Intellectual:** Uses specialized knowledge in practice
- **Scientific:** The person is having a body of scientific knowledge.
- Requires higher education
- **Essential:** Be vital to human and social welfare.
- **Self-governing:** Be able to provide leadership among members.
- **Service oriented:** Should put service first.

- **Continuous professional growth:** Should have planned opportunities for their professional development
- **Personal development:** able to work with a sense of knowing that they can make improvements and apply new ideas and methods.
- **Economic security:** having enough money to pay for essentials of life.

4. Enumerate functions of nurse.

Answer

Functions of Nurse

- Care provider
- Client Advocate
- Teacher
- Communicator
- Team member
- Leader

CONCEPTUAL REVISION

MULTIPLE CHOICE QUESTIONS

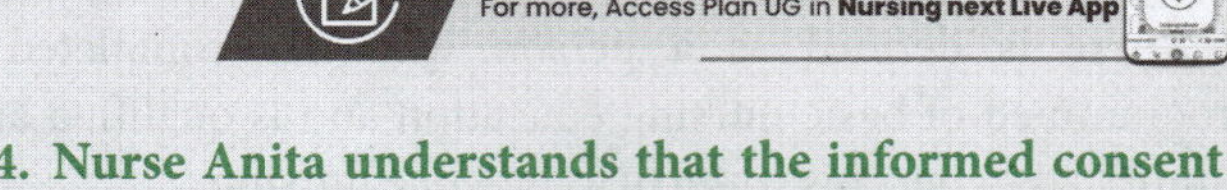

1. A child's immunization may cause discomfort during administration, but the benefits of protection from disease, both for the individual and society, outweigh the temporary discomforts. Which principle is involved in this situation?

a. Fidelity b. Beneficence
c. Non maleficence d. Respect for autonomy

Ans. b. Beneficence

2. The patient rights to refuse the treatment comes under which of the following heading?

a. Statutory law b. Common law
c. Regulatory law d. Civil law

Ans. b. Common law

3. A first-aid rescuer provides hands only CPR to a victim collapsed in front of him outside a coffee shop. Which of the following legal principle support the rescuer from being successfully sued for wrong doing?

a. Statutory law b. Misdemeanor
c. Good Samaritan laws d. Administrative law

Ans. c. Good Samaritan laws

4. Nurse Anita understands that the informed consent is based on ....ethical principle.

a. Justice b. Veracity
c. Fidelity d. Autonomy

Ans. d. Autonomy

5. All of the following descriptions come under the category of negligence; except:

a. Failure to follow standards of care
b. Failure to use equipment in a responsible manner
c. Breech of privacy
d. All of the above

Ans. c. Breech of privacy

6. The nurse is preparing a patient for the termination phase of the nurse-patient relationship. The nurse prepares to implement which nursing task that is most appropriate for this phase?

a. Planning short-term goals
b. Making appropriate referrals
c. Developing realistic solutions
d. Identifying expected outcomes

Ans. b. Making appropriate referrals

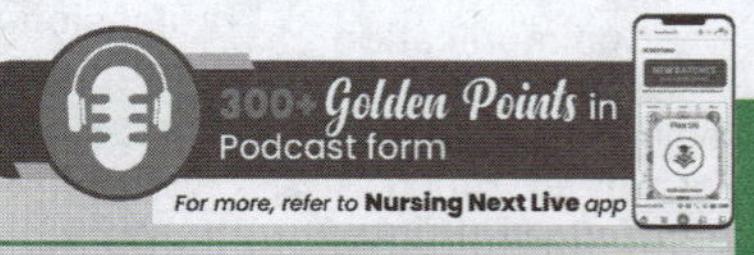

Golden Points

- Nursing is to bring healthy and those who are suffering from disease to a condition for nature to act for preserving health, preventing disease and injury and to restore health and cure disease.
- Nursing practice involves in Promotion of health and wellness, Prevention of illness, restoration of health and care for the dying or facilitating coping with Disability and Death
- The professional values in nursing are- Altruism, Autonomy, Human dignity, Integrity and Social justice
- The word Nurse is derived from a Latin word-nutrix which means to nourish.

CHAPTER

4

Communication and Nurse Patient Relationship

CONCEPTUAL THEORY

Terminology

150+ key terminologies for Quick Recall & Revision

Channel: Medium used in conveying of messages.
Communication: It is a process of exchanging information and generating and transmitting meanings between two or more individuals.
Message: Second component of communication process. It is a message itself which is said or written.
Meta communication: Broad term that refers to all factors that can affect the process of communication.
Non-verbal communication: Includes five senses and everything that does not involve the spoken or written words.
Receiver (decoder): It is the listener. Message is decoded by the receiver.
Response: Message that receiver sends to the sender either in the form of verbal, nonverbal or both.
Source (Encoder): Person or group that sends the information to the receiver.
Therapeutic nurse-patient relationship: This is a mutual learning experience and a corrective emotional experience for the patient. It is based on the underlying humanity of nurse and patient, with mutual respect and acceptance of sociocultural differences. In this relationship, the nurse uses personal attributes and clinical techniques in working with the patient to bring about insight and behavioral change.
Verbal communication: Uses spoken and written words that convey specific meaning through combination of the used words.

COMMUNICATION

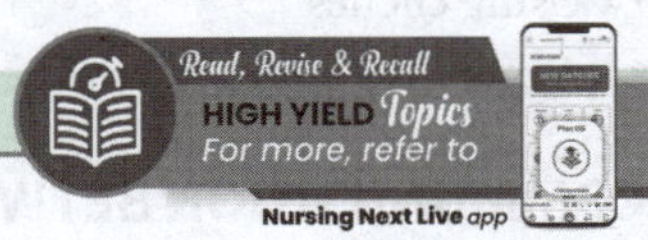

Communication is the process of exchanging information, and generating and transmitting meanings between two or more individuals.

Levels of Communication

Intrapersonal Communication

It is the communication that happens within the individual also called self-talk.

Interpersonal Communication

It occurs between two or more people with a goal to exchange messages.

Small-group Communication

It occurs when nurses interact with two or more individuals. It is used in small staff meeting, patient care conferences, teaching sessions or support groups.

Organizational Communication

It occurs when individuals and groups within an organization communicate to achieve established goals.

Communication Process

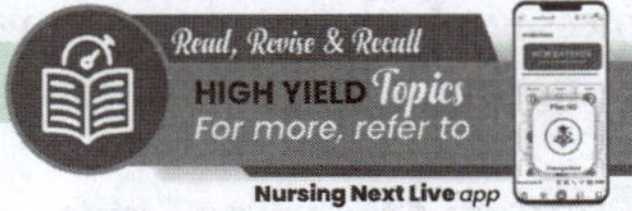

Source (Encoder, Sender)

The sender is a person or group that wishes to convey a message to another.

Message

Information to be convinced. Message itself is actually said or written.

Channel

The medium used to convey the message is the channel.

Receiver (Decoder)

The receiver is the listener, who must listen, observe and attend. The person is the decoder.

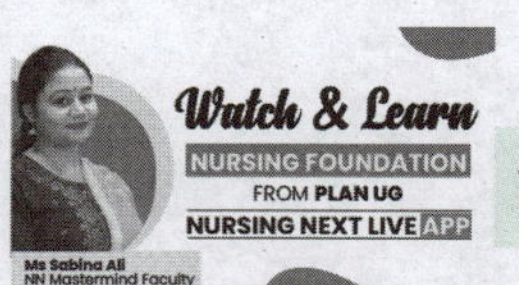

Response

It is also called **feedback**. It can be either verbal, nonverbal or both.

Modes of Communication

Communication is generally **verbal** and **nonverbal**.

Verbal Communication

Verbal communication is an exchange of information using words, including both spoken and written.

Nonverbal Communication

The transmission of information without the use of words is termed nonverbal communication, also known as body language.

Electronic Communication

Many health care agencies are moving toward electronic medical records where nurses document their assessments and nursing care.

Methods of Effective Communication

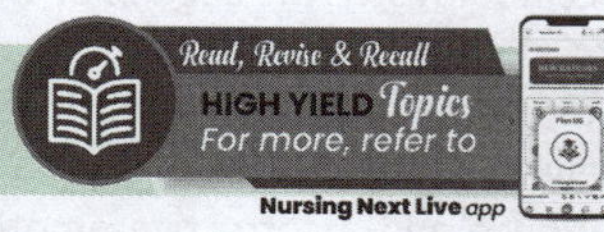

Therapeutic Communication

It is client- and goal-directed communication. It is important to understand how the client views the situation and feels about it before responding.

Attentive Listening

Attentive listening is an active process that requires energy and concentration. It involves paying attention to the total message, both verbal and nonverbal, and noting whether these communications are congruent.

Physical Attending Skills

- Face the other person
- Adopt an open posture
- Lean toward the person
- Maintain good eye contact
- Try to be relatively relaxed

Rapport Building Skills

Good rapport can be achieved by paying attention to the:

- Specific objectives
- Comfortable environment
- Privacy
- Confidentiality
- Using nursing observations
- Optimal pacing
- Respecting personal space

Empathy Skills

An empathetic nurse is sensitive to the patient's feelings and problems, but remains objective enough to help the patient attain positive outcomes.

Interviewing Skills

- Use of open-ended questions
- Use of closed questions
- Validating questions
- Clarifying questions
- Reflective questions
- Sequencing questions
- Summarizing
- Assertiveness skill

Barriers to Effective Communication

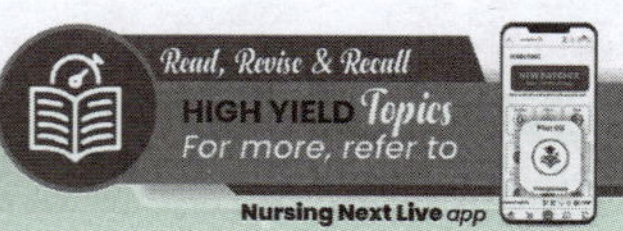

- Failure to perceive the patient as a human being
- Failure to listen
- Inappropriate comments and questions
- Giving false reassurances
- Changing the subject
- Judgmental response
- Being defensive
- Asking probing questions
- Giving advice
- Rejecting
- Using cliches
- Aggressive interpersonal behavior

COMMUNICATION BETWEEN HEALTH CARE TEAM

Communication within the health care team occurs through writing and reading nurse's notes, physician's orders, dietitian notes. Filling out a wide variety of forms for the laboratory, radiology, and other departments is another method of communication. Entering information on the computer is an essential tool for communication among hospital departments.

End-of-Shift Report

A full report on each patient should take one to three minutes. Give only essential information.

Documenting Communication

It helps to promote continuity of care because significant information must be passed on to others through nursing progress notes and care plans.

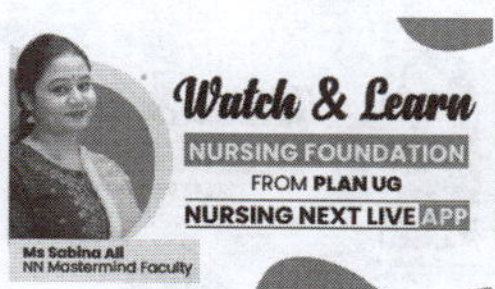

Hand-off Communication: SBAR Technique

Hand-off communication involves the accurate presentation of all patient-related information to another caregiver.

INTERPERSONAL RELATIONSHIP

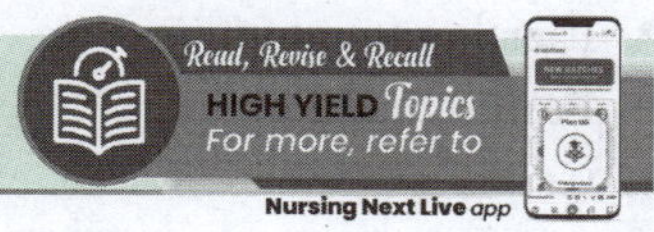

It develops and maintains effective relations steps with others. It brings people close and creates an open proudly and professional atmosphere. It has the following phases.

Preinteraction Phase

The nurse has information about the client before the first, face-to-face meeting.

Introductory Phase

Introductory phase or the pre-helping phase is important because it sets the tone for the rest of the relationship.

- **Structuring and formulating the contract:** In this stage, the nurse and client develop a degree of trust and verbally agree. The client may develop resistive behaviors which can be overcome by conveying a caring attitude, genuine interest in the client and competence.

Working Phase

It has two major stages:

1. Exploring and understanding thoughts and feelings
2. Facilitating and taking action.

Termination Phase

Nurse and client accept the end of the relationship without feelings of anxiety and dependence.

CONCEPTUAL EXERCISES

LONG ANSWER QUESTION

1. Define communication. Write the types of communication and explain the methods of effective communication. (DU, KUHS, MGR)

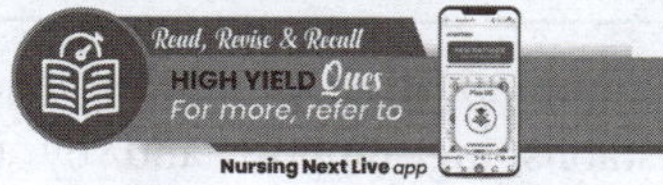

Answer

Communication

The word "Communication" has been is derived from a Latin word- communicare, which means to share.

Definition

- Communication is a process of sharing information using a set of common rules.

Or

- Communication is a process by which information is exchanged between individuals through a common system of symbols, signs or behavior.

Or

- Communication is a process of exchanging information and generating and transmitting meanings between two or more individuals.

Types of Communication

- **Verbal communication**
  - Uses spoken and written words that convey specific meaning through combination of the used words.
  - Most important aspects of verbal communication are:
    1. Vocabulary
    2. Denotative and connotative meaning
    3. Pacing
    4. Intonation
    5. Clarity and brevity
    6. Timing and relevance
- **Nonverbal communication**
  - It includes five senses and everything that does not involve the spoken or written words.
  - Most important aspects of nonverbal communication are:
    - Voice tone
    - Eye contact
    - Body position
    - Personal appearance
    - Posture and gait
    - Facial expression
    - Eye contact
    - Gestures
    - Sounds
    - Territoriality and personal space
- **Meta communication**
  - It is broad term that refers to all factors that can affect the process of communication.
- **Electronic communication**
  - E-mail is the most common mode of electronic communication used in health care industry to

communicate such as confirm appointments, report normal lab reports, etc.

Methods of Effective Communication

- **Attentive skills:** Listen actively using all senses. It is an active process that needs attention to the total message.
- **Rapport building:** It means the feeling of mutual trust. Good rapport can be achieved by paying attention to:
  - Specific objectives
  - Comfortable environment
  - Privacy
  - Confidentiality
  - Using nursing observations
  - Optimal pacing
  - Respecting personal space.
- **Empathy skills:** Identifying the way other feels. It is the basis used for setting up the trusting therapeutic relationships.
- **Physical attending skills:** Manner of being presented in a group or to another person. It involves five actions which show the posture of involvement:
  - Face the other person
  - Adopt an open posture
  - Lean toward the person
  - Maintain good eye contact
  - Try to be relaxed
- **Therapeutic communication:** Client-and goal oriented communication that promotes well established constructive relationship between nurse and the clients.
- **Interviewing skills:** These skills should be used to get the most accurate and thorough information. Various techniques used in the interview are discussed here:
  - Use of open-ended questions
  - Used of closed questions
  - Validation
  - Clarifying doubts
  - Reflective questions
  - Sequencing questions
  - Summarizing
  - Assertiveness skill

Criteria for Effective Verbal Communication

- Pace and Intonation
- Simplicity
- Clarity and brevity
- Timing and relevance
- Adaptability
- Credibility
- Humor

Criteria for Effective Nonverbal Communication

- Touch
- Eye contact
- Facial expression
- Posture and gait
- Gestures
- General physical appearance
- Mode of dress and grooming
- Sounds

Thus, communication can be enhanced by using attention skills, establishing rapport and by using empathy skills.

SHORT NOTES

1. Write a short note on communication and its types. (DU, KUHS, MGR)

Answer

For answer, refer to Long Question no. 1, pg. no. 577

2. Write a short note on methods of effective communication. (DU, KUHS, MGR)

Answer

Communication can be enhanced by using attention skills, establishing rapport and by using empathy skills. These methods are discussed here:

- **Attentive skills:** Listen actively using all senses. It is an active process that needs attention to the total message.
- **Rapport building:** It means the feeling of mutual trust. Good rapport can be achieved by paying attention to:
  - Specific objectives
  - Comfortable environment
  - Privacy
  - Confidentiality
  - Using nursing observations
  - Optimal pacing
  - Respecting personal space
- **Empathy skills:** Identifying the way other feels. It is the basis used for setting up the trusting therapeutic relationships.
- **Physical attending skills:** Manner of being presented in a group or to another person. It involves five actions which show the posture of involvement:
  - Face the other person
  - Adopt an open posture
  - Lean toward the person

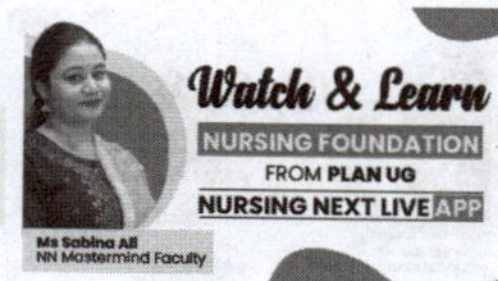

  - Maintain good eye contact
  - Try to be relaxed
- **Therapeutic communication:** client-and-goal oriented communication that promotes well established constructive relationship between nurse and the clients.
- **Interviewing skills:** These skills should be used to get the most accurate and thorough information. Various techniques used in the interview are discussed below:
  - Use of open-ended questions
  - Used of closed questions
  - Validation
  - Clarifying doubts
  - Reflective questions
  - Sequencing questions
  - Summarizing
  - Assertiveness skill

Criteria for Effective Verbal Communication

- Pace and Intonation
- Simplicity
- Clarity and brevity
- Timing and relevance
- Adaptability
- Credibility
- Humor

Criteria for Effective Nonverbal Communication

- Touch
- Eye contact
- Facial expression
- Posture and gait
- Gestures
- General physical appearance
- Mode of dress and grooming
- Sounds

3. Write a short note on barriers of communication. (DU, KUHS, MGR)

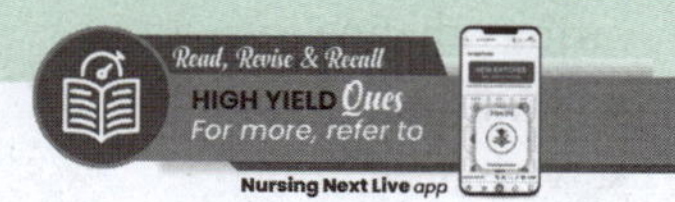

Answer

Barriers of Communication

Health care professionals need to identify these barriers to promote the communication effective in nature.

- Failure to perceive the patient as a human being
- Failure to listen
- Inappropriate comments and questions
- Giving false reassurances
- Changing the subject
- Judgmental response
- Being defensive
- Asking probing questions
- Giving advice
- Rejecting
- Using clichés
- Aggressive interpersonal behavior.

Categories of Barriers

- **Physiological barriers:** They include:
  - Poor retention
  - lack of attention
  - Discomfort due to illness
  - Poor sensory perception
  - Hearing problems
  - Poor listening skills
  - Information overload
  - Gender physiological differences
- **Environmental barriers:** They include:
  - Loud background noise
  - Poor lighting
  - Uncomfortable settings
  - Unhygienic surroundings
  - Very hot/cold room
  - Distance
- **Psychological barriers:** They include:
  - Misperception and misunderstanding
  - Distrust
  - Anger
  - Prejudice
  - Illness
  - Emotional disturbance
  - Fear
  - Anxiety
  - Confused thinking
- **Social barriers:** They include:
  - Social taboos
  - Different social strata
- **Cultural barriers:** They include:
  - Ethics
  - Religion
  - Values
  - Cultural Traditions
- **Semantic barriers:** They include:
  - Language barrier
  - Jargons

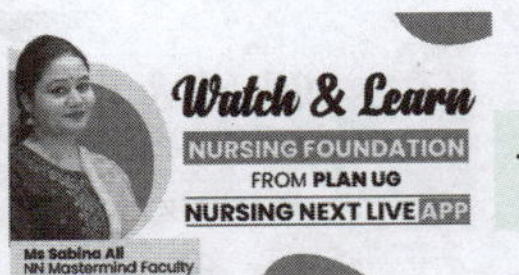

- Expression and perception
- Failure to listen
- **Organizational barriers:** They include:
  - Organizational policies and rules
  - Time pressure
  - Complexity of organizational structure
  - Size of unit
- **Communication process related barriers:** They include:
  - Unclear and conflicting messages
  - Stereotypical approach
  - Inappropriate channels
  - Lack of feedback

4. Write down the levels and elements of good communication. (RUHS, MGR, KUHS)

Answer

Levels of Communication

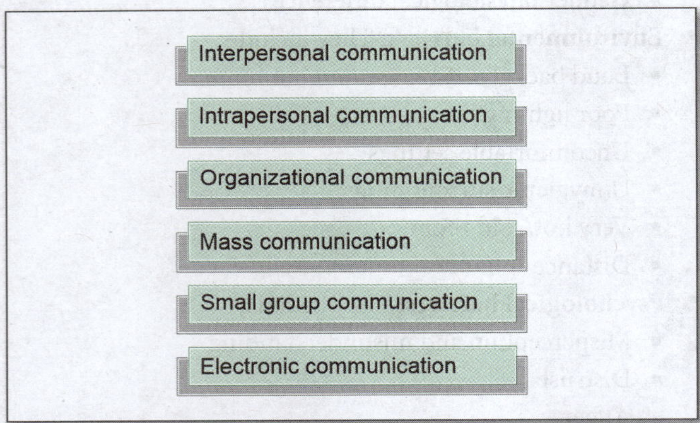

- **Intrapersonal communication** means internal thoughts and conversation happening inside the head, also called self-talk. In intrapersonal communication both the sender and receiver are the same person.
- **Interpersonal communication:** It is the communication, between two people.
- **Small group communication:** Small group communication between a small group, like small staff meeting.
- **Mass communication:** In this type of communication, communication occurs with a large group of people such as social media.
- **Organizational communication:** Occurs within the individuals and groups of an organization.
- **Electronic communication:** Use of technology to impart the information.

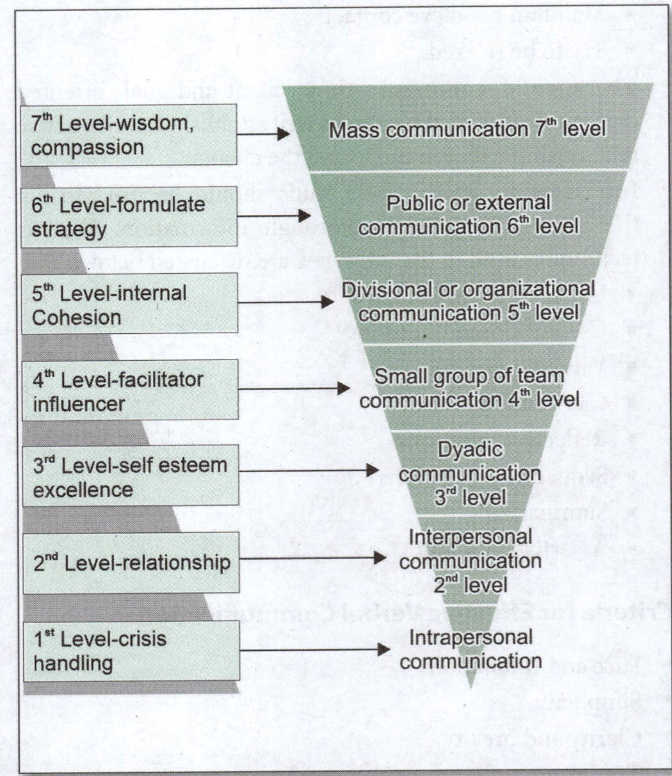

Adapted from: Karthikeyan C Karthikeyan C

Elements of Communication

Communication process is the process through which the exchange of information takes place between sender and receiver. This process involves:

- Source (encoder)
- Message
- Channel
- Receiver (decoder)
- Response or feedback
- **Source (Encoder):** Person or group that sends the information to the receiver.
- **Message:** Second component of communication process. It is a message itself which is said or written.
- **Channel:** Medium used in conveying of messages. The various channels used are:
  - Auditory
  - Visual
  - Kinethetic touch
- **Receiver (decoder):** It is the listener. Message is decoded by the receiver.
- **Response:** Message that receiver sends to the sender either in the form of verbal or nonverbal or both.

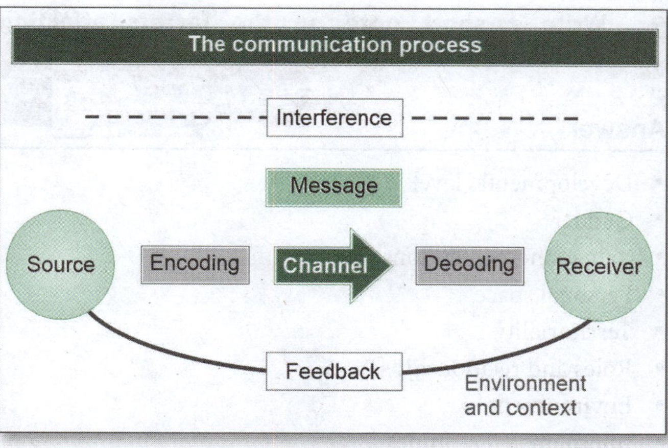

5. Write a short note on communication of nurse with health team members. (DU)

Answer

- According to Hannawa (2018), patient outcomes can improve when health care members communicate effectively. For effective therapeutic communication, the SACCIA technique is widely used. It stands for:
  - S – Sufficiency
  - A – Accuracy
  - C – Clarity
  - C – Contextualization
  - IA – Interpersonal Adaptation
- In order to communicate the information within the hospital settings, SBAR technique can improve the communication process. SBAR technique reveals:
  - S – Situation
  - B – Background
  - A – Assessment
  - R – Recommendation.
- Some organizations have also adopted the additional step of introduction in SBAR technique. This ISBAR technique is used when health care professionals do not know each other.
  - I – Introduction
  - S – Situation
  - B – Background
  - A – Assessment
  - R – Recommendation
- Communication of nurse with health team members occurs through:
  - End-of-shift report
  - Documenting communication
  - Hand-off communication- SBAR technique

6. Write a short note on nurse-patient relationship. (MGR, RUHS)

Answer

Therapeutic nurse-patient relationship is a mutual learning experience and a corrective emotional experience for the patient. It is based on the underlying humanity of nurse and patient, with mutual respect and acceptance of sociocultural differences. In this relationship, the nurse uses personal attributes and clinical techniques while working with the patient to bring about insight and behavioral change.

- It is the interpersonal relationship between nurse and patient.
- The nurse-patient relationship allows the attainment of health-related goals.
- It is the foundation of clinical nursing practice.
- It promotes the psychological climate which facilitates positive change and growth.
- It encourages narrative interaction.
- It includes a technique called motivational interviewing.
- This relationship has the following four phases.
  1. **Orientation**—problem defining phase
  2. **Identification**—selection of appropriate professional assistance
  3. **Exploitation**—phase of professional assistance for problem-solving alternatives
  4. **Resolution**—termination of professional relationship.

7. Write a short note on nonverbal communication. (DU)

Answer

- Nonverbal communication means the mode of communication without the use of words, and also known as body language.
- It represents the true meaning of message than verbal communication.
- Can be an incongruence between verbal and nonverbal message.
- It is considered to be the one that is more valid or true.
- Various forms of nonverbal communication are:
  - Touch
  - Eye contact
  - Facial expression
  - Posture and gait
  - Gestures
  - General physical appearance
  - Mode of dress and grooming
  - Sounds

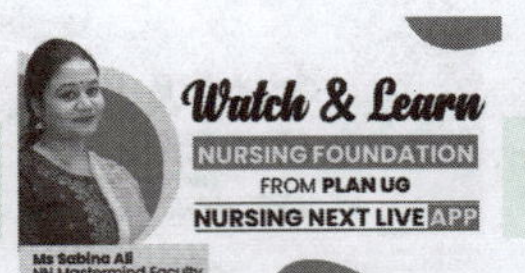

8. Write a short note on therapeutic communication. (MGR)

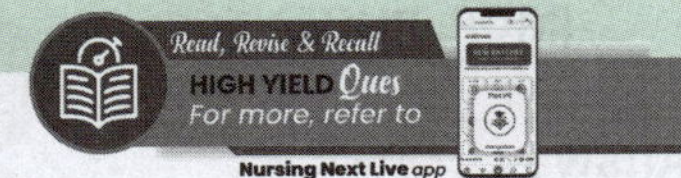

Answer

The therapeutic interaction between the nurse and the client will be helpful to develop mutual understanding between nurse and patient.

Definitions

- The nurse directs the communication toward the patient to identify his current health problems, plan, and implements and evaluates the action taken. **—Bimala kapoor, 2002**
- Promotes mutual understanding, establishes a constructive relationship between the nurse and the client. **—Kozier, 2004**
- It is a process in which the nurse utilizes a planned approach to learn about the client. **—Potter A, 1997**

Purposes

- To achieve self-realization and personal integration
- To formulate good IPR
- To achieve realistic personal goals
- To encourage family interaction process
- To treat communication problems
- To modify maladaptive behavior into adaptive behavior
- To motivate the client to utilize coping strategies
- To implement nursing process effectively

Elements of Therapeutic communication

- Courtesy
- Use of names
- Trustworthiness
- Autonomy
- Responsibility
- Assertiveness

Techniques used in Therapeutic Communication

- Observing
- Restating
- Validating
- Reflecting
- Clarifying
- Paraphrasing
- Pinpointing
- Linking
- Questioning
- Focusing
- Sharing
- Summarizing

9. Write a short note on the factors affecting communication. (RUHS)

Read, Revise & Recall HIGH YIELD Ques For more, refer to Nursing Next Live app

Answer

- Developmental level
- Gender
- Values and perceptions
- Personal space
- Territoriality
- Roles and relationships
- Environment
- Interpersonal attitudes
- Cultural diversity

- **Developmental level:** The message or the communication process can be modified as per client's age and knowledge level.
- **Gender:** Males and females possess different styles of communication. They also have different interpretation to the same conversation.
- **Values and perceptions:** These are the standards that can influence the behavior and perception. Each individual has its own personality traits and experiences of life.
- **Personal space:** People usually prefer the personal space during interactions. It involves:
  - Intimate distance (1.5 feet)
  - Personal distance (1.5–4 feet)
  - Social distance (4-12 feet)
  - Public distance(12–15 feet)
- **Territoriality:** Space and things that the people consider belonging to self.
- **Roles and relationships:** Roles, such as nursing student and instructor, child and parent, affect the process of communication.
- **Environment:** Internal as well as external environment both can affect the communication process. Comfortable environment can promote the effective communication. Some of the factors are time, place, poor lighting, long-distance barriers and noise.
- **Interpersonal attitudes:** Attitudes such as caring and worth, respect and acceptance can convey thoughts about people during the process of communication.
- **Cultural diversity:** It can also affect the process of communication between two people belonging to different cultural backgrounds.

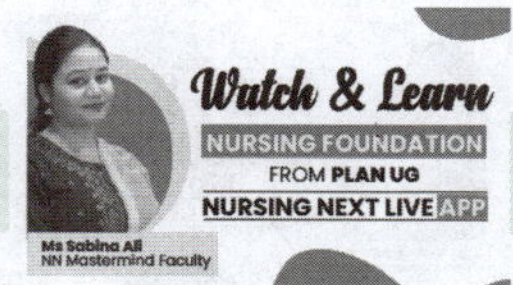

SHORT ANSWER QUESTIONS

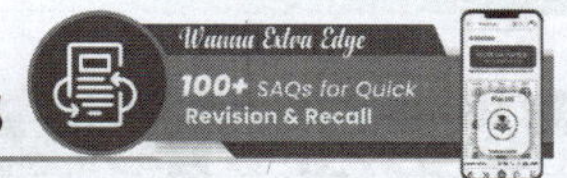

1. Define communication. (MGR)

Answer

The word "Communication" has been derived from a Latin word- communicare, which means to share.

Definition

- Communication is a process of sharing information using a set of common rules.

Or

- Communication is a process by which information is exchanged between individuals through a common system of symbols, signs or behavior.

Or

- Communication is a process of exchanging information and generating and transmitting meanings between two or more individuals.

2. Enumerate the type of communication and factors affecting communication. (MGR)

Answer

Types of Communication

- Verbal communication
- Nonverbal communication
- Meta communication
- Electronic communication

Factors Affecting Communication

- Developmental level
- Gender
- Values and perceptions
- Personal space
- Territoriality
- Roles and relationships
- Environment
- Interpersonal attitudes
- Cultural diversity

3. What are the methods of effective communication? (MGR)

Answer

- Attentive skills
- Rapport building
- **Empathy skills:** Identifying the way other feels. It is the basis used for setting up a trusting therapeutic relationship.
- **Physical attending skills:** Manner of being presented in a group or to another person.
- **Therapeutic communication:** Client- and goal- oriented communication that promotes well established constructive relationship between nurse and the clients.
- **Interviewing skills:** These skills should be used to get the most accurate and thorough information.

4. What are the elements of communication? (MGR)

Answer

Communication process is the process through which the exchange of information takes place between sender and receiver. This process involves:

- Source (encoder)
- Message
- Channel
- Receiver (decoder)
- Response or feedback

5. Define therapeutic communication. (MGR)

Answer

The therapeutic interaction between the nurse and the client will be helpful to develop mutual understanding between them.

Definitions

- The nurse directs the communication toward the patient to identify his current health problems, plan, and implements and evaluates the action taken. **—Bimala kapoor, 2002**
- Promotes mutual understanding, establishes a constructive relationship between the nurse and the client. **—Kozier, 2004**
- It is a process in which the nurse utilizes a planned approach to learn about the client. **—Potter A, 1997**

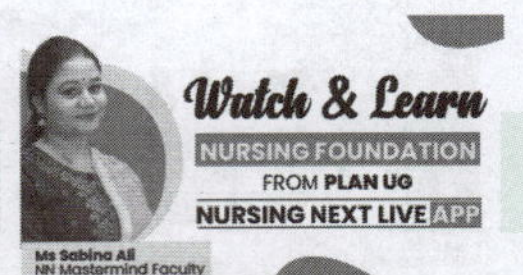

CONCEPTUAL REVISION

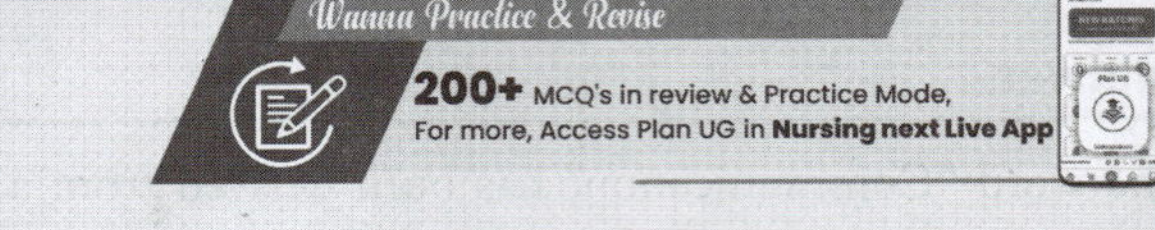

MULTIPLE CHOICE QUESTIONS

1. A patient needs to learn to use a walker. Which domain is required for learning this skill?

a. Affective domain b. Cognitive domain
c. Attentional domain d. Psychomotor domain

Ans. d. Psychomotor domain

2. Identify which method of delivery of nursing care is being used in the given below image?

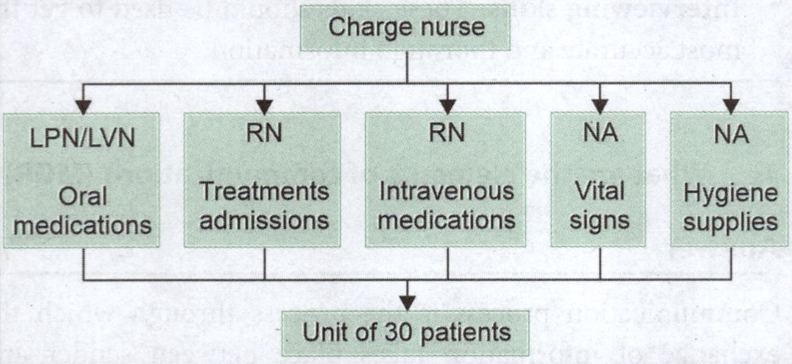

a. Primary Nursing care b. Functional Nursing care
c. Team Nursing d. Case method

Ans. b. Functional Nursing care

3. All of the following are levels of communication; except:

a. Small group communication
b. Electronic Communication
c. Interpersonal Communication
d. Verbal Communication

Ans. d. Verbal Communication

4. All of the following are the methods of effective communication; except:

a. Empathy b. Rapport building
c. Being sympathetic d. Attention skills

Ans. c. Being sympathetic

5. Who gave theory of interpersonal relationship?

a. Hildegard Peplau b. Virginia Henderson
c. Florence Nightingale d. Dorothy Johnson

Ans. a. Hildegard Peplau

6. This phase starts when the nurse meets the patient and identifies patient's problems and defines them:

a. Orientation phase b. Identification phase
c. Exploitation phase d. Resolution phase

Ans. a. Orientation phase

7. The client in the termination phase of the nurse-client relationship is being very confrontational. How should the nurse interpret this behavior?

a. This behavior is common for a client in the termination phase
b. The treatment should revisit the working phase
c. The patient should be admitted to the hospital
d. The nurse has done something to offend the client

Ans. a. This behavior is common for a client in the termination phase.

Golden Points

- Communication is the process of exchanging information, and generating and transmitting meanings between two or more individuals.
- Levels of communication are intrapersonal communication, interpersonal communication, small-group communication and Organizational communication.
- Communication process has Source (Encoder, Sender), Message, Channel, Receiver (Decoder) and Response (feedback) It can be either verbal, nonverbal or both.
- Therapeutic Communication is client- and goal-directed communication. It is important to understand how the client views the situation and feels about it before responding.
- Communication within the health care team occurs through writing and reading nurse's notes, physician's orders, dietitian notes.
- Filling out a wide variety of forms for the laboratory, radiology, and other departments is another method of communication.
- Entering information on the computer is an essential tool for communication among hospital departments.

CHAPTER

5

Documentation and Reporting

CONCEPTUAL THEORY

Terminology

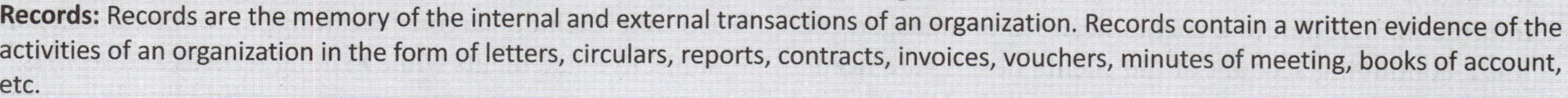

Documentation: It is the written or typed legal record of all pertinent interactions with the patient: Assessing, diagnosing, planning, implementing and evaluating.

Records: Records are the memory of the internal and external transactions of an organization. Records contain a written evidence of the activities of an organization in the form of letters, circulars, reports, contracts, invoices, vouchers, minutes of meeting, books of account, etc.

Report: It is a document containing information on organized in a narrative, graphic, or tabular form, prepared on ad hoc, periodic, recurring, regular, or as required basis. Reports may refer to specific periods, events, occurrences, or subjects and may be communicated or presented in oral or written form.

SBAR communication: (Situation, Background, Assessment, Recommendation) is a framework of communication between the members of the health care team about client's condition. It provides a consistent method for handing off communication that is clear, structured, and easy-to-use.

DOCUMENTATION

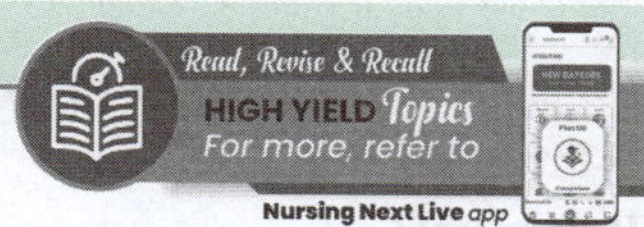

Documentation is the written or typed legal record of all pertinent interactions with the patient: Assessing, diagnosing, planning, implementing and evaluating.

The patient record is a compilation of patient's health information. Each health care institution has policies that specify the nurses' documentation responsibilities.

The patient's record is the only permanent legal document that details the nurse's interactions with the patient and is the nurse's best defense if a patient alleges nursing negligence. Health care personnel must not only maintain the confidentiality of the client's record but also meet legal standards in the process of recording.

SBAR Communication

SBAR communication (Situation, Background, Assessment, Recommendation) is a framework of communication between the members of the health care team about client's condition. It provides a consistent method for handing off communication that is clear, structured, and easy-to-use.

Do's and Don'ts of Nursing Documentation

Do's

- Check the correct file before you begin writing.
- Write legibly.
- Chart the time
- Record each phone call to a physician.
- Chart patient care at the time you provide it.

Don'ts

- Don't chart a symptom, such as "c/o pain,".
- Don't alter a patient's record.
- Don't use shorthand or abbreviations.
- Don't write imprecise descriptions.

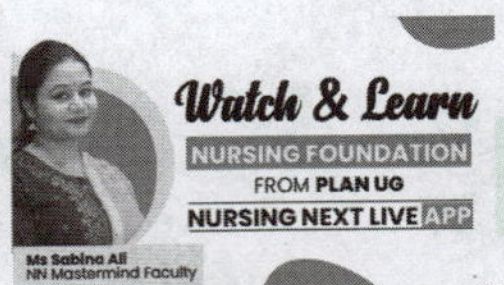

CONCEPTUAL EXERCISES

LONG ANSWER QUESTIONS

1. Define records and reports. Enlist the principles of maintaining records and characteristics of good reports. (KUHS, RUHS, DU)

Answer

Records and Reports

Records

- Records are the memory of the internal and external transactions of an organization. Records contain written evidence of the activities of an organization in the form of letters, circulars, reports, contracts, invoices, vouchers, minutes of meeting, books of account, etc. **—SL Geol, 2001**
- It is a written communication that permanently documents information relevant to a client's health care management. It is a continuing account of the client's health care needs. **—Sr Mary Lucita**

Report

- Report is a document containing information on organized in a narrative, graphic, or tabular form, prepared on ad hoc, periodic, recurring, regular, or as required basis. Reports may refer to specific periods, events, occurrences, or subjects and may be communicated or presented in oral or written form. Reports may refer to specific periods, events, occurrences, or subjects and may be communicated or presented in oral or written form. **—Basvanthappa bt. 2009**
- Reports are oral or written exchanges of information shared between care givers of workers in a number of ways. A report summarizes the service of the personnel and of the agency. ***—Jean b. 2002***

Principles of Maintaining Records

- The specific purpose of record and reports should be clearly understood.
- Items on forms and in registers should be grouped properly to make their completion easier.
- The wording should be easily understood.
- Records should permit freedom of expression.
- Records should be easily accessible.
- Person responsible for maintaining records should be aware of responsibility.
- Records should be up to date and accurate.
- There should be a provision for periodic review of all records.
- Adequate supply of stationery should be maintained.
- Sufficient number of filing cabinets and adequate, safe, fire proof storage arrangements must be present.

Characteristics of a Good Report

- Accuracy
- Conciseness
- Thoroughness
- Up to date
- Organization
- Confidentiality
- Objectivity
- Write up notes after an event within 24 hours.
- Make clear subsequent alterations or additions, if necessary.
- Do not include jargon, meaningless phrases, offensive subjective statements while making records and reports.

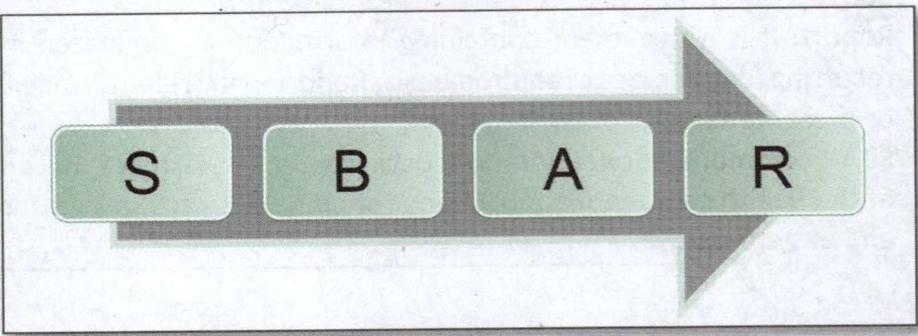

For effective reporting, SBAR communication can also be used:

S–Situation
B–Background
A–Assessment
R–Recommendation

- **Situation**—a concise statement of the problem
- **Background**—pertinent and brief information related to the situation.
- **Assessment**—analysis and considerations of options-what you found/think
- **Recommendation**—action requested/recommended-what you want.

SMART Model

- Specific
- Measurable
- Achievable
- Realistic
- Time-based

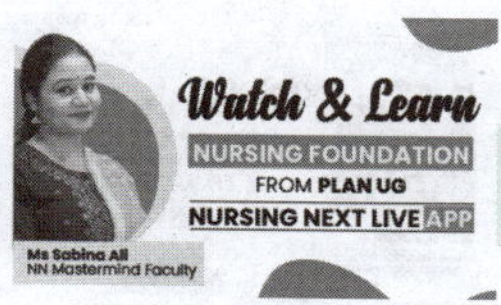

2. Discuss types of records. (DU, KUHS)

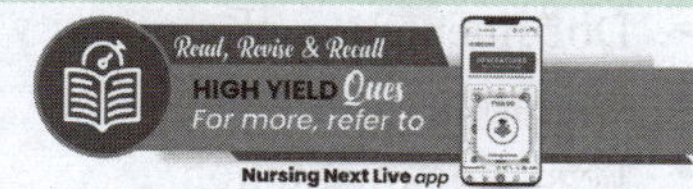

Answer

- **Records** are the memory of the internal and external transactions of an organization. Records contain a written evidence of the activities of an organization in the form of letters, circulars, reports, contracts, invoices, vouchers, minutes of meetings, books of account, etc.

  —SL Geol, 2001
- It is a written communication that permanently documents information relevant to a client's health care management. It is a continuing account of the client's health care needs.

  —Sr Mary Lucita

Classification of Records

- **Active Record:** Regularly referenced/required for use.
- **Inactive Record:** Still needed but not for current operations.
- **Electronic Record:** Recorded/formatted only by the use of computer.
- **Medical record:**
  - Admission history
  - Medical history
  - Family history
  - Consents
- **Nursing record:**
  - Nursing assessment
  - Nursing care plan
  - Kardex
  - Flow sheets
  - Graphic record
  - Progress notes.

Types of Records

- Patient's clinical records
- Individual staff records
- Ward records
- Administrative records with educational value

Patient's Clinical Records

It is the knowledge of events in the patient illness, progress in his or her recovery and the type of care given by the health care professionals.

- Scientific and legal
- Evidence to the patient case
- Avoids duplication
- Research
- Promotion of health and care
- Legal protection

Individual Staff Records

- A separate set of record for staff
- Details of their sickness and absences
- Carrier and development activities
- Personnel note

Ward Records

- Reduction or increase in the number of beds
- Change in staff for the ward
- The introduction and pattern of support

Administrative Records with Educational Value

- Treatments
- Admission
- Equipment losses and replacements
- Personnel performance
- Other administrative records

SHORT NOTES

1. Write a short note on purpose of documentation. (MGR, KUHS)

Answer

Documentation related to patients is considered a valuable source of information for all health care professionals. It facilitates the interdisciplinary communication within an organization. These are the following purposes of documentation:

- **Communication**—Necessary to be informed about the patient.
- **Diagnostic and therapeutic orders**—These orders are necessary to be implemented. Record should be duly signed, date and time should also be mentioned. In case of verbal records, concerned health care professional's name should be clearly mentioned.
- **Care planning**—Nurses, doctors, etc. use the patient record to plan the care required for the health promotion of the patient.
- **Quality review**—Clinical records are widely used for quality assurance. Various accreditation agencies such as NABH, JCI may review the patient record.
- **Health care analysis**—To maintain the utilized or underutilized hospital services. Can also be used in cost analysis of the inventory.
- **Education**—Health care professionals and students utilize the patient record in order to get the information about the disease process.

- **Legal documentation**—Can be used as an evidence in court.
- **Reimbursement**—Used to demonstrate to payers e.g. insurance companies.
- **Research**—For evidence based practice.

2. Write a short note on records and reports. (KUHS, RUHS)

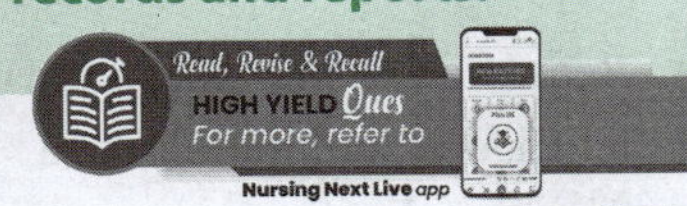

Answer

- Records are is a written communication that permanently documents information relevant to a client's health care management. It is a continuing account of the client's health care needs. —**Sr Mary Lucita**
- Reports are oral or written exchanges of information shared between care givers of workers in a number of ways. A report summarizes the service of the personnel and of the agency. —**Jean b. 2002**

Principles of Maintaining Records

- The specific purpose of record and reports should be clearly understood.
- Items on forms and in registers should be grouped properly to make their completion easier.
- The wording should be easily understood.
- Records should permit freedom of expression.
- Records should be easily accessible.
- Person responsible for maintaining records should be aware of responsibility
- Records should be up to date and accurate.
- There should be a provision for periodic review of all records.
- Adequate supply of stationery should be maintained.
- Sufficient number of filing cabinets and adequate, safe, fire proof storage arrangements must be present.

Characteristics of Good Record and Report

- Accuracy
- Conciseness
- Thoroughness
- Up to date
- Organization
- Confidentiality
- Objectivity

Purposes of Keeping Records

- Communication
- Aids diagnosis
- Education
- Documentation of continuity
- Research
- Legal documentation
- Individual case study

Uses of Records

- Show the health conditions.
- Prevents duplication of services
- Effectively helps in follow-up of services.
- Helps in evaluation of the care and the teaching Organization of work
- Serves as a guide for diagnosis treatment and evaluation
- Used in research
- The health assets and needs of the village area

3. Write a short note on characteristics of a good report. (DU)

Answer

Following are the characteristics of a good report.

- **Accuracy:** Accuracy is a crucial characteristic of a good report. It refers to the reliability and correctness of the information presented in the report.
- **Clear and concise:** Clarity and conciseness are essential in nursing reports to ensure effective communication. The information should be presented in a clear and understandable manner, avoiding unnecessary jargon or technical terms that may hinder comprehension. Use of appropriate headings, subheadings, and bullet points can enhance the readability and organization of the report.
- **Comprehensive:** A good nursing report provides a comprehensive overview of the patient's condition, including relevant medical history, current symptoms, diagnostic test results, medications, treatments administered, and any observed changes in the patient's status. It captures essential details to ensure a holistic understanding of the patient's health.
- **Timeliness:** Timeliness is crucial in nursing reports. They should be completed and shared promptly to ensure the timely communication of critical information to healthcare team members. Timely reports help in facilitating prompt interventions, continuity of care, and effective decision-making.
- **Organized and structured:** Nursing reports should follow a logical structure and organization. They should typically include an introduction or summary, background information, current assessment, interventions provided, and ongoing care plans. Consistent use of headings and

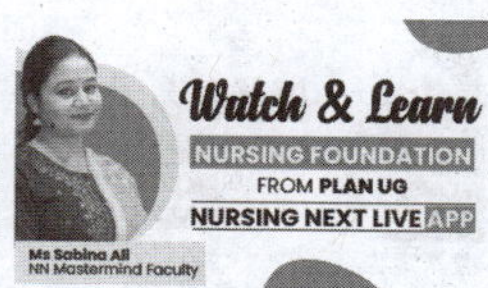

subheadings helps to guide the reader through the report and locate information easily.

- **Confidentiality and privacy:** Maintaining patient confidentiality and privacy is paramount in nursing reports. Adhere to ethical and legal guidelines regarding the protection of patient information. Avoid sharing sensitive information unnecessarily and ensure that the report is securely stored or transmitted according to institutional policies.
- **Objective and accurate:** Nursing reports should maintain objectivity and accuracy. Information documented should be based on factual observations, assessments, and measurements. Avoid personal opinions or assumptions, and ensure that the information presented is reliable and verifiable. Accurate documentation is critical for providing continuity of care and legal purposes.
- **Reflective and continuous improvement:** Nursing reports can serve as a tool for reflection and continuous improvement. Nurses should take the opportunity to reflect on the care provided, document any challenges or areas for improvement, and make suggestions for future care. This promotes a culture of learning and enhances the quality of nursing practice.
- **Interdisciplinary collaboration:** Nursing reports often serve as a means of communication among interdisciplinary healthcare team members. They should facilitate effective collaboration and information exchange, ensuring that relevant details are shared with other healthcare professionals involved in the patient's care.

4. Write a short note on importance of records. (KUHS)

Answer

- It is a written communication that permanently documents information relevant to a client's health care management. It is a continuing account of the client's health care needs.

—**Sr Mary Lucita**

Importance of Records

- Better access to information
- Enhanced quality of documentation through prompts.
- Reduced errors of omission
- Compliance with requirements of accrediting agencies
- Development of clinical database
- Concrete patient information

For the Individual and Family

- Serve the history of client
- Assist in continuation of care
- Evidence to support if legal issues arise
- Assess health needs, research and teaching

For the Doctor

- Serve guide for diagnosis, treatment, follow up and evaluation
- Indicate progress and continuity of care
- Self-evaluation of medical practice
- Protect doctor in legal issues
- Used for teaching and research

For the Nurses

- Document nursing service rendered
- Show progress
- Guide for professional growth
- Indicate plan for future
- Judge the quality and quantity of work done
- Planning and evaluation of service for future improvement
- Communication tool between nurse and other staff involved in the care

For Authorities

- Statistical information
- Administrative control
- Future reference
- Evaluation of care in terms of quality, quantity and adequacy
- Help supervisor to evaluate service
- Guide staff and students
- Legal evidence of service rendered by each employee
- Provide justification for expenditure of funds

5. Write a short note on principles of documentation. (MGR)

Answer

Documentation is the written legal record of all pertinent interactions with the client—Assessing, diagnosing, planning, implementing and evaluating.

- Specific purpose should be clearly understood.
- Items on forms and in registers should be conveniently grouped.
- The wording should be easily understood,
- Instructions to facilitate interpretation should be included.
- Records should permit some freedom of expression.
- Records should be easily accessible.
- Person responsible for maintaining records should be aware of his/her responsibilities.

- Keep records up to date and accurate.
- Provision for periodic review.
- Adequate supply of stationery to maintain records.
- Sufficient storage for the maintenance of records.
- Adequate, safe, fireproof storage arrangements.

6. Write a short note on types of client records.

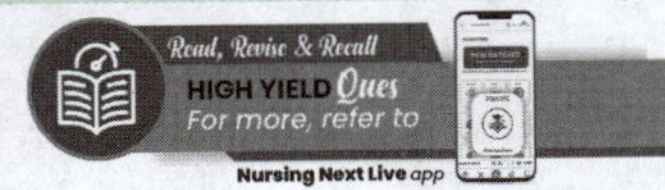

Answer

- **Medical record:**
  - **Medical record:** This record includes the patient's personal information, such as demographics, past medical conditions, surgical history, allergies, and family medical history. It provides important background information for healthcare providers.
  - **Admission records:** These records are created when a patient is admitted to the hospital and typically include information such as the reason for admission, initial assessment findings, and details of the admitting physician.
  - **Operative reports:** Operative reports are created after surgical procedures and provide a detailed account of the surgery, including pre-operative diagnosis, procedure performed, findings, complications, and post-operative care instructions.
  - **Discharge summary:** The discharge summary is created when a patient is discharged from the hospital. It includes a summary of the hospital stay, the patient's condition at discharge, prescribed medications, follow-up instructions, and recommendations for ongoing care.
  - **Consent forms:** Consent forms are legal documents that record a patient's informed consent for specific procedures, treatments, surgeries, or participation in clinical trials. They document the patient's understanding and agreement to undergo the recommended interventions.
  - **Diagnostic reports:** These reports include the results of various diagnostic tests and procedures performed on the patient, such as laboratory tests, imaging studies (X-rays, CT scans, MRIs), pathology reports, and other specialized tests. They provide crucial information for diagnosis and treatment planning.
- **Nursing record:**
  - **Physician orders:** Physician orders are written instructions from the attending physician regarding the patient's care, including medications, treatments, diagnostic tests, and dietary restrictions.
  - **Nursing notes:** Nursing notes document the ongoing assessments, observations, interventions, and evaluations performed by the nursing staff. These notes track changes in the patient's condition, responses to treatments, and any other pertinent information.
  - **Progress notes:** Progress notes are recorded by various healthcare professionals involved in the patient's care, including physicians, nurses, therapists, and consultants. They document the patient's progress, changes in condition, and responses to treatment.
  - **Medication administration records (MAR):** MARs document the administration of medications, including the drug name, dosage, route of administration, frequency, and nurse's signature. These records help ensure accurate and safe medication administration.

7. Write a short note on methods of recording and reporting. (MGR)

Read, Revise & Recall HIGH YIELD Ques For more, refer to Nursing Next Live app

Answer

Records

Recording is a written communication that permanently documents information relevant to a client's health care management. It is a continuing account of the client's health care needs. **—Sr Mary Lucita**

Reports

Reports are oral or written exchanges of information shared between care givers of workers in a number of ways. A report summarizes the service of the personnel and of the agency.

Methods of Recording

Some commonly used recording includes

- **SOAP (Subjective, Objective, Assessment, Plan):** A structured documentation format where subjective information, objective observations, professional assessment, and care plans are recorded.
- **PIE (Problem, Intervention, Evaluation):** Focuses on identifying patient problems, documenting nursing interventions, and evaluating outcomes.
- **Focus Charting (Data, Action, Response - DAR):** Centers on patient concerns or focus, using data to guide nursing actions and documenting patient responses.
- **Narrative Charting:** A free-text method that allows for detailed descriptions of patient events, observations, and interventions.
- **Flow Sheets/Checklists:** Templates used to document specific assessments or interventions, often used for routine or repetitive tasks.

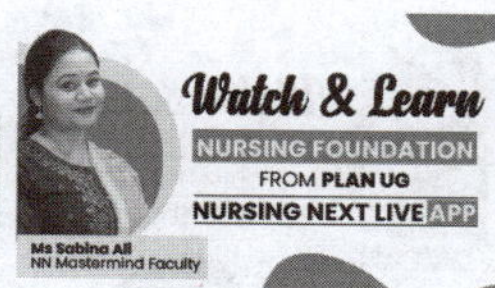

- **Graphic Charts/Vital Signs Charts:** Visual representations of vital signs and trends over time, providing a quick overview of the patient's condition.
- **Medication Administration Records (MAR):** Documents medication administration, including drug, dosage, route, time, and nurse's signature.
- **Nursing care plans:** Individualized plans outlining nursing diagnoses, goals, interventions, and evaluations to guide patient care.
- **Discharge summaries:** Summarizes the patient's stay, including diagnoses, treatments, follow-up instructions, and recommendations for post-discharge care.
- **Incident reports:** Documentation of any adverse events, errors, or incidents that occur in the healthcare setting to ensure proper investigation and follow-up.

Reporting Methods

There are various methods of reporting that ensure effective communication and continuity of care.

Some commonly used methods in Nursing care include:

- **ISBAR (Introduction, Situation, Background, Assessment, Recommendation):** Structured communication framework for clear and concise handoff reports and interprofessional communication.
- **SBAR (Situation, Background, Assessment, Recommendation):** Structured communication format primarily used for nurse-to-nurse or nurse-to-physician reporting, providing essential information about a patient's condition.
- **Handoff Reports:** Transfer of patient information during a shift change or transfer of care to ensure continuity and safety.
- **Change of Shift Reports:** Sharing relevant patient information during the transition between nursing shifts to ensure seamless care.
- **Rounds/Bedside Reporting:** Conducting patient rounds at the bedside to facilitate discussions, assessments, and updates among the healthcare team.
- **Verbal Orders and Verbal Reporting:** Communicating instructions or information verbally, often in emergencies or time-sensitive situations.
- **Telephone Reports:** Sharing patient-related information over the phone to ensure effective communication between healthcare providers.

Conclusion

The choice of method may vary depending on the healthcare setting, organizational policies, and specific communication needs. It's important for nurses to follow standardized approaches to ensure accurate and effective communication in patient care.

8. Write a short note on guidelines for reporting. (MGR)

Answer

The quality document should have five important characteristics:

1. Factual
2. Accurate
3. Complete
4. Current
5. Organized.

Some Important Guidelines for Reporting in Nursing

- **Use standardized reporting formats:** Utilize structured reporting formats such as ISBAR or SBAR to ensure consistent and comprehensive communication during handoffs and transfers of care.
- **Clear and concise:** Use clear and concise language to communicate important information, avoiding unnecessary jargon or abbreviations that may lead to misunderstandings.
- **Use effective communication techniques:** Practice active listening and encourage open communication during the reporting process. Clarify any uncertainties and ask for confirmation or clarification when needed.
- **Provide relevant and accurate information:** Include essential details about the patient's condition, vital signs, recent changes, medications, allergies, and any pending or completed interventions.
- **Use a systematic approach:** Organize your report in a logical and systematic manner, covering the patient's current situation, relevant background information, assessment findings, and recommendations for ongoing care.
- **Prioritize critical information:** Identify and prioritize critical or time-sensitive information
- **Include patient preferences and concerns:** Share any important patient preferences, concerns, or specific care instructions.
- **Document accurately:** After giving or receiving a report, ensure that all relevant information is accurately documented in the patient's medical record.
- **Maintain confidentiality and privacy:** Adhere to patient privacy and confidentiality standards during the reporting process, ensuring that sensitive information is shared only with authorized individuals.
- **Seek clarification and follow-up:** If there are any uncertainties or unanswered questions, seek clarification from the reporting nurse or healthcare provider.

9. Write a short note on guidelines for quality documentation. (DU, KUHS)

Answer

- **Sticking to the facts:** Document objective information and avoid subjective opinions or assumptions.
- **Writing in short sentences:** Use concise and clear sentences to convey information effectively.
- **Using simple language:** Use plain language that is easily understood by all healthcare professionals.
- **Using short words:** Choose words that are easy to comprehend and avoid unnecessary complexity.
- **Avoiding jargon:** Use terminology that is universally understood and avoid specialized healthcare jargon.
- **Date and time:** Include the date and time of each entry to provide a clear timeline of events.
- **Legibility:** Write in a clear and readable manner to ensure that documentation can be easily understood.
- **Permanence:** Ensure that documentation is permanent and resistant to alterations or tampering. E.g. avoid writing in pencil.
- **Accepted terminology:** Utilize standardized and accepted medical terminology to ensure consistency.
- **Correct spelling:** Maintain accurate spelling to avoid any misinterpretation or confusion.
- **Signature:** Sign each entry with your name and professional designation to take responsibility for the documentation.
- **Accuracy:** Document information accurately, reflecting the true condition and care provided.
- **Sequence, appropriateness:** Maintain a logical sequence of events and document information in a manner appropriate to the situation.
- **Completeness:** Include all relevant and essential information related to the patient's condition and care.
- **Conciseness:** Be concise in documenting information, focusing on essential details without unnecessary repetition or verbosity.

10. Write a short note on legal liabilities in record writing. (DU)

Answer

Patient records are legal documents that can be used as an evidence; thus, they play an important role in health care settings. Through effective record keeping, legal problems can be solved. Various problems are discussed below:

- When the content is not in accordance with organizational standards
- Content is incomplete and does not reflect patient's needs.
- Content does not include description of situation
- Tampering in documentation
- Illegibility
- Dates and times of entries omitted or inconsistent
- Improper nurse initials
- Transcription errors

11. Write a short note on nurses record. (MGR)

Answer

Nurses record is a record of treatments and nursing measures carried out by the nurse which reflects the observation of the client.

- **Admission nursing assessment:** for nursing assessment on admission.
- **Nursing care plans:** Patient's assessment, nursing diagnosis, nursing interventions and patient's evaluation.
- **Kardex:** method of making patient information quickly accessible to all health care teams.
- **Flow sheets:** It enables nurse to record nursing data quickly and concisely.
- **Graphic record:** Used for recording vital signs of patient.
- **Fluid-balance record:** Used for recording intake output of the patient.
- **Medication administration form:** Medication, order, name, dose, frequency route and initials.
- **Skin assessment form:** Skin, wound/bedsore assessment.
- **Progress notes:** Toward achieving desired goals.

Nurses Responsibilities

- Keep the records safe.
- No sheet should be separated
- Not accessible to patients/relatives
- Strangers are not permitted to read records
- Records no hand over of documents to the legal advisors without written permission of the administration.
- Handed carefully, not destroyed.
- Identify with bio-date of the patients such as name, age, admission number, diagnosis, etc.
- Records should never be sent outside of the hospital without the written permission.

Precautions

- Kept carefully
- Protected against termites and insects
- Good filling system
- Easily available on time
- Kept at a definite place
- Confidential

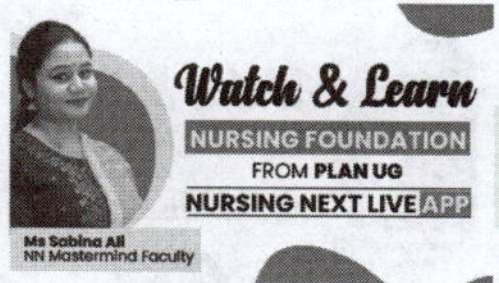

SHORT ANSWER QUESTIONS

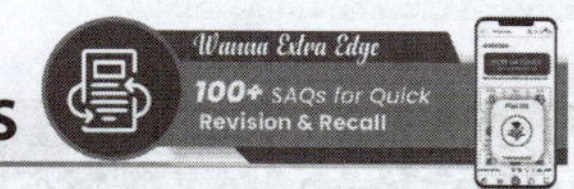

1. Enumerate purposes of documentation. (MGR, KUHS)

Answer

- Communication
- Diagnostic and therapeutic orders
- Care planning
- Quality review
- Health care analysis
- Education
- Legal documentation
- Reimbursement
- Research

2. Define records and reports. (KUHS, RUHS)

Answer

Records

Records are the memory of the internal and external transactions of an organization. Records contain a written evidence of the activities of an organization in the form of letters, circulars, reports, contracts, invoices, vouchers, minutes of meeting, books of account, etc. **—SL Geol, 2001**

Report

Report is a document containing information on organized in a narrative, graphic, or tabular form, prepared on ad hoc, periodic, recurring, regular, or as required basis. Reports may refer to specific periods, events, occurrences, or subjects and may be communicated or presented in oral or written form. Reports may refer to specific periods, events, occurrences, or subjects and may be communicated or presented in oral or written form. **—Basvanthappa bt. 2009**

3. Enumerate Characteristics of a good report. (DU)

Answer

- Accuracy
- Conciseness
- Thoroughness
- Up to date
- Organization
- Confidentiality
- Objectivity

4. Enumerate types of records. (DU, KUHS)

Answer

- **Medical record:**
  - Admission history
  - Medical history
  - Family record
  - Consents
- **Nursing record:**
  - Nursing assessment
  - Nursing care plan
  - Kardex
  - Flow sheets
  - Graphic record
  - Progress notes

5 Enumerate nurses record. (MGR)

Answer

- Admission nursing assessment
- Nursing care plans
- Kardex
- Flow sheets
- Graphic record
- Fluid-balance record
- Medication administration form
- Skin assessment form
- Progress notes

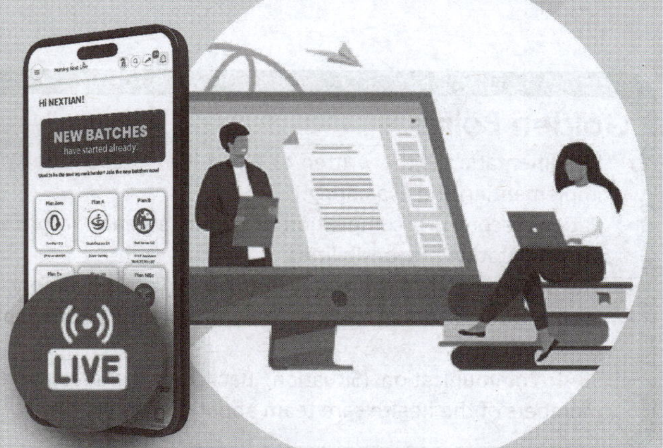

CONCEPTUAL REVISION

MULTIPLE CHOICE QUESTIONS

1. .... is a nursing action that produces a written account of pertinent patient data, nursing clinical decisions and interventions, and patient's responses in a health record.

a. Nursing Care Plan
b. Nursing Implementation
c. Documentation
d. Report

Ans. c. Documentation

2. Nursing documentation system needs to be flexible in all of the following; except:

a. Retrieve clinical data
b. Facilitate continuity of care
c. Track patient outcomes
d. Evaluating subordinates

Ans. d. Evaluating subordinates

3. All of the following are the purposes of medical record; except:

a. Interdisciplinary communication
b. Legal documentation
c. Reimbursement
d. Reducing hospital cost

Ans. d. Reducing hospital cost

4. All of the following are the mistakes in documentation that commonly result in malpractice; except:

a. Failing to record drug reactions
b. Failing to record nursing actions
c. Failing to document discontinued medications
d. Failing to record the observations

Ans. d. Failing to record the observations

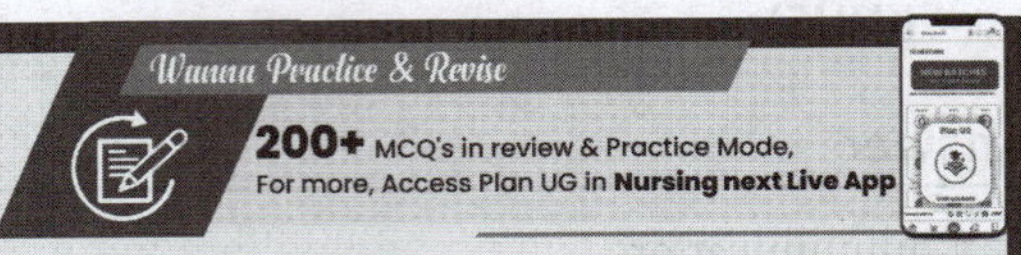

5. What does HIPAA stand for?

a. The Health Insurance Portability and Accountability Act
b. The Health Insurance Plan and Accessibility Act
c. Health Insurance Privacy and Accountability Act
d. Health Insurance Plan and Accountability Act

Ans. a. The Health Insurance Portability and Accountability Act

6. What does POMR stand for?

a. Problem oriented medical record
b. Progress oriented medical record
c. Problem oriented medical report
d. Progress objective medical record

Ans. a. Problem Oriented Medical Record

7. .... is a system of organizing documentation to place the primary focus on patient's individual problems.

a. Database
b. Problem list
c. Care plan
d. POMR

Ans. d. POMR

8. What does the acronym SOAP stand for?

a. Selected data, Objective data, Assessment, Plan
b. Subjective data, Objective data, Assessment, Plan
c. Subjective data, Objective data, Accountable, Plan
d. Subjective data, Objective data, Assessment, Problem

Ans. b. Subjective data, Objective data, Assessment, Plan

Golden Points

- Documentation is the written or typed legal record of all pertinent interactions with the patient: Assessing, diagnosing, planning, implementing and evaluating.
- Patient record is a compilation of patient's health information. Each health care institution has policies that specify the nurses' documentation responsibilities.
- The patient's record is the only permanent legal document.
- Health care personnel must not only maintain the confidentiality of the client's record but also meet legal standards in the process of recording.
- SBAR communication (Situation, Background, Assessment, Recommendation) is a framework of communication between the members of the health care team about client's condition.

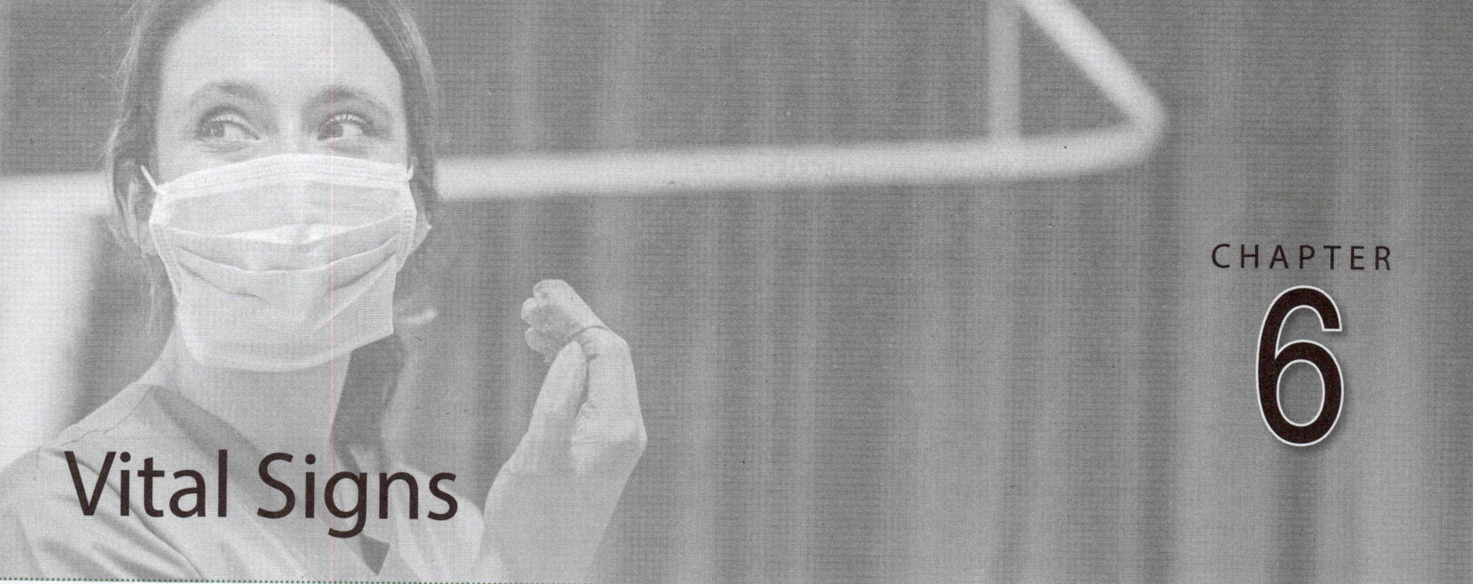

CONCEPTUAL THEORY

Terminology

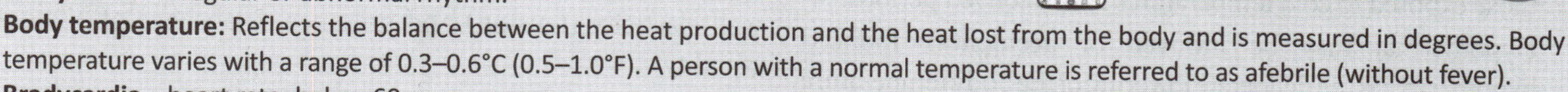

Arrhythmia—irregular or abnormal rhythm.
Body temperature: Reflects the balance between the heat production and the heat lost from the body and is measured in degrees. Body temperature varies with a range of 0.3–0.6°C (0.5–1.0°F). A person with a normal temperature is referred to as afebrile (without fever).
Bradycardia—heart rate, below 60.
Diastolic pressure: The diastolic pressure is the pressure when the ventricles are at rest.
Dyspnea: (difficult or labored breathing). So, effort required to breathe is referred to as labored breathing.
Eupnea: Breathing that is normal in rate and depth is called eupnea.
Hypothermia: It is defined as a core body temperature below the lower limit of normal.
Hypotension: A blood pressure that is below normal, i.e., 90/60 mm Hg is called hypotension.
Hypertension: A blood pressure that is persistently above normal is called hypertension. A systolic pressure above 140 mm Hg and a diastolic pressure above 90 mm Hg are regarded as being outside the normal range.
Induced hypothermia: It is the deliberate lowering of the body temperature whereas Accidental hypothermia can occur as a result of exposure to cold environment, immersion in cold water, lack of adequate clothing and absence of shelter of heat.
Korotkoff sounds: While measuring blood pressure, certain sounds may be heard that relate to the effect of the blood pressure cuff on the arterial wall. These sounds are called Korotkoff sounds.
Orthostatic hypotension: It is blood pressure that falls when the client sits or stands. It is usually due to peripheral vasodilatation, in which blood leaves the central body organs, especially the brain, and moves to the periphery causing the person to faint.
Pulse deficit: It is the difference between the apical and radial pulse rate.
Pulse rhythm: It is the pattern of the pulsations and the pauses between them. The pattern is normally regular. An irregular pattern of heart beats is called dysrhythmia.
Pulse pressure: The difference between the systolic pressure and diastolic pressure is called pulse pressure.
Pulse: The pulse is a wave of blood created by contraction of the left ventricle of the heart. Each time the heart contracts to force blood into the aorta, the arterial walls in the vascular system must expand to accept the increase in pressure. The pressure wave causing this expansion is called the pulse.
Pyrexia or fever: A body temperature above the usual range is called pyrexia or fever. A very high fever 41°C (105.8°F) is called hyperpyrexia. The client who has fever is referred to as febrile and one who does not have fever is called afebrile.
Respiration: It is the exchange of oxygen and carbon dioxide in the lungs and tissues and is initiated by the act of breathing. It is a combination of two processes: (1) External respiration and (2) Internal respiration.
Sphygmomanometer: Instrument with an occlusive cuff and the stethoscope is the most commonly used equipment for measuring blood pressure.
Systolic pressure: The systolic pressure is the pressure of the blood as a result of contraction of the ventricles.
Tachycardia—heart rate, above 100.
Wheezing—difficult breathing with high-pitched whistle sound during expiration.

VITAL SIGNS

- Recently, pain has been added as fifth vital sign. The vital signs are called so because they are important.
- Vital signs include **temperature, pulse, respiration and blood pressure.**
- Body temperature reflects the balance between the heat production and the heat lost from the body and is measured in *degrees*. The hypothalamus located between the cerebral hemispheres, acts as thermostat and controls body temperature.

- Body temperature varies with a range of 0.3–0.6°C (0.5–1.0°F). A person with a normal temperature is referred to as afebrile (without fever). There are two main alterations related to body temperature and these are pyrexia and hypothermia.
- A body temperature above the usual range is called *pyrexia* or fever. A very high fever 41°C (105.8°F) is called *hyperpyrexia*. The client who has fever is referred to as *febrile* and one who does not have fever is called *afebrile*.
- Hypothermia is defined as a core body temperature below the lower limit of normal.
- The thermal regulatory center in the hypothalamus is greatly impaired when the temperature of the body falls below 94°F (34.4°C). At this level, the activity of the cells is reduced, less heat is produced, and person may go into coma. Those at the risk of hypothermia include postoperative patients who are cooled during surgery, newborn infants whose skin is exposed to cool room temperatures, elderly or debilitated patients and those exposed to cold temperatures for prolonged periods.
- Hypothermia may be **induced** or **accidental**. Induced hypothermia is the deliberate lowering of the body temperature whereas **Accidental hypothermia** can occur as a result of exposure to cold environment, immersion in cold water, lack of adequate clothing and absence of shelter of heat.

COMMON SITES FOR ASSESSING BODY TEMPERATURE ORAL, RECTAL, AXILLARY AND TYMPANIC MEMBRANE

TABLE 6.1: Normal temperature for healthy adults at various sites

	Celsius	Fahrenheit
Oral temperature	37°C	98.6°F
Axillary temperature	36.5°C	97.7°F
Rectal temperature	37.5°C	99.5°F
Tympanic temperature	37.5°C	99.5°F
Forehead temperature	34.4°C	94.0°F

Clinical thermometer is used to measure body temperature. There are different types of thermometers available in the market such as **Glass Thermometer**, **Digital Thermometer**, **Tympanic Thermometers** and **Disposable Thermometers.**

- The pulse is a wave of blood created by contraction of the left ventricle of the heart. Each time the heart contracts to force blood into the aorta, the arterial walls in the vascular system must expand to accept the increase in pressure. The pressure wave causing this expansion is called the *pulse*. By counting each pulsation of the arterial wall, we can determine pulse rate.
- The pulse is regulated by the autonomic nervous system through the sinoatrial node (SA) (the pacemaker) of the heart. The pulse rate is expressed in beats per minute. It varies according to various factors such as Age, Gender, Exercise, Fever, Medication, Hypovolemia, Stress, Position change, Pathology, Pain, etc.

TABLE 6.2: Variation in pulse by age

Age	Pulse rate per minute
Newborn	120–160
1 year	110–120
5–8 years	95–100
Adult male	72–80
Adult female	76–80
Athletes	45–60

Common sites for measuring pulse are **Radial**, **Brachial**, **Temporal**, **Carotid**, **Apical**, **Femoral**, **Popliteal**, **Posterior Tibial**, **Dorsalis Pedis (Pedal)**. When assessing the pulse, the nurse collects the pulse rate, rhythm, volume, arterial wall elasticity (tension) and presence or absence of bilateral equality.

Pulse Rhythm is the pattern of the pulsations and the pauses between them. The pattern is normally regular. An irregular pattern of heart beats is called *dysrhythmia*

TABLE 6.3: Pulse rhythm

Regular rhythms

The pulse rhythms and the pauses occur similarly.

Description	Pattern
Normal	
Weak	
Bounding	

Dysrhythmias

The pulsations or lengths of pauses occur with no pattern or predictability.

Description	Pattern
Bisferiens	
Pulsus alternans	
Bigeminal	Premature contractions

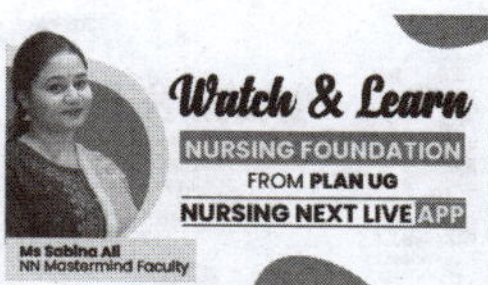

Pulse deficit is the difference in the apical and radial pulse rate.

Respiration is the exchange of oxygen and carbon dioxide in the lungs and tissues and is initiated by the act of breathing. It is a combination of two processes: (1) External respiration and (2) Internal respiration.

1. **External respiration:** It occurs in four ways:
   i. Ventilation, which is the mechanical movement of air in and out of the lungs.
   ii. Dispersion of air throughout the bronchial tree of the lungs.
   iii. Diffusion of oxygen and carbon dioxide molecules across the alveolar membrane.
   iv. Perfusion, the movement of blood through the lungs and tissues.
2. **Internal respiration:** It happens at the cellular level, oxygen is released from hemoglobin to the cell and the cell in turn releases carbon dioxide to the blood.

There are basically two types of breathing: (1) Costal (thoracic) breathing and (2) Diaphragmatic (abdominal) breathing.

- Respiratory centers in the medulla oblongata and the pons of the brain and chemoreceptors located centrally in the medulla and peripherally in the carotid and aortic bodies help in the control of respiration.
- Several factors influence respiratory rate. The ones that **increase** the respiratory rate include exercise, stress, increased environmental temperature and lowered oxygen concentration in increased altitudes. Factors that **decrease** the respiratory rate include decreased environmental temperature and certain medications, e.g., narcotics and increased intracranial pressure.
- Respiration is assessed every time, the full set of vital signs is assessed. The respiration should be counted for full minute. Breathing that is normal in rate and depth is called eupnea. Dyspnea (difficult or labored breathing). So, effort required to breathe is referred to as **labored breathing**.

TABLE 6.4: Pattern of respirations

	Description	Pattern	Associated features
Normal	12–20 breaths/min Regular		Normal pattern
Tachypnea	>24 breaths/min Shallow		Fever, anxiety, exercise, respiratory disorders
Bradypnea	<10 breaths/min Regular		Depression of the respiratory center by medications, brain damage
Hyperventilation	Increased rate and depth		Extreme exercise, fear, diabetic ketoacidosis (Kussmaul's respirations), overdose of aspirin
Hypoventilation	Decreased rate and depth; irregular		Overdose of narcotics or anesthetics
Cheyne-Stokes respiration	Alternating periods of deep, rapid breathing followed by period of apnea; regular		Drug overdose, heart failure, increased intracranial pressure, renal failure
Biot's respiration	Varying depth and rate of breathing followed by periods of apnea; irregular		Meningitis, severe brain damage

- Arterial blood pressure is a measure of the pressure exerted by the blood as it flows through the arteries.
- The **systolic pressure** is the pressure of the blood as a result of contraction of the ventricles. The **diastolic pressure** is the pressure when the ventricles are at rest.
- The difference between the systolic pressure and diastolic pressure is called *pulse pressure*. Blood pressure is measured in millimeters of mercury (mm Hg) and is recorded as a fraction of systolic pressure over the diastolic pressure. For a healthy adult, blood pressure is 120/80 mm Hg (pulse pressure of 40).

- A blood pressure that is persistently above normal is called *hypertension.* A systolic pressure above 140 mm Hg and a diastolic pressure above 90 mm Hg are regarded as being outside the normal range. A blood pressure that is below normal, i.e., 90/60 mm Hg is called *hypotension*.
- **Orthostatic hypotension** is blood pressure that falls when the client sits or stands. It is usually due to peripheral vasodilatation, in which blood leaves the central body organs, especially the brain, and moves to the periphery causing the person to faint.
- The sphygmomanometer with an occlusive cuff and the stethoscope is the most commonly used equipment for measuring blood pressure. Three types of manometers are generally used in clinical settings: (1) Mercury gauge sphygmomanometer, aneroid and digital.
- While measuring blood pressure, certain sounds may be heard that relate to the effect of the blood pressure cuff on the arterial wall. These sounds are called Korotkoff sounds.
- Doppler ultrasound stethoscopes (DUS) are also used to assess blood pressure. These are used when blood pressure sounds are difficult to hear, such as in infants, obese clients, and when clients are in shock. Systolic pressure may be the only blood pressure obtainable with this method.

CONCEPTUAL EXERCISES

LONG ANSWER QUESTIONS

1. Draw a nursing care plan of fever patient in medical ward. (RUHS)

Answer

Assessment	Nursing diagnosis	Expected outcome	Interventions	Evaluation
Subjective data: Patient says that he is having increased body temperature. **Objective data:** • Temperature-101°F. • Flushed skin • Skin warm to touch	**Hyperthermia** is related to infectious process as evidenced by increased body temperature above normal range (temperature of patient)	Patient maintains body temperature within normal range.	• Assess the general condition of patient. • Monitor vital signs of patient, especially temperature, as indicated. • Provide comfortable position to the patient. **Use of Nonpharmacological measures:** • Provide tepid sponging to the patient. • Encourage the patient for adequate fluid intake. • Encourage the use of a hypothermia blanket and wrap extremities with bath towels. • Maintain adequate bed rest to the patient. • Switch on the fan, open the windows of the room and maintain environmental temperature as tolerated by the patient. **Use of Pharmacological measures:** • Administer antipyretics such as paracetamol (IV/Oral) as prescribed by the physician. • Document the name, dose, route and frequency of the drug on drug chart. • Monitor and record the vital signs of the patient after medication administration.	After the interventions, patient was able to demonstrate body temperature within normal range as evidenced by the axillary temperature of 36.8°F

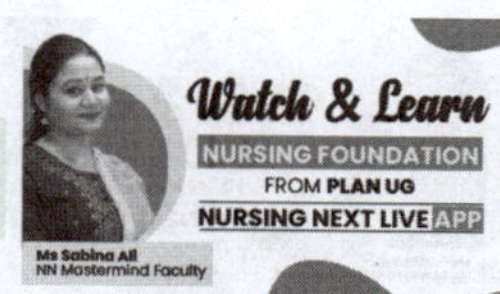

2. Mr X is admitted to medical ward with high fever and cough since three days. Answer the following heading: (DU)

a. **Sites and techniques of taking temperature**
b. **Factors affecting respiration**
c. **Guidelines for taking vital signs.**

Answer

Sites and Techniques of Taking Temperature

Common sites for assessing body temperature are:

- **Oral:**
  - Most accessible and convenient method.
  - Temperature should not be taken when client has had hot or cold fluid and even smoked. In these cases, nurses should wait for at least 20 minutes before taking temperature.
  - This site is not recommended in younger children as they may bite the thermometer.
  - Normal oral temperature is 37°C or 98.6°F.
- **Rectal:**
  - It is most reliable and accurate method of measuring body temperature.
  - It is contraindicated for patients who is diagnosed with myocardial infarction because it can stimulate vagus nerve which later on can cause life-threatening dysrhythmias.
  - It is also contraindicated in patients with diarrhea, having rectal surgeries, hemorrhoids, abnormal coagulating factors.
  - Normal rectal temperature is 37.5° or 99.5°F.
- **Axillary:**
  - It is safe method.
  - It is noninvasive in nature.
  - Most preferable site in children for measuring body temperature because it is accessible.
  - Normal axillary temperature is 36.5°C or 97.7°F.
- **Tympanic membrane:**
  - It is commonly used for estimating core body temperature.
  - Normal tympanic temperature is 37.5°C or 99.5°F.
- **Temporal artery:**
  - Temperature is measured on forehead.
  - Temperature is measured by using temporal artery thermometer.
  - It is safe.
  - It is noninvasive.
  - It is very quick method also.
  - Most useful in infants and children.
  - Equipment is expensive.
  - Normal temporal temperature is 34.4°C or 94.0°F.

Techniques of taking temperature:

Clinical thermometer is used to measure body temperature. There are different types of thermometers also.

- **Glass thermometer:**
  - It has a bulb containing mercury and a stem in which mercury rises. Stem also contains the scale for measuring temperature.
  - This scale can be calibrated in either in Celsius or Fahrenheit.
- **Digital thermometer:**
  - It is portable and battery-operated electronic thermometer.
  - It measures body temperature in seconds to 1 minute.
  - Temperature is displayed on a small screen on hand-held unit.
  - Reading is in tenth of a degree.
- **Tympanic thermometer:**
  - It is portable and battery-operated thermometer used in auditory canal.
  - It can measure temperature in 1–2 seconds.
  - It produces the reading of core temperature.
- **Disposable thermometer:**
  - This thermometer is temperature-sensitive tape.
  - It is paced on forehead or on abdomen.

b. **Factors affecting respiration**

Answer

The factors which can increase the respiration rate are:

- Exercise
- Stress
- Increased environmental temperature in response to metabolic alkalosis
- Lowered oxygen concentration in increased altitudes

The factors which can decrease the respiration rate are:

- Decreased environmental temperature
- Certain medications such as narcotics in response to metabolic acidosis
- Increased intracranial pressure

c. **Guidelines for taking vital signs**

Answer

Vital signs are the indicators for physiological functioning which help in reflection of health status of the individuals. It includes temperature, pulse, respiration and blood pressure. Pain is the fifth vital sign.

- Normal temperature is 98.6°F or 37°C

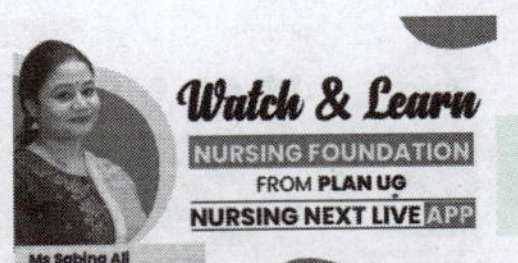

- Normal pulse is 72/min.
- Normal respiration is 12–20 breaths per minute
- Normal BP is 120/80 mm Hg.

Preparation and Environment

- Ensure a quiet and comfortable environment for the patient.
- Make sure the room is at a comfortable temperature.
- Wash your hands before approaching the patient to prevent cross-contamination.

Introduction and Communication

- Introduce yourself to the patient and explain what you'll be doing.
- Obtain informed consent before proceeding.
- Communicate clearly and reassure the patient to reduce anxiety.

Frequency

- Vital signs should be taken at appropriate intervals, depending on the patient's condition, the healthcare setting, and the physician's orders.
- It is commonly done on admission, at regular intervals (e.g., every 4 to 8 hours), and as needed based on the patient's condition.

Temperature (T)

- Use a clinically available appropriate thermometer for accurate temperature measurement.
- Oral, axillary, or tympanic routes are common. For some patients, other methods like rectal or temporal artery may be used.
- Avoid taking an oral temperature if the patient has recently consumed hot or cold fluids, as it may affect the accuracy.

Pulse (P)

- Assess the pulse rate (heart rate) by palpating the radial artery (wrist) or other appropriate sites (e.g., carotid or brachial).
- Count the number of pulse for one full minute, except emergency situations.

Respirations (R)

- Observe the patient's chest or abdomen rise and fall to count the respiratory rate.
- Count the number of breaths for 60 seconds. Especially in pediatric population respiration need to be counted for one full minute as they have irregular respiration.

Blood Pressure (BP)

- Use an appropriate-sized blood pressure cuff for accurate readings.
- Position the patient's arm at heart level.
- Inflate the cuff to about 30 mm Hg above the point where the pulse disappears (systolic) and deflate slowly while listening for the pulse to reappear (diastolic).
- Note the systolic and diastolic pressures in millimeters of mercury (mm Hg).

Pain Assessment

- Always assess the patient's pain level, using a pain scale that the patient can understand.
- Pain is considered the "fifth vital sign," and addressing pain management is an essential part of nursing care.

Recording and Documentation

- Record all vital signs accurately and promptly in the patient's medical chart.
- Include the date, time, and your name or initials with each measurement.
- Report any significant changes in vital signs to the appropriate healthcare team members.

Special Considerations

- Certain patient populations, such as infants, elderly, or critically ill patients, may require specific approaches or modifications in vital signs assessment.
- Always adhere to institutional policies and guidelines while performing any procedures and seek guidance from experienced nurses or healthcare providers when needed.

The various nursing responsibilities are discussed here:

- Monitor and document vital signs correctly. Nurse must be able to evaluate and interpret the values.
- Monitor and record vital signs during patient's admission process in any health care facility.
- Monitor vital signs in a hospital on a routine schedule as per physician's order and according to hospital policy also.
- Document the vitals monitoring chart effectively.
- Take vital signs before and after any invasive or noninvasive diagnostic procedures.
- Take vital signs before and after the administration of medications that affect the cardiovascular, respiratory and temperature control functions directly or indirectly.
- Record these signs when the patient's general condition changes. Also, always monitor all the vital signs in any emergency situation.

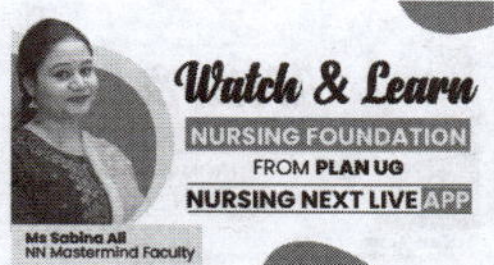

- Take vital signs when the patient reports physical distress, this time vital signs should be taken more frequently.
- Communicate all the abnormal findings related to vital signs to the concerned doctor in health care facilities.
- Nurses are also responsible in communicating the readings of vital signs in graphic flowsheet.
- Nurses should be competent enough to start the intervention, as indicated.

3. a. Describe the procedure step by step of taking blood pressure.
b. Write down the importance of vital signs. (RUHS)

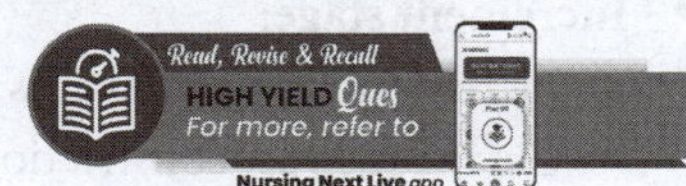

Answer

Step by Step Procedure of Taking Blood Pressure

Step by step procedure of measuring blood pressure:

- Stethoscope and sphygmomanometer, both are the equipment used for assessing the blood pressure.
- **Devices:** Aneroid, Mercury and Electronic devices.
- **Time of measurement:**
  - During the waking hours of the patient.
  - For those patient who are on antihypertensive medications, the blood pressure should be measured before administration of medications.
- Club together
- **Selecting the most accurate blood pressure cuff.**
- The length of the bladder—at least 80% of the circumference of the upper arm.
- The width of the bladder—approximately 40% of the circumference of the upper arm.

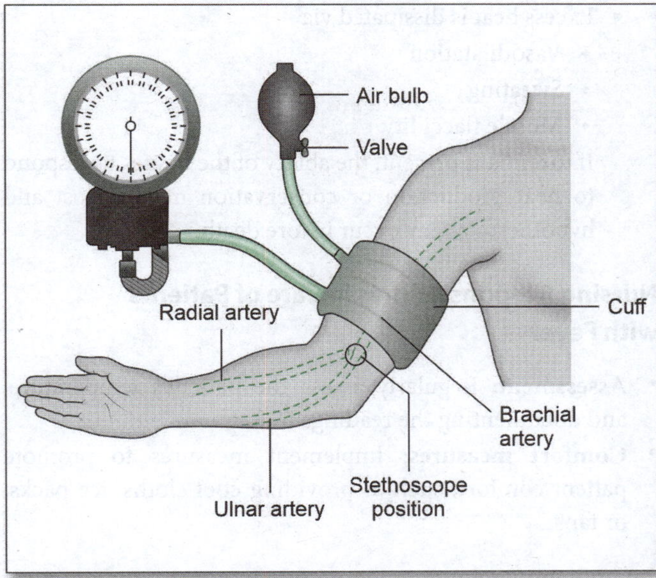

Materials Required

A tray containing:

- Stethoscope
- Sphygmomanometer
- Alcohol swabs
- Paper bag
- Vitals monitoring chart
- Pen

Procedure

- **Preparation:** Ensure the patient is in a relaxed and comfortable position, with their arm exposed and supported at heart level.
- **Position the cuff:** Wrap the cuff around the upper arm, approximately 2.5 cm (1 inch) above the antecubital fossa (the crease of the elbow). The cuff should be snug but not too tight.
- **Locate the brachial artery:** Palpate the brachial artery on the inside of the arm, just below the cuff's lower edge.
- **Position the stethoscope:** Place the earpieces of the stethoscope in your ears. Position the stethoscope's chest piece over the brachial artery, ensuring a good seal and contact with the skin.
- **Inflate the cuff:** Inflate the cuff rapidly by squeezing the bulb or activating the automated device. Inflate until the pressure is 30 mm Hg above the estimated systolic pressure.
- **Deflate the cuff:** Gradually release the pressure by opening the valve or releasing the button. The deflation should be done at a rate of 2–3 mm Hg per second.
- **Listen for Korotkoff sounds:** As the cuff pressure drops, listen through the stethoscope for the sounds of Korotkoff. The first sound indicates systolic pressure, and the point at which the sound disappears indicates diastolic pressure.
- **Record the blood pressure:** Note the systolic and diastolic pressure readings. It is important to record the arm used, cuff size, and patient's position during the measurement.
- **Repeat if necessary:** If the first measurement seems unusual or inconsistent, repeat the measurement after a brief rest period.

b. Write down the importance of vital signs.

Answer

- Vital signs are governed by vital organs.
- Vital signs are measures of physiological status and also help in assessing the most basic body functions.
- The values of vital signs can never be zero.
- Vital signs indicate that the individual is alive.
- All vital signs such as temperature, pulse, respiration and BP can be monitored, observed and documented.

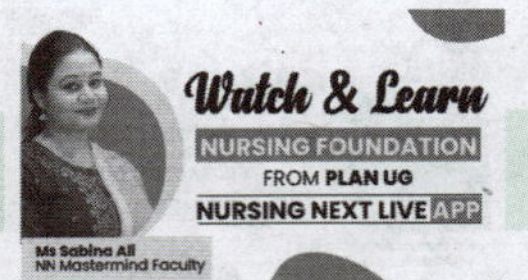

- Vital signs enable the assessment at which an individual is functioning.
- The normal ranges of vital signs can vary with age and medical condition also.
- Vital signs are useful in diagnosing and evaluating the medical problems.
- Vital signs can be measured in health care settings, at home, at the site of emergency, or elsewhere.

4. Explain the causes of fever and stages of pyrexia. (MGR)

Answer

Fever is defined as the increased body temperature above the normal range (37°C or 98.6°F). A person with fever is known as febrile.

Causes of Fever

- **Infection:** Fever occurs in response to cytokines produced by pathogens.
- It can also be caused by tissue injury-such as myocardial infarction, pulmonary emboli, cancer, trauma and any surgery.
- Its cause can be bacterial and viral also.

Etiology

- Infections most common
  - Sepsis
  - Enteric fevers
  - Tuberculosis
  - Infective endocarditis
  - Malaria
  - Fungal infections
  - Viral EBV, CMV, HIV
- Malignancy—20%
  - Leukemia
  - Lymphoma
  - Myeloma
  - Solid tumors
    - Renal
    - Liver
    - Stomach
    - Pancreas
- Tissue disorders—10%
  - Rheumatoid Arthritis
  - Temporal arteritis
  - PAN, SLE
  - Rheumatic fever
  - Still's disease
  - Polymyositis
- Miscellaneous 10%
  - Inflammatory bowel disease
  - Liver diseases
  - Sarcoidosis
  - Drug fever
  - Thyrotoxicosis
  - Hypothalamic lesions

Stages of Fever

- **Increment stage:**

  Increment stage of fever is characterized by
  - Cutaneous vasoconstriction
  - Absence of sweating
  - Cold skin and extremities
  - Reduced respiration
  - Muscle shivering
  - Reduced respiration
  - Oliguria
  - Rectal temperature is elevated.
- **Fastigium stage:**
  - It is the state of constant temperature.
  - The period of heat increment raises temperature to the new thermostatic level.
  - Cutaneous vasodilation to dissipate heat
  - Severe sweating
  - Diuresis (increased urine production)
  - Decreased ruminal motility
  - Increased metabolism and tissue wasting
- **Decrement stage:**
  - Excess heat is dissipated via
    - Vasodilatation
    - Sweating
    - Muscle flaccidity

  If toxemia is present, the ability of the tissues to respond to heat production or conservation may be lost and hypothermia may occur before death.

Nursing Responsibilities in Care of Patients with Fever

- **Assessment:** Regularly assess the patient's temperature, and documenting the readings
- **Comfort measures:** Implement measures to promote patient comfort, such as providing cool cloths, ice packs, or fans

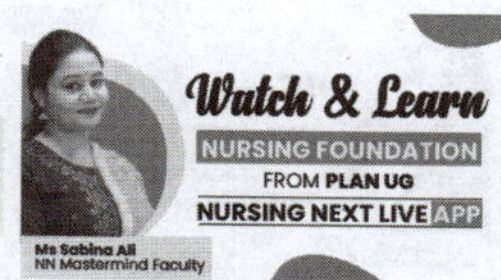

- **Fluid management:** Encourage the patient to increase fluid intake to prevent dehydration
- **Medication administration:** Administer antipyretic medications as ordered
- **Infection control:** Implement appropriate infection control measures to prevent the spread of infection.
- **Patient education:** Provide education to the patient and their family regarding fever management collaboration with the healthcare team.

5. Nitin was admitted in surgical ward with head injury after he met with a road traffic accident. Answer the following: (DU)

a. Explain the alterations in respiration.

b. Discuss the nursing responsibilities while taking vital signs of Nitin.

Answer

Alterations in Respiration

- **Eupnea:** Normal, unlabored breathing with a normal respiratory rate (12–20/min).
- **Tachypnea:** Increased respiratory rate (>20 breaths/min)
- **Bradypnea:** Decreased respiratory rate (<12 breaths/min)
- **Respiratory depth and rhythm:** The depth of respiration normally varies from shallow to deep.
- **Apnea:** No breathing, if apnea lasts longer than 4–6 minutes. It may lead to Brain damage and death.
- **Dyspnea:** Difficult or labored breathing. Dyspnea also reflects rapid and shallow respirations.
- **Orthopnea:** Ability to breathe only in upright position.
- **Stertorous:** Labored and snoring type of respiration due to obstruction of the airway.
- **Wheezing:** Noisy breathing accompanied by a whistle sound.
- **Stridor:** Shrill harsh sound due to laryngeal spasm.
- **Kussmaul's respiration:** Increase in rate and depth of the breathing pattern and is usually associated with diabetic ketoacidosis.

Refer to Table 6.4 explaining alterations in respiration pg. 597.

b. Nursing responsibilities while taking vital signs of Nitin

Answer

Vital signs are the indicators for physiological functioning which help in reflection of health status of the individuals. These are the basic components essential for assessment of physiological and psychological health. It includes temperature, pulse, respiration and blood pressure. Pain is the fifth vital sign.

Normal range of vitals signs are as follow:

- Normal temperature is 98.6°F or 37°C
- Normal pulse is 72/min.
- Normal respiration is 12–20 breaths/min
- Normal BP is 120/80 mm Hg.

The various nursing responsibilities are discussed here:

- **Prepare the environment:** Ensure the room is quiet, comfortable, and free from distractions.
- **Arrange necessary article at bedside:** Gather the necessary equipment, such as a thermometer, blood pressure cuff, and stethoscope.
- **Verify patient identification:** Confirm the patient's identity using two unique identifiers, such as their name and date of birth, to ensure accurate documentation.
- **Explain the procedure:** Communicate with the patient, explaining the purpose of taking vital signs and the process involved.
- **Assess baseline data:** Review the patient's medical history, current condition, and any relevant information that may impact the interpretation of vital signs. For eg, ask if patient had any hot drinks in the last 30 minutes before taking temperature.
- **Obtain temperature:** Use an appropriate thermometer to measure the patient's temperature orally, tympanically, or via other approved routes. Ensure proper technique and follow infection control protocols.
- **Measure pulse:** Assess the patient's pulse rate by palpating their radial, brachial, or carotid pulse. Note the rate, rhythm, and strength of the pulse.
- **Measure blood pressure:** Use a blood pressure cuff and sphygmomanometer or an automated blood pressure monitor to measure the patient's blood pressure. Apply the cuff correctly, follow proper technique, and record both systolic and diastolic pressures.
- **Assess respiratory rate:** Observe the patient's respirations, noting the rate, depth, and regularity. Count the number of breaths per minute.
- **Assess pain level:** Evaluate the patient's pain level using appropriate pain assessment tools, such as a numeric or visual analog scale.
- **Document and report findings:** Accurately record the patient's vital signs in their medical record, including the date, time, and any relevant observations. Report any significant changes or abnormal findings to the healthcare provider.
- **Provide comfort and support:** Ensure the patient's comfort and privacy during the vital sign assessment.

Offer reassurance, address any discomfort, and provide emotional support as needed.
- **Monitor trends and patterns:** Continually monitor and track the patient's vital signs over time to identify trends or changes that may indicate improvements or deterioration in their condition.

SHORT NOTES

1. Write short note on vital signs. (DU)

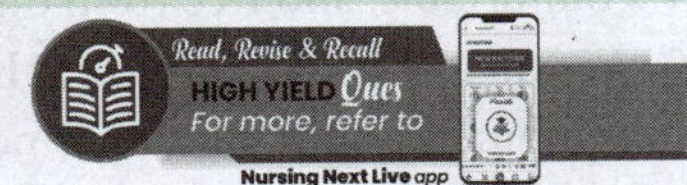

Answer

Vital signs are the indicators for physiological functioning which help in reflection of health status of the individuals. These are the basic components essential for assessment of physiological and psychological health. It includes temperature, pulse, respiration and blood pressure. Pain is the fifth vital sign.

Vital signs are also known as cardinal signs. They are called vital signs because:
- Governed by vital organs
- Changes in condition detected by vital signs
- Significant variations may indicate health-related problems.
- Specific information can be obtained for formulation of diagnosis.
- Normal temperature is 98.6°F or 37°C
- Normal pulse is 72/min.
- Normal respiration is 12–20 breaths/min
- Normal BP is 120/80 mm Hg.

Nursing responsibilities while taking vital signs:
- Prepare the environment
- Arrange necessary article at bedside
- Verify patient identification
- Explain the procedure
- Assess baseline data for any contraindications
- Obtain temperature
- Measure pulse.
- Measure blood pressure
- Assess respiratory rate
- Assess pain level
- Document and report findings
- Provide comfort and support
- Monitor trends and patterns.

2. Write the differences between hypothermia and hyperthermia. (MGR)

Answer

Body temperature—the balance between heat produced and heat lost by the body.
- Heat production is known as **thermogenesis** whereas Heat loss is **thermolysis.**

Characteristics	Hypothermia	Hyperthermia
Definition	It is defined as a core body temperature **below** the normal limit.	It is the body temperature above the normal range.
Temperature	Below 95°F or 35°C	More than 37°C or 98.6°F
Types	**Induced**—process of reducing the body temperature deliberately in order to reduce the need of oxygen by the tissues. **Accidental**—due to cold environment, lack of clothing etc.	**Intermittent**—temperature alternates at regular interval, e.g., malaria **Remittent**—wide range of fluctuations in terms of temperature (>2°C over 24 hours) **Relapsing**—short febrile phase, normal temperature of 2 days. **Constant-** always remains above normal, e.g., typhoid fever.
Management	• Warm environment • Adequate clothing such as cap or scarf • Use of warm blankets • Provide warm liquids (oral/IV)	• Adequate bed rest • Antipyretics • Provide cold liquids • Adequate hydration

3. Write short note on physiology and regulation of body temperature. (MGR)

Read, Revise & Recall
HIGH YIELD Ques
For more, refer to
Nursing Next Live app

Answer

Body temperature reflects the balance between the thermogenesis and thermolysis. It is measured in degrees. Body temperature has two kinds of temperature namely the core temperature and the surface temperature.

1. **Core temperature**—temperature of the deep tissues such as abdominal cavity and pelvic cavity.
2. **Surface temperature**—temperature of the skin, subcutaneous tissue and the fat.

As the by-product of metabolism, body continually produces heat. When the heat production is equal to the heat lost, that time the person is in heat balance.

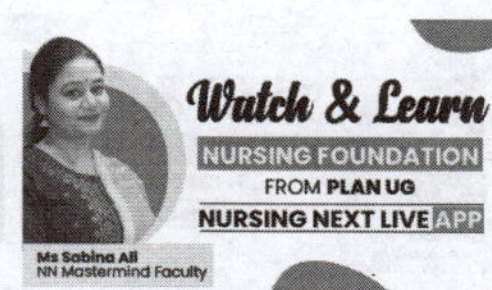

Physiology and Regulation of Body Temperature

- The hypothalamus located in the brain acts as thermostat which controls the body temperature through feedback mechanism.
- When the body heat rises, the hypothalamus sends out a signal through the nervous systems. It leads to vasodilatation, sweating, and inhibition of heat production.
- If the body temperature drops below the normal value, hypothalamus sends message for vasoconstriction of the blood vessels. It conserves heat and also helps in the induction of shivering which increases heat production.
- Heat loss occurs through radiation, conduction, convection and evaporation processes.
- Blood from the internal organs carries heat to the skin. Later on heat radiates to cooler objects in the vicinity of the person.
- When objects in the surroundings of the person are warmer, the heat from the object radiates to the body and gets absorbed.
- Similarly, when the warm skin touches a cool object, heat is lost to that object by the process of conduction.
- Air movement causes transfer of heat from the skin to the air molecules by convection.
- When the body temperature is high, sweat glands help in the loss of heat through the process of evaporation by secreting sweat in response to a message from the hypothalamus part of the brain.

4. Write about the heat production and heat losing mechanism in our body. (MGR)

Answer

Heat Production and Heat Losing Mechanism in Our Body

Body temperature—the balance between heat produced and heat lost by the body.

- **Heat production**
  - Heat production is known as thermogenesis whereas Heat loss is thermolysis.
  - The hypothalamus located in the brain acts as thermostat which controls the body temperature through feedback mechanism.
  - When the body heat rises, the hypothalamus sends out a signal through the nervous systems. It leads to vasodilatation, sweating, and inhibition of heat production.
  - If the body temperature drops below the normal value, hypothalamus sends message for vasoconstriction of the blood vessels. It conserves heat and also helps in the induction of shivering which increases heat production.
- **Heat production occurs through**
  - **Metabolism:** The primary source of heat production in the body is through metabolic processes.
  - **Muscular activity:** During exercise or movement, the increased metabolic activity of muscles produces heat.
  - **Hormonal activity:** Certain hormones, such as thyroxine, adrenaline, and noradrenaline, can increase metabolic rate and heat production in the body.
- **Heat loss**

  Heat loss occurs through following mechanisms:
  - **Radiation:** The transfer of heat through radiation occurs when the body radiates heat to its surroundings.
  - **Conduction:** Heat is transferred from the body to objects in direct contact with it. For example, when a person touches a cooler surface, heat is transferred from the body to that surface.
  - **Convection:** Convection involves the transfer of heat through the movement of air or fluid. When air or fluid passes over the body, it absorbs heat and carries it away, promoting cooling.
  - **Evaporation:** Sweat production and subsequent evaporation from the skin's surface provide a significant cooling effect. As sweat evaporates, it absorbs heat from the body, resulting in a cooling sensation
  - Blood from the internal organs carries heat to the skin. Later on heat radiates to cooler objects in the vicinity of the person.

5. Write the nursing responsibilities of patient with hyperthermia. (DU)

Answer

Assessment

- Monitor vital signs including temperature, pulse, respiration and BP.
- Assess hydration status and environment also (room is too cold or too hot).
- Monitor white blood cell count, hematocrit value.

Nursing Interventions

- Promote bed rest.
- Provide adequate nutrition to the patient. Consult dietitian, if necessary. Provide priority to the preferences/choices of the patient.
- Provide adequate fluids to the patient via either enteral or parenteral route.

- Prevent dehydration.
- Inspect the mouth of the patient for dry mouth. Provide oral hygiene to keep the mucous membranes moist.
- Reduce physical activity and encourage bed rest.
- Provide a tepid sponge bath to the patient.
- Provide dry and clean clothes and bed linens.
- Remove excess blankets when the client feels warm.
- Provide extra warmth or blankets when the client feels chilled.
- Monitor intake and output adequately for the patient.
- Use of pharmacological measures—administer antipyretics/ antibiotics to the patient, if indicated.

6. Write the nursing management of patient with hypothermia. (DU)

Answer

Assessment

- Monitor vital signs including temperature, pulse, respiration and BP.
- Assess hydration status and environment also (room is too cold or too hot).

Nursing Interventions

- Provide extra covering/layers of clothes and blankets.
- Regularly monitor the temperature of the patient.
- Cover the head, ears properly.
- Provide full sleeved clothes to the patient.
- Use of socks and cover the both extremities properly.
- Use heat retaining blankets.
- Keep patient's linen warm and dry.
- Control environmental temperature such as temperature of the room.
- Provide extra heat source such as heat lamp, radiant warmer, pads, etc.
- Carefully assess for hyperthermia or burn to prevent complications.
- Regulate heat source according to physical response of the patient.
- Provide warm fluids/liquids such as hot tea or coffee.
- Take measures to prevent all types of heat loss.
- Make sure that patient and environment is not wet to prevent evaporative heat loss.
- Close the doors and windows, switch off fan and AC to prevent convectional heat loss.
- Make sure that articles or object which are in close contact with the patient are warm to prevent conduction heat loss.
- Make sure that patient bed is away from wall and other cold object in the room to prevent radiation heat loss.

Management

- Continuous monitoring
- Rewarming
- Supportive care.

Rewarming

- **Passive:** Use of blankets.
- **Active:** The application of heat from outside.
  - **External:** Heat blanket/hot air system.
  - **Internal:** Introduction of warm fluids.

7. Write short note on remittent fever and intermittent fever. (KUHS)

Answer

- Fever or Hyperthermia is the body temperature above than normal.
- The person having fever is febrile.
- It is an elevation of body temperature.

Intermittent Fever

- Temperature returns to acceptable value at least once in 24 hours.
- The temperature curve returns to normal during the day and reaches its peak in the evening.
- E.g.: in septicemia.

Remittent Fever

- Fever spikes and falls without a return to the normal temperature levels.
- The temperature fluctuates but does not return to normal.
- E.g.: TB, viral diseases, bacterial infections.

8. What is temperature? Write about the types of temperature?

Answer

Temperature

- Body temperature is the degree of hotness or coldness of a body or environment.
- It is the somatic sensation of heat or cold. It is the degree of or intensity of heat of a body in relation to external environment.

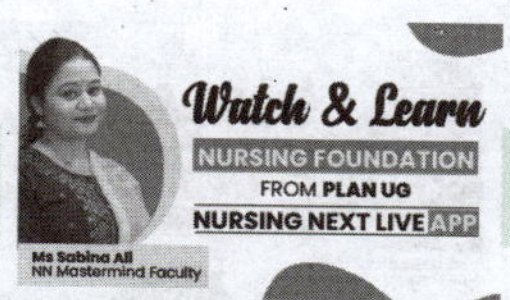

- The body temperature is the difference between the amount of heat produced by body processes and the amount of heat lost to the external environment.

Types of Temperature

Body temperature reflects the balance between the thermogenesis and thermolysis. It is measured in degrees. Body temperature has two kinds of temperature namely the core temperature and the surface temperature.

1. **Core temperature**—temperature of the deep tissues such as abdominal cavity and pelvic cavity.
2. **Surface temperature**—temperature of the skin, subcutaneous tissue and the fat.

As the by-product of metabolism, body continually produces heat. When the heat production is equal to the heat lost, that time the person is in heat balance.

Abnormality of Body Temperature

1. Hypothermia
2. Hyperthermia

Hypothermia

- It is defined as a core body temperature **below** the normal limit.
- Temperature range- below 94°F or 34.4°C.
- **Types:**
  - **Induced**—process of reducing the body temperature deliberately in order to reduce the need of oxygen by the tissues.
  - **Accidental**—due to cold environment, lack of clothing, etc.

Hyperthermia

- Body temperature above the normal range.
- Temperature range- more than 37°C or 98.6°F.
- **Types:**
  - **Intermittent:** Temperature alternates at regular interval, e.g., malaria
  - **Remittent:** Wide range of fluctuations in terms of temperature (more than 2 degrees Celsius over 24 hours).
  - **Relapsing:** Short febrile phase, normal temperature of 2 days.
  - **Constant:** Always remains above normal, e.g., typhoid fever.

9. Write short note on care of patient who is having rigor.

Read, Revise & Recall
HIGH YIELD Ques
For more, refer to
Nursing Next Live app

Answer

Rigor is defined as a sudden paroxysmal shaking chill occurring during a febrile illness.

Assessment

- Monitor vital signs including temperature, pulse, respiration and BP.
- Assess hydration status and environment also (room is too cold or too hot).

Nursing Interventions

- Provide extra covering/layers of clothes and blankets.
- Regularly monitor the temperature of the patient.
- Cover the head, ears properly.
- Provide full sleeved clothes to the patient.
- Use of socks and cover the both extremities properly.
- Use heat retaining blankets.
- Keep patient's linen warm and dry.
- Control environmental temperature such as temperature of the room.
- Provide extra heat source such as heat lamp, radiant warmer, pads, etc.
- Carefully assess for hyperthermia or burn to prevent complications.
- Regulate heat source according to physical response of the patient.
- Provide warm fluids/liquids such as hot tea or coffee.

Management

- Continuous monitoring
- Rewarming
- Supportive care.

Rewarming

- **Passive:** Use of blankets.
- **Active:** The application of heat from outside.
  - **External:** Heat blanket/hot air system.
  - **Internal:** Introduction of warm fluids.

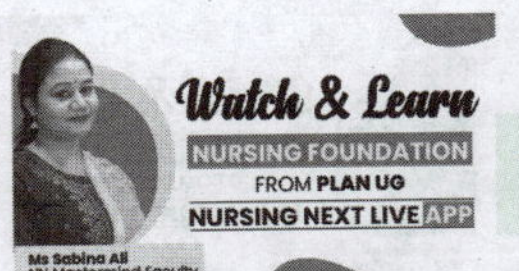

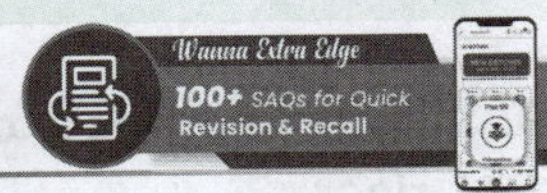

SHORT ANSWER QUESTIONS

1. Write the factors affecting respiration.

Answer

The factors which can increase the respiration rate are:

- Exercise
- Stress
- Metabolic acidosis
- Increased environmental temperature
- Lowered oxygen concentration in increased altitudes

The factors which can decrease the respiration rate are:

- Decreased environmental temperature
- Certain medications such as narcotics
- Metabolic alkalosis
- Increased intracranial pressure

2. Define fever and enumerate stages of pyrexia.

Answer

Fever

Fever is defined as the increased body temperature above the normal range (37°C or 98.6°F). A person with fever is known as febrile.

Stages of Pyrexia

- **Stage 1:** Increment stage
- **Stage 2:** Fastigium stage
- **Stage 3:** Decrement stage

3. Define pulse deficit and normal range of pulse rate. (MGR)

Answer

Pulse deficit: It is the difference between the apical and radial pulse rate. Pulse can be assessed by rate, rhythm, volume and elasticity of arterial wall through palpation and auscultation. The pulse deficit is usually zero.

Normal range of Pulse is **60–100** beats/min.

4. Write two differentiating features of dicrotic pulse and bigeminal pulse. (KUHS)

Answer

Dicrotic pulse	Bigeminal pulse
• It is defined as one peak during systole and another at the beginning of diastole. • It may be found in cardiac tamponade, severe heart failure, hypovolemic shock • Rarely presents in healthy individuals.	• It is known as a ventricular premature beat occurs after each normal systole. • It may be found in Ventricular premature beats in a patient with sinus rhythm, Mobitz type I (Wenckebach) second-degree atrioventricular block.

5. List four factors affecting blood pressure. (MGR, DU KUHS)

Answer

- **Circadian rhythms:** Predictable changes can be found in body temperature in the repeated cycle of time.
- **Age:** Infants are greatly influenced by the temperature of the environment and must be protected from extreme changes. Older people are at risk of hypothermia.
- **Biological sex:** Women usually experience more hormone fluctuations than men. Progesterone secretion at the time of ovulation raises body temperature by about 0.3°C to 0.6°C above basal temperature.
- **Physical activity/exercise:** Hard work or exercise can increase body temperature.

6. Mention the four characteristics of respiration. (MGR)

Answer

Respiration refers to the process of bringing oxygen to body tissues and removing carbon dioxide from it.

Characteristics of respiration are discussed here:

- **Respiration rate:** Number of times the person breathes in and out in 1 minute.
- **Depth:** It is observing the movement of chest during inspiration. It can be deep or shallow.
- **Rhythm:** The equal interval between two respirations.
- **Effort:** Effort by respiratory muscles.

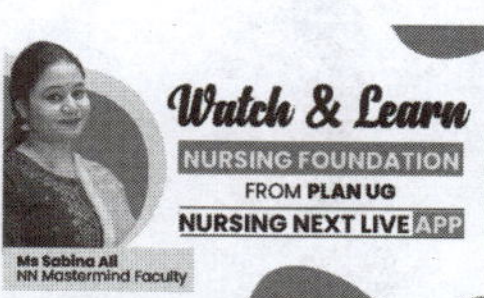

CONCEPTUAL REVISION

MULTIPLE CHOICE QUESTIONS

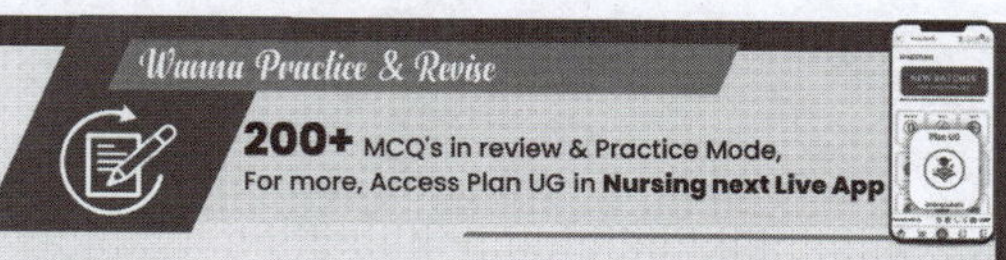

1. A patient presents in the clinic with dizziness and fatigue. The nursing assistant reports a slow but regular radial pulse of 44. What is your priority intervention?

a. Request that the nursing assistant repeat the pulse check
b. Call for a stat ECG
c. Assess the patient's apical pulse and evidence of a pulse deficit
d. Prepare to administer cardiac-stimulating medications

Ans. c. Assess the patient's apical pulse and evidence of a pulse deficit

2. A nurse assesses an oral temperature for an adult patient and records that the patient is "afebrile". What would be the nurse's best response to this finding?

a. Check the patient record for prescribed antipyretic medication
b. Report the finding to the primary care provider
c. Take the patient temperature using a different method
d. No action is necessary, this is a normal reading

Ans. d. No action is necessary, this is a normal reading

3. Upon assessment of a patient, the nurse determines that a patient is at risk of losing body heat through the process of convection. What would be the nurse's best response?

a. Turn off the overhead fan in the patient's room
b. Remove the patient's ice pack
c. Reduce the temperature in the room
d. Increase the temperature

Ans. a. Turn off the overhead fan in the patient's room

4. Pulse is a rhythmic beating in the body that signifies regular, recurrent expansion and contraction of an artery produced by the waves of pressure that are caused by the ejection of blood from which part of the part as it contracts?

a. Right ventricle
b. Right auricle
c. Left ventricle
d. Left auricle

Ans. c. Left ventricle

5. Which of the following statements about fever is not true?

a. Fever is a sign of illness.
b. It is the same as pyrexia or hyperthermia.
c. It is reflected through an increase of body temperature.
d. It does not do anything to defend the body.

Ans. d. It does not do anything to defend the body.

6. Acute pain and anxiety increase pulse rates because of what reason?

a. Sympathetic nerves are suppressed
b. Parasympathetic nerves are suppressed
c. Parasympathetic nerves are stimulated
d. Sympathetic nerves are stimulated

Ans. d. Sympathetic nerves are stimulated

7. A patient is experiencing dyspnea. What is the nurse's priority action?

a. Remove pillow's from under the head
b. Elevate the head of the bed
c. Elevate the foot of the bed
d. Take the blood pressure

Ans. b. Elevate the head of the bed

Golden Points

- Vital signs include **temperature, pulse, respiration and blood pressure**.
- Recently, pain has been added as fifth vital sign. The vital signs are called so because they are important
- Two main alterations of body temperature are pyrexia and hypothermia.
- **Pulse rhythm** is the pattern of the pulsations and the pauses between them.

CHAPTER 7

Equipment and Linen

CONCEPTUAL THEORY

Terminology

150+ key terminologies for Quick Recall & Revision

Audit: It is a periodic evaluation system to measure the quality of the medical equipment.
Ceramic: It is a material that is neither metallic nor organic. It may be crystalline, glassy or both crystalline and glassy. They are typically hard and chemically nonreactive and can be formed or densified with heat, e.g., nelson's inhaler, Mortar and pestle, Bowl, Plate, etc.
Critical device: It can be clean as soon as possible after using and sterilize by moist heat after cleaning.
Disposable product: A disposable product is a product designed for single use after which its recycled or is disposed as solid waste.
Enamel: Refers to a glassy, vitreous and usually opaque substance that is used in protective or decorative coating on metal, glass or ceramicware, e.g., trays, Kidney basins, Bowl, Funnel, Jars, Pint measures, Urinals, Bed pans, Enema cans, Buckets, Bath tubs, Dishes, etc.
Equipment: Refers to various devices, tools, instruments that are used in hospitals and health care works. Fixed or portable and non-expandable items used for the diagnosis, treatment, monitoring and direct care of patients.
Indent: It is an official order or requisition for medicine and supplies from the medical stores. Indent is a list of items made for availing in the ward.
Inventory: It is a detailed list of articles in the ward including its specification and the quantity available.
Medical calibration: Refers to the process of adjusting the accuracy of a medical display in line with regulatory standards.
Medical or surgical items: That are consumable, expendable, disposable or nondurable and that are used for the treatment or diagnosis of a patient's specific illness, injury or condition.
Noncritical device: Clean as necessary with discomfort and comes in contact with unbroken skin.
Reusable devices are the devices that can reprocess and reuse on multiple patients.
Semicritical device: It can be clean as soon as possible after using and sterilize by moist heat after cleaning.
Stainless steel: It is an alloy of steel with chromium and sometimes another element (such as nickel or molybdenum) that is practically immune to rusting and ordinary corrosion, e.g., Forceps, Scopes, Sharp instruments, etc.
Sterilization: It is the process by which both the pathogenic and nonpathogenic microorganisms including their spores are destroyed from objects.

Health care institution uses various items for diagnostic and therapeutic procedures. There are two types of equipment used in hospital settings:

- Disposable
- Reusable

DISPOSABLE

Equipment and items can be used only, not much care required and no need to be sterilized.

Example: Gloves, plastic syringes, cotton, etc.

REUSABLE

Items and equipment can be used for very long time. These are cleaned, disinfected and sterilized before and after each use.

More care should be given to reusable item than disposable items.

Various enamel articles used in hospitals include trays, kidney trays, basins, bowls, funnel, jugs, pint measure, urinals, bed pans, enema cans, buckets, bath tubs, sputum mugs, knife dish, soap dish, etc. These items include items mentioned under enamel items and the additional items are: **Forceps, different needles, different scopes, sharp instruments and miscellaneous items such as** spatulas, tongue depressors, tracheal airway, tube clamps, tracheostomy tubes, mouth gag, dilators, etc.

The head nurse/nurse manager is responsible for proper management of equipment and supplies required for patient care.

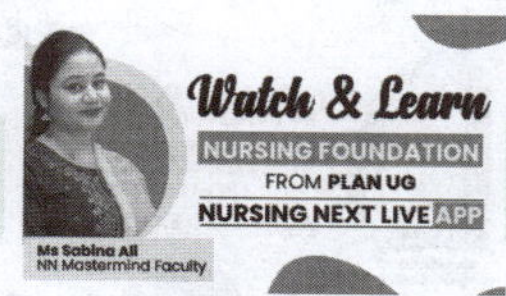

The following are the key activities of nurse managers:

- **Procurement:** It involves several steps:
  - Requirements must be established.
  - Send requisitions of the supplies and equipment through proper channels.
  - Place indent.
- **Receiving:** When the indent items arrive in workplace. They must be properly received, inspected and counted.
- **Storing:** The supplies and equipment are stored in appropriate place and in a correct way.

Nurse's managers must make sure that their nurses have the supplies they need. She distributes the supplies in the morning for the use to the operational level nurses. She also ensures that adequate supplies are there for evening and night staff.

Equipment found damaged must be sent for repair. The nurse manager should ensure the quality of equipment keeping in mind the safety of the patient.

CONCEPTUAL EXERCISES

LONG ANSWER QUESTION

1. Discuss the cleaning and disinfection of linen items in the hospital.

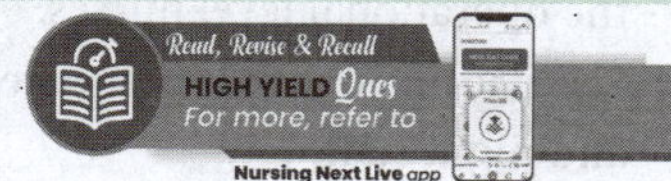

Answer

Common Linen Items Used in Hospital

- Bed sheets, draw sheets, counterpanes, pack sheets
- Cloth covers for pillow, mattress, blanket, IV fluid bottle, hot water bottle, ice collar, air cushion, inhaler cover, sandbag cover
- Pillows, blankets and mattresses
- Bath blankets
- Curtains
- Towels: face, bath, hand, dressing, treatment, anesthesia, doctors towel
- Wrappers for tray, dressing sets, bowls, syringes,
- Patients clothes—jacket gown, shirt, pyjama, leggings
- Staff clothes, shirt, pyjama, caps, head tie
- Binders
- Restraints—elbow, jacket, crib net and mittens
- Wringers
- Guard, spinal sheets
- Diet napkin, tray covers
- Dusters

Cleaning and Disinfection of Linen

- Dirty linen need to be sent to laundry for washing and ironing
- Regular dusting of mattresses using a piece of clean damp cloth
- Protect the mattress with mackintosh
- During therapeutic procedures, small rubber/plastic mackintosh over top linen
- Fresh stains need to be removed using an appropriate solvent
- Inspect and send torn linen for repair in time on regular basis to prevent further damage
- Always keep extra linen at hand
- Fold and keep different linen sorted out in cupboards with proper labels
- Periodically check the inventory and keep a proper record
- Always use laundry bags for used linen
- A record must be prepared of linen to laundry
- Store laundered linen in the cupboard neatly.

Note:

- Contaminated linen needs to be soaked in a big plastic bucket/drum with chlorine 0.5% solution minimum for 10 minutes for decontamination
- Rinse in cold water to prepare for autoclaving
- Dry in the sun
- Send for autoclaving and store neatly in appropriate cupboards
- While storing the linen in the sluice room for sending laundry, make sure that dry and wet linens are stored separately.

Types of Stains and Removal of Stains from the Linen

- **Tea, cocoa, coffee:**
  - Spread the cloth over a hole and pour boiling water from a reasonable height.
  - Rub lemon, boric powder over the stain and put for sunning. Wash with soap and water.
  - Milk and sodium carbonate can also be used to remove stains and then the cloth can be washed with soap and water.
- **Vegetable stains:**
  - Salt over the stain is applied and hot water poured from a height or else ammonia (NH_3) or Hydrogen peroxide (H_2O_2) solution is used .

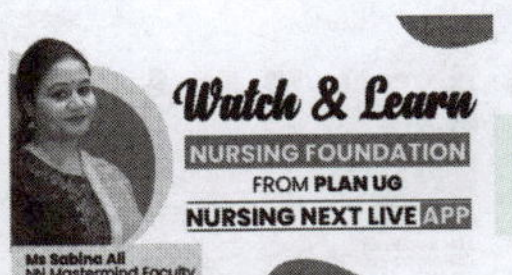

- **Gentian violet stain:**
  - Soak the stained area in a bowl/mug with raw milk for several hours then wash as usual.
- **Ink stain:**
  - Wet the stain area with cold water, sprinkle salt and rub lemon juice or apply NH_3 and wash as usual.
- **Medicine stain:**
  - Apply alcohol/spirit and wash.
- **Grease and oil:**
  - Soak the stained area in a mug filled with kerosene oil, rub it lightly, wash with soap and water and dry in the sun. Thereafter, put a blotting paper over the cleaned area of stain and iron it.
- **Paint and varnish:**
  - Same as grease and oil, turpentine can also be used to soak, in addition to kerosene oil.
- **Perspiration:**
  - Put a few drops of ammonia, over the stained area and wash as usual.

By the following these steps, cleaning and disinfection of linen items can be done in the hospital setting.

SHORT NOTES

1. Write the maintenance of inventory.

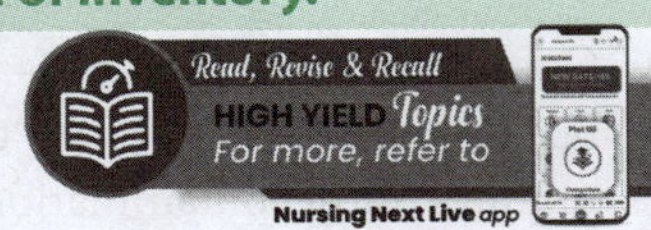

Answer

- Managing supplies and equipment involves much more than keeping the storage area neat.
- Managing a hospital's nursing department includes managing the supplies and equipment needed for patient care and treatment.
- The head nurse/nurse manager is responsible for proper management of equipment and supplies required for patient care.

The following are the key activities of nurse managers:

Procurement

It involves several steps:
- Requirements must be established.
- Send requisitions of the supplies and equipment through proper channels.
- Place indent by specifying a detailed description of equipment, specifications including whether this is fresh or additional or replacement.

Receiving

- When the indent items arrive in workplace.
- They must be properly received, inspected and counted.

Storing

- The supplies and equipment are stored in appropriate place and in a correct way.
- Group-wise and alphabetical arrangement helps in identification and retrieval.
- Monitor expiry date.

Issuing, Distribution and Maintaining Inventory

- Nurse's managers must make sure that their nurses have the supplies they need.
- She distributes the supplies in the morning for the use to the operational level nurses.
- She also ensures that adequate supplies are there for evening and night staff.
- She maintains the current inventory of equipment and inspects and then properly issues it for use.
- She is responsible for maintaining of supplies and distribution equipment.

Repairing and Disposal

- Equipment found damaged must be sent for repair.
- The nurse manager should ensure the quality of equipment keeping in mind the safety of the patient.
- She should conduct routine checking of equipment, label, isolate or remove faulty equipment to prevent injury.

SHORT ANSWER QUESTIONS

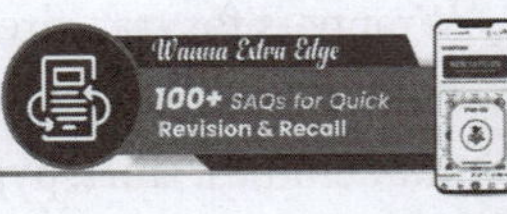

1. Write the steps for maintenance of inventory.

Answer

- Procurement
- Receiving
- Storing
- Issuing, distribution and maintaining inventory
- Repairing and disposal

CONCEPTUAL REVISION

MULTIPLE CHOICE QUESTIONS

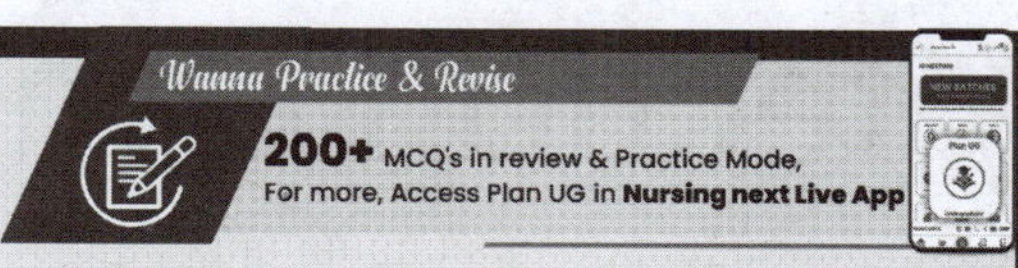

1. Ward furniture and instruments are an example of which type of equipment?

a. Fixed equipment b. Movable equipment
c. Hospital equipment d. Machinery

Ans. b. Movable equipment

2. ……………. aims to extend the life of the equipment and reduce failure rates.

a. Maintenance strategy
b. Performance inspection
c. Preventive maintenance
d. Corrective maintenance

Ans. c. Preventive maintenance

3. Which one of the following is not a purpose of Equipment maintenance?

a. Extend useful life of equipment
b. Prevention of wastage of consumables
c. Extend useful life of consumables
d. Readiness of equipment for emergency use

Ans. c. Extend useful life of consumables

4. Equipment maintenance process includes all; except:

a. Procurement b. Inventory
c. Maintenance d. Security

Ans. d. Security

5. Damp dusting is better than dry dusting because:

a. It saves time
b. It can be done less frequently
c. Dust easily flies out into the atmosphere
d. It reduces the efforts

Ans. c. Dust easily flies out into the atmosphere

6. …………..goods should be washed with mild soap, rinsed thoroughly and dried before putting away:

a. Rubber goods b. Linen
c. Glassware d. Enamelware

Ans. a. Rubber goods

7. Solvents, bleaches and absorbents are used for stain removal in cleaning which of the following material?

a. Rubber goods b. Linen
c. Glassware d. Enamelware

Ans. b. Linen

8. All of the following are the techniques of inventory management; except:

a. FIFO
b. Inspection of stock levels
c. Procurement
d. Security of stock

Ans. c. Procurement

9. Which of the following is one of the techniques of inventory management?

a. FIFO b. Procurement
c. Documentation d. Communication

Ans. a. FIFO

10. Which of the following is one of the equipment maintenance processes?

a. Procurement b. Documentation
c. Communication d. Security

Ans. a. Procurement

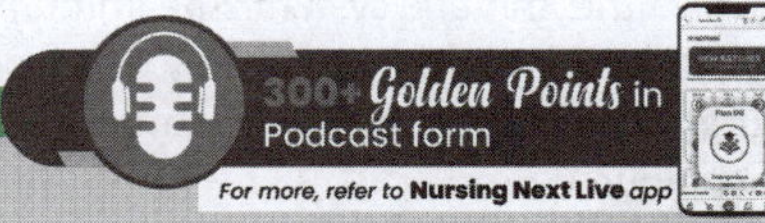

Golden Points

- Health care institution uses various items for diagnostic and therapeutic procedures.
- There are two types of equipment used in hospital settings: Disposable and Reusable.
- More care should be given to reusable item than disposable items.
- The head nurse/nurse manager is responsible for proper management of equipment and supplies required for patient care. Various key activities of nurse managers include Procurement, Receiving and Storing.
- The nurse manager should ensure the quality of equipment keeping in mind the safety of the patient.

Introduction to Infection Control in Clinical Setting Infection

CHAPTER

8

CONCEPTUAL THEORY

Terminology

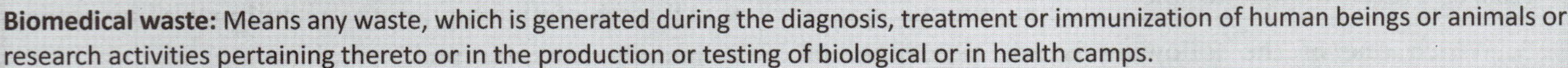

Antiseptics: It is are antimicrobial substances that are applied to living tissue/skin.

Biomedical waste: Means any waste, which is generated during the diagnosis, treatment or immunization of human beings or animals or research activities pertaining thereto or in the production or testing of biological or in health camps.

Disinfectants: It is are substances that are applied to nonliving objects to destroy microorganisms that are living on the objects.

Disinfection: Refers to chemical or physical processes used to reduce the numbers of pathogens from the object's surface. These processes do not necessarily remove all potential for infection, because spores may remain present.

Endogenous infection: When part of client's flora becomes altered and an overgrowth results, e.g., infections due to enterococci, yeasts streptococci, etc.

Exogenous infection: Infections caused by microorganisms external to the individual which do not exist as normal flora. E.g., *Clostridium tetani*

Iatrogenic infections: Infections caused by diagnostic or therapeutic procedures, e.g., CAUTI

Infection: An **infection** is the entry and multiplication of an infectious agent in the tissues of the host.

Isolation room: An **isolation room** is a specially constructed area in a hospital designed for housing patients with an infectious disease in order to prevent the spread of the disease in the hospital.

Isolation: It is the separation of infected persons from the non infected persons for the period of communicability under conditions which will prevent the transmission of infection to others.

Medical asepsis: Refers to all practices used to protect the patients and their environment from the transmission of disease-producing organisms that can transmit from one patient to another. In this clean technique is used.

Nonspecific: Defenses protect the person against all microorganisms regardless of prior exposure. Nonspecific defenses include anatomic and physiological barriers and the inflammatory response.

Nosocomial infections or Hospital acquired infections: Mean infections developed in the patient after admission in hospital, which was neither present nor in the incubation period at the time of hospital.

Pathogens: Disease-producing microorganisms are called **pathogens.**

Pathogenicity refers to the ability of a microorganism to produce disease.

Post-exposure prophylaxis or PEP: Refers to the comprehensive management following potential exposure to blood-borne pathogens (HIV, HBV, and HCV).

Specific defenses: Protect the person against identifiable bacteria, viruses, fungi or other infectious agents. Specific defenses of the body involve the immune system. The immune response has two components—Antibody-mediated defenses and cell-mediated defenses.

Sterilization: It is the process by which an object becomes free of all microorganisms.

Surgical asepsis: It refers to all procedures used to keep objects or areas sterile or completely free from all microorganisms, in this sterile technique is used.

Virulence: Refers to the frequency with which a pathogen causes disease.

INFECTION

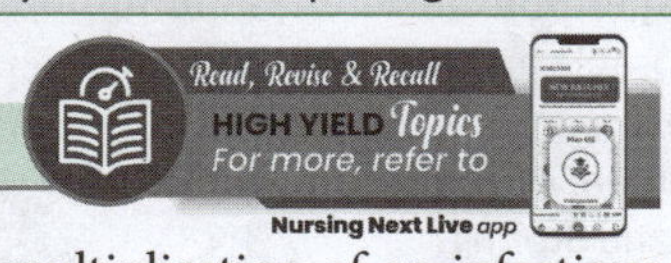

An infection is the entry and multiplication of an infectious agent in the tissues of the host. Disease-producing microorganisms are called pathogens **Pathogenicity** refers to the ability of a microorganism to produce disease. **Virulence** refers to the frequency with which a pathogen causes disease.

There are five types of microorganisms that can be pathogenic and these are: **bacteria, virus, fungi, protozoa and Rickettsia.**

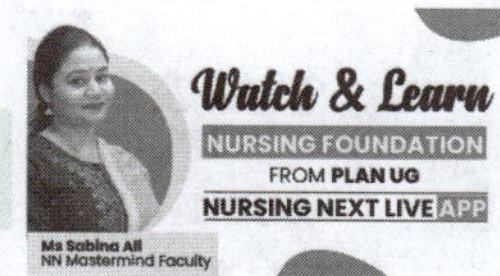

Development of an infection occurs in a cycle that depends on the presence of all of the following elements:

- An infectious agent or pathogen
- Reservoir or source for pathogen growth
- Portal of exit from the reservoir
- A mode of transmission
- A portal of entry to a host
- A susceptible host

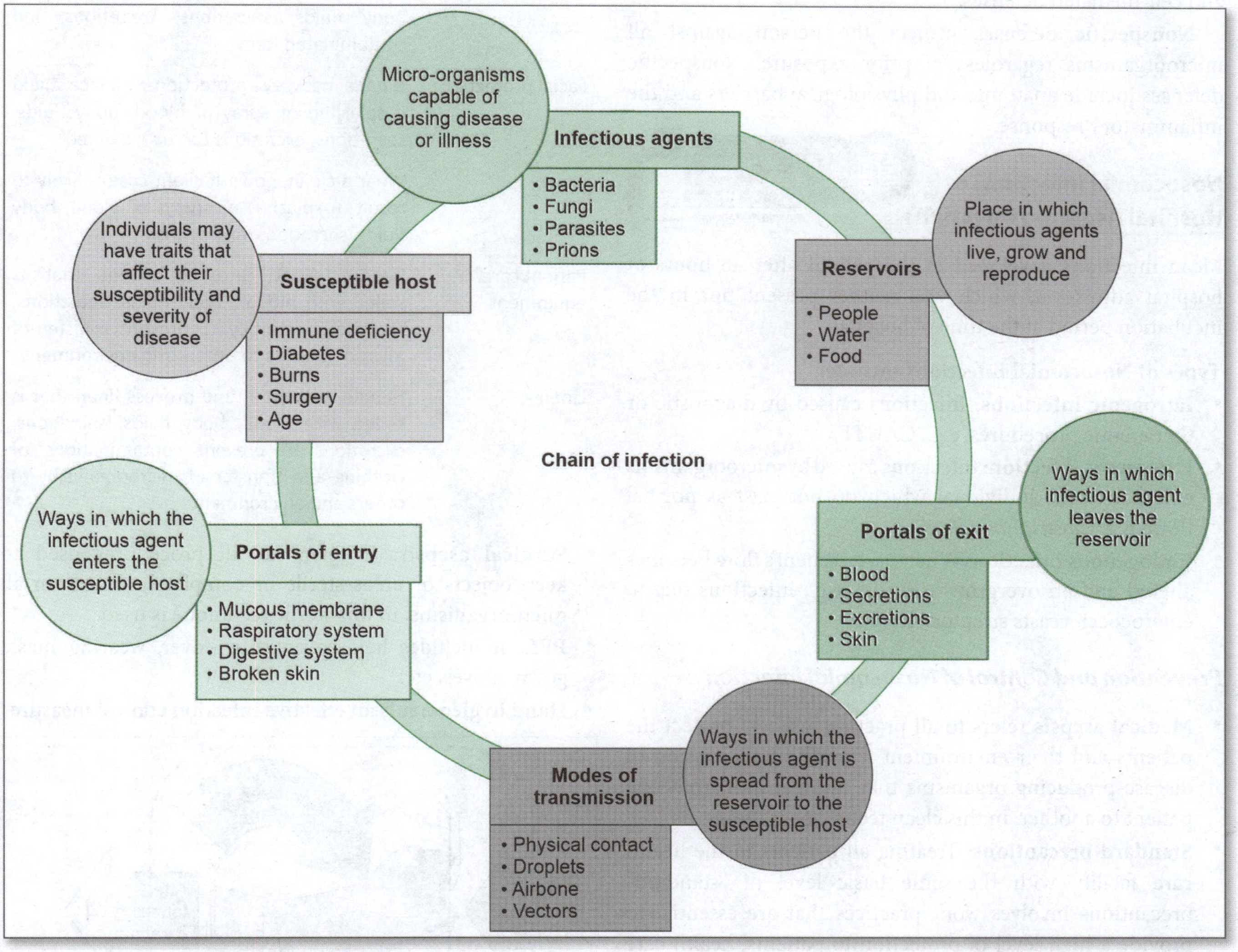

Stages of Infection

Stage	Description
Incubation period	Interval between entrance of pathogen into body and appearance of first symptoms, e.g., Chicken pox 2–3 weeks. Common cold for 1–2 days.
Prodromal stage	Interval from the onset of nonspecific signs and symptoms (malaise, low grade fever, fatigue) to more specific symptoms. Microorganisms grow and multiply and the client is more capable of spreading disease to others during this time.
Illness stage	Interval when the client manifests sign and symptoms specific to the type of infection (e.g., common cold, manifested by sore throat, rhinitis, sinus congestion, etc.)
Convalescence stage	Interval when acute symptoms of an infection disappear, length of recovery depends on severity of infection and the client's general state of health. Recovery may take several days to months.

Individuals normally have defenses that protect the body from infection. These defenses can be categorized as specific and nonspecific.

Specific defenses protect the person against identifiable bacteria, viruses, fungi or other infectious agents. Specific defenses of the body involve the immune system. The immune response has two components—Antibody-mediated defenses and cell-mediated defenses.

Nonspecific defenses protect the person against all microorganisms regardless of prior exposure. Nonspecific defenses include anatomic and physiological barriers and the inflammatory response.

Read, Revise & Recall
HIGH YIELD Topics
For more, refer to
Nursing Next Live app

Nosocomial Infections or Hospital Acquired Infections

Mean infections developed in the patient after 48 hours of hospital admission, which was neither present nor in the incubation period at the time of hospital.

Types of Nosocomial infections include:

- **Iatrogenic infections:** Infections caused by diagnostic or therapeutic procedures, e.g., CAUTI
- **Exogenous infection:** Infections caused by microorganisms external to the individual which do not exist as normal flora. E.g. *Clostridium tetani*
- **Endogenous infection**: When part of client's flora becomes altered and an overgrowth results, e.g., infections due to enterococci, yeasts streptococci, etc.

Prevention and Control of Nosocomial Infection

- **Medical asepsis** refers to all practices used to protect the patients and their environment from the transmission of disease-producing organisms that can transmit from one patient to another. In this clean technique is used.
- **Standard precautions:** Treating all patients in the health care facility with the same basic level of "standard" precautions involves work practices that are essential to provide a high level of protection to patients, health care workers and visitors.

  These include the following:
  - Handwashing and hand hygiene.
  - Use of personal protective equipment when handling blood, body substances, excretions and secretions.
  - Appropriate handling of patient care equipment and soiled linen.
  - Prevention of needle stick/sharp injuries.
  - Environmental cleaning of spills and appropriate handling of waste.
- **Universal precautions**

Universal precaution	Standard operational procedure (SOP)
Hand Hygiene	Wash hand after contact with blood, body fluids, secretion, and contaminated objects whether the gloves are warn on not
Gloves	Wear clean gloves when touching blood, body fluids, secretions, excretions and contaminated item
Facial protection	Wear a mask, eye protection, or a face shield if splashed or spray of blood, body fluids, secretions, excretions can be expected
Gown	Wear a clean, gown if client case is likely to result in splashes or sprays of blood, body fluids, secretions, excretions
Patient care equipment	Handle client care equipment that is soiled with blood , body fluids, secretions, excretions carefully to prevent transfer of microorganisms to others and environment
Linen	Handle, transport, and process linen that is soiled with blood, body fluids, secretions, excretions to prevent contaminations of clothing and transfer of microorganisms to others and environment

- **Surgical asepsis:** It refers to all procedures used to keep objects or areas sterile or completely free from all microorganisms, in this sterile technique is used.
- **PPE:** It includes hair cover, shoe cover, wearing mask, gown, gloves, etc.
- **Hand hygiene:** It is an effective infection control measure.

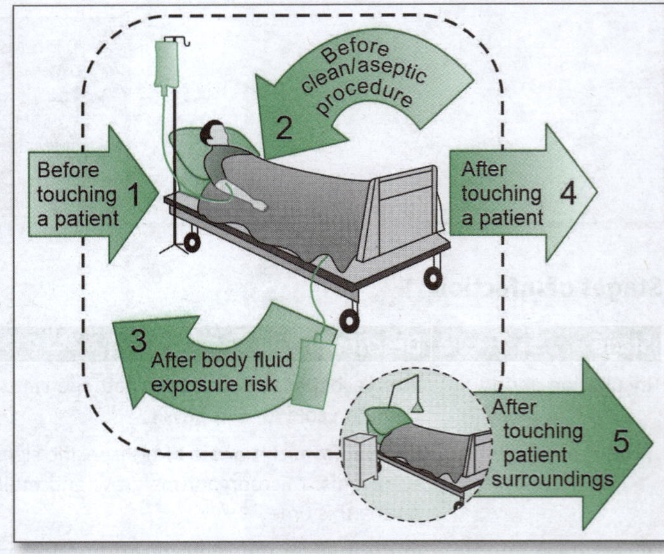

Figure 8.1: Moments of hand hygiene

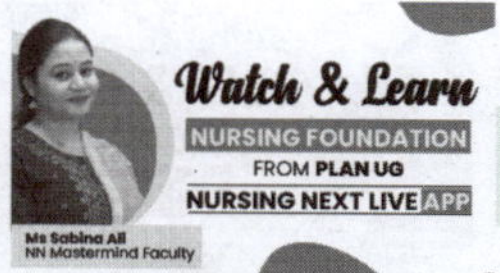

How to Hand Wash

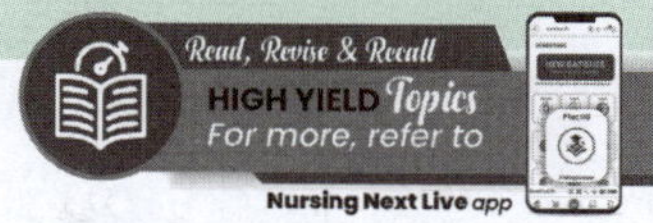

Wash hands when visibly soiled. Otherwise use handrub

Duration of the entire procedure: 40–60 seconds

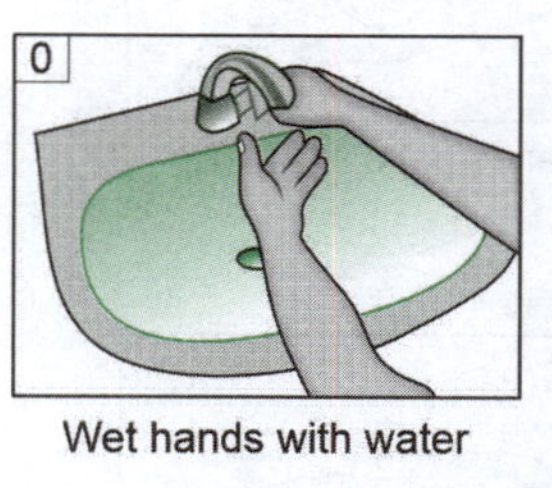

Wet hands with water

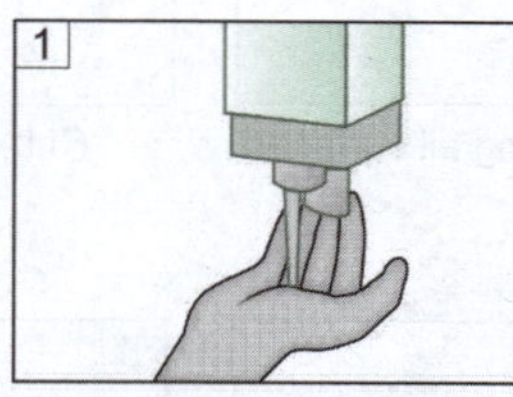

Apply enough soap to cover all hand surfaces

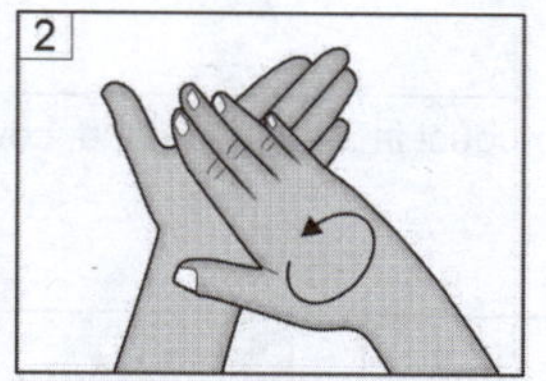

Rub hands palm to palm

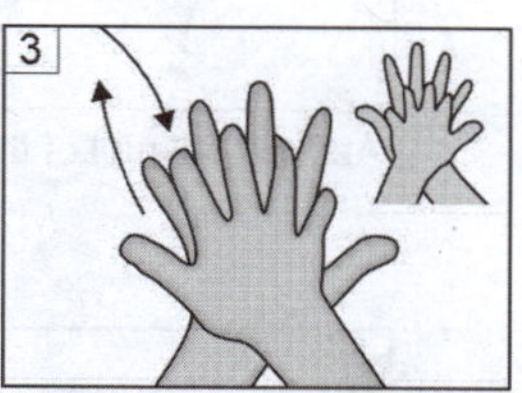

Right palm over left dorsum with interlaced fingers and vice versa

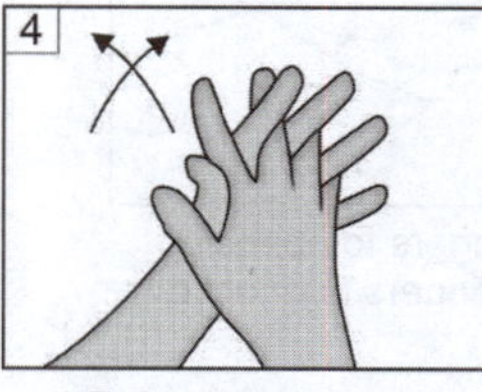

Palm to palm with fingers interlaced

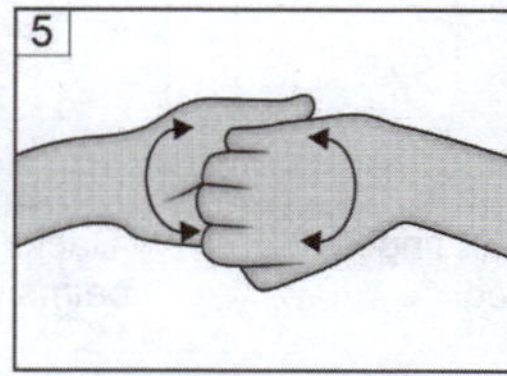

Backs of fingers to opposing palms with fingers interlocked

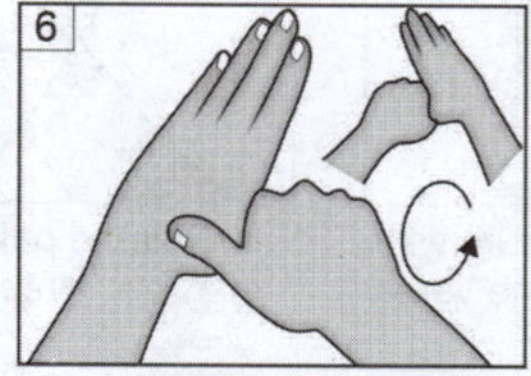

Rotational rubbing of left thumb clasped in right palm and vice versa

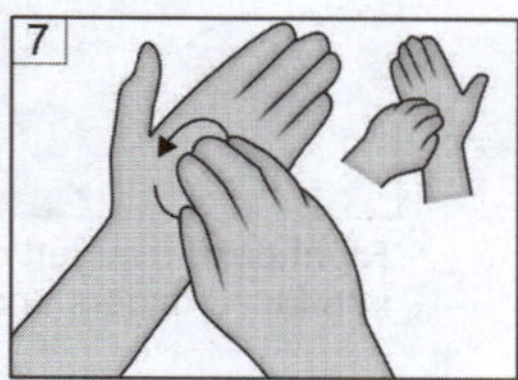

Rotational rubbing backward and forward with clasped fingers of right hand in left palm and vice versa

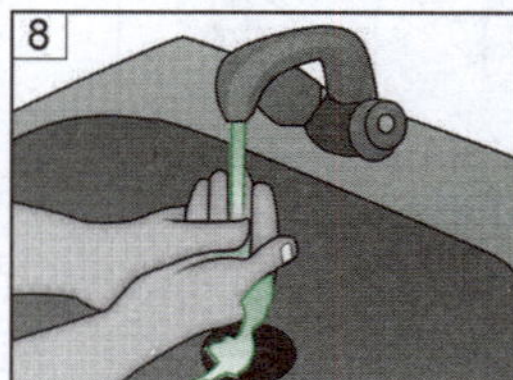

Rinse hands with water

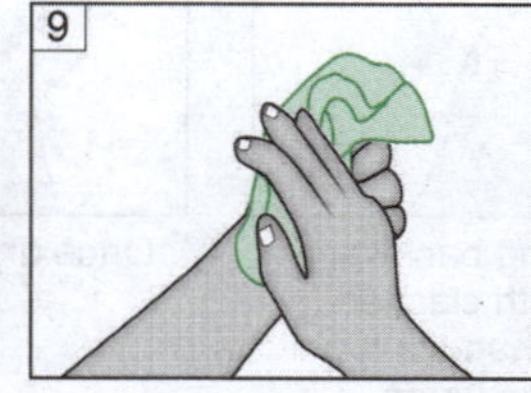

Dry thoroughly with a single-use towel

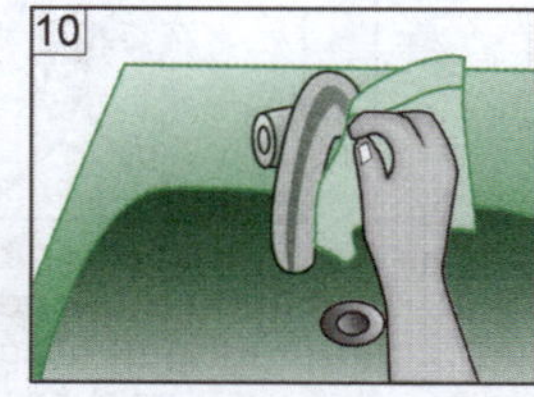

Use towel to turn off faucet

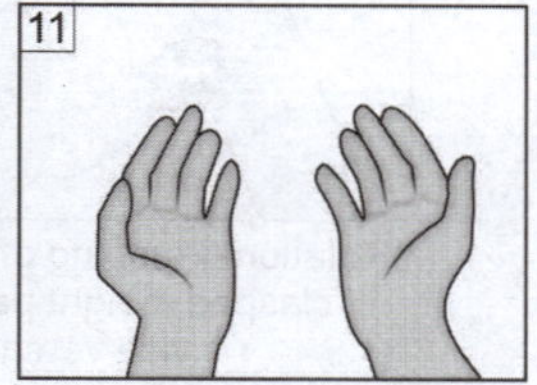

Your hands are now safe

Figure 8.2: Steps of hand hygiene

How to Handrub

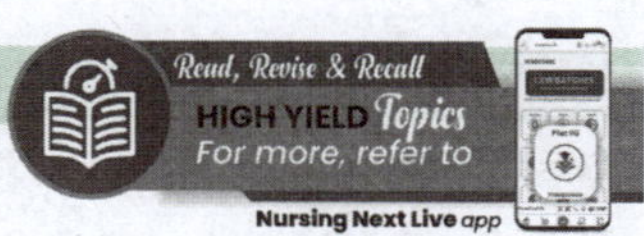

Rub hands for hand hygiene wash hand when visible soiled

Duration of the entire procedure: 20–30 seconds

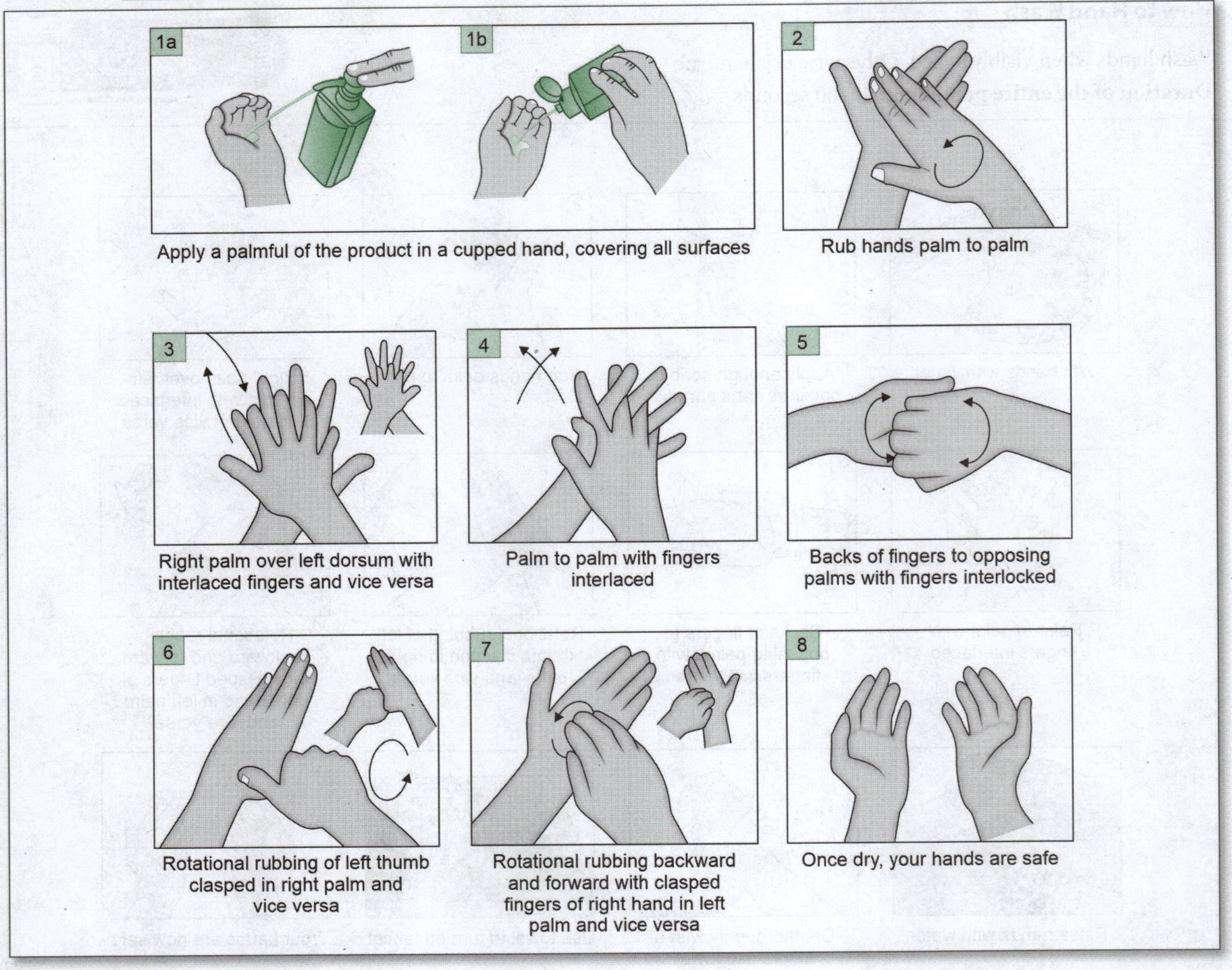

1a 1b
Apply a palmful of the product in a cupped hand, covering all surfaces

2
Rub hands palm to palm

3
Right palm over left dorsum with interlaced fingers and vice versa

4
Palm to palm with fingers interlaced

5
Backs of fingers to opposing palms with fingers interlocked

6
Rotational rubbing of left thumb clasped in right palm and vice versa

7
Rotational rubbing backward and forward with clasped fingers of right hand in left palm and vice versa

8
Once dry, your hands are safe

Figure 8.3: Steps of hand rub

An **isolation room** is a specially constructed area in a hospital designed for housing patients with an infectious disease in order to prevent the spread of the disease in the hospital. Isolation is the separation of infected persons from the non infected persons for the period of communicability under conditions which will prevent the transmission of infection to others.

Isolation room type	Isolation room use
Class S — Standard	Standard isolation used for isolating patients capable of transmitting infection by droplet or contact routes.
Class P — Positive pressure	Protective isolation used to isolate immunocompromised patients.
Class N — Negative pressure	Respiratory isolaton used to isolate patients capable of transmitting infection.
Class Q — Quarantine	A quarantine facility usually consists of the following components: **Quarantine room:** This is a designated space where individuals are isolated from the general population. It's typically a private room with its own facilities. **Amenities room:** This is a room equipped with essential amenities like bedding, toiletries, and other necessities for the individuals in quarantine. **Fumigation facilities:** These facilities are used to disinfect and sanitize the quarantine room and amenities room, helping to prevent the spread of the infectious agent to other areas.

Disinfection refers to chemical or physical processes used to reduce the numbers of pathogens from the object's surface. These processes do not necessarily remove all potential for infection, because spores may remain present.

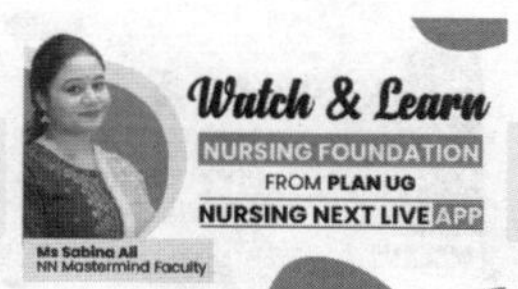

Disinfectants are substances that are applied to nonliving objects to destroy microorganisms that are living on the objects. Whereas **antiseptics** are antimicrobial substances that are applied to living tissue/skin. Disinfectants can be **Concurrent and terminal** type.

Sterilization is the process by which an object becomes free of all microorganisms. By sterilization both the pathogenic and nonpathogenic organisms are destroyed. There are various methods used for sterilization of articles such as direct **sun light, boiling, fumigation or gas sterilization, use of UV light, hot air sterilization, autoclaving, flaming, etc.**

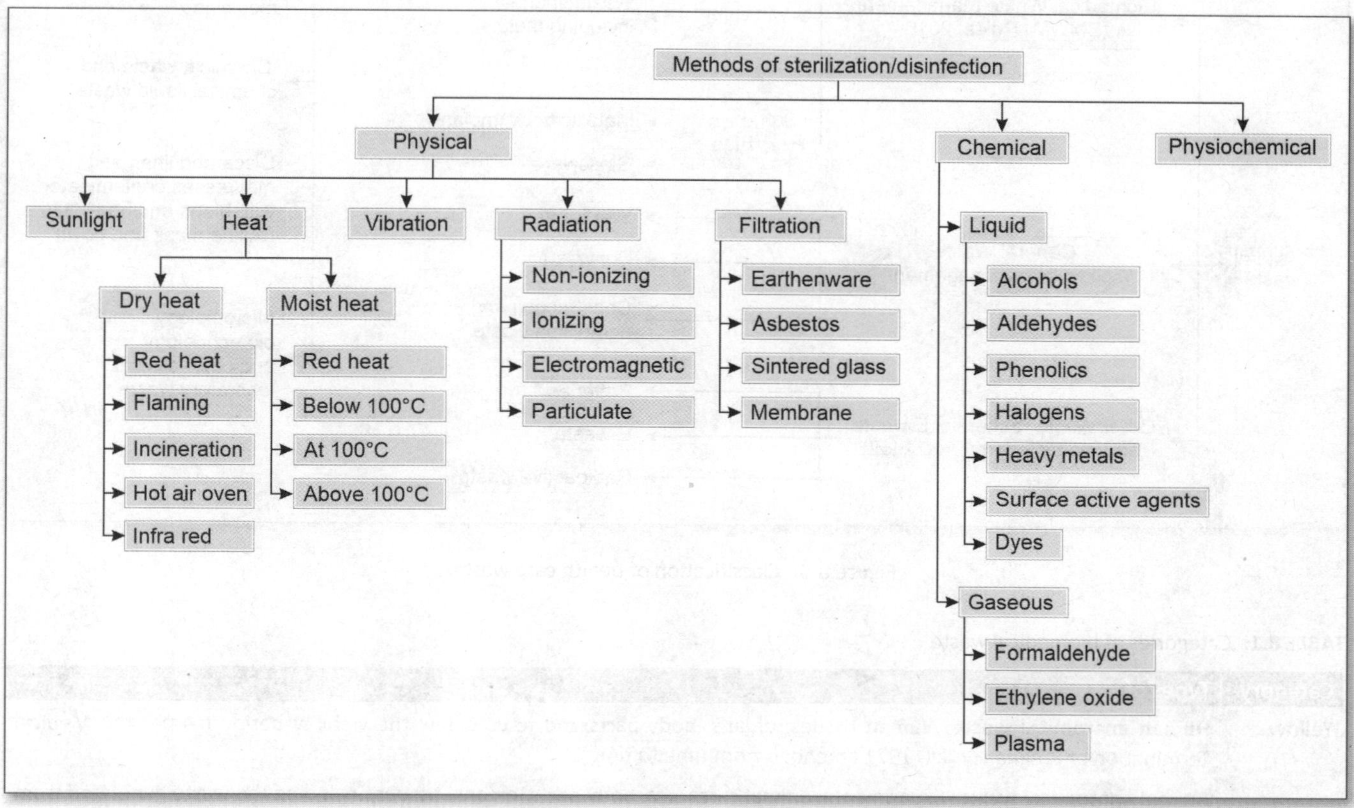

Figure 8.4: Methods of sterilization/disinfection

All hospitals have their Infection Control Committees, Infection Control Nurse (ICN) is the important member of this committee. It is the responsibility of the nurse and health care personnel for providing the clean and safe environment to the patients and enhance the effectiveness of infection control.

Health care facilities are primarily responsible for management of the health care waste generated within the facilities, including activities undertaken by them in the community. Waste generated from the health care facility is classified are into:

- **Biomedical waste** means any waste, which is generated during the diagnosis, treatment or immunization of human beings or animals or research activities pertaining thereto or in the production or testing of biologicals or in health camps.

Various types of biomedical waste are further assigned to each one of the categories, as detailed below:

- Yellow category
- Red category
- White category
- Blue category

General waste consists of all the waste other than biomedical waste and which has not been in contact with any hazardous or infectious, chemical or biological secretions and does not include any waste sharps.

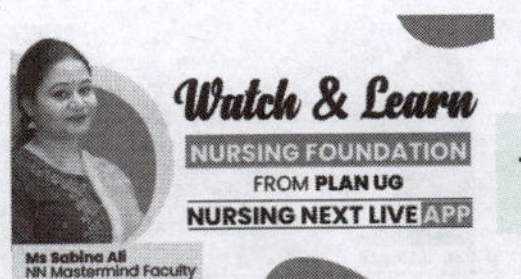

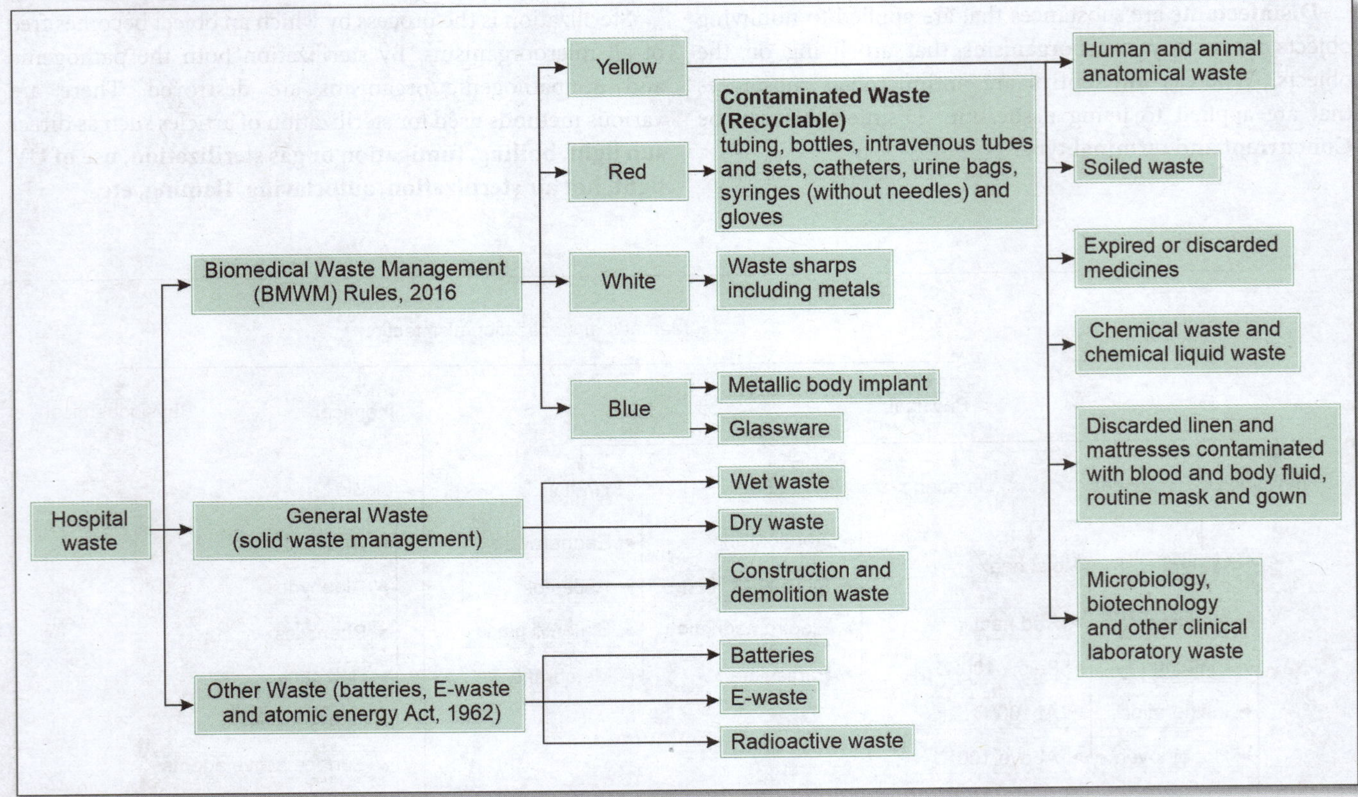

Figure 8.5: Classification of health care waste

TABLE 8.1: Categories of biomedical waste

Category	Types of waste
Yellow	**Human anatomical waste:** Human tissues, organs, body parts and fetus below the viability period (as per the Medical Termination of Pregnancy Act, 1971 amended from time to time).
	Animal anatomical waste: Experimental animal carcasses, body parts, organs, tissues, including the waste generated from animals used in experiments or testing in veterinary hospitals or colleges or animal houses.
	Soiled waste: Items contaminated with blood, body fluids like dressings, plaster casts, cotton swabs and bags containing residual or discarded blood and blood components.
	Discarded or expired medicine: Pharmaceutical waste like antibiotics, cytotoxic drugs including all items contaminated with cytotoxic drugs along with glass or plastic ampoules, vials, etc.
	Chemical waste: Chemicals used in production of biological disinfectants and used or discarded disinfectants
	Chemical liquid waste: Liquid waste generated due to use of chemicals in production of biological and used or discarded disinfectants, Silver X-ray film developing liquid, discarded Formalin, infected secretions. aspirated body fluids , liquid from laboratories and floor washings, cleaning, housekeeping and disinfecting activities, etc.
	Discarded linen, mattresses, beddings contaminated with blood or body fluid, routine mask and gown.
	Microbiology, biotechnology and other clinical laboratory waste (Pretreated): Blood bags, Laboratory cultures, stocks or specimens of microorganisms, live or attenuated vaccines, human and animal cell cultures used in research, industrial laboratories, production of biological, residual toxins, dishes and devices used for cultures.
Red	**Contaminated waste (recyclable):** Wastes generated from disposable items such as tubing, bottles, intravenous tubes and sets, catheters, urine bags, syringes without needles, fixed needle syringes with their needles cut, vacutainers and gloves.
White	Waste sharps including metals Needles, syringes with fixed needles, needles from needle tip cutter or burner, scalpels, blades, or any other contaminated sharp object that may cause puncture and cuts. This includes both used, discarded and contaminated metal sharps.
Blue	Broken or discarded and contaminated glass including medicine vials and ampoules except those contaminated with cytotoxic wastes and metallic body implants.

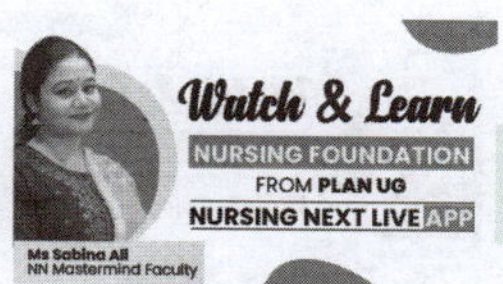

Other wastes consist of used electronic wastes, used batteries, and radioactive wastes which are not covered under biomedical wastes but have to be disposed as and when such wastes are generated as per the provisions laid down under E-Waste (Management) Rules, 2016, Batteries (Management and Handling) Rules, 2001, and Rules/guidelines under Atomic Energy Act, 1962 respectively.

Biomedical waste should be collected on daily basis from each ward of the hospital at a fixed interval of time. There can be multiple collections from wards during the day.

Health care facility should ensure collection, transportation, treatment and disposal of biomedical waste as per BMWM Rules, 2016 and health care facility should also ensure disposal of human anatomical waste, animal anatomical waste, soiled waste and biotechnology waste within 48 hours.

Biomedical waste collected by the staff, should be provided with personal protective equipment (PPE).

Color-coded waste bags and containers should be printed with the biohazard symbol, labeled with details such as date, type of waste, waste quantity, senders name and receiver's details as well as barcoded label for easy tracking till final disposal.

In-house transportation of biomedical waste from site of waste generation/interim storage to central waste collection center, within the premises of the hospital must be done in closed trolleys/containers preferably fitted with wheels for easy maneuverability. Such trolleys or carts are designated for the purpose of biomedical waste collection only. Patient trolleys must not be used for biomedical waste transportation. Size of such waste transport trolleys should be as per the volume of waste generated from the health care facilities.

Health care professionals are at risk of occupational exposure to blood and body fluids, which is a major risk factor in the transmission of infections such as human immunodeficiency virus (HIV), hepatitis B virus (HBV) and hepatitis C virus (HCV) through percutaneous and mucocutaneous routes.

In health care settings, injuries from needles or other sharp instruments are the number-one cause of occupational exposure to blood-borne infections.

The term "postexposure prophylaxis" or PEP refers to the comprehensive management following potential exposure to blood-borne pathogens (HIV, HBV, and HCV). The evaluation must be done rapidly, so as to start any treatment as soon as possible after the accident (ideally within 2 hours but certainly within 72 hours).

Risk of infection after needle stick from a patient with the infection:

- **HBV: 30% (30 in 100)**
- **HCV: 3% (3 in 100)**
- **HIV: 0.3% (3 in 1000)**

An exposed person should be advised to use precautions (e.g., avoid blood or tissue donations, breastfeeding, unprotected sex or pregnancy) to prevent secondary transmission, especially during the first 6–12 weeks following exposure.

Nurses are in tremendous risk of acquiring occupational exposure to blood, body fluids, needlestick and sharp injuries. Thus, it is of utmost importance for the nurses to have the knowledge and excellent practice on biosafety precautions and postexposure prophylaxis.

Postexposure prophylaxis helps to decrease the burden of HIV and HBV among the health care providers. PEP must be incorporated among the health care providers.

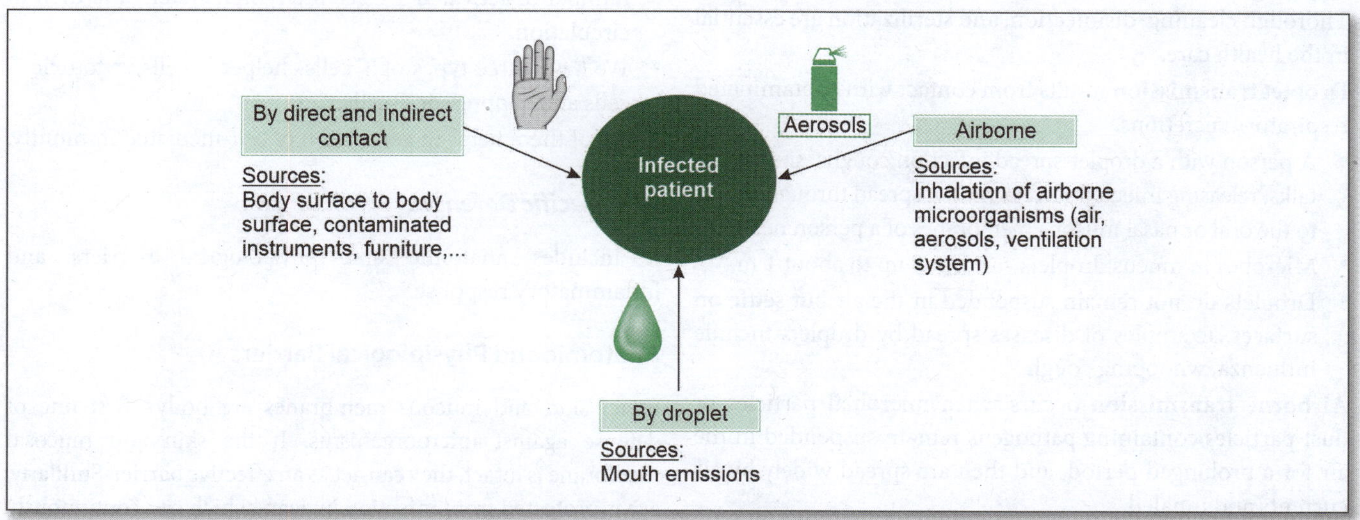

Figure 8.6: Modes of transmission of infection

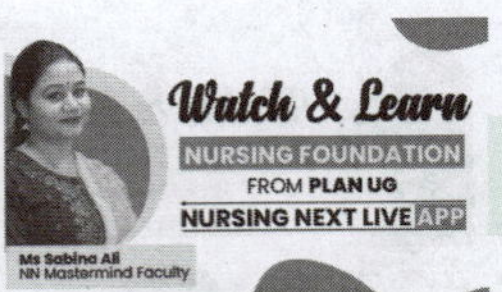

CONCEPTUAL EXERCISES

LONG ANSWER QUESTIONS

1. Define infection and describe the modes of transmission of infections. Explain the body defenses against infections. (KUHS)

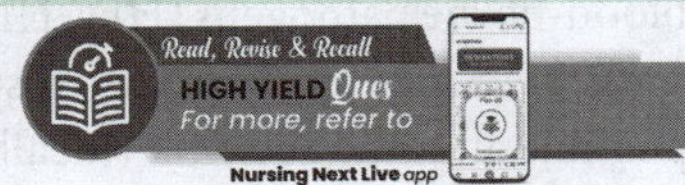

Answer

Infection is the entry and multiplication of an infectious agent in the tissues of the host. If the pathogen fails to cause injury to the cells or tissues, then the infection is asymptomatic. If the pathogen multiplies and causes clinical signs and symptoms, then the infection is symptomatic.

Mode of Transmission

- Contact transmission (direct and indirect)
- Droplet transmission (inhalation through respiratory tract)
- Airborne transmission
- Ingestion (through gastrointestinal tract)
- Inoculation (through accidental sharp injury or bites)
- Transplacental transmission (microbes may cross placenta from the mother to fetus).

Direct contact: It refers to the spread of microorganisms from one person to another through actual physical contact. Though unhealthy sexual practices can lead to sexual transmitted diseases.

Indirect contact: It occurs when a susceptible person comes in contact with a contaminated object. In health care settings, virtually any item could be contaminated with certain microorganisms, e.g., endoscopes, respiratory equipment, etc. Thorough cleaning, disinfection, and sterilization are essential in the health care.

Droplet transmission results from contact with contaminated respiratory secretions.

- A person with a droplet-spread infection coughs, sneezes, or talks, releasing infected secretions that spread through the air to the oral or nasal mucous membranes of a person nearby.
- Microbes in mucus droplets can travel up to about 1 m.
- Droplets do not remain suspended in the air but settle on surfaces. Examples of diseases spread by droplets include influenza, whooping cough.

Airborne transmission occurs when microbial particles or dust particles containing pathogens remain suspended in the air for a prolonged period, and then are spread widely by air currents and inhaled.

- The tiny particles remain suspended in the air for several hours and may cause infection when a susceptible person inhales them.
- Examples of diseases spread by the airborne include pulmonary tuberculosis and measles.

Body Defenses Against Infections

Humans have defense mechanism that can protect the body from infections. These are as follows:

- Specific defenses
- Nonspecific defenses

Specific defenses protect the individuals from specific viruses, bacteria, fungi, etc. While nonspecific type of defense mechanism protect the human body from all types of microorganisms.

Specific Defenses

This type of defense involves the immunity within the human body. An antigen is responsible for the generation of the immunity. This immune response has two components—antibody-mediated defenses and cell-mediated defenses.

Antibody-Mediated Defenses

- It is also known as humoral immunity.
- This type of immunity is mediated by B cells.
- Later on, B cells produce types of antibody molecules i.e., classes of immunoglobulins designated by IgG, IgM, IgD, IgA, IgE.

Cell Mediated Defenses

- It is also known as Cellular immunity.
- This type of immunity is mediated by T cells.
- On exposure to antigen, the lymphoid tissues release large number of activated T cells into lymph system and then in circulation.
- We have three types of T cells- helper T cells, cytotoxic T cells and suppressor T cells.
- All of them helps in generation of cell-mediated immunity.

Nonspecific Defenses

It includes anatomic and physiological barriers and inflammatory response.

Anatomic and Physiological Barriers

Intact skin and mucous membranes are body's first line of defense against microorganisms. If the skin and mucosal membrane is intact, they can act as an effective barrier. Similarly, eye is protected from infection by tears which can continuously wash out the microorganism and contain lysozyme also. High acidity of gastrointestinal (GI) system can prevent microbial growth. Vagina has natural defenses against infection.

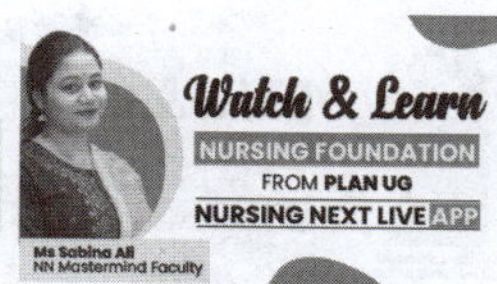

Inflammatory Response

It is a local and nonspecific defense which is adaptive mechanism that can destroy or deletes the injurious agent. It promotes repair of damaged tissue. It has vascular and cellular response, exudate production and reparative phase. It is characterized by:

- Dolor (Pain)
- Tumor (Swelling)
- Rubor (Redness)
- Calor (Heat)
- Impaired functions of body part.

2. Describe nosocomial infection and role of nurse in prevention of nosocomial infection in ICU. (RUHS, MGR, KUHS)

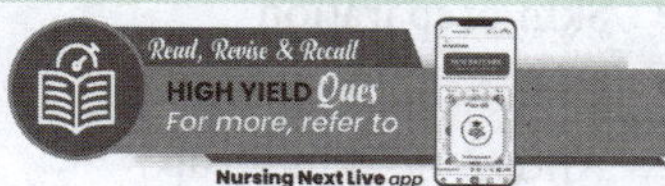

Answer

- Nosocomial infection derived from Greek words "**nosus**". disease and "**komeion**" — to take care of.
- Also known as **hospital acquired infection (HAIs)**.
- **Nosocomial infection** can be defined as an infection acquired by a patient during the process of care (including preventive, diagnostic and treatment services) in a hospital or other health-care facility, which was not present or incubating at the time of admission.
- HAIs can also occur after discharge of the patient.
- It can also be acquired by health care professionals, during health care delivery, and by the visitors.
- Infections are considered nosocomial if first appear **within 48 hours or more after hospital admission** or **within 30 days after discharge.**

Common types of hospital-acquired infections include:

- **Urinary Tract Infections (UTIs):** Due to the use of urinary catheters or improper hygiene practices.
- **Surgical Site Infections (SSIs):** SSIs develop at the site of a surgical incision.
- **Central Line-Associated Bloodstream Infections (CLABSIs):** CLABSIs occur when bacteria enter the bloodstream through a central venous catheter.
- Ventilator-Associated Pneumonia (VAP)

Causes

- Crowded hospitals
- New microorganisms
- Compromised immune system
- Increased bacterial resistance

Modes of Transmission

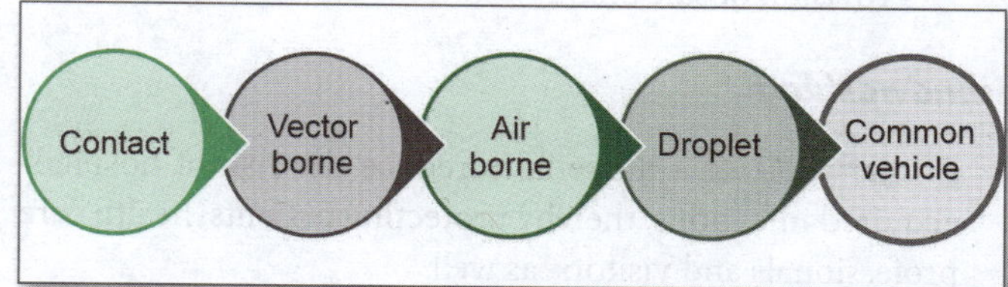

Role of Nurse in Prevention of Nosocomial Infection in ICU

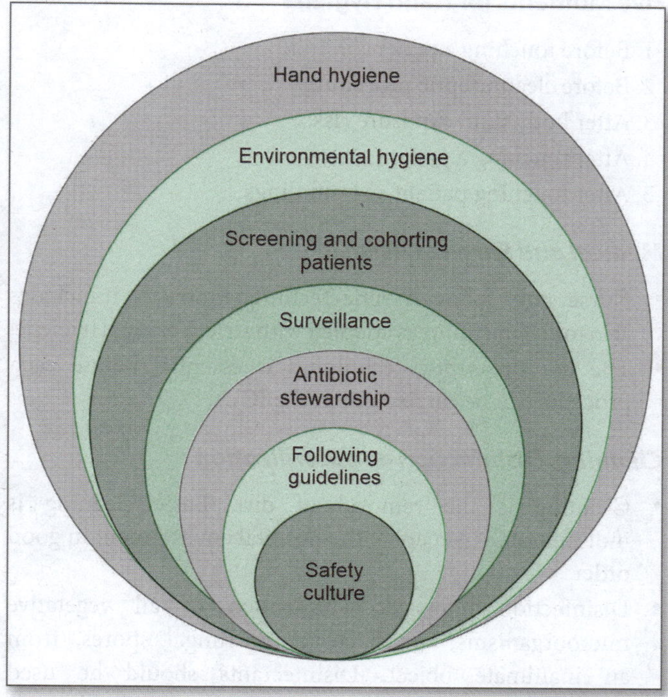

Figure 8.7: Strategies to prevent nosocomial infection

- Hospitals must have multidisciplinary Infection Control Committees. In this committee, infection control nurse is an important member. The nurse should be knowledgeable and competent in implementation of evidence-based practice to prevent and control infection in ICUs. She must be involved inservice/continuing education related to infection control practices.
- Various roles of Nurse in control and prevention of hospital acquired infections are mentioned below:
  - Handwashing
  - Use of medical and surgical asepsis
  - Cleaning and disinfection
  - Skin decontamination
  - Biomedical waste management
  - Use of PPE
  - Isolation
  - Personnel welfare

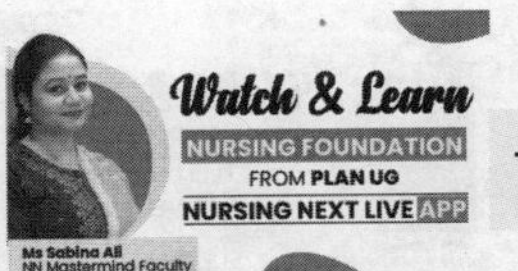

- Use of care bundles CLABSI, CAUTI, SSI, VAP
- Provision of safe blood

Handwashing

- Primary role of a nurse is to reduce the risk of hospital-acquired infections, thereby protecting patients, health care professionals and visitors as well.
- Thus, handwashing plays an important role in prevention of infection. Nurses should perform hand washing following 5 moments of hand washing.

Five Moments for Hand Hygiene

1. Before touching a patient
2. Before clean/aseptic procedure
3. After body fluid exposure risk
4. After touching a patient
5. After touching patient surroundings

Medical and Surgical Asepsis

- Nurse must follow Aseptic Techniques Strictly. It includes "No touch" techniques coupled with strict personal hygiene.
- The use of aseptic techniques is essential before each procedure to be carried out in the ICUs.

Cleaning, Disinfection and Sterilization

- Cleaning is the removal of dirt. Basic cleaning is indispensable in keeping the hospital environment in good order.
- Disinfection refers to elimination of all vegetative microorganisms; not bacterial or fungal spores, from an inanimate object. Disinfectants should be used according to laid down guidelines. Sodium hypochlorite is recommended for disinfection.
- Sterilization is the destruction of all forms of life including spores. Provision of sterile instruments, dressings and fluids is of fundamental importance. Sterilization practices alone will not prevent spread of infection if there is carelessness in its use.

Biomedical Waste Management

Follow the guidelines of biomedical waste management:

- Discard the waste in proper biomedical waste bins.
- Segregation of waste is essential.
- Discard the waste at the point of generation. The one who is generating the waste is also responsible for its proper disposal.

Skin Decontamination

- Thorough hand washing before and after any procedure is essential.
- Use of antiseptics may also be beneficial.
- Use of SSI bundle.

Use of Care Bundles

A care bundle is a set of interventions that, when used together, significantly improve patient outcomes. Nurses are responsible for using Care bundles in the ICUs. It includes:

- SSI (Surgical Site Infection) bundle
- CAUTI (Catheter Associated Urinary Tract Infection) Bundle
- CLABSI (Central Line Associated Blood Stream Infection) bundle
- VAP (Ventilator Associated Pneumonia) bundle

SSI Prevention Bundle

- Skin preparation
- Use of clipper
- Antiseptic skin scrub
- Normothermia
- Glycemic control
- Prophylactic antibiotic

CAUTI Bundles

- Hand washing
- Use of aseptic Techniques
- Continuity of flow
- Bag below the bladder level
- Cleaning of exit portal
- Catheter care

CLABSI Bundle

- Hand hygiene
- Maximum barrier precaution during insertion
- Selecting the vein
- Change of dressing

VAP Bundle

- Elevation of head of bed
- Daily sedation, vacation and readiness of patient to exudate
- Peptic ulcer prophylaxis
- Deep vein thrombosis prophylaxis
- Daily oral care with chlorhexidine

Personnel Welfare

- Pre-service screening and immunization where indicated.
- Provision of PEP when required.

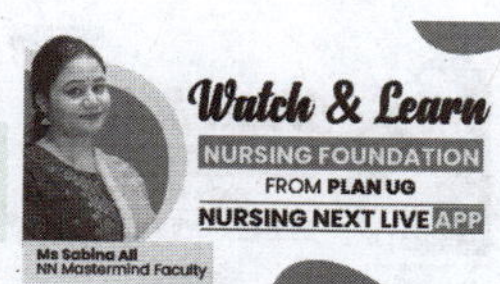

Provision of Safe Blood

- It is also a responsibility of a nurse to transfuse safe blood to the patient. It is essential to check details such as expiry date, blood group, screening of donor blood for transfusion transmissible infections like HIV, HBV, and HCV, etc.
- Documentation is also important.

SHORT NOTES

1. Write purpose of biomedical waste management. (MGR)

Answer

Biomedical waste means any waste, which is generated during the diagnosis, treatment or immunization of human beings or animals or in research activities pertaining thereto or in the production or testing of biologics. —***According to Biomedical Waste (Management and handling) rules,1998 of India***

Purposes

- To minimize the production/generation of infective waste.
- To recycle the waste after treating to the extent possible.
- To treat the waste by safe and environment friendly/acceptable methods.
- To prevent health care associated infections by adequate care handling.
- To follow safety precautions during handling the BMW.
- To prevent the harm resulting from waste.
- To minimize its volume.
- To retrieve reusable materials.
- To ensure safe economical disposal.

2. Write difference between disposable and reusable. (MGR)

Answer

Machinery and equipment are most basic and essential inventory tools used in hospitals for patient care. Handling of equipment in the hospitals is the most important responsibility of the nurses.

Machines and equipment are categorized in two ways:

1. Disposable
2. Reusable

Disposable	Reusable
• Disposable items can be used only once. • One disposable item is for one patient only. • All disposable articles should be discarded after use. • Each time new item is required for each patient. • Disposable articles are made up of a thinner material. • Cleaning, disinfection and sterilization are not meant for them.	• These items/equipment can be used for long time. • Single item can be used for multiple times and for many patients also. • Items can be cleaned, disinfected and sterilized before and after each use. No need to discard them. • Single item can be used for many patients after proper cleaning/disinfection process. • More care and maintenance is required. • Reuse items are made up of a stronger material than disposable products.

3. Write about barrier nursing. (MGR, DU, KUHS, RUHS)

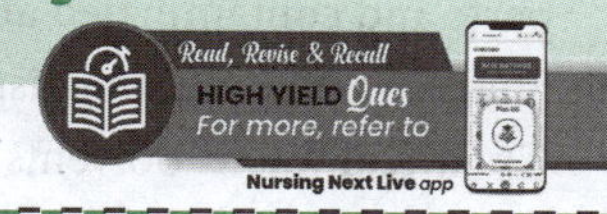

Answer

Definition

The nursing technique by which a patient with an infectious disease is prevented from infecting others is called barrier nursing.

It includes:

- Aseptic technique
- Isolation
- Safer handling of sharps
- Linen handling and disposal
- Waste disposal
- Handling biological spills
- Environmental cleaning
- Risk assessment
- Staff health
- Personal protective equipment (PPE)
  - Personal protective equipment, commonly referred to as "PPE", is equipment worn to minimize exposure to hazards that cause serious workplace injuries and illnesses result from contact with chemical, radiological, physical, electrical, mechanical, or other workplace hazards. PPE protects healthcare workers from Biological agents (virus, bacteria, etc.)
  - Health workers maintain close contact with patients. Thus, they need PPE that protects them from potential transmission. The use of Infection prevention and control (IPC) principles keep patients and health

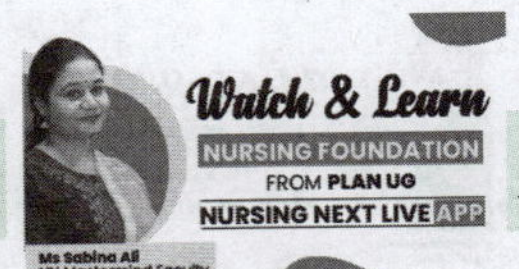

workers safe. IPC includes measures like: Hand hygiene, PPE use and waste management materials.

- Personal protective equipment include items such as gloves, gowns, shoe covers, head covers, masks, respirators, eye protection, face shields, and goggles.

Aseptic Technique

- **Medica asepsis (clean technique):** This is the procedure used to reduce and prevent spread of microorganisms. E.g., Hand washing.
- **Surgical asepsis (sterile technique):** The is procedure used to eliminate microorganisms.

Isolation

Source isolation of infected patients is to prevent airborne transmission *via* respiratory droplets, e.g., pulmonary tuberculosis, etc. and protective isolation is for immune-suppressed patient.

Safer Handling of Sharps

Prevention aspects—Handle with much care;correct disposal in appropriate container. Follow biomedical waste management protocol as per hospital policy.

Linen Handling and Disposal

- Bed making and linen changing techniques.
- Appropriate laundry bags.
- Hazards of on-site ward-based laundering.

Waste Disposal

- Clinical waste—High risk, Potentially/Actually contaminated waste including body fluids and human tissues. Discarded in yellow plastic sack, tied prior to incineration.
- Follow hospital policy.
- Handling biological spills.
- Cover areas with hypochlorite solution for several minutes.
- Clean areas with warm water and detergent, then dry.
- Treat waste as clinical waste—to be discarded in yellow plastic sack.

Environmental Cleaning

Encourage the effective protocol for environmental cleaning within the hospitals so that the cross infection can be prevented. Damp dusting should be used instead of dry dusting.

Risk Assessment

- No risk — routine care.
- Low or moderate risk — wear gloves and plastic apron.
- High risk (Contact/splashing) — wear gloves, plastic apron, gown, eye/face protection.

Staff Health

- Risk of acquiring and transmitting infection
- Immunization
- Cover lesions with waterproof dressings
- Restrict nonimmune/pregnant staff
- Transmitting infection
- Advice when caught infection
- Report accidents/untoward incidents
- Continuous Nursing Education Program
- Routine observation and feedback

4. Write different types of biomedical wastes and its hazards. (MGR, DU, KUHS, RUHS)

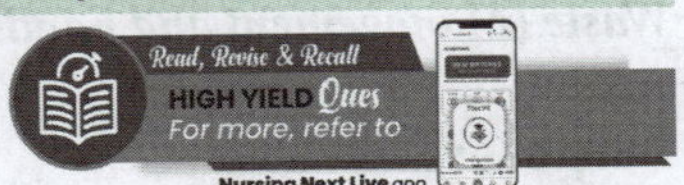

Answer

Types of Biomedical Waste

Biomedical waste means any waste, which is generated during the diagnosis, treatment or immunization of human beings or animals or in research activities pertaining thereto or in the production or testing of biologicals. *—According to Biomedical Waste (Management and handling) rules,1998 of India*

- **Infectious waste:** Waste contaminated with blood and other body fluids (e.g., from discarded diagnostic samples), cultures and stocks of infectious agents from laboratory work (e.g., waste from autopsies and infected animals from laboratories), or waste from patients with infections (e.g., swabs, bandages and disposable medical devices).
- **Pathological waste:** Human tissues, organs or fluids, body parts and contaminated animal carcasses.
- **Sharp waste:** Needles, disposable scalpels and blades, etc.
- **Chemical waste:** Solvents and reagents used for laboratory preparations, disinfectants, sterilants and heavy metals contained in medical devices (e.g., mercury in broken thermometers) and batteries.
- **Pharmaceutical waste:** Expired, unused and contaminated drugs and vaccines.
- **Genotoxic/Cytotoxic waste:** Wastes containing substances with genotoxic properties (i.e., highly hazardous substances that are, mutagenic, teratogenic or carcinogenic), such as cytotoxic drugs used in cancer treatment and their metabolites.
- **Radioactive waste:** Products contaminated by radionuclides including radioactive diagnostic material or radio therapeutic materials.

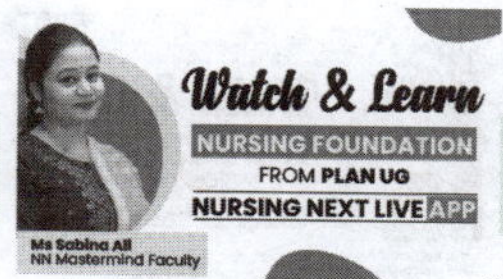

- **Nonhazardous or general waste:** Waste that does not pose any biological, chemical, radioactive or physical hazard.
- **Pressurized waste:** Gas cylinders, gas cartridges, aerosol cans.

Health Hazards

Health care waste can infect hospital patients, health care workers and the general public also. It may cause potential hazards due to drug-resistant microorganisms which can spread from hospitals to the environment.

According to WHO, various health hazards are as follows:

- Sharps-inflicted injuries.
- Toxic exposure to pharmaceutical products (antibiotics and cytotoxic drugs) and substances such as mercury or dioxins, during the handling or incineration of biomedical waste.
- Chemical burns can also occur due to disinfection, sterilization or other waste treatment related activities.
- Air pollution during medical waste incineration.
- Thermal injuries with open burning and incineration of medical waste.
- Radiation burns.

5. Write a short note on Segregation and transportation of hospital waste. (DU, RUHS)

Answer

Segregation

Segregation refers to the basic separation of different categories of waste generated at source and thereby reducing the risks as well as cost of handling and disposal.

Segregation is the most crucial step that ensures effective biomedical waste management.

Cat	Type of bag/container used	Type of waste	Treatment/disposal options
Yellow	Non-chlorinated plastic bags Separate collection system leading to effluent treatment system	• Human anatomical waste • Animal anatomical waste • Soiled waste • Expired or discarded medicines • Chemical waste • Micro, Bio-t and other clinical lab waste • Chemical liquid waste	Incineration or plasma pyrolysis or deep burial
Red	Non-chlorinated plastic bags or containers	**Contaminated waste (Recyclable)** tubing, bottles, intravenous tubes and sets, catheters, urine bags, syringes (without needles) and gloves	Autoclaving/microwaving/ hydroclaving and then sent for recycling not be sent to landfill
White	(Translucent) puncture, leak, tamper proof containers	**Waste sharps including metals**	Auto or dry heat sterilization followed by shredding or mutiation or encapsulation

Contd...

Cat	Type of bag/container used	Type of waste	Treatment/disposal options
Blue	Cardboard boxes with blue colored marking	**Glassware**	Disinfection or autoclaving, microwaving, hydroclaving and then sent for recycling

Importance

- Segregation helps in handling and treatment of specific waste only.
- Segregation prevents the mixing of medical waste with the general municipal waste.
- Prevents illegal reuse of medical wastes.
- Provides an opportunity for recycling after thorough disinfection that can be used for non-food grade applications.
- Reduces the cost of treatment and disposal.

Transportation

- The waste should be transported either in trolleys or in covered wheelbarrow for its management.
- Manual loading should be avoided.
- The biomedical waste bags should be tied/ lidded before its transportation.
- Before transporting, Nurse/ Doctor should document with a signed by mentioning date, shift, quantity and destination of the biomedical waste bag.
- Special vehicles must be used by the transportation operators.
- The transport containers should be closed properly.
- The driver must be trained in the management of an accidental spillage.
- Personnel safety devices should be made mandatory for all the personnel handling waste, e.g., **Gloves, Masks, Boots.**

6. Write a short note on care of sharps. (DU)

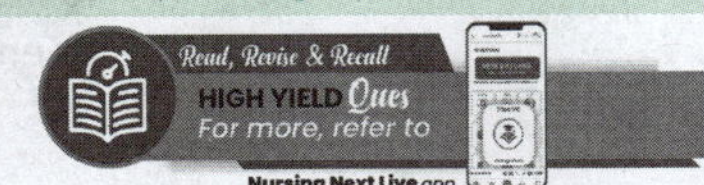

Answer

Care of Sharps

The proper handling and disposal of the used needles and syringes is necessary to prevent the transmission of HIV and other blood-borne diseases.

Collection of the Used Sharps

- A puncture proof container is to be used.
- The puncture proof container should be of such thickness that the deposited sharps should not able to pierce through it.
- The container should have a lid with a small opening.
- The container should be labelled 'BIOHAZARD' with biohazard sign or sticker.
- The box should be filled only till 3/4th of its total capacity.

DO's	DONT'S
• Pick up the sharps carefully. • Deposit the sharps only through the lid. • Collect all the deposited sharps in the thick plastic bag. • The bag should be marked with biohazard sign. • Always use long handed tong to pick up the sharps from the ground. • Always use the puncture proof container till 3/4th of its total capacity.	• Never Recap the needle. • Never hold the needle from its end, always use hub. • Never attempt to cut/ bend the needle before discarding in the puncture proof container. • Never collect the waste bare handed. • Avoid transfer of sharps from one container to another with hands. • Never use the puncture proof container beyond $3/4^{th}$ of its capacity.

7. Write about standard safety precautions. (DU)

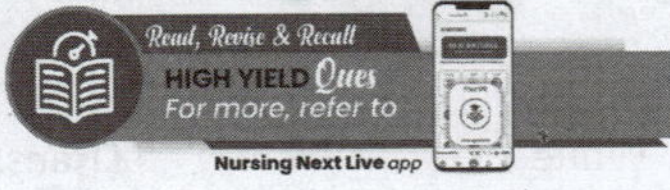

Answer

Standard Safety Precautions

Standard safety measures are a set of infection control practices used to prevent transmission of diseases that can be acquired by contact with blood, body fluids, nonintact skin (including rashes), and mucous membranes.

Standard safety measures are the minimum infection prevention practices that should be used in the care of all

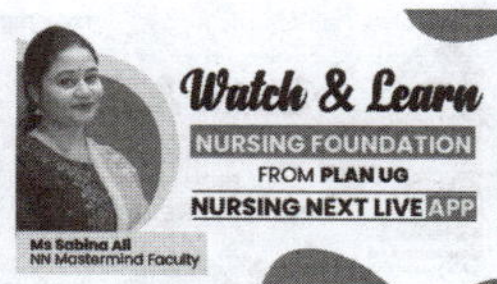

patients all of the time. These practices are designed to both protect the health care professionals and to prevent the health care professionals from the spreading infections among patients.

Elements of standard safety measures are as follows:

- **Hand hygiene:** The most important safety precaution of infection control.
- **Use of PPE:** Such as masks, gloves, gown, etc. act as protective barrier and help in infection control.
- **Needle stick and sharps injury prevention:** Helps in prevention of safety hazards such as transmission of blood-borne viruses (Hepatitis B, Hepatitis C and HIV).
- **Cleaning and disinfection:** To lower the number of cross-infections and also to prevent Health care-associated Infections (HAI).
- **Respiratory hygiene:** To prevent the transmission of all respiratory infections in health care settings.
- **Waste disposal:** *It is necessary to reduce the effect of waste on the environment* and health.
- **Safe injection practice:** *Aimed at maintaining quality care in the hospitals.*

8. Write a short note on principles of Biomedical waste management. (KUHS)

Answer

The principles of Biomedical Waste Management are as follows:

- **Identification of points of waste generation:** recognizing the specific areas or activities within a healthcare facility where biomedical waste is produced
- **Labeling of containers:** Each container or bag of biomedical waste should be clearly labeled with appropriate symbols or signage indicating the type of waste it contains.
- **Segregation at source:** Proper segregation of biomedical waste is crucial to minimize the risk of contamination and prevent the spread of infections.
- **Containment:** Biomedical waste should be stored and transported in leak-proof, puncture-resistant, and labeled containers to prevent spillage, exposure, or release of hazardous materials.
- **Handling and transportation:** Biomedical waste should be handled with proper precautions, including the use of personal protective equipment (PPE), such as gloves and masks.
- **Treatment and disposal:** Biomedical waste should undergo appropriate treatment methods based on its category and potential risks.
- **Waste Minimization and recycling of waste**

9. Write a short note on concurrent disinfection and terminal disinfection. (KUHS)

Answer

Concurrent Disinfection

Concurrent disinfection, also known as continuous disinfection or ongoing disinfection, refers to the practice of regularly and continuously disinfecting high-touch surfaces and equipment within a healthcare setting.

It is performed during routine patient care and is aimed at reducing the risk of transmission of pathogens between patients and healthcare providers.

E.g., disinfection of sputum, urine, feces, vomit, clothes, hands, dressings, apron, gloves.

Terminal Disinfection

Terminal disinfection, also known as discharge or terminal cleaning, is conducted after a patient is discharged or transferred from a healthcare facility. It involves a more comprehensive and thorough disinfection process to ensure that the environment is safe and ready for the next patient.

E.g., disinfection of patient's bed, walls of the room, furniture, etc.

10. Write a short note on source isolation and protective isolation. (KUHS)

Answer

Isolation is defined as the separation of a patient from others in order to control the spread of an infectious or communicable disease.

Source Isolation	Protective Isolation
• Source isolation is the type of isolation used to prevent spread of infection from the patient to other patients and hospital staff. • It requires AIIR (Airborne Infection Isolation Room) or negative pressure room. • It is implemented for patients with communicable disease. • E.g., TB positive patients, patients with SARS, H1N1, etc.	• Protective isolation is the type of isolation used to prevent contact between pathogens and uninfected persons with impaired resistance. • It requires Positive Pressure Room. • It is implemented for immunocompromised patients. • Sick people are not allowed to visit the patient. • Pets and plants are also prohibited. • E.g., oncology patient receiving chemotherapy, HIV patients, etc.

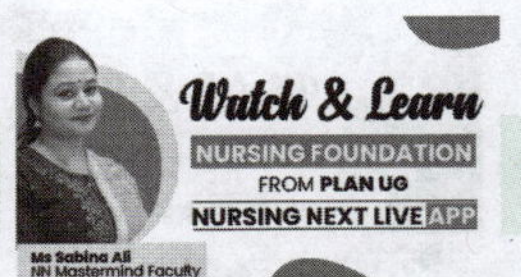

11. Mention the difference between medical and surgical hand washing. (MGR)

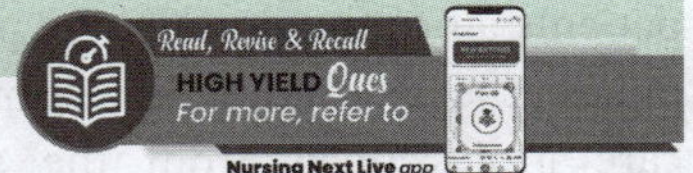

Answer

Difference between medical and surgical hand washing.

Criteria	Medical Hand Washing	Surgical Hand Washing
Purpose	Maintaining clean technique	Maintaining sterile technique
Time period	Hand wash: 40–60 sec, Hand rub: 20–30 sec	2–5 minutes
Number of steps	11 steps for hand wash, 8 steps for hand rub	17 steps
Hygiene	Basic hand hygiene performed	Sterile scrub performed
Field maintenance	Helps in maintaining a clean field	Helps in maintaining a sterile field
Usage	Can be performed before any procedure	Always performed in OTs and in all procedures where aseptic technique is needed

12. Write a short note on the principles of medical asepsis. (DU)

Read, Revise & Recall
HIGH YIELD Ques
For more, refer to
Nursing Next Live app

Answer

Medical asepsis refers to all the practices used to protect the patients and their environment from transmission of disease producing organisms that can transmit from one patient to another. In this, objects are referred to as clean thus, it is also known as clean technique.

Various **principles** of medical asepsis are discussed below:

Control or Elimination of Infectious Agents

- Proper cleaning by water and mechanical action with or without detergents
- Disinfection
- Sterilization of contaminated objects
- Handling linens in ways that prevents germs from spreading

Measures for Control or Elimination of Reservoirs of Infections

- Bathing with soap and water to remove secretion, drainage, perspiration, etc.
- Frequent change of dressings.
- Proper disposal of wastes and contaminated articles.
- Disposal of contaminated needles and syringes.
- Keep the patient's bedside unit clean, dry and biologically safe.
- Bottled solutions should be placed with tight caps as per the instructions.
- Keep drainage tubes and collection bags of the patient to prevent accumulation of serous fluid under the skin surface of surgical wounds.
- Drainage suction bottles should be emptied and disposed off as per the agency policy.

Control of Portals of Exit

- Practice aseptic precautions.
- Avoid talking directly into the client's face to prevent droplet infection.
- Wearing of masks is important as the nurse herself can have infection or may be dealing with clients suffering from infections.
- Careful handling of wastes, like urine, feces, emesis and blood is important.
- Disposable gloves should be worn to prevent direct contact with wastes or infected materials.

Control of Transmission of Infection

- Discourage sharing of bedpans, urinals, basins, eating utensils, etc.
- Use separate thermometers for infectious patients.
- Protect own clothing from direct contact with infected materials.
- Practice handwashing technique.

Control of Portals of Entry

- Maintain integrity of skin and mucous membranes.
- Proper positioning of tubings, etc. may prevent injuries and skin breakdowns.
- Regular skin care is essential with application of lubricants.
- Turning and positioning of debilitated clients help in preventing a skin breakdown.
- Ensure personal hygiene of clients regularly.
- Care should be taken while collecting and handling specimens.

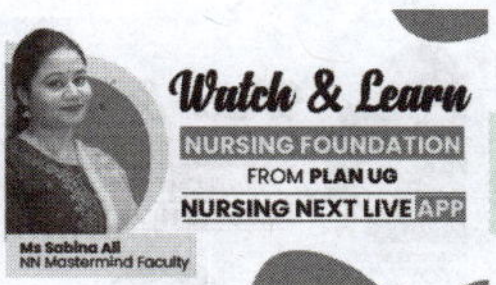

Protection of Susceptible Host

This involves protecting normal defense mechanisms by:

- Proper well-balanced diet.
- Regular oral hygiene.
- Maintaining an adequate fluid intake.
- Encouraging deep breathing and coughing exercises.
- Encouraging proper immunization of children and adult clients.

13. Write a short note on techniques used in surgical asepsis. (DU)

Answer

Techniques Used in Surgical Asepsis

- Always face the sterile field.
- Do not turn your back or side on a sterile field.
- Keep sterile equipment above your waist level or above table level.
- Do not speak, cough or sneeze over a sterile field. If it is necessary to do so, turn your head away from the sterile field.
- Never reach across a sterile field.
- Prevent excessive air currents around the sterile area. Air currents can be caused by moving fast, flapping the clothes and drapes and by closing doors, etc.
- Keep the unsterile objects away from the sterile field.
- Handle liquids cautiously near the sterile field or prevent drapes or wrappers from becoming wet.
- Keep the sterile field dry.
- The edge of the sterile field is considered unsterile.
- Each sterile supply should be clearly labelled as to its contents, time and date of sterilization.
- Never assume that an object is sterile. Always check the sterility, expiration date.
- Avoid sweeping and dusting when the sterile objects are opened.
- Wash hands and put on gowns, gloves and masks before handling the sterile supplies.
- Open the sterile packages in such a way that the edge of the wrapper is directed away from the worker.

Regarding Use of Transfer Forceps

- Hold the transfer forceps pointing downward.
- While removing the forceps from the container, lift it without touching the sides and the rim of the container.
- Keep the prongs (tip) of the forceps within the vision while using it.
- Gently tap the prongs together directly over the container to remove the excess solution.
- Transfer forceps and the container should be sterilized daily.

Regarding Use of Sterile Containers

- Remove the cover from the container when necessary and only for a short period of time.
- Lift the cover of the container in such a way that the inside of the lid is pointing down.
- Invert the cover when it is necessary to place it down.
- Consider the rim of the cover and the container to be contaminated.
- Do not return the unused sterile objects to the container, once it have been taken out.

14. Write a short note on principles of surgical asepsis. (KUHS)

Answer

Principles of Surgical Asepsis

- Operating room personnel must practice strict standard precautions (i.e., blood and body substance isolation).
- All items (e.g., instruments, needles, sutures, dressings, covers, solutions) used in the operating room must be sterile.
- All operating room personnel must perform a surgical scrub.
- All operating room personnel are required to wear specific, clean attire, with the goal of "shedding" the outside environment. Specific clothing requirements are prescribed and standardized for all operating rooms.
    - Operating room personnel must wear a sterile gown, gloves and special shoe covers.
    - Hair must be completely covered.
    - Masks must be worn at all times in the operating room for the purpose of minimizing airborne contamination; they must be changed between operations or more often if necessary.
- Any personnel who harbor pathogenic organisms (e.g., those with colds or infections) must report themselves unable to be in the operating room to protect the client from outside pathogens.
- Scrubbed personnel wearing sterile attire should touch only sterile items.
- Sterile gowns and sterile drapes have defined borders of sterility. Sterile surfaces or articles may touch other sterile surfaces or articles and remain sterile; contact with unsterile objects at any point renders a sterile area contaminated.

- The circulator and unsterile personnel must stay at the periphery of the sterile operating area to keep the sterile area free from contamination.
- The utmost caution and vigilance must be used when handling sterile fluids to prevent splashing or spillage.
- Anything that is used for one client must be discarded or, in some cases, re-sterilized.

15. Write a short note on personal protective equipment. (PPE, DU, KUHS)

Answer

- Personal protective equipment (PPE) refers to protective clothing, helmets, gloves, face shields, goggles, facemasks or other equipment designed to protect from injury or the spread of infection or illness.
- PPE is commonly used in health care settings and acts as a barrier between infectious agents and mucous membranes.
- PPE is equipment used to prevent or minimize exposure to hazards such as Biological hazards, Chemical hazards, Radiological hazards, etc.

Main characteristics of PPE include:

Category	Characteristic
Design feature	• Protects mucous membranes. • Minimizes the number of PPE element junctions. • Provides unobstructed range of vision. • Enables communication capability. • Use human factors design for size and comfort.
Material performance	• Able to protect for the duration of work period. • Able to withstand repeated disinfection. • Manufacture packaging to withstand tropical climate exposure.
Use desirability	• Standardize donning and doffing protocol with minimum steps. • Dispose PPE in nontoxic and environment-friendly manner.

Types of PPE

- **Gloves:** Gloves can protect the health care professionals against contamination with infectious material.
  - **Thick rubber:** Cleaning or housekeeping purposes.
  - **Clean gloves:** General contact with the patient and for the surroundings of the patients.
  - **Sterile gloves:** Maintain strict aseptic techniques during specimen collection and while performing any surgical procedure on patients.
- **Gowns** are generally for clothing, but aprons are used where contamination is limited.
- **Masks** should fully cover the nose and mouth. Masks should fit snugly.
- **Shoe covers** can be used to prevent contamination of footwear.
- **Goggles** provide barrier protection for the eyes and should fit snuggly over and around the eyes.
- **Face shield** can act as a substitute to wearing a mask or goggles. The face shield should cover the forehead, extend below the chin, and wrap around the side of the face.

16. What are the stages of infection? (MGR, DU, KUHS, RUHS)

Read, Revise & Recall HIGH YIELD Ques For more, refer to Nursing Next Live app

Answer

There are four stages of infection:

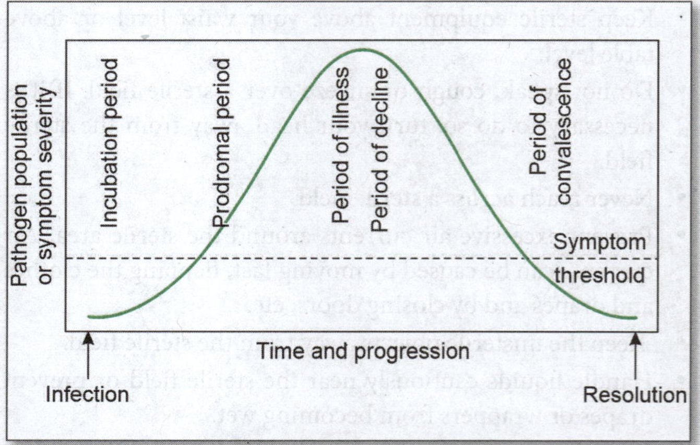

1. **Incubation period:** It is the time period between entrance of pathogen into body and appearance of first symptoms, e.g., Chicken pox 2–3 weeks. Common cold for 1–2 days.
2. **Prodromal stage:** Interval from the onset of nonspecific signs and symptoms to more specific symptoms. Microorganisms grow and multiply and the client is more capable of spreading disease to others during this time.
3. **Illness stage:** Interval when the client manifests sign and symptoms specific to the type of infection.
4. **Convalescence stage:** Interval when acute symptoms of an infection disappear, length of recovery depends on severity of infection and the client's general state of health. Recovery may take several days to month.

17. Write a short note on hazards and prevention of needle stick injury. (DU)

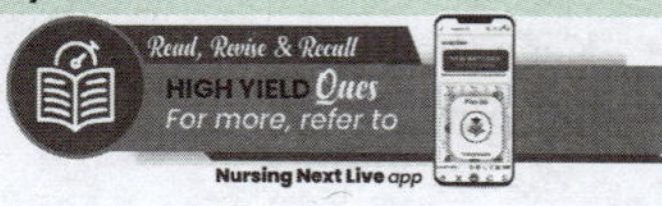

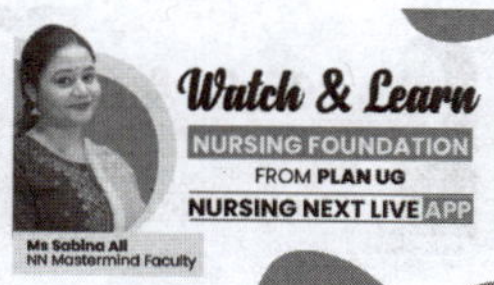

Answer

Needle Stick Injury

Needle stick and other sharps injuries are a serious hazard in any health care setting. Contact with contaminated needles, scalpels, broken glass, and other sharps may expose health care workers to blood that contains pathogens which pose a grave, potentially lethal risk.

Activities with Potential for Needlestick Injuries

Health care workers can be at risk for needle stick or sharps injuries when they:

- Handle needles that must be taken apart or discarded after use.
- Dispose of needles attached to tubing.
- Manipulate the needle in the client.
- Recap a needle.
- Use needles or glass equipment to transfer body fluid between containers.
- Fail to dispose off used needles in puncture-resistant sharps containers.
- Lack proper workstations for procedures using sharps.
- Work quickly.
- Bump into a needle, a sharp, or another worker while either person is holding a sharp.

Various Hazards Include

Most needle stick injuries (NSIs) involve doctors, nurses and laboratory staff. These injuries can transmit severe blood borne pathogens into your bloodstream. The list of pathogens includes:

- **Major Pathogens**
  - Hepatitis B virus (HBV)
  - Hepatitis C virus (HCV)
  - Human immunodeficiency virus (HIV)
- **Other Pathogens**
  - Human T-lymphotropic viruses (HTLV I and II)
  - Hepatitis D virus (HDV or delta agent, which is activated in the presence of HBV)
  - Hepatitis G virus (GB virus or GBV-C)
  - Cytomegalovirus (CMV)
  - Epstein-Barr virus (EBV)
  - Transfusion-transmitted virus (TTV)
  - West Nile virus (WNV)
  - Malarial parasites
  - Prion agents
  - Blastomycosis
  - Cryptococcosis
  - Diptheria
  - Ebola
  - Leptospirosis
  - *Mycobacterium tuberculosis*

Prevention of Needle Stick Injury

- Avoid recapping or bending needles that might be contaminated.
- Use standard-labeled, leak-proof, puncture-resistant sharps containers.
- Promptly dispose off used needle devices and sharps.
- Plan for the safe handling and disposal of needles before use.
- Store sharps containers out of the reach of children, pets, and others not needing access.
- Secure used sharps containers during transport to prevent spilling.
- Follow standard precautions, infection prevention, and general hygiene practices consistently.
- Participate in your employer's blood borne pathogens training program.
- Report any needle stick and other sharps injury immediately to the Infection Control Nurse.

After Needle Stick Injury, Immediately follow these Steps

- Wash with soap and water.
- Do not panic.
- Do not apply any emollient/antiseptics to the injured area.
- Flush splashes to the nose, mouth, or skin with water.
- Irrigate eyes with clean water, saline, or sterile irrigants.
- Report the incident to your supervisor.
- Immediately seek medical treatment.

18. Write a short note on modes of indirect transmission of infection. (KUHS)

Answer

Modes of Indirect Transmission

Indirect transmission can occur through vehicle-borne, vector-borne or airborne.

- **Vehicle-borne transmission:** Contaminated materials such as food, clothes, bedding and cooking utensils.

- **Vector-borne transmission:** Agent is carried by an insect or animal (the vector) to a susceptible host; the agent may or may not multiply in the vector.
- **Long-distance airborne transmission:** Dissemination of very small droplets to a suitable point of entry, such as respiratory tract. Dust particles also facilitate airborne transmission, for example- fungal spores.

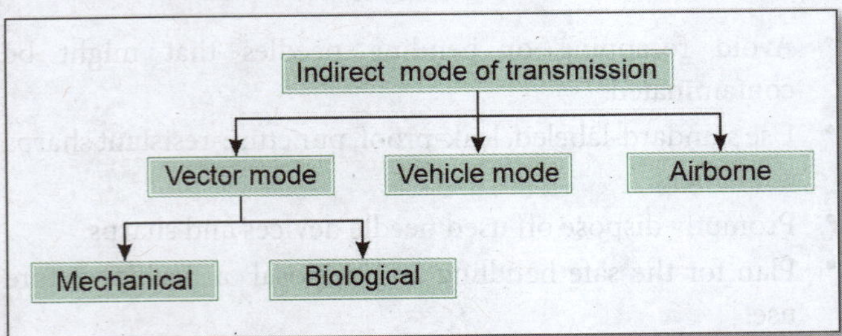

Vehicle-Borne Mode of Transmission

- Vehicles indirectly transmit an infectious agent (food, water, biological products (blood), and fomites (inanimate objects such as handkerchiefs, bedding, or surgical scalpels).
- A vehicle may passively carry a pathogen. Alternatively, the vehicle may provides an environment in which the agent grows, multiplies, or produces toxin.

Vectors-Borne Mode of Transmission

- Vectors such as mosquitoes, fleas, and ticks may carry an infectious agent. Mechanical means may support growth or changes in the agent such as flies carrying Shigella on their appendages and fleas carrying *Yersinia pestis*, the causative agent of plague, in their gut.
- In contrast, in biological transmission, the causative agent of malaria or guinea worm disease undergoes maturation in an intermediate host before it can be transmitted to humans.

Airborne transmission

- It occurs by dust or droplet nuclei suspended in the air.
- Droplet nuclei are dried residue of droplets, less than 5 microns in size.
- In contrast to droplets that fall to the ground within a few feet, droplet nuclei may remain suspended in the air for long periods of time and may be blown over great distances. For e.g., Measles disease.

19. Universal precautions. (MGR, DU, KUHS, RUHS)

Answer

Introduction

Universal precautions refer to the practice of avoiding contact with patients' body fluids, by means of the wearing nonporous articles (gloves, goggles, and face shields, etc.)

- This practice was introduced in 1985–88.
- In 1987, the practice of universal precautions was adjusted by a set of rules termed as Body substance isolation.
- Under universal precautions all patients are considered as possible carriers of blood-borne pathogens.
- Universal Precautions is applicable to all those patients who are infected with Blood borne pathogens. For Example: HIV, HbsAg, and HCV. In 1996, both practices were replaced by standard precautions.

Universal Precautions

- **Use barrier protection:** Cover up any wounds or sores before proceedings.
- **Wear gloves:** While handling body fluids or contaminated materials and other waste.
- Wear a face mask/gown
- Use caution When handling sharp objects, needles and waste.
- **Discard contaminated materials:** Follow biohazard procedures for disposal.
- Clean area thoroughly with disinfectant.
- Wash Hands thoroughly with soap and water for at least 20 seconds.
- Wash clothing in hot water.

Standard Precautions

The set of precautionary measures including good hand hygiene practices and use of protective barriers during routine patient care carried out by health care workers.

Standard precaution consists of:

- Hand washing
- Gloving
- Gowning
- Mask/protective eye wear/cap
- Shoe cover

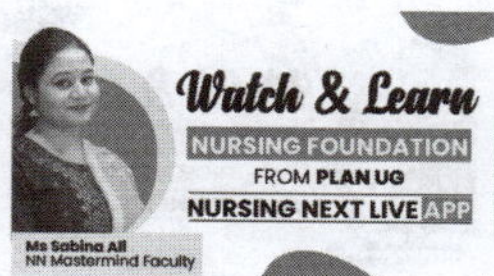

20. Write the differences between antiseptic and disinfectant. (MGR)

Answer

Differences between antiseptic and disinfectant

Parameter	Antiseptics	Disinfectants
Definition	Chemical agents applied to living tissues (animal and human tissues)	Chemical agents applied to inanimate objects or surfaces (floor, instruments, equipment, etc.)
Mode of action	Kill or inhibit growth of microorganisms on skin or wound	Kill or inhibit growth of microorganisms on surfaces
Examples	Hydrogen peroxide, Povidone-iodine, alcohol 70%	Bleaching powder, quaternary ammonium compounds, phenols,
Concentration	Lower concentration than disinfectants	Higher concentration than antiseptics
Toxicity	Generally less toxic than disinfectants	Generally more toxic than antiseptics
Safety for humans	Safe for use on human skin or wounds	Not always safe for use on human skin
Uses	Used for hand hygiene, wound cleaning, and skin preparation	Used for cleaning and disinfecting surfaces and objects

Examples:

- **Antiseptic:** Dettol and savlon
- **Disinfectant:** Hypochlorite solution and Lysol

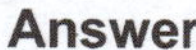

21. Write a short note on Infection control. (MGR, DU, KUHS, RUHS)

Answer

Infection

- Infection is defined as the invasion of tissue by pathogenic microorganisms that proliferate, resulting in tissue injury that can progress to disease.
- The invasion and multiplication of microorganisms (bacteria, viruses, and parasites) within the body.

Infection Control is the prevention of the transmission of microorganisms in a hospital from:

- Patient to patient
- Patient to staff member
- Staff member to patient
- Staff member to staff member

Breaking the chain of infection:

- The only way to prevent and control the infection is to break the chain of infection.
- Breaking the chain includes:
  - Rapid and accurate identification of organism.
  - Control or elimination of infectious agents including disinfection, environmental cleaning, handling of linen, pest control, visitors control.
  - Practice aseptic precaution, contact precautions, droplet precautions and airborne precautions.
  - Maintain integrity of skin and mucous membrane.
  - Ensure personal hygiene.
  - Proper waste disposal.
  - Maintaining healing process.

Various measures to control infection:

- Stop at the source
- Block the portal of exit
- Interrupt mode of transportation
- Protect portal of entry
- Increase host's defenses

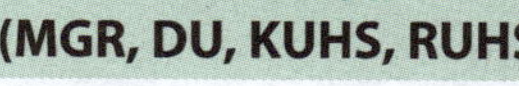

22. Mention four types of hospital wastes. (MGR, DU, KUHS, RUHS)

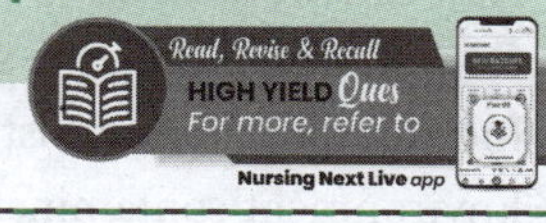

Answer

Four Types of Hospital Waste

1. Infectious wastes

- Human Anatomical waste
- Microbiology and biotechnology waste.
- Animal waste
- Laboratory waste

2. Chemical wastes/Pharmaceutical wastes

- Cytotoxic waste
- Discarded medicines.
- Incineration ash, any waste from disinfecting objects

3. Radioactive wastes (hazardous pharmaceutical wastes)
4. Sharp wastes

23. Write a short note on nosocomial infection. (MGR, DU, KUHS, RUHS)

Answer

Introduction

- Nosocomial infection derived from Greek words "**nosus**"- disease and "**komeion**" - to take care of.
- Also known as **hospital acquired infection** (HAI) of Health care-associated Infections **Nosocomial infection** can be defined as an infection acquired by a patient during the process of care (including preventive, diagnostic and treatment services) in a hospital or other health-care facility, which was not present or incubating at the time of admission.
- HAIs can also occur after discharge of the patient.
- It can also be acquired by health care professionals, during health care delivery, and by the visitors.
- Infections are considered nosocomial if first appear **after 48 hours or more after hospital admission** or **within 30 days after discharge**

Types

Common types of hospital-acquired infections include:
- Urinary tract infections (UTIs)
- Surgical site infections (SSIs)
- Central line-Associated Bloodstream Infections (CLABSIs)
- Ventilator-Associated Pneumonia (VAP)

Causes

- Crowded hospitals
- New microorganism
- Compromised immune system
- Increased bacterial resistance
- Environment contamination
- Poor hand hygiene or infection control practices
- Invasive medical procedures

Modes of Transmission

- Contact
- Vector borne
- Air borne
- Droplet
- Common vehicle

SHORT ANSWER QUESTIONS

1. Define Universal precautions and Standard precautions. (MGR, DU, KUHS, RUHS)

Answer

- **Universal precautions** refer to the practice of avoiding contact with patients' body fluids, by means of the wearing nonporous articles (gloves, goggles, and face shields, etc.)
- **Standard precautions** are the set of precautionary measures including good hand hygiene practices and use of protective barriers during routine patient care carried out by health care workers.

Standard precaution consists of:
- Hand washing
- Gloving
- Gowning
- Mask/protective eye wear/cap
- Shoe cover

2. What is bio-medical waste management and its purpose. (MGR)

Answer

Biomedical waste means any waste, which is generated during the diagnosis, treatment or immunization of human beings or animals or in research activities pertaining thereto or in the production or testing of biological. *—According to Biomedical waste (Management and handling) rules, 1998 of India*

Purpose of Biomedical Waste Management

- To minimize the production/generation of infective waste.
- To recycle the waste after treating to the extent possible.
- To treat the waste by safe and environment friendly/ acceptable methods.
- To prevent health care- associated infections by adequate care handing.
- To follow safety precautions during handling the BMW.
- To prevent the harm resulting from waste.
- To minimize its volume.
- To retrieve reusable materials.
- To ensure safe economical disposal.

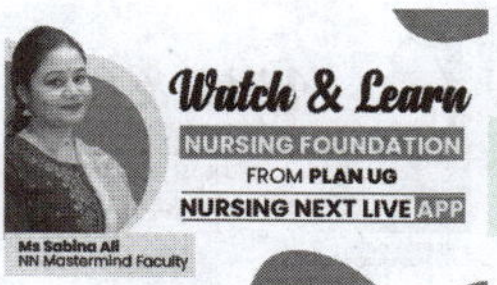

3. Define infection control. (MGR, DU, KUHS, RUHS)

Answer

Infection is defined as the invasion of tissue by pathogenic microorganisms that proliferate, resulting in tissue injury that can progress to disease.

- The invasion and multiplication of microorganisms (bacteria, viruses, and parasites) within the body.

Infection Control is the prevention of the transmission of microorganisms in a hospital from:

- Patient to patient
- Patient to Staff member
- Staff member to patient
- Staff member to staff member

4. Define barrier nursing. (MGR, DU, KUHS, RUHS)

Answer

Definition: The nursing technique by which a patient with an infectious disease is prevented from infecting others is called barrier nursing.

It includes:

- Aseptic technique
- Isolation
- Safer Handling of Sharps
- Linen handling and disposal, etc.

5. Define Surgical asepsis and Medical asepsis. (MGR, DU, KUHS, RUHS)

Answer

Surgical Asepsis

Surgical asepsis is a sterile technique. It is a state of being free from all pathogenic organisms and prevent entry of any organism into an open wound or sterile body cavity.

Medical Asepsis (Clean Technique)

Medical asepsis is the state of being free from disease causing microorganisms which is concerned with elimination of the spread of microorganisms through practices.

CONCEPTUAL REVISION

MULTIPLE CHOICE QUESTIONS

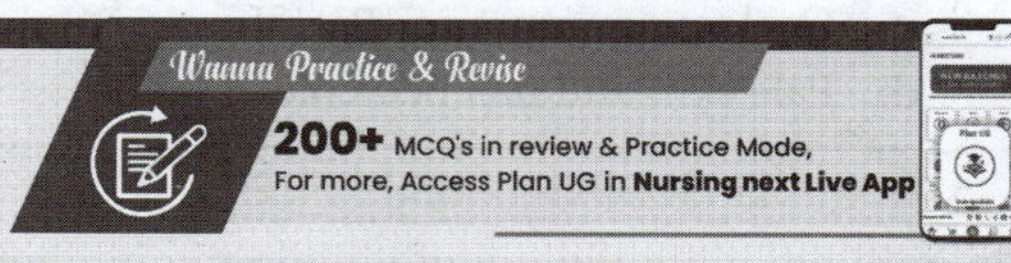

1. What is the most effective way to control transmission of infection?

a. Isolated precautions
b. Identifying the infectious agents
c. Hand hygiene practices
d. Vaccinations

Ans. c. Hand hygiene practices

2. A patient is diagnosed with methicillin-resistant *Staphylococcus aureus* (MRSA) pneumonia. Which type of isolation precaution is most appropriate for this patient?

a. Reverse isolation
b. Droplet precautions
c. Standard precautions
d. Contact precautions

Ans. b. Droplet precautions

3. When should a nurse wear a mask?

i. When patient's dental hygiene is poor.
ii. When the nurse is assisting with an aerosolizing respiratory procedure such as suctioning.
iii. When patient has AIDS and a congested cough.
iv. When patient is in droplet precautions.
v. When nurse is assisting a health care provider in the insertion of a central line catheter.

a. i, ii, v
b. ii, iii, iv
c. ii, iv, v
d. iii, iv, v

Ans. c. ii, iv, v

4. Put the following steps for removal of protective barriers after leaving an isolation room in order:

i. Remove mask
ii. Remove gloves
iii. Remove eyewear or goggles
iv. Remove gown

a. i, iii, iv, ii
b. i, ii, iii, iv
c. iii, i, ii, iv
d. ii, iv, iii, i

Ans. d. ii, iv, iii, i

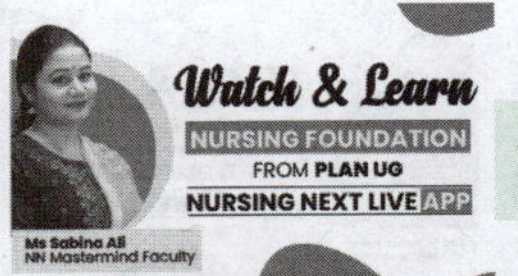

5. Which of the following statements are true regarding disinfection and cleaning?

i. Proper cleaning requires mechanical removal of all soil from an object or area
ii. General environmental cleaning is an example of medical asepsis
iii. When cleaning a wound, wipe around the wound edge first and then clean inward toward the center of the wound
iv. Cleaning in a direction from the least to the most contaminated area helps reduce infections.
v. Disinfecting and sterilizing medical devices and equipment involve the same procedures.

a. i, ii, iv
b. i, iii, v
c. ii, iii, iv
d. iii, iv, v

Ans. a. i, ii, iv

6. .... are type of HAI caused by an invasive diagnostic of therapeutic procedure.

a. Exogenous infection
b. Endogenous infection
c. Iatrogenic infection
d. Immunosenescence

Ans. c. Iatrogenic infection

7. Which physical assessment finding is most indicative of a systemic infection?

a. Nasal drainage
b. Bilateral 3+ pitting pedal edema
c. Oral temperature of 101.1°F
d. Pale skin and nail bed color

Ans. c. Oral temperature of 101.1°F

8. A patient is being admitted to a medical unit with a diagnosis of tuberculosis. Which type of room should this patient is assigned by the nurse?

a. Private room
b. Semiprivate room
c. Room with windows that can be opened
d. Negative airflow room

Ans. d. Negative airflow room

9. A surgical patient develops a wound infection during hospitalization. How is this type of infection classified?

a. Primary
b. Secondary
c. Superimposed
d. Nosocomial

Ans. d. Nosocomial

10. Autoclaving is also known as:

a. Dry heat sterilization
b. Moist heat sterilization
c. Flaming
d. Hot air oven

Ans. b. Moist heat sterilization

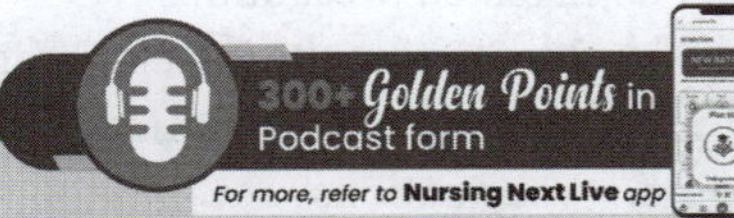

Golden Points

- An infection is the entry and multiplication of an infectious agent in the tissues of the host.
- Disease-producing microorganisms are called pathogens.
- Hospital acquired infections can be iatrogenic infections, exogenous infection and endogenous infection.
- Individuals normally have defenses that protect the body from infection. These defenses can be specific and nonspecific.
- Pathogenicity refers to the ability of a microorganism to produce disease.
- Virulence refers to the frequency with which a pathogen causes disease.
- Wastes can be Municipal waste, Biomedical waste and Hazardous waste. Moreover, the biomedical waste includes Infectious waste and Noninfectious waste.

CHAPTER

9

Comfort, Rest and Sleep and Pain

CONCEPTUAL THEORY

Terminology

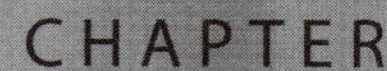

Admission bed: This is the bed prepared to receive a newly admitted patient.

Amputation/divided bed: It is a bed in which top linen is divided into two parts to visualize the amputed part of the lower limbs without disturbing the patient.

Bed: The bed is the equipment used most by a patient, therefore, it should be designed for comfort, safety and adaptability for changing positions.

Bed making: It is a procedure or technique in which different types of beds are prepared to make the patient comfortable according to the situations and procedures.

Bruxism: It is characterized by clenching and grinding of the teeth that occurs during stage II-NREM sleep.

Cardiac bed: A bed prepared for patients with cardiac diseases.

Central apnea occurs due to defect in the respiratory center of the brain.

Closed bed: It is an unoccupied or empty bed made to receive the patient and is fully covered with counter pane to protect it from dust and dirt. On admission of the patient, the closed bed is converted into an open bed.

Comfort devices: It is are the mechanical devices planned to provide optimal comfort to an individual.

Comfort: The absence of irritating stimuli that distract one's attention from the task at hand.

Dolorimeter: Instrument is used to measure pain threshold and pain tolerance.

Dysomnias: The sleep is normal but patient sleeps too little, too much, or may be at the incorrect time.

Enuresis or Bed-wetting usually occurs in children over 3-year-old and commonly 1 to 2 hours after falling asleep.

Fracture bed: It is a bed which is prepared for patients with fracture, bone diseases and deformity.

Hypersomnia: Refers to conditions that include sufficient sleep at night but still cannot stay awake during the day.

Insomnia: It is inability to fall asleep in which client remains awake and not feeling rested. Insomnia is the most common sleep complaint.

Insufficient Sleep/Sleep Deprivation is defined as the prolonged disturbance in quality and quantity of sleep.

Mixed apnea: It is combination of obstructive and central apnea.

Modulation: Modulation is the process of dampening or amplifying these pain-related neural signs. Modulation takes place primarily in the dorsal horn of spinal cord, but also elsewhere, with input from ascending and descending pathways.

Narcolepsy: It is a disorder of excessive daytime sleepiness. It is mainly occurring due to lack of the chemical hypocretin in CNS.

Obstructive apnea: Occurs when the anatomical structures of respiratory system such as pharynx or oral cavity block the air flow.

Occupied bed: This bed is made with the patient in it.

Open bed: It is a bed, made when it is about to be occupied by either a new patient or an ambulatory patient.

Pain scale: A **pain scale** measures a patient's pain intensity or other features. Pain scales are based on self-report, observational (behavioral), or physiological data.

Pain: The International Association for the Study of Pain (IASP) defines pain as a "sensory and emotional experience associated with tissue damage or described in terms of such damage."

Parasomnias: Something occurrence of abnormal during sleep itself, or during the times when the patient is falling asleep or waking up.

Perception: Perception refers to the subjective experience of pain that results from interaction of transduction, transmission, modulation, and the psychological aspects of the individual.

Periodic limb movement disorder (PLMD): In this condition, the legs jerk twice or thrice per minute during sleep.

Placebo effect: Occurs when a person responds to the medication or other treatment because of an expectation that the treatment will work rather than it actually does so.

Placebo: It is an inactive substance that looks like the drug or treatment being tested. Placebo has no therapeutic properties.

Contd...

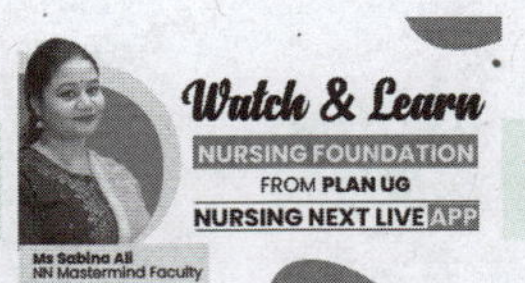

Postoperative bed: It is a bed prepared for a patient who is recovering from the effects of anesthesia following surgery.
Sleep apnea: It is characterized by frequent short breathing pauses or periods of apnea during sleep.
Sleep It is a state of rest accompanied by altered level of consciousness and relative inactivity and decreased perception to environment.
Sleep talking: In this, talking occurs during NREM sleep.
Sleepwalking or somnambulism occurs during stages III and IV of sleep cycle.
Transduction: It is the process by which afferent nerve endings participate in translating noxious stimuli into nociceptive impulses.
Transmission: Transmission is the process by which impulses are sent to the dorsal horn of spinal cord and then along the sensory tracts to the brain.

COMFORT

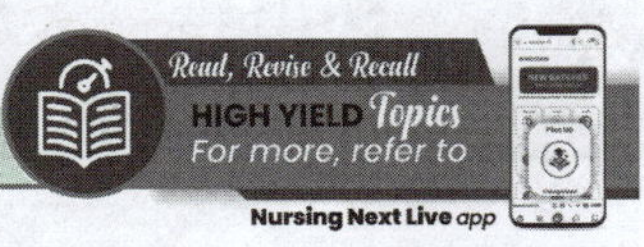

Nursing care meets all client's needs. The client's most important basic need is comfort.

The absence of irritating stimuli that distract one's attention from the task at hand. **Comfort devices** are the mechanical devices planned to provide optimal comfort to an individual. Various comfort devices are as follows:

- Pillows
- Back rest
- Bed cradle
- Cardiac table
- Mattresses
- Trapeze bar
- Footboard
- Trochanter rolls
- Sandbags
- Wedge/abductor pillow
- Knee rest
- Bed blocks
- Air cushion
- Rubber and cotton rings
- Hand rolls

Types of bed	Image	Description
Open bed	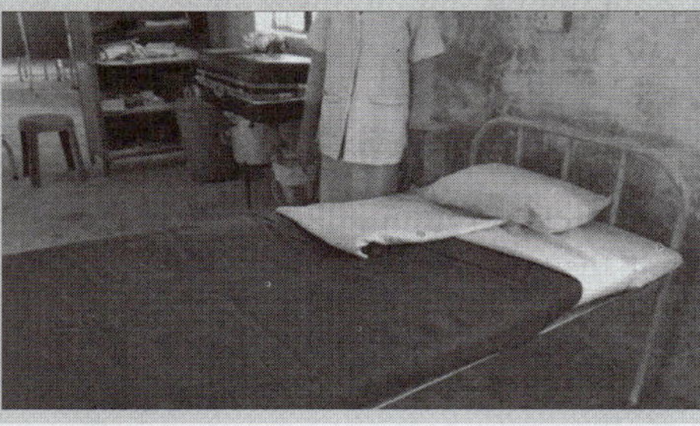	It is a bed, when it is about to be occupied by either a new patient or an ambulatory patient. Most beds are made when they are unoccupied.
Closed bed	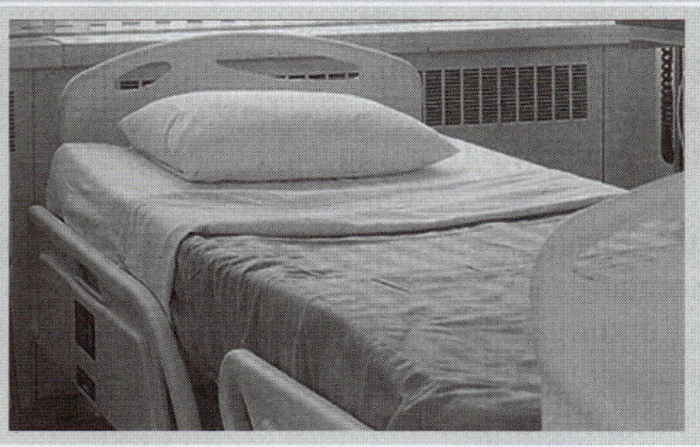	It is an unoccupied bed made to receive the patient and is fully covered with bed spread to protect it from dust and dirt. On admission of the patient, the closed bed is converted into an open bed.
Postoperative bed	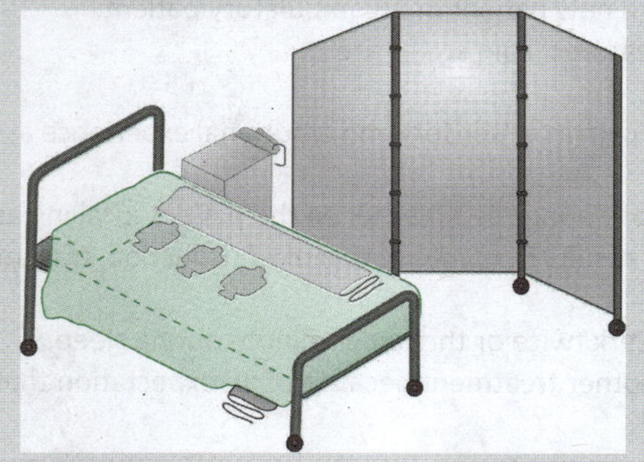	It is a bed prepared for a patient who is recovering from the effects of anesthesia following surgery.

Contd...

Types of bed	Image	Description
Cardiac bed	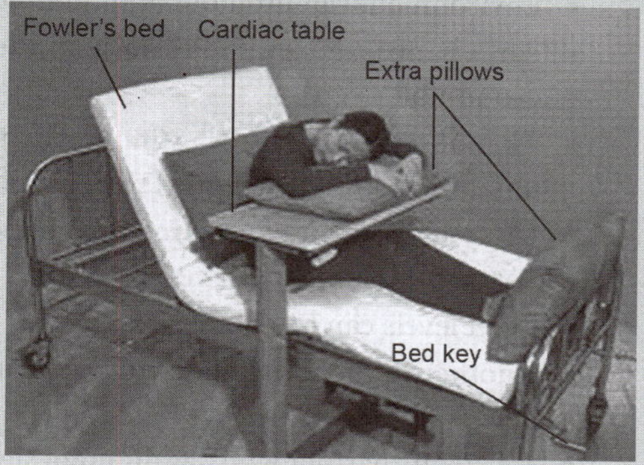	It is a bed prepared for patients with cardiac diseases
Amputation/ Divided/ Cradle bed	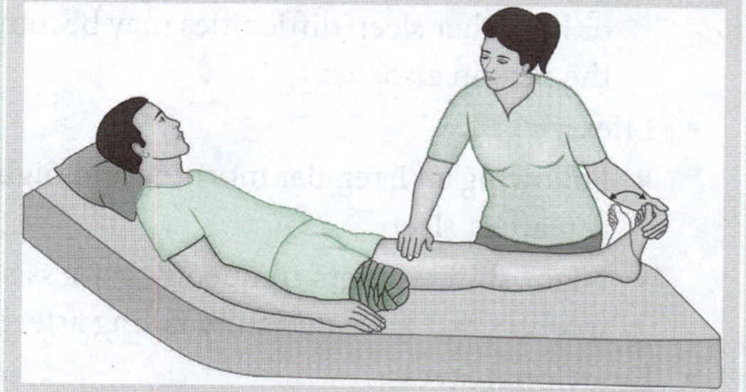	It is a bed in which top linen is divided into two parts to visualize the amputated part of the lower limbs without disturbing the patient.
Fracture bed	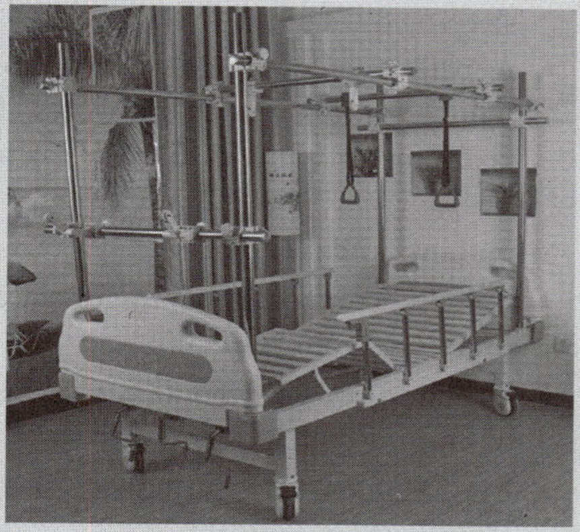	It is a bed which is prepared for patients with fracture, bone diseases and deformity.
Burn bed	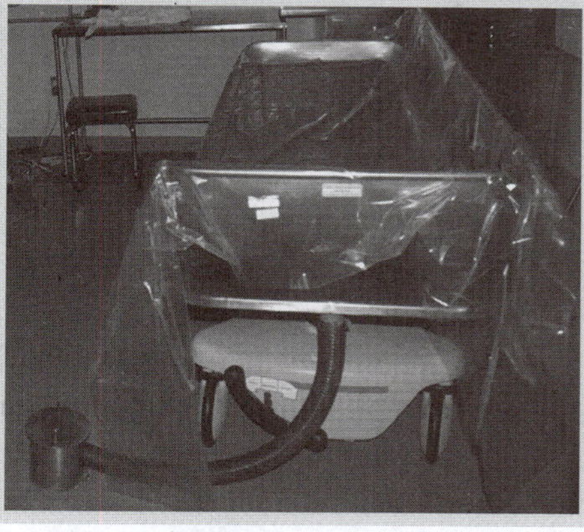	A burn recovery bed or burn bed is a special type of bed designed for patients who have severe skin burns across large portions of the body. It consists of a long bed cradle which takes of bed linen weight from all over the body.

Factors Influencing Comfort

Individual comfort and performance levels of a person are influenced by a number of factors such as:

- Physical Factors
- Environmental Factors
- Psychological Factors
- Sociocultural Factors

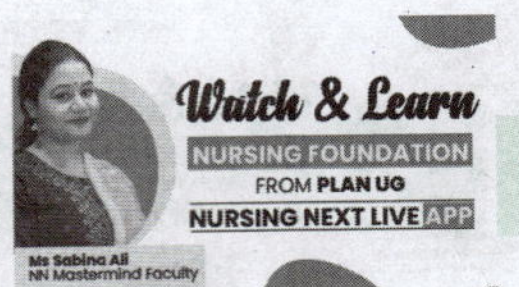

Physical Factors

- They involve all the aspects of an individual.
- They include need for food, water, oxygen, elimination of waste products from body.
- Physical factors such as mobility, personal care (cleanliness of body, oral care, hair, clean clothes), indulging in diversional activities, having a sound sleep of 6–8 hours, having a comfortable bed with clean and wrinkle free bed sheets adds to the physical comfort of a person.
- Other physical comfort measures are freedom from pain.
- Lack of exercise can be the source of discomfort.

Environmental Factors

- They involve the how hot or how cold the environment is.
- Human beings like to be in the range of 70–80°F, fresh air, decreased noise levels, humidity levels within comfortable limits. Too bright light and glares, unpleasant odors and any kind of radiation are some of the factors concerning environment.

Psychological Factors

It involve self-esteem, identity, sexuality, relationships, effective communication and sense of safety and security.

Inability to full fill these factors may be a source of discomfort to the client.

Sociocultural Factors

They involve family, societal and interpersonal relationships, traditions rituals and religious factors.

Information about the disease condition, interaction with hospital staff, family presence and support and friends influence the comfort of person.

SLEEP

Sleep is a state of rest accompanied by altered level of consciousness and relative inactivity, and decreased perception to environment.

Factors Affecting Sleep

Read, Revise & Recall HIGH YIELD Topics For more, refer to Nursing Next Live app

Both the quality and the quantity of sleep are affected by a number of factors.

Sleep quality is a subjective characteristic.

Quantity of sleep is the total time for which the individual sleeps.

- **Age**
- **Illness**: Illness that causes pain or physical distress (e.g., arthritis, back pain) or respiratory problems can result in sleep problem.
- **Environment**
  - Environment can promote or hinder sleep
  - Any change—for example, noise in the environment—can inhibit sleep.
  - The absence of usual stimuli or the presence of unfamiliar stimuli can prevent people from sleeping.
  - Discomfort from environmental temperature (e.g., too hot or cold) and lack of ventilation can affect sleep.
  - Light levels can be another factor.
  - Another influence includes the comfort and size of the bed.
  - A person's partner who has different sleep habits, snores, or has other sleep difficulties may become a problem for the person also.
- **Lifestyle:**
  - Following an irregular morning and night time schedule can affect sleep.
  - Night shift workers frequently get less sleep than other workers and have difficulty falling asleep.
- **Emotional Stress:**
  - Stress is considered to be the major cause of short-term sleeping difficulties
  - A person preoccupied with personal problems (e.g., school- or job-related pressures, family or marriage problems) may be unable to relax sufficiently to get to sleep.
- **Stimulants and Alcohol:**
  - Caffeine-containing beverages act as stimulants of the central nervous system (CNS).
  - Drinking beverages containing caffeine in the afternoon or evening may interfere with sleep.
  - Even though alcohol induces sleep, it disturbs REM sleep causing irritability.
- **Diet:** Certain foods induce sleep such as milk.
- **Smoking:**
  - Nicotine has a stimulating effect on the body, and smokers often have more difficulty falling asleep than non-smokers.
  - Smokers can be easily aroused.
- **Motivation:**
  - Motivation can increase alertness in some situations for example, during the time of examination browsing, internet in the late night.
- **Medications:**
  - Beta-blockers have been known to cause insomnia.
  - Narcotics, such as morphine, are known to suppress REM sleep and to cause frequent awakening and drowsiness.
  - Most hypnotics suppress REM sleep.

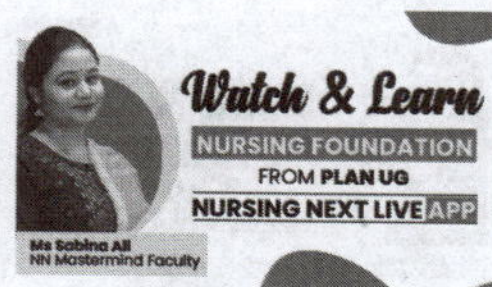

Stages of Sleep

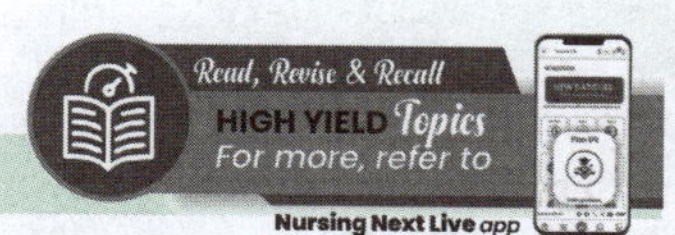

In order to identify stages of sleep, Electroencephalogram (EEG) patterns, eye movements and the muscle activity are widely used.

The stages of sleep are classified into two stages:

1. Nonrapid Eye Movement (NREM) Sleep
2. Rapid Eye Movement (REM) Sleep

Nonrapid Eye Movement (NREM) Sleep

- It is known as first stage of sleep.
- About 75% to 80% of sleep during a night is NREM sleep.

It consists of four stages:

Stage 1

- Stage 1 lasts for a few minutes.
- It is lightest level of sleep, characterized by gradual fall in vital signs and slowing of EEG frequency.
- Eyes tend to roll slowly from side to side.
- Sensory stimuli such as noise easily arouse person.
- Sleeper may also deny that he is sleeping.

Stage 2

- Stage 2 lasts for 10 to 20 minutes.
- Period of sound sleep in which relaxation progresses with slowing of EEG.
- Eye ball movements will be absent.
- Body functions continue to slow down.
- Arousal remains relatively easy.

Stage 3

- Stage 3 lasts for 15 to 30 minutes.
- Initial stage of deep sleep.
- Muscles are completely relaxed and large slow waves in EEG.
- Vital signs decline but regular.
- Difficult to arouse sleeper.

Stage 4

- Stage 4 lasts for approximately 15–30 minutes.
- It is deepest stage of sleep.
- Vital signs are significantly lower and slowing of EEG.
- Sleepwalking and enuresis (bed-wetting) sometimes occur.
- Very difficult to arouse sleeper.

REM Sleep

- Usually begins about 90 minutes after sleep has begun.
- Dreaming occurs in this stage.
- It involves rapid eyes movement, fluctuating heart rate, respiratory rates, blood pressure, loss of skeletal muscle tone, and increased gastric secretions.
- EEG pattern resembles awake state.
- Very difficult to arouse sleeper.

PAIN

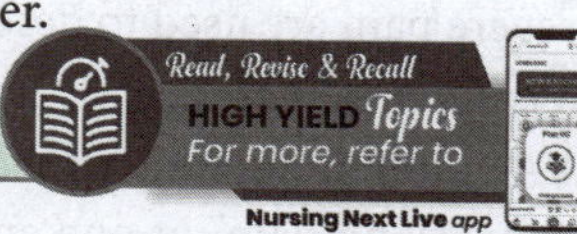
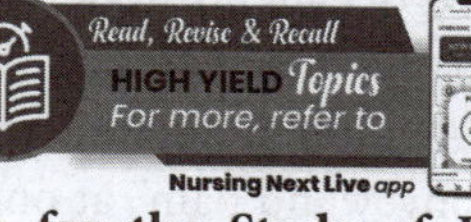

- The **International Association for the Study of Pain** (IASP) defines pain as a "sensory and emotional experience associated with tissue damage or described in terms of such damage."
- **McCaffery** defined pain as "whatever the experiencing person says it is and whenever he says it does (1979)."

Assessment of pain includes

A. Subjective Assessment

- **Pain history**
- **Onset and duration of occurrence**
- **Location**
- **Intensity**
  - Numerical rating scale
  - Verbal rating scale
  - Visual analog scale
  - Wong baker faces pain rating scale.

B. Objective Assessment

- **Behavioral effects:**
  - Assess verbalization, vocal response, facial and body movements and social interaction.
  - Facial expression is often first indication of pain and may be only one manifestation
  - Vocalization like moaning, groaning, crying, grunting, screaming is associated with pain.

Characteristics of Pain Assessment (PQRST)

- P – Provocation/Palliation.
- Q – Quality/Quantity. What does it feel like?
- R – Region/Radiation. Where is the pain located?
- S – Severity Scale.
- T – Timing

Pain Assessment Scales

Numerical Rating Scale

- A numerical rating scale with the range of 0 to 10 is another type of pain scale that is used.
- The word "no pain" appears by "0" and "worst pain possible" is found by "10".
- Patient is asked to choose a number from 0 to 10 that best reflects his/her level of pain

- Verbal rating scales
- Verbal pain scales as name suggests, use words to describe pain.
- Words such as no pain, mild pain, moderate pain and severe pain are used to describe pain levels.
- Visual analog scales
- VAS uses a vertical or horizontal line with words that convey "no pain" at one end and "worst pain" at opposite end - Patient is asked to place a mark along line that indicates his/her level of pain.
- Wong-Baker Faces pain rating scale
- With the Wong-Baker pain scale, six faces are used that are numbered 0 to 5 as follows:
  - Face 0 is a happy face
  - Face 2 is still smiling
  - Face 4 is not smiling or frowning
  - Face 6 is starting to frown
  - Face 8 is definitely frowning
  - Face 10 is crying

Physiology of Pain

Theories of Pain

Various modern theories of pain are mentioned as follows:

- Specificity theory
- Intensity theory
- Pattern theory
- Gate control theory

Specificity Theory

- Von Frey (1895) stated that the body has a separate sensory system for perceiving pain.

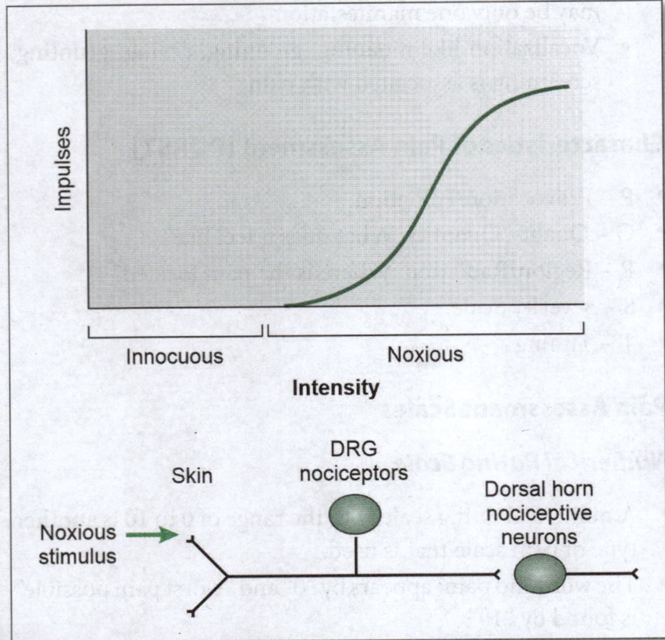

- This system contains its own special receptors for detecting pain stimuli, its own peripheral nerves and pathway to the brain, and its own area of the brain for processing pain signals.

Intensity Theory of Pain

- Relies on no distinct pathways for low- and high- threshold stimuli.
- Rather, the number of impulses in neurons determines the intensity of a stimulus.
- The primary afferent neurons synapse onto wide-dynamic range (WDR) 2nd-order neurons in the dorsal horn of the spinal cord, where low levels of activity encode innocuous stimuli, and higher levels of activity encode noxious stimuli.

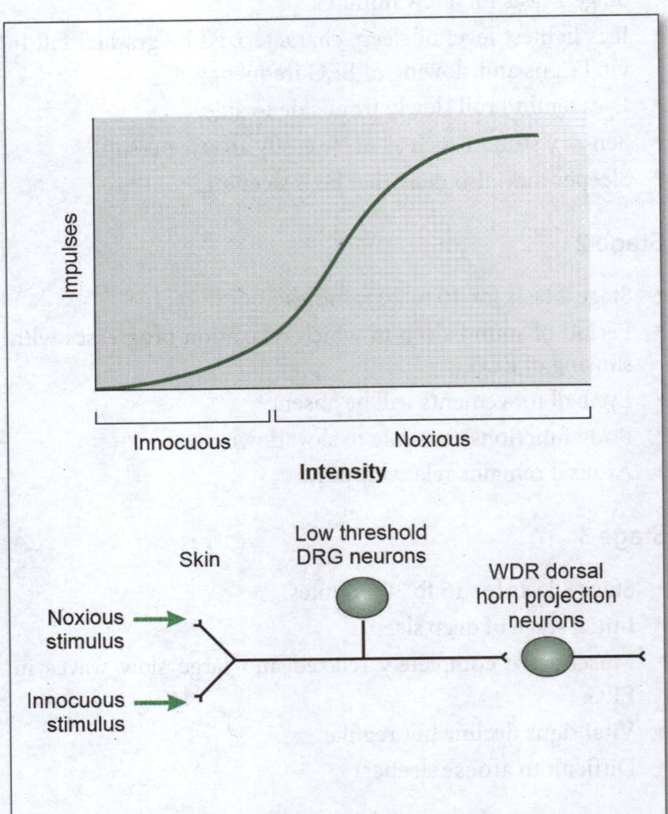

Pattern Theory

- Goldschneider (1920) proposed that there is no separate system for perceiving pain, and the receptors for pain are shared with other senses, such as of touch.
- According to this view, people feel pain when certain patterns of neural activity occur, such as when appropriate types of activity reach excessively high levels in the brain.

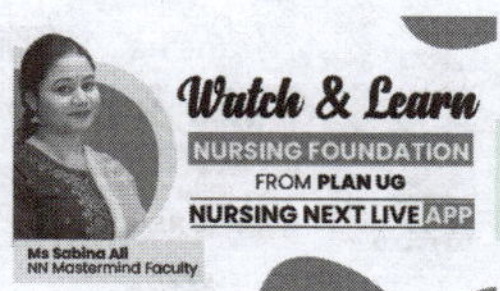

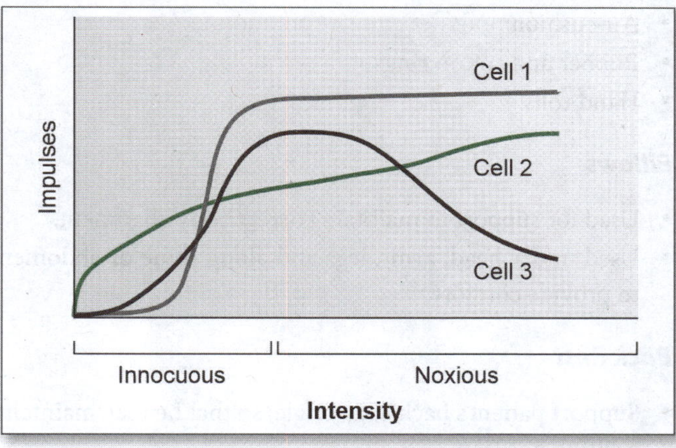

Gate Control Theory

- Ronald Melzack and Patrick Wall proposed the Gate Control Theory in 1965.
- Account for both "top-down" brain influences on pain perception as well as the effects of other tactile stimuli in appearing to reduce pain.
- There is a "gate" or control system in the dorsal horn of the spinal cord through which all information regarding pain must pass before reaching the brain.
- They can inhibit the communication of stimulation, while in other cases they can allow stimulation to be communicated into the central nervous system.

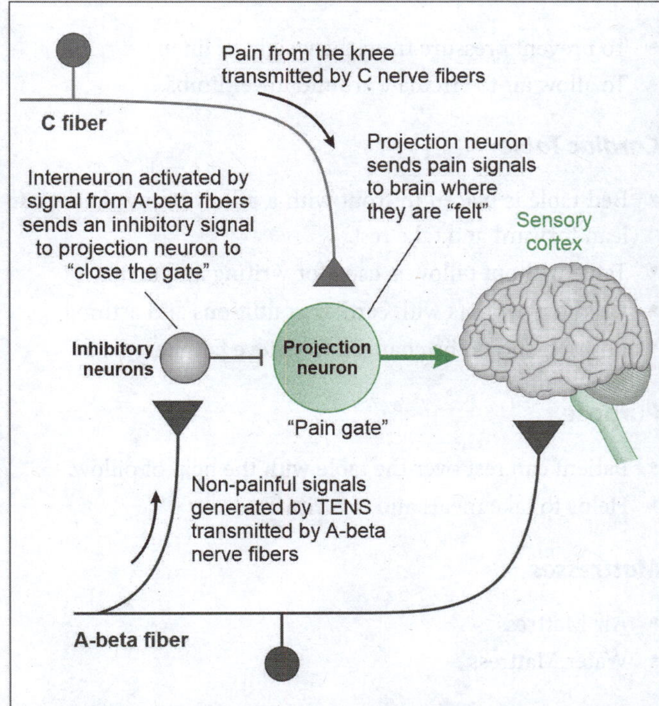

Acute pain is managed with medications such as analgesics and anesthetics. Management of chronic pain may require the pain management team, that includes medical practitioners, clinical psychologists, physiotherapists, occupational therapists, and nurse practitioners. Use of medications such as Paracetamol, NSAIDs, opioids, muscle relaxants, anticonvulsants, etc.

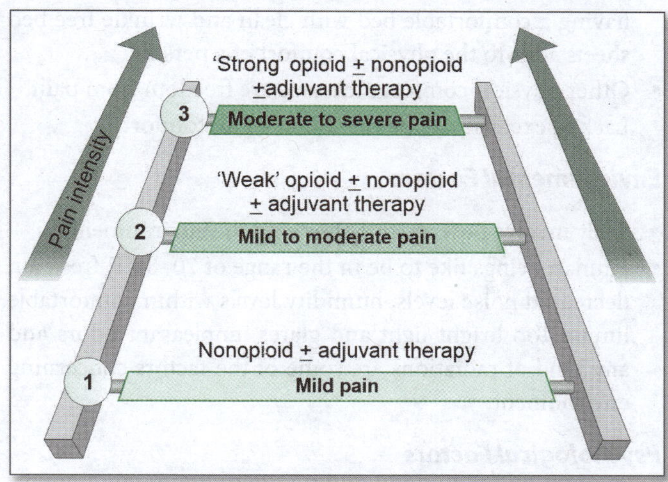

Placebo Effect

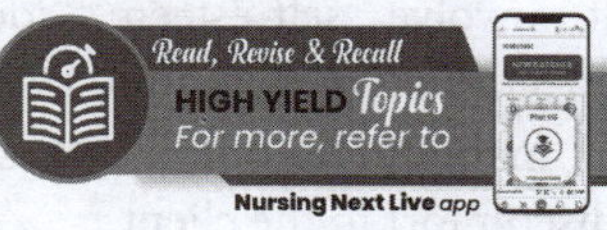

- A placebo is an inactive substance that looks like the drug or treatment being tested.
- Placebo has no therapeutic properties.
- The placebo effect occurs when a person responds to the medication or other treatment because of an expectation that the treatment will work rather than it actually does so.
- Placebo is more effective in intense pain than mild pain.

CONCEPTUAL EXERCISES

LONG ANSWER QUESTIONS

1. a. **Write the factors influencing comfort. (MGR, KUHS)**
   b. **Discuss comfort devices.**

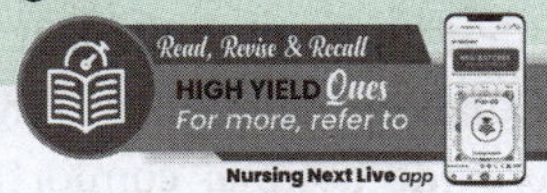

Answer

Factors Influencing Comfort

Individual comfort and performance levels of a person are influenced by a number of factors such as:

- Physical factors
- Environmental factors
- Psychological factors
- Sociocultural factors

Physical Factors

- They involve all the aspects of an individual.
- They include need for food, water, oxygen, elimination of waste products from the body.

- Physical factors such as mobility, personal care (cleanliness of body, oral care, hair, clean clothes), indulging in diversional activities, having a sound sleep of 6–8 hours, having a comfortable bed with clean and wrinkle free bed sheets adds to the physical comfort of a person.
- Other physical comfort measures are freedom from pain.
- Lack of exercise can be the source of discomfort.

Environmental Factors

- They involve how much hot or cold the environment is.
- Human beings like to be in the range of 70–80°F, fresh air, decreased noise levels, humidity levels within comfortable limits. Too bright light and glares, unpleasant odors and any kind of radiations are some of the factors concerning environment.

Psychological Factors

It involve self-esteem, identity, sexuality, relationships, effective communication and sense of safety and security.

Inability to full fill these factors may be a source of discomfort to the client.

Sociocultural Factors

- They involve family, societal and interpersonal relationships, traditions, rituals and religious factors.
- Information about the disease condition, interaction with hospital staff, family presence, support and **friends influence the comfort of person.**

b. Discuss comfort devices.

Answer

Comfort Devices

Comfort: The absence of irritating stimuli that distract one's attention from the task at hand.

Comfort devices are the mechanical devices planned to provide optimal comfort to an individual. Various comfort devices are as follows:

- Pillows
- Back rest
- Bed cradle
- Cardiac table
- Mattresses
- Trapeze bar
- Footboard
- Trochanter rolls
- Sandbags
- Wedge/abductor pillow
- Knee rest
- Bed blocks
- Air cushion
- Rubber and cotton rings
- Hand rolls

Pillows

- Used for support to maintain correct body alignment.
- Used under head, arms, legs and along spine or abdomen to provide comfort.

Back Rest

- Support patient's back at an angle, so that he may maintain a sitting position.
- Can be adjusted to desired angle.
- Extra pillows are needed.
- Arms of patient are well supported.
- Used for patients suffering from cardiac and pulmonary distress.

Bed Cradle

- It is a frame used to hold the bed linen from touching the patients.
- Cradle is a semicircular/rectangular frame of metal.
- In most cases, made of wood or bamboo.

Purpose

- To prevent pressure from the weight of linen.
- To allow air to circulate around lower limbs.

Cardiac Table

- Bed table is placed in front with a pillow on it, patient can lean forward and take rest.
- Table without pillow is used for writing and meals.
- Used for patients with cardiac conditions and asthma.
- Position should be changed to relieve fatigue.

Purpose

- Patient can rest over the table with the help of pillow.
- Helps to take meals and in writing.

Mattresses

- Air Mattress
- Water Mattress

Purpose

- To provide comfort.
- Used for very thin and very obese patients and for those who are prone to pressure sores.

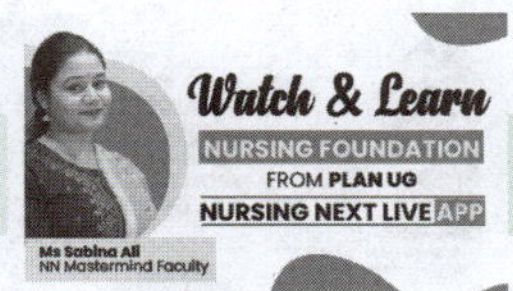

Trapeze Bar

Bar is suspended from an overhead frame to head of bed.

Purpose

Patient can grasp the bar to raise the trunk off the bed surface or to move up in bed.

Footboard

- Device that is placed toward the foot of patient's bed to serve as support for his feet.
- Usually made up of wood/plastic/heavy canvas.

Purpose

- To support patient's feet
- To prevent foot drop.

Trochanter Rolls

A cotton bath blanket/sheet is folded lengthwise to width extending from greater trochanter of femur to lower border of popliteal space.

Purpose

Prevent external rotation of legs when patient is in supine position.

Sandbags

- They are sand filled plastic bags that can be shaped to body contours.
- Can be used in place of or in addition to trochanter rolls.

Purpose:

- Provide support and shape to the body.
- Immobilize extremities and maintain specific body alignment.

Wedge/Abductor Pillow

It is a triangular shaped pillow made of heavy foam.

Purpose

Used to maintain legs in abduction following total hip replacement surgery.

Knee Rest

This is a device placed under the knees to provide comfort.

Purpose

This gives relaxation and thus, relieves pain on tendons beneath the knees.

Bed Blocks

Made up of wood or metal.

Purpose

These are used to raise the foot end or head end of the bed.

Air Cushion

Air cushions are made up of rubber and can be inflated with air.

Purpose

Used to take off the weight of the body and to relieve pressure on certain parts of the body.

Rubber and Cotton Rings

These are circular rings made of rubber or cotton.

Purpose

These are used to relieve pressure on certain parts of the body like elbow and heels.

Hand Rolls

- Made by folding a washcloth in half, rolling in lengthwise and securing roll with tape.
- Roll is placed against palmar surface of hand.

Purpose

- Maintain thumb in slightly adducted and in opposition direction to the fingers.
- Maintain fingers in slightly flexed position.

2. Write the following: (MGR, DU)

a. **Principles of bed making.**

b. **Nurse's role while preparing divided bed.**

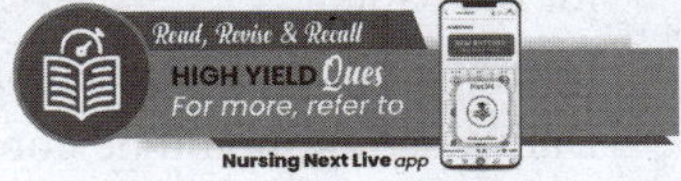

Answer

Bed making is a procedure or technique in which different types of beds are prepared to make the patient comfortable according to the situations and procedures.

Principle 1

Microorganisms are found everywhere on the skin, on the articles used by the patient and in the environment.

- The nurse takes care to prevent the transfer of microorganisms from source to the new host by direct or indirect contact or prevent the multiplication of organisms.
- The nurse washes her hands before and after bed making to protect the patient and herself from cross infection.
- Bed clothes are changed frequently to ensure cleanliness.
- While removing the bed linen, please make sure that linen does not touch the floor.
- Shake the linen gently to remove the dust. Flapping the bed clothes causes air motion, there by causing the transfer of bacteria along with the dust.
- Linen should be folded and held away from the nurse to prevent direct contact with the microorganisms.
- Dusting and thorough cleaning of the patient's bed and the unit daily to keep them free from infection.
- Dry dusting raises dust. Damp dusting is recommended.
- Do not interchange the patient linen.
- Nurses with respiratory infection should not attend the patient.
- Clean from less contaminated area to more contaminated area.
- Clean the bed first before cleaning the locker.
- Maintain reasonable distance from patient's face to prevent droplet infection.

Principle 2

A safe and comfortable bed will ensure rest and sleep and prevent several complications among bed ridden patients, e.g., bed sores, foot drop, etc.

- The nurse should make sure that the bed is wrinkle free and smooth to prevent bed sores due to friction between the skin and the mattress or wrinkled sheets.
- Pull the bottom sheet tightly so that there are no wrinkles.
- The linen should be tucked far enough under the mattress, keep it fixed, tight and smooth.
- Make sure the mattress remains flat and with firm and square corners.
- Remove unwanted wastes like cotton to avoid discomfort for the patient.
- Do not keep any wet linen on the bed.
- Daily dusting should be done to remove any food waste or hospital waste (like gauze, needles, cotton etc.)
- Expose the mattress and pillow to sunlight and air to keep them fresh.
- A bed should have enough space for free moving of the patient to prevent bed sores, stimulate circulation and maintain muscle tone.
- Use comfortable devices to provide additional comfort to the patient.

Principle 3

Good body mechanics maintain the body alignment and prevent fatigue.

- Maintain good body alignment while making bed (avoid bending, twisting, stretching).
- Use large muscles rather than back muscles.
- Work smoothly and rhythmically- two people can make beds together to save time and effort.
- If possible, raise the bed height to avoid bending and back strain.

Principle 4

- Client safety and comfort.
- Ensure that the locks of the bed are on.
- Ensure the height of the bed is adjusted to its proper height during the bed making.
- Make sure the bedside rails are on.
- Avoid areas of potential pressure on the bed.
- Promote comfort by having wrinkle free bed free from rough areas, creases, food crumbs and foreign bodies.

Principle 5

- Systematic ways of functioning save time, energy and material.
- Assemble all articles and arrange them conveniently before starting the procedure.
- Arrange the linen in reverse order.
- When stripping the bed, remove the bed linen one by one holding the open end toward the floor.
- The bed sheets are folded in such a way that they can be replaced easily.

General Rules

- Wash hands before and after the procedure.
- Do not expose the patient unnecessarily.
- Do not cover the patient's face while placing the linen.
- Do not mix clean linen with soiled linen.
- Never place the woolen blanket directly on the patient's body except for bed blanket.
- Always get extra help to make bed for helpless patients and to prevent them from falling.
- Never allow the patient to lie down on mackintosh directly.
- Do not let the linen touch your body or uniform.
- Maintain good body mechanics.
- Make the bed firm, smooth and wrinkle free.
- Practice economy of time, energy and material.

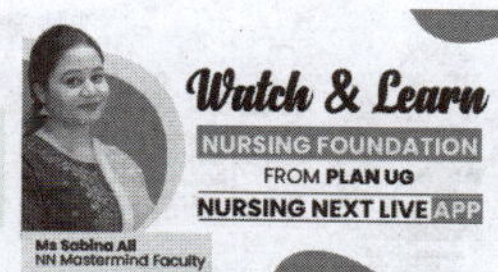

- Do not shake dirty linen to prevent spreading of germs around the room.
- Maintain privacy while making occupied bed making.
- Ensure patient safety and comfort during the procedure.
- The nursing principles such as individuality, comfort, safety and good relationship should be maintained.

b. Nurse's role while preparing divided bed

Answer

Divided Bed

- This bed is made to facilitate the dressing of the stump.
- To ensure that the stump is visible to the staff moving about the ward, so that at a glance any hemorrhage may be observed.
- It is commonly found that the stump quivers.

Requirement

- Mackintosh and dressing towels
- Two sand bags in covers
- A cradle
- A counterpane
- A bed linen
- The bed is modified depending upon where the amputation has occured.
- The bed is made up to the level of a simple bed.
- The flannelette sheet is placed over the patient's chest, trunk and the good leg.
- The dressing mackintosh and dressing towel are placed where the stump will lie.
- The cradle is then placed over the stump.
- The bed is now made up with the divide at the level of stump.
- Amputation bed below the knee.
- Requirement is as of amputation above knee.

Procedure

- The bed is made up to the level of simple bed until the flannelette sheet and the bed cradle is are position.
- The bed is then made up a of simple bed, but the top bed clothes at the stump side are turned back over the cradle.
- Amputation below knee
  - This is tucked in at the bottom on the other side, thus exposing the stump to view.

3. Write any four types of positioning and purposes. (MGR)

Read, Revise & Recall
HIGH YIELD Ques
For more, refer to
Nursing Next Live app

Answer

Positioning

Positioning is defined as the placement of person in such a way to perform therapeutic interventions for the purpose of preventive, promotive, curative and rehabilitative aspects of health.

Purpose of Positioning

- To provide comfort to the patient.
- To relieve pressure on various aspects and improve blood circulation.
- To prevent deformity and decubitus ulcers.
- To perform diagnostic and therapeutic procedures.
- To maintain good body mechanics.

Types of Positioning

- Dorsal position/supine position
- Dorsal recumbent position
- Lithotomy position
- Lateral position
- Prone position
- Sims position
- Knee-chest position
- Trendelenburg position
- Fowler's position

Dorsal position/supine position

- The patients lie on their back with head and shoulders slightly elevated.
- **Uses**
  - Comfortable position
  - Examination of head, neck, chest, abdomen and extremities
  - Surgery of anterior part of the body

Prone Position

- A patient lies flat on abdomen and head is turned to one side. Both the hands are held in a comfortable position.
- **Uses**
  - Examination of posterior trunk, spines and rectum.
  - Surgeries of back
  - To relieve pressure on areas such as sacrum, scapula and heel.
  - After anesthesia to prevent aspiration.

Lateral Position

Side lying position

- Patient lies on left side and most of the body weight is on the dependent hip and shoulders.
- **Uses**
  - Comfortable position
  - Relieve pressure on bony prominences
  - Used for enema, insertion of suppositories and for checking rectal temperature.

Sims Position

- Differ from side lying position in which weight is placed in the anterior ilium, humorous and clavicle.
- Patients lies on his left with left arm drawn behind the back.
- Right arm may be in any position.
- The right thigh is flexed against the abdomen.
- **Uses**
  - Vaginal and rectal examination.
  - To relieve pressure on the buttocks, scapula and heels.

Fowler's Position

- It is an upright position with the patient in a sitting position in the bed with legs resting on the bed.
- **Types**
  - **High fowler's:** 75–90°
  - **Semi fowler's**: 40–45°
  - **Low fowler's** position: 30°
- **Uses:**
  - Facilitates drainage of abdominal cavity.
  - Relieves breathing difficulty.
  - Relieves tension on the abdominal sutures.
  - Facilitates eating, reading, watching TV, etc.
  - Relaxes large muscles of the back.

Orthopneic Position

- High Fowler's position.
- Over table placed in front of the patient @ Patient to rest both hands on over bed table supported by pillows and lean forward to the table (facilitates respiration).
- **Uses**
  - Patient with severe dyspnea
  - Cardiac patients
  - Position for thoracentesis
  - Patient with chest drainage tubes

Lithotomy Position

- The patient lies on her back. The legs are separated and thighs are flexed on the abdomen.
- The buttocks are kept in the edge at the table and legs are supported by stirrups.
- Provides maximal exposure to genitalia.
- **Uses**
  - Vaginal examination
  - Pap smear
  - Position during delivery for many women
  - Surgical procedures of genitourinary system

Knee Chest Position

- Patient lies on the bed in such a way that the knees and the chest rest on the bed.
- The head is turned to one side.
- A small pillow can be placed under the chest.
- The weight of patient rests on chest and knees only.
- The knees are flexed and thighs are at right angle to legs.
- **Uses**
  - Examination of rectum and vagina
  - Postpartum exercise

Trendelenburg Position

- Head of the bed is lowered and the foot is raised in a straight incline.
- Patient lies on his back.
- Beds are available with electric control system.
- **Reverse Trendelenburg position:** Head end of the bed is raised.
- **Uses**
  - Promote venous circulation and venous return patient with poor peripheral perfusion.
  - Postural drainage
  - In OT examination and surgery in the pelvic organs

Dorsal Recumbent Position

- Patient lies on back, knees fully flexed and legs separated, thighs flexed and externally rotated and feet flat on the bed.
- Pillow is placed under the head.
- **Uses**
  - Examination of vagina and rectum
  - Catheterization and care
  - For doing procedures in the rectum, vulva and vagina

4. a. Define sleep. (MGR, KUHS, DU)

b. List down the various factors affecting sleep.

c. Discuss the stages of sleep and ways to promote rest and sleep.

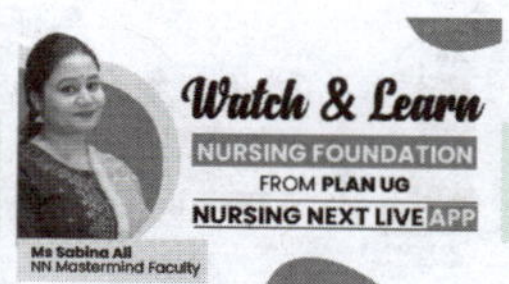

Answer

Sleep

- **Sleep** is a state of rest accompanied by altered levels of consciousness and relative inactivity, and decreased perception to environment.
- **Sleep** is defined as the physical and mental resting state in which a person becomes relatively inactive and unaware of the environment.

b. List down the various factors affecting sleep.

Answer

Factors Affecting Sleep

Both the quality and the quantity of sleep are affected by a number of factors.

Sleep quality is a subjective characteristic.

Quantity of sleep is the total time for which the individual sleeps.

- **Age:** With aging, various factors deteriorate the normal sleep process that is essential for the restoration of functional and physical performance.
- **Illness:** Illness that causes pain or physical distress (e.g., arthritis, back pain), respiratory distress can result in sleep problems.
- **Environment:**
  - Environment can promote or hinder sleep.
  - Any change—for example, noise in the environment—can inhibit sleep.
  - The absence of usual stimuli or the presence of unfamiliar stimuli can prevent people from sleeping.
  - Discomfort from environmental temperature (e.g., too hot or cold) and lack of ventilation can affect sleep.
  - Light levels can be another factor.
  - Another influence includes the comfort and size of the bed.
  - A person's partner who has different sleep habits, snores, or has other sleep difficulties may become a problem for the person also.
- **Lifestyle:**
  - Following an irregular morning and night time schedule can affect sleep.
  - Night shift workers frequently get less sleep than other workers and have difficulty falling asleep.
- **Emotional stress:**
  - Stress is considered to be the major cause of short-term sleeping difficulties.
  - A person preoccupied with personal problems (e.g., school- or job-related pressures, family or marriage problems) may be unable to relax sufficiently to get to sleep.
- **Stimulants and alcohol:**
  - Caffeine-containing beverages act as stimulants of the central nervous system (CNS).
  - Drinking beverages containing Caffeine in the afternoon or evening may interfere with sleep.
  - Even though alcohol induces sleep, it disturbs REM sleep causing irritability.
- **Diet:** Certain foods induce sleep such as milk.
- **Smoking:**
  - Nicotine has a stimulating effect on the body, and smokers often have more difficulty falling asleep than non-smokers.
  - Smokers can be easily aroused.
- **Motivation:**
  - Motivation can increase alertness in some situations for example, during the time of examination.
- **Medications:**
  - Beta-blockers have been known to cause insomnia.
  - Narcotics, such as morphine, are known to suppress REM sleep and to cause frequent awakening and drowsiness.
  - Most hypnotics suppress REM sleep.

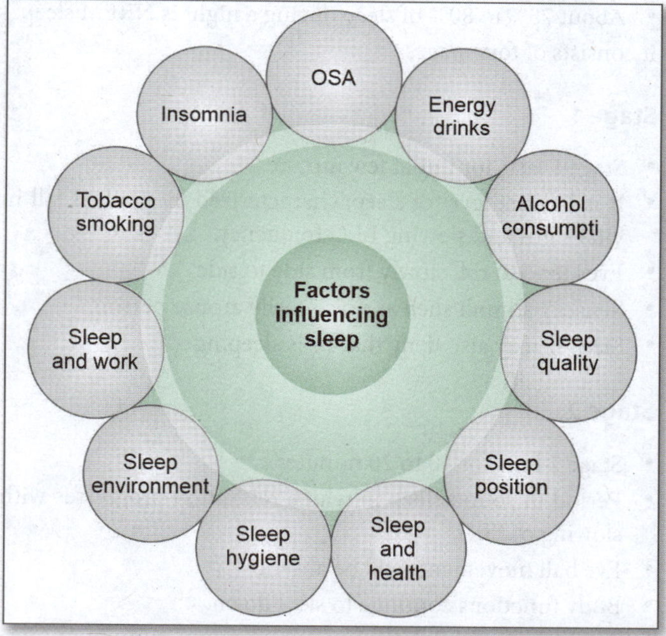

c. Discuss the stages of sleep and ways to promote rest and sleep.

Answer

Stages of Sleep

In order to identify stages of sleep, Electroencephalogram (EEG) patterns, eye movements and the muscle activity are widely used.

The stages of sleep are classified into two stages:

1. Nonrapid Eye Movement (NREM) Sleep
2. Rapid Eye Movement (REM) Sleep

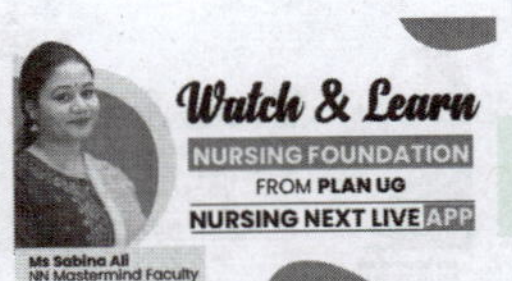

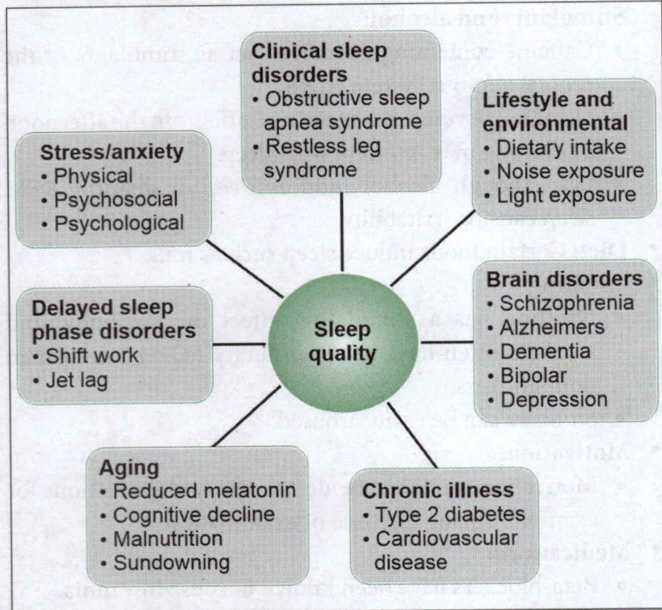

Nonrapid Eye Movement (NREM) Sleep

- It is known as first stage of sleep.
- About 75% to 80% of sleep during a night is NREM sleep.

It consists of four stages:

Stage 1

- Stage 1 lasts for initial few minutes.
- It is lightest level of sleep, characterized by gradual fall in vital signs and slowing EEG frequency.
- Eyes tend to roll slowly from side to side.
- Sensory stimuli such as noise easily arouse person.
- Sleeper may also deny that he is sleeping.

Stage 2

- Stage 2 lasts for 10 to 20 minutes.
- Period of sound sleep in which relaxation progresses with slowing of EEG.
- Eye ball movements will be absent.
- Body functions continue to slow down.
- Arousal remains relatively easy.

Stage 3

- Stage 3 lasts for 15–30 minutes.
- Initial stage of deep sleep.
- Muscles are completely relaxed and large slow waves are shown in EEG.
- Vital signs decline but regular.
- Difficult to arouse sleeper.

Stage 4

- Stage 4 lasts for approximately 15 to 30 minutes.
- It is the deepest stage of sleep.
- Vital signs are significantly lower and slowing of EEG is observed.
- Sleepwalking and enuresis (bed-wetting) sometimes occur.
- Very difficult to arouse sleeper.

REM Sleep

- Usually begins about 90 minutes after sleep has begun.
- Dreaming occurs in this stage.
- It involves rapid eyes movement, fluctuating heart rate, respiratory rates, blood pressure, loss of skeletal muscle tone, and increased gastric secretions.
- EEG pattern resembles awake state.
- Very difficult to arouse sleeper.

Ways to Promote Rest and Sleep

- Maintain a regular schedule of wake-up and bedtime.
- Eliminate day time naps.
- Instruct the client to go to bed when sleepy.
- Use warm bath and warm drinks before going to bed.
- Use relaxation techniques to reduce stress.
- Establish a relaxing bedtime routine before sleep such as reading a book, listening to soft music.
- Create a sleep-conducive environment.
- Sleep on a comfortable mattress and pillow.
- Avoid caffeine in late afternoon and evening.
- Take less fluid before 2 to 4 hours of sleep.
- Use sleeping medications only as a last resort.
- Consult physician about medications that may cause insomnia.

5. a. **Define pain. (MGR)**
b. **Discuss assessment of pain. (MGR)**
c. **Describe the role of nurse in management of pain. (MGR)**

Answer

Definition of Pain

- The **International Association for the Study of Pain** (IASP) defines pain as a "sensory and emotional experience associated with tissue damage or described in terms of such damage."

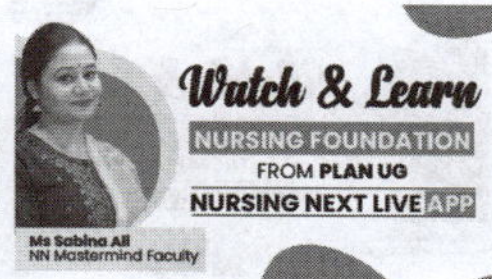

- **McCaffery** defined pain as "whatever the experiencing person says it is and whenever he says it does (1979)."
- The **American Pain Society** goes further by stating that it is "not the responsibility of clients to prove they are in pain; it is the nurse's responsibility to accept the clients' report of pain (2005)."

b. Discuss assessment of pain.

Answer

Assessment of Pain

Assessment of pain includes:

A. Subjective Assessment

- **Pain history:** While taking pain history, nurse must provide an opportunity for clients to express in their own words, how they view it and their situation. This will help the nurse to understand means of pain to client and how the client is coping with it.
- **Onset and duration of occurrence:** When did pain begin? How long has it lasted? Does it occur at same time each day? How often does it occur?
- **Location:** In which area it is felt? Does the area differ under different circumstances? If several parts of body are painful, do pain occur simultaneously? Is pain unilateral/bilateral? Ask the individual to point site of discomfort.
- **Intensity:** Use of pain intensity scale is an easy and reliable method of determining the clients' pain intensity. Most scales are either 0 to 5 or 0 to 10. Currently used scales are:
  - Numerical rating scale
  - Verbal rating scale
  - Visual analog scale
  - Wong baker faces pain rating scale.
  - **Numerical rating scale**
    - A numerical rating scale with the range of 0 to 10 is another type of pain scale that is used.
    - The word "no pain" appear by "0" and "worst pain possible" is found by "10".
    - Patients are asked to choose a number from 0 to 10 that best reflects his/her level of pain.
  - **Verbal rating scale:**
    - Verbal pain scales, as name suggests, use words to describe pain.
    - Words such as no pain, mild pain, moderate pain and severe pain are used to describe pain levels.
  - **Visual analogue scale:**
    - VAS uses a vertical or horizontal line with words that convey "no pain" at one end and "worst pain" at opposite end. - Patient is asked to place a mark along line that indicates his/her level of pain.
  - **Wong-Baker faces pain rating scale**

    With the Wong-Baker pain scale, six faces are used that are numbered 0 to 5 as follows.
    - Face 0 is a happy face.
    - Face 2 is still smiling.
    - Face 4 is not smiling or frowning.
    - Face 6 is starting to frown.
    - Face 8 is definitely frowning.
    - Face 10 is crying.

B. Objective Assessment

Behavioral Effects

- Assess verbalization, vocal response, facial and body movements and social interaction.
- Facial expression is often first indication of pain and may be only one manifestation.
- Vocalization like moaning, groaning, crying, grunting, screaming is associated with pain.

Characteristics of pain assessment (PQRST)

- P – Provocation/Palliation.
- Q – Quality/Quantity. What does it feel like?
- R – Region/Radiation. Where is the pain located?
- S – Severity Scale.
- T – Timing.

Pain Assessment Tool

A **pain scale** measures a patient's pain intensity or other features.

Pain scales are based on self-report, observational (behavioral), or physiological data.

- **Dolorimeter instrument** is used to measure pain threshold and pain tolerance.
- Dolorimeters apply steady pressure, heat, or electrical stimulation to some area, or move a joint or other body part and determine what level of heat or pressure or electric current or amount of movement produces a sensation of pain.

c. Describe the role of nurse in management of pain

Answer

Role of Nurse in Management of Pain

Identifying Goals for Pain Management

- The information obtained from the patient helps in identifying the goals for management.
- The goals are shared with the patient. For some patients, elimination of the pain might be the goal, whereas for some others, this may seem unrealistic.
- Another goal can be to reduce the intensity of pain. The goal for the patient may be accompanied by pharmacological or nonpharmacological means.

Establishing nurse-patient relationship and teaching:

- A positive nurse-patient relationship and teaching are keys to manage analgesia in patient with pain, because open communication and patient cooperation are essential to the success of pain management.
- The nurse also provides information by explaining how pain can be controlled.

Providing Physical Care

- The patient in pain may be unable to participate in the usual activities of the daily routine or usual self-care and may need assistance to carry out these activities.
- The patient is usually more comfortable when the physical and self-care needs have been met and efforts have been made to ensure as comfortable position as possible.

Managing anxiety related to pain:

- Anxiety may affect a patient's response to pain. The patient who anticipates pain may become very anxious. Teaching the patient about the nature of the impending painful experience and the ways to reduce it often decreases anxiety.
- Learning about the measures to reduce pain may lessen the threat of pain and give the person a sense of control.

Use of Pain Management Strategies

- Acute pain is managed with medications such as analgesics and anesthetics.
- Management of chronic pain may require the pain management team, which includes medical practitioners, clinical psychologists, physiotherapists, occupational therapists, and nurse practitioners.
  - **Pharmacological intervention:** Use of medications such as Paracetamol, NSAIDs, opioids, muscle relaxants, anticonvulsants etc.
  - **Use of nonpharmacological measures:** They include hot and cold applications, distraction, relaxation techniques, music therapy, use of acupuncture, cognitive behavioral therapy etc.

6. a. Physiology of pain. (MGR)
b. List the factors influencing pain. (MGR)
c. Discuss the nursing interventions for pain. (MGR)

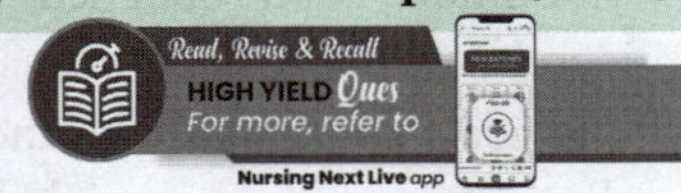

Answer

Physiology of Pain

The following is a brief review of the four basic concepts that are important to begin to understand the physiology of pain.

The concepts are:

- Transduction
- Transmission
- Modulation
- Perception

Transduction

It is the process by which afferent nerve endings participate in translating noxious stimuli into nociceptive impulses.

Transmission

Transmission is the process by which impulses are sent to the dorsal horn of spinal cord and then along the sensory tracts to the brain.

Modulation

Modulation is the process of dampening or amplifying these pain-related neural signs. Modulation takes place primarily in the dorsal horn of spinal cord, but also elsewhere, with input from ascending and descending pathways.

Perception

Perception refers to the subjective experience of pain that results from interaction of transduction, transmission, modulation, and the psychological aspects of the individual.

b. List the factors influencing pain.

Answer

Factors Influencing Pain

Pain is also known as 5th vital sign. It is an unpleasant sensory and emotional experience with actual or potential tissue damage, and described in terms of such damage.

Physiological Factors

- Organic origin
- Integrity of the nervous system including all endogenous opioids
- Concomitant physical influences (stress, fatigue)
- Age
- Type of pain
- Location
- Intensity
- Duration
- Frequency
- Quality
- Threshold
- Tolerance
- Genetics

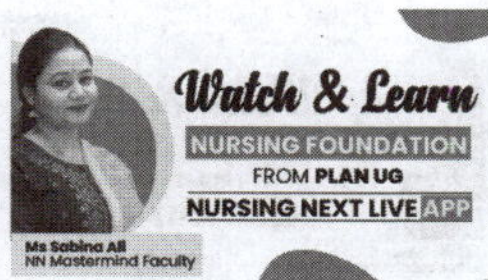

Affective Factors

- Distress of pain
- Depression
- Mood
- Anxiety, fear, worry

Psychological Influences

- Family and occupational roles
- Personal beliefs
- Spiritual belief system
- Cultural/social influences
- Sexual identity and stereotypes
- Demographic factors

Cognitive Factors

- Past experience
- Meaning of pain experience
- Attention paid to sensation/distraction
- Expectations
- Coping mechanisms
- Knowledge
- Values/attitudes
- Communication skills

c. Discuss the nursing interventions for pain.

Answer

Nursing Interventions for Pain

Interventions	Rationale	Outcomes
Reassure the patient that you know that the pain is real and will assist him/her in dealing with it	Fear that pain will not be accepted as it increases tension	Reports relief that pain is accepted as real and that he/she will receive assistance in pain relief
Use pain assessment scale to identify intensity of pain.	Provides baseline for assessing changes in pain level and evaluating interventions	• Reports lower intensity of pain and discomfort after interventions implemented • Reports less disruption from pain and discomfort after use of intervention
Assess and record pain and its characteristics: location, quality, frequency and duration.	Data assists in evaluating pain and pain relief and identifying multiple sources and types of pain	Uses pain medication as prescribed
Administer balanced analgesics as prescribed.	Administer early in pain cycle for more effectiveness	Identifies effective pain-relief strategies
Re-administer pain assessment scale.	Permits assessment of effectiveness of analgesia and identifies need for further action, if required	Demonstrates use of new strategies to relieve pain and reports their effectiveness
Document severity of patient's pain on chart.	Assists in demonstrating need for additional analgesics or alternative approach to pain relief	• Experiences minimal side effects of analgesia without interruption to treat side effects • Increases interactions with family and friends
Obtain additional prescription as needed.	Inadequate pain relief results in an increased stress response, suffering and prolonged hospitalization	
Identify and encourage patient to use strategies that have been successful with previous pain.	Encourages use of pain relief strategies familiar to and accepted by the patient	
Teach patient additional strategies to relieve pain and discomfort: distraction, relaxation, etc.	Use of these strategies along with analgesia may produce more effective pain relief	
Instruct patient and family about potential side effects of analgesics and their prevention and management.	Anticipating and preventing side effects enable the patient to continue analgesia without interruption because of side effects	

SHORT NOTES

1. Write a short note on nurses responsibilities while making an occupied bed. (DU)

Answer

- Some clients are unable to get out of bed as a result of their specific condition or generalized weakness.
- Changing bed linens with the client in the bed is known as making an occupied bed.
- Work quickly and disturb the client as little as possible.

Indications: Provide clean and comfortable bed with least disturbance to the patient in it.

Assessment

- Check the room/ward for the need of disinfection or hygiene.
- Explain the purpose and procedure to the client.
- Prepare all required equipment:
    - Trolley with –
    - Mattress (1)
    - Bed sheets (2):
    - Bottom sheet (1)
    - Top sheet (1)
    - Pillow (1)
    - Pillow cover (1)
    - Mackintosh (1)
    - Draw sheet (1)
    - Blanket (1)
- **A tray containing:**
    - 2 sponge cloth in hospital approved disinfectant.
    - Laundry bag or Bucket or hamper bag (1)
- Perform hand hygiene.
- Prepare all required equipment and bring the articles to the bedside.
- Remove the client's personal belongings from bedside and keep in locker/at any safe place.
- Lift the client's head and move pillow from center to the left side.
- Assist the client to turn toward left side of the bed.
- Adjust the pillow.
- Leave top sheet in place.
- Stand in right side
- Loose bottom bed linens.
- Fanfold (or roll) soiled linens from the side of the bed and wedge them close to the client.
- Wipe the surface of mattress by wet and dry sponge cloth.
- Moving the client as close to the other side of the bed as possible gives you more room to make the bed. Top sheet keeps the client warm and protects his or her privacy.
- Bottom sheet, mackintosh and draw sheet:
    - Place the clean bottom sheet evenly on the bed folded lengthwise with the center fold as close to the client's back as possible.
    - Adjust and tuck the sheet tightly under the head of the mattress, making the upper corners mitered.
    - Tighten the sheet under the end of the mattress and make the lower corners mitered.
    - Tuck in alongside.
    - Place the mackintosh and the draw sheet on the bottom sheet and tuck in them together.
- Assist the client to roll over the folded (rolled) linen to right side of the bed. Readjust the pillow and top sheet.
- Move to left side.
- Discard the soiled linens appropriately.
- Hold the soiled lines away from your uniform.
- Place the soiled lines in the laundry bag (or bucket).
- Wipe the surface of the mattress by wet and dry sponge cloth.
- Move the client to the bed's other side which can allow you to make the bed on that side.
- Soiled linens can contaminate your uniform, which may come into contact with other clients.
- Bottom sheet, mackintosh and draw sheet:
    - Grasp clean linens and gently pull them out from under the client.
    - Spread them over the bed's unmade side. Pull the linens taut.
    - Tuck the bottom sheet tightly under the head of the mattress and miter the corners.
    - Tighten the sheet under the end of the mattress and make the lower corners mitered.
    - Tuck in alongside.
    - Tuck the mackintosh and the draw sheet under the mattress.
- Assist the client back to the center of the bed. Adjust the pillow.
- Return to the right side.
- Clean top sheet, blanket.
    - Place the clean top sheet at the top side of the soiled top sheet.
    - Ask the client to hold the upper edge of the clean top sheet.
    - Hold both the top of the soiled sheet and the end of the clean sheet with right hand and withdraw to downward. Remove the soiled top sheet and put it into a laundry bag.

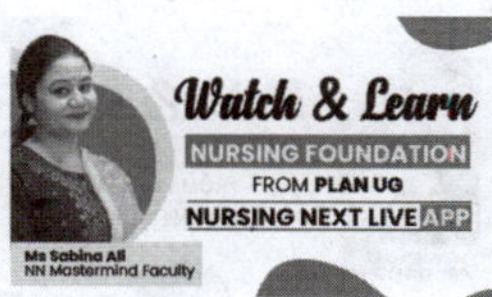

- Place the blanket over the top sheet. Fold top sheet back over the blanket over the client.
- Tuck the lower ends securely under the mattress. Miter corners.
- After finishing the right side, repeat the left side.

- Replace all equipment in proper place.
- Discard lines appropriately.
- Perform hand hygiene.

2. Write a short note on types of beds. (KUHS)

Answer

Bed making is a procedure or technique in which different types of beds are prepared to make the patient comfortable according to the situations and procedures.

Simple Bed or Unoccupied Bed

- Close bed (Admission bed)
- Open bed
- Postoperative bed/recovery bed/anesthetic bed

Occupied Bed

Special Bed

- Cardiac bed
- Fowler's bed
- Fracture bed
- Amputation bed/Stump bed/Divided bed
- Operation bed
- Blanket bed

Open Bed

It is a bed that is made when it is about to be occupied by either a new patient or an ambulatory patient.

Closed Bed

It is an unoccupied or empty bed made to receive the patient and is fully covered with counterpane to protect it from dust and dirt. On admission of the patient, the closed bed is converted into an open bed.

Purpose

- To keep the bed ready for occupancy.
- To provide a neat and tidy appearance to the unit.

Occupied Bed

This bed is made with the patient in it.

Purpose

- To make a bed with least possible discomfort to the patient.
- To handle the bed clothes skillfully while the patient is on bed, giving least disturbance to the occupant.
- To provide a neat, clean and tidy appearance.

Admission Bed

This is the bed prepared to receive a newly admitted patient.

Purpose

- To welcome the patient.
- To provide immediate care, safety and comfort.
- To protect the bed linen while giving bath on admission.

Postoperative Bed

It is a bed prepared for a patient who is recovering from the effects of anesthesia following surgery.

Purpose

- To receive the patient conveniently.
- To provide warmth and comfort.
- To prevent shock.
- To prevent injury.
- To prevent soiling of the bed.
- To meet any emergency.

Cardiac Bed

A bed prepared for patients with cardiac diseases.

Purpose

- To prepare the bed for the cardiac patients.
- To relieve dyspnea.

Amputation/Divided Bed

It is a bed in which top linen is divided into two parts to visualize the amputated part of the lower limbs without disturbing the patient.

Purpose

- To watch the stump for hemorrhage and apply tourniquet instantly.
- To take the weight of the bed clothes off the patient.
- To keep the stump in position.

Fracture Bed

It is a bed which is prepared for patients with fracture, bone diseases and deformity.

Purpose

- To prevent undue sagging of mattress.
- To immobilize the fractured part.
- To restrict sudden jerky movements.
- To keep the traction in position.

Renal/Rheumatism/Blanket Bed

It is a bed made for patients suffering from rheumatism or renal disease.

Purpose

- To carry the weight of the bed clothes off the painful joints.
- To keep the patient warm.
- To induce sweating.

3. Write a short note on physiology of sleep. (MGR)

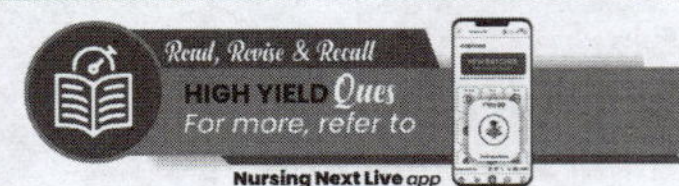

Answer

Sleep is a state of rest accompanied by altered level of consciousness and relative inactivity, and decreased perception to environment.

Physiology of Sleep

- The cyclic nature of sleep is thought to be controlled by centers located in the brain and by circadian rhythms.
- Reticular activating system (RAS) located at the brain stem and cerebral cortex plays an important role in sleep wake cycle.
- Sleep begins with the activation of the preoptic area of the anterior hypothalamus.
- Sleep promoting neurons act over wake promoting neurons by releasing Gamma Amino Butyric Acid (GABA).
- The inhibition of wake promoting neurons results in intensifying sleep process.
- Another key factor to sleep is exposure to darkness.
- Darkness and preparation for sleep (e.g., lying down, decreasing noise) cause a decrease in stimulation of the RAS.
- During this time, the pineal gland in the brain begins to actively secrete the natural hormone melatonin, and the person feels less alert.
- With the beginning of daylight, melatonin is at its lowest level in the body and the stimulating hormone cortisol is at its highest causing wakefulness.

4. Write a short note on sleep disorders. (KUHS)

Answer

Sleep disorders are commonly classified into three categories:

1. Dysomnias

- The sleep is normal but patient sleeps too little, too much, or may be at the incorrect time.
- It is associated with the quantity of sleep, its timing, and sometimes with quality of sleep also.
- Common dysomnias are:
  - Insomnia
  - Hypersomnia
  - Narcolepsy
  - Sleep Apnea
  - Insufficient Sleep/Sleep Deprivation

Insomnia is inability to fall asleep in which client remains awake and feels restless. Insomnia is the most common sleep complaint. It is of two types:

- Acute insomnia lasts for one to several nights and it is mainly due to personal stressors.
- Chronic insomnia persists for longer than a month.

Hypersomnia refers to conditions that include sufficient sleep at night but still cannot stay awake during the day.

Narcolepsy is a disorder of excessive daytime sleepiness. It mainly occurs due to lack of the chemical hypocretin in CNS.

Sleep Apnea is characterized by frequent short breathing pauses or periods of apnea during sleep. It is of three types based on the cause:

- Obstructive Apnea: occurs when the anatomical structures of respiratory system such as pharynx or oral cavity block the air flow.
- Central Apnea: occurs due to defect in the respiratory center of the brain.
- Mixed Apnea: is a combination of obstructive and central apnea.

Insufficient Sleep/ Sleep Deprivation is defined as the prolonged disturbance in quality and quantity of sleep.

2. Parasomnias

Some occurrence of any abnormal thing during sleep itself, or during the time when the patient is falling asleep or waking up. Most common disorders are:

- Bruxism
- Enuresis
- Periodic limb movement disorder
- Sleep talking
- Sleep walking

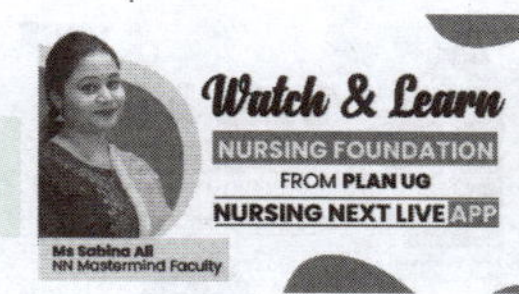

Bruxism is characterized by clenching and grinding of the teeth that occurs during stage II- NREM sleep.

Enuresis or Bed-wetting usually occurs in children over 3 years of age and commonly 1 to 2 hours after falling asleep.

Periodic limb movement disorder (PLMD): In this condition, the legs jerk twice or thrice per minute during sleep.

Sleep talking: In this, talking occurs during NREM sleep.

Sleepwalking or somnambulism occurs during stages III and IV of NREM sleep. It is episodic and usually occurs 1 to 2 hours after falling asleep.

3. Disorders Due to other Medical Conditions

These disorders are associated with illnesses including medical, psychiatric and other illnesses such as depression, thyroid dysfunction.

5. Write a short note on six physiologic changes during NREM sleep. (KUHS)

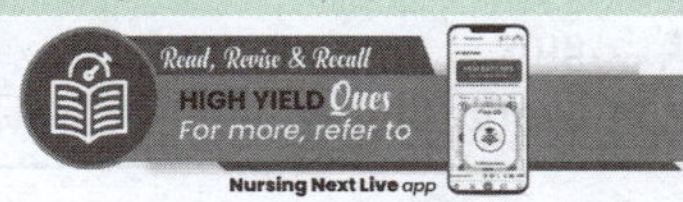

Answer

Physiologic changes during NREM Sleep

Physiological Process	During NREM
Brain activity	decreases from wakefulness
Heart rate	slows from wakefulness
Blood pressure	decreases from wakefulness
Blood flow to brain	does not change from wakefulness in most regions
Respiration	decreases from wakefulness
Airway resistance	increases from wakefulness
Body temperature	is regulated at lower set point than wakefulness; shivering initiated at lower temperature than during wakefulness
Sexual arousal	occurs infrequently

6. Write a short note on pain management. (MGR)

Answer

- Acute pain is managed with medications such as analgesics and anesthetics.
- Management of chronic pain may require the pain management team, which includes medical practitioners, clinical psychologists, physio-therapists, occupational therapists, and nurse practitioners.

Pharmacological Intervention

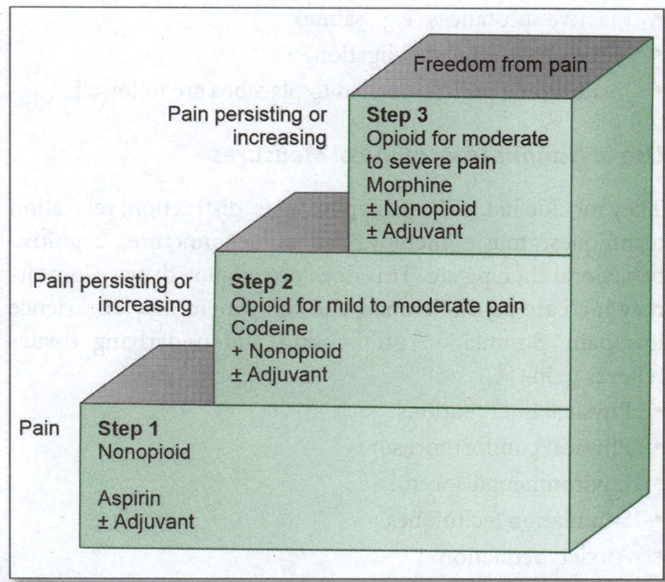

Figure 9.1: Pain management ladder

Use of medications such as paracetamol, NSAIDs, opioids, muscle relaxants, anticonvulsants etc.

Nonopioid Analgesics

- Aspirin, acetaminophen, and nonsteroidal anti-inflammatory drugs (NSAIDs) such as ibuprofen.
- Generally initial treatment of choice for mild pain.
- Act mostly on the peripheral nervous system.
- Antipyretic (fever-reducing), analgesic (pain-reducing), and/or anti-inflammatory (inflammation-reducing) properties.

Opioid Analgesics

- For moderate to severe acute pain, chronic cancer pain, and some other types of pain.
- Opioids: potency/duration of actions varies.
- Examples: codeine, methadone (Dolophine), hydromorphone (Dilaudid), meperidine (Demerol), morphine, and fentanyl.
- Routes of administration
  - Oral
  - Intramuscular
  - Sublingually
  - Intravenously
  - Epidural or intrathecal route

Placebos

- Inactive substances (e.g., saline)
- Nurses have ethical obligation.
- Institutional policies related to placebos are followed.

Use of Nonpharmacological Measures

They include hot and cold applications, distraction, relaxation techniques, music therapy, use of acupuncture, cognitive behavioral therapy etc. This does not employ drugs. Comfort may increase pain tolerance, and the patient may experience less pain. Stimulation of the skin and underlying tissues relieves pain.

- Physical interventions
- Physical comfort measures
- Environmental control
- Stimulation techniques
- Anxiety reduction
- Distraction
- Psychological interventions
- Relaxation
- Imagery

SHORT ANSWER QUESTIONS

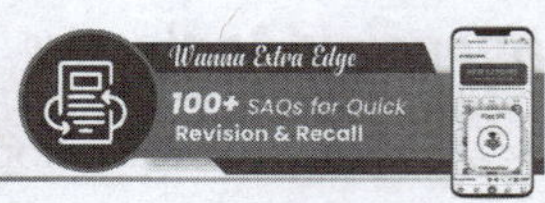

1. Define comfort devices and enumerate types of beds.

Answer

Comfort: The absence of irritating stimuli that distract one's attention from the task at hand.

Comfort devices are the mechanical devices planned to provide optimal comfort to an individual. Various comfort devices are pillows, mattresses etc.

Types of Beds

Simple Bed or Unoccupied Bed

- Close bed (Admission bed)
- Open bed
- Postoperative bed/recovery bed/anesthetic bed

Occupied Bed

Special Bed

- Cardiac bed
- Fowler's bed
- Fracture bed
- Amputation bed/ Stump bed/ Divided bed
- Operation bed
- Blanket bed

2. Define sleep and list the various factors affecting sleep.

Answer

Sleep is a state of rest accompanied by altered level of consciousness and relative inactivity, and decreased perception to environment.

Factors Affecting Sleep

- Clinical sleep disorders
- Stress/anxiety
- Lifestyle and environmental
- Delayed sleep phase disorders
- Sleep quality
- Brain disorders
- Aging
- Chronic illness

3. Define pain. (MGR)

Answer

- The **International Association for the Study of Pain** (IASP) defines pain as a "sensory and emotional experience associated with tissue damage or described in terms of such damage."
- **McCaffery** defined pain as "whatever the experiencing person says it is and whenever he says it does (1979)."
- The **American Pain Society** goes further by stating that it is "not the responsibility of clients to prove they are in pain; it is the nurse's responsibility to accept the clients report of pain (2005)."

4. Enumerate types of sleep disorder.

Answer

Sleep disorders are commonly classified into six categories:

1. **Insomnia:** Difficulty falling asleep, staying asleep, or both.
2. **Parasomnias:** abnormal behaviors or experiences that occur during sleep.
3. **Sleep apnea:** characterized by pauses in breathing during sleep.
4. **Narcolepsy:** excessive daytime sleepiness.
5. **Restless legs syndrome (RLS):** An urge to move the legs, often accompanied by unpleasant sensations.
6. **Circadian rhythm sleep disorders:** Problems with the body's internal clock.

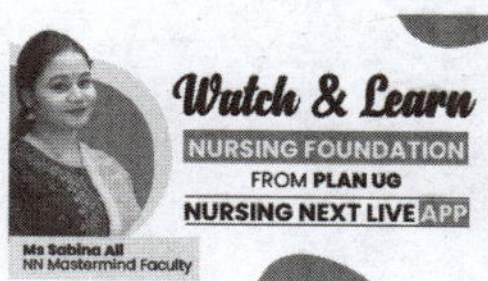

5. List the pharmacological management of pain.

Answer

Pharmacological Management

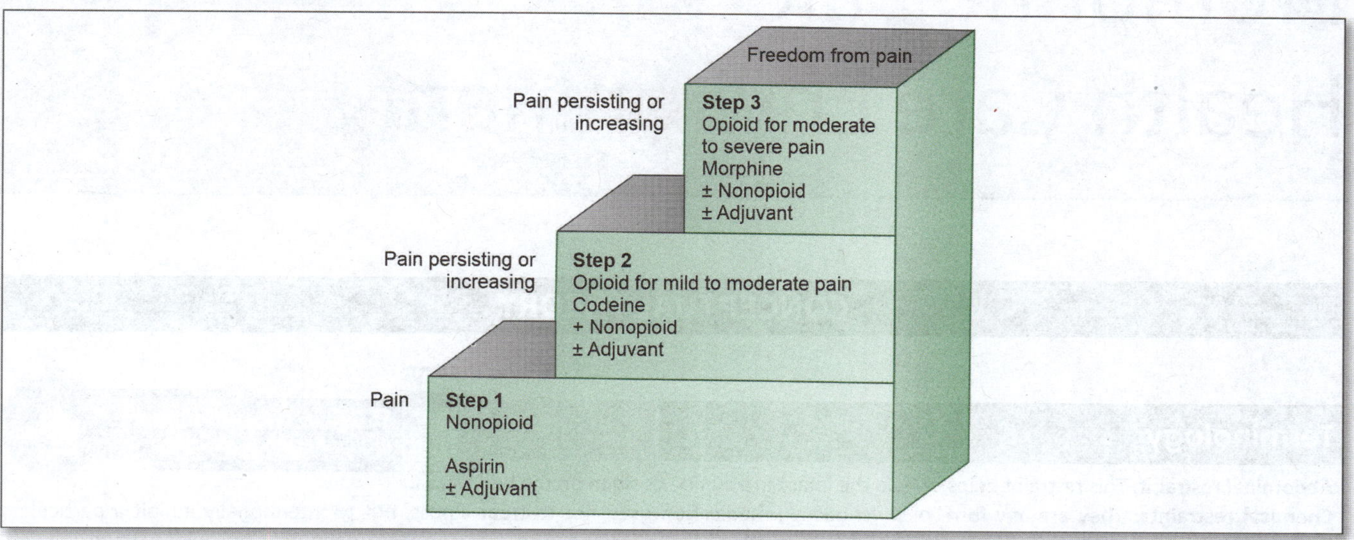

Figure 9.2: Pain management ladder

- **Nonopioid analgesics:** Aspirin, acetaminophen, etc.
- **Opioid analgesics:** Codeine, methadone (Dolophine), etc.

CONCEPTUAL REVISION

MULTIPLE CHOICE QUESTIONS

1. Choose the correct statement about circadian rhythm:
   a. Circadian Rhythm means everyday waking time
   b. Circadian Rhythm means everyday sleeping time
   c. Circadian Rhythm means cyclic psychological process
   d. Circadian Rhythm means 24-hour, day-night cycle

Ans. d. Circadian Rhythm means 24-hour, day-night cycle

2. Patient stated that, "I am worried about the healing process and pain after surgery. Last time I experienced a lot of pain." What will be the appropriate nursing action?
   a. Discussing the postoperative analgesic plan.
   b. Telling the patient not to worry
   c. Not paying attention to such complaints
   d. Explaining the cause of pain

Ans. a. Discussing the postoperative analgesic plan.

3. Nursing interventions that can help the patient to relax and sleep restfully include all of the following; except:
   a. Have the patient take a 30 to 60-minute nap in the afternoon.
   b. Turn on the television in the patient's room.
   c. Provide quiet music and interesting reading material.
   d. Massage the patient's back with long strokes.

Ans. a. Have the patient take a 30- to 60-minute nap in the afternoon.

4. Which of the following does not affect circadian rhythms?
   a. Social activities
   b. Work routines
   c. Light
   d. Food habits

Ans. d. Food habits

CHAPTER

10

Promoting Safety in Health Care Environment

CONCEPTUAL THEORY

Terminology

150+ key terminologies for Quick Recall & Revision

Abdominal restraint: This restraint helps to hold the infant in a supine position on the bed.

Chemical restraints: They are any form of psychoactive medication used not to treat illness, but to intentionally inhibit a particular behavior or movement. Chemical restraint is the administration of medications to control a patient's dangerous behavior with anxiolytics or sedatives.

Elbow restraint: This restraint is used to prevent flexion of the elbow and to hold the elbow in an extended position so that the infant cannot reach the face.

Environmental restraints: They control a client's mobility. E.g., a secure unit or garden, seclusion.

Extremity restraint: It is used to immobilize one or more extremities. One type of extremity restraint is clove-hitch restraint which is done with gauze bandage strip (2 inches wide) making figure-of-eight.

Mitten or finger restraint: Mitts are used for infants to prevent self-injury by hands in case of burns, facial injury or operations, eczema of the face or body. Mitten can be made wrapping the child's hands in gauze or with a little bag putting over the baby's hand and tie it on at the wrist.

Mummy restraint: It is a short-term type of restraint used on infants and small children during examinations and treatment of head and neck. It is used to immobilize the arms and legs of the child for a brief period of time.

Physical restraints: They limit a client's movement. E.g., table fixed to a chair or a bed rail that cannot be opened by the client.

Restraint: It is defined as 'the intentional restriction of a person's voluntary movement or behavior (Counsel and Care UK, 2002).

Safety devices: These devices are essential in the hospitals to separate people from dangerous zones or to reduce the risk of injury to others.

S – Sense the error
A – Act to prevent it
F – Follow safety guidelines
E – Enquire into accidents/deaths
T – Take appropriate remedial measure
Y – Your responsibility

Splints: These are prepared devices which are used to restrain the movements of extremities. These are made up of plastic, card- board, hard paper, and cotton and gauze pieces. These can be applied wherever needed.

Safety is a primary concern when caring for patients. Safety is needed to prevent accidents and possible injuries to patients, visitors, and health care personnel. The most common accidents among patients are falls, burns, cuts, and bruises. Fights with others, loss of personal possessions, choking and electric shock also occur.

In a Health care facility, nurses perform the following activities in promoting safe environment:

- Orient the patient and family
- Assess the patient's gait and risk for falling
- Keep the bed in a low position.
- Help the patient to go to toilet on a regular schedule
- Lock the bed wheels
- Provide a night light
- Answer call lights quickly
- Encourage the use of grab bars for the toilet, tub and shower.
- Stay with the patient who is confused, agitated, or unsteady.
- Restrict fluids after 6 pm so that patient does not have to get up frequently at night.

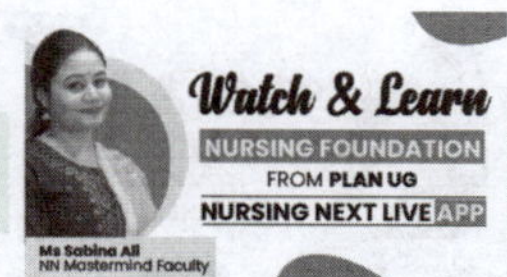

Nurses educate the patient/family member about the following points:

- Place a nonskid bath mat in the tub and shower
- Use of night light
- Installation of grab bars for bathroom/toilet
- Install door buzzers or bed alarms that sound when the patient leaves the bed.
- Encourage removal of extension cords because these may cause a fall.

Fall and injury prevention continues to be a considerable challenge across the care continuum. Morse scale is used as a fall risk assessment to find out if you have a low, moderate or high risk of falling.

SAFETY/PROTECTIVE DEVICES

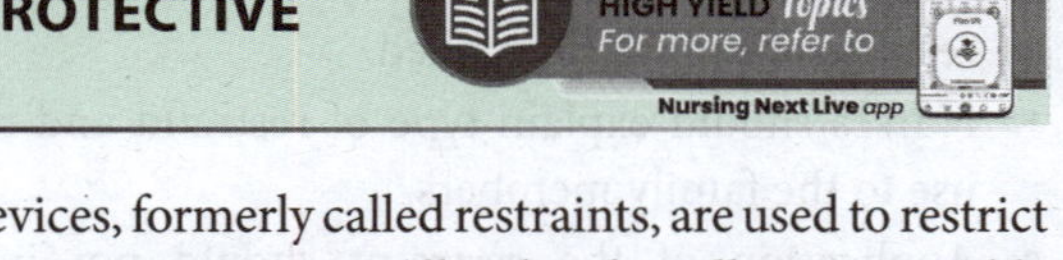

Protective devices, formerly called restraints, are used to restrict movement but at present it is an illegal and totally unacceptable practice that constitutes malpractice. Presently health care workers are encouraged to make frequent observations of the patient, which help to decrease the use of devices.

- The order must be written before applying a device. When the protective device is no longer needed, obtain an order to discontinue it. The usual time limit is 24–48 hours.
- The device should fit snugly when applied, but should not compromise the patient's neurovascular status. Nurses should be able to easily fit your index and middle fingers between the patient and the device.
- A device that is secured too tightly may cause injury.
- Active and passive exercises are performed for immobilized joints and muscles and remove the device at least every 2 hours. Check the area distal to the device every 15–30 minutes. Observe the signs of adequate circulation including pulse, distal to the device.

There are several kinds of restraints. The most common for adults are jacket restraint, belt restraint, a mitten or hand restraint and limb restraint; use of bed rails is also a restraint. Restraints for infants and children include mummy restraint, elbow restraint and crib knots.

There are three types of restraints: (1) Physical, (2) Chemical and (3) Environmental.

1. **Physical restraint:** Limit a patient's movement by use of certain devices.
2. **Chemical restraint:** It includes sedatives or antipsychotics for violent patients.
3. **Environmental restraint:** Control patients' mobility like confining them in a separate room.

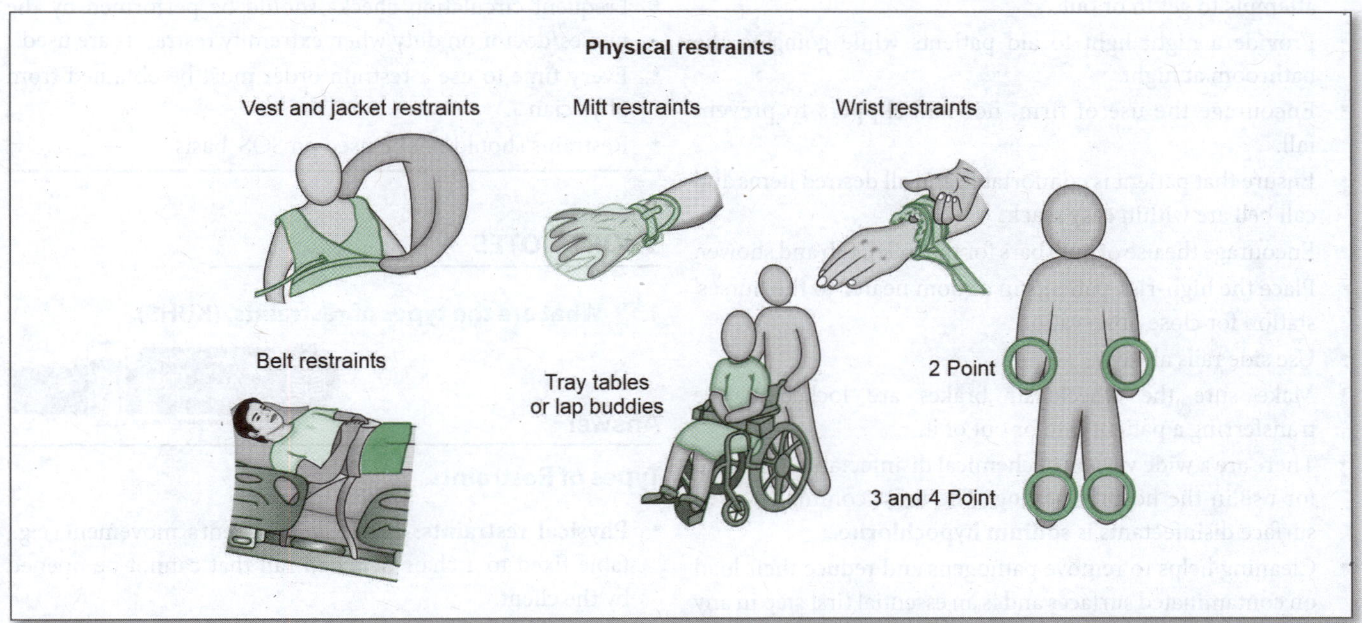

Other than restraints, there are a number of safety devices used in hospital to keep patient safe and secure. These devices are:

Side Rails, Grab Bars, Ambularm and Nonskid Slippers

Safety and security are main concern in nursing care. The responsibility of nurse is to provide safe and secure environment, and identify the harmful environment. Promoting safety and preventing injury are the primary concern in nursing.

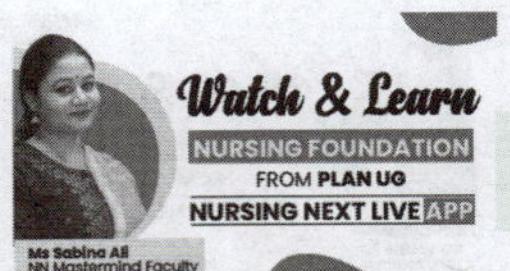

CONCEPTUAL EXERCISES

LONG ANSWER QUESTION

1. Write the responsibilities of nurse in providing clean and safe environment in hospital. Add a note on general principles for using restraints. (DU, MGR, KUHS, RUHS)

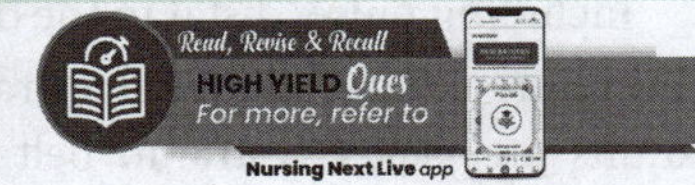

Answer

Nursing Responsibilities in Providing Clean and Safe Environment in Hospital

- On Admission, orient the patient and family members regarding call bell system, light controls, bed operation and television.
- Assess the patient's gait and risk for falling using Morse scale on admission.
- Keep the bed in a low position.
- Assist the patient to go to toilet in order to decrease the chances of accidental fall or fall-related complications such as brain injury, hemorrhage, fracture, etc.
- Lock the bed wheels to prevent the fall or when the patient attempts to get in or out.
- Provide a night light to aid patients while going to the bathroom at night.
- Encourage the use of firm, nonskid slippers to prevent fall.
- Ensure that patient is comfortable and all desired items and call bell are within easy reach.
- Encourage the use of grab bars for the toilet, tub and shower.
- Place the high-risk patients in a room nearer to the nurses' station for close observation.
- Use side rails always.
- Make sure the wheelchair brakes are locked before transferring a patient into or out of it.
- There are a wide variety of chemical disinfectants approved for use in the hospital setting. The most commonly used surface disinfectants is **sodium hypochlorite**.
- Cleaning helps to remove pathogens and reduce their load on contaminated surfaces and is an essential first step in any disinfection process. Cleaning with water, soap removes and reduces dirt, debris such as blood, secretions and excretions, but does not kill microorganisms. Therefore, a chemical disinfectant, such as chlorine or alcohol, should be applied after cleaning to kill any remaining microorganisms. Disinfectant solutions must be prepared and used according to the manufacturer's recommendations for volume and contact time.
- Enough disinfectant solution should be applied to allow surfaces to remain wet and untouched long enough for the disinfectant to inactivate pathogens, as recommended by the manufacturer.

General Principles for Using Restraints

- Restraints must be selected to reduce client's movement only.
- Before applying/using restraint, nurses should have consent from the doctor and from the family member also.
- Nurses should carefully inspect the site on which the restrains needs to be applied.
- Nurses should explain type of restraint and reason for its use to the family members.
- Application of the restraint should not interfere with treatment.
- Bony prominences should be padded before applying the restraint.
- They should be changed/discarded when they become soiled.
- Restraints should not be too tight or too loose. They should be able to release quickly.
- Frequent circulation checks should be performed by the nurses/doctor on duty when extremity restraints are used.
- Every time to use a restrain order must be obtained from physician
- Restrains should not be used on SOS basis.

SHORT NOTES

1. What are the types of restraints. (KUHS)

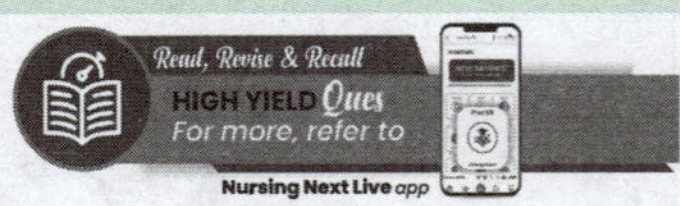

Answer

Types of Restraints

- **Physical restraints:** They limit a client's movement, e.g., table fixed to a chair or a bed rail that cannot be opened by the client.
- **Environmental restraints:** They control a client's mobility, e.g., a secure unit or garden, seclusion.
- **Chemical restraints:** They are any form of psychoactive medication used not to treat illness, but to intentionally inhibit a particular behavior or movement. Chemical restraint is the administration of medications to control a patient's dangerous behavior with anxiolytics or sedatives.

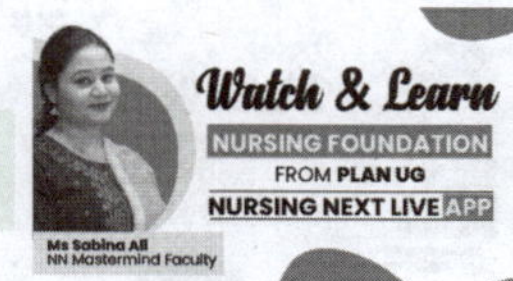

Types of Physical Restraints

- Mummy restraint
- Elbow restraint
- Extremity restraint
- Abdominal restraint
- Jacket restraint
- Mitten or finger restraint

Mummy Restraint

It is a short-term type of restraint used on infants and small children during examinations and treatment of head and neck. It is used to immobilize the arms and legs of the child for a brief period of time.

Elbow Restraint

This restraint is used to prevent flexion of the elbow and to hold the elbow in an extended position so that the infant cannot reach the face.

Extremity Restraint

It is used to immobilize one or more extremities. One type of extremity restraint is clove-hitch restraint which is done with gauze bandage strip (2 inches wide) making figure-of-eight.

The end of the gauze to be tied to the frame of the crib/bed.

This restraint should be used with padding of wrist or ankle.

Precautions to be taken to prevent tightening of the bandage.

Abdominal Restraint

This restraint helps to hold the infant in a supine position on the bed.

Jacket Restraint

These restraints are designed to limit a person's movement by wrapping around the individual's torso and arms, often resembling a jacket or vest, hence the name "jacket restraints.

Mitten or Finger Restraint

Mitts are used for infants to prevent self-injury by hands in case of burns, facial injury or operations, eczema of the face or body. Mitten can be made wrapping the child's hands in gauze or with a little bag putting over the baby's hand and tie it on at the wrist.

2. Write about the safety devices. (DU)

Answer

Safety devices are essential in the hospitals to separate people from dangerous zones or to reduce the risk of injury to others.

S – Sense the error

A – Act to prevent it

F – Follow safety guidelines

E – Enquire into accidents/deaths

T – Take appropriate remedial measure

Y – Your responsibility

Other than restraints, there are a number of safety devices used in the hospitals to keep the patients safe and secure. Various safety devices are discussed here:

- Side rails
- Grab bars
- Ambularm
- Nonskid slippers
- Safety belts
- Splints

Side Rails

The rails are made up of iron or steel. These can be raised when ever need arises and can be decreased as per convenience. The main purpose of side rails is to prevent from fall and can be used for other restraints. These are used for patients with convulsive disorders also.

Grab Bars

These are used to maintain balance. Lessen fatigue while standing and to grab onto in case of slip or fall. Grab bars increase patient safety and accessibility for anyone who has less mobility. These are often used in the washrooms of hospitals. These grab bars are also helpful in helping people using wheelchairs or walkers transfer to the toilet seat and back to the wheelchairs or walkers.

Ambularm

This is a position-sensitive electronic device that is an alternative to using restraints.

Nonskid Slippers

They are ideal to prevent falls. These slippers have latex-free rubber sole. These soles will need to dry before patient can walk unassisted as the wet soles will not grip properly.

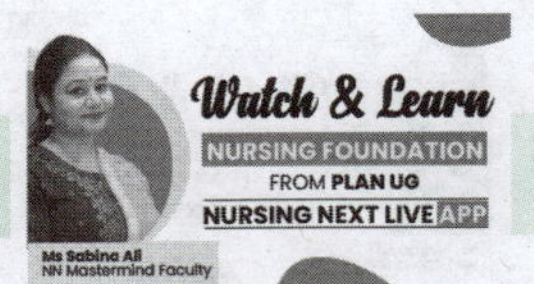

Safety Belts

These are made up of electrically nonconductive materials. These belts are used on stricter and operation labels to prevent the patients from fall. The belts go around the waist and tied to the frame of bed under the mattress.

Splints

These are prepared devices which are used to restrain the movements of extremities. These are made up of plastic, cardboard, hard paper, and cotton and gauze pieces. These can be applied wherever needed.

3. Write a short note on safe and clean environment. (DU)

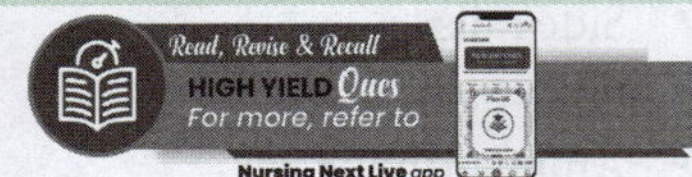

Answer

Safe environment contributes to patient's sense of well-being.

It is important for the nurse to ensure that bedside environment is clean, safe, and pleasant. The prime nursing responsibility is ensuring that necessary equipment and items are in their proper place and function properly.

On admission, the patient and the visitors should be oriented to the hospital environment, the equipment including the beds, call light, and the layout of the room and unit.

Arrange the equipment in the patient's room so that he or she is able to reach articles on his bedside locker like hearing aids, spectacles, crutch or cane, etc.

The nurse is responsible to allocate the type of bed/crib needed according to patient's age, needs, mental status and capabilities.

Safe bedside unit includes the following:

- Patient's call light should be functioning and always within reach.
- Bed should be positioned properly.
- Side rails and restraints are safely used.
- Provide uncluttered walk space.
- Attention to ventilation, odors, room temperature, lighting and noise.
- Odors may be decreased by promptly emptying bedpans, urinals and emesis basins, not to dispose of soiled dressing in client's room or near the bed.

SHORT ANSWER QUESTIONS

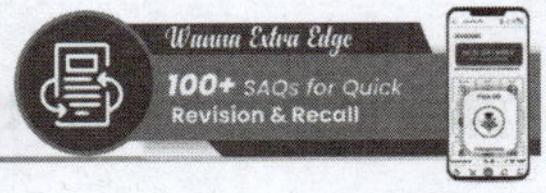

1. Define restraints and types of restraints. (MGR)

Answer

Restraints are physical, chemical or environmental measures used to control the physical/behavioral activity of patients or for his/her parts of the body.

Types of Restraints

Physical restraints: They limit a client's movement, e.g., table fixed to a chair or a bed rail that cannot be opened by the client.

Environmental restraints: They control a client's mobility, e.g., a secure unit or garden, seclusion.

Chemical restraints: Chemical restraint is the administration of medications to control a patient's dangerous behavior with anxiolytics or sedatives.

2. Define safety devices. (MGR)

Answer

Safety devices are essential in the hospitals to separate people from dangerous zones or to reduce the risk of injury to others. There are a number of safety devices used in the hospitals to keep the patients safe and secure. Various safety devices include:

- Side rails
- Grab bars
- Ambularm
- Nonskid slippers
- Safety Belts
- Splints

3. Give four examples of physical hazards. (MGR)

Answer

In a hospital setting, various physical hazards can pose risks to the safety and well-being of patients. This includes

- Falls
- Burns
- Smokes
- Fires

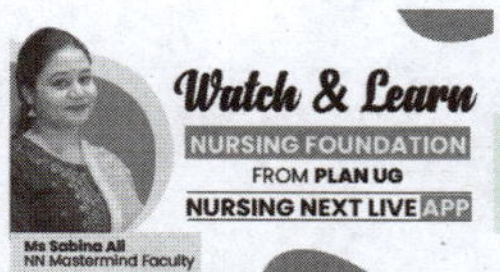

CONCEPTUAL REVISION

MULTIPLE CHOICE QUESTIONS

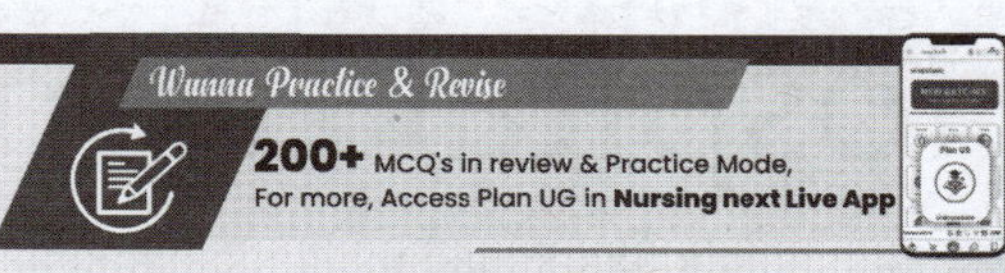

1. Which of the following is a risk factor for falls in the elderly?

a. Visual impairment
b. Decreased bone mineral density
c. Poor dental care
d. No orientation to the environment

Ans. a. Visual impairment

2. A nurse knows that the people most at risk for accidental hypothermia are: (Select all that apply)

i. People who are homeless
ii. People with respiratory conditions
iii. The very old
iv. People with cardiovascular conditions
v. People with kidney disorders

a. ii, iii, v b. ii, iv, v
c. i, iii, iv d. iii, iv, v

Ans. c. i, iii, iv

3. A fall risk assessment:

a. Promotes implementation of appropriate interventions based on need
b. Notifies all key health care staff of a patient's fall risk
c. Reduces potential of serious harm or even death through screening
d. All of the above
e. Only a and b

Ans. d. All of the above

4. In order to reduce the possibility of a patient fall, the optimal time to complete the initial fall risk assessment is:

a. <2 hours after admission to care unit
b. >4 hours after admission to care unit
c. Within 24 hours after admission to care unit
d. Sometime before discharge

Ans. a. <2 hours after admission to care unit

5. Nikhil, a healthy adolescent has meningitis and is receiving IV and oral fluids. The nurse should monitor this client's fluid intake because fluid overload may cause:

a. Dehydration b. Hypovolemic shock
c. Cerebral edema d. Heart failure

Ans. c. Cerebral edema

6. An infant is hospitalized for treatment of nonorganic failure to thrive. Which nursing action is most appropriate for this infant?

a. Encouraging the infant to hold a bottle
b. Keeping the infant on bed rest to conserve energy
c. Rotating caregivers to provide more stimulation
d. Maintaining a consistent, structured environment

Ans. d. Maintaining a consistent, structured environment

7. Identify which is considered as a beginning sign of a decubitus ulcers?

a. Numbness b. Discoloration
c. Swelling d. Peeling of skin

Ans. b. Discoloration

8. A nursing intern is providing care of a dying patient. She asked to the Registered Nursing Officer about the last sense in a dying client will be.

a. Hearing b. Sight
c. Taste d. Smell

Ans. a. Hearing

9. A 40-year-old male patient brought to the emergency department. Doctor confirms that the patient is experiencing the sickle cell crisis. The assigned nurse will place the patient in which of the following position?

a. Knee-chest b. Semi-Fowler's position
c. Trendelenburg position d. Supine position

Ans. b. Semi-Fowler's position

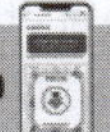

CHAPTER

11

Hospital Admission and Discharge

CONCEPTUAL THEORY

Terminology

Admission: It refers to the entry of a patient in a health care facility.

Assault: It is a threat or an attempt to do bodily harm.

Battery: It is physical contact with another person without that person's consent.

Consumer Protection Act (CPA) was passed by the Parliament in 1986 (INDIA) to provide better protection in the interest of consumers and focus on consumer justice through the establishment of consumer councils and other authorities for the settlement of consumer disputes and matters connected therewith. Under this act, consumer can complain in redressal forum.

Crime: It is a wrong act committed against a person or property or public good.

Defamation: It is communication that is false, or made with a careless disregard for the truth and results in injury to the reputation of a person.

Discharge or dismissal: It means the departure of the patient from the hospital. It can be a formal discharge of the patient by the attending doctor, when the patient's treatment is over.

Emergency admissions: Admissions for which there is no prior planning. Sudden illness, injury or abrupt worsening of an existing condition requires immediate admission

False imprisonment: It is the "unjustifiable detention of a person without legal warrant to confine the person."

Intentional torts: Include assault, battery, false imprisonment, invasion of privacy and defamation.

Invasion of privacy: It is a direct wrong of a personal nature.

Law: Can be defined as "the sum total of rules and regulations by which a society is governed." The law serves a number of functions in nursing:

Left Against Medical Advice (LAMA): In **Left Against Medical Advice (LAMA)**, due to personal reasons, the patient may abscond, i.e., leave the hospital without any prior information or the patient may expire during hospitalization.

Libel: It is defamation by means of print, writing or pictures.

Malpractice: It is the improper, injurious or faulty treatment of a client that results in illness or injury.

Negligence: It is defined as harm done to a client as a result of neglecting duties, procedures or ordinary precautions, e.g., performing nursing procedures that have not been taught, failing to follow standard protocols, failure to report, etc.

Nurse Practice Act (NPA): This law defines the scope of nursing practice, and provides for the regulation of the profession by a state board of nursing. The Nurse Practice Act in each state sets forth the scope of nursing for the registered professional nurse (RN), advanced practice nurses such as nurse practitioners and nurse anesthetists.

Routine admissions: Admissions which are scheduled in advance.

Slander is defamation by the spoken word, or stating unprivileged or false words by which a reputation is damaged, e.g., nurse telling a client that another nurse is incompetent.

The Occupational Safety and Health Act: It was passed in 1970 to improve the work environment in areas that affect worker's health or safety. It includes regulations for handling infections or toxic material radiation safeguards, and the use of electrical equipment. Health care agencies, as a result of OSHA requirements provide mandatory orientation and continuing education.

Tort is violation of a civil law, a wrong against an individual. The injury can be physical, emotional, or financial.

Transfer is the movement of a patient from one room to another, within the ward or from one unit to another or from one health care agency to another.

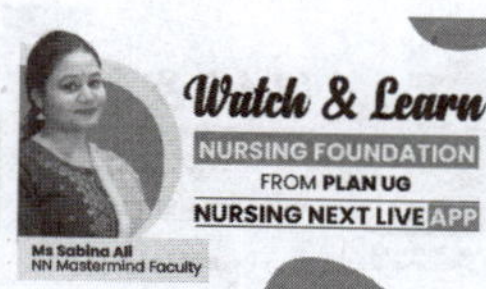

ADMISSION

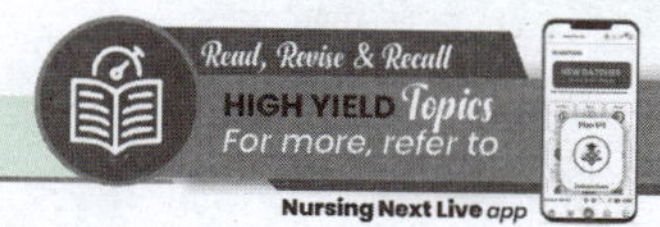

Admission refers to the entry of a patient in a health care facility. Admission is of two types:

1. Routine admission
2. Emergency admission

1. **Routine admissions** are those that are scheduled in advance.
2. **Emergency admissions** are those for which there was no prior planning. Sudden illness, injury or abrupt worsening of an existing condition requires immediate admission.

Admission Procedure

- Prepare the room
- Check the client's identification and greet the client and relatives and introduce self
- Observe the client's vital signs
- Check the physician's order for any treatment
- Provide privacy
- Demonstrate use of call-bell, over bed table use, lighting, TV, radio, telephone
- Explanation of hospital policies

Admission Formalities of Medical-legal Cases (MLC)

- Patient records should be kept confidential
- The records need to be properly labeled
- The chief medical officer and police need to be informed regarding admission

Transfer

Transfer is the movement of a patient from one room to another, within the ward or from one unit to another or from one health care agency to another.

Discharge or dismissal from the hospital means the departure of patient from the hospital. It can be formal discharge of the patient by the attending doctor, when the patient's treatment is over. In Left Against Medical Advice (LAMA), due to personal reasons, the patient may abscond, i.e., leave the hospital without any prior information or the patient may expire during hospitalization.

Safe nursing practice includes an understanding of the legal boundaries within which nurses must function. Nurses must understand the law to protect themselves from liability and to protect their client's rights. The laws are needed to ensure that the nurse's decisions and actions are consistent with current legal principles and to protect the nurse from liability.

Law

Law can be defined as "the sum total of rules and regulations by which a society is governed". The law serves a number of functions in nursing:

- It provides a framework for establishing which nursing actions in the care of clients are legal.
- It differentiates the nurses' responsibilities from those of other health professionals.
- It helps in establishing the boundaries of independent nursing action.
- It assists in maintaining a standard of nursing practice by making nurses accountable under the law.

Crime

Crime is a wrong committed against a person or property or public good.

A nurse may be liable if the client did not receive prescribed medications and was harmed (an act of omission).

Crimes of omission include failure to perform a prescribed treatment, failing to report child or elder abuse and failure to report a specified communicable disease.

TORT

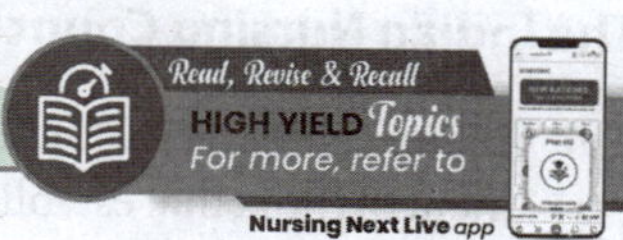

- Tort is violation of a civil law or, a wrong against an individual. The injury can be physical, emotional, or financial. It can be (i) Intentional or (ii) Unintentional.
  - **Intentional torts:** Include assault, battery, false imprisonment, invasion of privacy and defamation.
    - **Assault:** It is a threat or an attempt to do bodily harm.
    - **Battery:** It is physical contact with another person without that person's consent.
    - **False imprisonment**: It is the "unjustifiable detention of a person without legal warrant to confine the person."
    - **Invasion of privacy**: It is a direct wrong of a personal nature.
    - **Defamation:** It is communication that is false, or made with a careless disregard for the truth and results in injury to the reputation of a person. **Libel** is defamation by means of print, writing or pictures. **Slander** is defamation by the spoken word, or stating unprivileged or false words by which a reputation is damaged, e.g., nurse telling a client that another nurse is incompetent.
  - **Unintentional Tort:** It is (i) Negligence and (ii) Malpractice.
  - **Negligence:** It is defined as harm done to a client as a result of neglecting duties, procedures or ordinary precautions, e.g., performing nursing procedures that have not been taught, failing to follow standard protocols, failure to report, etc.
  - **Malpractice:** It is the improper, injurious or faulty treatment of a client that results in illness or injury.

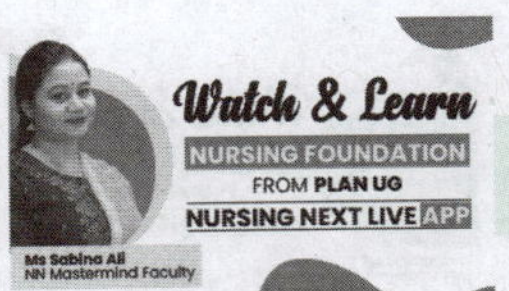

Target High Next Nursing **DECODE**

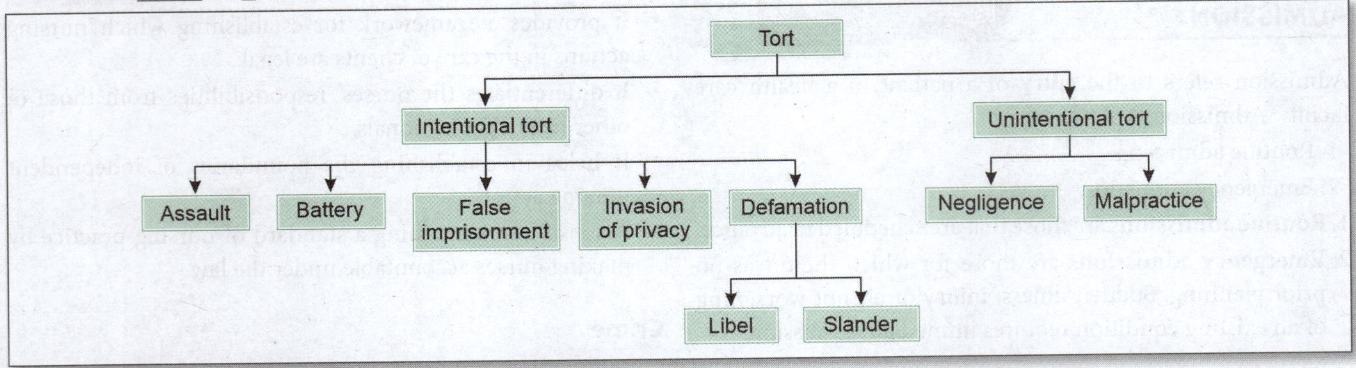

Figure 11.1: Classification of tort

LAWS RELATED TO THE PRACTICE OF NURSING AND LICENSURE

The Indian Nursing Council Act, 1947

The Indian Nursing Council Act, 1947 is an Act of the Parliament of India that establishes the Indian Nursing Council (INC), the national regulatory body for nursing in India. The Act sets out the qualifications and registration requirements for nurses in India, as well as the scope of practice for nurses. It also establishes a code of ethics for nurses and provides for disciplinary action against nurses who violate the act.

The Occupational Safety and Health Act, 1987 (OSHA)

OSHA is a central legislation in India that regulates the safety and health of employees in the workplace. The act was enacted in 1987 to provide a safe and healthy working environment for all employees in India. The OSHA sets out the minimum standards of safety and health that must be met by employers in India.

Consumer Protection Act (CPA)

Was passed by the Parliament in 1986 to provide better protection in the interest of consumers and focus on consumer justice through the establishment of consumer councils and other authorities for the settlement of consumer disputes and matters connected therewith. Under this act, consumer can complain in redressal forum.

Legal Protections in Nursing Practice

- Licensure and Certification
- Standards of Care
- Scope of Practice
- Documentation of care
- Confidentiality and privacy
- Indemnity insurance (Professional liability insurance)

CONCEPTUAL EXERCISES

LONG ANSWER QUESTION

1. Explain the nursing responsibilities for the following:

a. Admission of the patient

b. Inpatient Department (IPD)

c. Patient absconding and leaving hospital against medical advice (LAMA)

Read, Revise & Recall HIGH YIELD Ques For more, refer to Nursing Next Live app

Answer

Admission of the Patient

Nursing Responsibilities for Admission in Outpatient department:

- Receiving the client:
  - Nurses should greet the patient.
  - Nurses should make the patient feel comfortable.
  - Orient the client and relative to the healthcare facility.
- Recording of Social and Medical data:

Obtain the identification data of the patient such as name, age, sex, education, address, occupation, religion, income, marital status, telephone no, etc.

Medical Data

Diagnosis, provisional diagnosis, duration of illness, presence of comorbidities and their duration, drug history, family history, etc.

- Monitor and record the vital signs of the patient.
- Monitor the height and weight of the patient. Calculate the BMI if indicated.

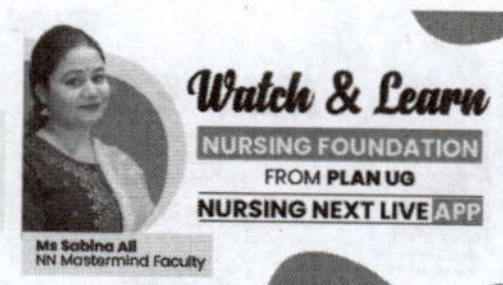

Medical Examination

- Assist the doctor in thorough physical examination of the patient.
- Maintain the privacy of the patient during physical examination.
- The necessary investigations such as X-ray, and lab test are need to be done.
- Orient the client to the different labs for diagnostic and therapeutic purposes.

b. Inpatient Department (IPD)

Answer

- Transporting the client from OPD to IPD through wheel chairs or stretchers.
- Arrange Patient's unit.
- Reception of the client by ward sister
- Nurses should introduce herself to the patient that she is her assigned nurse for the shift.
- Orient the client in terms of his/her room.
- Explain hospital policies such as no smoking policy, visiting hours, meal servings, doctor's visit, etc.
- Nurses are responsible for performing nursing assessment within 24 hours of the admission.
- Monitor and record vital signs.
- Perform the Morse scale and Braden scale on the day of admission in order to evaluate the patient in terms of fall risk assessment and presence of bedsores.
- If bedsore is present at the time of admission, it must be recorded, properly graded and informed to the head nurse and floor supervisor. These findings must be signed by the family member also.
- Check the doctor's orders that are to be carried out immediately.
- Give time to patient to change his dress with hospital dress.

Care of Valuables and Clothing

- Patient's clothing should be handed over to relatives.
- Encourage the client to send jewelry, money and other valuables such as watch to home with relatives.
- Apply identification band to the patient.
- Apply allergy band such as drug allergy and inform to physician also related to the same.
- Inform the concerned department related to the admission of the patient.
- Arrange diet, if applicable for the patient.
- Indent the consumables and prescribed medications for the patient.
- Complete patient's admission charts.

Medicolegal Issues at Admission and Discharge

- RTA
- Rail accidents
- Factory accidents or any other unnatural mishaps
- Suspected homicides
- Suicides
- Suspected or evident poisonings
- Alcohol intoxication
- Burn injuries due to any cause, electrocution
- Physical assault cases
- Animal attack, snake bite
- Mass food poisoning
- Cases of sexual assaults
- Suspected or evident criminal abortion
- Injury cases where foul play is suspected
- Injury cases where likelihood of death in near future
- Unconscious cases where cause of it is not clear
- Brought dead cases where foul play is suspected
- Cases referred from court

Brought Dead Cases

All the cases should be labeled as medicolegal and all the formalities must be done with informing the police constable on duty.

In the death certificate form against the column of cause of death, one should write "NOT KNOWN BROUGHT DEAD." In no case it should be mentioned that cause of death should be determined after postmortem.

Document in MLC register and inform the police of all cases of death on arrival/brought dead to casualty.

Tell the relatives/attendants about the legal issues and tell them that it is better to intimate police as autopsy is conducted to know the exact cause and manner of death.

- Informed consent not taken
- Advance directives
- Limitation of treatment (Do Not Resuscitate orders)
- Patient records should be kept confidential
- The record need to be properly labeled as medicolegal case.
- The chief medical officer and police need to be informed regarding admission of medicolegal case.

c. Patient Absconding and Leaving Hospital Against Medical Advice (LAMA)

Answer

LAMA

The patient's representative requests discharge from the hospital and the attending clinician considers that discharge may result in serious risk resulting in an adverse health outcome.

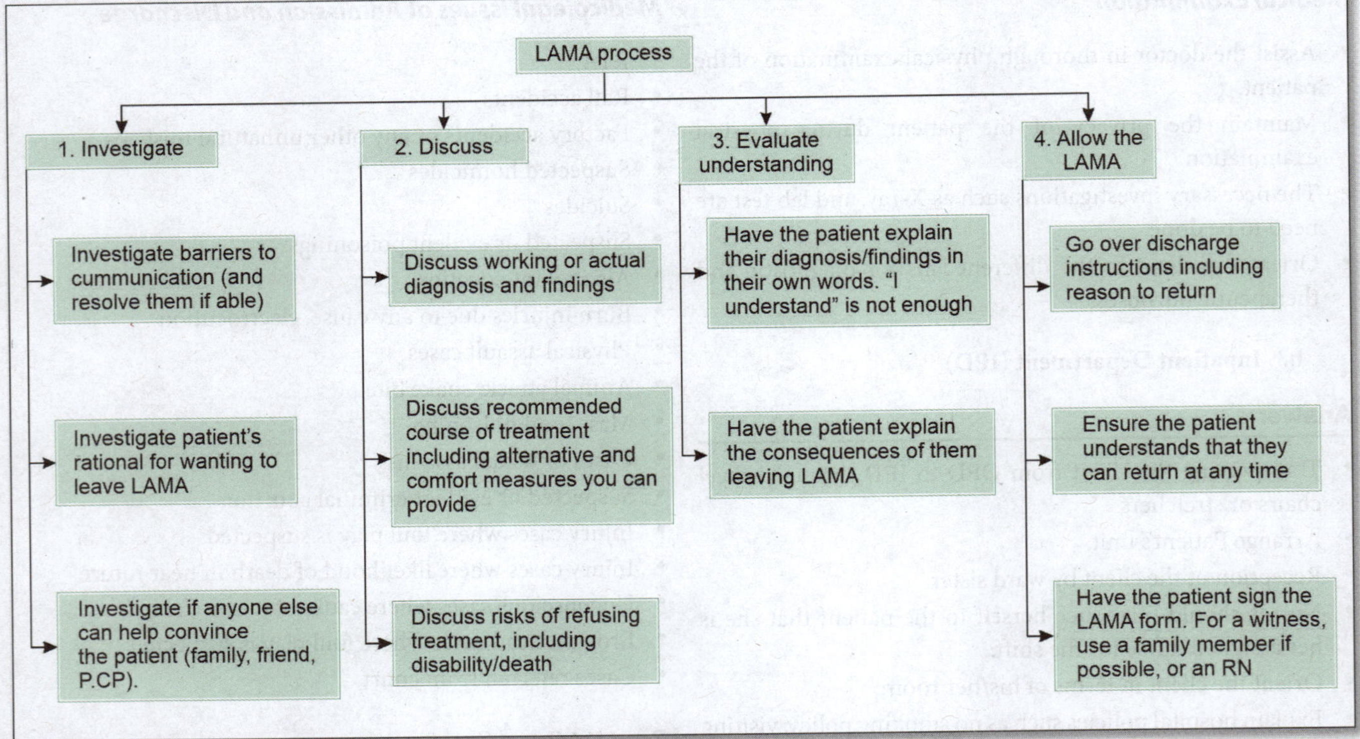

Figure 11.2: LAMA process

SHORT NOTES

1. Write a short note on patient transfer

Answer

Transfer of Patient

Transfer is the movement of a patient from one room to another, within the ward or from one unit to another or from one health care agency to another.

Reasons for Transfer

- For the implementation of diagnostic and therapeutic procedures.
- Changes (deterioration/improvement) in the patient's condition,
- For close monitoring (e.g., from procedural room to recovery room)
- After any minor/major surgery
- Transfer to long-term rehabilitation unit

Role of Nurse in Transfer

- Ensure that there is specific written order by the concerned doctor for the transfer of patients
- Inform the patient and family members for the reasons for transfer
- Assess the need of a patient whether a wheelchair or stretcher is required during transfer of patient.
- Notify the receiving unit of the time, date and condition of the patient before shifting.
- Notify the admission department about the room number of the shifting area so that patient's records can be updated.
- Document the transfer notes in nurse's notes both by the assigned nurse and the nurse receiving the patient with date/time and signature.
- Properly document the patient's chart for recording of vital signs, nursing care, treatment administered and assemble all the patient's documents, all lab reports and medications.
- Inform the dietician about transfer of patient.
- Document and inform the relatives about their belongings, valuables, glasses, contact lenses, dentures, hearing aids, watch, and jewellery, etc.
- Record the time, mode of transfer to the receiving unit.
- Accompany the patient while transferring.
- Introduce the patient to nursing staff of the receiving unit and handover the records, medication, etc.
- Collect the ward articles and return them to ward from where the patient was transferred

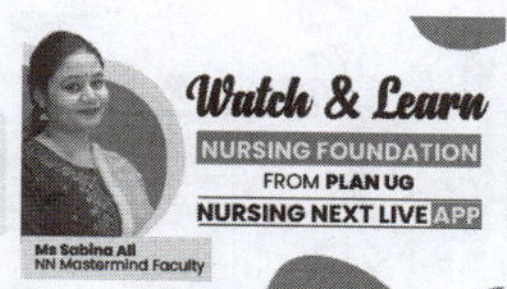

- Report to the nurse in charge regarding transfer.
- Document in census as per hospital policy.

2. Write a short note on discuss the nursing responsibilities while discharging the patient from hospital. (DU)

Answer

Discharge from the Hospital

Discharge means the departure of the patient from the hospital. It can be formal discharge, i.e., after the treatment of the patient. It can be LAMA (Leave Against Medical Advice) also i.e., discharge of the patient due to personal reasons and the patient may leave the hospital or abscond without any prior information. In the hospital, the discharge of the patient is also performed when the patient expires during hospitalization.

Discharge Planning

- Discharge planning is the systematic process for preparing the patient to leave the hospital for continuity of care. For effective discharge, planning has to start at the time of admission and it must be individualized.
- Preparation of patient and relatives
- During the discharge process, the physician writes a discharge order in patients file and also informs the head nurse or assigned nurse for the same.
- It is the responsibility of the nurse to make every effort during the discharge process also.
- Health teaching to the patient and to the family members ensures continuity of care.
- The patient needs to be instructed about diet, medication, activity, rest and follow-up.
- It is the responsibility of the concerned doctor to provide discharge information to the patient as well as to the family members.
- The patient and the relatives need to be psychologically prepared.
- Nurses should perform the proper arrangement for exit of the patient from the hospital either by wheelchair or stretcher.
- During discharge, one personnel as per hospital policy must be accompanied with the patient at the time of discharge.

Discharge Procedure

- Check the doctor's written order in patient's file for discharge.
- If the patient or relatives decide to take LAMA (leave the hospital against advice), doctor will take the signature either of the patient or of family member on LAMA form.
- Assist the patient to dress, check and pack belongings.
- Collect the discharge summary and prescriptions that the patient needs to bring for follow-up care.
- It should include the signature of the doctor and it should have complete necessary details of the patient.
- Complete the patient's record and discharge summary.
- Return all the unused consumables, all packed medicines, etc. to the pharmacy.
- Prepare the discharge file for the patient.
- Discharge file of the patient must include the discharge summary and reports of all investigations done in the hospital.
- Send the file to the billing section for clearance.
- Once the bill is settled, help the patient to obtain discharge his/her belongings.
- Instruct the family and patient for care, e.g., diet, medication, follow-up, etc.
- Nurses are responsible to communicate about the discharge to other departments of the hospital such as dietician, physiotherapist, etc.
- Accompany the patient up to the exit gate.
- Send the chart (in-patient) to the medical record department within 24 hours.

Special Considerations

- Patient's records or file should not be handed over to police or legal authority without a written permission of the treating physician.
- Name and address of the relative should be entered in hospital record with whom the patient has left the hospital.
- In case of death of the patient in hospital, physician should inform the chief medical officer and ensure that body is appropriately kept in mortuary for the postmortem examination as per hospital policy, if indicated.
- Unclaimed dead body must be handed over to police after due permission from the chief medical officer.
- The chief medical officer and police need to be informed regarding discharge of medicolegal case.

Care of Unit after Discharge

- Once the patient is discharged, the unit has to be prepared for next patient
- Remove the bed linen
- Clean the unit and wash the bed and locker with soap and water and use antiseptic lotion.

3. Write a short note on types of admission. (RUHS)

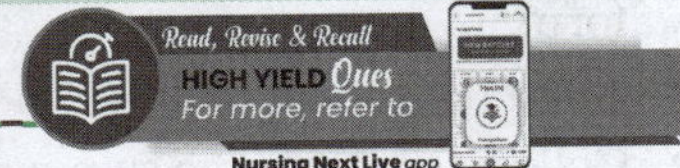

Answer

Introduction

Admission is defined as allowing a patient to stay in hospital for observation, investigation, treatment and care.

Admission is the entry of a patient into a hospital/ward for therapeutic/diagnostic purposes.

Types of admission:

- Emergency admission
- Routine admission

Emergency Admission

In this, patients are admitted in acute conditions requiring immediate treatment.

Examples are patient with RTA, poisoning, burns and cardiac or respiratory emergency.

Routine Aadmission

In this, patients are admitted for investigation, diagnostic and medical or surgical treatment. Treatment is given according to patient's problem.

E.g., Patient with hypertension, diabetes mellitus, etc.

Type	Explanation	Example
• **Inpatient**	**Length of stay generally more than 24 hours**	**Acute appendicitis, acute pneumonia.**
a. Planned (non urgent)	Is scheduled in advance	Elective surgery
b. Emergency admission	Unplanned, department and transferred to nursing unit	Unrelieved abdominal or chest pain
c. Direct admission	Unplanned, emergency department bypassed	Acute conditions as prolonged vomiting and diarrghea
• **Out patient**	Length of stay less than 24 hours	Minor surgery "Warts"
a. Observational	Monitoring required, need for inpatient admission determined within 23 hours	Head injury, RTA, FD

SHORT ANSWER QUESTIONS

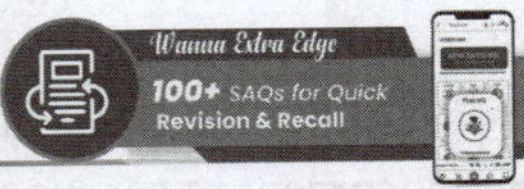

1. Define Admission and types of admission. (MGR)

Answer

Admission is the entry of a patient into a hospital/ward for therapeutic/diagnostic purposes.

Types of Admission

- **Emergency admission:** Patient with RTA, Poisoning, burns and cardiac or respiratory emergency.
- **Routine admission:** Patient with hypertension, diabetes mellitus, etc.

2. List the legal protections in nursing practice. (MGR)

Answer

- Licensure and certification
- Standards of care
- Scope of practice
- Documentation of care
- Confidentiality and privacy
- Indemnity insurance (professional liability insurance)

3. Define discharge and transfer of patient. (MGR)

Answer

Discharge or dismissal from the hospital means the departure of the patient from the hospital.

Transfer is the movement of a patient from one room to another, within the ward or from one unit to another or from one health care agency to another.

4. Define TORT.

Answer

Tort is violation of a civil law or a wrong against an individual. The injury can be physical, emotional, or financial. It can be (i) Intentional or (ii) Unintentional.

Intentional torts: Include assault, battery, false imprisonment, invasion of privacy and defamation.

Unintentional Torts: (i) Negligence and (ii) Malpractice

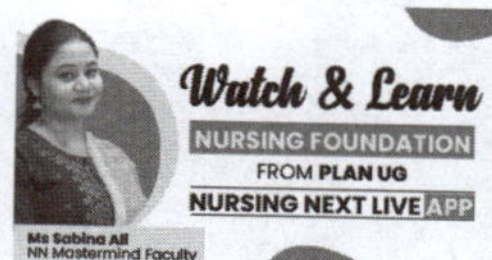

5. List down the admission procedures. (MGR)

Answer

Different types of admission procedures include:

- Emergency admission (to emergency dept.)
- Routine admission (to IPD)
  - Planned admission
  - Emergency (unplanned)
- Observational Admission (to OPD or Day care)

CONCEPTUAL REVISION

MULTIPLE CHOICE QUESTIONS

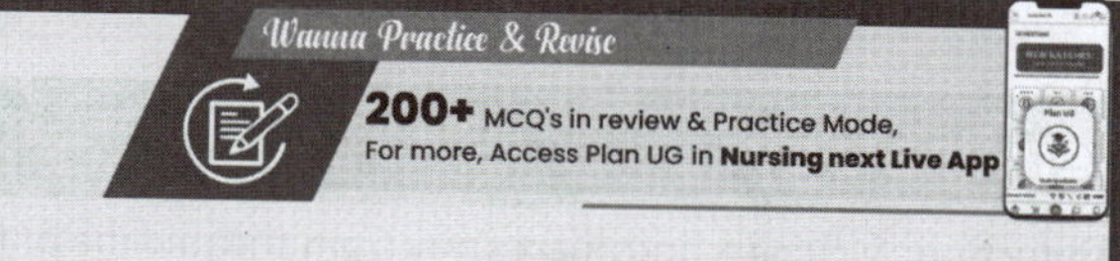

1. Admission of a patient means all of the following, except:

a. Allowing and facilitating a patient to stay in the hospital
b. Observation and investigation
c. Treatment and diagnosis
d. Rehabilitation

Ans. d. Rehabilitation

2. Which of the following is NOT the purpose of admission procedure?

a. Welcoming the patient
b. Providing comfort and safety to the patient
c. Involving patient and family in care
d. Ensuring patient and family understands the follow-up protocol

Ans. d. Ensuring patient and family understand the follow-up protocol

3. .... is done for clients suffering from acute conditions or life-threatening conditions like cardiac arrest, etc.

a. Routine admission b. Long term admission
c. Short term admission d. Emergency admission

Ans. d. Emergency admission

4. .... is planned for clients suffering from clinical disorders and who need to undergo any treatment modality or diagnostic procedure.

a. Routine admission b. Long term admission
c. Short term admission d. Emergency admission

Ans. a. Routine admission

5. .... required for clients suffering from pathological conditions having a long-term recovery period.

a. Routine admission b. Long term admission
c. Short term admission d. Emergency admission

Ans. b. Long term admission

6. .... is done for patient suffering from any medical condition requiring continuous medical care and are admitted to hospital for better management.

a. Routine admission b. Therapeutic admission
c. Short term admission d. Emergency admission

Ans. b. Therapeutic admission

7. .... is usually a short term admission meant to undergo some investigations.

a. Routine admission b. Diagnostic admission
c. Short term admission d. Emergency admission

Ans. b. Diagnostic admission

8. Which of the following is NOT a medicolegal issue related to admission?

a. Patient's OPD records must be kept under lock and key
b. Patient's record must be kept confidential
c. Patient's belongings should be kept under custody
d. Written consent is not necessary if patient unable to give consent.

Ans. d. Written consent is not necessary if patient is unable to give consent.

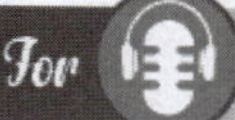

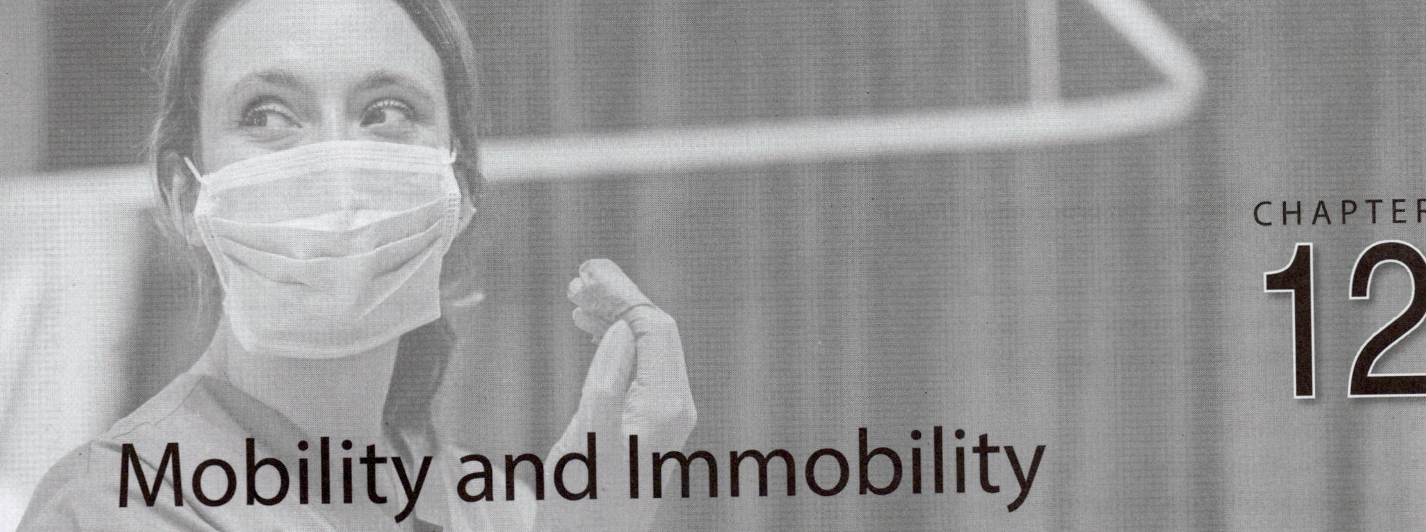

CHAPTER 12

Mobility and Immobility

CONCEPTUAL THEORY

150+ key terminologies for Quick Recall & Revision

Terminology

Abduction: Moving a body part away from the midline of the body.
Active range of motion: Exercises are highly independent, performed solely by the client.
Adduction: Moving a body part toward the midline of the body.
Aerobic exercise: Refers to sustained muscle movements that increase blood flow, heart rate, and metabolic demand for oxygen over time, promoting cardiovascular conditioning. Examples include swimming, walking, jogging, etc.
Ambulation: The ability to walk. This includes assistance from another person or an assistive device, such as a cane, walker, or crutches.
Bed mobility: The ability of a patient to move around in bed, including moving from lying to sitting and sitting to lying.
Body jacket cast: Encases the trunk
Cast: A **cast** is a rigid, temporary, immobilizing, and protective external device made of layers of plasters or fiberglass material molded to the body parts that it encases. Casting allows to perform normal activities of daily living and maintains stability.
Eversion: Turning the sole of the foot away from the midline.
Exercise: Active exertion of muscles involving the contraction and relaxation of muscle groups.
Extension: Straightening a body part.
External rotation: turning the joint outward.
Flexion: Bending a body part.
Functional mobility: It is the ability of a person to move around in their environment, including walking, standing up from a chair, sitting down from standing, and moving around in bed.
Immobility: Anything that disrupts this integrated process can lead to impaired mobility or immobility. Immobility can be caused by several physical and psychological factors, including acute and chronic diseases, traumatic injuries, and chronic pain.
Internal rotation: Turning the joint inward.
Inversion: Turning the sole of the foot toward the midline.
Isokinetic exercise involves muscle contraction with resistance. The resistance is provided at a constant rate by an external device.
Isometric exercise involves muscle contraction without shortening. Examples include contraction of quadriceps and gluteal muscles.
Isotonic exercise involves muscle shortening and active movement. Examples include carrying out activities of daily living (ADLs) independently performing range of motion exercises, and swimming, walking, jogging, and bicycling.
Long-arm cast: Extends from axilla to palm, with the elbow normally immobilized at a right angle.
Long-leg cast: Extends from the upper or middle thigh to the base of the toes.
Mobility is the ability of a patient to change and control their body position.
Passive range of motion: It is practiced on a joint that is inactive. The physical therapist may use this exercise on a client who is paralyzed or unable to mobilize a specific joint.
Plantar flexion: Bending the foot down at the ankle.
Positioning: It is defined as placing the person in such a way to perform therapeutic interventions for the purpose of preventive, promotive, curative and rehabilitative aspects of health.
Pronation: Turning the joint downward.
Range of motion (ROM) exercises are those in which a joint is moved through a full range of motion according to its capacity. It includes active exercises which are done by person himself and passive exercises which are carried with the help of another person. The main purpose is to improve muscle strength, prevent complications of immobility like contractures and to increase joint flexibility.
Rotation: Turning the joint.
Spica cast: Hip spica—a body cast that encases the trunk and one or both lower extremities; Shoulder spica—a body cast that encases the trunk, shoulder, and elbow.

Contd...

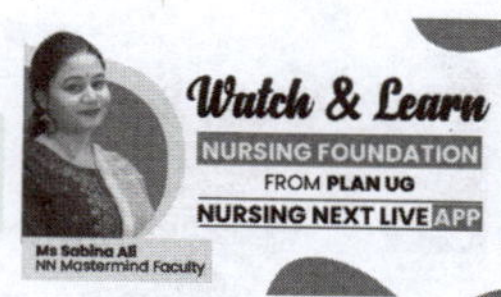

Short-arm cast: Extends from below the elbow to the palm.
Short-leg cast: Extends from below the knee to the base of the toes.
Splints: These are the devices used to support or immobilize a limb or joint. They are used as short-term treatment for any painful injury, which helps to prevent further injury.
Strength and endurance exercises are components of a variety of muscle building programs.
Stretching exercises: These exercises involve movements that allow muscles and joints to be stretched gently through their full range of motion, increasing flexibility, specific warm-up and cool down exercises.
Supination: Turning the joint upward.
Thumb spica: Extends from below the elbow to the palm and includes the thumb.
Transferring: The action of a patient moving from one surface to another. This includes moving from a bed into a chair or moving from one chair to another.

MOVEMENT OF THE BODY

Purposeful, coordinated movement of the body and maintenance of alignment require the integrated functioning of the musculoskeletal and nervous system.

Good posture or good body alignment is the alignment of body parts that permits optimal musculoskeletal balance and operation and promotes healthy physiologic functioning.

A body in correct alignment is balanced. An object is balanced when its center of gravity is close to its base of support, the line of gravity goes through the base of support and the object has wide base of support.

Active exertion of muscles involving the contraction and relaxation of muscle groups is termed exercise.

There are two types of exercises. One is based on the type of *muscle contraction* occurring during the exercise and second is based on the type of *body movement*.

On the Basis of Muscle Contraction

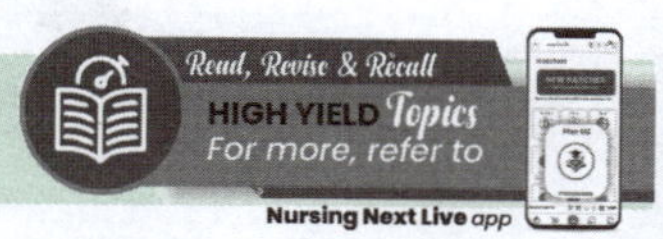

- **Isotonic exercise** involves muscle shortening and active movement. Examples include carrying out activities of daily living (ADLs) independently performing range of motion exercises, and swimming, walking, jogging, and bicycling.
- Isometric exercise involves muscle contraction without shortening. Isometric exercises are typically used to improve muscle strength and endurance.
- Examples include contraction of quadriceps and gluteal muscles.
- **Isokinetic exercise** involves muscle contraction with resistance. The resistance is provided at a constant rate by an external device.

On the Basis of Body Movement

Types of exercises involving body movement include aerobic exercises, stretching exercises, strength and endurance exercises, and movement and ADLs.

- **Aerobic exercise** refers to sustained muscle movements that increase blood flow, heart rate, and metabolic demand for oxygen over time, promoting cardiovascular conditioning. Examples include swimming, walking, jogging, etc.
- **Stretching exercises** involve movements that allow muscles and joints to be stretched gently through their full range of motion, increasing flexibility, specific warm-up and cool down exercises.
- **Strength and endurance exercises** are components of a variety of muscle building programs.
- **Range of motion (ROM) exercises** are those in which a joint is moved through a full range of motion according to its capacity. It includes active exercises which are done by person himself and passive exercises which are carried with the help of another person. The main purpose is to improve muscle strength, prevent complications of immobility like contractures and to increase joint flexibility.

These exercises include flexion, extension, hyperextension, abduction, adduction, circumduction, external rotation, internal rotation, pronation, supination, etc.

Many devices and equipment are available to aid in transferring, repositioning, and lifting patients. It is important to use the right equipment and appropriate device based on patient's assessment and desired movement Such as **Gait Belts, Stand Assist and Repositioning Aids, Lateral Assist Devices, Transfer Chairs, Powered Stand Assist** and **powered Full-body Lifts.**

Splints are the devices used to support or immobilize a limb or joint. They are used as short-term treatment for any painful injury, which helps to prevent further injury.

Purposes of Splinting

- To immobilize and stabilize extremity injuries to prevent further damage to soft tissues, blood vessels, nerves, or bones.
- To decrease pain from the impaired neurologic function or muscle spasm.
- To decrease swelling associated with injury by reducing blood and fluid loss into the soft tissues.
- To immobilize injured areas after burns, bites, or stings.
- To immobilize areas during the healing of infections or inflammatory processes and after the surgical repair of muscles or tendons.

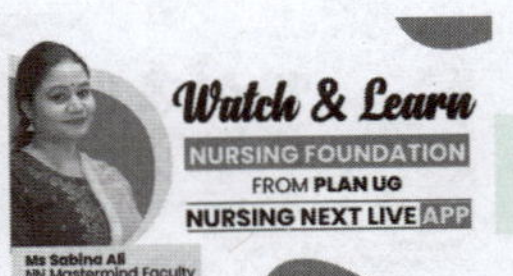

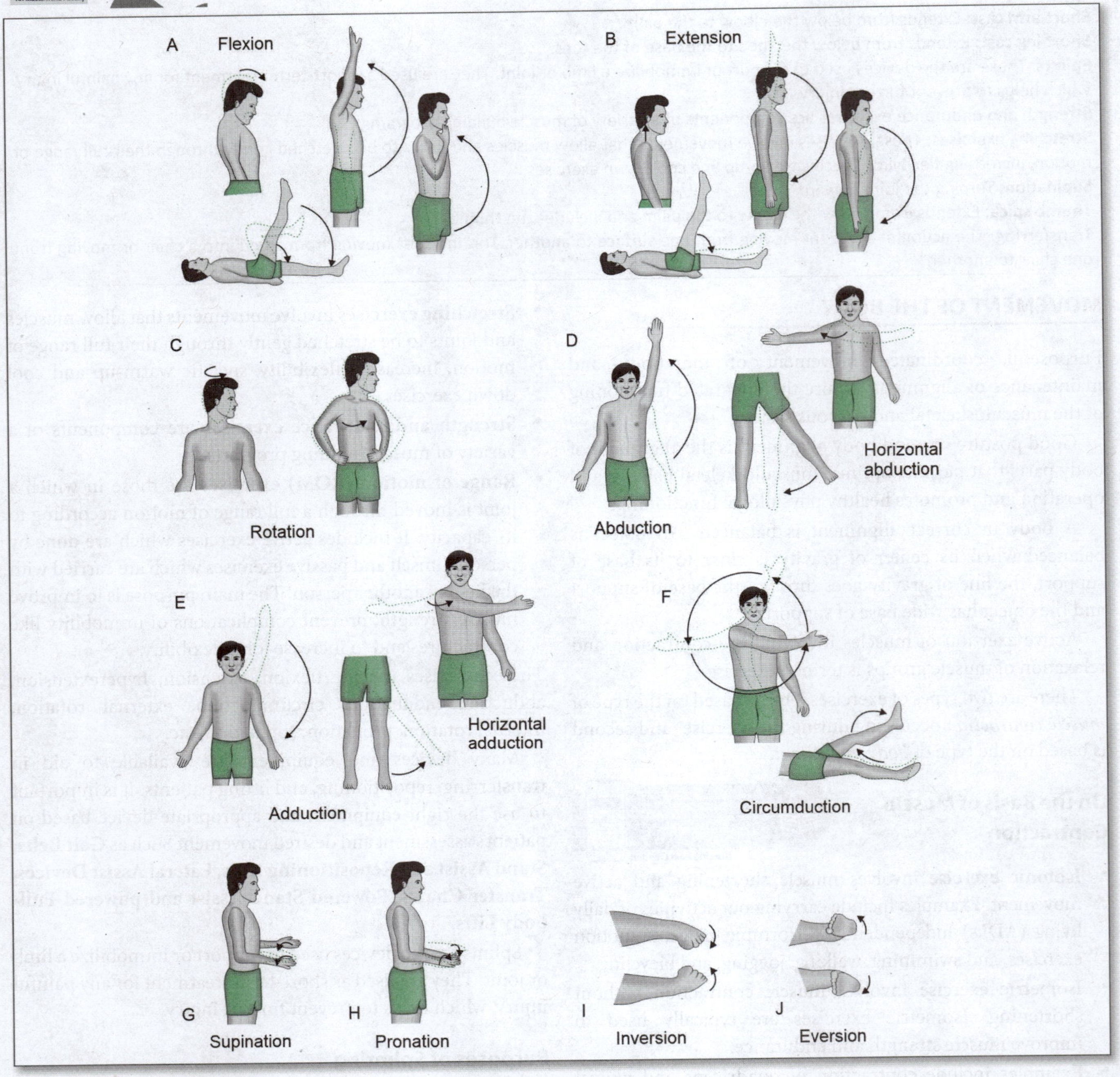

Figure 12.1: Body movements

Types of splints	Uses
Vacuum splint	To immobilize an injured extremity temporarily
Air splint (Pneumatic splint)	Temporarily immobilize injuries of the distal extremities – arm, lower leg, and ankle
Traction splint	Preferred splint for aligning and stabilizing a femur fracture (Thomas splint)
Posterior gutter splint	Used as a temporary stabilizing measure for knee injuries involving an angulated fracture and those requiring surgical intervention
Dorsal splint	For phalangeal fractures
Mallet finger splint	Used for alignment of crooked, arthritic fingers
Oval-8 finger splint	Used for interphalangeal joint stabilization

Contd...

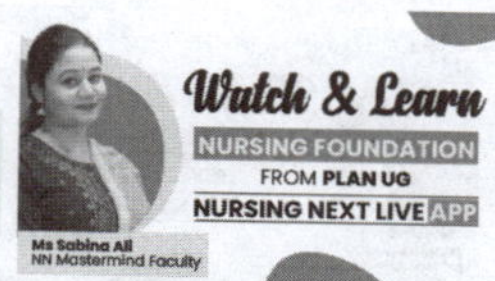

Types of splints	Uses
Thumb spica splint	Used for thumb fractures, tendonitis and arthritis to reliance
Volar splint (plaster, fiberglass, or aluminum splint)	Used for uncomplicated extra–articular fractures, sprains, and dislocations and for temporary immobilization, until operative reduction is accomplished
Internal fixation (Kirschner wire or pin or K wire)	Used for precise reduction with unstable or intra-articular fractures

Cast

A cast is a rigid, temporary, immobilizing, and protective external device made of layers of plasters or fiberglass material molded to the body parts that it encases. Casting allows to perform normal activities of daily living and maintains stability.

- **Short-arm cast:** Extends from below the elbow to the palm
- **Thumb spica:** Extends from below the elbow to the palm and includes the thumb
- **Long-arm cast:** Extends from axilla to palm, with the elbow normally immobilized at a right angle
- **Short-leg cast:** Extends from below the knee to the base of the toes
- **Long-leg cast:** Extends from the upper or middle thigh to the base of the toes
- **Body Jacket cast:** Encases the trunk
- **Spica cast:** Hip spica—a body cast that encases the trunk and one or both lower extremities; Shoulder spica—a body cast that encases the trunk, shoulder, and elbow

CONCEPTUAL EXERCISES

LONG ANSWER QUESTIONS

1. a. **Define mobility and immobility. (RUHS, KUHS)**
b. **Describe the principle of body mechanics. (RUHS, KUHS)**
c. **Describe various positions used in body alignment. (RUHS, KUHS)**

Answer

Mobility and Immobility

Mobility is defined as the ability to move freely, easily, rhythmically and purposefully in the environment.

Mobility is the ability of a patient to change and control their body position.

Functional mobility is the ability of a person to move around in their environment, including walking, standing up from a chair, sitting down from standing, and moving around in bed. The three main areas of functional mobility are as follows:

1. **Bed Mobility:** The ability of a patient to move around in bed, including moving from lying to sitting and sitting to lying.
2. **Transferring:** The action of a patient moving from one surface to another. This includes moving from a bed into a chair or moving from one chair to another.
3. **Ambulation:** The ability to walk. This includes assistance from another person or an assistive device, such as a cane, walker, or crutches.

Immobility

Anything that disrupts this integrated process can lead to impaired mobility or immobility. Immobility can be caused by several physical and psychological factors, including acute and chronic diseases, traumatic injuries, and chronic pain.

b. Describe the principle of body mechanics

Answer

Principles of Body Mechanics

Action	Principle
Assess the environment.	Assess the weight of the load before lifting and determine if assistance is required.
Plan the move.	Plan the move; gather all supplies and clear the area of obstacles.
Avoid stretching and twisting.	Avoid stretching, reaching, and twisting, which may place the line of gravity outside the base of support.
Ensure proper body stance.	Keep stance (feet) shoulder-width apart. Tighten abdominal, gluteal, and leg muscles in anticipation of the move. Stand up straight to protect the back and provide balance.
Stand close to the object being moved.	Place the weight of the object being moved close to your center of gravity for balance. Equilibrium is maintained as long as the line of gravity passes through its base of support. Hold objects close to your center of gravity.

Contd...

Action	Principle
Face direction of the movement.	Facing the direction prevents abnormal twisting of the spine.
Avoid lifting.	Turning, rolling, pivoting, and leverage requires less work than lifting. Do not lift if possible; use mechanical lifts as required. Encourage the patient to help as much as possible.
Work at waist level.	Keep all work at waist level to avoid stooping. Raise the height of the bed or object if possible. Do not bend at the waist.
Reduce friction between surfaces.	Reduce friction between surfaces so that less force is required to move the patient.
Bend the knees.	Bending the knees maintains your center of gravity and lets the strong muscles of your legs do the lifting.
Push the object rather than pull it, and maintain continuous movement.	It is easier to push an object than to pull it. Less energy is required to keep an object moving than it is to stop and start it.
Use assistive devices.	Use assistive devices (gait belt, slider boards, mechanical lifts) as required to position patients and transfer them from one surface to another.
Work with others.	The person with the heaviest load should coordinate all the effort of the others involved in the handling technique.

c. **Describe various positions used in body alignment.**

Answer

Various Positions used in Body Alignment

Positioning is defined as placing the person in such a way to perform therapeutic interventions for the purpose of preventive, promotive, curative and rehabilitative aspects of health.

The types of positioning are as follows:

Dorsal Position/Supine Position

The patients lie on their back with head and shoulders slightly elevated.

Uses

- Comfortable position
- Examination of head, neck, chest, abdomen and extremities
- Surgery of anterior part of the body

Prone Position

A patient lies flat on abdomen and head turned to one side. Both the hands to be held in a comfortable position.

Uses

- Examination of posterior trunk, spines and rectum
- Surgeries of back
- To relieve pressure on areas such as sacrum, scapula and heel
- After anesthesia to prevent aspiration

Lateral Position

- Side lying position
- Patient lies on left side and most of the body weight is on the dependent hip and shoulders.

Uses

- Comfortable position
- Relieves pressure on bony prominences
- Used for enema, insertion of suppositories and for checking rectal temperature

Sims' Position

- Differ from side lying position in which weight is placed in the anterior ilium, humerus and clavicle.
- Patients lies on his left with left arm drawn behind the back.
- Right arm may be in any position.
- The right thigh is flexed against the abdomen.

Uses

- Vaginal and rectal examination.
- To relieve pressure in the buttocks, scapula and heels.

Fowler's Position

It is an upright position with the patient in a sitting position in the bed with legs resting on the bed.

Types

- **High Fowler's position:** 75–90°
- **Semi fowler's position:** 40–45°
- **Low fowler's position:** 30°

Uses

- Facilitates drainage of abdominal cavity.

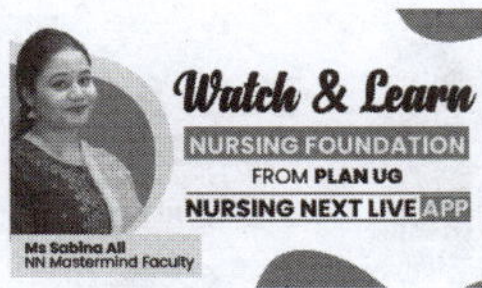

- Relieves breathing difficulty.
- Relieves tension on the abdominal sutures.
- Facilitating eating, reading, watching TV, etc.
- Relaxes large muscles of the back.

Orthopneic Position

- High fowler's position
- Over table placed in the front of the patient. Patient to rest both hands on over bed table supported by pillows and lean forward to the table (facilitates respiration)

Uses

- Patient with severe dyspnea
- Cardiac patients
- Position for thoracentesis
- Patient with chest drainage tubes

Lithotomy Position

- The patient lies on her back, the legs are separated and thighs are flexed on the abdomen.
- The buttocks are kept in the edge of the table and legs are supported by stirrups.
- Provides maximal exposure of genitalia.

Uses

- Vaginal examination
- Pap smear
- Position during delivery for many women
- Surgical procedures of genitourinary system

Knee-Chest Position

- Patient lies on the bed in such a way that the knees and the chest rest on the bed.
- The head is turned to one side.
- A small pillow can be placed under the chest.
- The weight of patient rests on chest and knees only.
- The knees are flexed and thighs are at right angle to legs.

Uses

- Examination of rectum and vagina
- Postpartum exercise

Trendelenburg's Position

- Head of the bed is lowered and the foot raised in a straight incline
- Patient lies on his back
- Beds are available with electric control system
- Reverse Trendelenburg's position: Head end of the bed is raised.

Uses

- Promotes venous circulation and venous return in patient with poor peripheral perfusion
- Postural drainage
- In OT examination and surgery in the pelvic organs

Dorsal Recumbent Position

- Patient lies on back, knees fully flexed and legs separated, thighs flexed and externally rotated and feet flat on the bed.
- Pillow is placed under the head.

Uses

- Examination of vagina and rectum
- Catheterization and care
- For doing procedures in the rectum, vulva and vagina

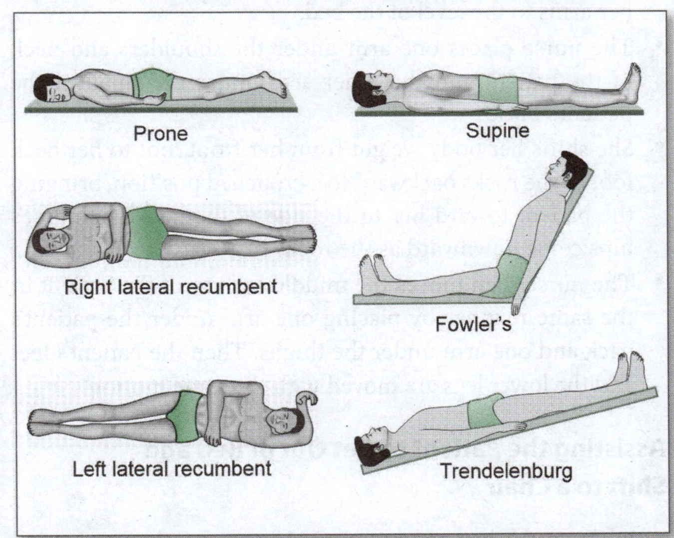

Figure 12.2: Various body positions

2. Explain the nurse responsibility for moving, lifting and transferring patients. (MGR)

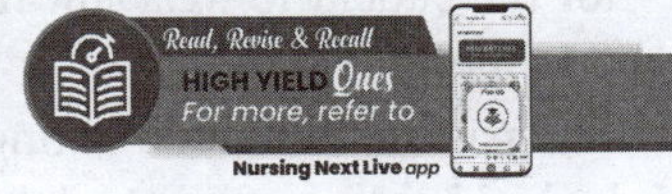

Answer

Turning the Patient in Bed

- The nurse stands on the side of the bed toward which the patient is to be turned.
- The patient places his/her far arm across his/her chest and his far leg over his/her near leg.

- The nurse checks that the patient's near arm is lateral to, and away from his/her body so that he/she does not roll upon it.
- The nurse stands opposite the patient's waist and faces the side of the bed with one-foot step in front of the other.
- The nurse places one hand on the patient's far shoulder and one hand on his/her far hip.
- As the nurse shifts her weight from her forward leg to her rear leg, the patient is turned toward her. The nurse's hips come downward during this motion.
- The patient is stopped by the nurse's elbows, which come to rest on the mattress at the edge of the bed.
- Helping the patient move to the side of the bed
- The nurse may require to move the patient to side of the bed. For example, if she is changing the dressing.
- The nurse stands facing the patient at the side of the bed toward which she wishes to move.
- She assumes a broad stance with one leg forward of the other and with her knees and hips flexed in order to bring her arms to the level of the bed.
- The nurse places one arm under the shoulders and neck of the patient and the other arm under the small of the patient's back.
- She shifts her body weight from her front foot to her back foot as she rocks backward to a crouched position, bringing the patient toward her to the side of the bed. The nurse's hips come downward as she rocks backward.
- The nurse then moves the middle section of the patient in the same manner by placing one arm under the patient's back and one arm under the thighs. Then the patient's feet and the lower legs are moved with the same motion.

Assisting the Patient to Get Out of Bed and Shift to a Chair

- In this procedure, the bed should be at a height from which patient can step naturally to the floor. If the bed cannot be lowered sufficiently, the nurse should obtain a footstool for the patient.
- The footstool must be stable and have a surface upon which the patient is unlikely to slip. Also, it is adjustable for the patient to wear low heeled shoes rather than loose on slippers.
- The patient assumes a sitting position on the edge of the bed and puts on shoes and dressing gown.
- A chair is placed at the side of the bed with its back towards the foot of the bed.
- The nurse stands facing the patient, her foot that is closer to the chair is a step in front of the other, to give her a wide base of support.
- The patient places her hands upon the nurse's shoulder, and the nurse grasps the patient's waist. The patient steps to the floor, and the nurse flexes her knees so that her forward knee is against the patient's knee. This prevents the patient's knee from bending involuntarily.
- The nurse turns with the patient while maintaining her wide base of support. She bends her knees as the patient sits in the chair.

Shifting the Patient from a Bed to a Stretcher (Three-Men Carry)

- To move a patient who must remain in the horizontal position from one place to another, for example, from a bed to a stretcher, three persons are usually needed.
- The tallest person should take the top-third of the patient, because she probably has the longest reach and can most easily support the patient's head and shoulders.
- The second person supports the middle-third of the patient, usually the heaviest part. She will be helped by the first and third person by putting their arms besides her. The shortest person supports the patient's legs.
- Before the patient is moved, a stretcher is placed at right angle to the bed, with the head of the stretcher almost touching the foot of the bed. The stretcher wheels should be locked. To coordinate their movement, the three persons must work by the numbers; the person who takes the head of the patient calls the numbers.
- The three who are to move the patient face the side of the patient's bed. Each assumes a broad stance, with her foot that is toward the stretcher being forward.
- At the call of "one", the three bend their knees and place their arms under the patient. The first person places one arm under the neck and shoulders and; the other arm under small of the patient's back. The middle person places one arm under the small of the patient's back and the other arm under his/her hips. The person at the foot of the bed places one arm under the patient's hips and the other arm under the patient's legs.
- At the call of "two" the patient is turned toward those who are lifting him/her. The patient's arms should not be allowed to dangle freely. The lifters hold him/her close to their bodies in order to avoid back strain.
- At the call of "three", they rise, step back (with the forward foot) and walk in unison to the stretcher.
- At the call of "four", they bend their knees and rest their elbows on the stretcher.
- At the call of "five", each lifter extends her arms so that the person rolls to his/her back at the middle of the stretcher. At the call of "six", each lifter withdraws her arms.
- In lifting the patient, the lifters should hold the patient close to their bodies. It is also important to lift and lower

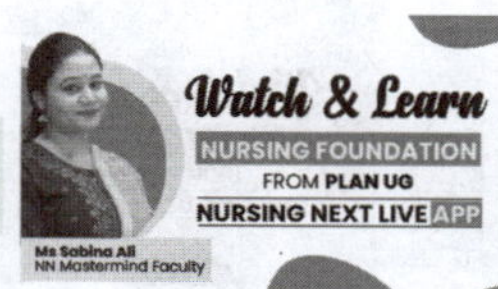

the patient with an easy smooth motion in order not to jar or frighten him/her.

Logrolling a Patient

- Provide privacy by closing door or bedside curtain. Explain the procedure to the patient.
- Raise the bed to a comfortable working height and lower the side rails.
- Have the patient cross his/her arms on the chest.
- Place a pillow between the knees.
- Have two nurses stand on one side of the bed opposite to the direction the patient will be turned. The third helper stands on the other side.
- Fanfold or roll the draw sheet tightly against the patient and carefully slide him or her to the side of the bed toward the two nurses.
- Have one helper, then move to the other side of the bed, so that two nurses are on the side to which the patient is turning.
- Face the patient. Holding the rolled draw sheet taut to support the body, turn the patient as a unit toward the two nurses. The patient's head, shoulders, spine, hips and knees should turn simultaneously.
- Use pillows to support the patient's back, buttocks, and legs in straight alignment in a side lying position.
- Raise the side rails, lower the bed, and place the call bell within patient's reach.

SHORT NOTES

1. State any four ROM exercises. (MGR)

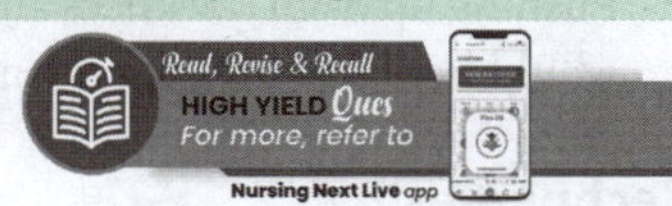

Answer

Range of motion (ROM) is the maximum amount of movement available at a joint in one of the three planes (Sagittal plane, Frontal plane, Transverse plane) of the body.

There are two types of range of motion:

1. Active range of motion
2. Passive range of motion

Active Range of Motion

- Exercises are highly independent, performed solely by the client.
- The physical therapists provide verbal clues.

Passive Range of Motion

- It is practiced on a joint that is inactive.
- The physical therapist may use this exercise on a client who is paralyzed or unable to mobilize a specific joint. This type of exercise, can help prevent stiffness from occurring. During this exercise the patient does not perform any movement, but the therapist is stretching the patient's soft tissues.
- **Flexion:** Decrease in the angle between circulating bones, e.g., Bending of head toward chest.
- **Extension:** Straightening a joint. There is increase in angle between circulating bones often to restore a part of the body to the anatomical position after it has been flexed, e.g., head in erect position.
- **Abduction:** Moving a joint or extremity away from midline of the body, e.g., moving of the palm laterally at wrist joint.
- **Adduction:** Moving a joint or extremity toward the midline of the body, e.g., bringing fingers together.

2. Mention the nursing intervention for impaired body alignment. (MGR)

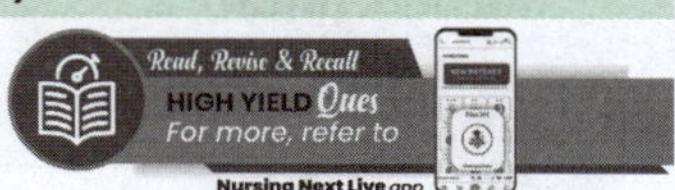

Answer

- If indicated pad bony prominences, soft-tissue areas (grain) and areas of skin-to-skin contact under the splint.
- If appropriate for the type of splint, measure against the unaffected extremity to determine the splint length.
- Grasp the extremity with both hands, one hand below and one hand above the injured site, and exert gentle longitudinal traction to straighten any angulation while the splint is applied.
- Align or straighten the extremity only enough to restore distal pulses. Altering or improving the splint to the extremity immobilize the joints above and below the injury site.
- Elevate the extremity as indicated and prescribed.
- Apply cold packs to the affected area for 10–20 minutes.
- Monitor the distal motor and neurovascular status.
- Prepare the patient who has an open fracture for operative intervention.

Documentation

- Distal motor and neurovascular status before and after splint application
- Type of splint applied and the patient's tolerance of the splinting procedure
- Skin condition of the extremity before and after splint application.

3. What are the complications of immobility? (MGR, KUHS)

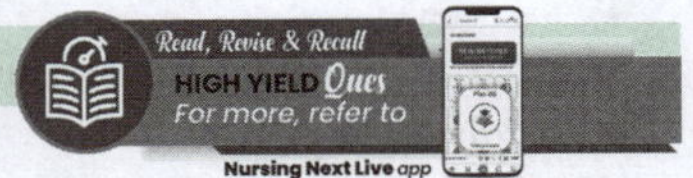

Answer

Complications of Immobility

Respiratory system	Gastrointestinal system	Circulatory system	Musculoskeletal system	Genitourinary system	Psychological
Pooling of mucus	Loss of appetite	Increased heart rate	Weakness	Incomplete bladder emptying	Anxiety
Decreased lung volume	Decreased peristalsis	Loss of plasma volume	Muscle atrophy	Formation of calculi in kidney and infection	Depression
Decreased oxygen saturation	Constipation	Development of DVT	Loss of calcium from bones		Delirium
Aspiration atelectasis	Increased risk of aspiration	Loss of orthostatic compensation	Increased risk of fall		Sensory deprivation
Less effective cilia			Loss of muscle strength		

4. Write the active exercises done by the clients on the bed. (MGR)

Answer

Active ROM exercises are those exercises which can be performed by the client independently.

- **Abduction:** Moving a body part away from the midline of the body.
- **Adduction:** Moving a body part toward the midline of the body.
- **Extension:** Straightening a body part.
- **Flexion:** Bending a body part.
- **Rotation:** Turning the joint.
- **Internal rotation:** Turning the joint inward.
- **External rotation:** Turning the joint outward.
- **Plantar flexion:** Bending the foot down at the ankle.
- **Pronation:** Turning the joint downward.
- **Supination:** Turning the joint upward.
- **Inversion:** Turning the sole of the foot toward the midline.
- **Eversion:** Turning the sole of the foot away from the mid line.

5. Mention the body mechanics for health care workers. (MGR)

Answer

Body mechanics is a broad term used to denote an effort coordinated by the muscles, bones and nervous system. It can either be good or bad and can be directly related to the occurrence of back pains.

Rules

- Keep the lower portion of your back in its normal position at all times.
- Move as close to the patient's bed as you can.
- Don't twist your body. Always do a side step or a pivot.
- Set your feet into a comfortable and solid wide base of support when lifting.
- Keep your abdominal muscles contracted, bow slightly using the hips and squat.
- Keep the head upright and hold your shoulders up.
- Pushing up from the knees and using your own momentum would help you lift the patient.

Techniques

Stable Center of Gravity

Maintain a stable center of gravity to evenly distribute your body weight.

- Keep your center of gravity low.
- Greater balance is met with a low center of gravity.
- Flex your knees and keep your body straight rather than bending.

Wide Base of Support

Maintain a wide base of support.

- Having a wide base of support gives your body more stability.

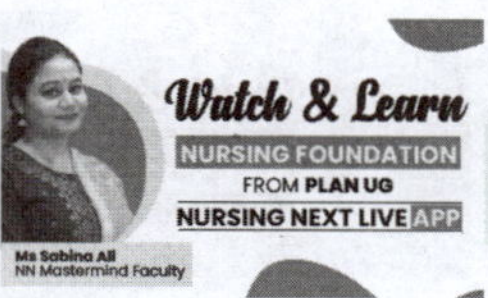

- Spread your feet apart to a reasonable distance.
- Flex your knees to move the center of gravity closer to the base of support.

Proper Body Alignment

Maintain Proper body alignment.

- Body alignment refers to the way the joints, tendons, ligaments and muscles are arranged when initiating a position.
- A line of gravity passing through your base of support maintains your balance.
- Equal activity balance in upper and lower parts of the body would reduce your risks of having back injury.
- When stronger muscle groups are involved, work can be safely done.
- Keep the back upright when performing interventions.

Moving Clients

Here are some guidelines for properly moving clients and other objects on the work area using proper body mechanics.

Pushing

- Stay close to the subject being pushed.
- Place one foot in front of the other.
- Place the hands on the subject, flex your elbows and lean to the subject.
- Place the weight from your flexor to the extensor portions of your leg.
- Apply pressure with the use of your leg muscles.
- To prevent fatigue, provide alternate rest periods.

Pulling

- Stay close to the subject being pulled.
- Place one foot in front of the other.
- Hold the subject, flex your elbows and lean your body away from the subject.
- Shift your weight away from the subject.
- Avoid any unnecessary movements.
- To prevent fatigue, provide alternate rest periods.

Lifting and Carrying

- Use squat position while facing the patients.
- Hold the patient and tighten your center of gravity.
- Use your dominant leg muscles for lifting.
- Hold the patient at waist height and close to the center of gravity.
- Always keep your back erect.

6. Write about four splints named after the surgeon. (MGR)

Answer

Internal fixation (Kirschner Wire or Pin or K Wire)

Used for precise reduction with unstable or intra-articular fractures.

Traction Splint (THomas Splint)

Preferred splint for aligning and stabilizing a femur fracture. (Thomas splint).

Structural Aluminum Malleable Splint (SAM)

It is a compact, lightweight, highly versatile device designed for immobilizing bone and soft tissue injuries in emergency settings. It consists of a layer of 0.16 inches (0.41 mm) strips of soft aluminum, with a polyethylene closed-cell foam coating.

Dynamic Traction Splint

Robert R Schenck develops a device for treating intra-articular fractures of the finger. The apparatus consists of a 6-inch-diameter circular splint that provides a rigid arc, with a 3-inch radius equidistant from the involved joint.

A wire is placed horizontally through the distal head of the middle phalanx. The wire is attached by rubber band to a movable component attached to the hoop of the splint. The amount of traction can be controlled by using different types of rubber bands or tying knots in them.

7. Write about the types of splints. (MGR)

Answer

Splints

Splints are the devices used to support or immobilize a limb or joint. They are used as short-term treatment for injury, which helps to prevent further injury.

Purposes of Splinting

- To immobilize and stabilize extremity injuries to prevent further damage to soft tissues, blood vessels, nerves, or bones.
- To decrease pain from the impaired neurologic function or muscle spasm.
- To decrease swelling associated with injury by reducing blood and fluid loss into the soft tissues.
- To immobilize injured areas after burns, bites, or stings.
- To immobilize areas during the healing of infections or inflammatory processes and after the surgical repair of muscles or tendons.

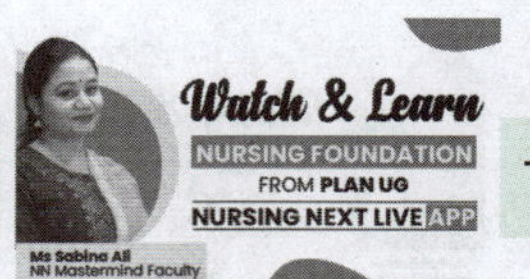

Types of Splints

Vacuum Splint

To immobilize an injured extremity temporarily.

Air Splint (Pneumatic Splint)

Temporarily immobilize injuries of the distal extremities-arm, lower leg, and ankle.

Traction Splint

Preferred splint for aligning and stabilizing a femur fracture. (Thomas splint).

Posterior Gutter Splint

Used as a temporary stabilizing measure for knee injuries in an angulated fracture and those requiring surgical intervention.

Dorsal Splint

For phalangeal fractures.

Mallet Finger Splint

Used for alignment of crooked, arthritic fingers.

Oval-8 Finger Splint

Used for interphalangeal joint stabilization.

Thumb Spica Splint

Used for thumb fractures, tendonitis and arthritis to reliance.

Volar Splint (Plaster, Fiberglass, or Aluminum Splint)

Used for uncomplicated extra-articular fractures, sprains, and dislocations and for temporary immobilization, until operative reduction is accomplished.

Internal Fixation (Kirschner Wire or Pin or K Wire)

Used for precise reduction with unstable or intra-articular fractures.

8. Write about the care of patient with impaired mobility. (DU)

Answer

Assessment

- Assess the patient's mobility limitations, strength, range of motion, and any specific challenges they face.
- Monitor changes in mobility status and evaluate the effectiveness of interventions.

Interventions

- **Positioning:** Help the patient maintain proper body alignment and positioning to prevent pressure ulcers, contractures, and discomfort. Use supportive devices like pillows, wedges, or cushions to provide stability and reduce the risk of skin breakdown.
- **Range of motion exercise:** Provide active or passive range of motion exercises (ROM) three times/day.
- **Activity of daily living:** Encourage activities of daily living (ADLs) as possible and progressively. Promote independence as much as possible.
- **Fall prevention:** Identify fall risks and implement preventive measures such as keeping the environment clutter-free, providing handrails or grab bars, and using alarms or monitoring systems. Educate the patient and their family on fall prevention strategies.
- **Assistive devices:** Provide therapeutic devices as needed. (Pillows, Footboard, Trochanter roll, Hand rolls, Trapeze bar).
- **Pain management:** Assess and address any pain or discomfort experienced by the patient related to their impaired mobility
- Consult appropriate health care provider (e.g. physician, physical therapist) if client's mobility and range of motion are more limited than expected.
- Provide foods rich in calcium.

9. Write a short note on hazards associated with immobility. (DU)

Answer

System	Complication
Respiratory	Pneumonia, atelectasis, pulmonary embolism
Cardiovascular	Postural hypotension, cardiac muscle atrophy, deep vein thrombosis
Skin	Pressure ulcers
Renal	Calculi, nephritis
Hematological	Anemia
Gastrointestinal	Constipation and fecal impaction
Metabolic	Glucose intolerance, negative nitrogen balance
Musculoskeletal	Osteoporosis, muscle atrophy, contractures
Neurological	Depression, psychosis

10. Write short note on active exercises and passive exercise. (DU)

Answer

Exercise is physical activity for conditioning the body, improving health, and maintaining fitness.

Exercise is classified into two forms:

1. Based on muscle contraction
2. Based on source of energy

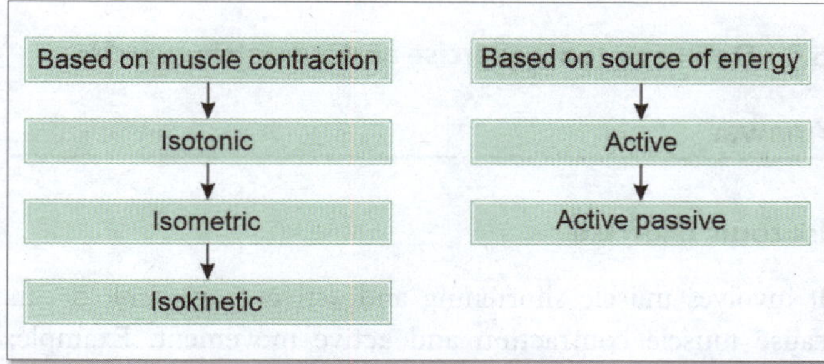

Active exercise is therapeutic activity that the client performs independently.

Passive exercise is therapeutic activity that the client performs with assistance and is provided when a client cannot move one or more parts of the body.

Range of motion exercises are the movement of a joint to the extent possible without causing pain.

Types of ROM exercises:

- **Active ROM exercises:** Exercises the client is able to perform independently.
- **Passive ROM exercises:** Exercises performed for the client by someone else.
- **Active assisted ROM exercises:** Performed by a client with some assistance. Client can move a limb partially through its ROM, but needs help completing the ROM.

11. Write the benefits of exercise. (KUHS)

Answer

Exercise is physical activity for conditioning the body, improving health, and maintaining fitness.

Benefits of Physical Exercise

- Improved cardiopulmonary function
- Reduced blood pressure
- Increased muscle tone and strength
- Greater physical endurance
- Increased weight loss
- Reduced blood glucose level
- Decreased low-density blood lipids
- Improved physical appearance
- Increased bone density
- Regularity of bowel elimination
- Promotion of sleep
- Reduce tension and depression

12. Write short note on isotonic exercise and isometric exercise. (KUHS)

Answer

Isotonic and isometric exercises are based on muscle contraction.

Isotonic Exercise

It involves muscle shortening and active movement. It can cause muscle contraction and active movement. Example: carrying out activities of daily living (ADLs) independently performing range of motion exercises and swimming, walking, aerobics and moving arms and legs.

Benefits

Increase muscle mass and strength, improve joint mobility, increased cardiac and respiratory function, etc.

Isometric Exercise

It involves muscle contraction without shortening, tightening or tensing of muscles without shortening (there is no movement). This increases muscle tension but does not change the length of muscle fibers. This type of exercise is typically used to improve muscle strength and endurance. Example: Rehabilitative exercises for knee and elbow injuries and lifting weights, contraction of gluteal muscles, etc.

Isotonic and isometric exercises can be combined to create a more effective strength training program.

SHORT ANSWER QUESTIONS

1. Define mobility and immobility. (RUHS)

Answer

Mobility is defined as the ability to move freely, easily, rhythmically and purposefully in the environment.

Immobility

Anything that disrupts this integrated process can lead to impaired mobility or immobility. Immobility can be caused by several physical and psychological factors, including acute and chronic diseases, traumatic injuries, and chronic pain.

2. State any four ROM exercises. (MGR)

Answer

- **Flexion:** Decrease in the angle between circulating bones, e.g., bending of head toward chest.
- **Extension:** Straightening a joint. There is increase in angle between circulating bones often to restore a part of the body to the anatomical position after it has been flexed, e.g., head in erect position.
- **Abduction:** Moving a joint or extremity away from midline of the body, e.g., moving of the palm laterally at wrist joint.
- **Adduction:** Moving a joint or extremity toward the midline of the body, e.g., bringing fingers together.

3. Write any four active exercises done by the clients on the bed. (MGR)

Answer

Active ROM exercises are those exercises the client is able to perform independently.

- **Abduction:** Moving a body part away from the midline of the body.
- **Adduction:** Moving a body part toward the midline of the body.
- **Extension:** Straightening a body part.
- **Flexion:** Bending a body part.

4. Name the four splints named after the surgeon. (KUHS)

Answer

- Internal fixation (Kirschner wire or pin or K wire)
- Traction splint
- SAM (Structural aluminum malleable) splint
- Dynamic traction splint

5. Define isotonic exercise and isometric exercise.

Answer

Isotonic Exercise

It involves muscle shortening and active movement. It can cause muscle contraction and active movement. Example: carrying out activities of daily living (ADLs) independently performing range of motion exercises and swimming, walking, aerobics, moving arms and Legs.

Isometric Exercise

It involves muscle contraction without shortening, tightening or tensing of muscles without shortening (there is no movement). This increases muscle tension but does not change the length of muscle fibers. Example: rehabilitative exercises for knee and elbow injuries and lifting weights, contraction of gluteal muscles, etc.

CONCEPTUAL REVISION

MULTIPLE CHOICE QUESTIONS

1. …………….. describes the coordinated efforts of the musculoskeletal and nervous systems.

a. Alignment b. Balance
c. Body mechanics d. Body alignment

Ans. c. Body mechanics

2. Which of the following postural abnormality is also called "genu valgum"?

a. Clubfoot b. Foot drop
c. Bowlegs d. Knock-knee

Ans. d. Knock-knee

3. Which of the following postural deformity is also known as "genu varum"?

a. Clubfoot b. Foot drop
c. Bowlegs d. Knock-knee

Ans. c. Bowlegs

4. Which plane of the body divides it into dorsal and ventral regions?

a. Transverse b. Axial
c. Coronal d. Sagittal

Ans. c. Coronal

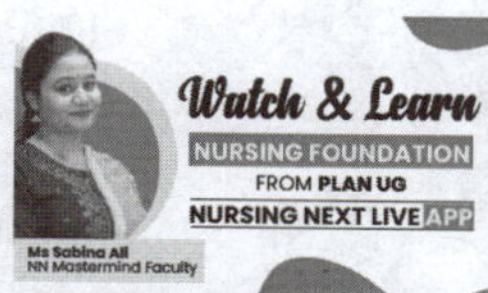

5. Identify the name of the position according to the image given here?

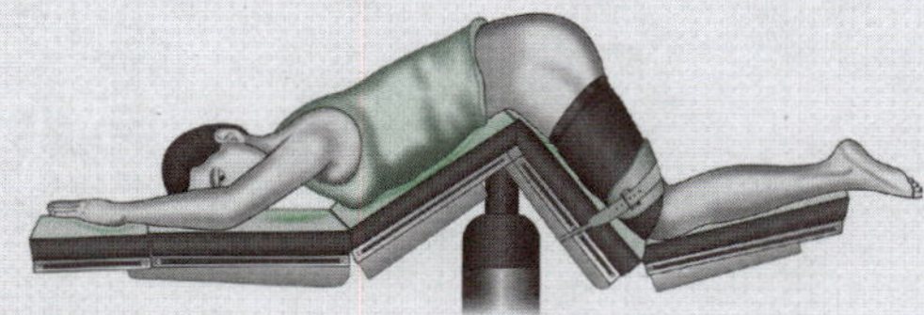

a. Jackknife position
b. Knee-chest position
c. Lloyd-Davies position
d. Rose position

Ans. a. Jackknife position

6. Identify the appropriate positioning of patient with increased intracranial pressure.

a. Elevate the head of the bed 30–45° and maintain the head in a midline.
b. Neutral position to facilitate venous drainage from the head.
c. Avoid extreme hip and neck flexion.
d. All of the above

Ans. d. All of the above

7. .... is more effective in treating physical ailments than in preventing disease or managing chronic illness.

a. Allopathic medicine
b. Complementary medicine
c. Alternative medicine
d. All of the above

Ans. a. Allopathic medicine

8. When bathing a patient's extremities, the nurse should use long, firm strokes from the distal to the proximal areas. This technique:

a. Provides an opportunity for skin assessment.
b. Avoids undue strain on the nurse.
c. Increases venous blood return.
d. Causes vasoconstriction and increases circulation.

Ans. c. Increases venous blood return.

9. The nurse puts elastic stockings on a patient following major abdominal surgery. The nurse teaches the patient that the stockings are used after a surgical procedure to:

a. Prevent varicose veins.
b. Prevent muscular atrophy.
c. Ensure joint mobility and prevent contractures.
d. Promote venous return to the heart.

Ans. c. Ensure joint mobility and prevent contractures.

10. The patient at greatest risk for developing multiple adverse effects of immobility is a:

a. 1-year-old child with a hernia repair.
b. 80-year-old woman who has suffered a hemorrhagic cerebrovascular accident (CVA).
c. 51-year-old woman following a thyroidectomy.
d. 38-year-old woman undergoing a hysterectomy.

Ans. b. 80-year-old woman who has suffered a hemorrhagic cerebrovascular accident (CVA).

Golden Points

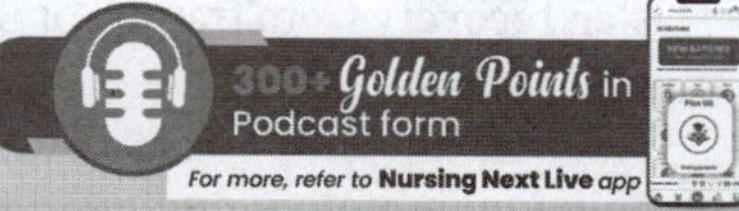

- Good posture or good body alignment is the alignment of body parts that permits optimal musculoskeletal balance and operation and promotes healthy physiologic functioning.
- Active exertion of muscles involving the contraction and relaxation of muscle groups is termed exercise.
- There are two types of exercises. One is based on the type of **muscle contraction** occurring during the exercise and second is based on the type of **body movement**.
- On the basis of Muscle contraction: Isotonic exercise, Isometric exercise and Isokinetic exercise
- Types of exercises involving body movement include Aerobic exercises, Stretching exercises, Strength and endurance exercises, and range of motion exercises.
- Range of motion (ROM) exercises are those in which a joint is moved through a full range of motion according to its capacity. These exercises include flexion, extension, hyperextension, abduction, adduction, circumduction, external rotation, internal rotation, pronation, supination, etc.
- Splints are the devices used to support or immobilize a limb or joint. They are used as short-term treatment for any painful injury, which helps to prevent further injury.
- A cast is a rigid, temporary, immobilizing, and protective external device made of layers of plasters or fiberglass material molded to the body parts that it encases.
- Casting allows to perform normal activities of daily living and maintains stability.

CHAPTER 13

Patient Education

CONCEPTUAL THEORY

Terminology

Patient education: It is the process of influencing the patient's behavior to effect changes in knowledge, attitudes and skills needed to maintain health.

Teaching Strategies: The techniques used by a teacher to promote learning are called teaching strategies. These are planned before the actual teaching session so that every content area and learning outcome can be matched with an effective teaching technique.

PATIENT EDUCATION

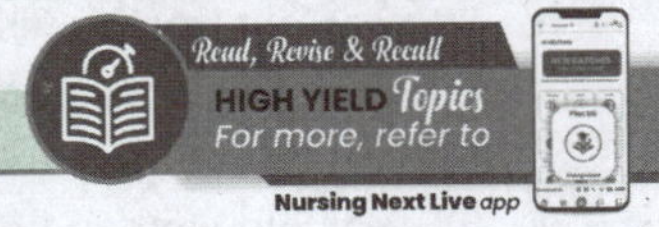

Patient education is the process of influencing the patient's behavior to effect changes in knowledge, attitudes and skills needed to maintain health. Teaching is done to:

- Assist in prevention of illness or promotion of wellness
- Care for self at home before discharge
- Help develop self-care abilities patients need
- Maximize their functioning and quality of life
- Hasten recovery from trauma or illness with minimal or no complications
- Enhance ability to adjust to developmental lifestyle changes
- Accept a the lifestyle changes necessitated by illness or disability.

Nurses play an important role in integrating teaching in nursing process by:

- Assessing learning needs and readiness to learn
- Diagnosing the patient's learning needs
- Developing learning outcomes
- Formulating a teaching plan
- Implementing teaching plan and strategies
- Evaluating learning

CONCEPTUAL EXERCISES

LONG ANSWER QUESTION

1. Define health education. Explain principles of health teaching. (MGR)

Answer

Health Education

Health education is the process of imparting information about health in such a way that the recipient is motivated to use that information for the protection or advancement of his own, his family's or his community's health.

Health education is an active learning process, which aims at favorably changing attitudes and influencing behavior related to health.

"Health education comprises consciously constructed opportunities for learning involving some form of communication designed to improve health literacy, including improving knowledge, and developing skills which are conducive to individual and community health"

—WHO Health Promotion Glossary

Health education is a process that informs, motivates, and helps people to adopt and maintain healthy practices and lifestyles, advocates environmental changes as needed to facilitate this goal and conducts professional training and research to the same end.

—**National Conference on Preventive Medicine in USA**

Principles of Health Teaching

Health education brings together the art and science of medicine and the principles and practice of general education.

Credibility

- Degree to which the message is perceived as trustworthy by the receiver.
- Scientifically proven
- Compatible with culture and social goals

Interest

- Listening
- Felt needs should be assessed

Participation

- Encourage participation
- Leads to acceptance

Motivation

- The fundamental desire for learning in an individual
- Primary motives- inborn desires
- Secondary motives- results of outside force

Comprehension

- Level of understanding of the receiver
- Determine the level of literacy and understanding of the audience
- Never use new or strange words
- Avoid technical or medical words, e.g., eat food items which are noncariogenic

Reinforcement

- Repetition
- Learning new things in short period is not possible
- Booster dose

Learning by Doing

- Learning process should be accomplished by doing
- E.g., brushing technique

Known to Unknown

- How much the people already know
- Existing knowledge can be used as a basic step
- **Setting an example** Should follow what he preaches, e.g., Anti-tobacco counseling

Good Human Relations

- Good personal qualities
- Maintain friendly relations with the people
- Help to clarify doubts of people.

Feedback

To find out if any modification is necessary to make program more effective

Community Leaders

Leaders will have a good rapport Familiar with people of their community Will have better understanding about the needs of their community E.g., Head of the village, headmasters.

Soil, Seed and Sower

- Soil- people
- Seeds- health facts (truthful)
- Sower- transmitting media (attractive, palatable and acceptable)

SHORT NOTES

1. Write a short note on patient teaching. (MGR)

Answer

Patient education is the process of influencing the patient's behavior to effect changes in knowledge, attitudes and skills needed to maintain health. Teaching is done to:

- Assist in prevention of illness or promotion of wellness.
- Care of self at home after discharge
- Help in developing the self-care abilities of the patient.
- Maximize their functioning and quality of life.
- Hasten recovery from trauma or illness with minimal or no complications
- Enhance ability to adjust to developmental lifestyle changes
- Accept the lifestyle changes necessitated by illness or disability.

Process of Patient Teaching

- Assess learning needs and readiness to learn
- Diagnose the patient's learning needs
- Develop learning outcomes

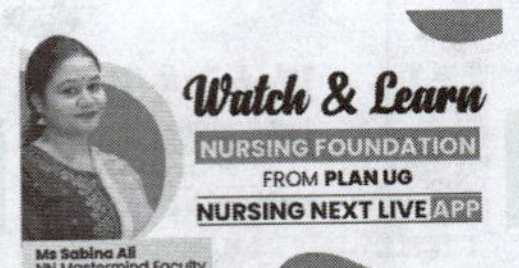

- Development of a teaching plan
- Implement teaching plan and strategies
- Evaluate the patient learning outcomes.

2. Write a short note on principles of health teaching. (MGR)

Answer

For answer, refer to pg. no. 691

3. Write a short note on health education. (MGR)

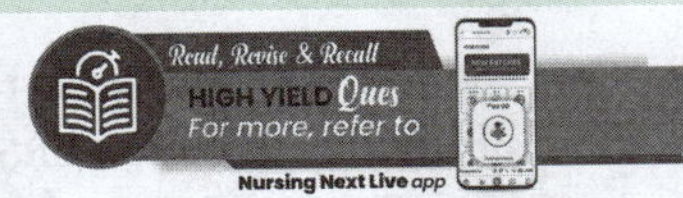

Answer

Health education is the process of imparting information about health in such a way that the recipient is motivated to use that information for the protection or advancement of his own, his family's or his community's health.

Health education is an active learning process, which aims at favorably changing attitudes and influencing behavior related to health.

"Health education comprises consciously constructed opportunities for learning involving some form of communication designed to improve health literacy, including improving knowledge, and developing skills which are conducive to individual and community health"

—WHO Health Promotion Glossary

Health education involves following:

- **Assessing learning needs:** Nurses assess the specific learning needs of individuals or groups by considering factors such as age, cultural background, literacy level, and health literacy.
- **Developing educational materials:** These materials should be culturally sensitive, language-appropriate, and visually appealing to enhance understanding.
- **Promoting health literacy:** Nurse ensure that individuals understand their health conditions, treatment plans, medication instructions, and preventive measures.
- **Health promotion:** Nurses encourage individuals to adopt positive health behaviors that contribute to overall well-being.
- **Creating awareness:** create awareness on self-care management

SHORT ANSWER QUESTIONS

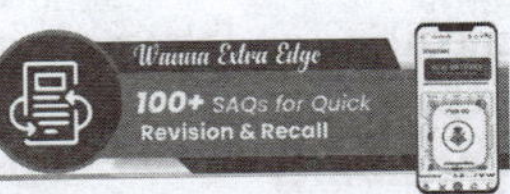

1. What is patient education? (MGR)

Answer

Patient education is the process of influencing the patient's behavior to effect changes in knowledge, attitudes and skills needed to maintain health.

2. What are the principles of health teaching? (MGR)

Answer

Health education brings together the art and science of medicine and the principles and practice of general education.

- Credibility
- Interest
- Participation
- Motivation
- Comprehension
- Reinforcement
- Learning by doing
- Known to unknown
- Setting an example
- Good human relations
- Feedback
- Community leaders
- Soil, seed, sower

3. Define health education. (MGR)

Answer

"Health education comprises consciously constructed opportunities for learning involving some form of communication designed to improve health literacy, including improving knowledge, and developing skills which are conducive to individual and community health"

—WHO Health Promotion Glossary

CONCEPTUAL REVISION

MULTIPLE CHOICE QUESTIONS

1. Comprehensive patient education includes three important purposes; except:

a. Maintenance and promotion of health and illness prevention
b. Enhance compliance with prescribed treatment plans
c. Restoration of health and impaired functions
d. Increase the health expenditure per person

Ans. d. Increase the health expenditure per person

2. A patient needs to learn to use a walker. Which domain is required for learning this skill?

a. Affective domain
b. Cognitive domain
c. Attentional domain
d. Psychomotor domain

Ans. d. Psychomotor domain

3. A patient with chest pain is having an emergency cardiac catheterization. Which teaching approach does the nurse use in this situation?

a. Telling approach
b. Selling approach
c. Entrusting approach
d. Participating approach

Ans. a. Telling approach

4. A patient who is hospitalized has just been diagnosed with diabetes. He is going to need to learn how to give himself injections. Which teaching method does the nurse use?

a. Simulation
b. Demonstration
c. Group instruction
d. One-on-one discussion

Ans. b. Demonstration

5. All of the following are the parameters of BRADEN risk assessment scale; except:

a. Mobility
b. Sensory perception
c. Activity
d. Upper limb movement

Ans. d. Upper limb movement

6. To be effective in meeting various ethnic needs, the nurse should:

a. Treat all clients alike.
b. Be aware of the client's cultural differences.
c. Act as if he or she is comfortable with the client's behavior.
d. Avoid asking questions about the client's cultural background.

Ans. b. Be aware of the client's cultural differences.

7. In …………….. approach, the nurse and patient set objectives and become involved in the learning process together.

a. Telling
b. Participating
c. Entrusting
d. Reinforcing

Ans. b. Participating

8. In …………….. approach, a stimulus is required to increase the probability of desired response.

a. Telling
b. Participating
c. Entrusting
d. Reinforcing

Ans. d. Reinforcing

9. In …………….. approach, limited teaching information is given.

a. Telling
b. Participating
c. Entrusting
d. Reinforcing

Ans. a. Reinforcing

Golden Points

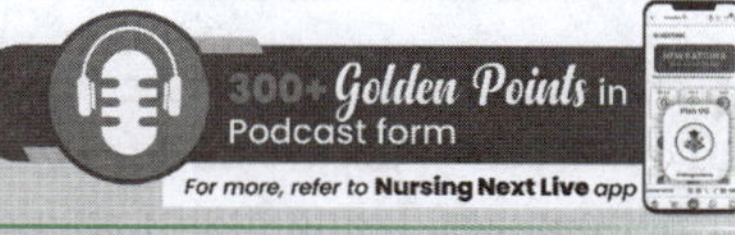

- Patient education is the process of influencing the patient's behavior to effect changes in knowledge, attitudes and skills needed to maintain health.
- Nurses play an important role in integrating teaching in nursing process by: Assessing learning needs and readiness to learn, diagnosing the patient's learning needs, developing learning outcomes, formulating and implementing a teaching plan and strategies and later on evaluating the learning.

CHAPTER 14

First Aid

CONCEPTUAL THEORY

Terminology

150+ key terminologies for Quick Recall & Revision

Asphyxia: It is a deficiency of oxygen in the blood and an increase of carbon dioxide in blood and tissues. It occurs due to an interruption in the normal exchange of oxygen and carbon dioxide between the lungs and atmospheric air.

Bandage is a piece of soft, usually absorbent gauze or other material applied to a limb or other part of the body as a dressing.

Burns are due to dry heat including friction, whereas scalds are due to wet heat. Burns and scalds are considered together as they produce severe type of injury.

Choking: Occurs due to blockage of the throat by foreign object. There is difficulty in speaking and breathing.

Dislocation: A dislocation is a separation of bones at a joints. Most common joint that can dislocate are shoulder, knees, jaw, thumb and finger joints.

First-aider: A **first-aider** is someone who has undertaken training appropriate to the circumstances.

First aid is an immediate temporary assistance given to a person who is injured or suddenly becomes ill, using facilities or materials available at that time before regular medical help is imparted.

Frost Bite: After being painfully cold, the affected parts become waxy white in appearance and feel quite numb. Whiteness and numbness are danger signals which must not be overlooked because prolonged freezing will do irreparable damage.

Heat Exhaustion: It is caused by too high temperature in the atmosphere directly by the sun or due to hard work and confinement in a close, hot atmosphere like factories, etc.

Manual Lift by One First-Aider: Casualty is carried by one first-aider using human crutch, drag method, cradle method, pick a back and fireman's lift and carry method.

Manual Lifting by Two First-Aiders: This can be done by two handed seat, four handed seat and fore and aft method. Manual lifting is the safe method for victim as well as for the first aider.

Poison: A **poison (or toxin)** is a substance which, if taken into the body in sufficient quantity, can cause temporary or permanent damage.

Poisoning: It is a condition caused by introduction of harmful substances or chemicals into the body by injection, inhalation or ingestion.

Sunstroke: It is caused by too high temperature in atmosphere by the sun rays.

Unconsciousness: It is a state in which a person is unable to respond to stimuli and appears to be asleep. Person may be unconscious for a few seconds as in fainting or for longer periods of time.

Wound: A **wound** is an injury in which the skin is cut or penetrated. If wound is deep, severe bleeding may occur, depending on how they are caused.

FIRST AID

An emergency is an unforeseen event which calls for prompt and quick action to save the life of a person or to prevent from further damage. Using basic first aid, you may be able to stop a minor mishap from getting worse.

First aid is an immediate temporary assistance given to a person who is injured or suddenly becomes ill, using facilities or materials available at that time before regular medical help is imparted.

The objectives of first aid are:

- To preserve life.
- To prevent further injury and deterioration of the condition.
- To prevent complications related to injury or illness or conditions.
- To make the victim as comfortable as possible to conserve the strength.
- To put the injured person under professional medical care at the earliest.

The following are the qualities which a trained first-aider should possess:

- Prompt and quick

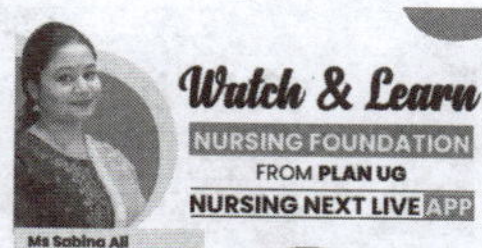

- Calm and controlled
- Wise and intelligent
- Resourceful
- Sweet tempered and sympathetic
- Skillful and tactful
- Dexterous and clever
- Confident and perseverant

When a first-aider comes across a seriously injured person, the following points should be taken into consideration:

- Make sure that scene is safe for you and prevent the further injury to the victim.
- If area is not safe move the victim to a safe place by avoiding further injury to the client.
- Make sure that victim's airway is not blocked by the tongue, secretions or some foreign body–restore respiration.
- Make sure that the person is breathing. If not, administer artificial respiration–restore respiration.
- Make sure that the patient has a pulse, if no pulse is felt, administer cardiopulmonary resuscitation (CPR)—for restoration of circulation.
- Check for bleeding–take measures to control bleeding.
- Act fast if the victim is bleeding severely or if he has swallowed poison or if the heart or breathing has stopped, every second counts for his survival.
- Arrange without delay for shifting of the victim to hospital for medical attention, although most injured persons can be safely moved. It is very important a not to move a person with serious neck and/or back injuries unless proper measures are taken to ensure him from further complications.
- Keep the victim/patient quiet and make him lie down. Turn the victim on his side to prevent choking if there is no danger of neck injury. Keep him warm with blanket.
- Have someone call for medical assistance while applying first aid. The person who summons help should explain the nature of the emergency and ask what should be done if the arrival of ambulance is pending.
- Examine the victim gently, cut clothing of necessary length.
- Reassure the victim, try to remain calm yourself. Your calmness can allay the victim's fear and panic.
- Do not give fluids to an unconscious or semiconscious victim.
- Do not try to arouse an unconscious person by slapping or shaking.
- Do not allow crowd to gather near the victim so that fresh air is allowed.
- Look for an emergency identification card for medical information related to victim.

The scope of first aid includes the diagnosis, the treatment and the disposal of the case.

Golden Rules of First Aid

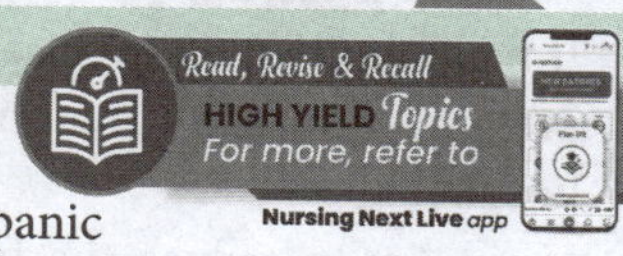

- Do first things first, quickly and quietly without fuss or panic
- Reassure the casualty through encouraging words
- Check ABC rule (airway, breathing, circulation)
- Open the airway by tilting the head
- Give artificial respiration, if breathing has stopped
- Perform chest compression, if the pulse is not present
- Stop bleeding, if any, by direct pressure
- Treat the shock
- Do not allow people to crowd around
- Do not remove clothes unnecessarily
- Arrange for transportation of the casualty
- Casualty should be sent to a hospital or doctor by quickest means of transport.
- Always inform the police and relatives about serious accidents.

First Aid for Sprain and Strain

Apply the principle Ricer: Rest, Ice, Compression, Elevation, Referral

- Provide rest to the casualty, raise the injured part
- Apply a compression bandage to injured part
- Apply ice pack to the area—apply for 20 minutes every 2 hours
- Seek medical advice

A dislocation is a separation of bones at a joint. Most common joints that can dislocate are shoulder, knees, jaw, thumb and finger joints.

Management of dislocation is very similar to that of a fracture and involves:

- Immobilization and support of injured part by use of slings or simple support measures.
- Application of ice or cold compress to the injured part to help reduce pain and swelling.
- Transporting injured person to nearby hospital at earliest.

First Aid Measures for the Fractures

When bones are broken, a good rule to follow is "Do not permit motion of the broken ends or of the joints near the injury." This prevents pain and further damage.

- For closed or simple fracture, place the limb in as natural position as possible without causing discomfort to the victim. Handle very gently; avoid all unnecessary movements of the injured part.
- Since the danger of infection is high in compound or open fractures, it is always better to get help from a doctor. While caring for the injury, clean the wound and apply dressing.

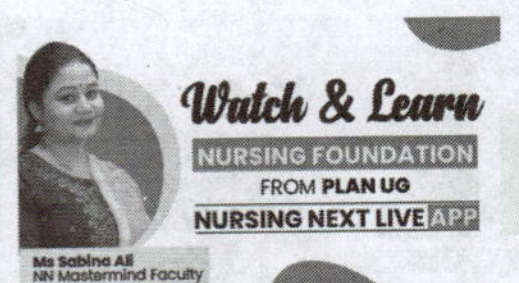

- If there is an excessive bleeding from open fracture, apply pressure dressing to control it. Transfer the patient to hospital.
- Never try to reduce the fracture, i.e., bringing bones to normal position (alignment).
- Before trying to move or carry a person with a broken bone, immobilize the broken ends with splints.
- Send the patient for medical aid as soon as possible.

For a first-aider, transportation of an injured person to a hospital is a vital step of action. Before transportation, it is important to check:

- Casualty's respiration is normal
- Pulse rate normal
- Any bleeding—should be arrested
- Injured part is well supported and immobilized
- Keeping the casualty warm
- Transportation must be done in a way so that no further injury occurs.

Methods of Transportation

- Manual lifting—by one first-aider and by two first-aiders
- Carry chair
- Stretchers
- Rescue by: Air helicopter
  Land—ambulance
  Water—boat

Manual lifting is the safe method for victim as well as for the first-aider.

Manual Lift by One First-Aider

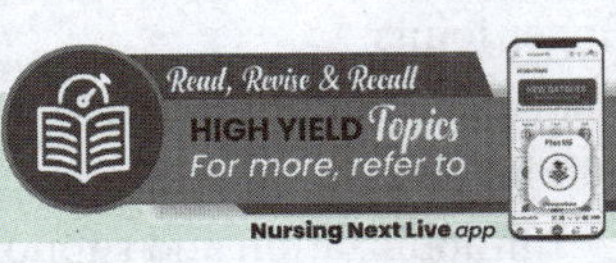

Casualty is carried by one first-aider using human crutch, drag method, cradle method, pick a back and fireman's lift and carry method.

- **Human crutch:** To assist the injured person in standing up, first, crouch down with your knees bent and back straight on the side of their injury. Help them sit up and place their arm over your shoulder. Slowly stand up together, allowing the injured person to bear weight on their good leg while supporting their weight on the side of the injury. Hold their hand around your shoulders with the hand furthest from them and place your other hand around their waist for added stability during the process.
- **Drag method:** The drag method is a safer alternative to lifting an injured person, benefiting both you and the casualty. Lifting increases the weight you need to support and poses a risk of falling for the injured person. When using the drag method, always pull slowly and steadily, aiming to move the person in a straight line to maintain proper alignment of their spine and prevent any unnatural twisting or bending, adapting the type of drag based on the person's specific injuries. Types of drag method includes leg drag, arm drag and clothing drag.
- **Cradle method:** This quick and easy method of lifting can be employed for children and individuals significantly smaller than the rescuer. However, it has limitations due to the rescuer bearing the person's entire weight, which may lead to fatigue quickly. To use this method, scoop the child up in front of you, supporting their back with one hand and their knees with the other. It's crucial to bend at the knees and maintain a straight back during the lift to minimize the risk of injuring your back, as a back injury would hinder your ability to provide effective help.
- **Carry like backpack:** The "pick-a-back" method is suitable for a conscious casualty who can assist with the lift. The first-aider stands behind the casualty, and after the casualty places their arms around the first-aider's neck and their legs around their waist, the first-aider lifts the casualty onto their back and carries them in this manner. This method is particularly useful when the casualty is conscious and cooperative, allowing for a more straightforward and supportive transfer.
- **Fireman's lift:** In this method, you position one shoulder into the person's midriff, lifting them so that their head, arms, and upper torso hang down your back. To maintain a secure grip, use one hand to hold their legs

Manual Lifting by Two First-Aiders

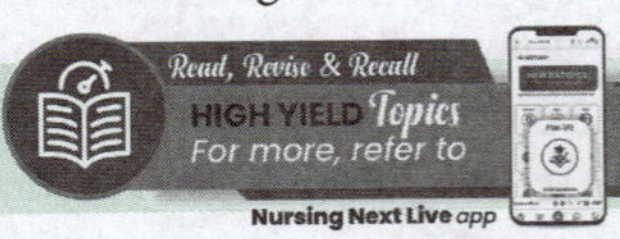

This can be done by two handed seat, four handed seat and fore and aft method.

- **Two handed seat:** In the two-handed seat method, both first-aiders stand facing each other and interlock their hands, creating a stable seat with their arms. The injured person sits on their hands, and the first-aiders lift them by standing up together. This method is typically used for shorter distances or when the person can bear some weight on their legs.
- **Four handed seat:** The four-handed seat method involves two first-aiders standing facing each other and placing their hands on their partner's wrists. The injured person sits on the hands of both first-aiders, and they lift the person by coordinating their movements. This method provides more stability and control than the two-handed seat.
- **Fore and aft method:** In the fore and aft method, one first-aider stands behind the injured person and supports their upper body by placing their arms under the person's armpits. The other first-aider stands in front, supporting the person's legs by holding them at the knees. Together, they lift the person as a team, providing support for both the upper body and the lower body.

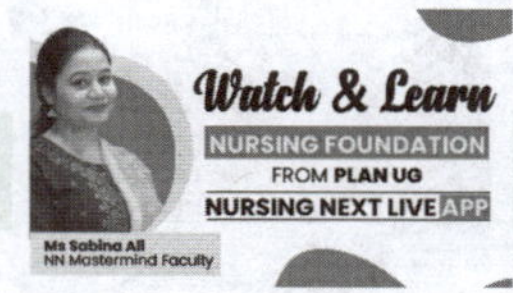

- **Carry chair:** It is a straightforward device designed for efficiently transporting a casualty. It features a seat, a backrest, and two handles. First-aiders place the casualty onto the carry chair and then lift it up, enabling them to walk forward while carrying the chair and safely transporting the casualty to a different location. This method is particularly useful when the casualty is unable to walk or requires swift and secure movement over a short distance.
- **Stretchers:** These are medical devices used to carry injured or immobilized individuals. They come in various designs, such as foldable or rigid stretchers, and may have wheels or handles for easier transport. Two first-aiders work together to position the person on the stretcher and then carry them to a safe location.

Individuals with certain health problems are at high risk. Patients suffering from cardiovascular diseases, obesity, diabetes mellitus, malnutrition, alcoholism are more vulnerable to heat related problems. Farmers, athletes, infants and elderly are also at high risk.

HEAT-RELATED PROBLEMS

There are three heat related problems which include heat stroke, heat exhaustion and heat cramp.

Sunstroke is caused by too high temperature in atmosphere by the sun rays.

First Aid Measures

- Move the patient to a dry and shady place, loosen collar and any tight clothes.
- Raise the head and sprinkle cool water on his body or wrap him in a thin wet sheet and fan him.
- Check temperature every 10 minutes.
- Do not allow the body temperature fall below 103°F.
- After this, wrap him in a dry sheet and keep fanning so that the temperature does not rise again.
- If the casualty is conscious, cool water mixed with salt and glucose can be given for drinking.
- Move the casualty to hospital.

Heat Exhaustion

It is caused by too high temperature in the atmosphere directly by the sun or due to hard work and confinement in a close, hot atmosphere like factories, etc.

First Aid Measures

- Move the casualty to a cool place.
- Place him flat on his back.
- Give him plenty of fluids with added salt or fruit juice.

These are intermittent, painful contractions of skeletal muscles. These cramps often occur in individuals who replace the fluid lost in sweat by drinking water, but do not replace sodium.

The treatment is to replace sodium with electrolyte solution. In severe cases, intravenous salt solutions may be required.

Effects of excessive cold are common in persons who live or work in a climate where temperature falls below 32°F or are in high altitudes. Extent of the injury caused depends on the degree of the temperature and the period of exposure to cold.

Frostbite

After being painfully cold, the affected parts become waxy white in appearance and feel quite numb. Whiteness and numbness are danger signals which must not be overlooked because prolonged freezing will do irreparable damage.

First Aid Measures

- Remove all wet or tight clothing from the frost bitten area.
- Carry the casualty to a closed room without fire and undress him carefully.
- Remove tight gloves, boots, socks, rings, etc.
- Do not rub the frozen part with snow.
- Cover the casualty with a dry sheet.
- Give him warm drinks.
- The hands and feet need to be wrapped in a blanket.
- Do not use hot water bottles or heat lamps.
- Do not allow the victim to walk, if the feet are affected.
- Do not allow the victim to smoke because the nicotine in tobacco may further constrict blood vessels.
- Send for the physician immediately.

Chocking

Choking occurs due to blockage of the throat by foreign object. There is difficulty in speaking and breathing.

First Aid Measures for Chocking (For Adult)

Heimlich Maneuver

- Reassure the casualty, bend the casualty forward so that the head is lower than the chest.
- Give up to five sharp blows to the back between the shoulder blades, with the palm of your hand.
- If back slaps fail, try abdominal thrust. The sudden pull up against the diaphragm compresses the chest, and may expel the obstruction.
- If abdominal thrust does not free the blockage, try again four times, then alternate five back blows with five thrusts.

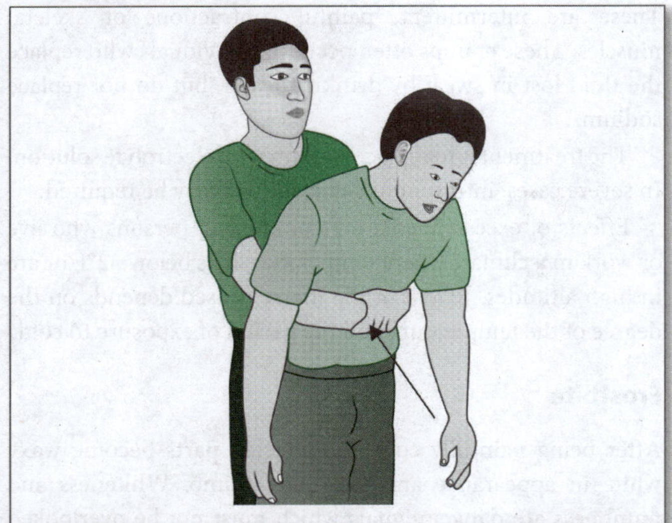

First Aid Measures (For Child)

- Place the child over your knee, head down, slap him between the shoulder blades using less force than for an adult.
- If back blow fails, use the abdominal thrust only if you have been trained to do on a child—otherwise, begin resuscitation.

First Aid Measures (For Baby)

- Lay the baby along your forearm.
- Slap the baby between the shoulder blades, using less force than for a child.
- If the baby becomes unconscious, begin resuscitation and do not use abdominal thrust.

Wound

A wound is an injury in which the skin is cut or penetrated. If wound is deep, severe bleeding may occur, depending on how it is caused.

First Aid Management of Wounds

- **Rest:** Make the casualty lie down still, so that amount of blood loss is less.
- **Elevation:** Elevate the wounded arm or leg above the level of the heart.
- **Direct pressure:** Apply firm pressure directly on the wound. Pressure is applied through a dressing which is bandaged firmly on the wound.
- **Indirect pressure:** If direct pressure is not possible to apply, then indirect pressure may be applied to a "pressure point" where a main artery runs close to a bone. It must not be applied for longer than 10 minutes.

Shock results due to the failure of the cardiovascular system to provide sufficient blood circulation to all parts of the body.

First Aid Measures

- Take measures to establish airway.
- Take steps to control bleeding if it is present.
- Take steps to reduce pain.
- Appropriate positioning of the victim in shock which is determined by the type and extent of injury.
- Maintain the victim's body temperature by keeping him dry and warm.
- Take measures to relieve pain.
- Give emotional support and reassurance.
- Do not let crowd gather around the patient.
- Arrange for transportation.

Unconsciousness

Unconsciousness is the state in which a person is unable to respond to stimuli and appears to be asleep. Person may be unconscious for a few seconds as in fainting or for longer periods of time.

First Aid Measures

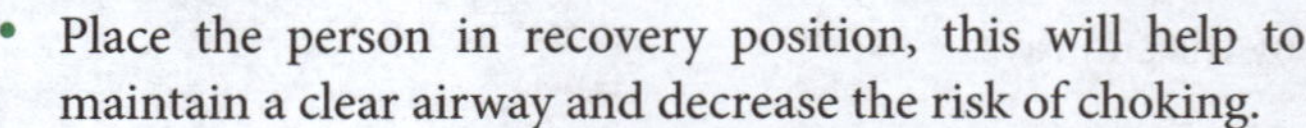

If person is breathing:

- Place the person in recovery position, this will help to maintain a clear airway and decrease the risk of choking.
- For providing recovery position, follow the instructions listed below: Kneel on the floor next to the person.
  - Take the arm that is closest to you and position it so that it is perpendicular to the person's body, forming a right angle. The head should be facing upward.
  - Take the person's other hand and position it so that the back of the hand is pressed against the cheek that is closest to you.
  - With your free hand, bend the person's knee that is farthest from you. His foot should be resting flat against the floor.
  - Help the person get onto his side by pulling on the bent knee. After you roll him over, ensure that his top arm is still helping to support the head.
  - Tilt the person's head back and lift the chin. This helps open airway.
  - Make sure there is no obstruction in the airway.
  - Keep an eye on the person's condition, and remain with him until emergency personnel arrives.

    If person is not breathing:
  - Call for help immediately and begin CPR.

Other First Aid Measures

- Do not try to arouse an unconscious person. Let him lie quiet.

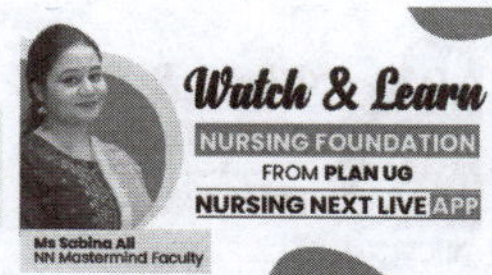

- Do not move the casualty unnecessarily, because of the possibility of spinal injury. Never attempt to make an unconscious person sit or stand.
- Do not let people gather around, give him fresh air.
- Loosen clothing at neck, chest and waist.
- Never give water to an unconscious person to drink, it might get into his windpipe.
- Apply specific treatment according to the cause of unconsciousness.

Fainting

This occurs most frequently in healthy young people, especially during hot weather, and while standing for long periods. People who are hungry, tired, emotionally upset, fearful may faint even though they are in good health. The cause is insufficient supply of blood to the brain.

First Aid Measures

- Keep the victim lying flat, and raise the legs to improve the blood flow to the brain.
- Loosen tight clothing at neck.
- Do not let the crowd gather and let there be plenty of fresh air.
- Consciousness will return in one or two minutes.
- After the victim recovers consciousness, a cup of tea or coffee may be given.
- If the victim does not recover, medical help is advised.

Burns

Burns are due to dry heat including friction, whereas scalds are due to wet heat. Burns and scalds are considered together as they produce severe type of injury.

Management of Burns

Stopping the burning process.

- Reduce pain.
- Providing life support–oxygenation, fluids, etc.
- Preventing complications.
- Restoration of functions.
- For stopping the burning process, do not allow the person to run about, as it increases the severity. Lay him flat on the ground, put any thick clothing which is available like blanket, carpet, shawl, etc. over the victim to extinguish flames. Do not try to remove the burning clothes.
- Immediately, immerse the burnt area under cool running water
- Assess airway breathing and circulation.
- Blisters should not be touched.
- All articles like bangles, belt, boot should be removed.
- Cover the burnt area with clean sheet over which blanket can be placed to maintain heat and prevent hypothermia.
- Give warm fluids to drink if casualty can take them and restrict the movement.
- In case of extensive burns, person may go into shock, then the first aid for shock is given and victim is rushed to a nearby hospital.
- In acid burns: Cool area with stream of plain water.
  - Remove acid soaked clothing.
  - Bathe affected part with alkaline solution of one table spoon of baking soda and 1 L of water.
  - Cover with clean linen.
  - Give analgesics for pain.
- **In alkali burns:** Flood burnt area with stream of plain water.
  - Remove alkali soaked clothing.
  - Bathe affected part with weak solution of vinegar and water in equal parts.
  - Cover with clean linen material only.
  - Give analgesics for pain.
- **In electrical burns:**
  - The passage of electrical current through the body may cause breathing problem and even heart to stop. A person while indoors may receive an electric shock, by touching a bare electric wire and the danger is greater if the floor is wet or one's body is wet.

Animal Bites

Animal bites always require medical attention because germs are harbored in the mouths of all animals. Bites from sharp, pointed teeth cause deep puncture wounds that carry germs to the tissues. They require prompt first aid followed by medical attention.

First Aid Measures

- Make the person lie down comfortably and reassure the casualty.
- Tie handkerchief or tourniquet at a distance away from the bitten area to avoid the venous blood flow toward the heart. Do not tie the tourniquet very tightly so that the blood flow to the organ is inhibited. Put an inch long cut over the snake bitten area and start sucking/removing out the blood mixed liquid coming out from the wound. Send the casualty for medical help.

Foreign Body

Foreign bodies in nose like pieces of betel nut, grains or peas or other seeds, crayon, etc. may be put by children in nose while playing.

First Aid Measures

- Do not probe at the object with a cotton swab or other tool.

- Don't try to inhale the object by forcefully breathing in. Instead, breathe through your mouth until the object is removed.
- Blow out of your nose gently to try to free the object but don't blow hard or repeatedly. If only one nostril is affected, close the opposite nostril by applying gentle pressure and then blow out gently through the affected nostril.
- Gently remove the object if it is visible and you can easily grasp it with tweezers. Don't try to remove an object that is not visible or easily grasped.
- Call for emergency medical assistance, if these methods fail.

Foreign Body in the Throat

A foreign body in the throat or upper part of the respiratory tract can cause choking and is a medical emergency that needs immediate attention.

First Aid Measures

- If the person is able to cough forcefully, the person should keep coughing. If the person is choking and cannot talk, cry or laugh forcefully, then the Red Cross recommends "five and five" approach in delivering first aid.
- Give five back blows. Stand to the side and just behind a choking adult. Place one arm across the person's chest for support. Bend the person over at the waist so that the upper body is parallel with the ground. Deliver five back blows between the person's shoulder blades with the heel of your hand.
- Perform five abdominal thrusts. Abdominal thrusts have been described in detail in first aid in asphyxia (also known as the Heimlich maneuver).
- Alternate between five blows and five thrusts until the blockage is dislodged.
- Call for help while you are performing first aid.

Foreign Body in Abdomen

Foreign bodies into the stomach are commonly found.
These may be accidently or intentionally swallowed.

- Ingested objects can pass through the digestive tract naturally and without any complications, but some patients may need assistance to remove the foreign body, if larger objects or sharp ones, such as tooth picks, chicken or fish bones, may get stuck in the esophagus or stomach.
- It can cause cramps, bloating, abdominal pain, nausea and vomiting.
- If sharp object pierces the esophagus, consequences may be serious; perforation may occur. It is a medical emergency.

Poisoning

Poisoning is a condition caused by introduction of harmful substances or chemicals into the body either by injection, inhalation or ingestion. A poison (or toxin) is a substance, which if taken into the body in sufficient quantity, can cause temporary or permanent damage.

First Aid for Poisoning

If the poison is swallowed:

- **If the person is alert:** Do not induce vomiting (in case of acid or alkali). Immediately rinse the mouth. Keep the product or medicine container handy for sending to lab.

On the skin:

- Carefully remove contaminated clothing and wash exposed areas with copious amounts of water.

In the eye:

- Rinse eyes with a slow gentle stream of water for 10 to 15 minutes. Allow the stream of water to flow from the inner corner across the eye to the outer corner.

Inhaled:

- Get the person to fresh air, without placing yourself at risk.
- Loosen any tight clothing at the neck.
- Avoid breathing fumes as you may become a victim yourself.

BANDAGE

- A bandage is a material used in medicine and first aid to cover, protect, and support wounds, injuries, or other affected areas of the body.
- It is typically made of cloth, gauze, or other flexible materials and is wrapped around the injured or affected body part to provide compression, prevent infection, and facilitate the healing process.
- Bandages come in various types and sizes, and they are an essential tool in wound care and injury management.

Classification of Bandaging

- Simple
- **Special:** Related to the organ to be bandaged.

Various Turns Used in Bandaging

- Circular turns
- Spiral turns
- Reverse spiral turns
- Recurrent turns
- Figure of eight turns

Circular Turn

- Hold the bandage in your dominant hand, with the roll on the upper side and unroll the bandage about 8 cm.
- Apply the end of the bandage
- Encircle the body part, each turn covering the previous turn, secure the end of the bandage with tape, metal clip or a safety pin.

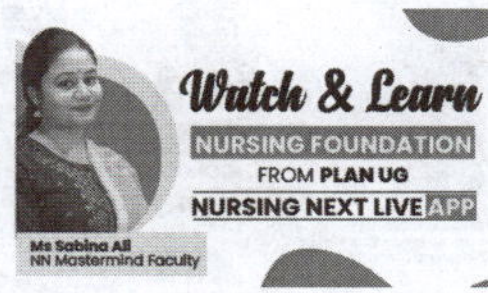

Spiral Turn

- Start with two circular turns and cover two-third and continue to wrap the bandage.
- Finish with two circular turns

Reverse Spiral Turn

- Start with two circular turns around the affected area
- Turn the bandage over so that side on top is now the bottom
- Continue to wrap around the affected area and finish with two circular turns

Recurrent Turns

- Start with two circular turns
- Then turns are made over and back
- Subsequent turns are folded alternatively

Figure of Eight Turns

- Anchor the bandage with two circular turns.
- Carry the bandage above the joint, around it and then below it making a figure of eight.
- Continue above and below the joint, overlapping the previous turn by two third the width of the bandage.
- Terminate the bandage above the joint with two circular turns and secure

SPECIAL BANDAGES

Eye Bandage

- Pad the affected eye. Take two circular turns around the head bandaging away from the injured eye.
- Carry the bandage, around the head until it reaches the eye on the affected side.

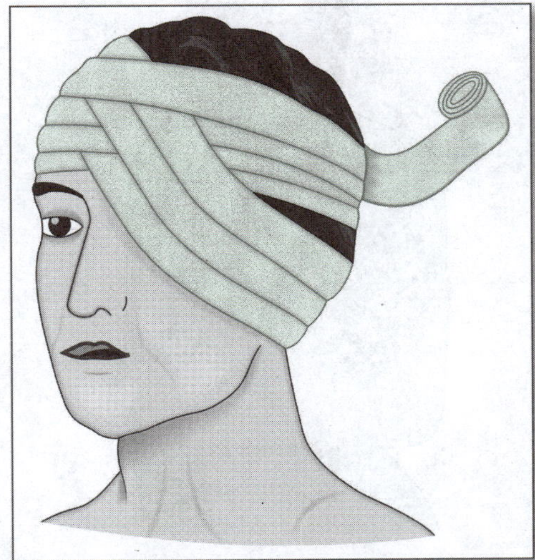

Figure 14.1: Eye bandage

- Take it obliquely to the back of the head and from there, bring it upward beneath the eye of the affected side.
- Repeat this turn two or three times until the dressing is covered.
- Secure the bandage with a tape.

Ear Bandage

- Secure the roller bandage with two circular turns around the forehead, and then down the nape of the neck.
- Repeat the turns with each turn being slightly higher than the previous one, continue the turns until the whole ear, on the affected side is covered and complete the bandage by two circular turns around the forehead.

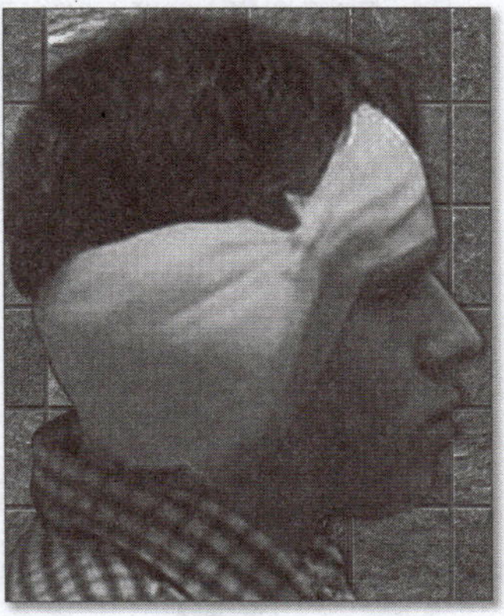

Figure 14.2: Ear bandage

Jaw Bandage Center: Four-Tailed

- Keep the center of the bandage at the chin.
- Take the upper tails on both the sides above the pinna and secure them at the occiput.
- Take the lower tails behind the ears and secure them on top of the head.

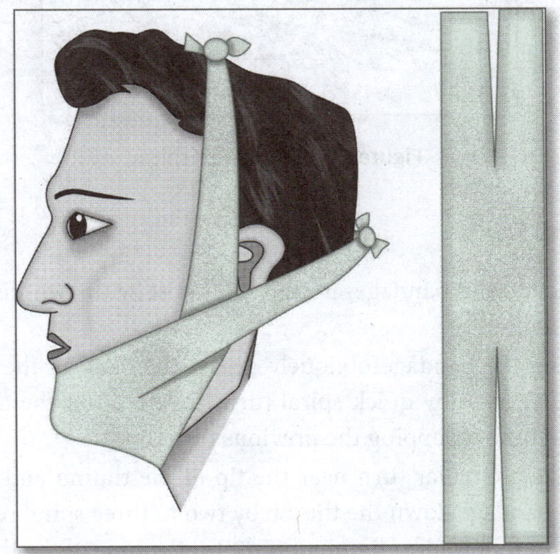

Figure 14.3: Jaw bandage

Jaw Bandage: Two-tailed

- Make a small slit at the center of the gauze and place it over the chin, take two ends above the head.
- Keep the bandage at the chin at the center slit and ears in the lateral slits.
- Secure the bandage at the top of the head.

Shoulder Spica

- Stand on the side where the bandage is to be applied; pad the axilla.
- Anchor the bandage around the upper arm near the axilla with two circular turns.
- For injury on the right side, carry around the arm and across the chest. For injury on the left side, take across the chest and through the opposite axilla and across the back to the injured arm, where it crosses the previous turns in mid line.
- Repeat the previous turns by overlapping one half to two-third width crossing it exactly in the midline and ascending toward the shoulder until covered.
- Secure the bandage in the front.

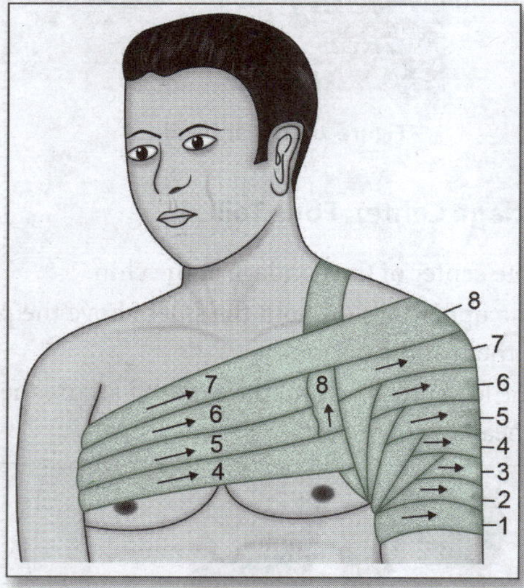

Figure 14.4: Shoulder spica

Thumb Spica

- Anchor the bandage around the wrist with two circular turns.
- Bring the bandage obliquely across the back of the hand and carry it by quick spiral turns to the tip of the thumb without overlapping the previous turns.
- Make a circular turn near the tip of the thumb and carry the bandage down the thumb by two to three spiral reverse turns, followed by figure of eight till the base of the thumb. Carry it to the dorsum of the thumb and then to the lateral aspect of the wrist and finish with two circular turns at the wrist.

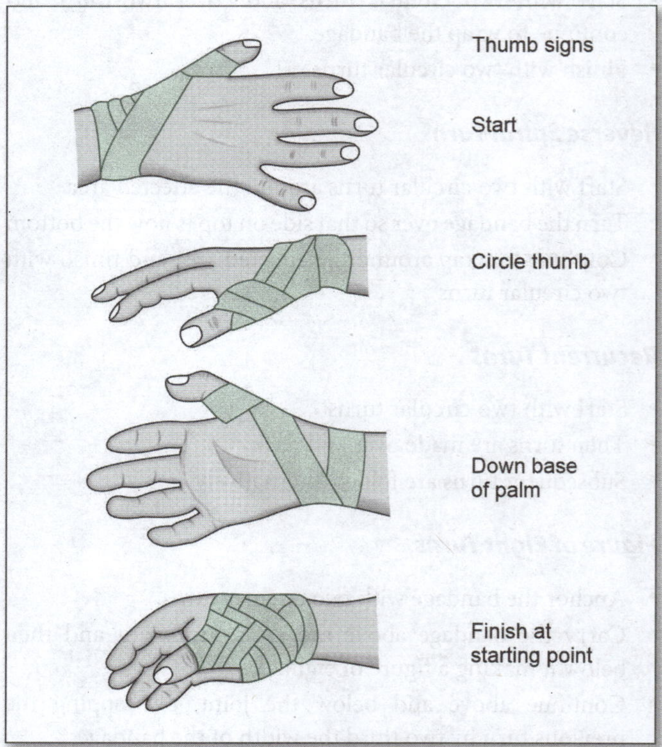

Figure 14.5: Thumb spica

Triangular Bandage

- This is used to support the arm, elbow and forearm and to prevent swelling of a hand.

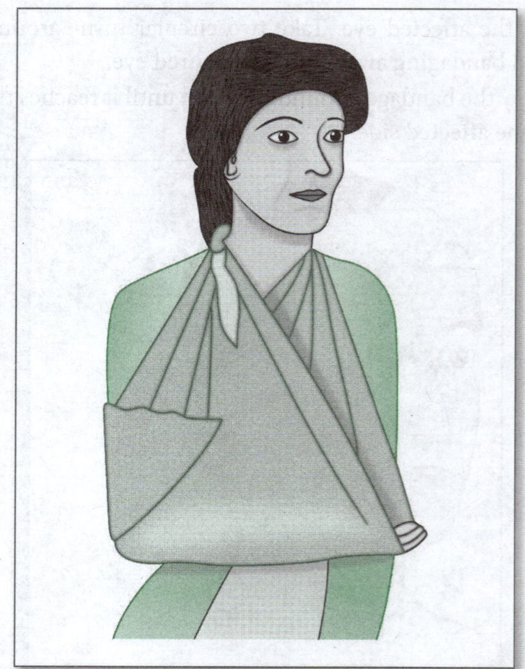

Figure 14.6: Triangular bandage

Binders: Abdominal Binder

- Position the patient in supine position with the binder in the middle and both straps should extend equally on both the sides.
- Begin at the lower end of the binder, bring alternate right and left straps tightly with slightly upward slant over the abdomen, covering half of the preceding strap, crossing at the midline.
- Hold the free end of the strap until the opposite strap secures it. Overlap final straps horizontally and secure with a clip or safety pin.

'T' Binder

- Secure the waist strap of the binder in the front with a pin.

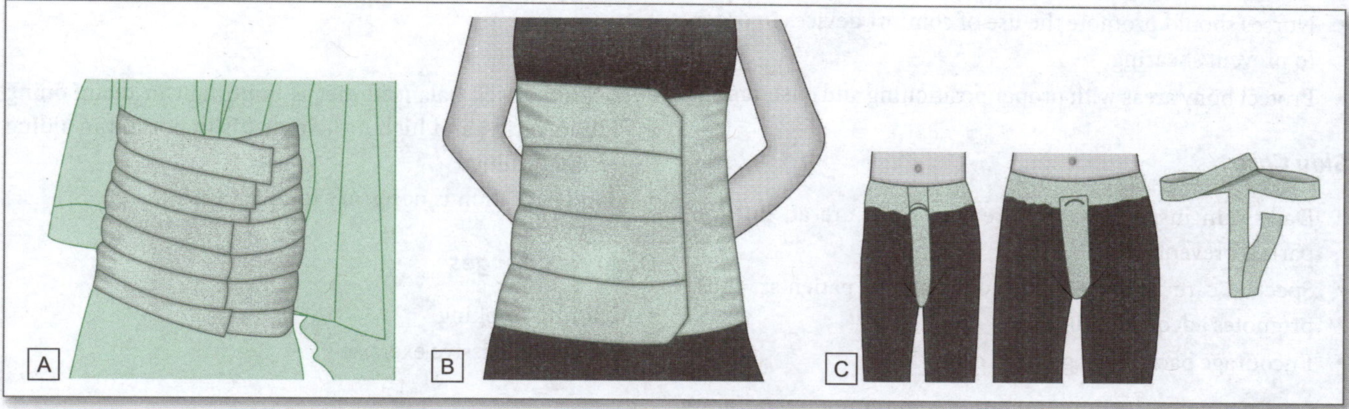

Figures 14.7A to C: 'T' Bandage. A and B. Abdominal binders; C. T-bandage

CONCEPTUAL EXERCISES

LONG ANSWER QUESTIONS

1. Define decubitus ulcer and list down the common sites of decubitus ulcer. Explain the nursing measures for the prevention of decubitus ulcer. (KUHS)

Answer

- Pressure ulcers are also called pressure sores or bedsores or decubitus ulcers. These are the localized injuries to the skin and underlying tissue, over a body prominence area resulting from prolonged pressure on the skin.

Common Sites of Decubitus Ulcer

- Bedsores commonly develop on the skin that covers bony areas of the body, such as the heels, ankles, hips and tailbone.
- People at high risk of bedsores are those with any medical condition that limits their ability to change positions or bed confined for a long time.

Pressure ulcers commonly occur over the:

- Sacrum
- Greater trochanter
- Ischial tuberosity
- Malleolus
- Heel
- Fibular head
- Scapula

While on a wheelchair, a pressure sore can develop on:

- Tailbone or buttocks
- Shoulder blades and spine
- The backs of arms and legs
- Feet

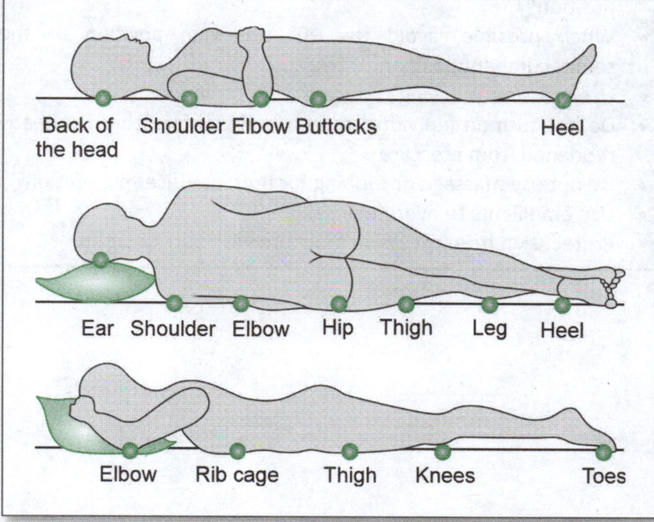

Nursing Measures for the Prevention of Decubitus Ulcer

The prevention of bedsores is easier than its management. Nurses play a vital role in the prevention of bedsores.

Repositioning in a Bed

- Change body position every two hours.
- Use of comfort devices such as air/water mattresses.
- Nurses should promote the use of comfort devices in order to prevent shearing.
- Protect bony areas with proper positioning and cushioning.

Skin Care

- Daily skin inspections for pressure sores are an integral part of prevention.
- Special care required for edematous patients; thus, promotes adequate skin care.
- Encourage back massage/back care.
- Avoid friction and shear.
- Clean the skin with mild soap and warm water. Pat dry gently.
- Apply lotion or coconut oil to dry skin.
- Change bedding and clothing whenever required.
- Manage incontinence to keep the skin dry.
- Prevent exposing the skin to moisture and microorganisms.
- Specially emphasized for unconscious patients, as they are more prone to pressure sores.

Nutrition

- A healthy well balanced diet is important in maintaining skin integrity; and high protein diet is important in aiding wound healing.
- Good hydration is necessary for healthy skin.

Lifestyle Changes

- Quitting smoking
- Active and passive exercise

Table 14.1: Instructions for prevention of decubitus ulcer according to National Pressure Injury Advisory Panel (NPIAP)

Structured risk assessment	Frequent skin assessment
Patients at risk of pressure ulcer development include all patients with alterations in intact skin, such as dry skin, excessive moisture, or redness • Patients with signs of altered nutrition (including anemia, low serum albumin, decreased intake, and/or body weight) • Older age • Increased friction and shear and/or altered mobility • Decreased sensory perception	Regularly assess each patient's skin for • Redness or change in color • Dryness or excessive moisture • Blanching response • Localized heat • Edema • Hardness (induration) • Areas of discomfort or pain that may be related to pressure • Medical devices pressing on skin
Skin care	**Nutrition for pressure ulcer prevention**
• Use frequent position changes to relieve and redistribute pressure • Avoid friction and shear (lift, don't drag) • Reposition using the 30° tilted side-lying position, or the prone position • When possible, avoid the 90° side-lying position or the semirecumbent position • Use pressure-relieving surfaces • Do not turn an individual onto a body surface that is already reddened from pressure • Do not use massage or rubbing for pressure ulcer prevention • Use emollients to hydrate dry skin • Protect skin from excessive moisture with barrier cream	• Use a team approach for nutrition risk assessment and intervention • If indicated for patients with nutritional risk, offer high-protein supplements between mealtimes in addition to the usual diet

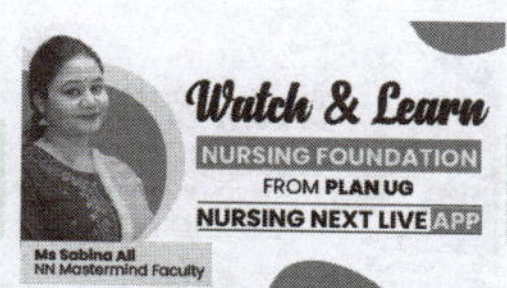

2. Define first aid and enumerate the qualities of a first-aider. Explain the first aid to a client with food poisoning. (KUHS)

Answer

First Aid

According to the **Red Cross Society of India**, first aid is the first assistance or treatment given to a casualty or a sick person for any injury or sudden illness before the arrival of an ambulance, a qualified paramedical or medical person or before arriving at a facility that can provide professional medical care.

A first-aider is the term describing any person who has received a certificate from an authorized training body indicating that he or she is qualified to render first aid.

Qualities of First-Aider

- Prompt and quick
- Calm and controlled
- Wise and intelligent
- Resourceful
- Sweet tempered and sympathetic
- Skillful and tactful
- Dexterous and clever
- Confident and perseverant

First Aid to a Client with Food Poisoning

- Wash your hands before providing first aid to the casualty. Use soap and water to wash hands.
- Use gloves to protect yourself.
- Try not to come in contact with the person's vomit.

First Aid Measures

- Assess the patient for vitals.
- Reassure the client.
- Advise the sick person to lie down.
- Promote adequate bed rest.
- Ensure adequate hydration. Prevent dehydration if the sick person suffers from vomiting and/or diarrhea.
- Prevent dehydration if the sick person suffers from vomiting and/or diarrhea.
- Carefully observe the client, if condition worsens, refer him/her to the nearest health care facility.
- Assist the doctor in obtaining history of the patient in the hospital.

3. Define wound. Classify the different types of wound. Explain the wound healing process in detail. (MGR)

Answer

Wound

Wound is a circumscribed injury which is caused by external force and it can involve any tissue and organ.

A wound is a break in the integrity of the skin or tissues often which may be associated with disruption of the structure and function. **—(SRB 4th edition)**

Classification of Wounds

Based on Types of Wound

- **Clean incised wound:** A well-defined, straight wound with smooth edges caused by a sharp object.
- **Lacerated wound:** A jagged, irregular-shaped wound with torn or ragged edges.
- **Bruising and contusion:** Discoloration and damage to underlying blood vessels due to blunt force trauma.
- **Puncture wound:** A small, deep wound caused by a sharp object penetrating the skin.
- **Abrasion:** A superficial wound caused by friction or scraping of the skin's surface.
- **Crush injury:** Occurs when a body part is subjected to significant force or pressure, causing damage to tissues, blood vessels, and potentially underlying structures.
- **Penetrating wounds:** Occur when an object enters the body and damages underlying tissues, organs, or structures.

Based on Thickness of Wound

- Superficial wound
- Partial thickness
- Full thickness
- Deep wounds
- Complicated wounds
- Penetrating wound

Types of Surgical Wounds

- Clean wound
- Clean contaminated wound
- Contaminated wound
- Dirty infected wound

Class I ***Clean***	An uninfected operative wound in which no inflammation is encountered and the respiratory, alimentary, genital, or uninfected urinary tract are not entered. In addition, clean wounds are primarily closed and, if necessary, drained with closed drainage. Operative incisional wounds that follow nonpenetrating (blunt) trauma should be included in this category if they meet the criteria.
Class II ***Clean-contaminated***	An operative wound in which the respiratory, alimentary, genital, or urinary tracts are entered under controlled conditions and without unusual contamination. Specifically, operations involving the biliary tract, appendix, vagina, and oropharynx are included in this category, provided no evidence of infection or major break in technique is encountered.
Class III ***Contaminated***	Open, fresh, accidental wounds. In addition, operations with major breaks in sterile technique (e.g., open cardiac massage) or gross spillage from the gastrointestinal tract, and incisions in which acute, nonpurulent inflammation is encountered are included in this category.
Class IV ***Dirty-infected***	Old traumatic wounds with retained devitalized tissue and those that involve existing clinical infection or perforated viscera. This definition suggests that organisms causing postoperative infection were present in the operative field before the operation.

Wound Healing Process

Stages of Wound Healing

I. Inflammatory Phase (Immediate to 2–5 days)

Hemostasis

- Damaged blood vessels start to constrict.
- Formation of platelet plug
- Activation of extrinsic and intrinsic clotting pathways.
- Formation of fibrin matrix

Early Events

- Fibrin and fibronectin form a lattice.
- Migration of inflammatory, endothelial, and mesenchymal cells.
- Neutrophilic infiltrate appears.
- Removal of dead tissues.
- Monocytes/macrophages follow neutrophils.
- Orchestrated production of growth factors and phagocytosis.

Late Events

- Entry of lymphocytes
- Appearance of mast cell

II. Proliferative Phase (2 days to 3 weeks)

- Granulation tissue formation (made up of fibroblasts, macrophages and endothelial cells)
- Angiogenesis- reconstructs vasculature in areas damaged by wounds.
- Wound edges pull together to reduce the defect.
- Epithelialization - Epithelial cells migrate to form a barrier between the wound and the environment.

III. Remodeling Phase (3 weeks to 2 years)

- New collagen forms the tensile strength of the wound.
- Cross links between collagen fibers increase dramatically.
- Remodeling continues for 12 months.

Wound healing is accomplished in one of the following three ways:

- **Healing by first intention:** Occurs in clean, incised wounds with good apposition of the edges, e.g., surgical incisions.
- **Healing by second intention:** Occurs in open wounds with significant loss of tissue, necrosis or large wounds with irregular margins.
- **Healing by tertiary healing intention:** Also known as **delayed primary wound healing.** This occurs when the healing (secondary intention) is intentionally interrupted and the wound is mechanically closed. This usually occurs after granulation tissue has formed.

4. Write the first aid measures you would provide in the following situations: (DU)

a. **While running on the road Ms Geeta had a wound on the right forearm with foreign body protruding out.**

b. **Ms Sagitha had a sunstroke/heat stroke while working under the sun.**

c. **Mr Andrew had asphyxia after drowning.**

d. **Mr Sanjay had fracture of collar bone while playing in the ground.**

e. **Ram had foot crush injury after road traffic accident.**

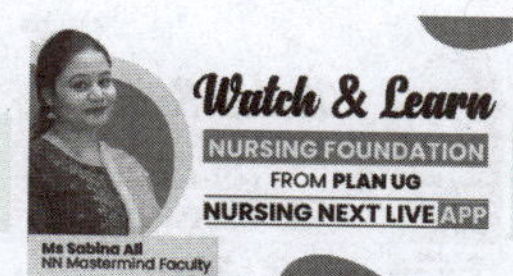

Answer

First Aid Measures for Ms Geeta's Wound

- **Ensure safety:** Ensure your safety and the safety of the injured person. Put on disposable gloves or use a clean cloth or towel to avoid direct contact with the wound.
- **Control bleeding:** Apply gentle pressure with a clean cloth or sterile dressing around the wound to control any bleeding. Do not remove any object protruding from the wound as it may be providing pressure to stop bleeding.
- **Stabilize foreign body:** Assess the foreign body and determine the position. If the foreign body is loose and easily removable without causing further harm, gently remove it using clean tweezers or forceps. Avoid pushing the foreign body further into the wound.
- **Cleanse the wound:** Use clean water or a saline solution to gently rinse the wound and remove any dirt or debris.
- **Cover the wound:** Place a sterile non-stick dressing or a clean cloth over the wound. Secure it in place with a bandage or adhesive tape to protect the wound from further contamination.
- **Seek medical attention:** Even if the bleeding is controlled and the wound appears superficial, it is important to seek medical attention for further evaluation, especially if the foreign body has been embedded or the wound is deep.
- **Comfort and reassurance:** Provide comfort and reassurance to the injured person to help reduce pain and anxiety.

b. Ms Sagitha had a sunstroke/heat stroke while working under the sun.

Answer

Sunstroke/Heatstroke

- **Move to a cool area:** Immediately move Ms Sagitha to a shaded or air-conditioned area away from direct sunlight and heat. Ensure good ventilation.
- **Call for help:** If Ms Sagitha is experiencing severe symptoms such as loss of consciousness, confusion, or difficulty breathing, call for emergency medical assistance.
- **Lower body temperature:** Remove any excess clothing and wet by sponging or showering her with cool water or use cool, wet towels on her forehead, neck, armpits, and groin area. Use fans or create air movement to promote evaporation and cooling.
- **Hydrate:** Encourage her to drink cool water or a rehydration solution if she is conscious and able to swallow.
- **Monitor vital signs:** Continuously monitor her vital signs, including her pulse rate, respiratory rate, and body temperature.
- **Elevate legs:** If the victim is conscious and not experiencing any leg injury, help her lie down and elevate her legs slightly to improve blood circulation.
- **Reassure and comfort:** Provide reassurance and keep the victim calm. Offer emotional support and comfort to help reduce anxiety.
- **Stay with the person:** Stay with victim until medical help arrives
- **Educate and prevent:** After the episode has resolved, educate Ms Sagitha about heat safety measures

First Aid *(When the Person Stops Breathing)*

- Perform CPR.
- Do not interrupt the resuscitation until:
  - The person starts to wake up,
  - Moves, opens his eyes and breathes normally;
  - Help (trained in CPR) arrives and takes over;
  - You become too exhausted to continue, or the scene becomes unsafe for you to continue.

c. Mr Andrew had asphyxia after drowning.

Answer

Safety First and Call for Help

- Make sure there is no danger of drowning.
- The person urgently needs help. Shout or call for help if you are alone but do not leave the person unattended. Ask a bystander to seek help or to arrange urgent transport to the nearest health care facility. Tell him to come back to you to confirm if help has been secured.

Moving the Victim Out of the Water

- Move the person rapidly and safely from the water, but do not place yourself into any danger by doing so.
- Try to throw a rope or something that the drowning person can hold onto (if he is still conscious and able to grasp the helpline).
- Once the person has been rescued from the water, do not try to remove water from his lungs.

What do I do if the Victim is Breathing?

- If the person is breathing, put him in the recovery position and cover him with a blanket or coat to keep him warm.
- Do not leave the victim alone and continue to observe him.

What do I do if the Victim is not Breathing or not Breathing Normally?

- Remove any cause of suffocation.
- If the person is not on his back, turn him on his back.
- Kneel down by the side of the person.
- Start CPR. Do not interrupt the resuscitation until the victim starts to wake up, moves, opens eyes and breathes normally; help (trained in CPR) arrives and takes over; you become too exhausted to continue; or the scene becomes unsafe for you to continue.

If the breathing starts again:

- Cover the victim.
- Arrange urgent transport to a hospital.
- Do not leave the victim alone and continue to observe him.
- If the breathing stops again, restart CPR.

d. Mr Sanjay had fracture of collar bone while playing in the ground.

Answer

Fracture of Collar Bone

The collar bone is normally broken when the person falls on the tip of the shoulder or on the palm of the outstretched hands.

First Aid Measures

- Support the arm of the injured side with the help of the casualty himself or an assistant.
- Do not remove the coat or bush coat.
- Place a pad in the armpit.
- Leave the forearm free, bandage the upper arm to the side of the chest with a broad bandage.
- Support the upper limb in the triangular sling and reassure him.
- Feel the pulse to make sure that circulation in the limb is free. Shock is not usually severe.
- The casualty may be transported even as a walking case.

e. Ram had foot crush injury after road traffic accident.

Answer

Foot crush injury is a condition where there is extensive damage to the skin, muscle and bone which are trapped under a heavy weight for a long time resulting in death of tissues which releases poisonous chemicals affecting the kidney's function extensively.

First Aid

Note: No time should be lost in treating a crush injury.

- Assure the casualty.
- Free the trapped limb immediately.
- Keep the part at rest and immobilize the limb.
- Stop bleeding (if any).
- Lay the casualty in flat position with his foot raised.
- Keep him warm with blanket or warm clothes.
- Elevate the affected limb and cover the wound.
- Do not allow him to drink anything.
- Treat for shock (if required).
- Monitor pulse, respiration and level of consciousness.
- Give CPR (if required).
- Transfer him to the hospital immediately.

5. Write the first aid measures you would provide in the following situations: (DU)

a. Anita was bitten by a snake.

b. Jaya had thermal burn injury while working in kitchen.

c. Rajiv had a cardiac arrest.

d. Sonu had bleeding from nose while playing in school playground.

e. Ritesh had fracture of right femur after he met with an accident.

f. Mr Britto sustained electrical shock while repairing a refrigerator.

Answer

The first aid recommended in case of snake bite:

First Aid Measures for Snakebite

- **Ensure safety:** Ensure your safety and the safety of others by moving away from the snake and keeping a safe distance.
- **Stay calm:** Encourage the victim to stay calm and still. Movement can increase the spread of venom throughout the body.
- **Call for help:** Dial emergency services or seek immediate medical assistance.
- **Immobilize the affected area:** Help Anita lie down and keep the affected part immobilized and at or below the level of the heart. This can help slow the spread of venom.
- **Remove constrictive items:** If there are any constrictive items, such as jewelry or tight clothing, near the bite site, gently remove them to prevent potential swelling.

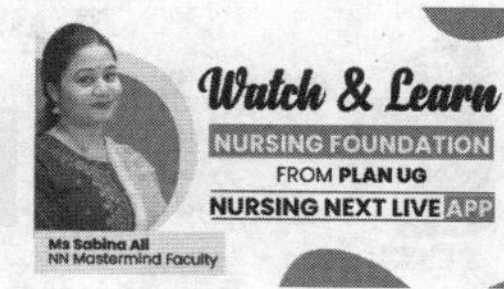

- **Cleaning the wound:** Clean the snakebite wound gently with soap and water, if available. Avoid scrubbing the wound, as it may cause further damage.
- **Apply a bandage:** Apply a loose sterile bandage or cloth over the snakebite wound. The bandage should be snug enough to limit the movement of the affected area but not too tight to restrict blood flow.
- **Keep the person still:** Advise the victim to avoid unnecessary movement and keep the affected limb as still as possible. Movement can increase the circulation of venom.
- **Monitor vital signs:** Monitor vital signs, such as breathing, pulse rate, and blood pressure.
- **Do not apply tourniquets or suck venom:** These measures can cause more harm than good and are not recommended.
- **Transport to medical facility:** Arrange for transportation to the nearest medical facility as soon as possible.

b. Jaya had thermal burn injury while working in kitchen.

Answer

- Cool the wound with water. Pour water on the burn for 10-15 minutes or until the burn stops hurting. Do not use very cold water for cooling the burns.
- Try not to touch her wound/blisters.
- Cover burn wounds with a clean cotton cloth.
- Do not open blisters – leave them intact
- Remove any clothing or jewellery that is not stuck to the burned skin. Do not remove parts of clothing or jewellery that are attached to the burn wounds.
- Do not apply any medicine, any pastes or creams to the burns.
- Make sure Jaya has sufficient fluids to drink.
- Refer the victim to a healthcare facility for further management.

c. Rajiv had a cardiac arrest.

Answer

- Ensure scene safety.
- Call for help
- Check carotid pulse (within 10 sec) and respiration
- Start CPR as soon as possible for effective results
- Follow:
  C – Circulation
  A – Airway
  B – Breathing

There are two versions of CPR

For Health care or First Aid Providers

Conventional CPR using chest compressions and mouth-to-mouth breathing at a ratio of **30:2** compressions-to-breaths.

- Chest compressions at a rate of **100 to 120/min.**
- Depth of compressions at least 2 inches (5 cm) for adults and children and 1.5 inches for infants.
- Initiate chest compressions (C-A-B rather than A-B-C).
- C- Compressions
- A- Airway
- B- Breathing
- Increase the depth of chest compressions to 2 inches for adults.

For the General Public or Bystanders, Who Witness an Adult Victim Suddenly Collapse:

- Compression-only CPR, or Hands-Only CPR.
- **Hands-Only CPR** is CPR without mouth-to-mouth breaths.
- It is recommended for use by people who see a teen or adult suddenly collapse in an out-of-hospital setting (such as at home, at work, or in a park).
- **High-Quality CPR**- Push hard and Push fast in the center of the chest. It has five critical components:
  - Minimize interruptions in chest compressions.
  - Provide compressions of adequate rate and depth.
  - Avoid leaning on the victim between compressions.
  - Ensure proper hand placement.
  - Avoid excessive ventilation.

Chain of Survival

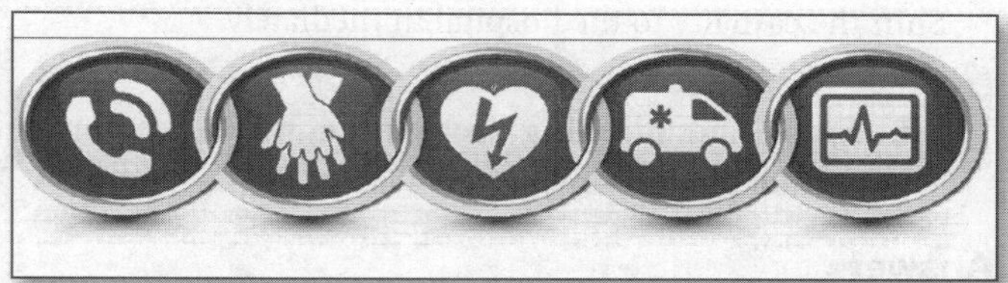

Adult CPR

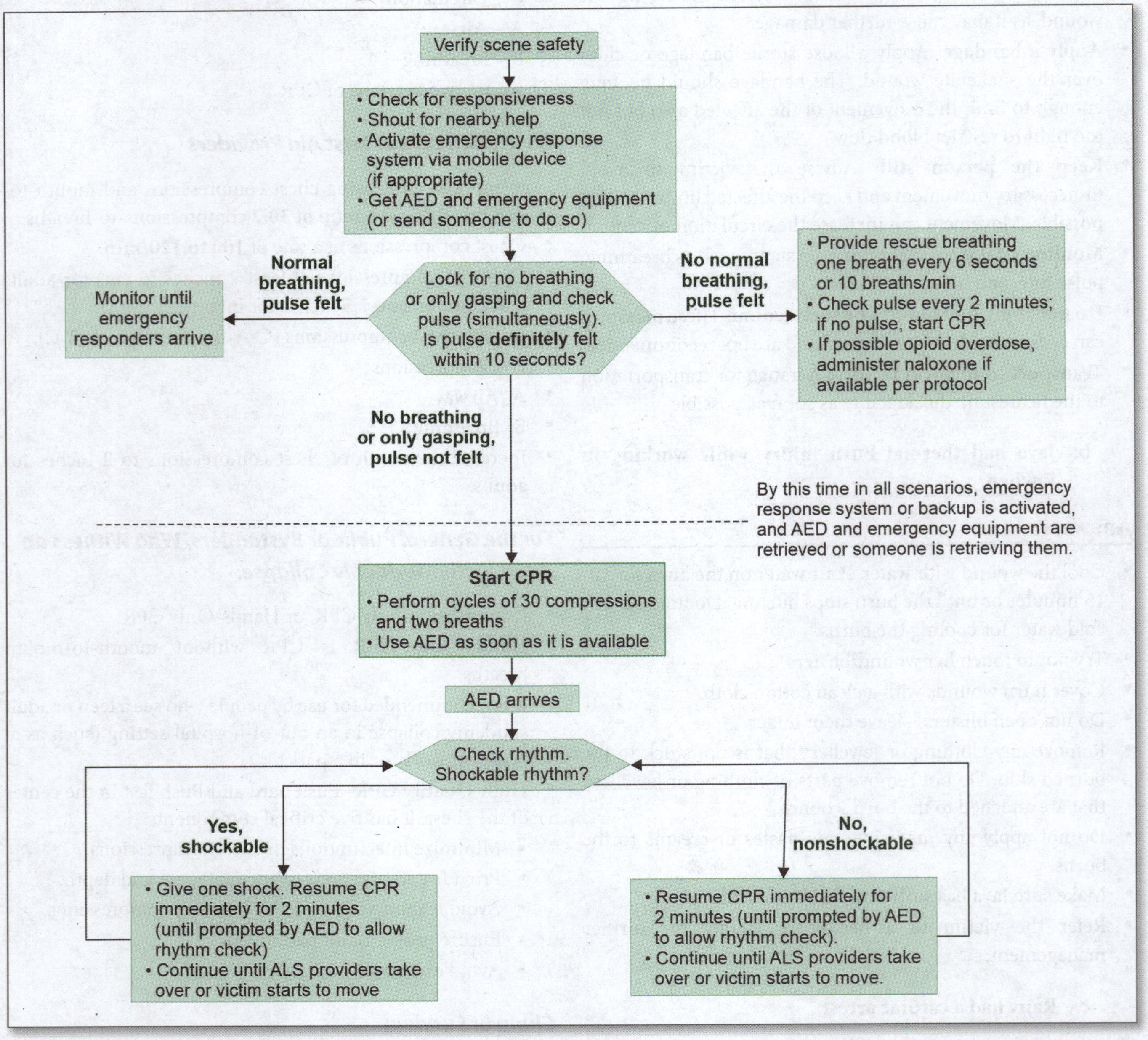

- Verify scene safety
- • Check for responsiveness • Shout for nearby help • Activate emergency response system via mobile device (if appropriate) • Get AED and emergency equipment (or send someone to do so)
- Look for no breathing or only gasping and check pulse (simultaneously). Is pulse **definitely** felt within 10 seconds?
  - **Normal breathing, pulse felt** → Monitor until emergency responders arrive
  - **No normal breathing, pulse felt** → • Provide rescue breathing one breath every 6 seconds or 10 breaths/min • Check pulse every 2 minutes; if no pulse, start CPR • If possible opioid overdose, administer naloxone if available per protocol
  - **No breathing or only gasping, pulse not felt** →

By this time in all scenarios, emergency response system or backup is activated, and AED and emergency equipment are retrieved or someone is retrieving them.

- **Start CPR** • Perform cycles of 30 compressions and two breaths • Use AED as soon as it is available
- AED arrives
- Check rhythm. Shockable rhythm?
  - **Yes, shockable** → • Give one shock. Resume CPR immediately for 2 minutes (until prompted by AED to allow rhythm check) • Continue until ALS providers take over or victim starts to move
  - **No, nonshockable** → • Resume CPR immediately for 2 minutes (until prompted by AED to allow rhythm check). • Continue until ALS providers take over or victim starts to move.

- Shift the casualty to the hospital immediately.

d. Sonu had bleeding from nose while playing in school playground.

Answer

- Ask to pinch the nose above the nostrils with the help of index finger and thumb.
- Instruct the victim to breathe through the mouth.
- Ask the injured person to lean forward and continue pinching the nose.
- Pinch the nostrils for 10 to 15 minutes.
- Apply a cold compress or ice pack to the bridge of your nose to constrict the blood vessels that can help in stopping the nosebleed.

e. Ritesh had fracture of right femur after he met with an accident.

Answer

First Aid Measures for the Fractures

- Assess the site of fracture.

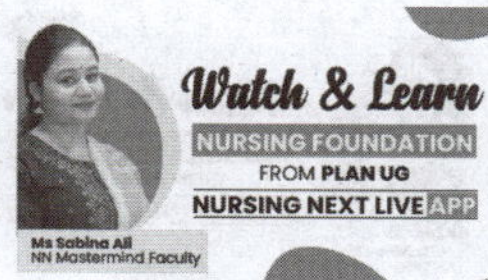

- Instruct him not to try to stand/move.
- **Immobilzation:** Immobilize the affected limb by keeping the leg still by bandaging or splinting one leg to the other non-broken/non-dislocated one.
- Carefully move the uninjured leg to the injured leg.
- Use suitable padding to fill between the legs.
- Use bandages to attach both legs together. Do not apply the bandages on the immediate site of the fracture
- The bandaging should be fairly firm so that there is no movement of the fracture ends, but it should not be too tight in which case the circulation of blood might be stopped.
- Ask Ritesh to keep still.
- Transport him to the nearest healthcare Facility.

 f. **Mr Britto sustained electrical shock while repairing a refrigerator.**

Answer

In Electrical Burns

- **Scene safety:** Look first and never touch him if still connected to an electrical source
- Immediately turn off the source of electricity first.
- Try to move him away from the source using a dry, non-conducting object such as cardboard, wood, etc.
- Shout or call for help
- Begin CPR if the person is not breathing, coughing or moving and doesn't have a pulse.
- If wound is present then cool down the burn wounds by using clean water for 10–15 minutes. Only do this, if there is no danger of further electrocution.
- Do not remove clothing or try to clean the burned area.
- Cover the wound with a sterile gauze bandage.
- Shift him to the nearest health care facility.

6. Discuss the first aid measures in the following situations: (DU)

 a. **Raghav suffered dog bite while playing in park with kids.**
 b. **Geeta had a fracture of pelvic bone in an accident.**
 c. **Kiran fell from a swing and is bleeding profusely at knee.**

Answer

First Aid for Dog Bite

- **Scene safety:** Ensure that the area is safe and dog cannot bite you or Raghav in the Park.
- Provide comfortable position to him
- Wear gloves if available and try not to come in contact with the injured person's blood or wound.
- **Wound cleaning:** Flush the wound immediately with the running tap water then wash it with soap and water for 10-15 minutes
- If still he is severely bleeding, stop the bleeding by applying pressure bandage to the wound.
- Cover the wound with a dry clean cloth or bandage.
- Refer Raghav to a healthcare facility immediately for further treatment

 b. **Geeta had a fracture of pelvic bone in an accident.**

Answer

- Assess the site of fracture.
- Instruct him not to try to stand/move.
- **Immobilzation:** Immobilize the affected limb by keeping the leg still by bandaging or splinting one leg to the other non-broken/non-dislocated one.
- Carefully move the uninjured leg to the injured leg.
- Use suitable padding to fill between the legs.
- Use bandages to attach both legs together. Do not apply the bandages on the immediate site of the fracture
- The bandaging should be fairly firm so that there is no movement of the fracture ends, but it should not be too tight in which case the circulation of blood might be stopped.
- Ask Ritesh to keep still.
- Transport him to the nearest healthcare Facility.

 c. **Kiran fell from a swing and is bleeding profusely at knee.**

Answer

- **Safety first and call for help:** Make sure there is no danger to you and Kiran also.
- Ask the injured to sit or lie down or provide her a comfortable position.
- Tell her to relax and rest.
- Try to stop or slow down the bleeding by press with both hands on the wound with a clean cloth or bandage.
- Later on cover the wound with clean bandages and continue to apply pressure until the bleeding stops. If the bandage becomes soaked in blood, do not remove it, but add another bandage on top of it and continue to apply pressure.
- Make sure the bandage is firm enough so it stops the bleeding but doesn't cut off all the blood flow.
- Keep checking for the bleeding and also check that she is conscious and breathing properly
- Transfer the victim as quickly as possible to a healthcare facility for further treatment.

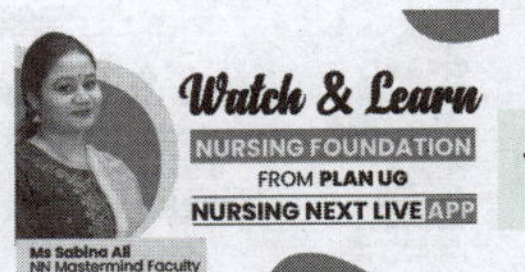

SHORT NOTES

1. Write a short note on the measures to control bleeding. (MGR)

Answer

There are four methods to control bleeding:

- Direct Pressure
- Elevation
- Indirect Pressure
- The Use of a Tourniquet

I. Direct Pressure

- Direct pressure is the most effective method.
- It includes application of pressure directly to the wound.
- Place a sterile dressing or clean cloth on the wound, tie a knot or adhere tape directly over the wound, tight enough to control bleeding.
- If bleeding does not stop, apply another dressing over the first on the wound.

II. Elevation

- Elevation of an injured arm or leg (extremity) above the level of the heart will help control bleeding.
- Elevation should be used together with direct pressure.
- Do not elevate an extremity if you suspect a broken bone (fracture) until it has been properly splinted.

III. Indirect Pressure

- In case where direct pressure and elevation are not controlling the bleeding.
- It involves applying pressure to the appropriate pressure point with the fingers, thumb, or heel of the hand.
- The brachial artery- used to control severe bleeding of the lower part of the arm.
- The femoral artery- used to control severe bleeding of the thigh and lower leg.
- Do not apply pressure to the carotid pressure points at one time, it can cause cardiac arrest.

IV. The Use of a Tourniquet

- A tourniquet should be used only as a last resort and only for extremities.
- A tourniquet can be a strap, belt, towel, or other similar item.

Application: Leave at least 2 inches of uninjured skin between the tourniquet and wound.

- Wrap the tourniquet twice.
- Never cover a tourniquet.
- Note the time at which tourniquet was applied.

2. Write a short note on the factors influencing wound healing. (MGR)

Answer

Factors Affecting Wound Healing

I. Local Factors

- Infection
- Presence of necrotic tissue and foreign body
- Poor blood supply
- Venous or lymph stasis
- Tissue tension
- Hematoma
- Large defect or poor apposition
- Recurrent trauma
- X-ray irradiated area
- Site of wound
- Underlying diseases such as osteomyelitis and malignancy

II. General Factors

- Age
- Obesity
- smoking
- Malnutrition
- Vitamin deficiency (Vitamin C, Vitamin A)
- Anemia
- Malignancy
- Diabetes
- HIV and immunosuppressive diseases
- Steroids and cytotoxic drugs

3. Write a short note on four complications of wound healing. (MGR, DU, KUHS, RUHS)

Answer

Wound dehiscence: It is the spontaneous opening of incision characterized by increased flow of serosanguineous drainage.

Wound evisceration: It is the protrusion of internal organ through incision wound.

Formation of contractures: Exaggeration of the normal contraction resulting in deformities of the wound and surrounding tissues is referred to as contractures. These are found in cases of severe burns.

Keloid: Due to excessive collagen accumulation and growth beyond the borders of the original wound. It is a raised abnormal scar . Do not regress.

4. Write a short note on causes of bed sore. (MGR)

Answer

Lack of sensory perception: Neurological disorders and other conditions can result in a loss of sensation. An inability to feel pain or discomfort can result in not being aware of warning signs and the need to change position. Medical conditions affect blood flow. Health problems that can affect blood flow, such as diabetes and vascular diseases, increase the risk of tissue damage.

Poor nutrition and hydration: Individuals need enough fluids, calories, protein, vitamins and minerals in their daily diet to maintain healthy skin and prevent the breakdown of tissues.

Moisture: Increased moisture for prolonged periods can cause skin maceration due to which skin is more prone to injury from pressure and other forces. In some cases moisture can be the primary cause of ulceration, even in the absence of any pressure.

Pressure: Constant pressure on any part of the body decreases the blood circulation to the body tissues.

Friction: Friction occurs when the skin rubs against clothing or bedding due to the fragile skin being more vulnerable to get injury, especially if the skin is also moist.

Shear: Shear occurs when two surfaces move in the opposite direction. For example, when a bed is elevated at the head, you can slide down in bed.

5. Write a short note on first aid for poisoning. (DU)

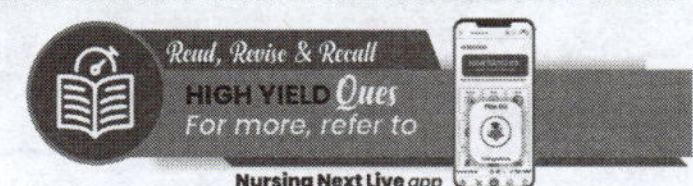

Answer

Assess the Person

- Assess the type and route of ingestion of poisoning.
- Check the level of consciousness of the person.

Remove Toxin/Poison from Contact

If the poisoning was caused by

Oral ingestion:

- If the person is alert, do not induce vomiting.
- If the person has ingested a corrosive substance such as a household cleaner or chemical, give them small sips of water or milk to help dilute the substance.

Contact with the Skin

- Carefully remove all the contaminated clothes.
- Wash the exposed area with water
- Transport the casualty to the nearest hospital

In the Eye

- Reassure the casualty
- Rinse the eyes with tap water for 10–15 minutes.
- Allow the water to flow from inner canthus to outer canthus.
- Transport the casualty to the nearest hospital

Inhaled

- Reassure the victim
- Get the person to the fresh air
- Avoid crowding
- Loosen the tighten clothes
- Transport the casualty to the nearest hospital

Call for help: Call for immediate medical attention.

Transport to medical facility: Immediately transport to medical facility for further evaluation and treatment.

6. Write a short note on the points to be kept in mind while doing wound dressing. (DU)

Answer

- Microorganisms are present in the environment, on the articles and on the skin also. Pathogenic organisms are transmitted from the source to the host both directly and indirectly.
- Bacteria travel along with the dust particles.
- Clean an area where there are less number of organisms before cleaning an area where there are more organisms; minimize the spread of organisms to the clean area. In surgical wound dressing, always clean inner to outer, while in dirty wound, clean outer to inner.
- A break in the skin and mucus membrane acts as the portal of entry for a various pathogenic organisms.
- Respiratory tract harbors microorganisms that can enter the wound. Nutrients and oxygen are carried to the wound via bloodstream and are essential for collagen formation.
- Moisture facilitates growth and movement of microorganisms.
- Fluid moves downward as a result of gravitational pull.
- Fluids move through materials by capillary action.
- Unfamiliar situations produce anxiety.
- Systematic ways of working save time, energy and material.

7. Write a short note on first aid for epistaxis. (KUHS)

Answer

For answer, refer to Long Question no. 5(d), pg. no. 709

8. Write a short note on first aid measures for fracture. (KUHS)

Answer

First Aid Measures for the Fractures

- When bones are broken, a good rule to follow is "Do not permit motion of the broken ends or of the joints near the injury." This prevents pain and further damage.
- For closed or simple fracture, place the limb in as natural position as possible without causing discomfort to the victim. Handle very gently; avoid all unnecessary movements of the injured part.
- Since the danger of infection is high in compound or open fractures, it is always better to get help from a doctor. In caring for the injury, clean the wound and apply dressing. If there is an excessive bleeding from open fracture, apply pressure dressing to control it. Transfer the patient to hospital.
- Never try to reduce the fracture, i.e., bringing bones to normal position (alignment).
- Before trying to move or carry a person with a broken bone, immobilize the broken ends with splints.
- Send the patient for medical aid as soon as possible.

9. Write a short note on the measures taken for prevention of bed sores or decubitus ulcers. (KUHS)

Answer

For answer, refer to Long Question no. 1, pg. no. 703

10. Write a short note on first aid for drowning. (KUHS)

Answer

Safety First and Call for Help

- Make sure there is no danger to you of drowning.
- The person urgently needs help. Shout or call for help if you are alone but do not leave the person unattended. Ask a bystander to seek help or to arrange urgent transport to the nearest health care facility. Tell him to come back to you to confirm if help has been secured.

Move the Victim Out of the Water

- Move the person rapidly and safely from the water, but do not place yourself into any danger by doing so.
- Try to throw a rope or something that the drowning person can hold onto (if he is still conscious and able to grasp the helpline).
- Once the person has been rescued from the water, do not try to remove water from his lungs.

What do I do If the Victim is Breathing?

- If the person is breathing, put him in the recovery position and cover him with a blanket or coat to keep him warm.
- Do not leave the victim alone and continue to observe him.

What do I do If the Victim is not Breathing or not Breathing Normally?

- Remove any cause of suffocation.
- If the person is not on his back, turn him on his back.
- Kneel down by the side of the person.
- Start CPR. Do not interrupt the resuscitation until: the victim starts to wake up, moves, opens eyes and breathes normally; help (trained in CPR) arrives and takes over; you become too exhausted to continue; or the scene becomes unsafe for you to continue.

If the breathing starts again:

- Cover the victim.
- Arrange urgent transport to a hospital.
- Do not leave the victim alone and continue to observe him.
- If the breathing stops again, restart CPR.

11. Write a short note on the qualities of a first-aider. (KUHS)

Answer

- **Prompt and quick:** As soon as an accident or injury takes place, the first aider should be prompt and quick, to render help to the victim, without delay.
- **Calm and controlled:** He should be a calm and controlled sort of person because he has to take immediate action, without any fuss or panic.
- **Wise and intelligent:** He should be intelligent and wise enough to decide the immediate treatment even before a complete diagnosis, especially in case of serious injuries and severe bleeding. Resourceful: He should be resourceful enough to make available his first aid material at once or get the required things on the spot, for giving immediate relief to the victim.

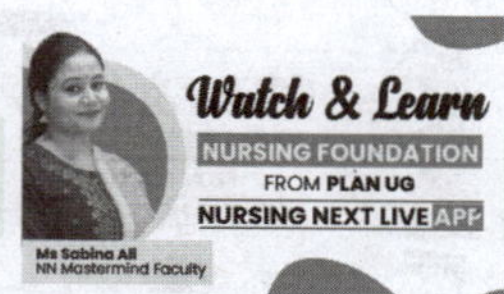

- **Sweet tempered and sympathetic:** The first-aider should use sweet and encouraging words to lessen the victim's distress. He should keep the victim as comfortable as possible and should be able to allay the victim's fears with sympathy.
- **Skillful and tactful:** The first-aider should be skillful and tactful to judge history of the case without wasting any time. If the need arises, he should be able to muster requisite support from the crowd.
- **Dexterous and clever:** Should be able to help the injured without causing and/or aggravating pain, and to use the appliances and/or procedure efficiently and effectively.
- **Confident and perseverant:** The first aider should have full faith in his skill to administer whatever assistance the situation demands, even if there is no response initially. He should have perseverance and should not give up. It may take time for the patient to respond to his handling.

12. Write a short note on the principles of bandaging. (KUHS)

Answer

- Select a bandage of proper size and suitable material.
- Put the patient in a comfortable position.
- Support the injured area while bandaging.
- If a joint is involved, flex it slightly.
- Face the patient while applying the bandage, except when applying it on the head.
- Hold the roll of the bandage in the right hand when applying the bandage on the left side.
- Always start bandaging from inner to outer aspect and far to near end
- While bandaging a joint, ensure flexibility of the joint (except if immobilization of joint is required).
- Always start and end with two circular turns.
- Cover the area 2 inches above and below the affected area.
- Overlap turns and slightly stretch the bandage.
- Cover 2/3 of the previous turn.
- Where possible, leave fingertips or toe tips exposed for observation.
- Do not end the bandage on the wound.

13. Write a short note on first aid for burns. (KUHS)

Answer

- Stopping the burning process.
- For stopping the burning process, do not allow the person to run about, as it increases the severity. Lay him flat on the ground, put any thick clothing which is available like blanket, carpet, shawl, etc. over the victim to extinguish flames. Do not try to remove the burning clothes.
- Immediately, immerse the burnt area under cool running water or cool moistened towels can be applied reduce pain and decrease the effect of transmission through the tissues.
- Assess airway breathing and circulation.
- Blisters should not be touched.
- All articles like bangles, belt, boot should be removed.
- Cover the burnt area with clean sheet over which blanket can be placed to maintain heat and prevent hypothermia.
- Give warm fluids to drink if casualty can take them and restrict the movement.
- In case of extensive burns person may go into shock then the first aid for shock is given and victim is rushed to a nearby hospital.

In Acid Burns

- Cool area with stream of plain water. Remove acid soaked clothing.
- Bathe affected part with alkaline solution of one table spoon of baking soda and 1 L of water.
- Cover with clean linen.

In Alkali Burns

- Flood burnt area with stream of plain water.
- Remove alkali soaked clothing.
- Bathe affected part with weak solution of vinegar and water in equal parts.
- Cover with clean linen material only.

In Electrical Burns

- Free the victim from the circuit immediately.
- Remove the wire from contact with the victim by taking a dry wooden stick, dry towel.
- Stand on dry insulating material-wooden, rubber or plastic mat or thick pile of newspapers.
- Call the fire department for outdoors electrocution.
- Start artificial respiration and continue till natural breathing is restored.

14. Write a short note on the risk factors for pressure ulcer. (KUHS)

Intrinsic factors	Extrinsic factors
Nutritional Status/Hydration	Pressure
Reduced mobility/immobility	Shearing

Contd...

Intrinsic factors	Extrinsic factors
Extremes of age	Friction
Sensory impairment	Moisture
Pain	Poor moving and handling
Chronic/acute/terminal illness	Medication
Vascular disease	
Mental health status	
Level of consciousness	
Previous history of pressure damage	

15. Write a short note on first aid for snake bite. (KUHS)

Answer

For answer, refer to Long Question no. 5(a), pg. no. 708

16. Write a short note on golden rules of first aid. (RUHS)

Answer

- Do first things first, quickly and quietly without fuss or panic
- Reassure the casualty through encouraging words
- Check ABC rule (airway, breathing, circulation)
- Open the airway by tilting the head
- Give artificial respiration if breathing has stopped
- Perform chest compression if the pulse is not present
- Stop bleeding, if any, by direct pressure
- Treat for shock
- Do not allow people to crowd around
- Don't remove clothes unnecessarily
- Arrange for transportation of the casualty
- Casualty should be sent to a hospital or doctor by quickest means of transport.
- Always inform the police and the relatives about serious accidents.

SHORT ANSWER QUESTIONS

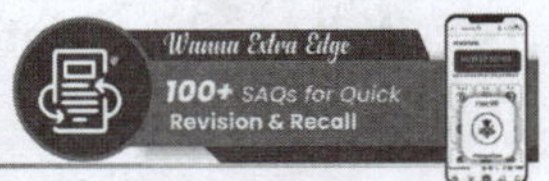

1. Define decubitus ulcer.

Answer

A pressure ulcer or pressure sore or decubitus ulcer or bedsore is localized injury to the skin or to the other underlying tissue, usually over a body prominence area , as a result of prolonged unrelieved pressure.

2. Define first aid.

Answer

As per Red Cross Society of India: First aid is the first assistance or treatment given to a casualty or a sick person for any injury or sudden illness before the arrival of an ambulance, the arrival of a qualified paramedical or medical person or before arriving at a facility that can provide professional medical care.

3. Enumerate the qualities of a first-aider.

Answer

Qualities of First-Aider

- Prompt and quick
- Calm and controlled
- Wise and intelligent
- Sweet tempered and sympathetic
- Skillful and tactful
- Dexterous and clever
- Confident and perseverant

4. Define wound.

Answer

Wound

A wound is a break in the integrity of the skin or tissues often which may be associated with disruption of the structure and function. —*(SRB 4th edition)*

A cut or break in the continuity of any tissue, caused by injury or operation. —*(Baillière's 23rd Ed)*

5. Define CPR. (MGR, DU, KUHS, RUHS)

Answer

CPR: Cardiopulmonary Resuscitation

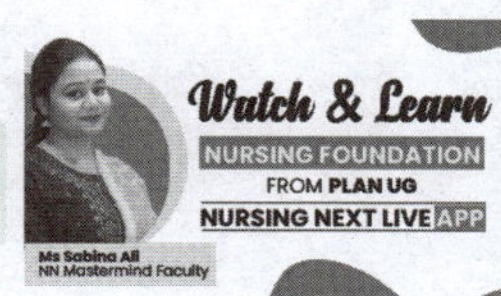

- According to AHA *(American Heart Association) Guidelines,* CPR – or Cardiopulmonary Resuscitation – is an emergency lifesaving procedure performed when the heart stops beating. Immediate CPR can double or triple the chances of survival after cardiac arrest.

6. Define CPR. (MGR, DU, KUHS, RUHS)

Answer

CPR: Cardiopulmonary Resuscitation

- According to AHA *(American Heart Association) Guidelines,* CPR – or Cardiopulmonary Resuscitation – is an emergency lifesaving procedure performed when the heart stops beating. Immediate CPR can double or triple the chances of survival after cardiac arrest.

CONCEPTUAL REVISION

MULTIPLE CHOICE QUESTIONS

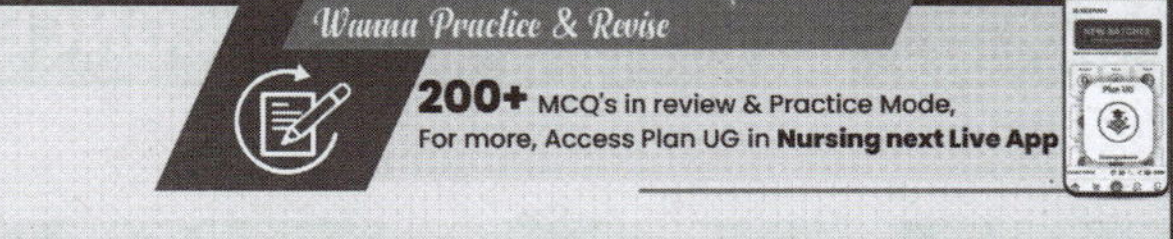

1. Which of the following is not a principle of first aid?

a. Preserve life
b. Response
c. Promote recovery
d. Prevent worsening
e. Provide transportation to nearest hospital

Ans. b. Response

2. The following options give the algorithm to provide first aid. Which of the following is written in correct order?

a. S- Safety, R- Response, A- Assistance, FA- First Aid
b. R-Response, S- Safety, A- Assistance, FA- First Aid
c. FA- First Aid, R-Response, A- Assistance, S- Safety
d. FA- First Aid, S- Safety, R-Response, A- Assistance

Ans. a. S- Safety, R- Response, A- Assistance, FA- First Aid

3. The mother of 11-month-old girl asks for the treatment of her baby hospitalized for choking. The nurse would explain the choking management as:

a. Abdominal thrust
b. Chest thrust
c. Five back blows, five chest thrusts
d. All of the above

Ans. c. Five back blows, five chest thrusts

4. A patient with deep partial-thickness burns would present with which of the following symptoms?

a. Redness with no blister formation
b. Exposed muscles, nerves, blackened skin, extremely painful
c. Oozing at the burnt site
d. Charred tissue

Ans. b. Exposed muscles, nerves, blackened skin, extremely painful

5. A child is bitten by a tick. Which of the following explanations given by the nurse is correct?

a. Tick bite can transmit Lyme disease
b. Tick leaves its sting behind in the victim which releases poison
c. It firmly attaches to the skin, and lays eggs
d. It does not cause any serious illness

Ans. a. Tick bite can transmit Lyme disease

6. Appropriate first aid measure of a snake bite includes:

a. Elevate the affected part
b. Immobilize the affected part
c. Place a tourniquet above 2 cm of bitten site
d. Apply ice over the bitten site

Ans. b. Immobilize the affected part

7. A first-aider is present at the site of swallowed poisoning. The victim swallowed acid. Which of the following actions is appropriate to perform?

a. Induce vomiting
b. Assess airway patency, breathing, and circulation.
c. Find out the ingested substance
d. Place the patient in a supine position

Ans. b. Assess airway patency, breathing, and circulation.

8. While applying a bandage to the patient's forearm, which movement the community health officer should use?

a. Distal to proximal
b. Median to lateral
c. Proximal to distal
d. Lateral to median

Ans. a. Distal to proximal

CHAPTER

15

Health Assessment

CONCEPTUAL THEORY

Terminology

Auscultation: It is the process of listening to sounds that are generated within the body by a stethoscope.

Health assessment: Health assessment is an organized systematic assessment of human body which involves the use of one's senses to determine the general physical and mental conditions of the body by collecting both subjective and objective data.

Inspection: It is the systematic visual examination by using sense of sight.

Palpation: It is the technique of using your hands/fingers based on sensation of touch to assess the body and further examine cues that were identified during inspection.

Percussion: It is a method of tapping body parts with fingers, hands, or small instruments as part of a physical examination. It is done to determine: the size, consistency, and borders of body organs. The presence or absence of fluid in body areas.

Physical examination: It is the systematic collection of objective information that is directly observed or is elicited through examination techniques.

PHYSICAL EXAMINATION

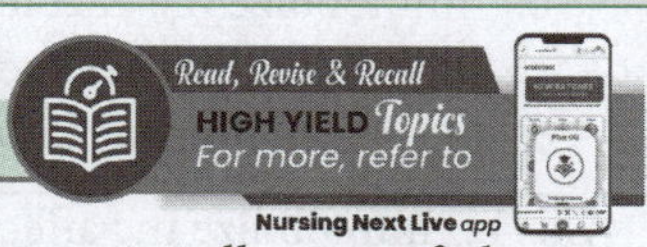

Physical examination is the systematic collection of objective information that is directly observed or is elicited through examination techniques.

- It is a systematic data collection method that uses the senses of sight, hearing, smell and touch to detect health problems.
- Physical examination is defined as a complete assessment of a patient's physical and mental status.

The **four methods** used in physical examination are explained as follows.

1. Inspection

It is the systematic visual examination by using sense of sight.

2. Palpation

Palpation is the technique of using your hands/fingers based on **sensation of touch** to assess the body and further examine cues that were identified during inspection.

3. Percussion

Percussion is a method of tapping body parts with fingers, hands, or small instruments as part of a physical examination. It is done to determine: the size, consistency, and borders of body organs. The presence or absence of fluid in body areas.

4. Auscultation

It is the process of listening to sounds that are generated within the body by a Stethoscope. The auscultation is performed for heart sounds, breath sounds and bowel sounds.

Positions used in Physical Assessment

Several positions are used during the physical examination of the patients. It depends upon the patient's ability to assume a position.

The five positions that can be used during physical examination are:

1. Dorsal Position/Supine Position

The patients lie on their back with head and shoulders slightly elevated.

Uses

- Comfortable position
- Examination of head, neck, chest, abdomen and extremities
- Surgery of anterior part of the body

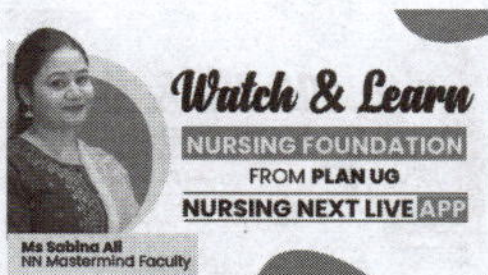

2. Prone Position

A patient lies flat on abdomen and head turned to one side. Both the hands held in a comfortable position.

Uses

- Examination of posterior trunk, spines and rectum
- Surgeries of back
- To relieve pressure on areas such as sacrum, scapula and heel
- After anesthesia to prevent aspiration

3. Sims' Position

- Differs from side lying position in which weight is placed in the anterior ilium, humerus and clavicle.
- Patients lies on his left with left arm drawn behind the back.
- Right arm may be in any position.
- The right thigh is flexed against the abdomen.

Uses

- Vaginal and rectal examination.
- To relive pressure in the buttocks, scapula and heels.

4. Lithotomy Position

- The patient lies on her back the legs are separated and thighs are flexed on the abdomen.
- The buttocks are kept in the edge of the table and legs are supported by stirrups.
- Provides maximal exposure of genitalia.

Uses

- Vaginal examination
- Pap smear
- Position during delivery for many women
- Surgical procedures of genitourinary system

5. Knee-Chest Position

- Patient lies on the bed in such a way that the knees and the chest rests on the bed.
- The head is turned to one side.
- A small pillow can be placed under the chest.
- The weight of patient rests on chest and knees only.
- The knees are flexed and thighs are at right angle to legs.

Uses

- Examination of rectum and vagina
- Postpartum exercise

HEALTH ASSESSMENT

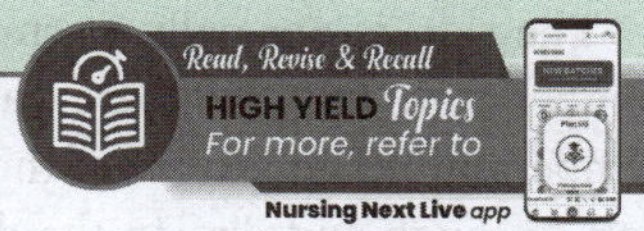

Health assessment is an organized systematic assessment of human body which involves the use of one's senses to determine the general physical and mental conditions of the body by collecting both subjective and objective data.

Types of Health Assessment

The types of health assessment depende on several factors like context of care, the patient's needs and the nurse's experience.

Comprehensive assessment: This involves a detailed history or physical examination performed at the onset of care in a primary care setting or an admission to a hospital or long-term care facility.

Problem-based/focused assessment: It involves a history and examination that are limited to a specific problem or complaint. This type of assessment is most commonly used in a walk in clinic or emergency department and outpatient departments.

Episodic/follow-up assessment: This type of assessment is usually done when a patient is following up with a health care provider for previously identified problem.

Shift assessment: When individuals are hospitalized, nurses conduct assessment each shift. The purpose is to identify changes in a patient's condition from baseline.

Screening assessment: It is a short examination focused on disease detection. It may be performed in a health care provider's office or at a health fair.

Process of Health Assessment

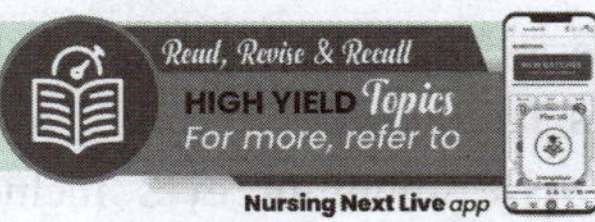

- Health history
- Physical examination: Inspection, Auscultation, Percussion and palpation
- General assessment
- System wise assessment
- Recording of health assessment

General examination: The examination is carried out in an orderly manner focusing upon one area of the body at a time.

Assessment of Each Body System

The integumentary system includes the skin, hair and nails. Assessing the integumentary structures provides information about the overall health status, as well as clues to local or systemic health problems.

Assessment of skin involves inspection and palpation.

The skin is inspected for vascularity, bleeding, or bruising. These signs might relate to a cardiovascular, hematologic, or liver dysfunction.

The skin is normally warm and dry. An increase in skin temperature and moisture can indicate an elevated body temperature. The texture of the skin varies from smooth and soft to tough and dry. In the dehydrated patient, the texture is dry, loose, and wrinkled, and the mucous membranes are cracked and dry. An excessive amount of perspiration, such as when the entire skin is moist, it is called diaphoresis.

The **nails** are inspected for shape, angle, texture and color. The nails should be somewhat convex and should follow the natural curve of the finger. The angle between the nail and its base should be about 160°.

Abnormal findings include indentations called Beau's lines (from acute illness), infection, painless separation of the nail plate from the nail bed (onycholysis), due to infection or trauma, (paronychia), increased brittleness or thickness and angulation (from anemia or iron deficiency anemia), and clubbing (from long-term lack of oxygenation).

Assess the **hair** for color, texture and distribution. The hair is normally resilient, evenly distributed, and neither excessively dry nor oily. Abnormal findings include an unusual balding (alopecia) and excessive amounts of hair on the face and body (hirsutism).

Assessment of the **head and neck** includes the skull, face, eyes, ear, nose and sinuses, mouth and pharynx, trachea, thyroid gland and lymph nodes.

Inspect and palpate the head for size and shape. Normal head size is referred to as normocephalic.

Abnormal findings include lack of symmetry or unusual size or contour of the skull and tenderness.

Inspect **face** for color, symmetry, and distribution of facial hair. Edema of the face, especially around the eye (periorbital edema) and involuntary facial movements (e.g., tics, fasciculation, tremors) are abnormal findings.

Assessment **of eyes** includes the external and internal eye structures, visual acuity, extraocular movements and peripheral vision.

Asymmetry of position and alignment of the eyes may be caused by muscle weakness or a congenital abnormality. The eyebrows should be equally distributed, the eyelashes should curl outward.

Abnormal findings include drooping of the upper lids (ptosis) which may be due to damage to oculomotor nerve, myasthenia gravis, or a congenital disorder, inward turning of the lower lid and lashes (entropion); outward turning of the lower lid (ectropion); and redness or drainage (from infection of the lid margins, conjunctivae, or hair follicles). Inspect and palpate the lacrimal glands for edema and pain.

Pupils equal round reactive to light and accommodation (PERRLA) is an acronym used to document a common pupillary response test. It stands for Pupils, Equal, Round, Reactire (to), Light and Accommodation. It is used to check the appearance and function of the pupil.

The internal eye is examined with the ophthalmoscope to assess the fundus, including the retina, optic nerve disk, macula, fovea centralis and retinal vessels.

Abnormal findings include cloudiness of the lens (cataract), changes in size and shape of blood vessels (from hypertension or arteriosclerosis), and changes in color and surface characteristics (from diabetes, hypertension, trauma, inflammation and detached retina).

Visual acuity is checked with **the Snellen chart.**

The **external ear** is assessed by inspection and palpation. The middle ear and tympanic membrane are assessed by inspection. An otoscope with the correct size of ear speculum is used to inspect the ear canal and tympanic membrane. A tuning fork and ticking watch are used to assess hearing acuity.

Tuning fork tests such as the Weber and Rinne tests help assess the type of hearing loss: conductive (the result of a problem with the transmission of sound waves through the outer and middle ear), sensorineural (from inner ear damage), or a combination of both.

Assessment of nose involves examining the external nose, the nares, and palpate the sinuses with the patient sitting with head slightly tilted back. Assess the nose for patency by occluding one nostril at a time and asking the patient to inhale and exhale through the nose. Inspect each nostril using an otoscope or nasal speculum and penlight. Examine the mucous membrane for color and presence of lesions, exudates, or growths. Inspect the nasal septum for intactness and deviation.

The **mouth and pharynx** include the lips, tongue, teeth, gums, hard and soft palate, salivary glands and tonsils. Equipment used to assess includes a penlight, tongue blade, gauze and gloves.

Assess the mouth and pharynx by inspecting the lips, gums and teeth, tongue and hard and soft palate. Make the patient sit with head tilted backward and mouth opened wide. Use palpation if any abnormalities are noted during inspection. Wear gloves when assessing patient's mouth and use gauze to hold tongue for palpation.

Abnormal findings are pallor, cyanosis, or redness and swelling of the mucous membranes, lesions of the mucosa and lips, swollen red tonsils indicate infection; swollen red, and bleeding gums; poorly aligned, missing or caries teeth; white coating on the tongue (from poor oral hygiene, irritation or smoking); a fissured tongue (due to dehydration); bright red tongue (seen in deficiency of vitamin B_{12} or niacin) or a black hairy tongue (from antibiotic use).

Assess the **neck** with the patient sitting and the neck slightly hyperextended, to assess range of motion.

The thorax comprises the lungs, rib cage, cartilage and intercostal muscles.

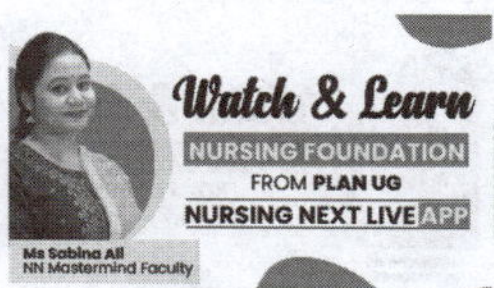

Inspect the patient's chest for color, shape or contour, breathing patterns and muscle development.

Abnormal findings include an increase in chest size and contour, abnormal breathing patterns with use of accessory muscles, unequal chest expansion and abnormal respirations.

Palpation is used to detect areas of sensitivity, chest expansion during respirations, and vibrations (fremitus). Use the palmar surface of the hands to palpate the anterior and posterior thoracic landmarks in a sequential pattern for temperature moisture, muscular development and any tenderness, or masses.

Auscultation is used to detect airflow within the respiratory tract.

Breath sounds vary over different parts of the lungs. **Bronchial sounds** heard over the trachea are harsh sounds, high-pitched, with expiration being longer than inspiration.

Bronchovesicular sounds are heard over the main stem bronchus and are moderate "blowing" sounds, with inspiration equal to expiration. **Vesicular breath sounds** are soft, low-pitched sounds heard best over the base of the lungs and lung periphery during inspiration, which is longer than expiration.

Adventitious breath sounds are not normally heard in lungs but, if present, they may be auscultated. **Stertorous breathing** is a general term used to refer to noisy, strenuous respiration. **Stridor** is harsh, high-pitched sound heard on inspiration, **crackles** are fine to coarse crackling sounds made as air moves through wet secretion: they are most often heard on inspiration.

Coarse crackles can also be documented as **rhonchi. Wheezes** are continuous sounds that originate in small air passages that are narrowed by secretions, swelling, or tumors. A **pleural friction** rub is a grating sound caused by an inflamed pleura rubbing against the chest wall.

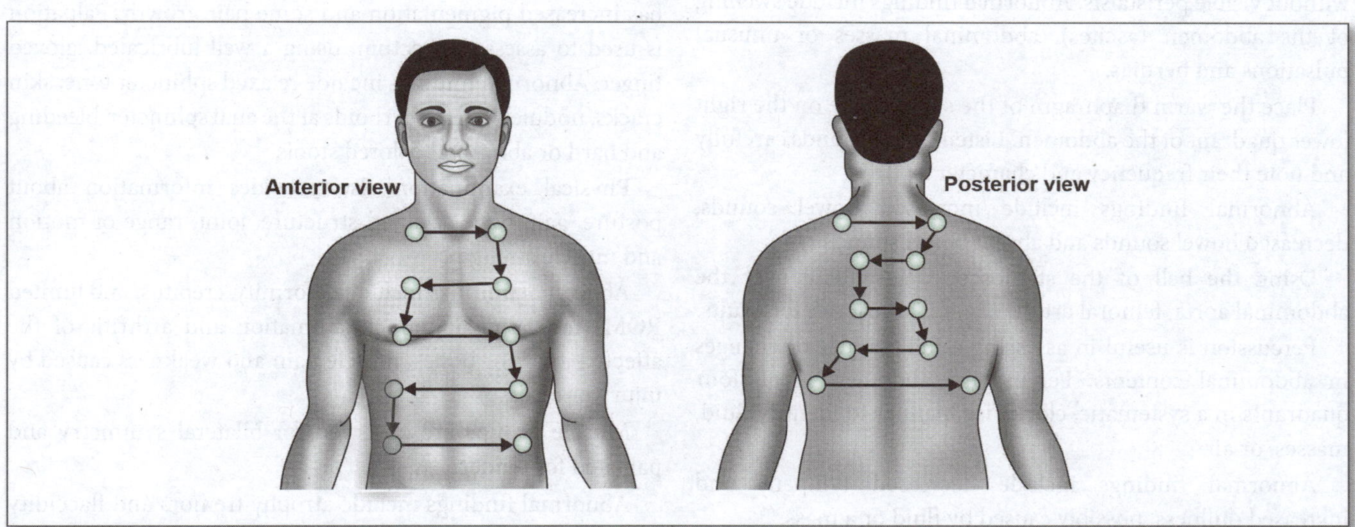

The techniques used for **cardiovascular assessment** are inspection, palpation and auscultation. Equipment includes a stethoscope and a sphygmomanometer.

Peripheral vascular assessment includes measuring the blood pressure and assessing the skin and perfusion of the extremities and the peripheral pulses.

Auscultation is used to determine the heart sounds caused by closure of the heart valves. Use systematic auscultation, beginning at the aortic area, moving to the pulmonic area, then to the Erb's point, then to the tricuspid area and finally to the mitral area. Use the diaphragm of the stethoscope first to listen high-pitched sounds. Then use the bell to listen to low-pitched **sounds.**

Abnormal findings include extra heart sounds at any of the cardiac landmarks and abnormal rate or rhythm.

Extra heart sounds may be S_3, S_4, murmurs, or bruits. Heart murmurs are caused by some disruption of blood flow through the heart.

In Palpating Peripheral Pulses

The amplitude of the pulses may be documented as 0 (absent), 1+ (weak), 2+ (normal), 3+ (increased), or 4+ (bounding).

Abnormal findings include an absent, weak, thready pulse a forceful or bounding pulse and an asymmetric pulse.

Assessing Peripheral Circulation through Allen's Test, Buerger's Test and Capillary Refill

Physical assessment of the **breasts and axillae** is primarily conducted to identify any lumps in the breasts or enlargement or pain in axillary lymph nodes; the breasts and axillae are assessed in both men and women using inspection and palpation.

Discharge from the breast nipples is an abnormal finding except in pregnancy. Other abnormal findings include dimpling, lesions, and asymmetry. Palpable lymph nodes are an abnormal finding.

The **abdominal cavity** contains the stomach, the small intestine, the large intestine, the liver, the gallbladder, the pancreas, the spleen, the kidneys, and the urinary bladder. The abdominal cavity also contains the female reproductive organs. Equipment needed are stethoscope and proper lighting.

To locate organs more easily the abdomen can be divided into four quadrants: right upper, right lower, left upper and left lower.

The sequence of techniques used to assess the abdomen is inspection, auscultation, percussion and palpation. Percussion and palpation are done after auscultation because they stimulate bowel sounds.

The abdomen should be evenly rounded or symmetric, without visible peristalsis. Abnormal findings include swelling of the abdomen (ascites), abdominal masses or unusual pulsations and hernias.

Place the warm diaphragm of the stethoscope on the right lower quadrant of the abdomen. Listen bowel sounds carefully and note their frequency and character.

Abnormal findings include increased bowel sounds, decreased bowel sounds and absent bowel sounds

Using the bell of the stethoscope, auscultate over the abdominal aorta, femoral arteries, and iliac arteries for bruits.

Percussion is useful in assessing a full bladder or changes in abdominal contents. Percuss the abdomen in all four quadrants in a systematic, clockwise manner to identify fluid, masses, or air.

Abnormal findings include decreased tympany and increased dullness, possibly caused by fluid or a mass.

The entire **liver** is not usually palpable, but the lower edge of the liver may be assessed with light palpation. To palpate bimanually, stand at the patient's right side and place your left hand under the patient's back at the level of 11th to 12th ribs.

Abnormal findings include a hard and firm liver edge nodularity and pain. If the liver border is more than 1–3 cm below the costal margin, it is considered enlarged.

The **external female genitalia** consist of mons pubis, labia majora and minora, clitoris, vestibular glands, vaginal vestibule, vaginal orifice, and urethral opening. During the physical assessment, the external genitalia may be examined and assessed for lesions, discharge, masses, and enlargement of internal organs. The rectum and anus may be assessed during part of this examination if a total health assessment is being performed.

The genitalia are assessed by inspection and palpation. Equipment required include a sterile vaginal speculum, water soluble lubricant and gloves. Inspect the external genitalia for color, size of the labia majora and vaginal opening, lesions, and discharge.

Abnormal findings include redness, swelling of glands, discharge, lesions and pain, which may indicate infection, an abscess, a polyp, or cancer.

The **male genitalia** include the penis, testicles, epididymis, scrotum, prostate gland and seminal vesicles. In addition, the inguinal area may be assessed as part of this assessment.

The external genitalia are inspected for size, placement, contour, appearance of the skin, redness, edema, and discharge. Abnormal findings include lesions, redness, edema, pain, discharge, fluid-filled masses in the scrotum (hydrocele), and displacement of the urinary meatus or difficulties with voiding.

Inspection and palpation are used to assess rectum and anus.

Inspection is used to assess the anal area, which normally has increased pigmentation and some hair growth. Palpation is used to assess the rectum, using a well lubricated, gloved finger. Abnormal findings include relaxed sphincter tone; skin cracks, nodules, or hemorrhoids at the anal sphincter, bleeding and hard or abnormal colored stools.

Physical examination also provides information about posture, gait, bone size and structure, joint, range of motion and muscle strength.

Abnormal findings include deformity, crepitus, and limited ROM (indicating injury, inflammation and arthritis of the affected joints or bones, muscle pain and weakness caused by injury or disease).

Muscle groups are observed for bilateral symmetry and palpated for tenderness.

Abnormal findings include atrophy tremors and flaccidity loss of strength and tone, decreased range of motion, swelling and pain

Neurologic assessment includes cerebral function, cranial nerve function, cerebellar function, motor and sensory function, and reflexes.

Assess the patient's mental status, memory, emotional status, cognitive abilities, and behavior. Evaluate cerebellar function by assisting the motor skills, coordination, and balance.

Equipment for a neurologic assessment includes vials of aromatic substances (for testing smell), a visual acuity chart, a penlight, a sharp object, cotton balls, vials of solution to test taste (sugar, salt), a tuning fork, a tongue depressor, a reflex hammer, and familiar objects, such as coin or key.

Mental status assessment includes level of consciousness, behavior and appearance, memory, abstract reasoning, and language. On initial contact, patient's orientation to person, place, and time, as well as cognitive abilities and affect.

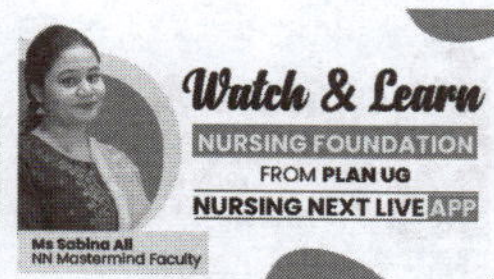

Assess awareness by evaluating orientation to time, place and person using Glasgow Coma Scale (GCS). The Glasgow Coma Scale is a standardized assessment tool that assesses level of consciousness.

Glasgow Coma Scale

Score ranges from 3 (deep coma) to 15 (normal)

Eye opening	Spontaneous	4
	To voice	3
	To pain	2
	No response	1
Best verbal response	Oriented	5
	Confused	4
	Inappropriate words	3
	Incomprehensible sounds	2
	No response	1
Best motor response	Obeys command	6
	Localizes pain	5
	Withdraws	4
	Abnormal flexion (Decorticate posturing)	3
	Abnormal extension (Decerebrate posturing)	2
	No response	1
Total		3 to 15

Interpretation of Glasgow coma scale score

- Best response : 15
- Mild brain injury: 13 or higher
- Moderate brain injury: 9–12
- Severe brain injury: 8 or less

The functions of the **12 cranial nerves** are assessed primarily during the neurological assessment. Each nerve has a specific function and is evaluated individually.

FUNCTIONS OF CRANIAL NERVES

Cranial nerve no.	Cranial nerve name	Procedure	Significant finding
I	Olfactory	With eyes closed, ask the patient to identify the odor (coffee). Test each nostril separately.	Loss of sense of smell (Anosmia)
II	Optic	Check near vision, far vision and peripheral visual field	• Decreased visual acuity • Blindness • Hemianopia: Loss of one half of the visual field.
III	Oculomotor	Inspect ability to move eyelids. Assess pupillary reflex Test for eye movement toward nose. Inspect for conjugate movement and nystagmus	• Inability to open the eyelids • Dilated pupil with or without impaired pupillary reaction to light. • Double vision • Dysconjugate gaze • Gaze weakness or paralysis.

Contd...

Cranial nerve no.	Cranial nerve name	Procedure	Significant finding
IV	Trochlear	Test for upward eye movement. Inspect for conjugate eye movement and nystagmus.	• Double vision • Dysconjugate gaze • Gaze weakness or paralysis.
V	Trigeminal	Ask patient to close eyes. And check for sensation by touching cotton to forehead, cheeks, and jaw. Check corneal reflex. Ask patient to clench and move the jaw from side to side. Palpate the masseter and temporal muscles and note the strength and equity.	• Facial numbness • Impaired or absent corneal reflex • Jaw weakness
VI	Abducens	Test eye for lateral eye movement; inspect for conjugate movement	• Double vision • Dysconjugate gaze • Gaze weakness or paralysis.
VII	Facial	Observe for symmetry while patient smiles, elevates eyebrows, frowns, tightly close eyelids against resistance (examiner attempts to open eyelids). Observe face for flaccid paralysis Ask patient to extend tongue. Test ability to discriminate between sugar and salt.	• Facial weakness • Inability to completely close the eyelid • Impaired taste
VIII	Auditory (Acoustic/ Vestibulocochlear)	Watch tick test Rinne test Weber test Romberg test	• Decreased hearing or deafness • Impaired balance
IX	Glossopharyngeal	Assess patient's ability to swallow Assess patient's ability to discriminate between sugar and salt.	• Difficulty swallowing • Impaired taste
X	Vagus	**Elicit gag reflex:** Depress a tongue blade on posterior tongue, or stimulate posterior pharynx Assess for hoarseness in voice. Check ability to swallow. Have patient say "ah" and observe for symmetric rise of uvula and soft palate.	• Weak or absent gag reflex • Difficulty swallowing • Aspiration • Hoarseness • Slurred speech (Dysarthria)
XI	Accessory	While patient shrugs shoulder against resistance, palpate and note the strength of trapezius muscle. As patient turns head against the opposing pressure of the examiner's hand, palpate and note strength of each sternocleidomastoid muscle.	• Weak or absent shoulder shrug • Inability to turn head to the side
XII	Hypoglossal	Ask patient to protrude the tongue and note any deviation or tremors. Test the strength of tongue by having patient move the protruded tongue from side to side against a tongue depressor.	• Difficulty in swallowing • Slurred speech (Dysarthria)

Evaluate **deep tendon reflexes** to determine the functional ability of specific spinal segment levels. Use the reflex hammer to elicit muscle contraction and reflexes. Reflex responses are usually graded on a scale of 0 to 5. A grade of 2 is considered normal or active response.

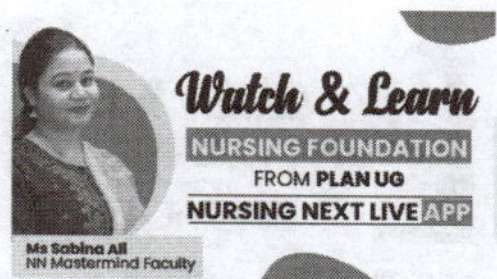

DEEP TENDON REFLEXES

Reflex	Procedure	Normal finding
Biceps	Support forearm with one arm while placing the thumb against the tendon and strike the thumb with reflex hammer.	Contraction of the biceps and flexion at the elbow
Triceps	Flex patient's forearm at the elbow and position in front of the chest. Palpate the triceps tendon by palpating 2.5 to 5 cm above the elbow and strike the tendon with the reflex hammer.	Contraction of the triceps muscle and extension of the elbow
Patellar	Place patient in a sitting position and strike the patellar tendon just below the patella.	Contraction of the quadriceps and extension of the knee
Achilles	Dorsiflex the foot at the ankle, strike the stretched Achilles ankle.	Plantar flexion of foot

Biceps Tendon

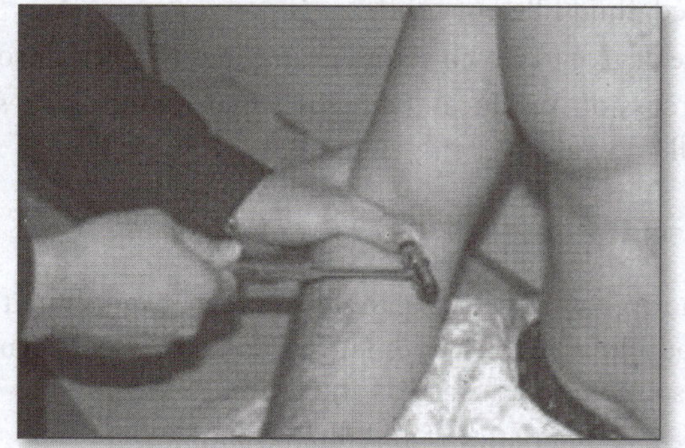

Achilles Tendon

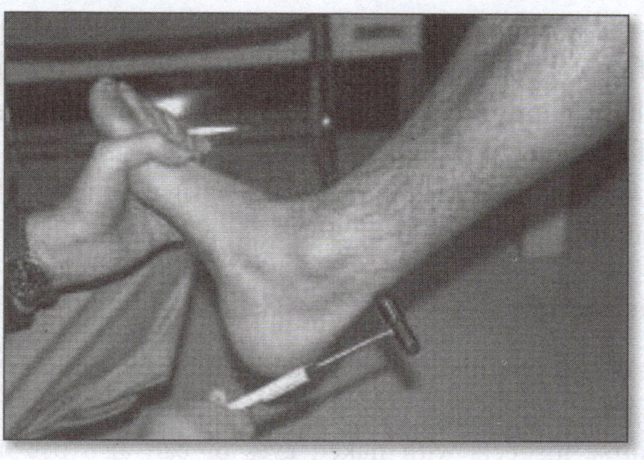

Triceps Tendon

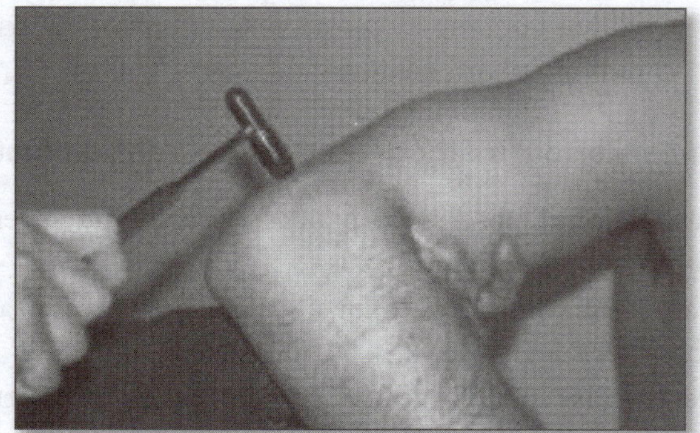

Plantar Reflex

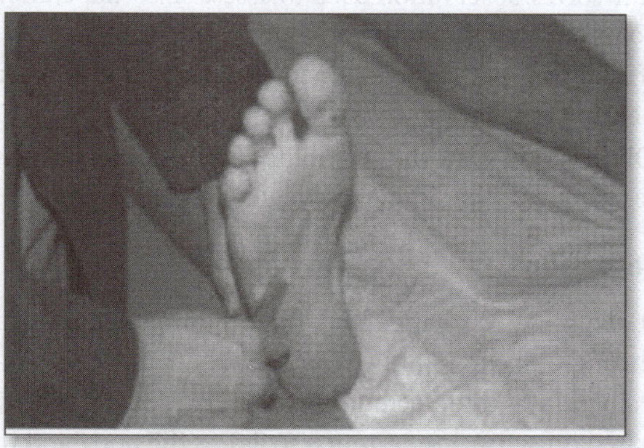

Patellar Reflex

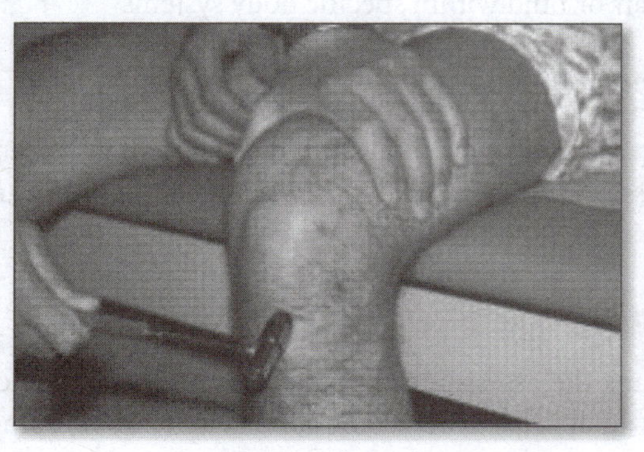

Grading of Deep Tendon Reflexes

0—No response
1+—Diminished (hypoactive)
2+—Normal
3+—Increased
4+—Hyperactive (Hyperreflexia/clonus)

After completing the nursing history and assessment, organize all assessment data to make nursing diagnosis, plan appropriate care, and evaluate the patient's responses to treatment.

CONCEPTUAL EXERCISES

LONG ANSWER QUESTIONS

1. Define physical examination. Explain the methods of physical examination. Describe the nurse's role in physical examination. (DU)

Answer

Physical Examination

- It is the systematic collection of objective information that is directly observed or is elicited through examination techniques.
- It is a systematic data collection method that uses the senses of sight, hearing, smell and touch to detect health problems.
- Physical examination is defined as a complete assessment of a patient's physical and mental status.

The four methods used in physical examination are explained as follows.

1. Inspection

- It is the systematic visual examination by using sense of sight.
- Nurse inspects with naked eyes or can also use lighted instrument such as ophthalmoscope.
- It involves observation used to assess size, shape, moisture, color and symmetry of body.
- It also uses the sense of smell to detect odor and sense of hearing to detect sounds.
- Observation can be combined with other assessment techniques.

2. Palpation

- It is use of the hands and fingers to gather information through touch.
- Palpation is the technique of using your hands/fingers based on **sensation of touch** to assess the body and further examine cues that were identified during inspection.
- It is feeling the body or a part with hands to note the size and position of the organs.
- The hands and fingers are sensitive tools and can assess temperature, turgor, texture, moisture, vibrations, size, position, masses and fluid.
- The dorsum (back) surfaces of the hand and fingers are used to measure temperature.
- The palmar (front) surfaces of the fingers and finger pads are used to assess texture, shape, fluid, size, consistency and pulsation.
- Vibration is palpated best with the palm of the hand.

3. Percussion

- Percussion is the act of striking one object against another to produce sound.
- Percussion is a method of tapping body parts with fingers, hands, or small instruments as part of a physical examination. It is done to determine: the size, consistency, and borders of body organs. The presence or absence of fluid in body areas.
- The sound waves produced by the striking action are known as percussion tones or percussion notes.
- Percussion is also used to determine if a structure is air filled, fluid filled or solid.
- The degree to which sound propagates is called Resonance.
- Percussion produces tympanic, hyperresonant, resonant, dull and flat.

4. Auscultation

It is the process of listening to sounds that are generated within the body by a Stethoscope. The auscultation is performed for heart sounds, breath sounds and bowel sounds.

- The characteristics of auscultated sound are:
  - Pitch—ranging from high to low
  - Loudness—ranging from soft to loud
  - Quality—gurgling
  - Duration—short, medium and long

Summary of four methods used in Physical Examination:

- **Inspection:** Observing patient visually for general appearance or specific details
- **Palpation:** Clinical touching of specific body areas to assess characteristics
- **Percussion:** Tapping technique with hands to determine condition of solid or air-filled body areas
- **Auscultation:** Using a stethoscope to assessment movement of air or fluid within specific body systems

Testing of Reflexes

The response to external stimuli is tested by means of a percussion hammer, safety pin, wisp of cotton or hot and cold water.

Olfaction

It means the assessment of patients with the source of body odor which helps to detect the abnormalities. For example, the presence of fruity smell from buccal cavity in case of diabetic ketoacidosis.

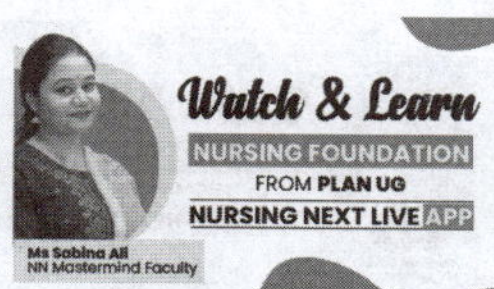

Nurse's Role in Physical Examination

- Nurses play an important role in physical examination procedure. They not also prepare the equipment required for the procedure but also assist the doctors in the physical examination.
- As per the instructions and the need of the procedure, they are also responsible for the recording and reporting of all the findings of the patients.

Preparation of Environment

Maintenance of Privacy

A separate examination room is needed, Keep the door closed. The relatives are not allowed.

Lighting

There should be Adequate Lighting (Natural Lighting)

Comfortable Bed or Examination Table

- The client should be placed comfortably throughout the examination.
  - It is necessary to prepare the environment before starting the assessment.
  - The time for the physical assessment should be convenient to both the client and the nurse.
  - The environment needs to be well lit and the equipment should be organized for timely use.
  - The room should be warm enough to be comfortable for the client. Providing privacy is important.

Preparation of the Equipment

- All equipment required for the health assessment should be clean, in good working order, and should be readily accessible.
- **Articles required:**
  - **Sphygmomanometer:** To measure BP.
  - **Stethoscope:** To listen the body sound
  - **Fetoscope:** To listen the FHR
  - **TPR tray:** To monitor the vital signs
  - **Tongue depressor:** To examine the mouth and throat
  - **Laryngoscope:** To examine the larynx
  - **Measuring tape:** To measure height, weight and abdomen circumference
  - **Flashlight:** To visualize body parts that need to be inspected
  - **Weighing machine:** To monitor the weight
  - **Ophthalmoscope:** To examine the inner parts of eyeball
  - **Otoscope:** To examine the ear
  - **Turning fork:** To test the hearing
  - **Nasal speculum:** To examine the nostrils
  - **Percussion hammer:** To test reflexes
  - **Vaginal speculum:** To examine the genitals in women
  - **Proctoscope:** To examine the rectum
  - **Surgical and clean gloves:** To examine
- Nurses are also responsible for cleaning, disinfection and sterilization of used equipment.
- Nurses for responsible for the maintenance of inventory of all the equipment used in the procedure of physical examination.

Preparation of the Client

- Preparation of client involves two processes:
  1. Physical preparation
  2. Mental preparation
     - Explain the procedure of physical examination to the client and its importance.
     - Instruct the client that all information gathered and documented is kept confidential and only accessible to health care professionals.
     - The nurse assists the client as needed to undress and put on a gown.
     - Clients should empty their bladder before examination.

Positioning

- Several positions are frequently required during the physical assessment.
- It is important to consider the client's ability to assume a position.
- Some positions are embarrassing and uncomfortable and therefore, should not be maintained for long.
- The assessment is organized so that several body areas can be assessed in one position, thus minimizing the number of position changes needed.

Draping

- Drapes should be arranged so that only the area to be assessed is exposed and other body areas are covered.
- Drapes provide not only privacy but also warmth. Drapes are made of cloth or bed linen, paper, etc.

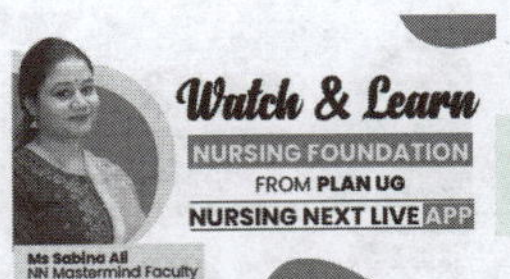

2. Geeta, 35-years, is admitted in surgical ward with c/o vomiting and pain abdomen since 2 days. Answer the following questions: (KUHS)

a. **Discuss assessment of gastrointestinal system.**

b. **Discuss recording of health assessment.**

Answer

Assessment of Gastrointestinal System

Gastrointestinal (GI) system performs the functions of ingestion, digestion, and elimination. Interruptions in any of these systems' functions can quickly affect the patient nutritionally and cause acid-base imbalances and later on whole body suffer.

Subjective Assessment

A focused gastrointestinal subjective assessment collects data about the signs and symptoms of GI diseases, including any digestive or nutritional issues, relevant medical or family history of GI health problems.

Objective Assessment

Physical examination of the abdomen includes inspection, auscultation, palpation, and percussion (Sequence differs for GI system than other systems) so that the accurate bowel sounds can be assessed.

- **Inspection**
  - The abdomen is inspected by providing supine position to the patient.
  - The head and knees should be supported with small pillows, arms should be at their side and not folded behind the head.
  - Ensure the patient is covered adequately to maintain privacy, while still exposing the abdomen as needed for a thorough assessment.
  - Visually examine the abdomen for overall shape, masses, skin abnormalities, and any abnormal movements.
  - Observe the general contour and symmetry of the entire abdominal wall. The contour of the abdomen is often described as flat, rounded, scaphoid (sunken), or protuberant (convex or bulging).
  - Assess for distention. Generalized distention of the abdomen can be caused by obesity, bowel distention from gas or liquid, or fluid buildup.
  - Assess for masses or bulges, which may indicate structural deformities like hernias or related to disorders in abdominal organs.
  - Assess the patient's skin for uniformity of color, integrity, scarring, or striae. Striae are white or silvery elongated marks that occur when the skin stretches, especially during pregnancy or excessive weight gain.
  - Note the shape of the umbilicus; it should be inverted and midline.
  - Carefully note any scars, and correlate these scars with the patient's recollection of previous surgeries or injury.
  - Document any abnormal movement or pulsations. Visible intestinal peristalsis can be caused by intestinal obstruction.
  - Pulsations may be seen in the epigastric area in patients who are especially thin, but otherwise should not be observed.
- **Auscultation**
  - Auscultation follows inspection for more accurate assessment of bowel sounds. Use a warmed stethoscope to assess the frequency and characteristics of the patient's bowel sounds.
  - Place the diaphragm of stethoscope in the right lower quadrant (RLQ). Move the stethoscope to the next quadrant in a clockwise motion around the abdominal wall.
  - Hyperactive bowel sounds may indicate bowel obstruction or gastroenteritis. Patient's bowel sounds without a stethoscope, often described as "stomach growling" or borborygmus. This is a common example of hyperactive sounds.
  - Hypoactive bowel sounds may be present with constipation, after abdominal surgery, peritonitis, or paralytic ileus. If heard, this finding should be reported.
- **Palpation**
  - Using the flat of the hand and fingers (not the fingertips) to detect palpable organs, abnormal masses, or tenderness.
  - Light palpation is to assess for musculature, abnormal masses, and tenderness.
  - Deep palpation is to assess for enlarged organs.
  - Lightly palpate the abdomen by pressing into the skin about 1 cm beginning in the RLQ. Continue to move around the abdomen in a clockwise manner.
  - Palpate the bladder for distention.
- **Percussion**
  - Percussion is to assess the liver and spleen or to determine if costovertebral angle (CVA) tenderness is present, which is related to inflammation of the kidney.

b. **Discuss recording of health assessment.**

Answer

Recording of Health Assessment

- Accurate recording is essential procedure and should include all relevant information collected related to the client health status.

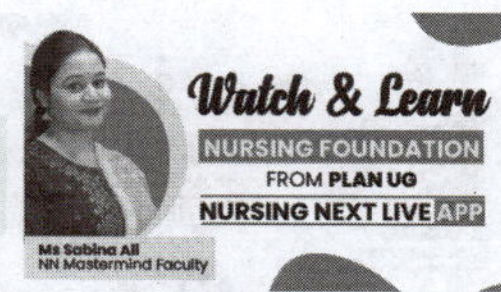

- The assessment is documented in the medical or nursing records of the patients.
- The documentation can be done on paper or as a part of the electronic medical record (HIS—Health Information System) which can be accessed by all members of the health care team or personel.

Purpose of Health Assessment Recording

- The main purpose of health assessment record is to provide a means of communication to facilitate the safe care and treatment of the clients.
- The health assessment record may also be used for communication with other health care personel.
- Establish a basis for screening or validation proposed diagnosis.
- Acts as a source of information to help diagnosis new problems
- Constitutes a permanent legal record
- Helpful in the medical or nursing research for educational purposes.

Guidelines for Recording Health Assessment

- Record patients own words
- Avoid generalizations – be specific
- Privacy and confidentiality
- Use correct grammar and spelling
- Record complete information and details for all client symptoms or experience
- Mention date and time of the procedure

SHORT NOTES

1. Write any four positions used in physical assessment.

Answer

Several positions are used during the physical examination of the patients. It depends upon the patient's ability to assume a position.

The five positions that can be used during physical examination are:

1. Dorsal Position/Supine Position

- The patients lie on their back with head and shoulders slightly elevated.

Uses

- Comfortable position
- Examination of head, neck, chest, abdomen and extremities
- Surgery of anterior part of the body

2. Prone Position

A patient lies flat on abdomen and head turned to one side. Both the hands held in a comfortable position.

Uses

- Examination of posterior trunk, spines and rectum
- Surgeries of back
- To relieve pressure on areas such as sacrum, scapula and heel
- After anesthesia to prevent aspiration

3. Sims' Position

- Differs from side lying position in which weight is placed in the anterior ilium, humerus and clavicle.
- Patients lies on his left with left arm drawn behind the back.
- Right arm may be in any position.
- The right thigh is flexed against the abdomen.

Uses

- Vaginal and rectal examination.
- To relive pressure in the buttocks, scapula and heels.

4. Lithotomy Position

- The patient lies on her back the legs are separated and thighs are flexed on the abdomen.
- The buttocks are kept in the edge of the table and legs are supported by stirrups.
- Provides maximal exposure of genitalia.

Uses

- Vaginal examination
- Pap smear
- Position during delivery for many women
- Surgical procedures of genitourinary system

5. Knee-Chest Position

- Patient lies on the bed in such a way that the knees and the chest rests on the bed.
- The head is turned to one side.
- A small pillow can be placed under the chest.
- The weight of patient rests on chest and knees only.
- The knees are flexed and thighs are at right angle to legs.

Uses

- Examination of rectum and vagina
- Postpartum exercise

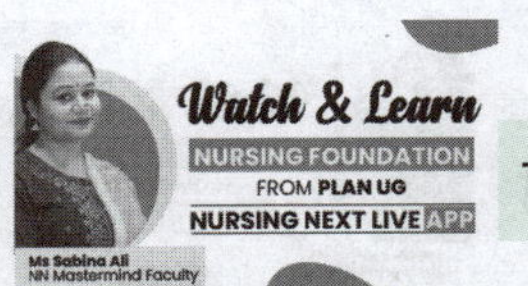

2. What are the techniques used for physical examination?

Answer

The basic techniques used in physical examination are explained in sequence as follows:

- Inspection
- Percussion
- Palpation
- Auscultation

Inspection

- It is the systematic visual examination by using sense of sight.
- Nurse inspects with naked eyes or with lighted instrument also such as ophthalmoscope.
- It is the process of performing deliberate purposeful observations in a systematic manner.
- It involves observation used to assess size, shape, moisture, color and symmetry of body.
- It also uses the sense of smell to detect odor and sense of hearing to detect sounds.
- Lighting should be adequate while performing inspection.
- Both artificial as well as natural lighting may be used during the process of inspection.
- Observation can be combined with other assessment techniques.

General Inspection

- Overall appearance of health or illness
- Signs of distress
- Facial expression and mood
- Body size
- Grooming and personal hygiene

Palpation

- It is use of the hands and fingers to gather information through touch.
- It is the assessment technique which uses sense of touch.
- It is feeling the body or a part with hands to note the size and position of the organs.
- The hands and fingers are sensitive tools and can assess temperature, turgor, texture, moisture, vibrations, size, position, masses and fluid.
- The dorsum (back) surfaces of the hand and fingers are used to measure temperature.
- The palmar (front) surfaces of the fingers and finger pads are used to assess texture, shape, fluid, size, consistency and pulsation.
- Vibration is palpated best with the palm of the hand.

Percussion

- It is the examination by tapping the fingers on the body to determine the condition of the internal organs by the sounds that are produced.
- Percussion is the act of striking one object against another to produce sound.
- The sound waves produced by the striking action are known as percussion tones or percussion notes.
- Percussion is also used to determine if a structure is air filled, fluid filled or solid.
- The degree to which sound propagates is called Resonance.
- Percussion produces tympanic, hyperresonant, resonant, dull and flat.

Auscultation

It is the process of listening to sounds that are generated within the body by a Stethoscope. The auscultation is performed for heart sounds, breath sounds and bowel sounds.

The characteristics of auscultated sound are:

- **Pitch:** Ranging from high to low
- **Loudness:** Ranging from soft to loud
- **Quality:** Gurgling
- **Duration:** Short, medium and long

Manipulation

It is the moving of a part of the body to note its flexibility.

Testing of Reflexes

The response to external stimuli is tested by means of a percussion hammer, safety pin, wisp of cotton or hot and cold water.

3. What are the types of health assessment?

Answer

The types of health assessment depend on several factors like context of care, the patient's needs and the nurse's experience.

- **Comprehensive assessment:** This involves a detailed history or physical examination performed at the onset of care in a primary care setting or an admission to a hospital or long-term care facility.
- **Problem-based/focused assessment:** It involves a history and examination that are limited to a specific problem or complaint. This type of assessment is most commonly used in a walk in clinic or emergency department and outpatient departments.

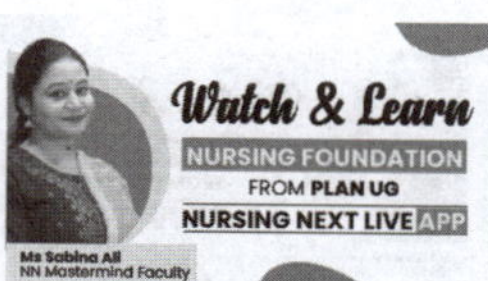

- **Episodic/follow-up assessment:** This type of assessment is usually done when a patient is following up with a health care provider for previously identified problem.
- **Shift assessment:** When individuals are hospitalized, nurses conduct assessment each shift. The purpose is to identify changes in a patient's condition from baseline.
- **Screening assessment:** It is a short examination focused on disease detection. It may be performed in a health care provider's office or at a health fair.
- **Emergency assessment:** This assessment is performed during emergency procedures, when it is crucial to evaluate the patient's airway, breathing and circulation, as well as the exact cause of the problem.

4. Write about adventitious breath sounds.

Answer

Adventitious lung sound	Explanation	Disorder
Crackles	**Crackles:** High-pitched, popping sound. Caused by air being forced through an airway. Heard during inspiration. • **Fine crackles:** Sound like hair rubbing together • **Course crackles:** Low gurgling sound	• Pneumonia • Pulmonary Edema • Acute respiratory distress syndrome (ARDS) • Heart failure
Wheeze	• **Wheezing:** High-pitched continuous musical sound • May occur during inspiration and/or expiration • Airway obstruction/narrowing/ constriction	Asthma
Rhonchi	• **Rhonchi:** Deep, low-pitched rumbling sound (sounds like a snore) • Caused by respiratory secretions. • Clears with cough	Chronic obstructive pulmonary disease (COPD)—bronchitis
Pleural friction rub	• **Pleural friction rub:** Low, deep, harsh grating sound • Caused by friction of inflamed and roughened pleural surfaces against one another during movement of the chest wall	Pleuritis

Contd...

Adventitious lung sound	Explanation	Disorder
Stridor Stridor	• **Stridor:** High-pitched, inspiratory wheezing. • Obstruction of upper airway	• Croup, epiglottitis • Foreign body aspiration

5. Discuss the methods of assessment of respiratory system.

Answer

Health History

- Identify risk factors for altered health during the health history by asking
- History of trauma to ribs or lung surgery
- Number of pillows used when sleeping
- History of chest pain with deep breathing
- History of persistent cough with or without sputum
- History of allergies, environmental exposure to chemicals, asbestos or smoke
- History of smoking (since how long and how many packs/day)
- History of lung disease in family members or self
- History of frequent or chronic respiratory infections

Physical Assessment

Equipment Needed

- Stethoscope
- Tape measure
- The environment should be warm and adequately lit.
- The techniques for assessment include: inspection, palpation. percussion and auscultation.

Inspecting the Thorax

- Inspect the patient's chest for color, shape or contour, breathing patterns and muscle development.
- The color should be even and consistent with the color of patient's face.
- The shape or contour should have a downward equal slope at the rib cage.
- The chest should be symmetric, with the transverse diameter greater than the anteroposterior diameter.

Palpation

- Palpation is used to detect areas of sensitivity, chest expansion during respirations, and vibrations (fremitus).
- Use the palmar surface of the hands to palpate the anterior and posterior thoracic landmarks in a sequential pattern for temperature moisture, muscular development and any tenderness, or masses. The skin should be warm and dry, with symmetric muscular development and no tenderness, masses or vibrations.

Chest expansion is determined by placing the hands over the posterior chest wall, with the fingers at the level of T9 or T10.

Ask the patient to take a deep breath, and observe the movement of your thumbs. The thorax should expand symmetrically.

Auscultation

- Ask the patient to breathe slowly and deeply through the mouth.
- Place the diaphragm of the stethoscope over the thoracic landmarks and auscultate breath sounds in the same sequential pattern as used for palpation.
- Normally, breath sounds result from the free movement of air into and out of all parts of the bronchial tree. Listen for the pitch, duration, and intensity of the sounds.
- Breath sounds vary over different parts of the lungs. Bronchial sounds heard over the trachea are harsh sounds, high-pitched, with expiration being longer than inspiration.
- Bronchovesicular sounds are heard over the main stem bronchus and are moderate "blowing" sounds, with inspiration equal to expiration.
- Vesicular breath sounds are soft, low-pitched sounds heard best over the base of the lungs and lung periphery during inspiration, which is longer than expiration.
- Adventitious breath sounds are not normally heard in lungs but, if present, they may be auscultated. Stertorous breathing is a general term used to refer to noisy, strenuous respiration.

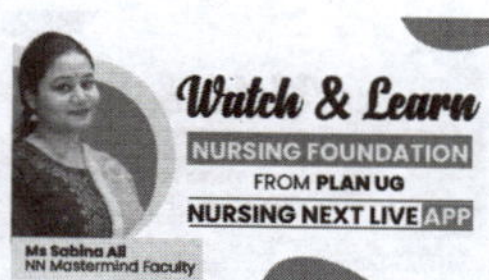

- Stridor is harsh, high-pitched sound heard on inspiration, when there is narrowing of the upper airway larynx or trachea.
- Crackles are fine to coarse crackling sounds made as air moves through wet secretion: they are most often heard on inspiration. Crackles are described as "fine" when they are made by air passing through moisture in small air passages and alveoli and as "coarse" when they are made by air passing through moisture in the bronchioles, bronchi and trachea.
- Coarse crackles can also be documented as rhonchi.
- Wheezes are continuous sounds that originate in small air passages that are narrowed by secretions, swelling, or tumors.
- A pleural friction rub is a grating sound caused by an inflamed pleura rubbing against the chest wall.

6. Write a short note on mention the neurological assessment.

Answer

Neurological assessment is the evaluation of the nervous system, which includes the brain, spinal cord, and peripheral nerves. It includes the following components:

- Mental status examination
- Level of consciousness
- Reflex examination
- Motor function examination
- Sensory function examination
- Cranial nerve examination

Mental Status

Orientation: Oriented to Time, Place, Person/ Disoriented
Behavior, mood, affect: Appropriate/Not
Level of consciousness: Unconscious/Conscious/Stupor/ Coma

Glasgow Coma Scale

Score ranges from 3 (deep coma) to 15 (normal)

Eye opening	Spontaneous	4
	To voice	3
	To pain	2
	No response	1
Best verbal response	Oriented	5
	Confused	4
	Inappropriate words	3
	Incomprehensible sounds	2
	No response	1
Best motor response	Obeys command	6
	Localizes pain	5
	Withdraws	4
	Abnormal flexion (Decorticate posturing)	3
	Abnormal extension (Decerebrate posturing)	2
	No response	1
Total		3 to 15

Contd...

Interpretation of glasgow coma scale score

- Best response : 15
- Mild brain injury: 13 or higher
- Moderate brain injury: 9–12
- Severe brain injury: 8 or less

Note:

- If patient is intubated and unable to speak they are evaluated only on the eye opening response and motor response and suffix "T" is added to their verbal response.
- If patient is hemiplegic, assess patient on the nonparalyzed side.

Deep Tendon Reflexes

Reflex	Procedure	Normal finding
Biceps	Support forearm with one arm while placing the thumb against the tendon and strike the thumb with reflex hammer.	Contraction of the biceps and flexion at the elbow
Triceps	Flex patient's forearm at the elbow and position in front of the chest. Palpate the triceps tendon by palpating 2.5 to 5 cm above the elbow and strike the tendon with the reflex hammer.	Contraction of the triceps muscle and extension of the elbow
Brachioradialis		
Patellar	Place patient in a sitting position and strike the patellar tendon just below the patella.	Contraction of the quadriceps and extension of the knee.
Achilles	Dorsiflex the foot at the ankle, strike the stretched Achilles ankle.	Plantar flexion of foot

Grading of Deep Tendon Reflexes

0—No response
1+—Diminished (hypoactive)
2+—Normal
3+—Increased
4+—Hyperactive (Hyperreflexia/clonus)

Motor Functions (Gross Motor and Fine Motor)

Gait: Normal/not
Standing on one foot: Able/not
Heel to toe walking: Able to walk in straight line/not
Finger to nose test: Normal/not
Supination of hands: Possible/not
Supination of hands—rotation of radius in-lateral direction, leaving thumbs moves and palms up or forward
Pronation of hands: Possible/not
Pronation of hands—rotation of radius in a medial direction, leaving thumbs moving medially and palms downward
Finger to nose and to the Nurse's finger: Normal/not
Fingers to thumb: Normal/not
Romberg test:

Sensory Function Test

Light touch sensation: Symmetrical/not
Pain, temperature, kinesthetic: Normal/not
Tactile—one-and two-point: Present/not
Stereognosis and extinction: Present/not

- **Kinesthetic:** A person's awareness of the position and movement of the parts of the body by means of sensory organs (proprioceptors) in the muscles and joints.
- **Stereognosis:** Ability to identify the shape and form of an object, and therefore its identity, with tactile manipulation of that object in the absence of visual and auditory stimuli.
- **Extinction:** Ability to perceive multiple stimuli of the same type simultaneously.

Functions of Cranial Nerves

Cranial nerve no.	Cranial nerve name	Procedure	Significant finding
I	Olfactory	With eyes closed, ask the patient to identify the odor (coffee). Test each nostril separately.	Loss of sense of smell (Anosmia)
II	Optic	Check near vision, far vision and peripheral visual field	• Decreased visual acuity • Blindness • Hemianopia: Loss of one half of the visual field.
III	Oculomotor	Inspect ability to move eyelids. Assess pupillary reflex Test for eye movement toward nose. Inspect for conjugate movement and nystagmus	• Inability to open the eyelids • Dilated pupil with or without impaired pupillary reaction to light. • Double vision • Dysconjugate gaze • Gaze weakness or paralysis.
IV	Trochlear	Test for upward eye movement. Inspect for conjugate eye movement and nystagmus.	• Double vision • Dysconjugate gaze • Gaze weakness or paralysis.
V	Trigeminal	Ask patient to close eyes. And check for sensation by touching cotton to forehead, cheeks, and jaw. Check corneal reflex. Ask patient to clench and move the jaw from side to side. Palpate the masseter and temporal muscles and note the strength and equity.	• Facial numbness • Impaired or absent corneal reflex • Jaw weakness
VI	Abducens	Test eye for lateral eye movement; inspect for conjugate movement	• Double vision • Dysconjugate gaze • Gaze weakness or paralysis.

Contd...

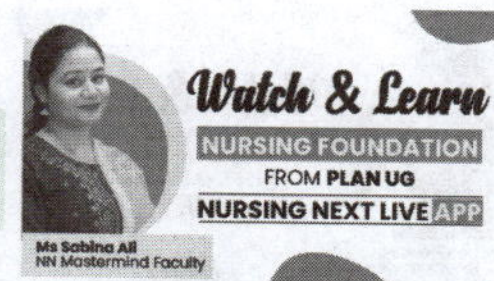

Cranial nerve no.	Cranial nerve name	Procedure	Significant finding
VII	Facial	Observe for symmetry while patient smiles, elevates eyebrows, frowns, tightly close eyelids against resistance (examiner attempts to open eyelids). Observe face for flaccid paralysis Ask patient to extend tongue. Test ability to discriminate between sugar and salt.	• Facial weakness • Inability to completely close the eyelid • Impaired taste
VIII	Auditory (Acoustic/ Vestibulocochlear)	Watch tick test Rinne test Weber test Romberg test	• Decreased hearing or deafness • Impaired balance
IX	Glossopharyngeal	Assess patient's ability to swallow Assess patient's ability to discriminate between sugar and salt.	• Difficulty swallowing • Impaired taste
X	Vagus	**Elicit gag reflex:** Depress a tongue blade on posterior tongue, or stimulate posterior pharynx Assess for hoarseness in voice. Check ability to swallow. Have patient say "ah" and observe for symmetric rise of uvula and soft palate.	• Weak or absent gag reflex • Difficulty swallowing • Aspiration • Hoarseness • Slurred speech (Dysarthria)
XI	Accessory	While patient shrugs shoulder against resistance, palpate and note the strength of trapezius muscle. As patient turns head against the opposing pressure of the examiner's hand, palpate and note strength of each sternocleidomastoid muscle.	• Weak or absent shoulder shrug • Inability to turn head to the side
XII	Hypoglossal	Ask patient to protrude the tongue and note any deviation or tremors. Test the strength of tongue by having patient move the protruded tongue from side to side against a tongue depressor.	• Difficulty in swallowing • Slurred speech (Dysarthria)

7. Describe the process of health assessment.

Answer

Process of health assessment includes:

- Health history
- Physical examination: inspection, auscultation, percussion and palpation
- General assessment
- System wise assessment
- Recording of health assessment
  - General examination: The examination is carried out in an orderly manner focusing upon one area of the body at a time.
    - Collecting subjective data: Subjective data are data that are elicited and verified only by the client obtained through complete health history which includes biographical data, family health history, reasons for seeking, previous hospitalizations and consultations, etc. and data directly observed or detectable by the examiner or can be tested by using an accepted standard.
    - The collection of data through physical examination involves inspection, percussion, palpation and auscultation.
- Head to toe examination
- Focused examination (system wise)
  - Documentation of data is an important step of assessment because it forms the database for the entire nursing process and provides data for all other members of the health care team.

- Nurse records all data collected about the client's health status.
- Data are recorded in a factual manner not as interpreted by the nurse.
- Record subjective data in client's word; restating in other words what client says might change its original meaning.

SHORT ANSWER QUESTIONS

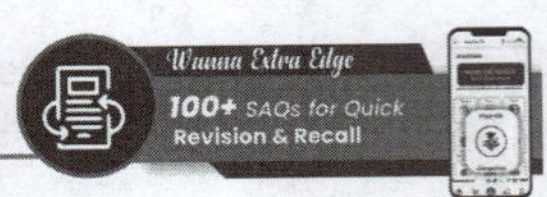

1. Define physical examination.

Answer

It is the systematic collection of objective information that is directly observed or is elicited through examination techniques.

- It is a systematic data collection method that uses the senses of sight, hearing, smell and touch to detect health problems.
- Physical examination is defined as a complete assessment of a patient's physical and mental status.

2. Define health assessment. (MGR)

Answer

Health assessment is an organized systematic assessment of human body which involves the use of one's senses to determine the general physical and mental conditions of the body by collecting both subjective and objective data.

3. Write the purpose of health assessment. (MGR)

Answer

- To establish a data base of client's normal abilities, risk factors that can contribute to dysfunction and any current alteration in function.
- To get a clear picture of a client's health status and health-related problems.
- To identify cause and extent of disease.
- To identify the problems at early stage.
- To determine the nature of treatment required for the client.
- To get a holistic view of the client.
- To contribute in medical research.
- To identify client's strength, weakness, knowledge, attitude, motivation, support systems and coping skills.
- To compare client's health status with an ideal status.

4. What are the techniques used for physical examination?

Answer

The basic techniques used in physical examination are explained as follows:

- **Inspection:** It is the systematic visual examination by using sense of sight.
- **Palpation:** Palpation is the technique of using your hands/ fingers based on sensation of touch to assess the body and further examine cues that were identified during inspection.
- **Percussion:** Percussion is a method of tapping body parts with fingers, hands, or small instruments as part of a physical examination. It is done to determine: the size, consistency, and borders of body organs. The presence or absence of fluid in body areas.
- **Auscultation:** It is the process of listening to sounds that are generated within the body by a Stethoscope. The auscultation is performed for heart sounds, breath sounds and bowel sounds.

5. What are the types of health assessment?

Answer

The types of health assessment depend on several factors like context of care, the patient's needs and the nurse's experience.

Types

- Comprehensive assessment
- Problem-based/focused assessment
- Episodic/follow-up assessment
- Shift assessment
- Screening assessment

CONCEPTUAL REVISION

MULTIPLE CHOICE QUESTIONS

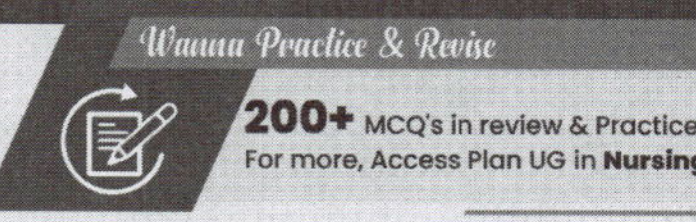

1. **The most important nursing intervention to correct skin dryness is:**
   a. Consult the dietitian about increasing the patient's fat intake, and take necessary measures to prevent infection.
   b. Ask the physician to refer the patient to a dermatologist, and suggest that the patient wear home-laundered sleepwear.
   c. Encourage the patient to increase his fluid intake, use nonirritating soap when bathing the patient, and apply lotion to the involved areas
   d. Avoid bathing the patient until the condition is remedied, and notify the physician.

Ans. c. Encourage the patient to increase his fluid intake, use nonirritating soap when bathing the patient, and apply lotion to the involved areas

2. **When bathing a patient's extremities, the nurse should use long, firm strokes from the distal to the proximal areas. This technique:**
   a. Provides an opportunity for skin assessment.
   b. Avoids undue strain on the nurse.
   c. Increases venous blood return.
   d. Causes vasoconstriction and increases circulation.

Ans. c. Increases venous blood return.

3. **A patient has just received 30 mg of codeine by mouth for pain. Five minutes later he vomits. What should the nurse do first?**
   a. Call the physician
   b. Remedicate the patient
   c. Observe the emesis
   d. Explain to the patient that she can do nothing to help him.

Ans. c. Observe the emesis

4. **The nurse is assessing a postoperative adult patient. Which of the following should the nurse document as subjective data?**
   a. Vital signs
   b. Laboratory test result
   c. Patient's description of pain
   d. Electrocardiographic (ECG) waveforms

Ans. c. Patient's description of pain

5. **A male patient has a soft wrist-safety device. Which assessment finding should the nurse consider abnormal?**
   a. A palpable radial pulse
   b. A palpable ulnar pulse
   c. Cool, pale fingers
   d. Pink nail beds

Ans. c. Cool, pale fingers

6. **Which of the following planes divides the body longitudinally into anterior and posterior regions?**
   a. Frontal plane
   b. Sagittal plane
   c. Midsagittal plane
   d. Transverse plane

Ans. a. Frontal plane

7. **A nurse has to perform an abdominal assessment on a patient who is complaining of having abdominal pain. What should be the order of the following techniques?**
   a. Percussion
   b. Palpation
   c. Inspection
   d. Auscultation
   1. a, c, d, b
   2. b, d, c, a
   3. c, d, b, a
   4. a, d, b, c

Ans. 3. c, d, b, a

8. **What should be the right position for breast examination to palpate for lumps or tumors?**
   a. Supine with both arms overhead with palm upward
   b. Sitting with hands clasped just above the umbilicus
   c. Supine with the right arm abducted and hand under the head and neck
   d. Lying on the right side, adducting the right arm on the side of the body

Ans. c. Supine with the right arm abducted and hand under the head and neck

9. **A nurse is going to assess level of consciousness in a neurological patient. Which is the best tool to measure the LOC?**
   a. Glasgow Coma Scale
   b. Neurological examination
   c. Checking motor response
   d. EEG

Ans. a. Glasgow Coma Scale

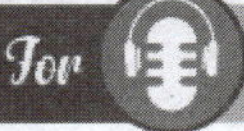
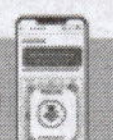

CHAPTER

16

Nursing Process

CONCEPTUAL THEORY

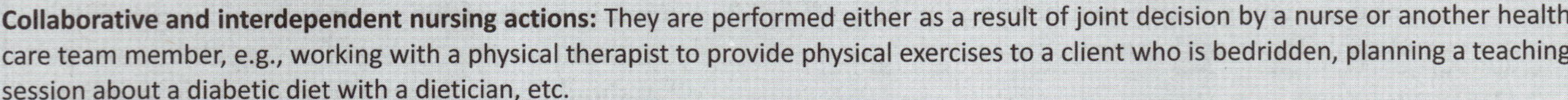

Terminology

Assessment: It is systematic and continuous collection, organization, validation, and documentation of data (information).

Collaborative and interdependent nursing actions: They are performed either as a result of joint decision by a nurse or another health care team member, e.g., working with a physical therapist to provide physical exercises to a client who is bedridden, planning a teaching session about a diabetic diet with a dietician, etc.

Dependent nursing actions: They are carried out according to specific routines, under the supervision of a physician, or as a result of an order by a physician, e.g., medication, injection or any other treatment modalities.

Emergency assessment: During emergency situation to identify any life-threatening situation.

Evaluation: It is an ongoing process which begins when the individual/family/community enters the health care system, until his/her exit from the system. To determine the client's progress toward meeting specified outcomes, the outcome statements present standards and criteria that are observable and measurable.

Health promotion diagnosis (also known as wellness diagnosis): It is a clinical judgment about motivation and desire to increase well-being. Health promotion diagnosis is concerned in the individual, family, or community transition from a specific level of wellness to a higher level of wellness.

Implementation: It consists of doing and documenting the activities. The process of implementation includes; implementing the nursing interventions and documenting nursing activities.

Independent nursing actions: They are initiated by the nurse based on nursing knowledge and skills.

Initial nursing assessment: Performed within specified time after admission to establish a complete database for problem identification.

Nursing diagnosis: It is a statement of client's health status or problem which can be solved by nursing actions. The process of arriving at a nursing diagnosis involves decision-making based on intuitive reasoning, experience and sound theoretical foundation in biological and social sciences.

Objective data: Refers to information based on observation of the nurse and examination of the patient.

Planning: It is basically a decision-making process mainly to decide appropriate nursing care for the problems of patients and prescribe nursing care in the form of written nursing instructions.

Problem-focused assessment: To determine the status of a specific problem identified in an earlier assessment.

Problem-focused diagnosis (also known as actual diagnosis): It is a client problem that is present at the time of the nursing assessment. These diagnoses are based on the presence of associated signs and symptoms.

Risk diagnosis: It is the clinical judgment that a problem does not exist, but the presence of risk factors indicates that a problem is likely to develop unless nurses intervene. The individual (or group) is more susceptible to develop the problem than others in the same or a similar situation because of risk factors.

Subjective data: It is obtained directly from the patient and elicits information.

Syndrome diagnosis: It is a clinical judgment concerned with a cluster of problem or risk nursing diagnoses that are predicted to present because of a certain situation or event.

Time-lapsed reassessment: Several months after initial assessment to compare the client's current health status with the data previously obtained.

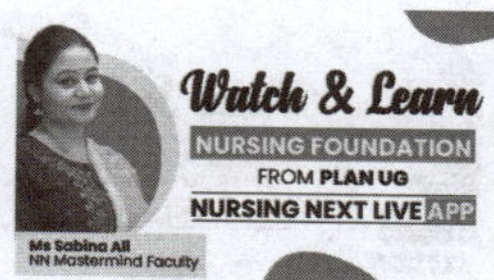

INTRODUCTION

Nursing process is a systematic and dynamic method of providing care to client; whether the client is an individual, group, family or community.

"The nursing process is an orderly systematic manner of determining the client's problem, making plan to solve them, initiating the plan or assigning others to implement it and evaluating the extent to which the plan was effective in resolving the problem identified." **—Yura, Helen and Walsh**

STEPS IN NURSING PROCESS

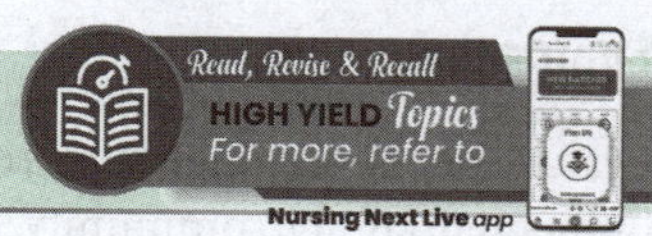

The steps in nursing process are patient-centered and outcome-oriented. It has five steps. Each of the five steps depends on the accuracy of the preceding step.

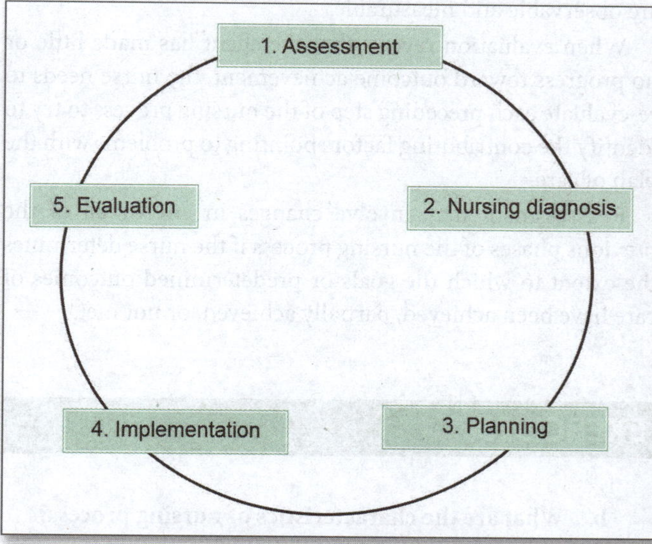

Figure 16.1: Five-step nursing process

Assessment

As far as collecting data relevant to nursing is concerned, subjective and objective data are collected to incorporate patient's perception of his problems and needs, along with observations, findings and results obtained by the nurse.

- **Subjective data:** It is obtained directly from the patient and elicits information.
- **Objective data:** Refers to information based on observation of the nurse and examination of the patient.

The data can be collected from patient, family members, records and reports.

Nursing Diagnosis

Nursing diagnosis is a statement of client's health status or problem which can be solved by nursing actions. The process of arriving at a nursing diagnosis involves decision-making based on intuitive reasoning, experience and sound theoretical foundation in biological and social sciences.

Nursing diagnosis is the most vital step in nursing process, since planning, implementation and evaluation depend on this. It is a clinical judgment about individual, family or community responses to actual health problems and potential health problems.

A nursing diagnostic statement consists of two parts:

1. Problem of the client
2. The related factor (contributing factor)

The problem is the statement identified by the nurse during the assessment phase.

The related factors are "Conditions or circumstances that can cause or contribute to the development of a diagnosis".

There are several ways to state nursing diagnosis. The widely accepted statement suggests PES of writing the nursing diagnosis.

- P stands for the **Problems**, in clear, concise statement of clients existing or potential health problem or unhealthy response. The statement of problem provides a clear indication of what needs to change.
- E stands for **Etiology**, explaining the factors believed to be related to or contributing to the health problem.
- S refers to the **Signs and symptoms** identified during assessment. These signs and symptoms form the basis for nursing inferences.

To facilitate the development of standard nursing language, the groups involved are: North American Nursing Diagnosis Association (NANDA), Nursing Interventions Classification (NIC) and Nursing Sensitive Outcomes Classification (NOC).

The four types of NANDA nursing diagnoses are—Actual (problem-focused) diagnosis, Risk diagnosis, Health promotion diagnosis and Syndrome diagnosis.

1. **Problem-focused diagnosis** (also known as actual diagnosis) is a client problem that is present at the time of the nursing assessment.
2. **Risk diagnosis** is a clinical judgment that a problem does not exist, but the presence of risk factors indicates that a problem is likely to develop unless nurses intervene.
3. **Health promotion diagnosis** (also known as wellness diagnosis) is a clinical judgment about motivation and desire to increase well-being.
4. **Syndrome diagnosis** is a clinical judgment concerning with a cluster of problems or risk of nursing diagnoses that are predicted to present because of a certain situation or event.

Planning

Planning is basically a decision-making process mainly to decide appropriate nursing care for the problems of patients

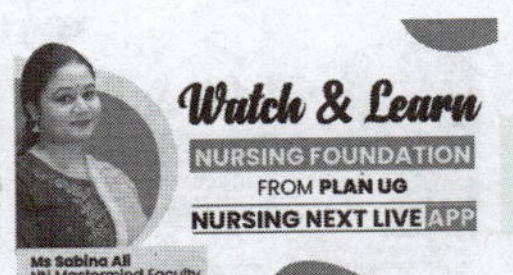

and prescribe nursing care in the form of written nursing instructions.

Planning the patient care involves four steps:

1. Establishing priorities.
2. Setting goals/Identifing outcomes.
3. Selecting nursing interventions.
4. Writing the plan of care.

Implementation

To implement the actions, nurses need to have cognitive, technical, interpersonal and ethical/legal skill, along with the willingness to use them creatively and critically when working with patients to promote or restore health, to prevent disease or illness, and to facilitate coping with altered functioning.

Nurses manipulate equipment skillfully to produce a desired outcome or result. Technically-skilled nurses are able to use technical equipment with sufficient competence and ease to achieve goals and adapt equipment and technical procedures to the needs of particular patients.

Independent nursing actions are initiated by the nurse based on nursing knowledge and skills.

Dependent nursing actions are carried out according to specific routines, under the supervision of a physician, or as a result of an order by a physician, e.g., medication, injection or any other treatment modalities.

Collaborative and interdependent nursing actions are performed either as a result of joint decision by a nurse or another health team member, e.g., working with a physical therapist to provide physical exercises to a client who is bedridden, planning a teaching session about a diabetic diet with a dietician, etc.

- Ongoing data collection during implementation step is important, this is done by:
  - Interacting with the client.
  - Measuring outcomes.
  - Observing responses.

Evaluation

Evaluation is an ongoing process which begins when the individual/family/community enters the health care system, until his/her exit from the system. Evaluation determines the client's progress toward meeting specified outcomes.

The outcome statements present standards and criteria that are observable and measurable.

When evaluation reveals that the client has made little or no progress toward outcome achievement, the nurse needs to re-evaluate each preceding step of the nursing process to try to identify the contributing factors pointing to problems with the plan of care.

Reassessment may involve changes in any or all of the previous phases of the nursing process if the nurse determines the extent to which the goals or predetermined outcomes of care have been achieved, partially achieved, or not met.

CONCEPTUAL EXERCISES

LONG ANSWER QUESTIONS

1. a. **Define nursing process. (MGR, DU, KUHS, RUHS)**
   b. **What are the characteristics of nursing process?**
   c. **Enumerate steps/components of nursing process.**

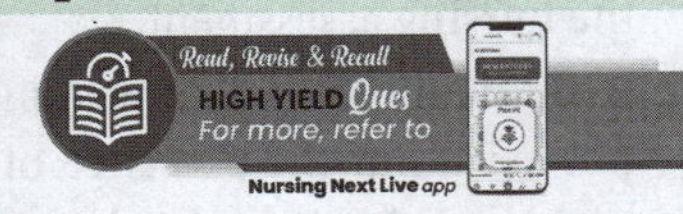

Answer

Nursing Process

Nursing process is a critical thinking process that professional nurses use to apply the best available evidence to caregiving and promoting human functions and responses to health and illness. —**American Nurses Association, 2010**

The nursing process is an orderly systematic manner of determining the client's problems, making plan to solve them, initiating the plan or assigning others to implement it and evaluating the extent to which the plan was effective in resolving the problem identified. —**Yura, Helen and Walsh**

b. **What are the characteristics of nursing process?**

Answer

Characteristics of Nursing Process

Systematic

Each nursing activity is part of an ordered sequence of activities. Each activity depends on the accuracy of the activity that precedes it and influences the actions that follow it. The nursing process directs each step of nursing care in a sequential and orderly manner.

Dynamic

There is a great interaction and overlapping among the five steps. No single step in the nursing process is one-time phenomenon; each step follows the next step. In some nursing situations, all five stages occur almost simultaneously.

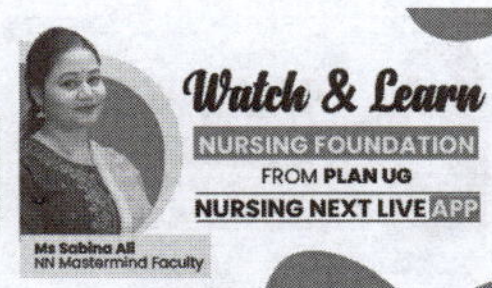

Interpersonal

The nursing process encourages nurses to work together to help patients use their strengths to meet all their human needs. Working intimately with patients helps nurses to explore their own strengths and limitations and to develop themselves personally and professionally.

Outcome-oriented

The nursing process offers means for nurses and patients to work together to identify specific outcomes related to health promotion, disease and illness prevention and coping with altered functioning; to determine which outcomes are most important to the patient; and to match them with appropriate nursing actions.

Universally Applicable in Nursing Situations

When nurses have a working knowledge of the nursing process, they find that they can practice nursing with healthy or sick people, young or old or in any type of practice setting.

Others:

- Cyclic
- Dynamic nature
- Client centeredness
- Focus on problem solving and decision making
- Use of critical thinking and clinical reasoning.

c. Enumerate steps/components of nursing process.

Answer

Steps/Components of Nursing Process

Nursing process is a critical thinking process that professional nurses use to apply the best available evidence to caregiving and promoting human functions and responses to health and illness.

It includes five components and they are:

1. Assessment

Assessment is the systematic and continuous collection, organization, validation, and documentation of data (information).

It includes:

- Subjective data
- Objective data

Subjective data are the symptoms or covert data and can be described only by the client.

Objective data are the signs or overt data that are detectable by an observer or can be measured/tested against an accepted standard obtained by physical examination.

The methods used to collect data are observation, interview and examination.

Observation: It is gathering data by using the senses. Vision, smell and hearing are used.

Interview: An interview is a planned communication or a conversation with a purpose.

Examination: The physical examination is a systematic data collection method to detect health problems. To conduct the examination, the nurse uses techniques of inspection, palpation, percussion and auscultation.

The nurse uses a systematic format that organizes the assessment data systematically.

2. Diagnosis

Diagnosis is the second phase of the nursing process.

In this phase, nurses use critical thinking skills and analyze the collected data accurately to interpret assessment data in order to identify client problems and use this problem to formulate the North American Nursing Diagnosis Association (NANDA) diagnosis. It is a clinical judgment concerning a human response to health conditions/life processes, or a vulnerability for that response, by an individual, family, group, or community.

NANDA nursing diagnosis has:

- **Problem:** Patient's health problem
- **Etiology:** Causes of health problem
- **Defining characteristics:** Signs and symptoms

3. Planning

Planning involves decision making and problem solving.

It is the process of formulating client goals and designing the nursing interventions required to prevent, reduce, or eliminate the client's health problems.

Planning includes:

- **Initial planning:** After the initial assessment
- **Ongoing planning:** Continuous planning.
- **Discharge planning:** Planning for needs after discharge

Planning involves:

- Setting priorities
- Establishing client goals/desired outcomes.
- Selecting prioritized nursing interventions.
- Writing these nursing interventions on care plans.

4. Implementation

- Implementation consists of doing and documenting the activities.
- Implementing the nursing interventions.
- Documentation of nursing interventions.

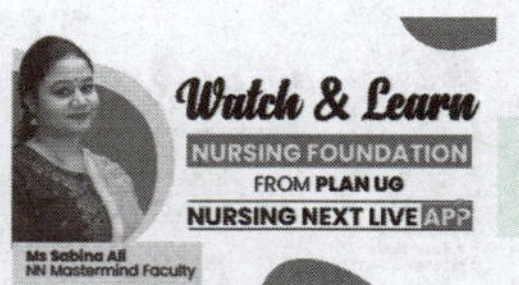

5. Evaluation

Evaluation is a planned, ongoing, purposeful activity in which the nurse determines:

- The client's progress toward achievement of goals/outcomes
- The effectiveness of the nursing care plan.
- Comparing the data with desired outcomes

Continuing, modifying, or terminating the nursing care plan.

2. Define nursing diagnosis and describe the types of nursing diagnosis. Explain the components of NANDA nursing diagnosis with suitable examples. Discuss nursing assessment in detail. (RUHS, KUHS)

Answer

Nursing Diagnosis

- Diagnosis is the second phase of the nursing process.
- In this phase, nurses use critical thinking skills to interpret assessment data to identify client's health problems.
- North American Nursing Diagnosis Association (NANDA) states the definition of nursing diagnosis.

The official NANDA definition of a nursing diagnosis is:

"A clinical judgment concerning a human response to health conditions/life processes, or a vulnerability for that response, by an individual, family, group, or community."

A nursing diagnosis is the statement of a patient's problem that is arrived by making inferences from the collected data.

Types of Nursing Diagnosis

The four types of NANDA nursing diagnoses are:

1. **Problem-focused diagnosis** (also known as actual diagnosis) is a client problem that is present at the time of the nursing assessment. These diagnoses are based on the presence of associated signs and symptoms.
   Examples are:
   It has eight components:
   - Nursing diagnosis
   - Related factors
   - Defining characteristics
   - Examples of actual nursing diagnosis are:
   - Ineffective breathing pattern
   - Anxiety
   - Acute pain
   - Impaired skin intergrity
2. **Risk diagnosis** is a clinical judgment that a problem does not exist, but the presence of risk factors indicates that a problem is likely to develop unless nurses intervene. The individual (or group) is more susceptible to develop the problem than others in the same or a similar situation because of risk factors.
   Examples are:
   - Risk for falls
   - Risk for injury
3. **Health promotion diagnosis** (also known as wellness diagnosis) is a clinical judgment about motivation and desire to increase well-being. Health promotion diagnosis is concerned in the individual, family, or community transition from a specific level of wellness to a higher level of wellness.
   Examples are:
   - Readiness for enhanced spiritual well-being
   - Readiness for enhanced family coping
4. **Syndrome diagnosis** is a clinical judgment concerning with a cluster of problems or risk of nursing diagnoses that are predicted to present because of a certain situation or event.
   Examples are:
   - Chronic pain syndrome
   - Frail elderly syndrome
   - Post-trauma syndrome

Components of a Nursing Diagnosis

A nursing diagnosis has three components:

1. The **problem statement** describes the statement identified by the nurse during assessment phase. It is the client's health problem.
2. The **etiology** component identifies causes of the health problem.
3. **Defining characteristics** are the cluster of signs and symptoms that indicate the presence of health problems.

Example:

Acute pain related to tissue ischemia as evidenced by pain rating of 8/10, grimacing, guarding behavior.

- **Acute pain:** Problem and diagnostic label
- **Tissue ischemia:** Etiology/related factor
- **Pain rating of 8/10, grimacing, guarding behavior:** Risk factors/defining characteristics

Nursing Assessment

- Assessment is the systematic and continuous collection, organization, validation, and documentation of data (information).
- Assessment involves data collection and analysis of data.
- It is the first step in nursing process.

Types of Assessment

There are four different types of assessments:

1. **Initial nursing assessment:**
   - The assessment is performed within specified time after admission to establish a complete database for problem identification.
   - For example, Nursing admission assessment

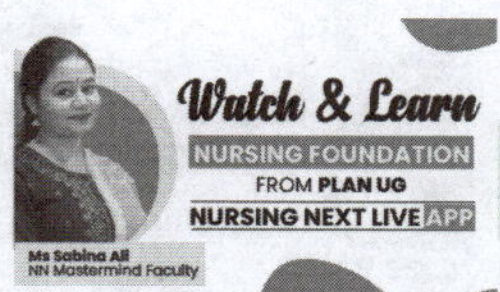

2. **Problem-focused assessment:**
   - This assessment is used to determine the status of a specific problem identified in an earlier assessment.
   - For example, Hourly checking of vital signs of fever patient
3. **Emergency assessment:**
   - During emergency situation in order to identify any life-threatening situation.
   - For example, Rapid assessment of an individual's airway, breathing status, and circulation during a cardiac arrest.
4. **Time-lapsed re-assessment:**
   - Several months after initial assessment.
   - To compare the client's current health status with the data previously obtained.

SHORT NOTES

1. Differences between medical diagnosis and nursing diagnosis. (MGR)

Answer

Differences between Medical Diagnosis and Nursing Diagnosis

Nursing diagnosis	Medical diagnosis
Care-focused	Etiology-focused
Identifies actual or potential health problems of the patient based on the assessment	Identifies a disease or condition based on medical test, symptoms and history.
Purpose is to identify patient needs to develop a nursing care plan	Purpose is to determine specific disease or condition to develop a treatment plan
Focuses on the signs and symptoms of the patient and his/her care givers	The medical diagnosis specifies the pathology
Focuses on the person and physiological/psychologic the responses to illness	Focuses on illness
E.g.: Ineffective denial related to difficulty coping with new diagnosis of "heart attack"	E.g.: Myocardial infarction

2. Subjective data and objective data. (KUHS)

Answer

Subjective data is also known as symptoms or covert data, are clear only to the person affected and can be described only by that person.

Itching, pain, and feelings of worry are examples of subjective data.

Objective data refers to signs or overt data, are detectable by an observer or can be measured or tested against an accepted standard. They can be seen, heard, felt, or smelled, and they are obtained by observation or physical examination.

For example, a discoloration of the skin or a blood pressure reading is objective data.

Subjective data	Objective data
What the patient tells to the physician	What physician detects on the examination
The history, from chief complaint through review of systems	All physical examination findings
Example: Mrs G is a 54-year-old hairdresser who reports pressure over her left chest "like an elephant sitting there," which goes into her left neck and arm.	Example: Mrs G is an older white female, deconditioned, pleasant, and cooperative. BP 160/80 HR 96 and regular, respiratory rate 24, afebrile.

3. Write a short note on the sources of data collection. (DU)

Answer

Types of Data

Subjective data: It is also known as symptoms or covert data, are clear only to the person affected and can be described only by that person.

Objective data: It refers to signs or overt data, are detectable by an observer or can be measured or tested against an accepted standard. They can be seen, heard, felt, or smelled, and they are obtained by observation or physical examination.

Sources of Data

Sources of data are **primary and secondary.**

- **Primary:**
  - It is the direct source of information.
  - The client is the primary source of data.
- **Secondary:**
  - It is the indirect source of information.
  - All sources other than the client are considered secondary sources.
  - Family members, health professionals, records and reports, laboratory and diagnostic results are secondary sources.

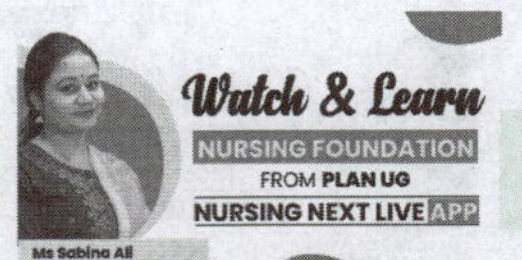

4. Define nursing process and characteristics of nursing process. (MGR, DU, KUHS)

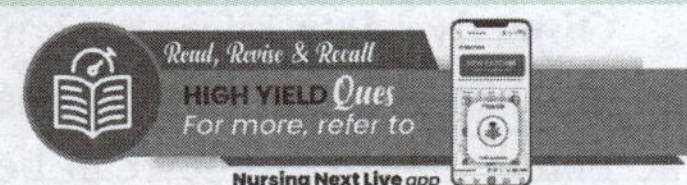

Answer

Nursing Process

Nursing process is a critical thinking process that professional nurses use to apply the best available evidence to caregiving and promoting human functions and responses to health and illness

—American Nurses Association, 2010

Characteristics of Nursing Process

- Systematic
- Dynamic
- Interpersonal
- Outcome-oriented
- Universally Applicable in Nursing Situations

Others:

- Cyclic
- Dynamic nature
- Client centeredness
- Focus on problem solving and decision making
- Use of critical thinking and clinical reasoning.

SHORT ANSWER QUESTIONS

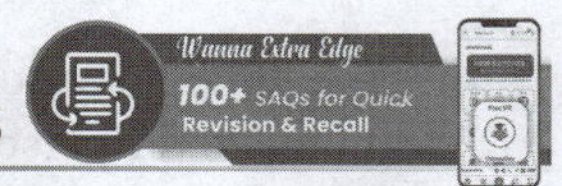

1. Enumerate methods of data collection.

Answer

The methods used to collect data are observation, interview and examination.

- **Observation:**
  - It is gathering data by using the senses.
  - Vision, smell and hearing are used.
- **Interview:**
  - An interview is a planned communication or a conversation with a purpose.
- **Examination:** The physical examination is a systematic data collection method to detect health problems. To conduct the examination, the nurse uses techniques of inspection, palpation, percussion and auscultation.

2. Define nursing diagnosis and enumerate types of nursing diagnosis.

Answer

Nursing Diagnosis

The official NANDA definition of nursing diagnosis is:

"A clinical judgment concerning a human response to health conditions/life processes, or a vulnerability for that response, by an individual, family, group, or community."

A nursing diagnosis is the statement of a patient's problem that is arrived by making inferences from the collected data.

Types of Nursing Diagnosis

The four types of NANDA nursing diagnoses are:

1. **Actual (problem-focused) diagnosis:** Examples are ineffective breathing pattern, anxiety, acute pain
2. **Risk diagnosis:** Examples are risk for falls, risk for injury
3. **Health promotion diagnosis:** Examples are readiness for enhanced spiritual well-being, readiness for enhanced family coping
4. **Syndrome diagnosis:** Examples are chronic pain syndrome, post-trauma syndrome, frail elderly syndrome

3. Enumerate steps of nursing process. (RUHS)

Answer

Nursing process includes five steps and they are:

1. Assessment
2. Diagnosis
3. Planning
4. Implementation
5. Evaluation

4. Define subjective data and objective data. (KUHS)

Answer

Subjective data is also known as symptoms or covert data, are clear only to the person affected and can be described only by that person.

Itching, pain, and feelings of worry are examples of subjective data.

Objective data refers to signs or overt data, are detectable by an observer or can be measured or tested against an accepted standard. They can be seen, heard, felt, or smelled, and they are obtained by observation or physical examination.

For example, a discoloration of the skin or a blood pressure reading is objective data.

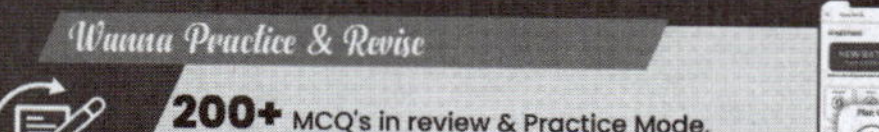

CONCEPTUAL REVISION

MULTIPLE CHOICE QUESTIONS

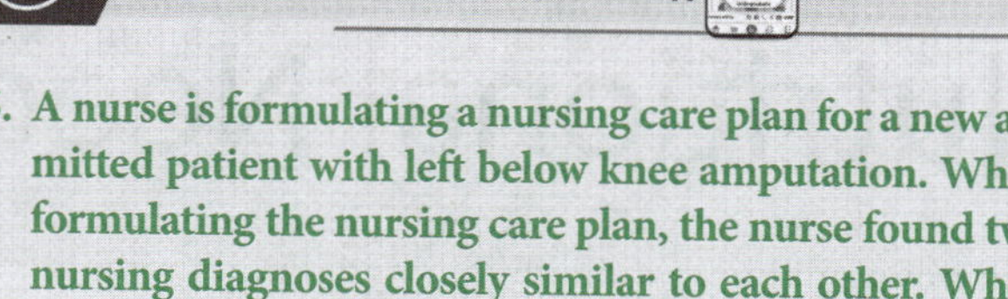

1. In which step of the nursing process does the nurse analyze data and identify patient's problems?

a. Assessment
b. Diagnosis
c. Planning outcomes
d. Evaluation

Ans. b. Diagnosis

2. The nurse documented the data obtained during nursing assessment. Identify which among the following is an example of data that should be validated?

a. The patient verbalizes "I'm having a feeling of fever" while measuring the body temperature the reading is 37°C.
b. Patient verbalizes that he has no difficulty in breathing and the nurse documented the respiratory rate of 18.
c. The patient verbalizes that he is having a history of hypertension and you recorded the BP 166/100 mm Hg.
d. The urinalysis report indicates there are white blood cells in the urine.

Ans. a. The patient verbalizes "I'm having a feeling of fever" while measuring the body temperature the reading is 37°C.

3. Identify the three components of problem focused Nursing diagnosis statement:

a. Problem, etiology and chracteristics
b. Diagnostic label, risk factors, signs and symptoms
c. Potential problem, related to and evidenced
d. Both a and b

Ans. d. Both a and b

4. A nursing intern is helping the assigned nurse in identifying the patient need. The assigned nurse after collecting the detailed history is making the nursing care plan for her patient according to patient needs. The nursing intern then asks the assigned nurse about the purpose of formulating the the nursing diagnosis?

a. Recognize the patient's response toward an illness
b. Center on disease and pathology
c. Offer the nurse's subjective and objective view of the patients
d. All of the above

Ans. a. Recognize the patient's response towards an illness

5. A nurse is formulating a nursing care plan for a new admitted patient with left below knee amputation. While formulating the nursing care plan, the nurse found two nursing diagnoses closely similar to each other. When two nursing diagnoses appeared closely related, what should the nurse do first to determine which diagnosis most accurately reflects the needs of a patient?

a. Analyze the secondary factors
b. Reassess the patient
c. Examine the related factors
d. Review the defining characteristics

Ans. d. Review the defining characteristics

6. Most widely used NANDA nursing diagnosis taxonomy is based on nine patterns of human responses. Identify the incorrect one among the following:

a. Exchanging
b. Choosing
c. Perceiving
d. Responsive

Ans. d. Responsive

7. Which term describes a way to organize and chart patient progress?

a. SOAP
b. POMR
c. PIE
d. All of these

Ans. a. SOAP

8. Match the following exmples of nursing diagnosis with their respectives types:

1. Ineffective airway clearance related to tracheal bronchial inflammation as evidenced by dyspnea, tachypnea, use of accessory muscles.	a. Syndrome diagnosis
2. Risk for infection related to inadequate primary defenses	b. Health Promotion
3. Readiness for enhanced urinary elimination	c. Problem-focused nursing Diagnosis
4. Neonatal abstinance syndrome related to opioids intoxication during pregnancy	d. Risk Diagnosis

a. 1-b, 2-d, 3-a, 4-c
b. 1-d, 2-c, 3-b, 4-a
c. 1-c, 2-d, 3-b, 4-a
d. 1-b, 2-d, 3-c, 4-a

Ans. c. 1-c, 2-d, 3-b, 4-a

CHAPTER 17

Nutritional Needs

CONCEPTUAL THEORY

Terminology

150+ key terminologies for Quick Recall & Revision

Bland diet: This diet is prescribed for patients with peptic ulcer. These patients are instructed to individualize their diet, omitting foods that tend to bother them. Eat small frequent meals in a relaxed environment.

Enteral nutrition (EN): Enteral feedings are administered through nasogastric and small bore feeding tubes, or through gastrostomy or jejunostomy tubes.

Essential nutrients: Some nutrients are considered essential because either they are not synthesized in the body or are made in insufficient amounts. Essential nutrients must be provided in the diet or through supplements.

High fiber diet: This diet is a variation of the regular diet and may be used therapeutically. It may be used as a treatment for some gastrointestinal (GI) disorders and may include a preventive effect against some diseases.

Macronutrients: Essential nutrients that supply energy and build tissue such as proteins, carbohydrates and fats are referred to as **macronutrients**.

Malnutrients: Failure to obtain sufficient nutrients causes **malnutrition**.

Micronutrients: These as vitamins and minerals, are required in much smaller amounts to regulate and control body processes.

Nagogastric (NG) tube is inserted through one of the nostrils, down the nasopharynx, and into the alimentary tract. The longer lumen of the tube allows delivery of liquids to the stomach or removal of gastric contents, the smaller vent lumen allows for an inflow of atmospheric air. When these tubes are used for feeding purpose it is called gastric gavage.

Nutrients are specific biochemical substances used by the body for growth, development, activity, reproduction, lactation, health maintenance, and recovery from illness or injury.

Nutrition: It is the biochemical and physiological process by which an organism uses food to support its life. It provides organisms with nutrients, which can be metabolized to create energy and chemical structures.

Nutritional assessment: A detailed, systematic evaluation of a patient's nutritional status conducted by healthcare providers in a team-based setting to diagnose malnutrition and identify underlying pathologies to plan intervention constitutes nutritional assessment.

Protein restricted diet: In the presence of defects in protein metabolism or excretion, protein intake should be reduced or controlled because of the buildup of protein waste products, dietary protein should be restricted.

Sodium restricted diet: This is given in patients suffering from hypertension, edema (water retention), congestive cardiac failure. In patients. Sodium restricted diets range from 2000 mg sodium to as little as 250 mg of sodium per day.

Therapeutic diet: It is a meal plan that controls the intake of certain foods or nutrients. It is part of the treatment of a medical condition

Total parenteral nutrition (TPN) is a method of delivering total nutrition through a catheter placed in a large central vein.

NUTRITION

Nutrition is vital for life and health, and poor nutrition can seriously decrease one's level of wellness, which makes it a vital component of nursing. It includes the study of nutrients and how they are handled by the body.

Nutrients are specific biochemical substances used by the body for growth, development, activity, reproduction, lactation, health maintenance, and recovery from illness or injury.

Some nutrients are considered **essential** because either they are not synthesized in the body or are not made in sufficient amount. Essential nutrients must be provided in the diet or through supplements. Essential nutrients that supply energy and build tissues such as proteins, carbohydrates and fats are referred to as **macronutrients. Micronutrients**, such as vitamins and minerals, are required in much smaller amounts to regulate and control body processes.

Out of six classes of nutrients, three nutrients supply energy, i.e., carbohydrates, proteins and fats, and three nutrients are needed to regulate body processes—vitamins, minerals and water.

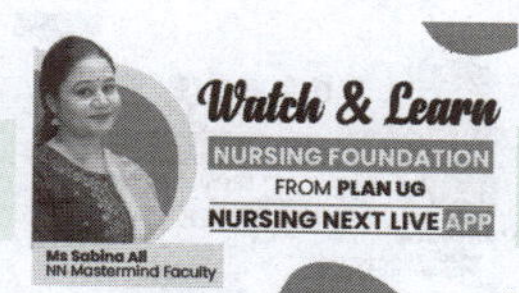

Energy:

1 g of carbohydrate = 4 Kcal

1 g of Protein = 4 Kcal

1 g of Fat = 9 Kcal

Nutritional assessment is for sick persons, good nutritional status can help to reduce risk for complications and speed up the recovery time. Conversely, poor nutritional status can increase the risk for illness or death.

NUTRITIONAL ASSESSMENT

Nutritional assessment involves:

- Obtaining a dietary history
- Collecting anthropometric measurements
- Clinical data
- Biochemical data

Diet History

Includes data about eating patterns and habits, food preferences and restrictions, daily fluid intake, use of vitamin or mineral supplements, any dietary problems such as problem in swallowing and chewing. It also covers data on food allergies or intolerances, concerns related to buying food, preparation, storage and type of diet.

The nurse elicits a 24-hour diet history which enables her to compare the data listed with recommended daily allowances or to determine whether the patient is receiving a nutritionally balanced diet.

Anthropometric Measurements

Include height, weight, triceps, skin-fold measurements, a measure of subcutaneous fat stores, mid-arm circumference, a measure of skeletal muscle mass and fat store. Body weight should be compared with BMI Standards.

Clinical Data

Assessment of nutritional status by various parameters like-appearance, weight, skin, nails, eyes, muscles, etc. help in identification of several nutritional problems.

Biochemical Data

Biochemical measurements - like protein status, hemoglobin, blood glucose, cholesterol, etc. are relative to nutritional status and help in identification.

Nutritional Need of Patients

Providing proper and adequate nutrition to the patient is a team effort. Diet is ordered by the doctor in the in-patient setting, sent to the dietician, and explained to the patient by the nurse. The nurse is also responsible for screening patients at home who are at nutritional risk.

Special diets are needed to treat a disease process such as diabetes mellitus, to prepare for a special examination or surgery, to increase or decrease weight, to restore nutritional deficits, or to allow an organ to rest and promote healing. Diets are modified in one or more of the following aspects: Texture, kilocalories, specific nutrients or consistency.

These diets include clear liquid, full liquid, soft diet and diet as tolerated. Many special diets may be prescribed to meet requirements for disease process or altered metabolism.

Whenever possible, the nurse should help incapacitated clients feed themselves rather than feed them. Sometimes, before surgery to prevent aspiration related to anesthesia and after surgery until bowel sounds return, patients are ordered nil per os (NPO) or nothing by mouth. NPO may also be necessary for patients undergoing certain medical tests, for patients experiencing severe nausea and vomiting, or inability to chew or swallow, those who are comatose and women during labor and delivery.

If patients are NPO for a short period, they can with-stand the stress of NPO. If they are well nourished but being NPO for an extended period of time, they may require nutritional support through **enteral nutrition**, (mustering nutrients directly into the stomach) **parenteral nutrition** (providing nutrition via intravenous (IV) therapy).

ENTERAL NUTRITION

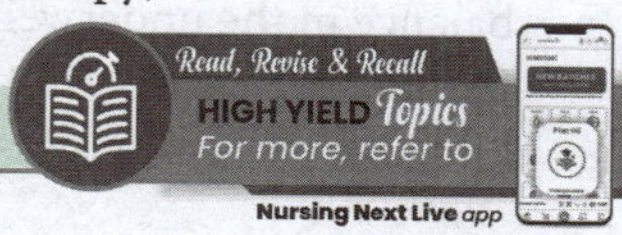

Enteral nutrition (EN) also referred to as total enteral nutrition (TEN). It is provided when the client is unable to ingest food or the upper gastrointestinal tract is impaired and the transport of foods to the small intestine is interrupted. Enteral feedings are administered through nasogastric and small bore feeding tubes, or through gastrostomy or jejunostomy tubes.

Nagogastric (NG) tube is inserted through one of the nostrils, down the nasopharynx, and into the alimentary tract. The longer lumen of the tube allows delivery of liquids to the stomach or removal of gastric contents, the smaller vent lumen allows for an inflow of atmospheric air. When these tubes are used for feeding purpose it is called gastric gavage.

Total parenteral nutrition (TPN) is a method of delivering total nutrition through a catheter placed in a large central vein. These options are used for patient receiving long-term therapy such as victims of massive burns, intestinal obstruction, inflammatory bowel disease, acquired immunodeficiency syndrome (AIDS) or cancer chemotherapy. Baseline levels of blood chemistry, vital signs, and nutritional status should be completed prior to beginning TPN infusion.

THERAPEUTIC DIETS

- **Bland diet:** This diet is prescribed for patients with peptic ulcer. These patients are instructed to individualize their diet, omitting foods that tend to bother them. Eat small frequent meals in a relaxed environment.

- **High fiber diet:** This diet is a variation of the regular diet and may be used therapeutically. It may be used as a treatment for some gastrointestinal (GI) disorders and may include a preventive effect against some diseases. High-Fiber diets are used in the treatment of constipation with adequate fluids, fiber can reduce constipation in the young as well as the elderly. High fiber diets are used to prevent diverticulitis, used in treating diabetes with other dietary controls to help regulate blood sugar. High fiber diets may also be used in the treatment of atherosclerosis.
- **Meal frequency modifications:** Especially in GI related disorders, small frequent meals will be used rather than three large meals. As many as 6–8 small meals or snacks may be consumed daily.
- **Kilocalorie modifications:** The body requires a specific amount of energy each day to carry out its tasks. Energy intake includes foods and beverages consumed daily.

  If energy intake is greater than output, positive energy balance results causing weight gain. On the other hand, if intake is less than output, negative energy balance occurs leading to weight loss.
  - **High kilocalorie and high protein diet:** Dietary treatment should aim at restoring energy balance in the normal weight patient or creating a positive energy balance in the underweight patient.

    If the patient is not able to consume adequate kilocalories or refuses to eat, nutritional support in the form of tube feedings or intravenous may be considered.
- **Carbohydrate modified diets**
  - **Insulin dependent diabetes mellitus (IDDM):** Meals and snacks should be eaten at about the similar time each day. The types and amounts of food eaten should be similar from day to day. This is necessary because the carbohydrate eaten must balance the insulin administered each day.
  - **Noninsulin dependent diabetes mellitus (NIDDM):** Many people with NIDDM are overweight, and one of the major dietary goals with this type of diabetes is weight control. Weight reduction can help control blood glucose and reduce the need for medication. Diet can also be adjusted to compensate for exercise.
- **Fat modified diets:** It is desirable for the treatment of atherosclerosis, heart disease, and hyperlipidemias. Diabetic diets also incorporate fat control. A fat-controlled diet limits both unsaturated and saturated fat intake.
- **Protein restricted diet:** In the presence of defects in protein metabolism or excretion, protein intake should be reduced or controlled because of the buildup of protein waste products, dietary protein should be restricted.
- **Sodium restricted diets:** This is given in patients suffering from hypertension, edema (water retention), congestive cardiac failure. In patients sodium restricted diets range from 2000 mg sodium to as little as 250 mg of sodium per day.

CONCEPTUAL EXERCISES

LONG ANSWER QUESTIONS

1. Elaborate:

a. The different methods of feeding. (MGR)

b. The factors affecting nutritional needs. (MGR)

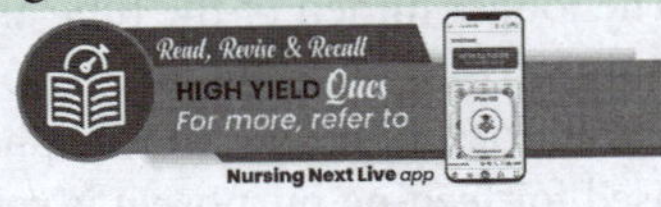

Answer

Different Methods of Feeding

Parenteral Nutrition

- It is the intravenous administration of nutrients directly into the systemic circulation bypassing the usual process of eating and digestion.
- It is the additional approach for nutrition intervention when nutritional needs cannot be met from the oral or enteral routes alone, or are contraindicated.
- The liquid mixture consists of protein, carbohydrates, fats, vitamins, minerals, and other nutrients, etc.
- Total parenteral nutrition (TPN) is a method of delivering total nutrition through a catheter placed in a large central vein.

Enteral Nutrition

- Enteral means administration of nutrition via gastrointestinal tract.
- It may be oral or via feeding tube
- **Oral nutrition:**
  - It is an effective and non-invasive way to meet the nutritional needs or increase their nutritional intake.
  - Requirement of extra nutrition along with regular diet to meet the nutritional requirement is fulfilled by oral nutrition.
- **Tube feeding:**

  When a patient is unable to take food/nutrients orally, enteral nutrition through tube feeding is the first option for administration of nutrition. Nutritional supplement administered directly into the gastrointestinal tract.

Feature	Enteral nutrition	Parenteral nutrition
Route of administration	Oral or *via* a tube inserted into the gastrointestinal tract	Intravenous (IV)
Nutrient source	Formula, food, or supplements	Nutrient solutions

Contd...

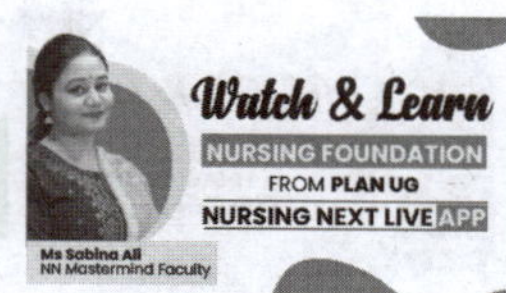

Feature	Enteral nutrition	Parenteral nutrition
Indications	Functional gastrointestinal tract, adequate absorption capacity	Malnourishment, inadequate absorption capacity, gastrointestinal dysfunction
Digestive process	Normal digestive process, absorption through the gastrointestinal tract	Bypasses the gastrointestinal tract, absorption through the bloodstream
Composition of feeding	Formulated to provide all essential nutrients	Customized to meet individual needs
Advantages	Promotes gut function, less invasive, less expensive	Can be used in patients with gastrointestinal dysfunction or malabsorption
Disadvantages	Risk of aspiration, limited access, may not meet all nutritional needs	Risk of infection, requires access to a central vein, more expensive
Examples of delivery methods	Oral, Nasogastric (NG) tube, Gastrostomy (G-tube)	Total parenteral nutrition (TPN)

b. The factors affecting nutritional needs.

Answer

Factors Affecting Nutritional Needs

Nutritional needs change in relation to growth, development activity, and age-related changes such as metabolism and body composition.

Developmental Stage

- Periods of intense growth and development such as during infancy, adolescence, pregnancy, and lactation cause an increase in nutritional needs.
- Nutritional needs stabilize during adulthood.
- Age influences not only nutrient requirements, but also food intake.
- The consistency of food consumed, eating patterns and the significance of food change with physical and psychosocial development.

Gender

Males require more nutrition due to differences in their body composition and due to their longer muscle mass.

State of Health

Illness, trauma and stress change the needs for nutrition due to indigestion, loss of appetite and hormonal changes which affect the metabolism of body.

Alcohol Abuse

Alcohol abuse alters the metabolism of body and their requirements. The toxic effects of alcohol on the intestinal mucosa interfere with normal nutrient absorption. Need of vitamin B increases because it is used to metabolize alcohol.

Medicines

Many medicines have the potential to influence nutrient requirements, nutrient absorption may be altered by drugs that:

- Change the pH of the gastrointestinal tract
- Increase the gastrointestinal motility
- Damage the intestinal mucosa
- Bind with nutrients, rendering them unavailable to the body

Factors that Influence Food Choices

Dietary choices are influenced by economic, culture, religion and personal feelings and meanings associated with food. The financial income can directly influence the ability to purchase sufficient food/or food of high nutritional value. Diverse lifestyles and eating habits directly impact the person's nutritional health. Religious belief restrictions, and cultural practices may affect the patient's acceptance with dietary therapies.

Sociocultural Factors

- Illiteracy
- **Language barrier:** Affects communication with healthcare professionals and understanding of food labels and instructions.
- Knowledge of nutrition
- Lack of caregiver or social support
- Social isolation
- Limited ability to obtain or purchase food
- Lack of or inadequate cooking preparation.

Combination of factors can affect an individual's nutritional intake. They can result in decreased food intake, leading to anorexia, underweight or increased food intake, leading to obesity.

2. Mrs A, a 50-year-old school teacher, is admitted in the ward with diabetes mellitus. She is getting 1500 cal, diabetic, nonvegetarian diet and on regular insulin. (MGR)

- **a What is therapeutic diet?**
- **b Explain the factors to be considered while planning a therapeutic diet.**
- **c Discuss in detail about her home care preparation/ health education.**

Answer

Therapeutic Diet

Therapeutic diet is part of the treatment of a medical condition and are normally prescribed by a physician and planned by a dietician. A therapeutic diet is usually a modification of a regular diet.

b. Factors to be considered while planning a therapeutic diet.

Answer

Therapeutic Diet

Therapeutic diets are planned to maintain or restore good nutrition in the patient.

Therapeutic diet is a normal diet, qualitatively and quantitatively modified as per the patient's special need and in line with the general principles of meal planning.

- The diet must be planned in relation to changes in metabolism occurring as a result.
- Diet must be planned according to habits of patient, culture, religion, socioeconomic status, personal preferences and disease condition.
- Whatever diet is prescribed, there should be variety for selection.
- Hot food should be served hot and cold should be as cold.

c. Discuss in detail about her home care preparation/ health education.

Answer

Health Education

- **Healthy eating and exercise**
  - Healthy eating and regular exercise can help prevent your blood sugar (glucose) from becoming too high or too low.
  - Improving your diet and becoming more active also help to keep your heart healthy, your weight down, and gives you more energy.
- **Eating right with diabetes**
  - What you eat can change your blood sugar. It is important to make healthy choices and to eat the right amount of food. Your meals should have a variety of healthy foods that contain protein, fats, and carbohydrates (starches).
  - Starch changes into sugar when eaten.
  - Simple carbohydrates, such as fruit juice, milk, and candy, can quickly raise your blood sugar.
  - Complex carbohydrates, such as whole grain bread, beans, potatoes, and oatmeal, are high in fiber and raise your blood sugar more slowly.
  - Fiber is also found in fruits and vegetable. Complex carbohydrates with lots of fiber are good for people with diabetes.
  - Your meals should have lots of vegetables and moderate amounts of protein (meat, fish, eggs) and starch.
  - Half of our plate should have vegetables.
  - Choose complex carbohydrates with lots of fiber, like beans, cereals, and brown rice.
  - Look for products that say "whole grain" on them.
  - Eat proteins with a small amount of fat, like lean meats, seafood, low-fat dairy products, and beans.
  - Avoid eating foods with lots of fat, like butter, whole milk, cooking oil, lard, red meat, and chicken skin because they are bad for your heart.
  - Do not eat too many sweets, like cakes, cookies, candy, soda, and fruit juice because they raise your blood sugar too high and can make you gain weight.
  - Be aware of portion sizes, but do not skip meals.
- Eating at regular mealtimes will help control your blood sugar. It is important to eat after taking insulin to make sure that your blood sugar does not get too low.
- Measuring your blood sugar 1–2 hours after your meal will help let you know how the types of food you eat can change your blood sugar.
- **Diabetes and exercise**
  - Exercise is an important part of your treatment, becoming more active can help lower blood sugar and keep your heart healthy. Exercise can also give you more energy and help to reduce your stress.
  - Try to pick activities that you like and will do often. A more active lifestyle can be a fun and easy way to stay healthy.
- Take the stairs instead of the elevator.
- Walk to the store instead of driving, or park farther away from the store and walk.
- Clean the house, work in the yard, wash the car, or walk the dog.
- Dance to your favorite music.
- Play sports of take a bike ride.
- Go for a walk around a mall.
- Check with your doctor before starting any new activities. Remember to check your blood sugar before and after increased activity.
- Wear good shoes and socks.
- Drink lots of water.
- Warm up and cool down before and after exercise.
- Bring a snack or juice to eat in case your blood sugar gets too low. A sugary snack, such as hard candy. Milk, or fruit, will help quickly raise your blood sugar.

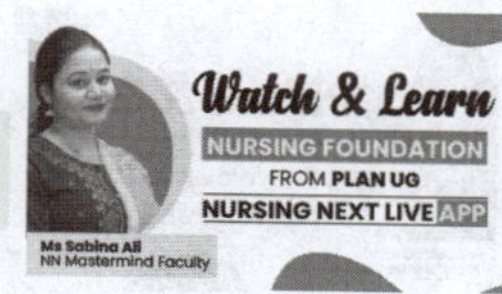

3. Explain the following: (MGR, KUHS)

a. **Gastric lavage.**
b. **Indications of gastric lavage.**
c. **Steps of procedure of gastric levage.**

Answer

Gastric Lavage

Gastric lavage, also commonly called stomach wash or gastric suction, is the process of cleaning out the contents of the stomach. It has been used for eliminating poisons from the stomach.

Stomach wash or gastric lavage means to wash out or irrigate the stomach with a solution. It is used most frequently as an emergency treatment in gastric dilatation and poisoning.

b. Indications of gastric lavage.

Answer

Indication of Gastric Lavage

- The patient who has ingested poison.
- Relieving pressure in someone who has blockage in the intestines.
- To relieve nausea and vomiting in case of acute dilatation of stomach, pyloric stenosis and intestinal obstruction.
- To cleanse the stomach as a preparation for surgery.
- To obtain casts of epithelial cells for bacteriological studies.

c. Steps of procedure of gastric levage.

Answer

Procedure

Requirement

- Nasogastric insertion equipments.
- Lavage fluid—Nacl or other prescribed solution.
- Syringe 20 mL for aspiration and 50 mL for lavage.
- Specimen container with lab request form.
- Kidney tray.

Steps

- Verify doctor's order.
- Assess patient level of consciousness.
- Greet patient and explain procedure.
- Provide privacy.
- Remove dental appliances and inspect oral cavity for loose teeth.
- Position patient in Semi-Fowler's.
- Insert NG tube as per procedure handout.
- Check placement of tube in stomach (3 times check).
- Aspirate stomach contents before instilling water or antidote. Keep specimen in container for analysis, if indicated.
- Remove 20 mL syringe and attach with 50 mL syringe to pour lavage solution into NG tube or attach with 50 mL syringe barrel.
- Pour or inject slowly 20 mL solution and wait for 1 minute.
- Aspirate (if use syringe) or siphon (if use barrel) gastric contents and discard it in kidney dish.
- Save samples of first two washings.
- Record input and output throughout procedures.
- Repeat step 10–14 until returns are clear. Usually requires a totalvolume of 2 liters.
- Remove NG tube as per procedure handout.
- Make patient comfortable.
- Label specimens and dispatch to lab immediately.
- Clean and clear equipment.
- Record and report findings.

Nursing Responsibilities

- Ensure procedure is carried out on correct client at correct site.
- Assess patient's level of consciousness.
- Ensure patient's comfort is maintained throughout the procedure.
  - Fowler's position.
- Perform procedure in a correct manner. Use appropriate solution.
- Monitor vital sign for pre, intra and post procedure.
- Monitor input and output.
- Send labeled specimens in appropriate container with lab request form, if indicated.
- Record and report findings.

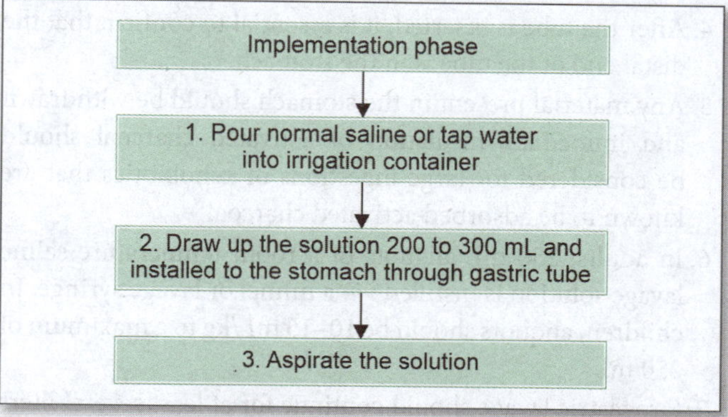

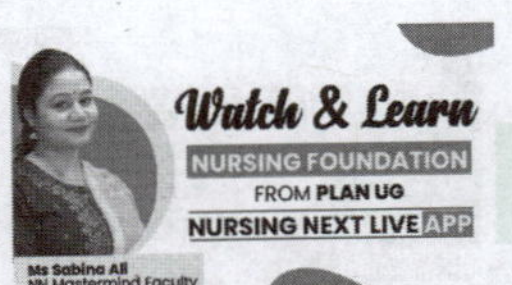

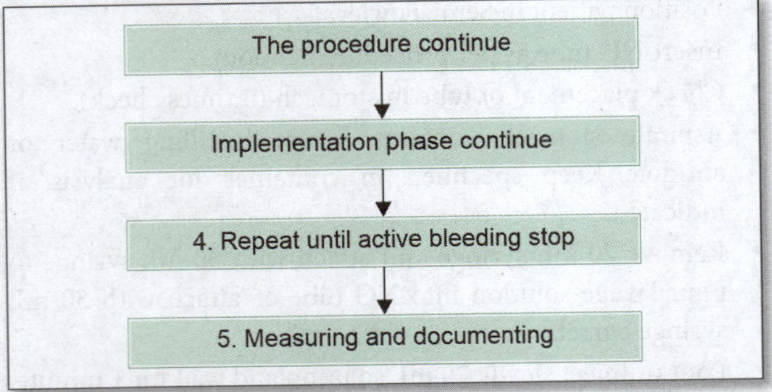

Implementation Phase

- Pour normal saline or tap water into an irrigation container.
- Draw up the solution 200–300 mL and installed to the stomach through gastric tube.
- Aspirate the solution.
- Repeat until active bleeding stop
- Measuring and documenting

Performing Orogastric Lavage

Select the correct tube size

Adults and adolescents: 36–40 French

Children: 22–28 French

Procedures

1. If there is potential airway compromise, endotracheal intubation should precede orogastric lavage.
2. The patient should be kept in the left lateral decubitus position. Because the pylorus points upward in this orientation, this positioning theoretically helps prevent the xenobiotic from passing through the pylorus during the procedure.
3. Before insertion, the proper length of tubing to be passed should be measured and marked on the tube. The length should allow the most proximal tube opening to be passed beyond the lower esophageal sphincter.
4. After the tube is inserted, it is essential to confirm that the distal end of the tube is in the stomach.
5. Any material present in the stomach should be withdrawn and immediate insulation of activated charcoal should be considered for large ingestions of xenobiotics that are known to be adsorbed activated charcoal.
6. In adults, 250 mL aliguots of a room temperature saline lavage solution is instilled *via* a funnel or lavage syringe. In children, aliquots should be 10–15 mL/kg to a maximum of 250 mL.
7. Orogastric lavage should continue for at least several liters in an adult and for at least 0.5–1.0 L in a child or until no particulate matter returns and the effluent lavage solution in clear.
8. After orogastric lavage, the same tube should be used to instill activated charcoal if indicated.

---

4. Write the nursing responsibilities in the following situations: (DU)

a. While providing Ryle's tube feeding.

b. Nursing responsibilities in nasogastric suction.

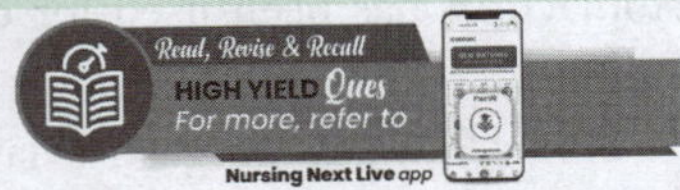

Answer

Nurse's Responsibility in Administering Ryle's Tube Feeding

Briefly describe about "indications for Ryle's tube feeding":

- Identify the client with name, bed no. etc.
- Check the doctor's orders for any specific precautions if any, regarding the tube feeding, movement of the client, positioning of the client, etc.
- Check the level of consciousness.
- Check whether the feed is ready at hand.
- Check the articles available in the client's unit.
- Assess the position of the tube correctly using any method example auscultation, aspiration, etc.

Preparation of the Client and the Unit

- Explain the procedure to the client, if the client is conscious, to gain his confidence and cooperation.
- Explain the sequence of procedure and explain how the client can cooperate with you.
- Provide privacy.
- Provide a safe and comfortable position for the client. If the general condition of the client permits, make the client sit on the chair or place him in a Fowler's position. If the general condition is weak, raise the head with extra pillows.
- Arrange the articles conveniently on the bedside locker.
- Give a rag piece in the client's hand to wipe the face and lips when necessary.
- Give a mouth wash and help him to clean the teeth.
- Clean the nostrils, if there is secretion or crust formation.

After Care of the Client and Articles

- Offer a mouthwash. Clean the face and hands and dry them.
- Remove the mackintosh and towel.
- Secure the ryles tube with adhesive tape if needed.
- Make the client comfortable in bed.

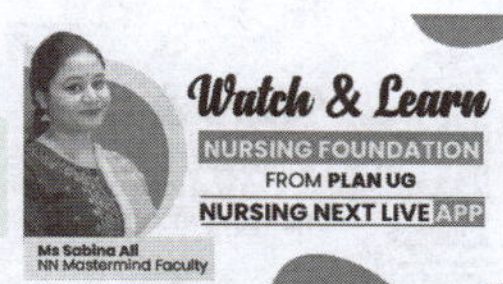

- Take all articles to the utility room. Discard the wastes and clean the articles with soap and water. Dry them. Replace them into their proper places.
- Wash hands.
- Record the time, date, amount of feed, the nature of the feed, the reaction of the client if any, in the nurse's record as well as in the intake and output chart.

b. Nursing responsibilities in nasogastric suction.

Answer

Nursing Responsibilities in Nasogastric Suction

- Assessment of tube every 2–4 hours for patency
- Irrigation of clogged tube according to Physician's instructions
- Monitoring of vacuum source setting
- Assessment of tubing connections and color, amount, consistency of gastric drainage
- Assessment of tube positioning
- Auscultation of bowel sound every 4 hours
- Assess abdomen for distention
- Assess patient for adverse effects every 2 hours
- Assess for passage of rectal flatus
- Provide mouth care every 2 hours and provide ice chips if not contraindicated
- Monitor I/O to prevent fluid deficit or overload
- Monitor serum K^+ level for hypokalemia

SHORT NOTES

1. Write any four purposes of Ryle's tube insertion. (MGR)

Answer

Four purpose of Ryle's tube are as follows:

1. **Used in the treatment of ileus or bowel obstruction:** Nasogastric decompression improves patient discomfort, minimizes recurrent vomiting and serve as a means to monitor the progress of conditions.
2. **Used for administration of medications:** Like oral contrast for computed tomography.
3. **Used to deliver enteral nutrition:** Nasogastric tubes are used to deliver enteral nutrition into the stomach (gastric feeding) or into the small intestine (Post-pyloric)
4. **Used for gastric lavage:** Lavage may be needed to remove blood or clots to facilitate endoscopy.

2. Write about indications of nasogastric feeding. (MGR)

Answer

Indications of Nasogastric Feeding

Medical

- Inflammatory bowel disease
- Hepatic failure
- Renal failure
- Respiratory failure

Neurological

- Cerebrovascular accident
- Motor neuron disease
- Acquired brain injury
- Brain tumor
- Parkinson's disease

Surgical

- Preoperative
- Postoperative
- Fistula
- Burns
- Sepsis
- Head and neck cancer
- Gastrointestinal tract cancer
- Gastrointestinal tract surgery
- Pancreatitis

Orthopedic

Trauma

Psychiatric

Anorexia nervosa

Pediatric

Cystic fibrosis

Miscellaneous

- Intensive care patients
- Short bowel
- Cachexia
- Transition from parenteral nutrition

3. Write a short note on intake output chart. (MGR)

Answer

Intake Output Chart

- Intake output chart is the most accurate 24 hours' measurement of a patient's fluid intake by mouth, feeding tubes or intravenous catheters and output from kidneys gastrointestinal tract, drainage tubes and wounds accurate.
- It is one of the most important aspect of patient assessment.
- Measurement of intake and output can monitor progress of treatment or of a disorder.
- This provides information about retention or loss of sodium and ability of the kidneys to concentrate or dilute urine in response to fluid change.

Intake and Output Record

Name:

Date:

Record for intake			Record for output		
Time	Intake amount	Type of intake	Time	Output amount	Type of output

Indication of Intake and Output Chart

- Fluid and electrolyte imbalance.
- Kidney impairment
- Dialysis
- Burns.
- Recent surgical procedure.
- Severe vomiting or diarrhea/dehydration
- Use of diuretics and corticosteroids.
- Congestive heart failure.
- Any bleeding.
- Excessive perspiration.
- Dark concentrated urine.
- How fluid output are measured. For, e.g., invisible fluid loss. how stool and urine, etc. are accounted for.

4. Write a short note on principles of Ryle's tube feeding. (MGR)

Answer

The Ryle's tube feeding procedure involves the insertion of a tube through the nose or mouth and into the stomach or small intestine. The following are the principles involved in Ryle's tube feeding:

Assessment of the patient's condition: Before the procedure, the patient's medical history, current medical condition, and nutritional status are to be assessed to determine the appropriate method and amount of feeding.

Placement of the tube: The tube is inserted through the nose or mouth and passed down the esophagus into the stomach or small intestine. The position of the tube is confirmed by X-ray or other imaging techniques.

Maintenance of the tube: The tube must also be checked regularly for patency and proper placement. The tube must be secured in place to prevent dislodgement or accidental removal.

Selection of the feeding formula: The type and amount of feeding formula are determined based on the patient's nutritional needs, medical condition, and any allergies or sensitivities.

Administration of the feeding: The feeding formula is administered through the tube using a syringe or pump. The rate and volume of feeding are carefully monitored to avoid complications such as aspiration or diarrhea.

Monitoring and management of complications: The patient's condition is closely monitored for any complications such as tube blockage, infection, or aspiration. Any complications that arise are promptly addressed and managed.

SHORT ANSWER QUESTIONS

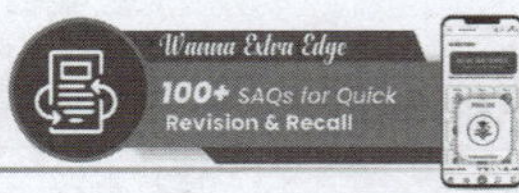

1. What is therapeutic diet?

Answer

Therapeutic diet is part of the treatment of a medical condition and is normally prescribed by a physician and planned by a dietician. A therapeutic diet is usually a modification of a regular diet.

Therapeutic diets are planned to maintain or restore good nutrition in the patient.

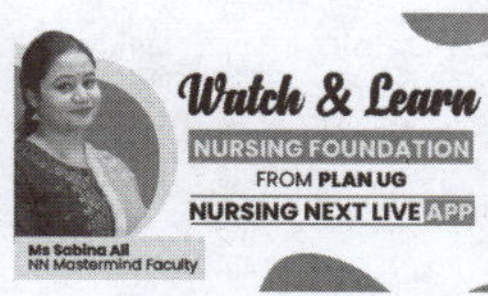

2. Define gastric lavage. (MGR, KUHS)

Answer

Gastric lavage, also commonly called stomach wash or gastric suction, is the process of cleaning out the contents of the stomach. It has been used for eliminating poisons from the stomach.

3. What is intake output chart? (MGR)

Answer

Intake output chart is the most accurate 24 hours' measurement of a patient's fluid intake by mouth, feeding tubes or intravenous catheters and output from kidneys gastrointestinal tract, drainage tubes and wounds accurate.

4. Write about nursing measures to improve appetite. (KUHS)

Answer

- Assist with food choices
- Refer to dietician if needed
- Provide comfortable environment
- Promote food hygiene
- Free of odors
- Promote appealing food presentation
- Hot/cold food as per patient preferences at bedtime can also be promoted
- Offer to open containers
- Assist with feeding as needed
- Make a schedule of diet serving

CONCEPTUAL REVISION

MULTIPLE CHOICE QUESTIONS

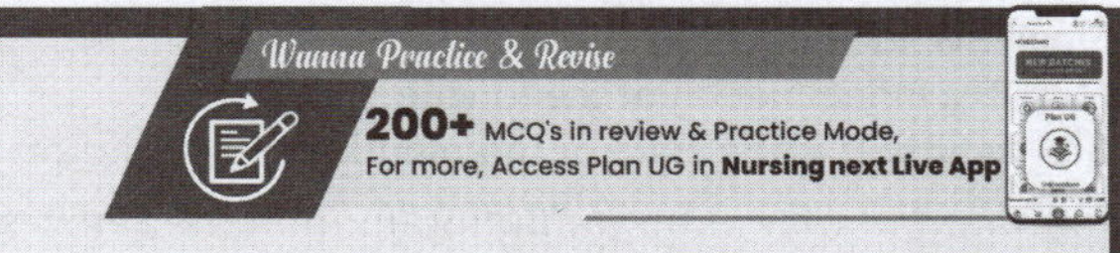

1. A nurse is taking care of a patient with severe COPD. What type of diet would best suit this patient's needs?

a. Fried chicken, french fries, and pudding
b. Cut apples, fresh broccoli, and grilled chicken
c. Pureed sweet potatoes, ground turkey and gravy with mash potatoes
d. Green beans, boiled carrots, and steamed fish

Ans. c. Pureed sweet potatoes, ground turkey and gravy with mash potatoes

2. A patient is diagnosed with Congestive Heart Failure and must follow a specific diet. Which spices are okay for the patient to use daily?

a. Onion salt and garlic powder
b. Sea salt and pepper
c. Ginger and bay leaves
d. Garlic sodium and nutmeg

Ans. c. Ginger and bay leaves

3. Which of the following match of foodborne disease and organism is incorrect?

a. Botulism—*E. coli*
b. Listeriosis—*Listeria monocytogenes*
c. Salmonellosis—*Salmonella typhi*
d. Shigellosis—*Shigella dysenteriae*

Ans. a. Botulism—*E.coli*

4. A patient with gout should follow what type of diet?

a. High-calcium diet
b. Low-purine diet
c. Renal diet
d. Potassium-modified diet

Ans. b. Low-purine diet

5. A patient with anemia would benefit from which diet?

a. Legumes, organ meat, and dark green leafy vegetables
b. Nuts and seeds, fruits, and soy products
c. Grains, berries, and organic vegetables
d. Vegetables, fish, and pasta

Ans. a. Legumes, organ meat, and dark green leafy vegetables

6. The patient is on a low potassium diet that includes food such as applesauce, green beans, cabbage, lettuce, grapes, and raspberries. What type of patient would you expect to be on this type of diet?

a. A patient with heart disease
b. A patient who recently had gastric bypass surgery
c. A patient with osteoporosis
d. A patient with Addison's disease

Ans. d. A patient with Addison's disease

CHAPTER

18

Hygiene

CONCEPTUAL THEORY

Terminology

Anorexia: Loss of appetite
Effleurage/stroking: Long, firm, slow, rhythmic and sweeping movement should be done with palm.
Friction: Deep massage by using palm, finger or thumbs in circular motion in a defined small part of the back. Controlled pressure use to be applied.
Gingivitis: Inflammation of gum.
Glossitis: Inflammation of the tongue
Oral health: It is the state of the mouth, teeth and orofacial structures that enables individuals to perform essential functions such as eating, breathing and speaking, and encompasses psychosocial dimensions such as self-confidence, well-being and the ability to socialize and work without pain, discomfort and embarrassment.
Oral hygiene: It means brushing the client's teeth or cleaning the dentures according to the client's usual routine.
Parotitis: Inflammation of the parotid gland.
Perineal hygiene: Involves cleaning the external genitalia and surrounding area.
Petrissage (Kneading): Deeper massage technique than effleurage. Here with the help of thumb, fingers or palm, large grasping of the skin, subcutaneous tissue and muscles is done.
Pyorrhea: Pus formation in the sockets of the teeth.
Stomatitis: Inflammation of the mucous membrane of mouth.
Tapotements: This is used at the end of other kinds of strokes of massage. Light, stimulating and repetitive massage produced via wrist, fists, fingers and sides of the hands.
Vibrating: Fine vibrating movements should be given by fingertips, produced by contraction and relaxation of the muscles of forearm.

INTRODUCTION

Hygiene is the practice of cleanliness that is conducive to the preservation of health. Assisting the patient with hygiene and personal care activities is an essential nursing function. Proper care of the skin, hair, teeth and nails promotes good health by protecting the body from infection and disease.

PURPOSES OF PERSONAL HYGIENE

- To prevent illness
- To promote good health
- To improve the standard of health
- To maintain quality life of an individual
- To promote mental well-being
- To promote social and spiritual health
- To improve self-esteem in society
- To maintain resistance and prevent from illness

FACTORS AFFECTING HYGIENE

- Social practices
- Personal preferences
- Body language
- Socioeconomic status
- Health belief and motivation
- Cultural variables.
- Physical condition

MOUTH CARE

Mouth is an ideal place for multiplication of germs as there is warmth, moisture and food. Therefore, to prevent infection, it

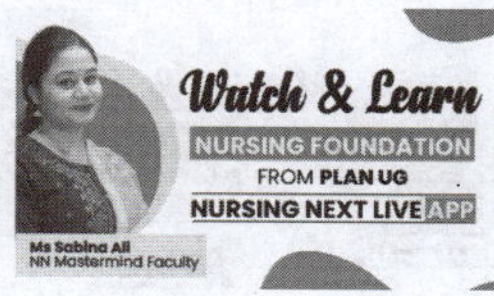

should be kept clean. Oral care is care of mouth and teeth of a patient that prevents many diseases because bacteria can enter the stomach and lungs through the mouth.

According to WHO, oral health is the state of the mouth, teeth and orofacial structures that enables individuals to perform essential functions such as eating, breathing and speaking, and encompasses psychosocial dimensions such as self-confidence, well-being and the ability to socialize and work without pain, discomfort and embarrassment.

Purposes of Mouth Care

- To prevent VAP (Ventilator associated Pneumonia) in mechanical ventilated patients
- To keep the oral cavity clean, moist and intact
- To prevent local and systemic infection
- To help maintain and improve patient's appetite.
- To promote self-esteem and comfort.
- To prevent complications due to poor oral hygiene.

Common Problems of Oral Cavity

Local Problems

- Halitosis
- Dental caries
- Dental plaque
- Calcus or tartar
- Bottle mouth syndrome
- Periodontal diseases or pyorrhea
- Sordes
- Cheilosis
- Bleeding gums
- Glossitis
- Root abscess
- Cancrum oris
- Stomatitis

Infections of Neighboring Areas

- Parotitis
- Sinusitis
- Otitis media
- Adenitis
- Tonsillitis

Systemic Infections

Presence of pus in pulp cavity can spread to distal areas of the body via bloodstream and can cause:

- Rheumatic arthritis
- Bacterial endocarditis
- Nephritis
- Gastritis
- Anorexia

An unconscious patient should be provided full mouth care at least once every 8 hours. If the patient is mouth breathing, care should be done every 4 hours.

CARE OF SKIN

Bathing

The type of cleansing bath depends on the patient's physical capabilities and the degree of hygiene required. The nurse is responsible for assessing what type of bath is most appropriate for the patient's need.

Types

- **Complete bed-bath:** This is administered to patients who are totally dependent. The nurse gives the bath to the patient in bed and the entire body is cleaned.
- **Partial bed-bath:** Consists of bathing only those body parts that would cause discomfort if left unbathed such as hands, face, axillae and perineal care. Dependent patients in need of partial hygiene or bed-ridden patients who are unable to reach all body parts receive partial bed-bath.
- **Tub bath:** The patient is immersed in a tub of water. The tub bath allows thorough washing and rinsing than a bed-bath. The patient may still require the nurse's assistance.
- **Shower:** Here, the patient sits or stands under a continuous stream of water. The shower provides thorough cleansing than a bed bath.
- **Therapeutic baths:** Therapeutic means having healing or medicinal qualities such as Sitz bath. The bath promotes healing and relieves pain and discomfort. It is commonly used after delivery and vaginal or rectal surgery.

Key Points for Bathing a Patient

- Safety must be maintained
- Fully drawn curtains around the bed to maintain privacy
- Draping prevents chills and promotes warmth and comfort. Closing the patient's door and windows provides warmth by decreasing drafts of air.
- Encourage the patient to be independent, but offer assistance as needed. Depending on the patient's activity and ability level, you may plan to give either partial or complete bath.

CARE OF OTHER BODY PARTS

Nail Care

Nail care includes regular trimming. Cleaning under the nails and cuticle care are usually done with the bath. Soak the nails

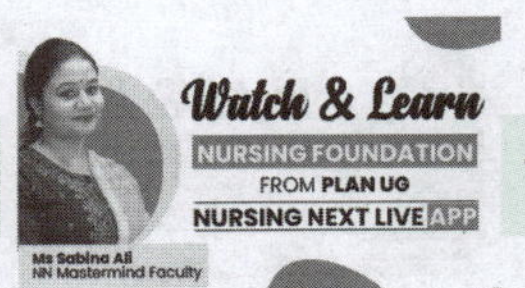

in warm soapy water for 5–10 minutes. Push cuticles back gently and use nail clippers to cut the toe nails straight across to prevent them from growing into the skin along the sides.

Eye Care

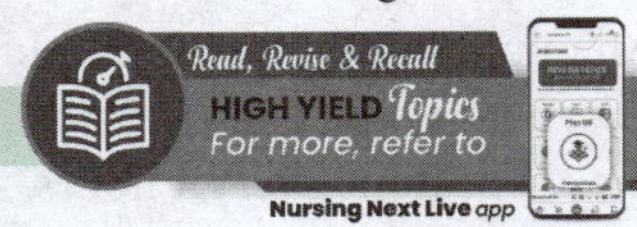

Assess eyes of patients for drainage, crusting or redness. Unconscious patients may need more frequent eye care. Patients with diminished or absent blink (corneal) reflex and patients whose eyelids remain open require frequent eye care, at least every 4 hours. If the eye is not kept moist, corneal ulceration may result from excessive drying of the eye.

Nursing measures include using saline or artificial tears, to lubricate the eye and a protective shield to keep the eye closed.

If a patient wears **contact lenses** but cannot remove them, the nurse is responsible for removing them. Leaving contact lenses in place for long periods could result in permanent eye damage.

Ear Care

Hearing acuity may be affected if cerumen or foreign material collects in the external ear canal. Remove these materials by gently washing the external ear canal with a warm washcloth. If wax is dried or excessive, there is a need to irrigate the ear after notifying the physician.

After the ears are washed, dry them carefully with a soft towel so that water and cerumen (wax) are removed by capillary action. Use of hairpins, paper clips, or finger nails to remove wax from the ear is extremely dangerous because they may injure or puncture the eardrum.

If the patient uses a hearing aid, check the batteries routinely and clean the earpiece or ear mold daily, with mild soap and water.

Providing Nose Care

The best way to clean the nose is to blow it gently. Both nostrils should be open while doing this.

If the external nares are crusted, applying a warm, moist compress helps to soften and remove the crusts. Disposable paper tissues are recommended for nasal secretions. Never introduce the applicator into the nares.

Hair Care

Hair needs to be brushed and combed daily and washed, as needed, to keep it clean. Nurses may need to provide hair care for clients who cannot meet their own self-care needs. A nurse should use a clean brush or comb and brush from the scalp toward the hair ends.

Care of Hands and Feet

Patients with diabetes mellitus or peripheral vascular disease should be observed for adequate circulation of the feet.

Care of the Feet

- Inspect the feet daily including the top and soles and the area between the toes.
- Wash and soak the feet daily using lukewarm water (37°C)
- If the feet perspire, apply a foot powder.
- If dryness is noted along the feet, apply soft oil and rub gently into the skin.
- File the toe nails straight across and square.
- Avoid wearing elastic stockings.
- Wear clean socks daily.
- Do not walk barefoot.
- Wear properly fitted shoes.
- Exercise regularly to improve circulation to the lower extremities
- Immediately wash minor cuts and dry them thoroughly. Mild antiseptics may be applied to the skin.

Back Care

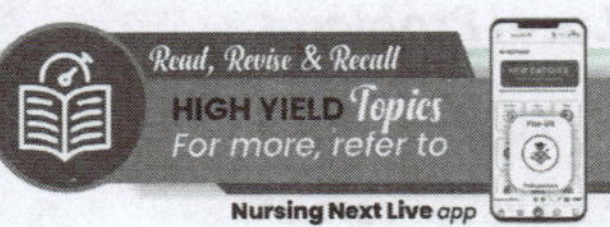

"Back care is cleaning and massaging, individual's back as therapeutic and comfort measure."

- Agents used for back massage:
  - Lotions or emollients
  - Rubbing alcohol:
  - Powder

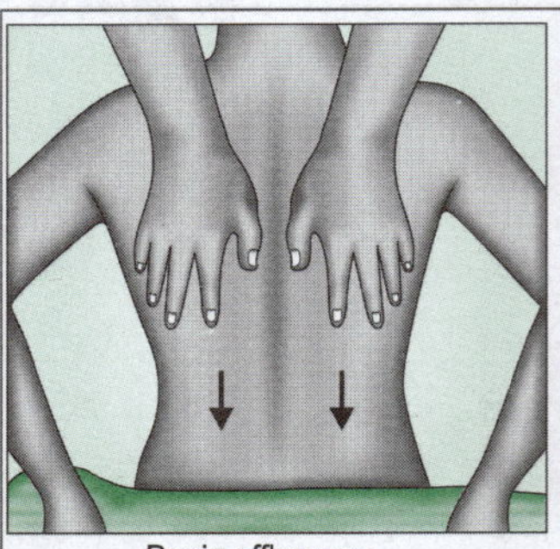
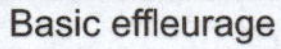
Basic effleurage

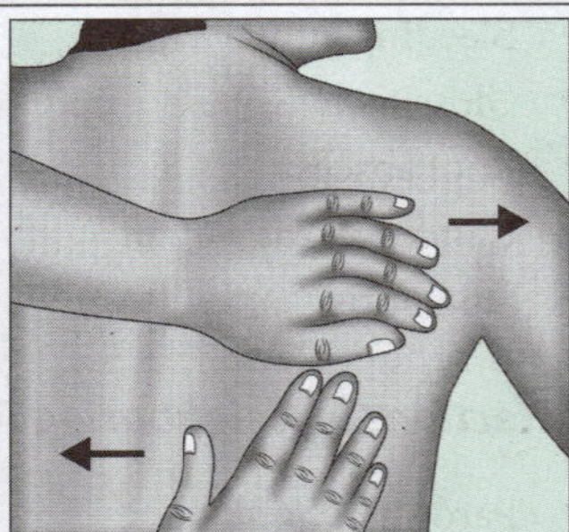
Rolling petrissage

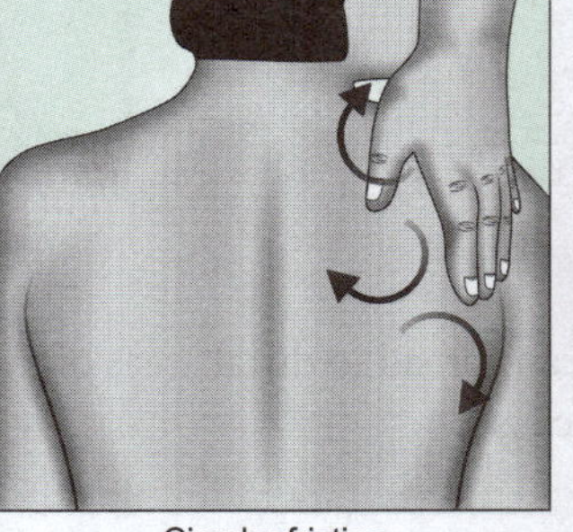
Circular friction

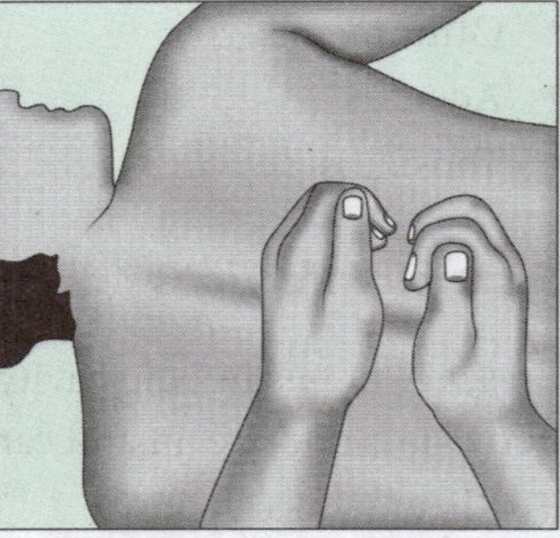
Beating percussion

- **Effleurage/stroking**
- **Petrissage (Kneading)**
- **Friction**
- **Vibrating**
- **Tapotements**

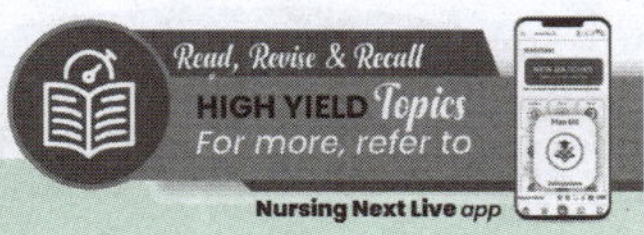

PRESSURE ULCERS

- A Pressure Ulcer or Pressure Sore or Decubitus Ulcer or Bedsore is localized injury to the skin and other underlying tissue, usually over a body prominence, as a result of prolonged unrelieved pressure.
- Pressure ulcer is also called pressure sores or Bed sores or decubitus ulcer. These are the injuries to skin and underlying tissue resulting from prolonged pressure on the skin.

Risk Factors for Pressure Ulcers

Table 18.1: Risk factors for pressure ulcers

Major factors	
• Bed or chair confinement • Inability to move • Loss of bowel and bladder control	• Poor nutrition • Lowered mental awareness
Contributing factors	
• Dehydration • Obesity • Excessive diaphoresis	• Extreme due to age fragile skin • Edema

Common Sites of Pressure Ulcer

- Bedsores most often develop on skin that covers bony areas of the body, such as the heels, ankles, hips and tailbone.
- People most at risk of bedsores are those with a medical that limits their ability to change positions or are confined to bed confined for a long time.

Pressure ulcers commonly occur over the:

- Sacrum
- Greater trochanter
- Ischial tuberosity
- Malleolus
- Heel
- Fibular head
- Scapula

While on a wheelchair, a pressure sore develops on:

- Tailbone or buttocks
- Shoulder blades and spine
- Backs of arms and legs
- Feet

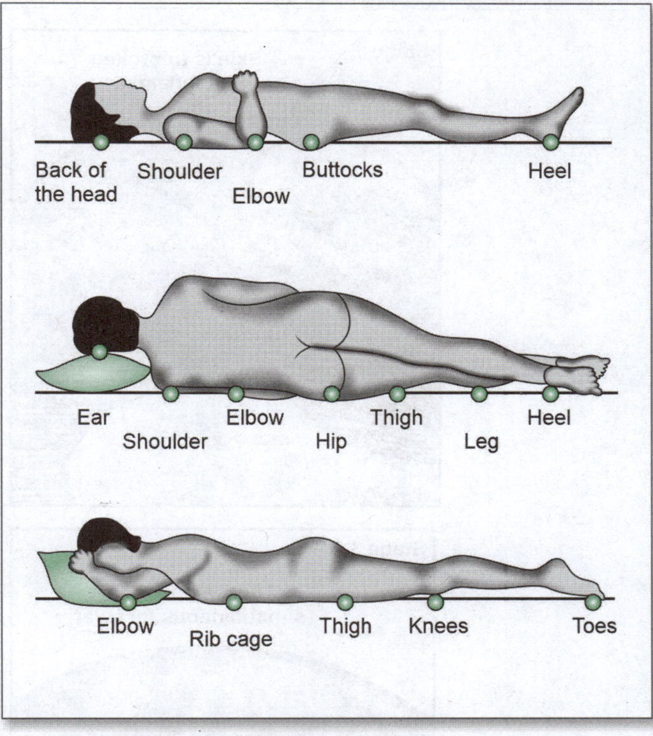

Figure 18.1: Common sites for pressure uncles

Pressure Uncles

A commonly used tool is the Braden scale for predicting pressure sore risk.

Prevention of Pressure Ulcers

- Assessment and reassessment of skin status
- Position changing every 2nd hourly.
- Use pressure reducing devices such as air mattress
- Back care. Do not massage reddened skin.
- Provide adequate nutrition and fluid intake

Care for Pressure Ulcers

The most effective method of pressure ulcer treatment is through a team approach.

The initial care of a pressure ulcer involves debridement, wound cleansing and the application of dressings.

For cleaning ulcers, use only normal saline and apply light mechanical force with sponges or irrigation fluid to prevent damage to granulation tissue.

Cover the wound with a dressing.

Thin film dressings are used on **stage I ulcers** to protect them from shearing forces and to keep them moist.

For stage II ulcers that are non-infected, use a hydrocolloid dressing that can be left on for up to a week.

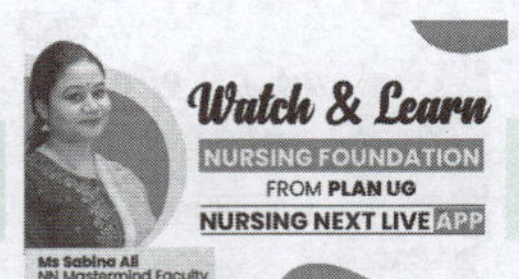

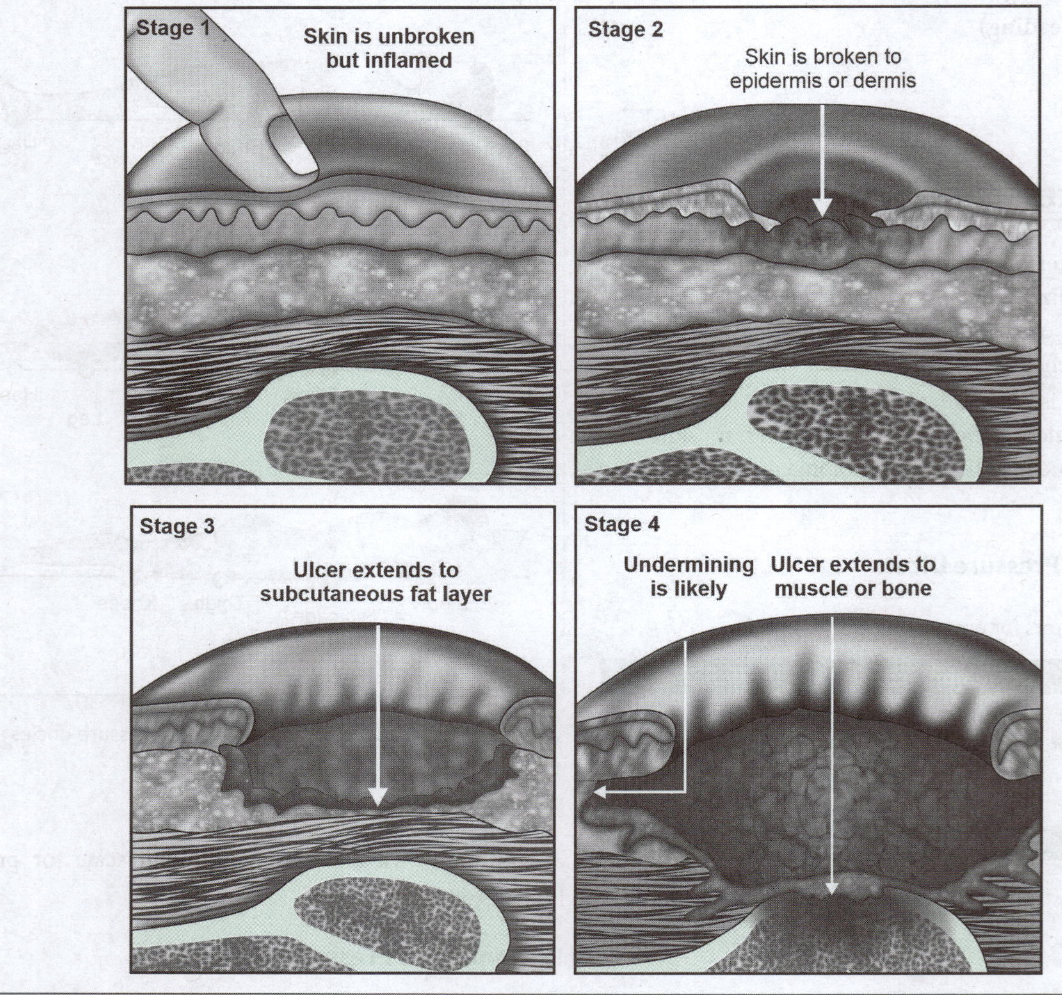

Figure 18.2: Stages of pressure ulcer

For stage III ulcer that is draining, use a dressing that will absorb exudate and maintain a moist environment. For infected ulcers, a non-occlusive dressing is always used.

Chemical enzyme formulas may be used in the wound to help debride eschar in **stage IV ulcers**. A wet to dry dressing may also be applied to help the sloughing of necrotic tissue.

Hydrocolloid dressings are dressings with complex formulations of colloids, elastomer and adhesive components. The wound contact layer of this dressing forms a gel as fluid is absorbed and maintains a moist healing environment. These dressings support healing in clean granulating wound.

Hydrogel dressings are impregnated with water or glycerin-based amorphous gel. This type of dressing hydrates wounds and absorbs smaller amounts of exudate. It is useful for partial thickness and full thickness wounds, deep wounds with some exudate, necrotic wounds, burns and radiation-damaged skin.

CONCEPTUAL EXERCISES

LONG ANSWER QUESTION

1. a. **Define oral hygiene. (MGR)**
   b. **Common problems of oral cavity. (MGR)**
   c. **Prevention of complication arising from negligence of oral care. (MGR)**

Answer

Oral Hygiene

- Oral hygiene means brushing the client's teeth or cleaning the dentures according to the client's usual routine. Oral hygiene is provided to maintain the integrity of client's teeth, gums, mucous membrane and lips.

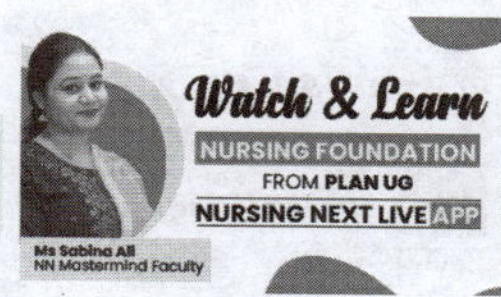

- According to WHO, Oral health is the state of the mouth, teeth and orofacial structures that enables individuals to perform essential functions such as eating, breathing and speaking, and encompasses psychosocial dimensions such as self-confidence, well-being and the ability to socialize and work without pain, discomfort and embarrassment. Oral health varies over the life course from early life to old age, is integral to general health and supports individuals in participating in society and achieving their potential.
- Oral hygiene is the practice of keeping your mouth clean and disease-free.

b. Common problems of oral cavity.

Answer

Common Problems of Oral Cavity

Local Problems

- Halitosis
- Dental caries
- Dental plaque
- Calcus or tartar
- Bottle mouth syndrome
- Periodontal diseases or pyorrhea
- Sordes
- Cheilosis
- Bleeding gums
- Glossitis
- Root abscess
- Cancrum oris
- Stomatitis

Infections of Neighboring Areas

- Parotitis
- Sinusitis
- Otitis media
- Adenitis
- Tonsillitis

Systemic Infections

Presence of pus in pulp cavity can spread to distal areas of the body via bloodstream and can cause:

- Rheumatic arthritis
- Bacterial endocarditis
- Nephritis
- Gastritis
- Anorexia

c. Prevention of complication arising from negligence of oral care.

Answer

- Adequate and correct brushing technique promotes good oral hygiene; it is advised to follow brushing of teeth in the morning as well as in the evening. The mouth should be rinsed after every meal to dislodge any food particle left between the teeth.
- All persons who are unable to attend to the mouth should be assisted to clean the mouth.
- Frequent mouth care for all dependent patients, i.e., mouth care every 2 hours or 4 hours to prevent the development of complications.

  All patients with ryles tube should be focused for oral hygiene.
- Prevent dehydration of the tissues by the administration of enough fluids.
- Care must be taken in brushing the teeth, not to cause any injury to the gums by the hard bristles. For the patients having any bleeding tendency, brushes with soft bristles should be used for oral care.
- Care must be taken to select a good dentifrice. Dentifrices clean the mouth through mechanical action rather than by chemical action on the bacteria.
- Brushing of the teeth should be done in such a way that the brush reaches all five surfaces of every tooth the inner surface, the outer surface, the two sides (right and left), the lower surfaces of the upper row and the upper surface of the lower row. Brushing is done from the gum to the enamel.
- The use of emollients such as cream, aids in softening the dry lips and prevent cracking of the lips.
- Simple and inexpensive mouth washes may be used to prevent or treat unpleasant odors of the mouth.
- For healthy teeth and gums, a well-balanced diet is necessary.
  - A regular check up by a dental surgeon can minimize the complications.
  - The nurse should use every opportunity to teach the clients and their relatives about oral hygiene.

SHORT NOTES

1. Write a short note on complications of neglected mouth. (MGR)

Answer

For answer, refer to Long Question no. 1(c), pg. no. 761

2. Write a short note on purpose of mouth care. (MGR)

Answer

- To prevent VAP (Ventilator associated Pneumonia) in mechanical ventilated patients
- To keep the oral cavity clean, moist and intact
- To alleviate pain
- To remove and prevent the build-up of debris related to food particles
- To increase general well-being.
- To prevent local and systemic infection
- To help maintain and improve patient's appetite.
- To promote self-esteem and comfort.
- To prevent complications due to poor oral hygiene.
- To avoid bad odor while talking.

3. Write a short on techniques of back massage. (KUHS)

Answer

Effleurage/stroking: Long, firm, slow, rhythmic and sweeping movement should be done with palm.

Petrissage (Kneading): Deeper massage technique than effleurage. Here with the help of thumb, fingers or palm, large grasping of the skin, subcutaneous tissue and muscles is done.

Friction: Deep massage by using palm, finger or thumbs in circular motion in a defined small part of the back. Controlled pressure use to be applied.

Vibrating: Fine vibrating movements should be given by fingertips, produced by contraction and relaxation of the muscles of forearm

Tapotements: This is used at the end of other kind of strokes of massage. Light, stimulating and repetitive massages are produced via wrist, fists, fingers, sides of the hands.

4. Write a short note on purposes of personal hygiene. (KUHS)

Answer

Purposes of personal hygiene include the following:

- **To prevent illness:** Good personal hygiene practices and cleanliness can prevent the spread of pathogens and reduce the risk of infections.
- **To promote good health:** Regular personal hygiene practices such as bathing and oral care can promote physical health and prevent health problems.
- **To improve the standard of health:** Personal hygiene practices can improve the overall standard of health in individuals.
- **To maintain quality life of an individual:** Personal hygiene practices can contribute to a better quality of life by reducing the risk of infections and promoting physical health.
- **To promote mental well-being:** Personal hygiene practices can help boost self-esteem, reduce stress and anxiety, and promote mental well-being.
- **To promote social and spiritual health:** Good personal hygiene practices can promote social and spiritual health by enhancing personal relationships and promoting a positive outlook on life.
- **To improve self-esteem in society:** Maintaining good personal hygiene can improve an individual's self-esteem, which can lead to increased confidence.
- **To maintain resistance and prevent from illness:** Personal hygiene practices can improve the body's ability to resist infections and other illnesses.

5. Write a short note on factors affecting hygiene. (KUHS)

Answer

Social practices: Social groups influence the type of personal care and during childhood, hygiene is influenced by family customs.

Personal preferences: Each person has individual desires and preferences about when to bathe, shave and perform hair care. Individuals select different product according to personal preference, needs and financial resources.

Body language: Body image is a person's subjective concept of his or her physical appearance. These images can change frequently. When an individual undergoes surgery, illness or a change in functional status, body image can change dramatically.

Socioeconomic status: A person's economic resources influence the type and extend of hygiene practices used. Socioeconomic status may influence his/her ability to regularly maintain hygiene.

Health belief and motivation: Knowledge about importance of hygiene and its implication for well-being influences hygiene practices. However, knowledge alone is not enough. The individual must be motivated to maintain self-care as well.

Cultural variables: An individual's cultural belief also affects hygienic care. People from diver cultural backgrounds follow different self-care practices. Culturally, maintaining cleanliness may not hold the same importance for some ethnic group as it does for other.

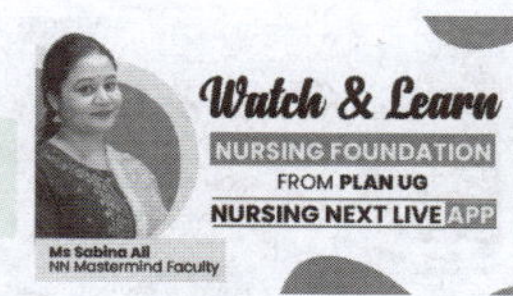

Physical condition: Person with certain types of physical limitations or disabilities often lack physical energy and dexterity to perform hygienic care.

6. Write a short note on menstrual hygiene. (DU)

Answer

Menstrual Hygiene

Menstrual hygiene refers to the practices and behaviors that individuals undertake during menstruation to maintain cleanliness, prevent infection, and promote physical, mental, and emotional well-being.

Purposes of Menstrual Hygiene

- To prevent infections
- To promote physical health
- To maintain reproductive health
- To reduce social stigma and exclusion
- To promote mental health
- To improve quality of life

UNICEF works in four key areas for improved menstrual health and hygiene:

1. Social support
2. Knowledge and skills
3. Facilities and services
4. Access to absorbent materials and supportive supplies

Measures to Maintain Menstrual Hygiene

- Change the sanitary pad frequently
- Try to use cotton sanitary pads. No use of dirty clothes.
- Maintain perineal care
- Eat balanced diet
- Stress management
- Wear comfortable and clean undergarments
- Discard used sanitary products properly
- Consult a Gynecologist, if necessary

7. Write a short note on perineal care. (DU, MGR)

Answer

Perineal Care

Use sterile gauze/cotton for each stroke separately. For female patients separate labia and start cleaning from pubic area toward anal region. For male patients, clean the tip of penis first in a circular motion from meatus outward. Wash the shaft of the penis using strokes in the downward direction towards the pubic area. Always proceed from least contaminated area to most contaminated area.

- Indication
- Articles required.
- Procedure and
- Role of nurses

8. Write the nursing responsibilities in below mentioned situation. (DU)

a. **While providing mouth care to an unconscious patient**
b. **While giving cold sponge**

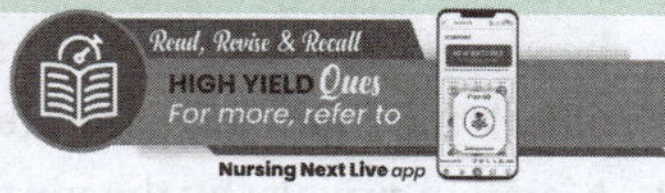

Answer

During Mouth Care on Unconscious Patient

- Before providing oral care, arrange all the articles properly in a tray.
- Keep the tray required for oral care at bedside.
- Greet the patient and explain the procedure to the patient.
- Maintain proper privacy.
- Wear gloves while providing oral care to the unconscious patient.
- Inspect the oral cavity for any complications.
- Place the patient in a side lying position toward the defended side.
- Place the mackintosh and towel under the patient's face and chin.
- Always keep the kidney tray close to the chin.
- Use chlorhexidine solution for oral care.
- Do not pour water in the mouth. Use tongue depressor, if needed.
- Wrap a swab/gauze (as per hospital policy) around the forceps covering the lips completely and clean the mouth systematically.
- Clean the mouth in the following manner inside cheeks, gums, teeth, roof of the mouth, lips.
- Use SINGLE swab/gauze for single stroke till the mouth is clean.
- When the teeth and tongue are cleaned well, stop the procedure, wipe the lips and face with towel.
- Apply emollient after performing oral care to prevent cracked lips.
- Remove all equipment from the bedside and replace in a proper place.
- Make the patient comfortable.
- Record the procedure with date, time and signature. Document the inspection of oral cavity and its finding also.

- Report any abnormal condition to the nurse incharge and physician immediately.

b. While giving cold sponge

Answer

- Check the physician's orders.
- Assess the patient's body temperature
- Explain the purpose and need of the procedure to the client
- Keep the unnecessary items away from the work area

Articles Required

- Place the articles needed, conveniently on the bedside table
- Adjust the height of the bed to the comfortable working height of the nurse
- Check the room temperature
- Maintain privacy by the means of curtains
- Offer bedpan or urinal if necessary, before sponge bath
- Keep the client flat if the condition permits. Remove extra pillows and back rest.
- Remove the personal clothing and cover the client with the bath blanket. If the client has IV, remove the gown from the arm without IV first, then lower the IV bottle, slide gown up the IV tubing and over the IV container.
- Reassess the temperature after sponge bath
- Rechange the IV container and check the rate of flow.

SHORT ANSWER QUESTIONS

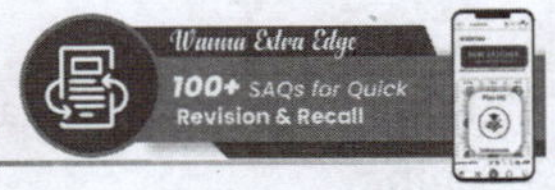

1. Define oral hygiene. (MGR)

Answer

According to WHO, Oral health is the state of the mouth, teeth and orofacial structures that enable individuals to perform essential functions such as eating, breathing and speaking, and encompasses psychosocial dimensions such as self-confidence, well-being and the ability to socialize and work without pain, discomfort and embarrassment.

2. List four indications of perineal care. (MGR)

Answer

The following are the indications for perineal area:

- Bedridden patients.
- Unconscious patients
- Incontinence
- All patients with indwelling catheters

3. List four purposes of mouth care. (MGR)

Answer

Four Purposes of Mouth Care

1. To keep the oral cavity clean, moist and intact
2. To prevent local and systemic infection
3. To help maintain and improve patient's appetite.
4. To prevent complications due to poor oral hygiene.

4. List six factors affecting hygiene. (KUHS)

Answer

1. **Social practices:** Type of personal care; during childhood, hygiene is influenced by family customs.
2. **Personal preferences:** Each person has individual desires and preferences about when to bathe, shave and perform hair care.
3. **Body language:** Body image is a person's subjective concept of his or her physical appearance.
4. **Socioeconomic status:** Socioeconomic status may influence his/her ability to regularly maintain hygiene.
5. **Health belief and motivation:** Knowledge about importance of hygiene and its implication for well-being influences hygiene practices.
6. **Cultural variables:** People from diverse cultural backgrounds follow different self-care practices.

5. Define Perineal care. (DU)

Answer

Perineal hygiene involves cleaning the external genitalia and surrounding area. The perineal area is conducive to the growth of pathogenic organisms because it is warm, moist and is not well ventilated. Since there are many orifices (urinary meatus, vaginal orifice and the anus) situated in this area, the pathogenic organisms can enter into the body.

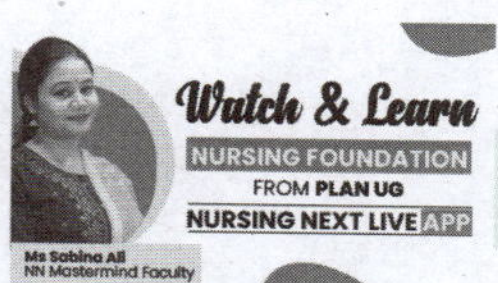

CONCEPTUAL REVISION

MULTIPLE CHOICE QUESTIONS

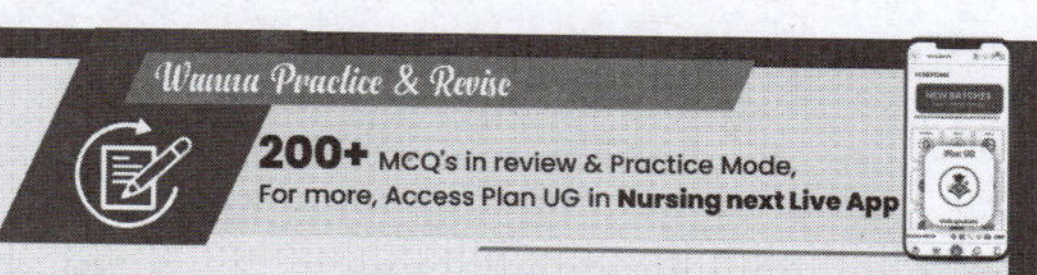

1. When bathing a patient's extremities, the nurse should use long, firm strokes from the distal to the proximal areas. This technique:

a. Provides an opportunity for skin assessment.
b. Avoids undue strain on the nurse.
c. Increases venous blood return.
d. Causes vasoconstriction and increases circulation.

Ans. c. Increases venous blood return

2. The most important purpose of cleansing bed bath is:

a. To cleanse, refresh and give comfort to the client who must remain in bed.
b. To expose the necessary parts of the body.
c. To develop skills in bed-bath.
d. To check the body temperature of the client in bed.

Ans. a. To cleanse, refresh and give comfort to the client who must remain in bed.

3. It refers to the preparation of the bed with a new set of linens:

a. Bed-bath
b. Bed making
c. Bed shampoo
d. Bed lining

Ans. b. Bed making

4. Back care is best described as:

a. Caring for the back by means of massage.
b. Washing of the back.
c. Application of cold compress at the back.
d. Application of hot compress at the back.

Ans. a. Caring for the back by means of massage.

Golden Points

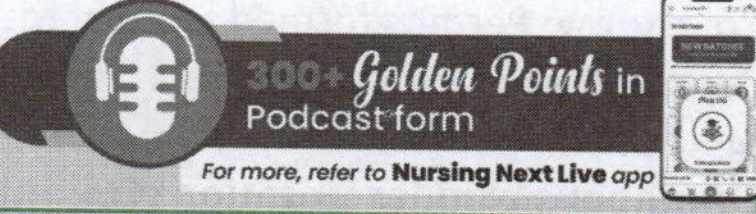

- A Pressure Ulcer or Pressure Sore or Decubitus Ulcer or Bedsore is a localized injury to the skin and other underlying tissues, usually over a body prominence, as a result of prolonged unrelieved pressure.
- An unconscious patient should be provided full mouth care at least once every 8 hours. If the patient is mouth breathing, care should be done every 4 hours.
- Back care is the cleaning and massaging of an individual's back as a therapeutic and comfort measure. The steps involved in back care are Effleurage/stroking, Petrissage (Kneading), Friction, Vibrating and Tapotements.
- Bedsores most often develop on skin that covers bony areas of the body, such as the heels, ankles, hips and tailbone. People at risk of bedsores are those with a medical condition that limits their ability to change positions or are confined to bed for a long time.
- Braden scale is used for predicting pressure sore risk. Stages of bedsores can be grade 1 to 4.
- Hygiene is the practice of cleanliness that is conducive to the preservation of health.
- If the patient uses a hearing aid, check the batteries routinely and clean the earpiece or ear mold daily, with mild soap and water.
- Mouth is an ideal place for multiplication of germs as there is warmth, moisture and food.
- Patients with diabetes mellitus or peripheral vascular disease should be observed for adequate circulation of the feet.
- Patients with diminished or absent blink (corneal) reflex and patients whose eyelids remain open require frequent eye care, at least every 4 hours. If the eye is not kept moist, corneal ulceration may result from excessive drying of the eye. If a patient wears, contact lenses but cannot remove than, a nurse should remove than.
- Pressure ulcers commonly occur over the: Sacrum, Greater trochanter, Ischial tuberosity, Malleolus, Heel, Fibular head, Scapula, etc.
- The cleansing bath depends on the patient's physical capabilities and the degree of hygiene required. It can be Complete bed-bath, Partial bed-bath, Tub bath, Shower and Therapeutic bath also.
- The most effective method of pressure ulcer treatment is through a team approach. The initial care of a pressure ulcer involves debridement, wound cleansing and the application of dressings.

CHAPTER 19

Elimination Needs

CONCEPTUAL THEORY

Terminology

Anesthetic enema: It is a retention enema containing an anesthetic drug to produce anesthesia in client.

Anthelmintic enema: To destroy and expel the worms from the intestines, e.g., Carminitive enema (antispasmodic).

Astringent enema: It lessens the amount of mucus discharge & gives a temporary relief in the inflamed area.

Bowel elimination: The term bowel refers to the intestine. Bowel elimination, the excretion of solid waste, is the final step in the process of digestion.

Bowel incontinence: Also called fecal incontinence, refers to the loss of voluntary ability to control fecal and gaseous discharges through the anal sphincter.

Cold enema (ice enema): To decrease the body temperature in hyperpyrexia and heat stroke.

Colostomy: Permits formed feces in the colon to exit through the stoma.

Constipation: May be defined as fewer than three bowel movements per week. This infers the passage of dry, hard stool or the passage of no stool.

Continuous bladder irrigation (CBI): May be ordered when a blood clot or other debris threatens to block the catheter. Closed system irrigation is recommended to prevent entry of pathogens into the bladder.

Diarrhea: Refers to the passage of liquid feces and an increased frequency of defecation.

Dysuria: It means voiding that is either painful or difficult.

Emollient enema: Introduction of bland solution into the rectum for the purpose of checking diarrhea or soothing & relieving irritation on an inflamed mucus membrane.

Enema: It is the introduction of fluid into the rectum and colon by means of a tube. Enemas are given to stimulate peristalsis and the urge to defecate or to wash out the waste products or feces. The action of an enema is to distend the intestine and sometimes to irritate the intestinal mucosa, thereby increasing peristalsis and the excretion of feces and flatus.

Enuresis: Enuresis is involuntary urination in children beyond the age when voluntary bladder control is normally acquired, usually 4 or 5 years of age. Nocturnal enuresis or bedwetting is the involuntary passing of urine during sleep.

Evacuant enema: Evacuant enema is designed to prompt the bowel to expel fecal matter or flatus, together with the contents of the enema. Phosphate and sodium citrate are the most common types.

Fecal impaction: It is a mass or collection of hardened feces in the folds of the rectum. Impaction results from prolonged retention and accumulation of fecal material.

Flatulence: It is the presence of excessive flatus in the intestines that leads to stretching and inflation of the intestines.

Functional incontinence: Urine loss caused by the inability to reach the toilet because of environmental barriers, physical limitations, loss of memory or disorientation.

Ileostomy: Allows liquid fecal content from the ileum of the small intestine to be eliminated through the stoma.

Irrigation: The flushing of a tube canal or area with solution is called irrigation.

Nocturia: It is voiding urine two or more times at night.

Contd...

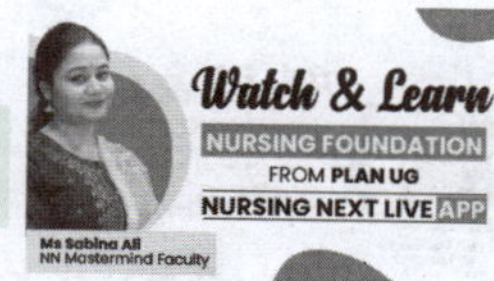

Nutrient enema: It is a retention enema to supply food and fluids to the body.
Oil enema: To soften fecal matter in case of severe constipation. It should be retained for half an hour to 1 hour to soften the feces followed by a soap and water enema to open the bowels.
Oliguria and anuria: Oliguria is low urine output, usually less than 500 mL a day or 30 mL an hour for an adult.
Ostomy: It is a term used for surgical opening from the inside of an organ to the outside. The intestinal mucosa is brought out to the abdominal wall and a stoma, the part of the ostomy that is attached to the skin, is formed by suturing the mucosa to the skin.
Overflow incontinence: The involuntary loss of urine associated with over distension and overflow of the bladder.
Polyuria or diuresis: It is the production of abnormally large amounts of urine by the kidneys.
Purgative enema: To contrast actively and to evacuate its contents.
Rectal suppositories: Consist of concentrated food, soap, glycerine, plain or medicated cocoa butter, prepared in the shape of a cone. They retain this shape at ordinary room temperature but when introduced into the rectum, these suppositories are dissolved by body heat and the drugs contained in them are then released.
Reflex incontinence: Clients with this incontinence, experience emptying of bladder without the sensation of the need to void.
Retained enema: This enema type is for people whose stool has hardened. This type of enema softens the stool.
Sedative enema: Sedative medication is administered through enema which induces sleep.
Simple Evacuant enema: To stimulate defecation and to treat constipation.
Sitz bath: It is a method of applying tepid or warm water to the pelvic or rectal area by sitting in a tub, special chair or basin filled with sufficient water to reach the umbilicus at the desired temperature. The legs and feet remain out of the water.
Stimulant enema: Used in treatment of shock and collapse.
Stress incontinence: It occurs when there is involuntary loss of urine related to increase in intra-abdominal pressure.
Total incontinence: A continuous and unpredictable loss of urine, resulting from surgery, trauma or physical malformation.
Transient incontinence: It appears suddenly and lasts for 6 months or less.
Urge incontinence: The involuntary loss of urine that occurs soon after feeling an urgent need to void (urgency).
Urinary diversion: It is the surgical rerouting of urine from the kidneys to a site other than the bladder. There are two categories of diversions: Incontinent and continent.
Urinary frequency: Voiding at frequent intervals, i.e., more than 6 times per day.
Urinary incontinence: It is any involuntary leakage of urine that is widely under reported and undiagnosed. It is more prevalent in women and increases with age.
Urinary retention: When emptying of the bladder is impaired, urine accumulates and the bladder becomes over-distended, giving rise to a condition known as urinary retention.

URINARY ELIMINATION

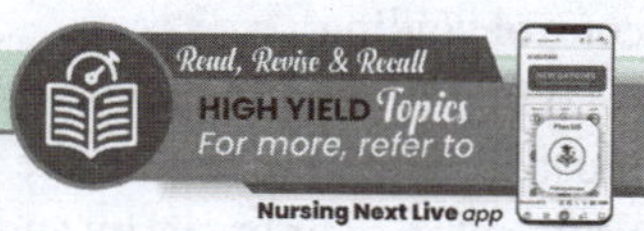

Elimination from the urinary tract helps the body to get rid of the waste products and materials not needed by the body. Urinary elimination depends on effective functioning of the kidneys and ureters; and the urinary bladder, urethra and pelvic floor.

Despite normal urine production, a number of factors or conditions can affect urinary elimination.

- **Polyuria or diuresis:** It is the production of abnormally large amounts of urine by the kidneys.
- **Oliguria and anuria:** Oliguria is low urine output, usually less than 500 mL a day or 30 mL an hour for an adult.
- **Urinary frequency:** Voiding at frequent intervals, i.e., more than 6 times per day.
- **Nocturia:** It is voiding urine two or more times at night.
- **Urgency:** It is the sudden desire to void.
- **Dysuria:** It means voiding that is either painful or difficult.
- **Enuresis:** Enuresis is involuntary urination in children beyond the age when voluntary bladder control is normally acquired, usually 4 or 5 years of age. Nocturnal enuresis or bedwetting is the involuntary passing of urine during sleep.

When emptying of the bladder is impaired, urine accumulates and the bladder becomes over-distended, giving rise to a condition known as ***urinary retention***.

URINARY INCONTINENCE

Urinary incontinence is any involuntary leakage of urine that is widely under reported and undiagnosed. It is more prevalent in women and increases with age.

Types of Urinary Incontinence

- **Transient incontinence:** It appears suddenly and lasts for 6 months or less.

  Stress incontinence: It occurs when there is involuntary loss of urine related to increase in intra-abdominal pressure.

  Urge incontinence: The involuntary loss of urine that occurs soon after feeling an urgent need to void (urgency).

  Overflow incontinence: The involuntary loss of urine associated with over distension and overflow of the bladder.
- **Functional incontinence:** Urine loss caused by the inability to reach the toilet because of environmental barriers, physical limitations, loss of memory or disorientation.

- **Reflex incontinence:** Clients with this incontinence, experience emptying of bladder without the sensation of the need to void.
- **Total incontinence:** A continuous and unpredictable loss of urine, resulting from surgery, trauma or physical malformation.

Treatment for Incontinence

- Bladder training
- Habit training:
- Pelvic muscle exercises (PME)

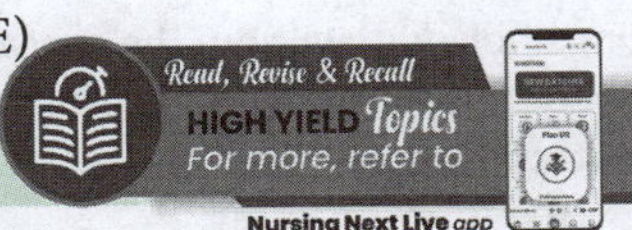

Urinary Catheter

The application of a **urinary catheter** connected to a urinary drainage system can be used for incontinence. Urinary catheterization is the introduction of a catheter into the urinary bladder. This is usually performed only when absolutely necessary, because there are chances of introducing microorganisms into the bladder. Thus, strict sterile technique is used for catheterizations. Another hazard is trauma with urethral catheterization, particularly the male client, whose urethra is longer and more tortuous.

Nursing care of the client with an indwelling catheter and continuous drainage is largely directed toward preventing infection of the urinary tract and encouraging urinary flow through the drainage system.

It includes encouraging large amounts of fluid intake, changing retention catheter and tubing, maintaining the patency of the drainage system and preventing contamination of the drainage system.

CAUTI Bundle Care

- Maintain strict aseptic technique which insertion of urinary catheter.
- Perform hand hygiene before and after client contact.
- Wear gloves to manipulate the catheter and/or the drainage system.
- Urinary catheter should be anchored by a stabilization device (to the upper thigh in women – upper thigh or lower abdomen in men).
- Catheter should be continuously connected to tubing and drainage system. If catheter was disconnected from the drainage tube, clean the connection site prior to reconnection of tubing.
- Always keep the drainage bag below the level of the bladder and not in contact with the floor.
- Drainage bag should be emptied regularly into a separate clean container dedicated for client use only. There should be no contact between the nonsterile container and the drainage bag spout when emptied.
- Perform catheter care at least once daily and after each bowel movement.
- Record the date and time of insertion as well as removal of catheter in nurses notes.

URINARY DIVERSION

A **urinary diversion** is the surgical rerouting of urine from the kidneys to a site other than the bladder. There are two categories of diversions: Incontinent and continent.

Incontinent Diversion

The most common urinary diversion is the **ileal conduit** or ileal loop. In this, a segment of the ileum is removed and the intestinal ends are reattached. One end of the portion removed is closed with sutures to create a pouch and the other end is brought out through the abdominal wall to create a stoma. The ureters are implanted into the ileal pouch.

Continent Diversion

With continent diversion, a continence mechanism is created giving control to client over the passage of urine either by intermittent catheterization of the internal reservoir (Koch pouch) or by strained voiding (neobladder). This is used when the bladder is diseased or damaged. This new bladder is sutured to the functional urethra. Clients with these can control voiding.

When caring for clients with a urinary diversion, the nurse must **accurately assess intake and output**, note any changes in urine color, odor or clarity and frequently assess the condition of the stoma and surrounding skin.

The flushing of a tube canal or area with solution is called irrigation. **Irrigation** may be intermittent or continuous depending on the need for keeping the drainage system patent.

CONTINUOUS BLADDER IRRIGATION

Continuous bladder irrigation (CBI) may be ordered when a blood clot or other debris threatens to block the catheter. Closed system irrigation is recommended to prevent entry of pathogens into the bladder.

For doing continuous bladder irrigation, a triple lumen catheter is used, on which one port is attached to the irrigating fluid with drip chamber, second port is used for inflating the balloon and third port is used for drainage purpose. Hang the bladder irrigant on IV pole and release clamp on irrigation tubing and regulate flow at determined flow rate.

Noting down the intake and output records and comparing them from day to day indicates whether fluid intake is sufficient and output is adequate.

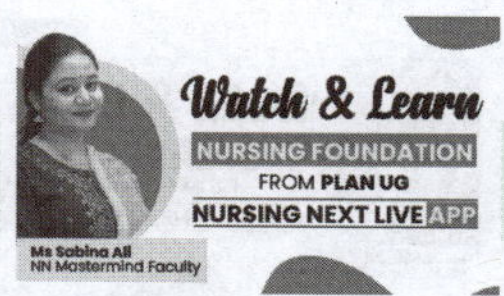

BOWEL ELIMINATION

The term *Bowel* refers to the intestine. Bowel elimination is the excretion of solid waste, and is the final step in the process of digestion.

Four common problems are related to fecal elimination: constipation, diarrhea, bowel incontinence and flatulence.

1. **Constipation** may be defined as fewer than three bowel movements per week. This infers the passage of dry, hard stool or the passage of no stool. **Fecal impaction** is a mass or collection of hardened feces in the folds of the rectum. Impaction results from prolonged retention and accumulation of fecal material.
2. **Diarrhea** refers to the passage of liquid feces and an increased frequency of defecation.
3. **Bowel incontinence** also called *fecal incontinence*, refers to the loss of voluntary ability to control fecal and gaseous discharges through the anal sphincter.
4. **Flatulence** is the presence of excessive flatus in the intestines that leads to stretching and inflation of the intestines.

Enema

An **enema** is the introduction of fluid into the rectum and colon by means of a tube. Enemas are given to stimulate peristalsis and the urge to defecate or to wash out the waste products or feces. The action of an enema is to distend the intestine and sometimes to irritate the intestinal mucosa, thereby increasing peristalsis and the excretion of feces and flatus.

Enemas are classified into cleansing and retention enemas.

Evacuant Enema

An Evacuant enema is designed to prompt the bowel to expel fecal matter or flatus, together with the contents of the enema. Phosphate and sodium citrate are the most common types.

Retained Enema

This enema type is for people whose stool has hardened. This type of enema softens the stool.

Sitz Bath

Sitz bath is a method of applying tepid or warm water to the pelvic or rectal area by sitting in a tub, special chair or basin filled with sufficient water to reach the umbilicus at the desired temperature. The legs and feet remain out of the water.

A sitz bath is recommended to:

- Relieve pain in the rectal or perineal area
- Reduce inflammation
- Relieve painful hemorrhoids
- Encourage voiding
- Decrease congestion of blood in the pelvic area
- Promote drainage from wound
- Relieve renal colic
- Help remove slough.

Rectal Suppositories

Rectal suppositories consist of concentrated food, soap, glycerine, plain or medicated cocoa butter, prepared in the shape of a cone. They retain this shape at ordinary room temperature but when introduced into the rectum, these suppositories are dissolved by body heat and the drugs contained in them are then released.

Types of Suppositories

- Evacuating suppositories such as glycerine
- Astringent suppositories such as tannic acid, belladonna and glycerine—used in dysentery and diarrhea
- Suppositories containing opium or barbital are used for sedation
- Anodyne are used for hemorrhoids, dysentery and diarrhea
- Ice suppositories are used to treat local bleeding.

Surgical Procedures to Help Elimination Needs

Sometimes patients undergo surgical procedures to create an opening into the abdominal wall for fecal elimination. **Ostomy** is a term used for surgical opening from the inside of an organ to the outside. The intestinal mucosa is brought out to the abdominal wall and a **stoma**, the part of the ostomy that is attached to the skin, is formed by suturing the mucosa to the skin.

An **ileostomy** allows liquid fecal content from the ileum of the small intestine to be eliminated through the stoma. A **colostomy** permits formed feces in the colon to exit through the stoma.

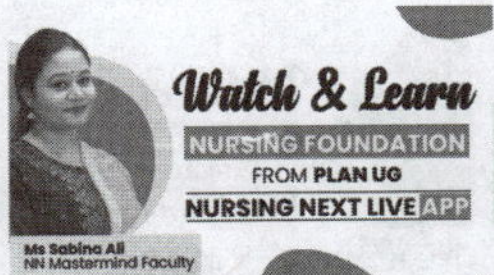

CONCEPTUAL EXERCISES

LONG ANSWER QUESTIONS

1. **Mr S, a 60-year-old man is admitted in the ward with the complaints of abdominal discomfort and constipation for four days. (MGR)**
   a. **List the causes of constipation.**
   b. **List the contraindications for enema.**
   c. **Explain the Nursing responsibilities while administering enema to the patient.**

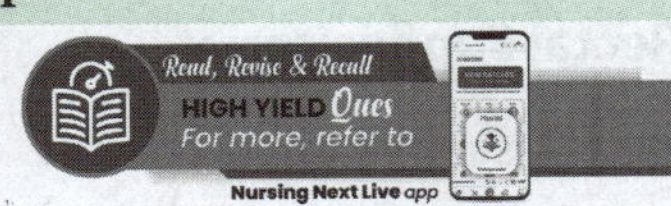

Answer

Causes of Constipation

Mechanical
Benign and malignant tumor
Stricture (e.g., inflammatory, ischemic, anastomotic)
Endometriosis
Uterine fibroids
Volvulus
Metabolic
Diabetes mellitus
Thyroid abnormalities
Mitochondrial disorders
Heavy metal toxicity
Neurological
Multiple sclerosis
Parkinson's disease
Spinal cord injury
Severe cognitive dysfunction
Connective tissue disorders
Systemic sclerosis
Amyloidosis
Mixed connective tissue disease, overlap syndrome
Medications
Opioids
Anticholinergics (e.g., selected antiemetics, antispasmodics)
Calcium-channel blockers
Antihistamines
Anticonvulsants
Diuretics
Motility/functional
Dietary change
Immobility
Colonic inertia
Hirschsprung's disease
Dyssynergic defecation
Irritable bowel syndrome
Chronic idiopathic constipation

b. **List the contraindications for enema.**

Answer

Contraindications for Enema

- **Loose sphincter:** Weak or loose sphincter muscle could result in difficulty retaining the enema solution.
- **Painful and bleeding hemorrhoids:** Enema administration can worsen hemorrhoids or cause bleeding, leading to discomfort and potential complications.
- **Fistula in anus:** An abnormal passage (fistula) near the anus may exacerbate the condition and lead to infection.
- **Painful skin lesions around anus:** Enema usage can cause irritation or damage to painful skin lesions or sores surrounding the anus.
- **Massive carcinoma or tumors of the rectum:** It may cause further obstruction or complications.
- **Acute inflammation of the colon:** Acute inflammation of the colon, such as in cases of severe colitis, as they can worsen the condition.
- **Ulcer:** Enemas should be avoided in patients with ulcers in the rectal or colonic area due to the risk of aggravating the ulcer and causing pain or bleeding.

c. **Nursing responsibilities while administering enema to the patient**

Answer

Preliminary Assessment

- Check the doctor's order and indications as well.
- Check the conscious level, abilities and limitations concerning movement.
- Check the nature of enema ordered and special precautions, if any, to be followed.
- Inspect the rectal and perineal area for any lesion.
- Keep the articles available in the client's unit such as bedpan.

Preparation of the Client and the Unit

- Explain the procedure to the client to win his confidence and cooperation.
- Explain the discomfort caused by the enema fluid and the need for retaining the solution for some time.
- Maintain privacy
- Place the mackintosh and towel under the client's buttocks to protect the bed and the linen.
- Provide left lateral position/sims position to the patient.
- Remove bottom garments or raise it above the waist level.
- Drape the client immediately before giving the enema.

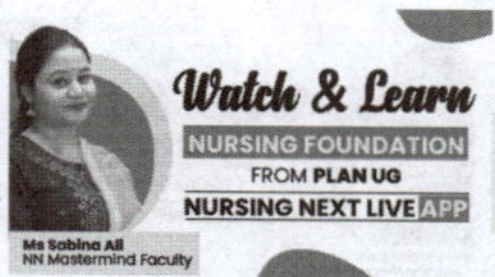

- Fold back a small portion of the sheet or the bath blanket, covering the client to expose only the anus.

General Instructions for Giving Enema

- Use the appropriate size catheter or rectal tube
- The rectal tube needs to be atraumatic
- Use lubricant
- Follow the temperature of solution
- Follow the amount of the solution
- Maintain the correct patient position
- Maintain the height of the enema bag
- Follow the depth of the introduction of rectal tube
- Follow the time of retention of solution in intestines
- Good condition equipment
- Follow the flow speed of fluid
- Prevent air from entering into the rectum
- Observe the patient's condition during the procedure.

After Care of the Client and Articles

- Encourage the clients to retain the fluid for 10 to 15 minutes.
- Encourage slow breathing with open mouth for relaxation.
- Turn the client on the back and assist him onto toilet, commode or bedpan.
- Explain the client that he may need to evacuate the bowel several times in the next few hours.
- Record the type of enema, the result, the untoward results observed, if any, with date and time on the nurse's record.

2. Define urinary retention. Explain the principles of urinary catheterization. Describe the nurse's role in urinary catheterization. (KUHS)

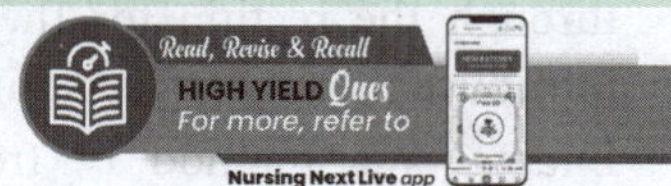

Answer

Urinary Retention

- When the natural process of elimination of the urine from bladder is impaired, urine gets accumulated into the bladder which results into over distention, giving rise to a condition known as urinary retention.
- Over-distention of the bladder causes poor contractibility of the detrusor muscle which further impairs the process of urination.
- In urinary retention, urine production continues but the accumulated urine is not excreted from the bladder.

Principles of Urinary Catheterization

Principles	Rationale
Microorganisms are present in the environment on the articles and on the skin.	Pathogenic organisms are transmitted to a host directly or by contaminated articles.
Always clean from less contaminated to more contaminated area	To minimize the spread of organisms to clean area.
Urinary bladder is a sterile cavity and the urinary meatus acts as a portal of entry for pathogenic organisms.	Strict aseptic techniques are necessary to prevent entry of organisms.
A break in the integrity of the skin and mucous membrane provides ready entrance for microorganisms. Skin and mucous membranes can be injured by chemical, mechanical, thermal and microbial agents.	To prevent injury to the urethra
Lubrication reduces friction.	To prevent injury to the urethra and easy insertion without much discomfort.
Thorough knowledge of anatomy and physiology of the genitourinary system facilitates catheterization of the urinary bladder.	To reduce the difficulties that may arise during insertion of catheter.
Systematic ways saves time, energy and material. Any unfamiliar situations produce anxiety.	Energy can be conserved, can improve the efficiency of nurses and promote better care for the patients.

Nurse's Role in Urinary Catheterization

- Wash hands and wear appropriate PPE before doing urinary catheterization.
- Help the patient to get comfortable in a supine position and drape him/her properly to ensure patient's privacy.
- Assess the need and indication of catheterization.
- Select urinary catheter of appropriate size.
- Catheter insertion is done using strict aseptic technique. Thus, do not touch the sterile field. Use sterile catheter for insertion.
- Clean the perineal area with povidone iodine before urinary catheterization.
- Only after confirmation, fix the catheter
- Place and secure the catheter drainage bag below the level of the bladder and off the floor.
- Remove gown and gloves and wash hands.

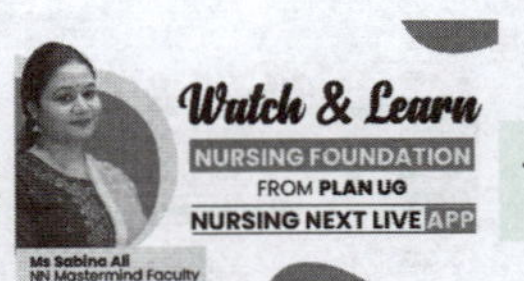

CAUTI Bundle Care

- Maintain strict aseptic technique during insertion of urinary catheter.
- Perform hand hygiene before and after client contact.
- Wear gloves to manipulate the catheter and/or the drainage system.
- Urinary catheter should be anchored by a stabilization device (to the upper thigh in women – upper thigh or lower abdomen in men).
- Catheter should be continuously connected to tubing and drainage system. If catheter was disconnected from the drainage tube, clean the connection site prior to reconnection of tubing.
- Always keep the drainage bag below the level of the bladder and not in contact with the floor.
- Drainage bag should be emptied regularly into a separate clean container dedicated for client use only. There should be no contact between the nonsterile container and the drainage bag spout when emptied.
- Perform catheter care at least once daily and after each bowel movement.
- Nursing role with an indwelling catheter is largely directed toward preventing infection of the urinary tract and encouraging urinary flow through the drainage system.
- It includes encouraging large amounts of fluid intake, changing retention catheter and tubing, maintaining the patency of the drainage system and preventing contamination of the drainage system.

Core Measures for Prevention

- Placement only for appropriate indications.
- Leave catheters in place only as long as needed.
- Ensure that only properly trained persons insert and maintain catheters.
- Insert catheters using aseptic technique and sterile equipment
- Follow aseptic insertion, maintain a closed drainage system
- Maintain unobstructed urine flow.
- Maintain hand hygiene and standard precautions.

Fluids

The client with a retention catheter should drink up to 3,000 mL/day if permitted. Large amounts of fluid intake ensures a large output, which keeps the bladder flushed out and decreases the likelihood of urinary stasis and infection. It also minimizes the risk of sediment obstructing the drainage tubing.

Dietary Measures

Acidifying the urine of clients with a retention catheter may reduce the risk of urinary tract infection and calculus formation. Foods such as eggs, cheese, meat and poultry, whole grains, plums and tomatoes tend to increase the acidity of urine.

Perineal Care

Routine hygienic care is necessary for clients with retention catheter as per hospital practice.

Changing the Catheter and Tubing

Collection of sediments in the catheter or tubing or impaired urine drainage are indicators for changing the catheter and drainage system. When this occurs, the catheter and drainage system are removed and discarded, and a new sterile catheter and closed drainage system is inserted.

Removing Indwelling Catheters

- Indwelling catheters are removed after their purpose has been achieved. If the catheter has been in place for a short time, the client usually has little difficulty regaining normal urinary elimination patterns.
- Clients who have had a retention catheter for a prolonged period may require bladder retraining to regain bladder muscle tone.
- With an indwelling catheter in place, the bladder muscle does not stretch and contract regularly as it does when the bladder fills and empties by voiding.
- A few days, before removal, the catheter may be clamped for specified periods of time (2–4 hours) then released to allow the bladder to empty. This allows the bladder to distend and stimulate its musculature.

SHORT NOTES

1. Write a short note on types of enema. (MGR, KUHS)

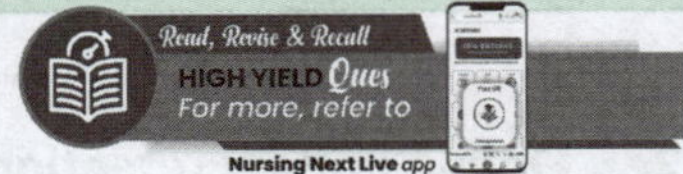

Answer

- An enema is an introduction of fluid into the lower bowel through the rectum for the purpose of cleansing or to introduce medication or nourishment.
- Enema is a method of treatment in which liquid is introduced into the rectum and colon through the anus, then it is flushed out through the bowels.

Evacuant Enema

An Evacuant enema is designed to prompt the bowel to expel fecal matter or flatus, together with the contents of the enema. Phosphate and sodium citrate are the most common types.

- **Simple evacuant enema:** To stimulate defecation and to treat constipation
- **Oil enema:** To soften fecal matter in case of severe constipation. It should be retained for half an hour to

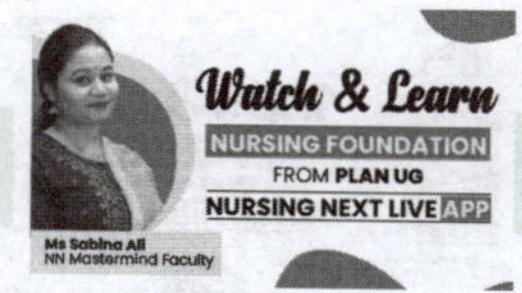

1 hour to soften the feces followed by a soap and water enema to open the bowels

- **Purgative enema:** To contrast actively and to evacuate its contents
- **Anthelmintic enema:** To destroy and expel the worms from the intestines, e.g., Carminitive enema (antispasmodic)
- **Astringent enema:** It lessens the amount of mucus discharge and gives a temporary relief in the inflamed area.
- **Cold enema (ice enema):** To decrease the body temperature in hyperpyrexia and heat stroke

Retained Enema

This enema type is for people whose stool has hardened. This type of enema softens the stool.

- **Stimulant enema:** Used in treatment of shock and collapse
- **Sedative enema:** To induce sleep

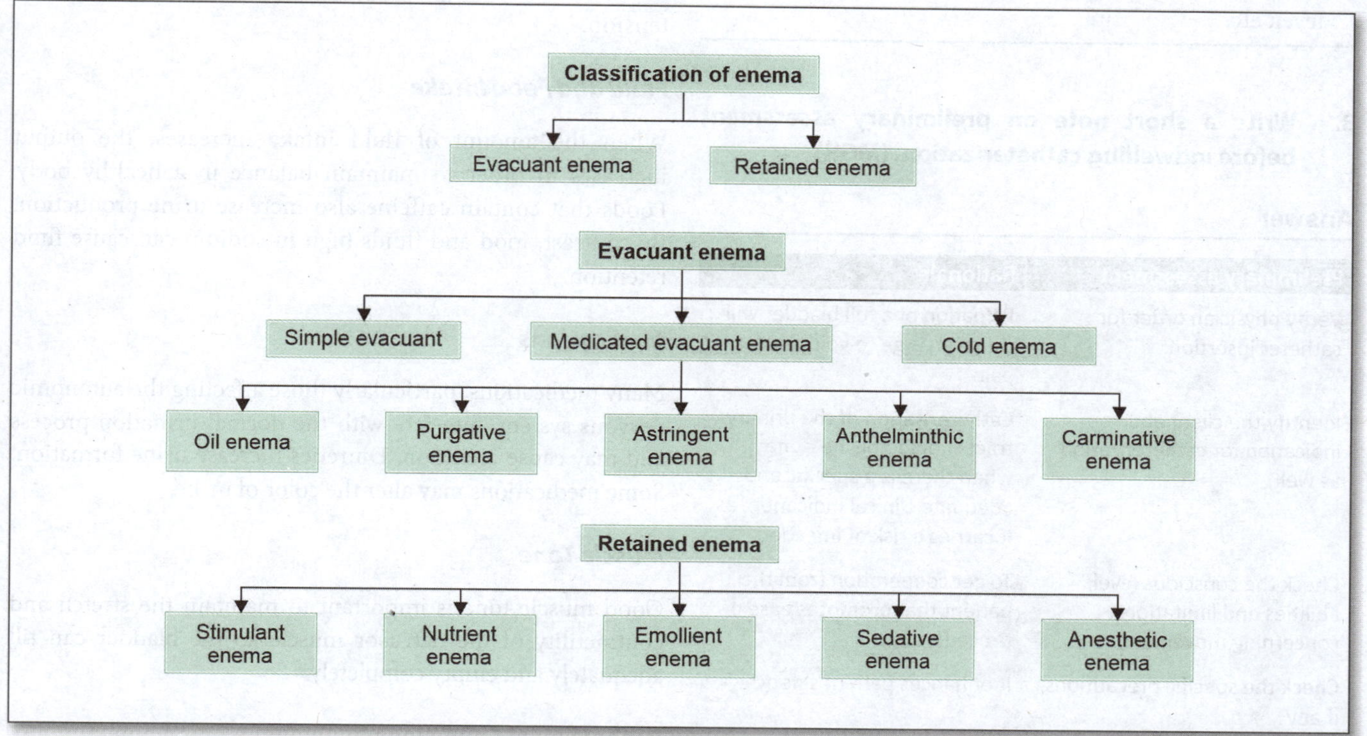

Figure 19.1: Classification of enema

- **Emollient enema:** Introduction of bland solution into the rectum for the purpose of checking diarrhea or soothing and relieving irritation on an inflamed mucus membrane.
- **Anesthetic enema:** It is a retention enema containing an anesthetic drug to produce anesthesia in client
- **Nutrient enema:** It is a retention enema to supply food and fluids to the body

2. Write a note on types and etiology of hematuria. (MGR)

Answer

Hematuria is defined as the presence of 5 or more red blood cells (RBCs) per high-power field in 3 of 3 consecutive centrifuged specimens obtained at least one week apart.

Types

According to the amount of RBC in the urine, hematuria can be classified as:

- **Gross** (i.e., overtly bloody, smoky, or tea-colored urine)
- **Microscopic** > 5 RBCs /HPF

According to timing (when it occurs during urination):

- **Early (initial) hematuria:** Urethral origin, distal to external Sphincter
- **Terminal hematuria:** Bladder neck or prostate origin
- **Diffuse (total) hematuria:** Source is in the bladder or upper urinary tract

Etiology

- Glomerulonephritis
- Renal cystic diseases

- Acute pyelonephritis tuberculosis
- Renal allograft rejection
- Malignancy
- Trauma
- Cystitis/Urethritis/Prostatitis
- Arterial emboli or thrombosis
- Renal vein thrombosis
- Hemophilia, ITP (idiopathic thrombocytopenic purpura), infective endocarditis, Septicemia, epidemic hemorrhagic fever, etc.

3. Write a short note on preliminary assessment before indwelling catheterization. (MGR)

Answer

Preliminary assessment	Rationale
Verify physician order for catheter insertion	Palpation of a full bladder will cause an urge to void and/or pain.
Identify the client and indication for catheterization as well	Catheterisation of the urinary tract should only be done when there is a specific and adequate clinical indication, as it carries a risk of infection.
Check the conscious level, abilities and limitations concerning movement	To get cooperation from the patient that promotes ease of procedure.
Check the specific precautions, if any	It enhances patient safety.
Inspect the perineal area before insertion	Assessment of perineal area allows for determination of perineal condition and position of anatomical landmarks to assist with insertion.
Perform the part preparation	Preparation ahead of time enhances patient comfort and safety.
Provide perineal care before insertion and maintain CAUTI bundle	Cleaning removes any secretions, urine, and feces, and reduces risk of CAUTI.
Keep the articles available in the client's unit	This step ensures preparation and organization for procedure.

4. Write a short note on factors affecting normal urinary elimination. (MGR)

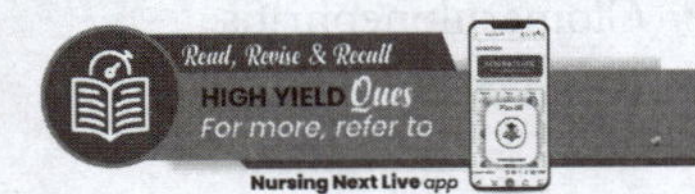

Answer

Factors Affecting Normal Urinary Elimination

Psychosocial Factors

For many people, a set of conditions helps stimulate the micturition reflex. These conditions include privacy, normal position, sufficient time, and occasionally, running water. Circumstances that do not allow for the client's accustomed conditions may produce anxiety and muscle tension.

Fluid and Food Intake

When the amount of fluid intake increases, the output increases in order to maintain balance in a healthy body. Foods that contain caffeine also increase urine production. By contrast, food and fluids high in sodium can cause fluid retention.

Medications

Many medications, particularly those affecting the autonomic nervous system, interfere with the normal urination process and may cause retention. Diuretics increase urine formation. Some medications may alter the color of urine.

Muscle Tone

Good muscle tone is important to maintain the stretch and contractility of the detrusor muscle so the bladder can fill adequately and empty completely.

Pathological Conditions

Diseases of the kidney may affect the ability of nephrons to produce urine.

5. Write a short note on bowel wash and flatulence. (MGR)

Answer

Bowel Wash

Washing out of colon with large quantities of solution, to clear colon of feces.

Procedure

The procedure typically involves using a special enema kit or equipment to introduce the cleansing solution into the rectum. The solution may consist of water, saline, or a specific bowel cleansing agent.

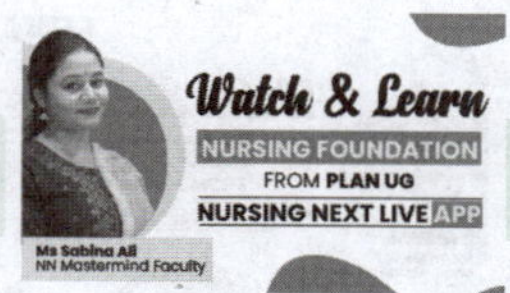

As the liquid is introduced, it travels up the colon, softening and dislodging stool and debris, which is then expelled from the body along with the liquid.

Purposes

- To prepare colon for specific surgical or diagnostic procedures
- To dilute and remove toxic agents that may be present in large intestine
- To reduce temperature in hyperpyrexia and heat stroke
- To supply fluid and electrolytes that are absorbed from intestine
- To stimulate peristalsis
- To keep the individual clean in case of fecal incontinence

Contraindications

- Bleeding hemorrhoids
- Chronic diarrhea
- Rectal surgeries
- Intestinal obstruction
- Rectal polyps, etc.

Flatulence

- Flatulence is the accumulation of excessive amount of gas (flatus) in the gastrointestinal tract, leading to distention of the abdomen
- This is also known as tympanites.

6. Write a short note on factors affecting bowel elimination. (MGR)

Answer

Factors Affecting Bowel Elimination

Age

Must be of a certain age or physical maturity to be able to control your bowels. Humans also can lose control of their bowels after a certain age.

Diet

There many different ways that diet can affect bowel elimination e.g., high fiber diets and fruits promote regularity, while cheese causes constipation.

Fluid Intake

The more fluid you take in, the less likely you are to become constipated.

The less fluid you take in, the more likely you are to become constipated.

Physical Activity

Higher activity rate lessens the chances of constipation.

Psychological Factor

- Usually the source of ulcerative colitis or crohn's disease
- Depression causes peristalsis to decrease

Positions

Normal positioning for bowel elimination is sitting or squatting.

Pain

Person may be hesitant about going if they think it will cause them pain, usually due to hemorrhoids, rectal surgery, or abdominal surgery.

Medications

Different medications affect bowel elimination differently. Some medications increase the process and others may inhibit it or stop it completely.

Diagnostic Tests

These affect the patient because they usually require them to be NPO prior to it which will limit their food intake and in turn will limit bowel elimination or stop them completely.

7. Write a short note on purposes of bladder irrigation. (MGR, DU)

Answer

Purposes of bladder irrigation are:

- To clean the bladder from decomposed urine, bacteria, excess of mucus, pus and blood clots.
- To maintain the patency of the urinary catheter.
- To relieve congestion and pain in case of inflammatory conditions by the application of heat.
- To promote healing.
- To prevent the clot formation in case of bladder surgeries.
- To prevent and treat infections.
- To arrest bleeding.

8. Write a short note on patient with urinary incontinence. (DU)

Answer

A number of measures can be used to reduce the problem of incontinence:

- **Urinary incontinence:** It is any involuntary leakage of urine that is widely under reported and undiagnosed. It is more prevalent in women and increases with age.
- Establish a regular voiding schedule for the client, e.g., every 2 hours whether he or she feels the urge or not.
- Increase the physical activity. This will improve the muscle tone, thus helping the client to control voiding.
- Perineal exercises: These increase the tone of muscles concerned with the micturition, in particular, the perineal and abdominal muscles. Periodic tightening of the perineal muscles, intentionally stopping and then starting the urine stream, etc., can help in gaining voiding control.
- Arrange for toilet or bedpan within the easy reach of the client. If the incontinent client can get into a toilet or bedpan quickly, this will gradually help him to gain confidence in his control of the bladder.
- Medical and surgical correction of the causative factors, e.g., treatment of the urinary tract infections, correction of the anatomic problem.
- **Bladder training program:** An exercise program is started to strengthen the involved muscles. The client is placed on the commode or toilet every 1 to 2 hours depending on the frequency of micturition. The intervals are lengthened as the program progresses.
- **Skin care:** The major problem caused by incontinence is skin irritation and maceration. The skin that is constantly bathed in moisture, becomes macerated. The skin should be kept clean and dry.
- **Condom drainage:** A male client with incontinence of urine can be safely managed with a condom drainage.

9. Write a short note on patient with ileostomy. (DU)

Answer

Assessment

- Identify the type and location of ostomy in the patient.
- Assess the skin integrity around the stoma and appearance.
- Note the amount and character of fecal material in pouch.

Procedure

- Arrange all the necessary articles.
- Explain the procedure to the patient.
- Provide privacy and assist patient to a comfortable position.
- Wash hands and wear gloves to prevent infection.
- Spread Mackintosh and draw sheet to protect linen
- Remove used pouch and skin barrier gently by pushing the skin away from the barrier.
- Reduces trauma, and jerking, that irritate skin and can cause tear.
- Remove clamp and empty the contents into the bedpan.
- Rinse the pouch with tepid water or normal saline to minimize the odor and growth of microbes
- Discard the disposable pouch in paper bag.
- Observe stoma for color, swelling, trauma and healing. Stoma should be moist and pink
- Cover the stoma with a gauze piece to prevent the contact of fecal matters from contacting with skin
- Clean stoma gently with warm tap water using gauze pad.
- Do not scrub the skin, dry completely by patting the skin with gauze.
- Remove gauze and clean stoma with gauze and pat dry.
- Measure the stoma using measuring guide.
- Ensure accuracy in determining correct pouch size needed.
- Trace same circle behind the skin barrier, using scissors, cut an opening 1/16th to 1/8th inch larger than stoma before removing the wrapper over adhesive part.
- Put skin barrier and pouch over the stoma, and gently press on to the skin, for 1–2 minutes.
- Use the pouch if it is drainable using a clamp or clip
- Remove gloves and wash hands.
- Make the patient comfortable
- Clean the area and replace all articles.

10. Write a short note on Urinary retention and incontinence. (KUHS)

Answer

Urinary Retention

- When emptying the bladder is impaired, urine accumulates and the bladder becomes over-distended, giving rise to a condition known as urinary retention.
- Over-distention of the bladder causes poor contractibility of the detrusor muscle which further impairs urination.
- In urinary retention, urine production continues but the accumulated urine is not released from the bladder.

Assessment

Assess the client's normal voiding pattern, frequency, appearance of urine, presence of any urinary diversions. Percussion of the bladder and if there is a need of inspection of urethral meatus for any swelling, discharge and inflammation.

In case of urinary retention, bladder will be found firm, distended and may be displaced to one side of midline.

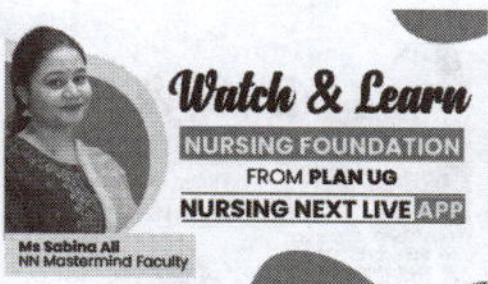

Intervention

Assisting the client with providing a urinal for men and women use bedpan for the same. In order to initiate voiding, urinary catheterization may be necessary to empty the bladder completely. Maintain normal voiding habits by providing adequate position, relaxation and use of usual times of voiding. Provide the warm bed pan, assist them with toileting and preventing UTIs.

Urinary Incontinence

- Urinary incontinence is the inability of the urinary sphincters to control the passage of the urine from the bladder.
- **Complete incontinence** indicates total emptying of bladder
- **Partial incontinence** means dribbling of urine without total drainage of the bladder.

Types of Incontinence

- Stress incontinence: Due to increased abdominal pressure under stress
- Urge incontinence: Due to involuntary contraction of bladder muscles
- Overflow incontinence: Blockage of urethra
- Neurogenic incontinence: Impaired functioning of the nervous system

Assessment

Review the client's record to determine a pattern of voiding and other pertinent data. Assess the condition of skin on penis and urethral meatus also. Assessment of physical and psychological factors should also keep in mind as the etiology of urinary incontinence.

Intervention

It is one of the most common chronic health problems. Various interventions include

- **Bladder training:** Voiding may be encouraged every 2–3 hours except during sleep and then every 4–6 hours. A vital component of bladder training is inhibiting the urge-to-void sensation.
- **Habit training** or scheduled toileting, attempts to keep clients dry by having them void at regular intervals.
- **Pelvic muscle exercises or Kegel exercises** help to strengthen pelvic floor muscles and can reduce or eliminate episodes of incontinence. The incontinent person requires meticulous **skin care**. The application of a **condom or external catheter** connected to a urinary drainage system can be used for incontinent males.

11. Write the procedure for giving enema to a patient. (KUHS)

Answer

Assessment

- Assess bowel movement of patient
- Determine the level of consciousness and understanding, provide privacy
- Explain the purpose of the procedure to the patient
- Assemble articles, wash hands and don gloves
- Raise the bed to appropriate height
- Assist patient to side lying position (sim's position)
- Place mackintosh under hip and buttocks
- Cover the patient exposing only anal area, clearly visualizing anus
- Place bedpan or commode in an easily accessible position

Articles Required

- Enema container and tubing with clamp
- Bedpan or bedside commode
- Lubricant
- Gloves
- Enema solution
- Bath blanket
- Tissue wipes
- Mackintosh
- Kidney tray
- Paper bag

Procedure

- Remove plastic cap from rectal tip and lubricate the tip
- Gently separate the buttocks and locate the anus. Instruct the patient to relax by breathing out through mouth.
- Insert tip of the tube gently into rectum: Adult: 7.5 cm, Child: 5–7.5 cm, Infant: 2.5–3.7 cm
- Squeeze the container until all solution has entered rectum and sigmoid colon while squeezing container roll it up as fluid is instilled
- Place toilet tissue around the anus and withdraw the tube
- Discard the disposable items in proper receptacle
- Assist the patient to toilet or help to position on bedpan
- Observe the fecal matter and expelled solution
- Remove gloves and discard, wash hands.
- Assess condition of patient's abdomen, cramping or rigidity which can indicate problems.
- Record the enema given and characteristics of result.
- Report any problem if noticed.

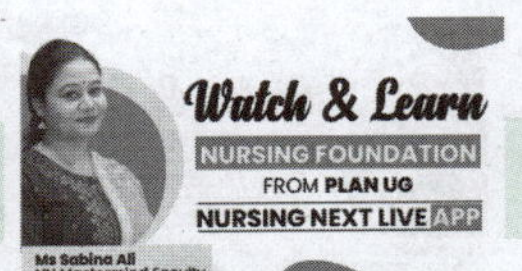

12. Write a short note on oliguria and anuria. (KUHS)

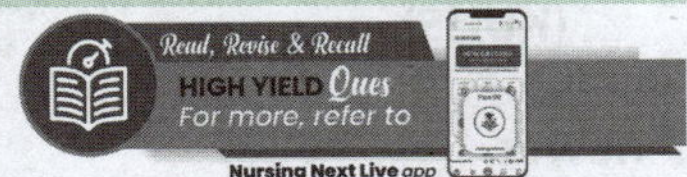

Answer

Oliguria

- Oliguria is urine output <1 mL/kg/h in adults and < 0.5 mL/ kg/h in children.
- Oliguria is not a clinical diagnosis but a sign that indicates an underlying disorder.
- Oliguria, if left untreated may lead to acute renal failure and its sequelae, including hyperkalemia, acidosis, and fluid overload.

Anuria

- Anuria is the production of urine <50 mL/day.
- There are numerous causes of anuria, such as renal impairment, urinary tract obstruction (kidney stones), pharmaceutical agents or severe infections (septicemia).
- Anuria is a symptom, not a disease.
- The patient often complains about weakness, fatigue, lack of appetite, vomiting tendency and dyspnea.

13. Write a short note on colostomy and gastrostomy. (KUHS)

Answer

Colostomy

Colostomy is an artificial opening (stoma) in the large intestine brought to the surface of the abdomen for the purpose of evacuation of bowel.

Classification

According to Time

- Temporary Colostomy
- Permanent Colostomy

According to Stoma site

- Ascending Colostomy
- Transverse Colostomy
- Descending Colostomy

According to Stoma Number and Type

- Single-barrel colostomy
- Loop colostomy
- Double-barrel colostomy

Indications

- Colon cancer
- Ulcerative colitis
- Hirschsprung's disease
- Polyps in intestine

Gastrostomy

Gastrostomy is defined as an opening in the stomach made surgically, usually connecting the stomach to the outside of the abdomen so that a feeding tube or gut decompression tube can be passed into the stomach.

Indications for Gastrostomy

- Neurological swallowing disorders, e.g., cerebral palsy, multiple sclerosis, etc.
- Esophageal stricture or atresia
- Esophageal cancer
- Gastric outlet or small bowel obstruction
- Major neck surgeries

14. Write a short note on constipation and faecal impaction. (KUHS)

Answer

Constipation

Constipation occurs when stool moves through the large intestine too slowly or remains in the large intestine for too long. Constipation is referred to the person's normal defecation pattern and involves a change in stool consistency (harder and drier than usual) and a change in defecation frequency (less than usual).

Causes

- Intestinal obstruction
- Intestinal tumor, adhesions, stenosis, etc.
- Insufficient fluid intake
- Lack of exercise and prolonged bedrest
- Use of certain drugs, e.g., sedatives and beverages such as coffee, tea, etc.
- Embarrassment about using a bedpan.
- Fecal impaction
- Insufficient intake of roughage

Management

- Adequate intake of diet
- Adequate intake of roughage in diet
- Encourage squatting position while defecation
- Regular exercise
- Adequate amount of fluid intake
- Use of laxatives, suppositories and enemas, if indicated
- Use of relaxation technique to reduce stress that interferes with defecation reflex
- Establish a healthy eating habit pattern

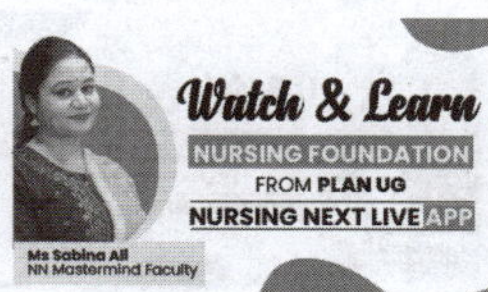

Fecal Impaction

Fecal impaction is the accumulation of hardened feces in the rectum, and the patient is unable to voluntarily evacuate the stool.

Fecal impaction must be suspected:

- History of constipation for 3–5 days or more followed by passage of liquid or liquid stool.
- Passage of semi-liquid stool from the seepage of unformed fecal tests around the impacted stool in the rectum, the pressure from the large mass of accumulated fecal contents.

Signs and Symptoms

- Fullness of rectum and abdomen
- Bloating
- An urge for defecation but unable to pass
- Malaise
- Anorexia
- Nausea or vomiting
- Abdominal distension

Management: Laxatives, enema and digital evacuation

SHORT ANSWER QUESTIONS

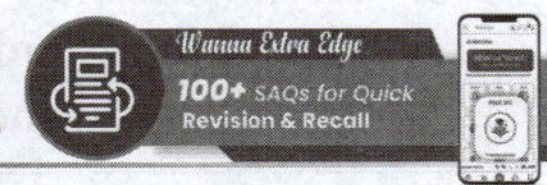

1. List the contraindications for enema.

Answer

- Loose sphincter
- Painful and bleeding hemorrhoids
- Fistula in anus
- Painful skin lesions around anus
- Massive carcinoma or tumors of rectum
- Bleeding piles
- Acute inflammation of colon
- Ulcer

2. Define urinary retention.

Answer

When emptying the bladder is impaired, urine accumulates and the bladder becomes over-distended, giving rise to a condition known as urinary retention.

3. What is enema? List types of enema. (MGR)

Answer

An enema is the introduction of fluid into the lower bowel through the rectum for the purpose of cleansing or to introduce medication or nourishment.

Enema is a method of treatment in which liquid is introduced into the rectum and colon through the anus, then flushed out through the bowels.

- Classification of eneme
- Evacuant enema
- Retained enema

4. Enumerate purposes of bladder irrigation. (MGR, DU)

Answer

- To clean the bladder from decomposed urine, bacteria, excess of mucus, pus and blood clots.
- To maintain the patency of the urinary catheter.
- To relieve congestion and pain in case of inflammatory conditions by the application of heat.
- To promote healing.
- To prevent the clot formation in case of bladder surgeries.
- To prevent and treat infections.
- To arrest bleeding.

5. Define urinary retention and incontinence. (KUHS)

Answer

Urinary Retention

When emptying the bladder is impaired, urine accumulates and the bladder becomes over-distended, giving rise to a condition known as urinary retention.

Urinary Incontinence

It is the inability of the urinary sphincters to control the passage of the urine from the bladder.

6. What is hematuria? (MGR)

Answer

Hematuria is defined as the presence of 5 or more red blood cells (RBCs) per high-power field in 3 of 3 consecutive centrifuged specimens obtained at least one week apart.

CONCEPTUAL REVISION

MULTIPLE CHOICE QUESTIONS

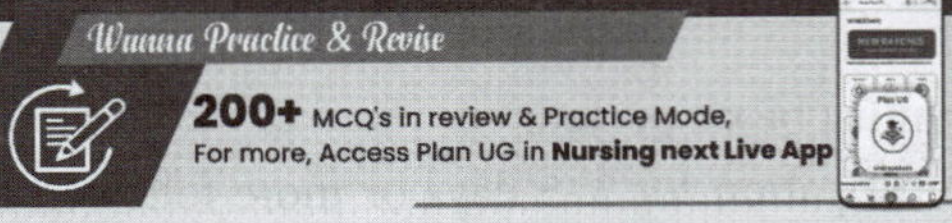

1. The nurse administers a cleansing enema. The common position for this procedure is:

a. Sims left lateral b. Dorsal Recumbent
c. Supine d. Prone

Ans. a. Sims left lateral

2. Immobility impairs bladder elimination, resulting in such disorders as:

a. Increased urine acidity and relaxation of the perineal muscles, causing incontinence
b. Urine retention, bladder distention, and infection
c. Diuresis, natriuresis, and decreased urine specific gravity
d. Decreased calcium and phosphate levels in the urine

Ans. b. Urine retention, bladder distention, and infection

3. While a nurse is administering a cleansing enema, the client reports abdominal cramping. Which of the following is the appropriate intervention?

a. Have a client hold his breath briefly.
b. Discontinue the fluid installation.
c. Remind the client that cramping is common at this time.
d. Lower the enema fluid container.

Ans. d. Lower the enema fluid container.

4. A nurse is preparing to administer a cleansing enema to an adult client in preparation for a diagnostic procedure. Which of the following are appropriate steps for the nurse to take? Select all that apply.

i. Warm the enema solution prior to installation.
ii. Position the client on the left side with the right leg flexed forward.
iii. Lubricate the rectal tube or nozzle.
iv. Slowly insert the rectal tube about 2 inches.
v. Hang the enema container 24 inches above the client's anus.

a. i, ii, iii
b. ii, iii, iv
c. iii, iv, v
d. i, iii, v

Ans. a. i, ii, iii

5. A nurse is caring for a client who has diarrhea for the past four days. When assessing a client, the nurse should expect which of the following findings? Select all that apply.

i. Bradycardia ii. Hypotension
iii. Fever iv. Poor skin turgor
v. Peripheral edema

a. ii, iii, iv b. i, ii, v
c. ii, iv, v d. iii, iv, v

Ans. a. ii, iii, iv

6. A nurse is talking with a client who reports constipation. When the nurse discusses dietary changes that can help prevent constipation, which of the following foods should the nurse recommend?

a. Macaroni and cheese
b. Fresh food and whole-wheat toast
c. Rice pudding and ripe bananas
d. Roast chicken and white rice

Ans. b. Fresh food and whole-wheat toast

7. A nurse discourages a patient from straining excessively when attempting to have a bowel movement. What physiological response primarily may be prevented by avoiding straining on defecation?

a. Incontinence b. Dysrhythmias
c. Fecal impaction d. Rectal hemorrhoids

Ans. b. Dysrhythmias

8. A practitioner orders a return flow enema (Harris flush drip) for an adult patient with flatulence. When preparing to administer this enema, the nurse compares the steps of a return flow enema with cleansing enemas. What should the nurse do that is unique to a return flow enema?

a. Lubricate the last 2 inches of the rectal tube.
b. Insert the rectal tube about 4 inches into the anus.
c. Raise the solution container about 12 inches above the anus.
d. Lower the solution container after instilling about 150 mL of solution.

Ans. d. Lower the solution container after instilling about 150 mL of solution.

CHAPTER 20

Diagnostic Testing

CONCEPTUAL THEORY

Terminology

150+ key terminologies for Quick Recall & Revision

Arthroscopy: Examines joint structures, primarily the knee. It is a surgical procedure used to visualize, diagnose, and treat problems inside a joint.

Bone marrow biopsy: A small sample of bone marrow (usually from the hip) is removed via a slender needle. This type of biopsy helps to diagnose diseases such as leukemia.

Bronchoscopy: Examines the bronchus and bronchial tree.

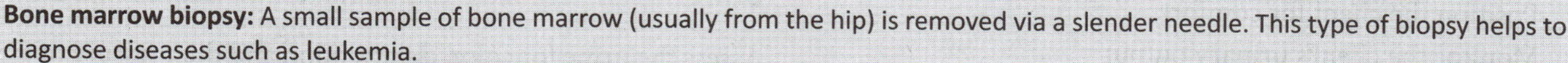

Cardiac Ultrasonography (Echocardiography): This test checks both the heart valves and the movement and thickness of the heart walls.

Chest X-ray: This test determines the heart's size and position, and whether the lungs are functioning properly.

Colonoscopy: Examines the large intestine.

Colposcopy: Examines the cervix and vagina following a positive Pap smear.

Colposcopy-directed biopsy: A colposcope is a small microscope used to examine a woman's cervix while a tissue sample is taken. This biopsy is usually performed to investigate the reasons for an abnormal Pap test result.

Cystoscopy: To examine the bladder and ureter openings.

Electrocardiogram (ECG): This test evidences the characteristics and duration of the heart's electrical activity. It is a test to measure the electrical activity of the brain.

Endoscopic biopsy: The endoscope is a flexible tube that can be inserted into an orifice (such as the mouth or anus) or through a small skin incision. Once the lump is reached, cutting tools are threaded through the endoscope so that a sample of tissue can be taken.

Esophagogastroduodenoscopy (EGD): Examines the esophagus, stomach, and upper duodenum.

Excisional biopsy: This type of biopsy may be used for breast lumps.

Holter ECG: A portable recording device monitors the time of occurrence of the extra- systoles over twenty-four hours.

Incisional biopsy: This type of biopsy may be used for lumps located in connective tissue such as muscle.

Invasive: Means that the body's tissues, organs, or cavities are accessed through some type of instrument.

Laparoscopy: Examines the peritoneal cavity: pelvis and abdomen.

Non-invasive: Means that the body is not entered with any type of instrument; the skin and other body tissues, organs, and cavities remain intact.

Proctoscope: To examine the lower rectum and anal canal.

Urethroscopy: To examine the bladder neck and the urethra

Urine testing: Refers to laboratory analysis on a routine or clean voided specimen or a specimen obtained from catheter to perform a routine or microscopic examination of urine.

TYPE OF DIAGNOSTIC TESTS AND THE ROLE OF NURSE

Diagnostic tests are of two types: noninvasive and invasive. Noninvasive means that the body is not entered with any type of instrument; the skin and other body tissues, organs, and cavities remain intact. Invasive means that the body's tissues, organs, or cavities are accessed through some type of instrument.

The nurse teaches the client, family and significant others to prepare for the specific tests and the care required after the test.

The nurse plays a key role in scheduling and preparing for diagnostic testing. Nurses establish baseline, vital signs, identify known allergies, and assess teaching effectiveness. Nurse advises the client about the things to expect during the procedure and the outcomes to decrease anxiety.

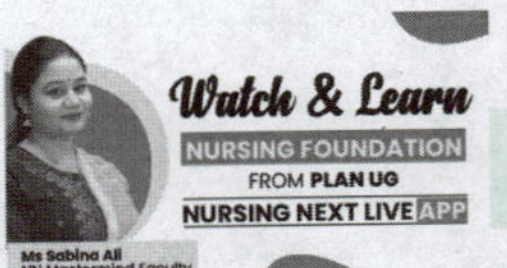

Care of the Client During Preparation

- Ensure that the client is wearing an identification band
- Review the medical record
- Monitor vital signs
- Monitor level of hydration and weakness implement NPO status,
- Document in the record regarding preparation

Care of the Client During Diagnostic Testing

- Use of standard precautions
- Label all specimens
- Prepare the procedure room, supplies, testing of equipment
- Assist the client to a comfortable, safe position
- Document the details of test

Care of the Client after Diagnostic Testing

- Assess the client closely for any bleeding, vital signs, pain, respiratory distress
- Position the client for comfort
- Monitor the client's urinary output
- **Teach the client and the family members about:**
  - Dietary or activity restrictions
  - Medications to be taken
- **Document in the client's medical record:** Achievement of expected outcomes

It is the responsibility of the nurse that the specimens are accurately obtained, labeled in appropriate container and transported to the laboratory on time.

It includes:

- **Blood tests such as**
  - Type and Cross Match
  - Blood biochemistry
  - Complete hemogram
- **Culture and sensitivity tests**
  - Sputum culture
  - Blood culture
  - Throat culture

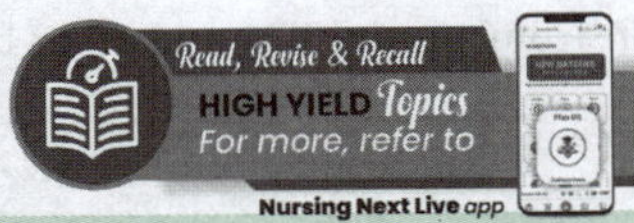

OBSERVATION OF SPECIMENS

Specimens

A specimen is a small sample or part taken to show the nature of the whole as a small quantity of urine, stool, vomitus or a small fragment of tissue for a microscopic study.

The specimens collected for various examinations are urine, stool and sputum.

TABLE 20.1: Specimen and types of examination

Specimen	Type of examination
Urine	• Collection of mid-stream urine • Routine examination • Culture and sensitivity • 24-hour urine • Pregnancy test • Double voided specimen
Stool	• Routine microscopic and culture • Occult blood • Ova and cyst
Sputum	• Microscopic acid fast bacilli • Culture

Urine testing refers to laboratory analysis on a routine or clean voided specimen or a specimen obtained from catheter to perform a routine or microscopic examination of urine. **It includes: Urinary pH, Specific Gravity, Urine Sugar, Acetone, Albumin, etc.**

Urine

Assess the urine for color, clarity, odor, and the pressure of any sediment. Monitor the pH and specific gravity of the urine and check the urine for abnormal constituents such as proteins, blood, glucose, ketone bodies and bacteria.

Stool

Examination of stool helps in diagnosis of gastrointestinal tract problems and worm infestation.

Sputum

Its observation helps to detect the function of respiratory system and any disease process.

Vomitus

Observation of vomitus helps to detect gastric and intestinal disorders, poisoning and irritation to vomiting centers due to increased intracranial pressure.

Radiological Studies

- **Electrocardiogram (ECG):** This test evidences the characteristics and duration of the heart's electrical activity.
- **Electroencephalography (EEG):** It is a test to measure the electrical activity of the brain.
- **Holter ECG:** A portable recording device monitors the time of occurrence of the extrasystoles over twenty-four hours.

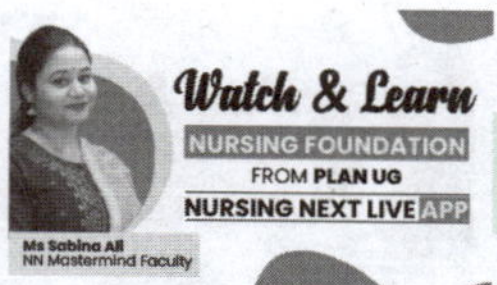

- **Chest X-ray:** This test determines the heart's size and position, and whether the lungs are functioning properly.
- **Cardiac Ultrasonography (Echocardiography):** This test checks both the heart valves and the movement and thickness of the heart walls.

Invasive Diagnostic Tests

- **Endoscopic procedures** include the followings:
  - **Arthroscopy:** Examines joint structures, primarily the knee. It is a surgical procedure used to visualize, diagnose, and treat problems inside a joint.
  - **Bronchoscopy:** Examines the bronchus and bronchial tree.
  - **Colonoscopy:** Examines the large intestine.
  - **Colposcopy:** Examines the cervix and vagina following a positive Pap smear.
  - **Cystourethroscopy:** Uses two instruments:
    - **Cystoscope:** To examine the bladder and ureter openings
    - **Urethroscope:** To examine the bladder neck and the urethra
  - **Esophagogastroduodenoscopy (EGD):** Examines the esophagus, stomach, and upper duodenum.
  - **Laparoscopy:** Examines the peritoneal cavity: pelvis and abdomen.
  - **Proctoscope:** To examine the lower rectum and anal canal.
- **Biopsy procedures:** There are various kinds of biopsy procedures, including:
  - **Bone marrow biopsy:** A small sample of bone marrow (usually from the hip) is removed via a slender needle. This type of biopsy helps to diagnose diseases such as leukemia.
  - **Colposcopy-directed biopsy:** A colposcope is a small microscope used to examine a woman's cervix while a tissue sample is taken. This biopsy is usually performed to investigate the reasons for an abnormal Pap test result.
  - **Endoscopic biopsy:** The endoscope is a flexible tube that can be inserted into an orifice (such as the mouth or anus) or through a small skin incision. Once the lump is reached, cutting tools are threaded through the endoscope so that a sample of tissue can be taken.
  - **Excisional biopsy:** This type of biopsy may be used for breast lumps.
  - **Incisional biopsy:** This type of biopsy may be used for lumps located in connective tissue such as muscle.
  - **Needle biopsy:** This type of biopsy may be used to diagnose conditions of the liver or thyroid.
  - **Punch biopsy:** This type of biopsy can help diagnose various skin conditions.
  - **Stereotactic biopsy:** This type of biopsy is usually performed whenever the lump is hard to see or feel.
- **Lumbar puncture:** CSF is withdrawn through a needle inserted in to the subarachnoid space of the spinal canal between L3 and L4 or between L4 and L5

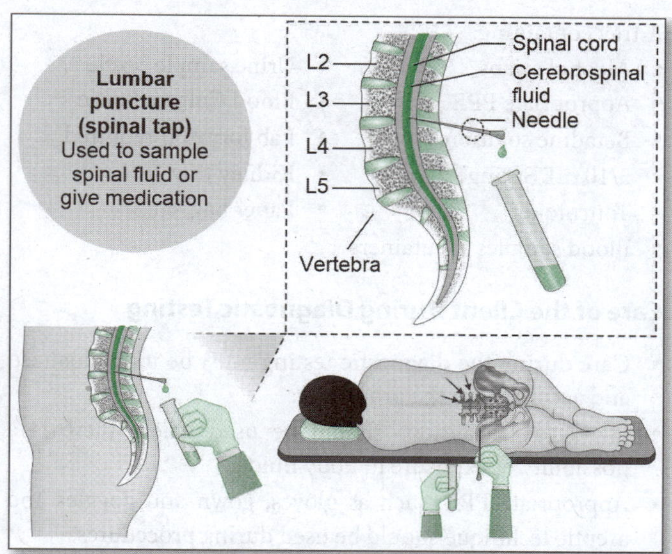

CONCEPTUAL EXERCISES

LONG ANSWER QUESTION

1. Write the nursing responsibilities for diagnostic testing. (MGR)

Answer

Introduction

- Nurse plays a vital role in scheduling the date and time of sample collection and preparing the patients/clients for sample collection or diagnostic testing.
- The nursing responsibility varies depends on the type of diagnostic test being performed.
- The diagnostic test may be invasive or non-invasive.
- The invasive diagnostic proceudres includes Biopsy, Endoscopy, Cardiac catheterization, Lumbar puncture, Angiography, Bronchoscopy, Colonoscopy, Cystoscopy, Arthroscopy, Laparoscopy.
- Non-Invasive Diagnostic Procedures include X-ray, MRI, CT scan, Ultrasound, ECG, EEG, Spirometry, Doppler ultrasound, USG, Mammogram, PET scan, etc.

During Preparation and Assessment of Clients/ Patients by the Nurse

- Ensure that the patient is wearing an identification band.
- Review the medical record for any known allergies and any drug-related adverse reactions.
- Collect the consent form from the concerned doctor.
- Check-Doctors order.
- Monitor the vital signs of the patient including pain to get the baseline data.
- Monitor the hydration status of the patients/clients.
- As per the instructions of the concerned doctor for the diagnostic test, implement NPO, status administration of laxatives, establishing IV access and teaching relaxation techniques, etc.
- Collect the barcode of all samples.
- Document all the necessary findings of patient for diagnostic test, e.g., allergies, etc.

Articles Required

A tray containing:

- Alcohol swabs
- Appropriate PPE
- Betadine solution
- 5/10 mL Syringe
- Tourniquet
- Blood samples vacutainers
- Urine sample bottle
- Blood Culture bottle
- Lab forms, if required
- Kidney tray
- Paper bag, etc.

Care of the Client During Diagnostic Testing

- Care during the diagnostic testing must be individualized and according to the procedure.
- Standard precautions should be used where there is a possibility of exposure to body fluids.
- Appropriate PPE, such as gloves, gown and goggles and aseptic technique should be used during procedures.
- Label all specimens correctly with the client's name, date, time and specimen.
- Follow all the instructions properly applicable for the storage and transportation of samples to lab.
- Prepare the procedure room, all required articles and testing of equipment.
- Provide comfortable and safe position to the patients.
- Document the details of tests in the record chart such as the HCPs who performed the procedure, indications for the procedure, type of anesthesia used, dye and medications administered during the procedure.
- Continuous monitoring of vital signs and other parameters, if indicated.
- Monitor for complications during the procedure.
- Assist the doctor during the procedure.

Care of the Client after Diagnostic Testing

- Recording and monitoring of vital signs after the procedure.
- Assess the patients for any signs of bleeding, pain, respiratory distress, etc.
- Position the client as per comfort or as per the instructions.
- Monitor and record the urinary output.
- Dismantle all the articles used. Send for cleaning/ disinfection/sterilization as per need.

Teach the client and the family members about:

- Dietary pattern
- Signs and symptoms or early warning signs that should be reported immediately to the physician
- Medications to be administered and their side effects also.

Principles of Specimen Collection

- Contaminated and improperly collected specimens will produce false results which will adversely affect the diagnosis and treatment of clients.
- Specimens allowed to remain at the room temperature for a long time will give a false result.
- Blood chemistry is not uniform throughout the day; it varies with the food intake.
- The accuracy and reliability of findings depend upon the correct method of collection, transportation of the specimens to the laboratory and recording of reports. Inaccurate results may mislead the physician in the diagnosis and treatment of clients.
- Specimens serve as a media for transmission of disease producing organisms to the personnel who handle them carelessly.

SHORT NOTES

1. Discuss the different methods of urine collection with the purposes of respective methods.

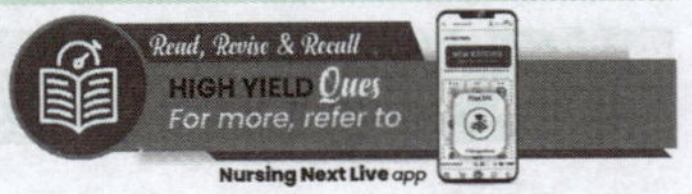

Answer

Methods of Collection of Urine Specimens

- There are various methods of urine sample collection, depending on the purpose of the test and the specific requirements.

Types of urine specimens:

- **Random sample:** Sample which is collected anytime during the day for routine screening
- **First voided specimen:** Sample also referred to as a first morning specimen collected the first time in the morning. A first voided specimen is the preferred specimen for

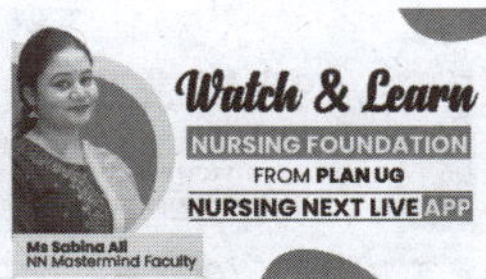

pregnancy testing, bacterial cultures and microscopic examinations.

- **Timed specimen:** These specimens requires urine samples to be taken at specific intervals during the day. Twenty-four (24) hour urine specimens are required for creatinine clearance tests and other hormone studies.
- **Clean-catch midstream specimen:** This sample type is collected and examined for bacterial growth or used for cytology.
- **Dirty collection:** This specimen used for DNA testing and the FIRST part of the voided stream is collected.
- **Catheterized specimen:** These specimens are obtained by inserting a catheter/sterile flexible tube into the bladder via the urethra to withdraw urine.

24-hour Urine Specimen

For 24-hour urine specimen, the collection is initiated at a specified time from 6 am to 6 am of next day in a receptacle.

- After 24 hours are over, the specimen is collected and preservatives are added as per the institutional policy to prevent decomposition and multiplication of bacteria.
- The specimen is labeled before the start of collection of urine and sent to laboratory.

2. Write a short note on collection of stool specimen. (MGR, DU)

Answer

It is the responsibility of the nurse that the specimens should be obtained from the patient properly, sent to the lab properly; as well as the reporting and recording of the findings of the patient.

Precautions

- Wash hands before and after the procedure
- Always wear gloves
- Always use disposable supplies whenever possible.

Specimen	Type of examination
Stool	• Routine microscopic and culture • Occult blood • Ova and cyst

Collection of Stool Specimen

- Explain the procedure to the client to gain cooperation. Ask the client to pass urine so that stool does not mix with urine.
- Ask the patient to defecate into clean bedpan. It is easy to collect and transfer stool into the specimen container by using a wooden spatula.
- Wear gloves and with a clean wooden spatula, lift up a portion of the stool from the center of the mass and place it directly into the labeled specimen container.
- Send the specimen to the laboratory.

Stool for Ova and Parasites

- Stool for ova and parasites is collected as per the steps above to detect intestinal infections.
- The client should be instructed to avoid things such as mineral oil, castor oil or antidiarrheal compounds, which may alter the feces.
- The client should be informed that stool specimens are to be given for three consecutive days.

Stool Culture

- This is carried out to identify pathogenic organisms in the gastrointestinal tract.
  If the client has been on antibiotics recently, it has to be reported. It should be collected using sterile technique in a sterile stool container for three consecutive days.

Stool for Occult Blood

- Stool examinations for occult blood help to detect gastrointestinal bleeding and early diagnosis of colorectal cancer. The guaiac or ortho toluidine test is commonly used.
- If the ortho toluidine test is used, the client is instructed to eat high-fiber diet for 48–72 hours before the collection of stool specimen.
- The client should avoid red meat, poultry, fish and turnips.
- This may create a false positive result. The following medications should be withheld for 48-72 hours before the test such as iron preparation, bromides, steroids, colchicine and vitamin C, which can produce a negative result.
- Usually three specimens over consecutive days are required.

Stool for Lipids

- Excessive secretion of fecal fats may occur in various digestive and absorption disorders.
- Normally, dietary lipids are completely absorbed in the small intestine.
- The client should be instructed to have extra high fat diet and refrain from alcohol for three days before the test and during the collection period.
- The client should avoid drugs that interfere with the test such as mineral oil, neomycin and potassium chloride.

3. Write a short note on collection of sputum specimen. (DU)

Read, Revise & Recall HIGH YIELD Ques For more, refer to Nursing Next Live app

Answer

Sputum is a material from mucus lining of trachea and bronchi which is coughed out through mouth.

Sputum Culture Sample Collection

It includes:

Culture: Sputum samples are often used for culture tests to identify the bacteria causing respiratory infections such as pneumonia, bronchitis, or tuberculosis. The sample should be collected in the morning before eating or drinking anything and after brushing teeth and washing the mouth. The sample should be collected in a sterile container and transported to the laboratory as soon as possible.

Smear: Sputum samples can be used for smear tests to look for bacteria, fungi, or abnormal cells in the respiratory tract. The sample should be collected in the morning before eating or drinking anything and after brushing teeth and washing the mouth. Sputum can be refrigerated if not sent to the lab.

Sputum cytology: Sputum samples can also be used for cytology tests to look for abnormal cells in the respiratory tract, such as cancer cells. The laboratory will examine the sputum sample under a microscope to identify abnormal cells.

Collection of Sputum Sample

- Instruct the patient to rinse the mouth with plain water.
- Avoid brushing of teeth and intake of food before sample collection.
- A wide mouth container or sputum mug should be used for the collection of the sample.
- A wax-lined disposable paper cup should be taken for the process of sample collection.
- Instruct the patient to cough up for the morning specimen after deep breathing in the container.
- Outer and inner surface of the container should not be spoiled.
- Label the container properly and send to the lab as soon as possible.

4. Write a short note on test for albumin in urine. (KUHS)

Answer

The purpose of the test is to identify the albumin in the urine. It includes:

Dipstick Test

- A dipstick test performed on a urine sample can detect the presence of albumin in the urine.
- For the test, a nurse or technician places a dipstick, a strip of chemically treated paper, into the urine.
- The dipstick changes color if albumin is present in the urine.

Hot Test

- It is a qualitative test used to detect the presence of albumin in urine
- Firstly, filter the urine specimen.
- Fill 2/3rd of a test tube with filtered urine.

Heat the upper 1/3rd of urine over a flame.

- If upper 1/3rd becomes cloudy, add few drops of acetic acid.
- If cloudy appearance disappears, it shows the presence of phosphates.
- If cloudy appearance does not disappear, it shows the presence of albumin.

Cold Test

- Pour 2 mL of concentrated nitric acid in a test tube.
- Pour 2 mL of filtered urine in another test tube.
- With a dropper, pour the urine gently along the sides of first test tube.
- A white ring at the junction of the two fluids indicates the presence of albumin.

SHORT ANSWER QUESTIONS

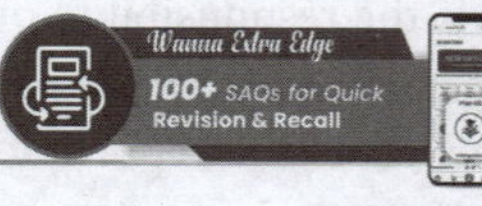

1. Observation of sputum. (MGR, DU)

Answer

Characteristic	Normal	Special considerations
Amount	Normally, no sputum very little is expectorated	Amount may vary according to the diseases, e.g., asthma or bronchitis
Color	It is colorless and translucent	• Yellowish: bacterial infection • Blackish: carbon pigment, e.g., smoking • Bright red/dark red and tarry color indicate blood • Greenish: bronchiectasis; brown: gangrenous condition of lungs.

Contd...

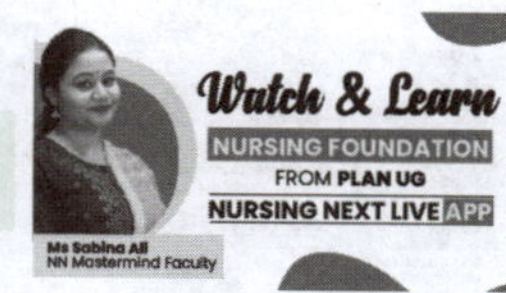

Characteristic	Normal	Special considerations
Odor	Odorless	Unpleasant odor indicates lung abscess, lung cancer, lung gangrene
Consistency		Frothy-watery, tenacious and thick depending on the type of condition

2. **Collection of stool specimen. (MGR, DU)**

Answer

Steps of collection of stool sample:

- Obtain a clean, leak-proof container.
- Collect a representative sample from different areas of the bowel movement.
- Avoid urine or water contamination.
- Securely close the container.
- Label with your name and date.
- Transport to the designated laboratory or healthcare facility promptly.

CONCEPTUAL REVISION

MULTIPLE CHOICE QUESTIONS

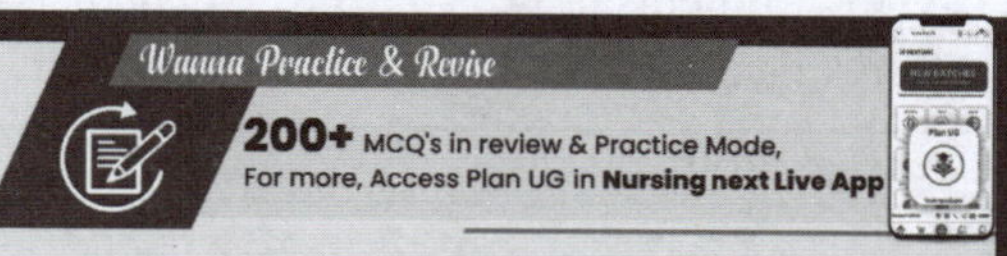

1. A patient recently started on phenytoin (Dilantin) to control simple complex seizures is seen in the outpatient clinic. Which information obtained during his chart review and assessment will be of greatest concern?

a. Patient occasionally forgets to take the phenytoin until after lunch.
b. The gums appear enlarged and inflamed.
c. Patient wants to renew his driver's license in the next month.
d. The white blood cell count is 2,300/mm

Ans. d. The white blood cell count is 2,300/mm

2. Best time to collect the specimen for microbiological examination of urine of a hospitalized adult is:

a. An early morning specimen, collected from midstream urine
b. Collected from the first portion of an early morning specimen
c. A catheter specimen in a afternoon
d. Collected in the morning after consuming water

Ans. a. An early morning specimen, collected from midstream urine

3. Which of the following laboratory values is expected for a patient just diagnosed with chronic lymphocytic leukemia?

a. Elevated sedimentation rate
b. Uncontrolled proliferation of granulocytes
c. Thrombocytopenia and increased lymphocytes
d. Elevated aspartate aminotransferase and alanine aminotransferase levels

Ans. c. Thrombocytopenia and increased lymphocytes

4. The doctor ordered for a complete blood count. After the test, nurse received the result from the laboratory. Which laboratory values will confirm the diagnosis of appendicitis?

a. RBC = 5.5 106/mm^3
b. WBC = 13,000/mm^3
c. Hct = 44%
d. Hgb = 15 g/dL

Ans. b. WBC = 13,000/mm^3

5. Which laboratory finding is the primary diagnostic indicator for pancreatitis?

a. Elevated aspartate aminotransferase (AST)
b. Elevated blood urea nitrogen (BUN)
c. Elevated serum lipase
d. Increased lactate dehydrogenase (LD)

Ans. c. Elevated serum lipase

6. Which of the following assessment is essential in administering total parenteral nutrition (TPN)?

a. Evaluation of the peripheral IV site
b. Confirmation that the tube is in the stomach
c. Assess the bowel sound
d. Fluid and electrolyte monitoring

Ans. d. Fluid and electrolyte monitoring

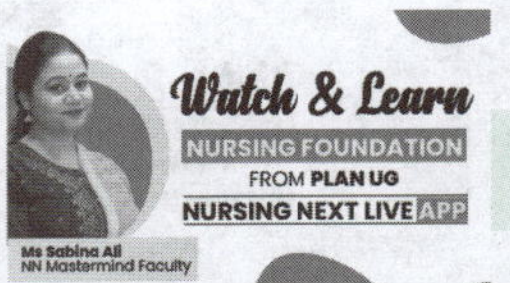

7. Assessing the laboratory findings, which result would the nurse most likely expect to find in a patient with chronic renal failure?

a. BUN 35 to 40 mg/dL, potassium 3.5 mEq/L, pH 7.35, decreased serum calcium
b. Decreased serum calcium, blood pH 7.2, potassium 6.5 mEq/L
c. BUN 10 to 30 mg/dL, potassium 4.0 mEq/L, creatinine 0.5 to 1.5 mg/dL
d. BUN 15 mg/dL, increased serum calcium, creatinine 1.0 mg/dL

Ans. b. Decreased serum calcium, blood pH 7.2, potassium 6.5 mEq/L

8. The test to detect acetone in urine is:

a. Rothera's test
b. Benedicts's test
c. Fehling's test
d. Cold test

Ans. a. Rothera's test

9. Hey's Test is done for:

a. Detection of bile
b. Detection of sugar in urine
c. Detection of albumin
d. Detection of acetone

Ans. a. Detection of bile

10. Barium enema is a type of:

a. Endoscopy
b. Electrodiagnostic study
c. Radiological study
d. Biochemical study

Ans. c. Radiological study

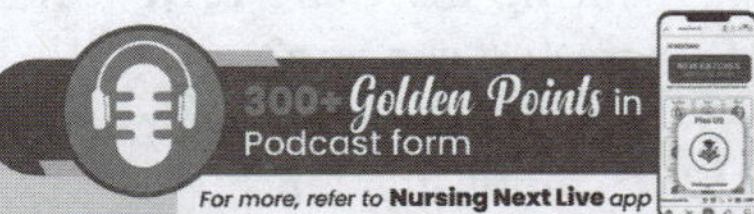

Golden Points

- A specimen is a small sample or part taken to show the nature of the whole as a small quantity of urine, stool, vomitus or a small fragment of tissue for a microscopic study. The specimens usually collected for various examinations are urine, stool and sputum.
- Diagnostic tests are blood tests, various examination tests and radiological tests.
- Diagnostic tests are of two types: Noninvasive and invasive.
- Endoscopic procedures include arthroscopy, bronchoscopy, colonoscopy, cystoscopy, endoscopic retrograde cholangiopancreatogram (ERCP) and sigmoidoscopy
- Invasive means that the body's tissues, organs, or cavities are accessed through some type of instrument.
- It is the responsibility of the nurse that the specimens are accurately obtained, labeled in appropriate container and transported to the laboratory on time.
- Noninvasive means that the body is not entered with any type of instrument; the skin and other body tissues, organs, and cavities remain intact.
- Nurses establish baseline, vital signs, identify known allergies and document in the client's medical record.
- Radiological studies include X-ray, CT, MRI, USG, Mammography, Barium studies etc. Electrocardiogram, Electroencephalogram, Electromyography (EMG), Halter monitor, Stress test, etc. are electrodiagnostic studies.
- Stool and sputum samples can be sent for culture and sensitivity as well as for microscopic examination.
- The nurse plays a key role in scheduling and preparing for diagnostic testing.
- Urine testing refers to laboratory analysis on a routine or clean voided specimen or a specimen obtained from catheter to perform a routine or microscopic examination of urine. It includes: Urinary pH, Specific Gravity, Urine Sugar, Acetone and Albumin.

CHAPTER 21

Oxygenation Needs

CONCEPTUAL THEORY

Terminology

A tracheostomy: It is an opening into the trachea through the neck. A tube is usually inserted through this opening and an artificial airway is created.

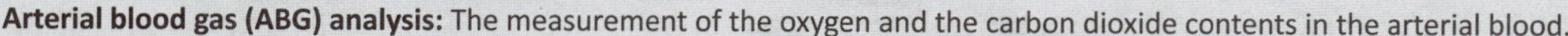

Arterial blood gas (ABG) analysis: The measurement of the oxygen and the carbon dioxide contents in the arterial blood.

Basic life support (BLS) defines sequences of procedures performed to restore the circulation of oxygenated blood after a sudden pulmonary or cardiac arrest until they can be given full medical care at a hospital. BLS does not include the use of drugs or invasive skills.

Endotracheal tubes (ETTs) are most commonly inserted in clients who have had general anesthetics or in those who are in emergency situations where mechanical ventilation is required. It is inserted through the mouth or nose and into the trachea with the help of laryngoscope. The tube terminates just superior to the bifurcation of the trachea into the bronchi.

Incentive spirometers also referred to as sustained maximal inspiration (SMI) devices, measure the flow of air inhaled through the mouthpiece and are used to: Improve pulmonary ventilation and expand collapsed alveoli

Nebulization is a process of administration of medication via inhalation. By this method, the medication is dispersed in the form of mist and delivered into the respiratory tract with the help of device called nebulizer.

Oxygen therapy or oxygenation is the administration of oxygen as a medical intervention, which can be for a variety of purposes in both chronic and acute patient care.

Pulse oximetry is the noninvasive measurement of arterial oxygen saturation done with the help of pulse oximeter.

Ventilation refers to the process of moving air in and out of the lungs (respiration).

OXYGENATION

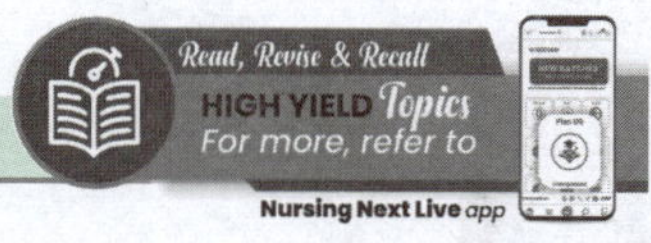

Oxygen therapy or oxygenation is the administration of oxygen as a medical intervention, which can be for a variety of purposes in both chronic and acute patient care.

- Oxygen is essential for cell metabolism, and in turn, tissue oxygenation is essential for all normal physiological functions.
- Oxygen therapy is used when hypoxemia is present.
- Oxygen administered in different ways from a nasal cannula to hyperbaric oxygen inside a closed chamber.

Nursing Interventions in Oxygenation

- Nursing interventions to facilitate pulmonary ventilation may include—**ensuring a patent airway, positioning, encouraging deep breathing and coughing, and ensuring adequate hydration.**
- Other nursing interventions helpful in ventilation are—**suctioning, lung inflation techniques, administration of analgesics before deep breathing and coughing, postural drainage, and percussion and vibration.**
- Many dependent nursing interventions such **as oxygen therapy, tracheostomy care, and maintenance of a chest tube are also to be included in maintaining oxygenation.**

Pharmacological Measures to Improve Oxygenation

- **Bronchodilators**
- Anti-inflammatory drugs
- Expectorants and cough suppressants
- **Incentive spirometers** also referred to as sustained maximal inspiration (SMI) devices, measure the flow of air inhaled through the mouthpiece and are used to:
- Improve pulmonary ventilation
- Expand collapsed alveoli.

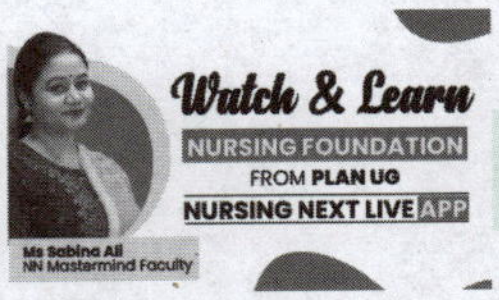

Indications of Oxygen Administration

Indications for Oxygen Therapy

- Cyanosis
- Breathlessness and labored breathing
- High altitudes
- Anemia
- Any respiratory illness/distress
- Poisoning
- Shock and circulatory failure
- Hemorrhage and air hunger
- Patients under anesthesia and postoperatively
- Patients who are critically ill
- Patients with psychologically induced breathlessness
- Asphyxia
- Neurological conditions such as status epilepticus

Different Methods of Oxygen Administration

Oxygen device type	Device appearance	% Fio_2 obtained
Nasal Cannula	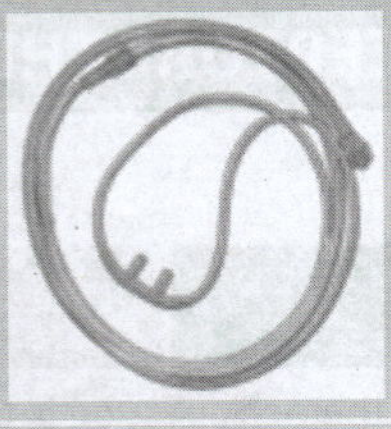	24–40% FiO_2
Oxymizer	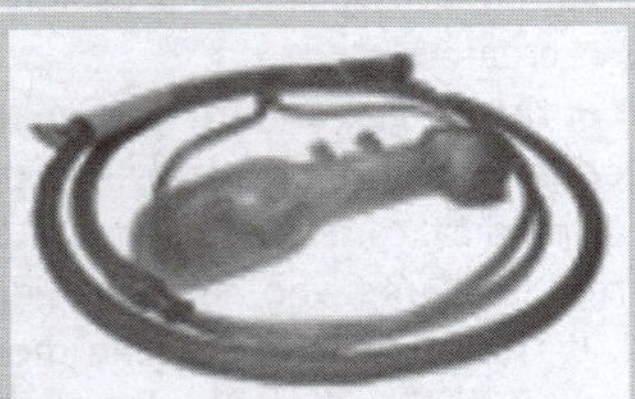	24–40% FiO_2
Simple Face Mask	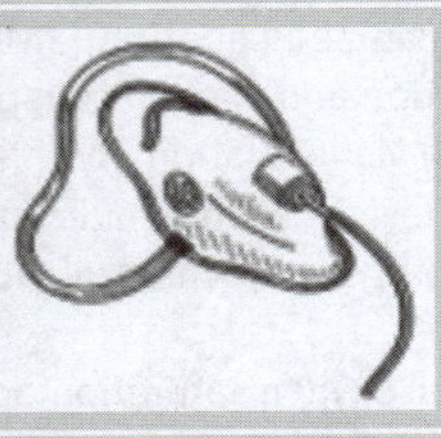	35–55% FiO_2
Venturi Face Mask	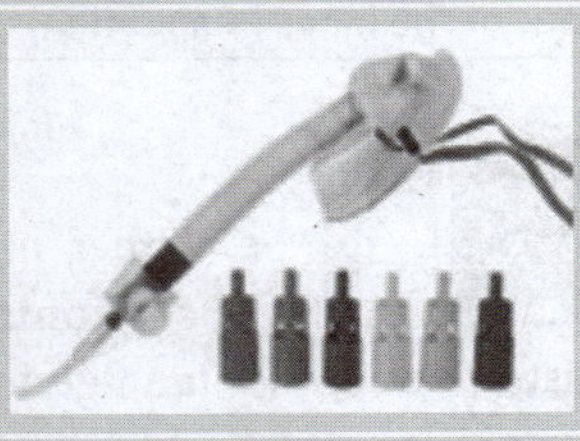	24–60% FiO_2
Nonrebreather	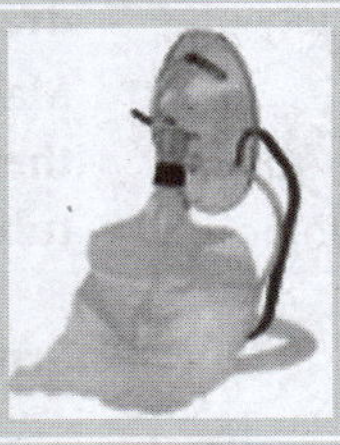	60–95% FiO_2
High-Flow Nasal Cannula	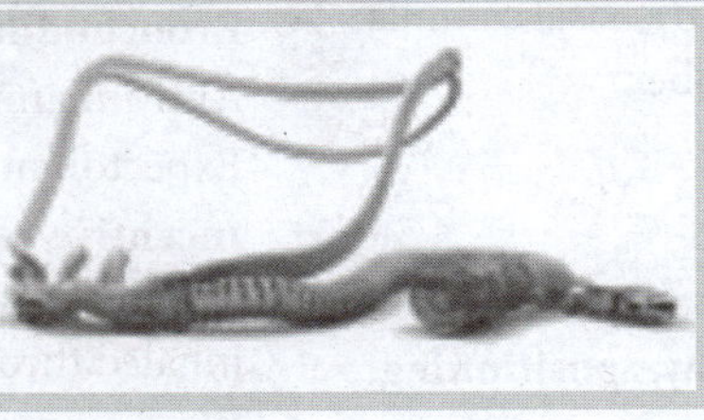	20–100% FiO_2

Contd...

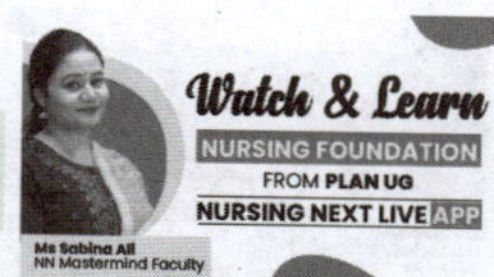

Oxygen device type	Device appearance	% FiO_2 obtained
BiPAP		35–100% FiO_2
Endotracheal Intubation		35–100% FiO_2

Hazards of Oxygen Inhalation

- Infection
- Combustion (fire)
- Drying of the mucous membranes of the respiratory tract
- Oxygen-toxicity
- Atelectasis
- Oxygen-induced apnea
- Retrolental fibroplasia
- Asphyxia

ARTIFICIAL AIRWAY

- Oropharyngeal airway
- Nasopharyngeal airway

Endotracheal tubes (ETT) are most commonly inserted in clients who have had general anesthetics or in those who are in emergency situations where mechanical ventilation is required. It is inserted through the mouth or nose and into the trachea with the help of laryngoscope. The tube terminates just superior to the bifurcation of the trachea into the bronchi.

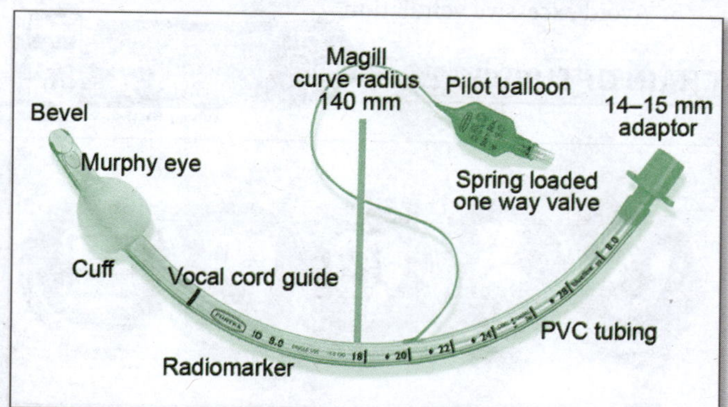

Clients who need long-term airway support may have a tracheostomy.

A tracheostomy is an opening into the trachea through the neck. A tube is usually inserted through this opening and an artificial airway is created. Tracheotomy is done by using one of the two techniques: The traditional open surgical method or a percutaneous insertion. The percutaneous method can be done at the bedside in a critical care unit. The open technique is done in the operating room, and surgical incision is made in the trachea just below the larynx. A curved tracheostomy tube is inserted to extend through the stoma into the trachea. Tracheostomy tubes may be either plastic or metal and are available in different sizes.

PULSE OXIMETRY

- Pulse oximetry is the noninvasive measurement of arterial oxygen saturation done with the help of pulse oximeter.
- Pulse oximetry is used for any patient who is at risk of hypoxia. With the pulse oximeter (machine to measure oxygen saturation of the blood), changes in arterial oxygen saturation can be continuously monitored. It is one of the valuable tools to measure arterial oxygen saturation. The device measures oxygen saturation by determining the percentage of hemoglobin that is bound with oxygen.
- A sensor or probe is attached to an appendage of the patient on earlobe, fingertip, toe, through which infrared and red light can reach the capillary vascular bed. Oxyhemoglobin absorbs more infrared than red light. A microprocessor in the monitor receives the information from the sensor-probe, computes the saturation value, and displays it on the monitor screen.

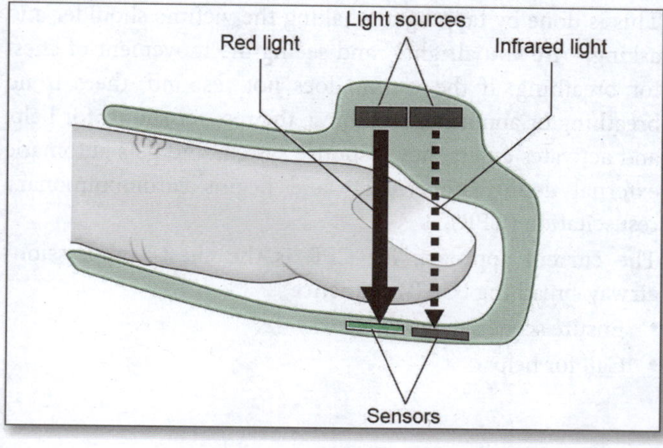

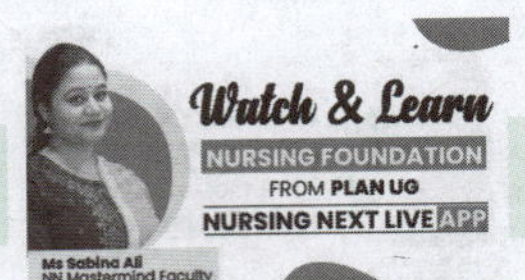

Principle

- Pulse oximetry works on the principle of spectral analysis for measurement of oxygen saturation, i.e. the detection and quantification of components in solution by their unique light absorption characteristics.
- Pulse oximeters combine the principle of spectrophotometry and plethysmography to noninvasively measure the oxygen saturation in arterial blood.

Sites for Pulse Oximetry

Fingers, forehead, nose, foot, ears and toes.

Nursing Responsibility

- Assess the previous SPO_2 level to have baseline data and determine the site for sensor probe placement.
- Compare SPO_2 levels with previous baseline and acceptable levels of SPO_2.
- Record the date, time, site of probe placement and the reading. Specify the type and amount of oxygen, if the patient is on oxygen flow and report any abnormalities.
- Nails should be free of nail polish.

NEBULIZATION

Nebulization is a process of administration of medication via inhalation. By this method, the medication is dispersed in the form of mist and delivered into the respiratory tract with the help of device called nebulizer.

- Monitor the response to the therapy
- Auscultate the lung fields to see the effectiveness of the therapy.

BASIC LIFE SUPPORT

Basic life support consists of a series of actions and skills performed by the rescuer based on assessment findings. The first actions the rescuer performs on finding an adult victim are to assess for responsiveness and to look for signs of breathing. This is done by tapping or shaking the victim's shoulder and asking, "Are you alright?" and seeing the movement of chest for breathing. If the victim does not respond, there is no breathing or abnormal breathing, the rescuer shouts for help, and activates emergency response system and gets automatic external defibrillator (AED) and begins cardiopulmonary resuscitation (CPR).

The current approach for CPR is the chest compression-airway-breathing **(CAB) sequence**

- Ensure scene safety.
- Call for help
- Check carotid pulse (within 10 seconds) and respiration
- Start CPR as soon as possible for effective results
- Follow:

C- Circulation

A- Airway

B- Breathing

For health care or first aid providers:

CPR using chest compressions and mouth-to-mouth breathing at a ratio of **30:2** compressions-to-breaths.

- Chest compressions at a rate of **100 to 120/min**
- Depth of compressions at least 2 inches (5 cm) for adult and children and 1.5 inches for infants.
- Initiate chest compressions (C-A-B rather than A-B-C)
  C- Compressions
  A- Airway
  B- Breathing
- Increase the depth of chest compressions to 2 inches for adults.
- **For the general public or bystanders who witness the sudden collapse of an adult victim:**
  - Compression-Only CPR, or Hands-Only CPR.
  - **Hands-Only CPR** is CPR without mouth-to-mouth breaths.
  - It is recommended for use by people who see a teen or adult suddenly collapses in an out-of-hospital setting (such as at home, at work, or in a park).
- **High-Quality CPR:** Push hard and Push fast in the center of the chest. It has five critical components:
  1. Minimize interruptions in chest compressions
  2. Provide compressions of adequate rate and depth
  3. Avoid leaning on the victim between compressions
  4. Ensure proper hand placement
  5. Avoid excessive ventilation

CHAIN OF SURVIVAL

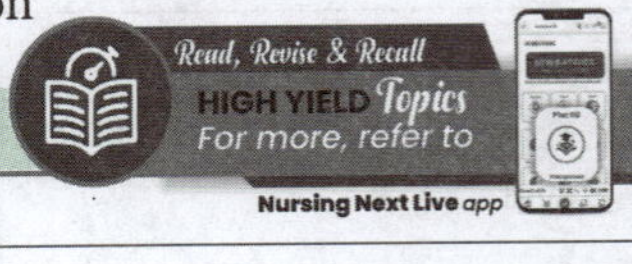

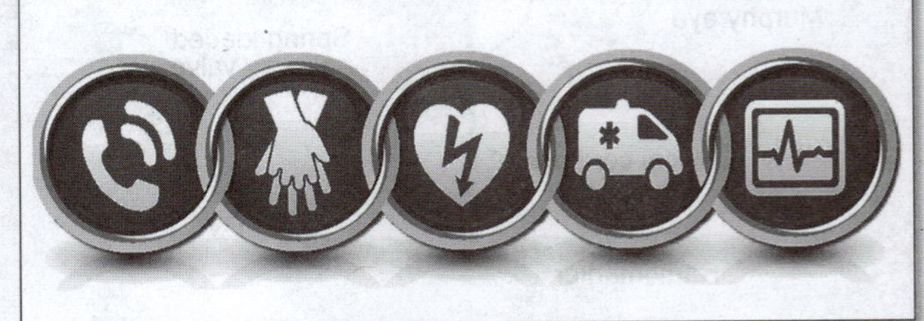

Adult CPR

For flow chart, refer to Chapter 14, Page no. 710

CONCEPTUAL EXERCISES

LONG ANSWER QUESTIONS

1. Define oxygenation. Explain about nursing interventions in oxygenation. (MGR)

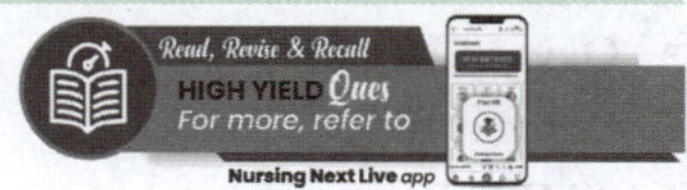

Answer

Oxygenation

- Oxygen therapy or oxygenation is the administration of oxygen as a medical intervention, which can be for a variety of purposes in both chronic and acute patient care.
- Oxygen is essential for cell metabolism, and in turn, tissue oxygenation is essential for all normal physiological functions.
- Oxygen therapy is used when hypoxemia is present.
- Oxygen administered in different ways from a nasal cannula to hyperbaric oxygen inside a closed chamber.

Nursing Interventions in Oxygenation

Preliminary Assessment

- Before administering oxygen therapy, check the identification data of the patient including bed number.
- Check the indication and the need for oxygen therapy.
- Check the doctor's orders for the dosage (liter/minute), etc.
- Assess the patient for any signs of clinical hypoxia, e.g., cyanosis.
- Assess the patient's vital signs and the breathing patterns carefully before starting the therapy.
- Check the results of arterial blood gas analysis.
- Note any signs of pulmonary dysfunction.
- Inspect the anterior nares for encrustation and irritation.
- Inspect the skin on the nose and the surrounding areas for any skin lesions. Clean the nostrils, if any crust is present.
- Check the articles available in the unit. Check the oxygen cylinder and its accessories for their functions, (e.g., check for any leakage of oxygen).
- Choose the right method of oxygen deliery:
- Check the prescription order for the mode of delivery.
- The manner in which oxygen is administered or delivered to the client depends upon the condition of the patient, the concentration desired, the facilities available and the preference of the doctor. Oxygen can be administered by following methods:
  - Nasal Cannula
  - Simple Mask
  - Partial re-breather Mask
  - Non re-breather Mask (NRBM)
  - Venturi Mask
  - Oxygen Hood
  - Oxygen Tent
  - AMBU Bag
  - Transtracheal
  - T-piece

Preparation of the Patient and the Environment

- Explain the procedure to the patient.
- Instruct the patient, the family members and the visitors, if any, about the safety precautions required during the oxygen therapy.
- Put up the instruction regarding fire precautions in the unit. Remove the inflammable articles from the patient's unit.
- Assemble the equipment and arrange them conveniently in the unit.
- Place the patient in a comfortable position (Fowler's position) to help in the expansion of the lungs.

Aftercare of the Patient and the Articles

- Stay with the patient till he is at ease.
- Assess the vital signs very frequently. Assess the breathing pattern as well.
- Record the procedure with date and time on the nurse's record. In the record, mention the method of oxygen delivery or oxygen device used.
- Check the apparatus for its good working condition and the safety measures.
- Take the sample for blood gas analysis at specified intervals, if indicated.
- Assess the mucous membrane of the nostril, oral cavity frequency for its dryness.
- Discard the used oxygen device properly as per BMW guidelines.
- Monitor the patient for any deteriorating symptoms after the removal of oxygen inhalation.

2. a. List the principles related to oxygen administration.
b. Discuss the indications of oxygen administration.
c. Explain the different methods of oxygen administration.
d. Describe the hazards/complications of O_2 therapy.

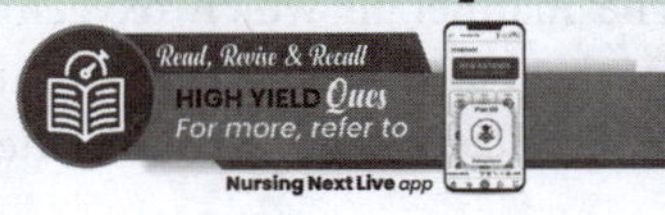

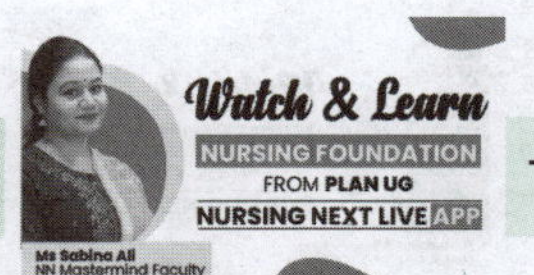

Answer

Principles Related to Oxygen Administration

- Since oxygen acts as a drug, it must be prescribed and administered in specific dose as per doctor's order in order to avoid oxygen toxicity.
- When using an oxygen cylinder, use a regulator and humidifier to control the pressure of the oxygen in the cylinder to a safer level. The humidifier helps to prevent the drying of the mucous membranes of the respiratory tract.
- Oxygen apparatus should be clean to prevent infection.
- During the administration of oxygen, the valve controlling the rate of flow should not be handled. If any alteration is to be made in the flow of oxygen, first take out the catheter from the nose and then adjust the valve.
- Oxygen administration must never be stopped until the factors that caused hypoxia are reversed.
- When oxygen therapy is discontinued, it should be weaned by reducing the dosage and then administering it intermittently.
- For all patients receiving oxygen inhalation, the oxygen saturation temperature should be monitored and recorded accurately.
- Assess the patients receiving oxygen therapy continuously to detect the early signs of oxygen toxicity.
- Since oxygen supports combustion, fire precautions are to be taken when the oxygen is on flow.

b. Indications for oxygen therapy

Answer

- Cyanosis
- Breathlessness and labored breathing
- High altitudes
- Anemia
- Any respiratory illness/distress
- Poisoning
- Shock and circulatory failure
- Hemorrhage and air hunger
- Patients under anesthesia and postoperatively
- Patients who are critically ill.
- Patients with psychologically induced breathlessness
- Asphyxia
- Neurological conditions such as status epilepticus

c. Different Methods of Oxygen Administration

Answer

The manner in which oxygen is administered or delivered to the client depends upon the condition of the patient, the concentration desired, the facilities available and the preference of the doctor. Oxygen can be administered by following methods:

- Nasal Cannula
- Simple Mask
- Partial re-breather Mask
- Non re-breather Mask (NRBM)
- Venturi Mask
- Oxygen Hood
- Oxygen Tent
- AMBU Bag
- Transtracheal
- T-piece

Classification of Oxygen Delivery Systems

- Low flow systems
  - Contribute partially to inspired gas client breathes
  - E.g.: nasal cannula, simple mask, non re-breather mask, Partial rebreather mask
- High flow systems
  - Deliver specific and constant percentage of oxygen independent of client's breathing
  - E.g.: Venturi mask, trach collar, T-piece

Nasal Cannula

A nasal cannula is a simple comfortable device. The two cannula about 1.5 cm (1/2 inch) long, protrude from the center of a disposable tube and are inserted into the nares. Oxygen is delivered via the cannula with a flow rate of up to 4 L/min. Higher flow rates dry air mucosa and do not further increase inspired oxygen concentrations.

Oxygen by Nasal Catheter

This is the most common method of administering oxygen to the patients in the hospital wards. The nasal catheter is inserted into the nostril reaching up to the uvula and is held in place by adhesive tapes.

Oxygen by Mask

- An oxygen mask is a device used to administer oxygen, humidity or heated humidity. It is shaped to fit snugly over the mouth and nose and is secured in place with a strap.
- There are two primary types of masks, high and low concentration. Masks are advantageous for patients who are unable to breathe through the nose.

Oxygen Tent

An oxygen tent consists of canopy over the patient's bed that may cover the patient fully or partially and it is connected to

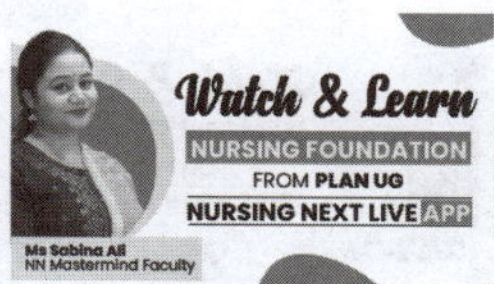

a supply of oxygen. The canopies are transparent and enables the nurse to observe the patient. The lower part of the canopy is tucked under the bed to prevent the escape of oxygen.

Transtracheal Oxygen

This is a method of oxygen delivery for clients, with chronic lung diseases, in which a small intravenous size catheter is inserted directly into the trachea through a surgical tract in the lower neck. Oxygen is delivered directly into the trachea.

Oxygen delivery devices			
Device		Flow rate	% Oxygen delivered (approx.)
Nasal Cannula		1 L/min	24%
		2 L/min	28%
		4 L/min	36%
Venturi Valve and Mask	Blue	2–4 L/min	24%
	White	4–6 L/min	28%
	Yellow	8–10 L/min	35%
	Red	10–12 L/min	40%
	Green	12–15 L/min	60%
Non-rebreather Mask		15 L/min	85%

d. **Hazards of Oxygen Inhalation**

Answer

- Infection
- Combustion (fire)
- Drying of the mucous membranes of the respiratory tract
- Oxygen toxicity
- Atelectasis
- Oxygen-induced apnea
- Retrolental fibroplasia
- Asphyxia

SHORT NOTES

1. Write about the types of oxygen delivery devices. (MGR)

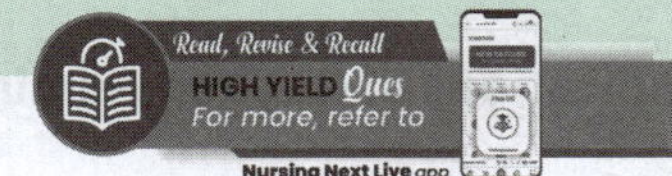

Answer

Nasal Cannula

Also called nasal prong, this oxygen delivery device is most commonly used in clinical settings. The nasal cannula has two plastic protruding prongs that are inserted into the nostrils. The cannula is connected to an oxygen source (flow meter and a humidifier). It can provide oxygen by both a low-flow and high-flow system.

- **Low flow system:**
  Flow rate- 1–6 L/min
  FiO_2 — 22–44%
- **High flow system:**
  Flow rate—up to 60 L/min
  FiO_2 — 21–100%

Simple Face Mask

The simple face mask is connected to oxygen tubing, a humidifier, and a flow meter. This mask has vents on its sides that allow exhaled carbon dioxide to escape. It is used when an increased delivery of oxygen is needed for short periods.

Flow rate — 6–10 L/min
FiO_2 — 40–60%

Partial Rebreather Mask

The partial rebreather mask is equipped with a reservoir bag for the collection of exhaled air and is mixed with 100% oxygen for the next inhalation. Thus, the patient rebreathes about one-third of the expired air from the reservoir bag. This type of mask permits the conservation of oxygen.

Flow rate — 8–11 L/min
FiO_2 — 50–75%

Nonrebreather Mask

The nonrebreather mask delivers the highest concentration of oxygen via a mask that has two one-way valves. These valves prevent the patient from rebreathing exhaled air. The reservoir bag is filled with oxygen that enters the mask on inspiration. Exhaled air escapes through side vents.

Flow rate — 12–15
FiO_2 — 80–95%

Venturi Mask

The Venturi mask delivers the most precise concentrations of oxygen according to the prescription. It is also known as an air-entrainment to deliver on controlled oxygen therapy.

Flow rate — 2–15 L/min
FiO_2 — 24–60%

2. Write the nursing responsibilities on the following. (DU)

a. **Nebulization**

b. **Oxygen administration by nasal cannula**

Answer

Nebulization

Nursing Responsibilities

- Position the patient appropriately, allowing optimal ventilation (semi-Fowler's position).
- Assess and record breath sounds, respiratory status, pulse rate and other significant respiratory functions.
- Teach patient the proper way of inhalation.
- Prepare equipment at hand.
- Check doctor's orders for the medication, prepare thereafter
- Place the medication in the nebulizer (can add amount of saline solution if ordered).
- Offer assistance to the patient until he is able to perform proper inhalation [if unable to hold the nebulizer (pediatric/ geriatric/special cases)].

Aftercare

- Each time it is used, wash the nebulizer chamber in warm water or clean with a spirit swab and then rinse thoroughly with clean water.
- Reconnect the nebulizer chamber to the tubing and blow air from it.
- Disconnect the nebulizer chamber from the tubing and allow it to dry completely.

b. **Oxygen Administration by Nasal Cannula.**

Answer

Preliminary Assessment

- Before administering oxygen therapy, check the identification data of the patient including bed number.
- Check the indication and the need for oxygen therapy.
- Check the doctor's orders for the dosage (L/min), etc.
- Assess the patient for any signs of clinical hypoxia, e.g., cyanosis.
- Assess the patient's vital signs and the breathing patterns carefully before starting the therapy.
- Check the results of arterial blood gas analysis.
- Note any signs of pulmonary dysfunction.
- Inspect the anterior nares for encrustation and irritation.
- Inspect the skin on the nose and the surrounding areas for any skin lesions. Clean the nostrils, if any crust is present.
- Check the articles available in the unit. Check the oxygen cylinder and its accessories for their functions (e.g., check for any leakage of oxygen).

Preparation of the Patient and the Environment

- Explain the procedure to the patient.
- Instruct the patient, the family members and the visitors, if any, about the safety precautions required during the oxygen therapy.
- Put up the instruction regarding fire precautions in the unit. Remove the inflammable articles from the patient's unit.
- Assemble the equipment and arrange them conveniently in the unit.
- Place the patient in a comfortable position (Fowler's position) to help in the expansion of the lungs.

Aftercare of the Patient and the Articles

- Stay with the patient till he is at ease.
- Assess the vital signs very frequently. Assess the breathing pattern as well.
- Record the procedure with date and time on the nurse's record. In the record, mention the method of oxygen delivery or oxygen device used.
- Check the apparatus for its good working condition and the safety measures.
- Take the sample for blood gas analysis at specified intervals, if indicated.
- Assess the mucous membrane of the nostril, oral cavity frequency for its dryness.
- Discard the used oxygen device properly as per BMW guidelines.
- Monitor the patient for any deteriorating symptoms after the removal of oxygen inhalation.

SHORT ANSWER QUESTIONS

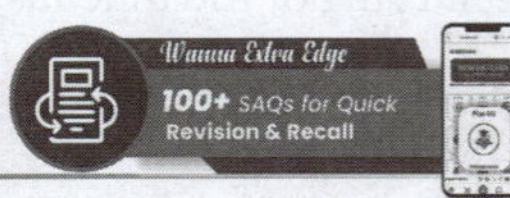

1. Define oxygenation. List the indications of oxygen administration.

Answer

Oxygen therapy or oxygenation is the administration of oxygen as a medical intervention, which can be for a variety of purposes in both chronic and acute patient care.

Indications of Oxygen Administration

- Cyanosis
- Breathlessness and labored breathing
- High altitudes

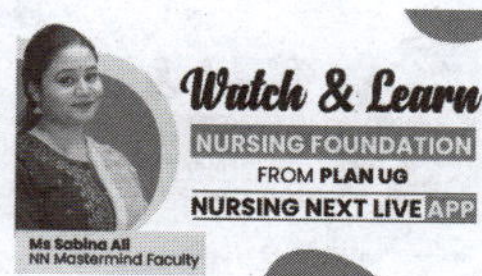

- Anemia
- Any respiratory illness/distress
- Poisoning
- Shock and circulatory failure
- Hemorrhage and air hunger
- Patients under anesthesia and postoperatively
- Patients who are critically ill
- Patients with psychologically induced breathlessness
- Asphyxia
- Neurological conditions such as status epilepticus

2. List the different methods of oxygen administration.

Answer

- Nasal Cannula
- Simple Mask
- Partial re-breather Mask
- Non re breather Mask (NRBM)
- Venturi Mask
- Oxygen Hood
- Oxygen Tent
- AMBU Bag
- Transtracheal
- T-piece

3. Define dyspnea.

Answer

Dyspnea derives from Greek for "hard breathing". It is often also described as "shortness of breath".

This is a subjective sensation of breathing, from mild discomfort to feelings of suffocation.

4. Describe the hazards/complications of O_2 therapy.

Answer

Hazards of Oxygen Inhalation

- Infection
- Combustion (fire)
- Drying of the mucous membranes of the respiratory tract
- Oxygen toxicity
- Atelectasis
- Oxygen-induced apnea
- Retrolental fibroplasia
- Asphyxia

CONCEPTUAL REVISION

MULTIPLE CHOICE QUESTIONS

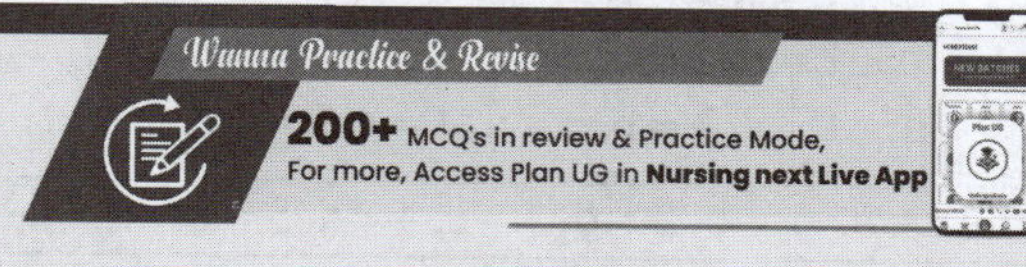

1. A prescribed amount of oxygen is needed for a patient with COPD to prevent:
a. Cardiac arrest related to increased partial pressure of carbon dioxide in arterial blood ($PaCO_2$)
b. Circulatory overload due to hypervolemia.
c. Respiratory excitement.
d. Inhibition of the respiratory hypoxic stimulus.

Ans. d. Inhibition of the respiratory hypoxic stimulus.

2. The nurse explains to a patient that a cough:
a. Is a protective response to clear the respiratory tract of irritants.
b. Is primarily a voluntary action.
c. Is induced by the administration of an antitussive drug.
d. Can be inhibited by "splinting" the abdomen.

Ans. a. Is a protective response to clear the respiratory tract of irritants.

3. To prevent airway obstruction in the postoperative patient who is unconscious, the nurse should perform which of the following action?
a. Encourages deep breathing
b. Positions the patient in a side-lying position
c. Use of incentive spirometry
d. Administers oxygen per mask

Ans. b. Positions the patient in a side-lying position

4. What is the full form of FFP in relation to a respirator?
a. Filtering Face Piece
b. Filtrating Frozen Particles
c. Fixed Filtration Pearls
d. Focused Filtering Pouch

Ans. a. Filtering Face Piece

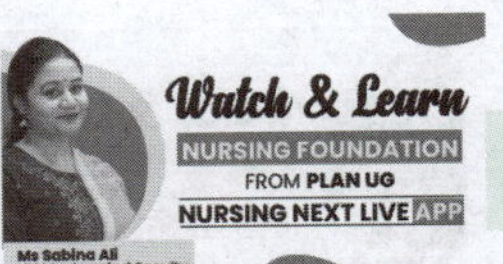

5. Ms Benny, a registered nurse is assigned to provide care to a patient with the diagnosis of right lower lobe pneumonia in the medicine ward. While monitoring the vital sign, the nurse auscultates the right lower lobe. What findings of breath sounds the nurse would expect to note?

a. Breath sound will be absent
b. Vesicular
c. Bronchial
d. Bronchovesicular

Ans. c. Bronchial

6. Match the following abnormal breathing patterns with their respective condition?

1. Irregular respiratory rate and depth with alternating periods of apnea and hyperventilation	a. Apneustic respiration
2. Periods of rapid respirations of near equal depth followed by regular or irregular periods of apnea	b. Cheyne-stroke respiration
3. A type of labored or hyperventilation characterized by a consistently deep and rapid respiratory pattern	c. Ataxic respiration
4. Have a prolonged inspiratory phase followed by a prolonged expiratory phase	d. Biot's respiration
5. Completely irregular breathing pattern with irregular pauses and increasing episodes of apnea	e. Kussmaul's respiration

a. 1 = b, 2 = d, 3 = e, 4 = a, 5 = c
b. 1 = e, 2 = c, 3 = b, 4 = a, 5 = d
c. 1 = d, 2 = a, 3 = e, 4 = c, 5 = b
d. 1 = c, 2 = b, 3 = a, 4 = e, 5 = d

Ans. a. 1 = b, 2 = d, 3 = e, 4 = a, 5 = c

7. A patient has exacerbation of chronic obstructive pulmonary disease (COPD) manifested by shortness of breath; orthopnea: thick, tenacious secretions; and a dry hacking cough. An appropriate nursing diagnosis would be:

a. Ineffective airway clearance related to thick, tenacious secretions
b. Ineffective airway clearance related to dry, hacking cough
c. Ineffective individual coping to COPD
d. Pain related to immobilization of affected leg

Ans. a. Ineffective airway clearance related to thick, tenacious secretions.

8. The assigned nurse has monitored the patient's vital signs and recorded in the patient TPR chart. Identify which of the following values of vital signs would the nurse address first to the doctor?

a. Blood pressure = 150/89 mm Hg
b. Temperature = 37.2°C, tympanic
c. Oxygen saturation = 89%
d. Respiratory rate = 27 breaths/minute

Ans. c. Oxygen saturation = 89%

9. All of the following can cause tachycardia; except:

a. Fever
b. Exercise
c. Sympathetic nervous system stimulation
d. Parasympathetic nervous system stimulation

Ans. d. Parasympathetic nervous system stimulation

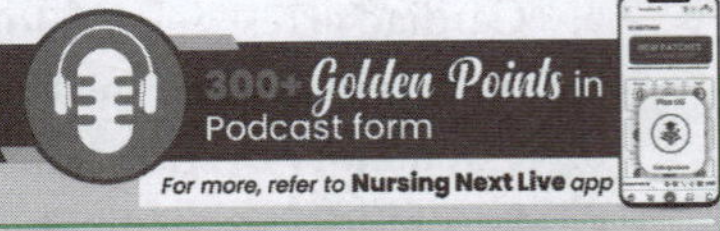

Golden Points

- Oxygen therapy or oxygenation is the administration of oxygen as a medical intervention, which can be for a variety of purposes in both chronic and acute patient care.
- Oxygen is essential for cell metabolism, and in turn, tissue oxygenation is essential for all normal physiological functions.
- Pulse oximetry is the noninvasive measurement of arterial oxygen saturation done with the help of pulse oximeter.
- Oxygen administered in different ways from a nasal cannula to hyperbaric oxygen inside a closed chamber.
- In maintaining oxygenation, various pharmacological measures are also used. It includes Bronchodilators, Anti-inflammatory drugs, Expectorants and cough suppressants.
- Incentive spirometers also referred to as sustained maximal inspiration (SMI) devices, measure the flow of air inhaled through the mouthpiece and are used to improve pulmonary ventilation and also help in expanding collapsed alveoli.
- Clients who need long-term airway support may have a tracheostomy.
- Nebulization is a process of administration of medication via inhalation. By this method, the medication is dispersed in the form of mist and delivered into the respiratory tract with the help of device called nebulizer.

CHAPTER

22

Fluid and Electrolyte Imbalance

CONCEPTUAL THEORY

Terminology

Hypercalcemia: Hypercalcemia or total serum calcium levels >10.5 mg/dL, or an ionized calcium level of >5.0 mg/dL, most often occurs when calcium is mobilized from the bony skeleton. This may be due to malignancy or prolonged immobilization.

Hyperkalemia: It is a potassium excess or a serum potassium level >5.0 mEq/L.

Hypermagnesemia: It is present when the serum magnesium level rises above 2.5 mEq/L. It is due to increased intake or decreased excretion. It is often iatrogenic, that is, it occurs as a result of overzealous magnesium therapy.

Hypernatremia: It is excess sodium in ECF or serum sodium of >145 mEq/L. Because the osmotic pressure of ECF is increased, fluid moves out of the cells into the ECF.

Hypocalcemia: It is defined as calcium deficit, or a total serum calcium level of <8.5 mg/dL or an ionized calcium level of <0.4 mg/dL. Severe depletion of calcium can cause tetany with muscle spasms and paresthesias (numbness and tingling around the mouth and hands and feet) and can lead to convulsions.

Hypokalemia: It is a potassium deficit or a serum potassium level of <3.5 mEq/L

Hypomagnesemia: It is defined as magnesium deficiency, or a total serum magnesium level of <1.5 mEq/L. It occurs more frequently than hypermagnesemia. Chronic alcoholism is the most common cause of hypomagnesemia. Magnesium deficiency may also aggravate the manifestation of alcohol withdrawal, such as delirium tremens.

Hyponatremia: It is a sodium deficit, or serum sodium level of <135 mEq/L, and is, in acute care settings, a common electrolyte imbalance.

ELECTROLYTES

Electrolytes are minerals in our blood and other body fluids that carry an electric change. Some electrolytes present in the body are sodium, potassium, calcium, magnesium, chloride, bicarbonate and phosphorus.

Regulation and Functions of Electrolytes

Electrolyte	Regulation	Functions
Sodium (Na^+)	• Renal reabsorption and/or excretion • Aldosterone increases Na^+ reabsorption in collecting ducts of nephrons	• Regulating ECF volume and distribution • Maintaining blood volume • Transmitting nerve impulses and contracting muscles
Potassium (K^+)	• Renal excretion and conservation • Aldosterone increases K^+ excretion • Movement into and out of cells • Insulin helps move K^+ into cells; tissue damage and acidosis shift K^+ out of cells into ECF	• Maintaining ICF osmolality • Transmitting nerve and other electrical impulses • Regulating cardiac impulses transmission and muscle contraction • Skeletal and smooth muscle function • Regulating acid-base balance

Contd...

Electrolyte	Regulation	Functions
Calcium (Ca^{2+})	• Redistribution between bones and ECF • Parathyroid hormone and calcitriol increases serum Ca^{2+} levels; calcitonin decreases serum levels	• Forming bones and teeth • Transmitting nerve impulses • Regulating muscle contraction • Maintaining cardiac pacemaker (automaticity) • Blood clotting • Activating enzymes such as pancreatic lipase and phospholipase
Magnesium (Mg^{2+})	• Conservation and excretion by kidney • Intestinal absorption increased by vitamin D and parathyroid hormone	• Intracellular metabolism • Operating sodium-potassium pump • Relaxing muscle contraction • Transmitting nerve impulses • Regulating cardiac functions
Chloride (Cl^{-})	• Excreted and reabsorbed along with sodium in the kidney • Aldosterone increases chloride reabsorption with sodium	• HCl production • Regulating ECF balance and vascular volume • Regulating acid-base balance • Buffer in oxygen-carbon dioxide exchange in RBCs
Phosphate (PO_4^{3-})	• Excretion and reabsorption by the Kidney • Parathyroid hormone decreases serum levels by increasing renal excretion • Reciprocal relationship with calcium; increased serum calcium level decreases phosphate levels; decreased serum calcium increases phosphate	• Forming bones and teeth • Metabolizing carbohydrate, protein and fat • Cellular metabolism; producing ATP and DNA • Muscle, nerve and RBC function • Regulating acid-base balance • Regulating calcium levels
Bicarbonate (HCO^{3-})	• Excretion and reabsorption by the Kidney • Regeneration by the kidney	• Major body buffer involved in acid-base regulation

Sodium

Sodium: It is the most abundant cation in the extracellular fluid (ECF).

Hyponatremia

Hyponatremia is a sodium deficit, or serum sodium level <135 mEq/L, and is, in acute care settings. It is a common electrolyte imbalance.

Hypernatremia

Hypernatremia is excess sodium in extracellular fluid (ECF) or serum sodium level >145 mEq/L. Because the osmotic pressure of ECF is increased, fluid moves out of the cells into the ECF.

Potassium

Potassium is vital to normal neuromuscular and cardiac functions. Normal renal function is important for maintenance of potassium balance as 80% of potassium is excreted by the kidneys. Potassium must be replaced daily to maintain its balance. Normally, potassium is replaced in food.

Hypokalemia

Hypokalemia is a potassium deficit or a serum potassium level <3.5 mEq/L.

Hyperkalemia

Hyperkalemia is a potassium excess or a serum potassium level >5.0 mEq/L. Hyperkalemia is less common than hypokalemia and rarely occurs in clients with normal renal function. It is, however, more dangerous than hypokalemia and can lead to cardiac arrest.

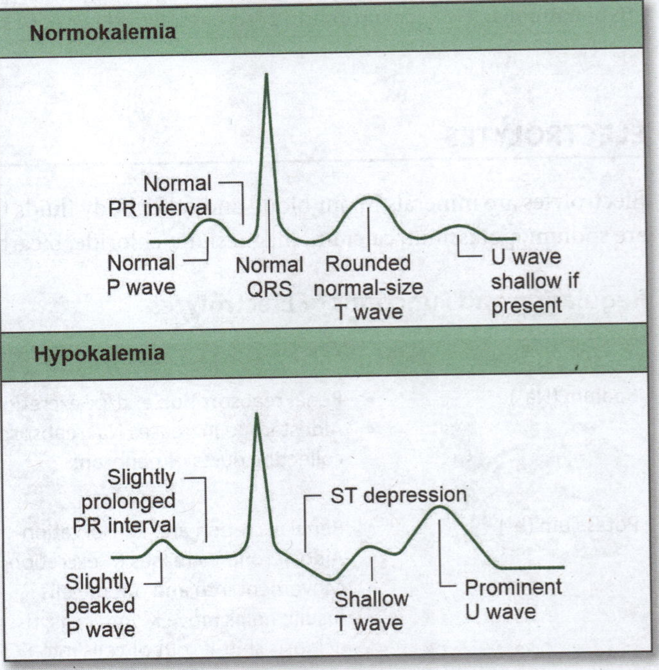

Contd...

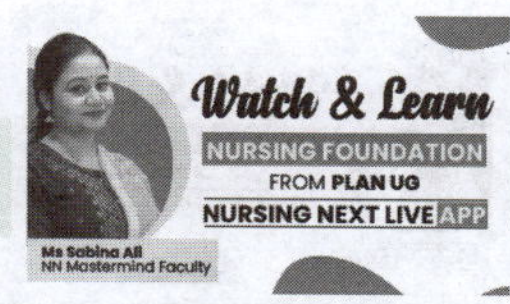

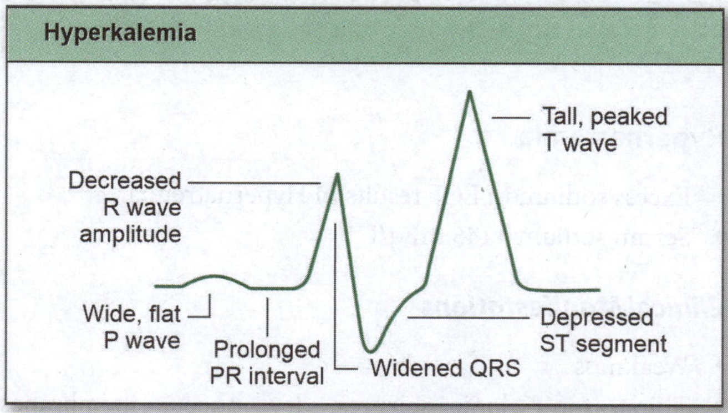

Calcium

Hypocalcemia

Hypocalcemia is defined as calcium deficit, or a total serum calcium level <8.5 mg/dL or an ionized calcium level less than 0.4 mg/dL. Severe depletion of calcium can cause tetany with muscle spasms and paresthesias (numbness and tingling around the mouth and hands and feet) and can lead to convulsions.

Hypercalcemia

Hypercalcemia is a calcium excess or total serum calcium levels >10.5 mg/dL, or an ionized calcium level of >5.0 mg/dL, most often occurs when calcium is mobilized from the bony skeleton. This may be due to malignancy or prolonged immobilization.

Magnesium

Hypomagnesemia

Hypomagnesemia is defined as magnesium deficiency, or a total serum magnesium level <1.5 mEq/L. It occurs more frequently than hypermagnesemia. Chronic alcoholism is the most common cause of hypomagnesemia. Magnesium deficiency may also aggravate the manifestation of alcohol withdrawal, such as delirium tremens.

Hypermagnesemia

It is present when the serum magnesium level rises above 2.5 mEq/L. It is due to increased intake or decreased excretion. It is often iatrogenic, that is, it occurs as a result of overzealous magnesium therapy.

Fluid Therapy

Intravenous Fluid Comparison

Type	Solution	Uses	Special Considerations
Isotonic	Dextrose 5% in water (D5W)	• Fluid loss • Dehydration • Hypernatremia	• Use cautiously in renal and cardiac patients • Can cause fluid overload
Isotonic	0.9% sodium chloride (Normal Saline) (NaCl)	• Shock • Hyponatremia • Blood transfusions • Resuscitation • Fluid challenges • DKA	• Can lead to overload • Use with caution in patients with heart failure or edema
Isotonic	Lactated Ringer's (LR)	• Dehydration • Lower GI fluid loss • Acute blood loss • Hypovolemia due to third spacing	• Contains potassium, do not use with renal failure patients • Do not use with liver disease, cannot metabolize lactate
Hypotonic	0.45% sodium chloride (1/2 normal saline)	• Water replacement • DKA • Gastric fluid loss • From NG or vomiting	• Use with caution • May cause cardiovascular collapse or increased intracranial pressure
Hypotonic	Dextrose 5% in ½ normal saline	• Later in DKA treatment	• Use only when blood sugar falls below 250 mg/dL
Hypertonic	Dextrose 5% in normal saline	• Temporary treatment for shock if plasma expanders aren't available • Addison's crisis	• Do not use in case of cardiac or renal patients
Hypertonic	Dextrose 10% in water	• Water replacement • Conditions where some nutrition with glucose is required	• Monitor blood sugar levels

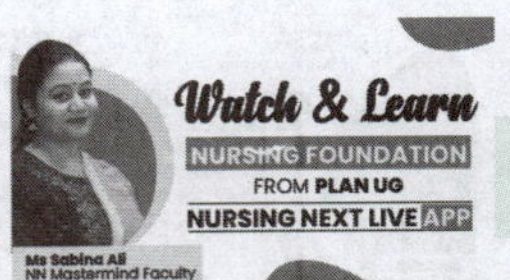

CONCEPTUAL EXERCISES

LONG ANSWER QUESTIONS

1. Discuss electrolytes imbalances in detail.

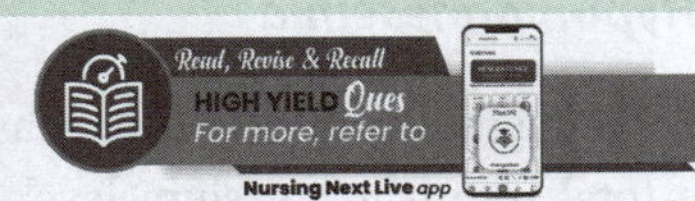

Answer

Electrolyte Imbalances

When the level of electrolytes like- sodium, potassium, calcium, etc. are too low or high in the body results into electrolyte imbalance.

Hyponatremia

- Hyponatremia is a sodium deficit or serum sodium level <135 mEq/L.
- It is a common electrolyte imbalance.

Clinical Manifestations

- Dry skin, ↓ saliva + BP, seizures, coma, headache, muscle twitching.
- Lethargy, confusion and apprehension
- Muscle twitching
- Abdominal cramps

Nursing Management

Assessment

- Assess clinical manifestations.
- Obtain thorough diet and medical history, including use of over-the-counter drugs and herbal drugs.
- Daily weight monitoring.
- Assessment of the skin and mucous membrane.
- Monitor lung sounds every 2–4 hours.
- Assess vital signs and peripheral vein filling every 4–8 hours.
- Monitor fluid intake and output.
- Monitor laboratory data (e.g., serum sodium).
- Assess client closely if administering hypertonic saline solutions.

Interventions

- Identify patients at risk of hyponatremia.
- Assess fluid intake and output.
- Assess the patient for signs and symptoms of hyponatremia.
- Restrict fluid intake.
- Administer isotonic IV fluids. That ensure appropriate fluid and sodium intake.

Hypernatremia

- Excess sodium in ECF results in Hypernatremia.
- Serum sodium >145 mEq/L.

Clinical Manifestations

- Weakness
- Thirst, tonic-clonic seizures, dry mucous membranes ↑HR+ BP+ temperature
- Tongue: red, dry and swollen

Nursing Management

Assessment

- Monitor fluid intake and output.
- Obtain detailed diet and medical history, including use of corticosteroids, over-the-counter drugs and herbal drugs.
- Daily weight monitoring.
- Assess the skin and mucous membrane.
- Monitor lung sounds every 2–4 hours.
- Assess vital signs and peripheral vein filling every 4–8 hours.
- Monitor behavioral changes (e.g., restlessness, disorientation).
- Monitor laboratory findings (e.g., serum sodium).

Interventions

- Identify patients at risk of hypernatremia.
- Assess the patient for fluid losses.
- Assess the patient for signs and symptoms of hypernatremia.
- Consult with a nutritionist to determine
- Encourage the patient to increase his fluid intake but decrease his sodium intake.
- Teach the patient and his family how to prevent, recognize, and treat hypernatremia

Hypokalemia

It is a potassium deficit with serum potassium level <3.5 mEq/L.

Clinical Manifestations

- Muscle weakness, leg cramps, depressed deep tendon reflexes
- Fatigue and lethargy
- Decreased bowel sounds and decreased bowel mobility
- Cardiac dysrhythmias
- Weak irregular pulses
- T-wave flattening and ST segment depression on ECG

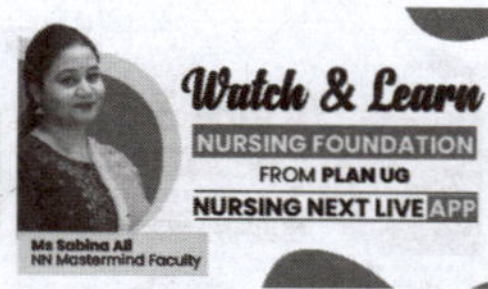

Nursing Management

Assessment

- Obtain history related to dietary intake, condition promoting potassium loss and use of diuretics, cortisone, over-the-counter drugs and herbal medications.
- Assessment of heart rate and rhythm.
- Assess the apical pulse. If irregular, assess for pulse deficit.
- Review of laboratory potassium level.
- Assess cardiac and renal functions every hour for client with severe hypokalemia and 8-hourly when the conditions improve.
- Assess neuromuscular and bowel functions every 4–8 hours.
- Monitor clients receiving digitalis (e.g., digoxin) closely, because hypokalemia increases risk of digitalis toxicity.

Interventions

- Identify patients at risk for hypokalemia.
- Assess the patient's diet for a lack ofpotassium.
- Assess the patient for signs and symptoms of hypokalemia.
- Administer a potassium replacement as prescribed.
- Encourage intake of potassium rich foods, such as bananas, dried fruit, and oran juice.
- Monitor the patient for complications.
- Have emergency equipment available for cardiopulmonary resuscitation and cardiac defibrillation.

Hyperkalemia

Hyperkalemia is a potassium excess or a serum potassium level >5.0 mEq/L.

Clinical Manifestations

- Gastrointestinal hyperacidity and diarrhea
- Irritability, apathy and confusion
- Cardiac dysrhythmias or arrest
- Muscle weakness, areflexia (absence of reflexes)
- Decreased heart rate
- Irregular pulse, paresthesias and numbness in extremities

Nursing Management

Assessment

- Assess the vital signs, bowel functions, urine output, peripheral edema and lung sounds every 4–8 hours.
- Closely monitor cardiac status and ECG.
- Monitor serum K^+ levels and BUN carefully; a rapid drop may occur as potassium shifts into the cells.
- Assess the apical pulse.

Interventions

- Identify patients at risk for hyperkalemia.
- Assess for signs and symptoms of hyperkalemia.
- Have emergency equipment available.
- Administer calcium gluconate to decrease myocardial irritability.
- Administer insulin and IV glucose to move potassium back into cells.
- Carefully monitor serum glucose levels.
- Administer sodium polystyrene sulfonate
- (Kayexalate) with 70% sorbitol to exchange sodium ions for potassium ions in the intestine

Hypocalcemia

It is called as calcium deficit, or a total serum calcium level of less than 8.5 mg/dL.

Clinical Manifestations

- Positive Trousseau's and Chvostek's signs
- Confusion, anxiety, possible psychosis, Tetany, seizures
- Numbness, tingling of the extremities and around the mouth
- Confusion, anxiety, possible psychosis

Nursing Interventions

- Assess the patient for signs and symptoms of hypocalcemia, especially changes in cardiovascular and neurologic status and in vital signs
- Administer IV calcium as prescribed
- Administer a phosphate-binding antacid
- Take seizure or emergency precautions as needed
- Encourage the patient to increase his intake of foods that are rich in calcium and vitamin D.

Hypercalcemia

Hypercalcemia is calcium excess or total serum calcium level >10.5 mg/dL

Clinical Manifestations

- Bone pain
- Anorexia, nausea, vomiting
- Constipation
- Polyuria, hypercalciuria
- Flank pain secondary to urinary calculi
- Lethargy, weakness

Nursing interventions

- Assess the patient for signs and symptoms of hypercalcemia.
- Encourage ambulation.
- Move the patient carefully to prevent fractures.
- Administer phosphate to inhibit GI absorption of calcium.
- Administer a loop diuretic to promote.
- Calcium excretion.
- Reduce dietary calcium.

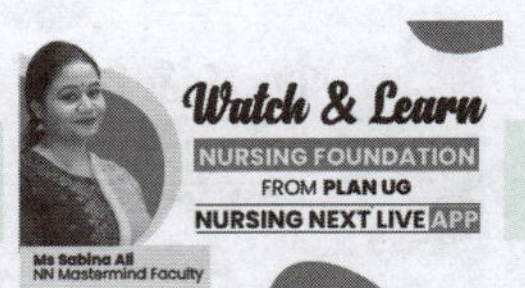

Hypomagnesemia

Hypomagnesemia is called as magnesium deficiency, or a total serum magnesium level of <1.5 mEq/L.

Clinical Manifestations

- Neuromuscular irritability with tremors
- Increased reflexes, tremors, convulsions
- Positive Chvostek's and Trousseau's signs
- Tachycardia, elevated blood pressure, dysrhythmias
- Disorientation, confusion and vertigo
- Anorexia, dysphagia
- Respiratory difficulties

Nursing Interventions

- Assess the patient for signs and symptoms of hypomagnesemia.
- Administer IV magnesium as prescribed.
- Encourage the patient to consume magnesium-rich foods.
- If the patient is confused or agitated, take safety precautions.
- Take seizure precautions as needed.
- Teach the patient and his family how to prevent, recognize, and treat hypomagnesemia

Hypermagnesemia

Hypermagnesemia is present when the serum magnesium level rises above 2.5 mEq/L.

Clinical Manifestations

- Peripheral vasodilation, flushing
- Hypotension, bradycardia
- Respiratory depression, coma
- Respiratory and cardiac arrest
- Prolonged QT interval, prolonged PR interval, widened QRS complexes and tall T wave on ECG

Nursing Interventions

- Review all medications for a patient with renal failure.
- Assess the patient for signs and symptoms of hypermagnesemia.
- Assess reflexes; if absent, notify the practitioner.
- Administer calcium gluconate.
- Prepare the patient for hemodialysis if prescribed.
- If the patient is taking an antacid, a laxative, or another drug that contains magnesium, instruct him to stop.
- Teach the patient and his family how to prevent, recognize, and treat hypermagnesemia

Chloride

- Hypochloremia is decreased serum chloride level, in adults a level below 95 mEq/L
- Conditions that cause sodium retention also can lead to high serum chloride level or hyperchloremia, in adults a level above 108 mEq/L

Phosphate

- The phosphate anion PO_4^{3-} is found in both ICF and ECF.
- Most of the phosphorus (P) in the body exists as PO_4^{3-}.
- Phosphate imbalance is frequently related to therapeutic interventions of other disorders.
- Manifestations of hypophosphatemia include paresthesias, muscle weakness and pain, mental changes, and possible seizures
- Hyperphosphatemia is defined in adult as total serum phosphate level >4.5 mg/dL

SHORT NOTES

1. Write difference between fluid volume excess and deficit. (MGR, DU)

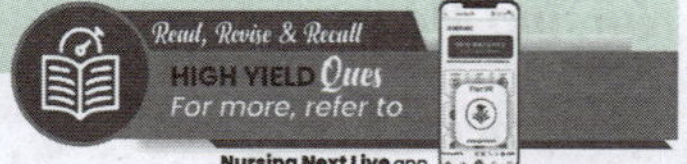

Answer

	Fluid deficit	Fluid overload
Definition	A decrease in intravascular, interstitial, and/or intracellular fluid. "Dehydration, water loss alone without change in sodium" (Wayne, 2019, para. 1).	Hypervolemia, or fluid overload, is the medical condition where there is too much fluid in the blood.
Causes/Risk Factors	• Abnormal bleeding • Diarrhea • Diuresis • Electrolyte and acid-base imbalance • Edema or effusion • Inadequate fluid intake, increased metabolic rate	• Heart failure • Kidney failure • Cirrhosis • Nephrotic syndrome • Premenstrual edema Pregnancy • Decreased cardiac output

Contd...

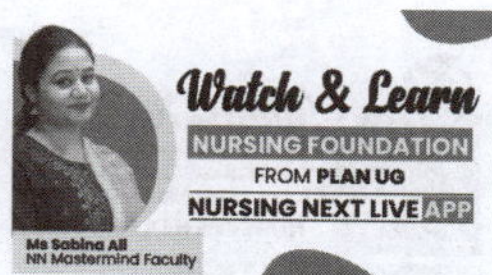

	Fluid deficit	Fluid overload
Causes/Risk Factors		• Chronic or acute heart disease • Excessive fluid intake Excessive sodium intake • Head injury • Hormonal disturbances • Liver disease • Low protein intake Malnutrition • Renal Insufficiency Severe stress • Steroid therapy
Clinical Manifestations (Including laboratory data)	• Alterations in mental state • Concentrated urine • Decreased skin turgor • Urine output <30 mL/hr • Dry mucous membranes, Hypotension • Sudden weight loss • Tachycardia • Thirst • Monitor BUN—if elevated, this can determine fluid deficit.	Symptoms of fluid overload Include: • Weight gain 2 lb./24 hours High BP • Normal temperature • Full bounding pulse • Moist labored respirations light yellow urine • Cool pale moist skin pitting and dependent edema • Distended jugular neck • Veins anxious

Management

Fluid deficit	Fluid overload
• Assess vital signs including heart rhythm, respiratory rate, monitor oxygen saturation. • Monitor CBC and serum electrolytes • Administer Supplemental oxygen, if needed. • Check neurological status to determine level of consciousness • Infuse Isotonic Infusions: 0.9% NS, LR. • Maintain I and O; encourage oral fluids, if tolerated by the patient. • Alert if urine output is <30 mL/ hr. report to the physician immediately.	• Observe RR, symmetry, effort. • Auscultate breath sounds for crackles • Assess the grade of edema • Strictly monitor intake and output of the patient. • Administer Supplemental oxygen, if needed • Administer diuretics as per doctor's order. • Support arms and legs to decrease dependent edema. • Reposition the patient.

2. Write a short note on dehydration. (MGR)

Answer

Dehydration

Dehydration is also known as hyperosmolar imbalance. A condition that occurs when the body loses too much water and other fluids that it needs to work normally.

Risk Factors

- GI loss-vomiting, NG suction, diarrhea
- Diaphoresis
- Diuretics, diabetes insipidus, CKD
- Peritonitis, intestinal obstruction, ascites, burns
- Excessive loss from wound
- Hemorrhage
- Altered intake dehydration
- Hyperventilation
- Prolonged fever
- DKA
- Enteral feeding w/o water

Signs and Symptoms

- Hypothermia
- Tachycardia
- Thready pulse
- Hypotension
- Orthostatic hypotension
- Decrease CVP
- Tachypnea
- Hypoxia
- Dizziness, syncope, confusion, weakness, fatigue
- Thirst, dry mouth, dry tongue, anorexia, weight loss
- Oliguria
- Diminished cap refill, cool clammy skin, diaphoresis, flattened neck veins, decreased skin turgor

Management

- Observe Respiratory rate, monitor for shortness of breath, dyspnea
- Check KFT, O_2 saturation, CBC, electrolytes
- Supplemental oxygen as per need with appropriate oxygen device
- Monitor vital signs, especially BP for hypotension
- Check neurological status to determine level of consciousness
- Assess heart rhythm
- Isotonic Infusions: 0.9% NS, RL, D5W
- Monitor and document I and O; encourage oral fluids also
- Alert if <30 mL/hr urine

Nursing Management

- **Intake include:** Water, juice, tea and coffee, IV fluid, NG feeding
- **Output include:** Urine, emesis, NG drainage, and blood drainage.
- Record all fluid intake in the sheet and calculate the total at the end of each shift.
- If intake (I) more than Output (O) look for signs of edema
- If intake (I) less than Output (O) look for signs of dehydration.
- Observations vital signs, such as pulse, blood pressure and respiratory rate, will change when a patient becomes dehydrated.
- Assess the skin status also for dehydration.
- Administer isotonic solutions if dehydration occurs as per orders of doctor.

3. Write nursing intervention for fluid and electrolyte imbalance. (MGR)

Answer

Different electrolyte imbalances in body are given below:

- **Hyponatremia:** Hyponatremia is a sodium deficit or serum sodium level <135 mEq/L.
- **Hypernatremia:** Serum sodium >145 mEq/L results in hypernatremia
- **Hypokalemia:** Serum potassium level <3.5 mEq/L.
- **Hyperkalemia:** Serum potassium level >5.0 mEq/L.
- **Hypocalcemia:** It is called as calcium deficit, or a total serum calcium level of <8.5 mg/dL.
- **Hypercalcemia:** Hypercalcemia is calcium excess or total serum calcium level >10.5 mg/dL
- **Hypomagnesemia:** Total serum magnesium level of <1.5 mEq/L.
- **Hypermagnesemia:** serum magnesium level above 2.5 mEq/L.
- **Hypochloremia:** Decreased serum chloride level, in adults a level below 95 mEq/L
- **Nursing Interventions:** Identify the patients who are at risk of fluid and electrolyte imbalances.
- Monitor serum electrolytes.
- Have emergent management available.
- Obtain IV access and maintain strict I/O status of the patient.
- Restrict fluid intake in case of excess
- Provide most appropriate fluid to the patient as per replacement therapy.
- In case of potassium imbalances, report the ECG to the doctor. Administer medications as per order.
- Monitor the patient carefully in terms of cardiopulmonary status especially.

4. Differentiate between respiratory acidosis and respiratory alkalosis. (DU, KUHS)

Answer

Respiratory acidosis	Respiratory alkalosis
Characterized by an increase in arterial CO_2 concentration and a decrease in pH	Characterized by a decrease in arterial CO_2 concentration and an increase in pH
Causes include hypoventilation, respiratory depression, chronic obstructive pulmonary disease (COPD), and airway obstruction	Causes include hyperventilation, anxiety, pulmonary embolism, and high altitude
Symptoms may include headache, confusion, lethargy, drowsiness, and shortness of breath	Symptoms may include light-headedness, tingling or numbness in the extremities, confusion, and seizures
Treatment may include supplemental oxygen, mechanical ventilation, bronchodilators, and corticosteroids	Treatment may include breathing into a paper bag, relaxation techniques, treating the underlying condition, and adjusting mechanical ventilation settings
In severe cases, respiratory acidosis can lead to cardiac arrhythmias, seizures, and coma	In severe cases, respiratory alkalosis can lead to cardiac arrhythmias, hypokalemia, and seizures

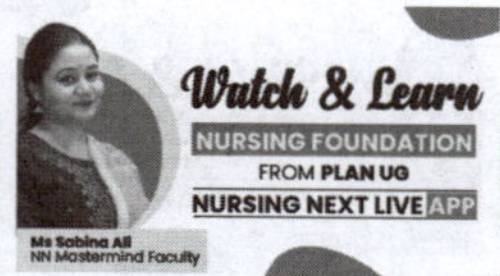

SHORT ANSWER QUESTIONS

1. Enumerate a difference between fluid volume excess and deficit. (MGR, DU)

Answer

	Fluid deficit	Fluid overload
Definition	A decrease in intravascular, interstitial, and/or intracellular fluid. "Dehydration, water loss alone without change in sodium" (Wayne, 2019, para. 1).	Hypervolemia, or fluid overload, is the medical condition where there is too much fluid in the blood.

2. Write the formula used for calculating drops per minute in IV infusions. (MGR)

Answer

$$\frac{\text{Volume (mL)}}{\text{Minutes}} \times \frac{\text{Door Factor}}{\text{(gtt/mL)}} = \frac{\text{Flow Rate}}{\text{(gtt/min.)}}$$

CONCEPTUAL REVISION

MULTIPLE CHOICE QUESTIONS

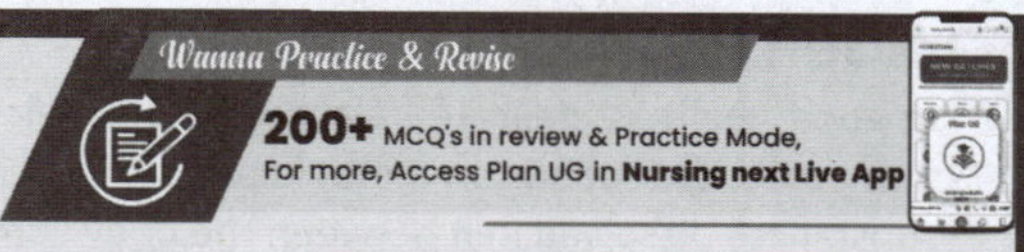

1. Which electrolyte would the nurse identify as the major electrolyte responsible for determining the concentration of the extracellular fluid?

a. Potassium
b. Phosphate
c. Chloride
d. Sodium

Ans. d. Sodium

2. A patient has a potassium level of 6.5 mEq/L, which medication would the nurse anticipate?

a. Potassium supplements
b. Kayexalate
c. Calcium gluconate
d. Sodium tablets

Ans. b. Kayexalate

3. A client is diagnosed with metabolic acidosis, which would the nurse expect the health care provider to order?

a. Potassium
b. Sodium bicarbonate
c. Serum sodium level
d. Bronchodilator

Ans. b. Sodium bicarbonate

4. A patient with tented skin turgor, dry mucous membranes, and decreased urinary output is under nurse Mark's care. Which nursing intervention should be included in the care plan of Mark for his patient?

a. Administering IV and oral fluids.
b. Clustering necessary activities throughout the day.
c. Assessing color, odor, and amount of sputum.
d. Monitoring serum albumin and total protein levels.

Ans. a. Administering IV and oral fluids

5. A first year nursing student, was rushed to the clinic department due to hyperventilation. Which nursing intervention is the most appropriate for the client who is subsequently developing respiratory alkalosis?

a. Administering sodium chloride IV
b. Encouraging slow, deep breaths.
c. Preparing to administer sodium bicarbonate.
d. Administer low-flow oxygen therapy.

Ans. b. Encouraging slow, deep breaths.

6. Lab tests revealed that patient's [Na^+] is 170 mEq/L. Which clinical manifestation would nurse Natty expect to assess?

a. Tented skin turgor and thirst
b. Muscle twitching and tetany
c. Fruity breath and Kussmaul's respirations
d. Muscle weakness and paresthesia

Ans. a. Tented skin turgor and thirst

7. Which client situation requires the nurse to discuss the importance of avoiding foods high in potassium?

a. A 14-year-old who is taking diuretics.
b. A 16-year-old with ileostomy.
c. A 16-year-old with metabolic acidosis.
d. An 18-year-old who has renal disease.

Ans. d. An 18-year-old who has renal disease.

8. A 36-year-old male client is about to be discharged from the hospital after 5 days due to surgery. Which intervention should be included in the home health care nurse's instructions about measures to prevent constipation?

a. Discouraging the client from eating large amounts of roughage-containing foods in the diet.
b. Encouraging the client to use laxatives routinely to ensure adequate bowel elimination.
c. Instructing the client to establish a bowel evacuation schedule that changes every day.
d. Instructing the client to fill a 2-L bottle with water every night and drink it the next day.

Ans. d. Instructing the client to fill a 2-L bottle with water every night and drink it the next day.

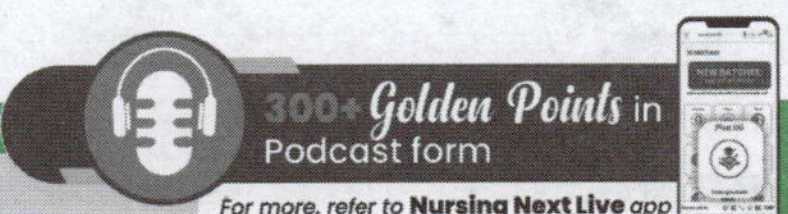

Golden Points

- In good health, a delicate balance of fluids, electrolytes, acids and bases is maintained in the body. This balance, or physiologic homeostasis, depends on multiple physiologic processes that regulate fluid intake and output, and the movement of water and the substances dissolved in it between the body compartments.
- An ion is an atom or molecule carrying an electrical charge. Substances capable of breaking into electrically charged ions when dissolved in a solution are called electrolytes. Water is the primary solvent in the body. The solutes are electrolytes and nonelectrolytes.
- The milliequivalent (mEq) is the unit of measurement that describes the chemical activity of electrolytes. For homeostasis, the total cations in the body are normally equal to the total anions.
- Potassium, glucose and urea are the primary contributors to the osmolality of intracellular fluid. Fluids are normally found in three spaces: inside the cells (intracellular), around the cells (interstitial), and in the blood stream (intravascular).
- The term tonicity maybe used to refer to the osmolality of a fluid. Solutions may be termed isotonic, hypertonic, or hypotonic.
- Isotonic fluid volume deficit (FVD) occurs when the body loses both water and electrolytes from the ECF in similar proportions.
- If the dehydration is not corrected, fluid is shifted from the cells into the vascular system. When the fluid loss is severe or life threatening, intravenous (IV) fluids are used for replacement. The type of solution used is based on the type of fluid loss from the body. Generally, isotonic, hypertonic and hypotonic solutions are used.
- Fluid volume excess (FVE) occurs when the body retains both water and sodium in similar proportions to normal ECF. This is commonly referred to as hypervolemia (increased blood volume).
- In fluid volume excess, both intravascular and interstitial spaces have an increased water and sodium content. Excess interstitial fluid is known as edema. Edema can be caused by several different mechanisms
- Electrolytes, charged ions capable of conducting electricity, are present in all body fluids and fluid compartments.
- Most electrolytes enter the body through dietary intake and are excreted in the urine.
- Some electrolyte, such as sodium and chloride, are not stored by the body and must be consumed daily to maintain normal levels.
- An electrolyte disorder is an imbalance of certain ionized salts (i.e., bicarbonate, calcium, chloride, magnesium, phosphate, potassium, and sodium) in the blood.
- The kidneys play a major role in maintaining fluid and electrolyte balance and renal disease is a significant cause of imbalance.

Administration of Medications

CHAPTER 23

CONCEPTUAL THEORY

Terminology

150+ key terminologies for Quick Recall & Revision

Adverse side effects: Although therapeutic effect is the desired outcome in administration of medicine, sometimes secondary undesirable effects occur. Undesirable effects other than the desired effects of a drug are known as adverse side effects.

Drug: A drug or medication is any substance that modifies body functions when taken into the body.

Intradermal route: The intradermal (ID) route, which deposits small amount of drug solution into the dermal layer, is used extensively for skin testing, such as tuberculin, on the inner surface of the fore arm.

Oral administration is the most common, least expensive and most convenient route for most clients. In oral administration, the drug is swallowed, therefore, the skin is not broken as in case of injection. Oral administration is also a safe method

Parenteral route: The **parenteral route** is defined as other than through the alimentary or respiratory tract that is by needle.

Pharmacology: The study that deals with chemicals that affect the body's functioning is called Pharmacology.

Pharmacokinetics: It is the effect of the body on the drug. It is the movement of drug molecule in the body in relation to the drug's absorption, distribution, metabolism, and excretion.

Subcutaneous route: The subcutaneous (SC) route is used for injecting medication into the tissues below the dermal layer of the skin usually in the upper portion of the upper outer arm, the anterior surface of the thigh, or the abdomen where there are no major vessels or nerves.

Topical applications are those applied to a circumscribed surface area of the body.

ADMINISTRATION OF MEDICATION

One of the basic nursing functions is the medication administration that involves skillful technique and consideration of the patient's development, health status, and safety.

A drug or medication is any substance that modifies body functions when taken into the body. One drug can have as many as four kinds of names.

The study that deals with chemicals which affect the body's functioning is called **Pharmacology**.

Drugs are available in many forms, or preparations. Drug preparations are available for oral, topical, and parenteral administration.

Pharmacokinetics: It is the effect of the body on the drug. It is the movement of drug molecule in the body in relation to the drug's absorption, distribution, metabolism, and excretion.

Although therapeutic effect is the desired outcome in administration of medicine, sometimes secondary undesirable effects occur. Undesirable effects other than the desired effects of a drug are known as **adverse side effects**. It is important to monitor adverse effects of drug therapy.

The adverse effects include allergic effects, drug tolerance, toxic effects, idiosyncratic effects, and drug interactions.

Serious adverse reactions must be documented according to agency policy and should be reported.

An allergic effect is an immune system response that occurs when the body interprets the administered drug as a foreign substance and forms the antibodies against it. Drug allergies can be manifested in a variety of symptoms ranging from minor to serious. The reaction can occur immediately after the patient receives the drug or may be delayed for hours and days.

The most serious allergic effect is called an **anaphylactic reaction** (anaphylaxis). It is life-threatening and results in respiratory distress, sudden severe bronchospasm, and cardiovascular collapse. This reaction is treated with

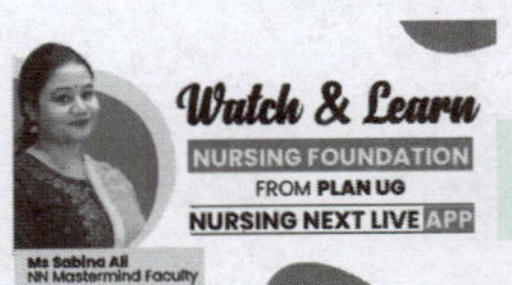

vasopressors, bronchodilators, corticosteroids, oxygen therapy, intravenous fluids, and antihistamines.

Drug tolerance occurs when the body becomes accustomed to the effects of a particular drug over a period of time. Larger doses of the drug must be taken to produce the desired effect.

Toxic effects are specific groups of symptoms related to drug therapy that carry risk for permanent damage or death. The organ or system affected by the toxicity is used to name the toxicity as in hepatotoxicity, or damage to the liver. Toxicities can occur from a cumulative effect. A cumulative effect occurs when the body cannot metabolize one dose of a drug before another dose is administered.

An idiosyncratic effect is an unusual or peculiar response to a drug that may manifest itself by over response, under response, or even the opposite of the expected response.

Drug interactions occur when one drug is affected in some way by another drug, a food or another substance that is taken at the same time. Drug interactions may be advantageous when a medication is given to decrease the adverse effects of a drug or increase its therapeutic effects. In a drug-drug interaction, the combined effect of two or more drugs acting simultaneously produces an effect either less than that of each drug alone (antagonist effect) or greater than that of each drug alone **(synergistic effect).**

Types of Medication Administration

Oral Administration

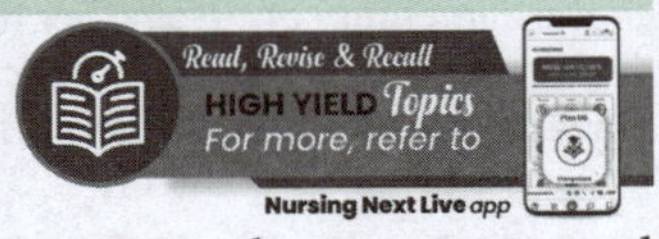

Oral administration is the most common, least expensive and most convenient route for most clients. In oral administration, the drug is swallowed, therefore, the skin is not broken as in case of injection. Oral administration is also a safe method.

Sublingual Administration

In sublingual administration, drug is placed under the tongue where it dissolves. In a relatively short time, the drug is largely absorbed into the blood vessels on the underside of the tongue. The medication should not be swallowed.

Buccal Administration

Buccal means "pertaining to the cheek". In buccal administration, a medication is held in the mouth against the mucous membranes of the cheek until the drug dissolves. The drug may act locally on the mucous membranes of the mouth or systemically when it is swallowed in the saliva.

Parenteral Route

The **parenteral route** is defined as other than through the alimentary or respiratory tract that is by needle. The following are some of the most common routes for parenteral administration:

- **Subcutaneous (hypodermic):** Into the subcutaneous tissue just below the skin.
- **Intra-muscular:** Into a muscle
- **Intradermal:** Under the epidermis (into the dermis)
- **Intravenous:** Into a vein
- **Intraarterial:** Into an artery
- **Intracardiac:** Into the heart muscle
- **Intraosseous:** Into a bone
- **Intrathecal or Intraspinal:** Into the spinal canal
- **Intrapleural:** Into the pleural space
- **Epidural:** Into the epidural space
- **Intra-articular:** Into a joint

Topical Applications

Topical applications are those applied to a circumscribed surface area of the body. They affect only the area to which they are applied. Topical applications include the following:

- Dermatological preparations
- Instillations and irrigations
- Inhalations: Administered

No medication may be given to a patient without a medication order from a licensed practitioner. Each health agency has its own policies. Usually the order is written, although telephone and verbal orders are also acceptable in a number of agencies.

For safer practice, the nurse should follow only a written or typed order or an order entered into a computer order entry system as these types of orders are less likely to result in error or misunderstanding. Under certain circumstances, such as in emergency a verbal order from the physician may be given to a registered nurse or a pharmacist.

TYPES OF MEDICATION ORDERS

There are four common medication orders which are as follows:

1. A stat order
2. The single order
3. The standing order
4. A PRN or as needed order permits

ESSENTIAL PARTS OF A DRUG ORDER

The medication order consists of seven parts:

1. Patient's name
2. Date and time at which the order is written
3. Name of the drug to be administered
4. Dosage of the drug
5. Route by which the drug is to be administered
6. Frequency of administration of the drug
7. Signature of person writing the order.

Drugs should be administered punctually as ordered.

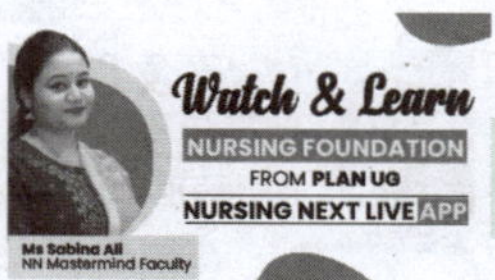

MEASUREMENT SYSTEMS FOR ADMINISTERING MEDICATIONS

Nurses are legally responsible for the drugs they administer. Any drug order suspected to be an error should be questioned. The suspected error may be in any part of the order.

It is important to understand that the patient's safety is a primary objective in the administration of medication:

Nurses need to be proficient in the use of weight and measures as well as system of measurement to calculate drug dosage and prepare medication for administration.

Three systems of measurement are used for administering medications:

- Metric system
- Apothecary system
- Household system

The **metric system** is the most widely accepted and convenient system. The basic units of measurement are the meter (linear), the liter (volume), and the gram (weight). The metric system is a decimal system, in which each unit can be divided into multiples of 10 (10, 100, 1000). Calculation of the metric system often involves moving the decimal point to the right or left.

The **apothecary system** is less convenient and precise than the metric system and is infrequently used. The basic unit of weight is the grain. The minim, dram, ounce, pint and quart are used for volume. In this system, Roman numerals are used to express numbers (grains X) and quantities less than one are written in fraction form (grains 1/4).

Household system is the least accurate system of measurement and is not widely used except in home setting. Teaspoon, tablespoon, teacup, and glass are commonly used household measures.

Sometimes drugs are prepared and supplied in the amount ordered by the prescriber, and the nurse can see while checking the medication label that no calculation is necessary. At other times, drugs are not prepared and supplied in the exact quantities called for in the medication order, and the nurse must do a dosage calculation to determine what quantity of medication the patients is supposed to receive.

Calculating Dosages

Several formulas can be used to calculate drug dosages. Formula to calculate the ratio:

$$\frac{\text{Dose on hand}}{\text{Quantity on hand}} = \frac{\text{Desired dose}}{\text{Quantity desired } (\times)}$$

Dosages for Children

The formula is the ratio of the child's body surface area to the surface area of an average adult (1.7 square meters, or 7.7 m^2), multiplied by the normal adult dose of the drug:

$$\text{Child's dose} = \frac{\text{Surface area of child } (m^2)}{1.7\ m^2} \times \text{Normal adult dose}$$

SAFETY IN DRUG ADMINISTRATION

Safety is of utmost importance in preparing and implementing drug administration. **Medication errors** are defined as the preventable inappropriate use of medications. These errors occur when medications are ordered, transcribed, dispensed, administered, and monitored. Medication errors can occur with almost any type of drug. There are many interventions that can minimize the risk of medication errors.

Three Checks and the Rights of Medication Administration

Observe the three checks and the rights of medication administration while administering medications to ensure medications are being administered safely: Check the label on the medication package of container three times during medication preparation and administration. The label should be read:

1. When the nurse reaches for the container or unit dose package.
2. After retrieval from the drawer and compared with the computerized medication administration record (CMAR) and before pouring from a multi-dose container
3. While replacing the container to the drawer or shelf or before giving the unit dose medication to the patient.

The rights of medication administration can help to ensure accuracy while administering medications. Ensure the following:

- Right medication
- Right patient
- Right dosage
- Right route
- Right time
- The right reason
- The right documentation
- Right to refuse
- Right assessment
- Right evaluation

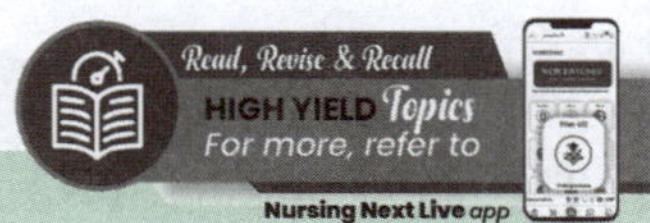

Safety Precautions

- Medication dispensing rooms should be locked.
- Controlled substances are kept in a locked drawer or container as an added safety measure, providing for a "double locked" system.
- Narcotics or controlled substances may be ordered only by physicians, and in some states, nurse practitioner, who are registered with Department of Justice, Bureau of Narcotics, and Dangerous Drugs.

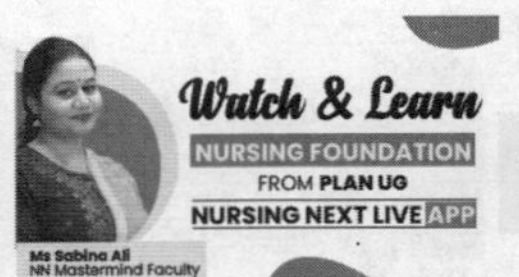

According to federal law, a record must be kept for each narcotic drug that is administered. The following information is required in the record:

- Name of the patient receiving the narcotic drug
- Amount of the narcotic drug used
- Hour of administering the narcotic drug
- Name of the physician who prescribed the narcotic
- Name of the nurse who administered the narcotic

The amount of narcotics on hand is counted, and each used narcotic must be accounted for ion the narcotic record.

PARENTERAL THERAPIES

The word 'parenteral' means outside the intestines or alimentary canal. It requires the use of syringe and needle, or intravenous catheter, to introduce medications into the body tissues or fluids.

Medications that are given parenterally must be sterile, non-allergenic to the patient and readily absorbable.

ROUTES

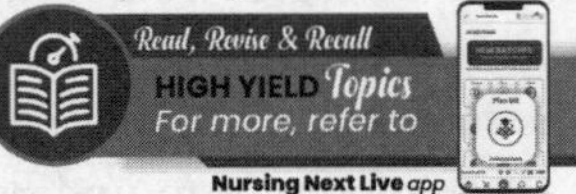

- **The intradermal (ID) route**, which deposits small amount of drug solution into the dermal layer, is used extensively for skin testing, such as tuberculin, on the inner surface of the forearm.

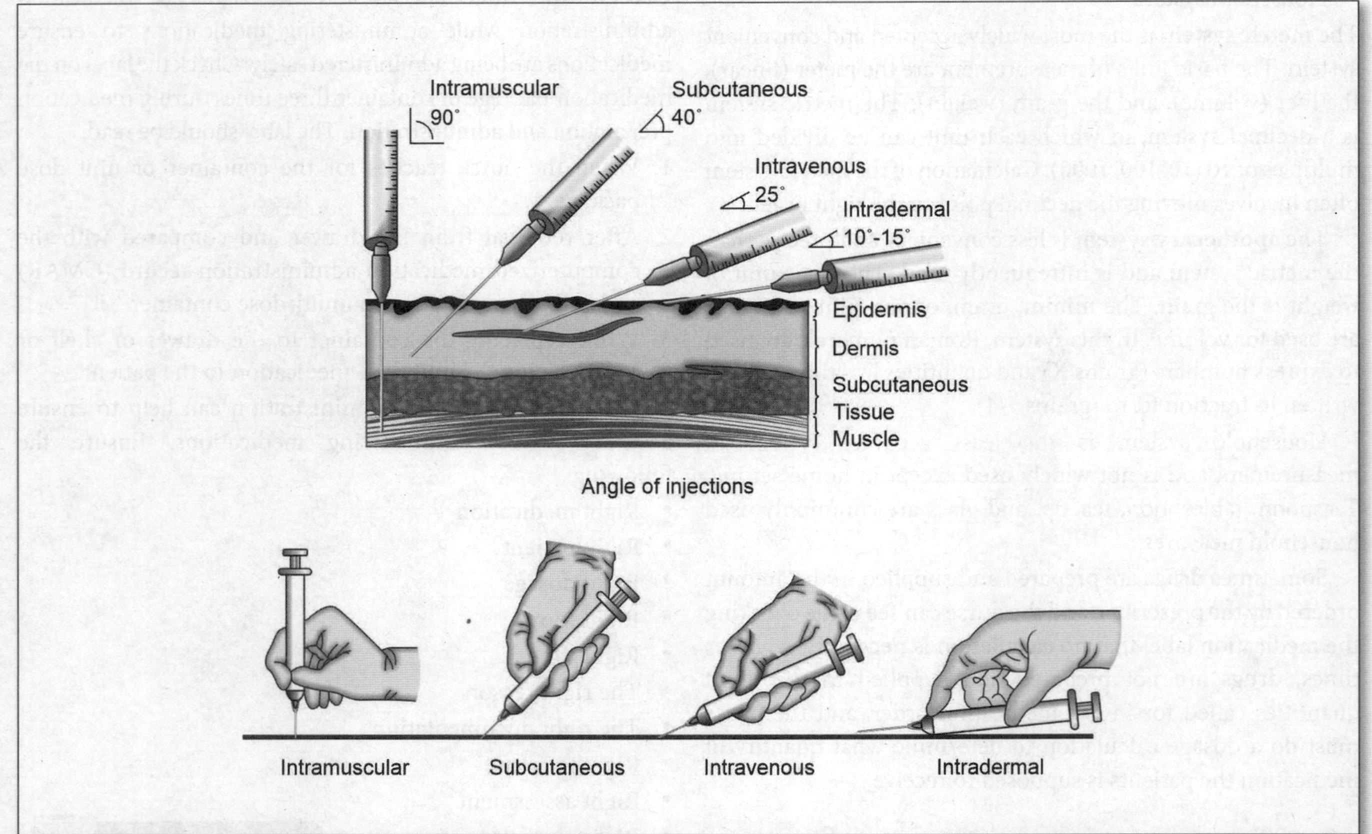

- **The subcutaneous (SC) route** is used for injecting medication into the tissues below the dermal layer of the skin usually in the upper portion of the upper outer arm, the anterior surface of the thigh, or the abdomen where there are no major vessels or nerves.

  Small amounts of solution (0.05–1.0 mL) are injected subcutaneously with either a tuberculin or insulin syringe which is inserted at a 45 or 90° angle depending on the needle length and the size of the individual.

- **The intramuscular (IM) route** means medication is injected in the muscular layer.

  The most frequently used IM sites are the deltoid, dorsogluteal, ventrogluteal, vastus lateralis, and rectus femoris of the thigh. The angle of injection is 90°, and depending on the size of the patient, a needle from 1 inch to 3 inches in length is utilized. Up to 3 mL can be safely injected in these sites in any patient.

Anterior
Posterior
Back
Lateral aspects of the lower part of the upper arm
Posterior aspects of the upper arm
Abdomen in the umbilical region
Thighs
Lower loins

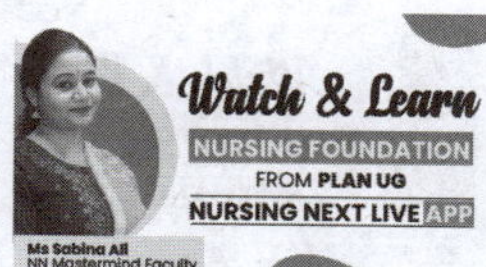

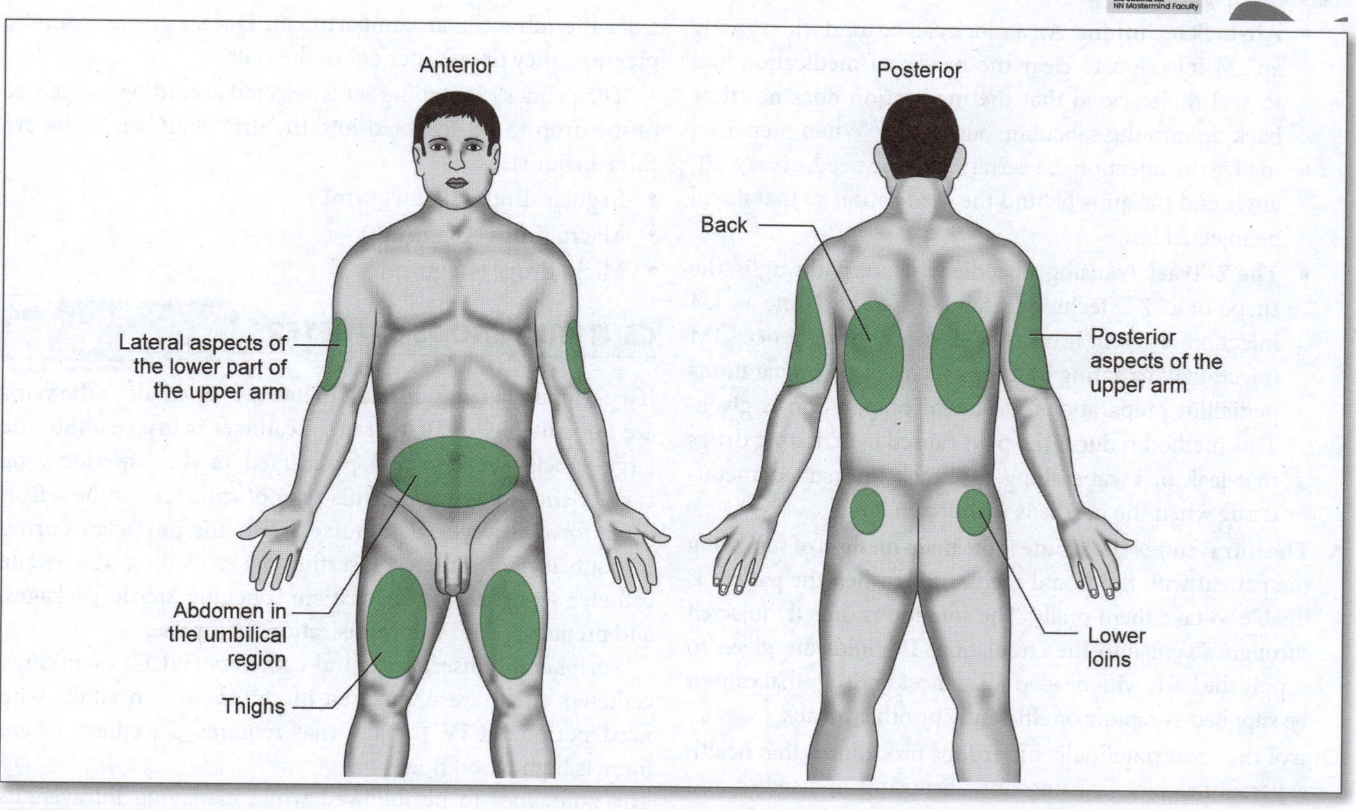

Deltoid
Deltoid muscle
Scapula
Deep brachial artery
Radial nerve
Humerus
Vastus lateralis and rectus femoris
Greater trochanter of femur
Rector femoris
Vastus lateralis
Vastus medialis
Dorsogluteal (not recommended)
Posterior superior iliac spine
Gluteus medius
Gluteus maximus
Greater trochanter of femur
Sciatic nerve
Ventrogluteal
Iliac crest
Anterior superior iliac spine
Gluteus medius
Greater trochanter of femur

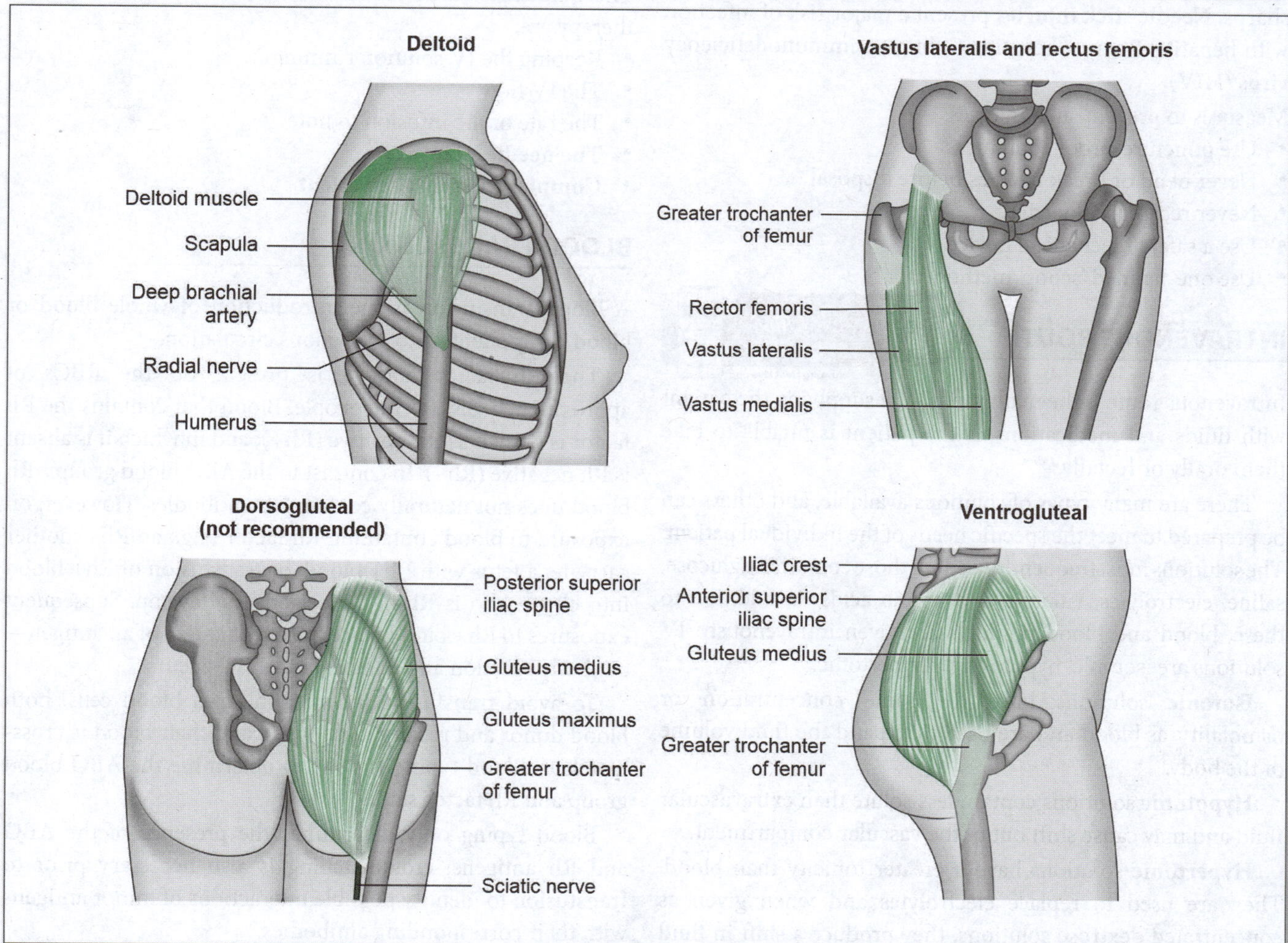

- **Air-lock technique:** An air lock can be used when giving an IM injection to clear the needle of medication and to seal the track so that the medication does not flow back up into the subcutaneous tissues. When preparing to give the injection, be certain that the needle is at a 90° angle and the air is behind the medication so that it will be injected last.
- **The Z-Track** (causing a needle track, or pathway, in the shape of a "Z") technique can be used any time an IM injection is given. It must be used whenever a deep IM injection of irritating solutions such as Iron preparations penicillin preparations, oil-based preparation is given. This method reduces the pain caused by irritating drugs that leak or escape along the track into subcutaneous tissue when the needle is withdrawn

- **The intravenous (IV) route** is the main method of supplying the patient with fluids and medications when the patient is unable to take them orally. The solution is directly injected through a vein into the circulation. IV fluids are given to supply the body with needed substances or drugs that cannot be supplied as rapidly or efficiently by other means.

One of the most potentially hazardous procedures that health care personnel face is using and disposing of needles and sharps. **Needle stick injuries** present a major risk of infection with hepatitis B virus, hepatitis C, human immunodeficiency virus (HIV).

Measures to prevent such injuries:

- Use puncture-proof containers
- Never bend or break needles before disposal
- Never recap used needles
- Use a safety mechanical device
- Use one-handed 'scoop' method.

INTRAVENOUS ROUTE

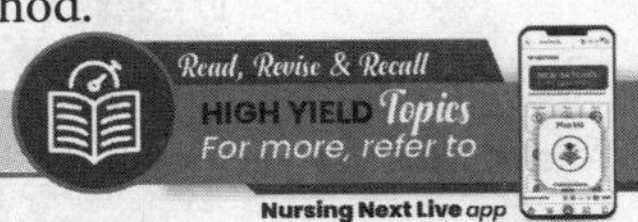

Intravenous route is the main method of supplying the patient with fluids and medications, if the patient is unable to take them orally or rectally.

There are many types of solutions available, and others can be prepared to meet the specific needs of the individual patient. The solutions most frequently used are those containing glucose, saline, electrolytes, vitamin, and amino acids. In addition to these, blood and blood products are given intravenously. IV solutions are isotonic, hypotonic or hypertonic.

Isotonic solutions have the same concentration or osmolality, as blood and are used to expand the fluid volume of the body.

Hypotonic solutions contain less solute than extravascular fluid and may cause shift out of the vascular compartment.

Hypertonic solutions have a greater tonicity than blood. They are used to replace electrolytes and when given as concentrated dextrose solutions, they produce a shift in fluid from the intracellular compartment. Due to greater osmotic pressure, they draw water out of the cells.

The primary IV tubing set is selected according to the size of the drop to be delivered into the drip chamber. There are three major sizes:

- Regular drops (10–20 gtt/mL)
- Macro drops (10 gtt/mL)
- Micro drops (60 gtt/mL)

CENTRAL VENOUS CATHETERS

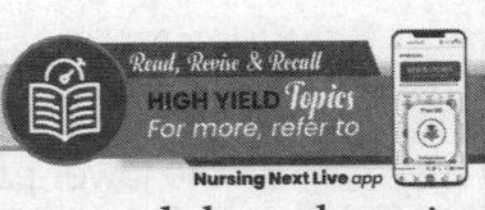

If a peripheral vein is difficult to locate in an adult or the veins are not suitable for IV therapy, a catheter is inserted into the large subclavian vein and positioned in the superior vena cava or the right atrium. This type of catheter can be left in place for 6–8 weeks. The nurse assists the physician during the subclavian catheter insertion by providing the sterile catheter tray, draping the patient, opening sterile packages, and preparing the IV administration set for use.

Peripherally inserted central catheters (PICC) or midline catheters (ML) are often used in children or in adults who need peripheral IV therapy that requires placement where there is high blood flow.

The guidelines to be followed while managing intravenous therapy are:

- Keeping the IV solution running
- The IV flow
- The rate of the infusion to note
- **The needle site**
- **Complaints from the patient**

BLOOD TRANSFUSION

A blood transfusion is the introduction of whole blood or blood components into the venous circulation.

The Rh factor antigen is present on the RBCs of approximately 85% of the people. Blood that contains the Rh factor is known as Rh positive (Rh+); and in which it is absent is Rh negative (Rh–). In contrast to the ABO blood groups, Rh blood does not naturally contain Rh antibodies. However, on exposure to blood containing Rh factor (e.g., an Rh– mother carrying a fetus with Rh+ blood, or transfusion of Rh+ blood into client who is Rh–), Rh antibodies develop. Subsequent exposures to Rh+ blood place the client at risk of an antigen—antibody reaction and hemolysis of RBC occurs.

To avoid transfusing incompatible red blood cells, both blood donor and recipient are typed and their blood is cross-matched. Blood typing is done to determine the ABO blood group and Rh factor status.

Blood typing only determines the presence of the ABO and Rh antigens, crossmatching is also necessary prior to transfusion to identify possible interactions of minor antigens with their corresponding antibodies.

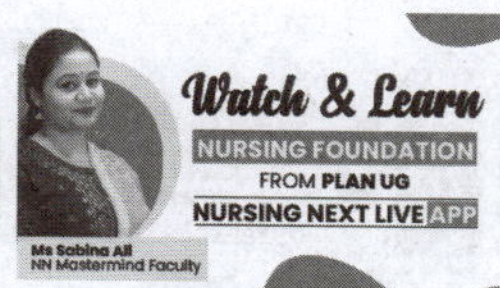

Screening of blood donors is rigorous.

Criteria are:

- Blood donors are unpaid volunteers.
- Donor is free from disease.
- Donor should not have history of heart disease, cancer, severe asthma, bleeding disorders, convulsions, malaria or hepatitis, pregnancy, surgery, anemia, high or low blood pressure and certain drugs.
- Potential donors are questioned about their lifestyle and health history, including questions about diseases, past surgeries, tattoos, body piercing, travel, sex and drug use.
- Donors may give blood only if their blood count, Hb level, temperature, pulse, respiration, blood pressure, and weight are within normal limits.

In other situations, only plasma is required, in case of low plasma protein or the blood clotting factors. **Fresh frozen plasma** is particularly useful in emergencies for immediate restoration of fluid because serum transfusion presents no compatibility problems and time need not be lost seeking donors and matching blood.

Platelet infusion is indicated for the treatment or prevention of bleeding associated with deficiencies in the number or function of patient's platelets. Platelet infusion is indicated in certain diseases such as Dengue fever in which the platelet count goes down.

Transfusion of ABO or Rh incompatible blood can result in hemolytic transfusion reactions with destruction of the transfused RBCs and subsequent risk of kidney damage or failures. Other forms of transfusion reactions may also occur, including febrile, allergic, circulatory overload and sepsis.

- Once a transfusion is ordered, obtain the blood from the blood bank just before starting the transfusion.
- Do not store the blood in the refrigerator in the nursing
- Blood is usually administered through 18–20-gauge intravenous needle.
- A Y-type blood transfusion set with filter is used while administering blood.
- Saline is used to prime the set and flush the needle before administering blood. It also provides a means to keep the vein open if a transfusion reaction occurs. No other IV solution should be administered with blood; it may cause the blood cells to clump or cause clotting.

TOPICAL APPLICATIONS

Topical medications are administered directly to the skin and mucous membrane by painting or spreading it over an area, applying moist dressing or soaking body parts in a solution.

They are applied to produce local effects, but certain topical preparations have systemic effects since they are absorbed through the skin and mucous membrane.

Systemic effects will be more if skin is very thin, if the drug concentration is high or if skin contact is prolonged.

Percutaneous routes are those by which medicines are absorbed through the skin or mucous membranes. They include:

- **Topical:** Applied to the skin
- **Instillation:** To the mucous membranes
- **Sublingual:** Under the tongue
- **Buccal:** In the cheek
- To the mucous membranes of eye, ear, nose and vagina
- **Inhalation:** Aerosolized liquids or gases

Different forms of Skin Applications

- **Ointments, lotion, paste and creams:** Smear lightly and evenly onto the skin's surface. Do not rub over the area.
- **Liniment:** Applied by rubbing it gently but firmly into the skin
- **Powder:** It is dusted lightly to cover the affected area with a thin layer.

Eye Drop Instillation

Read, Revise & Recall
HIGH YIELD Topics
For more, refer to
Nursing Next Live app

- For instillation of eye drops, hands should be thoroughly washed and gently shake the bottle to gently mix the content of the bottle. Using index finger, gently pull down your lower eyelid to form a pocket and instill one drop eye drop into the pocket ensuring the tip of the bottle doesn't touch eye, eyelid or eyelashes. Gently wipe away excess eye drops and perform punctal occlusion.
- Eye irrigation is the method of washing the conjunctival sac by a stream of liquid. The liquid used for irrigation should flow from inner canthus to outer canthus to prevent forcing the infection into the nasolacrimal duct.

Ear Irrigation

Ear irrigation is the washing of the external auditory canal with a stream of liquid.

- To remove the earwax
- To remove foreign bodies (except hygroscopic substances)
- To cleanse the ear in case of purulent discharge caused by middle ear infection
- To provide antiseptic effect
- To apply heat
- To evaluate vestibular functions

Solutions Used

- Boric Acid (2–4%)
- Sodium bicarbonate solution (1%)
- Normal saline
- Hydrogen peroxide (2%)
- Sterile water

CONCEPTUAL EXERCISES

LONG ANSWER QUESTIONS

1. List the various routes of medication administration. Explain the nurses' responsibility in ensuring medication safety. (KUHS)

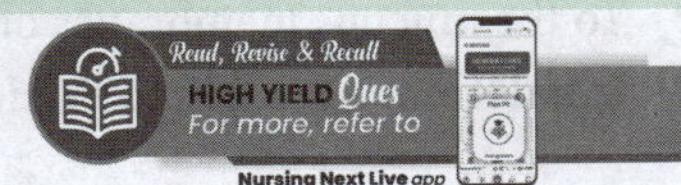

Answer

Routes of Medication Administration

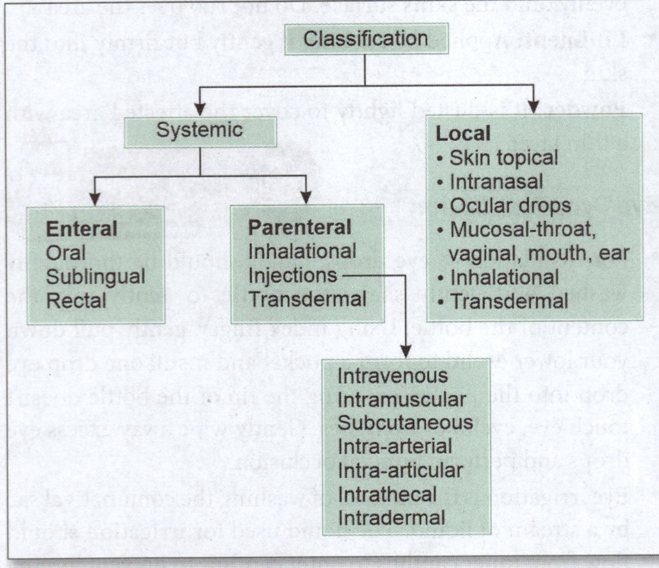

Nurses' Responsibility in Ensuring Medication Safety

- **During preparation of medications**
  - Read the physician's orders before preparing the drug. No medicine should be prepared without the doctor's written orders. Verbal orders are carried out only in emergency.
  - Check the medicine card against the physician's orders. Be sure that the medicine check is copied correctly on the medicine card and the nurse's record.
  - Concentrate on the preparation of medicines. Avoid conversations during the preparation of medicines.
  - Calculate the fractions of dosage accurately.
  - Give the medication only from a clearly labeled container.
  - Read the label of the container and compare it with the medicine card thrice:
    - Before the medicine container is taken from the shelf.
    - Before pouring the drug.
    - Before replacing the container in the shelf.
  - Always use a calibrated measure in order to measure the accurate dose.
  - Make sure that the medicine glasses are clean and dry before the medicine is taken.
  - Shake the fluid medication before pouring it into the ounce glass.
  - Wipe the mouth of the bottle, close it tightly and keep the bottle in a proper place after use.
  - Pour the medicine from the bottle on the side opposite to the label.
  - Hold the ounce glass at eye level and place the thumb on the mark on the ounce glass to which the medicine is to be poured. Read the lower meniscus of the fluid level in the medicine glass.
  - When taking tablets and capsules, do not touch them with hand. Drop the tablets or capsules from the container to its lid and then into the medicine cup to be taken to the bedside.
  - Once the medication is poured out of a bottle, it should not be poured back into the same bottle to prevent contamination of the whole medicine.
  - Do not use the medicine that differs in color, taste, odor and consistency.
  - Prepare the drug just before the time of administration of medicine. Never leave the drug in the medicine tray without proper identification.
- **Regarding the administration**
  - Observe ten rights
  - Observe the symptoms of overdosage of the drugs before they are administered, e.g., bradycardia observed in the clients getting digoxin tablets.
  - Identify the client correctly- by the bed number, room number, calling the name of the client, asking the client to repeat his name, asking others who know the client.
  - Give the drugs one by one.
  - Stay with the client until he has taken the medication completely.
  - Observe any contraindications in oral administration of medicine such as nausea, vomiting, unconsciousness, etc., whether the drug can safely be administered through the oral route.
  - Always give the medicine you have prepared yourself.
  - Remove the unpleasant taste of medicines from the mouth by the use of orange syrups, lemon juice or by mouthwash.
  - Do not allow the medicine glass to touch the mouth of the client when the medicine is administered to the client.

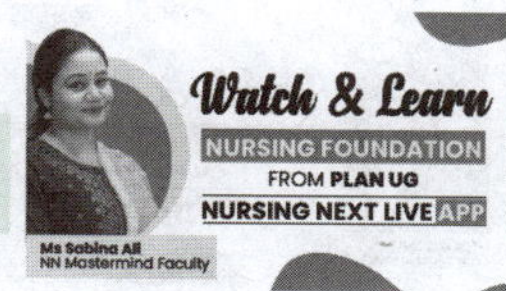

- Always provide a glass of fresh water to the client after giving an oral medicine.
- Report an error in medication immediately to the charge nurse and the physician.
- Do not leave the medicine with the client. Prepare a fresh dose of medicine, if the medication is to be given later.
- The drugs that stimulate appetite should be given before food. The drugs that are irritant to the gastric mucosa should be given only after meals. The drugs given for the local effect in the stomach (e.g., an antacid) should be given after meals to prevent quick absorption of the drug.
- Never give water after administering the cough syrups as they leave a soothing effect on the throat and prevent coughing sensation.
- If the client has a nasogastric tube for feeding purposes, the nurse can powder the medication and dissolve it in a solution and feed the client. The capsules can be opened to mix the powder with the other medications.
- Enteric coated tablets should never be chewed or broken or crushed for ease of administration, because they have irritating effect on the mucosa of the stomach. Some drugs are destroyed by the action of the gastric juice.
- The lozenges are to be sucked and not chewed until they are completely dissolved in the mouth.

- **Regarding the documentation of drug administration**
  - Record each dose of medicine soon after it is administered.
  - Use standard abbreviations in recording the medications.
  - Record only those medicines which you have administered.
  - Record the date, time, name of the drug administered, the dose of the medicine and the strength.
  - Never record a medication before it is given to the client.
  - Record the effect observed, the local and systemic effects, the side effects, the symptoms of toxicity etc.
  - Record the medications that are vomited by the client, refused by the client and those drugs that are not administered to the client and the reason for not giving the medication,
- **Ethical and legal aspects**
  - Under the law, nurses are responsible for their own actions regardless of a written order.
  - The nurse should know the law about the use of narcotics.
  - Narcotics should be stocked only by the persons/ institutions who possess licence to do so. (Narcotics are controlled because of the problems of drug addiction).
  - The nurse's responsibility includes prevention of medication errors by observing the "Ten rights" of giving medications.
  - Charting the administration of medication or its omission is the legal responsibility of the person who gives the medication.
  - The nurse should know what is and what is not acceptable practice in her own institution, e.g., leaving medications at the bedside of the client is strictly prohibited in certain institutions; in others, certain medications may be left with the clients.
  - Nurses have legal obligation to be fully informed about any investigational medications which she will be administering to a client.

2. Explain the nurse's responsibility in storage and maintenance of drugs in the hospital. (KUHS)

Answer

Responsibility of Nurse in Storage and Maintenance of Drugs in the Hospital

- To stock the medicines, each ward should be provided with a medicine cabinet, which should be large enough to accommodate all drugs to be stocked in the ward.
- As far as possible, the medicine cabinet should be kept in a separate room adjacent to the nurse's room.
- A washing sink with running water should be provided in that room for hand washing facilities.
- Adequate lighting should be provided within the cabinet to read the labels clearly.
- There should be separate compartments for different categories of drugs - for mixtures, tablets, powders etc.
- Drugs used for external use should be kept separate from the drugs used for internal use.
- The containers should be arranged alphabetically, so that it is easy to find them.
- Poisonous drugs should be kept in a separate cupboard with lock and key. Cupboard should be labeled properly- "poison" in red ink.
- A senior nurse should have responsibility for inventory maintenance and care of all poisonous medicines in the cupboard. A register should be maintained to keep the account of the poisonous drugs.
- A daily inventory should be taken to prevent theft of narcotics.
- No drug should be stored without labels, even for a day. All the containers should have labels written neatly and legibly. The labels should contain the name of the drug, the ingredients, the strength, the dose, etc.

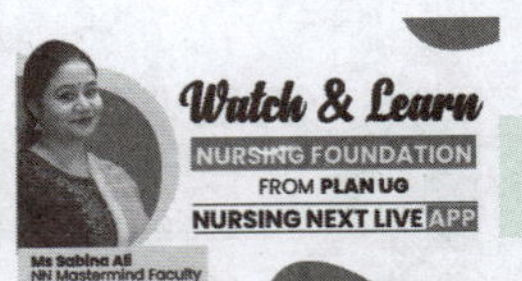

- All medicine containers should be kept closed always. The containers keeping the capsules, alcoholic preparations, volatile drugs, etc., should have airtight caps. The tablets and pills tend to disintegrate if exposed to air.
- The drugs that are unusual in color, odor and consistency should be returned to the pharmacy and replaced with fresh ones.
- Check the expiry date of every drug and make use of it before its expiry date is over or send it to the dispensary and get it replaced.
- The drugs which are destroyed at the room temperature such as vaccines, sera, antibiotics, etc., should be kept in the refrigerators.
- Emergency drugs should be kept in a place where they are readily obtainable for emergency use.
- When indenting for drugs, indent only the required quantity: the request for new supply of medicines should be signed by the ward sister. All medicines should be checked and signed as they are received from the dispensary.
- The medicine cabinet should always be kept neat and clean and kept locked and only doctors and nurses should have access to it.

3. Explain the procedure of intramuscular medicine administration. (KUHS)

Answer

Preliminary Assessment

- Check the doctor's order and identification data of the client.
- Check the indication of the injection.
- Recheck the physician's orders for the type of injection, the dosage, the time and the route of administration.
- Check the nurse's record to find the time at which the last dose was given.
- Check any history of allergic reactions and necessity for giving test dose.
- Check the site of injection where the last dose was given and the site where the next dose is to be given.
- Check the areas for redness, pain, itching, induration, skin lesions, sloughing, abscess formation. If any one of the symptoms present, report it to the charge nurse and rotate the site.

Preparation of the Client and Environment

- Identify the client correctly.
- Explain the procedure to the client to win his confidence and cooperation. Explain the sequence of the procedure and tell the client how he can cooperate in the procedure.
- Provide privacy with curtains and drapes, if needed.
- Restrain the site of the injection, in case of children.
- As far as possible avoid meal timings.
- Keep the attention of the client away from the injection by friendly conversations and curious articles.
- Place the client in a comfortable and relaxed position suitable for the type of injection.
- **Sites for IM injections are:**
  - Ventrogluteal
  - Dorsogluteal
  - Vastus Lateralis
  - Deltoid

Steps of Procedure

- Select the medication
- Wash hands
- Prepare the medication
  - Select appropriate needle and syringe
- Keep the syringe with medication in the sterile tray and cover it
- Make sure that the right dose and right drug was taken. Confirm using three checks.
- Carry medication to the patient in sterile tray
- Identify the right patient
- Maintain privacy of the patient.
- Prepare the site of injection
- Clean the site with alcohol swab.
- Inject the medication by correct technique. Needle is inserted at 90° and aspirate. If no blood comes give the medication slowly
- Remove the needle gently. Place the dry swab at injection site.

Aftercare of the Client and Articles

- Inspect the area for bleeding. If bleeding takes place, apply pressure, but do not massage.
- Help the client to dress up and take a comfortable position.
- Ask the client to take rest for 15 min to 1 hour especially when the drug is expected to produce some form of allergic reaction in the client.
- Ask the client to move the limbs to check whether any nerve injury has taken place.
- Monitor signs and symptoms of allergic reactions.
- If the client develops numbness or weakness walking, it may be due to nerve injury. Ask him to take rest, and inform the doctor.
- If the client develops pain, redness, induration, etc., at the site of injection, apply warmth. Inspect the area for abscess formation. The nurse can prevent these complications using correct method of injection and by rotation of sites.

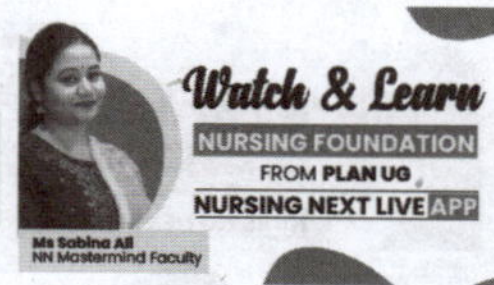

- Discard the needle and syringe as per protocol of biomedical waste management of the hospital.
- Clean all other articles and replace them in their proper places.
- Wash hands.
- Document the procedure on the nurse's record, with date and time.

4. Define therapeutic effects of medication. Describe the principles followed during administration of medications. (KUHS)

Answer

Therapeutic Effects

- Therapeutic effect is the effect which is desired or the reason a drug is prescribed. Therapeutic effects are the medication's desired and intentional effects.
- These effects vary with the nature of medications, the length of time the client has been receiving them and the client's physical condition. Interaction with other drugs can also affect a drug's therapeutic action.

The drugs are administered for the following purposes:

- **To promote health:** Drugs are given to the individual to increase the resistance against diseases, e.g., vitamins,
- To prevent diseases; e.g., vaccines and anti-toxins.
- **To diagnose disease:** e.g., helium used in the X-ray studies.
- **To alleviate diseases:** Certain drugs are given for the palliative effect or for the temporary relief of distressing symptoms but does not remove the cause or cure the disease, e.g., analgesics.
- **To treat or cure a disease:**
  - By restoring normal functions, e.g., digoxin
  - By supplying a substance that is deficient in the body, e.g., insulin.
  - By destroying the causative organisms, e.g., Quinine in malaria,
  - By counteracting with a toxic substance circulating in the body e.g., antidotes.
  - By stimulating the functions of an organ or a system, e.g., stimulants.
  - By depressing the functions of an organ or a system, e.g. sedatives

Principles Followed During Administration of Medications

The ten rights of Medications:

1. Right Patient
2. Right Medication
3. Right Dosage
4. Right Route
5. Right Time
6. Right Documentation
7. Right Client Education
8. Right to Refuse
9. Right Assessment
10. Right Evaluation

Three Checks of Medication Administration

Check the label on the medication package of container three times during medication preparation and administration. The label should be read:

1. When the nurse reaches for the container or unit dose package.
2. After retrieval from the drawer and compared with the computerized medication administration record (CMAR) and before pouring from a multi-dose container.
3. While replacing the container to the drawer or shelf or before giving the unit dose medication to the patient.

Principles	Rationale
• The knowledge of anatomy and physiology of the body is essential for safe administration of injection.	• To avoid injury, minimize pain and aid in absorption of drug.
• If carelessly given, injections become means of introducing infection into the body.	• Syringes and needles must be sterile to prevent infections and bloodborne diseases.
• Drugs that change the chemical composition of the blood will endanger life of the client, if not given properly.	• To promote proper functioning of vital signs.
• Any unfamiliar situation causes anxiety.	• Explain the procedure to the client.
• Once a drug is injected it is irretrievable. Antidote may be available for particular medications but the best antidote is prevention.	• Check ten rights of medications
• Organization and planning result in economy of time, material and comfort.	• It enhances manual and technical skills of the nurses.

5. Write the nursing responsibilities in the following scenarios: (MGR)

a. **Oral medication**
b. **Patient undergoing eye drop instillation**
c. **Patient undergoing eye irrigation**
d. **Intradermal injection**

Answer

Preliminary Assessment

- Check the doctor's order and identification data of the client.
- Check the indication of the oral medication.
- Recheck the physician's orders for the type of injection, the dosage, the time and the route of administration.
- Check the nurse's record to find the time at which the last dose was given.
- Check any history of allergic reactions, etc.
- If any adverse effects are present, report it to the charge nurse and doctor on duty immediately.

Preparation of the Client

- Explain the procedure to the client. Discuss the need for medication.
- Assist the client to a sitting position, if possible. A lateral position is the next safest and easiest, because a person lying on the back may aspirate the drug and fluids when swallowing. Unless contraindicated, raise the head end with extra pillows to provide a propped up position.
- Give a mouthwash, if necessary.
- If the medication is ill tasting, prepare a drink (e.g., lemon juice) to mask the taste of the medication.
- Protect the bed clothes and garments with a towel placed under the chin across the chest.

Aftercare of the Client and Articles

- Remove the towel and wipe the face with it.
- Position the client for good body alignment. Tidy up the bed.
- Take all articles to the utility room. Wash and dry all articles and place them in their proper places.
- Wash hands.
- Record medications given and omitted on the nurse record. Record the reason for omission. Record any reactions observed after the administration of the medicines.
- Return to the client to observe any expected and unexpected reactions, Report any errors, problems, omissions and untoward reactions to the appropriate person immediately.
- Return the medication cards to the storage area.

b. Patient Undergoing Eye Drop Instillation

Answer

Preliminary Assessment

- Check the name, bed number and identification of the patient.
- Check the diagnosis and the purpose of the eye irrigation.
- Check the doctor's order for specific instructions regarding type of solution, and the temperature at which it is to be used.
- Assess the patient's abilities and limitations.
- Assess the patient's mental state to follow instructions.
- Assess the need for any restraints.
- Check the articles available in the patient's unit.

During the Procedure

- Place the patient in a back lying position with the head hyper extended with a pillow under the shoulders.
- Ask the patient to look upwards while the nurse separates the lower lid by pressing it against the cheek bone.
- The drops are taken in a dropper holding the dropper from 1 to 2 cm above the eye.
- Instill a number of drops in the center of the lower lid.
- If ointment is to be applied, apply it from the inner aspect to the outer aspect.
- Ask the patient to close the eyelids and move the eyeballs from side to spread the medications all over the conjunctiva.
- Wipe off the excess medication that remains on the eye with a clean cotton swab.
- The nurse discards a small amount of ointment on a sterile cotton ball and wipes the top of the tube before she replaces the cap.
- Be certain that you have the right patient, right medication and the right eye.
- Check the doctor's orders to see what medication is to be instilled in which eye.
- Never instill any medication into the eye, unless it is ordered by the physician.
- Check the expiry date of the medications.
- Ophthalmic solutions should be sterile and are prevented from contamination during the preparation or administration.
- Use separate eye droppers for separate medications.
- Neither substitute a solution or medication of one strength with that of another strength nor substitute one medication for another, without permission from the doctor.
- Never use any solution or ointment which is unlabeled to instill in the eye.

After Procedure

- Take all articles to the utility room, clean and keep them to their proper places
- Wash hands.
- Record the procedure on the nurses record with date and time.

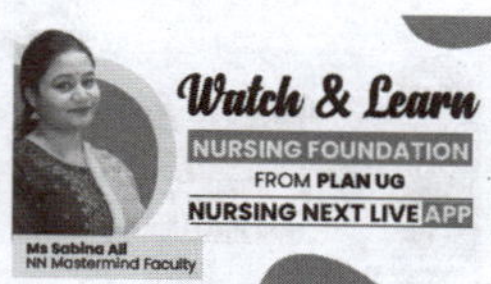

- Record the solutions used, medications instilled, the condition of the eye before and after the procedure.
- Repeat the procedure at the specified interval.

c. Patient undergoing eye irrigation

Answer

Preliminary Assessment

- Check the name, bed number and identification of the patient.
- Check the diagnosis and the purpose of the eye irrigation.
- Check the doctor's order for specific instructions regarding type of solution, and the temperature at which it is to be used.
- Assess the patient's abilities and limitations.
- Assess the patients mental state to follow instructions.
- Assess the need for any restraints.
- Check the articles available in the patient's unit.

During the Procedure

- Explain the procedure to the patient to win his confidence and cooperation.
- Explain the sequence of the procedure and tell him how he can cooperate in the procedure.
- Have the patient lying on his back with the head turned slightly to the side to be irrigated.
- If the patient is a child or uncooperative, restrain the movement to prevent any interference with the procedure.
- Protect the patient's garments and the bedding with a mackintosh and a towel.
- Arrange the light in a way to provide adequate light.
- Ask the patient, if appropriate, to hold the kidney tray to receive the return flow.
- Arrange the articles conveniently in the patient's unit.
- Wash hands
- Clean the eyelids and eyelashes using the wet swabs.
- Wipe the lids from the inner corner of the eye to the outer corner using one swab for one stroke.
- Irrigate the eye using an appropriate irrigator, don't apply pressure on the eyeball but press against the cheek and eyebrow.
- Irrigate the eye until the desired effect is achieved.
- Repeat the procedure on the other side, if necessary using separate articles and solutions.
- Wipe the discharge, if any, from the eyelids and clean thoroughly.
- Inspect the eyes for the effect of the irrigation. If the irrigation was carried out to treat inflammatory conditions, no pus should be seen when the procedure is completed.
- Instill the eye drops or ointments, if ordered.
- Apply dressings, if ordered.

After Procedure

- Take all articles to the utility room, clean and keep them at their proper places
- Wash hands.
- Record the procedure on the nurses record with date and time.
- Record the solutions used, medications instilled, the condition of the eye before and after the procedure.
- Repeat the procedure at the specified interval.

d. Intradermal injection

Answer

Preliminary Assessment

- Check the doctor's order and identification data of the client.
- Check the indication of the injection.
- Recheck the physician's orders for the type of injection, the dosage, the time and the route of administration.
- Check the nurse's record to find the time at which the last dose was given.
- Check the necessity for giving ID dose.
- Check the site of injection where the last dose was given and the site where the next dose is to be given.
- Check the areas for redness, pain, itching, induration, skin lesions, sloughing, abscess formation. If any one of the symptoms is present, report it to the charge nurse and rotate the site.

Preparation of the Client and Environment

- Identify the client correctly.
- Explain the procedure to the client to win his confidence and cooperation. Explain the sequence of the procedure and tell the client how he can cooperate in the procedure.
- Keep the attention of the client away from the injection by friendly conversations and curious articles.
- Place the client in a comfortable and relaxed position suitable for the type of injection.

Aftercare of the Client and Articles

- Discard the needle and syringe as per protocol of biomedical waste management of the hospital.
- Clean all other articles and keep them in their proper places.
- Wash hands.

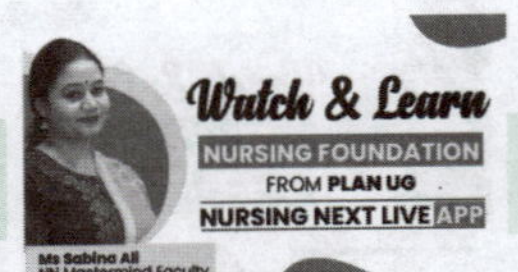

- Document the procedure on the nurse's record, with date and time.

Observation of the Site After Intradermal Injections

- If tuberculin test is done (PPD) ask the client to report after 48 hours. Instruct the clients not to compress the injection site, don't rub the site and don't apply any ointment, etc.
- If a test dose is given for penicillin injection, observe the area for reactionary changes after 20 min to 1 hour. The area will be reddened; the wheel will be increased in case of reactionary changes.
- Any unusual symptoms observed should be reported to the charge nurse and the physician.
- Any client who is developing increased pulse rate, respiration rate, giddiness, vomiting, wheezing, itching, cyanosis, etc., should be treated immediately.

SHORT NOTES

1. Write a note on complications of injections. (KUHS)

Answer

Complications of Injections

- **Allergic reactions:** Certain drugs, e.g., penicillin, sera etc., can produce allergic reactions in the client. Allergic reactions can be prevented by a test dose.
- **Infections:** Infections may be introduced through the careless handling and improper sterilization of syringes, needles and the fluids used for injections. It can lead to abscess formation and sloughing of the tissues.
- **Pyrogenic reactions** (producing fever): For example, the clients getting intravenous fluids may develop fever due to the pyrogens present in the fluids.
- **Tissue trauma:**
  - Repeated injections on the same spot can lead to induration of the skin, scar formation, etc.
  - Injury to the periosteum.
  - Injury to the nerves, e.g., injury to the sciatic nerve due to faulty intragluteal injections.
  - Injury to the walls of the blood vessels.
  - Psychic trauma especially in children.
- **Pain.**
- Accidental intravascular injections.
- Foot drop, persistent paralysis of the limbs etc., due to the nerve injury.
- Air embolism due to the introduction of air into the blood vessels.
- Overdose and underdose of the medication.
- Errors in the administration of medicines.
- Circulatory overload when large quantities of fluids are introduced into the body within short time.
- **Serum hepatitis:** Infectious hepatitis has been attributed to improperly disinfected syringes and needles. Inoculation of 0.0004 mL of the infected blood may transmit the serum hepatitis.

2. Write a short note on Idiosyncratic effect and synergistic effect. (KUHS)

Answer

Idiosyncratic Effect

Uetrecht and Naisbitt defined an idiosyncratic drug reaction as "an adverse reaction that does not occur in most patients treated with a drug and does not involve the therapeutic effect of the drug… they are unpredictable and often life threatening."

- This effect is unrelated to established pharmacological effects
- The effect may lead to serious organ damage
- There is a poor relationship to dose
- Uncommon
- Difficult to detect in drug development
- Cannot be avoided
- Patient idiosyncrasy is a major factor

Synergistic Sffect

The interaction of two or more drugs when their combined effect is greater than the sum of the effects seen when each drug is given alone.

- A synergistic effect occurs when a user takes two or more drugs/medicines which cause an effect that is far greater and potentially dangerous than if the medicines were taken separately.
- Mixing depressant drug such as alcohol and anti-depressants (Valium, Zoloft, Lexapro, Prozac) can cause respiratory distress and ultimately death from relaxing the respiratory system to the point that it can't function.

3. Write a note on sites of intramuscular injection. (KUHS)

Answer

Sites for IM injections are:

- Ventrogluteal
- Dorsogluteal
- Vastus Lateralis
- Deltoid

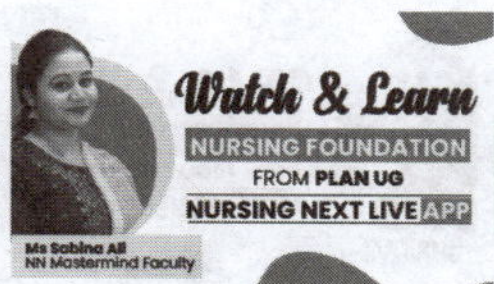

Ventrogluteal Site

- Injection is given to gluteus medius muscle.
- Position client in prone or side lying position with the knee bent and raised slightly toward the chest. The nurse places the heel of the hand on the client's greater trochanter, with the fingers pointing toward the client head.
- Point the thumb toward the patient's groin and the index finger toward the anterior superior iliac spine; extend the middle finger back along the iliac crest toward the buttock. The index finger, the middle finger, and the iliac crest form a V-shaped triangle; the injection site is the center of the triangle.

Dorsogluteal Site

- Injection is given to the gluteus maximus muscle.
- Position the client in prone position. Draw an imaginary line to divide the buttocks into four equal quadrants. The injection site is upper outer quadrant.

Vastus Lateralis

- The muscle is located on the anterior lateral aspect of the thigh.
- The landmark is established by dividing the area between the greater trochanter of the femur and the lateral femoral into thirds and selecting the middle third.

Deltoid Site

- It is found on the lateral aspect of the upper arm. Locate the site by placing four fingers across the deltoid muscle, with the top finger along the acromion process.
- The injection site is then three finger widths below the acromion process.

4. Write a short note on types of medication error. (KUHS)

Answer

A medication error is a drug error that may or may not reach the patient.

- It is usually preventable.
- It is usually unintentional.
- May or may not cause harm.
- A medication error that causes death is called a sentinel event by the Joint Commission. When a sentinel event occurs, the institution is required to perform a root cause analysis.

Types of Medication Error

- **Prescribing Errors:** Occurs when prescriber orders drug for a specific patient.
- **Omission Errors:** Failure to administer an ordered dose (not late dose).
- **Wrong Time Errors:** Administering the medication at least 60 minutes early or late.
- **Unauthorized Drug Errors:** Administration of medication to patient without proper authorization by prescriber
- **Improper Drug Errors:** Dose that is greater or less than prescribed dose.
- **Wrong Dose Form Errors:** Doses administered in different form than ordered.
- **Wrong Dose Preparation Errors:** Using Bacteriostatic normal saline instead of sterile water.
- **Wrong Administration Technique Errors:** Drug administered IV instead of subcutaneous/intramuscular
- **Deteriorated Drug Errors:** Refrigerated drugs stored at room temperature may decompose and lose efficacy.
- **Monitoring Errors:** Inadequate drug therapy review.
- **Compliance Errors:** Failure to adhere to prescribed drug regimen.

5. Write about nurse's responsibilities while administering blood. (DU, MGR)

Answer

Preparation for the Procedure

Identify the patient and check doctor's order.

Send blood sample for grouping and cross matching, it must be labelled correctly. A request form should accompany the specimen.

Blood bag received from the blood bank should be verified independently by a registered physician. Blood bag should be returned to the blood bank if there is any discrepancy.

It is recommended to use 18 gauge needle for infusion and care is to be taken to prevent introduction of air into the apparatus.

Rinse the blood transfusion set with normal saline before starting the solution.

Before the administration of blood, the patient's vital signs should be recorded correctly.

Offer bedpan before starting the procedure and as necessary.

Keep the medications (Avil, Adrenaline and Hydrocort) ready as per doctor's order.

Nursing Care During the Transfusion

Adjust the rate of flow to 5–10 mL per minute during the first 30 minutes of transfusion. Give the blood at a slower rate.

Transfuse the blood/blood products at room temperature.

Monitor the vitals during blood transfusion and record in the monitoring chart.

Watch the patient carefully for the onset of any complications.

In case of any adverse reactions developed in the patient, should be reported to the charge nurse and the physician immediately.

In case of any complication, administer the medications as per doctor's order. Send the sample to the lab and start infusion of NS. Send the blood bag with IV set to the Blood bank.

Document the incident report and report for further action.

Documentation and After Care

Record on the nurse's record with date and time (Starting and ending time)

- The amount of blood administered.
- The group and the type of blood administered.
- The rate of flow.
- Any reactions observed.
- Any medications administered e.g., antihistamines.

When leaving the ward, the charge nurse should report the following to the relieving nurse:

- The name and the bed number of the patient receiving the blood transfusions.
- The time at which the drip has started.
- The type of blood that is given.
- Amount of blood that is administered and the quantity to be given more.
- Any specific precautions to be followed.
- The specified rate of flow.
- Any reactions observed.
- Any medications administered.
- General condition of the patient.

SHORT ANSWER QUESTIONS

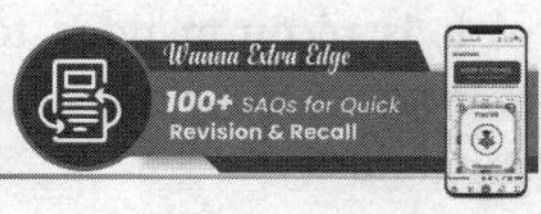

1. Write down the meaning of the following abbreviations: (DU)

Answer

- **NPO:** Nil Per Oral
- **Rx:** Take thou/take, prescription
- **BD:** Bis in Die (Twice a day)
- **s/c:** Subcutaneous
- **HS:** Hora somni (At bedtime)
- **alt.h:** Alternate hours

2. Write the ten rights for drug administration.

Answer

The ten rights for drug administration are:

- Right client
- Right drug
- Right dose
- Right time
- Right method
- Right patient education
- Right documentation
- Right to refuse
- Right assessment
- Right evaluation

3. Enlist various routes of parenteral therapy.

Answer

The following are the major sites of injection:

- **Intradermal (ID):** Injection into the dermis just under the epidermis.
- **Subcutaneous (SC):** Injection into tissues just below the dermis of the skin.
- **Intramuscular (IM):** Injection into a muscle.
- **Intravenous (IV):** Injection into a vein.
- **Intra-arterial:** Into the artery
- **Intracardiac:** Into the cardiac muscles
- **Intrathecal or intraspinal:** Into the spinal cavity
- **Intraosseous:** Into the bone marrow
- **Intraperitoneal:** Into the peritoneal cavity.

4. Define irrigation, instillation and inunction. (KUHS)

Answer

Irrigation

Irrigation is the washing or flushing of an area, using a large volume of fluid in order to cleanse, to apply heat or to apply medications.

Instillation

Instillation is putting a drug in liquid form into a body cavity such as urinary bladder or into a body orifice such as ears, eyes.

Inunction (Topical application)

Inunction is the application of the drug to the skin usually by friction, e.g., ointment. Many drugs are applied topically such as astringents, emollients, antiseptics, etc.

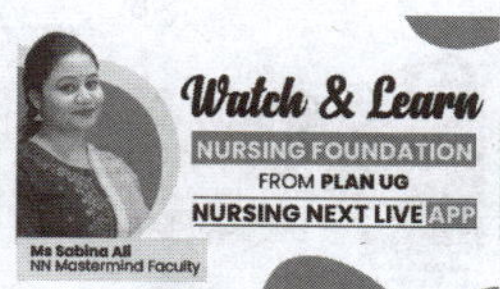

5. Define side effects and toxic effects. (KUHS)

Answer

Side Effects

- Side effects are minor adverse effects. Side effects can be harmful or harmless.
- These are the effects other than the principal action desired.
- Various side effects observed due to the administration of drugs are: dyspnea, rashes, dry mouth, etc.

Toxic Effects

- Toxic effects are specific groups of symptoms related to drug therapy that carry risk of permanent damage or death.
- The organ or system affected by the toxicity is used to name the toxicity as in hepatotoxicity, or damage to the liver.

CONCEPTUAL REVISION

MULTIPLE CHOICE QUESTIONS

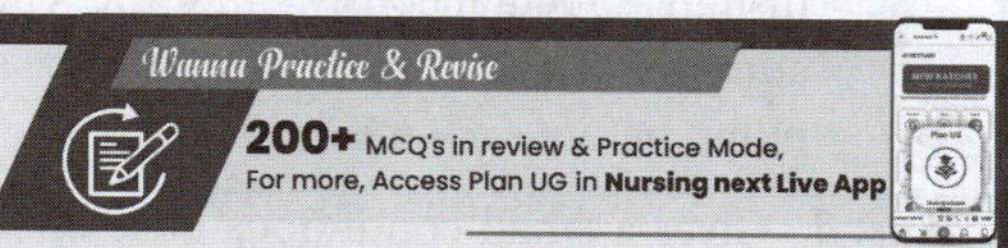

1. The best way of determining whether a patient has learned to instill ear medication properly is for the nurse to:

a. Ask the patient if he/she has used ear drops before.
b. Have the patient repeat the nurse's instructions using her own words.
c. Demonstrate the procedure to the patient and encourage to ask questions.
d. Ask the patient to demonstrate the procedure.

Ans. d. Ask the patient to demonstrate the procedure

2. All of the following nursing interventions are correct when using the Z-track method of drug injection; except:

a. Prepare the injection site with alcohol.
b. Use a needle that's at least 1" long.
c. Aspirate for blood before injection.
d. Rub the site vigorously after the injection to promote absorption.

Ans. d. Rub the site vigorously after the injection to promote absorption.

3. The correct method for determining the vastus lateralis site for IM injection is to:

a. Locate the upper aspect of the upper outer quadrant of the buttock about 5 to 8 cm below the iliac crest.
b. Palpate the lower edge of the acromion process and the midpoint lateral aspect of the arm.
c. Palpate a 1" circular area anterior to the umbilicus.
d. Divide the area between the greater femoral trochanter and the lateral femoral condyle into thirds, and select the middle third on the anterior of the thigh.

Ans. d. Divide the area between the greater femoral trochanter and the lateral femoral condyle into ...

4. The mid-deltoid injection site is seldom used for IM injections because it:

a. Can accommodate only 1 mL or less of medication.
b. Bruises too easily.
c. Can be used only when the patient is lying down.
d. Does not readily absorb parenteral medication.

Ans. a. Can accommodate only 1 ml or less of medication

5. Diclofenac sodium, 50 mg PO, is ordered. Diclofenac sodium is available as 100 mg per tablets. How many tablets would the nurse administer?

a. 0.25
b. 0.5
c. 1
d. 2

Ans. b. 0.5

6. You are posted in community health centre and assisting the OPD doctor. The doctor asked you to give 20 mL syrup to the client by using the teaspoon available at OPD. How much teaspoon of syrup the nurse will give to the client?

a. 1
b. 2
c. 4
d. 5

Ans. c. 4

7. Which of the following statements is true in relation to skin fold technique used for insulin administration in an adult patient?

a. If the needle is longer than 4 mm
b. Skin fold technique is used to avoid the risk of injecting insulin into the muscles
c. The best way of skin fold technique is to use thumb of both the hands.
d. When administering the insulin through pen, there is no need to perform skin folding technique

Ans. b. Skin fold technique is used to avoid the risk of injecting insulin into the muscles

8. Which of the following statements is correct in relation to an insulin infusion pump?

a. Is timed to release programmed doses of short-duration or NPH insulin into the bloodstream at specific intervals
b. Continuously infuses small amounts of NPH insulin into the bloodstream while regularly monitoring blood glucose levels
c. Is surgically attached to the pancreas and infuses regular insulin into the pancreas, which in turn releases the insulin into the bloodstream
d. Gives a small continuous dose of short-duration insulin subcutaneously, and the client can self-administer a bolus with an additional dose from the pump before each meal

Ans. d. Gives a small continuous dose of short-duration insulin subcutaneously, and the client can…

9. The physician has ordered Digoxin 0.1 mg every day PO What kind of medication order is this?

a. Stat
b. Standing
c. PRN
d. All of the above

Ans. b. Standing

10. Which of the following is not included among the 5 Moments for Medication Safety as per the World Health organization (WHO) Global Patient Safety Challenge?

a. Starting a medication
b. Adding a medication
c. Purchasing my medication
d. Reviewing my medication

Ans. c. Purchasing my medication

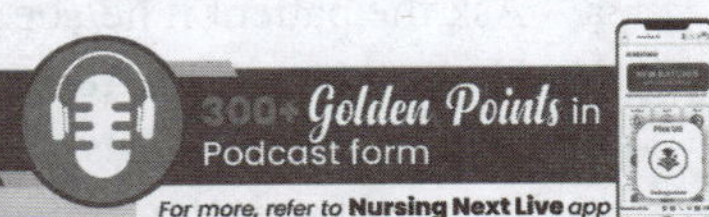

Golden Points

- One of the basic nursing functions is the medication administration that involves skillful technique and consideration of the patient's development, health status, and safety.
- A drug or medication is any substance that modifies body functions when taken into the body. One drug can have as many as four kinds of names.
- The study that deals with chemicals which affect the body's functioning is called Pharmacology.
- Pharmacokinetics: It is the effect of the body on the drug. It is the movement of drug molecule in the body in relation to the drug's absorption, distribution, metabolism, and excretion.
- Although therapeutic effect is the desired outcome in administration of medicine, sometimes secondary undesirable effects occur. Undesirable effects other than the desired effects of a drug are known as adverse side effects.
- The adverse effects include allergic effects, drug tolerance, toxic effects, idiosyncratic effects, and drug interactions.
- Drugs are available in many forms or preparations. Drug preparations are available for oral, topical, and parenteral administration.
- Oral administration is the most common, least expensive and most convenient route for most clients. In oral administration, the drug is swallowed, therefore, the skin is not broken as in case of injection. Oral administration is also a safe method.
- In sublingual administration, drug is placed under the tongue where it dissolves.
- Buccal means "pertaining to the cheek". In buccal administration, a medication is held in the mouth against the mucous membranes of the cheek until the drug dissolves.
- Topical applications are those applied to a circumscribed surface area of the body.
- The parenteral route is defined as other than through the alimentary or respiratory tract, that is by needle.
- Intradermal, subcutaneous, intramuscular and intravenous routes are used for parenteral medication administration.
- The intradermal (ID) route, which deposits small amount of drug solution into the dermal layer, is used extensively for skin testing, such as tuberculin, on the inner surface of the fore-arm.
- The subcutaneous (SC) route is used for injecting medication into the tissues below the dermal layer of the skin usually in the upper portion of the upper outer arm, the anterior surface of the thigh, or the abdomen where there are no major vessels or nerves.
- The intramuscular (IM) route means medication is injected in the muscular layer. The most frequently used IM sites are the deltoid, dorsogluteal, ventrogluteal, vastus lateralis, and rectus femoris of the thigh.
- In IM, the angle of injection is 90°, and depending on the size of the patient, a needle from 1 inch to 3 inches in length is utilized. Up to 3 mL can be safely injected in these sites in any patient
- The intravenous (IV) route is the main method of supplying the patient with fluids and medications when the patient is unable to take them orally. The solution is directly injected through a vein into the circulation.
- There are four common medication orders which are stat order, single order, standing order, PRN or as needed order permits.
- Nurses are legally responsible for the drugs they administer. Any drug order suspected to be an error should be questioned. The suspected error may be in any part of the order.

CHAPTER

24

Sensory Needs

CONCEPTUAL THEORY

Terminology

150+ key terminologies for Quick Recall & Revision

Coma: The patient who appears to be asleep and at the same time in incapable is responding, is in a state of coma. Coma may vary in degree from light to medium to deep. In deepest stage, no reaction of any type from the patient. Corneal, pupillary, pharyngeal, tendon and plantar reflexes are absent. Coma may last for can be obtained few days to few weeks.

Confusion state: It is a state in which the patient cannot take into account all elements of his/her immediate environment, implying an element of sensorial clouding. Apathy and drowsiness are often prominent and accompanied by disorientation primarily for time, less often for place and rarely for self.

Consciousness: It is defined as a state of awareness of self, time and of environment, as well as a state of responsiveness to that environment or adaptation to the external stimuli.

Delirium: It is characterized by a fluctuating disturbance in consciousness and change in cognition that develop over a period of time. It is generally accompanied by increased morbidity and subsequent functional decline.

Obtundation: It is characterized by reduced alertness and hypersomnia (a state of excess of sleep). When awakened from an obtunded state, the patient remains drowsy and confused and wakefulness can only be maintained by continuous verbal and painful stimuli.

Sensory Deficit: Inadequate functioning or impairment in any of the senses is known as sensory deficit, e.g., impairment of hearing and vision, taste alterations, and numbness. Such sensory deficits may be present at the time of birth or may develop suddenly due to any illness. These deficits may be permanent or temporary, reversible or irreversible.

Sensory Perception: This is the conscious process of selecting, organizing and interpreting data from the senses into meaningful information. Perception is influenced by the intensity, size, change or representation of stimuli, as well as by past experiences, knowledge and attitudes.

Sensory Reception: It is the process of receiving data about the external and internal environment through the senses. The senses by which individuals maintain contact with the external environment are vision (visual), hearing (auditory), smell (olfactory), taste (gustatory) and touch (tactile). Individuals orient themselves internally by the kinesthetic and visceral senses.

Stupor: It is unresponsiveness from which the patient can only be aroused by vigorous repeated painful stimuli. **The patient** is unable to localize the site of the painful stimuli.

Unconsciousness: It is a condition in which the patient is unresponsive and unaware of environmental stimuli. Impairment of consciousness indicates dysfunction of reticular activating system (RAS). It can be brief, lasting for few seconds, hours, days or longer.

INTRODUCTION

A person's senses are vital for the survival, growth and development and the experience of environmental stimuli. The sensory experience consists of two components: Reception and perception.

Sensory Reception

Sensory reception is the process of receiving data about the external and internal environment through the senses. The senses by which individuals maintain contact with the external environment are vision (visual), hearing (auditory), smell (olfactory), taste (gustatory) and touch (tactile). Individuals orient themselves internally by the kinesthetic and visceral senses.

Sensory Perception

Sensory perception is the conscious process of selecting, organizing and interpreting data from the senses into meaningful information. Perception is influenced by the intensity, size, change or representation of stimuli, as well as by past experiences, knowledge and attitudes. Four conditions must be met to receive data:

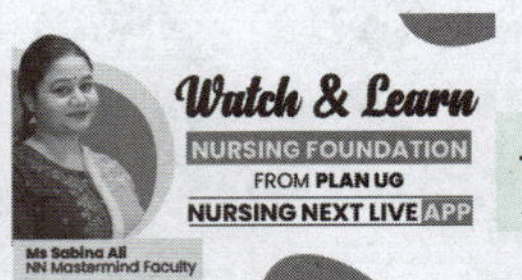

1. A stimulus
2. A receptor
3. Nerve impulse
4. A particular area in the brain must receive and translate the impulse into a sensation.

To receive stimuli and respond appropriately, the brain must be alert or aroused. The reticular activating system (RAS) that extends from the hypothalamus to the medulla, mediates arousal. Nerve impulses from all the sensory tracts reach the RAS, which then selectively allow certain impulses to reach the cerebral cortex and be perceived. The RAS serves to monitor and to regulate incoming sensory stimuli, thus maintaining, enhancing, or inhibiting cortical arousal.

Sensory Deficit

Inadequate functioning or impairment in any of the senses is known as sensory deficit, e.g., impairment of hearing and vision, taste alterations, and numbness. Such sensory deficits may be present at the time of birth or may develop suddenly due to any illness. These deficits may be permanent or temporary, reversible or irreversible.

A person's senses are vital to the survival, growth and development and the experience of environmental stimuli.

The sensory experience consists of two components: Reception and perception.

Arousal Mechanism

To receive stimuli and respond appropriately, the brain must be alert or aroused. The reticular activating system (RAS) that extends from the hypothalamus to the medulla, mediates arousal. Nerve impulses from all the sensory tracts reach the RAS, which then selectively allows certain impulses to reach the cerebral cortex and be perceived. The RAS serves to monitor and to regulate incoming sensory stimuli, thus maintaining, enhancing, or inhibiting cortical arousal. States

- Factors influencing sensory function:
- Developmental Consideration
- *Drugs*
- *Personality and Lifestyle*
- *Stress and Illness*

In normal situations, individuals are adjusted to a certain level of sensory stimulation which varies both, in quantity and quality as compared to individuals who get admitted in hospital. Patients in hospitals, are confronted with the different stimuli which directly or indirectly influence the sensory stimulation in several ways and can lead to sensory alterations. Carefully observing the factors which have impact on the hearing, visual and tactile stimulation of patients can help the patients in reducing the sensory disturbance.

Sensory Deficit

Inadequate functioning or impairment in any of the senses is known as sensory deficit-impairment of hearing and vision, taste alterations, and numbness. Such sensory deficits may be present at the time of birth or may develop suddenly due to any illness. These deficits may be permanent or temporary, reversible or irreversible.

Sensory Deprivation

- Decreased sensory input leads to insufficient quantity or quality of stimuli, which is known as sensory deprivation.
- The decreased sensory input disables reticular actively system (RAS) to an extent where RAS does not project a normal level of activation of the brain.
- Sensory deprivation can cause cognitive, emotional and perceptual damage to the person.

Sensory Overload

Sensory overload refers to the condition. When five senses—sight, hearing, smell, touch, and taste take in more information than your brain can process. Common symptoms include: Difficulty focusing, extreme irritability restlessness and discomfort, stress, fear, anxiety about surroundings.

PROMOTING MEANINGFUL COMMUNICATION

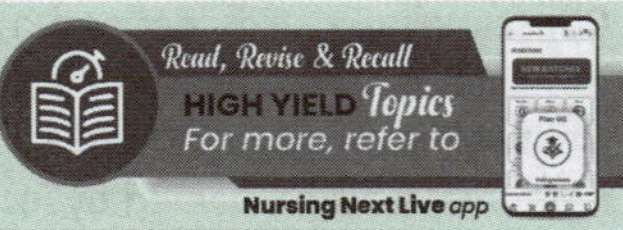

Communicating with Hearing-Impaired Client

- Speak very clearly and do not shout
- Speak slowly and keep voice pitch at mid-range
- Get the person's attention, making sure that the person is aware of communication taking place.
- The best distance for speaking to a hearing-impaired person is 2½–4 ft. Face the person at eye level. Never speak directly into the person's ear.
- Be aware of the nonverbal communication. Facial expressions, gestures, lip and body movements all give cues to the meaning of message.
- Use short, simple sentences. Rephrase the statement if the patient does not understand.
- Give time to the person to respond to questions.
- Ask for rephrasing to make sure the patient has understood important information.

Communicating with Visually-Impaired Client

- Acknowledge your presence in the patient's room.
- Identify yourself by name.
- Speak in a normal tone
- Explain the reason for touching the patient before doing so.

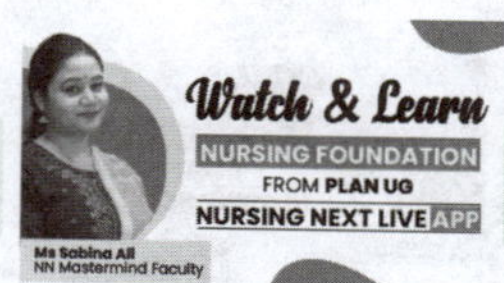

- Indicate to the patient, when the conversation has ended and when you are leaving the room.
- Keep a call bell within easy reach of patient.
- Orient the patient to room
- Be sure eyeglasses are clean, intact or contact lenses are in place.

Communicating with the Aphasic Person

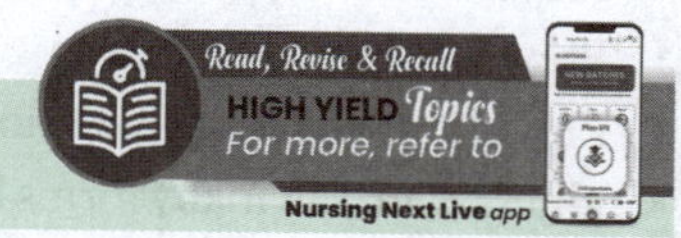

Aphasic person has difficulty expressing or understanding language.

- Make the environment relaxed and quiet.
- Assume that the patient can understand what is heard.
- Talk to the patient and do not talk to someone else in the room, about the patient.
- Face the patient, establish eye contact, and speak slowly and distinctly, do not shout.
- Frame questions so that they can be answered in Yes or No.
- Give the person time to respond to questions.
- Ask only one question at a time, be patient and wait for an answer.
- If there is a need for repetition, use the same words the second time.
- Use body language to enhance the message.
- Allow one person to speak at a time. Be patient.

Communicating with Patient having Artificial Airway

Patients with artificial airways like endotracheal intubation and tracheostomy tube require certain communication. Use nonverbal communication aids to communicate for such patients so that they can express their needs or symptoms.

- Use any voice enabling communication aid to produce any word which can be understood.
- Speech generating augmentative and alternatives communication aids are basically sound-based communication that does not have patients' own voice.
- Use nonverbal language to make patient understand
- Be calm and patient while handing such patients
- Talk in simple and short sentences with the patients
- Provide an alternate method to communicate like provide writing pad or mobile to type and convey the message.

LEVELS OF CONSCIOUSNESS

Consciousness is defined as a state of awareness of self, time and of environment, as well as a state of responsiveness to that environment or adaptation to the external stimuli.

Unconsciousness is a condition in which the patient is unresponsive and unaware of environmental stimuli. It can be brief, lasting for few seconds, hours, days or longer.

Impairment of consciousness indicates dysfunction of reticular activating system (RAS).

Confusion state is a state in which the patient cannot take into account all elements of his/her immediate environment, implying an element of sensorial clouding. Apathy and drowsiness are often prominent and accompanied by disorientation primarily for time, less often for place and rarely for self.

A severely confused person is usually unable to carry out more than a few simple commands.

Delirium is characterized by a fluctuating disturbance in consciousness and change in cognition that develop over a period of time. It is generally accompanied by increased morbidity and subsequent functional decline.

Obtundation is characterized by reduced alertness and hypersomnia (a state of excess of sleep). When awakened from an obtunded state, the patient remains drowsy and confused and wakefulness can only be maintained by continuous verbal and painful stimuli.

Stupor is unresponsiveness from which the patient can only be aroused by vigorous repeated painful stimuli. The patient is unable to localize the site of the painful stimuli.

CARE OF UNCONSCIOUS PATIENTS

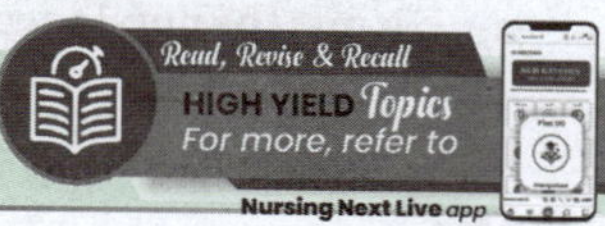

Introduction and Definition

The patient who appears to be asleep and at the same time is incapable of responding, is in a state of coma. Coma may vary in degree from light to medium to deep. In deepest stage, no reaction of any type can be obtained from the patient. Corneal, pupillary, pharyngeal, tendon and plantar reflexes are absent. Coma may last few days to few weeks.

Assessment

- Level of consciousness is assessed through Glasgow Coma Scale.
- Client's response is rated from 3 to 15. **Less than 3 indicates unconsciousness due to neurological impairment.**
- Unconscious comatose clients are completely dependent on others because their consciousness and protective reflexes are impaired. Therefore, they require aggressive nursing intervention. Nurses are responsible for meeting basic needs and preventing the complications associated with unconsciousness.
- For the effective care, nurse should perform frequent assessment of comatose client, plan the care and implement the care.
- Assess vital signs (temperature, pulse, blood pressure respiration) of the patient 4 hourly or as required to plan the care, prevent complications and manage early signs of any deviation in normal functioning.

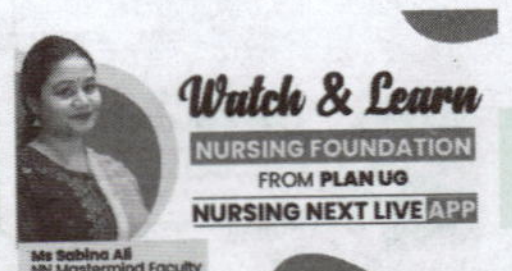

NURSING MANAGEMENT OF UNCONSCIOUS PATIENT

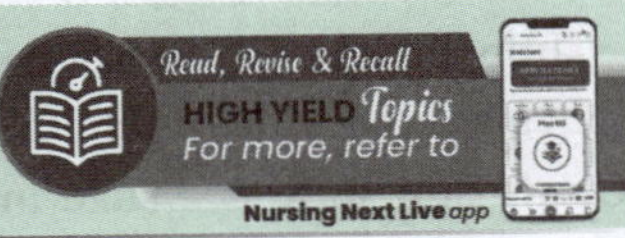

- Nursing care for maintaining patent airway
- Nursing care for protecting the client from injury
- Nursing care for maintaining optimum fluid volume state
- Nursing care for maintaining nutritional status
- To maintain body temperature
- Maintain oral hygiene
- Tracheostomy care
- To maintain eyes integrity
- To maintain hygiene
- Preventing urinary retention
- For prevention of complications
- Prevention of contracture and joint deformity and muscle wasting
- Prevention of deep vein thrombosis
- Prevention of hypostatic pneumonia/aspiration
- Prevention of constipation
- Providing sensory stimulation

Kindness comes in many forms but it has to be always from the heart. Therefore, be kind and caring on your part to promote health and prevent illness in unconscious patients as they are fully dependent on you.

CONCEPTUAL EXERCISES

LONG ANSWER QUESTIONS

1. a. **Define unconsciousness. (MGR)**
   b. **List the common causes of unconsciousness. (MGR)**
   c. **Discuss the nursing care of unconscious patient. (MGR)**

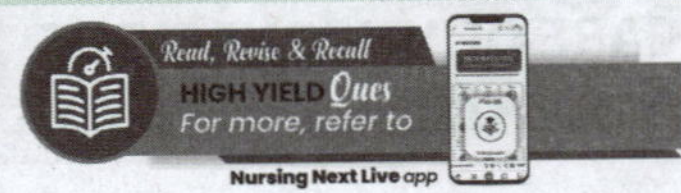

Answer

Unconsciousness

- Unconsciousness is an abnormal state in which a patient is totally unaware of both self and external surroundings, and is unable to respond meaningfully to external stimuli. It can range from a brief episode of fainting to the prolonged unconsciousness of coma from which the person cannot be aroused, even with vigorous external stimuli.
- When someone's consciousness level decreases, his or her state of alertness gradually declines from somnolence to coma.

b. List the common causes of unconsciousness.

Answer

Continuum of Unconsciousness

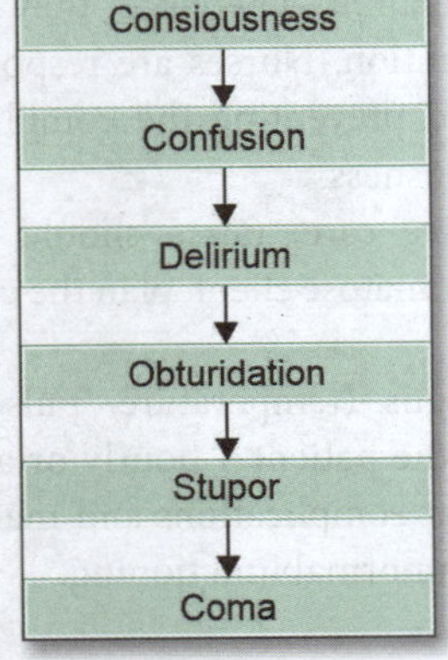

Common Causes of Unconsciousness

Brain-derived causes

- Brain injury
- Cerebral hemorrhage
- Cerebral infarction
- Brain tumor
- Central nervous system infections
- Status epilepticus

Systemic Causes

- Metabolic causes (e.g., ketoacidosis, electrolyte imbalance)
- Cardiovascular causes (e.g., cardiac arrest, arrhythmia, shock)
- Hypoxic-ischemic (e.g., drowning, choking)
- Severe infections (e.g., sepsis)
- Pulmonary diseases (e.g., aspiration, foreign object in respiratory tract)
- Intoxication (e.g., carbon monoxide, medicines, ethanol, cyanide)
- Medicine disadvantage (e.g., opioids, antipsychotics)

Common Causes

- Interruption of energy substrate delivery
- Hypoxia
- Ischemia
- Hypoglycemia
- Alteration of neurophysiologic responses of neuronal membranes
- Drug intoxication
- Alcohol intoxication
- Epilepsy

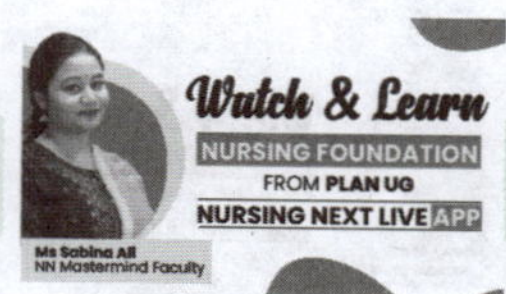

- Abnormalities of osmolality
- Diabetic ketoacidosis
- Nonketotic hyperosmolar state
- Hyponatremia
- Hepatic encephalopathy
- Hypertensive encephalopathy
- Uremic encephalopathy
- Hypercapnia
- Hypothyroidism
- Hypothermia
- Hyperthermia

c. Discuss the nursing care of unconscious patient.

Answer

Nursing Care of Unconscious Patient

Goals of Nursing Care

- Maintain ABC (Airway, Breathing and circulatory pattern) of the patient
- Maintain adequate cerebral tissue perfusion
- Maintain normal body temperature
- Attain maximal cognitive, motor and sensory function
- Prevent complications

Assessment

- Assess the conscious level of the patient using GCS Assessment scale
- Assess patent airway and ABG levels periodically
- Assess neurological status of the patient including pupillary reaction.
- Assess vital signs the continuously including oxygen saturation
- Assess the skin status of the patient
- Assess nutritional status of the patient.
- Assess the patency of all invasive lines used in hemodynamic monitoring of the patient
- Assess intake/output of the patient

Physical Assessment

- Voluntary movement – Strength and asymmetry in the upper extremities
- Deep tendon reflexes – biceps, triceps and patella
- Pupillary light reflex (pupil size)
- Corneal blink reflex
- Gag swallowing reflex

Nursing Diagnosis

- Ineffective airway clearance related to inability to clear respiratory secretions as evidenced by unclear lung sounds, unequal lung expansion, noisy respiration, presence of stridor, cyanosis or pallor
- Ineffective cerebral tissue perfusion related to effects of increased ICP as evidenced by papilledema, vomiting.
- Imbalanced nutrition: Less than body temperature, related to inability to eat and swallow as evidenced by weight and other nutritional parameters less than normal.
- Altered oral mucous membrane related to ET insertion, absence of pharyngeal reflex, inability to ingest fluid as evidenced by dryness, inflammation, crusting and halitosis.
- Self-care, deficit-bathing, feeding, grooming, toileting related to unconscious state as evidenced by unkempt and poorly nourished look, bed soiling.
- Ineffective thermoregulation related to damage to hypothalamic center as evidenced by persistent elevation of body temperature, warm and dry skin, flushed appearance of skin.
- Risk for complications: Pressure sore, contractures, DVT, hypostatic pneumonia, constipation – related to immobility.
- Risk of injury related to unconscious state.
- Risk for fluid volume deficit related to inability to ingest fluids, dehydration from osmotic diuretics.
- Interrupted family process related to chronic illness of a family member as evidenced by anger, grief, non-participation in client care.

Nursing Interventions

Maintaining a Patent Airway

- Use an oral/nasal artificial airway to maintain patency
- The breath sounds must be assessed every 2 hourly using auscultation.
- ABG results must be interpreted to determine the degree of oxygenation provided by the ventilators or oxygen.
- Assess for cough and swallow reflexes
- Tracheostomy/endotracheal intubation and mechanical ventilation may be necessary.

Preventing Airway Obstruction

- Provide fowler's position to the patient. Maintain the neck in a neutral position
- Periodically change the position (every 2nd hourly) on alternate sides to prevent accumulation of secretions in the airway.
- Periodic suctioning must be performed under asepsis to remove the accumulated secretions.
- Chest percussion and postural drainage may be performed by the nurses/physiotherapists to assist in the removal of tenacious secretions.
- Encourage oral care in each shift to prevent VAP and promote oral hygiene.

Ineffective Cerebral Tissue Perfusion

- Assess the GCS, SPO_2 level and ABG of the patient.
- Monitor the vital signs of the patients (increased temperature)
- Head elevation of 30 degrees, neutral position maintained to facilitate venous drainage.
- Follow VAP bundle
- Schedule care so that harsh activity [suctioning, bathing, turning] are not grouped together, with breaks between care for recovery.
- Administer laxatives, antitussives and antiemetics as ordered
- Maintain body temperature with antipyretics and cooling measures.
- Prevent seizure by administering anticonvulsants.
- Administer mannitol 25–50 g IV bolus if ICP >20, as prescribed.
- Pre-oxygenation before suctioning should be mandatory, and each pass of the catheter limited to 10 seconds, with appropriate sedation to limit the rise in ICP.

Imbalanced Fluid and Electrolyte

- Maintain strict Intake/output charting hourly.
- Assess the serum electrolytes of the patient.
- Correct the dehydration and electrolyte imbalances as per doctor's order.
- Provide adequate nutrition to the patient as per dietician. Enteral as well as parenteral feed can be indicated as per condition of the patient.
- Assess the fluid volume overload or deficit by assessment and documentation of grading of edema
- Diuretics may be prescribed to correct fluid overload and reduce edema.

Impaired Skin Integrity

- The nurse should provide intervention for all self-care needs including bathing, hair care, skin and nail care.
- Frequent back care should be given.
- Comfort devices should be used.
- Positions should be changed.
- Special mattresses or airbeds to be used.
- Adequate nutritional and hydration status should be maintained.
- Patient's nails should be kept trimmed.
- Protective eye shields can be applied or the eyelids closed with adhesive strips if the corneal reflex is absent to prevent corneal abrasions and ulcers.
- Inspect the oral cavity. Frequent oral hygiene every 4 hourly.

Impaired Bowel/Bladder Functions

- Assess for constipation and bladder distention.
- Auscultate bowel sounds.
- Administer stool softeners or laxatives as per doctor's order.
- Bladder catheterization care should provide under aseptic techniques using CAUTI bundle.
- Monitor the urine output and color.
- Initiate bladder training as soon as consciousness has been regained.

Self-Care Deficit

- Attending to the hygiene needs of the unconscious patient should not be compromised.
- Involve the family in self-care needs
- Care should be taken to examine the skin properly, noting any areas which are red, dry or broken.
- Fingernails and toenails also need to be assessed for oxygenation.
- Personal hygiene includes bed bath, hair care, oral hygiene (chlorhexidine-based solution), eye care, nasal care perineal care, back care, etc.

Risk for Infection

- Perform all procedures under aseptic techniques.
- Use all care bundles.
- Send the cultures under aseptic technique and report the findings to the physician.
- Perform hand hygiene
- Inspect the site of invasive lines in each shift.
- Follow standard precautions for the patient.
- Follow safe injection practices.

Risk for Injury

- Side rails must be kept whenever the patient is not receiving direct care.
- Seizure precautions must be taken.
- Adequate support to limbs and head must be given when moving or turning an unconscious patient. Protect from external sources of heat.
- Over sedation should be avoided – as it impedes the assessment of the level of consciousness and impairs respiration.
- Assess the need for restrain

Risk for Contractures

- Maintain the extremities in functional positions by providing proper support.
- Remove the support devices every four hours for passive exercises and skin care.
- Foot support should be provided.

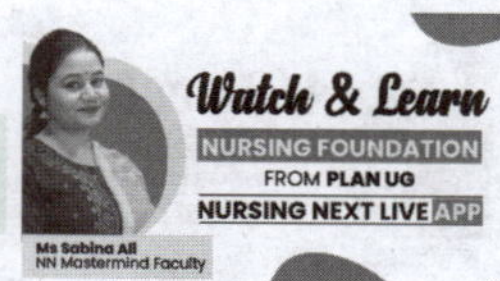

Nurses Responsibility

- Show respect
- Encourage family to contribute to the care of their loved ones
- Afford the privacy for both the client and family deserve
- Encourage stimulation by: Massage, combing/washing hair, playing music/radio/CD/TV, reading a book, etc.
- Include the family members in patient care.
- Communicate frequently with the family members.
- Use external support systems like professional counselors, religious clergy, etc.

Points to Remember

- Put airway if Patient is unconscious.
- Tracheostomy – if airway obstruction.
- Suction equipment available.
- Assess breath sound 1-2 hourly.
- Never give fluid / food to shallow.
- Position changing of patient
- Perineal care.
- Examine abdomen for distention.
- Involve family in care (general wards).

SHORT NOTES

1. Writ a short note on maintenance of patent airway.

Answer

Interventions to Maintain Patent Airway

Provide comfortable position to the client (fowler's position provides maximum lung expansion which helps in easing breathing difficulty)

- Removal of foreign bodies
- Always check the airway for any sign and symptom of blockage. If the blockage is due to any foreign object and it is clearly visible, then remove it but if it is not or partially visible then in that case do not perform the blind finger sweep to remove it.
- Airway maneuvers like jaw thrust or head tilt chin lift (add image)
- Invasive airway management
  - Assist the patient in performing deep breathing and coughing exercises.
  - Optimal positioning (sitting position)
  - Use of abdominal muscles for more forceful cough
  - Use of Incentive Spirometry
  - Encourage adequate intake of fluids to prevent dehydration.
  - Administer bronchodilators and expectorants medications as ordered
  - Consult for chest physiotherapy
  - Provide steam inhalation to clear the thick mucus secretions
  - Removal of foreign bodies with the help of megalis forceps
  - Provide recovery position to prevent aspiration.

Airway Maneuvers

- Head-tilt chin-lift
- Jaw-thrust maneuver

Artificial Airways

Most common invasive airways are:

- Oropharyngeal airway
- Nasopharyngeal airway
- Tracheal intubation: Use of Endotracheal tube
- Surgical management: Use of Tracheotomy

2. Write a short note on nursing care of patient with altered sensorium.

Answer

Impairment of vision related to aging (cataract long sight), vitamin A deficiency (night blindness) leading to difficulty in reading, accidental falls, etc.

Nursing Implications

- Provide bright light for reading.
- Use lamps that do not have glare.
- Use dim light burning in bedrooms and bathrooms all through the night.
- Provide safety rails at the sides of the bed to protect the client from falls.
- Place the furniture in a convenient place away from the passages especially in corridors.
- Regular eye check up and correction of eye glasses (spectacles) with appropriate lens for short sight and long sight.
- Treatment of infections of the eyes in their early stages.

Impairment of hearing related to aging process, disease conditions, toxicity of drugs.

Nursing Implications

- Face the client while speaking so as to enable the client for lip reading.

- Talk slowly and distinctly.
- Use simple language and short sentences.
  - Lower the pitch of the voice.
- Use nonverbal communication (facial expressions, use of hands, writings, etc.).
- When giving instructions, get feedback from the client to make sure that the client has received the same message that you wanted to communicate.
- Get the cleaning of the auditory canal to remove accumulation of ear wax (cerumen).
- Periodical check up to detect other problems causing impairment of hearing (e.g., otitis media). Teach the traffic rules to prevent road accidents while walking on busy roads.

Inability to recognize the temperature variations of the liquids (e.g., water) and other hot articles causing burns and scalds.

- Check the temperature of the water/liquids before giving to the clients for drinks, bath, enema, hot and cold applications on the skin (e.g., hot water bottles).
- Daily observation of the skin for its color, integrity (break in the continuity of the skin).
- Do not apply hot applications directly over the skin.
- Do not apply any type of pressure on the skin that may cause ulcer or blister on the skin.

Alterations in smell and taste. Inability to recognize the presence of bad smell, poisonous gas, spoiled food articles, etc. related to aging, environmental factors, smoking, certain medications, decreased salivation.

- Create the meal time as a pleasant occasion. Avoid conflicts.
- Provide the food with good flavor to increase the appetite, thus reducing the problem of anorexia.
- Create a pleasant atmosphere by maintaining the client's unit as clean as possible. For example, remove the bedpans from the sight of the client.
- Serve the food attractively. Remember that the appetite is increased by the sight and smell of the food.
- Check the gas leaks from the gas cylinders. Clients with decreased sensation of smell are prone to poisoning if gas cylinders are kept open.
- Maintain good oral hygiene. Care is taken to clean the mouth before and after food intake.
- Administer vitamins, particularly vitamin B complex to those clients taking broad antibiotics.

SHORT ANSWER QUESTIONS

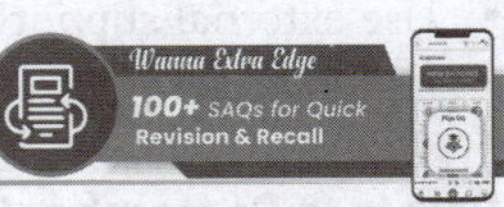

1. a. Define unconsciousness.
b. List the common causes of unconsciousness

Answer

- "Unconsciousness is an abnormal state in which a patient is totally unaware of both self and external surroundings, and unable to respond meaningfully to external stimuli." It can range from a brief episode of fainting to the prolonged unconsciousness of coma from which the person cannot be aroused, even with vigorous external stimuli.

b. List the common causes of unconsciousness

Answer

Common Causes of Unconsciousness

- Shock
- Head injury
- Fainting
- Imbalance of heat
- Heart attack
- Stroke
- Asphyxia
- Diabetes
- Epilepsy

CONCEPTUAL REVISION

MULTIPLE CHOICE QUESTIONS

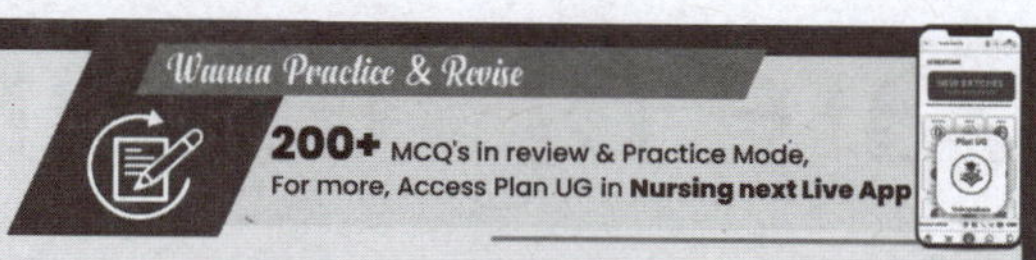

1. The nurse is assessing the motor function of an unconscious client. The nurse would plan to use which of the following to test the client's peripheral response to pain?

a. Sternal rub
b. Pressure on the orbital rim
c. Squeezing the sternocleidomastoid muscle
d. Nail bed pressure

Ans. d. Nail bed pressure

2. Which of the following is the best nursing intervention when communicating with a patient who has expressive aphasia?

a. Ask open ended questions
b. Speak to the patient as if he or she is a child
c. Use a dry-erase board or paper and pen for writing messages
d. Avoid use of gestures and other nonverbal forms of communication

Ans. c. Use a dry-erase board or paper and pen for writing messages

3. An elderly patient with bilateral hearing loss wears a hearing aid in her left ear. Which of the following approaches best facilitates communication with her?

a. Talk to the patient at a distance so he or she may read your lips
b. Keep your arms at your side; speak directly into the patient's left ear.
c. Face the patient when speaking; demonstrate ideas you wish to convey.
d. Position the patient so the light is on his or her face when speaking

Ans. c. Face the patient when speaking; demonstrate ideas you wish to convey.

4. This is a type of loss, where people learn that life changes are normal, expected, and often positive:

a. Maturational loss
b. Situational loss
c. Necessary loss
d. Perceived loss

Ans. c. Necessary loss

5. This is the type of grief a person experiences before the actual loss or death occurs:

a. Anticipatory grief
b. Normal grief
c. Complicated grief
d. Exaggerated grief

Ans. a. Anticipatory grief

6. All of the following relates to Rando's "R" Process Model, except:

a. Recognizing
b. Reacting
c. Responding
d. Relinquishing

Ans. c. Responding

Golden Points

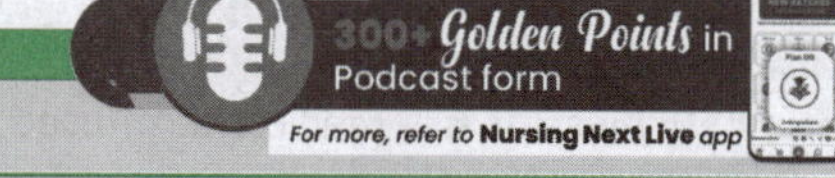

- Sensory Reception is the process of receiving data about the external and internal environment through the senses.
- The senses by which individuals maintain contact with the external environment are vision (visual), hearing (auditory), smell (olfactory), taste (gustatory) and touch (tactile). Individuals orient themselves internally by the kinesthetic and visceral senses.
- Sensory Perception is the conscious process of selecting, organizing and interpreting data from the senses into meaningful information.
- Inadequate functioning or impairment in any of the senses is known as sensory deficit. These deficits may be permanent or temporary, reversible or irreversible.
- Impairment of consciousness indicates dysfunction of reticular activating system (RAS).
- The patient who appears to be asleep and at the same time incapable of responding, is in a state of coma. Coma may vary in degree from light to medium to deep. In deepest stage, no reaction of any type is obtainable from the patient. Corneal, pupillary, pharyngeal, tendon and plantar reflexes are absent. Coma may last few days to few weeks.
- Unconscious comatose clients are completely dependent on others because their consciousness and protective reflexes are impaired.
- Nurses are responsible for meeting basic needs and preventing the complications associated with unconsciousness.

CHAPTER 25

Care of Terminally Ill Patient

CONCEPTUAL THEORY

Terminology

150+ key terminologies for Quick Recall & Revision

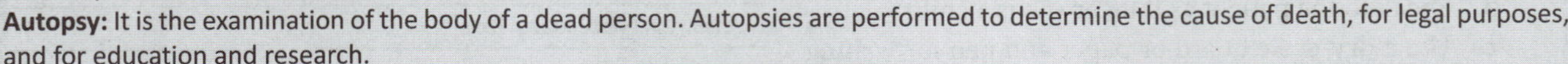

Algor mortis: Temperature decreases by a few degrees each hour. The skin loses its elasticity and will tear easily.

Autopsy: It is the examination of the body of a dead person. Autopsies are performed to determine the cause of death, for legal purposes, and for education and research.

Biological death: It occurs four–six minutes after clinical death. This is due to the fact that the heart is the main pumping machine of the body, and without the blood coming from the heart, the brain gradually ceases to function until it achieves irreversible damage.

Clinical death: It is the medical term for cessation of blood circulation and breathing, the two necessary criteria to sustain life. This is called cardiopulmonary arrest, a period when a person's heartbeat and breathing stop, but can still be revived if early medical attention is given.

Death: It is defined as, "cessation of heart-lung function, or of whole brain function, or of higher brain function, either irreversible cessation of circulatory and respiratory functions or irreversible cessation of all functions of the entire brain, including the brain stem."

Embalming: It is the art and science of preserving human remains by treating them with chemicals to forestall decomposition.

Hospice care: It is a coordinated program of interdisciplinary services provided by professional caregivers and trained volunteers to patients with serious illness. In hospice setting, the patient and family together are a unit of care.

Hospice care team: It typically includes doctors, nurses, home health aides, spiritual counselors, social worker, pharmacists and bereavement counselors.

Livor mortis: Bluish color of death, also known as hypostasis, is the discoloration of the skin due to the pooling of blood in the dependent part of body following death.

Palliative care: It means taking care of the whole person: body, mind and spirit, heart and soul. This mode of care, looks at dying as something natural and personal.

Rigor mortis: Body becomes stiff within 4 hours after death as a result of decreased adenosine triphosphate (ATP) production. ATP keeps muscles soft and supple.

Terminal illness: It is a medical term used to describe a disease that cannot be cured or adequately treated and that is reasonably expected to result in the death of the patient within a short period of time.

INTRODUCTION

Terminal illness is a medical term used to describe a disease that cannot be cured or adequately treated and that is reasonably expected to result in the death of the patient within a short period of time.

The family and significant others of terminally ill patients should be encouraged to participate in planning the patient's care. Health care personnel should be available to discuss the patient's condition with the family members.

Loss is anything that is perceived as such by the individual. Throughout our lives, from birth to death, we form attachments and suffer losses. Loss is defined as the experience of parting with an object, person, belief or relationship that one values.

The object may be animate or inanimate, a relationship or situation, or even a change or a failure (real or perceived).

TYPES OF LOSS

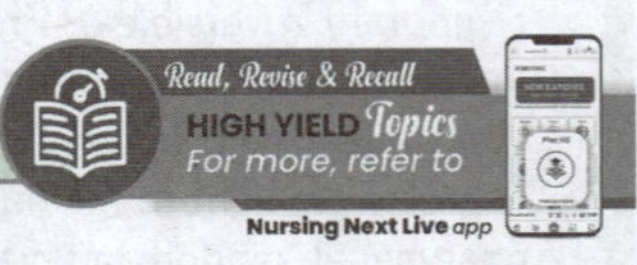

- Actual loss – can be recognized by others as well as the person sustaining the loss Perceived loss– sense of loss felt by the individual but not tangible to others
- Physical loss – loss of a part or aspect of the body

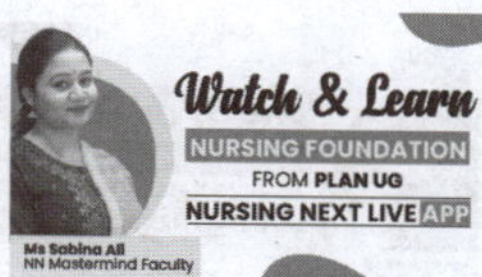

- Physiological loss – emotional loss
- Anticipatory loss – a person displays loss and grief behaviors for a loss that has not yet taken place. It is often seen in families of terminally ill patients.
- Grief is a characteristic pattern of psychological and physical responses experiencing after the loss of significant person, object, belief, or relationship.
- Bereavement is a state of desolation that occurs as a result of loss, particularly death of a significant other.
- Mourning encompasses socially prescribed behaviors after the death of other (vary as per culture)

STAGES OF DYING

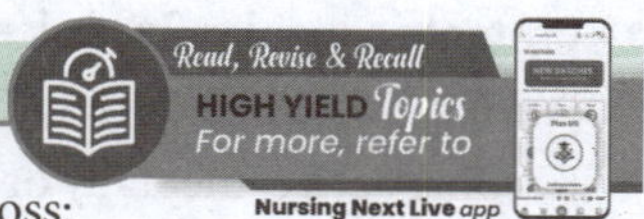

Psychiatrist Elisabeth Kübler-Ross:

- **Denial:** In denial and isolation stage, the patient denies that he or she will die, may repress what is discussed, and may isolate himself or herself from reality.
- **Anger:** In anger stage, patient expresses rage and hostility and adopts, a why me attitude.
- **Bargaining:** In the bargaining stage, the patient tries to barter for more time. Many patients put their own personal affairs in order, make wills and fulfill last wishes.
- **Depression:** The patient goes through a period of grief before death. The grief is characterized by crying and not speaking much. For example patient thinks, "I just don't know how my wife will get along after l am gone."
- **Acceptance:** The patient feels tranquil. He or she has accepted death and is ready to die, having no regrets.

FACTORS INFLUENCING LOSS AND GRIEF RESPONSE

- Significance of loss such as Age of the person, Value placed on the lost person and Degree of change required because of loss
- **Culture:** In includes the Customs of expression of grief, Family structure, Family and social roles
- **Spiritual beliefs:** Practice related to dying, death rituals
- **Sex role:** Gender differences
- **Socioeconomic status:** it affects support system available
- Coping skills in terms of previous experiences of loss, Emotional stability and Physical health

COMPONENTS FOR CARE OF TERMINALLY ILL PATIENTS

There are three essential components for care of terminally ill client:

1. Teamwork and partnership
2. Assessing and to care for the needs
3. Psychosocial support

Care for Physiological Needs

Pain

- Patients who have an established regimen of analgesics should continue to receive those medications as they approach the end of life.
- The route of administering the drugs should be considered.
- Assess the pain periodically and change the doses as required.
- In case of opioids, a regimen to combat constipation should be implemented.
- Patient controlled analgesia (PCA) pumps can provide the patient with a sense of independence and manage the pain at the same time.
- Provide distractions and verbal analgesia.

Dyspnea

- Anti-anxiety agent, bronchodilators, Corticosteroids should be provided.
- Treat underlying pathology (cardiovascular disease or respiratory disease).
- Administer blood products and erythropoietin as prescribed.
- Administer prescribed diuretics and monitor fluid balance.
- Provide oxygen therapy.
- Maintain high Fowler's position.
- Ensure drainage of secretions, provide steam inhalation and chest physiotherapy.
- Periodic suctioning is necessary.
- Maintain adequate ventilation in the room.
- Avoid overcrowding around the patient.

Skin and Mucus Membrane

- Patients should be comfortably placed and their position should be frequently changed in the bed.
- Frequent skin care should be given to the patient.
- Perineal care should be given to the patient.
- Catheterization has to be done.
- Protect the eyes from corneal ulceration with protective ointment.
- Prevent drying of lips and skin breakdown.
- Provide daily bath.
- Assist in elimination and keep the area clean.
- Assist the patient in mobilization.
- Prevent fall and injury.
- Maintain skin integrity, especially in old patients.
- Change the bed linen and clothes whenever soiled.
- Assist in active and passive exercise.
- Keep the skin moist and clean.

Nausea and Vomiting

- Provide small frequent meals.
- Allow the patient to choose favorite foods and fluids.
- Monitor the weight of the patient.
- Provide Fowler's position and make the patient to sit upright after food intake, for at least 15 minutes.
- Provide anti-emetics half an hour before the meals.
- Provide adequate fluid intake.
- Provide intravenous IV fluids if oral intake is inadequate.
- Provide oral care after vomiting episodes.
- Provide antacids.

Altered Nutrition

- Maintain a strict input and output chart.
- Provide meals as per the taste of the client.
- Provide a pleasant environment while meals are served.
- Serve the foods as per the appropriate temperature.
- Provide IV, fluids and Total Parenteral Nutrition (TPN) parenteral nutrition (TPN) in case the patient is not tolerating orally.
- Maintain adequate hydration.
- Provide a well-balanced diet.
- Do not force-feed the patient.
- Provide home-cooked food if allowed.
- Prevent gas forming foods.

Anorexia (Desire, Appetite)

- Offer small portions of food.
- Cold foods may be better tolerated than hot foods.
- Place nutritious food at bedside (fruit juices, fruits, etc.).
- Schedule meals.
- Avoid arguments.
- Assist the patient to maintain a schedule of oral care. Rinse the mouth.

Bowel and Bladder Care

Constipation

- Provide small frequent meals and increased fluid intake.
- Provide increased roughage in the diet.
- Provide stool softeners.

Diarrhea

- Provide meticulous skin care during diarrhea to prevent skin breakdown.
- Provide medications as prescribed to prevent diarrhea.
- The food served should be properly cooked.
- Proper handwashing should be done.
- Keep the anal area dry and clean.
- Change the linen and clothes when wet and soiled.

Bladder Care

- Maintain an intake and output chart.
- Ensure adequate hydration.
- Provide privacy.

Sleep Disturbances

- Promote a regular fixed sleeping pattern.
- Staying out of bed during the day should be practiced.
- Keeping active, mentally or physically during the day.
- Avoid stimulants like coffee at night.
- Treat potential causes contributing to impaired sleep
- Minimizing night time disruptions.
- A sedative or hypnotic can be given to the patient.

Care of Psychological Needs

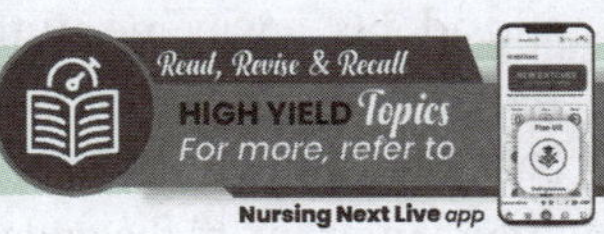

Delirium

Delirium is one of the most common complications seen in clients with advanced illness.

- Treat the underlying causes such as hypoxia, dehydration, hypercalcemia, hyponatremia, sepsis, etc.
- Teach the family how to interact with the patient.
- Provide safety to the patient.
- Spiritual intervention is required.
- Avoiding harsh lighting or very dim lighting.
- The presence of familiar faces and gentle reorientation and reassurance are also helpful.

Depression

- Emotional and spiritual support.
- Control of physical distressing symptoms.
- Presence of relatives.
- Provide space and time for family.
- Pharmacological intervention.

Psychosocial Needs

Spiritual Needs

- Spiritual coping strategies enhance self-empowerment.
- Assessing the desire for spiritual counseling and support.
- Obtain information regarding significant religious rituals, beliefs and practices.
- Encourage their practise to the maximum extent possible.
- Foster the insights.

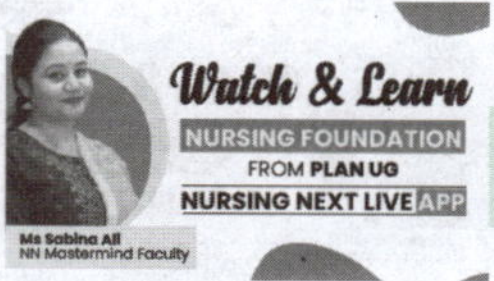

Palliative Care

Palliative care, means taking care of the whole person: body, mind and spirit heart and soul. This mode of care looks at dying as something natural and personal. The goal of palliative care is to give patients the best quality of life they can have by the aggressive management of symptoms.

Palliative care, by definition of its derivative is to palliate, a type of care that focuses on alleviation of a patient's symptoms and not to cure.

Hospice Care

Hospice care is a coordinated program of interdisciplinary services provided by professional caregivers and trained volunteers to patients with serious illness. In hospice setting, the patient and family together are a unit of care. Hospice care can take place:

- At home
- At a hospice center
- In a skilled nursing facility

A hospice care team typically includes doctors, nurses, home health aides, spiritual counselors, social worker, pharmacists and bereavement counselors.

DEATH

Death is defined as, "cessation of heart-lung function, or of whole brain function, or of higher brain function, either irreversible cessation of circulatory and respiratory functions or irreversible cessation of all functions of the entire brain, including the brain stem."

Clinical Death

Clinical death is the medical term for cessation of blood circulation and breathing, the two necessary criteria to sustain life. This is called **cardiopulmonary arrest**, a period when a person's heartbeat and breathing stop, but can still be revived if early medical attention is given.

Biological Death

It occurs four-six minutes after clinical death. This is due to the fact that the heart is the main pumping machine of the body, and without the blood coming from the heart, the brain gradually ceases to function until it achieves irreversible damage.

Immediate Signs of Death

- The respiration becomes labored, irregular, rapid or very slow, noisy breathing (death rattle) sound of secretions moving in the airway.
- There is a weak thready pulse and falling blood pressure.
- The heart rate decreases.
- As the oxygen supply to the brain decreases, the patient may become restless.
- The skin becomes pale and cool.
- The extremities are cold to touch.
- The sight gradually fails. The pupils fail to react to light.
- Mental confusion arises.
- Urinary output may decrease.
- There may be incontinence of urine and distension in bladder because of loss of sphincter control.
- Difficulty in talking or swallowing.

Changes in Body after Death

- **Rigor mortis:** Body becomes stiff within 4 hours after death as a result of decreased adenosine triphosphate (ATP) production. ATP keeps muscles soft and supple.
- **Algor mortis:** Temperature decreases by a few degrees each hour. The skin loses its elasticity and tears easily.
- **Livor mortis:** Bluish color of death, also known as hypostasis is the discoloration of the skin due to the pooling of blood in the dependent part of body following death.

Postmortem Care

- Immediate notification should be the officials.
- General consideration for other patients in the ward.
- Preparation of the body for transfer to home/morgue.
- The nurse notifies the physician and the ward sister immediately if the patient has ceased breathing.
- It is the duty of physician to declare death of the client.
- When the death occurs following certain communicable diseases such as smallpox, the body requires special attention to prevent the spread of the disease.
- The personal care needs to be carried out within 2–4 hours after death, to preserve the appearance, condition and dignity of the person dying.
- Pack personal property.
- **Organ donation:** Once brain death has been confirmed, the patient will remain connected to the ventilator while members of the medical team speak with the person's family about donation.
- **The medicolegal case:** If death is caused by accident, suicide, homicide, etc., it should be brought to the notice of legal authorities. The body should not be handed over to the relatives without the permission of the legal authorities.
- **Autopsy:** It is the examination of the body of a dead person. Autopsies are performed to determine the cause of death, for legal purposes, and for education and research.
- **Embalming:** Embalming is the art and science of preserving human remains by treating them with chemicals

to forestall decomposition. The intention is to keep them suitable for public display at a funeral, for religious reasons, or for medical and scientific purposes such as their use as "anatomical specimens".

The first step in the **embalming process** is *surgical*, in which bodily fluids are removed and are replaced with formaldehyde-based chemical solutions. The second step is *cosmetic*, in which the body is prepared for viewing by styling the hair, applying make-up, and setting the facial features.

Mortuary is an important integral part of every hospital as it deals with the preservation of the dead body. Bodies may be viewed and identified and bodies may be kept until burial can be arranged.

Mortuary complex consists of Autopsy room/ postmortem room, and preservation room (Cold storage room) for dead body.

The **pronouncement** is a terminology that denotes the time when an individual is found to be legally dead. This is the specific date and time an individual is found to be legally dead. The declaration can be made by a physician, medical examiner, or coroner

The **death certificate** is a public record that can be accessed by the decedent's family and should document the immediate cause of death, which can be an event or a clinical condition. The main purpose of death certification is for governmental agencies to compile vital statistics.

Grief counselling is also known as bereavement therapy intended to help and cope with loss, the death can cause both emotional and physical pain that can sometimes impair the ability to function.

CONCEPTUAL EXERCISES

LONG ANSWER QUESTIONS

1. Define euthanasia and state clinical signs of death. Add a note on stages of dying. (MGR, RUHS, DU, KUHS)

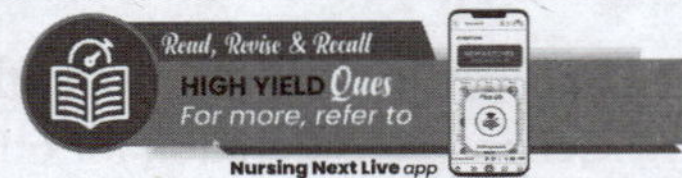

Answer

Euthanasia

Euthanasia is derived from 2 Greek words:

- Eu (good) and Thanatos (death) means "Good Death"
- It can also be defined as the act of inducing an easy death.
- Euthanasia is also defined as "mercy killing".
- It is the act or practice of ending a life of a person either by a lethal injection or suspension of medical treatment.

According to the *World Medical Association* euthanasia means:

Deliberate and intentional action with a clear intention to end another person's life under the following conditions:

- The subject is a competent informed person with incurable illness.
- Who voluntarily asked for ending his life.
- The person who is acting, knows about the state of this person and about his wish to die and is doing this action with an intention to end life of this person.
- The action is done with compassion and without any personal profit.

Clinical Signs of Death

- Absence of pulse, heart beat and respiration.
- Fixed Pupil (not reacting to light).
- Absence of refluxes.
- Rigor mortis (Stiffing of the body after death).
  The extremities (both upper and lower) cannot be bent/ straightened during rigor mortis unless the tendons are torn.
- Post-mortem hypostasis- Dark red or bluish discoloration of the body.

Stages of Dying

Dying means approaching death.

The stages of the Kubler-Ross theory include:

- **Denial**
- **Anger**
- **Bargaining**
- **Depression**
- **Acceptance**

MNEMONIC: "DABDA"

Stage 1: Denial

- Refusing about probable death occurrence.
- There is initial reaction of shock.
- Patient isolates himself/herself.
- Do not seek treatment or any medical assistance.
- Also refuses hospital admission.
- Patient appears to be superficially happy to deny the truth of diagnosis.

Stage 2: Anger

- After Recognition of loss or of death – the patient/family members may become angry, frustrated and irritable.

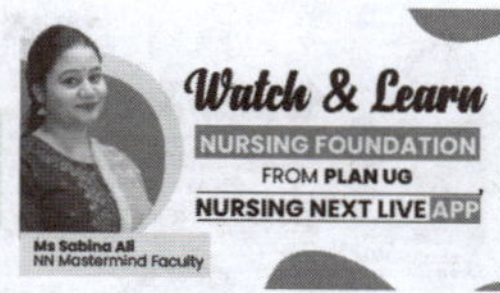

- Patient may show anger at the doctors, nurses, family members, self, on fate etc.
- Patent may blame everybody for misfortunes- death/loss.
- Allow the patient/ family members to express the emotions as they are in the grieving process.

Stage 3: Bargaining

- Attempts to make deal to prevent loss.
- Deep sense of yearning at this stage.

Stage 4: Depression

- At this stage, bargaining turns into depression.
- Realizes death.
- It is the normal process of preparing to die.
- Patient shows clinical signs of depression such as psychomotor retardation, sleep disturbances, hopelessness, etc.

Stage 5: Acceptance

- From the stage of depression, patient/family members night move into the phase of acceptance.
- Realizes the death and accepts its universality.
- Patients begin to write a will, start, completing financial arrangements for their family, gives up the personal possessions, etc.

SHORT NOTES

1. Write a short note on care of dying/terminally ill patient. (MGR, DU)

Answer

Care of Dying

- To provide effective care of dying patient, nurses should have reconciled their own feelings and must be aware of the phases of grief and dying.
- Nurse must understand the concept of dignified death while providing care to the dying patients.
- It is the responsibility of the nurse to maintain good communication with family members and also allow them to assist in care.

Assessment

- Thorough assessment of the state of patient for the awareness of family members, to communicate freely and to assist the family in grieving process.
- Assessment of the physiological signs of approaching death such as drowsiness, mental confusion, withdrawal and decreased socialisation, loss of bowel and bladder control, irregular breathing pattern, myoclonus, change in heart rate, loss of reflexes, etc.

Meeting the Needs of Dying Individual

- Hospice care
- Physical care
- Psychological care
- Social care
- Spiritual care

Hospice Care

Hospice care is a coordinated program of interdisciplinary services provided by professional caregivers and trained volunteers to patients with serious illness. In hospice setting, the patient and family together are a unit of care.

Physical Care

- Providing comfort to the patient.
- Perform interventions to relieve pain.
- Careful and regular observations for control of pain and agitation.
- Provide mouth care.
- Family members can be encouraged to give sips of water
- Moisten the patient's mouth.
- Provide comfortable position to the patient to facilitate drainage of secretions.
- Provide eye care.
- Maintain personal hygiene.

Psychological Care

- Assess the patients' insight of their condition.
- Communicate with the dying person and hear them. Never force communication.
- Fulfill the need of privacy.
- Acknowledge them, honor their wishes.
- Provide a caring touch or hand holding in order to provide the psychological support to the patient.

Social Care

- Prepare the family members for the expected change.
- Use therapeutic communication to facilitate their expression of feelings.
- Allow the presence of loved ones and time to share with spouse/children.

- Show empathetic and caring attitude with patients as well as with family members.
- The nurse must have a calm and patient manner to provide information as repeated information may be needed as the family members are in the grieving process.

Spiritual Care

- Specific interventions such as facilitating expressions of feelings, performing prayers according to religion, meditation and discussion with clergy man or a spiritual advisor.
- Nurses play a vital role in meeting their cultural/spiritual/individual needs at the time of death.

2. Write a short note on grief and grieving process or Stages of Dying. (DU, KUHS)

Answer

For answer, refer to Long Question no. 1, pg. no. 840

3. Write a short note on difference between Algor mortis and Livor mortis. (KUHS)

Answer

Algor Mortis	Livor Mortis
• **Algor mortis** is defined as the reduction in body temperature after death. It shows a steady decline with no presence of ambient temperature.	• **Livor mortis:** Dependent lividity due to settling of the blood in the lower portion of the body.
Characteristics: • Loss of 1.4 degrees F per hour (for the 1st 12 hours) after death. • 1.4 degrees'/hour x 12 hours =16.8 F lost • After 12 hours- loss of 0.7 degrees per hour	**Characteristics:** • Livor Mortis begins after 2 hours of death. • Lividity is defined as the pooling of blood in the parts of the body that are lowest to the ground. • It becomes permanent after 8 hours. • If the skin is discolored but turns white when touched, lividity is not complete.

4. Write a short note on care of dead body. (KUHS)

Answer

Care of Dead Body

Death is an irreversible cessation of circulatory, respiratory function or the irreversible cessation of all functions of the entire brain, including the brainstem.

After death, the body undergoes many physiological changes so it's necessary to provide dead body care so that tissue damage/disfigurement of the body can be prevented.

Purposes of Dead Body Care

- To prepare for the morgue.
- To prevent discoloration/deformity of the body.
- To protect from post mortem discharge.

Procedure

- Care of dead body depends on the customs and religious beliefs of patient's family.
- Nurses should provide care with dignity and sensitivity to the client and family members.

Nursing Interventions

- Various nursing interventions are as follows:
- Check doctor's orders for any sample collection, if indicated.
- Remove all equipment's such as ventilator support/breathing devices, invasive lines/tubes.
- Provide sponge to the patient.
- Apply clean sheets.
- Use clothes such as hospital gown or patient's clothes (as per family requests).
- Brush/provide oral care. Remove all the oral secretions properly.
- Comb the hair.
- Keep the eyelids closed.
- Dentures, if any should be kept in the mouth to maintain facial alignment.
- Mouth should be closed and all the orifices such as nose ears should be closed.
- Remove all the ornaments/accessories of the patient.
- Absorbent pads or diapers can be used for muscle sphincter relaxation.
- Cover the body with a clean sheet.
- Apply name tag properly.
- Allow the family members to view the dead body. The body should be wrapped in a large plastic or cotton material.
- Identification is then applied outside of the wrapper.
- Hand over all the belongings of the patient to the relatives.
- Document the time of death on patients tag.
- In the nurse's notes, record the name of the doctor who announced death. Also document all the items handed over to family members.
- Hand over the dead body to the relatives, if possible. If not sent the dead body to the mortuary.

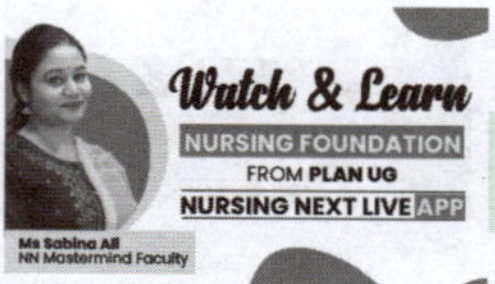

SHORT ANSWER QUESTIONS

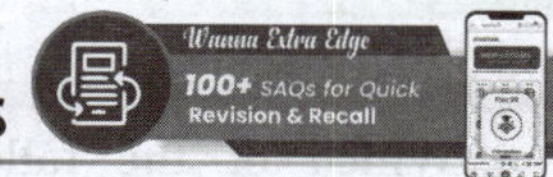

1. Enumerate changes in body after death.

Answer

- **Rigor mortis:** Body becomes stiff within 4 hours after death as a result of decreased adenosine triphosphate (ATP) production. ATP keeps muscles soft and supple.
- **Algor mortis:** Temperature decreases by a few degrees each hour. The skin loses its elasticity and can tear easily.
- **Livor mortis:** Bluish color of death, also known as hypostasis is the discoloration of the skin due to the pooling of blood in the dependent part of body following death.

2. Define Hospice care

Answer

Hospice is a coordinated program of interdisciplinary services provided by professional caregivers and trained volunteers to patients with serious illness. In hospice setting, the patient and family together are a unit of care. Hospice care can take place:

- At home
- At a hospice center
- In a skilled nursing facility

3. Enumerate stages of dying.

Answer

- **Denial:** Patient denies impending death, isolates themselves, and avoids discussing the situation.
- **Anger:** Patient expresses anger and hostility, questioning "why me?"
- **Bargaining:** Patient attempts to negotiate for more time and may focus on personal matters like making wills or fulfilling last wishes.
- **Depression:** Patient experiences grief, characterized by crying and withdrawal, and may worry about loved ones' well-being after their passing.
- **Acceptance:** Patient reaches a state of tranquility, accepting death without regrets.

4. Define terminal illness.

Answer

- Terminal illness is a medical term used to describe a disease that cannot be cured or adequately treated and that is reasonably expected to result in death of the patient within a short period of time.
- The family and significant others of terminally ill patients should be encouraged to participate in planning the patient's care.

5. Define Embalming.

Answer

Embalming is the art and science of preserving human remains by treating them with chemicals to forestall decomposition. The intention is to keep them suitable for public display at a funeral, for religious reasons, or for medical and scientific purposes such as their use as "anatomical specimens".

CONCEPTUAL REVISION

MULTIPLE CHOICE QUESTIONS

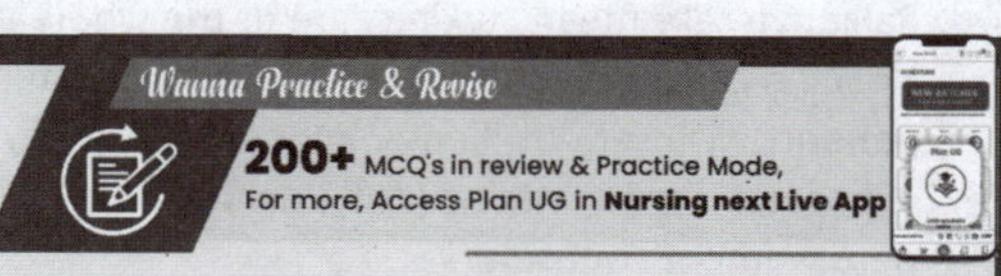

1. Which of the following is a common physical symptom experienced by terminally ill patients?

a. Fever
b. Diarrhea
c. Fatigue
d. All of the above

Ans. c. Fatigue

2. Which of the following is an example of spiritual care for a terminally ill patient?

a. Administering pain medication
b. Providing emotional support
c. Assisting with hygiene
d. Facilitating a visit with a spiritual leader

Ans. d. Facilitating a visit with a spiritual leader

3. Which of the following is a common ethical dilemma encountered when caring for terminally ill patients?

a. Deciding when to withhold life-sustaining treatment
b. Deciding when to discharge the patient
c. Deciding when to transfer the patient to another facility
d. Deciding when to increase the frequency of vital sign checks

Ans. a. Deciding when to withhold life-sustaining treatment

4. Which of the following is an appropriate communication technique when discussing end-of-life care with a terminally ill patient?

a. Using medical jargon to explain the patient's condition
b. Offering false hope to the patient
c. Allowing the patient to express their feelings and concerns
d. Avoiding the topic of death altogether

Ans. c. Allowing the patient to express their feelings and concerns

5. Which of the following is a common spiritual need of terminally ill patients?

a. A desire for physical comfort
b. A desire to be surrounded by loved ones
c. A desire to find meaning and purpose in life
d. A desire for financial security

Ans. c. A desire to find meaning and purpose in life

6. Which of the following is a common cultural consideration when caring for terminally ill patients?

a. Dietary restrictions
b. Language barriers
c. Religious practices
d. All of the above

Ans. d. All of the above

7. Which of the following is a common legal consideration when caring for terminally ill patients?

a. Obtaining informed consent for treatment
b. Administering medications without the patient's knowledge
c. Refusing to provide pain management
d. All of the above

Ans. a. Obtaining informed consent for treatment

8. Which of the following is a common physical intervention for managing pain in terminally ill patients?

a. Surgery
b. Physical therapy
c. Heat therapy
d. Opioids

Ans. d. Opioids

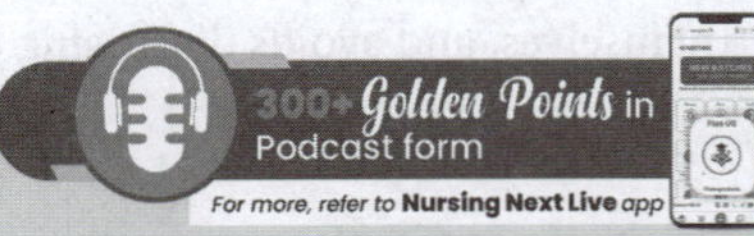

Golden Points

- Terminal illness is a medical term used to describe a disease that cannot be cured or adequately treated and that is reasonably expected to result in the death of the patient within a short period of time.
- Stages of dying are Denial, Anger, Bargaining, Depression, Acceptance
- Palliative care means taking care of the whole person: body, mind and spirit and heart and soul.
- Hospice care is a coordinated program of interdisciplinary services provided by professional caregivers and trained volunteers to patients with serious illness. In hospice setting, the patient and family together are a unit of care.
- A hospice care team typically includes doctors, nurses, home health aides, spiritual counselors, social worker, pharmacists and bereavement counselors.
- Clinical death is the medical term for cessation of blood circulation and breathing, the two necessary criteria to sustain life. This is called cardiopulmonary arrest, a period when a person's heartbeat and breathing stop, but can still be revived if early medical attention is given.
- Biological Death occurs four–six minutes after clinical death.
- Changes in Body after Death includes Rigor mortis, Algor mortis and Livor mortis
- Once brain death has been confirmed, the patient will remain connected to the ventilator while members of the medical team speak with the person's family about donation.
- Autopsy is the examination of the body of a dead person. Autopsies are performed to determine the cause of death, for legal purposes, and for education and research.
- Embalming is the art and science of preserving human remains by treating them with chemicals to forestall decomposition.

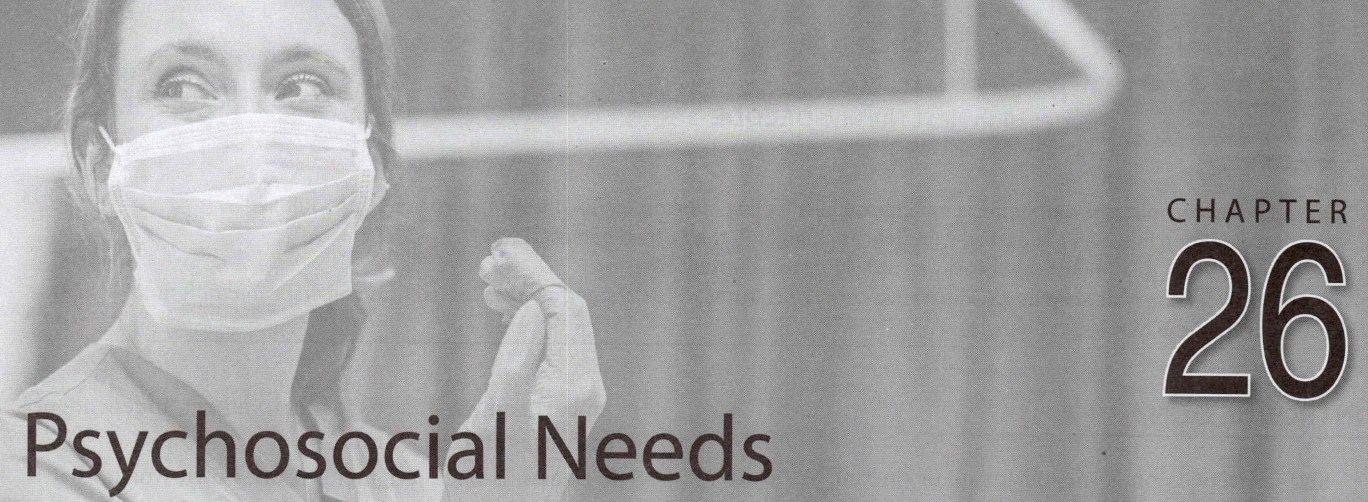

Psychosocial Needs

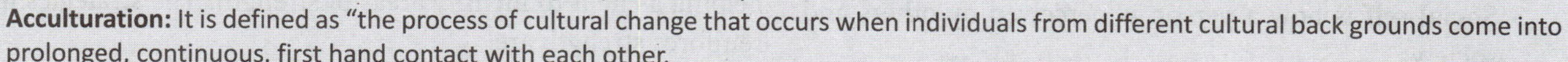

CONCEPTUAL THEORY

Terminology

150+ key terminologies for Quick Recall & Revision

A dominant group: It is the group that has the most ability to control the values and sanctions of the society. It is usually the largest group in a society.

Acculturation: It is defined as "the process of cultural change that occurs when individuals from different cultural back grounds come into prolonged, continuous, first hand contact with each other.

Cultural assimilation occurs when a minority group lives with a dominant group.

Culture may be defined as a shared system of beliefs, values, and behavioral expectations that provides social structure for daily living.

Defense mechanisms are strategies that protect us from increasing anxiety. Defense mechanisms reduce both anxiety and the secretion of stress hormones. Defense mechanisms are used to maintain and improve our self-esteem. They can be overused in a maladaptive way as well.

Ethnicity is a sense of identification with a collective cultural group, largely based on the group's common heritage.

Minority groups usually have same physical or cultural characteristics such as race, religion, beliefs or occupation that identify the people within groups as different from the dominant group.

Personal identity is the conscious sense of individuality and uniqueness that is continually evolving throughout life.

Physiological stressors are stressors that exert strain on human body.

Psychosocial stressors are events, situations, individuals, or anything a person explicate as negative, threatening or fearful.

Quid pro quo means something given or withered in exchange for something else.

Role ambiguity occurs when expectations are unclear, and people do not know what to do or how to do it and are unable to predict the reactions of others to their behavior.

Role development involves socialization into a particular role.

Role mastery means that the person's behaviors meet social expectations. Expectations or standards of behavior of a role, are set by society.

Role performance relates what a person in a particular role does to the behaviors expected of that role.

Self-concept is one's mental image of oneself. A positive self-concept is essential to a person's mental and physical health. Individuals with a positive self-concept are better able to develop and maintain interpersonal relationships. An individual possessing a strong self-concept.

Self-esteem is one's judgment of one's own worth, that is, how that person's standards and performances compare to others and to one's ideal self. If a person's self-esteem does not match with the ideal self, then low self-concept results.

Self-expectation is what one expects of oneself; may be a realistic or unrealistic expectation.

Self-knowledge is the knowledge that one has about oneself, including insights into one's abilities, nature and limitations.

Sexual abuse, also referred to as sexual assault or sexual violence or molestation, is abusive sexual behavior by one person upon another. It includes unwanted sexual touching, forced oral sex and rape, among other sexual acts.

Sexual harassment is unwelcome behavior that is sexual or gender-based in nature.

Sexual health may be defined as the integration of the somatic, emotional, intellectual, and social aspects of sexual being, in ways that are positively enriching and that enhance personality, communication, and love.

Sexuality is an integral part of a person's identity and is present in one's demeanor through actions, communications and physical experiences.

Sexually transmitted diseases (STDs) or venereal diseases are infections that spread from one person to another primarily through sexual contact. Common types of STIs are: Acquired immunodeficiency syndrome (AIDS), Chlamydia, Cytomegalovirus (CMV), Syphilis, Gonorrhea, Human papillomavirus (HPV).

Social self is how a person is perceived by others and society.

Spiritual distress refers to a challenge to the spiritual well-being or to the belief system that provides strength, hope, and meaning to life.

Contd...

Spiritual health or spiritual well-being is manifested by a feeling of being "generally alive, purposeful, and fulfilled".
Stress is a condition in which the person experiences changes in the normal balanced state.
Stressor is an event or stimulus that causes an individual to experience stress.
Transcultural nursing is defined as a comparative study of cultures to understand similarities (culture universal) and differences (culture specific) beyond the human groups.

INTRODUCTION

- **Self-concept** is one's mental image of oneself. A positive self-concept is essential to a person's mental and physical health. Individuals with a positive self-concept are better able to develop and maintain interpersonal relationships. An individual possessing a strong self-concept.
- There are four dimensions of self-concept:
  1. **Self-knowledge** is the knowledge that one has about oneself, including insights into one's abilities, nature and limitations.
  2. **Self-expectation** is what one expects of oneself; may be a realistic or unrealistic expectation.
  3. **Social self** is how a person is perceived by others and society.
  4. **Appraisal of oneself** in relationship to others, events or situations.

There are four components of self-concept:

1. Personal identity
2. Body image
3. Role performance
4. Self-esteem.

- **Personal identity** is the conscious sense of individuality and uniqueness that is continually evolving throughout life.
- The image of physical self is **body image** that how a person perceives the size, appearance, and functioning of the body and its parts. Body image has both cognitive and affective aspects.
- A role is a set of expectations about how the person occupies one position or behaves. **Role performance** relates what a person in a particular role does to the behaviors expected of that role.
  - **Role mastery** means that the person's behaviors meet social expectations. Expectations or standards of behavior of a role, are set by society.
  - **Role development** involves socialization into a particular role.
  - **Role ambiguity** occurs when expectations are unclear, and people do not know what to do or how to do it and are unable to predict the reactions of others to their behavior.

    Self-concept is also affected by role strain and role conflicts.
  - **Role conflicts** arise from opposing or incompatible expectations. In an interpersonal conflict, people have different expectations about a particular role. Role conflicts can lead to tension, decrease in self-esteem and embarrassment if needs for achievement, independence and recognition are unmet.
- **Self-esteem** is one's judgment of one's own worth, that is, how that person's standards and performances compare to others and to one's ideal self. If a person's self-esteem does not match with the ideal self, then low self-concept results. There are two types of self-esteem: (1) Global and (2) Specific.
  - **Global self-esteem** is how much one likes oneself as a whole.
  - **Specific self-esteem** is how much one approves of a certain part of oneself.

Nursing interventions to promote positive self-concept include helping a client to identify areas of strength. The strategies to reinforce strength are:

- Stress on positive thinking rather than self-negation
- Notice and verbally reinforce client strengths
- Encourage the setting of attainable goals
- Acknowledge goals that have been attained
- Provide honest, positive feedback.

SEXUALITY

Sexuality is an integral part of a person's identity and is present in one's demeanor through actions, communications and physical experiences.

Sexual health may be defined as the integration of the somatic, emotional, intellectual, and social aspects of sexual being, in ways that are positively enriching and that enhance personality, communication, and love.

- Sexual development in infancy—birth to 2 years
  - Infants have many sensual experiences, including sucking on fingers and toes.
- Sexual development in early childhood—age: 3–7 years. By age 3, children's genitals play a role in gender differentiation.
  - Increased curiosity for sexual exploration
  - More social interaction
  - Recognize gender difference
- Sexual development in preadolescence—age: 8–12 years. Age 8–12 reflects a transition from childhood to adolescence.
  - Most children of this age attain puberty.
  - According to the Freud's psychosexual theory, children transfer this repressed libidinal energy into asexual pursuits such as school, athletics, and same sex friendships.

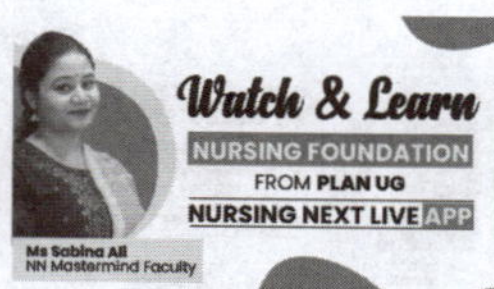

- Sexual development in adolescence—age: 13–19 years
  - Sexual maturation
  - Increasing hormone levels
  - Prepare for adult roles
  - May have sexual experience
  - Need for sex education
- Sexual development in adulthood—age: 21–40 years
  - Most active sexual life
  - Choose life partner
  - Experiment with sexual expression
- Sexuality in late adulthood—age more than 41 years and older
  - Menopause in females
  - Decreased testosterone in males
  - Fear of loss of sexual abilities

SEXUALLY TRANSMITTED DISEASES (STDS)

Sexually transmitted diseases (STDs) or venereal diseases are infections that spread from one person to another primarily through sexual contact. Common types of STIs are: Acquired immunodeficiency syndrome (AIDS), Chlamydia, Cytomegalovirus (CMV), Syphilis, Gonorrhea, Human papillomavirus (HPV).

Prevention of STD

- The best measure to prevent is to avoid sexual contact.
- Use of condom correctly and consistently
- Have a mutually monogamous sexual relationship with an uninfected partner.
- Use sterile needles if injecting intravenous medications
- Avoid multiple partners
- Stop intravenous drug abuse
- To have regular checkup for STIs even in the absence of symptoms or having sex with new partner.
- Indulge in natural form of intercourse (vaginal) and use a condom.
- If diagnosed with STI, reduce the risk of transmission to partner or from mother to baby
- If diagnosed with STI, notify all recent sex partners and urge them to go for screening
- Stop all sexual activity while being treated for STI
- Do not donate blood if diagnosed with STI

SEXUAL HARASSMENT

Sexual harassment is unwelcome behavior that is sexual or gender-based in nature.

This type of harassment usually occurs in an asymmetrical relationship where one person has more power than the other, "Quid pro quo" and environmental harassment.

Quid pro quo means something given or withered in exchange for something else. This occurs when an individual's employment or well-being is dependent on agreeing to unsolicited and unwelcome demands.

Quid pro quo harassment is a clear cut abuse of power and is legally, morally, and ethnically wrong.

Sexual abuse, also referred to as sexual assault or sexual violence or molestation, is abusive sexual behavior by one person upon another. It includes unwanted sexual touching, forced oral sex and rape, among other sexual acts.

Steps of dealing with inappropriate sexual behavior include:

- Talk about behavior
- Provide feedback about behavior

STRESS AND ADAPTATION

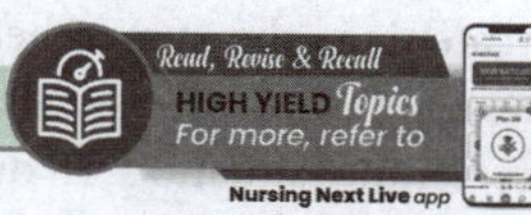

Stress is a condition in which the person experiences changes in the normal balanced state.

A stressor is an event or stimulus that causes an individual to experience stress.

There are many sources of stress. They can be broadly classified as internal or external stressors, or developmental or situational stressors.

- *Internal stressors* originate within a person,
- *External stressors* originate outside the individual,
- Developmental *stressors* occur at *predictable* times throughout an individual's life.
  - *Situational stressors* are unpredictable and may occur at any time during life.
  - *Situational stress* may be positive or negative

Stressor can also be classified as physiological or psychosocial also:

- **Physiological stressors** are stressors that exert strain on human body. They have both specific as well as generalized impact. The specific impact includes an alteration of normal body structure and function, whereas general impact includes response to the stress. Primary physiological stressors include physical agents, chemical agents, infections agents, genetic disorders, and immune disorders.
- **Psychosocial stressors** are events, situations, individuals, or anything a person explicate as negative, threatening or fearful. They involve both real and perceived threats.

Adaptation to Stress

Coordination of the central nervous system, autonomic nervous system, and the endocrine system is required for the body to adjust, adapt and maintain equilibrium.

The central nervous system consisting of the brain and spinal cord, coordinates adaptation within the body. Cortex, the thinking part of the brain, communicates with the midbrain and brain stem, which contains many of the structures involved in adaptation and maintenance of physiologic functions.

The reticular-activating system (RAS), a bundle of nerve fibers in the brain stem, transmits messages to the cortex from the sensory receptors of the body and carries messages back to the hypothalamus in the midbrain to regulate physiologic functions. The hypothalamus helps regulate the autonomic nervous system and the secretion of hormones by the endocrine system.

The autonomic nervous system regulates physiologic functions that are essentially automatic and beyond voluntary control. It is divided into the sympathetic and parasympathetic nervous systems. When the brain perceives a stimulus as threatening, the sympathetic nervous system stimulates the physiologic functions needed for fight or flight. Once the threatening situation is over, the parasympathetic nervous system works to restore equilibrium.

As long as the body's capacity is not over-taxed, the central nervous system, autonomic nervous system, and endocrine systems regulate body systems to maintain homeostasis.

If the body overreacts in defending itself, there is surplus of hormones that are favorable to the development of inflammation, etc. may develop. When the body underreacts, too many inflammatory hormones are circulating and serious infection or peptic ulcers may result.

General Adaptation Syndrome (GAS)

Selye states that a General adaptation syndrome (GAS) occurs in response to long-term exposure to stress.

The stages are: **the alarm stage**, the **stage of resistance** and the **stage of exhaustion**.

Alarm Stage

During the **alarm stage**, hormone released mobilizes the body's defenses. Nonspecific signs of illness such as slight rise on temperature, a loss of energy, decreased appetite and a general feeling of malaise occur.

Resistance Stage

During the second stage, **the stage of resistance**, the body is battling for equilibrium. If this stage is excessive or prolonged, the response becomes maladaptive and a pathologic condition occurs, which may be in the form of a stress-related disorder.

Exhaustion Stage

The **stage of exhaustion** occurs if the stressor is severe enough or is present over a long enough period of time to deplete the body's resources for adaptation. Critical illness or death results. Stressor that causes the GAS includes trauma, burns, infection, severe cold, and emotional upsets.

The body adapts to local stressors also in similar ways. The local response is called the Local adaptation syndrome (LAS). This takes place within a single organ or area of the body, such as injury or cut finger become inflamed.

Coping Mechanism

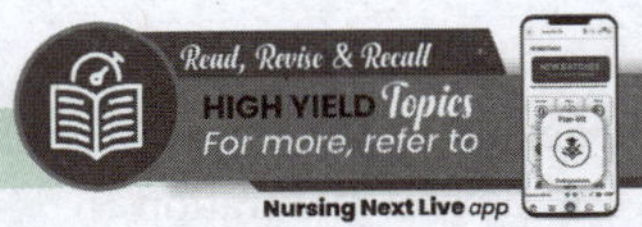

Coping mechanisms help us to resist and master stressors. Coping mechanisms are learned and once used successfully, they become part of our psychological defense armor.

There are three types of coping responses:

1. Actions or thoughts that change the situation so it is no longer stressful.
2. Alteration of thoughts to control the meaning of the situation before it triggers a stress response.
3. Control of thoughts and actions to stop a stress reaction.

Defense mechanisms are strategies that protect us from increasing anxiety. Defense mechanisms reduce both anxiety and the secretion of stress hormones. Defense mechanisms are used to maintain and improve our self-esteem. They can be overused in a maladaptive way as well.

There are various stress reduction techniques that help reduce stress and anxiety in patients such as recreational and diversional therapies.

CONCEPTS OF CULTURAL DIVERSITY AND SPIRITUALITY

Culture may be defined as a shared system of beliefs, values, and behavioral expectations that provides social structure for daily living. Culture defines roles and interactions with others as well as within families and communities, and is apparent in the attitudes unique to particular groups. (Andrew and Bowles, 2008)

There are **subcultures** within most cultures. A subculture is a large group of people who are members of an even larger cultural group, but who have certain ethnic, occupational, or physical characteristics that are not common to the larger culture.

Societies include dominant culture groups and minority culture groups.

A dominant culture group is the group that has the most ability to control the values and sanctions of the society. It is usually the largest group in a society.

Minority culture groups usually have same physical or cultural characteristics such as race, religion, beliefs or occupation that identify the people within groups as different from the dominant group.

Cultural assimilation occurs when a minority group lives with a dominant group

Acculturation: It is defined as "the process of cultural change that occurs when individuals from different cultural backgrounds come into prolonged, continuous, first hand contact with each other. *—Redfield, Linton and Herskovits (1936)*

Culture shock refers to the feelings, a person experiences when placed in a different culture perceived as strange. Culture

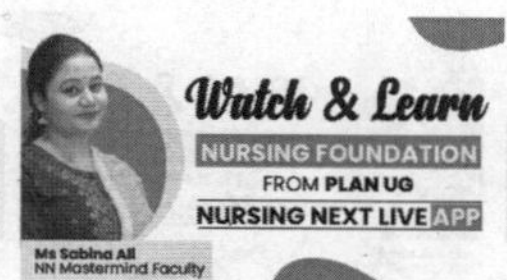

shock may result in psychological discomfort or disturbances, as the patterns of behavior a person found acceptable and effective in his or her culture may not be adequate or even acceptable to the new one.

Ethnicity is a sense of identification with a collective cultural group, largely based on the group's common heritage. One belongs to a specific ethnic group either by birth or through adaption of certain characteristics of that group. People within the ethnic group generally share unique cultural and social beliefs and behavior patterns, including languages. Ethnicity largely develops through day-to-day life with family and friends within the community.

Race: The term "Race" is often used interchangeably with ethnicity, these terms are not the same. Racial categories are typically based on specific physical characteristics such as skin pigmentation, body stature, facial features, and hair texture.

People from different cultures may also have different beliefs about best way to treat an illness or disease.

TRANSCULTURAL NURSING

Transcultural nursing is defined as a comparative study of cultures to understand similarities (culture universal) and differences (culture specific) beyond the human groups.

—**Leininger (1991 and 2002)**

Transcultural nursing is a distinct nursing specialty, which focuses on global cultures and comparative cultural caring, health and nursing phenomena. The transcultural nurse focuses to respond to the imperative for developing a global prospective within the nursing field in an increasingly globalized world of interdependent and interconnected nations and people.

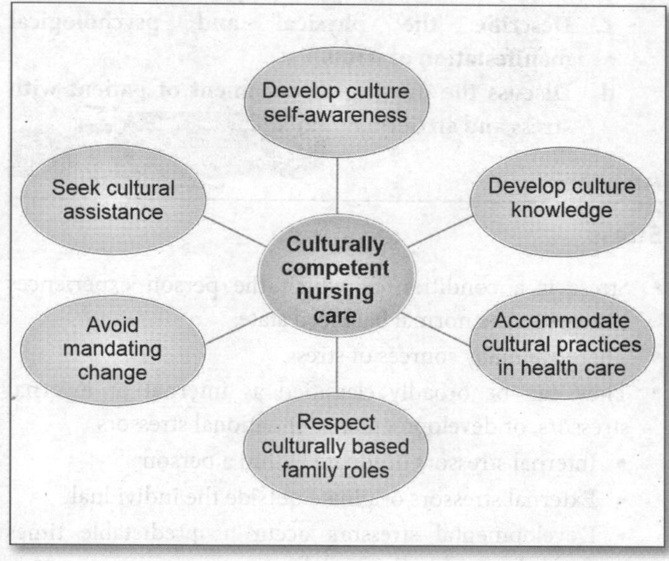

Figure 26.1: Culturally competent nursing care

SPIRITUAL HEALTH OR SPIRITUAL WELL-BEING

Spiritual health or spiritual well-being is manifested by a feeling of being "generally alive, purposeful, and fulfilled".

People nurture or enhance their spirituality in many ways. Some focus on development of the inner self, others focus on the expression of their spiritual energy with others or the outer world.

Spiritual distress refers to a challenge to the spiritual well-being or to the belief system that provides strength, hope, and meaning to life. Some factors that may be associated with or contribute to a person's spiritual distress include physiologic problems, treatment-related concerns, and situational concerns.

The focus on spiritual needs of patients along with meeting physical, social and psychological needs so that quality of life can be enhanced.

One simple guide is Anandarajah and Hight's (2001). HOPE acronym:

H : Sources of hope, comfort, strength, peace, love and connection
O : Organized religion
P : Personal spirituality and practice
E : Effects of spiritual belief and practice on medical care and end of life issue

Nursing interventions for spiritual care:

- Offer supportive or healing presence
- Facilitating the spiritual practices
- Nurturing spirituality
- Praying with patients
- Performing spiritual counseling
- Resolving conflicts between spiritual beliefs and medical treatments

CONCEPTUAL EXERCISES

LONG ANSWER QUESTION

1. a. **Define Stress.**
   b. **Discuss General Adaptation Syndrome**
   c. **Describe the physical and psychological manifestation of stress**
   d. **Discuss the nursing management of patient with stress and anxiety.**

Answer

Stress

- Stress is a condition in which the person experiences changes in the normal balanced state.
- There are many sources of stress.
- They can be broadly classified as internal or external stressors, or developmental or situational stressors.
  - Internal stressors originate within a person
  - External stressors originate outside the individual,
  - Developmental stressors occur at predictable times throughout an individual's life.
  - Situational stressors are unpredictable and may occur at any time during life.

b. **General Adaptation Syndrome**

Answer

- Selye states that a General adaptation syndrome (GAS) occurs in response to long-term exposure to stress.
- The stages are: **the alarm stage**, the **stage of resistance** and the **stage of exhaustion.**
- **Alarm stage:** During this stage, hormone released mobilizes the body's defenses. Nonspecific signs of illness such as slight rise on temperature, a loss of energy, decreased appetite and a general feeling of malaise occur.
- **Resistance stage:** During this **stage**, the body is battling for equilibrium. If this stage is excessive or prolonged, the response becomes maladaptive and a pathologic condition occurs, which may be in the form of a stress-related disorder.
- **Exhaustion stage:** it occurs if the stressor is severe enough or is present over a long enough period of time to deplete the body's resources for adaptation. Critical illness or death results. Stressor that causes the GAS includes trauma, burns, infection, severe cold, and emotional upsets.

c. **Physical and Psychological Manifestation of Stress:**

Answer

- Physical manifestation of stress may be short-term and long-term.
- Short term symptoms include dry mouth, increased sweating, increased heart rate and pulse rate, cold hands and feet, diarrhea headache, etc.
- Long term symptoms include intense tiredness, insomnia, change in appetite, etc.
- Psychological manifestation of stress results in memory issues, negative thoughts, loss of focus, lack of self-confidence, hopelessness, irritation, change in mood, loss of happiness, etc.

d. **Nursing management of patient with stress and anxiety**

Answer

Nursing Assessment

- Assess and recognize patient's level of anxiety
- Assess the client's perspective of a stressful situation.
- Assess patient's physical reactions to anxiety such as pain, nausea, weakness, or dizziness and patient's coping mechanisms for anxiety
- Observe how the client uses coping techniques and defense mechanisms to cope with anxiety.

Nursing Interventions and Rationales

- Recognize awareness of the client's anxiety. Use presence, touch (with permission), verbalization to remind clients that they are not alone and to encourage expression or clarification of needs, concerns, unknowns, and questions.
- Familiarize the client with the environment and new experiences or people as needed.
- Interact with the client in a peaceful manner.
- Accept the client's defenses; do not dare, argue, or debate.
- Converse using simple language and brief statements.
- Reinforce the client's personal reaction to or expression of pain, discomfort, or threats to well-being (e.g., talking, crying, walking, and other physical or nonverbal expressions).
- Lessen sensory stimuli by keeping a quiet and peaceful environment; keep "threatening" equipment out of sight.
- Allow the client to talk about anxious feelings and examine anxiety-provoking situations if they are identifiable.
- If the situational response is rational, use empathy to encourage the client to interpret the anxiety symptoms as normal.

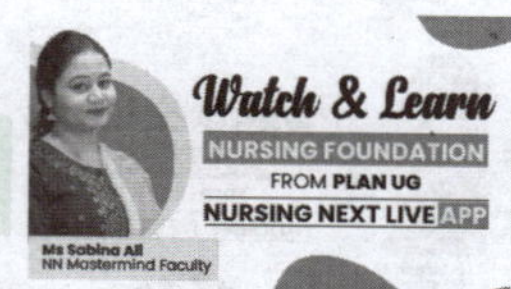

Recommend client to keep a log of episodes of anxiety

- Consider the client's use of coping strategies that the client has found effective in the past.
- Avoid unnecessary reassurance; this may increase undue worry.
- Assist the client in developing new anxiety-reducing skills (e.g., relaxation, deep breathing, positive visualization, and reassuring self-statements).
- Intervene when possible to eliminate sources of anxiety.
- Assist the client in strengthening problem-solving abilities.
- Explain all activities, procedures, and issues that involve the client; use non-medical terms and calm, slow speech. Do this in advance of procedures when possible, and validate the client's understanding.
- Administering anxiolytics and providing pharmacological support
- Instruct the client on the appropriate use of antianxiety medications.

Provide massage and backrubs for the client to reduce anxiety.

- Provide the client with a means to listen to the music of their choice.

Rule out withdrawal from alcohol, sedatives, or smoking as the cause of anxiety.

Educate the client and family about the symptoms of anxiety.

Teach the client to visualize or fantasize about the absence of anxiety or pain, successful experience of the situation, resolution of conflict, or outcome of the procedure.

Educate about and assist the client with breathing exercises, recreational therapy, etc.

Provide information regarding psychotherapy.

Arrange referrals or consultations with a psychiatrist, psychologist, and other medical professionals

- Ensure the client's safety during panic-level anxiety.

SHORT NOTES

1. What are the nurses role in meeting psychosocial needs of the patient?

Answer

There are three psychological needs (**autonomy, competence, relatedness**) that are universally important for psychological well-being and autonomous motivation.

- The first step to meet the psychological need of the individual is to facilitate and enhance the coping and adaptation mechanism.
- The nursing interventions are depending upon the severity of presence of any stressors.
- Effective techniques that can promote the psychological status of the individuals are:

Healthy lifestyle: Exercise, rest, and good nutrition are important components of stress reduction.

Exercise: Regular exercise maintains physical and emotional well-being. It also helps in releasing the endorphins which further promotes a feeling of well-being.

Rest and sleep: It helps in maintaining the homeostasis within the body and also promotes the restoration of energy levels.

Relaxation techniques and meditation: Various techniques can be used, but most involve rhythmic breathing, and recreational/diversional therapies

Diet: Foods should include well-balanced diet and healthy eating pattern and to avoid or limit saturated and trans fats, added sugar, excessive sodium intake.

Support systems: Family and good support systems provide emotional support that helps a person to identify and verbalize feelings associated with stress.

Using management techniques: These techniques include exercise, prayer, art therapy, music therapy, massage, therapeutic touch, biofeedback, yoga, meditation.

Anticipatory guidance: It focuses on psychologically preparing a person for an unfamiliar or painful event.

Creating therapeutic environment: It can promote positive healthy intrapersonal and interprofessional relationships to prevent stressful environment.

Measures to Reduce Stress and Anxiety in Patients

- Explain everything—hospital routine, TV, lights, curtains, procedures, and diagnostic tests
- Listen carefully to the patient; answer questions.
- Provide privacy and maintain confidentiality
- Treat the patient with respect
- Answer of all call bells promptly
- Check on the patient frequently
- Provide uninterrupted rest and sleep periods: coordinate care and treatments
- Keep visitors within acceptable numbers and time limits per patient's desire
- Keep noise to a minimum and Keep the room temperature adjusted to patient's comfort.

2. Write a short note on nurses role in meeting recreational need of the patient.

Answer

Recreation is anything which diverts, stimulates or refreshes our mind and body.

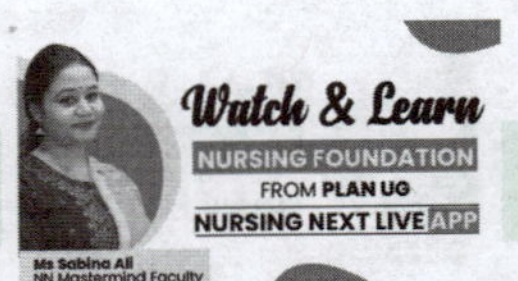

Common recreation therapies are reading a book or magazine, watching TV, playing musical instrument, swimming, walking on beach, art and crafts, meditation, gardening, etc.

Various nurses' role is discussed here:

- Promoting social interaction among patients to improve quality of life.
- Encourage the patient to increase their activity tolerance.
- Cognitive simulation.
- Providing opportunities to learn new skills and maintain current level of functioning.
- Offering leisure education opportunities.
- Community resource planning for patients being discharged.
- Provide opportunities for community involvement while in hospital.
- Nurses encourage opportunities for self-expression.

3. Write the spiritual needs of the patient. (DU)

Answer

Meeting the client's spiritual needs can help in decreasing the suffering and thus promotes the physical and mental healing of the individual.

Nurses need to be competent in establishing a trusting nurse-patient relationship for meeting the spiritual needs.

She should possess a healthy spiritual self-awareness.

She should be able to identify the need of spiritual care and be empathetic toward the spiritual concerns of clients/patients.

Nurses also need to be aware of the diverse spiritual beliefs and practices that the various patients may possess.

Each client's spiritual needs to be approached as unique needs.

Nurses can implement spiritual care therapeutics to promote spiritual and emotional health, coping and adjustment, or assist one to face a more peaceful death.

Various spiritual needs are:

Needs related to the self:

- Need for meaning and purpose
- Need for express creativity
- Need for hope
- Need to transcend life challenges
- Need for personal dignity
- Need for gratitude
- Need for vision
- Need to prepare for and accept death

Needs related to others:

- Need to forgive others
- Need to cope with loss of loved ones

Needs related to the ultimate other:

- Need to be certain there is a God or ultimate power in the universe
- Need to believe that God is loving and personally present
- Need to worship

Needs among and within groups:

- Need to contribute or improve one's community
- Need to be respected and valued
- Need to know what and when to give and take.

4. Write a short note on spiritual care. (KUHS)

Answer

Nurses should focus on spiritual needs of patients along with physical, social and psychological needs so that the overall quality of life can be improved.

Nursing assessment of the patient's spirituality including spiritual beliefs and practices, their effect on day to day living and health, spiritual distress, and spiritual needs should be addressed in nursing history collection. One simple guide is HOPE acronym:

H : Sources of hope, comfort, strength, peace, love and connection

O : Organized religion

P : Personal spirituality and practice

E : Effects of spiritual belief and practice on medical care and end of life issue

Assess for signs of spiritual distress: Sudden changes in spiritual practices (neglect, rejection, fanatical devotion), mood changes (anger, frequent crying, apathy, depression), sudden interest in spiritual matters (reading religious books or watching religious programs, visit to clergy, etc.) and disturbed sleep.

Interventions

A number of interventions are available to help the patients to meet their spiritual needs such as:

- Offer supportive or healing presence
- Facilitating the spiritual practices
- Nurturing spirituality
- Praying with patients
- Performing spiritual counseling
- Resolving conflicts between spiritual beliefs and medical treatments
- Develop mutually caring relationships
- Help the patients to move toward a healthy acceptance of the current situation: illness, pain, suffering, impending death

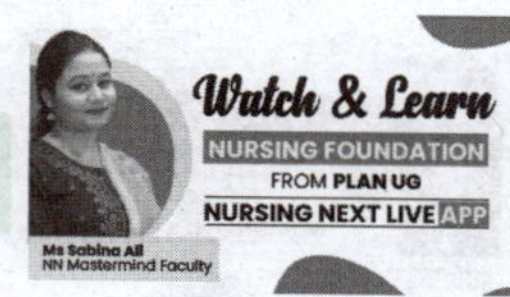

- Reconcile an interpersonal differences causing the patients' anguish
- Encourage the patients in expressing peaceful acceptance of limitations and failures
- Encourage the patients in expressing the ability to forgive others and to live in the present.

SHORT ANSWER QUESTIONS

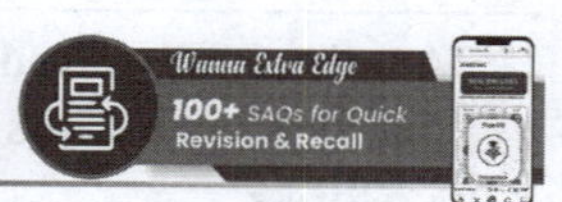

1. Define self-concept. Enumerate four dimensions of self-concept.

Answer

Self-concept is one's mental image of oneself. A positive self-concept is essential to a person's mental and physical health. Individuals with a positive self-concept are better able to develop and maintain interpersonal relationships. An individual possessing a strong self-concept.

There are four dimensions of self-concept:

1. Self-knowledge
2. Self-expectation
3. Social self
4. Appraisal of oneself

2. Define stress and its types.

Answer

Stress

Stress may be defined as a real or interpreted threat to the physiological or psychological integrity of an individual that results in physiological and/or behavioral responses.

Types

- Acute stress: a short-term stress that occurs in response to immediate challenges or demands
- Chronic Stress: a long-term stress that persists over an extended period.
- Psychological or Emotional Stress
- Environmental stress
- Work-related stress
- Relationship stress

3. Define culture.

Answer

Culture may be defined as a shared system of beliefs, values, and behavioral expectations that provides social structure for daily living. Culture defines roles and interactions with others as well as within families and communities, and is apparent in the attitudes unique to particular groups. (Andrew and Bowles, 2008).

CONCEPTUAL REVISION

MULTIPLE CHOICE QUESTIONS

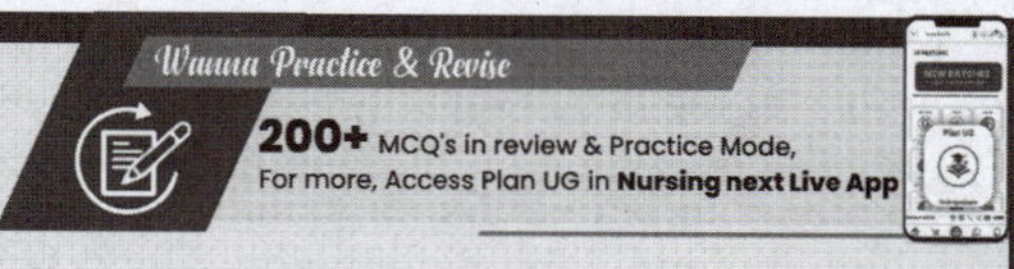

1. A female patient with a terminal illness is in denial. Indicators of denial include:

a. Shock and dismay
b. Numbness
c. Stoicism
d. Preparatory grief

Ans. a. Shock and dismay

2. Which of the following reflects as the dimension of the holistic approach?

a. Physical, Mental, Emotional, Spiritual and Social
b. Physical, Vocational, Spiritual, Cultural and Emotional
c. Social, Spiritual, Emotional and Religious
d. Social, Cultural, Emotional, Spiritual and Mental

Ans. a. Physical, Mental, Emotional, Spiritual and Social

3. When a hospitalized patient dies, his wife stares blankly at the nurse and states, "It can't be." The nurse assesses this as indicating:

a. Despair and protest
b. Shock and disbelief
c. Anger and hostility
d. Disorganization and confusion

Ans. b. Shock and disbelief

4. A teen is grieving the loss of her pet dog. She states to her mother, "I miss my dog so much, but I know that if I start crying, I will never stop." The teen is expressing a fear of:

a. Losing control over her emotions
b. Appearing emotionally immature
c. Embarrassing herself by crying in public
d. Losing the support of her friends and family

Ans. a. Losing control over her emotions

5. Dimensions of self-concept include:

a. Self-knowledge
b. Social self
c. Self-expectation
d. All of these

Ans. d. All of these

6. Coping means:

a. Solving or adjusting challenges
b. Adapt to respond to change
c. State of equilibrium
d. None of the above

Ans. a. Solving or adjusting challenges

7. Anything perceived as demanding or challenging that triggers a stress reaction is:

a. Stress
b. Stressor
c. Adaptation
d. Coping

Ans. b. Stressor

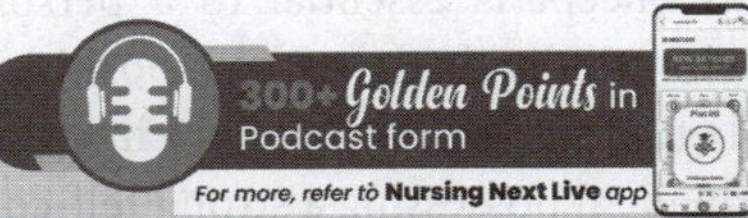

Golden Points

- **Self-concept** is one's mental image of oneself.
- A positive self-concept is essential to a person's mental and physical health.
- There are four dimensions of **self-concept: Self-knowledge, Self-expectation, Social self** and **appraisal of oneself** in relationship to others, events or situations.
- The Four components of self-concept: **Personal identity, body image, role performance and self-esteem.**
- Self-concept is also affected by role strain and role conflicts.
- Sexuality is an integral part of a person's identity and is present in one's demeanor through actions, communications and physical experiences.
- Sexual health may be defined as the integration of the somatic, emotional, intellectual, and social aspects of sexual being, in ways that are positively enriching and that enhance personality, communication, and love.
- Sexual harassment is unwelcome behavior that is sexual or gender-based in nature. Sexual abuse, also referred to as sexual assault or sexual violence or molestation, is abusive sexual behavior by one person upon another.
- **Stress** is a condition in which the person experiences changes in the normal balanced state. **A stressor** is an event or stimulus that causes an individual to experience stress.
- **Stressor can also be classified as Physiological or Psychosocial also**. Coordination of the central nervous system, autonomic nervous system, and the endocrine system is required for the body to adjust, adapt and maintain equilibrium.
- As long as the body's capacity is not over-taxed, the central nervous system, autonomic nervous system, and endocrine systems regulate body systems to maintain homeostasis.
- Selye states that a General adaptation syndrome (GAS) occurs in response to long-term exposure to stress.
- The stages are: **the alarm stage, the stage of resistance** and **the stage of exhaustion.**
- The body adapts to local stressors also in similar ways. The local response is called the Local adaptation syndrome (LAS). This takes place within a single organ or area of the body, such as injury or cut finger become inflamed.
- Coping mechanisms help us to resist and master stressors. Coping mechanisms are learned and once used successfully, they become part of our psychological defense armor.
- **Defense mechanisms** are strategies that protect us from increasing anxiety.
- Defense mechanisms reduce both anxiety and the secretion of stress hormones. Defense mechanisms are used to maintain and improve our self-esteem. They can be overused in a maladaptive way as well.
- Culture may be defined as a shared system of beliefs, values, and behavioral expectations that provides social structure for daily living.
- There are **subcultures** within most cultures. A subculture is a large group of people who are members of an even larger cultural group, but who have certain ethnic, occupational, or physical characteristics that are not common to the larger culture.
- **Acculturation:** It is defined as "the process of cultural change that occurs when individuals from different cultural backgrounds come into prolonged, continuous, first hand contact with each other.
- Culture shock refers to the feelings, a person experiences when placed in a different culture perceived as strange. Culture shock may result in psychological discomfort or disturbances, as the patterns of behavior a person found acceptable and effective in his or her culture may not be adequate or even acceptable to the new one.

CHAPTER 27

Nursing Theories

CONCEPTUAL THEORY

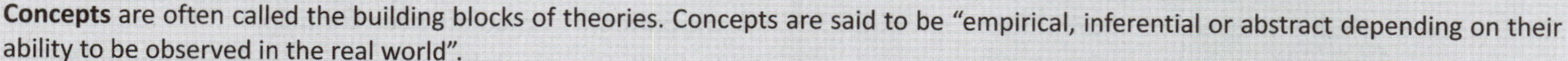

Terminology

150+ key terminologies for Quick Recall & Revision

Abstract concepts: These ideas are difficult to be observed directly or indirectly, such as stress, state of health, etc.
Concepts are often called the building blocks of theories. Concepts are said to be "empirical, inferential or abstract depending on their ability to be observed in the real world".
Conceptual framework: It is a group of related ideas, statements, or concepts.
Empirical concepts: Refer to what we can observe directly in the real world.
Environment: The internal and external surroundings that affect the client.
Health: The degree of wellness or well-being that the client experiences.
Inferential concepts: Refer to the ones that are indirectly observed.
Model: A model is an idea that explains by using symbolic and physical visualization. Models are pictorial or diagrammatically representation of a proposition where propositions are explained as the statements that explain relationship between the concepts.
Nursing: The attributes, characteristics, and actions of the nurse providing care on behalf of or in conjunction with the client.
Paradigm: It refers to a pattern of shared understandings and assumptions about reality and the world.
Person or client: The recipient of nursing care includes individuals, families, groups and communities.
Theory: It has been defined as a supposition or system of ideas that is proposed to explain a given phenomenon. Theories are also used to describe, predict and control phenomenon.

NURSING THEORIES

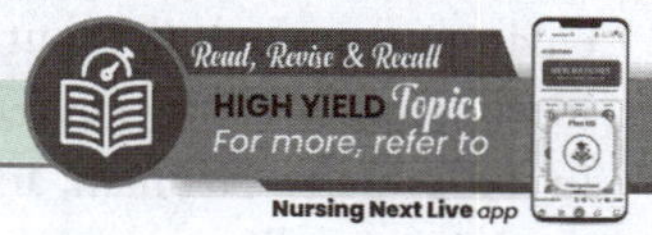

As a profession, nursing is involved in identifying its own unique body of knowledge essential to nursing practice. To identify this knowledge base, nurses must develop and recognize concepts and theories that are specific to nursing.

Concepts are often called the building blocks of theories. Concepts are said to be "empirical, inferential or abstract depending on their ability to be observed in the real world".

Empirical Concepts

Refer to what we can observe directly in the real world.

Inferential Concepts

Refer to the ones that are indirectly observed.

Abstract Concepts

These ideas are difficult to be observed directly or indirectly, such as stress, state of health, etc.

Conceptual Framework

It is a group of related ideas, statements, or concepts.

Theory

These are attempts to explain relationships between concepts.

Theory has been defined as a supposition or system of ideas that is proposed to explain a given phenomenon. Theories are also used to describe, predict and control phenomenon.

Model

A model is an idea that explains by using symbolic and physical visualization. Models are pictorial or diagrammatically representation of a proposition where propositions are explained as the statements that explain relationship between the concepts.

Paradigm

It refers to a pattern of shared understandings and assumptions about reality and the world.

THE METAPARADIGM FOR NURSING/CONCEPTS IN NURSING THEORY

In the late 20th century, most of the theoretical work in nursing was focused on articulating relationships among four major concepts: (1) Person, (2) Environment, (3) Health and (4) Nursing. They are sometimes collectively referred to as metaparadigm for nursing.

These four concepts are central to nursing.

1. **Person or client:** The recipient of nursing care includes individuals, families, groups and communities.
2. **Environment:** The internal and external surroundings that affect the client.
3. **Health:** The degree of wellness or well-being that the client experiences.
4. **Nursing:** The attributes, characteristics, and actions of the nurse providing care on behalf of or in conjunction with the client.

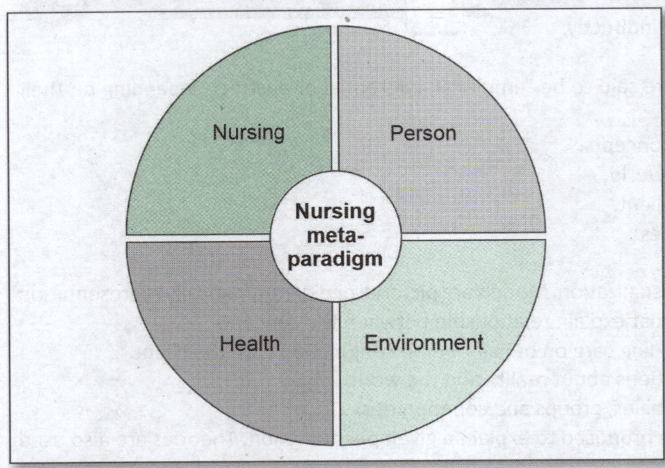

Importance of Theories in Nursing

- Theory provides nurse with a sound basis to describe, explain and predict factors that influence nursing care.
- Nursing theory is a source of professional autonomy and power.
- It guides nursing education, research and practice and differentiates nursing practice from other disciplines.

HISTORY OF NURSING THEORIES

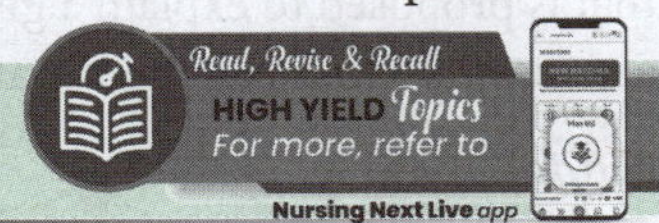

The first nursing theories appeared in the late 1800s when a strong emphasis was placed on nursing education.

- **In 1860**, Florence Nightingale defined nursing in her "Environmental Theory" as "the act of utilizing the patient's environment to assist him in his recovery."
- In the 1950s, there is a consensus among nursing scholars that nursing needed to validate itself through the production of its own scientifically tested body of knowledge.
- In 1952, Hildegard Peplau introduced her Theory of Interpersonal Relations that emphasizes the nurse-client relationship as the foundation of nursing practice.
- In 1955, Virginia Henderson conceptualized the nurse's role as assisting sick or healthy individuals to gain independence in meeting 14 fundamental needs. Thus, her Nursing Need Theory was developed.
- In 1960, Faye Abdellah published her work "Typology of 21 Nursing Problems," which shifted the focus of nursing from a disease-centered approach to a patient-centered approach.
- In 1962, Ida Jean Orlando emphasized the reciprocal relationship between patient and nurse and viewed nursing's professional function as finding out and meeting the patient's immediate need for help.
- In 1968, Dorothy Johnson pioneered the Behavioral System Model and upheld the fostering of efficient and effective behavioral functioning in the patient to prevent illness.
- In 1970, Martha Rogers viewed nursing as both a science and an art as it provides a way to view the unitary human being, who is integral with the universe.
- In 1971, Dorothea Orem stated in her theory that nursing care is required if the client is unable to fulfill biological, psychological, developmental, or social needs.
- In 1971, Imogene King's Theory of Goal attainment stated that the nurse is considered part of the patient's environment and the nurse-patient relationship is for meeting goals toward good health.
- In 1972, Betty Neuman, in her theory, states that many needs exist, and each may disrupt client balance or stability. Stress reduction is the goal of the system model of nursing practice.
- In 1979, Sister Callista Roy viewed the individual as a set of interrelated systems that maintain the balance between these various stimuli.
- In 1979, Jean Watson developed the philosophy of caring, highlighted humanistic aspects of nursing as they intertwine with scientific knowledge and nursing practice.

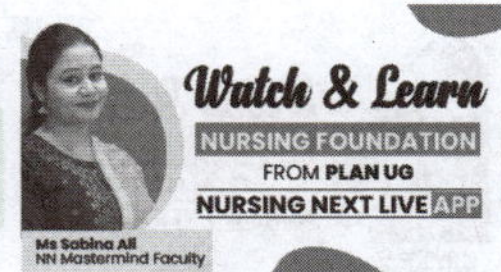

NURSING METAPARADIGM OF DIFFERENT NURSE THEORIES

	Person	Health	Nursing	Environment
Nightingale	Human beings were not defined by Nightingale specifically.	Nightingale (1859/1992) did not define health specifically.	"What nursing has to do... is to put the patient in the best condition for nature to act upon him" (Nightingale, 1859/1992)	Nightingale's writings reflect a community health model in which all that surrounds human beings is considered in relation to their state of health.
Orem	Humans are defined as "men, women, and children cared for either singly or as social units," and are the "material object" of nurses and others who provide direct care.	Health is "being structurally and functionally whole or sound".	Nursing is an art through which the practitioner of nursing gives specialized assistance to persons with disabilities which makes more than ordinary assistance necessary to meet needs for self-care.	The environment has physical, chemical and biological features. It includes the family, culture, and community.
Henderson	Individuals have basic needs that are component of health and require assistance to achieve health and independence or a peaceful death.	Health was taken to mean balance in all realms of human life.	"The unique function of the nurse is to assist the individual, sick or well, in the performance of those activities contributing to health or its recovery that he would perform unaided if he had the necessary strength, will or knowledge. And to do this in such a way as to help him gain independence as rapidly as possible."	No explicit definition of the environment, though she stated that: "maintaining a supportive environment conducive for health is one of the elements of her 14 activities for client assistance."
Peplau	An organism that "strives in its own way to reduce tension generated by needs".	Health is defined as "a word symbol that implies forward movement of personality and other ongoing human processes in the direction of creative, constructive, productive, personal, and community living."	Hildegard Peplau considers nursing to be a "significant, therapeutic, interpersonal process".	Although Peplau does not directly address society/ environment, she does encourage the nurse to consider the patient's culture and mores when the patient adjusts to hospital routine.
Rogers	A person is defined as an indivisible, pandimensional energy field identified by a pattern, and manifesting characteristics specific to the whole, and that can't be predicted from knowledge of the parts.	Rogers defines health as an expression of the life process	Nursing aims to assist people in achieving their maximum health potential.	It is the study of unitary, irreducible, indivisible human and environmental fields: people and their world.
King	Individuals are social beings who are rational and sentient. Humans communicate their thoughts, actions, customs, and beliefs through language.	Health is dynamic life experience of a human being, which implies continuous adjustment to stressors in the internal and external environment through optimum use of one's resources to achieve maximum potential for daily living.	Environment is the background for human interactions. It is both external to, and internal to, the individual.	Nursing is a process of action, reaction, and interaction whereby nurse and client share information about their perceptions in the nursing situation.

Contd...

	Person	Health	Nursing	Environment
Watson	Human being is a valued person to be cared for, respected, nurtured, understood, and assisted; in general a philosophical view of a person as a fully functional integrated self.	Health is the unity and harmony within the mind, body, and soul; health is associated with the degree of congruence between the self as perceived and the self as experienced.	Society provides the values that determine how one should behave and what goals one should strive toward.	Nursing is a human science of persons and human health-illness experiences that are mediated by professional, personal, scientific, esthetic, and ethical human care transactions.

CONCEPTUAL EXERCISES

LONG ANSWER QUESTION

1. **Write in detail about two systems theory. (MGR)**

Answer

Introduction

- First proposed as General Systems theory by Ludwig von Bertalanffy.
- General systems theory refers to as a general science of "wholeness".
- The application of system theory is in developing nursing theories and in conducting nursing research also.

Characteristics of Systems Theory

- Systems—self-regulating systems.
- Systems—self-correcting through feedback.
- Systems have a structure. Structure is having its parts and processes.
- Systems—generalizations of reality.
- The parts of a system have functional and structural relationships between each other.
- Systems function in the same way.
- Every living organism is an open system.

Examples of Systems Theory

- Neuman's Systems Theory
- Rogers' Theory
- Roy's Adaptation Model
- Imogene King's Theory of Goal Attainment
- Orem Self-care Deficit Theory
- Johnson's Behavior System Model

Imogene King's Theory of Goal Attainment

Imogene King's Goal Attainment theory states that the nurse is considered part of the patient's environment and the nurse-patient relationship is for meeting goals toward good health.

King Toward a Theory for Nursing

- In 1964, Imogene M King published a paper discussing problems and prospects to the development of nursing knowledge.
- In 1968, she first identified several concepts, she later used in her conceptual system and continued to discuss the need for a nursing knowledge base.
- King identified her work as a conceptual system. The function of a conceptual system is to give support for arranging ideas or concepts into group that provides meaning.
- As the theory of goal attainment is derived from the conceptual system, the conceptual system and its assumptions and concepts are presented first and then the goal attainment theory.

King's Conceptual System

- Concepts are necessary to Nursing as a discipline
- Provides the derivation of theories
- Provides an organizing structure for Nursing Curriculum
- Supports quality care in all settings in which Nursing occurs

Essential elements

- Goal
- Structure
- Functions
- Resources
- Decision-making

Conceptual system

- Personal system
- Interpersonal system
- Social system

This theory focuses on the process to aid nurses in the Nurse-Patient Relationship, helping the patients to meet the goals they have set for their health.

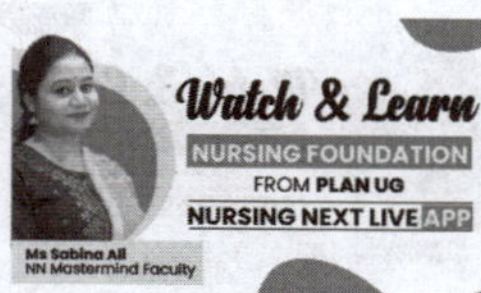

The theory's focus on interpersonal systems reflects that the practice of nursing and is differentiated from that of other health professions by what nurses do with and for individuals.

The interpersonal system in which two people who are usually strangers come together in a health care organization to help and be helped to maintain a state of health that permits functioning in roles.

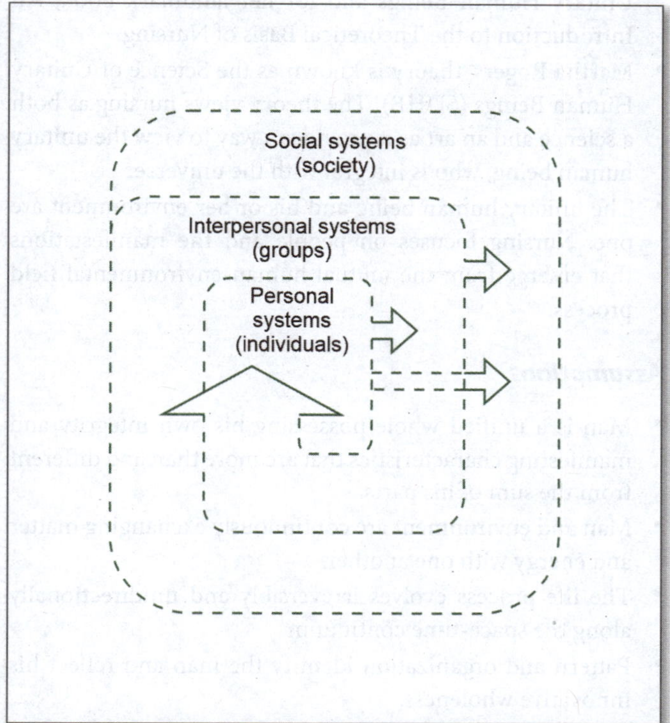

Interaction: Observable verbal and nonverbal goal-directed behavior and judgment or decision to act and then each reacts to the other.

Perception: Reality as seen by each individual and exporting information in the form of observable behaviors.

Communication: Exchange of information may occur within a person as well as between people.

Transaction: Series of exchange and represent the aspect of human interactions in which values are apparent.

Decision-making: The process of making choices and then evaluating the results in relation to goals achieved.

Law of Nurse-Patient Interaction

"Nurses and patients are in mutual presence, interacting purposefully, make transactions in nursing situations based on each individual's perceptions, purposeful communication and valued goals."

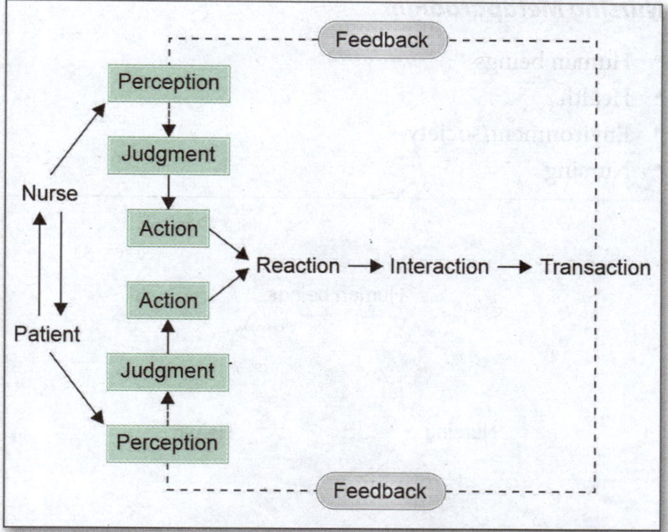

Assumptions

- Nursing focus is the care of human being.
- Nursing goal is the health care of individuals and groups
- Human beings: are open systems interacting constantly with their environment.
- Nurse and client communicate information, set goal mutually and then act to attain those goals.
- Each human being perceives the world as a total person in making transactions with individuals and things in environment.
- Transaction represents a life situation in which perceiver and thing perceived are encountered and in which person enters the situation as an active participant and each is changed in the process of these experiences"

Propositions

- If perceptual interaction accuracy is present in nurse-client interaction, transaction will occur.
- If nurse and client make transaction, goal will be attained.
- If goals are attained, satisfaction will occur.
- If transactions are made in nurse-client interactions, growth and development will be enhanced.
- If role expectations and role performance as perceived by nurse and client are congruent, transaction will occur.
- If role conflict is experienced by nurse or client or both, stress in nurse-client interaction will occur
- If nurse with special knowledge skill communicates appropriate information to client, mutual goal setting and goal attainment will occur.

Nursing Metaparadigm

- Human beings
- Health
- Environment/society
- Nursing

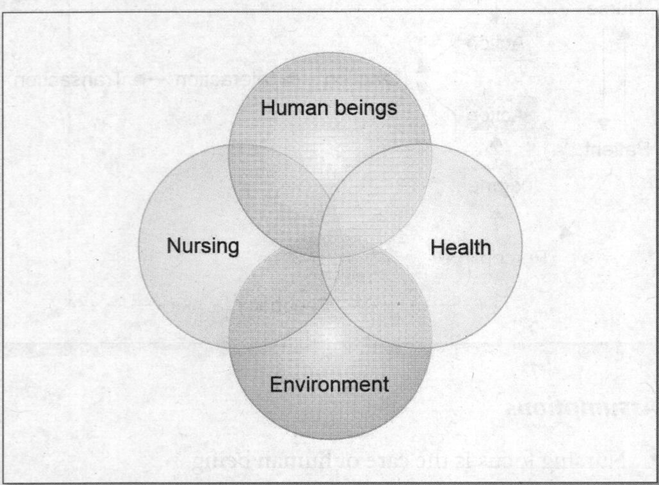

Utilization of the Theory

- Provides a theoretical base for Nursing process.
- Demonstrates a way for Nurses to interact purposefully with patients.

Strengths

- Easily understood.
- Clear and conceptually defined from research literature at the time when the theory was developed.

Limitations

- Social system is not clearly connected to the theory, which leads to limitations of utilizing the theory in nursing care with groups, families and communities.
- King's theory presents nine major concepts, thus making theory complex.
- King's theory has been criticized for having limited application in areas of nursing where patients are unable to interact with the nurse in case of unconscious and psychiatric patients.
- King took learning and control as a subconcept but does not define it.

Rogers' Theory

Introduction

- First introduced by Martha Rogers in 1970, the Rogerian model is an abstract system of ideas from which to approach the nursing care of unitary human beings.
- Her ideas were revolutionary and challenged nursing to approach care from a holistic and dynamic, constantly evolving energy fields, rather than as homeostatic beings. Variation is expected and embraced within this homeodynamic perspective.
- **Martha Elizabeth Rogers (May 12, 1914–March 13, 1994):** She was an American nurse, researcher, theorist, and author widely known for developing the Science of Unitary Human Beings and for her landmark book, An Introduction to the Theoretical Basis of Nursing.
- Martha Rogers' theory is known as the Science of Unitary Human Beings (SUHB). The theory views nursing as both a science and an art as it provides a way to view the unitary human being, who is integral with the universe.
- The unitary human being and his or her environment are one. Nursing focuses on people and the manifestations that emerge from the mutual human-environmental field process.

Assumptions

- Man is a unified whole possessing his own integrity and manifesting characteristics that are more than and different from the sum of his parts.
- Man and environment are continuously exchanging matter and energy with one another.
- The life process evolves irreversibly and unidirectionally along the space-time continuum
- Pattern and organization identify the man and reflect his innovative wholeness.
- Man is characterized by the capacity for abstraction and imagery, language and thought sensation and emotion.

Major Concepts

- Energy field
- Openness
- Pattern
- Pandimensional

Energy Field

- The energy field is the fundamental unit of both the living and the nonliving.
- It provides a way to view people and the environment as irreducible wholes.
- The energy fields continuously vary in intensity, density, and extent.

Openness

- There are no boundaries that stop energy flow between the human and environmental fields, which is the openness in Rogers' theory.

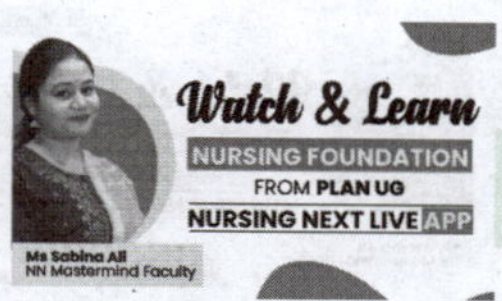

- It refers to qualities exhibited by open systems; human beings and their environment are open systems.

Pattern:

- Rogers defined the pattern as the distinguishing characteristic of an energy field seen as a single wave. It is an abstraction and gives identity to the field.

Pandimensional:

- Pandimensionality is defined as "nonlinear domain without spatial or temporal attributes".
- The parameters that humans use in language to describe events are arbitrary, and the present is relative; there is no temporal ordering of lives.

Hemodynamic Principles

- Hemodynamics refers to the balance between the dynamic life process and environment. These principles help to view human as unitary human being.
- The three principles of hemodynamics are:
  1. **Resonance:** Wave patterns are continuously changing in environmental and human energy fields.
  2. **Helicy:** The nature of change is unpredictable, continuous, and an innovative.
  3. **Integrality:** Energy fields of humans and environment are in a continuous mutual process.

Metaparadigm of Martha Rogers' Nursing Theory

- Person
- Environment
- Health
- Nursing

Strengths

- Martha Rogers' concepts provide a worldview from which nurses may derive theories and hypotheses and propose relationships specific to different situations.
- Rogers' theory is not directly testable due to lack of concrete hypotheses, but it is testable in principle.

Weaknesses

- Rogers' model does not define particular hypotheses or theories for it is an abstract, unified and highly derived framework.
- Testing the concepts' validity is questionable because its concepts are not directly measurable.
- Rogers claimed that nursing exists to serve people; however, nurses' roles were not clearly defined.
- The purpose of nurses is to promote health and well-being for all persons wherever they are. However, Rogers' model has no concrete definition of health state.

SHORT NOTES

1. Write a short note on Betty Neuman's stress model. (MGR, KUHS, DU)

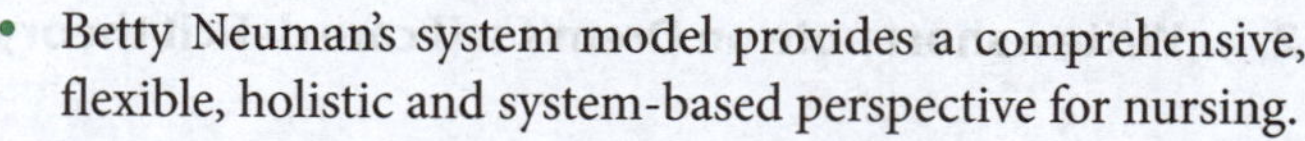

Answer

- Betty Neuman's system model provides a comprehensive, flexible, holistic and system-based perspective for nursing.
- It focuses attention on the response of the client system to actual or potential environmental stressors.
- The model was published in 1972 as "A Model for Teaching Total Person Approach to Patient Problems" in nursing research.
- It was refined, and subsequently published in the first edition of Conceptual Models for Nursing Practice, in 1974, and in 1980 (Second edition).

Major Concepts of Neuman's Theory

- **Person**
- **Environment**
- **Health**
- **Nursing**

1. Person

Each layer is of five person variables or subsystems:

- **Physiological**—physiochemical structure and function of the body.
- **Psychological**—mental processes and emotions.
- **Sociocultural**—relationships; and social/cultural expectations and activities.
- **Spiritual**—influence of spiritual beliefs.
- **Developmental**—processes related to development over the life span.

2. Environment

- The internal environment exists within the client system.
- The external environment exists outside the client system.
- A created environment—environment that is created and developed unconsciously by the client and is symbolic of system wholeness.

3. Health

- Health/wellness is defined as the condition in which all parts and subparts (variables) are in harmony with the whole of the client (Neuman, 1995).

- The client system moves toward wellness when more energy is available than is needed; and it moves toward illness and death when more energy is needed than its availability.

4. Nursing

- Action which assist individuals, families and groups to maintain a maximum level of wellness.
- Primary aim is stability of the patient/client system with the help of nursing interventions to reduce stressors.

2. Write a short note on Orem's self care deficit theory

Answer

- Dorothea Elizabeth Orem was American nursing theorists who developed the *Self-Care Deficit Nursing Theory, also known as the Orem Model of Nursing.*
- According to her, Nursing is "The act of assisting others in the provision and management of self-care to maintain or improve human functioning at the home level of effectiveness.
- Dorothea Orem's Self-Care Deficit Theory focuses on each *"individual's ability to perform self-care, defined as 'the practice of activities that individuals initiate and perform on their own behalf in maintaining life, health, and well-being."*
- The Self-Care or Self-Care Deficit Theory of Nursing is composed of three interrelated theories: (1) **the theory of self-care,** (2) **the self-care deficit theory,** and (3) **the theory of nursing systems**, which is further classified into wholly compensatory, partially compensatory and supportive-educative.

3. Write a short note on Peplau Interpersonal relation theory.

Answer

Hildegard Elizabeth Peplau was an American nurse who is well-known for her *Theory of Interpersonal Relations* and also known to many as the *"Mother of Psychiatric Nursing"* and the *"Nurse of the Century."*

Hildegard Peplau's Interpersonal Relations Theory emphasized the nurse-client relationship as the foundation of nursing practice. Peplau form an interpersonal model emphasizing the need for a partnership between nurse and client as opposed to the client passively receiving treatment and the nurse passively acting out doctor's orders.

The four components of the theory are **person**, which is a developing organism that tries to reduce anxiety caused by needs; **environment**, which consists of existing forces outside of the person and put in the context of culture; **health**, which is a word symbol that implies a forward movement of personality and **nursing**, which is a significant therapeutic interpersonal process that functions cooperatively with another human process that makes health possible for individuals in communities.

SHORT ANSWER QUESTIONS

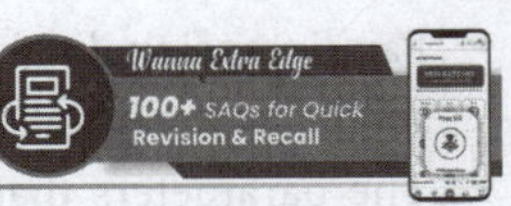

1. Give the examples of systems theory. (MGR)

Answer

Examples of Systems Theory

- Neuman's Systems Theory
- Rogers' Theory
- Roy's Adaptation Model
- Imogene King's Theory of Goal Attainment
- Orem Self-care Deficit Theory
- Johnson's Behavior System Model

2. Define nursing theory and enlist different theories in nursing. (RUHS)

Answer

Nursing theories are organized bodies of knowledge to define what nursing is, what nurses do, and why do they do it.

Different Theories in Nursing.

- Florence Nightingale's Environment theory
- Betty Neuman's System model
- Dorothea Orem - Self-care theory
- Hildegard Peplau's Interpersonal theory
- Virginia Henderson's Need Theory
- Sister Calista Roy's Adaptation theory
- Fay Abdella's Twenty One Nursing Problems
- Ida Jean Orlando's Nursing Process theory
- Martha Rogers's-Unitary Human beings
- Imogene King's Goal Attainment theory
- Jean Watson's Philosophy and Caring Model

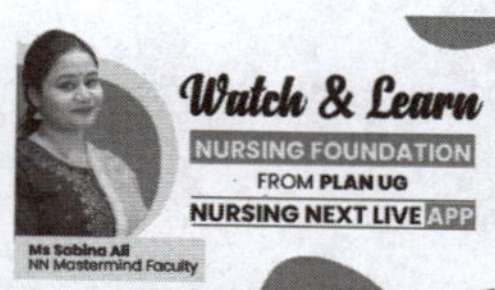

CONCEPTUAL REVISION

MULTIPLE CHOICE QUESTIONS

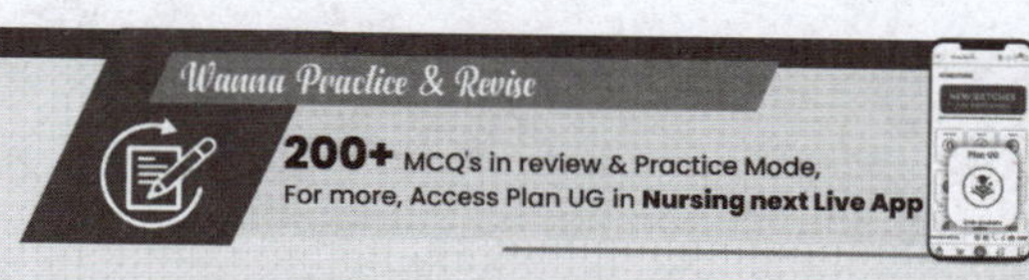

1. Which of the following cluster of data belongs to Maslow's hierarchy of needs?

a. Love and belonging
b. Physiological needs
c. Self-actualization
d. All of the above

Ans. d. All of the above

2. Which of the following is included in Orem's theory?

a. Maintenance of a sufficient intake of air.
b. Self-perception.
c. Love and belongingness.
d. Physiologic needs.

Ans. a. Maintenance of a sufficient intake of air

3. Select which among the following Nursing theory describes the nurse -patient relationship concepts?

a. Leininger
b. Dorothea Orem
c. Hildegard Peplau
d. Betty Neuman

Ans. c. Hildegard Peplau

4. Which of the following principles of primary nursing has proven the most satisfying to the patient and nurse relationship?

a. Autonomy and authority for planning are best delegated to a nurse who knows the patient well
b. Accountability is clearest when one nurse is responsible for the overall plan and its implementation.
c. The holistic approach provides for a therapeutic relationship, continuity, and efficient nursing care.
d. Dividing the role and responsibility among the staff nurses will have better patient oriented outcome.

Ans. c. The holistic approach provides for a therapeutic relationship, continuity, and efficient nursing care.

5. The four main concepts common to nursing that appear in each of the current conceptual models are:

a. Person, nursing, environment, medicine
b. Person, health, nursing, support systems
c. Person, health, psychology, nursing
d. Person, environment, health, nursing

Ans. d. Person, environment, health, nursing

6. Self-care deficit theory was proposed by:

a. Virginia Henderson
b. Betty Neuman
c. Imogene King
d. Dorothea Orem

Ans. d. Dorothea Orem

7. Environmental theory was given by:

a. Orem
b. Peplau
c. Nightingale
d. Henderson

Ans. c. Nightingale

8. Using Malsow's hierarchy of needs, identify the priority for a patient who is experiencing chest pain and difficulty breathing.

a. Self-actualization
b. Air, water, and nutrition
c. Safety
d. Esteem and self-esteem needs

Ans. b. Air, water, and nutrition

9. How are critical thinking skills and critical thinking attitudes similar?

a. Both influence the nurse's problem-solving and decision-making.
b. Both are like feelings rather than cognitive activities.
c. Both are cognitive activities rather than feelings.
d. Both are applicable in all aspects of a person's life.

Ans. a. Influences on the nurse's problem-solving and decision-making.

10. A nurse has received a 75-year-old female patient into the surgical ward with the diagnosis of osteoarthritis. On admission, the nurse has given a room orientation to the patient and placed her on bed with side rails up. This action of the nurse is justifying which level of Maslow-Hierarchy for the patient?

a. Esteem need
b. Physiological need
c. Safety and security need
d. Self-actualization need

Ans. c. Safety and security need

Nursing Care Plan

NURSING CARE PLAN—ANEMIA (FATIGUE)

Assessment	Diagnosis	Outcome	Intervention	Rationale	Evaluation
Subjective data: The client says, "Inability to maintain usual level of physical activity and Report of fatigue and lack of energy" **Objective data:** On assessment, exertional discomfort or dyspnea	Fatigue related to decreased hemoglobin and diminished oxygen-carrying capacity of the blood as evidenced by decreased exercise tolerance level.	Client will demonstrate a reduction in fatigue, as evidenced by reports of increased energy levels and ability to perform desired activities.	Assist the patient in setting a daily exercise and rest regimen. Emphasize the need of taking frequent breaks **Educate energy-conservation techniques** • Educate the patient about medicines that can increase RBC synthesis in the bone marrow. • As needed, use supplemental oxygen therapy. • Suggest occupational therapy to patient.	• To make strategy that integrates periods of activity with intervals of rest can assist the patient in completing targeted activities without increasing fatigue levels • To teach organization and time management might assist the patient in conserving energy and minimizing fatigue. • Hematological growth factor, recombinant human erythropoietin increases hemoglobin and reduces the requirement for RBC transfusions. • To ensure oxygen saturation level is sustained at 90% or higher. • To educate the patient on the use of assistive equipment for extra energy-saving measures in the house.	The patient verbalizes his or her understanding of energy conservation principles and showed increased energy level and better performance in activities.

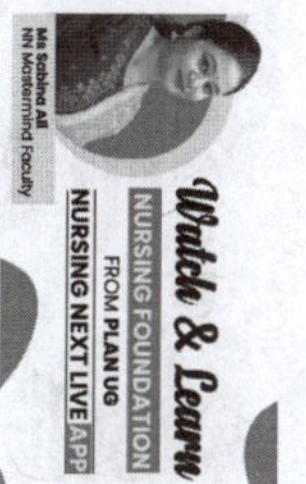

NURSING CARE PLAN—RENAL FAILURE (FLUID VOLUME EXCESS)

Assessment	Diagnosis	Outcome	Intervention	Rationale	Evaluation
Subjective data: Patient says, "I have swollen extremities and body and I feel very weak" **Objective data:** Generalized edema, Fatigue	Fluid volume excess related to compromise regulatory mechanism (renal failure) as evidenced by generalized edema.	The client's fluid volume will be within normal limits within 8 hours.	• Record accurate intake and output (I&O). • Weigh daily at same time of day, on the same scale, with same equipment and clothing. • Assess skin, face, dependent areas for edema. • Plan oral fluid replacement with patient, within multiple restriction.	• Accurate I&O is necessary for determining renal function and fluid replacement needs and reducing risk of fluid overload. • Daily body weight is best monitor of fluid status. • Edema occurs primarily in dependent tissues of body (e.g.- hands, feet). • Helps avoid periods without fluids and reduces sense of deprivation.	Goal met, patient has displayed appropriate urinary output near normal, stable weight, vital signs within normal range and absence of edema.

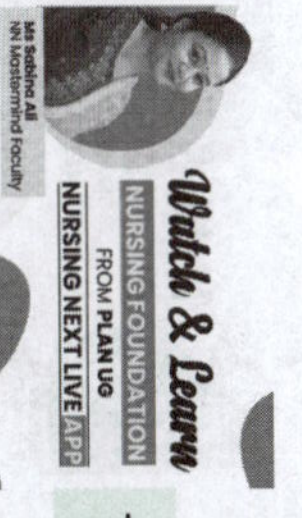

NURSING CARE PLAN—SURGERY/POSTOPERATIVE CONDITION (ACUTE PAIN)

Assessment	Diagnosis	Outcome	Intervention	Rationale	Evaluation
Subjective data: The client says, " I am having pain at the surgical site" **Objective data:** On assessment pain rating scale, patient had score of 6. **Temperature:** 98° Celsius **Pulse:** 88 b/min **BP:** 130/88 mm Hg **Respiration:** 22br/min	**Acute pain** related to surgical incision and tissue trauma as evidenced by reports of 6 out of 10 pain in a scale of 1/10 at abdomen, grimacing, and difficulty moving secondary to cholecystectomy surgery.	• Client will demonstrate satisfactory pain control less than 3 to 4 on a rating scale of 0 to 10 • Patient will display improved well-being such as baseline levels for pulse, BP, respirations, and relaxed muscle tone or body posture.	• Client pain was of moderate intensity, at surgical site and vitals are stable. • Distraction therapy was provided to the client that is watching TV or listening to music and drawing therapy. • Deep breathing exercises were taught. • Pillow and back rest were provided. • Cold application was given to the client. • Injection tramadol in 100 mL NS was administered and inj. Emset was also given before this. • Comfortable position was provided to the client. • Pain and vitals sign were assessed again at regular intervals.	• To identify intensity, onset, duration of pain and, physiological changes in the vital signs. • Distraction therapy, guided imagery can be provided to the client. • To allow proper circulation of oxygen in the blood. • Comfort devices will help the client to maintain the body posture. • Cold application reduces pain, inflammation and muscle spasticity by reducing the release of pain inducing chemicals. • Analgesics and opioids block the pain receptors and release of pain inducing chemicals. • So, that client can take rest and to reduce the discomfort. • To determine the effectiveness of the interventions provided to the client.	Client showed reduced pain on the pain scale that is 3 out of 10 on pain rating scale and vital parameters are also stable.

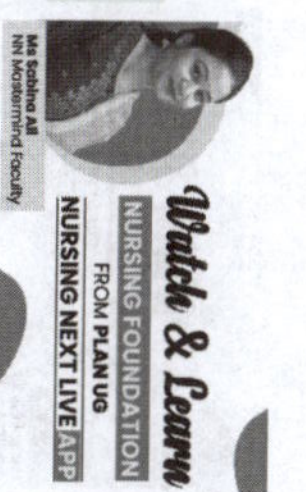

NURSING CARE PLAN—INVASIVE PROCEDURE LIKE IV CANNULATION OR URINARY CATHETER ASSOCIATED INFECTION (RISK FOR INFECTION)

Assessment	Diagnosis	Outcome	Intervention	Rationale	Evaluation
Subjective data: The client says, "Inability to maintain usual level of physical activity and Report of fatigue and lack of energy" **Objective data:** On assessment Exertional discomfort or dyspnea.	Risk of infection related to invasive procedures and exposure to pathogens.	After providing the interventions individual risk factors and measures to lower the risk of infection will be identified by the client and they will keep an aseptic environment.	• Examine the skin for symptoms of infection, such as breaks or discomfort. • Examine laboratory blood reports for signs of systemic infections. • Follow the infection control, sterilization, and aseptic policies and procedures of the facility. • Maintain dependent gravity drainage of indwelling catheters, tubes, and/or parenteral or irrigation lines under positive pressure. • Antibiotics should be given as directed.	• Skin disruptions at or near the surgical site are sources of wound contamination. • An elevated WBC count may indicate an ongoing infection, which the surgical operation will treat. • To create strategies for infection prevention. • Prevents bodily fluid stasis and reflux. • Prophylactic administration for suspected illness or contamination.	Client showed reduced risk of infection after interventions.

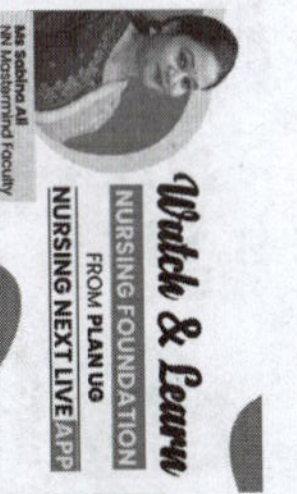

NURSING CARE PLAN—DEPRESSION OR LOSS OF INSIGHT (SELF-CARE DEFICITS)

Assessment	Diagnosis	Outcome	Intervention	Rationale	Evaluation
Subjective data: The client says, "Inability to maintain usual level of personal hygiene and self-care" **Objective data:** On assessment patient was not willing to do any self-care activity	Self-care deficits related to depression or loss of insight as evidenced by unable to do the self-care activities like bathing, brushing, etc.	Patient will demonstrate self-care activities Independently.	• Assess the level of self-care • Establish short-term goals with the patient. • Assist the patient in maintaining the personal hygiene • Teach the patient to coordinate diaphragmatic breathing with activity. • Encourage patient to begin to bathe self, walk and do some self-care activities	• To know the insight of patient • To help the patient with setting realistic goals will reduce frustration. • The patient's capacity for self-care measures may fluctuate frequently over time, necessitating regular evaluations. • To provide diversion and relaxation therapy • To help patient accept both temporary and permanent dependence	Patient is Independent in self-care activities as manifested by performing self-care activities and maintaining the personal hygiene

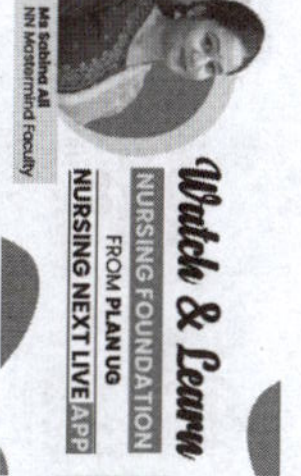

NURSING CARE PLAN—PREOPERATIVE CONDITION (ANXIETY)

Assessment	Diagnosis	Outcome	Intervention	Rationale	Evaluation
Subjective data: Patient says, "I am having anxiety about my disease condition and surgical procedure" **Objective data:** On assessment, patient has inadequate information regarding the disease condition and surgical procedure	Anxiety related to upcoming surgical procedure as evidenced by excessive sweating and shaking of hands.	The patient will remain free from anxiety to maximum extent.	• Assess the level of anxiety. • Maintain the IPR with the client. • Collect knowledge regarding the disease condition and about the surgery. • Educate the client regarding the disease condition and surgical procedure. • Teach client deep breathing techniques, guided imagery, progressive muscle relaxation and meditation • Provide calm and quite environment to the client • Provide the client comfort devices • Encourage the client to ask questions and clear the doubt of the client.	• To collect the baseline information and classify the level by mild, moderate and severe anxiety. • To build trust of the client. • To understand the level of knowledge regarding the similar objective • To make client understand about the disease condition as well as the surgical procedure need to be performed. • To increase the oxygen circulation and reduce the anxiety • To reduce the factors that can lead to anxiety • To provide comfort to the client • To reduce the anxiety	Anxiety was reduced to the maximum extent

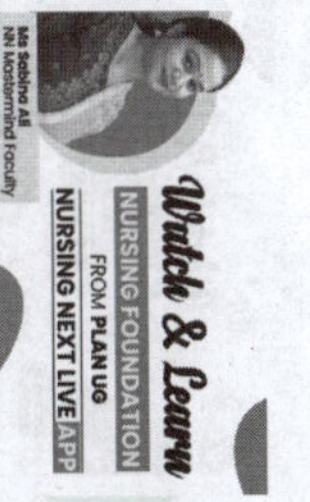

NURSING CARE PLAN—MUSCULOSKELETAL INJURY/FRACTURE/SPINAL INJURY (RISK FOR INJURY)

Assessment	Diagnosis	Outcome	Intervention	Rationale	Evaluation
Subjective data: Patient says, "I am having pain in legs and I am unable to walk" **Objective data:** On assessment patient has disturbed gait and pain due to injury	Risk of injury related to musculoskeletal impairment.	Patient will remain free from injury and fall.	• Assess the level of pain and impairment. • Maintain the IPR with the client. • Collect knowledge regarding the disease condition and about the surgery. • Educate the client regarding the disease condition and surgical procedure. • Position extremities so they may be periodically checked for safety, circulation, nerve pressure, and alignment. • Provide calm and quite environment to the client • Provide the client comfort devices • Encourage the client to ask questions and clear the doubt of the client.	• To collect the baseline information and classify the level by mild, moderate and severe pain and musculoskeletal. • To build trust of the client. • To understand the level of knowledge regarding the similar objective • To make client understand about the disease condition as well as the surgical procedure need to be performed. • Monitor peripheral pulses, skin color, and temperature. • To reduce the factors that can lead to anxiety • To provide comfort to the client • To reduce the anxiety related to risk for injury	Clients risk for injury was reduced to the maximum extent

NURSING CARE PLAN—ASTHMA/COPD/PULMONARY EDEMA (INEFFECTIVE BREATHING)

Assessment	Diagnosis	Outcome	Intervention	Rationale	Evaluation
Subjective data: The client says, "Inability to maintain usual breathing pattern and have lack of energy" **Objective data:** On assessment there is changes in respiratory rate and depth and reduced vital capacity	Ineffective breathing pattern related to decreased lung expansion or energy	The client will establish effective respiratory pattern that is free of hypoxia.	• Listen for breath sounds. Look for gurgling, wheezing, or crowing. • Examine breathing rate and depth, chest expansion, usage of accessory muscles, nose retraction or flaring. • Monitor vital signs continuously. • Suction whenever necessary. • Encourage the usage of breathing assistance with an incentive spirometer.	• To assess lack of breath sounds that indicates mucus or tongue obstruction, which can be remedied by positioning and/ or suctioning. • Determines the effectiveness of respirations quickly so that corrective actions can be taken. • Hypoxia is indicated by increased breathing, tachycardia, and/or bradycardia. • Airway obstruction can occur as a result of blood or mucus in the throat or trachea. • Maximum respiratory effort lowers the risk of atelectasis and infection.	The patient verbalizes he or she is able to breathe effectively, showed increased energy level and better performance in activities

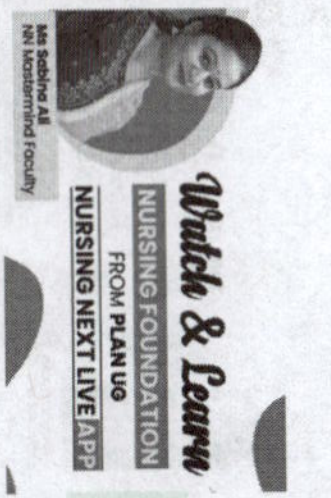

NURSING CARE PLAN—LACK OF KNOWLEDGE REGARDING ANY DISEASE CONDITION OR ANY CLINICAL PROCEDURE (KNOWLEDGE DEFICIT)

Assessment	Diagnosis	Outcome	Intervention	Rationale	Evaluation
Subjective data: Client says, "I don't know what has happened to me" **Objective data:** On assessment, client has less knowledge regarding their own condition of disease.	Knowledge deficit related to disease condition as evidenced by asking questions regarding the disease condition.	The patient will have improved knowledge and understanding regarding the disease condition and clear doubts.	• Assess the level of knowledge. • Assess motivation and willingness of patient to learn. • Provide clear, thorough, and understandable explanations and demonstrations. • Educate the client regarding the disease condition. • Teach client deep breathing techniques, guided imagery, progressive muscle relaxation and meditation • Provide calm and quite environment to the client • Provide the client comfort devices • Encourage the client to ask questions and clear the doubt of the client.	• To collect the baseline information and knowledge regarding the disease condition. • Learning requires energy. Patients must see a need or purpose for learning. • Patients are better able to ask questions when they have basic information about what to expect. • To make client understand about the disease condition. • To increase the oxygen circulation and reduce the anxiety • To reduce the factors that can lead to anxiety • To provide comfort to the client • To reduce the anxiety	Knowledge was improved to the maximum extent

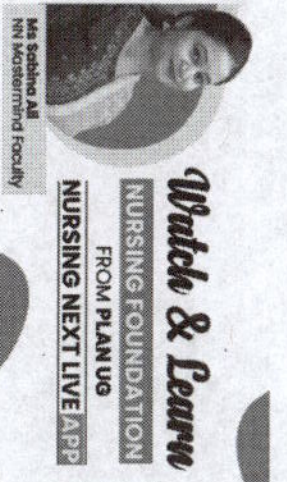

NURSING CARE PLAN—DEHYDRATION (ALTERED LEVEL OF CONSCIOUSNESS)

Assessment	Diagnosis	Outcome	Intervention	Rationale	Evaluation
Subjective data: Client says, "I am not aware of things around me and feel agitated and restless" **Objective data:** On assessment, client shows impaired awareness and attention and do not participate in daily living activities.	Altered level of consciousness related to electrolyte imbalance as evidenced by confusion, agitation, disorientation secondary to dehydration.	The client regains normal reality orientation and level of consciousness and participated in daily living activities.	• Assess the level of consciousness. • Conduct an accurate mental status examination using assessment tools. • Evaluate and report possible physiological changes like infection or fluid and electrolyte imbalances. • Monitor laboratory values noting level of electrolyte for imbalances. • Prevent injury and maintain patient safety. • Promote effective communication.	• To collect the baseline information and knowledge regarding the client condition. • The confusion assessment method and tools will help to quantify the illness. • Such alterations may be causing confusion and must be addressed. It is critical to verify that the illness is not caused by other neurocognitive reasons when diagnosing acute confusion. • Once acute confusion has been identified, the linked underlying causes must be identified and treated. • As mental status impairment can lead the patient to fall and can hamper the patient safety. • To give client support.	Client regains normal reality orientation and level of consciousness and participated in daily living activities.

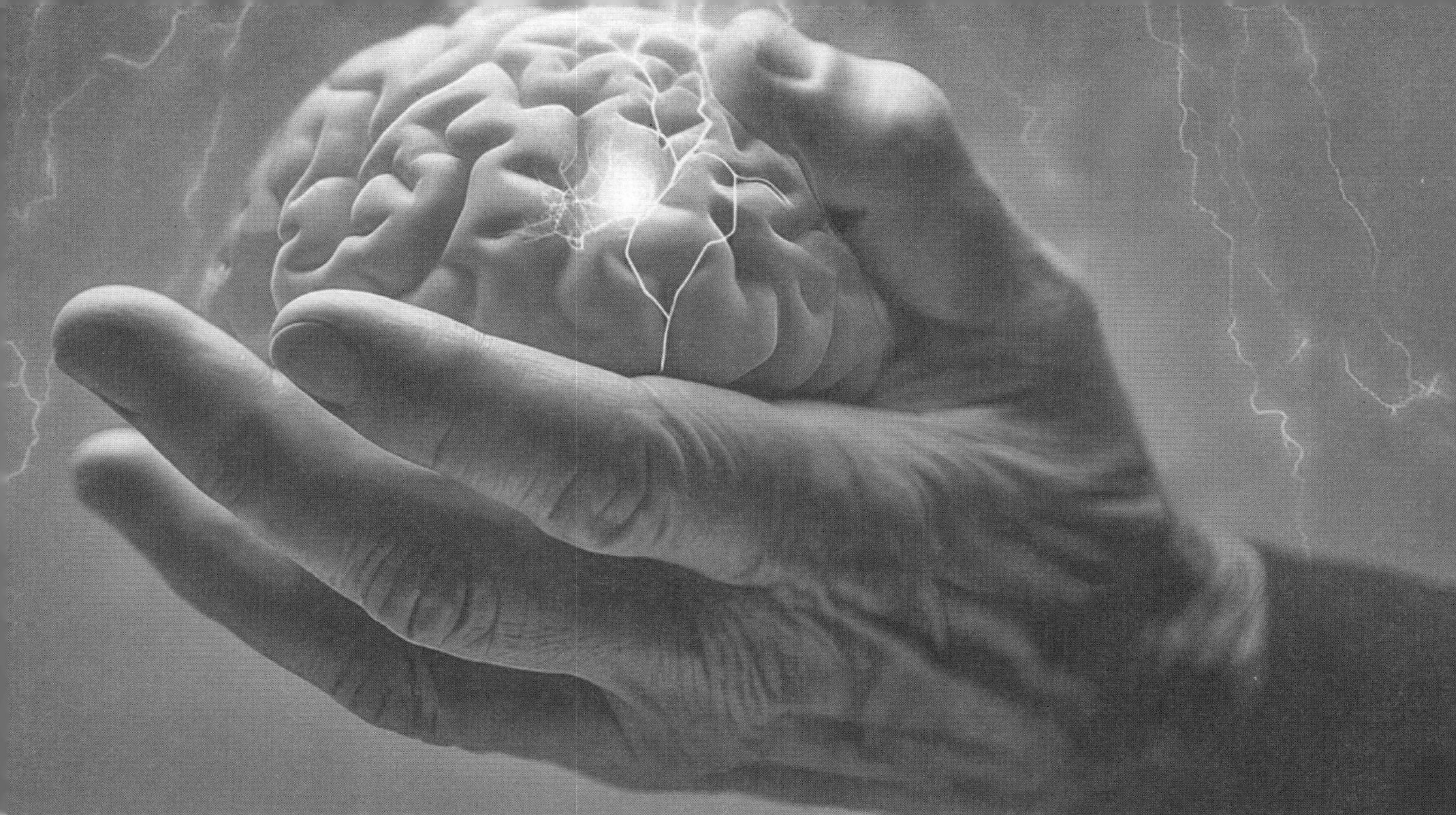

Applied Psychology

Unit Outline

CHAPTER

1

Introduction

CONCEPTUAL THEORY

Terminology

150+ key terminologies for Quick Recall & Revision

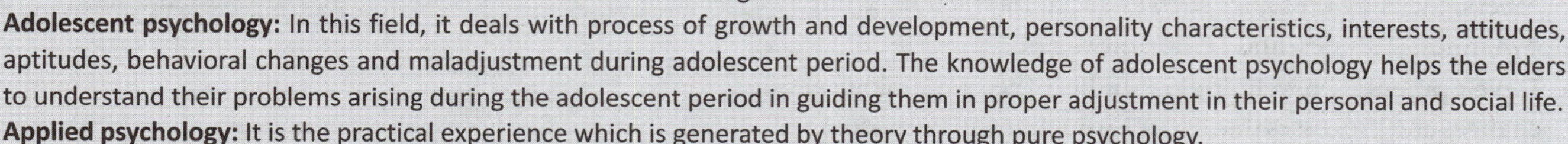

Abnormal psychology: It is that branch of psychology which deals with the abnormal behavior of an individual in relation to the surroundings.

Adolescent psychology: In this field, it deals with process of growth and development, personality characteristics, interests, attitudes, aptitudes, behavioral changes and maladjustment during adolescent period. The knowledge of adolescent psychology helps the elders to understand their problems arising during the adolescent period in guiding them in proper adjustment in their personal and social life.

Applied psychology: It is the practical experience which is generated by theory through pure psychology.

Child psychology: It describes the development of behavior of the children from birth to the adolescent period (age up to 12 years).

Clinical psychology: It refers to a study to understand the unhealthy people's behavior who take treatment in different areas, such as hospital, clinic, nursing home, dispensary.

Developmental psychology: It describes about the growth and development of behavior pattern, such as motor skills, intelligence, thinking, emotion and their personality in each and every stage of human beings from conception to death.

Educational psychology: It is the educational psychology which deals with the application of psychological theories, principles and techniques with human behavior in relation to educational situations.

Gestalt psychology: This School of Psychology was founded in Germany around 1912 by Max Wertheimer (1880–1943) and his colleagues. These psychologists felt that structuralism was faulty in thinking of the mind as being made up of elements. They argued that mind could be thought of as arising from the whole pattern of sensory activity and the relationships and organizations within this pattern.

Introspection: The behavior was analyzed through a method of self-examination or self-observation.

Mental health: An adjustment of human beings to the world and to each other with a maximum of effectiveness and happiness.

Parapsychology: It explains the alleged psychic phenomena such as extra sensory perceptions which are present in telepathy, precognition, etc., and paranormal claims (e.g., near death experiences or re-birth).

Psychology: It is the science of human and animal behavior which includes the application of the science to getting solution for human behavior.

MEANING AND DEFINITION OF PSYCHOLOGY

The word, 'psychology,' is derived from Greek words *psyche* means soul and *logos* means study, known as "the study of soul". Hence, it is defined as the study of soul or spirit.

"It is the science of human and animal behavior which includes the application of the science to getting solution for human behavior."

—**Clifford T Morgan**

HISTORY OF PSYCHOLOGY

Wundt was the first to calculate human behavior accurately and is known as the Father of Psychology.

According to William James, Wilhelm Wundt and other psychologists, psychology is considered the study of mind. These schools of thought were called the schools of psychology.

BRANCHES OF PSYCHOLOGY

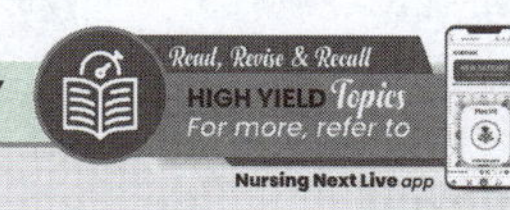

Two main divisions:

1. **Pure psychology:** Focuses on the theoretical understanding and study of fundamental psychological principles and concepts.
2. **Applied psychology:** Applies psychological principles, theories, and research findings to solve practical problems

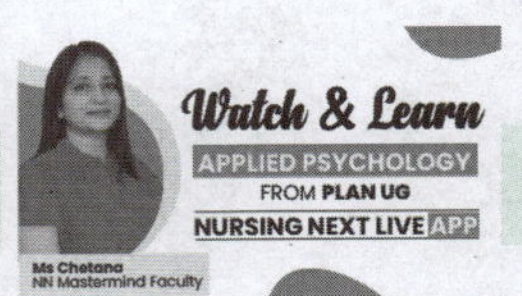

and address real-world issues in various domains such as education, industries, law, military, etc.

Pure Psychology can be further classified into:

- **General psychology:** Focuses on the fundamental principles and concepts of psychology, covering various areas of human behavior and mental processes
- **Experimental psychology:** Involves the scientific study of behavior and mental processes through controlled experiments, aiming to understand the underlying mechanisms and processes
- **Physiological psychology:** Explores the relationship between the brain, behavior, and mental processes, investigating how physiological factors impact psychological functioning
- **Abnormal psychology:** Focuses on the study of abnormal behavior, psychological disorders, and psychopathology, aiming to understand the causes, symptoms, and treatment of mental illnesses
- **Social psychology:** Examines how individuals' thoughts, feelings, and behaviors are influenced by the presence of others, focusing on topics such as social interaction, group dynamics, attitudes, and conformity.
- **Developmental psychology:** Studies the psychological changes and processes that occur throughout an individual's lifespan, from infancy to old age
- **Geopsychology:** Investigates the influence of the environment, particularly geographical factors, on human behavior and mental processes
- **Para psychology:** Explores phenomena that are outside the scope of conventional psychology, such as telepathy, precognition, and psychic abilities

Applied psychology may be classified into:

- **Educational Psychology:** Focuses on understanding and improving educational processes and systems, studying topics such as learning, motivation, instructional methods, and assessment.
- **Clinical psychology:** Involves the assessment, diagnosis, and treatment of mental disorders and psychological distress
- **Industrial psychology:** Applies psychological principles and research to optimize workplace environments, employee performance, job satisfaction, and organizational effectiveness
- **Legal psychology:** Examines the intersection of psychology and the legal system, covering areas such as forensic assessment, eyewitness testimony and the psychology of criminal behavior.
- **Military psychology:** Focuses on psychological principles and interventions specific to the military context, e.g., combat stress, personnel selection and training.
- **Political psychology:** Investigates the psychological factors that influence political behavior, attitudes, and decision-making at individual and group levels.

METHODS OF PSYCHOLOGY

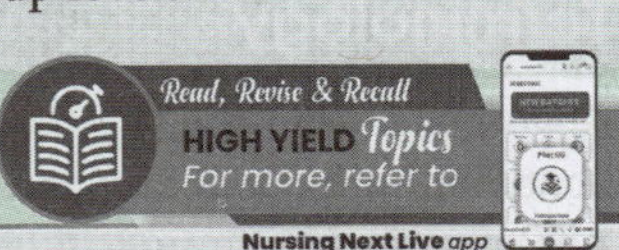

Major methods of psychology:

- Introspection method
- Observation method
- Experimental method
- Survey method
- Case history or clinical method
- Developmental method

SIGNIFICANCE OF PSYCHOLOGY IN NURSING

Psychology plays a significant role in understanding the patient, relatives, others, understanding of self and understanding of Psychometric Assessment.

CONCEPTUAL EXERCISES

LONG ANSWER QUESTIONS

1. Define psychology. Explain different methods of psychology. (MGR)

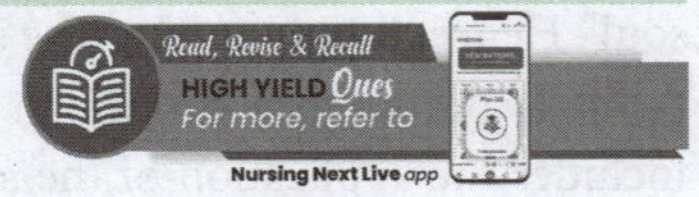

Answer

Definition

- Psychology is the scientific study of human behavior.
- Psychology is defined as a science which aims to give us better understanding and control of the behavior of the organism as a whole.

—William McDoughall 1949

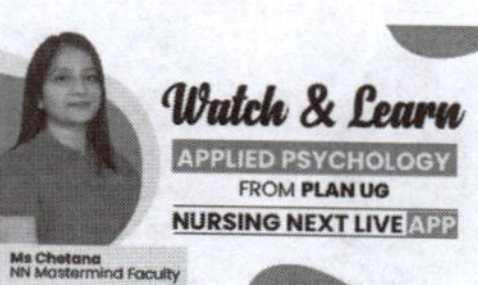

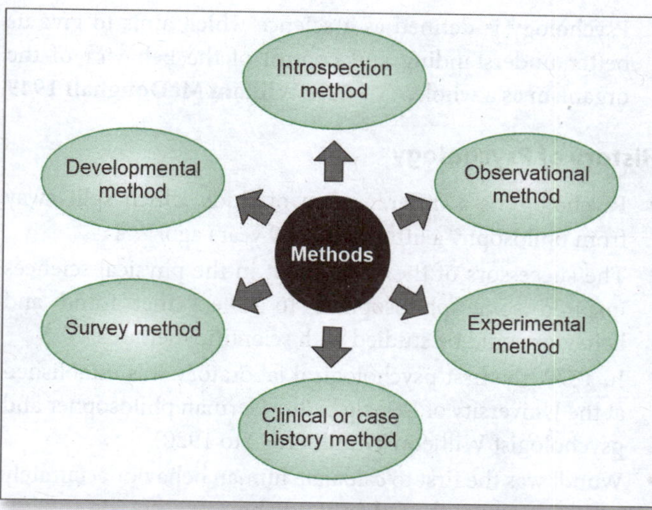

Figure 1.1: Methods of psychology

Methods of Psychology

Introspection method

Introspection means to look within. This method is also known as self-observation method.

Merits	Demerits
Fundamental method of psychology	Not applicable for children or animals or mentally retarded people as they cannot introspect or look within.
It gives direct, immediate and exact knowledge of mental processes	It is very private and cannot be observed
Enables us to fully understand the behavior of others	If patients do not have insight, then they cannot use it accurately.
Inexpensive, easy and does not require any laboratory	This method requires power of alertness.

Observation Method

- In this method, observation is used to study the behavior of individuals. It is an objective method.
- In this method, there is one observer who observes and collects the data, e.g., when nurse makes observation regarding patient's behavior, or vital signs, etc.
- **Steps in observation method:**
  - Observation of behavior
  - Noting of observer
  - Interpretation and analysis of behavior
  - Generalization
- **Merits**
  - This method is natural and flexible and inexpensive.
  - The data can be analyzed and interpreted.
  - The results of the analysis can be verified.
  - This method is suitable for many situations like in case of small children where it is not feasible to use any other method.
- **Demerits**
  - It can be biased because of the observer's characteristics, likes and dislikes.
  - It requires more time and energy.
  - It cannot be repeated because natural situations can occur only once.
  - It is not possible to establish cause and effect relationship.

Experimental Method

- In this, experiments are used to study the human behavior. This method is used to study the cause-and-effect relationship regarding the nature of human behavior. Psychologists use objective observations under controlled conditions to observe actions or behaviors of individuals.
- **Steps in experimental method:**
  - Stating the problem: The problem is stated in the first step.
  - Formulating hypothesis: Hypothesis is formed before studying the problem.
  - Identifying study subjects: Study subjects need to be identified. To establish cause and effect relationship and to do experiments study subjects are required.
  - Allotting the subjects to treatment and control groups: For experiments, two groups are allotted. One group is for the experiment and the other is for comparison or control.
  - Measuring the dependent variable: In this step, independent variable is manipulated and the effect is studied on dependent variable.
  - Comparing the results of the two groups: The effect on dependent variable is compared for both groups and based on that the hypothesis may be approved or disapproved.
- **Merits:**
  - Establishes cause-and-effect relationship
  - Retention is possible
  - Maximum control of phenomena
- **Demerits**
  - All problems cannot be studied by this method as experiments are not possible for all problems.
  - Costly and time consuming

Clinical or Case History Method

- This method is used by clinical psychologists and psychiatrists.
- The aim of this method is to study the cause and basis of people's anxieties, fears and personal maladjustments.

- In this, the information is collected from the memory of the individual, his parents, family members, friends, teachers and all other available sources.
- **Merits:**
  - This will give the clinician an insight into the cause of the problem and help him suggest possible solutions.
  - Case studies can be good sources of ideas for future investigation by other methods. They can form a basis for other investigations.
- **Demerit:**
  - This method depends on the memory which may be over interpreted.

Survey Method

- It includes collection or gathering of information from a large number of people by using questionnaires, inventories, checklists, rating scales and interviews.

Merit	Demerit
A large amount of data can be collected in short period of time.	The behavior is not directly observed.

Developmental Method

- Psychologists study not only the behavior of an individual at a particular time but also his development from birth to death.
- They study the influence of heredity and environment in the development of the person and conditions favorable and unfavorable for normal and abnormal behavior, e.g., to study the learning behavior of an adult, the study will start from the childhood and adolescence.
- This can be done in two ways:
  1. Cross-sectional study in which the children of different age groups are studied simultaneously.
  2. Longitudinal study in which the same child is studied at different stages of life.
- **Merit**
  - This is a more useful method to understand the behavior from point of view of heredity and environmental influences.
- **Demerit**
  - This method requires more time and energy.

2. Define the term psychology and discuss the history of psychology. (MGR)

Answer

Definition

- Psychology is the scientific study of human behavior.
- Psychology is defined as a science which aims to give us better understanding and control of the behavior of the organism as a whole. **—William McDoughall 1949**

History of Psychology

- Psychology is a different area of study which split away from philosophy a little over 1000 years ago.
- The successors of the experiment in the physical sciences inspired some philosophers to reflect that mind and behavior could be studied with scientific methods.
- In 1879, the first psychological laboratory was established at the University of Leipzig by the German philosopher and psychologist Wilhelm Wundt (1832 to 1920).
- Wundt was the first to calculate human behavior accurately and is known as the father of psychology.
- William James, Wilhelm Wundt and other psychologists of the time thought of psychology as the study of mind.
- In the first decade of the 20th century, psychologists came across quite various uses about the nature of mind and the finest ways to study it.
- Schools of thought were framed by these psychologists.
- The schools of thought were called the schools of psychology.

Schools of psychology are:

- Structuralism school of thought
- Functionalist school of thought
- Gestalt school of thought
- Behaviorist school of thought
- The psychoanalytic school of thought

Structuralism School of Thought

- Structuralism is widely regarded as the first school of thought in psychology.
- Major thinkers associated with structuralism include Wilhelm Wundt and Edward Titchener.
- The focus of structuralism was on reducing mental processes down into their most basic elements.
- The structuralists used techniques such as introspection to analyze the inner processes of the human mind.
- The introspective experimental technique used by the structuralists involved trained observers examine the inner responses.
- Using this approach, also known as experimental self-observation, experimenters like Wundt trained people to analyze their thoughts as carefully and objectively as possible.
- While these methods were understandably not the most empirically rigorous, the structuralist school of thought played an important role in the development of experimental psychology.

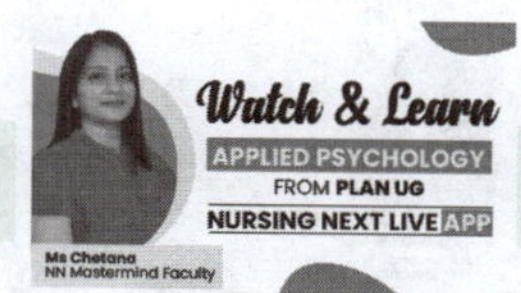

Functionalist School of Thought

- Functionalism formed as a reaction to the theories of the structuralist school of thought and was heavily influenced by the work of William James. It functioned on the mind's functions and adaptations.
- Instead of focusing on the mental processes themselves, functionalist thinkers were interested in the role that these processes play.
- In a functionalist approach, for example, instead of trying to understand the underlying processes that cause mental states, the focus would be on understanding the function that those states serve.
- The functionalist school was interested in the purpose of thoughts and behaviors, whereas structuralism was concerned with the elements that make up consciousness.
- While functionalism largely disappeared as a school of thought, its influence persisted in applied psychology, behaviorism, and educational psychology.

Gestalt School of Thought

- Gestalt psychology was a school of psychology based upon the idea that people experience things as unified wholes.
- This approach to psychology began in Germany and Austria during the late 19th century in response to the molecular approach of structuralism.
- Some thinkers associated with the Gestalt school of thought included Max Wertheimer, Wolfgang Köhler, and Kurt Koffka.
- Instead of breaking down thoughts and behavior to their smallest elements, the Gestalt psychologists believed that you must look at the whole of experience.
- According to Gestalt thinkers, the whole is greater than the sum of its parts, a philosophy known as holism.

Behaviorist School of Thought

- Behaviorism became a dominant school of thought during the 1950s. It was based upon the work of thinkers such as John B. Watson, Ivan Pavlov, and BF Skinner.
- Behaviorism suggests that all behavior can be explained by environmental causes rather than by internal forces. Behaviorism is focused on *observable behavior*. Examples of behavioral theories that emerged during this time include:
  - **Classical conditioning:** This is a type of learning that involves associating a previously neutral stimulus with a stimulus that naturally and automatically triggers a response. For example, pairing the sound of a bell with the presentation of food. After an association is formed, the previously neutral stimulus will produce the same response as the natural stimulus.
  - **Operant conditioning:** This type of learning involves using rewards and punishments to create an association between the behavior and the consequences of that behavior.

The Psychoanalytic School of Thought

- Psychoanalysis is a school of psychology founded by Sigmund Freud. This school of thought emphasized the influence of the unconscious mind on behavior.
- Other major psychoanalytic thinkers included Anna Freud and Otto Rank and neo-Freudians such as Erik Erikson, Alfred Adler, and Karen Horney.
- Freud believed that the human mind was composed of three elements: the id, ego, and superego.
  - **The id** consists of primal urges.
  - **The ego** is the component of personality responsible for dealing with reality.
  - **The superego** is the part of the personality that holds all the ideals and values we internalize from our parents and culture.
- Freud believed that the interaction of these three elements led to all of the complex human behaviors.

3. Define Psychology. Why is it called a science subject? (MGR)

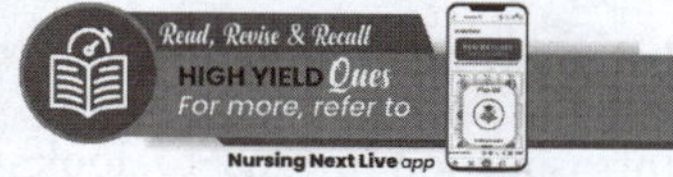

Answer

Definition

Psychology is defined as a science which aims to give us better understanding and control of the behavior of the organism as a whole. **—William McDoughall 1949**

Psychology is called a science subject:

Psychology is considered a science subject for several reasons. The reasons for psychology to be considered sciences are as follows:

Deals with living organisms: Psychology is focused on understanding the complexities of human behavior and mental processes. Psychology deals with living organisms and the intricacies of the human mind.

Scientific methods used for experimentation: Like other sciences, psychology involves making predictions about how variables will interact and then systematically testing those predictions through experimentation and observation.

Objectivity: Psychology strives for objectivity in its research. This means that psychologists attempt to remove their personal biases and opinions from their research and instead rely on empirical evidence to draw conclusions.

Systematic observation: Psychology uses systematic observation to gather data about human behavior and mental processes. This involves observing and measuring behavior in a controlled and structured way, and using standardized instruments and methods to ensure consistency and accuracy.

Data analysis: Psychology uses statistical methods to analyze data and test hypotheses.

Theory development: Psychology is also focused on developing theories that help to explain and predict human behavior and mental processes. These theories are based on empirical evidence and are constantly refined and updated as new evidence becomes available.

Replication: In another way, psychology is a science which has the importance of replication. Replication involves conducting studies with the same methodology to see if the results are consistent. This is an essential part of the scientific process because it helps researchers determine the reliability and validity of their findings.

In conclusion, these aspects of psychology demonstrate how it is a science subject that uses systematic and empirical methods to study human behavior and mental processes.

SHORT NOTES

1. Define the term introspection. (MGR)

Answer

Introspection Methods

Introspection means to look within. This method is also known as self-observation method.

Merits	Demerits
Fundamental method of psychology	Not applicable for children or animals or mentally retarded people as they cannot introspect or look within.
It gives direct, immediate and exact knowledge of mental processes	It is very private and cannot be observed
Enables us to fully understand the behavior of others	If patients do not have insight then, they cannot use it accurately.
Inexpensive, easy and does not require any laboratory	This method requires power of alertness.

2. Write a short note on abnormal psychology. (MGR)

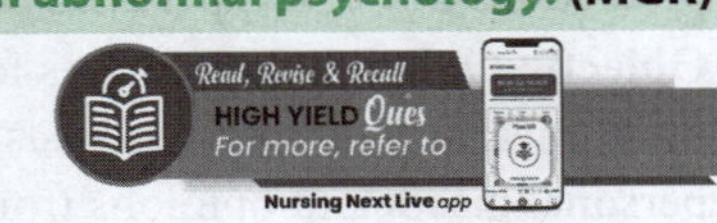

Answer

Abnormal Psychology

- Abnormal psychology is the branch of psychology that studies unusual patterns of behavior, emotion, and thought, which could possibly be understood as a mental disorder.
- Although many behaviors could be considered abnormal, this branch of psychology typically deals with behavior in a clinical context.
- Abnormal psychology focuses on the patterns of emotion, thought, and behavior that can be signs of a mental health condition.
- Rather than the distinction between normal and abnormal, psychologists in this field focus on the level of distress that behaviors, thoughts, or emotions might cause.
- If a behavior is creating problems in a person's life or is disruptive to other people, then this would be an "abnormal" behavior. In such cases, the behavior may require some type of mental health intervention.

Concepts of Abnormality

- **Statistical abnormality:** When a certain behavior/ characteristic is relevant to a low percentage of the population.
- **Psychometric abnormality:** Psychometric abnormality implicates abnormality as a deviation from a statistically determined norm, such as the population average IQ of 100.
- **Deviant behavior:** This is not always a sign of mental illness, as mental illness can occur without deviant behavior, and such behavior may occur in the absence of mental illness.
- **Combinations:** Including distress, dysfunction, distorted psychological processes, inappropriate responses in given situations, and causing/risking harm to oneself.

Examples

There is a wide range of mental disorders that are considered to be forms of abnormal psychology. These include, but are not limited to:

- **Schizophrenia:** Schizophrenia can be described as a disorder that causes extreme loss of touch with reality.
- **Attention deficit hyperactivity disorder (ADHD)** is characterized by high amounts of inattention and hyperactive impulsiveness.
- **Antisocial personality disorder:** Antisocial personality disorder can be described as a cluster of personality traits that lead to specific outcomes, and violate the rights of other people. These personality traits include callousness, deceitfulness, lack of remorse, apathy, manipulation of others, impulsiveness, and grandiosity.
- **Dissociative identity disorder:** Dissociative identity disorder (DID) involves one individual having multiple personalities.
- **Social anxiety disorder:** Those with social anxiety disorder (SAD) have a very intense fear of social situations. This

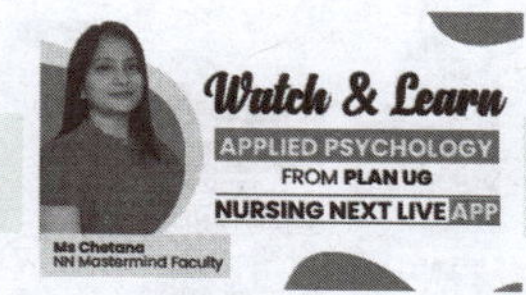

fear stems from the belief that the person will be evaluated negatively, or embarrass themselves. SAD is also considered to be one of the more disabling mental disorders.

- **Generalized anxiety disorder:** It is characterized by a constant, chronic state of worry and anxiety that is related to a large variety of situations, and is difficult to control.
- **Specific phobia:** Individuals with specific phobias have an extreme fear and avoidance of various objects or situations.
- **Post-traumatic stress disorder:** It is described as physical and mental distress related to past traumatic experiences.

3. Write short note on any four branches of applied psychology. (MGR)

Answer

Applied Psychology

Applied psychology deals with the practical part. It deals with the application of theories and principles generated in pure psychology.

Branches of Applied Psychology

Applied psychology has the following branches.

1. Educational Psychology

- Educational psychology is the study of how people learn, including teaching methods, instructional processes, and individual differences in learning.
- It is the branch of psychology concerned with the scientific study of human learning.
- The study of learning processes, from both cognitive and behavioral perspectives, allows researchers to understand individual differences in intelligence, cognitive development, affect, motivation, self-regulation, and self-concept, as well as their role in learning.
- The field of educational psychology relies more on quantitative methods, including testing and measurement, to enhance educational activities related to instructional design, classroom management, and assessment, which serve to facilitate learning processes in various educational settings across the lifespan.

2. Clinical Psychology

- Clinical psychology is branch of psychology concerned with the practical application of research methodologies and findings in the diagnosis and treatment of mental disorders.
- Clinical psychology is the psychological specialty that provides continuing and comprehensive mental and behavioral health care for individuals, couples, families, and groups; consultation to agencies and communities; training, education and supervision; and research-based practice.
- It is a specialty in breadth — one that addresses a wide range of mental and behavioral health problems— and marked by comprehensiveness and integration of knowledge and skill from a broad array of disciplines within and outside of psychology proper.
- The scope of clinical psychology encompasses all ages, multiple diversities, and varied systems.

3. Industrial Psychology

- Industrial and organizational psychology focuses on scientifically-based solutions to human problems in work and other organizational settings.
- The specialty of industrial-organizational psychology (also called I/O psychology) is characterized by the scientific study of human behavior in organizations and the work place.
- The specialty focuses on deriving principles of individual, group and organizational behavior and applying this knowledge to the solution of problems at work.

4. Legal Psychology

- Legal Psychology is a modern term that refers to the study and use of psychology as it applies to the legal system and people who come into contact with the legal system.
- People who work in the area of legal psychology work with methods of understanding, evaluating and questioning suspects, evaluating jury candidates, investigating crimes and crime scenes, forensic investigation and other legally related situations.
- The term legal psychology is used to differentiate this field of applied psychology from the more theoretically based clinical psychology.

4. Write a short note on principles of psychological tests. (MGR)

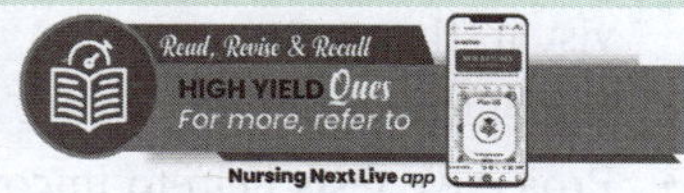

Answer

Psychological Assessment/Tests

- A psychological assessment or test can be defined as structured technique to produce selected behavior.
- It is an objective and standardized measure, the results of which are used to deduce the individual's behavior.

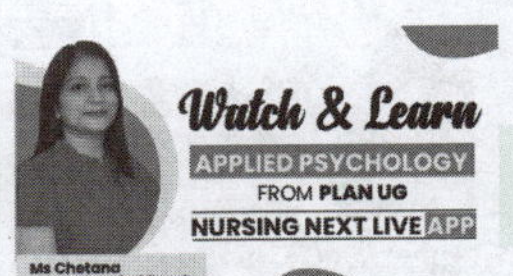

- Several attributes and traits can be judged by means of testing.

Psychological tests are used in:

- Making decisions about one's behavior
- Research
- Personal development
- Psychological assessment

Assessment includes tests, interviews, case studies, behavior observation, and other techniques.

Techniques vary according to the goal of the assessment and the client.

Principles of Psychological Assessment

- Psychological assessments or test should have some components that make it feasible for anybody to administer the test anytime. These are standard content and the procedure.
- Apart from all the previously described essential characteristics, a good test must have norms to compare an individual score to that of a known group against whom the test has been calibrated.
- Test items are constructed by experts tested and selected on the basis of difficulty differentiation and relationship between specifications.
- Directions for administration must be stated concisely and clearly in order to ensure uniformity in test methodology.
- Attached manual must be provided along with which acts as a guide for administration, scoring, influence and results

5. Write a short note on projective test. (MGR)

Answer

Projective Techniques

- Projective techniques involve visual stimuli, incomplete sentences or story creation by the subjects, which are interpreted with high precision and skill.
- The therapist presents ambiguous visual stimulus to patient and asks to respond with whatever comes to the mind.
- The psychologist will interpret the client's answer to the visual stimulus.
- It requires lots of experience and it is an art.
- Projective tests help to uncover the unconscious concern, fears, conflict, desires and urges that affect the client's conscious behavior.
- This test is very useful in the diagnosis of personality disturbance.
- It is highly subjective and may not be accurate sometimes.
- The projective techniques are as follows:

Rorschach inkblots:

- This test was developed by Hermann Rorschach in 1921.
- He used 10 ink blots, 5 in black on white background and 5 in colored inks on a white background.
- The patients were asked to look at each inkblot and they had to say whatever came to their mind by looking at those ink blots.
- Scores were given based on color, shape, figures in the blot and response to the whole or to details.
- This technique is very useful in describing personality, diagnosing mental illnesses and in prediction of behavior.

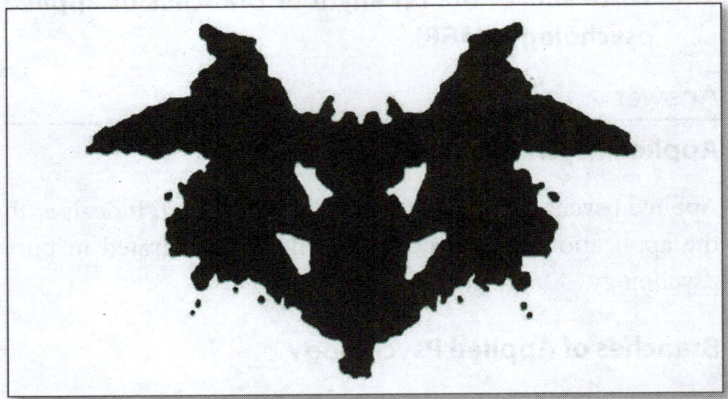

Thematic apperception test

- This test was developed by Morgan and Henry Murray in 1935. In this technique, 31 pictures (black and white) were shown to clients.
- The patients were asked to tell a story about the person in the picture.
- The patient had to explain themes which were shown. The story told by the patient is interpreted for projection.

6. Write a short note on health psychology. (MGR)

Answer

Health psychology is a field of psychology that focuses on the psychological and behavioral factors that contribute to health, illness, and health care. It is concerned with understanding how people's thoughts, feelings, and behaviors affect their health and well-being, as well as how social, cultural, and environmental factors impact health.

Types of Health Psychology

There are four main types of health psychology careers (i) clinical health psychology, (ii) community health psychology, (iii) occupational health psychology, (iv) public health psychology.

Purposes of Health Psychology

- Health psychology has several practical purposes in life.

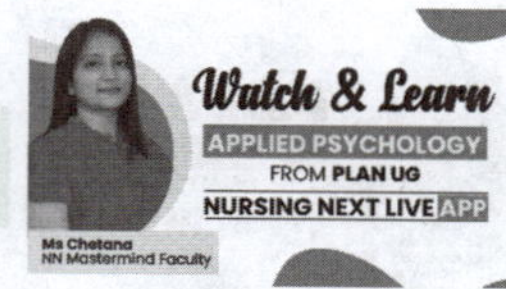

- First of all, it can help doctors take better care of their patients' health.
- By understanding the mental, emotional, and socioeconomic factors that might lead to certain illnesses, doctors can also have a better understanding of how to prevent these illnesses.
- Health psychology also plays a role in helping medical professionals understand the mental and emotional effects of certain illnesses.
- This not only refers to the effects of certain symptoms on patients, but also the behavioral, social, and economic ramifications that illnesses might have as well.
- Research conducted in the field of health psychology can also help improve the relationships between medical doctors and their patients.
- Improving communication between these two sets of people — the professional and the layperson — can lead to a higher percentage of patients following through with their treatments and less physical illnesses.

7. Write a short note on Observation method. (MGR)

Answer

Observation Method

- In this method, observation is used to study the behavior of individuals. It is an objective method. In this method, there is one observer who observes and collects the data, e.g., when nurse makes observation regarding patient's behavior, or vital signs, etc.

Steps in observation method:

Step 1: Adequate and proper planning beforehand for observing an individual

Step 2: Observation of the behavior as planned in the preparation

Step 3: Recording of the behavioral activities using camera or telescope

Step 4: Interpretation and analysis of behavior

Step 5: Generalization of the observed behavior

- **Merits**
  - This method is natural and flexible and inexpensive.
  - The data can be analyzed and interpreted.
  - The results of the analysis can be verified.
  - This method is suitable for many situations like in case of small children where it is not feasible to use any other method.
- **Demerits**
  - It can be biased because of the observer's characteristics, likes and dislikes.
  - It requires more time, energy.
  - It cannot be repeated because natural situations can occur only once.
  - It is not possible to establish cause and effect relationship.

8. Write about the goals in psychology. (MGR)

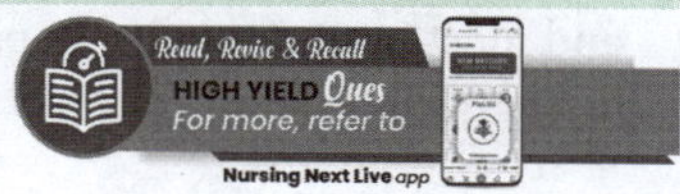

Answer

The four goals of psychology are to describe, explain, predict, and control behavior and mental processes.

Describe

- The first goal of psychology is to describe the actual phenomenon in which humans and animals behave in different situations.
- By describing a problem, an issue, or behavior, psychologists can distinguish between normal and abnormal behavior, allowing them to gain a better understanding and a more accurate perspective of human and animal behavior, thoughts, and actions.
- To achieve this goal, psychologists use a variety of research methods, including surveys, case studies, natural observation, and self-assessment tests.
- Through these scientific methods, behavior can be described in minute details and as objectively as possible. Once the action has been described, the information gathered is used as basis to further study the behavior that just occurred.

Explain

- Once a specific behavior has been described, psychologists then attempt to go beyond the obvious and explain why people act the way they do.
- Through a series of rigorous tests, scientific experiments, and observations, psychology expounds on the reason behind someone's actions.
- Explaining behavior provides answers to why people behave the way they do under different circumstances.
- Some of the well-known theories that explain all aspects of human psychology include Pavlov's theory of classical conditioning, which refers to a learning procedure where two kinds of biologically potent stimuli are linked together to produce a newly-acquired learning response from an animal or a person.

Predict

- Making predictions based on how people previously thought and acted is the third goal of psychology.

- By analyzing past observed behavior, psychological studies aim to predict and anticipate how a certain behavior will appear again in the future.
- This allows psychologists to form a pattern of behavior and better understand the underlying causes of people's actions.
- Successfully predicting behavior is important to the last and most important goal in psychology, which is to control or change behavior.

Control

- Besides treating mental illnesses and enhancing well-being, changing or controlling human behavior is a huge focus of psychology.
- Various psychological studies about human behavior are used to influence, change, or control behavior using previously gathered data about human behavior.
- In psychology, there are a number of theories that deal with changing or controlling people's behavior.
- Whether behavior can be successfully changed or controlled largely depends on one's ability to accurately define a behavioral issue, assess the fundamental causes of these problems, and develop and implement theory and evidence-based interventions.

9. What is the relevance of psychology to nursing? (DU)

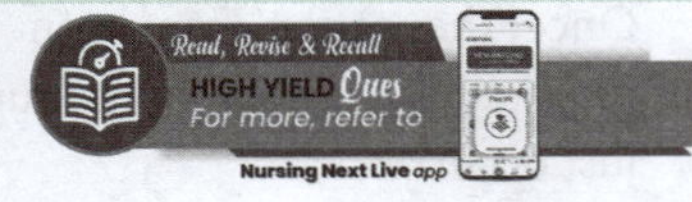

Answer

Introduction:

- Psychology comes from Greek words, *'psychi'* and *'logos'*.
- *'Psychi'* means 'soul' and *'logos'* means the study of knowledge or study of soul.
- Psychology is defined as the systematic study of human and animal 'behavior'.

Relevance of Psychology to Nursing

Nurses need psychology because they work in a setting that requires interaction with patients and other professionals to provide quality care.

- It helps them to understand the way other people behave and act in particular situations.
- Psychological skills come into play because all the people come from different backgrounds which affect the way they behave.
- Psychology helps nurses in these ways:
  - **To understand herself:** Gaining insight into her own emotions, feelings, weaknesses, and strengths.
  - **To understand patients:** It enables nurses to understand their patient's behavior. The patient may be suffering with worries and tensions. Nurses will be able to understand the hidden emotions, feelings and motives and will be able to help their patients.
  - **To understand other people around:** Nurse will be able to realize the individual differences and will be able to coordinate better with other team members.
  - **To recognize abnormal behavior:** It enables nurses to understand normal and abnormal behaviors. This will help nurses to differentiate between normal and abnormal.
  - **To provide quality care:** By having knowledge of psychology, nurses will be able to provide quality care to patients.

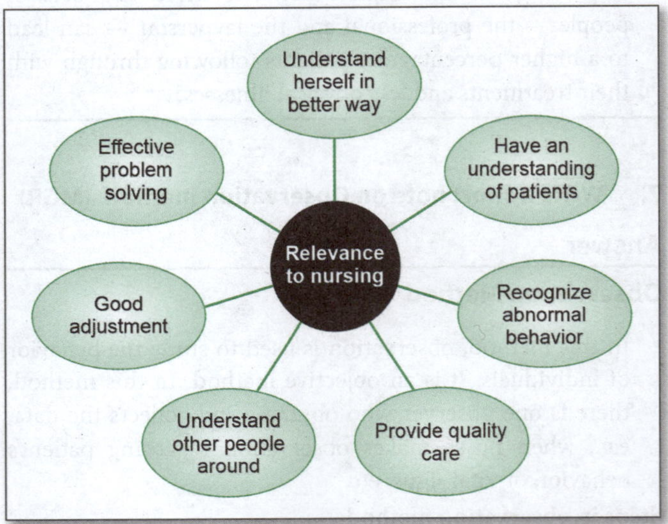

- **Good adjustments:** Nurse will be able to help her patients in major adjustments in life after an illness and disability.
- **Effective problem solving:** Psychology helps us to be an effective problem solver and decision maker.

SHORT ANSWER QUESTIONS

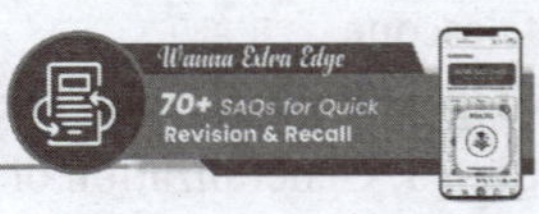

1. Define the terms 'introspection' and 'free-association. (MGR)

Answer

Introspection Methods

Introspection means to look within. This method is also known as self-observation or self-examination method which helps an individual to perceive, analyze or assess and reports his own feelings that has taken part in his mind during the time of mental act.

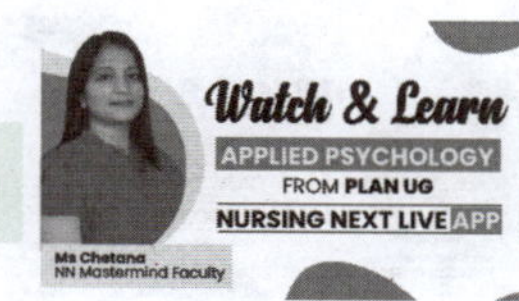

Free Association

- Free association is the expression (as by speaking or writing) of the content of consciousness without censorship as an aid in gaining access to unconscious processes.
- The technique is used in psychoanalysis (and also in psychodynamic theory) which was originally devised by Sigmund Freud out of the hypnotic method of his mentor and colleague, Josef Breuer.

2. Name any four branches of applied psychology. (MGR)

Answer

Four branches of applied psychology:

1. Educational psychology
2. Legal psychology
3. Political psychology
4. Clinical psychology

3. Name the schools of psychology. (MGR)

Answer

Schools of psychology are:

- Structuralism
- Gestalt psychology
- Functionalism
- Behaviorism
- Psychoanalysis

4. Meaning of observation method. (MGR)

Answer

Observation Method:

It is collection of data by observing an individual's behavior by other individual and analyzing the behavior and interpretation of the perceived behavior

5. List out the methods used in psychology. (MGR)

Answer

Methods used in Psychology:

- Introspection method
- Observation method
- Clinical method
- Survey method
- Experimental method
- Testing method

6. List the contributions made by Wilhelm Wundt to the field of psychology. (MGR)

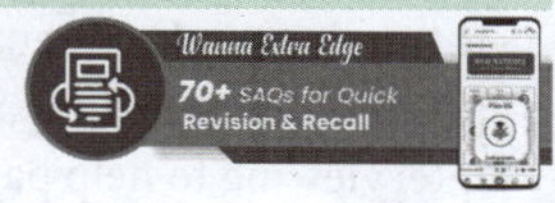

Answer

Wilhelm Wundt (1832–1920) is considered the father of experimental psychology and made numerous contributions to the field of psychology.

The following are some of the major contributions of Wilhelm Wundt:

- Wundt founded the first laboratory for experimental psychology at the University of Leipzig in 1879.
- Wundt developed the technique of introspection.
- Wundt developed a comprehensive theory of psychology.
- Wundt conducted experiments on sensation and perception.
- He conducted studies on language, mythology, and other cultural phenomena.

7. Psychology and nursing. (MGR)

Answer

- Psychology is the scientific study of human behavior and mental processes. It includes a wide range of areas, like perception, cognition, emotion, personality, social behavior, and development.
- Psychology has various methods, such as experiments, surveys, and observations, to study human behavior and mental processes.
- Nursing is a health care profession focused on promoting and maintaining health, preventing illness, and providing care and support to individuals, families, and communities.
- Nurses play a critical role in patient care, working alongside other health care professionals to provide physical, emotional, and psychological support to patients.
- Nurses who have a solid understanding of psychology can better care for their patients, communicate effectively with them, and provide support for their emotional and mental well-being.

Psychology and nursing fields are closely related and both focus on the study and care of human behavior, cognition, and emotions. Psychology is an essential component of nursing care, helping nurses provide holistic and patient-centered care. Psychology plays a crucial role in nursing care, as it helps nurses understand and address the mental and emotional needs of their patients.

Some applications of psychology in nursing are as follows:

- **Building rapport:** Nurses use their knowledge of psychology to build rapport with patients. This includes active listening, empathy, and nonjudgmental attitudes toward patients.
- **Understanding patient behavior:** Nurses use psychology to understand patient behavior and help them make positive changes. For example, nurses can use motivational interviewing to help patients quit smoking or improve their diet.
- **Identifying mental health issues:** Nurses use their psychological knowledge to identify mental health issues such as depression, anxiety, and PTSD. This helps them to refer patients to mental health professionals for further evaluation and treatment.
- **Managing anxiety and stress:** Nurses use psychological techniques to help patients manage anxiety and stress, such as relaxation techniques, guided imagery, and cognitive-behavioral therapy.
- **Enhancing patient education:** Nurses use psychology to enhance patient education by using strategies such as modeling, role-playing, and teaching patients to self-monitor their symptoms.

CONCEPTUAL REVISION

MULTIPLE CHOICE QUESTIONS

1. Psychoanalytic therapy was developed by:
a. Sigmund Freud
b. Eugene Bleuler
c. Alfred Adler
d. Abraham Maslow

Ans. a. Sigmund Freud

2. Select the correct match:
a. Sigmund Freud-Theory of cognitive development
b. Jean Piaget-Founder of psychoanalysis
c. Eugene Bleuler - 4A's of schizophrenia
d. All of the above

Ans. c. Eugene Bleuler - 4A's of schizophrenia

3. Psychology is said to be the scientific study of _____ and ______.
a. Behavior, mental processes
b. Mental illness, Mental health
c. Physical states, mental states
d. None of these

Ans. a. Behavior, mental processes

4. Who is the father of Experimental psychology?
a. Wilhelm Wundt
b. G. Jung
c. Sigmund Freud
d. None of these

Ans. a. Wilhelm Wundt

5. Individual Psychology was proposed by:
a. Adolf Meyer
b. Alfred Adler
c. Carl Jung
d. Harry Stack Sullivan

Ans. b. Alfred Adler

6. The branch which deals with the physical environment:
a. Geo-psychology
b. Industrial psychology
c. Educational psychology
d. Political psychology

Ans. a. Geo-psychology

7. First psychology lab was established by:
a. Wilhelm Wundt
b. RS Woodworth
c. Sigmund Freud
d. Max Wertheimer

Ans. a. Wilhelm Wundt

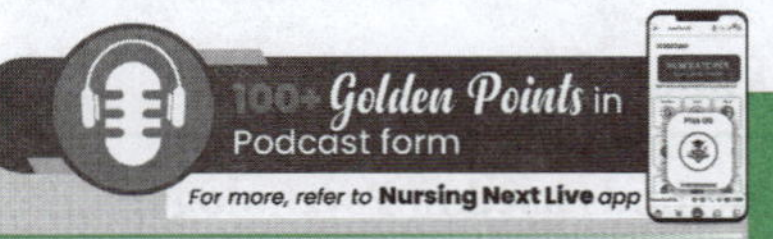

Golden Points

- Applied psychology has categories like educational psychology,
- Applied psychology includes the practical application of theoretical knowledge derived from pure psychology.
- Industrial psychology, legal psychology, military psychology.
- Political psychology, and clinical psychology.
- Psychology and applied psychology.
- Psychology can be divided into two main branches: pure

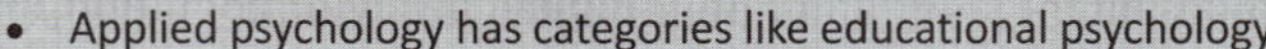

CHAPTER

2

Biological Basis of Behavior

CONCEPTUAL THEORY

Terminology

Behavioral Genetics: The study of effects of hereditary on behavior is called behavioral genetics.
Body-mind Relationship: According to modern psychology, "interdependent relationship between body and mind as they continue to influence each other.
Endocrine system: Endocrine system is a series of glands that produce chemical substances known as hormones.
Glands: Activated body structures responsible for human behavior are known as glands.
Neuron: Basic functional units of the nervous system.
Neurotransmitter: Neurotransmitters are the chemical messengers of the body. They carry messages from one nerve cell across a space to the next nerve, muscle or gland cell.
Synapse: Junction or gap between the neurons is called synapse.

BIOLOGICAL BASIS OF BEHAVIOR

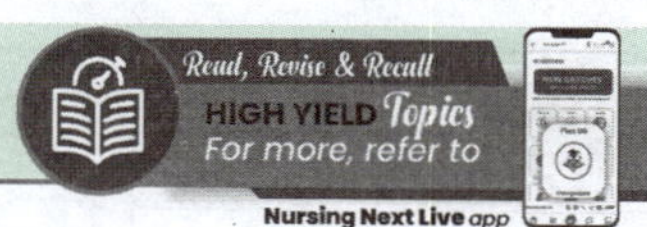

Body-mind Relationship

- The study of connection between the human body and mind has gained significant attention in recent times.
- From the era of Charles Darwin, who is known as the Father of Evolution, understanding behavior has relied heavily on the physiological basis of psychology.
- Behavior is seen as an integrated concept that encompasses various elements and cannot be separated from physical processes.

The Endocrine System

- Human behavior involves the activation of specialized organs called glands. Glands can be categorized into two types: endocrine glands and exocrine glands.
- Exocrine glands release chemical substances that are transported through ducts or tubes, such as tear glands. On the other hand, endocrine glands secrete hormones directly into the bloodstream.
- The endocrine system plays a crucial role in regulating various aspects of behavior. Hormones such as serotonin, dopamine, and norepinephrine, which are produced by the endocrine system, play a vital role in regulating mood, emotions, and overall mental well-being.

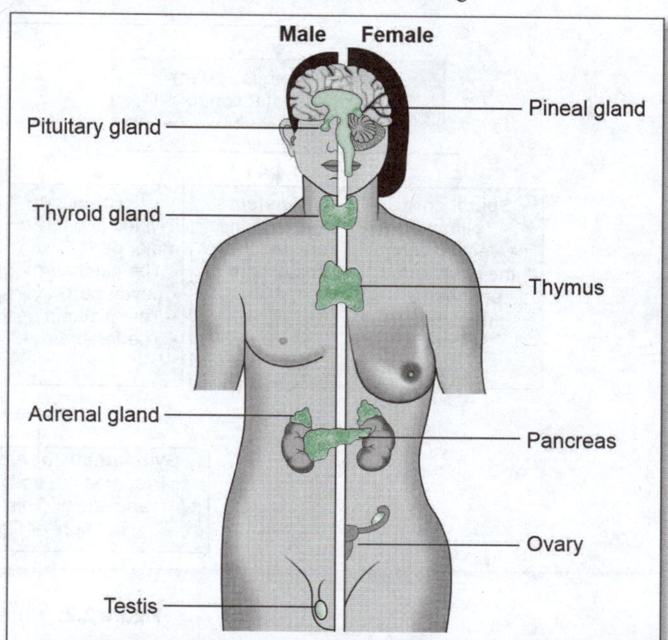

Figure 2.1: Glands in human body

- The hypothalamus and pituitary gland, along with the adrenal glands, play a significant role in the body's stress

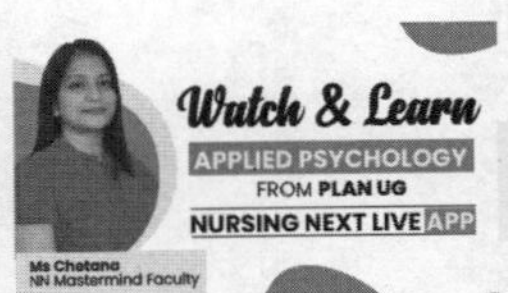

response. It is also responsible for sexual behavior and reproduciton.

Role of Genetics in Behavior

- Nature implies that our genetic composition determines our behavior.
- Personality traits and intellectual abilities are thus in our 'nature' and inherited just like the physical traits.
- Nurture theory argues that our environment, upbringing and experiences shape our behavior by and large.
- The study of effects of heredity on behavior is called behavioral genetics.
- The earliest findings on genetics were laid through the work of Mendel. Mendel's theory enumerated genes as well as the dominant and recessive nature of genes.

Inheritance

- Behavior can influence genetic expression in humans as well as animals right from prenatal development.
- Some factors that determine the role of behavior on genetics are as follows:
  - **Drugs and alcohol**: Exposure to substances such as drugs and alcohol prenatally has negative implications on the fetus.
  - **Light:** Exposure to light influences genetic behavior. Morgan experiment led to the conclusion that light exposure influenced genes and a caterpillar actively seeking out light will appear different to one that avoids light.
  - **Nutrition:** Nutrition is vital in shaping behavior and genes in humans. Prenatal malnutrition as well as malnutrition in the first three years of development can alter genetic makeup.

BRAIN AND BEHAVIOR

- The brain and behavior have a close relationship.
- The brain is the central command center of the body, responsible for controlling and coordinating various bodily functions, including behavior.
- It receives and processes sensory information, integrates it with existing knowledge and emotions, and generates appropriate responses and actions.
- Changes in brain structure or function can impact behavior, while behavior and experiences can also shape the structure and function of the brain through neuroplasticity.
- The brain and behavior are interconnected, influencing each other in a complex and dynamic manner.

Nervous System

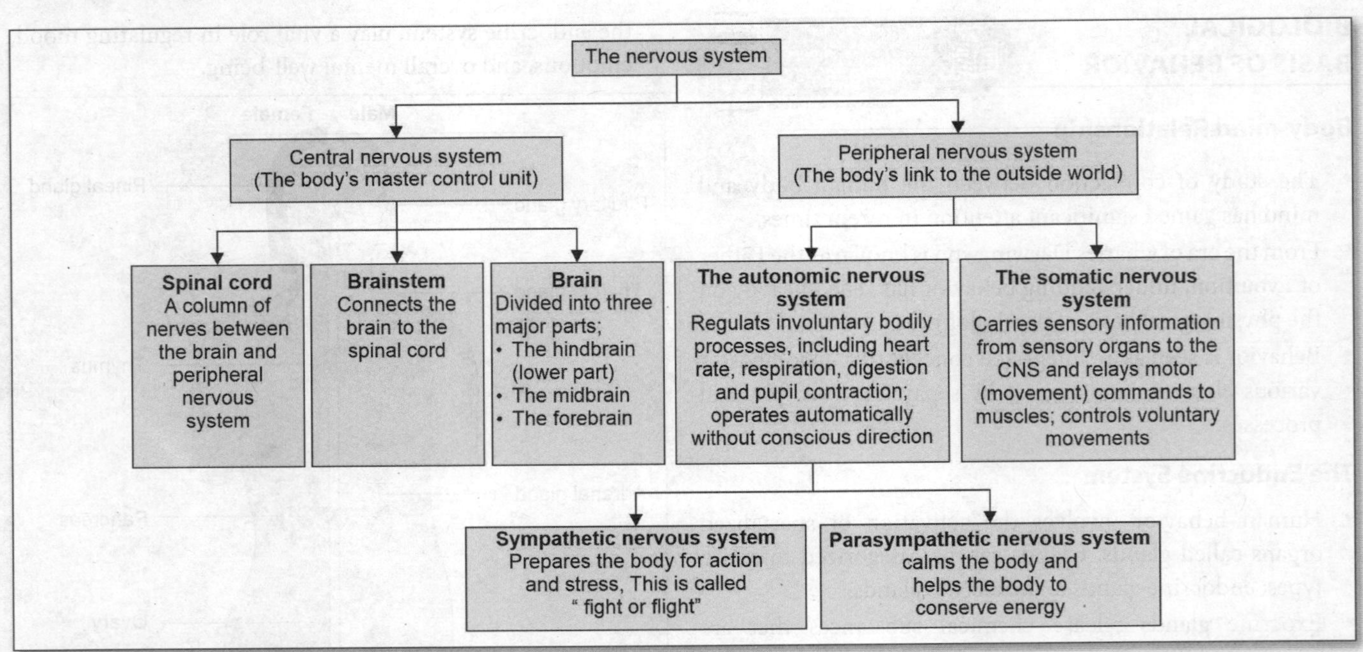

Figure 2.2: Human nervous system

- The nervous system is divided into two parts: The central nervous system (CNS) and the peripheral nervous system (PNS).
- The CNS consists of the brain and the spinal cord, encased within the bony skull and vertebral column. Parts outside of the CNS form the PNS.

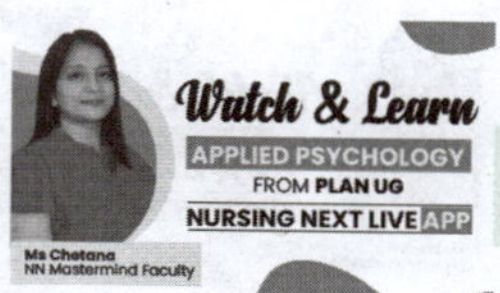

Neurons

Neuron is the basic unit and prime information carrier of the nervous system.

Nerve Impulses

A nerve impulse is similar to a lightning strike occurring due to differences in electrical charge across the plasma membrane of a neuron.

Synapses and Neurotransmitters

- The spaces or connections between neurons are referred to as synapses.
- Neurons are separated by a small gap called the synaptic cleft.
- Synapses consist of small button-like structures called boutons, which are located at the axonal endings of the transmitting or presynaptic neuron.
- These boutons contain vesicles containing neurotransmitters, which are chemicals.
- When a neuronal impulse occurs, the chemicals within these vesicles are released into the synaptic cleft.
- The neurotransmitter then binds to specific receptor molecules on the receiving neuron.

Central Nervous System and Behavior

- All complex actions that involve organization and coordination of activities of different parts of the body, learning and memory are functions of the higher centers of the CNS.

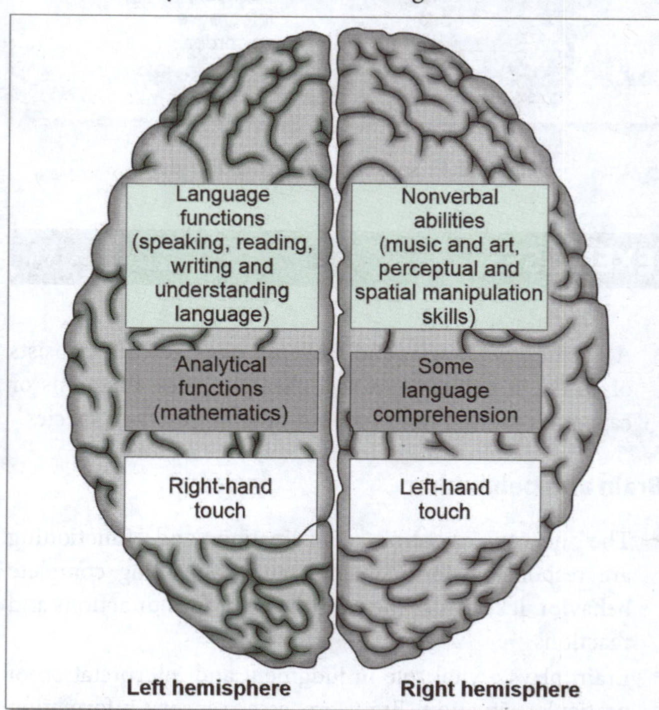

Figure 2.3: Left hemisphere and right hemisphere of brain

- The brain includes the cerebrum, cerebellum, thalamus and the brainstem or medulla oblongata.

Psychology and sensation – sensory process – normal and abnormal

- Sensations are experiences that are closely linked to our bodies and are the basis of all experiences.

SENSATIONS

- There are eight basic sensations experienced by human beings involving eight sense organs and eight different sensory experiences.

Table 2.1: Kinds of sensations along with sense organs and sensory experiences

Sensation	Sense organ involved	Sensory experience
Vision	Eye-retina	Light, color, shape, etc.
Audition	Ear-basilar membrane	Sounds
Taste	Tongue-taste buds	Sweet, sour, bitter, spicy, salty
Olfaction	Nose-nasal receptors	Odor
Cutaneous	Skin receptors	Temperature, pain pressure
Kinesthetic	Muscle receptors	Push/pull, strain, etc.
Organic/ Interception	Receptors and muscles in internal organs	Hunger, nausea, etc.
Static sense	Ear-semi-circular canals	Equilibrium, dizziness, etc.

Kinds of sensations

Influence of Light on Behavior in Humans

Light is a crucial regulator of the circadian rhythms. Exposure to bright light in the morning promotes alertness and wakefulness during the day and better sleep at night. Light exposure influences the regulation of sleep and wakefulness. Disruptions in the natural light-dark cycle can lead to disturbances to circadian rhythm and sleep pattern.

Seasonal affective disorder (SAD) is a type of depression that typically occurs during specific seasons, most commonly in winter months when daylight is reduced.

Sensory Process: Vision

- Vision is concerned with the eyes; visual stimuli occur as light rays.
- Vision plays a crucial role in human behavior. Our visual system allows us to perceive and interpret the surrounding world, influencing various aspects of behavior.

- It influences perception and environmental awareness, attention, emotional responses, learning and cognitive development, aesthetics and preferences.

Sensory Process: Audition

- The sense of hearing, also known as auditory sensation, is a significant sensory process.
- Auditory perception and experiences significantly shape human behavior and interactions with the world around us.
- The auditory system and the sense of hearing play a vital role in communication, environmental awareness, emotional responses, attention, movement, and cultural influences.

Sensory Process: Olfaction

- The receptors responsible for detecting smells are highly sensitive to chemical substances.
- These olfactory receptors are located in small clusters on both sides of the nasal passage.
- Our olfactory experiences shape our perceptions, choices, and responses, contributing to our overall behavior and well-being.
- Sense of smell has significant influences on human behavior, including emotions, memory, food preferences, avoidance, social interactions, environmental perception, and conditioning.

Sensory Process: Taste

- Taste receptors, also known as taste buds, are groups of specialized cells responsible for detecting different tastes.
- The sensory process of taste, or gustation, has significant influences on human behavior, particularly in relation to food preferences, dietary choices, and eating behavior.

Sensory Process: Cutaneous Sensations

- The skin is the human body's largest organ.
- The somatosenses, also known as skin senses, play a crucial role in informing us about the sensations occurring on the surface of our bodies.
- Cutaneous sensations refer to the sensory processes associated with the skin, including touch, pressure, temperature, and pain perception.
- These sensations play a vital role in human behavior and influence various aspects of our daily lives including pain perception, thermal sensations, haptic perception, sensory integration, and emotional/social influences.

Normal and Abnormal Sensory Processes

- Sensory processing disorders (SPDs) are neurological disorders that result in difficulties to process information from the five primary sense organs, sense of movement or positional sense.
- SPDs are divided into four categories.

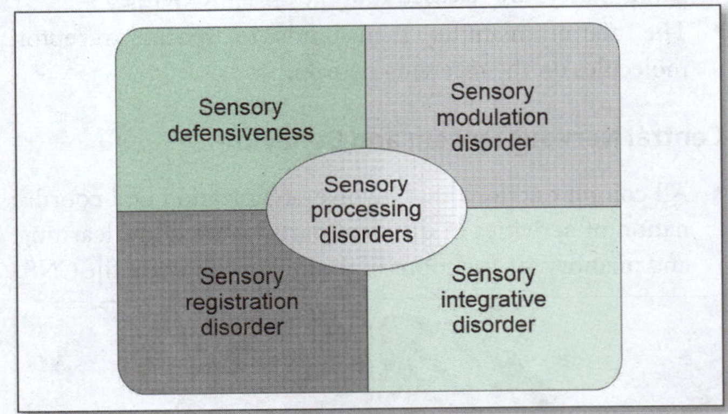

Figure 2.4: Sensory processing disorders

CONCEPTUAL EXERCISES

LONG ANSWER QUESTIONS

1. Define heredity. Explain the relation between brain and behavior. (KUHS)

Answer

Heredity

- Heredity is considered 'the sum total of inborn individual traits.'
- Biologically, it has been defined as 'the sum of traits potentially present in the fertilized ovum.'
- According to Douglas and Holland, 'one's heredity consists of all the structures, physical characteristics, functions or capacities derived from parents, other ancestry or species.'

Brain and behavior

- The nervous system's coordination and functioning are responsible for managing and controlling complete behavior. It serves as the control center for our actions and reactions.
- Brain plays a vital role in judgment and interpretation of particular situation. Brain processes sensory information and helps us make sense of the world around us.

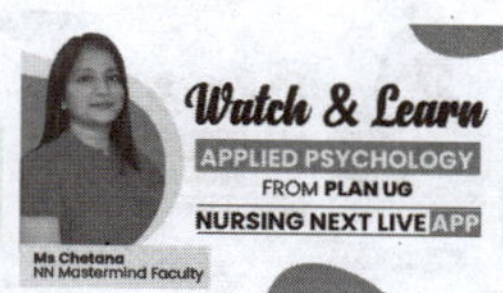

- Sense impressions received through our sense organs, such as sight, hearing, taste, touch, and smell, are given meaning by the nervous system. It allows us to perceive and understand the sensory input.
- Learning is significantly influenced by the nervous system. It enables the acquisition of knowledge, skills, and behaviors through various cognitive processes.
- The proper growth and development of nerve tissues and nervous system as a whole help in proper intellectual development.
- Any defect in the spinal cord or the brain seriously affects the intellectual growth.
- The emotional behavior is also influenced by the nervous system, especially at the time of anger, fear and other emotional changes.
- During emotional outbursts, nerve tissues cause a change in the secretion of hormones by some glands and consequently influence the emotional behavior of an individual.
- The process of growth and development is also directly and indirectly controlled by the functioning of the nervous system.
- Human behavior involves the body-mind interaction of various bodily factors.
- The most important are:
  - The sense organs called receptors.
  - The muscles and endocrine glands called effectors.
  - The nervous system known as the connecting or integrating mechanism.

2. Describe role of heredity and environment in development of human behavior. (KUHS)

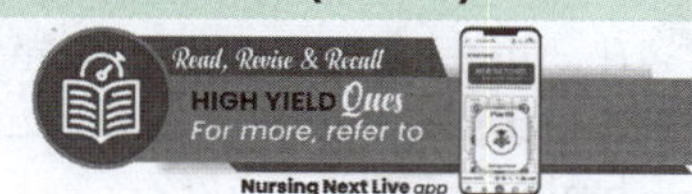

Answer

Heredity

- Heredity is considered 'the sum total of inborn individual traits'.
- Biologically, it has been defined as 'the sum of traits potentially present in the fertilized ovum'.
- According to Douglas and Holland, 'one's heredity consists of all the structures, physical characteristics, functions or capacities derived from parents, other ancestry or species.'

Role of Genetics in Behavior

Genetics plays an important role in the development of behavior. The works of Gregor Mendel were instrumental in establishing the role of genetics in development of behavior.

Modern genetics research has identified a wide range of genes that are associated with various behavioral traits, including personality traits, mental health conditions and even intelligence.

Genes provide the blueprint for physical and psychological characteristics.

Genes can influence everything from the height and eye color to the personality traits and predisposition to certain mental health conditions of an individual.

Genes help to determine the structure and function of our brain cells, including how they communicate with one another. This can have an impact on a wide range of behaviors, including the ability to learn, emotional responses and social interactions of an individual.

Genetics can also influence behavior by shaping our personality traits. For example, research has shown that certain genes are associated with traits such as extroversion, introversion and neuroticism.

Genetics can contribute to the development of mental health conditions such as schizophrenia, depression and anxiety.

Methods of Studying Heredity

- **Pedigree method:** Traits and characteristics spanning across generations in a family are studied to make inferences about heredity transmission of the characteristics.
- **Cytological studies:** Blood cells are studied using appropriate equipment to make inferences about the transmission of disorders. The conditions responsible for Down's syndrome were discovered through this method.
- **Breeding experiments:** The most common method used in studying genetic transmission. This method is useful within animal studies as well as in studying the role of environment although the feasibility is limited in human subjects.
- **Twin studies:** The most relevant method from a psychological point of view. Twins are the most natural and convenient subjects to study the role of heredity in behavior.

Role of Environment in the Development of Behavior

The environment plays a critical role in the development of behavior. The role of environment in the development of behavior can be discussed under intrauterine and extrauterine environment.

Intrauterine Environment

- Intrauterine environment refers to the environment inside the uterus during fetal development.
- It Includes factors such as maternal nutrition, exposure to toxins and maternal stress.

- Intrauterine environment can have a profound impact on fetal development, affecting everything from physical growth to cognitive development and emotional well-being.
- Inadequate maternal nutrition during pregnancy has been linked to cognitive deficits and behavior problems in children.
- Exposure to toxins such as lead and mercury during pregnancy can increase the risk of developing behavior problems and personality disorders.

Extrauterine Environment

- Extrauterine environment refers to the environment outside the womb after birth.
- It includes physical, biological and psychosocial factors that can have an impact on an individual's development and behavior.
- **Physical environment:** This refers to the physical surroundings that an individual is exposed to after birth. This includes factors such as air quality, temperature, and access to natural resources. For example, exposure to air pollution is associated with a range of negative outcomes, including cognitive deficits and mood disorders.
- **Biological environment:** This refers to the biological factors that an individual is exposed to after birth. This includes factors such as nutrition, exposure to toxins and physical health. For example, malnutrition during childhood can increase the risk of developing behavioral problems and personality disorders, while exposure to environmental toxins such as lead can lead to cognitive deficits and behavioral problems.
- **Psychosocial environment:** It refers to the social and psychological factors that an individual is exposed to after birth. This includes factors such as parenting practices, social support and exposure to stress and trauma. For example, positive parenting practices such as warmth, responsiveness and consistency can promote healthy emotional development and reduce the risk of behavioral problems in children, while exposure to stress and trauma can have a negative impact on mental health and behavior.

3. Write about Psychology of sensation. (KUHS)

Answer

Psychology of Sensation

The psychology of sensation refers to the study of how our senses gather and process information from the environment, leading to our subjective experience of sensory stimuli.

It is a branch of psychology that is concerned with the physiological and psychological processes involved in sensation.

The five main senses and their receptors are as follows:

Senses	Location/organ	Receptors
Vision	Retina of the eye	Photoreceptors
Audition or hearing	Cochlea of the inner ear	Hair cells
Taste or gustatory	Tongue	Taste buds
Smell or Olfactory	Olfactory epithelium of nose	Olfactory receptors
Touch or tactile	Skin	Tactile receptors

Factors Influencing Sensory Perception

- There are many factors that can influence the way we perceive sensory information, including our:
  - **Attention:** Attention is the process of focusing on specific stimuli in the environment. If we are not paying attention to a stimulus, we are less likely to perceive it.
  - **Expectations:** If we expect to see a certain thing, we are more likely to see it even if it is not actually there. For example, if we are expecting to see a red apple, we are more likely to see a red apple even if it is actually green.
  - **Past experiences:** If we have had a bad experience with a certain food, we are more likely to perceive that food as being less appealing.

The following are the key concepts in the psychology of sensation:

- **Sensory systems:** Five main sensory systems include vision, audition, taste (gustatory), smell (olfactory) and touch (tactile). Each sensory system has specialized receptors that detect specific types of stimuli and transmit signals to the brain.
- **Sensory perception:** Perception is the process of interpreting sensory information. It is a complex process that involves the brain, the senses, and the environment.
- **Sensory threshold:** Sensory thresholds are the minimum amount of stimulation that is required to detect a stimulus. There are three types of sensory thresholds: absolute threshold, difference threshold, and just noticeable difference. The absolute threshold is the lowest intensity of a stimulus that can be detected.
- **Sensory adaptation:** Sensory adaptation is the process by which our sensitivity to a stimulus decreases over time. This is why we stop noticing the smell of our perfume after a while.
- **Bottom-up and top-down processing:** Bottom-up processing refers to the analysis of sensory information starting from the basic sensory receptors. Top-down

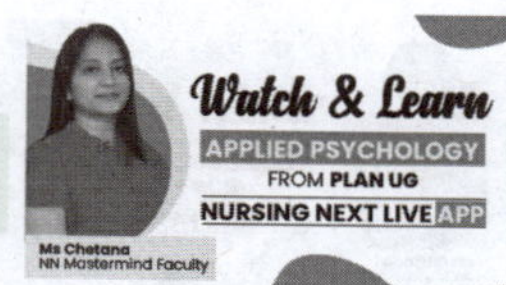

processing involves using our existing knowledge, experiences, and expectations to interpret sensory input and guide our perception.

- **Perceptual organization:** The brain organizes sensory input into meaningful perceptual experiences using figure-ground segregation, grouping and depth perception.
- **Multisensory integration:** Our sensory systems work together to create a unified perception of the world. Brain has ability to combine information from different sensory organs.
- **Individual differences:** Sensory perception can vary across individuals due to factors such as genetic predispositions, prior experiences, attentional processes, and cultural influences.

In conclusion, psychology of sensation helps us understand how we experience and make sense of the world through our senses.

SHORT NOTES

1. Explain the types of environment. (MGR)

Answer

- Environment covers all the outside factors that have acted on the individual, since he began life. —**Woodworth**

Types of Environment

The following are different types of environment that affect an individual directly or indirectly:

Intracellular Environment

It relates to embryonic development. The cytoplasm is in the intercellular environment because the genes surrounded by it are influenced by and in turn influence its characteristics.

Intrauterine Environment

- Intrauterine environment shelters the baby during perinatal life.
- In the womb, the growing organism is surrounded by amniotic fluid and attached to the mother by the umbilical cord.
- The physiological and psychological states of the mother during pregnancy, her habits and interest, etc. all influence the development of the child.

External Environment

Three types: Physical environment, biological environment and psychosocial environment

1. **Physical environment:** Nonliving things, like water, air, housing, soil, climate, heat, light, radiation, noise, etc. form the physical environment. These affect the body and mind of the growing child.
2. **Biological environment:** It refers to the living component of man's external environment, which consists of plants, animals, insects, bacteria, viruses. It is necessary that the child should be allowed to grow in a good healthy biological environment.
3. **Psychosocial environment:** It includes cultural values, customs, habits, beliefs, attitudes, morals, religion, education, occupation, social and political organization, etc. Parents, members of the family, friends, classmates, neighbors, teachers, mass communication and recreation are also included in this environment.

2. Muscular and glandular controls of behavior. (DU)

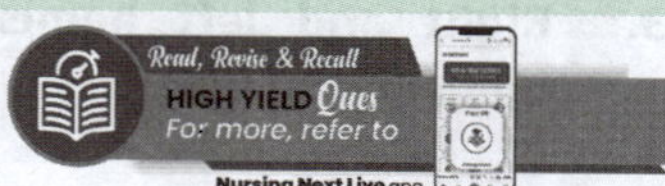

Answer

Human behavior involves the body-mind interaction of various bodily factors. The most important are:

- The sense organs called receptors
- The muscles and endocrine glands called effectors
- The nervous system known as the connecting or integrating mechanism

The Muscles and Endocrine Glands (Effectors)

- Effectors are termed the organs of responses.
- What is received through the sensory organs in the form of sensory input is responded through bodily reactions and motor activities carried out through muscles and glands, particularly the hormones secreted by the ductless glands which are responsible for most of our behavior patterns.
- The underactivity or over activity of these glands causes deficiency or excess of hormonal secretion.
- This affects the entire personality makeup of the individual.

Muscles

- There are mainly three types of muscles: smooth muscles, cardiac muscles and skeletal muscles.
  - **Smooth muscles:** Involved in the process of digestion, excretion and blood circulation.
  - **Cardiac muscles:** Function smoothly in a rhythmic fashion but when one is emotionally upset, their normal functioning is disturbed causing heart trouble.

- **Skeletal or striped muscles:** Voluntary activities like running walking to the fine psychomotor skills, like typing, etc.

Glands

- There are two types of glands:
  - **Duct glands:** These glands release their hormones in little ducts into the body cavities or on the surface of the body.
    - E.g., salivary glands, gastric glands, sweat glands, etc.
  - **Ductless or endocrine glands:** These secrete hormones directly into bloodstream. They play an important role in the determination of human personality.
    - E.g., pituitary gland, thyroid gland, parathyroid gland, adrenal gland, pancreas, etc.

3. Right and left hemisphere related to human behavior (KUHS)

Answer

- The human brain is divided into two hemispheres: the left hemisphere and the right hemisphere. Each hemisphere is responsible for different functions, and they are connected by a bundle of nerve fibers called the corpus callosum.
- The left hemisphere is generally associated with logical thinking, language processing and analytical skills. It is also involved in controlling the right side of the body. People with strong left-brain dominance tend to be logical, analytical and verbal.
- The right hemisphere is generally associated with creativity, intuition and spatial awareness. It is also involved in controlling the left side of the body. People with strong right-brain dominance tend to be creative, artistic and spatially aware.
- The left and right hemispheres of the brain are also not completely separate. There is a large bundle of nerve fibers called the corpus callosum that connects the two hemispheres. This allows the hemispheres to communicate with each other and to work together to perform complex tasks.
- It is important to note that the left and right hemispheres of the brain work together in a complex way. There is no single brain region (left or right) that is exclusively responsible for any particular function. For example, language processing is typically associated with the left hemisphere of the brain. However, there are also some language processing areas in the right hemisphere.

4. Neurons and synapse. (RUHS)

Answer

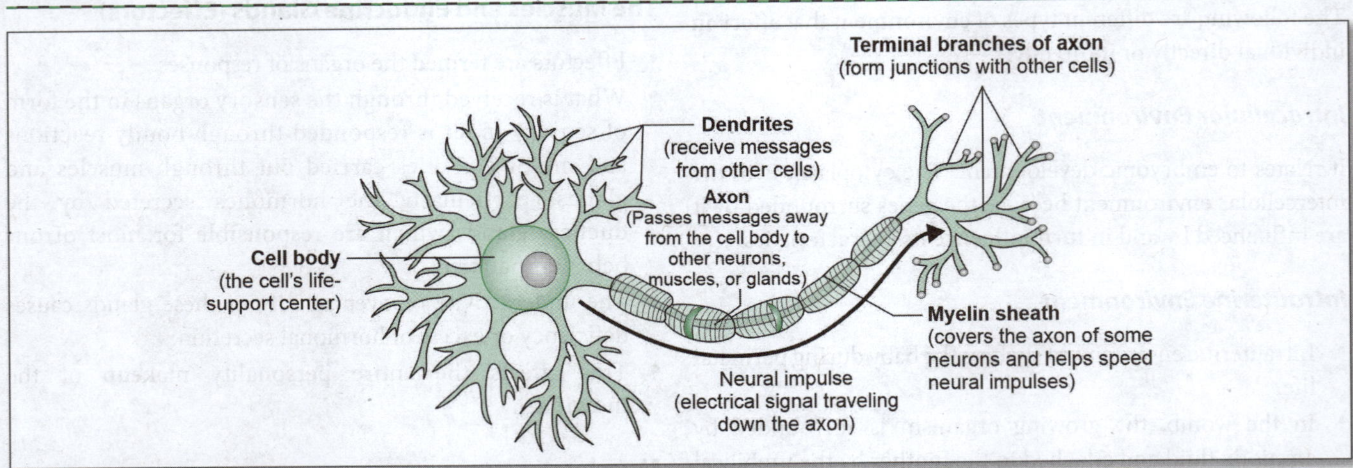

Figure 2.5: Structure of neuron

Neuron

- Neuron is the basic unit and prime information carrier of nervous system.
- Neurons carry information through the electrochemical signals.
- Neurons vary in shape, size, chemical composition and function but share some common features.
- A neuron has three fundamental structures: Soma, dendrite and axon.
- Axon conducts nerve impulses to other neurons.

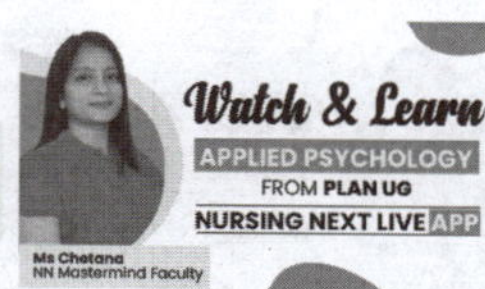

Synapse

- A synapse is a small gap or junction between two neurons (nerve cells) or between a neuron and a muscle cell or gland. It is the point at which these cells communicate with each other by transmitting chemical or electrical signals.

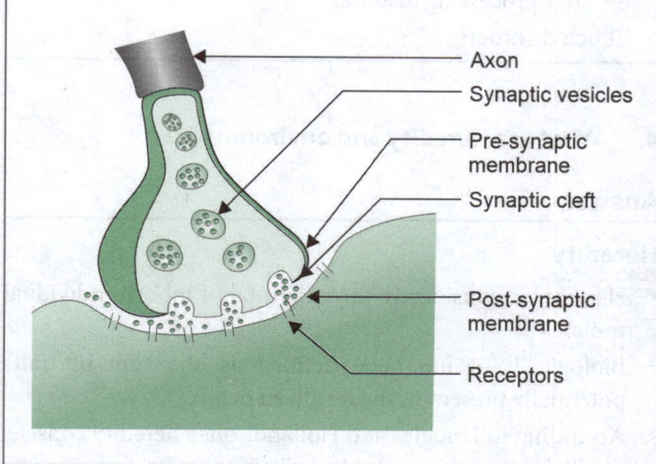

- Chemical synaptic transmission involves the release of a neurotransmitter from the pre-synaptic neuron, and neurotransmitter binding to specific post-synaptic receptors.
- Electrical synapse transmission involves the transfer of electrical signals through gap junctions.
- The synapse plays a critical role in many important functions of the nervous system, including learning, memory and muscle contraction.
- It also provides a site of action for many drugs that affect the nervous system by altering the release, uptake or effects of neurotransmitters.
- Disruptions in synaptic function have been implicated in a wide range of neurological and psychiatric disorders, such as Alzheimer's disease, Parkinson's disease, depression and schizophrenia.

5. Explain the cortical functions. (RUHS)

Answer

Cortical areas and their functions

Cortical area	Function
Primary motor cortex	Execution of voluntary movement
Primary somatosensory cortex	Receives tactile information, pain, pressure, position, movement and temperature

Contd...

Cortical area	Function
Motor association	Co-ordination of complex movements
Speech center (Broca's area)	Speech production and articulation
Auditory cortex	Auditory perception and hearing
Auditory association area	Complex processing of auditory information
Sensory association area	Processing of multisensory information
Visual association area	Primary visual perception
Wernicke's area	Comprehension of spoken

6. Define neuron. Explain the structure and function of neuron. (RUHS)

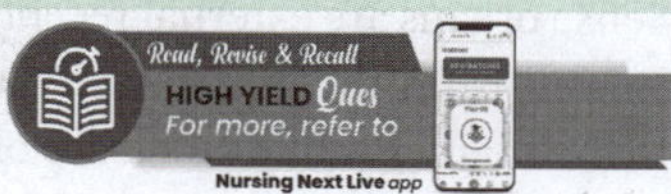

Answer

Neuron

- Neuron is the basic unit and prime information carrier of the nervous system. Neurons carry information through electrochemical signals. *(Please refer to Figure 2.5)*
- Neurons vary in shape, size, chemical composition and function but share common features.
- All neurons consist of three fundamental elements: Soma, dendrites and axon.
  - **Soma:** The soma, also known as the cell body, contains the protoplasm. Soma houses the nucleus.
  - Dendrites: They receive stimulation from other neurons. They are short and branched.
  - Axons: Axons are often long. Axons connect the toes and the spinal cord, measure about a meter in length.
  - Axons conduct nerve impulses to other neurons, muscles or glands.
  - Dendrites and soma receive information that is then conducted along the axon.

Neuron are of three types:

Sensory neurons	Motor neurons	Associative neurons
Found in the nerves that carry information from the peripheral organs to the CNS	Found in the nerves carrying messages from various centers of the CNS to various peripheral parts	Transport impulses from motor neurons to the central nervous system (CNS).
Information flows from the receptor organs to the centers	Information flows from the centers to effector organs	Coordination and integration of functions of the sensory and motor neurons

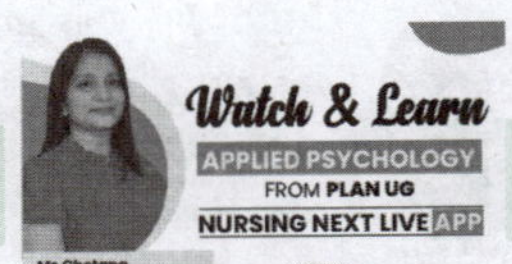

SHORT ANSWER QUESTIONS

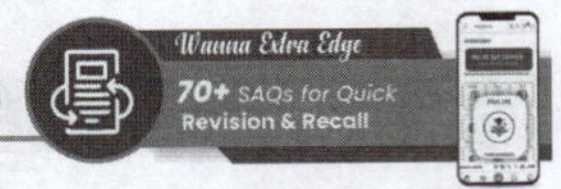

1. Define Chromosomal abnormalities.

Answer

Chromosomal abnormalities are genetic conditions that occur when there are errors in the number or structure of chromosomes. Examples Down syndrome, Turner syndrome, Klinefelter syndrome.

2. What are Sense organs?

Answer

Sense Organs/External Receptors

Sense organs are external receptors that detect various types of stimuli from the environment and transmit this information to the brain. Each of our sense organs has a distinct function to perform. The five main sense organs are as follows:

1. Eyes – for vision
2. Ears – for hearing
3. Nose – for olfaction (smell)
4. Tongue – for taste
5. Skin – for touch

3. What are Sensory disorders?

Wanna Extra Edge
70+ SAQs for Quick Revision & Recall

Answer

Here are some common sensory disorders:

- Hearing loss
- Vision loss
- Taste and smell disorders
- Sensory processing disorder
- Touch disorders

4. What are Heredity and environment?

Answer

Heredity

- Heredity is considered 'the sum total of inborn individual traits.'
- Biologically, it has been defined as 'the sum of traits potentially present in the fertilized ovum.'
- According to Douglas and Holland, 'one's heredity consists of all the structures, physical characteristics, functions or capacities derived from parents, other ancestry or species.'

Environment

- Environment covers all the outside factors that have acted on the individual, since he began life. —**Woodworth**
- **Types of environment:** Internal (Intercellular and Intrauterine) and external environment

CONCEPTUAL REVISION

MULTIPLE CHOICE QUESTIONS

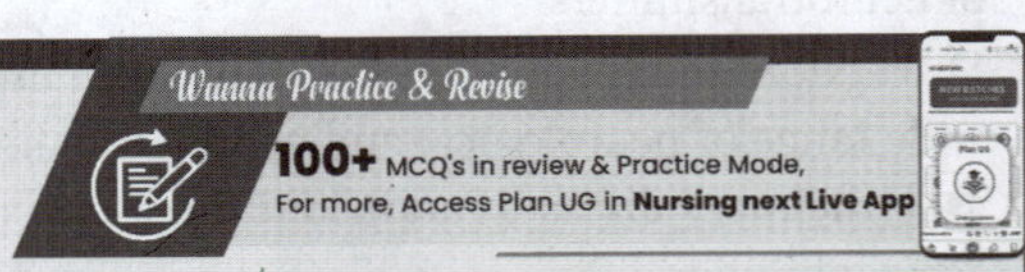

1. According to Sigmund Freud, we have a barrier in our mind called repression. This function is done by:

a. The conscious part of our mind
b. The preconscious part of our mind
c. The unconscious part of our mind
d. Both b and C

Ans. b. The preconscious part of our mind

2. Besides hearing, the auditory system is involved with:

a. Hemostasis
b. Gait
c. Smell
d. Kinesthetic

Ans. b. Gait

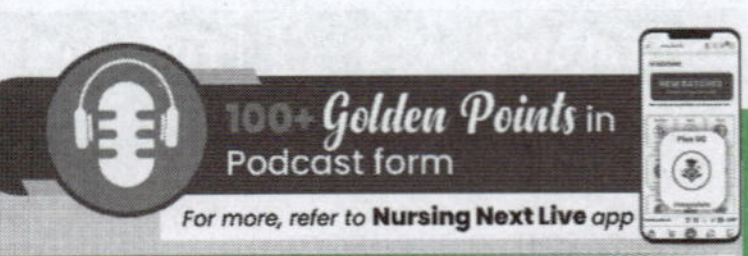

Golden Points

- Human behavior involves activation of body structures called glands.
- Modern psychology is concerned with the interdependent relationship between body and mind as they continue to influence each other.

CHAPTER

3

Mental Health and Mental Hygiene

CONCEPTUAL THEORY

Terminology

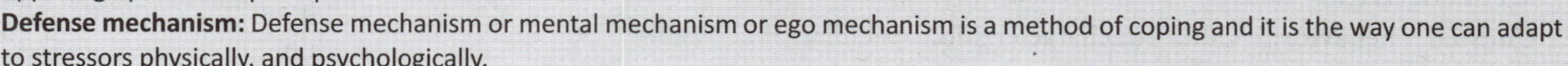

Conflict: Conflict may be defined as an active disagreement between people with opposing opinions or principles.
Defense mechanism: Defense mechanism or mental mechanism or ego mechanism is a method of coping and it is the way one can adapt to stressors physically, and psychologically.
Denial: The individual refuses to accept or face the reality.
Displacement/transference: Displacement or transference is the transfer of negative feelings from one person or thing to another.
Dissociation: Dissociation is inability of an individual to perceive the association between an action and its consequences.
Frustration: Frustration can be described as a sense of discontent that arises when a person is unable to accomplish his/her objectives.
Mental Health: Mental health is a state of well-being in which an individual can realize his or her own potential, cope with the normal stresses of life, work productively and make a contribution to the community. (WHO)
Mental Hygiene: A science which suggests measures for prevention of mental illness and restoration of mental health by the cure of mental illness.(APA)

MENTAL HEALTH

- Karl Menninger (1947) defined mental health as, "An adjustment of human beings to the world and to each other with a maximum of effectiveness and happiness."
- Mental health is a state of well-being in which an individual can realize his or her own potential, cope with the normal stresses of life, work productively and make a contribution to the community. —WHO

MENTAL HYGIENE

A science which suggests measures for prevention of mental illness and restoration of mental health by the cure of mental illness. —APA

Characteristics of a Mentally Healthy Person

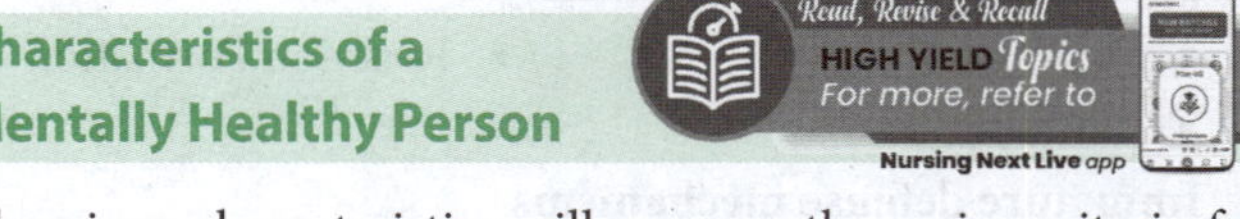

The given characteristics will serve as the major criteria for optimum mental health.

- A mentally healthy person is well-adjusted with adequate understanding and awareness of his motives, desires, his weaknesses, and strengths. He knows himself and can evaluate his own behavior.
- He has self-confidence and self-esteem. He is able to face all the challenges and accepts responsibilities.
- He always shows interest and pleasure in working with his age group.
- He has a sense of personal security. He has self-respect and respects people in group.
- A mentally healthy person is always optimistic and has ability to succeed. He follows his own philosophy of life.
- He adjusts with others in all difficult situations. He does not avoid responsibilities given to him.
- A mentally healthy individual develops his own philosophy of life and gives meaning on his own for his daily activities.
- He can be able to think wisely and independently.
- He takes appropriate decisions at required situations.
- A mentally healthy person knows when to say 'yes' and 'no'

Warning Signs of Poor Mental Health

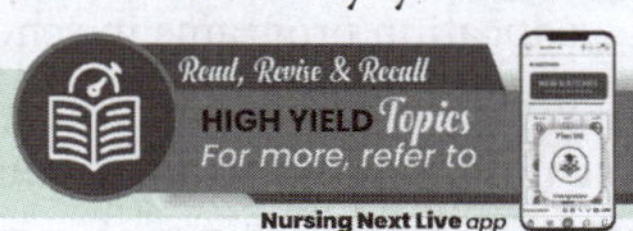

- **Sleep or appetite changes:** Dramatic sleep and appetite changes or decline in personal care.
- **Mood changes:** Rapid or dramatic shifts in emotions or depressed feelings, greater irritability.

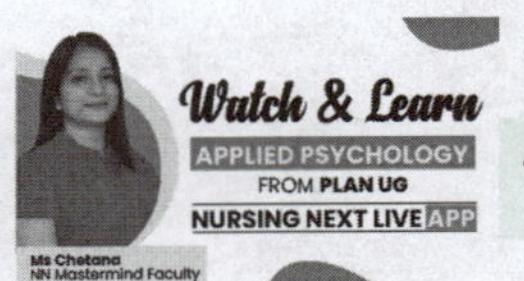

- **Withdrawal:** Recent social withdrawal and loss of interest in activities previously enjoyed.
- **Drop in functioning:** An unusual drop in functioning, at school, work or social activities, such as quitting sports, failing in school or difficulty performing familiar tasks.
- **Problem thinking:** Problems with concentration, memory or logical thought and speech that are hard to explain.
- **Increased sensitivity:** Heightened sensitivity to sights, sounds, smells or touch; avoidance of over-stimulating situations.
- **Apathy:** Loss of initiative or desire to participate in any activity.
- **Feeling disconnected:** A vague feeling of being disconnected from oneself or one's surroundings; a sense of unreality.
- **Illogical thinking:** Unusual or exaggerated beliefs about personal powers to understand meanings or influence events; illogical or "magical" thinking typical of childhood in an adult.
- **Nervousness:** Fear or suspiciousness of others or a strong nervous feeling.
- **Unusual behavior:** Odd, uncharacteristic, peculiar behavior.
- **Changes in school or work:** Increased absenteeism, worsening performance, difficulties in relationships with peers and co-workers.

Promotive and Preventive Mental Health Strategies and Services

There are some levels of promotion and prevention:

Primordial prevention: It aims to create conditions and promote behaviors that prevent the emergence of risk factors and promote overall health and well-being.

- It aims to prevent the initial development of risk factors in a population.
- For example: The promotion of a healthy lifestyle from early childhood. By encouraging healthy eating habits, regular physical activity, and avoiding tobacco and alcohol use, individuals can reduce the risk of developing various chronic diseases later in life, such as obesity, cardiovascular diseases, and diabetes.

Primary prevention: It involves interventions and strategies aimed at preventing mental health illnesses and promoting mental health and well-being in the population.

- **For example:** Implementing comprehensive mental health education programs in schools can be an effective primary prevention strategy.

Secondary prevention: It aims to identify individuals who are in the early stages of mental illness or at high risk and provide timely interventions to prevent further complications or mitigate the impact of the condition.

- **For example:** Routine screenings and early detection programs.
- Implementing routine mental health screening programs in various settings, such as healthcare facilities, schools, or workplaces, can help identify individuals with mental illnesses.

Tertiary prevention: It aims to prevent complications, manage symptoms, and provide rehabilitation and support to those who have experienced a disease or health condition.

- **For example:** Psychosocial rehabilitation programs are designed to assist individuals with severe and persistent mental illnesses in their recovery and reintegration into the community.

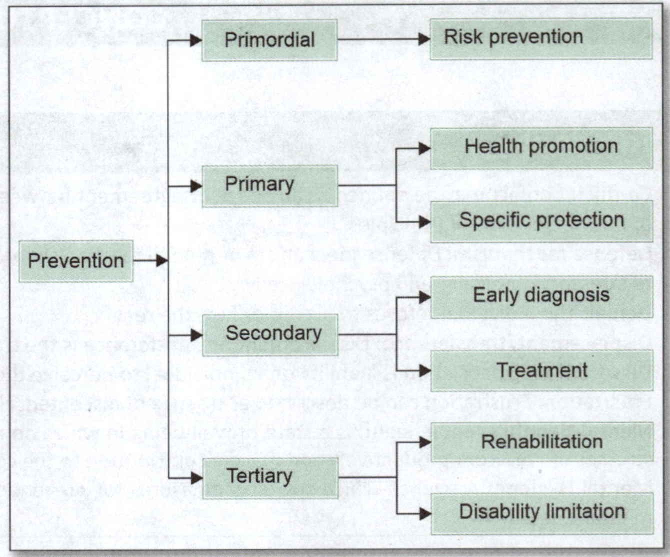

Figure 3.1: Levels of prevention

DEFENSE MECHANISM

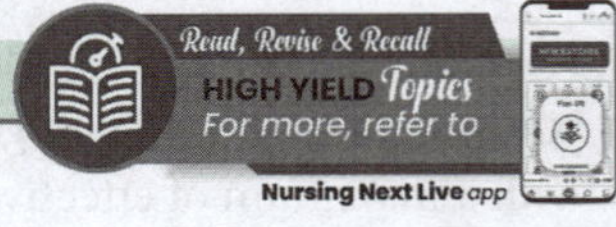

Defense mechanism or mental mechanism or ego mechanism is a method of coping and it is the way one can adapt to stressors physically, and psychologically.

Defense mechanisms are psychological strategies that are unconsciously used to protect a person from anxiety arising from unacceptable thoughts or feelings.

- **Mature defense mechanisms**
  - Sublimation
  - Suppression
- **Neurotic defense mechanisms**
  - Repression
  - Undoing
  - Reaction Formation
- **Immature defense mechanisms**
  - Projection
  - Denial
  - Displacement
  - Dissociation
  - Rationalization

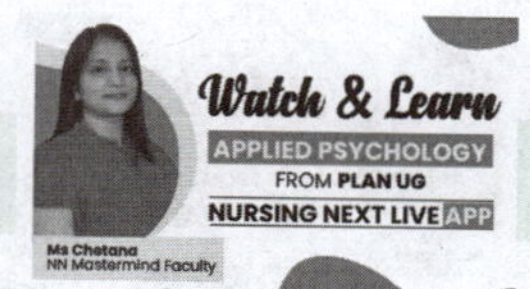

Types of Defense Mechanism

Note: Explained in Q and A section (Defense mechanism, Description and Example)

FRUSTRATION

Frustration can be described as a sense of discontent that arises when a person is unable to accomplish their objectives. It occurs when individuals face insurmountable goals, aspirations, and motivations.

Sources of Frustration

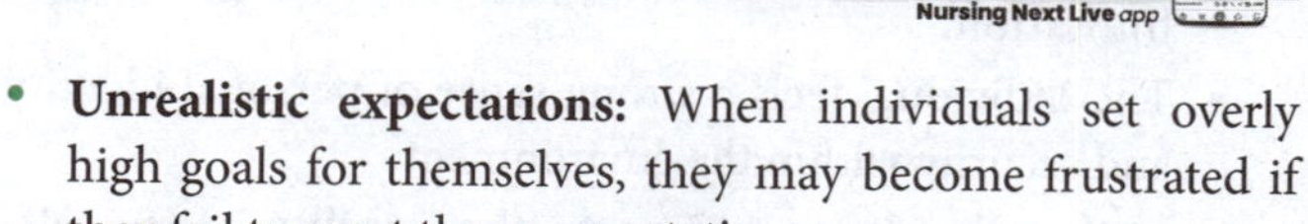

- **Unrealistic expectations:** When individuals set overly high goals for themselves, they may become frustrated if they fail to meet those expectations.
- **Lack of control:** Feeling helpless or having limited control over a situation can lead to frustration. This can occur in personal relationships, work environments, or other areas of life where individuals feel powerless.
- **Obstacles and setbacks:** Facing continuous obstacles, setbacks, or failures in pursuing one's goals can be frustrating. It can feel disheartening when progress is impeded or when unexpected challenges arise.
- **Unclear or ambiguous goals:** When goals or objectives are not clearly defined or understood, it can lead to confusion and frustration.
- **Lack of resources or support:** Insufficient resources, such as time, money, or information, can hinder progress and create frustration.
- **Conflict and interpersonal issues:** Difficulties in personal relationships, whether it's with family, friends, or colleagues, can contribute to frustration. Conflicts, misunderstandings, or unmet expectations within these relationships can generate feelings of dissatisfaction and frustration.
- **External factors and circumstances:** Certain external factors beyond an individual's control, such as traffic, weather conditions, or bureaucratic processes, can also be sources of frustration. These external circumstances can impede progress or create additional challenges.

CONFLICT

Conflict may be defined as an active disagreement between people with opposing opinions or principles.

Types of Conflict

- **Approach-approach conflict:** Conflict within a person where he or she needs to decide between two appealing goals
- **Avoidance-avoidance conflict:** Deciding between two equally undesirable choices
- **Approach-avoidance conflict:** There is one goal that has both positive and negative effects which make the goal appealing and unappealing simultaneously
- **Multiple approach-avoidance conflict:** It refers to a situation in which an individual is faced with multiple options or goals that have both positive and negative aspects.

Role of Nurse in Reducing Frustration and Conflict and Enhancing Coping

- **Cultivate the practice of taking deep breaths:** Develop the habit of engaging in breathing exercises, coughing exercises, practicing yoga, and spending time in refreshing natural environments.
- **Envision and express your aspirations:** Visualize your goals realistically and adopt a positive approach toward achieving them.
- **Embrace laughter:** Recognize the healing power of laughter and make an effort to laugh as much as possible.
- **Share humor:** Infuse your surroundings with liveliness by frequently sharing jokes and fully embracing each moment.
- **Embrace your silliness:** Engage in funny activities and adopt a lighthearted approach to handle situations and minimize frustration.
- **Delight a beloved child:** Express your affection by playfully tickling a child you care about, allowing the joy of love to thrive.
- **Acknowledge your choices:** Remember that you always have options and don't feel discouraged by initial attempts. Keep trying to reach greater heights.
- **Learn to decline when necessary:** Understand that you cannot take on everything you are asked to do. Sometimes it's important to say no, which can bring a sense of tenderness. Avoid overwhelming yourself with burdensome tasks.
- **Practice gratitude:** Express appreciation to the people who spend time with you and make a point to share valuable moments with them. Gratitude is a symbol of love.
- **Practice inactivity:** Frequently, remaining silent allows individuals to engage in thoughtful reflection and experience a sense of freedom from anxiety and depression.
- **Cultivate the skill of meditation and release frustration:** Regular meditation promotes mental tranquility. Therefore, make it a habit to meditate and let go of frustration.
- **Enjoy the therapeutic effects of music:** Music undeniably influences mental well-being. Take the time to listen to music and benefit from its positive impact on your state of mind.

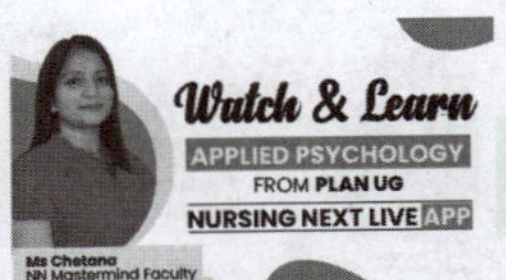

CONCEPTUAL EXERCISES

LONG ANSWER QUESTIONS

1. Define mental hygiene. Describe the concepts of mental health and mental hygiene in detail. (KUHS, MGR)

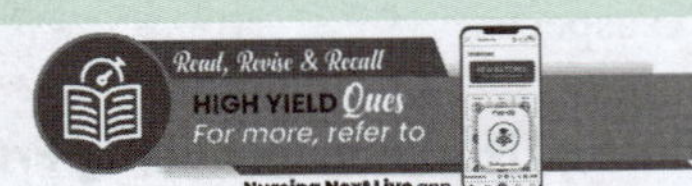

Answer

Mental Hygiene

Mental hygiene is the science which studies laws and means of curing and preventing mental diseases, personality disorders and other abnormalities for balancing adjustment and healthy development of personality.

Definition

Mental hygiene consists of measures to reduce the incidence of mental illness through prevention and early treatment and to promote mental health. —**Singh and Tiwari- 1971**

Concept of Mental Hygiene

- **Prevention**
  Here comes prevention of mental illness by the following methods:
  - Identify the cause
  - Telling ways and means to stay healthy and achieve balance
  - Methods of resolving conflicts and frustration
  - Getting rid of anxieties and tension
- **Preservation**
  - Preserving or marinating mental health to stay healthy and enjoy life by the following methods:
    - Develop inner potential
    - Emotional maturity
    - Sense of security: personal and social
    - Promote healthy relationships
- **Curative measures**
  Here come the methods to cure mental illness:
  - First comes awareness regarding mental illness and diseases
  - Various therapies
  - Proper treatment
  - Methods of rehabilitation
- **Balanced development of the personality**
  - One should have a well-balanced life for enjoying it to the fullest. Lack of balance results in maladjustment and diseases.
- **Leading happy and contented life**
  - If a person is in a good mental health, he can lead a happy and contented life. An individual must maintain his mental hygiene to have a good mental health.

Concept of Mental Health – Jahoda (1958)

- **A positive attitude toward health**
  - This includes an objective view of self-including knowledge and acceptance of strengths and limitation.
  - The individual feels a strong sense of personal identity and security within the environment.
- **Growth, development and the ability for self-actualization**
  - Growth, development and the ability for self-actualization indicator correlates with whether the individual successfully achieves the tasks associated with each level of development.
- **Integration**
  - It includes the ability to adaptively respond to the environment and the development of a philosophy of life, both of which help the individual maintain anxiety at a manageable level in response to stressful situations.
- **Autonomy**
  - It refers to the individual's ability to perform in an independent self-directed manner; the individual makes choices and accepts responsibility for the outcomes.
- **Perception of reality**
  - It includes perception of the environment without distortion, as well as the capacity for empathy and social sensitivity-a respect and concern for the wants and needs of others.
- **Environmental mastery**
  - It suggests that the individual has achieved a satisfactory role within the group, society and environment.
  - He is able to love and accept the love of others.

2. Define mental health. Explain the characteristics of a mentally healthy person. (MGR)

or

Discuss the characteristics of a mentally healthy person and the signs of poor mental health. (MGR, RUHS, KUHS)

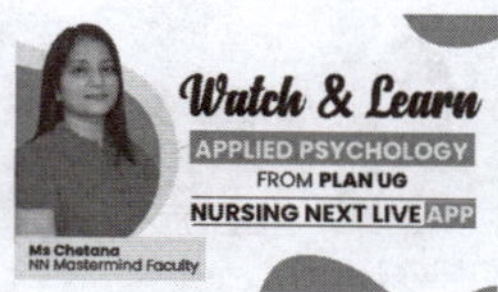

Answer

Definition of Mental Health

- "Mental health is a state of mental well-being that enables people to cope with the stresses of life, realize their abilities, learn well and work well, and contribute to their community." **—WHO**
- "An adjustment of human beings to the world and to each other with a maximum of effectiveness and happiness." **—Karl Meninger (1947)**

Characteristics of a Mentally Healthy Person

- He feels good about himself.
- He can make adjustments whenever required.
- He has a sense of self-worth and feels important and worthwhile.
- He does not become overwhelmed by emotions, such as fear, anger, love, jealousy, guilt, or anxiety.
- He has a sense of personal security.
- He has a sense of responsibility.
- He lives in a world of reality rather than fantasy.
- He shows emotional maturity.
- He is able to express empathy.
- He has variety of interest and hobbies to enjoy life.
- He has lasting and satisfying personal relationships.
- He feels comfortable with other people.
- He can laugh at himself and with others.
- He has respect for himself and for others even if there are differences.
- He is able to accept life's disappointments.
- He can meet life's demands and handle problems when they arise.
- He makes his own decisions.
- He has developed his own philosophy of life that gives meaning to his life.
- He shapes his environment whenever possible and adjusts to it when necessary.

Signs of Poor Mental Health

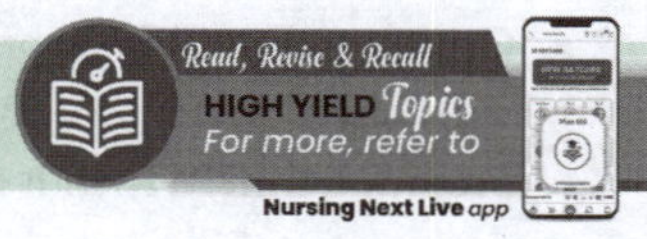

- There are some signs that indicate poor mental health and must be taken into consideration for further referral or treatment.
  - **In younger children**
    - School performance goes down
    - Change in grades
    - Change in behavior
    - Change in eating patterns
    - Irritable behavior or aggressive behavior
    - Not obeying the authorities
    - Temper tantrums
    - Hyperactivity
    - Nightmares
  - **In older children and adolescents**
    - Aggressive behavior
    - Inobedience
    - Change in eating and sleeping pattern
    - Missing school
    - School performance going down suddenly
    - Withdrawn behavior
    - Abuse of drugs and alcohol
    - Excessive complaint so physical problems
    - Intense fear of gaining weight
    - Negative mood
    - Thoughts of death
    - Frequent outburst of anger
  - **In adults**
    - Confused thinking
    - Low/sad mood
    - Irritability
    - Hopelessness
    - Social withdrawal
    - Strong feelings of anger
    - Suicidal thoughts
    - Changes in eating and sleeping patterns
    - Excessive fear or worrying
    - Abuse of drugs or alcohol

3. Describe the promotive and preventive mental health strategies and services. (RUHS)

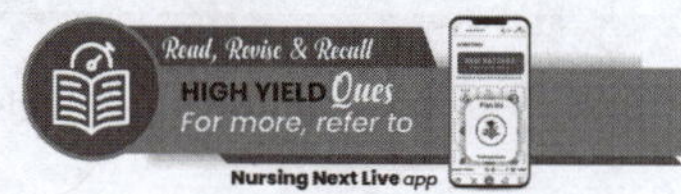

Answer

Promotive Mental Health Strategies (Primordial Prevention)

Promotive mental health strategies aim to improve overall mental well-being and create a supportive environment for mental health. They include:

- **Education and awareness:** Raising awareness of mental health and its importance through education and awareness programs
- **Providing supportive environment:** Creating environments that are supportive of mental health, such as schools, workplaces, and communities
- Promoting healthy lifestyle factors that support mental health
- Identifying and strengthening protective factors, such as social support, coping skills, and resilience.

Preventive Mental Health Strategies (Primary, Secondary and Tertiary Prevention)

Preventive mental health strategies aim to reduce the risk of developing mental health problems. They include:

- **Screening:** Screening for mental health problems in at-risk populations, such as children and adolescents.
- **Early intervention:** Providing early intervention for people who are at risk of developing mental health problems. This can help to prevent the onset of a mental health problem or reduce its severity.
- **Treatment:** Early treatment of mental illnesses to improve the prognosis.
- Rehabilitation of mentally ill patients.
- Gerald Caplan described levels of prevention specific to psychiatry.

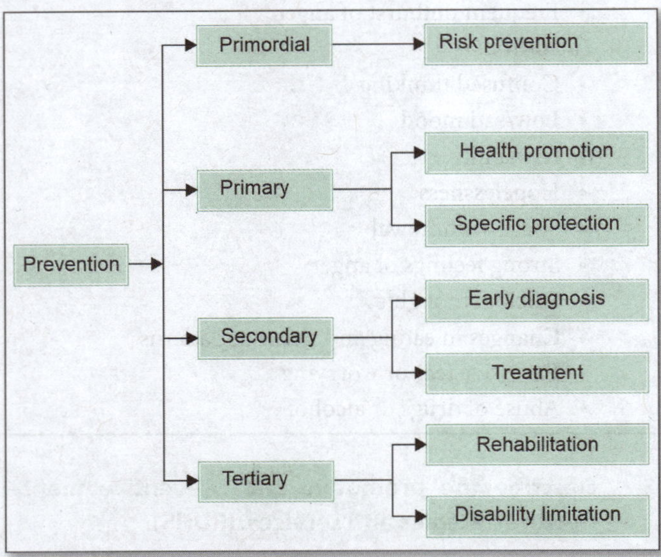

Figure 3.2: Levels of prevention

Primordial Prevention

- It aims to create conditions and promote behaviors that prevent the emergence of risk factors and promote mental health and well-being.
- It aims to prevent the initial development of risk factors in a population.

Strategies in primordial prevention:

- The promotion of a healthy lifestyle from early childhood
  - By encouraging healthy eating habits
  - Regular physical activity
  - Avoiding tobacco and alcohol use

Primary Prevention

- Primary prevention focuses on preventing the occurrence of mental disorders by doing health promotion and specific protection of individuals, families, and communities.
- **Interventions in primary prevention:**
  - Making people aware regarding mental health and mental illness.
  - Spreading the awareness regarding early signs and symptoms of mental illness in different age groups.
  - Encouraging individuals to adopt healthy lifestyle so that occurrence of mental illnesses can be prevented.
  - Strengthening social support system
  - Encouraging families to have an open communication
  - Teaching ill effects of substance, especially to adolescents
  - Encouraging people to stop abusing drugs
  - Encouraging harmonious relationship in families
  - Spreading awareness regarding mental hygiene
  - Strengthening mental health workers by training and education programs.

Secondary Prevention

- Secondary prevention focuses on individuals who experience early symptoms of disease and can regain premorbid state with proper treatment.
- **Interventions in secondary prevention**
  - Early diagnosis and identification of patient. Through screening, early signs and symptoms of suspected patients can be identified.
  - Early referral for treatment should be done. Educate individuals regarding early signs and symptoms of diseases.
  - Screening programs are carried out to rule out the new cases. On time screening will help in early identification.
  - Training of health personnel should be provided so that they can be updated with knowledge. Adequate knowledge of health workers will enable them to work more efficiently with the community.
  - Consultation services, like guidance and consultation should be provided to vulnerable people at risk.
  - Crisis intervention is provided to individuals who met with some crisis in their life. If crisis intervention is not provided timely, then it can lead to maladjustments and many mental illnesses.

Tertiary Prevention

- Tertiary prevention in mental health focuses on reducing the long-term consequences and improving the quality of life for individuals who already have been diagnosed with mental health conditions.
- **Interventions in tertiary prevention**
  - Disability limitation is done in tertiary rehabilitation.

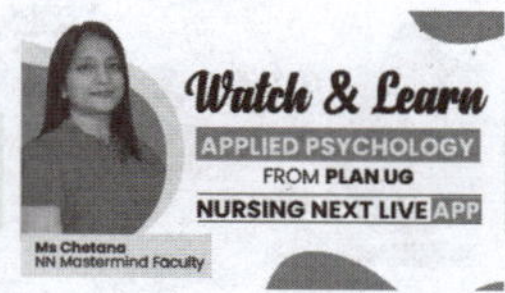

- Rehabilitation is done to preserve the remaining potential in the patient.
- Occupational and recreational therapies are provided.
- There should be constant communication between the nurse and family members after the discharge from the hospital.
- Preparing patients to shift back to his own community after getting discharged from the hospital.

4. Describe the factors affecting personal and social adjustment. State different defense mechanisms. (RUHS)

Answer

Definition

Adjustment means the modification to compensate for or meet special conditions.

Personal Adjustment

- An individual tries to be in harmony with his/her environment.
- The individual puts efforts to make his own place in society and environment and tries to fulfil all his needs.
- The adjustment is highly selective process.

Social Adjustment

- Social adjustment is a process of making adjustments in the society we live.
- It involves adjusting to the norms and values of the society.
- It also involves coping with the rules, regulations and trends of the society.
- This means getting along with other members of the society.
- One has to behave according to the society's expectations.

Factors Affecting Personal and Social Adjustment

There are many factors that can influence an individual's personal and social adjustment, which include the following:

- **Biological factors:** Biological factors such as genetics, and health can have an impact on an individual's personal and social adjustment. For example, a person with a genetic predisposition to anxiety may find it difficult to cope with stressors, while a person with a physical illness may experience social isolation and difficulties with daily activities.
- **Individual factors:** Individual factors such as education, employment, and socioeconomic status can affect the personal and social adjustment. An individual with an access to education, having a good job may be able to adjust easily while a person from low socioeconomic background may face barriers in adjustment.
- **Environmental factors:** Environmental factors such as family, society and culture can also influence personal and social adjustment. For example, a person who comes from a dysfunctional family may struggle with interpersonal relationships.
- **Psychological factors:** Psychological factors such as self-esteem, coping skills, and personality traits can also impact personal and social adjustment. For example, a person with low self-esteem may have difficulty asserting himself in social situations, while a person with poor coping skills may be unable to handle stressors effectively.
- **Life events:** Life events such as trauma, loss, and major life changes can also affect personal and social adjustment. For example, a person who experiences a traumatic event such as a natural disaster or a car accident may struggle with anxiety and depression, while a person who experiences a major life change such as a divorce or job loss may experience financial difficulties and social isolation.

5. Define defense mechanisms. Explain various types with suitable examples. (RUHS, KUHS, MGR)

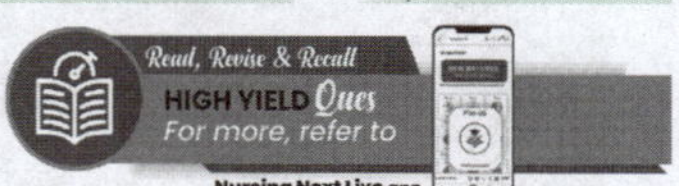

Answer

Introduction

- Defense mechanisms are also known as mental mechanisms or ego mechanisms and they are the method of coping and the way one can adapt to stressors physically and psychologically.
- Sigmund Freud, the "Father of modern psychiatry," coined the term defense mechanism.
- He defined defense mechanism as unconscious processes that defend a person against anxiety.

Definition

Defense mechanisms are psychological strategies that are unconsciously used to protect a person from anxiety arising from unacceptable thoughts or feelings.

Table 3.1: Types of defense mechanisms—description with examples

Sr. no.	Defense mechanism	Description	Example
1.	Fantasy or day dreaming	It is both an escape and compensatory mechanism and a kind of withdrawing reaction. Conquering hero Suffering hero	Imagination of success without putting any effort or working on it. Intellectually brilliant Feels lack of appreciation from others.
2.	Dissociation	Dissociation is inability of an individual to perceive the association between an action and its consequences.	Adult forgets everything about his childhood sexual abuse.
3.	Suppression	Consciously decides to exclude an idea, desire or feeling. It is one of the self-control methods.	Suppression of feelings and tries to adjust with the present situation.
4.	Seclusiveness	To reduce the frustration, an individual withdraws himself from painful situation, stimuli, or difficult situation, as he cannot face the problems in real life.	Not appearing for exams as the individual fails to prepare for it and feels anxious.
5.	Reaction formation/ reversal formation	Reaction formation is a method of protecting self by expressing opposite of what one really feels.	Parents of unwanted child show more concern toward others.
6.	Displacement/ transference	Dissociation is doing something as a substitute for something. Displacement to physiological symptom (e.g., breathing difficulty) Displacement to change stimuli/sensitivity (e.g., phobias)	Students get scolding from teacher for misbehaving. Instead of showing anger, she diverts.
7.	Projection	Projection is pointing out on others or blaming others who does the same thing. It helps to reduce the feeling of guilt.	A student may blame his teacher for the mistake he has done. "It's my math teachers' fault, and I failed in test."
8.	Sublimation	It is one of the most advanced, highly developed, and constructive mechanisms. It modifies the undesirable motives into substitute reaction.	A person who is getting aggressive thoughts will engage oneself in the sports actively.
9.	Denial	It is one of the primitive defense mechanisms. The individual will refuse to accept or face the reality. If this denial is used excessively, it leads to difficulties in health and lifestyle.	Hearing the news of death of a loved one is painful and the individual will deny accepting it.
10.	Regression	Regression is an immature way of responding to stress and returning to previous state.	When an individual becomes older, he acts like a child.
11.	Undoing	This is a defense mechanism in which the person asks excuses for wrong deeds.	Giving a gift to an individual with a dislike feeling toward him.
12.	Compensation	A person uses this mechanism only when he is unsuccessful in a direction to minimize the frustration due to lack of success, the individual may try some other object. Use of this mechanism avoids inferiority and inadequacy feelings. **Direct compensation:** Putting effort on the same field. **Indirect compensation:** The person may satisfy his desires by seeing in others. **Overcompensation:** An individual will mold his out-standing weaknesses to an outstanding achievement.	A student may fail in an exam and later achieves in the same exam is the example of direct compensation. When a father cannot become a doctor, he tries to prepare his daughter to become a doctor is an example of indirect compensation. When a person is poor in English language, he may achieve by becoming a poet is an example of overcompensation.
13.	Rationalization	It is called **excuse making defense mechanism.** Giving reasons as they are painful. Special forms: Sour- grape mechanism Sweet- lemon mechanism	The person will say whatever happens, happens for the best. He loses all his properties and says, God gave to enjoy life.

Contd...

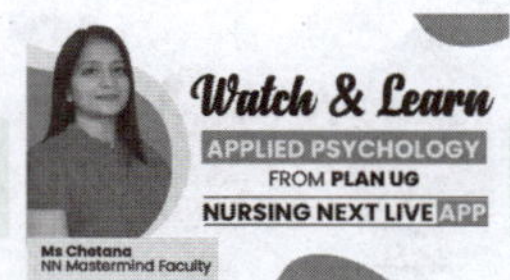

Sr. no.	Defense mechanism	Description	Example
14.	Identification	Psychological act of taking other person's achievement as their own to derive satisfaction and success.	Teenage children will see their teacher as their role-model or hero worshipping.
15.	Negativism	The use of this defense mechanism draws attention of others. It is both defense and escape mechanism. This is mostly used by toddlers and adults.	Children who are discouraged may develop uncooperative and disobedient behavior.
16.	Repression/motivated forgetting/selective forgetting	Unconscious mechanism by ego to keep disturbing thoughts from becoming conscious. It is not a very successful mechanism in long-term as repressed memories may manifest in subconscious means such as dreams or 'Freudian slips'	Oedipus complex

6. Define mental health and discuss the importance of defense mechanism in mental health. (MGR)

Answer

Definition of Mental health

- "Mental health is a state of mental well-being that enables people to cope with the stresses of life, realize their abilities, learn well and work well, and contribute to their community." **WHO**
- "An adjustment of human beings to the world and to each other with a maximum of effectiveness and happiness." **Karl Meninger (1947)**

Importance of Defense Mechanisms in Mental Health

- Defense mechanisms serve as psychological strategies to manage and reduce anxiety, discomfort, or distress.
- Defense mechanisms help in resolving conflicts.
- Defense mechanisms help individuals strike a psychological balance.
- When faced with traumatic experiences or overwhelming emotions, defense mechanisms provide a protective shield that allows individuals to distance themselves from distressing thoughts or memories. E.g., Suppression and Repression.
- Defense mechanisms can aid in adapting to challenging circumstances and coping with difficult emotions.
- Defense mechanisms help safeguard an individual's self-concept and identity by minimizing threats to their self-esteem.
- They help in coping with unfavorable situations
- They are healthy if used in moderation.
- Defense mechanisms help deal with disappointments and frustrations of daily life.
- They help in relieving tensions.
- These mechanisms can prove to be unhealthy if used frequently.
- Excessive use of defense mechanism does not solve problems.
- Excessive use does not let us change the problem behavior that causes tension or anxiety.
- Too much use can make us incapable of solving or facing problems.

7. Define conflict. Explain various types of conflict with suitable examples. (RUHS,MGR)

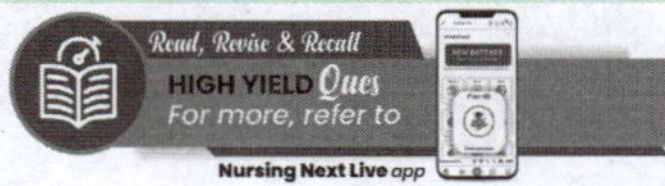

Answer

Definition of Conflict

- Conflict means a painful emotional state which results from a tension between opposed and contradictory wishes. **—Douglas and Holland**
- Conflict may be defined as an active disagreement between people with opposing opinions or principles.
- According to Joe Kelly, "Conflict is defined as opposition or dispute between persons, groups or ideas."

Types of conflicts

Conflict is of different types. There may be conflict between two persons, person with his environment or the person within himself.

- **The conflict between two persons**: This type of conflict is very common, e.g., conflict between parents and children, conflict between employer and employee.
- **The conflict between person and his environment**: This type of conflict occurs when a person becomes powerless in the situation of any environmental problem, for example, floods, earthquakes, etc.
- **The conflict within a person**: This is also described as internal conflict. The conflict within a person comprises the following types:
    - **Approach-approach conflict**: In this type of conflict, there is a conflict within a person where he or she needs

to decide between two appealing goals, for example, a student wishes to pursue a graduate degree and has been accepted into two graduate programs and needs to decide about which one to attend.

- **Avoidance-avoidance conflict**: This type of conflict refers to deciding between two equally undesirable choices, for example, deciding between doing a homework assignment and doing house work.
- **Approach-avoidance conflict:** This type of conflict occurs when there is one goal that has both positive and negative effects or characteristics which make the goal appealing and unappealing simultaneously, for example, marriage is a momentous decision that has both positive and negative aspects.
- **Multiple approach avoidance conflict:** This refers to a situation in which an individual is faced with multiple options or goals that have both positive and negative aspects. For example, an individual getting job offers from two companies and admission for higher education from a reputed university will have this type of conflict.

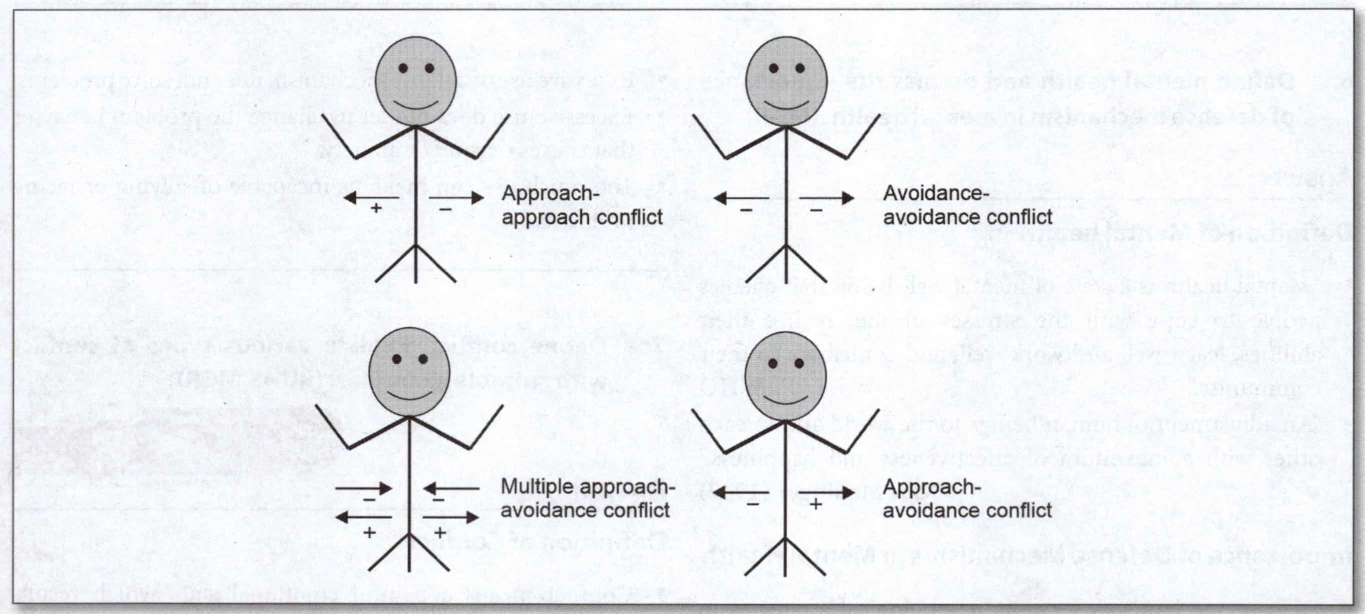

Figure 3.4: Types of conflict

SHORT NOTES

1. Write a short note on Mental hygiene and Mental health. Add a note on characteristics of mentally healthy person. (RUHS, MGR, KUHS)

Answer

"Please refer to Q. 1 and Q. 2 of Long Answer Questions, pg. no. 902

2. Warning signs of poor mental health. (RUHS, MGR, KUHS, DU)

Answer

Warning Signs of Poor Mental Health

There are some signs that indicate poor mental health and must be taken into immediate consideration for further referral or treatment.

In Younger Children

- School performance goes down
- Change in grades
- Change in behavior
- Change in eating patterns
- Irritable behavior or aggressive behavior
- Not obeying the authorities
- Temper tantrums
- Hyperactivity
- Nightmares

In Older Children and Adolescents

- Aggressive behavior
- Inobedience
- Change in eating and sleeping pattern
- Missing school
- School performance going down suddenly
- Withdrawn behavior

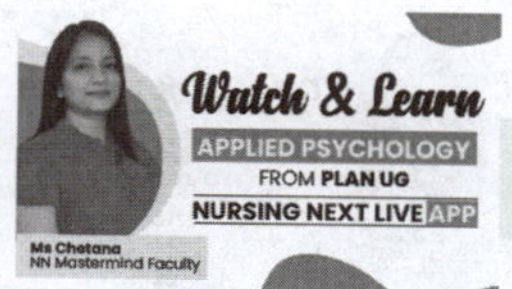

- Abuse of drugs and alcohol
- Excessive complaint so physical problems
- Intense fear of gaining weight
- Negative mood
- Thoughts of death
- Frequent outburst of anger

In Adults

- Confused thinking
- Low/sad mood
- Irritability
- Hopelessness
- Social withdrawal
- Strong feelings of anger
- Suicidal thoughts
- Changes in eating, sleeping patterns
- Excessive fear or worrying
- Abuse of drugs or alcohol

3. Explain the steps in prevention of mental and emotional disturbance. (MGR, KUHS, DU)

Answer

Levels of Preventive Psychiatry

There are three levels of prevention used to preventing **mental and emotional disturbance**. The levels are: primary prevention, secondary prevention, tertiary prevention.

Primary Prevention

Primary prevention focuses on preventing the occurrence of mental disorders by doing health promotion and specific protection on individuals, families, and communities.

Interventions in Primary Prevention

- Making people aware regarding mental health and mental illness.
- Spreading the awareness regarding early signs and symptoms of mental illness in different age groups.
- Encouraging individuals to adapt healthy lifestyle so that occurrence of mental illness can be prevented.
- Strengthening social support system
- Encouraging families to have an open communication
- Teaching ill effects of substance, especially to adolescents
- Encouraging people to stop abusing drugs
- Encouraging harmonious relationship in families
- Spreading awareness regarding mental hygiene
- Strengthening mental health workers by training and education programs.

Secondary Prevention

Secondary prevention focuses on individuals who experience early symptoms of disease and can regain premorbid state with proper treatment.

Interventions in Secondary Prevention

- Early diagnosis and identification of patient. Through screening, early signs and symptoms of suspected patients can be identified.
- Early referral for treatment should be done. Educate individuals regarding early signs and symptoms of mental illnesses.
- Screening programs are carried out to rule out the new cases of mental illness. On time screening will help in early identification.
- Training of health personnel should be provided so that they can be updated with knowledge.
- Consultation services, like guidance and consultation should be provided to such patients who suffer with conditions, like anxiety, peptic ulcer, postpartum psychosis, etc.
- Crisis intervention is provided to individuals who met with some crisis in their life.

Tertiary Prevention

Tertiary prevention focuses on individuals who have advanced stage mental illness. The goal here is to reduce the severity, discomfort and disability associated with their illness.

Interventions in Tertiary Prevention

- Disability limitation is done in tertiary rehabilitation.
- Rehabilitation is done to preserve the remaining potential in the patient.
- Occupational and recreational therapies are provided.
- There should be constant communication between the nurse and family members after the discharge from the hospital.
- Preparing patients to shift back to his own community after getting discharged from the hospital.

4. Id, Ego and Superego. (MGR, RUHS, DU)

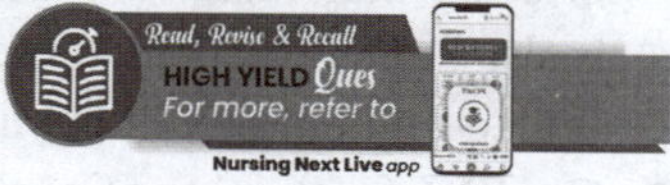

Answer

Structure of Mind

According to Freud, there are three structures of mind: Id, ego, and superego.

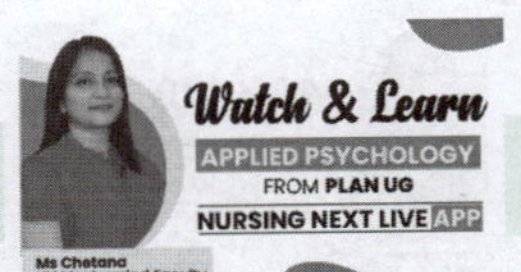

Target High Next Nursing **DECODE**

Id

- It works on the pleasure principle.
- It is the most primitive part and contains all biological based drives.
- It includes all physiological drives.
- The human behavior that originates from Id is impulsive, pleasure-oriented and disconnected from reality.
- Demands of id are impulsive and irrational.

Ego

- It works on the reality principle.
- It is that part of the human personality which is in closest contact with reality.
- It maintains harmony between id, external demands of world and superego.
- Ego is able to postpone the demands until there is appropriate place or time for need fulfilment.
- Ego acts as a mediator.
- Ego-driven behavior is more mature and adaptive.

Superego

- Superego works on perfection principle.
- It contains values, legal and moral regulations and social expectations that stop free expression of those behaviors which are pleasure seeking.
- It is important in the socialization of the individual as it assists the ego in the control of id impulses.

5. Sources of frustration. (MGR)

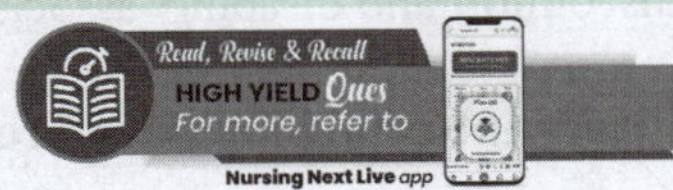

Answer

Sources of Frustration

- **Environmental frustration:** Frustration may also occur from the surroundings like workplace or dwellings.
  - Our surroundings might be responsible in most of the cases for frustration in an individual's mind. When an individual faces any unfavorable environment, it makes him/her frustrated at that moment.
- **Personal frustration:** Every individual has few expectations and personal needs. Qualities and abilities of every individual vary and the capability of the person is also limited. So, with these limited capabilities, no one is able to fulfill the expectations of one's life.
- **Conflict frustration:** Conflict exists between the owner and workers and it may also occur among the workers. The conflict may make the industrial workers gloomy and nervous. The incidence might create more psychological pressure among the workers and because of this, the workers may experience conflicting frustration.
- **Motivational conflict:** Motivation is said to be a type of power which helps the individual to work in a delightful manner. Positive motivation encourages an individual to work. The motivation also reduces the mental pressure of the person.

SHORT ANSWER QUESTIONS

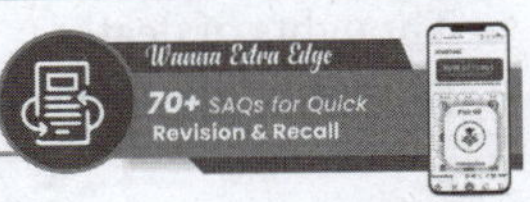

1. Frustration. (MGR)

Answer

Frustration is a state of being upset or disappointed due to an obstacle or barrier that prevents an individual from achieving his/her goals or fulfilling his/her needs or desires. It can result from internal factors, such as personal limitations or conflicting motivations, or external factors, such as environmental constraints or social pressure.

2. Any two solutions for frustration. (MGR)

Answer

There are various ways to deal with frustration. Two of them are mentioned here:

- Take a break: Sometimes, taking a break and stepping away from the source of frustration can help clear the mind and provide a fresh perspective. This can be as simple as taking a few deep breaths, going for a walk, or engaging in a relaxing activity.
- Problem-solving: Identifying the source of frustration and finding a way to address it can be a helpful approach. This can involve brainstorming possible solutions, seeking advice or feedback from others, or breaking down the problem into smaller, more manageable tasks.

3. Types of conflicts. (MGR)

Answer

Types of conflicts are:

- Approach-approach conflict
- Avoidance-avoidance conflict
- Approach-avoidance conflict
- Multiple approach avoidance conflict

4. Mental hygiene. (MGR)

Answer

Mental Hygiene

Mental hygiene is the science which studies laws and means of curing and preventing mental diseases, personality disorders

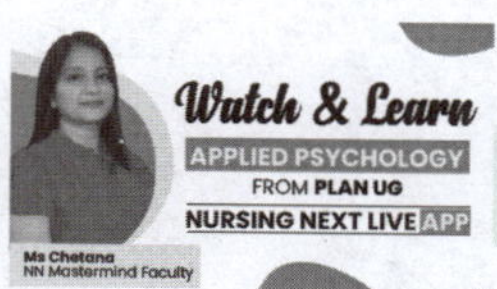

and other abnormalities for balancing adjustment and healthy development of personality.

Definition

Mental hygiene consists of measures to reduce the incidence of mental illness through prevention and early treatment and to promote mental health. **Singh and Tiwari- 1971**

5. Name any four defense mechanisms. (MGR)

Answer

Four Defense Mechanisms

1. Denial
2. Sublimation
3. Displacement
4. Reaction formation

6. Conflict resolution. (RUHS, MGR)

Answer

Some methods for conflict resolution are:

- Identify the source of conflict.
- Try to change the situation.
- Decide your priority before making any decision.
- Check everything carefully. Consider and think every possible consequence of your decision before making it.
- Review the situation again.
- Seek advice from others.
- Accept all the negative and positive outcomes.
- Stick with decisions and forget about other choices.

CONCEPTUAL REVISION

MULTIPLE CHOICE QUESTIONS

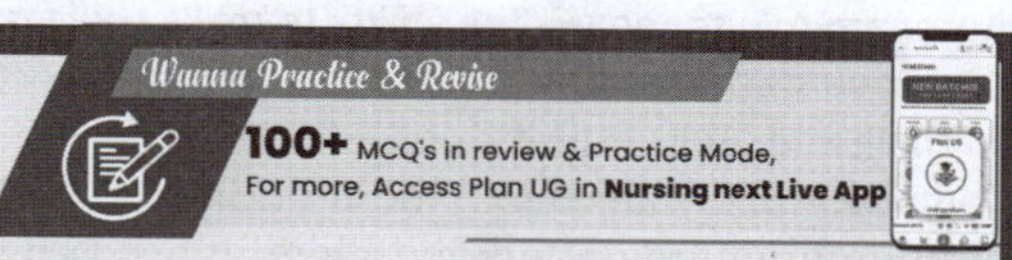

1. Creative thinking comprises four stages. Choose the correct sequence of stages.

a. Incubation, preparation, verification, illumination
b. Preparation, incubation, illumination, verification
c. Incubation, preparation, illumination, verification
d. Preparation, illumination, incubation, verification

Ans. b. Preparation, incubation, illumination, verification

2. Which of the following is an example of sublimation?

a. Blaming the teacher for failing in exams
b. A woman has no memory of being sexually assaulted as a child
c. Child starts bedwetting after the birth of sibling
d. A young man who is dealing with aggression by playing football

Ans. d. A young man who is dealing with aggression by playing football

3. Which of the following is a fear of an object, place, situation, feeling or animal?

a. Mania
b. Phobia
c. Conversion disorder
d. Depression

Ans. b. Phobia

4. Which of the following principles is matched correctly with the part of the mind it works on? (mental health and mental hygiene)

a. **Id**-Principle of reality, in the conscious domain
b. **Ego**-Principle of pleasure, in the unconscious domain
c. **Superego**-Principle of idealism, both in the conscious and unconscious domains
d. **Id**-Defense mechanism, in the unconscious domain

Ans. c. Superego-Principle of idealism, both in the conscious and unconscious domains

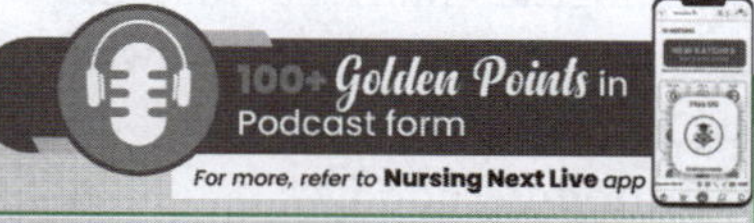

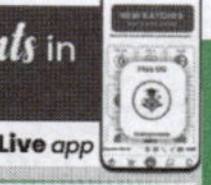

Golden Points

- Conflict is defined as opposition or dispute between persons, groups or ideas.
- Counseling is the interaction process between the counselee (seek help) and counselor (provide help)
- Defense mechanism or mental mechanism or ego mechanism is a method of coping and it is the way one can adapt to stressors physically, and psychologically.

CHAPTER 4

Developmental Psychology

CONCEPTUAL THEORY

Terminology

Adolescence: Transitional phase of growth and development between childhood and adulthood.

Adulthood: It is a developmental phase in which an individual focuses on family, career and strives for stability in life.

Autonomy: Autonomy is the ability to make choices yourself rather than having them made for you by other people.

Cognitive development: Advances in mental processes associated with perception, memory, reasoning, problem solving, language, learning and other aspects.

Competence: Competence is the ability to exert control over one's life, to cope with specific problems effectively, and to make changes to one's behavior and one's environment, as opposed to the mere ability to adjust or adapt to circumstances as they are.

Grief: The term "grief " is defined as a response to the loss of someone who has died, to which the emotional bonding or affection was formed.

Infancy: A period when a child is born and is termed " newborn" in its first month of birth.

Psychological need: Psychological need, as defined by Dr Ryan (1995), is "a psychological nutrient that is essential for individuals' adjustment, integrity, and growth".

Resilience: Resilience is an ongoing and fluid process or phenomenon that enables children and young individuals to flourish, endure and perform effectively despite encountering hardships.

INTRODUCTION

According to the World Health Organization (2004), mental health can be described as a state of overall well-being where individuals recognize and utilize their own capabilities, effectively manage typical life pressures, engage in productive and meaningful work, and actively contribute to their communities.

Psychological Needs

Psychological need, as defined by Dr Ryan (1995), is "a psychological nutrient that is essential for individuals' adjustment, integrity, and growth".

Psychological needs in infant/toddlerhood (0–2 years) for maintenance of health and during sickness

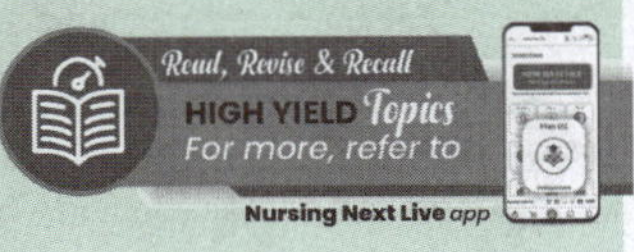

- **Secure attachment:** Infants and toddlers require a nurturing and responsive caregiving environment that promotes a secure attachment bond.
- **Responsive communication:** Frequent and meaningful interactions with caregivers, such as eye contact, facial expressions, and vocalizations, are vital for infants and toddlers.
- **Sensory stimulation:** Infants and toddlers explore and make sense of their environment through their senses.
- **Basic needs:** Meeting the basic physiological needs of infants and toddlers, including proper nutrition, hydration, sleep, and hygiene, is essential for their physical health and well-being.
- **Play and exploration:** Play is a primary way through which infants and toddlers learn about themselves and the world around them.
- **Emotional regulation:** Infants and toddlers are still developing their ability to regulate their emotions. They rely on caregivers to provide a safe and supportive environment, respond to their emotional cues, and help them manage and express their feelings in healthy ways.
- **Responsive caregiving:** Providing responsive and sensitive caregiving is essential for promoting the psychological well-being of infants and toddlers.

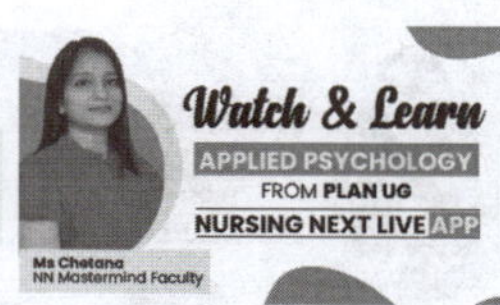

The psychological needs in childhood (2–12 years) for maintenance of health and during sickness

- **Emotional support:** Children require emotional support from their caregivers to foster a sense of security and well-being.
- **Social interaction and relationships:** Children have a fundamental need for social interaction and the development of positive relationships.
- **Autonomy and independence:** Encouraging children's autonomy and independence is crucial for their psychological well-being.
- **Physical activity and play:** Engaging in regular physical activity and play is essential for children's physical health and mental well-being.
- **Educational stimulation:** Providing educational stimulation and opportunities for learning is important for children's cognitive development and overall well-being.
- **Clear and consistent boundaries:** Children thrive in an environment with clear and consistent boundaries. Establishing age-appropriate rules, expectations, and consequences helps children develop self-discipline, a sense of security, and an understanding of acceptable behavior.
- **Positive reinforcement and encouragement:** Offering positive reinforcement, praise and encouragement helps children develop a positive self-image and motivation.
- **Emotional regulation skills:** Teaching children emotional regulation skills is important for their overall well-being.

Resilience

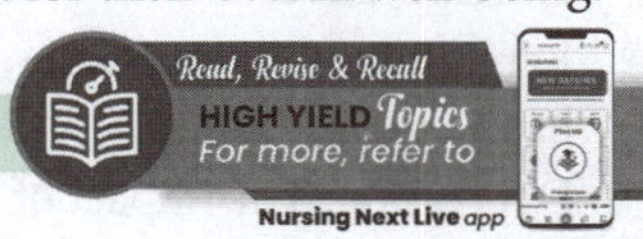

- Resilience is an ongoing and fluid process or phenomenon that enables children and young individuals to flourish, endure, and perform effectively despite encountering hardships.
- It empowers them to embrace risks and successfully navigate the daily obstacles of their lives.

The psychological needs in adolescence (12–19 years) for maintenance of health and during sickness

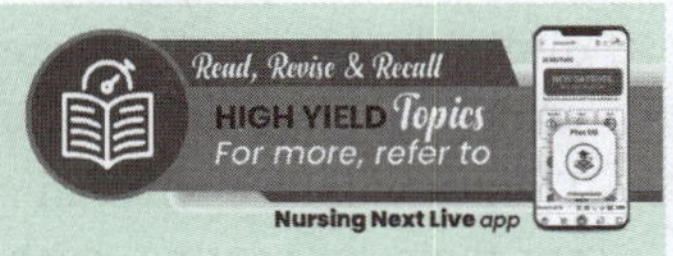

- **Identity and self-expression:** Adolescents have a strong need to develop a sense of identity and to express themselves. They strive to understand who they are, their values, beliefs, and aspirations.
- **Autonomy and independence:** Adolescents have a growing need for autonomy and independence. They seek opportunities to make decisions, take responsibility for their actions, and assert their individuality.
- **Social interaction and belongingness:** Adolescents have an increased need for social interaction and a sense of belonging. They seek acceptance, support, and connection with peers, family, and community.
- **Emotional well-being and regulation:** Adolescents experience a wide range of emotions, and they need support in understanding and regulating their emotions effectively.
- **Purpose and future orientation:** Adolescents need a sense of purpose and direction in their lives. They require opportunities to explore their interests, set goals, and work toward a meaningful future.
- **Physical health and self-care:** Adolescents need to prioritize their physical health and engage in self-care practices. This includes maintaining a balanced diet, engaging in regular physical activity, practicing good hygiene, and getting sufficient sleep.

The psychological needs in adulthood (19–65 years) for maintenance of health and during sickness

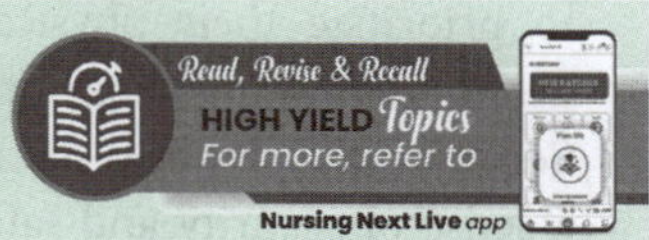

- **Self-esteem and self-worth**: Adults have a need for self-esteem and a sense of self-worth. They require recognition, respect, and validation from themselves and others.
- **Personal Growth and Development**: Adults have a need for personal growth and continued development. They seek opportunities for learning, acquiring new skills, and pursuing meaningful goals.
- **Autonomy and control**: Adults have a need for autonomy and a sense of control over their lives.
- **Social connection and support**: Adults have a need for social connection and support. They require meaningful relationships, social interaction, and a sense of belonging.
- **Purpose and meaning**: Adults have a need for a sense of purpose and meaning in their lives. They seek fulfillment through meaningful work, relationships and contributions to society.
- **Emotional well-being and resilience**: Adults have a need for emotional well-being and resilience. They require emotional awareness, regulation and coping strategies to navigate life's challenges.
- **Work-life balance**: Adults have a need for a healthy work-life balance. They require opportunities to engage in leisure activities, spend time with family and friends, and take care of their personal well-being.
- **Health promotion and self-care:** Adults have a need to prioritize their physical and mental health through health-promoting behaviors and self-care practices.

The psychological needs in adulthood (65 years and above) for maintenance of health and during sickness

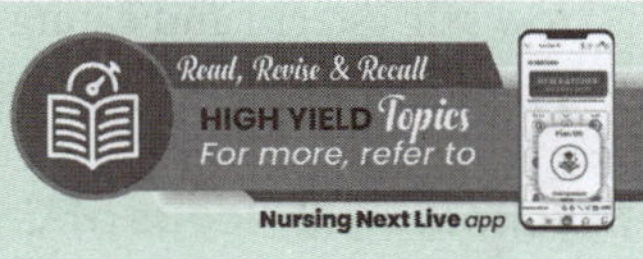

- **Autonomy and independence:** Older adults have a need to maintain a sense of autonomy and independence. They value their ability to make decisions, engage in activities they enjoy, and have control over their lives.
- **Social connection and relationships:** Older adults have a need for social connection and meaningful relationships.

Maintaining social interactions with family, friends and the community is vital for their mental health.

- **Sense of purpose and meaning:** Older adults have a need for a sense of purpose and meaning in their lives.
- **Emotional well-being and resilience:** Older adults have a need for emotional well-being and resilience. They may face unique challenges, including loss, health issues and life transitions.
- **Cognitive stimulation:** Older adults have a need for cognitive stimulation to maintain mental acuity and overall cognitive health.
- **Health promotion and self-care:** Older adults have a need to prioritize their physical and mental health through health-promoting behaviors and self-care practices.
- **Sense of security and safety:** Older adults have a need for a sense of security and safety. This includes having a safe and supportive living environment, access to necessary resources, and protection from abuse or exploitation.
- **Access to supportive services:** Older adults may require access to supportive services that cater to their specific needs. This includes health care services, assistance with daily activities, transportation and community programs.

Introduction to Child Psychology

- Children's psychology, also known as developmental psychology, is a significant field within psychology that specifically concentrates on the emotional and behavioral aspects of children as they progress from infancy through puberty.
- By studying children's emotional and behavioral problems, developmental psychologists aim to promote healthy development and provide interventions and support to enhance children's well-being.

Symptoms of Vulnerable Individuals and Role of Nurse

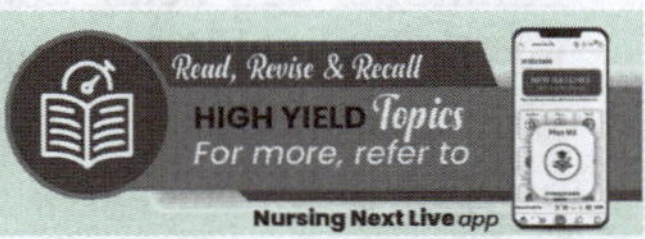

Vulnerable Individuals are:

- Patients who are suffering from chronic disease or illness
- Patient's caregivers during the course of illness
- Patients who are undergoing loss, grief and mourning
- Women who are vulnerable, suffer from depression due to early pregnancy, infertility, sexual abuse, domestic violence, low self-esteem and eating disorders.
- Physically and mentally challenged individuals

Psychological Needs of Caregivers During Illness

- During the duration of a family member's illness, caregivers often experience feelings of depression, stress or anxiety.
- When negative emotions, such as anger, are expressed between the caregiver and the patient, it can have detrimental effects on the patient's psychological well-being.
- Caregivers should be advised not to openly display their emotions such as crying or expressing anger in front of the patient.

Psychological Needs of Individual during the State of Loss or Grief

In 1965, Glaser and Strauss identified three different levels of awareness experienced by the dying person and their family members.

These states of awareness include:

- Closed awareness: In this state, neither the patient nor family members are aware of the impending death.
- Mutual pretense: This state occurs when both the patient and family members are aware of the poor prognosis and the impending death.
- Open awareness: In this state, both the patient and family members are fully aware of the impending death.

Grief

The term "Grief" is defined as a response to the loss of someone who has died, to which the emotional bonding or affection was formed.

Kubler-Ross (1969) postulated the theory of grief as follows:

- Denial: Refusal that it has not happened to me.
- Anger: Expression of anger toward higher power due to the loss happened.
- Bargaining: Bargain with higher power that why did it happen to me?
- Depression: The impact of loss has been felt by patient and so depressed.
- Acceptance: Feeling of accepting the loss.

Psychological Needs of Physically/Mentally Challenged Individuals

- Individuals experiencing low self-esteem may exhibit a diminished sense of self-worth in comparison to individuals who do not face such challenges.
- They may lack interest in engaging in daily activities that are typically routine, such as eating, dressing, brushing teeth and bathing.
- In some cases, they may express feelings of anger toward their family members.
- Individuals who have experienced loss of sight, speech and hearing may feel isolated and choose to withdraw from social interactions, avoiding interaction with others.

Psychological Needs of Women

- **Domestic violence**: The nurse needs to remove the patient from the violent situation and also, counseling session has to be planned to promote self-esteem.

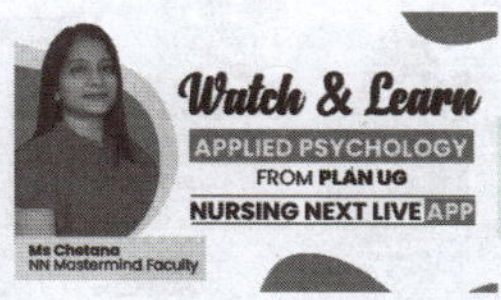

- **Lack of assertive behavior**: The nurse needs to provide the assertiveness training to the women to enhance the assertive behavior.
- **Body image:** This behavior has higher risk of self-injury. So, the nurse needs to render interventions and psychological counseling to promote the right perception of positive body image.
- **Early and unwanted teen pregnancy:** Unwanted teen pregnancy causes psychological trauma among women. So, the nurse needs to teach the right coping strategies based on the situation.
- **Infertility:** Women will be fulfilled as a complete woman when she becomes mother; if not, there will be high social pressure on the women.
- **Sexual abuse or rape:** Women who are victims of rape by the stranger or family member might experience the psychological trauma called Rape Trauma syndrome. Women will have low self-esteem and self-blame.

CONCEPTUAL EXERCISES

LONG ANSWER QUESTIONS

1. Discuss stages of development with special reference to psychology of each stage. (RUHS)

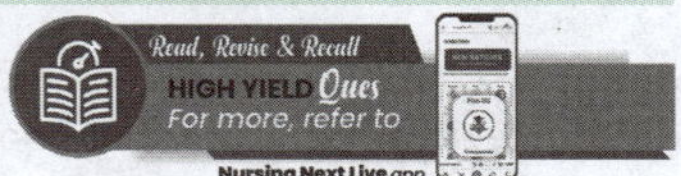

Answer

Stages of Development

Developmental psychology explains the processes and factors that influence the growth and development in relation to the behavior of an individual from birth to old age.

Stages of development explained by two theories:

- Psychosexual stages of development by Sigmund Freud
- Psychosocial stages of development by Erik Erikson

Freud's Psychosexual Stages of Development

Stage	Age	Psychology of the stage
Oral stage	0–1-year-old	Children derive pleasure from oral activities, including sucking and tasting. They like to put things in their mouth. Psychological consequences may include oral fixation or dependency issues later in life. Individuals may seek oral gratification through activities such as overeating, smoking, or nail-biting.
Anal stage	2–3-year-old	Children begin potty training. Psychological consequences may include issues related to control, orderliness, and autonomy. Individuals may develop anal-retentive or anal-expulsive personality traits.
Phallic stage	6-year-old to puberty	Children spend more time and interact mostly with same sex peers. Psychological consequences may involve the development of gender identity and the formation of the superego. Failure to resolve conflicts during this stage may lead to difficulties in relationships or issues related to sexuality and identity.
Genital stage	Beyond puberty	Individuals are attracted to opposite sex peers. Psychological consequences include the capacity for mature sexual relationships, the ability to form intimate connections, and the development of a strong sense of identity and purpose.

Erikson's Stages of Psychosocial Development

Stage	Age range	Psychology of the stage
Trust vs. Mistrust	Infancy (birth to 18 months)	Infants learn to trust or mistrust the world based on their caregiving experiences. Developing a sense of trust is crucial for forming secure relationships and a positive worldview. Mistrust can lead to difficulties in relationships and a sense of insecurity.
Autonomy vs. Shame	Early Childhood (18 months -3 years)	Toddlers strive for independence and autonomy, asserting control over their bodies and exploring their environment. Successful navigation of this stage leads to a sense of autonomy and self-confidence. Feelings of shame and doubt can arise if autonomy is discouraged or punished.
Initiative vs. Guilt	Preschool (3–5 years)	Preschoolers engage in purposeful play and take on new tasks. They develop a sense of initiative, setting goals and planning activities. If their initiative is met with excessive criticism or control, they may experience guilt and a lack of confidence in their abilities.

Contd...

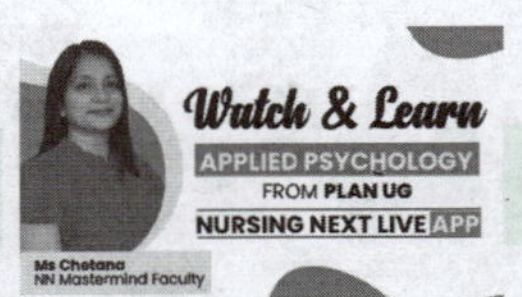

Stage	Age range	Psychology of the stage
Industry vs. Inferiority	School Age (5–12 years)	Children focus on acquiring new skills and competencies. They develop a sense of industry and accomplishment through schoolwork, hobbies, and social interactions. If they experience consistent failure or receive inadequate support, they may develop feelings of inferiority and incompetence.
Identity vs. Role Confusion	Adolescence (12–18 years)	Adolescents explore their identities, including personal values, beliefs, and career aspirations. Successful identity formation leads to a clear sense of self and direction. Role confusion can arise if individuals struggle to establish a stable identity, resulting in uncertainty and difficulties in decision-making.
Intimacy vs. Isolation	Young adulthood (19–40 years)	Young adults seek close, intimate relationships and develop long-term commitments. Achieving intimacy involves the ability to share oneself authentically and establish deep connections. Failure to do so may lead to feelings of isolation and loneliness.
Generativity vs. Stagnation	Middle adulthood (40–65 years)	Middle-aged adults focus on contributing to society, nurturing relationships, and leaving a positive impact on future generations. Generativity involves activities such as parenting, mentoring, and career accomplishments. Stagnation can occur if individuals feel a lack of purpose or fail to contribute meaningfully.
Ego Integrity vs. Despair	Late adulthood (65+ years)	Older adults reflect on their lives and evaluate their achievements. Ego integrity involves accepting the past, finding meaning, and embracing the reality of mortality. Failing to achieve ego integrity may lead to feelings of despair and regret.

2. Explain the psychological and emotional changes occurring during adolescence. (RUHS)

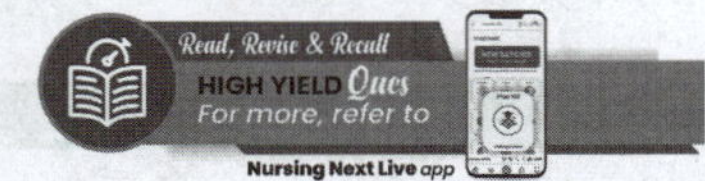

Answer

Adolescence (12–19 Years)

Adolescence is a developmental stage between childhood and adulthood, characterized by significant changes in physical, psychological, and emotional domains.

According to psychosocial theory of Erik Erikson, adolescents go through the stage of identity versus role confusion.

Here are some of the key changes that occur during adolescence:

- **Puberty:** Adolescence is marked by the onset of puberty, which involves a series of physical changes such as growth spurts, the development of secondary sex characteristics, and hormonal changes. These changes can have a significant impact on an adolescent's self-image and self-esteem.
- **Cognitive development:** Adolescents also experience significant cognitive changes, including improvements in abstract reasoning, problem-solving, and critical thinking skills. This allows them to think more deeply about complex topics and develop their own beliefs and values.
- **Emotional regulation:** Adolescents often experience heightened emotions and struggle with regulating their emotions. This can lead to mood swings, intense feelings of happiness or sadness, and conflicts with others.
- **Identity formation:** Adolescents begin to develop a sense of identity, which involves exploring their own beliefs, values and interests. This process can be challenging and confusing, as adolescents try to balance their own desires and values with the expectations of others.
- **Social development:** Adolescents begin to form more complex social relationships and develop a sense of identity within their peer group. They may also experience conflicts with parents or authority figures as they strive for more independence and autonomy.
- **Risk-taking behavior:** Adolescents may engage in risk-taking behavior, such as substance use, sexual activity or dangerous driving. This may be due to a combination of factors, including a desire for novelty and excitement, peer pressure, and a lack of experience and judgment.

Overall, adolescence is a time of significant change and growth in many domains. While these changes can be challenging, they also provide opportunities for personal growth, self-discovery and the development of important life skills.

3. What psychological and emotional changes occur during adolescent stage and early adulthood stage of life cycle? (RUHS)

Answer

Psychological and emotional changes that occur during adolescent stage:

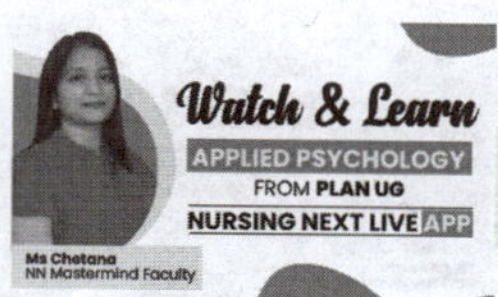

For answer, refer to Long Question 2.

Psychological and emotional changes that occur during early adulthood stage:

Early adulthood is a developmental stage that generally spans from ages 18 to 40, and it is characterized by a variety of psychological and emotional changes.

Erik Erikson's psychosocial theory of development suggests that the psychosocial stage of early adulthood is Intimacy versus Isolation. During this stage, individuals face the challenge of forming intimate, meaningful relationships or experiencing feelings of isolation. Successful resolution of this stage leads to the development of a strong sense of intimacy and the ability to form lasting connections with others. Here are some examples of common changes that occur during early adulthood:

- **Identity development:** Early adulthood is a time when people often explore and experiment with different identities, both in terms of personal and professional goals. This process can lead to a sense of clarity and purpose, but it can also be challenging and uncertain.
- **Increased autonomy:** Early adulthood is a time when people typically become more independent and self-reliant, as they move away from their family of origin and establish their own lives. This can be empowering, but it can also be stressful and overwhelming.
- **Changes in relationships:** Early adulthood is a time when people often experience changes in their social networks, including changes in friendships and romantic relationships. This can be a time of growth and expansion, but it can also be a time of loss and heartbreak.
- **Career development:** Early adulthood is a time when people often focus on building their careers and establishing themselves in the workforce. This can be a time of excitement and opportunity, but it can also be a time of stress and uncertainty.
- **Emotional regulation:** Early adulthood is a time when people typically become better at regulating their emotions and coping with stress. This can lead to greater emotional stability and resilience, but it can also be a time of vulnerability and insecurity.

Overall, early adulthood is a time of great change and growth, with both opportunities and challenges.

SHORT NOTES

1. Period of old age. (MGR)

Answer

- **Late adulthood (60 years and above)**
  - This is considered old age
  - Period of retirement from work
  - Impairment of sensory functioning
  - Slowing down of motor functions
  - Impairment in muscle coordination
  - Gradual decline in mental functioning
  - Cardiovascular diseases
  - Old age related diseases: arthritis, osteoporosis, loss of hearing and vision

Psychological Needs of Late Adulthood

According to Erik Erikson's psychosocial theory, the stage of late adulthood is referred to as "Ego Integrity vs. Despair." During late adulthood, individuals face the psychosocial challenge of reflecting on their lives and coming to terms with the choices they have made.

- Improvement in self-image happens during adulthood.
- There is a need for normal roles and relationships
- There is a need for love and relatedness
- Individual becomes hopeful and develops a sense of hopefulness
- There is a need for accomplishment of tasks

Role of a Nurse

- Nursing care of elderly is called geriatric nursing
- Elderly should feel respected and valued
- Insecurities and apprehensions should be taken care of. Proper explanation to the patient and family should be provided during hospitalization.
- Elderly might need frequent hospitalization.
- Nurses should be prepared to provide terminal illness care
- Allow elderly to express their emotions and feelings
- Observe the patient for hearing and vision loss
- Prevent bed sores
- Close observations
- Take care of eating and sleeping habits
- Provide warmth and emotional support
- Take care of bowel habits
- In case of mental function decline, give them frequent orientation and observe them
- Protect from injuries and harm
- Keep the side rails up
- Health education

2. The period of infancy. (MGR)

Answer

Infancy

- Infancy period is from birth till one year of life.
- Infant develops rapid motor development during this age

- Learns to sit, stand and begins to walk.
- Weight also triples by the age of one year.
- Length increases by almost 50% from birth.

Psychological Needs

According to Erik Erikson's psychosocial theory, the infancy stage of development is referred to as the "Trust vs. Mistrust" stage (from birth to 18 months). This stage is crucial in the development of a child's sense of trust and sets the foundation for their future psychosocial development.

- There is a need for security in infants
- Infants need love, affection and warmth so that they can develop trust
- Infants are dependent on caregivers and there is a need of comfort
- Infants need to feel a sense of acceptance to develop trust
- Need of physical contact
- Basic need fulfillment like hunger, thirst, hygiene, etc.

During Hospitalization

- Fearful, angry
- Separation anxiety
- Distressing
- Fear of strange medical and surgical procedures
- Stranger anxiety
- There may be excessive clinging on returning home
- Nightmares
- Emotional disturbance may be present

3. Psychological needs of adolescence. (MGR)

Answer

Adolescence (12–19 Years)

- Adolescence is a period of rapid physical, intellectual, emotional and social growth.
- According to Erikson, adolescence is a stage of development that occurs during the transition from childhood to adulthood. This stage is characterized by the psychosocial crisis known as "Identity vs. Role Confusion."
- Successful resolution of this stage leads to the development of a clear and stable sense of identity. If adolescents struggle to establish a sense of identity or feel overwhelmed by conflicting expectations and roles, they may experience role confusion and uncertainty about who they are.
- The psychological needs of adolescence include:
  - **Identity development:** Adolescents have a strong need to explore and develop their own identity.
    - Sex consciousness develops.
    - Extremely sensitive and self-conscious
  - **Autonomy and independence:** Adolescents have a growing desire to make decisions for themselves, take on more responsibilities, and have a sense of control over their own lives.
  - **Peer-relationship and belonging:** They seek connections with peers, form friendships, and desire acceptance and support from their social groups.
  - **Emotional regulation:** They strive to express themselves authentically and navigate the complexities of their emotional experiences.
  - **Privacy and personal space:** They require privacy and personal space to explore their thoughts, reflect on their experiences, and establish a sense of individuality.
  - Need for proper guidance in selecting a vocation

4. Developmental needs of adolescent. (DU)

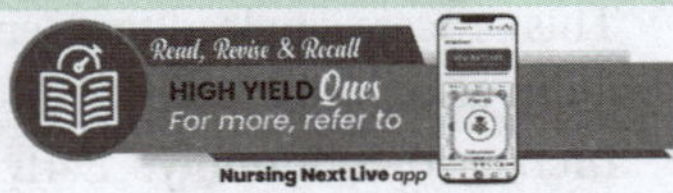

Answer

Adolescence (12–19 Years)

- **Physical developmental needs:**
  - It is a period of rapid physical, intellectual, emotional and social growth.
  - Sex organs mature and secondary sexual characteristics develop
  - Rapid increase in height
  - Changes in weight and body shape, voice
  - Presence of pubic, facial hair and external sex characteristics
  - Growth spurt in girls begins two years earlier than that in boys
- **Psychological needs:**
  - As per Erikson, this stage is characterized by the psychosocial crisis known as "Identity vs. Role Confusion."
  - Successful resolution of this stage leads to the development of a clear and stable sense of identity. If adolescents struggle to establish a sense of identity or feel overwhelmed by conflicting expectations and roles, they may experience role confusion and uncertainty about who they are.
  - **Identity development:** Adolescents have a strong need to explore and develop their own identity.
    - Sex consciousness develops.
    - Extremely sensitive and self-conscious
  - **Autonomy and independence:** Adolescents have a growing desire to make decisions for themselves, take on more responsibilities, and have a sense of control over their own lives.

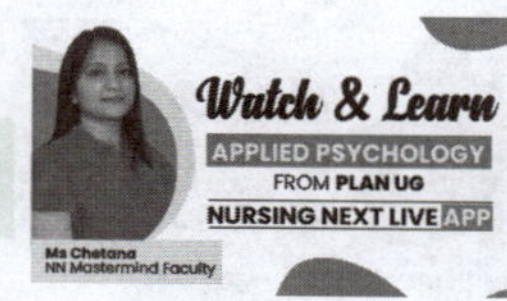

- **Peer-relationship and belonging:** They seek connections with peers, form friendships, and desire acceptance and support from their social groups.
- **Emotional regulation:** They strive to express themselves authentically and navigate the complexities of their emotional experiences.
- **Privacy and personal space:** They require privacy and personal space to explore their thoughts, reflect on their experiences, and establish a sense of individuality.
- Need for proper guidance in selecting a vocation.

5. Psychology of vulnerable individuals. (MGR)

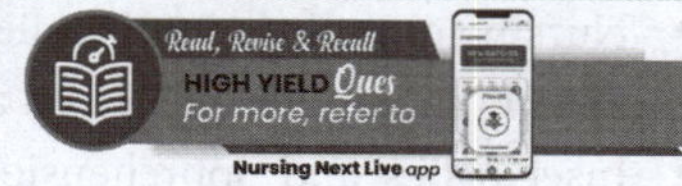

Answer

Psychology of Vulnerable Individual

Vulnerable individual refers to someone who is at a higher risk of experiencing harm, mistreatment, or negative outcomes due to various factors, e.g., challenged individuals (differently abled), women, children, sick individuals and their caregivers, elderly, etc.

- **Psychology of challenged individuals**
  - Challenged individual refers to a person with physical, intellectual, sensory, or developmental disabilities.
  - Permanent disability patients become angry and sometimes anger can turn inward
  - Sometimes anger may turn toward family members and staff nurses
  - Patients can experience low self-esteem
  - Patient loses interest in his surroundings
  - Patient may pretend to be positive because he doesn't want to make the relatives psychologically disturbed
- **Psychology of women**
  - Women are more likely to be affected by depression than men.
  - Mood changes especially in premenstrual stage and during menopause
  - Mood changes during childbirth and postpartum period
  - Infertility also affects psychology of women as they have feeling of incompleteness if they are not able to conceive.
  - Verbal, emotional or physical abuse also makes women vulnerable. Women lose their sense of worth and dignity.
  - Rape victim has low self-esteem, lot of self-blame and self-attack.
- **Psychology of children**
  - Children require a safe and secure environment that protects them from harm, abuse, and neglect.
  - Children need affection, care, and nurturing from caregivers
  - Children require emotional support to understand and regulate their emotions.
  - Need for social interaction and the development of social skills
  - Children have a natural curiosity and need opportunities for exploration, play, and learning
- **Psychology of sick person**
  - Patients during hospitalization experience different kinds of emotions.
  - People will have stressful and anxious situations due to the long-lasting illness.
  - Patient might refuse to meet anyone.
  - This might lead to high progressive low self-esteem and loss of interest in self as well as the surroundings.
  - The chronic illness that may lead to disability provokes extreme depression in such patients.
  - Some patients might pretend to be positive because they do not want to give any psychological distress to their relatives.
  - Some patients with sensory disabilities may feel isolated and they may experience disorientation and confusion.
  - Psychology of chronic illness patients is highly dependent on their attitude.
- **Psychology of caregivers during illness**
  - Emotional disturbance
  - Burnout syndrome among caregivers is a common issue.
  - May have feelings of guilt for not observing the symptoms earlier
  - They are anxious about their patient's condition
  - Financial strain
  - They may detach themselves and not want to speak
  - They may experience loss and grief in case of loss of family member.
- **Psychology of elderly**
  - Aging can bring cognitive changes, including slower processing speed, mild memory decline, and potential challenges in attention.
  - Some individuals may experience cognitive impairments, such as dementia or Alzheimer's disease.
  - Elderly often experiences loss of loved ones. This leads to feelings of grief, adjustment difficulties.
  - Social isolation and loneliness can be significant challenges for the elderly.

6. Explain different developments at infancy stage (KUHS)

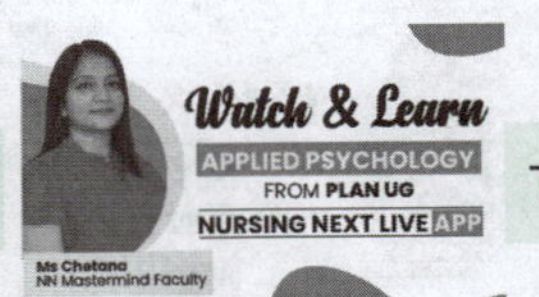

Answer

Infancy is the first stage of human development, spanning from birth to 18 months of age. During this time, a number of key developmental changes occur. Here are some examples of different developments that take place during infancy:

- **Physical development:** Infants undergo rapid physical development during the first two years of life. They gain weight, increase in height, and develop their motor skills, such as rolling over, sitting up, crawling, and eventually walking.
- **Cognitive development:** Infants begin to explore and learn about the world around them through their senses and interactions with others. They develop object permanence (the understanding that objects still exist even when they are out of sight) and start to form mental representations of people, objects and events.
- **Social and emotional development:** Infants begin to form attachments to caregivers and develop a sense of trust in their environment. They learn to recognize and respond to facial expressions and emotional cues, and they start to develop their own emotional responses.
- **Language development:** Infants start to communicate through nonverbal cues, such as crying and cooing, and eventually start to use words and gestures to communicate. They also begin to understand the meaning of words and simple phrases.
- **Sensory and perceptual development:** Infants develop their sensory and perceptual abilities, including vision, hearing, touch, taste and smell. They learn to discriminate between different sounds, sights, and textures, and to respond to their environment in more sophisticated ways.

Overall, infancy is a time of rapid growth and development, with a wide range of changes taking place in physical, cognitive, social, emotional and sensory domains. These early experiences lay the foundation for later development and can have a lasting impact on an individual's overall health and well-being.

7. Psychological needs of old age (DU)

Answer

Old Age (60 Years and Above)

- Impaired sensory function.
- Slowing down motor functions.
- Aging can bring cognitive changes, including slower processing speed, mild memory decline, and potential challenges in attention.
- Some individuals may experience cognitive impairments, such as dementia or Alzheimer's disease.
- Elderly often experiences loss of loved ones. This leads to feelings of grief, adjustment difficulties.
- Social isolation and loneliness can be significant challenges for the elderly.

Psychological Needs of Elderly

- Improvement in self-image
- Need for normal roles and relationships
- Need for love and relatedness
- Sense of hopefulness
- Need for accomplishment of tasks

Role of a Nurse

- Nursing care of elderly is called geriatric nursing
- Elderly should feel respected and valued
- Insecurities and apprehensions should be taken care of. Proper explanation to the patient and family should be provided during hospitalization.
- Elderly might need frequent hospitalization.
- Nurses should be prepared to provide terminal illness care
- Allow elderly to express their emotions and feelings
- Observe the patient for hearing and vision loss
- Prevent bed sores
- Close observations
- Take care of eating and sleeping habits
- Provide warmth and emotional support
- Take care of bowel habits
- In case of mental function decline, give them frequent orientation and observe them
- Protect from injuries and harm
- Keep the side rails up
- Health education

8. Four kinds of emotions noticed during hospitalization.

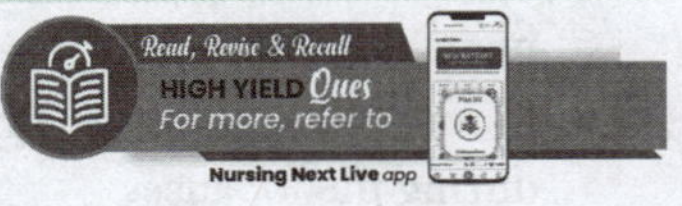

Answer

Hospitalization can be a stressful and emotional experience for patients, and there are several common emotions that patients may experience during their stay.

Four common emotions that are often noticed in patients during hospitalization are as follows:

Fear: Patients may experience fear related to their illness or medical procedures, as well as fear of the unknown. They may worry about their future health, their ability to return to normal life, and their relationships with loved ones.

Anxiety: Hospitalization can also lead to feelings of anxiety, which can manifest as nervousness, restlessness or worry.

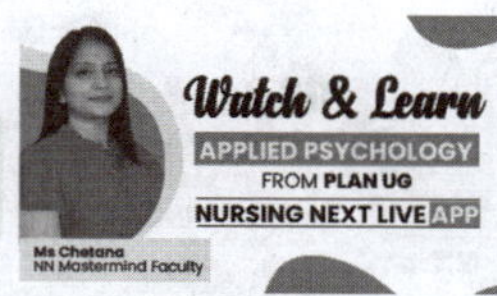

Patients may feel anxious about their medical condition, the hospital environment, and the care they are receiving.

Sadness: Hospitalization can be isolating and can cause patients to feel sad or depressed. They may feel disconnected from their normal routines, social support networks, and may lack sense of purpose. Patients may also feel grief and loss related to their illness or medical condition.

Frustration: Patients may feel frustrated with their medical condition, the hospital environment, and the care they are receiving. They may feel like they have lost control over their lives and their health, and they may feel misunderstood or ignored by health care providers.

SHORT ANSWER QUESTIONS

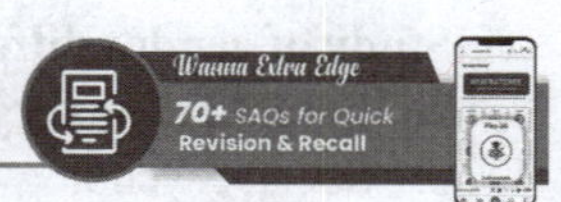

1. Define the term adolescence. (MGR)

Answer

Adolescence is the transitional period between childhood and adulthood, typically starting around the age of 10 to 12 and ending around the age of 18 to 21. It is a time of significant physical, emotional and cognitive development, as individuals undergo rapid changes in their bodies, minds and social roles.

2. Name the vulnerable individuals. (MGR)

Answer

Vulnerable individuals are those who are at higher risk of harm or disadvantage due to various factors that may affect their physical, psychological or social well-being. Some examples of vulnerable individuals include:

- Children
- Elderly
- Pregnant women and new mothers
- Individuals with disabilities
- Individuals with chronic illnesses
- Individuals with mental illness, etc.

3. Name any four psychosocial stages. (MGR)

Answer

- **Stage I:** Trust versus Mistrust (Birth to 1 year)
- **Stage II:** Autonomy versus shame and doubt (1–3 years)
- **Stage III:** Initiative versus guilt (3–6 years)
- **Stage IV:** Industry versus inferiority (6–12 years)
- **Stage V:** Identity versus role confusion (12–18 years)
- **Stage VI:** Intimacy versus isolation (19-25 years)
- **Stage VII:** Generativity versus stagnation (25–64 years)
- **Stage VIII:** Ego integrity versus despair (65 years to death)

4. Psychological reactions to emotions. (MGR)

Answer

Some common psychological reactions to emotions may include:

- Cognitive appraisal
- Physiological arousal
- Subjective experience
- Behavioral expression
- Regulation

5. Mention psychosexual stages by Sigmund Freud (MGR)

Answer

Stage	Age
Oral stage	0–1-year-old
Anal stage	1–3-year-old
Phallic stage	3–6-year-old to puberty
Latent stage	6 to Puberty
Genital stage	Beyond puberty

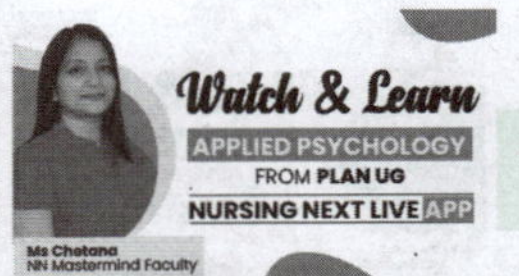

CONCEPTUAL REVISION

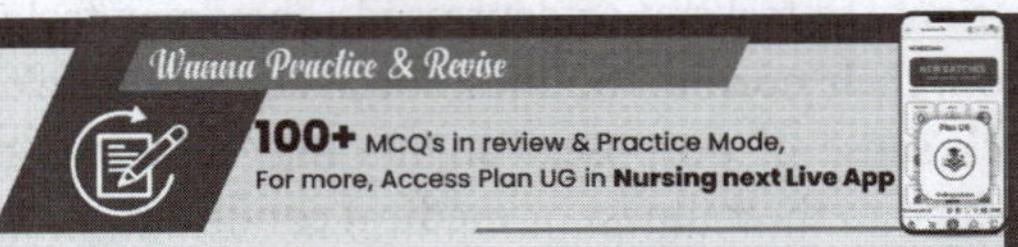

MULTIPLE CHOICE QUESTIONS

1. Oedipus complex (given by Sigmund Freud) is seen in:

a. Boys of 1–3 years of age
b. Girls of 1–3 years of age
c. Boys of 3–5 years of age
d. Girls of 3–5 years of age

Ans. c. Boys of 3–5 years of age

2. If parents encourage their child to ask question, use her imagination and choose some of her activities, they are encouraging:

a. Industry b. Identity
c. Generativity d. Initiative

Ans. d. Initiative

3. Which is not a key feature of resilient child?

a. Pessimistic b. Negative thinking
c. Poor coping skills d. All of these

Ans. d. All of these

4. Ego integrity assessment scale was given by:

a. Freud b. Cattell
c. Allport d. Ryff and Heincke

Ans. d. Ryff and Heincke

5. Which of the following is not seen during the operational period of cognitive development?

a. Reversibility b. Transitivity
c. Conservation d. Animism

Ans. d. Animism

6. Major part of developmental psychology is devoted to the understanding of behavior of:

a. Children b. Adolescents
c. Women d. Old people

Ans. a. Children

7. Study of gender difference is the subject matter of:

a. Industrial and organizational psychology
b. Social psychology
c. Developmental psychology
d. Clinical psychology

Ans. c. Developmental psychology

8. Gaining pleasure through activities of discovering the different properties of tools and materials is defined as:

a. Following rules in play b. Explorative play
c. Dramatic play d. Constructive play

Ans. b. Explorative play

9. Basic psychological needs described by Michael Borg-Laufs are:

a. Orientation and Control
b. Gain of pleasure or control of distress
c. Both a and b
d. None of these

Ans. c. Both a and b

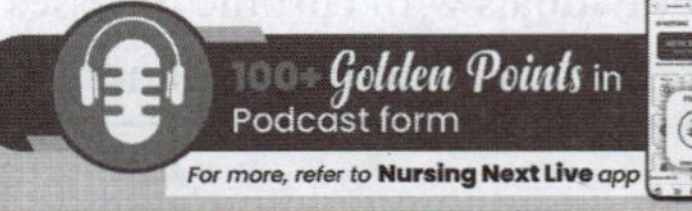

Golden Points

- During childhood (2–12 years), psychological needs for maintaining health and well-being, both in sickness and in health, include cognitive development through play, working memory and recall, activation, controlling emotions, internalizing language, complex problem-solving, emotional development, socialization, and building resilience.
- Early adulthood is characterized by psychological needs for stable, intimate, and positive interpersonal relationships, generativity, and the search for meaning in life.
- Erikson has given developmental stages, wherein a human being has different sets of needs and upon fulfilment of those needs he/she enjoys a joyous, comfortable and psychologically healthy and self-satisfactory life.
- In adolescence, psychological needs for maintaining health and well-being encompass developing a sense of identity, self-acceptance, autonomy, competence, and relatedness.
- Late adulthood involves psychological needs for ego integrity, social support, and spiritual growth to maintain health and well-being, regardless of sickness or wellness.

CHAPTER

5

Personality

CONCEPTUAL THEORY

Terminology

Conscious: All memories that remain in an individual's awareness.
Defense Mechanism: It is the tactic developed by the ego for protection against anxiety.
Ego: It works on reality principle. Ego denies Id's desire and it is unpleasant for the individual.
Extrovert: Person is sociable, friendly, not easily upset by difficulties and is a man of action.
Id: It includes all basic biological drives such as hunger, thirst, self-preservation and sex. It works on pleasure principle.
Introvert: Person is shy and reserved, and prefers to work alone and avoids social contacts.
Melancholic: Individual is sad, depressed, pessimistic, dejected, deplorable and self-involved.
Personality: Personality refers to the deeply ingrained patterns of behavior, which include the way one relates to, perceives and thinks about the environment and oneself. —American Psychological Association (APA), 1987.
Sanguine: Individual is optimistic, happy, hopeful, accommodating, light-hearted and cheerful.
Superego: It is the moral aspect of the personality. It is learned from the society from preschool age onward such as rules, customs, values.

DEFINITION

Personality refers to the deeply ingrained patterns of behavior, which include the way one relates to, perceives and thinks about the environment and oneself.

—**American Psychological Association (APA), 1987**

Personality is the dynamic organization within the individual of those psychophysical systems that determine his unique adjustments to the environment. —**Allport G 1937**

Determinants of Personality

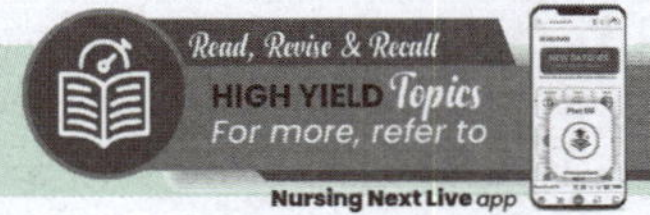

Genetics and Heredity

Physique

Someone with a pleasing physical appearance tends to possess self-assurance, composure and independence.

Biological

Biological factors, including brain structure, neurochemical processes, and hormonal influences, can impact personality.

Environment

Environmental factors, such as family, peers, and socio-cultural influences, contribute to personality development.

Society

Social values and norms play a crucial role in teaching a child to be compliant, respectful and capable of socializing effectively.

Psychological Factors

Factors including motives, interests, attitudes, intellectual abilities, reasoning skills, attention span, perception, imagination, decision-making capabilities, etc. influence the personality in a broad manner.

Society

- Society has a significant impact on one's personality.
- Social values and norms play a crucial role in teaching a child to be compliant, respectful and capable of socializing effectively.

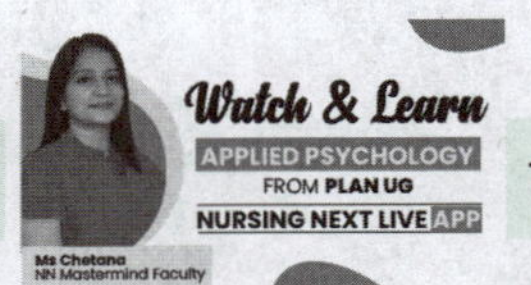

Psychological

The development of personality is influenced by a wide range of factors, including motives, interests, attitudes, intellectual abilities, reasoning skills, attention span, perception, imagination, decision-making capabilities, problem-solving aptitude, adjustment skills, and the ability to maintain healthy relationships.

Topography of Personality

Freud divided the structure of mind into three levels, such as the conscious, the preconscious or the subconscious and the unconscious.

Conscious: All memories that remain in an individual's awareness. It comprises smaller portion in which the events or experiences are easily remembered and retrieved.

Preconscious: All memories that have been forgotten or are not present in present awareness, but with attention can readily be recalled into consciousness.

Unconscious: The unconscious mind stores all memories that are inaccessible to conscious awareness. Memories are suppressed and can only be brought to the surface through therapeutic methods, hypnosis, or substances that modify awareness and have the ability to reorganize repressed memories.

Classification of Personality

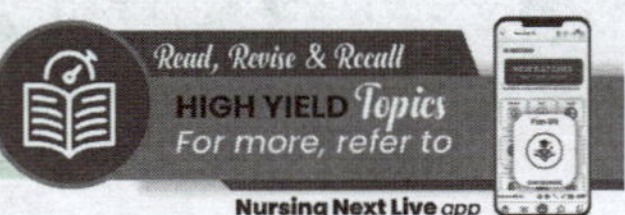

Sr. no.	Classification	Types	Description
1.	Hippocrates	Sanguine	Blood as the body fluid. Optimistic, happy, hopeful, accommodating, light-hearted and cheerful.
		Phlegmatic	Phlegm as the body fluid. Cold, calm, slow and indifferent.
		Melancholic	Black bile as the body fluid. Sad, depressed, pessimistic, dejected, deplorable and self-involved
		Choleric	Yellow bile as the body fluid. Irritable, hot tempered, passionate, strong, active, imaginative
2.	Bhagavad Gita	Tamasik (tamoguna)	Arrogant and self-centered
		Rajasik (rajaguna)	Passionate, active and dynamic
		Satvik (satvaguna)	Wise, knowledgeable with pure soul, believes in good deeds
3.	Kretschmer	Pyknic	Obese, may be sociable, jolly, easy-going, and good natured
		Athletic	A balanced body, energetic, optimistic, aggressive and adjustable.
		Asthenic	Lean and thin, may exhibit characteristics such as reserved, unsociable, shy and pessimistic.
4.	Sheldon	Endomorphic	Highly developed viscera, but weak somatic structure, appears fat, soft and round (like pyknic type). Easy going, sociable, affectionate and fond of eating.
		Mesomorphic	Balanced development of viscera and strong somatic structure muscular (like athletic type). Craving for muscular activity, self-assertive, loves risk and adventure, energetic and bold tempered.
		Ectomorphic	The individual has weak somatic structure as well as underdeveloped viscera, thin, long, fragile (like leptosomatic type). Pessimistic, unsociable, reserved, brainy, artistic and introvert.
5.	Allport	Ascendant	They tend to dominate a situation. Outgoing and interested in the world.
		Descendant	Submissive, self-critical, self-analytical and indecisive. Daydreaming and withdraws from social or competitive situations.

Contd...

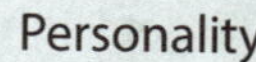

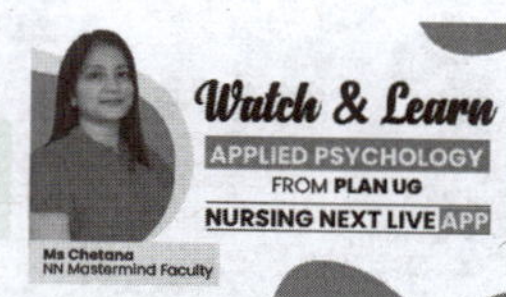

Sr. no.	Classification	Types	Description
6.	Carl Jung	Extrovert	Sociable, friendly, not easily upset by difficulties and are the men of action.
		Introvert	Have their own feelings, emotions and reactions and are found aloof and withdrawn. Shy and reserved and prefer to work alone and avoid social contacts
7.	According to Type A and Type B	Type A personality	Hardworking and competitive, live under high pressure, largely of their own making, seek recognition and advancement, function well as alert, competent, efficient
		Type B personality	Easy going, noncompetitive, placid, unflappable and can bear stress easily

Dynamics of Personality

Id: It includes all basic biological drives such as hunger, thirst, self-preservation and sex. It works on pleasure principle.

Ego: It works on reality principle. Ego denies Id's desire and it is unpleasant for the individual.

Superego: It is the moral aspect of the personality. It is learned from the society from preschool age onward such as rules, customs, values.

Psychosocial Theory of Personality Development

Refer to theory section chapter 4 pg. 912

Maslow's Humanistic Theory of Personality

Abraham Maslow states that people achieve their full potential by meeting their needs, moving from basic needs to self-actualization.

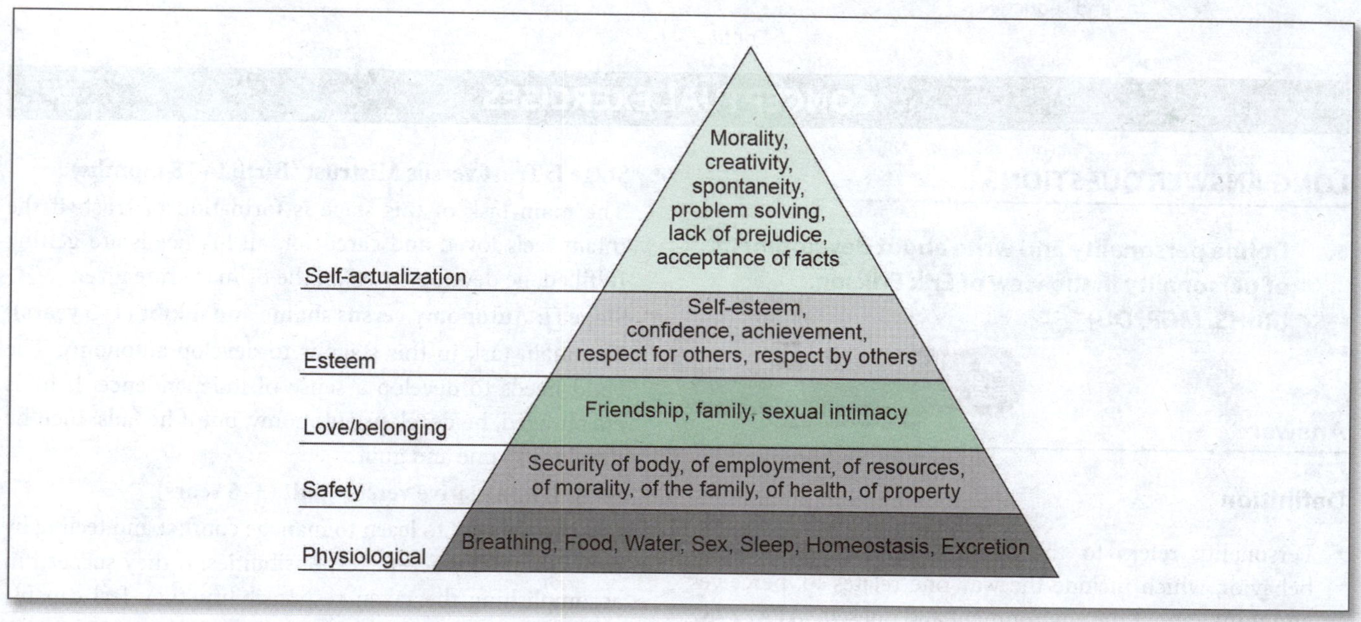

Figure 5.1: Maslow's hierarchy of needs

PSYCHOMETRIC ASSESSMENTS OF PERSONALITY

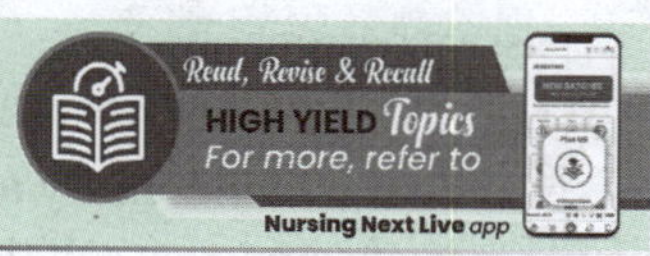

Personality test:
Interviews
Projective tests:
Rorschach
Thematic apperception test

Contd...

Behavioral assessments:
Direct observation
Rating scales
Frequency counts
Personality inventories:
The Minnesota multiphasic personality inventory (MMPI)
Millon clinical multiaxial inventory (MCMI)
California psychological inventory (CPI)
Myers-Briggs Type Indicators (MBTI)
Cattell's 16 Personality Factor (16PF)

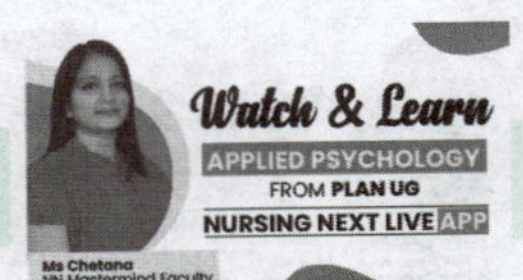

ALTERATIONS IN PERSONALITY

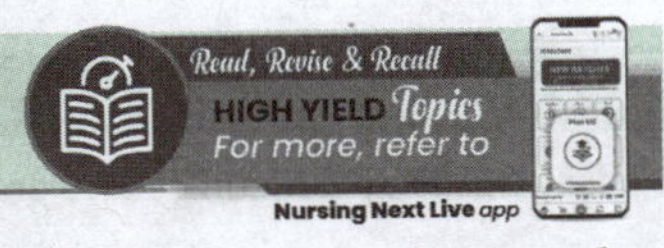

DSM-IV defines a personality disorder in terms of personality traits that are "inflexible and maladaptive and that cause significant functional impairment and subjective distress."

DSM 5 category	Primary characteristics
Cluster A: The odd or eccentric cluster of personality disorders	
Schizoid	Being isolated from others, with absence of emotional expression
Paranoid	Suspicious, being lonely, envious, chronically hostile, tense
Schizotypal	Odd mannerisms or appearances or experiences; often detached from other persons
Cluster B: The dramatic/emotional/erratic cluster of personality disorders	
Histrionic	Often seeks attention of others, shallow in nature, shows exaggerated emotions and seductive

Contd...

DSM 5 category	Primary characteristics
Narcissistic	High self-esteem, low empathy toward others, feels entitled toward the special privileges
Antisocial	Violating rights of others, being manipulative, absence of honest behavior, does not feel guilt for his/her actions.
Borderline	Lack of stable mood, impulsive behavior, angry, interpersonal turmoil, lack of a coherent sense toward the self
Cluster C: Anxious or fearful disorders	
Avoidant personality disorder	Social inhibition, feelings of inadequacy, extreme sensitivity to negative evaluation and avoidance of social interaction.
Dependent personality disorder	Pervasive psychological dependence on other people.
Obsessive-compulsive personality disorder	Characterized by rigid conformity to rules, moral codes and excessive orderliness

CONCEPTUAL EXERCISES

LONG ANSWER QUESTIONS

1. Define personality and write about development of personality in the view of Erik Erikson. (RUHS, MGR, DU)

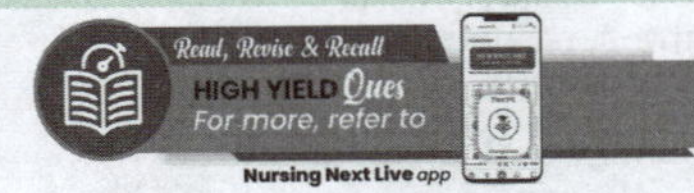

Answer

Definition

- Personality refers to the deeply ingrained patterns of behavior, which include the way one relates to, perceives and thinks about the environment and oneself. **APA, 1987**
- Personality is the dynamic organization within the individual of those psychophysical systems that determine his unique adjustments to the environment. **Allport G, 1937**

Development of Personality in the View of Erik Erikson

Psychosocial Stages of Personality Development

- Psychosocial theory was proposed by Erik Erikson (1902–1994), who was a German psychoanalyst. He did not believe in the involvement of sexual pleasure in development of personality.
- He said that social relationship, parents and peers and others play an important role in the personality development. He explained stages of psychosocial development.
- **Stage I: Trust versus Mistrust (Birth to 18 months)**
  The main task of this stage is formation of trust. If the infant feels loved and cared for, all his needs are getting fulfilled, he develops trust on the primary care giver.
- **Stage II: Autonomy versus shame and doubt (1–3 years)**
  The main task in this stage is to develop autonomy. The child needs to develop a sense of independence. If he is encouraged, he develops autonomy, but if he fails, then he develops shame and guilt.
- **Stage III: Initiative versus guilt (3–6 years)**
  Preschoolers try to learn to manage conflict and feeling by their own. They accept responsibilities, if they succeed in accomplishing the taken responsibility, they feel capable and develop initiative. If they fail in taking responsibility, they feel irresponsible, anxious and guilty and become passive personality.
- **Stage IV: Industry versus inferiority (6–12 years)**
  In this stage, children try to learn new skills and they have a sense of competence. If they successfully learn new skills, they develop a sense of industry, competence and self-esteem. If children fail to develop new abilities, they feel incompetent, inadequate, unmotivated and inferior.
- **Stage V: Identity versus role confusion (12–18 years)**
  Adolescent wants to develop a self-identity. Successfully completing this stage leads to a strong sense of self that will remain throughout life. If it is unsuccessful resolution, they become rebellion, resort to substance abuse, have difficulty keeping personal relationship.

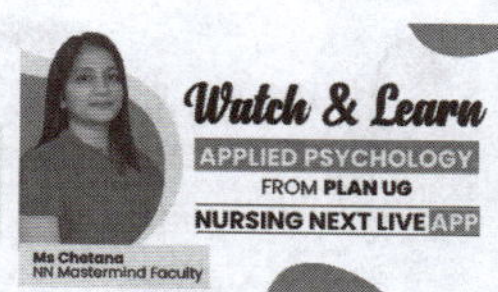

- **Stage VI: Intimacy versus isolation (18–25 years)**
  This stage involves development of intimate, meaningful and loving relationships with other people. Success at this stage leads to close personal relationships, and failure, on the other hand, can result in emotional immaturity, feelings of loneliness and isolation.
- **Stage VII: Generativity versus stagnation (26–64 years)**
  The middle adults are involved in caring and nurturing their children. They will be creative and productive. Successful adults will contribute to family and the society. Stagnation occurs if they fail to contribute, and are unable to show concern for anyone except self.
- **Stage VIII: Ego integrity versus despair (65 years to death)**
  Older adults look back on the life they have lived and come away with either a sense of fulfillment from a life that is well lived or a sense of regret and despair over a life of failures. They accept responsibility for their own self and life.

Table 5.1: Erikson's Psychosocial stages summary chart

State	Basic conflict	Important events
Infancy (birth to 18 months)	Trust vs. Mistrust	Feeding/Comfort
Early Childhood (18 months to 3 years)	Autonomy vs. Shame and Doubt	Toilet Training/Dressing
Preschool (3–6 years)	Initiative vs. Guilt	Exploration/Play
School age (6–12 years)	Industry vs. Inferiority	School/Activities
Adolescence (12–18 years)	Identity vs. Role Confusion	Social Relationship/Identity
Young adult (19–40 years)	Intimacy vs. Isolation	Intimate Relationships
Middle adulthood (40–65 years)	Generativity vs. Stagnation	Work and Parenthood
Maturity (65+ years)	Ego Identity vs. Despair	Reflection on life

2. How personality is developed according to psychoanalytic theory? (MGR, DU)

Answer

Definition

- Personality refers to the deeply ingrained patterns of behavior, which include the way one relates to, perceives and thinks about the environment and oneself.
  —**APA, 1987**
- Personality is the dynamic organization within the individual of those psychophysical systems that determine his unique adjustments to the environment.
  —**Allport G, 1937**

Personality Development in the View of Sigmund Freud

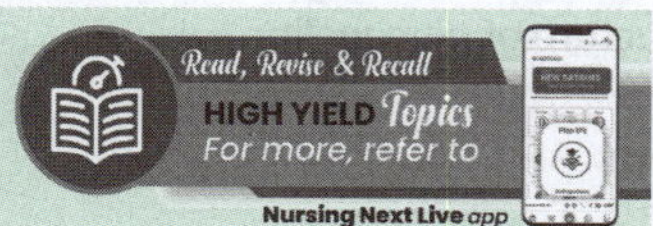

- **Topography of personality:** Sigmund Freud compared the mind with iceberg. He divided the structure into three levels. The levels are the conscious, the preconscious or the subconscious, and the unconscious.
  1. **Conscious:** This level of mind consists of all memories that remain in an individual's awareness. It comprises smaller portion; the events and experiences can be easily remembered and retrieved.
  2. **Preconscious:** This level consists of all the memories that have been forgotten or they are not present in present awareness but with attention they can be readily recalled into consciousness.
  3. **Unconscious:** This level consists of all memories that one is unable to bring to conscious awareness. It is the largest ocean that contains unpleasant or nonessential memories that have been repressed and can be brought back only through therapy, hypnosis and with substances that alter awareness and have the capacity to restructure replaced memories. It is an important determining factor for human behavior and personality. Freudian slip or slip of the tongue is a phenomenon in which words appear to be spoken accidentally but provide a clue to individual's unconscious urges or wishes.
- **Psychoanalytical or Psychosexual theory of personality development**
  - **Dynamics of personality**
- **Id**
  - It works on the pleasure principle.
  - It includes all physiological drives.
  - The human behavior that originates from id is impulsive, pleasure oriented and disconnected from reality.
  - Demands of id are impulsive and irrational.
- **Ego**
  - It works on reality principle.

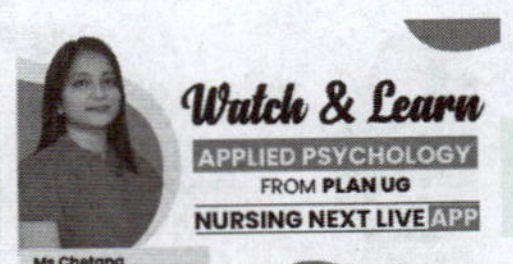

- It is that part of the human personality which is in closest contact with reality.
- It maintains harmony between id, external demands of world and superego.
- Ego is able to postpone the demands until there is appropriate place or time for need fulfillment.
- Ego acts as a mediator.
- Ego-driven behavior is more mature and adaptive.

- **Superego**
  - Superego works on perfection principle.
  - It contains values, legal and moral regulations and social expectations that stop free expression of those behaviors which are pleasure seeking.
  - It is important in the socialization of the individual as it assists the ego in the control of id impulses.

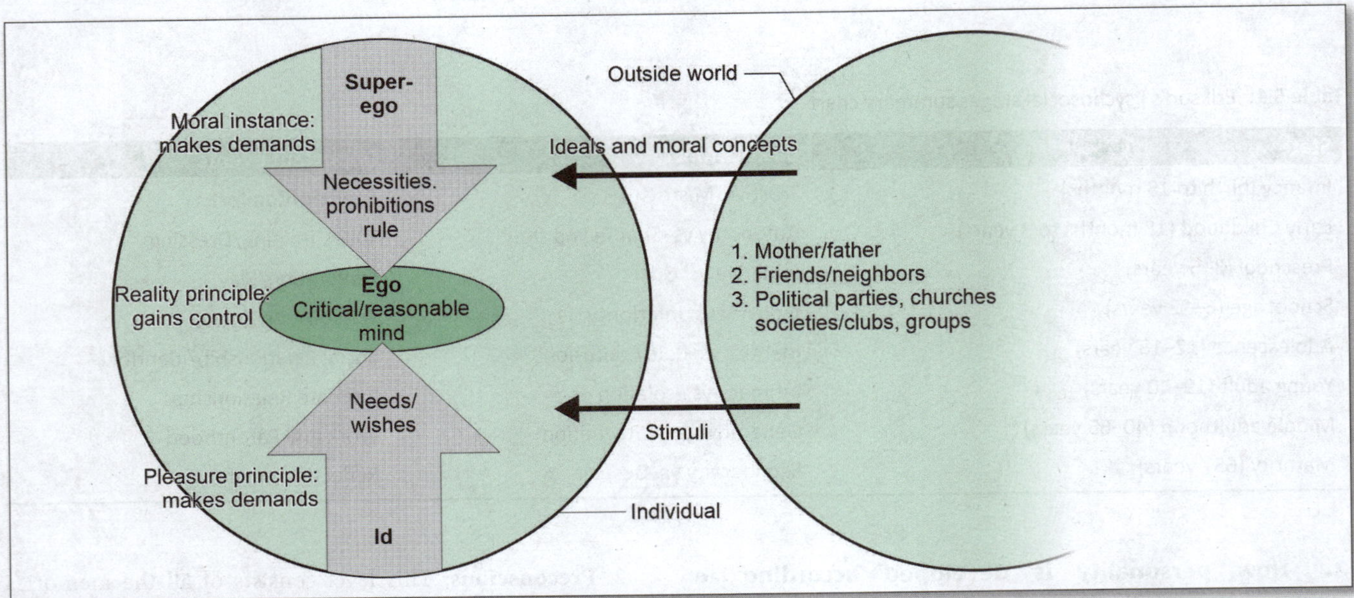

Figure 5.2: Functioning of personality components

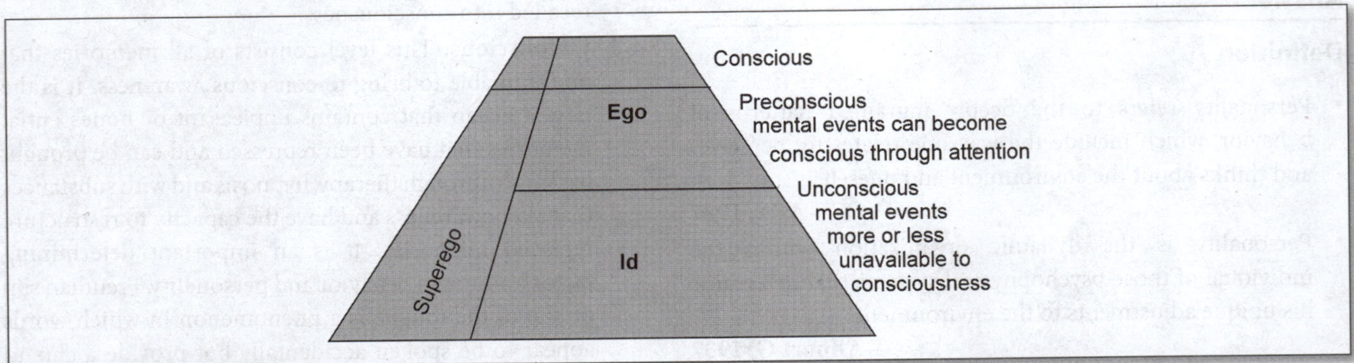

Figure 5.3: Freud's structure of personality

Freud's Psychosexual Stages of Personality Development

Stage	Age range	What happens at this stage?
Oral stage	0–1-year-old	Children derive pleasure from oral activities, including sucking and tasting. They like to put things in their mouth.
Anal stage	2–3-year-old	Children begin potty training.
Phallic stage	3–6-year-old	Boys are more attached to their mother, while girls are more attached to their father.
Latency stage	6-year-old to puberty	Children spend more time and interact mostly with same sex peers.
Genital stage	Beyond puberty	Individuals are attracted to opposite sex peers.

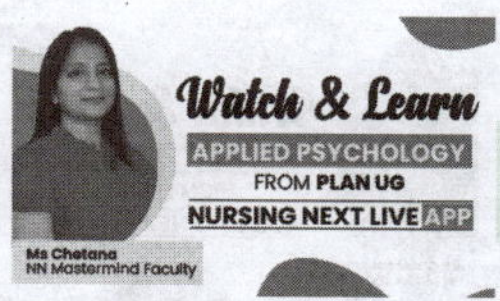

3. **Discuss personality and its classification. (RUHS, MGR, KUHS)**

Answer

Definition

- Personality refers to the deeply ingrained patterns of behavior, which include the way one relates to, perceives and thinks about the environment and oneself.

  —APA, 1987

- Personality is the dynamic organization within the individual of those psychophysical systems that determine his unique adjustments to the environment.

  —Allport G, 1937

  - The term "personality" is derived from Latin word, Persona (mask worn by actors to indicate role of villain or hero in drama).
  - It is the total quality of an individual behavior which will be reflected in his habits, thinking, attitudes, interests, the manner of acting and the personal philosophy of life.
  - It is the sum total of ways in which an individual reacts and interacts with others.
  - Personality is a pattern of stable states and characteristics of a person that influences his or her behavior toward goal achievement. It is the sum total of an individual's traits and characteristics.

The Types of Personality by Various Theorists

Hippocrates Classification of Personality

- **Sanguine:** Blood as the body fluid. The individual will be optimistic, happy, hopeful, accommodating, light-hearted and cheerful.
- **Phlegmatic:** Phlegm as the body fluid. The person will be cold, calm, slow and indifferent.
- **Melancholic:** Black bile as the body fluid. The person will be sad, depressed, pessimistic, dejected, deplorable and self-involved.
- **Choleric:** Yellow bile as the body fluid. The person will be irritable, hot tempered, passionate, strong, active, imaginative.

Classification of Personality According to Sheldon

Sheldon (1954) Classified Personality Based on the Physical Structure

- **Endomorphic:** The person who has highly developed viscera, but weak somatic structure, appears fat, soft and round (like pyknic type). The person will be easy going, sociable, affectionate and fond of eating.
- **Mesomorphic:** The individual has balanced development of viscera and strong somatic structure-muscular (like athletic type). The characteristics of this type of personality are craving for muscular activity, self-assertive, loves risk and adventure, energetic and bold tempered.
- **Ectomorphic:** The individual has weak somatic structure as well as underdeveloped viscera, thin, long fragile (like leptosomatic type). The individual is pessimistic, unsociable, reserved, brainy, artistic and introvert.

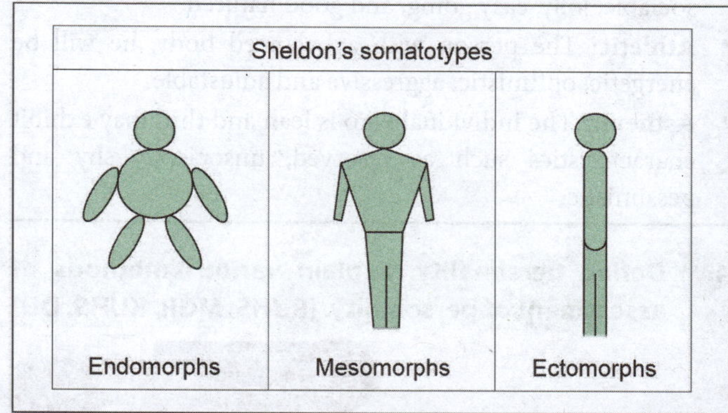

Allport (1961) Classification

Ascendant: They tend to dominate a situation. They are outgoing and interested in the world around them.

Descendant: They are submissive, self-critical, self-analytical and indecisive. They are day dreaming and withdraw from social or competitive situations.

Carl Jung classification:

Extrovert: They are the individuals who are interested in the world around them. They are sociable, friendly, not easily upset by difficulties and are the men of action.

Introvert: They show interest in themselves, they have their own feelings, emotions and reactions and are found aloof and withdrawn. Their nature is shy and reserved and prefer to work alone and avoid social contacts.

Type A and Type B Personality

Type A personality: The individuals are hardworking and competitive, live under high pressure, largely of their own making, seek recognition and advancement, function well as alert, competent, efficient (get things done).

Type B Personality: They are easy going, noncompetitive, placid, unflappable and can bear stress easily. They are likely to live longer than Type A persons and work harder when a deadline is given.

Classification of Personality According to Bhagavad Gita

- **Tamasik (tamoguna):** The individual is arrogant and self-centered
- **Rajasik (rajaguna):** The individual is passionate, active and dynamic

- **Satvik (satvaguna):** The individual is wise, knowledgeable with pure soul, believes in good deeds

Classification of Personlaity According to Kretschmer

Kretschmer (1925) classified personality based on the body structure.

- **Pyknic:** It means the individual who is obese, may be sociable, jolly, easy going, and good natured.
- **Athletic:** The person with a balanced body, he will be energetic, optimistic, aggressive and adjustable.
- **Asthenic:** The individual who is lean and thin may exhibit characteristics such as reserved, unsociable, shy and pessimistic.

4. Define personality. Explain various methods of assessment of personality. (RUHS, MGR, KUHS, DU)

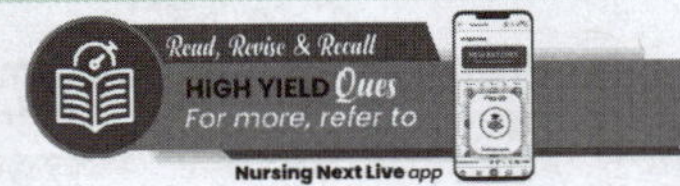

Answer

Definition

- Personality refers to the deeply ingrained patterns of behavior, which include the way one relates to, perceives and thinks about the environment and oneself.

  —**APA, 1987**

- Personality is the dynamic organization within the individual of those psychophysical systems that determine his unique adjustments to the environment.

  —**Allport G, 1937**

Various methods of Personality Assessment

Psychometric Assessments of Personality

There are various techniques which are available to assess the personality. Personality assessment techniques may differ according to the purpose in which they are conducted.

The following are the various methods of personality assessment:

- Interview
- Projective tests
- Behavioural assessments
- Personality inventories
- **Interview:**
  - It involves the face to face interaction between the psychologist and the client.
  - The psychologist or therapist asks questions to the client and allows the client to answer either in a structured or unstructured manner.
  - Client reports innermost feelings, urges and concerns.
  - The main drawback of this technique is that the clients may lie, vanish the truth, misremember or else give the information what they think is said to be a socially acceptable one instead of providing true information.
  - It means that their information can be biased and the psychologist or therapist has to rely on the information provided by them.
  - Psychologists can also form favorable impressions of someone in the first meeting.
- **Projective tests:**
  - The therapist presents an ambiguous visual stimulus to the patient and asks to respond with whatever comes to the mind.
  - The psychologist will interpret the patient's answer to the visual stimulus.
  - It requires lots of experience and it is an art.
  - Projective tests help to uncover the unconscious concerns, fears, conflicts, desires and urges that affect the patient's conscious behavior.
  - This test is very useful in the diagnosis of personality disturbance.
  - It is highly subjective and may not be accurate sometimes.
  - The projective techniques are as follows:
    - **Rorschach inkblots:** This test was developed by Hermann Rorschach in 1921. He used 10 inkblots, 5 in black ink on white background and 5 in colored ink on a white background. The patients were asked to look at each inkblot and they had to say whatever came to their mind by looking at those inkblots. Scores were given based on color, shape, figures in the blot and response to the whole or to details. This technique is very useful in describing personality, diagnosing mental illnesses and in prediction of behavior.
    - **Thematic apperception test:** This test was developed by Morgan and Henry Murray in 1935. In this technique, 31 pictures (black and white) were shown to patients. The patients were asked to tell a story about the person in the picture. The story or interpretation that patient gave about the picture revealed something about their past experience and feelings. These interpretations by patients projected their attitudes, conflicts or any kind of fear.
- **Behavioral assessments:** This is an objective observation of a patient's behavior. These are the techniques used to detect behavioral problems such as inability to pay attention lack of time management skills and impulsivity, etc. The drawbacks may be the observers effect and no control over external environment.
  - **Direct observation:** Direct observation is used to assess someone's behavior. This means observing the individual's behavior to have a correct understanding.
  - **Rating scales:** A Behavior Rating Scale (BRS) is *a tool that can be used to quantitatively measure behavior.* Likert scale is an example.

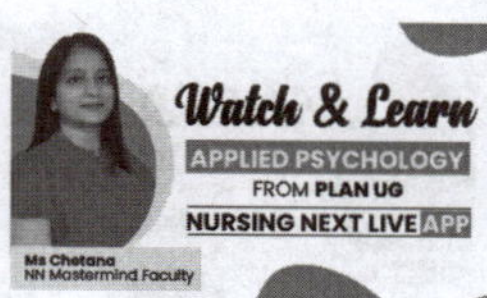

- **Frequency count:** Frequency (or event) recording is *a way to measure the number of times a behavior occurs within a given period.*

- **Personality inventories:** A questionnaire that has a standard list of questions and only requires certain specific answers such as "yes or no" and "cannot decide". It does not have open-ended answers. It is more objective and reliable than projective test. It is a form of self-report. Following are the examples:
  - **MMPI:** The Minnesota Multiphasic Personality Inventory (MMPI) is **a psychological test that assesses personality traits and psychopathology**. It is primarily intended to test people who are suspected of having mental health or other clinical issues.
  - **CPI:** The California Psychological Inventory (CPI) is **a self-report questionnaire** designed to measure normal-range human behavior. It consists of 434 true/false items representing concepts—such as Tolerance, Responsibility, Integrity, Empathy and Self-Control—that are commonly used to describe and understand human behavior.
  - **MBTI:** The Myers–Briggs Type Indicator is an introspective self-report questionnaire indicating differing psychological preferences in how people perceive the world and make decisions.
  - **Cattell's 16 personality factor questionnaire:** The Sixteen Personality Factor Questionnaire (16 PF) measures personality on two hierarchical levels, primary and secondary traits, and has been developed as a result of extensive factor analyses of large arrays of behavioral items.

---

5. Define personality. Describe various theories of personality. (RUHS, KUHS)

Answer

Definition

Personality refers to the deeply ingrained patterns of behavior, which include the way one relates to, perceives and thinks about the environment and oneself. —**APA, 1987**

Theories of Personality

- Personality theories are frameworks that attempt to explain and understand the patterns of thoughts, feelings, and behaviors that make up an individual's personality.
- Personality theories provide different perspectives on how personality develops and how it influences behavior.
- **These theories include**
  - Psychodynamic theory (Sigmund Freud)
  - Psychosocial theory (Erik Erikson)
  - Behaviorist theory (learning and conditioning)
  - Humanistic Theory (E.g., Carl Roger's person centered approach)
  - Trait theory
  - Biological theory
  - Cognitive theory

Psychodynamic Theory

- Freud's psychodynamic theory suggests that personality is shaped by unconscious processes and childhood experiences.
- It emphasizes the importance of the unconscious mind, early childhood experiences, and the interplay between different components of personality, such as the id, ego, and superego.

Psychosocial Theory

- Erik Erikson's theory of personality development describes the psychological and social challenges individuals face throughout their lifespan.
- Erikson proposed eight stages of psychosocial development from infancy to old age, each characterized by a specific conflict or crisis that individuals must successfully resolve to achieve healthy personality development.
- These stages include infancy (trust vs mistrust), Autonomy vs. Early Childhood (Shame and Doubt), Preschool age (Initiative vs. Guilt), School age (Industry vs Inferiority), Adolescence (Identity vs Role confusion), Young adulthood (Intimacy vs Isolation), Middle adulthood (Generativity vs Stagnation), Late adulthood (Integrity vs Despair).

Behaviorist Theory

- Behaviorist theories, rooted in the works of psychologists such as Ivan Pavlov, John B. Watson, and BF Skinner, focus on explaining personality and behavior through the principles of learning and conditioning, e.g., Classical conditioning and Operant conditioning
- They suggest that behavior is influenced by environmental factors, such as rewards and punishments.
- **Classical conditioning:** Classical conditioning (by Ivan Pavlov) suggests that behaviors can be learned through associations between stimuli.
- **Operant conditioning:** Operant conditioning (by BF Skinner) focuses on how behavior is shaped by its consequences. According to this theory, behaviors that are followed by desirable consequences are more likely to be repeated, while behaviors followed by undesirable consequences are less likely to recur.

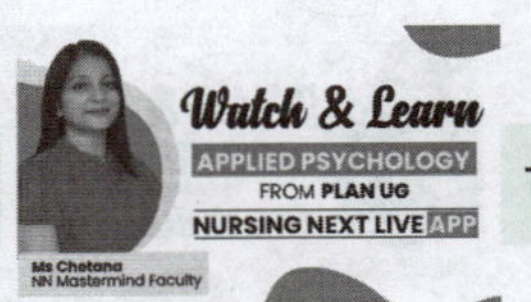

Humanistic Theory

- Humanistic theories, including Carl Rogers' person-centered approach, focus on the subjective experiences and the unique qualities of individuals.
- These theories emphasize the inherent worth and capacity for personal growth within each person.
- Key concepts of this theory include self-concept, self-actualization, and promoting person-centered approach.

Trait Theory

- Trait theories propose that personality consists of a set of stable traits or characteristics that describe and predict an individual's behavior.
- Traits are consistent patterns of thoughts, emotions, and behaviors that tend to be relatively stable over time and across different situations.
- One of the most widely recognized and researched models of trait theory is the Big Five model of personality.
- The Five trait theory or Five-Factor Model (FFM), consists of five broad dimensions of personality that are believed to capture the fundamental traits of individual. it includes Openness to experience, Conscientiousness, Extraversion, Agreeableness, and Neuroticism (OCEAN).

Biological Theory

- Biological theories propose that genetics and physiological factors have a significant impact on the development and expression of personality.
- Biological theories explore the influence of genetic predisposition, brain structure and function, and neurotransmitter on the personality of an individual.
- Twin studies have found that identical twins, who share 100% of their genes, tend to have more similar levels of extraversion than fraternal twins, who share approximately 50% of their genes.

Cognitive Theory

- Cognitive theories focus on how thoughts, beliefs, and perceptions influence personality and behavior.
- These theories emphasize how cognitive processes, such as perception, memory, attention, and problem-solving, influence the way individuals interpret and interact with the world.

6. Define personality and explain the various factors influencing it. (MGR, KUHS)

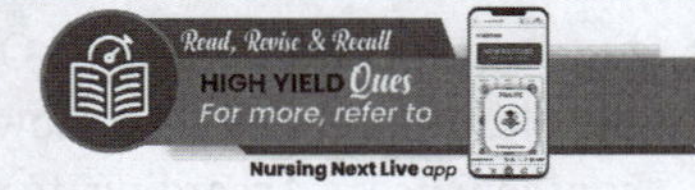

Answer

Definition

- Personality refers to the deeply ingrained patterns of behavior, which include the way one relates to, perceives and thinks about the environment and oneself. —**APA, 1987**
- Personality is the dynamic organization within the individual of those psychophysical systems that determine his unique adjustments to the environment. —**Allport G, 1937**

Factors Influencing Personality

The factors affecting personality can be classified into heredity and environment.

Genetics and Heredity

Physique

- The personality of an individual is influenced by his/her size and strength.
- Someone with a pleasing physical appearance tends to possess self-assurance, composure and independence.
- A strong physique reflects powerful and commanding qualities.

Biological

- Biological factors, including brain structure, neurochemical processes, and hormonal influences, can impact personality. For example, variations in neurotransmitter levels or hormonal imbalances may contribute to differences in temperament or emotional stability.
- A decrease in triiodothyronine (T3) and tetraiodothyronine (T4) levels can result in sluggishness and reduced mental sharpness..

Environment

- Environmental factors, such as family, peers, and socio-cultural influences, contribute to personality development.
- Early childhood experiences, parenting styles, cultural norms, and socialization processes shape an individual's beliefs, values, and behavioral patterns.
- **Home environement:** When a child grows up in an environment characterized by peace, love, understanding, harmony, and respect, the child tends to develop a sense of self-confidence and security.
- If the child is subjected to excessive discipline or overprotection, it may result in the development of a dependent personality.
- **School environment:** Educational experience, extracurricular activities, discipline measures at school, and academic performances can influence the personality.

Society

- Society has a significant impact on one's personality.
- Social values and norms play a crucial role in teaching a child to be compliant, respectful and capable of socializing effectively.

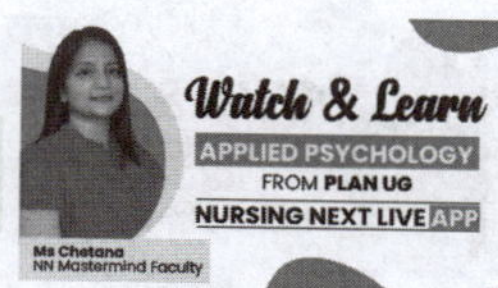

Psychological

The development of personality is influenced by a range of factors, including motives, interests, attitudes, intellectual abilities, reasoning skills, attention span, perception, imagination, decision-making capabilities, problem-solving aptitude, adjustment skills, and the ability to maintain healthy relationships.

SHORT NOTES

1. Mention any four personality inventories. (MGR)

Answer

- **Personality inventories:** A questionnaire that has a standard list of questions and only requires certain specific answers such as "yes or no" and "cannot decide". It does not have open ended answers. It is more objective and reliable than projective test. It is a form of self-report.
- Following are the examples:
  - **MMPI:** The Minnesota Multiphasic Personality Inventory (MMPI) is **a psychological test that assesses personality traits and psychopathology**. It is primarily intended to test people who are suspected of having mental health or other clinical issues.
  - **CPI:** The California Psychological Inventory (CPI) is **a self-report questionnaire** designed to measure normal-range human behavior. It consists of 434 true/false items representing concepts—such as Tolerance, Responsibility, Integrity, Empathy and Self-Control—that are commonly used to describe and understand human behavior.
  - **MBTI:** The Myers–Briggs Type Indicator is an introspective self-report questionnaire indicating differing psychological preferences in how people perceive the world and make decisions.
  - **Cattell's 16 personality factor questionnaire:** The Sixteen Personality Factor Questionnaire (16 PF) measures personality on two hierarchical levels, primary and secondary traits, and has been developed as a result of extensive factor analyses of large arrays of behavioral items.

2. Name four projective tests of personality. (MGR)

Answer

Psychometric Assessments of Personality

- There are various techniques which are available to assess the personality. Personality assessment techniques may differ according to the purpose in which they are conducted.
- **Projective tests:**
  - The therapist presents an ambiguous visual stimulus to the patient and asks to respond with whatever comes to mind.
  - The psychologist will interpret the patient's answer to the visual stimulus.
  - It requires lots of experience and it is an art.
  - Projective tests help to uncover the unconscious concerns, fears, conflicts, desires and urges that affect the patient's conscious behavior.
  - This test is very useful in the diagnosis of personality disturbance.
  - It is highly subjective and may not be accurate sometimes.
  - The projective techniques are as follows:
- **Rorschach inkblots:**
  - This test was developed by Hermann Rorschach in 1921.
  - He used 10 inkblots, 5 in black ink on white background and 5 in colored inks on a white background.
  - The patients were asked to look at each inkblot and they had to say whatever came to their mind by looking at those inkblots.
  - Scores were given based on color, shape, figures in the blot and response to the whole or to details.
  - This technique is very useful in describing personality, diagnosing mental illnesses and in prediction of behavior.
- **Thematic Apperception Test:**
  - This test was developed by Morgan and Henry Murray in 1935.
  - In this technique, 31 pictures (black and white) were shown to clients.
  - The patients were asked to tell a story about the person in the picture. The story or interpretation that patient gave about the picture revealed something about their past experience and feelings.
  - These interpretations by patients projected their attitudes, conflicts or any kind of fear.
- **Sentence completion test is a** type of semi-structured projective technique. Sentence completion tests provide patients with beginnings of sentences, referred to as "stems", and patients then complete the sentences in ways that are meaningful to them. The responses are believed to provide indications of attitudes, beliefs, motivations, or other mental states.

  Therefore, sentence completion technique, with such advantage, encourages the patients to disclose their concealed feelings.
- **The Draw-a-Person test** is a psychological projective personality or cognitive test in which the test subject uses simple art supplies to produce depictions of people. It is used to evaluate children and adolescents for a variety of purposes.

3. Extrovert personality. (KUHS)

Answer

According to psychologists like Carl Jung, extroversion or extraversion is a personality type that feels energized in the company of others. Extroverts feel a sense of purpose when they interact with new people or participate in networking events. They are outgoing and cheerful.

Characteristics of an Extrovert

Here are some characteristics of an extrovert:

1. Enjoy social gatherings and events

People with extrovert personality enjoy social gatherings and events. They initiate conversations, crack jokes and break the ice among a group of strangers. They are like life of the party. They're more likely to host events and flock from one group to another to include everyone in the conversation.

2. Love to talk to people

Extroverts love to talk and have long conversations with other people. They seek out new people so that they can get to know them and exchange thoughts and opinions.

Extroverts are not afraid to talk about their feelings and may even reach out to people, if they need help.

Facing their problems head-on and finding creative solutions are some of the things that come easily to them.

3. Engage in group activities

People with extrovert personality engage in group activities. In school children with extrovert personality take part in group projects and get involved in planning. They are the ones who bring other people together as a group. They enjoy participating in debates on various topics. They can light up a room with their energy, which may even energize others.

4. Not afraid to take risks

People with extrovert personality are not afraid to take risks and experience new things. They like to explore and do some adventure. They're the ones who volunteer to go up on stage during a performance or a magic show. They aren't afraid of judgment or concerned with what people might think.

4. Theories of personality. (KUHS)

Answer

Theories of Personality

For answer, refer to Q. 5 Long Answer Questions

5. Sheldon's theory of personality – explain.

Answer

Sheldon (1954) Classified Personality Based on the Physical Structure

- **Endomorphic:** The person has highly developed viscera, but weak somatic structure, appears fat, soft and round (like pyknic type). The person will be easy going, sociable, affectionate and fond of eating.
- **Mesomorphic:** The individual has balanced development of viscera and strong somatic structure-muscular (like athletic type). The characteristics of this type of personality are craving for muscular activity, self-assertive, risk and adventure, loving, energetic and bold tempered.
- **Ectomorphic**: The individual has weak somatic structure as well as underdeveloped viscera, thin, long fragile (like leptosomatic type). The individuals is pessimistic, unsociable, reserved, brainy, artistic and introvert.

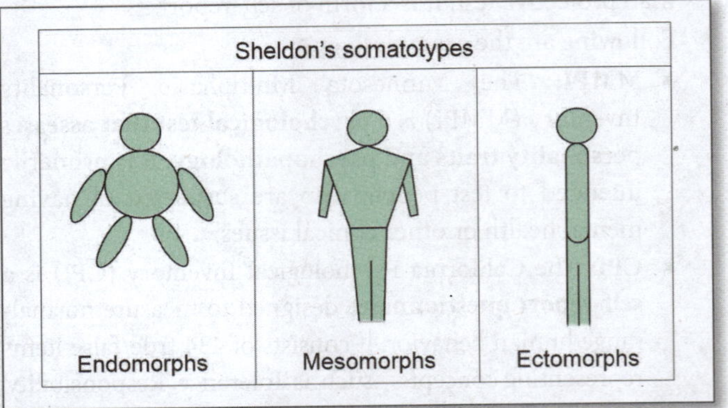

SHORT ANSWER QUESTIONS

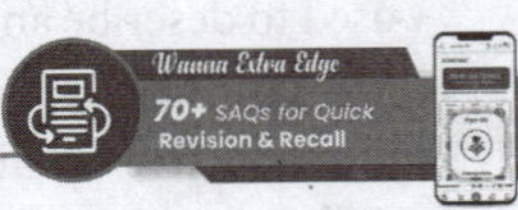

1. Types of personality.

Answer

Hippocrates classification of personality	Sanguine, Phlegmatic, Melancholic, Choleric
Bhagavad Gita	Tamasik (tamoguna), Rajasik (rajaguna), Satvik (satvaguna)
Kretschmer	Pyknic, Athletic, Asthenic
Sheldon	Endomorphic, Mesomorphic, Ectomorphic
Allport	Ascendant, Descendant
Carl Jung classification	Extrovert, Introvert
Type A and Type B personality	Type A and Type B

2. Define CPI.

Answer

CPI: The California Psychological Inventory (CPI) is **a self-report questionnaire** designed to measure normal-range human behavior. It consists of 434 true/false items representing concepts—such as Tolerance, Responsibility, Integrity, Empathy, and Self-Control—that are commonly used to describe and understand human behavior.

3. Rorschach inkblot test.

Answer

Rorschach inkblots

- This is a projective test which works on projection principle.
- This test was developed by Hermann Rorschach in 1921.
- He used 10 inkblots, 5 in black on white background and 5 in colored inks on a white background.
- The patients were asked to look at each inkblot and they had to say whatever came to their mind by looking at those inkblots.
- Scores were given based on color, shape, figures in the blot and response to the whole story or to details.
- This technique is very useful in describing personality, diagnosing mental illnesses and in prediction of behavior.

4. Define MMPI.

Answer

MMPI: The Minnesota Multiphasic Personality Inventory (MMPI) is **a psychological test that assesses personality traits and psychopathology**. It is primarily intended to test people who are suspected of having mental health or other clinical issues.

5. Any four ego mechanisms.

Answer

- **Denial**
- **Sublimation**
- **Displacement**
- **Reaction formation**

6. Four projective techniques.

Answer

Projective Techniques

- Rorschach inkblot test
- Thematic apperception test
- Word association test
- Sentence completion test

7. Define BAI.

Answer

BAI stands for "Beck Anxiety Inventory." It is a self-report questionnaire that measures the severity of anxiety symptoms in adults and adolescents.

- The BAI is used by mental health professionals to diagnose anxiety disorders and to monitor treatment progress.
- It consists of 21 items that assess physical, cognitive and emotional symptoms of anxiety, such as nervousness, worry and fear.
- Each item is rated on a scale of 0 to 3 based on the severity of symptoms experienced in the past week. The total score ranges from 0 to 63, with higher scores indicating more severe anxiety symptoms.

8. Any four methods of studying behavior.

Answer

- Observation
- Self-report
- Experiments
- Case Studies

9. Define TAT.

Answer

Thematic Apperception Test (TAT)

- This is one of the projective techniques.
- This test works on projection principle and reveals hidden thoughts, fears and beliefs of the examinee.
- This test was developed by Morgan and Henry Murray in 1935.
- In this technique, 31 pictures (black and white) are shown to examinee.

- Then the examinee is asked to tell a story about the person in the picture.
- The story told by the examinee reveals something about their past experience and feelings.
- The whole exercise is noted by the examiner and then interpretations are made.
- Then examiner interprets the examinee's personality based on the findings.

10. Definition of Personality.

Answer

Personality refers to the deeply ingrained patterns of behavior, which include the way one relates to, perceives and thinks about the environment and oneself. —**APA, 1987**

Personality is the dynamic organization within the individual of those psychophysical systems that determine his unique adjustments to the environment. —**Allport G, 1937**

11. Meaning of defense mechanism.

Answer

- Defense mechanism is also known as mental mechanism or ego mechanism and it is a method of coping and the way one can adapt to stressors physically and psychologically.
- Sigmund Freud, the "Father of modern psychiatry", coined the term defense mechanism.
- He defined defense mechanism as unconscious processes that defend a person against anxiety.

12. Name the four principles of classical conditioning.

Answer

The four principles of classical conditioning are:

1. Unconditioned stimulus (UCS)
2. Unconditioned response (UCR)
3. Conditioned stimulus (CS)
4. Conditioned response (CR)

13. Define ego.

Answer

Ego

- It works on reality principle.
- It is that part of the human personality which is in closest contact with reality.
- It maintains harmony between id, external demands of world and superego.
- Ego is able to postpone the demands until there is appropriate place or time for need fulfillment.
- Ego acts as a mediator.
- Ego-driven behavior is more mature and adaptive.

14. Classical conditioning

Answer

Classical conditioning is a type of learning that was first described by Ivan Pavlov. The process of classical conditioning involves repeated pairing of the neutral stimulus (conditioned stimulus-CS) with the unconditioned stimulus (UCS) until the neutral stimulus alone elicits a response (CR) similar to the unconditioned response (UCR). This association is known as conditioned learning.

15. Mention any four personality inventories.

Answer

- **Personality inventories:** A questionnaire that has a standard list of questions and only requires certain specific answers such as "yes or no" and "cannot decide". It does not have open ended answers. It is more objective and reliable than projective test. It is a form of self-report. Following are the examples:
    - **MMPI:** The Minnesota Multiphasic Personality Inventory
    - **CPI:** The California Psychological Inventory (CPI)
    - **MBTI:** The Myers-Briggs Type Indicator
    - **Cattell's 16 personality factor questionnaire**

CONCEPTUAL REVISION

MULTIPLE CHOICE QUESTIONS

1. Which of the following is not a defense mechanism?

a. Self-esteem b. Regression
c. Projection d. Sublimation

Ans. a. Self-esteem

2. The MMPI is used to measure:

a. Leadership potential
b. The Big Five traits
c. Personality and psychological disorders
d. Unconscious drives

Ans. c. Personality and psychological disorders

3. Which of the following personality test works on the principle of projection?

a. Thematic apperception test
b. MMPI
c. Interview method
d. Observation method

Ans. a. Thematic apperception test

4. Sheldon proposed the traits that would best describe a football player would be:

a. Ectomorph b. Endomorph
c. Mesomorph d. Activomorph

Ans. c. Mesomorph

5. Which of the personality types best describes sociable and easy-going characteristics according to Kretschmer's classification?

a. Athletic b. Pyknic
c. Leptosomatic d. Endomorph

Ans. b. Pyknic

6. In which of the following personality types, philosophers and scientists fall according to Jung's classification?

a. Extrovert b. Introvert
c. Mesomorph d. Pyknic

Ans. b. Introvert

7. All of the following are the three levels of awareness; except:

a. Conscientiousness b. Conscious
c. Preconscious d. Unconscious

Ans. a. Conscientiousness

8. One trait that dominates a personality so much that it influences nearly everything a person does is a:

a. Global Trait b. Central Trait
c. Specific Trait d. Cardinal Trait

Ans. d. Cardinal Trait

9. Most subjective method for measuring personality of a child is:

a. Projective method b. Interview method
c. Questionnaire method d. Sociometry method

Ans. c. Questionnaire method

10. Thematic Apperception Test (TAT) of measuring personality is a:

a. Subjective technique
b. Objective technique
c. Projective technique
d. Experimental technique

Ans. c. Projective technique

Golden Points

- A personality disorder is an enduring pattern of inner experience and behavior that is extremely inflexible, deviates markedly from the expectations of a person's culture, and causes personal distress or behavioral impairment.
- Cluster A: The Odd or Eccentric Cluster of Personality Disorders – Schizoid, Paranoid, Schizotypal type.
- Cluster B: The Dramatic/Emotional/Erratic Cluster of Personality Disorders – Histrionic, Narcissistic, Antisocial and Borderline type.
- Cluster C: Anxious or fearful disorders - Avoidant personality disorder, Dependent personality disorder and Obsessive-compulsive personality disorder.
- Psychometric assessments of personality include projective tests (Rorschach inkblot test, Thematic Apperception Test), Behavioral Assessments (Direct Observation, Rating Scales and Frequency Counts), Personality Inventories (The Minnesota Multiphasic Personality Inventory, Millon Clinical Multiaxial Inventory, California Psychological Inventory (CPI), Myers-Briggs Type Indicator (MBTI), and Cattell's 16 Personality Factor questionnaire.

CHAPTER

6

Cognitive Process

CONCEPTUAL THEORY

Terminology

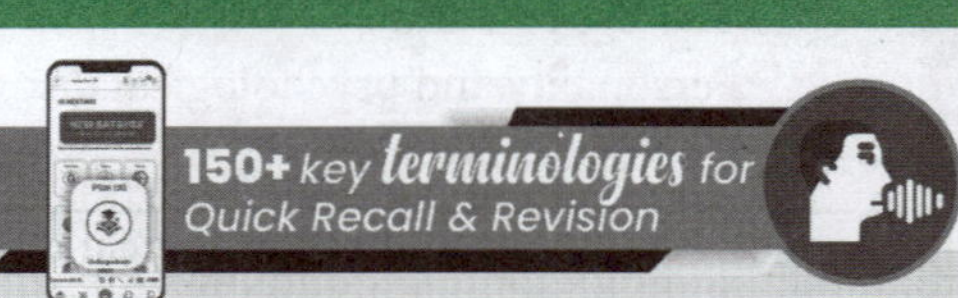

Aptitude: Aptitude refers to a person's innate or acquired capacity or potential to perform certain tasks, skills, or activities.

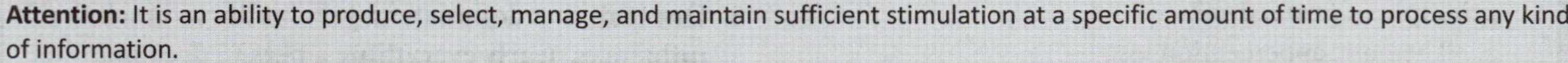

Attention: It is an ability to produce, select, manage, and maintain sufficient stimulation at a specific amount of time to process any kind of information.

Bloom's taxonomy levels of thinking: According to the theory, thinking process consists of six categories, knowledge, comprehension, application, analysis, synthesis and evaluation.

Cognition: Cognition is a basic mental process like sensation, attention, perception and complex mental operations such as intelligence, reasoning, decision-making, memory and problem-solving.

Forgetting: According to Munn (1967), forgetting is the loss of permanent or temporary memory. It is the ability to recall or recognize something learned earlier.

Intelligence: Intelligence is the aggregate or global capacity of the individual to think rationally, to act purposefully and to deal effectively with the environment. —Wechsler 1994

Learning: Learning is the conservation of new behavior or the strengthening and weakening of old behavior as a result of experience. —Henry Smith

Memory: Memory is the faculty of the brain by which data or information is encoded, stored and retrieved when needed.

Perception: Perception is the process of organization, identification and interpretation of sensory stimulus in order to represent and understand the current information or environment.

Thinking: Thinking is a mental activity in its cognitive aspect or mental activity with regard to psychological aspects. (Rose)

ATTENTION

Definition

Attention is an ability to produce, select, manage, and maintain sufficient stimulation at a specific amount of time to process any kind of information.

Types of Attention

- **Selective attention**
  - This refers to the ability to focus on a specific stimulus while ignoring other irrelevant stimuli.
  - Selective attention allows individuals to prioritize and concentrate on relevant information.
- **Divided attention**
  - Divided attention involves the ability to allocate and sustain attention across multiple tasks or stimuli simultaneously.
  - It is the capacity to attend to and process multiple sources of information simultaneously.
- **Sustained attention**
  - Sustained attention is the ability to maintain focus and concentration on a particular task or stimulus over an extended period.
  - It is often associated with tasks that require vigilance and continuous mental effort.
- **Visual attention**
  - Visual attention pertains to the selection and processing of visual stimuli in the environment.
  - It involves the ability to give direct attention to specific visual features or locations.
- **Auditory attention**
  - Auditory attention involves the selection and processing of auditory stimuli.
  - It refers to the ability to focus on specific sounds or voices while filtering out irrelevant auditory information.

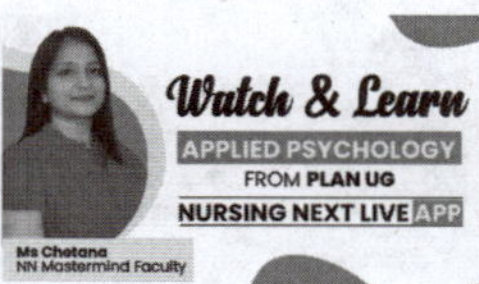

- **Executive attention**
  - Executive attention involves higher-level cognitive processes that facilitate goal-directed behavior, decision-making, and inhibitory control.
  - It plays a crucial role in tasks requiring planning, problem-solving, and cognitive flexibility.
- **Bottom-up and top-down attention**
  - Bottom-up attention refers to attentional processes that are driven by the sensory characteristics of stimuli, such as salience or novelty.
  - Top-down attention, on the other hand, involves attentional processes guided by cognitive factors, such as expectations, goals, and prior knowledge.

PERCEPTION

Meaning

Perception is the process of organization, identification and interpretation of sensory stimulus in order to represent and understand the current information or environment.

Principles of Perception

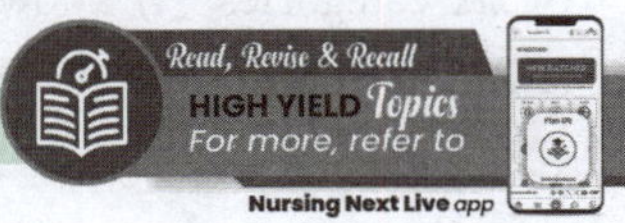

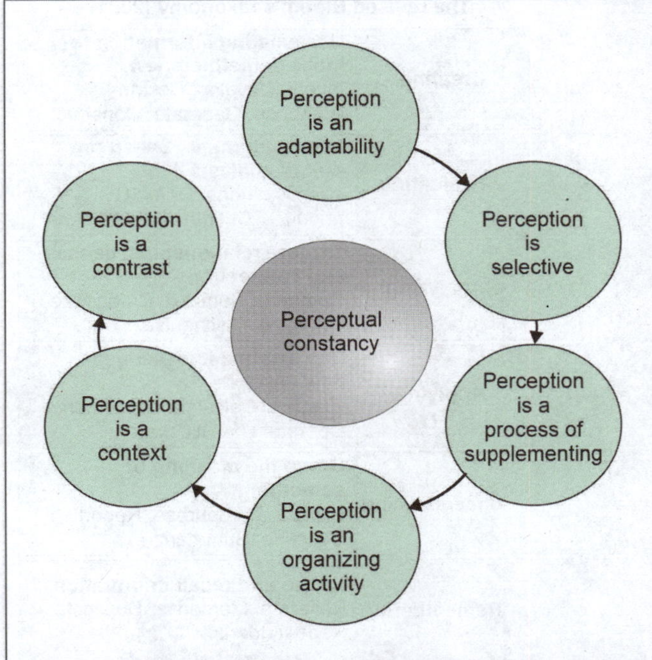

LEARNING

Definition

Learning is the conservation of new behavior or the strengthening and weakening of old behavior as a result of experience. **—Henry Smith**

Learning Process

Steps in Learning Process:

- **Step 1:** Motivation within the learner.
- **Step 2:** An attractive goal or goals related to motivation.
- **Step 3:** A block or barrier to attainment of the goal.
- **Step 4:** An appropriate line of action to reach goal.
- **Step 5:** Selection of appropriate action and practice and termination of inappropriate action.

MEMORY

Meaning

Memory is the faculty of the brain by which data or information is encoded, stored and retrieved when needed.

Memory consists of remembering what has previously been learned. **—Woodworth**

Methods of Memorizing and Forgetting

- **Whole and part method:** This method involves learning and memorizing information as a whole or breaking it down into smaller parts.
- **Space and unspaced repetition:** Spaced repetition involves studying and reviewing information at spaced intervals over time. Unspaced repetition refers to studying and reviewing information without intervals.
- **Memory pegs:** Memory pegs are mnemonic devices or associations that act as reminders for the information you want to remember.
- **Method of loci:** Greek word *loci* means location or place. This method involves associating information with specific locations or places in a familiar environment.
- **Grouping and rhyming:** Grouping and rhyming of the word also facilitate learning and help in memory process.
- **PQ4R:** It is a specific technique which is used for memorizing.

P – Preview Q – Question 4Rs – Read, Reflect, Result, Review

- **SQ3R:** It is also a technique: S – Study Q – Question 3Rs – Read, Recite, Review

FORGETTING

Meaning

According to Munn (1967), forgetting is the loss of permanent or temporary memory. It is the ability to recall or recognize something learned earlier.

Types

- **Natural forgetting (trace dependent)**

  Forgetting due to lapse of time and without intention of the individual. It is not quite common type of forgetting process.

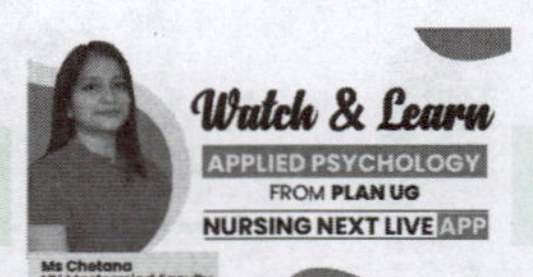

- **Morbid forgetting (abnormal)**
  It has two subtypes:
  1. **General forgetfulness:** Individual tries to forget the total event.
  2. **Specific:** Individual tries to forget some specific part of the total event.
- **Cue dependent forgetting**
  The inability to retrieve information from memory occurs when there are inadequate cues both internally and externally, leading to a difficulty in recalling stored information.
- **State dependent**
  - The phenomenon of remembering something more easily when an individual is in a similar emotional and physical state as he/she was during the initial learning experience is known as state-dependent memory.
  - In the absence of this state-dependent recall, the person may encounter difficulties in retrieving the information.
- **Motivated forgetting**
  - Deliberate or intentional forgetting happens when individuals actively choose or desire to forget something.
  - In our everyday lives, many instances of forgetfulness can be attributed to motivated forgetting.

THINKING

Definition

Rose: Thinking is a mental activity in its cognitive aspect or mental activity with regard to psychological aspects.

Types of Thinking

Perceptual Thinking (or) Concrete Thinking

- Perceptual is a foundation for all forms of thinking.
- It involves the interpretation of sensations based on an individual's prior experiences.

Conceptual (or) Abstract Thinking

This type of thinking involves the ability to concentrate on the underlying meanings of concepts and theories.

Creative Thinking

Creative thinking is linked to an individual's capacity to generate fresh, original, or unconventional ideas.

Logical or Reflective Thinking

Logical or reflective thinking necessitates the integration of all pertinent experiences into specific situations and involves the removal of obstacles rather than simply relying on previous experiences, ideas, or concepts.

Critical Thinking

- Critical thinking is a mental activity which is the analysis of facts to form a judgment.
- It helps to develop individual skills.
- It consists of several steps as follows:
  - Conceptualization
  - Interpretation
  - Analysis
  - Synthesis
  - Evaluation

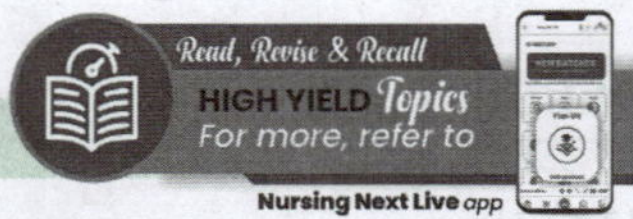

Levels of Thinking

Bloom's Taxonomy Levels of Thinking

- Bloom created Bloom's taxonomy levels of thinking.
- According to the theory (1984), thinking process consists of six categories, (i) knowledge, (ii) comprehension, (iii) application, (iv) analysis, (v) synthesis and (vi) evaluation.

The revised Bloom's taxonomy (2001)

Creating	**Use existing information to make something new** Invent, Develop, Design, Compose, Generate, Construct
Evaluating	**Make judgments based on sound analysis** Assess, Judge, Defend, prioritize, Critique, Recommend
Analyzing	**Explore relationships, causes, and connections** Compare, Contrast, Categorize, Organize, Distinguish
Applying	**Use existing knowledge in new contexts** Practice, Calculate, Implement, Operate, Use, Illustrate
Understanding	**Grasp the meaning of something** Explain, Paraphrase, Report, Describe, Summarize
Remembering	**Retain and recall information** Reiterate, Memorize, Duplicate, Repeat, Identify

Errors in Thinking

- **All-or-nothing thinking:** Perceiving things as either one extreme or its opposite—such as white or black, good or bad, success or failure. In doing so, we avoid considering the various degrees of possibilities that lie in between.

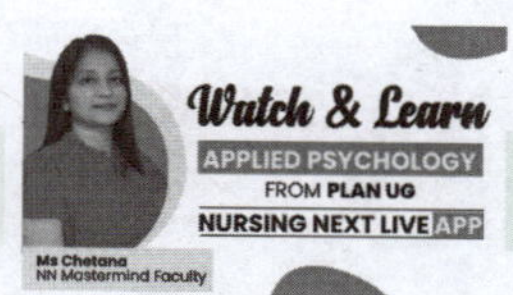

- **Overgeneralization:** By focusing on a singular event, we tend to make generalizations that extend to the entirety of our life.
- **Filtering out the positive:** It involves disregarding the positive aspects, which can hinder the development of a realistic perspective on a situation.

INTELLIGENCE

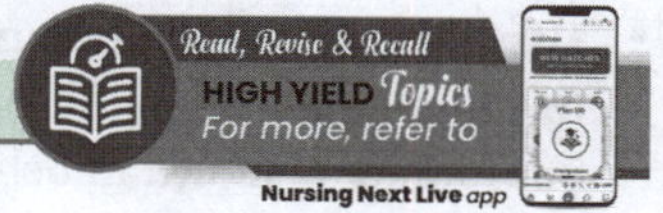

Definition

Intelligence is the aggregate or global capacity of the individual to think rationally, to act purposefully and to deal effectively with the environment. —**Wechsler 1994**

Intelligence Quotient (IQ)

IQ = Mental Age/Chronological Age × 100

For example: 15-year-old girl scores a mental age of 20. IQ = 20/15 × 100 IQ = 133

APTITUDE

- Aptitude refers to a person's innate or acquired capacity or potential to perform certain tasks, skills, or activities.
- Aptitude can be seen as a combination of inherent qualities, such as intelligence, creativity, problem-solving skills, and the ability to acquire knowledge quickly.

INDIVIDUAL DIFFERENCES

Definition

Individual differences stand for the variations or deviations among individuals in regard to a single characteristic or number of characteristics. —**Carter B Good**

PSYCHOMETRIC ASSESSMENT OF COGNITIVE PROCESSES

Definition

Psychometric assessment of cognitive processes refers to the use of standardized and objective measures to evaluate an individual's cognitive abilities, skills, or processes.

It involves the administration of tests or assessments that are designed to assess various aspects of cognition, such as memory, attention, reasoning, problem-solving, and decision-making.

ALTERATION IN COGNITIVE PROCESSES

Alteration in Attention

- Attention Deficit Hyperactivity Disorder (ADHD) is a neurodevelopmental disorder that typically begins in childhood and can persist to adulthood.
- It is characterized by a persistent pattern of inattention, impulsivity, and hyperactivity that interferes with daily functioning and quality of life.

Alterations in Sensation

- **Anesthesia:** Loss of sensation or feeling.
- **Hyperanesthesia:** Heightened sensitivity to stimuli.
- **Paresthesia:** Abnormal sensations like tingling or numbness.
- **Dysesthesia:** Unpleasant or abnormal sensations.
- **Allodynia:** Painful response to non-painful stimuli

Alteration in Perception

- **Hallucination:** False perception without a real stimulus. E.g., A person hears a voice when there is no one in the room.
- **Illusion:** Misperception of a real stimulus. E.g., A person perceive a rope on streat as snake.

Alteration in Learning

- **Dyslexia:** Reading disorder
- **Dyscalculia:** Mathematical disorder
- **Dysgraphia:** Disorder of written expression

Alteration in Memory

- **Amnesia:** Memory loss or inability to recall past events.
- **Dementia:** A decline in cognitive function, including memory, thinking, and reasoning.
- **Agnosia:** Difficulty in interpreting sensory information despite intact sensory abilities.
- **Alzheimer's disease:** Progressive decline in memory and cognitive ability.
- **Hyperthymestic syndrome:** Exceptionally vivid and detailed autobiographical memory.
- **Wernicke-Korsakoff syndrome:** Memory and cognitive impairment due to thiamine deficiency.

Alteration in Thinking

- Dementia
- **Delirium:** Acute state of confusion and disorientation.

Alteration in Intelligence

Intellectual Disability (formerly known as Mental Retardation)

- Mild (50–70)
- Moderate (35–50)
- Severe (20–35)
- Profound (less than 20)

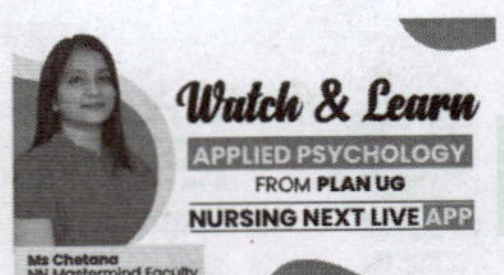

CONCEPTUAL EXERCISES

LONG ANSWER QUESTIONS

1. Define attention. Explain factors or determinants affecting attention and various types of attention. (RUHS, MGR, KUHS)

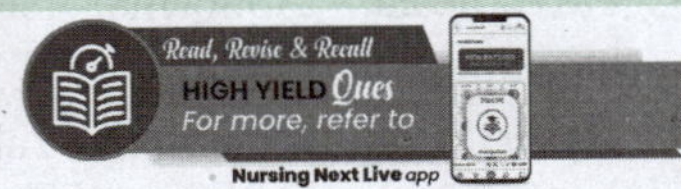

Answer

Definition of Attention

Attention is defined as an ability to produce, select, manage, and maintain sufficient stimulation at a specific amount of time to process any kind of information.

Factors/Determinants affecting attention can be divided mainly into two:

1. Internal factors
2. External factors

Internal Factors

- **Instincts:** Instincts help us to critically analyze the situation and pay attention before making any decision. So, it enhances our attention process.
  For example: Whether to go alone or not to an unfamiliar place.
- **Motives:** They are basic drives and urges of the people which are more important to raise attention like thirst, hunger, sex, curiosity. For example: We pay attention to our health when our motive is to stay healthy.
- **Habit:** A person develops a habit of attending to important things and a habit of not attending to the unimportant things. For example: Eating healthy to stay healthy.
- **Interests:** Attention will be dragged by an individual in which he or she is interested to perform the task. For example: Small children pay attention to toys in the market as they are interested in playing.
- **Mood:** The mood state of the individual determines the attention which the person will put to any certain stimuli. For example: We tend to ignore some things when we are in good mood.
- **Aim:** The personal aims of the person also guide his ability to attend certain stimuli. For example: A student will pay attention to studies if he aims to score good in exams.
- **Mindset:** A person always attends to one subject which the mind has set. For example: Paying attention to a project because mind is set to complete that in time.
- **Past experiences:** Previous experiences and learning felicitate attention. If we find that certain things have been beneficial in the past, we give more attention to it in the present. For example: If we know the taste of ice cream by our past experiences, we pay attention to wherever it is available.
- **Disposition and temperament:** Both are essential factors to promote attention. Disposition is the natural aspect of one's mind as shown in behavior and in relationships with others like happy disposition. Temperament refers to the specific emotional balance determining a person's character like artistic temperament. For example: A man having moral disposition will attend the moral stories sessions.

External Factors

These are the factors present in our environment.

- **Size of the stimulus:** The objects that are larger and bigger than others grab our attention. At the same time, very small object against a huge background will attract attention. For example: In seminars or conferences, emphasis is placed on bold and large font for audio-visual presentation.
- **Intensity of the stimulus:** Our attention is focused on a stimulus that is constantly present and intense.
- **Environmental changes:** Well-focused attention requires sound environment like noise free. The individual focusing ability depends upon the nature of external stimuli. If any changes in environment and family dynamics, it may affect the attention ability. Examples: Rise in temperature, disturbance in the food chain, changes in climatic conditions, family cohesion.
- **Movement of the stimulus:** The object that is moving catches out attention easily. For example: Animation or moving pictures on PowerPoint presentations catch attention easily.
- **Contrast of the stimulus:** Any stimulus that is strikingly different from its surrounding will tend to stand out and attract attention. It is a focus that shifts on the unusual things. For example: Red dot in black and white or a spot on clean dress or a smudge on a clear wall.
- **Novelty:** Novelty means something different or new. Any object which is different from routine makes a powerful appeal. For example: Any thing new in a room grabs attention immediately.
- **Repetition of the stimulus:** A stimulus that is repeatedly present in the environment easily grabs attention. For example: A table kept at the same place in a room grabs attention.
- **Definite form of the object:** A cleared defined object attracts more than vague and indefinite object. The figure attracts our notice more than the background because the latter is less defined and less sharp than the former. For example: Arrow mark in the traffic signals.

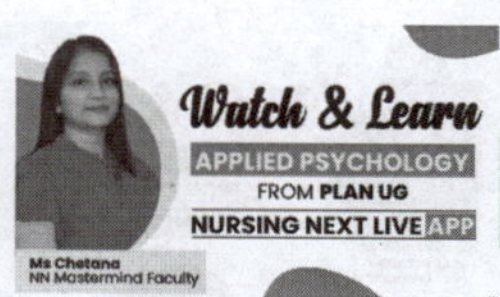

- **Location of the stimulus:** A note placed on wall to memorize grabs attention because we are repeatedly seeing it and we are able to memorize it easily.
- **Isolation:** A stimulus isolated is easily attended. Like a student sitting alone in the corner of the class is seen first.

Types of Attention

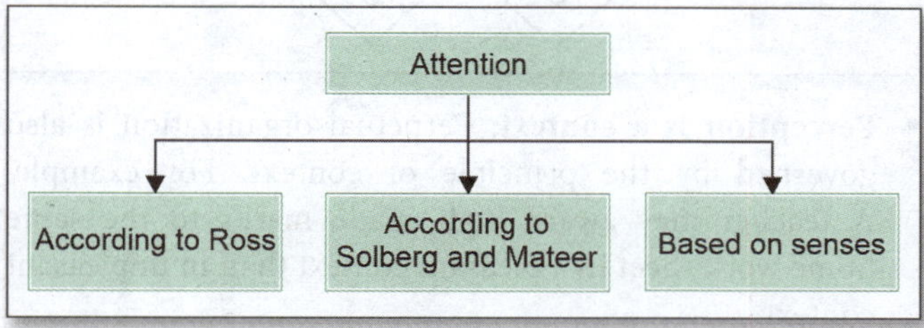

According to Ross

- **Volitional (Voluntary) Attention:** It requires will and deliberate efforts for arriving at a solution. This type of attention is not spontaneous. For example: Listening to a long lecture.
  - **Implicit:** A single act of will is enough to arouse this attention. For example: Teacher has given some project to complete.
  - **Explicit:** It is obtained by repeated acts. Here repeated attempts are made to bring the attention. For example: Making a child to sit and do his homework during holidays.
- **Nonvolitional (Involuntary) Attention:** It does not require role of will or conscious effort. It is aroused either by instincts or our sentiments. It is divided into:
  - **Spontaneous attention:** Nonvolitional attention aroused by sentiments is called spontaneous attention. For example: Parents pay attention to their kids whenever they are outside.
  - **Enforced attention:** It is aroused by our instincts. For example: Attention given to the other gender.

According to Solberg and Mateer

- **Selective attention:** It is the ability to attend to a specific stimulus or specific activity in the presence of other distracting stimulus. For example: Keep oneself from getting distracted by irrelevant stimuli while driving.
- **Divided attention:** It is the ability to attend different stimuli or activity at the same time. For example: Need to carry out all the necessary activities for driving like using the pedals, turning the wheel, and changing gears is dividing attention.
- **Alternating attention:** It is the ability to change focus and attention between two or more stimuli. For example: Doing multitasking in the kitchen.
- **Sustained attention:** It is the ability to attend or a stimulus or activity over a long period of time. For example: Need to pay attention for long period of time while driving or stay focused on studying for hours.
- **Arousal attention:** It refers to our activation level and level of alertness whether one is tired or energized. For example: Driving for long hours and staying alert.
- **Focused attention:** It refers to the ability to focus attention on a stimulus. For example: To stay focused while driving.
- **Executive attention:** Executive attention refers to the cognitive ability to allocate and manage attentional resources in a flexible and goal-directed manner.

Based on Senses

- **Auditory attention:** It pays attention only to the hearing senses. For example: Listening to PODCAST.
- **Visual attention:** It pays attention to the details or inputs which are received by eyes only and no attention to other stimuli present in the environment. For example: Reading a book.
- **Habitual attention:** It arises from attitude, habits, and interests. For example: The attention that a mother gives to her kid while they are outside.

2. Define perception. Describe the perceptual organization in detail. (MGR, DU)

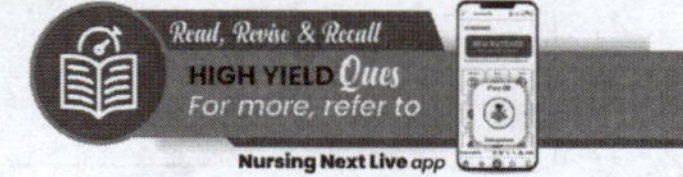

Answer

Definition of Perception

Perception is the process of organization, identification and interpretation of sensory stimulus in order to represent and understand the current information or environment.

Principles of Perception (Perceptual Organization)

Gestalt theorist followed the basic principle that the whole is greater than the sum of its part. Here are some principles that explain how our mind perceive things differently.

- **Perception is selective:** We perceive selective things in our environment. Different people perceive different things.
- **Perception is a process of supplementing:** We perceive the full objects even there are no corresponding sensory impressions and only some isolated sensation is received. For example: We hear sound at a distance and perceive that a train is approaching.
- **Perception is an organizing activity**
- **This principle is explained in following types:**

Principle of Figure-ground Relationship

- **Figure and ground:** It states that we instinctively perceive objects as either being in the foreground or the background. They either standout prominently in the front (the figure) or recede into the back (the ground). The perception of the object or figure in terms of color, size, shape and intensity, etc. depends upon the figure-ground relationship, a proper figure-ground relationship is quite important from the angle of perception of the figure or the ground.

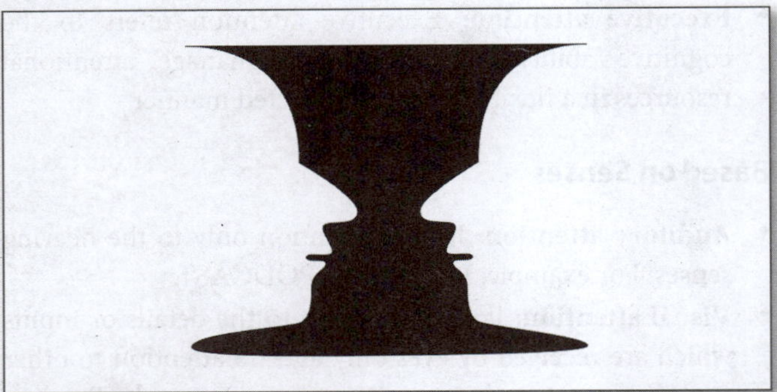

- **Principle of proximity:** When objects are close to each other. The tendency is to perceive them together is more rather than separate.

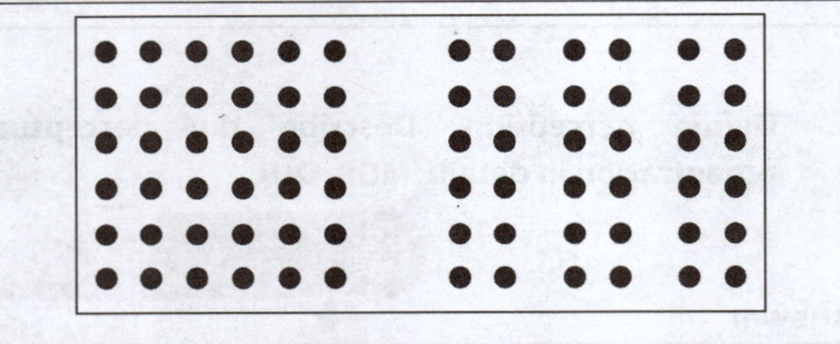

- **Principle of continuity:** We perceive continuous patterns easily. The things arranged in some patterns are perceived faster than things that are not arranged.

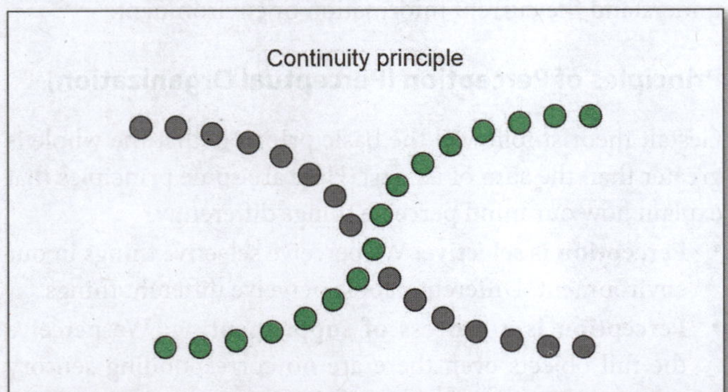

- **Principle of closure:** Figures or patterns that are closed tend to be perceived easily.
- **Principle of similarity:** Objects that are having symmetrical shape.

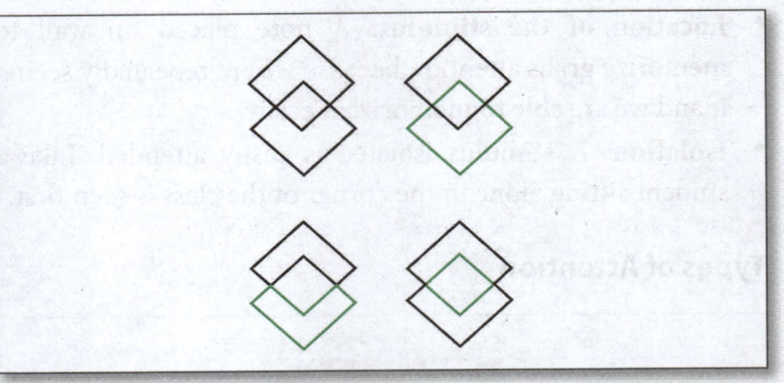

- **Perception is a context:** Perpetual organization is also governed by the principle of context. For example: A teacher may award high grade marks to the same home work sheet in a pleasant context than in unpleasant context.
- **Perception is a contrast:** It states that external stimuli that stand out against the background, will receive attention. Perpetual organization is very much affected through contrast effects as the stimuli that are in sharp contrast to nearby stimuli may drew our maximum attention and carry different perpetual effects.
- **Perception is an adaptability:** Good perceptual organization depends upon the stimuli and the adaptability of the perceiver to perceive similar stimuli. For example: A person who adapts himself to work before an intense bright light will perceive normal sunlight as quite dim.
- **Perceptual constancy:** Perceptual constancies refer to our tendency to perceive object as relatively stable and unchanging despite changing information. For example: Due to size constancy leads us to perceive that the aeroplane we see at a distance is a large one even though we see its tiny image as it flies across the vast sky.

3. Define intelligence. Explain theories of intelligence and various intelligence tests used for measurement of intelligence. (RUHS, MGR)

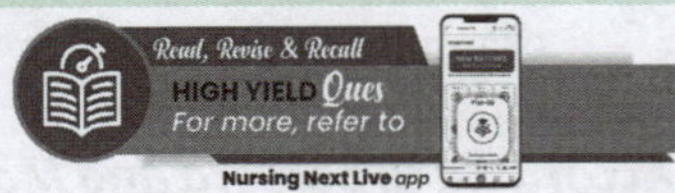

Answer

Definition of Intelligence

Intelligence is the aggregate or global capacity of the individual to think rationally, to act purposefully and to deal effectively with the environment. **—Wechsler 1994**

Intelligence is the ability to master the knowledge or skills needed to succeed within a particular culture. **—Lolurto 1991**

Theories of Intelligence

Different researchers proposed a variety of theories to explain the nature of intelligence.

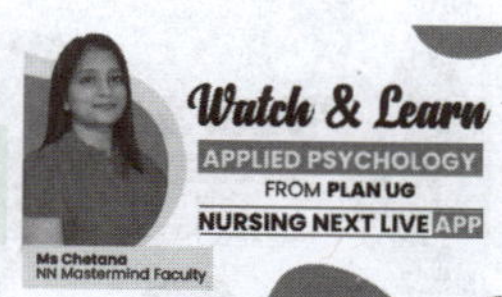

The different types of theories are:

- **General Intelligence Theory** by Charles Spearman
- **Primary Mental Abilities Theory** by Louis L Thurstone
- **Theory of Multiple Intelligence** by Howard Gardner
- **Piaget Theory, 1970** by Piaget
- **Brunner's Theory, 1973** by Brunner

General Intelligence Theory

- General Intelligence Theory was described by Charles Spearman.
- It refers to general intelligence or G-factor. Spearman concluded that scores on this test were remarkably similar.
- People who perform well in one test tend to perform well in other tests. While who scores badly in one test, tend to give other test also badly.
- So, he concluded that intelligence is a general cognitive ability that can be measured and numerically expressed.

Primary Mental Abilities Theory

Primary Mental Abilities Theory was described by Louis L Thurstone (1887–1955). It is not a single ability and is focused on seven different primary mental abilities.

They are as follows:

1. **Associative memory:** It is an ability to memorize and recall.
2. **Numerical ability:** It is an ability to solve arithmetic problems.
3. **Perceptual speed:** The ability to see differences and similarities in objects.
4. **Reasoning:** The ability to find rules.
5. **Spatial visualization:** It is ability to visualize relationship.
6. **Verbal comprehension:** The ability to define and understand words.
7. **Word fluency:** The ability to produce words rapidly.

Theory of Multiple Intelligence

Theory of Multiple Intelligence was proposed by Howard Gardner.

He explained the traditional idea of intelligence based on IQ test is not an accurate theory that depicts a person's abilities. He proposed eight different intelligences based on skills and abilities that are valued in variety of cultures. They are as follows:

1. **Bodily kinesthetic intelligence:** Ability to control body movement and handle objects skillfully.
2. **Interpersonal intelligence:** Capacity to detect and respond to moods and desires of others appropriately.
3. **Intrapersonal intelligence:** Self-awareness of values and beliefs.
4. **Logical mathematical intelligence:** Logical and numerical pattern.
5. **Musical intelligence:** Appreciate rhythm, pitch and timbre.
6. **Naturalistic intelligence:** Categorize animal, plants and other object.
7. **Verbal linguistic:** To reason, solve problems, and learn using language.
8. **Visual spatial:** Images and pictures.

Piaget Theory, 1970

According to Piaget, intelligence is an adaptive process involving interplay of biological, material and interaction with the environment. He viewed that it is an evolution of cognitive processes like nature, principles of grammar and mathematical rules.

Brunner's Theory, 1973

According to Brunner, intelligence is growing dependence on interpersonal representatives of objects or situations. It is influenced by reinforcement like rewards and punishments.

Assessment of Intelligence

Intelligence can be assessed with the help of psychological tests. Alfred Binet was the first psychologist to construct an intelligence test.

There are two main broad categories of intelligence test:

1. **Individual test:** Classified as verbal test and nonverbal test
2. **Group test:** Classified as verbal test and nonverbal test

Individual Test

Individual Verbal Tests

Individual verbal tests are the tests where only one individual is tested at a time. This type of test involves use of language. For example: Stanford-Binet Scale.

Individual Nonverbal Tests

Individual nonverbal tests use nonverbal approach. They involve manipulation of items like picture arrangement or picture completion, etc. These types of tests are conducted for individuals who are not able to understand language like small kids, in case of language barrier. For example: Bhatia's battery of performance test.

Group Test

Group Verbal Test

Group verbal test can be applied to a group at a time. For example: Army general classification test.

Group Nonverbal Intelligence Tests

Some activities are given to perform. The group can perform such activities together. Here no verbal component is involved. Activities like draw a picture, complete a figure, etc.

Some Scales of Measuring the Intelligence

- **Stanford-Binet intelligence scale:** This is one of the oldest and most widely used intelligence tests. It is a standardized test that assesses a person's cognitive abilities, including verbal and nonverbal reasoning, memory, and spatial awareness. This test assesses intelligence across different age groups
- **Wechsler adult intelligence scale:** This is a popular intelligence test used to measure cognitive ability in adults. It includes several subtests that assess different aspects of intelligence, including verbal comprehension, perceptual reasoning, working memory, and processing speed.
- **Kaufman assessment battery for children:** This test is designed to measure the cognitive abilities of children aged 2.5 to 12.5 years. It includes subtests that assess different areas of intelligence, including fluid reasoning, visual-spatial processing, and working memory.
- **Raven's progressive matrices:** This is a nonverbal intelligence test that measures abstract reasoning ability. It consists of a series of visual puzzles that require the test-taker to identify the missing piece in a pattern.
- **Differential ability scales:** This test is designed to measure cognitive ability in children and young adults. It includes subtests that assess different areas of intelligence, including verbal comprehension, visual spatial ability, and processing speed.
- **Woodcock-Johnson tests of cognitive abilities:** This test is designed to measure cognitive ability in children and adults. It includes subtests that assess different areas of intelligence, including verbal comprehension, visual spatial ability, and processing speed.

4. Describe learning process. Explain instrumental learning with examples. (RUHS, MGR, KUHS)

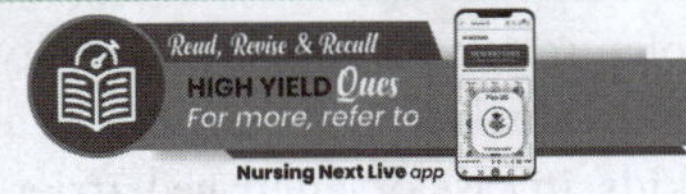

Answer

Definition of Learning

Learning is the conservation of new behavior or the strengthening and weakening of old behavior as a result of experience.
—**Henry Smith**

Learning is the acquisition of habits, knowledge and attitude.
—**Crow and Crow**

Learning Process

Learning process is a process of acquiring new understanding, knowledge, behavior, skills, values, attitude and preferences.

Some learning is immediate which is induced by single event. Like being burnt by hot stove but still knowledge accumulates from repeated experiences.

Steps in Learning Process

Step 1: Motivation within the learner.
Step 2: An attractive goal or goals related to motivation.
Step 3: A block or barriers to attainment of the goal.
Step 4: An appropriate line of action to reach goal.
Step 5: Selection of appropriate action and practice and termination of inappropriate action.

Step 1: Motivation within the Learner

Motives are the dynamic forces that energize behavior and compel the individual to learn something. They depend upon the strength of internal and external motives, the outcome exists. Example: A boy has a strong internal motivation to learn how to play the guitar because he always admired musicians

Step 2: An Attractive Goal

A predetermined goal arises interest within the individual for learning and also make path to find various methods or techniques to achieve a task. Example: The boy sets a goal to be able to play their favorite song on the guitar.

Step 3: Block or Barriers to Attainment of the Goal

Barriers are the obstacles for learning. If the person faces no difficulties in attaining goal, then he won't change their attitude.

But if the person faces any difficulties in attainment of goal, then she/he learns to modify her/his behavior and finds new behavior which helps to achieve tasks.

Effective learners can overcome the barriers in learning process and reach the goal. Example: The boy initially struggles with finger coordination and finds it difficult which serves as a barrier to achieving his goal.

Step 4: An Appropriate Action

In this step, the learner searches for an appropriate line of action to reach goal by many trial and error. For this, individual readiness is very important to find appropriate one.

To promote readiness, learner's reinforcement, integration and learning situations are necessary. A variety of actions take place based on needs and problems in this stage. Example: The boy seeks out various resources such as online tutorials and

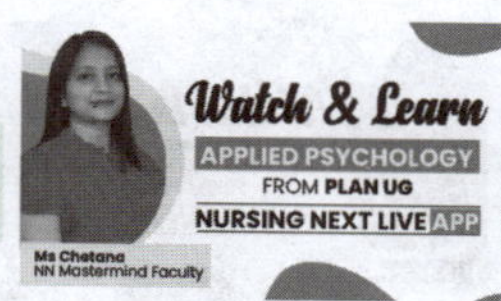

practice exercises to find effective techniques and methods to improve his finger coordination.

Step 5: Selection and Practice of Appropriate Action

At last, the most appropriate action is selected and practiced which strengthens the individual. At the same time, inappropriate behavior is dropped which weakens the learner. Learning process does not end only with the acquisition of certain skills or knowledge. It is a continuous process and never-ending process in human being. Example: After experimenting with different finger positioning and practice techniques, the boy finds a specific finger placement and a consistent practice routine that helps him improve coordination.

Instrumental Learning

- Instrumental learning is also known as operant conditioning. This type of learning was introduced by B. F Skinner.
- Instrumental conditioning is an association between a stimulus and a response. It helps the individual to adjust his or her behavior. For example: Training your dog to shake hands would involve offering a reward every time the desired behavior occurs.
- In instrumental conditioning, positive or negative reinforcement is used to either increase or decrease the probability that a behavior will occur again in the future.
- There are two types of reinforcement used to establish a desired behavior or disappear an unwanted behavior pattern. They are positive reinforcement and negative reinforcement.
  - **Positive reinforcement** is the stimulus that is presented after a behavior. In this, a desired response or behavior is strengthened by adding the praise or reward. **Example**: If a child keeps his things organized and he is rewarded, probability of repeating this behavior is increased.
  - **Negative reinforcement** refers to the use of punishment after the display of unwanted behavior. For example: If a child does not keep his things organized, then not letting him watch his favorite cartoon. This decreases the probability of not leaving his things unorganized.

---

5. Define learning. How a reflex is going to be learnt according to Pavlov classical conditioning? (RUHS,MGR)

Answer

Definition

Learning is the conservation of new behavior or the strengthening and weakening of old behavior as a result of experience.

—**Henry Smith**

Learning is the acquisition of habits, knowledge and attitude.

—**Crow and Crow**

Pavlov's Classical Conditioning

Pavlov's classical conditioning experiment explains that how behavior can be changed by using conditioning. Pavlov did an experiment with a dog that explains how a reflex is learnt.

Pavlov's Dog Experiment

- The dogs were placed in separate room with restraint. In front of them, a food bowl was placed to feed them.
- A device was used to measure the rate of saliva which is secreted by the dogs.
- Pavlov observed that dogs naturally salivate when presented with food (unconditioned stimulus) as a reflexive response.
- Pavlov introduced a neutral stimulus, such as ringing a bell, before presenting the food to the dogs. The bell had no natural connection to salivation.
- The dogs naturally salivated in response to the food (unconditioned stimulus), which is an unconditioned response.
- Pavlov repeatedly paired the neutral stimulus (bell) with the unconditioned stimulus (food) by ringing the bell before presenting the food.
- Over time, the dogs began to associate the sound of the bell with the food. As a result, the bell alone started to elicit salivation, even without the presence of food. This salivation in response to the bell became a conditioned response.
- The bell, which originally had no connection to salivation, became a conditioned stimulus that triggered the conditioned response of salivation.
- Same as the dog's response was conditioned, any reflex can be learnt or conditioned with the use of conditioned stimulus.
- **A reflex can be learnt by** using Pavlov conditioning. In Pavlov conditioning, there is an association between two stimuli like:
  - Conditioned stimulus (CS)
  - Unconditioned stimulus (US).

  By making an association and pairing the two stimulus, a reflex can be learnt.
- **Principles of Pavlov conditioning:** The principles of learning by classical conditioning can be used for the following areas:
  - **Developing good habits:** Cleanliness, respect elders
  - **Breaking of bad habits:** Fear and anxiety in maladjusted person
  - **Training of animals:** Training for police dog

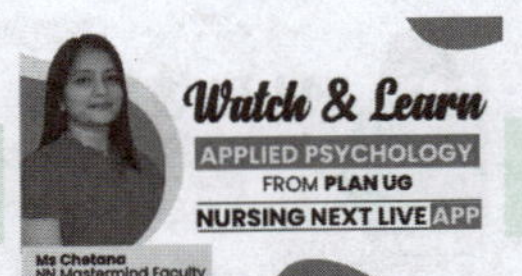

- **Use in psychotherapy:** Deconditioning abnormal emotions
- Used to develop favorable and unfavorable attitude toward learning.

---

6. **What are the types of learning? How classical conditioning is different from operant conditioning? (RUHS, KUHS)**

Answer

Definition

Learning is the conservation of new behavior or the strengthening and weakening of old behavior as a result of experience. **—Henry Smith**

Learning is the acquisition of habits, knowledge and attitude. **—Crow and Crow**

Types of Learning

Based on underlying process/mechanism, the major types of learning are as follows:

- **Learning through association (classical conditioning):**
  - This type of learning is based on the association between stimuli.
  - It focuses on the pairing of a neutral stimulus with a naturally occurring stimulus to create a learned response.
- **Learning through consequences (operant conditioning):**
  - This type of learning is based on the consequences that follow a behavior.
  - It emphasizes the relationship between behavior and its outcomes, such as reinforcement (increasing the likelihood of the behavior) or punishment (decreasing the likelihood of the behavior).
- **Learning through trial and error method:**
  - Trial and error learning is an experimental approach where individuals try out different behaviors until they find one that produces a desired outcome.
- **Learning through observation (modeling/observational learning):**
  - This type of learning is based on observing and imitating others.
  - It involves acquiring new behaviors, attitudes, or knowledge by observing the actions and outcomes of others without directly experiencing the consequences.

On the basis of degree of complexity, Robert M Gagne described eight types of learning as per the hierarchy as explained here. The first four levels of learning focus on behavioral aspects of learning and last four levels focus on the cognitive aspects of learning.

- **Signal carrying/learning (classical conditioning):**
  - It is the simplest form of learning, also known as "classical conditioning".
  - The learner associates a conditioned stimulus with a desired response that would not occur naturally.
  - **Example:** Training a dog to salivate at the sound of a bell by pairing the bell with food.
- **Stimulus-response learning (operant conditioning):**
  - This is second level of learning, also known as operant conditioning.
  - The learner engages in voluntary behavior that is reinforced by the examiner.
  - **Example:** Giving a child a toy as a reward for completing homework on time.
- **Chain learning:**
  - The learner connects multiple previously learned behaviors in a specific order.
  - **Example:** Learning to ride a bicycle by sequentially coordinating pedaling, balancing, and steering.
- **Verbal association:**
  - The learner makes associations using verbal units, contributing to language development.
  - **Example:** Learning medical terminology and applying it in a clinical setting.
- **Discrimination learning:**
  - The learner differentiates and responds differently to similar situations.
  - **Example:** Differentiating post-surgery fever from other types of fever based on specific symptoms.
- **Concept learning:**
  - The learner consistently responds to different stimuli related to a specific concept.
  - **Example:** Teaching a child about colors and having them consistently identify different colors.
- **Rule learning:**
  - The learner learns and applies multiple concepts in various situations.
  - **Example:** Understanding privacy and confidentiality principles and applying them appropriately in different health care scenarios.
- **Problem-solving learning:**
  - The learner engages in complex problem-solving, using a systematic approach to address challenges.
  - **Example:** Applying the nursing process (assessment, diagnosis, planning, implementation, evaluation) to solve patient problems.

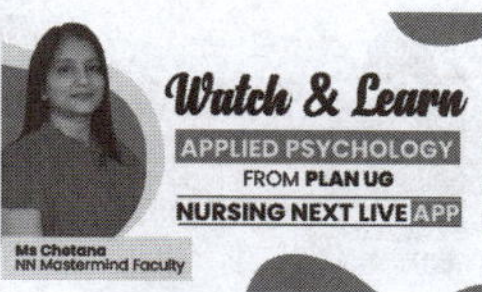

Differences Between Classical Conditioning and Operant Conditioning

Classical Conditioning

Classical conditioning explains that a behavior response can be conditioned.

Operant Conditioning

Operant conditioning suggests the use of positive or negative reinforcement for establishing a desired behavior.

Basis for comparison	Classical conditioning	Operant conditioning
Meaning	Classical conditioning is a process in which learning is possible by forming association between two stimuli.	Operant conditioning refers to the learning in which the organism studies the relation between responses and its consequences.
Nature of behavior	Involuntary, reflexive responses	Voluntary behaviors
Stresses on	What precedes response?	What follows response?
Based on	Involuntary or reflexive behavior	Voluntary behavior
Responses	Under control of stimulus	Under control of organism
Role of stimuli	Conditioned stimulus paired with unconditioned stimulus	Consequences of behavior influence likelihood of behavior
Occurrence of unconditioned stimulus	Controlled by experimenter.	Controlled by organism.

7. What is learning? Enlist the characteristics of learning. Explain trial and error theory of learning. (RUHS, MGR)

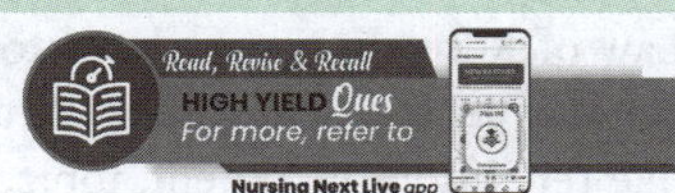

Answer

Definition

Learning is the conservation of new behavior or the strengthening and weakening of old behavior as a result of experience. —**Henry Smith**

Learning is the acquisition of habits, knowledge and attitude. —**Crow and Crow**

Characteristics of Learning

- Learning is a continuous process. It is not a product effect.
- Learning is a complex process that involves changes in behavior, knowledge, and skills.
- Learning is an active process. It requires the learner to be engaged and involved in the learning process.
- Learning is about change. It involves acquiring new knowledge, skills, or behaviors.
- Learning is a consistent process. It requires repeated exposure to new information or experiences
- Learning is transferable. What is learned in one context can be applied to other contexts.
- Learning can be permanent. When learning is well-established, it can last for a lifetime
- Learning is goal-directed. Learners are motivated to learn because they want to achieve a particular goal.
- Learning is constructive. Learners actively construct their own knowledge by making connections between new and existing information.
- Learning is social. Learners learn from each other and from their environment.
- Learning is emotional. Learners' emotions can affect their ability to learn. For example, if learners are feeling anxious or stressed, they may not be able to learn as effectively.

Trial and Error Theory of Learning

- This theory was proposed by Edward Lee Thorndike (1874–1949).
- The trial and error theory of learning, also known as the learning by doing theory, proposes that learning occurs through repeated trial and error experiments, and gradually refining behavior based on the results of those experiments.
- This theory suggests that humans and animals learn new behaviors by making mistakes and adjusting their actions accordingly until they achieve the desired outcome.
- The trial and error theory of learning can be observed in many different settings, including academic learning, athletic training, and problem-solving. In this theory, the individual tries various methods until they find one that works and achieves the desired outcome. If the first attempt is unsuccessful, they will try again, perhaps modifying their approach or trying a completely new approach.
- Through repeated experimentation, the individuals learn what works and what doesn't, and eventually, they develop an effective strategy for achieving their goals.

- The trial and error theory of learning is closely related to the concept of reinforcement. Positive outcomes, or rewards, encourage the individual to continue their behavior, while negative outcomes, or punishments, discourage that behavior.
- In this way, the individual learns to associate certain behaviors with specific outcomes, and modifies their behavior accordingly to achieve the desired results.
- Overall, the trial and error theory of learning suggests that learning is an active and iterative process that involves experimentation, modification, and adaptation based on the outcomes of those experiments.

Major theoretical principles which form the basis of Thorndike trial and error theory of learning are:
- Learning involves trial and error
- Learning is a result of the formation of connections
- Learning is improvement in performance not insightful
- Learning is direct, not mediated by ideas

8. What is learning? Explain laws of effective learning. (RUHS, MGR, DU)

Answer

Definition of Learning

Learning is the conservation of new behavior or the strengthening and weakening of old behavior as a result of experience. **—Henry Smith**

Learning is the acquisition of habits, knowledge and attitude. **—Crow and Crow**

Laws of Effective Learning

Edward Thorndike, a psychologist, conducted a series of experiments on trial and error method of learning by animals. He formulated certain laws for effective learning.
They are as follows:

Law of Readiness

Learning takes place when a person is ready to learn something. A mindset or some sort of preparatory attitude is necessary for effective learning. If the individual is not ready, he or she can't learn anything.
For example: If the person is ready to learn English, he will learn quickly.

Law of Affect

Any response which is successful will strengthen the individual and tend to be repeated the same and unsuccessful responses will demotivate the individual and tend to be not repeated again. So, pleasure and pain have a particular effect on learning.

Law of Exercise/Use

Exercise means repetition of act. It is based on law of use and disuse. The repetition of the act will be strengthened, the individual will give rewards or make desirable changes in his behavior. The individual tend to reuse the act again and again.

Law of Disuse

The repetition of the act will weaken the individual or give pain or punishment. The individual will tend to disuse or withdraw the act.

Law of Frequency

More frequency of the act strengthens the individual and helps to attain a task easily or quickly. On the first act, which is successful, it makes a strong bond between stimulus and response. On the second act, the individual becomes stronger. On the third act, furthermore stronger and more frequencies can promote faster learning.

Law of Recency

Law of Recency is correlated to law of disuse. A very recent act may decrease the interest of the learner in learning activity like repetition of content, topic, method, etc. The weakening of response gradually makes learning ineffective.

Law of Primacy

The first experience gains more attention from the individual. It attracts very fast like the first day of college, first love, and first act of solving the puzzles. So, novelty promotes the learner to learn effectively. Like virtual training attracts more than PPT.

Law of Purpose

Clear and defined goals may influence learning process. Purposive learning always gains effectiveness like studying for examination.

Law of Association

Law of Association is based on association of ideas from one to another. The connectivity between two stimuli makes it easier to learn. For example: When we talk about Taj Mahal, we think about it as a symbol of love, constructed by Shah Jahan in memory of his wife Mumtaz Mahal. This law governs the association of ideas as follows:
- Law of similarity
- Law of contract

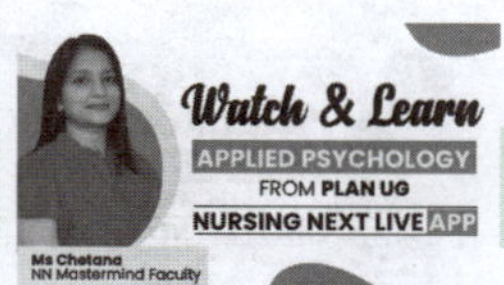

9. What is a memory? Discuss various theories of memory and factors influencing memory. (RUHS)

Answer

Definition of Memory

Memory is the faculty of the brain by which data or information is encoded, stored and retrieved when needed.

Memory consists of remembering what has previously been learned. —**Woodworth**

Theories of Memory

Developmental Theories of Memory

Theories related to memory explain regarding exact representations of memory process. Many authors explain about memory.

Multistore Model (Atkinson and Shiffrin, 1968)

- According to this model, information exists in one of the three states of memory—the sensory, short-term, and long-term stores.
- **Sensory memory:** It is the initial stage of memory where information from the senses is briefly registered. It holds sensory information for a very brief period. Examples: the flashing visual memory of an image or the echoic memory of a sound that quickly fades away.
- **Short-term memory:** It is also known as working memory, is the temporary storage system where information is actively processed and maintained for a short duration. Example: remembering a phone number just long enough to dial it.
- **Long-term memory:** It is the storehouse of information that has been encoded from short-term memory for long-term retention. It can hold memories for long period, ranging from days to years or even a lifetime. Example: remembering significant life events, own name, date of birth, etc.

Levels of Processing (Craik and Lockhart, 1972)

- This theory was proposed by Fergus Craik and Robert Lockhart. It was based on the levels of processing effect.
- Our memory has two types of processing, Shallow processing and Deep processing (semantic).
  1. **Shallow processing:** It considers the overall appearance about something. It leads to forget soon. For example: On the way to office, we see many people in the street but unable to remember even a single face at afternoon.
  2. **Deep processing:** It involves elaborative rehearsal focusing on a stimulus in a more considered way. It includes meaning of the word and consequences of the event. For example: Reading a novel is a shallow processing. Characters in a story and remembering the childhood memory is a deep processing of memory.

Working Memory Model (Baddeley and Hitch, 1974)

The Working Memory Model, proposed by Baddeley and Hitch in 1974, is a theoretical framework that explains how information is stored and processed in short-term memory. The model consists of three main components: The central executive, the phonological loop, and the visuospatial sketchpad.

- **Central executive:** The central executive is the control center of the working memory system. It is responsible for coordinating the activities of the other two components and for directing attention to specific tasks. It is also involved in **decision** making, problem solving, and planning.
- **Phonological loop:** The phonological loop is responsible for the **processing** and temporary storage of verbal information. It is made up of two subcomponents: the phonological store and the articulatory loop. The **phonological** store holds auditory information in a passive, nonverbal form for a short period of time, while the articulatory loop is responsible for the rehearsal of this information through subvocalization or inner speech.
- **Visuospatial sketchpad:** The visuospatial sketchpad is responsible for the **processing** and temporary storage of visual and spatial information. It is involved in mental imagery, navigation, and visual memory tasks.

Miller's Magic Number

- George A Miller proposed Magic Number theory which explains about capacity of short-term memory or limits.
- According to his experiments, he concluded that the average short-term memory capacity is 7 chunks of information (+ or –) before the leading process to LTM like people is able to remember 9-digit mobile number and struggle to remember 10-digit numbers (registration numbers).
- Finally, he described the number 7 (+ or –) as a magical number in our understanding of memory. When we want to encode more letter words, our brain encodes the list of 7 letters separately.

Memory Decay (Peterson and Peterson, 1959)

- Memory decay theory states that memories fade over time if they are not practiced or rehearsed.
- In their experiments, participants were given lists of meaningless trigrams (e.g., UPM, PRS, STU) to remember. After presenting the trigrams, participants were distracted

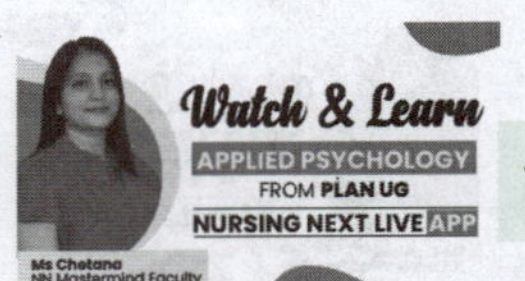

with a counting task, which prevented rehearsal of the trigrams. The researchers then measured the participants' ability to recall the trigrams at different time intervals.

- The findings revealed that initially, participants could easily recall the assigned meaning to the trigrams due to encoding. However, as time passed without rehearsal, the accuracy of recall declined rapidly. Within a short period of around 18 seconds, the recall accuracy dropped to approximately 10%. This demonstrates the brief life span of memories in short-term memory (STM) before decay impacts our ability to retrieve them.

Factors Influencing Memory

The factors are divided into two categories: Intrinsic and Extrinsic factors

Intrinsic Factors

Age: Aging is one most important and obvious factor that affects our memory. Our memory function declines as we age. Elderly people are at a risk of developing dementia.

Maturity: Younger child cannot remember and also encode complex material. For example: Pre-schooler cannot do multiplications in Maths.

Interest and attention: If an individual is interested and paying attention, chances to memorize that thing are high. Individual interest and desire are essential for new learning and focusing ability is needed for sustaining in learning process. Without interest, we cannot learn even simple things. For example: With full interest, school going children can learn a full-page poem.

Level of intelligence: Intelligence is a more enhancing factor for memory. More intelligent person has good memory than less intelligent one. For example: Children with intellectual disability are not able to memorize as compared to other children of their age.

Will to learning: Willingness to learn influences our memory. If we are willing to learn then we will be able to memorize. So, individual will promote to recall the encoded information later. For example: A student who has will to learn Maths, he learns very fast.

Rest and sleep: Continuous learning interrupts the memory process. A break in the middle enhances good memory. At the same time, adequate sleep promotes fresh mind which helps to learn fast. Dullness and fatigue decrease the capacity to learn and affect memory process.

Extrinsic Factors

Practice:

- Memory is a skill which can be improved by repeated practices and healthy habits.
- Many people exercise their working memory through practice daily and they can store it for execution function.
- Practice is nothing but to do repeated exercises for proficiency. It enhances the memory process effectively.
- **For example:** Pick a new challenging activity to learn (poem), practice a few minutes of exercise daily and along with it maintain a sleep schedule and eat healthy food.

Feedback: Feedback can influence encoding strategies of memory and also help to establish specific memory goals by shaping individual motivation and awareness of memory target.

- It also reduces false memories effectively.
- **For example:** Parents wrongly think that their children become ill by consuming certain variety of food items and then lead to judge their children's preference for the food and question more negatively and reduce their willingness to have and actually consume it.

Task classification: Task classification is a division of tasks by certain facets that identify different aspects, properties or characteristics of every task.

- There are several task classifications.
- It may be visual, psychomotor and kinesthetic.
- Based on the nature of the task, memory process is enhanced effectively in that visual tasks are easily memorized than other types.
- **For example:** Visual story boards.

10. Define thinking. Explain various types of thinking, steps in creative thinking along with the characteristics of a creative person. (MGR)

Answer

Definition of Thinking

Thinking is the mental activities involved in processing information, solving problems, making decisions, and forming judgments, using both conscious and unconscious cognitive processes.

—Kahneman, 2011

Types of Thinking

Thinking is an important cognitive process. It can be classified into several types:

Perceptual Thinking (or) Concrete Thinking

- Perceptual thinking is a simple form of thinking.
- Perceptual is basic for all types of thinking.
- This starts with the interpretation of sensation and previous experiences.

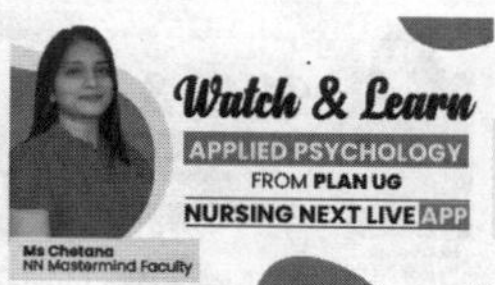

- When we look at an object or a person, we start integrating with our previous experiences.
- It is more common among animals and children. For example: Ability to discriminate different shades of colors.

Conceptual (or) Abstract Thinking

- Conceptual thinking is superior to perception thinking.
- It is an ability to use our concept to make understanding of generalizations and connect to the events, objects or items.
- It involves focusing ability to hidden meaning of concepts and theories. It also economizes efforts in understanding and problem solving. For example: Understanding about Maslow hierarchy theory.

Creative Thinking

- Creative thinking is associated with one's ability to create something new, novel or unusual. It finds new relationship and association to interpret the nature of things, events, or situations.
- Here the creative thinker usually formulates the tools for its solution. For example: Discovering the attractive way to present answer sheet.
- It is not connected with any pre-established concept. Skinner states that the creative thinking is one that expresses new ideas, new observations, new predictions and new inferences.

Logical or Reflective Thinking

- Reflective thinking helps in solving complex problems.
- It requires reconnection of all relevant experiences to situations or removing obstacles instead of relating with those experiences or ideas, concept, etc.
- It is an insightful (deep understanding) cognitive approach for solving problems.
- **For example:** A Maths teacher spends two hours in teaching about a complex sum.

Critical Thinking

Critical thinking is a mental activity which is the analysis of facts to form a judgment. It helps to develop individual skills. It consists of several steps as follows:

- Conceptualization
- Interpretations
- Analysis
- Synthesis
- Evaluation

Critical thinking helps the individual to step aside from his own beliefs, projects and opinions to sort out the faith and helps to discover the truth.

Examples for Critical Thinking

- Analytical thinking
- Good communication
- Creative thinking
- Open-mindedness
- Ability to solve problems
- Asking thoughtful questions

Analytical Thinking

Analytical thinking is the ability to break any situation into parts and then examine or learn about it. For example: Being observer, take a walk around the classroom and observe the students by using many of your senses, see what's happening around you.

Divergent Thinking

- Divergent thinking is a multi-aspect thinking process.
- It refers to an ability to generate creative ideas by exploring many possible solutions in an effort to find one that works.
- It brings ideas and knowledge from various sources to solve problems and make decisions. For example: Giving a child a stack of blocks and asking him to see how many shapes they have create with those blocks.

Convergent Thinking

Convergent thinking is an ability to put a number of different aspects or perspectives of topic together in an organized manner which is logical to find a single answer. It focuses on a single solution or result rather than multiple solutions. For example: All types of tests such as multiple-choice test, standardized test, quizzes, spelling test, etc.

Sequential (Linear) Thinking

- Sequential thinking is a type of thinking to the ability to process information or ideas in orderly prescribed manner. It involves step-by-step manner.
- Before moving to another step, previous step progression is needed to solve a problem or make a decision. For example: When assembling a table, a sequential thinker would follow the step-by-step directions.

Holistic (Nonlinear) Thinking

- Holistic thinking is a form of thinking ability to see the big picture and recognize the interconnectedness of various components that form the largest system.
- It helps to expand our thought process in various directions rather than one direction. For example: A novel method of digital presentation created by the folks.

Controlled Thinking

In controlled thinking, the process of thinking is controlled and regulated. It is related to achievement of a specific goal. The individual is able to stop and think deeply about himself or herself and society. For example: Writing a letter to your friend or answering to questions in interview.

Free Thinking

Free thinking is automatic. There is no restriction and control in thinking process, freethinkers are able to achieve a certain goal which is realistic.

For example: Free thinking is imagination, daydreaming and dreaming.

Steps in Creative Thinking

- Creative thinking is associated with one's ability to create something new, novel or unusual. It finds new relationship and association to interpret the nature of things, events, or situations.
- Here the creative thinker usually formulates the tools for its solution. For example: Discovering the attractive way to present answer sheet.

Stages of Creative Thinking

Stage I-Preparation

This stage is related to all the preparation that is needed to solve a problem.

All the needed information to understand the problem is gathered by the thinker. The creative thinker finds out that the problem cannot be solved in a short duration of time and he just moves away from it either voluntarily or involuntarily.

Stage II-Incubation

The thinker moves away from the problem. The ideas that were not letting the problem to be solved also start to reduce. The thought process is working unconsciously. The person moves to third stage.

Stage III-Insight (Illumination)

The solution suddenly illuminates and generates an insight in the creative thinker.

Stage IV-Verification (Evaluation)

This stage refers to the evaluation of the solution. If the solution can solve the problem effectively, then the creative thinker moves to the next stage and if the solution is not effective, then the thinker goes back and starts thinking again.

Stage V-Revision

This stage refers to any revision or modification that is needed in the solution.

Characteristics of a Creative Person

- **Curious:** Curiosity generates the creativity. A curious person can be a creative thinker. He can find solutions to his problem in a creative way. He can create the solutions.
- **Playful:** Creative people enjoy the playfulness. They play with different ideas and solutions before reaching to the final solution. It means they try different methods and solutions before reaching to the final one.
- **Open-minded:** They are open to new experiences and ideas. They are not afraid to try new alternatives to solve the problems. They are receptive and nonjudgmental.
- **Flexible:** Creative people are always ready to change. They are not rigid. They can adapt to changes easily.
- **Sensitive:** This sensitivity can help creative people in many areas of life, both personally and professionally. Sensitive people tend to appear more approachable to others and willing to listen to their thoughts or feelings.

11. Define learning. Discuss the factors influencing learning and theories of learning. (MGR, KUHS)

Answer

Definition of Learning

Learning is the conservation of new behavior or the strengthening and weakening of old behavior as a result of experience. **—Henry Smith**

Learning is the acquisition of habits, knowledge and attitude. **—Crow and Crow**

Factors Influencing Learning

Learning is central to all our behavior as we learn to speak, write, think and perceive. Effective learning process depends upon the major factors as follows:

- Nature of the learner
- Nature of the learning material
- Nature of the learning situations
- Learner's perception.

Nature of the Learner

- **Organic defects:** The individual cannot perceive the stimulus properly from the environment in presence of any organic defect.

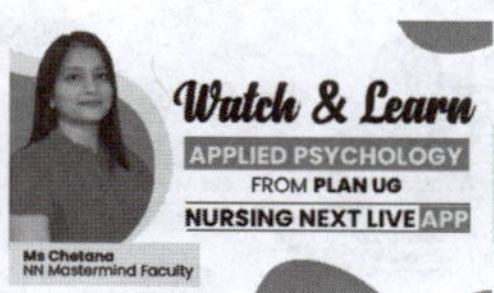

- **Learner's interest and attention:** Interest is the mother of attention. It is an important factor for individuals to receive certain stimulus. Interest is nothing but our likes and dislikes toward stimulus.
- **Learner's maturation:** Learning process depends upon individual's maturation. It means maturation of the central nervous system and other physiological systems of our body. The learning process starts at birth and continues till death.
- **Learner's motivational levels:** Motivation is the internal drive or force which is needed for individuals to learn something new. With strong and clear motivation, we can learn very difficult tasks but without motives, we cannot learn even simple things.
- **Fatigue:** Some of the factors, like loneliness, compulsion, restlessness may cause physiological and mental fatigue which lead to an ineffective learning process. For example: Studying in dark rooms, less ventilated.
- **Time of the day:** There is no variation in efficiency of learning throughout the day. But some environmental factors, like noise, excessive heat can overcome learners' will power which affect learning.
- **Age and learning:** Aging process affects learning. The capacity to learn improves up to 22–24 years after 48 declines.
- **Mental health:** Mental health and mental well-being is necessary for learning. With worries, fears, inferiority, loneliness, we cannot learn new things. If learners have no self-confidence, self-reliance, self-respect due to the attitude of teachers or others, it is very difficult for him or her to learn well.
- **Basic potentials:** Learner's innate abilities and capacities are needed for learning.

The following potentials are necessary for effective learning:

- General Intelligence.
- Knowledge, understanding skills, interest, attitudes and aptitude.

Nature of the Learning Material

- **Quality of teaching:** High quality of learning materials and teaching always promotes an effective learning process. It is done only by effective utilization of resources.
- **Availability of learning material:** Learning materials are basic tools for learning. They enhance the desirable changes in learners like text books, laboratory facilities, projects, learning aids, etc.
- **Availability of conducive environment:** Sound environment is an important external factor for learning. It motivates the learners to learn effectively.

The conducive environment is calm, noise free, proper seating arrangement, absence of distractions, etc.

Nature of the Learning Methods

Learning methods influence process of learning:

- **Nature of learning experiences:** Nature of the subject matter can influence the learning process. It may be:
  - Formal or informal
  - Incidental or well-planned
  - Direct or indirect
- Methodology also affects the learning techniques and tools.
  - Link the reason of learning with past
  - Correlate one area with another
  - Utilization of maximum number of resources
  - Revision and practice
  - Proper feedback and reinforcement
- **Meaningfulness of material**

  It promotes faster learning like:
  - **Goal:** It should be clear and strong.
  - **Knowledge:** It promotes frequent regular review of the amount of progress being made toward the goals.
- **Amount and length**

  It depends upon:
  - Distribution of practice period (shorter)
  - Whole versus part method
  - Rest (between two studies)
  - Over learning or repetitions (at regular interval)

Theories of Learning

There are two broad classifications of learning theories: general theories and specific theories.

1. **General theories:** General theories provide a broader framework for understanding learning, e.g., behaviorism, constructivism, cognitive, humanism, and connectivism.
2. **Specific theories:** Specific theories focus on particular aspects of learning, such as how new information is organized or how learning transfers from one situation to another, e.g., Apperception Theory, Theory of Identical Elements, Theory of Generalization, Transposition of Theory of Transfer, and Theory of Ideals.

General Theories

Behaviorism (classical conditioning and operant conditioning): This theory emphasizes the role of environmental stimuli and reinforcement in shaping behavior. It suggests that learning is the result of conditioning and the association between stimuli and responses.

Cognitive theory: Cognitive theories focus on the mental processes involved in learning, such as perception, memory, attention, and problem-solving. They highlight the role of cognitive structures and information processing in acquiring knowledge and skills.

Constructivism: Constructivist theories propose that learning is an active process where learners construct their own understanding and knowledge through experiences and interactions with the environment. They emphasize the importance of prior knowledge and social interactions in learning.

Humanism: Humanistic theories emphasize the individual's personal agency, self-directed learning, and the importance of meeting psychological needs such as autonomy, competence, and relatedness in the learning process.

Connectivism: Connectivism is a relatively newer theory that highlights the significance of networked connections and digital technologies in learning. It emphasizes the role of social networks, information sources, and technology in knowledge acquisition and learning.

Specific Theories

Apperception Theory

- This theory states that learning is a process of organizing new information into existing schemas.
- According to this theory, reference of learning occurs due to previous experiences and storage of ideas in one's unconscious mind. It is strengthening with repetition of ideas and it leads to transfer automatically in the current learning situation.
- For example: A rich girl and a poor girl are eating same number of idlis together. The bill is around ₹50. The rich girl says it is not very much money and the poor girl says it is too much of cost.
- The difference lies in how they apperceive the same bill. The knowledge of previous experience through which they value the money.

Theory of Identical Elements

- Theory of identical elements was introduced by Thorndike and Wordsworth.
- It states that the level of training transfer depends upon the level of similarity between training and performing environment like dual – tasks, rapid decision making and attention control.
- Transfer of content from one situation to another to the extent that the same content or component are found in different situations. It is enhanced through:
  - **Similarity of content:** Same components between two learning.
  - **Similarity in technique:** Same element or techniques between two learning. For example: The study of Tamil helps one with the study of Malayalam to an extent as the two languages contain identical vocabularies.

Sometime less transfer occurs when an individual does not notify similarity between the two. But transfer is not an automatic process here.

Theory of Generalization

- Generalization provokes that transfer occurs as a result of common features or general principles which one learns in a situation.
- As a result, one is able to apply those learned generalizations to a new situation.
- At the same time, generalization is not applicable for all situations. It is positively related to the learner's intelligence.
- For example: A person who is extremely methodological in office work may be quite disorderly and chaotic in her house.

Transposition of Theory of Transfer

- Transposition theory was introduced by Gestalt field psychologists. According to this concept, transfer of learning implies that what is learnt in one situation can be shifted directly to another situation.
- For example: Students who learned the procedure of intramuscular injection on dummy can perform it on the real patients during their clinical postings.
- The process of gaining and developing insight into the use of concepts and generalization in one situation and applying it afterwards in another situation is called transposition.
- For example: Administration of injections after watching injection demonstration by teacher.

Theory of Ideals

- Theory of ideals was introduced by Bagley. He believed that ideals are deeper than generalization. Ideals are the basis of transfer of learning.
- Ideals once adopted in one situation are applicable to all situations. Ideals give proper weightage to the development of desired attitudes and ideas about the things or situations. For example: Being honest in studies and classroom influences the student's behavior and decisions across various situations outside school setting.

SHORT NOTES

1. Error of perception. (RUHS, MGR)

Answer

Errors of perception refer to distortions, inaccuracies, or abnormalities in the processing of sensory information, resulting in a perception of the external environment that differs from the objective reality. These errors can occur in any of the five senses (sight, hearing, taste, touch, and smell) and can vary in severity from subtle to profound.

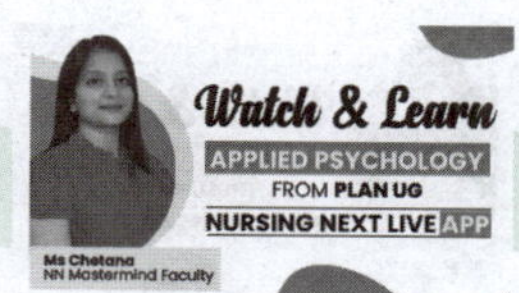

The errors in perception can be divided mainly into two types:

1. **Hallucination:** It is defined as sensory perception in the absence of any external sensory stimuli. It is of many types:
   - **Visual hallucination:** A visual hallucination is a sensory experience in which a person perceives something that is not actually present in the external environment.
   - **Auditory hallucination:** A sensory experience in which a person hears sounds or voices that are not actually present in the external environment.
   - **Tactile hallucination:** A sensory experience in which a person feels sensations on their skin or internally that are not actually present in the external environment.
   - **Olfactory hallucination:** A sensory experience in which a person smells odors that are not actually present in the external environment.
   - **Gustatory hallucination:** A sensory experience in which a person tastes flavors that are not actually present in the external environment.
2. **Illusion:** It is a misinterpretation of actual perception. For example: A rope in dark is perceived as a snake.

2. What is shaping? (MGR)

Answer

- Shaping is a behavioral learning process that involves gradually modifying and reinforcing behavior to achieve a desired outcome.
- It is based on the principles of operant conditioning and is often used in behavior modification and training.
- Shaping is often used to train animals, such as dogs, to perform specific behaviors, but it can also be used to help humans learn new skills or behaviors.
- The process typically involves breaking down the target behavior into smaller, more manageable steps and reinforcing each step as it is accomplished.
- For example, when training a dog to sit on command, the trainer might initially reward the dog for simply looking at them when they say "sit." Once the dog has mastered this step, the trainer might then require the dog to take a step forward, and reward the dog for doing so. Over time, the trainer would gradually require more and more of the behavior until the dog is sitting on command.
- Shaping can be an effective technique for teaching complex behaviors because it allows the learner to build confidence and motivation by achieving small successes along the way.
- It can also help the learner to generalize the behavior to other contexts, making it more likely that they will continue to perform the behavior even in new situations.
- There are two types of reinforcement used to establish a desired behavior or disappear an unwanted behavior pattern.
  1. Positive reinforcement
  2. Negative reinforcement

3. The classification of intelligence. (MGR)

Answer

Definition of Intelligence

Intelligence is the aggregate or global capacity of the individual to think rationally, to act purposefully and to deal effectively with the environment. **—Wechsler 1994**

Intelligence is the ability to master the knowledge or skills needed to succeed within a particular culture. **—Lolurto 1991**

Classification of Intelligence

Concrete intelligence

Concrete intelligence is applicable for using concrete materials like machines, tools and instruments. Human being uses this intelligence in the operation of tools like engineers. For example: All dogs are friendly.

Social intelligence

Social intelligence is an ability to understand social situations in daily life. Human being uses social intelligence to understand people and act wisely in human relationship to know the art of winning friends and influence them. For example: Leaders, Ministers and Salesmen use social intelligence.

Abstract Intelligence

Abstract intelligence is an ability to respond to words, numbers and letters. Abstract intelligence is required for study of books or literature. For example: Jury members of the competition might find that person who danced well.

Emotional Intelligence

Emotional intelligence is also called social intelligence. It is the ability to perceive, express, understand and, regulate emotions. For example: An upset employee finds a compassionate ear.

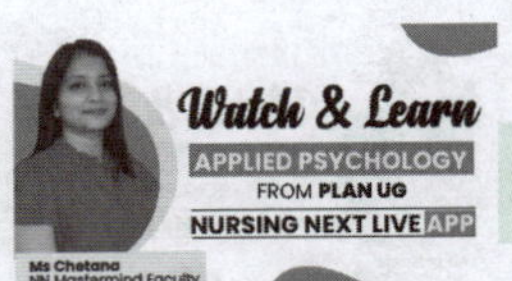

Another Classification of Intelligence: Gardner's Multiple Intelligence

According to Howard Gardner, there are eight major kinds of intelligence:

1. Musical intelligence: It is a form of intelligence with skills in tasks involving music.
2. Bodily-kinesthetic intelligence: Human being have skills of using whole body or various portions of it in the solution of problems or in the construction of products.
3. Logical mathematical intelligence: It is a special skill in problem solving and scientific thinking.
4. Spatial intelligence: Skills involving spatial configurations used.
5. Interpersonal intelligence: Skills in human interactions like temperament, sensitivity, motivations and intentions.
6. Linguistic intelligence: It is a skill used in production and use of language. Linguistic intelligence helps the individual become public speakers, good spellers, writers and literature. For example: literature.
7. Intrapersonal intelligence: It is a knowledge of the internal aspect of oneself; access to once own emotions and feelings.
8. Naturalistic intelligence: It is an ability to identify and classify patterns in nature.

4. Discuss the usefulness of study habits. (MGR)

Answer

Study habits: Study habits refer to the practices and routines that individuals adopt to facilitate effective learning and academic success.

These habits encompass various strategies and behaviors that contribute to efficient studying, comprehension, and retention of information.

Usefulness of study habits: The usefulness of study habits are as follows:

- **Build knowledge and confidence:** Study habits increase knowledge, confidence, competence and self-esteem
- **Reduce anxiety:** Study habits reduce anxiety about tests and deadlines.
- **Effective utilization of resources:** Good study habits help individuals utilize their time and resources more effectively.
- **Enhanced retention and understanding:** Effective study habits promote better comprehension and long-term retention of information.
- **Increased focus and attention:** Study habits involve creating a conducive study environment and minimizing distractions.
- **Better organization and preparedness:** Creating a study schedule, breaking down complex topics into manageable chunks, and using Audio-Visual aids contribute to a structured and approach to learning.
- **Self-discipline and motivation:** Developing study habits cultivates self-discipline and motivation.
- **Worthwhile:** Students who use effective study skills may feel their work and effort is more worthwhile.

5. Types of forgetting and theories of forgetting. (MGR)

Answer

Types of Forgetting

Forgetting is an inability to recall something. There are various types of forgetting:

- **Natural forgetting (trace dependent):** Forgetting due to lapse of time and without intention of the individual. It is a quite common type of forgetting process.
- **Morbid forgetting (abnormal):** Person deliberately tries to forget something. It may be anxiety procedure, emotional threatening, or unpleasant one.

  It has two subtypes:

  1. **General forgetfulness:** Individual tries to forget the total event.
  2. **Specific:** Individual tries to forget some specific part of the total event.
- **Cue dependent forgetting:** It is an inability to recall information stored in memory due to insufficient internal and external generated cues.
- **State dependent:** It is a tendency to remember something when one is in the same emotional and physical state as during the original learning experience. Without it the person has difficulty in recalling.
- **Motivated forgetting:** Forgetting occurs with individual purpose or wishes. Many lapses occur due to motivated forgetting in our daily life. This is due to not to our liking or not interested to do. For example: Forget the names of the people whom we hate or we forget to buy some eatable which your partner asked to buy.

Theories of Forgetting

Consolidation Theory

- Consolidation theory explains about faulty memory process, that means learning without understanding.

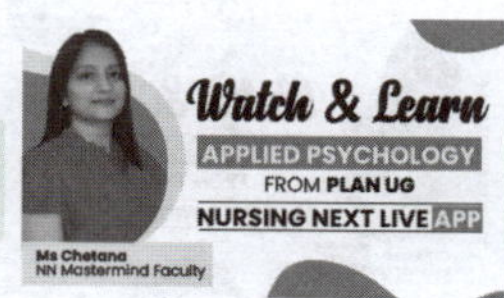

- Certain materials may be simplified or changed during encoding.

Memory Trace Decay Theory

- Forgetting occurs due to decay of memory trace with the lapse of time.
- According to this theory, when we learn something, a memory trace is formed because of neurological changes in brain.
- Gradually it fades away, if the imprint is not occasionally reactivated. With proper retrieval, we can keep the stress active.
- As aging processes, the individual memory stores begin to regenerate and a lot of encoded materials are lost.

Repression Theory

Repression theory is also called morbid forgetting. It is an ego defense that automatically hides, emotionally threatens and produces anxiety in the unconscious mind. It is not recalled voluntarily.

Interference Theory

- Mechanism of interference is responsible for forgetting. It means one learning affects another one. We forget something due to the following interference:
- **Proactive inhibition**: It is a prior learning interference with the learning of new. For example: Learnt material in car driving affects your current learning of bus driving.
- **Retroactive inhibition**: It is a backward process. It is a new learning interfering with materials previously learnt. For example: If you learn one chapter in research and then you learn one chapter in statistics then you try to recall the research chapter but you unable to recall because of interference of statistics.

6. Write a short note on Memory disorders. (MGR)

Answer

Memory Disorders

Memory disorder is defined as an inability to encode and recall the information. It is caused by some neuroanatomical damages or organic disorders. It may vary according to the individual differences. Some common memory disorders are:

- **Amnesia:** It is an abnormal mental state in which memory and learning are affected out of all proportion to other cognitive functions.
- **Dementia:** It refers to a chronic, persistent disorder of mental processes characterized by progressive deterioration of thinking ability, memory disorder, personality changes and impaired reasoning.
- **Agnosia:** It is the loss of ability to recognize objects, persons, places and voices.
- **Alzheimer disease:** Due to aging process, progressive degeneration of brain cells causes cognitive impairment.
- **Hyperthymestic syndrome or Hyperthymesia or piking:** It is characterized by extremely detailed autobiography memory. The individual possesses superior autobiographical memory that is the individual can recall the vast majority of personal experiences and events of life.
- **Wernicke-Korsakoff syndrome:** It is a severe neurological disorder caused by vitamin B_1 deficiency. It is characterized by confusion, amnesia, memory loss, impairment in new learning, inattentiveness and agitation.

7. Define thinking and explain the favorable elements in thinking. (MGR)

Answer

Definition of Thinking

Thinking is the mental activities involved in processing information, solving problems, making decisions, and forming judgments, using both conscious and unconscious cognitive processes. —**Kahneman, 2011**

Favorable Elements of Thinking

There are many favorable elements that can help an individual to be a better thinker. These includes:

Open-mindedness: Being open-minded allows for the consideration of new ideas, perspectives, and information. It promotes intellectual growth, expands knowledge, and encourages a more comprehensive understanding of complex issues..

Critical thinking: Critical thinking is the ability to think carefully and rationally about information. It enables individuals to assess the validity of arguments, identify biases, and make informed decisions based on evidence and reasoning.

Flexibility: Flexibility in thinking entails the willingness to consider different perspectives, adapt to new situations, and revise one's beliefs or strategies when necessary

Creativity: Creativity involves thinking outside the box, generating innovative ideas, and approaching problems from unique angles. It fosters originality, resourcefulness, and adaptability in finding solutions to challenges.

Problem-solving skills: Problem-solving skills are the ability to identify and solve problems. This includes being able to break down problems into smaller parts, as well as being able to think creatively about solutions.

Metacognition: Metacognition refers to the awareness and understanding of one's own thinking processes.

Curiosity: Curiosity drives a thirst for knowledge and a desire to explore and understand the world.

8. Explain efficient methods of memorizing. (DU, KUHS, MGR)

Answer

There are various effective methods of memorizing:

- **Whole and part method:** Breaking a long paragraph or learning material into parts for memorizing easily.
- **Space and unspaced:** Spaced means taking a break in between memorizing a whole thing and unspaced means memorizing the whole thing at once without any break.
- **Memory pegs**: Memory pegs are the reminder cues called memory pegs to hang that to be remembered items. For example: VIBGYOR — rainbow colors of violet, indigo, blue, green, yellow, orange and red.
- **Method of loci:** This method is about using power of visualization. 'Loci' means location. It uses visualization to organize and recall the information. For example: Visualizing checking reflexes with reflex hammer in a patient.
- **Grouping or rhyming:** Memorizing a phone number or account number by grouping. For example: Small children learn alphabets by grouping them. This is an easy and effective method.
- **Repetition and practice:** By repeating again and again, chances of memorizing the concept are higher. For example: Sticking things on the wall and repeating them.
- **Use of principle of association:** Associating the learning material with other things help in memorizing. For example: Caution for AIDS.
- **Make a story:** It is a form of elaborative encoding. Doing this gives coherence and meaning to the otherwise unrelated items.
- **Keyword techniques:** If you have any complicated items to remember like any other language, unknown words, new words, you can make a keyword which consists of item that is very easy to encode and recall when needed.
- **Flashbulb memory:** It is memorizing of specific events that are so clear that they seem like snapshots of the events or situations. For example: Flash bulb events are September 11th, assassination of Kennedy.

  PQ4R: It is a specific technique which is used for memorizing.
  - P – Preview
  - Q – Question
  - 4Rs – Read, Reflect, Result, Review

  SQ3R: It is also a technique:
  - S – Study
  - Q – Question
  - 3Rs – Read, Recite, Review
- **Funnel approach:** It means learning general concepts before moving onto specific details. For example: Learning tables in Maths before moving into Maths problems.
- **Acronym:** Acronym is a word name or set of letters created as an abbreviation of longer phrases or sentences. For example, DABDA-Stages of grief
- **Utilization of senses:** It uses many senses in memorizing. For example: Signal board in road traffic
  - Red – Stop
  - Yellow – Get ready
  - Green– Go

9. Definition and causes of forgetting. (DU)

Answer

Definition of Forgetting

According to Munn (1967), forgetting is the loss of permanent or temporary memory. It is the ability to recall or recognize something learned earlier.

Causes

- Inadequate attention at the time of learning
- Lapse of time
- Interference: There are two types:
  1. **Proactive interference:** When something learnt earlier disturbs recall of something you are learning now that means past learnt things interfere in recalling newly learnt material. For example: Inability to recall the recently watched movie with interference of past watched movie with the same hero.
  2. **Retroactive interference:** It means recently learnt materials interfere in recalling of past learnt material.
- Lack of rest and sleep
- Raised emotions
- Poor physical and mental health
- Nature of learning material
- Methods used to learn

10. Explain the levels of thinking. (DU, KUHS)

Answer

Levels of Thinking

In 1956, Benjamin Bloom created Bloom's taxonomy levels of thinking. According to the theory, thinking process consists of six categories: (i) knowledge, (ii) comprehension, (iii) application, (iv) analysis, (v) synthesis and (vi) evaluation.

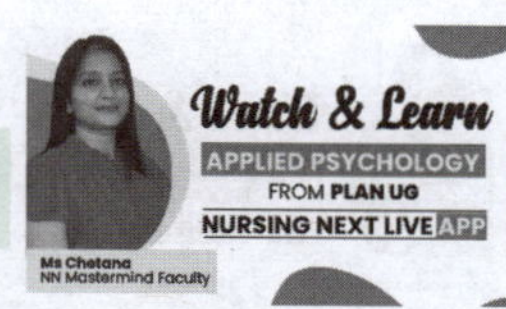

Level 1: Knowledge

Knowledge is the basic level of thinking that involves recall of concepts. Knowledge helps individual to recall the pattern, structure or setting principles and theories. This level helps the individual to identify and understand about objects like when, where, how, define.

Level 2: Comprehension

Comprehension is the second level of thinking. This involves understanding something that we have learnt in first level. Comprehension means understanding something by organizing, interpreting, comparing, and describing.

Level 3: Application

Application is the third level that means applying the knowledge that we have learnt and understood. This level of thinking helps in problem solving and applying new strategies, techniques, facts, rules in different ways in problem solving. Simply it refers to use of abstractions in particular or concrete situations.

Level 4: Analysis

Analysis is the fourth level that consists of breaking of information or ideas into small parts and making relationships, facts, finding evidence to support generalization. Analysis promotes hierarchy of ideas and its relationships. This level of thinking in individual helps to find out causes and risk factors about the situations.

Level 5: Synthesis

Synthesis is the fifth level that involves the putting together of elements and parts so as to form a whole. It is connecting all the information together and to find out new way or technique to solve problem or proposing many alternative solutions. It is promoted by array of materials used in thinking process.

Level 6: Evaluation

Evaluation is a process of making comparison and judgment. It involves evaluating the outcomes after judging the ideas. Effectiveness of this level of thinking is based on effective materials. It is the final level in effective thinking process.

11. Describe the process of 'Transfer of Learning'. (KUHS)

Answer

Transfer of Learning

Transfer of learning means the use of previously acquired knowledge and skills in new learning or problem-solving situations. Transfer of learning refers to the process by which knowledge, skills, or strategies learned in one context can be applied or transferred to another context.

There are two types of transfer: Positive and Negative transfer

1. **Positive transfer:** In this, previously learned information enhances learning or performance on a new task.
2. **Negative transfer:** In this, previously learned information interferes with learning or performance on a new task.

Process of Transfer of Learning

The process of transfer of learning can be described through following steps:

Initial learning: Transfer of learning begins with the acquisition of knowledge or skills in a specific learning context.

Recognition of similarities: The learner must identify the similarities or common elements between the original learning context and the new context where transfer is desired.

Abstraction and generalization: The learner extracts the essential features or principles from the original learning context. Generalization allows the learner to apply the acquired knowledge or skills to a broader range of situations that share similar characteristics.

Mapping and mapping adjustments: The learner maps or matches the abstracted knowledge or skills onto the new context.

Application and practice: The learner actively applies the transferred knowledge, skills, or strategies in the new context. This could involve problem-solving, decision-making, or performing tasks

Feedback and evaluation: The learner receives feedback on their performance in the new context.

Consolidation and reinforcement: Successful transfer of learning leads to consolidation and reinforcement of the transferred knowledge or skills.

12. Explain Spearman's two-factor theory of intelligence.

Answer

This theory was proposed by Charles Spearman in 1904.

- According to this theory, intelligence includes two factors and they are General Intelligence and Specific Intelligence.
- General intelligence (g) refers to a broad, underlying factor that influences performance on a wide range of cognitive tasks, such as reasoning, problem-solving, and abstract thinking.
- According to Spearman, g is the primary source of individual differences in cognitive ability across different domains.

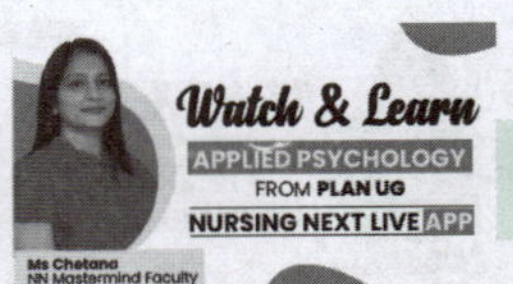

- Specific intelligence (s) refers to more specialized abilities that are specific to particular tasks or domains, such as musical ability or language proficiency.
- These specific abilities are unique to each individual and are not necessarily related to their level of general intelligence.
- Spearman believed that all intellectual tasks involve both g and s factors, with g providing a common factor that underlies performance on all tasks, and s providing unique factors that are specific to particular tasks. He proposed that the relationship between g and s could be expressed as a mathematical formula:

Performance on a specific task = g + s

SHORT ANSWER QUESTIONS

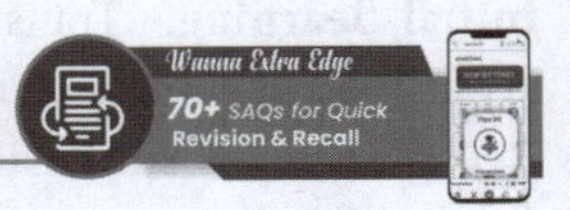

1. Name the different steps in creative thinking.

Answer

Creative thinking is a process that involves coming up with new and original ideas or solutions to problems.

- Preparation
- Incubation
- Inspiration
- Ideation
- Evaluation
- Refinement
- Implementation

2. What are the three types of intelligence?

Answer

Three types of intelligence are:

1. Linguistic intelligence
2. Logical-mathematical intelligence
3. Spatial intelligence

3. Causes of forgetting. (DU)

Answer

Causes

- Inadequate attention at the time of learning
- Lapse of time
- Interference
  - **Proactive interference:** For example: Inability to recall the recently watched movie with interference of past watched movie with the same hero.
  - **Retroactive interference:** It means recently learnt materials interfere in recalling of past learnt material.
- Lack of rest and sleep
- Raised emotions
- Poor physical and mental health
- Nature of learning material
- Methods used to learn

4. What is the formula used for measuring intelligence quotient?

Answer

Intelligence quotient is calculated by using this formula.

Here mental age is calculated by using psychological tests by psychologists.

IQ = Mental age/Chronological age × 100

5. What is illusion?

Answer

Illusion is a misinterpretation of actual perception. For example: A rope in dark is perceived as a snake.

6. Write the subtests of Bhatia's battery of intelligence scale.

Answer

Bhatia's Battery of Intelligence Scale (BBIS) is a popular intelligence test developed by N. S. Bhatia, an Indian psychologist. The BBIS includes several subtests that assess different aspects of intelligence. Some of the subtests of the BBIS are:

- Verbal intelligence test
- Performance intelligence test
- Abstract reasoning test
- Mechanical reasoning test
- Spatial intelligence test
- Memory test
- Numerical ability test

7. Name three laws of learning.

Answer

Learning can be defined as the process of acquiring new knowledge, skills, behaviors, or attitudes through study,

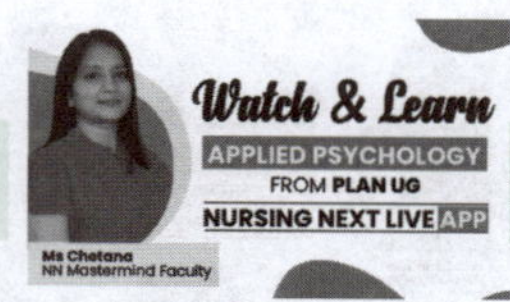

experience, or instruction. It involves a change in an individual's mental representations, behaviors, or ways of thinking, which result from experiences and interactions with the environment. Three laws of learning are:

1. Law of effect
2. Law of readiness
3. Law of exercise

8. Write a few external determinants of attention.

Answer

External factors: These are the factors present in our environment.

- Size of the stimulus
- Intensity of the stimulus
- Environmental changes
- Movement of the stimulus
- Contrast of the stimulus
- Novelty
- Repetition of the stimulus
- Definite form of the object
- Location of the stimulus
- Isolation

9. SQ3R – Write the expansion form.

Answer

SQ3R: It is also a technique of memorizing.

- S – Study
- Q – Question
- 3Rs – Read, Recite, Review

10. Write the five types of intelligence.

Answer

Five types of intelligence:

1. Linguistic intelligence
2. Logical-mathematical intelligence
3. Spatial intelligence
4. Bodily-kinesthetic intelligence
5. Musical intelligence

11. Define sensation and attention.

Answer

Sensation is the process by which sensory receptors in the body detect and respond to external stimuli, such as light, sound, touch, taste, and smell. It is the initial process that allows us to perceive the world around us and involves the conversion of physical energy (such as light or sound waves) into neural signals that can be processed by the brain.

Attention is defined as an ability to produce, select, manage, and maintain sufficient stimulation at a specific amount of time to process any kind of information.

12. Write about laws of learning by Thorndike.

Answer

Laws of Learning by Thorndike

Law of effect: Behaviors that are followed by positive outcomes (such as rewards) are more likely to be repeated, while behaviors that are followed by negative outcomes (such as punishments) are less likely to be repeated.

Law of readiness: Learning is most effective when the learner is motivated and ready to learn. The learner should be prepared intellectually, emotionally, and physically to engage with the material being taught.

Law of exercise: Repetition and practice are essential for learning and skill development. The more a behavior or skill is practiced, the more likely it is to become automatic and be retained over time.

13. Explain transfer of learning.

Answer

Transfer of Learning

Transfer of learning is the process by which prior knowledge or skills influence the acquisition or performance of new knowledge or skills.

There are two types of transfer: Positive and Negative transfer

14. Name the different intelligent tests.

Answer

Intelligent Tests (IQ tests):

- Stanford-Binet intelligence scale
- Wechsler adult intelligence scale
- Kaufman assessment battery for children
- Raven's progressive matrices
- Differential ability scales
- Woodcock-Johnson tests of cognitive abilities

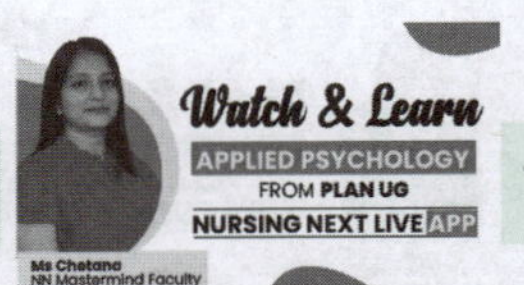

15. Types of memory. (MGR, RUHS)

Answer

Types of Memory

There are major three types of memory:

1. **Immediate or sensory memory:** It is a brief and temporary memory system that retains information from the environment for a very short duration. It includes iconic memory (visual sensory memory) and echoic memory (auditory sensory memory).
2. **Short-term memory:** STM can retain a small amount of information for a short period of time (20–30 seconds).
3. **Long-term memory:** LTM can retain memory for a very long time. It can store information up to days, months, or years. We can retain memory of our lifetime in our LTM. For example: Always remembering your names, date of birth.

16. Emotional intelligence.

Answer

- Emotional intelligence (EQ) is also called social intelligence.
- It is the ability to perceive, express, understand and, regulate emotions. Some studies show that EQ is a greater predictor for future success than IQ.
- It is basic for empathy to others like social skills and self-awareness. For example: An upset employee finds a compassionate ear.

17. Expand WAIS and WISC.

Answer

- The Wechsler Adult Intelligence Scale (WAIS) is a clinical instrument used to measure adult and adolescent intelligence.
- The Wechsler Intelligence Scale for Children (WISC) is developed to measure general cognitive ability and intellectual functioning in Verbal Comprehension (VC), Perceptual Reasoning (PR), Working Memory (WM) and Processing Speed (PS).

18. Insight learning.

Answer

Insight learning is a type of learning that occurs when an individual suddenly solves a problem or achieves a goal through a sudden realization or understanding of a previously unseen or hidden relationship between the elements of the problem. It involves a cognitive process that allows an individual to see a problem in a new light, leading to a sudden solution.

19. Types of attention.

Answer

Definition of Attention

Attention is defined as an ability to produce, select, manage, and maintain sufficient stimulation at a specific amount of time to process any kind of information.

Types of Attention

According to Ross

- Volitional (Voluntary) Attention
- Nonvolitional (Involuntary) Attention

According to Solberg and Mateer

- Selective attention
- Divided attention
- Alternating attention
- Sustained attention
- Arousal attention
- Focused attention

Types of Attention Based on Senses

- Auditory attention
- Visual attention
- Habitual attention

20. Long-term memory.

Answer

Long-term memory (LTM) can retain memory for a very long time. It can store information up to days, months, or years. We can retain memory of our lifetime in our LTM. For example: Always remembering your names, date of birth.

Long-term memory can be categorized into:

- **Declarative memory:** Semantic memory, Episodic memory
- **Procedural memory**

21. Concept of IQ.

Answer

The concept of IQ, or Intelligence Quotient, refers to a score of an intelligence test that is designed to measure an individual's cognitive abilities and potential for success in various areas of life.

The IQ score is typically obtained through standardized tests that measure various aspects of intelligence, including verbal and nonverbal abilities, working memory, processing speed, and problem-solving skills.

CONCEPTUAL REVISION

MULTIPLE CHOICE QUESTIONS

1. Stimulus operating on our nervous system is termed:

a. Sensation b. Observation
c. Attention d. Perception

Ans. a. Sensation

2. Which of the following factors influence an individual's perception?

a. Motives and needs b. Learning
c. Person's mental status d. All of these

Ans. d. All of these

3. According to which principle of perception, there is tendency to perceive objects of a similar size and shape or color as a unit or figure?

a. Similarity b. Proximity
c. Continuity d. Closure

Ans. a. Similarity

4. According to which of the principles, items which are closer together in space of time tend to be perceived as belonging together or forming an organized group?

a. Similarity b. Proximity
c. Good figure d. Closure

Ans. b. Proximity

5. A common type of perceptual error found in a psychotic patient is:

a. Illusion b. Hallucination
c. Delusion d. Thought disorder

Ans. b. Hallucination

6. Concentration of consciousness upon one object rather than upon another is called:

a. Observation b. Sensation
c. Attention d. Perception

Ans. c. Attention

7. A relatively enduring behavioral change brought about by an experience is called:

a. Learning b. Habituation
c. Growth d. All of these

Ans. a. Learning

8. Memory images or traces are present in the mind in the form of:

a. Pictures b. Engrams
c. Signals d. Diagrams

Ans. b. Engrams

9. Thinking which aims at solving complex problems is:

a. Perceptual thinking b. Reflective thinking
c. Abstract thinking d. Creative thinking

Ans. b. Reflective thinking

10. All of the following are the stages of creative thinking, except:

a. Preparation b. Reflection
c. Incubation d. Insight

Ans. b. Reflection

Golden Points

- A psychological test is any procedure on the basis of which influences are made concerning a person's capacity, propensity or liability act, react, experience or to structure order thought or behavior in particular ways.
- Aptitude is a combination of characteristic indicative of an individual capacity to acquire some specific knowledge, skills or set of organized responses.
- Attention is an ability to produce, select, manage, and maintain sufficient stimulation at a specific amount of time to process any kind of information.
- Bloom's Taxonomy levels of thinking consist of six categories such as knowledge, comprehension, application, analysis, synthesis and evaluation.
- Cognition is a basic mental process like sensation, attention, perception and complex mental operations such as intelligence, reasoning, decision-making, memory and problem-solving.
- Forgetting is the loss of memory, permanent or temporary, of the ability to recall or recognize something learned earlier.
- Intelligence is the aggregate or global capacity of the individual to think rationally, to act purposefully and to deal effectively with the environment.
- Learning is the conservation of new behavior or the strengthening and weakening of old behavior as a result of experience.

CHAPTER

7

Motivational and Emotional Process

CONCEPTUAL THEORY

Terminology

Adaptation: Adaptation takes place when an individual's physical or behavioral reaction to any alteration in their internal or external surroundings leads to the preservation of personal well-being and a return to a state of balance.

Attitude: Attitude can be described as an individual's perspective and assessment of something or someone, representing their inclination or inclination to respond favorably or unfavorably to a specific concept, entity, individual, or circumstance

Coping: Coping styles refer to the predominant behaviors individuals frequently employ to manage and navigate stress and distress in various situations.

Emotions: Emotion refers to a subjective experience that occurs alongside overall internal adaptation and heightened mental and physiological states within an individual. (Lester D. Crow and Alice D)

Motivation: Motivation refers to the states within a person or animal that drive behavior toward some goals. —(Morgan and King)

Motives: A motive is a rather specific process, which has been learned. It is directed toward goal. —(Carol-1969)

Stress: Stress is a biological, psychological, social or chemical factor that causes physical or emotional tension and may be a factor in the etiology of certain illnesses.

MOTIVATION

Definition

Motivation refers to the states within a person or animal that drive behavior toward some goals. **—Morgan and King**

Motivation Cycle

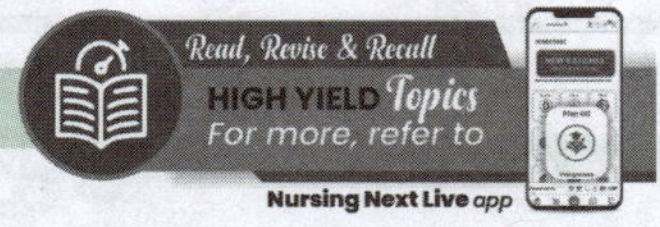

The motivation cycle refers to the process by which individuals become motivated to pursue a goal or engage in a particular behavior. It involves a series of psychological and physiological events that drive and sustain motivation.

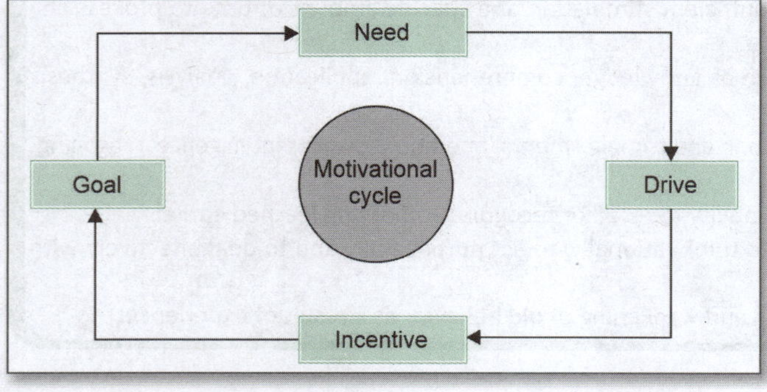

MOTIVES

A need gives rise to one or more motives. A motive is a rather specific process, which has been learned. It is directed toward goal. **—Carol-1969**

Types of Motives

- Primary Motives or Physiological Motives or Biological Motives
- Secondary Motives/Psychosocial Motives/Social Learned Motives

Primary Motives or Physiological Motives or Biological Motives

- Need for oxygen, food and water
- Temperature, rest and sleep
- Sex
- Elimination of waste

Secondary Motives/Psychosocial Motives/ Social Learned Motives

- Need for achievement

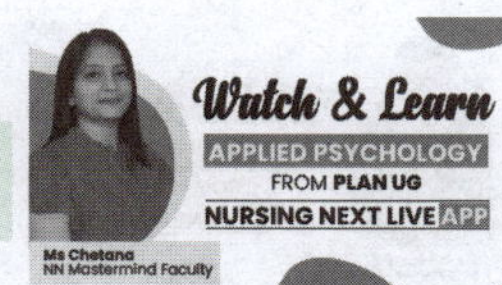

- Need for power
- Need for affiliation

Intrinsic motivation: Intrinsic motivation refers to engaging in behavior for the inherent satisfaction, enjoyment, or personal interest it brings. The driving force comes from within the individual, and the activity itself is rewarding, e.g., hobbies, solving puzzle, etc.

Extrinsic motivation: Extrinsic motivation involves engaging in behavior to attain external rewards or to avoid punishments. The motivation stems from external factors rather than inherent interest in the activity itself. e.g., Training in sports for recognition and trophies.

THEORIES OF MOTIVATION

Maslow's Hierarchy of Needs

Maslow's hierarchy of needs is a psychological theory proposed by Abraham Maslow.

- **Physiological needs:** At the base of the hierarchy are the physiological needs, which include basic biological requirements for survival such as food, water, shelter, sleep and clothing. These needs must be met in order to maintain physical well-being.
- **Safety needs:** Once physiological needs are fulfilled, individuals seek safety and security. This includes personal security, financial stability, a stable and secure environment, access to health care and protection from harm.

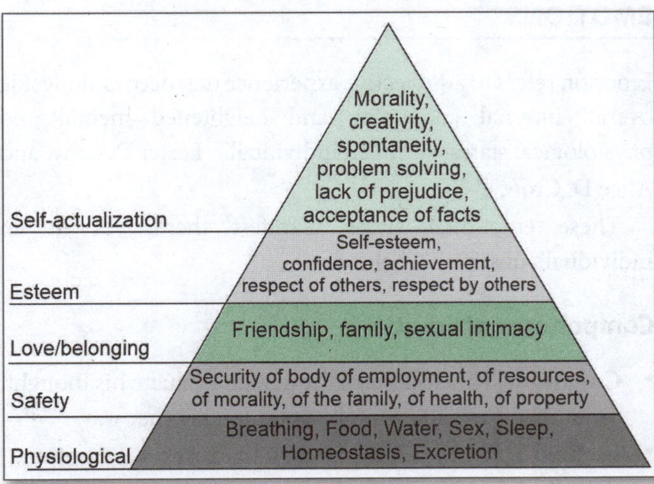

- **Love and belongingness needs:** Once safety needs are met, individuals have a need for love, affection and a sense of belonging. This involves forming meaningful relationships, having a sense of community, and feeling accepted and valued by others.
- **Esteem needs:** After fulfilling the lower-level needs, individuals seek to develop self-esteem and gain recognition and respect from others. This includes gaining self-confidence, achieving personal goals, and receiving appreciation and acknowledgment for one's accomplishments.
- **Self-actualization needs:** At the top of the hierarchy is the need for self-actualization, which refers to fulfilling one's full potential and achieving personal growth. This involves pursuing individual talents, creative endeavors, personal development, and a sense of purpose and meaning in life.

Drive-reduction Theory of Motivation

- The concept was initially formulated by Clark Leonard Hull, who is considered the "Father of Drive Reduction Theory," in 1943.
- It posits that the needs of individuals can generate psychological drives, which subsequently guide their behavior in order to maintain homeostasis.

Arousal Theory of Motivation

- According to the Arousal Theory, individuals have an optimal level of arousal that is most conducive to their performance and well-being.
- This optimal level varies from person to person and can differ depending on the task or situation.
- Some individuals may prefer higher levels of arousal, while others may prefer lower levels.

Incentive Theory of Motivation

- The theory emphasizes that individuals evaluate the potential outcomes or incentives associated with different actions or goals and choose to engage in behaviors that offer the greatest perceived rewards or incentives.
- Positive incentives increase the likelihood of behavior repetition, while negative incentives or punishments decrease the likelihood of behavior.

Herzberg's Two Factor Theory (1959)

- Herzberg's Two Factor Theory, proposed in 1959 by Frederick Herzberg, suggests that job satisfaction and dissatisfaction are influenced by two sets of factors: hygiene factors and motivators.
- Hygiene factors, such as salary, job security, work conditions, and company policies, are extrinsic factors that, when absent or inadequate, can lead to dissatisfaction.

McClelland's Achievement Theory (1988)

- According to the theory, individuals possess varying degrees of three primary needs: achievement, affiliation and power.
- The need for achievement refers to the desire to excel, set and accomplish challenging goals, and receive recognition for one's accomplishments.

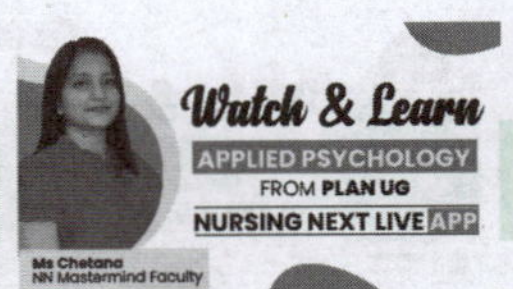

- The need for affiliation pertains to the desire for positive social relationships and belongingness.
- The need for power involves the desire to influence and control others or the environment.

STRESS

Stress is a normal reaction in our body.

Stress is a physiological and psychological response to a real or perceived threat to physical or psychological integrity of an individual. Stress can be triggered by both positive and negative events in our lives.

Models of Stress

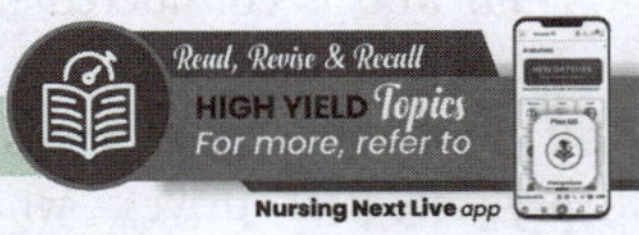

Response-based Model

Selye called this general reaction of the body to stress as general adaptation syndrome (GAS). He described the reaction in three distinct stages.

1. **Alarm reaction stage:** In the alarm reaction, there are two responses to the stress such as flight response and fight response.
2. **Stage of resistance:** Resistance reaction allows the body to fight with the stressors for a long time and copes with the stressful situation.
3. **Stage of exhaustion:** In this stage, tissues start to die and organs get weaken due to the long-time resistance and create higher demand on lungs, heart, blood vessels and gastrointestinal system.

ADAPTATION

Adaptation takes place when an individual's physical or behavioral reaction to any alteration in internal or external surroundings leads to the preservation of personal well-being and a return to a state of balance.

COPING

Coping styles refer to the predominant behaviors individuals frequently employ to manage and navigate stress and distress in various situations.

Types of Coping

Lazarus and Folkman (1984) defined three types of coping as:

1. **Problem-focused coping:** It refers to the approach of actively addressing the stressor at hand by utilizing coping strategies to tackle a specific problem.
2. **Emotion-focused coping**: It involves employing coping strategies to manage and address the emotions that arise from problems or challenges.
3. **Cognitive-focused coping**: It entails employing coping strategies that rely on existing knowledge and understanding to effectively manage and address stress.

Stress Management

- Stress management entails utilizing coping mechanisms that are beneficial in effectively handling and mitigating stress.
- Coping strategies are considered adaptive as they serve to shield individuals from harm and enhance their capacity to navigate challenging situations.
- These adaptive strategies aid in restoring balance within the body and prevent the onset of diseases.

Stress Busters

- Planning
- Find the right solution
- Coping practice
- Spirituality
- Getting connected
- Meditation
- Biofeedback
- Massage
- Drugs
- Hypnosis
- Pet therapy

EMOTIONS

Emotion refers to a subjective experience that occurs alongside overall internal adaptation and heightened mental and physiological states within an individual. - Lester D. Crow and Alice D. Crow.

These emotional states manifest themselves in an individual's observable behavior.

Components of Emotion

- **Cognition:** This will make the person evaluate his thought, prompting ways to express emotion in another way.
- **Feeling:** This will help the person to express his emotion.
- **Behavioral:** Various behavioral responses to express emotions, facial expressions, posture and gestures.

Alteration of Emotions

External Alterations

External modifications in emotions, also known as physiological changes, encompass various aspects:

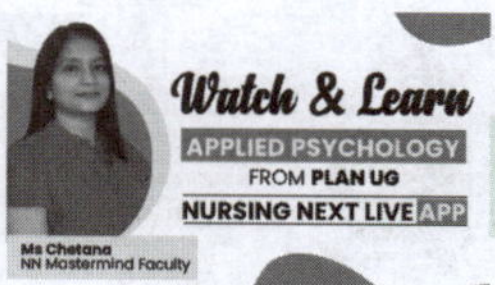

- Studies conducted on voice modulation have confirmed that emotions can induce alterations in vocal characteristics.
- Facial expressions are subject to changes as well.
- Body language can exhibit signs of emotion, such as muscle stiffness.
- Emotions can trigger physical responses like sweating and the appearance of facial wrinkles, particularly on the forehead.

Internal Alterations

Internal transformations within emotions take place as part of the fight-or-flight response, which occurs when an individual encounters a critical situation and has the choice to either confront it (fight) or escape from it (flight).

In such instances, specific internal organ changes occur, including:

- The brain receives the stimulus, leading to a response from various areas, particularly the amygdala, resulting in the release of adrenaline.
- The heart rate escalates.
- Blood pressure elevates.
- There is an increase in sugar levels within the body.

Role of Nurses in Emotionally Sick Patients

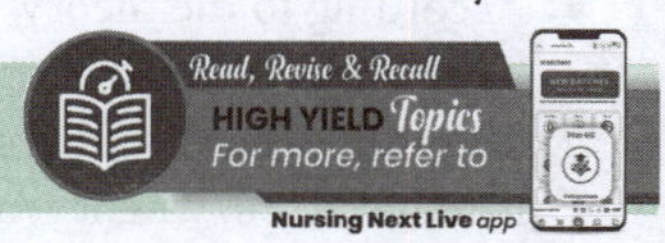

- **Imparting knowledge about the illness:** It is the responsibility of nurses to provide patients with information about their illness.
- **Assisting patients in adjusting to the hospital environment:** Helping patients acclimate to the hospital setting can be challenging, as they often experience fear and anxiety related to hospitals and medications.
- **Addressing patients' psychological stress:** Nurses should accompany patients, helping them overcome psychological pressure and fostering positive emotions.
- **Seeking assistance from professionals:** It is important to seek the help of professionals such as clinical psychologists, medical social workers and occupational therapists as they possess a deeper understanding of patients' emotions and feelings.
- **Preparing patients for discharge:** Nurses should provide clear explanations about medication regimens and ensure that all routine test dates are clearly communicated to patients.

ATTITUDE

Attitude can be described as an individual's perspective and assessment of something or someone, representing their inclination or inclination to respond favorably or unfavorably to a specific concept, entity, individual, or circumstance.

Types of Attitudes

- **Positive attitude:** Individuals with a positive attitude often strive to excel and achieve success in society. They have a strong motivation to perform well and seek recognition and appreciation for their efforts.
- **Negative attitude:** A negative attitude is a mindset or disposition characterized by pessimistic thoughts, emotions, and behaviors.
- **Neutral attitude:** A neutral attitude refers to a mindset or disposition that is neither positive nor negative. It is characterized by a lack of strong emotional or evaluative leaning toward a particular person, object, idea, or situation.

Role of Attitude in Health and Sickness

Attitude can influence an individual's well-being, coping mechanisms, and overall health outcomes.

- **Health promotion:** Individuals with a positive attitude are more likely to engage in healthy habits such as regular exercise, balanced nutrition and preventive health care practices.
- **Resilience and coping:** A positive attitude can enhance an individual's ability to adapt to and cope with challenging health conditions.
- **Treatment adherence:** Individuals with a positive attitude are more likely to follow medical recommendations, take medications as prescribed, attend appointments, and engage in self-care activities.
- **Psychological well-being:** Positive attitudes are associated with lower levels of stress, anxiety and depression, leading to improved mental health and a positive impact on physical health.
- **Healing and recovery:** A positive attitude can contribute to better outcomes in terms of healing, pain management and overall recovery.

CONCEPTUAL EXERCISES

LONG ANSWER QUESTIONS

1. Define motivation. Explain various theories of motivation. (RUHS, MGR, KUHS)

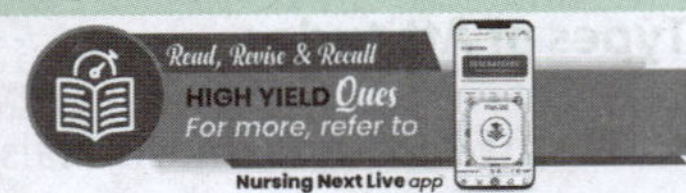

Answer

Definition of Motivation

Motivation refers to the states within a person or animal that drive behavior toward some goals. —**Morgan and King**

Motivation is the class of operations used to produce or measure the changes in performance and changes in energy. —**Underwood**

Theories of Motivation

- **Evolutionary theory of motivation:** Evolutionary theory takes long-term look at the emergence of the human species. According to this theory, the genes are passing from generation to generation. This feature has contributed to survival and reproductive success.
- **Maslow's hierarchy of needs**

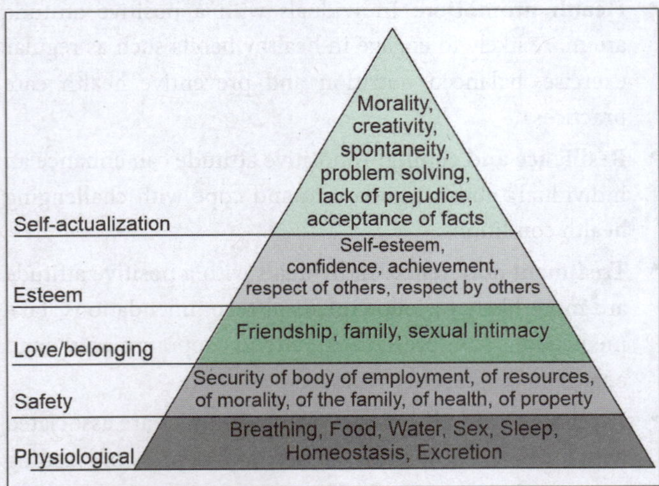

Figure 7.1: Maslow's hierarchy of needs

Maslow identified certain levels of hierarchy of needs. Before moving to the next level of need, first level of need must be fulfilled.

Physiological needs: This level includes basic needs. Need for food, water, warmth, rest and shelter are some examples. Whenever a person needs to fulfill these basic needs, he is motivated and all behavior is directed toward that. But once these needs are fulfilled, they are no longer a motivation.

Safety needs: After fulfilling basic needs, then comes safety, security needs. Human beings are always motivated toward feeling secure and safe.

Belongingness and love needs: These needs come at third level. Needs include intimate relationship, friends. Human beings need to feel loved and wanted. Human beings are social beings and they need to have friends and family.

Esteem needs: This level includes needs like prestige, feeling of accomplishment. Human beings have desire for being respected and appreciated. They need to have feelings of importance.

Self-actualization: This is the highest-level need. In this level, human beings achieve full potential, including creative activities, new challenges, and achievements of the life goals. Only a few people actually lead to the self-actualized state.

- **Drive-reduction theory of motivation: Clark Leonardo Hull (1943) developed this theory.** Drive-reduction theory says that the primary idea behind all human behavior is to reduce 'drives.'
  - A 'drive' is a state of arousal or discomfort which is triggered by a person's physiological or biological needs such as hunger, thirst and the need for warmth.
  - According to the theory, when a person's drive emerges, he/she will be in an unpleasant state of tension which causes him/her to behave in such a way that this tension is reduced. So, whenever there is an unmet need within the body, human beings begin to behave in a manner that allows them to address this need, reduce the drive and achieve a state of balance.
  - Drive-reduction theory suggests that human behavior is a result of wanting to reduce the drives we have.
  - The drives can be: **primary and secondary drives.**
  - **Primary drives** are innate biological needs such as being hungry or thirsty.
  - **Secondary drives** are those learned through conditioning or association with a primary drive, such as money and social acceptance.
- **Arousal theory of motivation:** The Arousal Theory of Motivation was first proposed by Henry Murray in 1938. Murray's theory was based on his observations of humans' needs for achievement, power and affiliation. He believed that these needs were motivated by a desire to reduce one's levels of arousal.

  The Arousal Theory of Motivation suggests that individual's levels of arousal play an important role in determining level of motivation.

  This theory says that when an individual experiences low levels of arousal, they seek out stimulation, but if they get too highly aroused, they will feel unmotivated.

  The arousal theory of motivation suggests that every individual has some kind of arousal to work and it is different for everyone. The theory also suggests that we

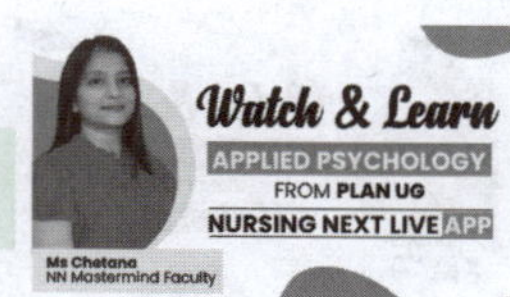

tend to seek for our own stimulation in order to maintain our optimal level of arousal.

- **Incentive theory of motivation:** This theory suggests that human being's behavior is motivated by some extrinsic factors. Human beings feel motivated toward the goal in presence of some incentive.

  For example: A child gets motivated to organize his room if parents say that he will get to watch his favorite TV show.
- **Alderfer's existence, relatedness and growth theory (1969)** Existence, relatedness and growth theory is compared with needs of Maslow's hierarchy of needs.

  E-Existence needs (Primary needs of Maslow's theory)

  R-Relatedness needs (Safety, security, love and belongingness of Maslow's theory)

  G-Growth needs (Self-esteem and self-actualization of Maslow's theory)
- **Herzberg two-factor theory (1959):** The two factors are hygiene or maintenance factors and motivators or growth factors.
- **Hygiene factors:** Hygiene factors are those job factors which are essential for existence of motivation at workplace. These do not lead to positive satisfaction for long-term. But if these factors are absent/if these factors are non-existent at workplace, then they lead to dissatisfaction.
- **Motivational factors:** According to Herzberg, the hygiene factors cannot be regarded as motivators. The motivational factors yield positive satisfaction. These factors are inherent to work. These factors motivate the employees for a superior performance.
- **McClelland's achievement theory (1988)**
  - McClelland's Theory of Three Needs mentions the three desires that an individual can have. Each person is motivated by power, affiliation or achievement.
  - Each human being strives to get the power, affiliation or achievement.
  - Power: Capacity to influence others
  - Affiliation: Capacity to interact with others
  - Achievement: Individual having a strong desire to achieve
- **Adams' equity theory (1965):** There should be a balance between the input and output so that the individual gets motivated. This theory talks about balance and equity.

  There should be a balance between input and output. For example: If an employee gives his maximum efforts, then he expects appreciation and promotion in return.
- **Vroom's expectancy theory (1964):** According to Vroom's Expectancy Theory, the employee will put in the efforts to complete a task only if he thinks that his task is achievable and doable. If the employee feels that a particular task is doable, he will be motivated to perform and put his best efforts in anticipation of the bonus (Expectancy).

  The employee must also believe that the effort he puts in will get the desired outcome (Instrumentality), so the organization must deliver on the outcomes it promises.
- **Locke's goal setting theory (1968):** According to this theory, goal setting is more important to achieve a task than motivation or reward. When individuals establish goals, they become committed to aligning their thoughts, actions, and behavior towards accomplishing those goals.
- **Reinforcement theory of motivation:** Reinforcement theory was proposed by BF Skinner. According to this theory, positive reinforcements play a very important role in establishing a good behavior. A positive behavior that is rewarded is likely to be repeated but if a negative behavior is associated with negative reinforcements, it is not repeated and gradually disappears.

2. What is motivation? Classify motives and explain any three motives. (RUHS, MGR, KUHS)

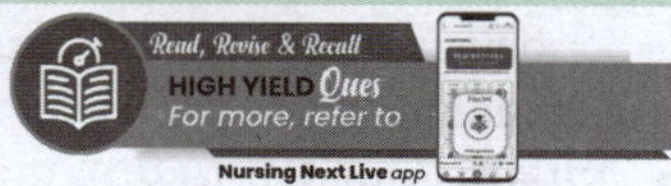

Answer

Definition of Motivation

Motivation refers to the states within a person or animal that drive behavior toward some goals. **—Morgan and King**

Motivation is the class of operations used to produce or measure the changes in performance and changes in energy.

—Underwood

Classification of Motivation

- Primary motives
- Secondary motives
- Stimulus motives
- Personal motives
- Unconscious motives

Primary Motives/Biological Motives

Primary or biological needs are important for all living organisms. Such motives are triggered when there is imbalance in the body. The body always tends to maintain a state of equilibrium called "Homeostasis"- in many of its internal physiological processes.

These are:

- **Need for oxygen, food and water:** These are the basic needs and are required for survival. If these needs are not fulfilled, the survival is threatened.
  - These needs motivate individual to act in order to fulfill.
  - Oxygen is required for survival. No one can survive without regular supply of oxygen.

- Lack of oxygen supply may lead to serious consequences like damage to brain or death. In order to fulfill the motives of hunger and thirst, an individual performs the action.

- **Temperature, rest and sleep:**
  - An individual can suffer from hypo or hyperthermia, if temperature is not maintained. If a person does not get proper rest and sleep, he can become sick.
  - Minimum of 7–8 hours sleep is required by an individual to feel refreshed and rejuvenated. If he does not take proper sleep, he will always have low energy and tiredness.
  - He will have low level of mental alertness. Body and mind need rest to again be ready to work. If a person is not taking adequate rest, it will be difficult for him to concentrate.
- **Sex:**
  - Sex is also a basic need for human beings.
  - Sex need is not essential for the survival of an individual, but it is essential for the survival of the species. Human beings need to reproduce from one generation to another.
- **Elimination of waste:**
  - Elimination is also a basic need.
  - If bowel and bladder are not emptied on time, discomfort arises. An individual needs to feel comfort by eliminating the waste.

Secondary Motives/Social Learned Motives

Social motives are those motives that have social importance. These are called social motives because they are learnt in social groups as a result of interaction with the family and society.

Some of the common social motives are:

- **Need for achievement:** This refers to the need of some achievement. People desire to achieve something significant in their field, e.g., a student wants to achieve good rank in class.
- **Need for power:** People with need for power want to influence and control people. They want to take up jobs where they can exert their power on their subordinates.
- **Need for affiliation:** People want to be affiliated with other people. For example: elderly people need to get associated with other elderly in their community to spend time with them.
- **Social approval:** People need social approval. We all want to have a social approval for our actions and behavior.

Stimulus Motives

There are some internal stimuli that make us to perform some actions. We tend to do something new because our internal stimulus is stimulating or motivating us to do so.

Personal Motives

Personal motives, as the name suggests are personalized and individualized. They are different for everyone.

These are:

- **Force of habits:** This means the actions we perform because of our habits. Our habits can be healthy or unhealthy. For example: Healthy habits like eating well balanced meal, doing regular exercise etc. These habits will motivate us to act on those good and healthy habits.
- **Goals of life:** Our life goals motivate us for actions. They may be related to education, occupation, income, sports, acquisition of property, public service, social service, etc. Once a goal is set, he will be motivated to fulfill that goal.
- **Levels of Aspirations:** Every individual has a goal in his life and strives to achieve that goal. But the effort to attain that goal varies from one individual to another. The amount of satisfaction he gains depends upon his level of aspiration.
- **Attitude and interest:** Our attitudes and interests influence our actions and behaviors. These are also individualized. Attitudes and interest of every individual are different.

3. Discuss motivation. Describe nature and types of motivation with examples. (RUHS, MGR, KUHS)

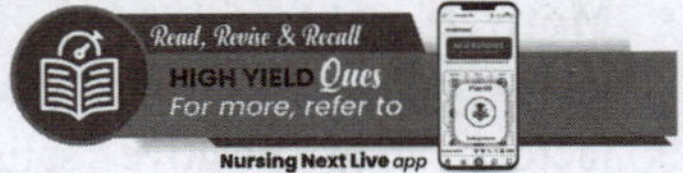

Answer

Definition of Motivation

Motivation refers to the states within a person or animal that drive behavior toward some goals. **—Morgan and King**

Motivation is the class of operations used to produce or measure the changes in performance and changes in energy. **—Underwood**

Theories of Motivation

Maslow's Hierarchy of Needs

Maslow's hierarchy of needs is a psychological theory proposed by Abraham Maslow.

Drive-reduction Theory of Motivation

The concept was initially formulated by Clark Leonard Hull, who is considered the "Father of Drive Reduction Theory," in 1943.

Arousal Theory of Motivation

According to the Arousal Theory, individuals have an optimal level of arousal that is most conducive to their performance and well-being.

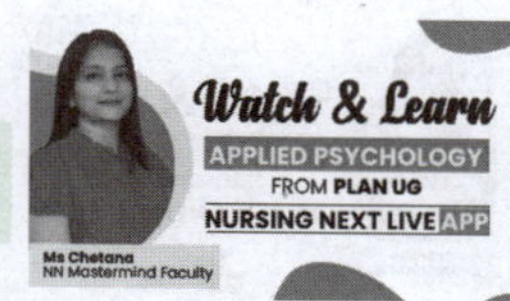

Incentive Theory of Motivation

The theory emphasizes that individuals evaluate the potential outcomes or incentives associated with different actions or goals and choose to engage in behaviors that offer the greatest perceived rewards or incentives.

McClelland's Achievement Theory (1988)

According to the theory, individuals possess varying degrees of three primary needs: Achievement, affiliation and power.

Other theories are: Adams equity theory (1965), Vroom's expectancy theory (1964), Reinforcement theory of motivation and Locke's goal setting theory (1968).

Nature of Motivation

- Motivation in psychology refers to the process by which internal and external factors stimulate, sustain and direct behavior toward achieving a specific goal or outcome.
- Motivation can be driven by a variety of factors, including physiological needs (such as hunger and thirst), social needs (such as affiliation and recognition), cognitive needs (such as curiosity and achievement) and emotional needs (such as pleasure and avoidance of pain).
- Motivation is often described as a dynamic and fluctuating state that can change over time, depending on a person's current goals, environment and level of satisfaction with their current situation.
- Motivation can be intrinsic (arising from within oneself) or extrinsic (arising from external rewards or incentives), and can vary in strength and direction depending on a range of individual and situational factors.
- Motivation is a key determinant of human behavior and plays a critical role in driving individuals toward achieving their goals and fulfilling their needs.
- Motivation is invisible force and the energizing force within us. We act when we feel motivated toward a goal. Our behavior is also influenced by our motives.

Classification of Motivation

For answer, refer to Long Question no. 2, pg. no. 971

4. Explain stress in detail. (RUHS, RUHS, MGR)

Answer

Definition of Stress

Stress is biological, psychological, social or chemical factor that causes physical or emotional tension and may be a factor in the etiology of certain illnesses.

Stress is a physiological and psychological response to a real or perceived threat to physical or psychological integrity of an individual. It is a bodily or mental tension resulting from the factors that tend to alter an existing equilibrium.

Types of Stress

Distress: This type of stress occurs when the demand is excess and it creates a disequilibrium. This disequilibrium can cause physical and mental damage. For example: Loss of a loved one.

Eustress: This type of stress produces feelings of confidence, satisfaction and excitement. An optimal amount of stress is required for normal health and growth. For examle: Prepared for exam and feeling confident.

Stressors

Stressor is defined as an event or situation or person which causes stress.

- **Internal stressors:** Stressors that arise from within, e.g., hunger, thirst, sex.
- **External stressors:** Stressors that arise from outside, e.g., pressure of studying well.

Models of Stress

Transaction-based Model

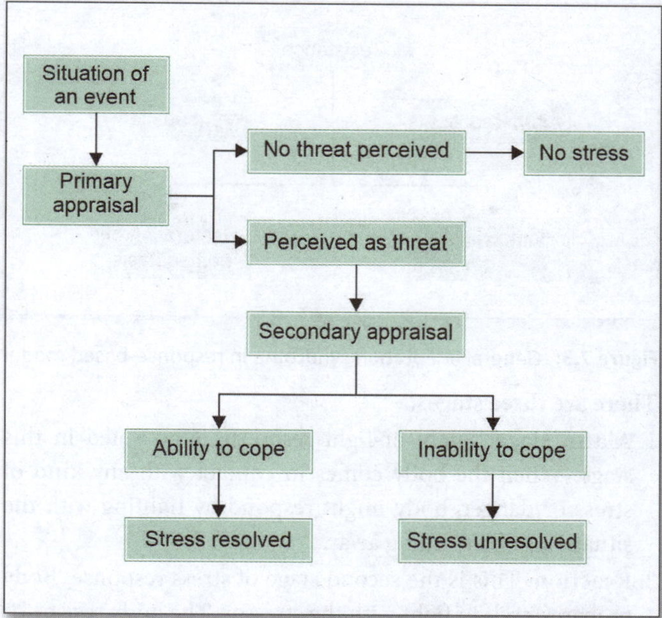

Figure 7.2: Transaction model of stress

- The Transactional Model of Stress and Coping Theory is a framework which emphasizes appraisal to evaluate harm, threat and challenges, which results in the process of coping with stressful events (Lazaurus, 1966; Lazarus & Folkman, 1984).

- The level of stress experienced in the form of thoughts, feelings, emotions and behaviors, as a result of external stressors, depends on appraisals of the situation which involves a judgment about whether internal or external demands exceed resources and ability to cope when demands exceed resources (Lazarus & Folkman, 1984).

Stimulus-based Model

- Stimulus-based model defines stress as a stimulus, a life event or a set of circumstances that arouses physiological and/or psychological reactions that may increase the individual's vulnerability to illness.
- In this, Holmes and Rahe (1967) assigned a numerical value to 43 life changes or events. The most recent version of that scale includes 77 items (Miller and Rahe, 1997), and a shortened version (54 items, full stress and coping inventory completed in 15 minutes).
- The scale of stressful life events is used to document a person's relatively recent experiences, such as divorce, pregnancy and retirement. In this view, both positive and negative events are considered stressful.

Response-based Model/General Adaptation Syndrome

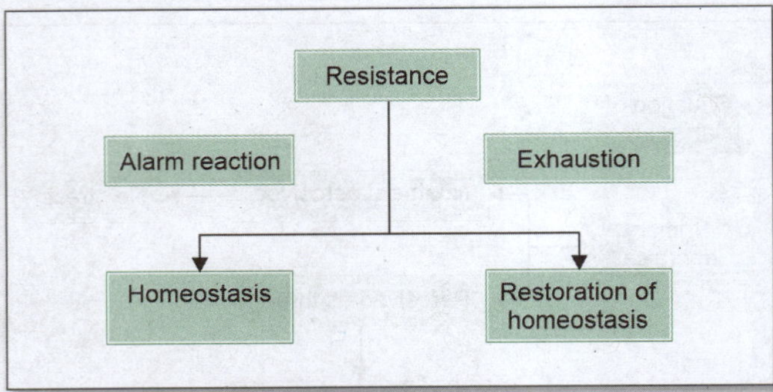

Figure 7.3: General adaptation syndrome in response-based model

There are three stages:

1. **Alarm stage:** Flight-or-fight response is activated in this stage. When the body comes in contact with any kind of stress or danger, body might respond by fighting with the situation or by running away.
2. **Reaction:** This is the second stage of stress response. Body prepares itself to fight with the stressor. The body resists for a long time and copes with the situation. If this mechanism fails, then the body moves to the next stage, i.e., exhaustion.
3. **Exhaustion stage:** In this stage, body starts to get exhausted because of the long-term stress. Tissues start to die and organs become weak due to the long-time resistance to carry out the functions. This extreme demand on the organs results in organ failure.

Acute stress responses: Acute stress is a short-term response to a stressful event.

Acute stress can cause a number of physical and psychological symptoms, including:

- Increased heart rate and blood pressure
- Rapid breathing
- Sweating
- Muscle tension
- Feelings of anxiety, fear, or panic

Chronic stress responses: Chronic stress is long-term stress that lasts for months or even years. It is often caused by ongoing stressors.

Chronic stress can have a various negative effects on the body and mind, including:

- Increased risk of heart disease, stroke, and other health problems
- Weakened immune system
- Sleep problems
- Digestive problems
- Depression
- Anxiety

Role of Nurses in Stress Management

Nurses play an important role in stress management, both for their patients and for themselves.

Identifying the sources of stress: Nurses can help patients to do this by asking them about their daily lives and identifying the things that are causing them stress.

Teaching stress management techniques: Once the sources of stress have been identified, nurses can teach patients about stress management techniques.

Providing support: Nurses can also provide support to patients who are struggling to manage stress. This support can take many forms, such as listening to patients, offering advice, and providing encouragement.

5. Explain attitude and factors affecting behavior and attitude. (RUHS, MGR)

Answer

Attitude means behavior or emotion for a particular person or object. It can be negative or positive.

Definition of Attitude

"An attitude is a mental and neutral state of readiness, organized through experience, exerting a directive or dynamic influence upon the individual's response to all objects and situations with which it is related." **—Gordon Allport**

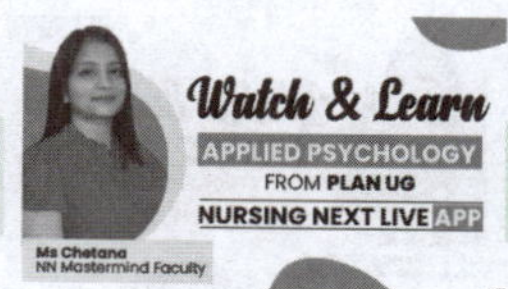

Factors Affecting Attitude

Social factors: Social factors like family and religion influence our attitude toward any object or event. These factors are associated with society in which we belong to. Our attitude is influenced by the common thoughts and beliefs we share as a society, the cultures and trends we follow in our family.

Direct instruction: Direct instructions from any other person can change our attitude toward something.

Family: Family has a strong influence in shaping our attitude. The family environment in which we live since birth shapes the way our beliefs form.

Prejudices: Prejudices mean having a feeling of dislike for someone or a group. Feeling of dislike or false belief about someone also affects our attitude.

Personal experiences: Our experiences also have an impact on our attitude. We perceive things based on our past experience.

Media: Media puts a strong impact on our way of thinking. The way media showcases the things, event or any person we also start believing in that way only.

Educational and religious institutions: Our education and religion form our attitude and beliefs from the very beginning. Every religion and culture have different values and perspectives that are transferred to the individual.

Physical factors: Our attitude toward any person, object or event is also influenced by physical appearance and style. For example: Our attitude toward a person is impacted by his looks and confidence level.

Factors Affecting Behavior

Behavior is affected by factors relating to the person, including:

- **Physical factors:** These include age, health, illness, pain, influence of a substance or medication. For example: If we have pain, we cannot behave in joyful manner.
- **Personal and emotional factors:** These include personality, beliefs, expectations, emotions, mental health. Our behavior is deeply impacted by our beliefs. For example: We do something for our friend and we expect something in return, but if he fails to fulfill our expectations, we will behave differently.
- **Life experiences:** These include family, culture, friends, life events. Our perception depends on our past experiences and our behavior depends how we perceive things around us. For example: If we perceive that the trends that are followed by our elderly do not have any logic, then we will not accept those trends and will behave in opposite manner.
- Needs and wants also influence our behavior. For example: A child wants to watch his favorite cartoon, he will behave as per his parents expectations so that parents allow him to watch the cartoon.

Behavior is also Affected by Environment

- Event happening around. For example: If there is a gathering around, our behavior changes according to that event.
- The environment itself- heat, light, noise, privacy.
- The response of other people, which is affected by their own physical factors, personal and emotional factors, life experiences, wants and needs.

6. Explain sources of stress. (MGR)

Answer

Definition of Stress

Stress is a physiological and psychological response to a real or perceived threat to physical or psychological integrity of an individual. It is a bodily or mental tension resulting from the factors that tend to alter an existing equilibrium.

Sources of Stress

Sources of stress are known as stressors.

Stressor is defined as an event or situation or person which causes stress. Stressor is the stimuli proceeding or precipitating a change. Internal and external are two types of stresses.

1. **Internal stressors:** Stressor which arises from inside, e.g., hunger, sex.
2. **External stressors:** Stressor which arises from outside, e.g., parents forcing their children to study well.

Internal Sources of Stress

Internal sources of stress refer to thoughts, feelings and behaviors that can cause **stress**. Here are some examples:

- **Negative self-talk:** This is when individuals engage in self-critical or self-**defeating** thoughts, such as "I'm not good enough" or "I'll never be able to do this." These thoughts can lead to feelings of anxiety and stress.
- **Perfectionism:** When individuals set unrealistic standards for themselves, they **may** experience stress when they feel they are falling short of those standards.
- **Rumination:** This is when individuals repeatedly focus on negative thoughts or past experiences, which can lead to feelings of stress and **anxiety**.
- **Procrastination:** When individuals delay taking action on important tasks or **responsibilities**, they may experience stress as the deadline approaches.

- **Lack of assertiveness:** When individuals have difficulty expressing their needs or standing up for themselves, they may experience stress in social situations or in their relationships.
- **Unrealistic expectations:** When individuals have unrealistic expectations for themselves or others, they may experience stress when those **expectations** are not met.
- **Overthinking:** This is when individuals excessively analyze or worry about a **situation**, which can lead to feelings of stress and anxiety.
- **Poor time management:** When individuals struggle to manage their time **effectively**, they may experience stress due to deadlines or feeling overwhelmed by their workload.

External Sources of Stress

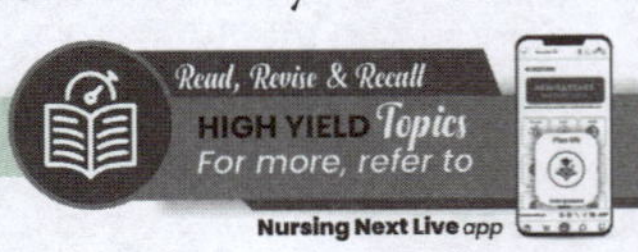

External sources of stress refer to environmental or situational factors that can cause stress. Here are some examples:

- **Work-related stress:** This includes job demands, long working hours, job insecurity, work overload and conflicts with coworkers or supervisors.
- **Financial stress:** This includes financial difficulties, such as debt, unemployment and financial insecurity.
- **Family-related stress:** This includes conflicts with family members, parenting responsibilities, and caregiving for elderly or ill family members.
- **Health-related stress:** This includes chronic illness, injury, disability and other health problems.
- **Environmental stress:** This includes natural disasters, pollution, noise and other physical factors in the environment that can cause stress.
- **Academic stress:** This includes academic demands, test anxiety and other factors related to the educational environment.
- **Social stress:** This includes interpersonal conflicts, social isolation, discrimination and other social factors that can cause stress.
- **Life changes and transitions:** This includes major life events such as divorce, death of a loved one, relocation or the birth of a child.

7. Define emotions. Discuss the theories of emotions and emotions in health and illness. (KUHS, MGR, RUHS)

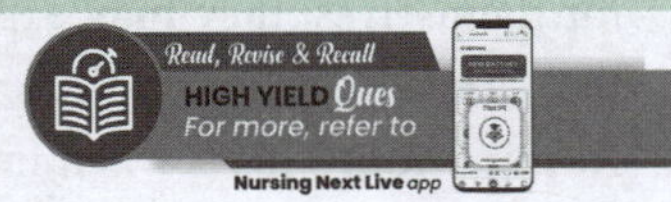

Answer

Definition of Emotion

Emotion is an affective experience that accompanies generalized inner adjustment and mental and physiological stirred up states in the individual and that shows itself in his overt behavior.

—**Crow and Crow**

Theories of Emotion

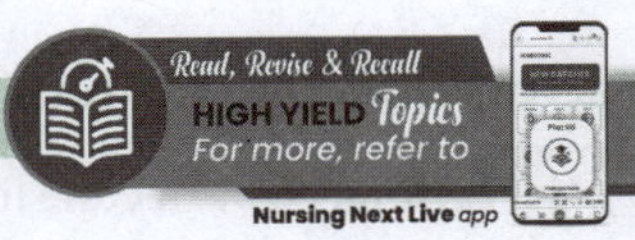

There are five theories:

1. **Evolutionary theory:** This theory was proposed by Charles Darwin.
   - According to this theory, emotion has a motivational role as it understands other people's emotion.
   - The evolutionary theory of emotion is rooted in the work of Charles Darwin, who argued that emotions are universal across cultures and have a biological basis.
   - Darwin believed that emotions evolved through natural selection, with those that provided a survival advantage being passed down to future generations.
2. **James-Lange theory (1880):** The James-Lange theory of emotion suggests that physical changes in the body happen first, which then leads to the experience of emotion. The James-Lange theory suggests that emotions are a direct result of physiological changes in the body.
   - According to this theory, when we experience a stimulus, our body responds with a physical reaction, which then triggers an emotional response. For example, we might feel afraid because our heart is racing and we are trembling.
3. **Cannon-Bard theory (1920):** This theory was given by Walter Cannon and Philip Bard.
   - This theory states that when we come across a situation before the emotion, then it creates a physical impact on our body very quickly. The Cannon-Bard theory suggests that emotions and physiological responses occur simultaneously, rather than one causing the other.
   - According to this theory, when we experience a stimulus, our brain simultaneously processes the stimulus and produces an emotional response, as well as a physiological response. For example, we might feel afraid and experience a racing heart at the same time.
4. **Schachter-Singer theory (1962):** This theory was proposed by Schachter and Singer.
   - The Schachter-Singer theory explains that emotion is formed from physiological arousal and a cognitive label.
   - This theory also explains that a person's emotional response is formed from an interpretation of immediate environment. According to this theory, when we experience a stimulus, our body responds with a physiological reaction, which is then interpreted and labeled by our cognitive processes.
   - The emotions we experience are a result of this interpretation. For example, we might interpret our racing heart and trembling as fear because we have learned to associate those physical responses with the emotion of fear.
5. **Cognitive appraisal theory:** Cognitive theory is based on the sequence of events which finally leads to emotion. At

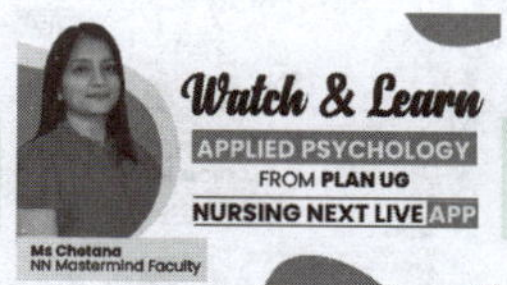

first, the response occurs and then the body reacts to this and finally emotion occurs.

Emotions in health and illness

- Emotions are greatly impacted by our health state. If we are healthy, we experience good emotions; but if we are not in a good health state, we feel frustrated, depressed and disappointed.
- Strong and unpleasant emotions affect our health. We cannot stay healthy if we are experiencing unhealthy emotions for a long time. We become sick.
- Unpleasant and bad emotions make our immune system weak and make us prone to get frequent infections like common cold.
- Emotions play a very important role in our health states. Long-term intense emotions make us prone to peptic ulcers.
- Emotions can cause inflammation, headache and increased BP.
- Research has shown that negative emotions, such as stress, anxiety and depression, can increase the risk of developing a variety of health problems, including cardiovascular disease, diabetes and chronic pain.
- Emotions can also affect the progression of existing illnesses, with some studies indicating that positive emotions can improve immune system functioning and enhance recovery from illness.
- It is very much required for a nurse to understand these emotions and to teach patient and family to handle emotions in such situations.

8. Physiology of emotion. (KUHS, MGR, RUHS)

Answer

- The physiology of emotions refers to the physical changes that occur in the body in response to an emotional experience.
- Physiology of emotions is based on the changes that occur because of autonomic nervous system and the endocrine gland system.
- The autonomic nervous system has two divisions: Sympathetic nervous system and parasympathetic nervous system.
- Emotion puts impact on the brain especially on amygdala, which plays role in the creation of emotion.
- Emotions or emotional behavior can trigger the release of neurotransmitters.
- Dopamine provides a sense of pleasure and motivation by regulating the release of endorphins.
- Serotonin makes oneself feel peaceful and promotes sleep.
- Glutamate is helpful in long-term learning, retention of memory and pain tolerance.
- Research evidences state that negative emotions such as anger, aggression, sadness, anxiety, fright, shocked, nervousness, etc. also affect the physical health.
- Sympathetic nervous system prepares the body for any state of emergency.
- SNS causes the release of adrenaline in blood that causes changes like:
  - Increased BP and heart rate
  - Changes in the rate of respiration
  - Dilation of pupils
  - Increased blood sugar level
  - Muscular tensions and tremors
- Parasympathetic nervous system calms down the body after a period of intense emotions.
  - Reduces heart rate and BP
  - Normalizes the blood circulation
  - Conserves body's energy
- There are some internal, external and physiological changes that occur due to change in emotional state. Physiological changes occur during intense emotional periods.

SHORT NOTES

1. Motivational cycle. (MGR)

Answer

Definitions

Motivation refers to the states within a person or animal that drive behavior toward some goals. **—Morgan and King**

Motivation is the class of operations used to produce or measure the changes in performance and changes in energy.

Motivation Cycle

- Need is the desire to do a particular thing, e.g., biological need, i.e., the requirement of food by the internal organs of the body.
- Drive is the internal motivation created by the need, e.g., hunger drive. Arousal refers to mental alertness or mental attentiveness.
- Arousal leads to goal-directed behavior, e.g., cooking or buying the food from the shop.
- Goal-directed behavior leads to the achievement of task, e.g., eating the food.
- After achievement, the reduction of arousal takes place.

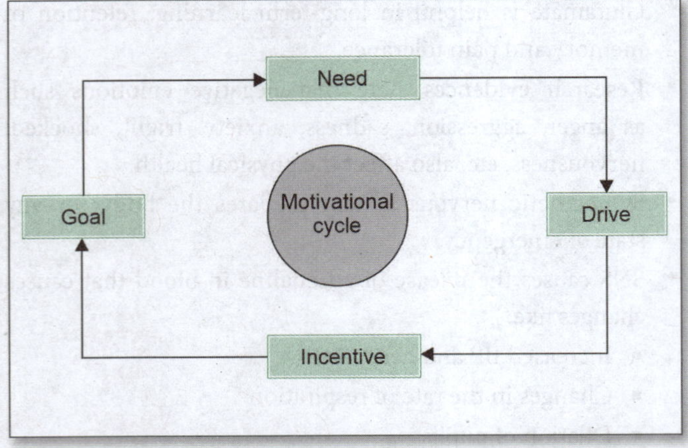

2. Four secondary motives. (MGR)

Answer

Secondary Motives/Psychosocial Motives/Social Learned Motives

- Secondary motives come after fulfillment of primary motives.
- These are acquired through external demands and learned from others and lead to change or mold our behavior.
- These secondary motives are achievement, power, need for social approval.
- Social motives or urges have social importance and performance in our relationship with other people.
- Social motives are learned from groups, family and other social interaction.
  - **Need for achievement:** It refers to individual's desire to acquire significantly in a particular field, e.g., want to achieve 'ranker' in the class.
  - **Need for power:** Power to influence others and want to take control of others, e.g., legislative power, political power, police power.
  - **Need for affiliation:** It denotes the need to be with others. The child wants to play with other children. People live together and form a family.
  - **Social approval:** Children and adolescents want to accept their behavior by approving other person's behavior like nodding head, eyes movement, e.g., hairstyle, dress code.

3. Components of emotion. (RUHS)

Answer

According to Woodworth, "emotion is a conscious stirred up state of human organism."

The three components of a emotions are:

1. **Cognition:** This component will make the person evaluate his thought, prompting ways to express emotion in another way.
2. **Feeling:** Feeling is considered an instant emotional response and this will help the person to express his emotion.
3. **Behavioral:** The behavioral response is noticed by:
   - **Facial:** Our facial expressions change because of our emotional state.
   - **Postural:** Our posture changes with emotions. For example, if we are happy and joyful, we will look very energetic and active. We will be sitting straight. But if we are sad, we will not stand or sit straight.
   - **Gestural:** Our gestures also change with emotions. Our gestures show our excitement and joy whenever we are happy and excited.

These are the various ways of expressing emotion in a behavioral way.

4. Stress-related physical illnesses. (MGR)

Answer

Stress-related physical illnesses are known as psychosomatic problems. The appearance of physical symptoms that have psychological basis and lack medical evidence.

This is explained by psychosomatic model of stress.

Psychosomatic Model of Stress

Udupa explained the concept of psychosomatic model of stress. It has four phases. (i) psychic phase, (ii) psychosomatic phase, (iii) somatic phase and (iv) organic phase.

Table 7.1: Phases as per psychosomatic model of stress

Phases	Description	Example
Psychic phase	Psychological symptoms are predominant	Craving for alcohol
Psychosomatic phase	Psychological conditions alter the bodily function	Alcohol causes liver damage
Somatic phase	Impairment of the bodily function damages the organ	Liver damage persists
Organic phase	Damage of an organ leads to disease	Hepatic dysfunction

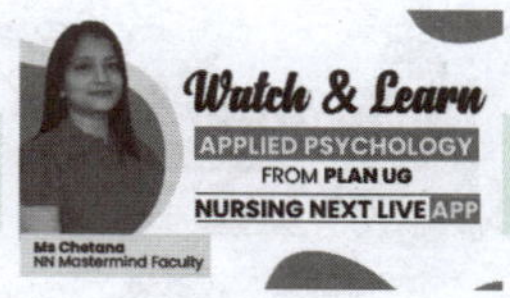

Stress-related Physical Illnesses

Acute stress responses: Acute stress can cause a number of physical illnesses, including:

- Increased heart rate and blood pressure
- Rapid breathing
- Sweating
- Muscle tension
- Aches and pains, back pain
- Headaches and migraine
- Stomach ulcers
- Skin rash

Chronic stress responses: Chronic stress is long-term stress that can have various physical illnesses, including:

- Increased risk of heart disease, stroke, and other health problems
- Weakened immune system
- Sleep problems (insomnia)
- Digestive problems
- Gastrointestinal problems
- Erectile dysfunction
- Headaches and migraine

5. Discuss the nature of attitude and attitude change. (MGR)

Answer

Definition of Attitude

According to Gordon Allport, "an attitude is a mental and neutral state of readiness, organized through experience, exerting a directive or dynamic influence upon the individual's response to all objects and situations with which it is related."

Nature of Attitude

- Attitude is a combination of various components like values, behaviors, etc.
- Attitude is displayed under any situation and under any scenario.
- Attitude is held by all people with difference of intelligence.
- If an attitude is sometimes internal it can be clearly displayed outside.
- Attitude may force us to behave differently toward a person or an object.
- An attitude can predict the future behavior of the person.
- Attitude has different faces according to the scenario.
- An attitude tells the inner feelings of a person.
- Attitude strongly influences behavior and its effects in different situations.
- Attitude may be frequently used for various situations.

Ways of Changing Attitude

There are various ways of changing the attitude. A person will be sticking to an attitude and then he will showcase it to everyone. Due to various factors, there are some changes in the attitude, which are:

- A new information changes the attitude
- Experiences which are direct affect and change the attitude.
- Attitude changes through law.
- Fear is also a cause of change in attitude.
- Situations also change attitude.

6. Write a note on attitude and its components. (MGR)

Answer

Attitude

According to Gordon Allport, "an attitude is a mental and neutral state of readiness, organized through experience, exerting a directive or dynamic influence upon the individual's response to all objects and situations with which it is related."

Attitudes are formed through a combination of personal experiences, social influences and cultural factors. They can be explicit or implicit, conscious or unconscious, and can influence a person's behavior and decision-making.

Components of Attitude

- Cognitive Component
- Affective Component
- Behavioral Component

Cognitive Component

- The cognitive component of attitude refers to the beliefs, thoughts and attributes that we would associate with an object.
- It is the opinion or belief segment of an attitude. It refers to that part of attitude which is related to general knowledge of a person.
- Typically these come to light in generalities or stereotypes, such as: all babies are cute, smoking is harmful to health, etc.

Affective Component

Affective component is the emotional or feeling segment of an attitude.

- It is related to the statement which affects another person.
- It deals with feelings or emotions that are brought to the surface about something, such as fear or hate. Using the above example, someone might have the attitude that

they love all babies because they are cute or that they hate smoking because it is harmful to health.

Behavioral Component

- Behavioral component of attitude consists of a person's tendencies to behave in a particular way toward an object.
- It refers to that part of attitude which reflects the intention of a person in the short-run or long- run.
- Using the above example, the behavioral attitude maybe- I cannot wait to kiss the baby, or we better keep those smokers out of the library, etc.

7. Psychosomatic disorders of emotion. (MGR)

Answer

- The term "psychosomatic" refers to the mind-body connection, which suggests that emotional experiences can have an impact on physical health. Here are some examples of psychosomatic disorders related to emotion:
- **Irritable Bowel Syndrome (IBS):** This is a gastrointestinal disorder that is associated with stress and anxiety. Symptoms can include abdominal pain, bloating and changes in bowel habits.
- **Asthma:** Asthma is a respiratory condition that can be triggered or exacerbated by stress, anxiety or strong emotions.
- **Migraines:** Migraines are a type of headache that can be triggered by stress, anxiety or emotional experiences.
- **Dermatological conditions:** Skin conditions such as eczema, psoriasis and acne can be influenced by emotional factors such as stress, anxiety and depression.
- **Hypertension:** High blood pressure can be caused or exacerbated by stress, anxiety and emotional factors.
- **Cardiovascular disease:** Emotional factors such as stress and anxiety have been linked to an increased risk of cardiovascular disease.
- **Chronic pain:** Chronic pain conditions such as fibromyalgia and chronic fatigue syndrome are often associated with emotional factors such as stress, anxiety and depression.

8. Enumerate the nurse's role in managing negative emotions. (KUHS)

Answer

Role of Nurse in Managing Negative Emotions

- Identify patient's negative emotions
- Make patient aware of negative emotions. For example, in some situations, patients are not at all aware of the intense emotions that are causing health issues.
- Nurses should help patients deal with their symptoms by providing emotional support to them.
- By meeting their patients' physiological and emotional needs, nurses also improve the healing process and help patients feel safe and more empowered with managing their own recovery.
- Once the patient has developed insight of the emotional issues, it is nurse's responsibility to encourage patient to deal with emotions.
- It is always therapeutic to face and deal with emotions rather than ignoring them and denying with the intense emotions.
- This is not the healthy way to deal with them because if we deny to address the emotions, they will become the basis for psychosomatic disorders.
- It is nurses' responsibility to encourage patient for healthy resolution of emotional issues.
- Make patient aware of psychosomatic issues that have a psychological basis.
- Encourage patients to maintain mental hygiene so that they can prevent mental illnesses and maintain their mental health.

9. Assessment of emotion. (KUHS)

Answer

Psychometric Assessment of Emotions

- Psychometric assessments of emotions are tools and techniques used to measure and evaluate various aspects of emotions in individuals.
- These assessments aim to provide quantitative data about an individual's emotional experiences, traits, or tendencies. They help in understanding emotional states, identifying emotional strengths and weaknesses, and assessing emotional well-being.
- The most common way in the assessment of emotion is known as the emotional intelligence test. Some of the psychometric tests for emotional intelligence are:
- EQ appraisal (Dr Travis Bradberry): This is a skill-based method that depends on:
  - Self-awareness
  - Self-management
  - Social awareness
  - Relationship management

This EQ appraisal consists of 28 performance-based items and assesses both the EQ and the four factors.

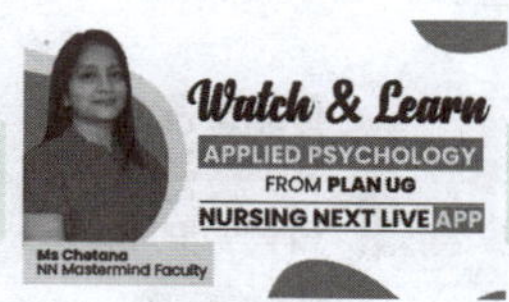

- The emotional quotient inventory (Australian Council for Educational Research)—This is a widely used inventory.
- Profile of emotional competence (Brasseur and Mikolajczak)—This is used to measure intrapersonal and interpersonal emotional intelligence.

These are the common psychometric assessments for the emotional quotient, the EQ range is:

- The average - EQ score is 90–100
- Perfect - EQ score is –160.

10. Write a short note on aptitude and types of aptitude with a brief difference between attitude and aptitude. (RUHS, MGR)

Answer

Definition of Aptitude

Freeman defined, an aptitude is a combination of characteristic indicative of an individual's capacity to acquire some specific knowledge, skills or set of organized responses. For example: Ability to speak language, become a musician, etc.

An aptitude is a component of competence to do certain kind of works at a certain level. It may be physical or mental talent. It is an inborn potential to do some work whether developed or undeveloped.

Types of Aptitude

- **General aptitude:** It is an ability to do something. It may be innate or acquired. Like comprehension, reading and writing.
- **Special aptitude:** It is a special ability to do something very effectively and fast.
- **Manual aptitude:** It is a motor ability or skills required for semi-skilled occupation.
- **Mechanical aptitude:** It is an ability to understand and solve problems like repair of machine.
- **Clerical aptitude:** It is some special ability like perception, intellectual, mental and motor skills. Other types of aptitude may be musical, scholastic and professional.

Attitude	Aptitude
An attitude is one's opinion or standpoint about something. It can be described as "a set of emotions, beliefs, and behaviors toward a particular object, person, thing, or event". Attitudes are based on a person's experiences, values, beliefs, and emotions.	An aptitude is a combination of characteristic indicative of an individual's capacity to acquire some specific knowledge, skills or set of organized responses. For example: Ability to speak language, become a musician, etc.
	Aptitude measures an individual's mental strength to learn any new skill.
Attitude is related to personality	Aptitude is related to capabilities. It is considered talent.
Attitude is always at mental level	Aptitude can be at mental as well as at physical level.

SHORT ANSWER QUESTIONS

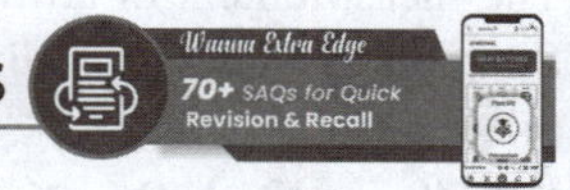

1. Any four physiological changes of emotion.

Answer

Emotions

Emotion is an affective experience that accompanies generalized inner adjustment and mental and physiological stirred up states in an individual and that shows itself in his overt behavior.

Four Physiological Changes of Emotions

1. Increased heart rate
2. Activation of sympathetic nervous system
3. Changes in skin conductance
4. Activation of HPA axis

2. Define stress.

Answer

Stress is a physiological and psychological response to a real or perceived threat to physical or psychological integrity of an individual. It is a bodily or mental tension resulting from the factors that tend to alter an existing equilibrium.

3. Name the theories of emotion.

Answer

Theories of Emotion

- Evolutionary theory
- James-Lange theory (1880)
- Cannon-Bard theory (1920)

- Schachter-Singer theory (1962)
- Cognitive appraisal theory

4. Motivational cycle.

Answer

Motivation Cycle

It includes need, drive, incentive and goal.

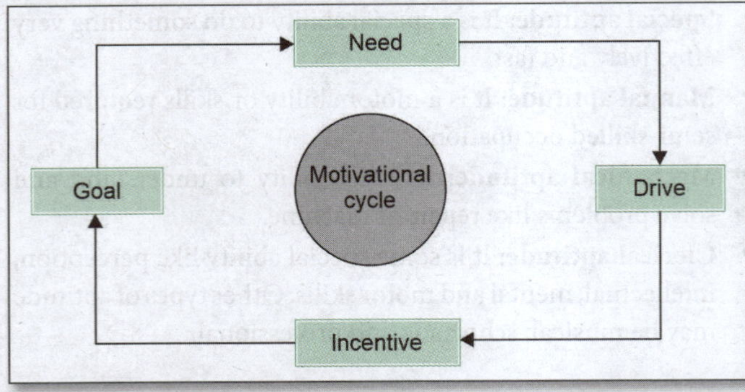

5. Which period is called "Storm and Stress" period?

Answer

"Storm and Stress" refers to a period of psychological and emotional upheaval that occurs during adolescence. This term was first coined by German psychologist G. Stanley Hall in the late 19th century.

During the "storm and stress" period, adolescents experience intense emotions, including anxiety, confusion and mood swings. They may also engage in risk-taking behaviors and question authority and societal norms. This period is characterized by the struggle for identity, independence and autonomy.

6. Define general adaptation syndrome.

Answer

GAS stands for General Adaptation Syndrome, which is a concept introduced by Hans Selye, a pioneering stress researcher. The GAS theory describes the body's response to stress and how it adapts to stressors over time.

Three stages: Alarm, Resistance and Exhaustion

7. Define motivation.

Answer

Definition of Motivation

Motivation refers to the states within a person or animal that drive behavior toward some goals. **—Morgan and King**

Motivation is the class of operations used to produce or measure the changes in performance and changes in energy. **—Underwood**

8. Enlist primary motives.

Answer

Primary Motives/Biological Motives

Primary or biological needs are important for all living organisms. Such motives are triggered when there is imbalance in the body. The body always tends to maintain a state of equilibrium called "Homeostasis"- in many of its internal physiological processes.

These are:

- **Need for oxygen, food and water**
- **Temperature, rest and sleep**
- **Sex**
- **Elimination of waste**

9. Measurement of attitude. (RUHS)

Answer

The measurement of attitudes involves assessing individuals' thoughts, beliefs, and feelings toward specific objects, people, or concepts.

- **Self-reported Questionnaires:** Most common method for measuring attitudes. Participants are presented with a series of statements or questions related to the attitude to rate their agreement or disagreement on a Likert scale.
- **Implicit measures:** Implicit measures assess attitudes indirectly by examining automatic or unconscious associations. Example, Implicit Association Test (IAT) and the Affect Misattribution Procedure (AMP).
- **Behavioral observations:** Attitudes can also be inferred from an individual's observable behavior.

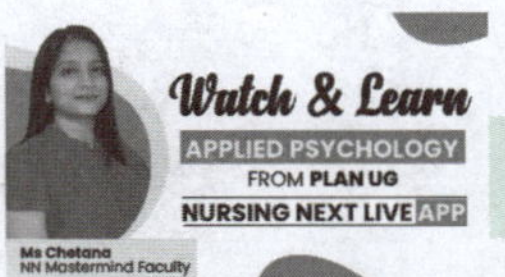

CONCEPTUAL REVISION

MULTIPLE CHOICE QUESTIONS

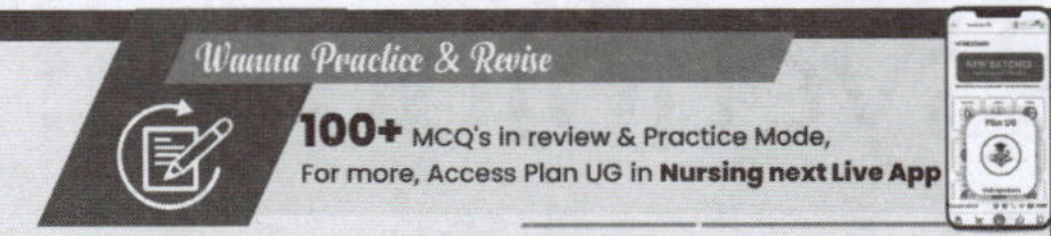

1. The forces that help in initiation and persistence of behavior are called:

a. Emotions
b. Drives
c. Motives
d. Intellect

Ans. c. Motives

2. Other name for primary drive is:

a. Biological drive
b. Socio-psychological drive
c. Secondary drive
d. Drives

Ans. a. Biological drive

3. The types of needs that are necessary for the survival of the individual are:

a. Biological needs
b. Psychosocial needs
c. Physiological needs
d. Secondary needs

Ans. a. Biological needs

4. Anything that encourages a person and works as an reinforcing agent:

a. Motives
b. Drives
c. Incentives
d. Needs

Ans. c. Incentives

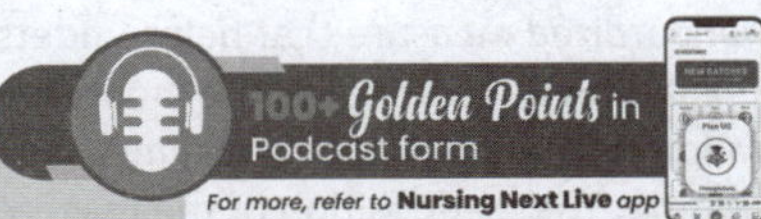

Golden Points

- An attitude is a mental and neutral state of readiness, organized through experience, exerting a directive or dynamic influence upon the individual's response to all objects and situations with which it is related.
- Emotion is an affective experience that accompanies generalized inner adjustment and mental and physiological stirred up states in the individual and that shows itself in his overt behavior.
- Factors that influence the attitude are Social factors, Direct instruction, Family, Prejudices, Personal experiences, Media, Educational and religious institutions and Physical factors.
- Motivation refers to the states within a person or animal that drives behavior toward some goals.
- Reduction Theory of Motivation, Arousal Theory of Motivation, Incentive Theory of Motivation, Alderfer's Existence, Relatedness and Growth Theory (1969), Herzberg Two Factor Theory (1959), Mc-Clelland Achievement Theory (1988), Adams' Equity Theory (1965), Vroom's Expectancy Theory (1964) and Locke's Goal Setting Theory (1968).
- Stress is a biological, psychological, social or chemical factor that causes physical or emotional tension and may be a factor in the etiology of certain illnesses.
- Theories of attitude are Cognitive consistency theory, Congruity theory and Affective cognitive consistency theory.
- Theories of Motivation are Evolutionary Theory of Motivation, Maslow's Hierarchy of Needs, Drive
- Types of attitudes are positive attitude, negative attitude and neutral attitude.
- Types of emotions are happiness, sadness, fear, disgust, anger, surprise, etc.
- Types of Motives - Primary Motives (oxygen, food, water, temperature, rest, sleep, elimination of waste, sex), Secondary Motives/ Psychosocial Motives/Social Learned Motives (Need for achievement, Need for Power, Need for affiliation and social approval) and Stimulus motives.
- Types of stress are eustress and distress. Types of stressors are internal and external.

CHAPTER

8

Psychological Assessment and Tests

CONCEPTUAL THEORY

Terminology

Convenience: Cost-effectiveness, equipment and training required.
Planning: Adequate planning and a clear vision are necessary before creating a test measure.
Psychological test: Psychological tests refer to structured methods designed to elicit specific behaviors, providing an objective and standardized measure that helps understand an individual's behavior.
Reliability: Consistency in the measurement results.
Validity: Extent to which a test measures what it claims to measure.
Writing: The composition of the test requires careful writing. The author must have in-depth knowledge of the subject matter.

PSYCHOLOGICAL TEST

- Psychological tests refer to structured methods designed to elicit specific behaviors, providing an objective and standardized measure that helps understand an individual's behavior.
- These tests assess various attributes and traits and serve multiple purposes, such as informing decisions about behavior, aiding research, and facilitating personal growth.

Principles of Psychological Test

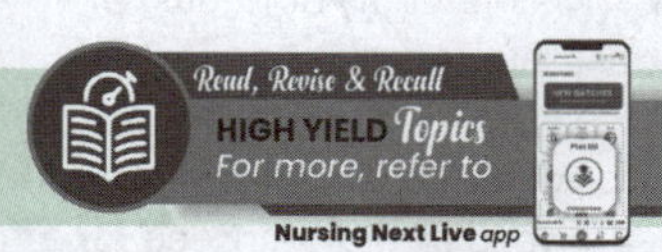

- Psychological tests need to possess certain elements that allow anyone to administer them at any given time. These components include Standardization, Content, and Procedure.
- A reliable test should include norms that enable the comparison of an individual's score to that of a known group against whom the test has been calibrated.
- Test items are created by experts, tested, and chosen based on factors like difficulty, differentiation, and the relationship between specifications.
- Clear and concise directions for test administration are essential to ensure consistency in the testing process.
- A comprehensive test manual should be provided, serving as a guide for test administration, scoring, drawing inferences, and interpreting results.

Development of Psychological Tests

- **Planning:** Adequate planning and a clear vision are necessary before creating a test measure.
- **Writing:** The composition of the test requires careful writing. The author must have in-depth knowledge of the subject matter.
- **Establishment of norms:** A Establishing the reliability and validity of psychometric tests is crucial to ensure their effectiveness and accuracy in measuring psychological constructs.
  Reliability refers to the consistency and stability of test scores over time, while validity refers to the extent to which a test measures what it claims to measure.
- **Preparation of manual:** A test manual includes information on the psychometric properties of the test, instructions for administration and scoring, a scoring key that may be categorized for different groups (e.g., age, gender), and references.

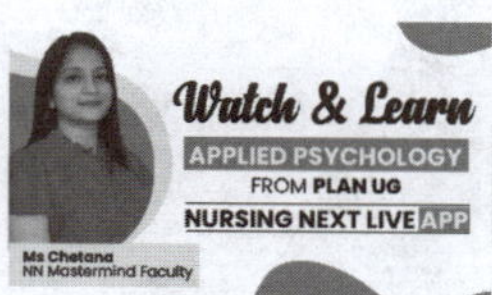

Classification of Psychological Tests

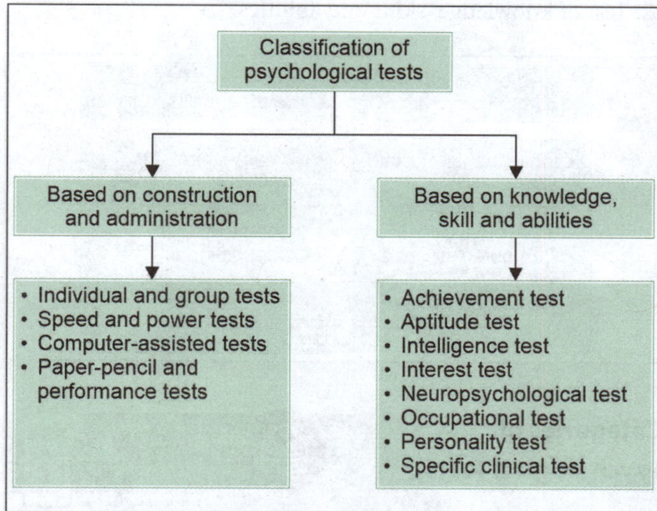

Role of Nurse in Psychological Assessment

Nurses play a crucial role in psychological assessment as part of their overall patient care responsibilities. While nurses may not have the specialized training of a psychologist or psychiatrist, they often perform initial assessments and screenings as part of patient care to identify potential psychological issues in patients.

CONCEPTUAL EXERCISES

LONG ANSWER QUESTIONS

1. Explain the role of nurse in psychological assessment. (KUHS)

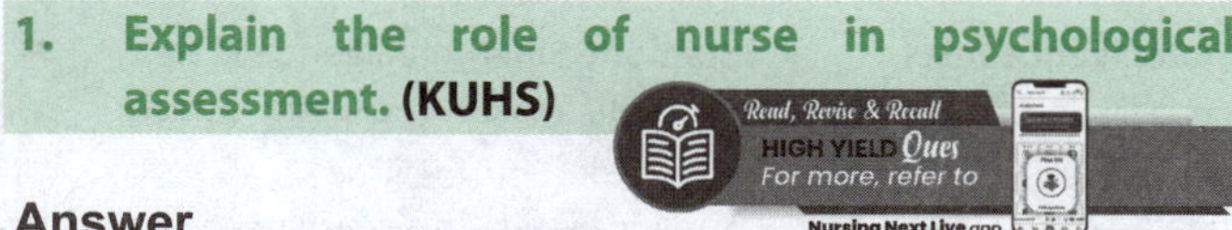

Answer

Role of Nurse in Psychological Assessment

- Nurses play a crucial role in psychological assessment as part of their overall patient care responsibilities.
- While they may not have the specialized training of a psychologist or psychiatrist, nurses often perform initial assessments and screenings to identify potential psychological issues in patients.
- Nurses are expected to have adequate knowledge about the psychological tests.
- Nurses should be aware of the safety of the test and utility of findings by the designated personnel and confidentiality of data are essential.
- Some key roles of nurses in psychological assessment:
  - **Support and Education**
    - Nurses play an essential role in briefing the patients/clients and their family caregivers about the psychological assessment.
    - Nurses are the primary contact between psychologists and patient, so nurses must be able to clarify doubts and queries related to the disease conditions and about any psychological test the patient has to take.
    - Nurse provides emotional support and education to patients and their families.
    - Nurses are responsible to identify and allay any anxiety related to the tests by answering their doubts.
  - Initial Screening
    - Nurses are often the first health care professionals to interact with patients. They conduct initial screenings to identify any psychological concerns or symptoms that may require further evaluation.
    - By asking relevant questions and observing the patient's behavior, nurses can gather information about potential mental health issues.
    - If significant concerns are identified during the initial assessment, nurses will typically refer the patient to a mental health professional for further evaluation and diagnosis.
  - Psychosocial Assessment
    - As part of the nursing assessment, nurses gather comprehensive data about a patient's psychological and social well-being.
    - They assess the patient's emotional state, coping mechanisms, support systems, and any psychosocial stressors that may be impacting their mental health.
  - Mental Health History
    - Nurses gather information about the patient's mental health history, including previous diagnoses, treatments, hospitalizations, and medications. Helps in determining appropriate interventions.
  - Symptoms Monitoring
    - In an in-patient setting, Nurses exposed to patients for the longest period of time in comparison to other clinical staff.
    - The nurse thus observes changes in the patient's behavior, mood fluctuations, sleep patterns, undertakes risk assessments and notifies/updates the mental health team.
    - The nurse is responsible to observe behavioral changes and improvement in behavior.
    - It is the nurse's duty in most hospitals to observe changes, inform the respective departments and record changes in the case file.
  - Collaboration with Mental Health Professionals
    - Nurses collaborate with psychologists, psychiatrists, and other mental health professionals to facilitate comprehensive assessments.

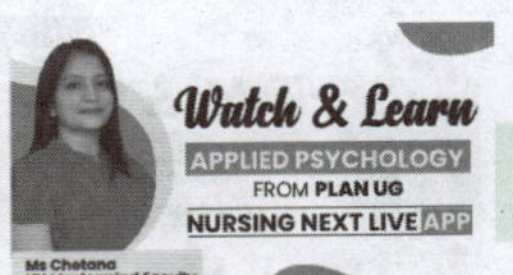

- They may share their observations, assessment findings, and collaborate on the development of treatment plans.

2. Describe psychological tests. (KUHS, RUHS)

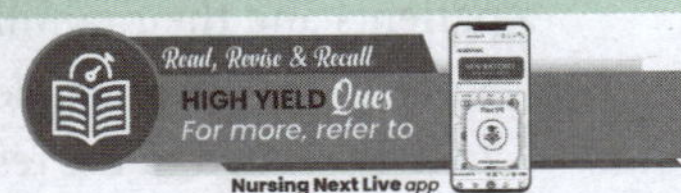

Answer

Definition of Psychological Test

A psychological test can be defined as a structured technique to produce selected behavior. It is an objective and standardized measure, the results of which are used to deduce the individual's behavior. Several attributes and traits can be judged by means of testing. Psychological tests are used in:

- Making decisions about one's behavior
- Research
- Personal development

Principles of Psychological Test

- Psychological tests should have some components that make it feasible for anybody to administer the test anytime. These are Standard, Content and the Procedure.
- A good test must have norms to compare an individual's score to that of a known group against whom the test has been calibrated.
- Test items are constructed by experts, tested and selected on the basis of difficulty, differentiation and relationship between specifications.
- Directions for administration must be stated concisely and clearly in order to ensure uniformity in test methodology.
- A test manual must be provided along with which acts as a guide for administration, scoring, inference and results.

Characteristics of Good Psychological Test

- **Validity:** Validity refers to the extent to which a test measures what it claims to measure.
- **Reliability:** Reliability refers to the consistency in the measurement results.
- **Convenience:** Cost-effectiveness, equipment and training required.
- **Uniformity:** Uniformity in administration, measurement and scoring.
- **Standardized norms:** Implementation of technical standards to ensure objectivity and consistency in testing.
- **Objectivity:** Minimal room for bias. It means the test is bias free.

Types of Psychological Tests

Psychological tests can be classified on the basis of two categories:

1. Construction and administration
2. Test of knowledge, skills and abilities.

Based on construction and administration	Based on test of knowledge, skills, abilities
• Individual and group tests • Speed and power tests • Computer-assisted tests • Performance and paper-based tests	• Achievement • Aptitude • Intelligence • Cognitive abilities • Occupational • Neuropsychological • Personality • Clinical

Categories of Psychological Tests

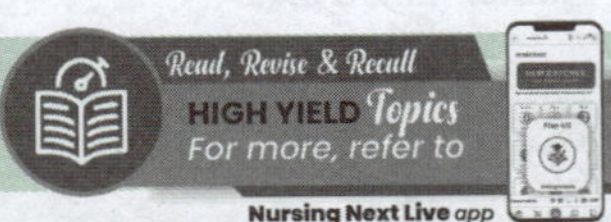

Psychological test are categorized into:	
Personality tests	• Minnesota Multiphasic Personality Inventory, Eysenck's Personality Inventory, State-Trait Personality Test
Aptitude tests	• Scholastic assessment test, Differential aptitude test, Tests of numerical reasoning, logical ability, verbal ability
Achievement tests	• Iowa Test of Basic Skills, Ohio Graduation Test, Stanford Achievement Test, Weschler Individual Achievement Test
Attitude test	• The Empathy Questionnaire, The Scale of Locus of Control, Marital Satisfaction Scale
Intelligence tests	• Stanford-Binet Intelligence Scale, WAIS-III, WAIS-IV, Pass Along test, Matrices
Neuropsychological tests	• Luria-Nebraska Battery, NIMHANS Neuropsychological Battery, Mini Mental State Examination
Projective tests	• Rorschach's inkblot, Thematic Apperception Test, Draw a person test
Observation tests	• Direct Observation, Participant observation, Structured Observation, Case Studies

Utility of Psychological Tests

Psychological tests have multiple utilities to clinical practitioners as well as academicians. Some common uses are as follows:

- The administration of test and getting information is easy as compared to clinical interviews.
- The tests can be used for making clinical diagnosis, for example: Rorschach Inkblot Test
- Information from tests are more scientifically consistent in comparison to clinical interview

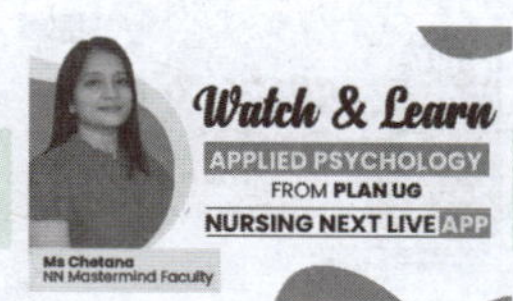

- They assist in the formulation of psychopathology and identification of areas of stress and conflict. Example: Thematic appreciation test
- The tests enable to determine the deficiency present. Example: cognitive neuropsychological assessments.
- They help in assessing severity of psychopathology and response to treatment. Example: Hamilton rating scale for depression, brief psychiatric rating scale.
- They help in assessing general characteristics of the individual. Example: assessment of intelligence, assessment of personality.
- These tests are also used for forensic evaluations regarding litigation, family court issues or criminal charges.
- These tests assess the level of functioning or disability, help direct treatment and assess treatment outcome.

Limitations of Psychological Tests

There are a few limitations also to the application of these tests:

- Indiscriminating usage
- Forgery and counterfeit
- Attitude toward testing and its negative implications
- Ethical concerns
- Privacy and data protection
- Interpretation

SHORT NOTES

1. Projection test of personality. (KUHS, MGR)

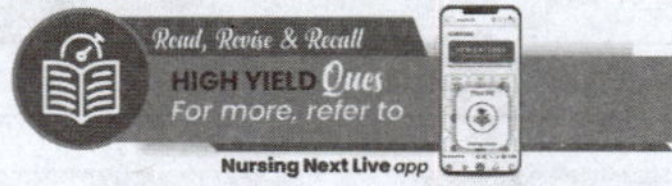

Answer

Projective Test

A projective test is a personality test that is designed to assess hidden emotions and conflicts. These hidden conflicts are projected by the person during the test and then interpretations are made by the psychologists. Projective tests work on projection principle.

- It requires lots of experience and it is an art.
- Projective tests help to uncover the unconscious concern, fears, conflict, desires and urges that affect the client's conscious behavior.
- This test is very useful in the diagnosis of personality disturbance.
- It is highly subjective and may not be accurate sometimes.
- The projective techniques are as follows:
- **Rorschach inkblots**
  - This test was developed by Hermann Rorschach in 1921.
  - He used 10 ink blots, 5 in black on white background and 5 in colored inks on a white background.
  - The patients were asked to look at each inkblot and they had to say whatever came to their mind by looking at those ink blots.
  - Scores were given based on color, shape, figures in the blot and response to the whole story or to details. This technique is very useful in describing personality, diagnosing mental illnesses and in prediction of behavior.
- **Thematic apperception test:**
  - This test was developed by Morgan and Henry Murray in 1935.
  - In this technique, 31 pictures (black and white) were shown to clients.
  - The patients were asked to tell a story about the person in the picture. The story or interpretation told by the patient about the picture reveals something of their past experience and feelings.
  - These interpretations by patients project their attitudes, conflicts or any kind of fear.
- **Word association test**
  - In this, the person is asked to say the first word that comes to his mind after listening to a series of words from the examiner.
  - The examinee has to say one word at a time immediately.
  - There is nothing wrong or right answer, just the first word that comes to mind.
  - The examiner records the whole exercise and then interprets the findings.
  - **For example:** Examiner says 'mother' and the examinee has to say the first word that comes to his mind after hearing 'mother'.
- **Sentence completion test**
  - In this test, the examinee is asked to complete a sentence told by the examiner.
  - The examiner says an incomplete sentence.
  - This test reveals the hidden attitudes and thoughts of the examinee.
  - Here, the examinee is asked to answer in more than one word.
  - Replying in more than one word gives a more wider opportunity to make interpretations.

SHORT ANSWER QUESTIONS

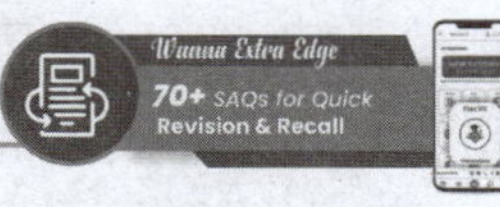

1. Enlist characteristics of Psychological tests.

Answer

Characteristics of Psychological Tests

- Validity
- Reliability
- Uniformity
- Objectivity

- Convenience
- Standardized norms
- Specificity
- Applicability

2. Define reliability and validity of psychological test.

Answer

Reliability

Refers to the consistency of results. A psychological test is said to be reliable when it gives same results on different occasions.

For example: A questionnaire gives same results when administered to same population on different occasions.

Validity: Validity refers to the ability to the extent to which a test measures what it claims to measure. For example: A knowledge questionnaire should measure knowledge about the particular phenomenon what it is supposed to measure.

CONCEPTUAL REVISION

MULTIPLE CHOICE QUESTIONS

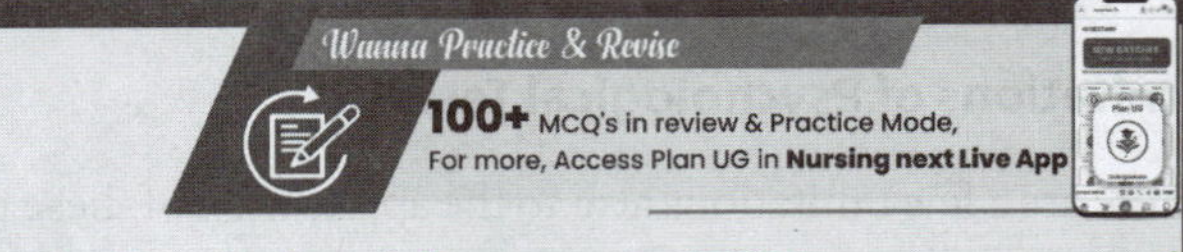

1. Which of the following methods like most other attitude measurement techniques relies on the self-report of the respondents?

a. Physiological measures
b. Public opinion polling
c. Interview
d. Case study

Ans. b. Public opinion polling

2. What is Rorschach's Projective Test designed to measure?

a. Unconscious intentions
b. Dreams
c. Conscious desires
d. Brain size

Ans. a. Unconscious intentions

3. Which of the following is NOT a property of psychological assessment?

a. Problem-focused
b. Trained personnel
c. Individually administered
d. Objective measure

Ans. d. Objective measure

4. Which of the following is NOT a characteristic of good psychological test?

a. Validity
b. Reliability
c. Uniformity
d. Subjectivity

Ans. d. Subjectivity

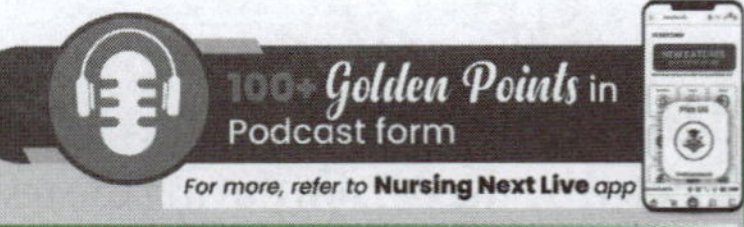

Golden Points

- A nurse should be able to reassure the patient and support with making informed decisions and obtaining consent.
- A nurse should ideally possess sufficient knowledge about the psychological tests in practice. Hospitals and trusts follow selected routine tests and assessment patterns within the system, and it is important that all clinical staff working with patient are aware of these.
- A psychological test can be defined as a structured tool to assess selected behavior. It is an objective and standardized measure, the results of which are used to deduce the individual's behavior. Several attributes and traits can be judged by means of testing.
- Being the most common and primary contact between the patient, caregivers and the medical system, a nurse plays an important role in communication. Knowing about tests enable the nurse to clarify doubts of any party involved regarding any psychological test the patient has to undergo.
- Characteristics of Good Psychological Test are Validity, Reliability, Uniformity, Standardized norms, and Objectivity.
- **Reliability:** Consistency in the measurement results.
- **Validity:** The extent to which a test measures what it claims to measure.

CHAPTER 9

Application of Soft Skill

CONCEPTUAL THEORY

Terminology

150+ key terminologies for Quick Recall & Revision

Assertiveness: Being assertive is an essential skill both personally and interpersonally, encompassing the ability to effectively express emotions, desires, needs, and preferences.

Conflict resolution: Conflict resolution in nursing refers to the process of addressing and resolving conflicts or disagreements that may arise among nurses, or between nurses and other health care professionals, patients, or their families.

Emotional intelligence: Emotional intelligence refers to the aptitude to acknowledge and comprehend one's own emotions and behaviors, and how they impact others.

Interpersonal skills: Interpersonal skills encompass a diverse set of abilities that involve effective communication, such as active listening and articulate speaking, as well as the capacity to regulate and handle emotions.

Resilience: Resilience is the ability to adjust and thrive in the presence of challenges, difficult situations, or high levels of stress

Self-motivation: Self-motivation refers to the internal drive, determination, and initiative to pursue goals, take action, and persist in the face of challenges, without relying solely on external factors or rewards.

Soft skills: Soft skills (also known as noncognitive skills) are "patterns of thought, feelings, and behavior" that are socially determined and can be developed throughout one's lifetime to produce value, according to the United Nations Educational, Scientific, and Cultural Organization (UNESCO).

SOFT SKILLS

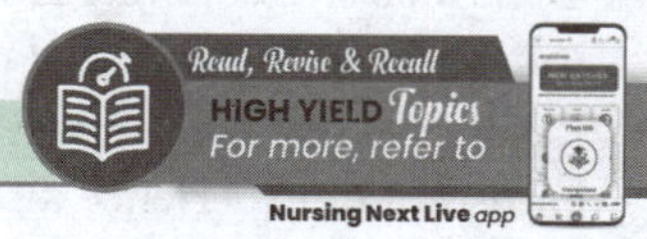

Soft skills (also known as noncognitive skills) are, "patterns of thought, feelings, and behavior," that are socially determined and can be developed throughout one's lifetime to produce value. —UNESCO

Soft skills refer to a set of personal attributes, qualities, and abilities that enable individuals to effectively interact with others, navigate social situations, and perform well in various professional and personal settings.

Categories of Soft Skills

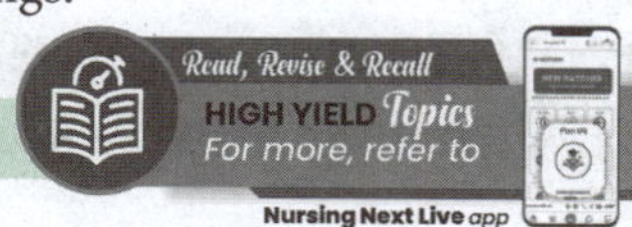

There are various soft skills required by nurses:

- **Communication skills:** Active listening, clear and empathetic verbal communication, nonverbal communication, and the ability to adapt communication styles to different individuals and situations.
- **Empathy and compassion:** Being sensitive to patients' needs, displaying kindness, and demonstrating a caring attitude.
- **Teamwork and collaboration:** Ability to collaborate, cooperate, and effectively contribute to a multidisciplinary team is essential for providing comprehensive patient care.
- **Problem-solving and critical thinking:** Assess and analyze information, make informed decisions, and think quickly on their feet. Nurses should be able to anticipate and respond to potential issues and find appropriate solutions.
- **Adaptability and flexibility:** Nurses need to be adaptable, flexible, and able to handle changing priorities, unexpected events, and varying patient needs.
- **Time management and organization:** Efficiently balancing patient care responsibilities, documentation, medication administration, and other duties to ensure optimal patient outcomes.
- **Emotional intelligence:** Nurses with high emotional intelligence can handle stressful situations, navigate conflicts, and maintain professional relationships with patients, families, and colleagues.

- **Cultural competence:** Understanding and respecting different cultural beliefs, customs, and practices, and delivering care that is responsive to individual patient needs.
- **Professionalism and ethics:** Demonstrate professionalism in their interactions, appearance, and ethical decision-making.
- **Patient education and advocacy:** Providing clear explanations, teaching self-care techniques, promoting health literacy, and advocating for patients' needs and preferences.

SELF-MOTIVATION

- Self-motivation refers to the internal drive, determination, and initiative to pursue goals, take action, and persist in the face of challenges, without relying solely on external factors or rewards.
- It is the ability to find intrinsic motivation and derive satisfaction and fulfillment from within oneself, rather than relying on external pressures or incentives to stay motivated.

CONFLICT RESOLUTION

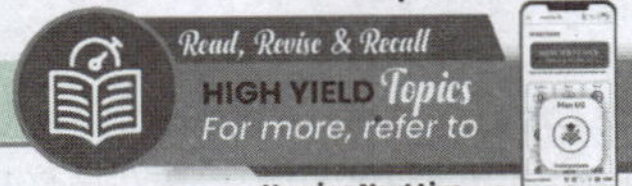

- Conflict resolution in nursing refers to the process of addressing and resolving conflicts or disagreements that may arise among nurses, or between nurses and other health care professionals, patients, or their families.
- Effective conflict resolution in nursing is crucial for maintaining a harmonious work environment, promoting teamwork, and ensuring the delivery of safe and quality patient care.

ASSERTIVENESS

- Being assertive is an essential skill both personally and interpersonally, encompassing the ability to effectively express emotions, desires, needs, and preferences.
- Assertiveness enables individuals to communicate themselves clearly, openly, and reasonably in various interactions, whether in personal or professional settings.
- This approach allows for effective communication with employers, customers, co-workers, and individuals at home, without compromising the rights of oneself or others.

EMOTIONAL INTELLIGENCE

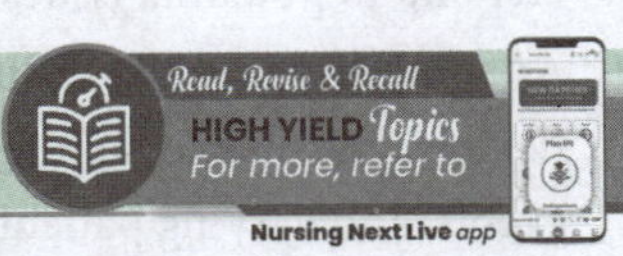

- Emotional intelligence refers to the aptitude to acknowledge and comprehend one's own emotions and behaviors, and how they impact others.
- It also entails valuing and attending to the goals and needs of others, along with the ability to empathize and connect with them on multiple levels.
- Emotional intelligence, also known as EQ, encompasses the capacity to perceive, understand, manage, and reason with emotions.

INTERPERSONAL RELATIONSHIP

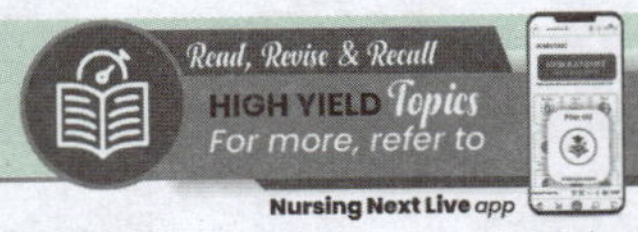

- Interpersonal relationships are a type of soft skill which are essential for nurses.
- Interpersonal relationships are essential for nurses for effective communication and rapport building with patients.
- Hildegard Peplau (1952) formulated an interpersonal model which emphasizes the need of partnership between the nurse and patient as opposed to patient passively receiving the treatment and the nurse who passively acts out as per the Physician's orders.

INTERPERSONAL SKILLS

- Interpersonal skills encompass a diverse set of abilities that involve effective communication, such as active listening and articulate speaking, as well as the capacity to regulate and handle emotions.
- In the workplace, the ability to collaborate effectively with others is commonly known as interpersonal skill. These skills are often referred to as social skills, people skills, or life skills.

RESILIENCE

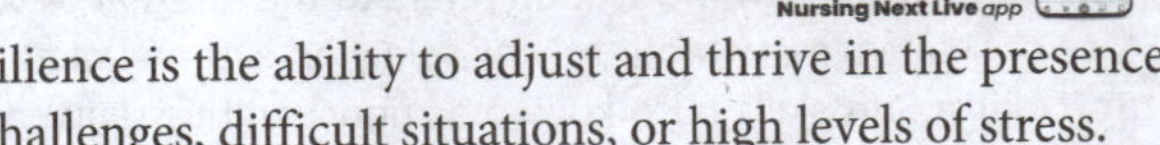

- Resilience is the ability to adjust and thrive in the presence of challenges, difficult situations, or high levels of stress.
- This includes adversity, trauma, tragedy, threats, as well as various stressors like family issues, health problems, or work-related and financial pressures.
- Resilience does not imply that one will not encounter hardships or experience distress.
- Rather, it signifies the capacity to effectively cope and bounce back from setbacks and difficulties.

CONCEPTUAL EXERCISES

LONG ANSWER QUESTIONS

1. What are soft skills? How are the soft skills beneficial in nursing?

Read, Revise & Recall HIGH YIELD Ques For more, refer to Nursing Next Live app

Answer

Soft Skills

- Soft skills are nontechnical skills which are a person's interpersonal skills.

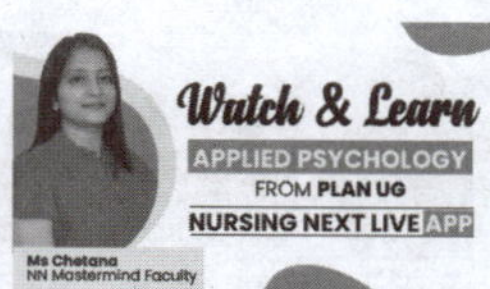

- These skills are character traits and interpersonal skills that characterize a person's relationship with other people.
- Soft skills are complementary to hard skills.
- Soft skills refer to a set of personal attributes, qualities, and abilities that enable individuals to effectively interact with others, navigate social situations, and perform well in various professional and personal settings.
- Some common examples of soft skills include:
  - **Communication:** The ability to convey information, listen actively and express with others
  - **Problem solving ability:** Ability to analyze complex situations and think critically.
  - Empathy and compassion
  - **Time management:** Manage time and balance multiple responsibilities
  - **Adaptability:** Willingness to be flexible and adopt new situations.
  - **Collaboration/team-work:** Capacity to work as a member of the team
  - **Creativity:** Innovative and out of box thinking
  - **Leadership:** Ability to guide and mentor
  - **Emotional intelligence:** Capacity to understand and manage own emotions
  - **Conflict resolution:** Skills to navigate conflicts and find resolutions
  - Assertiveness

Benefits of Soft Skills in Nursing

- **Patient-centered care:** Soft skills such as empathy, compassion, and active listening are critical for building strong connections with patients. These skills enable nurses to understand and respond to patients' emotional and psychological needs, leading to more personalized and patient-centered care.
- **Effective communication:** Nurses with excellent verbal and nonverbal communication skills can effectively build good rapport, provide clear instructions to patients and their families, and collaborate with interdisciplinary health care teams. Effective communication minimizes the risk of errors, misunderstandings, and enhances patient safety.
- **Collaboration and teamwork:** Nursing is a collaborative profession that requires effective teamwork. Soft skills like collaboration and conflict resolution enable nurses to work as an effective member of health care team along with physicians, therapists, and support staff.
- **Patient education:** Nurses who possess strong communication and teaching abilities can explain complex medical information in a clear and understandable manner to patients and family members.
- **Emotional support:** Soft skills like empathy and compassion allow nurses to provide emotional support to patients and their families during difficult times, e.g., situations involving grief, end-of-life care, chronic illnesses, or significant life changes.
- **Conflict resolution:** Nurses often work in high-stress environments where conflicts may arise. Having the ability to address conflicts constructively and find resolutions fosters a healthier work environment and improves team dynamics.
- **Leadership and advocacy:** Soft skills such as leadership, advocacy, and assertiveness empower nurses to take on leadership roles, advocate for their patients' rights, and contribute to improvement of health care practices.

Types of Soft Skills

Types of soft skills		
Visual communication skills	Aural communication skills	Communication skills
1. Projection equipment	1. Sign language	1. Vocal
2. Black board or whiteboard	2. Tactile communication	2. Visually
3. Videos	3. Braille	3. Nonverbal
4. Powerpoint presentation	4. Large print	4. Written
5. Handout	5. Audio	
6. Print	6. Accessible multimedia	
7. Object		

Figure 9.1: Types of soft skills

SHORT NOTES

1. Why is aural communication a soft skill?

Answer

Aural Communication

Aural communication is a soft skill because it is a personal attribute that enables people to interact effectively and harmoniously with others through listening.

- Aural communication means communicating through any means like using sign language, human reader, tactile communication, Braille, large print, audio, accessible multimedia and any other augmentative or alternative mode inclusive of accessible information and communication technology.
- Aural communication involves the transmission of information through the auditory sensory system, the system of speaking and hearing.
- It usually encompasses both verbal communication and paralinguistic communication to convey meaning.
- Aural communication can be used to transmit information independently or in combination with visual communication.
- When conducting surveys, the mode of data collection determines whether information can be transmitted aurally, visually, or both.
- Whether survey information is transmitted aurally or visually, it influences how respondents first perceive and then cognitively process information to provide their responses.
- Aural communication relies heavily on verbal language when information is transmitted through spoken words.

2. How one can overcome interpersonal barriers?

Answer

Interpersonal Barriers

- Interpersonal barrier means having poor self-esteem, social anxiety and any other issue which can make it difficult for people to feel comfortable in opening up to others.
- **Emotional barrier and taboos**
  - People might feel difficult to express emotions and some topics out of their comfort zone or taboo.
  - By taboo we mean difficult topics that may include politics, religion, disabilities (mental and physical), sexuality and sex, racism and any opinion that may be seen as unpopular.
  - To overcome it, one should keep himself away from communication until he feels confident enough to collect his thoughts, think clearly and hold back undue comments. Relaxation exercises will strengthen mental health.
- **Lack of participation**
  - It is nearly impossible to communicate with someone who is not interested. The lack of desire to participate in the communication is a significant barrier.
  - One can overcome this by the usage of simple words to convey the message, learning the art of listening, keeping composure while communicating and by providing constructive criticism.
- **Different perspectives and viewpoint**
  - It's tough to communicate when someone refuses to explore different points of view, opinions or ideas about the world.
  - One can overcome this barrier by analyzing your own perception, working to improve your own perception and by focusing on others.
- **Language differences**
  - Misunderstandings may happen within workers who don't have the same primary language.
  - When the sender and the receiver of the message speak different languages, interpersonal communication can go away.
  - Note everyone understands the slang, jargon and acronyms, instead of seeking clarification one might misunderstand the meaning of the message.
  - To overcome the language barrier, simple words with fewer syllables should be used. Translation of all relevant documents into the primary languages of employees should be done. Visual communication should be used more often and not to raise voice or over-enunciate words.
- **Cultural differences**
  - Cultural misunderstanding, mis-perception, bias and stereotypical beliefs can affect interpersonal communication adversely.
  - To overcome cultural barriers, one should determine whether a specific behavior or attribute is required for the job.
  - Identify whether you can accommodate the cultural differences or not. Learn about other cultures, ask your employees for insight.

3. How are aural and nonverbal communication different?

Answer

Aural communication refers to the exchange of information through spoken words or sound. It involves using the voice to convey a message, which can be heard and interpreted by the listener. Nonverbal communication, on the other hand, refers to the exchange of information through facial expressions, body language, gestures, and other forms of communication that do not involve words.

Here are some of the key differences between aural and nonverbal communication:

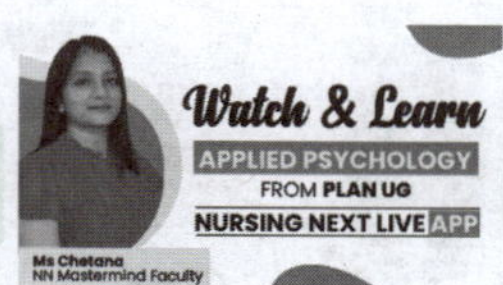

- **Medium:** Aural communication uses the spoken word, while nonverbal communication uses visual cues like body language, gestures, and facial expressions.
- **Channel:** Aural communication is typically transmitted through the airwaves or other auditory channels, while nonverbal communication is usually transmitted through visual cues.
- **Complexity:** Aural communication is typically more complex than nonverbal communication, as it involves the use of words, tone of voice, and other verbal cues. Nonverbal communication, on the other hand, is usually simpler and more straightforward.
- **Ambiguity:** Aural communication can be ambiguous, as words can be interpreted in different ways depending on the context and the listener's interpretation. Nonverbal communication can also be ambiguous, but it is usually easier to interpret than aural communication, as it is based on visual cues.
- **Cultural differences:** Aural communication can be influenced by language, while nonverbal communication can be influenced by culture. Different cultures may interpret nonverbal cues differently, leading to misunderstandings.

4. What are the most common issues faced by the nurses?

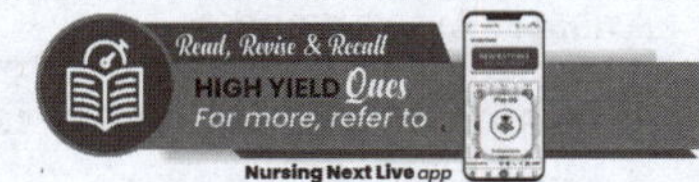

Answer

There are various issues that are faced by nurses on daily basis. The issues are as follows:

- **Inadequate staffing**
  - Staff shortage is a very common issue among nurses. This causes burden on nurses. But in nursing, inadequate staffing can be a matter of life and death.
  - "Staff shortages are brought about by cost-cutting decisions, an aging population, increased patient complexity and need, and an aging workforce places stress on working conditions for nurses and affects patient care and overall outcomes," the ANA says. "An increasing body of evidence shows appropriate nurse staffing that contributes to improved patient outcomes and greater satisfaction for both patients and staff."
- **Stress**
  - The emotional and physical demands of caring for others place another burden on nurses.
  - "Healthy nurses are great role models for their patients, colleagues, families, and neighbors," the ANA says.
  - Stress can cause burnout and results in poor quality of patient care.
- **Safety on the job**
  - Many factors are necessary to create a safe work environment. ANA initiatives to improve workplace safety include:
    - Safe patient handling
    - Safe needles
- **Workplace Violence**
  - "Health care and social service workers face an increased risk of work-related assaults resulting primarily from violent behavior of their patients, clients, and/or residents," the Occupational Safety and Health Administration (OSHA) writes in *Guidelines for Preventing Workplace Violence for Health care and Social Service Workers.*

SHORT ANSWER QUESTIONS

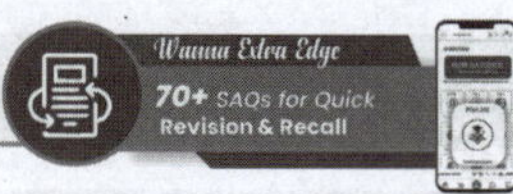

1. Define soft skills.

Answer

Soft Skills

- Soft skills are nontechnical skills which are a person's interpersonal skills.
- These skills are character traits and interpersonal skills that characterize a person's relationship with other people.
- Soft skills are complementary to hard skills.

2. Define IPR.

Answer

Interpersonal relationship refers to the social connection or association between two or more individuals. It involves the exchange of information, emotions, and experiences through verbal and nonverbal communication. Interpersonal relationships can take many forms, including romantic partnerships, friendships, family relationships, and professional relationships.

3. Enlist types of soft skills.

Answer

Types of soft skills are:

Visual communication skills:

- Projection equipment
- Black board/white board

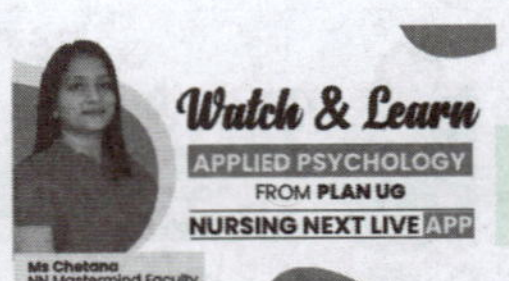

- Videos
- PowerPoint presentation
- Handout
- Print
- Object

Aural communication skills:
- Sign language
- Large print
- Braille
- Audio
- Tactile communication

Communication skills:
- Vocal
- Nonverbal
- Written
- Visual

4. Define work-life balance.

Answer

Work-life balance is the state of equilibrium where a person equally prioritizes the demands of one's career and the demands of one's personal life and for a healthy work environment , work-life balance is important because it reduces stress and it prevents burnout at work place.

CONCEPTUAL REVISION

MULTIPLE CHOICE QUESTIONS

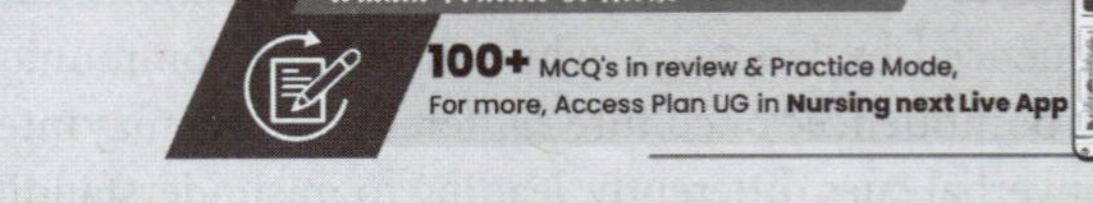

1. Nontechnical skills which are also known as interpersonal skills are known as:

a. Hard skills　b. Soft skills
c. Emotional Intelligence　d. Intelligence quotient

Ans. b. Soft skills

2. The qualities which are also known as Transferable qualities:

a. Hard skills
b. Soft skills
c. Emotional Intelligence
d. Intelligence quotient

Ans. b. Soft skills

3. The ability that involves being able to adequately communicate sentiments, wishes, needs, and desires are:

a. Communication skills　b. Conflict resolution
c. Assertiveness　d. Accountability

Ans. c. Assertiveness

4. Which of the following is NOT a category of soft skills?

a. Visual communication skills
b. Aural communication skills
c. Communication skills
d. Leadership skills

Ans. d. Leadership skills

100+ Golden Points in Podcast form
For more, refer to Nursing Next Live app

Golden Points

- Building and maintaining relationships require a lot of patience and understanding of client and society.
- Each aspect helps a person to communicate effectively in any position.
- Soft skills are personal attributes that enhance an individual's interactions, career prospects and job performance.
- There are various types of soft skills, like visual communication, aural communication and communication skill.
- There are various ways by which one can communicate, i.e., writing, verbal, nonverbal, visual, etc. and it is beneficial in establishing a relationship among clients as well as society.
- To build interpersonal relationship, you should have interpersonal skill. It is embedded into our behavior so it's important to maintain a positive personality. So, to survive into a workplace or in society, you should have an ability to manage time, cope stress, have resilience and know how to balance between work and personal life.
- We should have a good hold on our soft skills for this. It is essential for building interpersonal relationship which is a progressive trait in society as well as workplaces.

CHAPTER

10

Self-Empowerment

CONCEPTUAL THEORY

Terminology

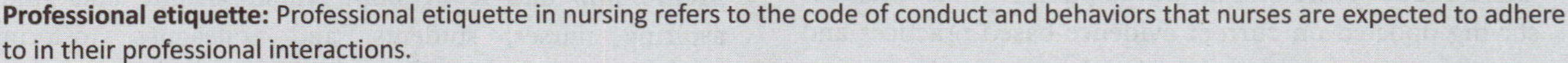

Continuous professional development: This includes staying updated on current evidence-based practices and participating in relevant educational opportunities.

Professional etiquette: Professional etiquette in nursing refers to the code of conduct and behaviors that nurses are expected to adhere to in their professional interactions.

Self-empowerment: Self-empowerment refers to the ability to make decisions and have a variety of options available, rather than being limited to a simple "yes" or "no."

INTRODUCTION

- Self-empowerment refers to the ability to make decisions and have a variety of options available, rather than being limited to a simple "yes" or "no."
- It involves being assertive, having a sense of hope that individuals can make a difference, developing critical thinking skills, adopting different perspectives, respecting the rights of others, taking initiative, embracing continuous personal growth and change, and making a positive impact on others.

DIMENSIONS OF SELF-EMPOWERMENT

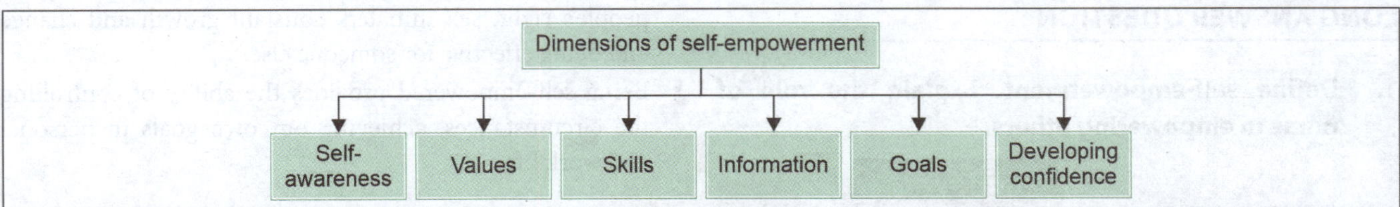

IMPORTANCE OF WOMEN'S EMPOWERMENT IN SOCIETY

- Development of nation
- Overall development of society
- Reduced domestic violence
- Poverty reduction
- Unemployment or underemployment
- Equally competent and intelligence
- Talented
- Irreplaceable

PROFESSIONAL ETIQUETTE

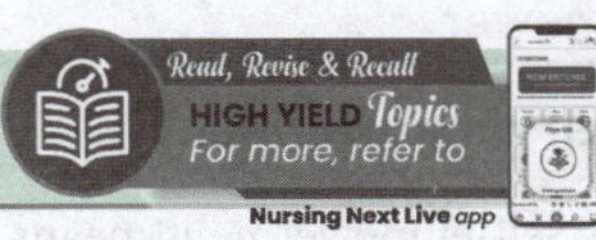

Professional etiquette in nursing refers to the code of conduct and behaviors that nurses are expected to adhere to in their professional interactions.

There is a set of guidelines and principles that promote professionalism, respect, and effective communication:

- **Respect and courtesy:** Includes using appropriate language, being attentive and responsive, and valuing diversity and cultural differences.
- **Professional appearance:** Nurses should maintain a professional appearance by adhering to the dress code and

grooming standards of their health care facility to create a positive impression and fosters trust and confidence in patients and colleagues.

- **Confidentiality and privacy:** This involves safeguarding patient's information and refraining from discussing patient details in public or with unauthorized individuals.
- **Effective communication:** Nurses should be respectful, empathetic, and sensitive when interacting with patients and their families.
- **Punctuality and reliability:** Nurses should be on time for shifts, meetings, and appointments, and fulfilling commitments and obligations in a timely manner.
- **Collaboration and teamwork:** Nurses involve effective communication, mutual respect, and a willingness to contribute to a positive work environment and the overall patient care experience.
- **Ethical conduct:** Nurses must maintain integrity, honesty, and accountability, and adhere to professional standards and regulations.
- **Continuous professional development:** This includes staying updated on current evidence-based practices and participating in relevant educational opportunities.
- **Conflict resolution:** This involves active listening, effective communication, and seeking mutually beneficial solutions.

ROLE OF NURSE IN EMPOWERING OTHERS

- **Patient education:** Providing information and resources, nurses empower individuals to actively participate in their own health care decisions and take control of their well-being.
- **Advocacy:** Nurses advocate for their patients' rights, preferences, and needs within the health care system.
- **Health promotion and disease prevention:** Nurses empower others by promoting healthy lifestyles and preventive measures.
- **Emotional support:** Nurses provide emotional support to patients and their families during challenging times.
- **Collaborative decision-making:** Nurses involve patients and their families in health care decisions through shared decision-making processes.
- **Health empowerment programs:** These programs provide tools and resources to empower individuals to take charge of their own well-being.
- **Community engagement:** By participating in health promotion activities, conducting screenings, and providing education, nurses empower individuals and communities to make informed choices for their health.
- **Mentorship and leadership:** Nurses inspire and guide aspiring nurses, students, and colleagues, fostering professional growth and confidence in others.

CONCEPTUAL EXERCISES

LONG ANSWER QUESTION

1. Define self-empowerment. Explain the role of nurse in empowering others.

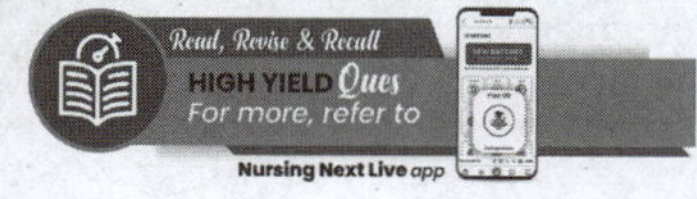

Answer

Self-empowerment

- Self-empowerment means having control on your life and not letting someone else overpower you. Empowerment means being powerful.
- Being powerful always consists of building self-esteem and confidence.
- Self-empowerment is power of making decisions, having range of options from which you can make choices not just yes or no, being assertive, having hope that a difference could be made by an individual, learning to think critically, seeing things in a different way, understanding other people's right, self-initiated, constant growth and change and being effective for someone else.
- Being self-empowered provides the ability of controlling the circumstances, achieving our own goals in personal and work life.

Role of Nurse in Empowering others

Nurses play a vital role in empowering others, including patients, families, and fellow health care professionals.

Empowerment involves supporting individuals to gain control over their own lives, make informed decisions, develop their strengths, and take actions that positively impact their well-being.

Nurses contributes to the empowerment of patients, family members and other health care professionals in the following ways:

- **Patient education:** Nurses empower patients by providing them with accurate and understandable health information.

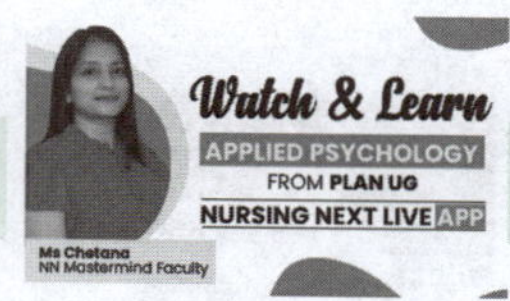

They educate patients about their medical conditions, treatment options, and self-care practices. By enhancing health literacy, nurses enable patients to actively participate in their care, make informed decisions, and take control of their health.

- **Encouraging self-care:** Nurses empower individuals by promoting self-care practices and providing guidance on maintaining optimal health. They educate patients about healthy lifestyle choices, disease prevention, and strategies to manage chronic conditions.
- **Collaborative decision-making:** By involving patients in their care plans and treatment decisions, nurses empower them to actively participate in their health care journey. Nurses engage in shared decision-making with patients and their families, considering their perspectives, values, and goals.
- **Mentoring and leadership:** Nurses can empower their colleagues by serving as mentors and leaders. They share their knowledge, expertise, and experiences, supporting the professional growth and development of others.
- **Advocacy:** Nurses act as advocates for their patients, ensuring their voices are heard and their rights are respected. They provide support, information, and resources to help patients navigate the health care system.
- **Health promotion and community engagement:** Nurses empower individuals and communities by promoting health and engaging them in activities that improve their well-being.
- **Emotional support:** Nurses empower others by providing emotional support and empathy. They create safe spaces for patients, families, and colleagues to express their concerns and emotions openly.

SHORT NOTES

1. Professional etiquette

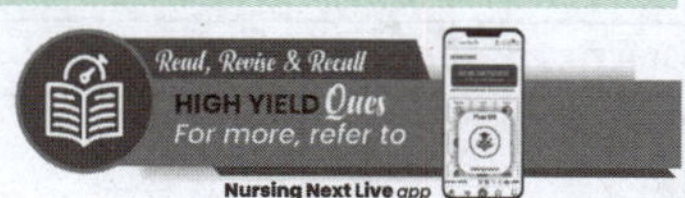

Answer

Professional etiquette refers to the set of behaviors and norms that are expected of individuals in a professional setting. It involves demonstrating respect, **courtesy**, and professionalism in all interactions with colleagues, clients, and other stakeholders. Here are some key principles of professional etiquette:

- **Dress appropriately:** Dress professionally and appropriately for the **workplace**. Understand the dress code and adhere to it.
- **Punctuality**: Be punctual and arrive on time for meetings and appointments.
- **Communication:** Use clear and concise language in all written and oral **communication**. Use proper grammar, spelling, and punctuation.
- **Respect:** Demonstrate respect for colleagues, clients, and other **stakeholders** at all times. Treat everyone with courtesy and professionalism.
- **Listening:** Practice active listening by paying attention to what others are **saying** and demonstrating that you are engaged in the conversation.
- **Confidentiality:** Respect confidentiality by keeping sensitive information private and only sharing it with those who have a need to know.
- **Professionalism:** Act professionally at all times and avoid engaging in behavior that is inappropriate or unprofessional.
- **Conflict resolution:** Handle conflicts and disagreements in a professional and respectful manner. Use diplomacy and tact to resolve conflicts and avoid escalating the situation.
- **Respect diversity:** Demonstrate respect for diversity in all its forms, **including** race, gender, age, religion, and culture.
- **Follow up:** Follow up on commitments and promises in a timely manner.

2. Self-empowerment.

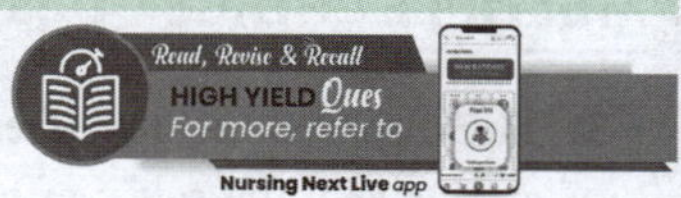

Answer

Self-empowerment

Self-empowerment refers to the process of gaining control over one's own life and achieving a sense of personal power, confidence, and autonomy.

It involves **developing** a strong sense of self-awareness, identifying one's strengths and weaknesses, and taking action to improve one's life circumstances. Here are some key strategies for self-empowerment:

- **Self-reflection:** Take time to reflect on your thoughts, feelings, and actions. This can help you gain a better understanding of your values, goals, and aspirations.
- **Positive self-talk:** Use positive self-talk to boost your confidence and self-**esteem**. Focus on your strengths and accomplishments, and use affirmations to encourage yourself.
- **Goal setting:** Set realistic goals for yourself and work toward achieving them. Break down larger goals into smaller, more manageable steps.
- **Skill development:** Identify areas where you can improve your skills and knowledge, and take action to develop new skills or improve existing ones.
- **Mindfulness:** Practice mindfulness and meditation to help manage stress and **improve** focus and concentration.
- **Healthy habits:** Develop healthy habits, such as exercise, good nutrition, and regular sleep, to improve your physical and mental well-being.

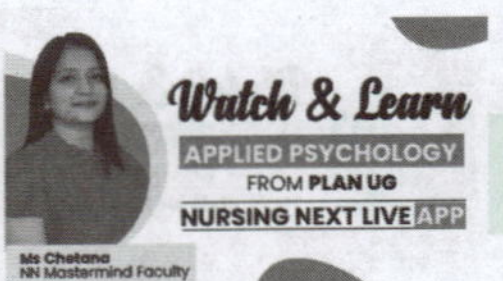

Target High Next Nursing **DECODE**

- **Support network:** Build a support network of family, friends, and colleagues who can provide encouragement, advice, and support.
- **Take action:** Take action to make positive changes in your life. This may **involve** stepping out of your comfort zone and taking calculated risks.

SHORT ANSWER QUESTIONS

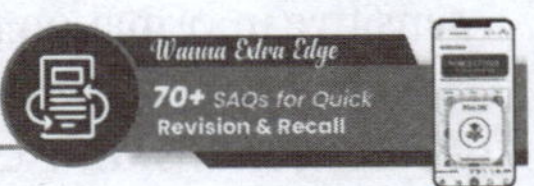

1. Dimensions of self-empowerment.

Answer

Self-empowerment refers to the process of taking control of one's life and becoming more self-aware, confident, and capable. There are several dimensions of self-empowerment, including:

- Self-awareness
- Self-confidence
- Self-efficacy
- Self-determination

2. Define self-empowerment.

Answer

Self-empowerment

- Self-empowerment means having control on your life and not letting someone else overpower you. Empowerment means being powerful.
- Being powerful always consists of building self-esteem and confidence.

CONCEPTUAL REVISION

MULTIPLE CHOICE QUESTIONS

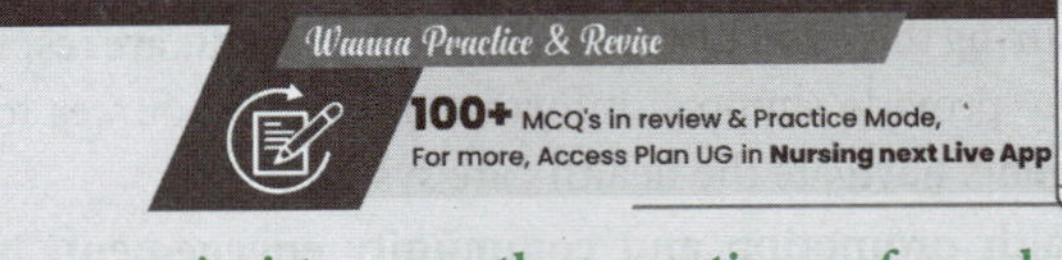

1. The dimensions of self-empowerment include:

a. Developing self-confidence
b. Values
c. Skills and goals
d. All of the above

Ans. d. All of the above

2. Which of the following is the first step of self-empowerment development?

a. Knowing yourself
b. Develop skills
c. Identify your goals
d. Enhance leadership

Ans. a. Knowing yourself

3. _________ insists on the creation of such an environment where decision making is easy for women.

a. Women empowerment b. Self-awareness
c. Advocate social change d. Enhance leadership

Ans. a. Women empowerment

4. _________ enhances self-confidence, communication skills, personal and professional image.

a. Professional etiquette b. Personal grooming
c. Empowerment d. Body language

Ans. b. Personal grooming

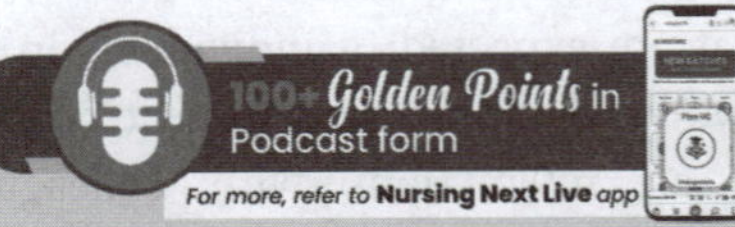

Golden Points

- Empowerment necessitates interventions at multiple levels, including societal/structural changes, improvements in service provision and professional growth, and fostering empowerment on individual and societal levels.
- External conditions and internal qualities are vital for achieving empowerment goals, including hope, respect, reclaiming one's life, understanding and exercising rights, learning essential skills, transitioning from secrecy to transparency, and embracing ongoing self-initiated growth and change.
- Recognizing that mental health issues provide opportunities for learning, growth, and development, and bringing additional skills and qualities is essential for individuals with mental health challenges and society as a whole.
- Self-awareness is linked to increased focus, continuous learning from mistakes and personal experiences, and the conscious pursuit of a better life.
- To foster the strength and prosperity of a nation, it is crucial to empower women, enabling them to embrace their rights and achieve independence in all aspects of their growth and development.

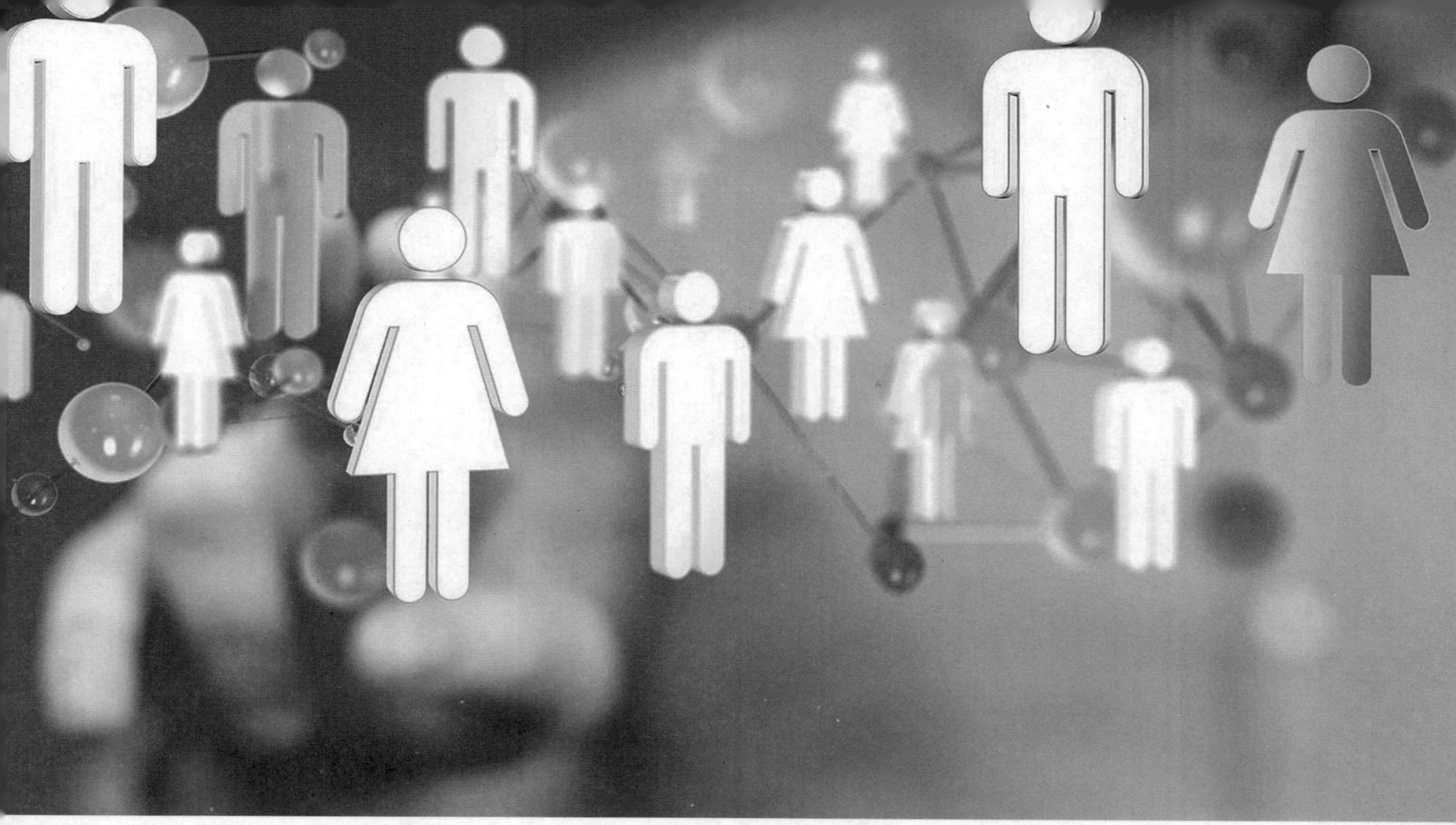

Applied Sociology

Unit Outline

CHAPTER 1

Introduction to Sociology

CONCEPTUAL THEORY

Terminology

Applied sociology: The use of sociological information, principles, methods, concepts, and theories to solve contemporary social problems. Sociology has practical applications in dealing with social pathologies.
Conflict theory: A conflict perspective holds that social behavior is best understood through conflict or tension between competing groups.
General sociology: General sociology is the study of the structural and dynamic features and uniformities that are shared by all social and cultural processes.
Ideal type: A concept or paradigm that is ideal for analyzing specific instances.
Macrosociology: Sociological research focusing on large-scale phenomena or entire civilizations.
Manifest function: A manifest function is one that is open, expreszed, and conscious.
Microsociology: A sociological approach that emphasizes the study of small groups, frequently using experimental methods.
Natural science: Natural science is the study of natural physical properties and how they interact and change.
Sociological imaginations: Understanding of the relationship between an individual and society as a whole.
Sociology: Sociology is the systematic study of human groupings and social behavior.
Special sociology: Special sociology is the study of a specific sociocultural phenomenon that has been chosen for in-depth investigation.
Theory: In sociology, a theory is a series of claims that attempts to explain situations, actions, or behavior.
Verstehen: A German word for "understanding" or "insight"; used to emphasize the subjective understanding of a society on its own terms, and not from an outsider's prospective.

ORIGIN OF THE TERM "SOCIOLOGY"

- The term "Sociology" was coined by a French philosopher Auguste Comte in 1839 (Saint Simon).
  He is known as the "Father of Sociology".
- The word "sociology" has been derived from a Latin word "Societus", which means society, association, togetherness or companionship and a Greek Word "Logos", which means "study" or "science".
- Literal meaning is to "speak about" or "word".
- Therefore, sociology in simpler terms means "study of society" or "science of society".
- It includes patterns of social relationships, social interaction, and culture.
- Four main paradigms:
  1. Structural-functional
  2. Functionalist paradigm
  3. Conflict paradigm
  4. Symbolic interactionist paradigm

DEFINITIONS

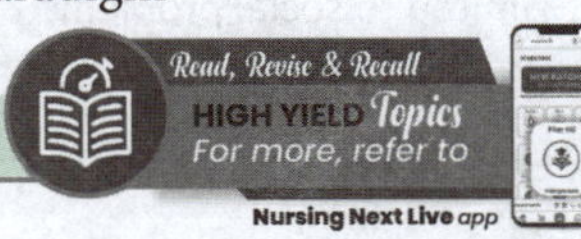

Auguste Comte, the founding father of sociology, defines sociology as the science of social phenomena "subject to natural and invariable laws, the discovery of which is the object of investigation".

Kingsley Davis says, "Sociology is a general science of society."

Emile Durkheim: "Science of social institutions."

Max Weber defines sociology as " the science which attempts the interpretative understanding of social action in order thereby to arrive at a causal explanation of its course and effects".

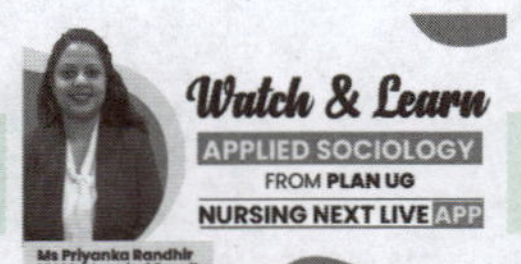

MEANING OF SOCIOLOGY

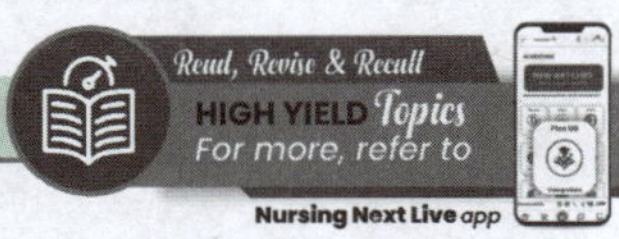

- Sociology basically means the study of social activities of humans, how humans live in society and how they interact with each other.
  Example: In a cricket stadium (feeling of connection + you interact like saying excuse me, please, etc.).
- In other countries/areas, it is difficult to identify crowd and you do not feel yourself as part of the crowd. You do not know how to behave.
- Within the same crowd, there may be different groups with different behaviors. Example: In a class room lecture, some are actively participating, while others are just listening or observing and some are not even bothered about what is going on.
- **Example:** Cricket (People react differently)
- **Main focus:** Being in group changes one's behavior
- Sociology gives answer to the following questions:
  - Why an individual feels and acts differently in different types of social situations?
  - Why people of a single group exhibit different behaviors in same situation?
  - Why people acting similarly do not feel connected to others who have same behavior?

NATURE OF SOCIOLOGY

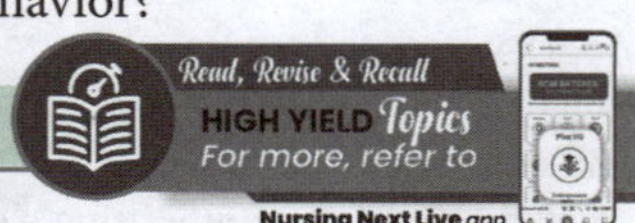

- Sociology is generalized in nature.
- Robert Bierstedt in his book " The Social Order "analyzed the characteristics of sociology as:
  - Independent science
  - Social science
  - Categorical and not normative (what is not what ought to be)
  - Pure science not applied science
  - Abstract not concrete
  - Generalizing science not particular
  - Both rational and empirical
- The nature of sociology can be divided into:
  - **Macro:** Macro-level sociology deals with the analysis of large-scale social structures, systems, and patterns that influence societies and nations as a whole. It focuses on understanding broad phenomena such as social institutions, economic systems, political structures, and global processes, exploring how these factors shape the behavior and interactions of individuals and groups within a society.
  - **Meso:**
    Meso-level sociology examines intermediate-sized social structures and organizations, such as communities, organizations, and subcultures. It delves into the interactions and relationships within these smaller units, exploring how they contribute to the functioning of larger societal systems and how they can influence the behaviors and identities of individuals within them.
  - **Micro:**
    Micro-level sociology focuses on the individual-level interactions and behaviors within social contexts. It explores the intricacies of everyday life, personal relationships, and small-group dynamics. This perspective seeks to understand how individuals interpret symbols, communicate, make decisions, and construct their identities through their interactions with others, ultimately contributing to the formation of larger societal patterns.

SCOPE OF SOCIOLOGY

Read, Revise & Recall HIGH YIELD Topics For more, refer to Nursing Next Live app

- Specialistic or formalistic school
- Synthetic school

Formalistic school	Synthetic school
• Limited to social problems	• Study as a whole (Auguste Comte compares it with human body)
• Narrow or Micro	• Broad or Macro
• Emanual Kant laid its basis	• General (Emile Durkheim says it is science of collective representation)
	• Durkheim asks to Borrow subjects like suicide (from psychology), DOL (from economics example: Varna system)
• Subjective understanding of objective reality. Example: Most people are from Germany	• General (family, religion) and specific sociology (caste, race) by Pitrim Sorokin • Karl Manheim says to discuss the structure and broader ideas (example, PK movie)
• Interpretive school by Weber	• Hobhouse says that sociology is a synthesis of many social studies
• Forms of Interaction (Formal Vs Informal) by George Simmel (different behavior)	• Alex Inkele's (social analysis, primary concept of social life, basic social institutions, social process)
• Alfred Vierkandt (sum total of social + psychic behavior = SOCIOLOGY) how to talk to someone	• JB Mckee's (social action, social structure, social institution, social process all should be included in scope)

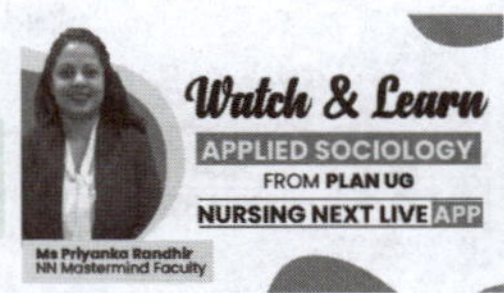

SIGNIFICANCE OF SOCIOLOGY IN NURSING

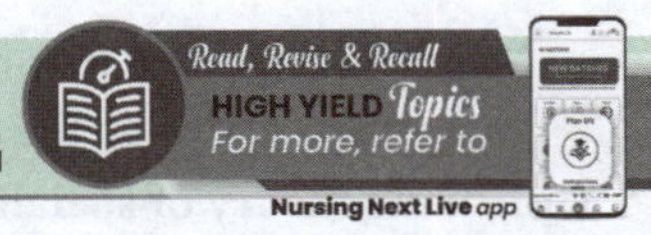

- Understanding human nature is the key benefit of studying sociology for nursing students.
- Nurses are capable of understanding their patients' issues through learning about their own ideas and habits.
- This enables them to carry out their nursing responsibilities in a way that is advantageous to them and the patient.
- Psychology is useful to nursing, but so is sociology. Similar to how psychology does, sociology aids a nurse in understanding what makes individuals "tick."
- The only distinction is that sociology approaches it from the standpoint of a "group" or "community."
- These are crucial since a nurse also needs to be kind, sensitive, and caring in addition to having medical knowledge. Patients' families exist.
- Even a superficial understanding of the information included in those fields could help nurses become more compassionate and gentle.
- Additionally, sociological research can help answer some of the ethical issues that are currently prevalent in medicine.
- While some sociologists prioritize improving the theoretical knowledge of social processes, many sociologists aim to perform research that can be immediately applied to social policy and welfare.
- From the micro level of individual agency and interaction to the macro level of systems and the social structure, a variety of topics are covered.
- In nursing, sociology helps in:
  - Scientific study of society
  - Understanding role of social institutions in forming society
  - Understanding and planning society
  - Finding out solution to social problems
  - Telling us the worth and dignity of humans
  - Developing new outlook
  - Contributing to human culture
  - Studying health
  - Determining social causes of disease
  - Understanding patient
  - Necessity to change environment
  - Knowledge of family
  - Helps in understanding community
  - Understands social position
- There are various educational options for nurses, including the Registered Nurse (RN, frequently gained after a bachelor's degree), the Licensed Vocational Nurse (LVN), and the Bachelor of Science in Nursing (BSN Nurses can also pursue advanced degrees in their field, such as a Master of Science in Nursing (MSN) or a Doctor of Nursing (DN) degree.

CONCEPTUAL EXERCISES

LONG ANSWER QUESTIONS

1. Explain the theories of socialization.

Answer

Socialization: "Socialization is a learning that enables the learner to perform social roles." —**Harry M Johnson**

Theories of Socialization

There are four famous theories of socialization and these are:

1. **Freud's theory of socialization:** In the viewpoint of **Sigmund Freud,** "basic biological instincts combine with societal factors to shape personalities."
   - Sigmund Freud's theory of socialization is based on his theory of personality, which he called psychoanalysis.
   - Freud emphasizes that a significant portion of a person's personality develops throughout childhood and is then developed and refined over the rest of his/her life.
   - Sigmund Freud classified the human mind into three main regions:
     i. **Consciousness:** The conscious part of the mind connects the person with his/her current circumstances and actions.
     ii. **Preconsciousness:** Preconscious region stores up memories, which easily enter consciousness.
     iii. **Unconsciousness:** All of the suppressed urges and unpleasant experiences that the conscious mind finds unacceptable are kept in the unconscious region.
   - The interaction of the "id", "ego", and "superego" is what gives a person's personality a particular shape.
2. **Cooley's theory of socialization**
   - Charles Horton Cooley said, 'people form their self-images through interaction with other people'.
   - That means our significant others help to shape who we are.

- Someone we value and who has the power to shape our thinking, particularly about ourselves, is a significant other.
- The idea of the looking-glass self is part of Cooley's theory of socialization.
- A self-image that is dependent on how we believe others see us is referred to as the Looking-Glass Self.
- Cooley proposed a three-step procedure for self-development:
- **Step I:** Visualizing how we would appear to someone else. (We assume that a significant other has a particular perception of us.)
- **Step II:** His judement of that appearance in his imagination. (We assume that based on that perception, he or she will judge us.)
- **Step III:** A feeling of one's own, such as pride or shame. (Our self-image is shaped by how we believe our significant other perceives us.)

3. **Mead's theory of socialization (symbolic interactionism)**

- Mead's theory of the social self is founded on the ideas that the self develops through social interactions, including:
  - Observing and engaging with others
  - Reacting to others' judgments of oneself
  - Internalizing external opinions and internal sentiments about oneself.
- Mead believes that the self is not there at birth but rather develops gradually as a result of social interactions and activities.
- Mead proposed that three activities—languages, play, and games—develop the self.

4. **Goffman's theory of socialization**

- Goffman's theory of socialization is based on the idea that social interaction is like a performance.
- Goffman identifies two main types of social interaction: frontstage and backstage.
- Frontstage interactions are those that occur in public, where we are aware that others are watching us. We use impression management to create a favorable impression of ourselves. We do this by carefully controlling our appearance, our behavior, and our speech. For example, if we are giving a presentation at work, we will dress professionally, speak clearly and confidently, and try to make eye contact with our audience.
- Backstage interactions are those that occur in private, where we can relax and be ourselves.
- In backstage interactions, we can relax and be ourselves. We do not have to worry about controlling our impressions, because we are not aware that others are watching us. We can let our hair down, be informal, and talk about anything we want.
- Here are some of the key concepts in Goffman's theory of socialization: Front stage, back stage, impression management, setting and role.

Table 1.1: Approach to self and interaction

Perspective	Approach to self and interaction	Case study: Identity in childhood
Psychoanalysis	Freud's theory of the unconscious mind as composed of an interrelated system (id, ego, superego) that underlines human behavior; personality develops through psychosexual stages.	Parents instill a conscience (superego) in children through rules that govern their instinctual behavior (id) until children mature and are self-governing (ego).
Looking-Glass self	Cooley's theory of the self-concept; our sense of self is derived from how we imagine others see us, and the feelings about ourselves based on the perceived judgments of others.	Parents and significant others serve as a reflection to children, who develop a sense of self based on their appraisals, real or imagined.
Mind, self, and society	Mead's theory of the self that develops through three stages (preparatory, play, and game); in role taking the particular or generalized other, we learn to see ourselves as others do.	Children gain a sense of self through imitation, play, and games, in which they learn various roles and take on the perspectives of others.
Dramaturgy	Goffman's theory of the presentation of self; we are like actors on a stage, whose performance strategies aid in impression management.	Children learn the art of impression management and may present a different self to their parents than to other children or to teachers.

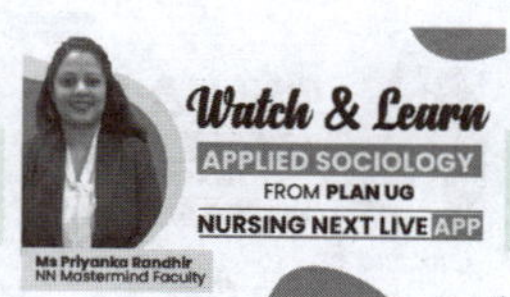

2. Explain the importance of sociology in nursing.

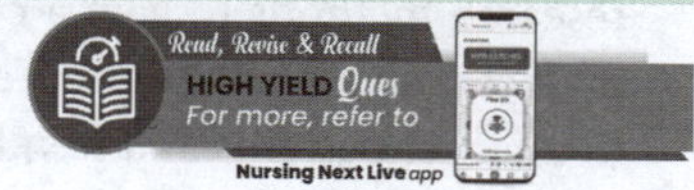

Answer

- **Sociology:** "Sociology is about social relationships, the network of relationships we call society".

  —MacIver and Page

- **Nursing:** The field of nursing is concerned with how people react to current and potential health issues. Human reactions to acute and chronic health issues, health promotion, health maintenance, and nursing treatments are the core topics of current nursing research.

Importance of Sociology in Nursing

- Understanding human nature is the key benefit of studying sociology for nursing students.
- Nurses are capable of understanding their patients' issues through learning about their own ideas and habits.
- This enables them to carry out their nursing responsibilities in a way that is advantageous to them and the patient.
- Psychology is useful to nursing, and so is sociology. Similar to how psychology does, sociology aids a nurse in understanding what makes individuals "tick."
- The only distinction is that sociology approaches it from the standpoint of a "group" or "community."
- These are crucial since a nurse also needs to be kind, sensitive, and caring in addition to having medical knowledge. Patients' families exist.
- Even a superficial understanding of the information included in those fields could help nurses become more compassionate and gentle.
- Additionally, sociological research can help answer some of the ethical issues that are currently prevalent in medicine.
- While some sociologists prioritize improving the theoretical knowledge of social processes, many sociologists aim to perform research that can be immediately applied to social policy and welfare.
- From the micro level of individual agency and interaction to the macro level of systems and the social structure, a variety of topics are covered.
- In nursing, sociology helps in:
  - Understanding scientific study of society
  - Understanding role of social institutions in forming society
  - Understanding and planning society
  - Finding out solution to social problems
  - Telling us the worth and dignity of humans
  - Developing new outlook
  - To provide Cultural-competent care: Sociology helps nurses develop cultural competence by providing insights into diverse social and cultural backgrounds. Understanding societal norms, beliefs, and values helps nurses provide culturally sensitive and appropriate care to patients from different background.
  - Studying health
  - Social Determinants of Health: Sociology helps nurses recognize the impact of social factors on health outcomes. By understanding social determinants of health such as poverty, education, housing, and access to healthcare, nurses can address these factors and advocate for policies and interventions that promote health equity.
  - Understanding patient
  - Necessity to change environment
  - Knowledge of family
  - Helps in understanding community
  - Understands social position
- Advocacy and social justice: Sociology equips nurses with the knowledge and tools to advocate for social justice and address healthcare disparities.
- Health promotion and education: Sociological knowledge allows nurses to understand how social factors influence health behaviors.
- Ethical decision making: Sociology provides a foundation for ethical decision making in nursing practice. By examining societal values, norms, and ethical frameworks, nurses can make informed choices that promote social well-being.
- Interprofessional collaboration: Understanding the social context in which healthcare is delivered allows nurses to work collaboratively to address complex health and social issues.

3. How can you prove that the sociology is a science?

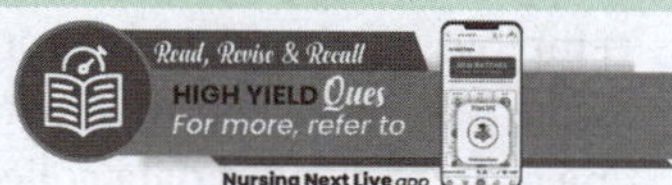

Answer

Introduction

- The science of sociology is the study of people and their cultures. It combines the methodical study of the development, composition, connections, and attitudes of ordered social groups of people. Scientists, social scientists, and activists can better understand society with the help of sociology. Additionally, it aids in raising the standard of living for members of society.
- **Definition:** Sociology is the science of social phenomena 'subject to natural and invariable laws, the discovery of which is the object of investigation'. **—Auguste Comte**

Sociology as a Science

- The definition of sociology as a science is currently up for debate.

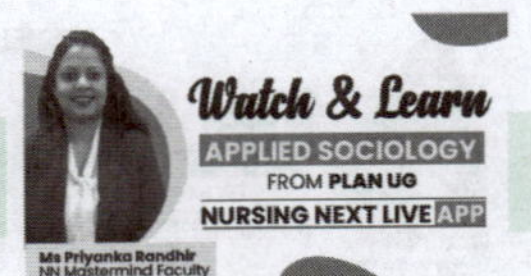

- The idea that sociology should be treated as a science like all other social sciences is opposed by some skeptics.
- Since it uses unbiased and organized methods for analysis and evaluation, sociology can be regarded as a science.
- In addition, it can be judged as a social reality using empirical evidence and justification.
- However, as human behavior is not comparable to natural sciences, it cannot be directly compared to them.
- At least two definitions of science are possible:
  - An organized, validated body of information that has been established via scientific research
  - A research technique that results in the discovery of a body of organized and validated information
- However, if the first definition is accepted, sociology can be referred to as a science on the basis of the theory that it does so after conducting a body of organized and validated information.
- According to American sociologist W F Ogburn, sociology is a science.
- According to him, science should be evaluated using the following three criteria:
  - The reliability of its body of knowledge
  - Its structure
  - Its methodology
- Sociology is considered a science based on several characteristics and principles that align with scientific inquiry. While the social sciences, including sociology, may differ from the natural sciences in some ways, they still adhere to scientific principles.
- Here are some ways in which sociology demonstrates its scientific nature:
- **Empirical approach:** Like other sciences, sociology employs an empirical approach to studying the social world. It relies on systematic and objective observation, measurement, and data collection. Sociologists gather data through various methods, such as surveys, interviews, experiments, and observations, to test hypotheses and analyze patterns and relationships.
- **Theory and hypothesis testing:** Sociology develops and tests theories to explain social phenomena. Theories in sociology are based on empirical evidence and logical reasoning. Sociologists formulate hypotheses derived from these theories and subject them to empirical testing to evaluate their validity and refine understanding.
- **Use of scientific methods:** Sociology applies scientific methods and research techniques to study social phenomena. This includes formulating research questions, designing research studies, collecting and analyzing data, and drawing conclusions based on evidence. Sociologists strive for objectivity and rigor in their research methodologies.
- **Systematic observation:** Sociologists systematically observe social phenomena and collect data to draw conclusions. They employ both qualitative and quantitative research methods to gain a comprehensive understanding of social phenomena, often employing statistical analyses to uncover patterns and trends.
- **Replication and peer review:** Like other scientific disciplines, sociology encourages replication and peer review. Replication involves repeating research studies by different researchers to verify the findings and enhance the reliability of the results. Peer review involves subjecting research findings to scrutiny and evaluation by other experts in the field to ensure the quality and validity of the research.
- **Theoretical and conceptual frameworks:** Sociology utilizes theoretical frameworks and concepts to organize and explain social phenomena. These frameworks provide a foundation for understanding and predicting social behavior.
- **Cumulative knowledge:** Through ongoing research and the accumulation of empirical evidence, sociology contributes to a body of knowledge that expands over time.
- While sociology may not adhere to all the methodologies of natural sciences due to the complexity of social phenomena, it shares fundamental principles of scientific inquiry, including systematic observation, empirical testing, theory development, and the accumulation of knowledge.

4. Explain how sociology is playing a major role in health services.

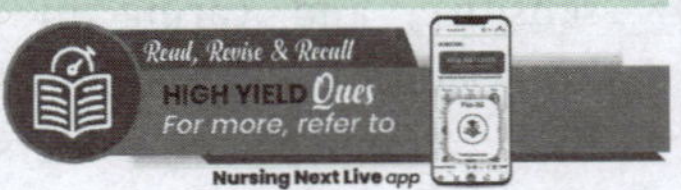

Answer

Sociology is a very important subject particularly in the fields of nursing education, practice, and service.

Major Role in Health Services

- **Focusing on transcultural concept:** It is crucial to understand the patients' cultures in a place like India where individuals belong to many castes, tribes, faiths, and communities. To better the medical and nursing services, it must be known before treating patients, and sociology study is required for this.
- **Helps in adjustment:** The ability to adapt to conditions in the hospital setting including the doctor-nurse-patient interaction, nurse administration and doctor relations, and doctor-nurse and public relations will be aided by sociological knowledge on the part of the doctor or nurse.
- **Importance of sociological factors:** The entire health care system can benefit greatly from medical sociology which helps in understanding the importance of social factors in health, such as changes in cognitive function. It is necessary to address social processes like motivation and health values, i.e., changes to effective processes.

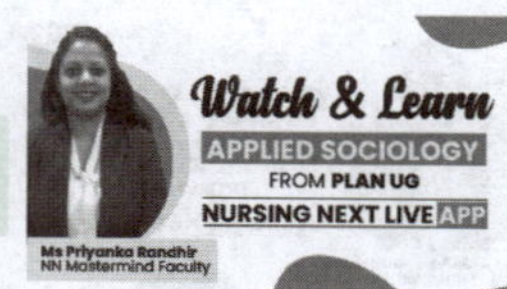

- **Disease prevention:** In addition to providing patient care, nurses should aid in disease prevention. In other words, they ought to encourage neighborhood health. The study of sociology will aid nurses in determining the patients' social backgrounds.
- **Improving treatment quality:** The study of sociology enables nurses to recognize patients' sociopsychological issues, which enhances the effectiveness of care.
- **Relationships between several social life components:** The study of sociology enables nurses to comprehend how many facets of social life—such as those that are economic, political, moral, religious, and intellectual—relate to one another and to particular disorders.
- **In government policies:** The study of sociology also enables nurses to assist the government in a variety of social planning initiatives, such as the family health program and welfare of the government, which can only be executed successfully with the active involvement of nurses.
- **Care of vulnerable:** The study of sociology aids nurses in providing better care to vulnerable populations such as children, the elderly, persons with physical or mental disabilities, those living with HIV/AIDS, etc. These diseases can be effectively treated, only by having a thorough understanding of the patients' varied cultural origins.
- **Family Welfare Programs:** The study of sociology aids nurses in raising the standard of the government's Family Welfare Programs and Community Health Services.
- **Health care:** A wide range of people with diverse behaviors must be interacted with by nurses, including patients, doctors, other family members, management, the government, and society at large. Understanding these behavioral tendencies will help to advance health care, which will benefit from the study of sociology.
- **IPR:** The use of preventative, curative, and promotional aspects of health in the community benefits from the development of interpersonal relationships between patients, medical staff, and paramedical employees.
- **Good citizen:** In order to be responsible citizens in the advancement of health education in the nation, nurses must have a good understanding of sociology.

5. Describe the social factors that affect the health status in taking treatment, hospitalization and rehabilitation.

Answer

Introduction

There are a lot of things besides health care that affect our health. Only 10–20 percent of what keeps us healthy is related to health treatment. The health of an individual and society is influenced by a variety of social factors in addition to genetics and lifestyle choices. Up to 40% of what keeps us healthy is attributed to social variables like housing, social relationships, money, and education.

Social Factors that Affect the Health Status

These factors include:

- **Monthly income:** Where we live, what we eat, and what we do for leisure might all depend on our income or financial situation. Higher-income individuals typically have longer lifespans and better general health. They can spend easily on treatment, hospitalization and rehabilitation as compared to those with low socio-economic status. Example: people with low socioeconomic status do not have ample money for seeking medical care.
- **Educational status:** Higher income and the capacity to comprehend what keeps us healthy are both correlated with education. Together, education and income play a significant role in determining our health as well as the health of our families, communities, and our society. It also helps in determining the decision to seek treatment, hospitalization and rehabilitation. Example: Most of the illiterate people come un-booked and un-investigated at the time of delivery in the labor room.
- **Social interactions:** People can cope with difficult circumstances by maintaining positive social contacts. Health issues may be reduced or avoided with the help of friends, family, coworkers, sports teams, or faith-based organizations.
- **Housing:** The availability of affordable housing in good neighborhoods with good transit options can have a big impact on someone's health and well-being. Absence of such factors prevents the people to seek treatment, hospitalization and rehabilitation.
- **Access to healthy food:** "Food security" refers to regular access to wholesome foods that satisfy dietary and cultural requirements and promote excellent health. Poor health is more prevalent in people who can't afford good food on a daily basis.
- **Type of community:** As the health facilities are more centralized in urban areas, it becomes difficult for the people residing in rural areas to seek treatment, hospitalization and rehabilitation.
- **Gender:** In general, health care needs of women is much more than men due to many reasons besides reproductive health. However, traditional gender roles and expectations can impact health-seeking behaviors and treatment adherence. For example, societal expectations of stoicism in men may discourage seeking help for mental health issues.
- Gender disparities in access to healthcare can affect health outcomes. Women may face barriers due to financial

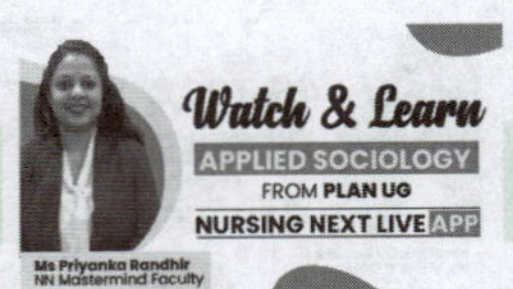

constraints, lack of insurance coverage, or limited availability of gender-specific services.

- **Age group:** Working-age people and older adults are the ones who often seek treatment, hospitalization and rehabilitation as compared to other age groups. In addition, different age groups may have varying levels of health literacy, understanding of treatment options, and ability to make informed decisions. Age-related factors, such as cognitive decline in older adults, can affect treatment adherence.
- **Race and ethnicity:** Racial and ethnic minorities may face systemic discrimination and bias within healthcare systems, affecting their experiences and health outcomes. This can lead to disparities in access, treatment quality, and patient-provider communication.
- Cultural beliefs, values, and practices can influence treatment preferences and adherence. Understanding and respecting diverse cultural perspectives can improve healthcare delivery and outcomes.
- **Linguistic differences:** Language difficulties and minimal or no ability in speaking, reading, or understanding English/Hindi/Regional language are common among people who belong to racial and ethnic minorities. These obstacles can pose significant difficulties for both patients and providers in a health care context.
- **Sociodemographic characteristics:** There are several significant differences between rural and urban residents that are associated with their use of health care. Rural people have a low socioeconomic status and low income, there by limiting their access to treatment, hospitalization and rehabilitation.
- **Risk Factors:** Compared to urban populations, rural residents have a larger percentage of various risk factors for poorer health. For instance, self-reported obesity rates vary according to urbanization and rise as rurality increases. Women in the most rural counties had the greatest age-adjusted prevalence of obesity in 2010 - 2011, compared to persons living in center counties of large urban regions nationwide (Meit et al., 2014). But lack of awareness about this prevents the rural people from seeking treatment, hospitalization and rehabilitation.
- **Geographic practice patterns:** Across geographic areas, health care services, and through time, there is persistent geographic variance in spending and utilization.
- **Access:** A literature assessment on the availability and accessibility of health care in rural areas of the United States was done by Douthit et al. (2015). Their findings show to a reluctance to seek medical attention due to cultural and economic restrictions, which are frequently exacerbated by a lack of services, a shortage of qualified doctors, inadequate public transportation, and a lack of broadband Internet service availability. In comparison to metropolitan areas, residents of rural areas were shown to have worse health, and rural communities had more difficulties in accessing physicians.
- **Utilization:** Adults residing in nonmetropolitan areas generally exhibit higher rates of healthcare utilization compared to those living in metropolitan areas. This indicates that individuals in nonmetropolitan areas are more likely to seek medical care and utilize healthcare services at a greater frequency.

SHORT NOTES

1. Scope of sociology.

Answer

Sociology

Auguste Comte, the founding father of sociology, defines sociology as the science of social phenomena "subject to natural and invariable laws, the discovery of which is the object of investigation".

Scope of Sociology

Regarding the scope of sociology, there are many different perspectives. There are, however, two opposing viewpoints regarding the range of sociology.

- A group of authors led by the German sociologist George Simmel clearly identify sociology from other social science disciplines and limit it to the study of specific, predetermined characteristics of human relationships.
- The opposing party argues that there needs to be specialization and division of labor if any progress is to be made because the subject of social inquiry is too broad for any one science.

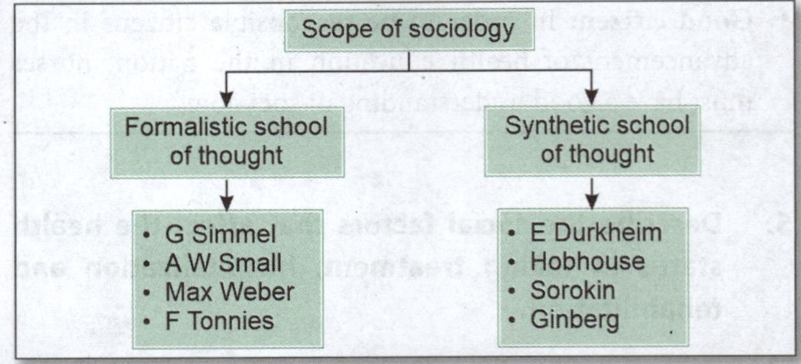

Formalistic school	Synthetic school
• Limited to social problems	• Study as a whole (Auguste Comte compares it with human body)
• Narrow or micro	• Broad or macro

Contd...

Formalistic school	Synthetic school
• Emanual Kant laid its basis	• General (Emile Durkheim says it is science of collective representation)
	• Durkheim asks to Borrow subjects like suicide (from psychology), DOL (from economics example: Varna system)
• Subjective understanding of objective reality Example: Most people are from Germany	• General (family, religion)and specific sociology(caste, race) by Pitrim Sorokin
	• Karl Manheim says to discuss the structure and broader ideas (example, PK movie)
• Interpretive school by Weber	• Hobhouse says that sociology is a synthesis of many social studies
• Forms of Interaction (Formal Vs Informal) by George Simmel (different behavior)	Alex Inkele's (social analysis, primary concept of social life, basic social institutions, social process)
• Alfred Vierkandt (sum total of social + psychic behavior = SOCIOLOGY) how to talk to someone	J.B Mckee's (social action, social structure, social institution, social process all should be included in scope)

2. Nature of sociology.

Answer

Nature of Sociology

- Sociology, in a wide sense, is the study of human relationships, including their causes and effects. It is a branch of science that uses methodical and objective investigative approaches.
- It leads to the development of social truth, which is founded on empirical data and interpretation.
- However, because human behavior is a peculiar phenomenon, it cannot be solely based on natural sciences.
- Additionally, it varies from scientific sciences in that human behavior shows fluctuations and flexibility, whereas the contents of natural sciences are stable.
- As a field of study, sociology has its own distinctive features. In certain ways, it differs from other sciences.
- One can better comprehend its primary traits by analyzing internal logical characteristics, which are as follows:
  - **Sociology is an independent science:** It is not viewed as a subset of any other science and is not studied as such. It has its own topic of research, limit, and methodology as an autonomous science.
  - **Sociology is a social science and not a physical science:** It concentrates on man, his social behavior, social activities, and social existence because it is a social science. History, political science, economics, and other social sciences are all tied to it.
  - **Sociology is a categorical and not a normative discipline:** Sociology does not assign any sort of value to anything. Its strategy is amoral rather than moral or immoral. It is morally impartial. It doesn't offer any recommendations regarding social policy, legislation, or programs. Problems of good and evil, right and wrong, moral and immoral behavior, cannot be addressed by sociology.
  - **Sociology is a pure science and not an applied science:** Pure science's primary goal is knowledge accumulation, regardless of whether the knowledge is practical or usable. On the other hand, applied science integrates learned information into daily living.
  - **Sociology is relatively abstract and not concrete science:** It has no interest in actual human events as they occur in the world. It is more interested in the structure and patterns of human occurrences. For instance, sociology is more interested in generic social processes as forms of social conflict than it is in wars and revolutions explicitly.
  - **Sociology is not based on particular subjects or individuals, but is a general science:** Sociology looks for overarching rules or principles governing human behavior, associations, and the makeup, composition, and organization of social groups. It takes a broad stance based on an analysis of a few chosen occurrences.
  - **Sociology is a rational and empirical science:** Empiricism and rationalism are two major approaches to scientific knowledge. Empiricism places a strong emphasis on observations and facts that come from experiment and observation. Rationalism places a strong emphasis on logic, reason, and theories that follow from it. Both have importance in sociological research.

SHORT ANSWER QUESTIONS

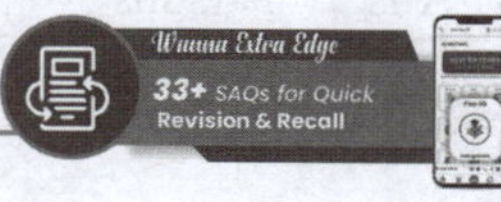

1. Define sociology.

Answer

The word 'sociology' has been derived from the Latin word ***societus***, meaning 'society', and the Greek word ***logos***, meaning 'study' or 'science'.

"Science of social phenomena, subject to natural and invariable laws, the discovery of which is the object of investigation" Comte identified three basic methods for discovering these invariant laws: Observation, experimentation, and comparison.

2. Who is the father of sociology?

Answer

Auguste Comte (1798–1857), a French philosopher, is considered the father of sociology. In 1839, Auguste Comte coined the term "sociology". Auguste Comte believed that a theoretical science of society and a systematic investigation of behavior were needed to improve society.

3. Write two differences between sociology and social anthropology.

Answer

Sociology	Social anthropology
Sociology is the study of society and its proceses, like social class, caste, social institutions	Anthropology is the study of humanity which focuses on cultural practices, human behavior and environment and its changes as time passes.
Area of focus is civilized society	Area of focus is primitive society

CONCEPTUAL REVISION

Wanna Practice & Revise
50+ MCQ's in review & Practice Mode,
For more, Access Plan UG in **Nursing next Live App**

MULTIPLE CHOICE QUESTIONS

1. In sociology, society refers to:
- a. Members of specific in-groups
- b. Patterns of the norms of interaction
- c. Congregation of people
- d. People with laws and customs

Ans. b. Patterns of the norms of interaction

2. Society is the total social heritage of folkways, mores and institutions, of habits, sentiments and ideals. This is a ________view of society:
- a. Structural
- b. Cultural
- c. Functional
- d. None of these

Ans. b. Cultural

3. Who among the following has given the functional view of society?
- a. Giddings
- b. Cooley
- c. Parsons
- d. Morris Ginsberg

Ans. c. Parsons

4. The relationship between fire and smoke is not a social one as the very relationship is not in any way determined by:
- a. Cooperation
- b. Mutual awareness
- c. Integration
- d. Stability

Ans. b. Mutual awareness

5. The increasing population is reduced by:
- a. By increasing agricultural production
- b. By giving higher education
- c. By reducing poverty
- d. All of the above

Ans. b. By giving higher education

6. Name the community which is larger in area where thousands of occupations are there, where population and complex relations are there:
- a. Urban community
- b. Rural community
- c. Tribal community
- d. None of these

Ans. a. Urban community

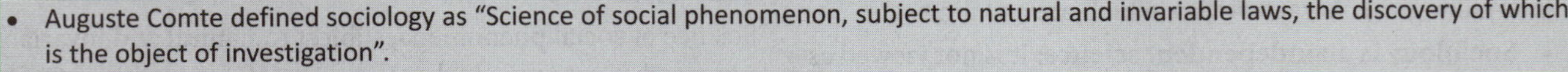

Golden Points

- Auguste Comte defined sociology as "Science of social phenomenon, subject to natural and invariable laws, the discovery of which is the object of investigation".
- Sociology is the science of society.
- The term Sociology was coined by a French philosopher, named Auguste Comte in 1839.

CHAPTER

2

Social Structure

CONCEPTUAL THEORY

Terminology

150+ key terminologies for Quick Recall & Revision

Accommodation: The term "accommodation" refers primarily to the process by which man achieves a sense of harmony with his environment."

Achieved status: Achieved status is obtained primarily by our own efforts and hard work.

Agrarian societies: Agrarian communities or societies originated around 5,000 years ago as the final stage of preindustrial development. An agrarian society's relative permanency and greater surpluses allow or permit individuals to produce artefacts such as statues, public monuments, and art pieces and pass them down from one generation to the next.

Ascribed status: An ascribed status is one that society bestows on a person without regard or consideration for the person's unique qualities or attributes. This assignment usually occurs at birth, therefore, a person's racial background, gender, and age are all considered ascribed statuses.

Assimilation: Assimilation is defined as "the process by which individuals or groups that were once distinct or diverse in nature become similar and identified in their interests and outlook."

Association: An association is a structured group. People band together to complete certain tasks or to achieve short- and long-term goals.

Community: A community is a social group that has a 'we feeling' and lives in a certain place.

Competition: "Competition is the striving of two or more persons for the same goal that is limited in such a way that all cannot share."

Conflict: "Conflict is a process of economic development, a revolutionary change brought about by class struggle between labors and capitalists."

Cooperation: Cooperation is defined as "the continuous and common effort of two or more people to perform a task or reach a common goal."

Gemeinschaft: The Gemeinschaft is a common feature of rural life. It is a tiny community with comparable backgrounds and life experiences. Almost everyone knows everyone else, and social interactions are intimate and familiar, almost as if they were among kinfolk (nearest and dearest).

Gesellschaft: The Gesellschaft is a model community that embodies modern urban life. Most inhabitants in this neighborhood are strangers who have little in common with the other residents. Relationships are governed by social roles that emerge from immediate or imminent tasks, such as purchasing a product or scheduling a business meeting.

Group: A group is any number of people who share similar standards, attitudes, and expectations and who engage or act together on a regular basis.

BASIC CONCEPT OF SOCIETY, COMMUNITY, ASSOCIATION AND INSTITUTION

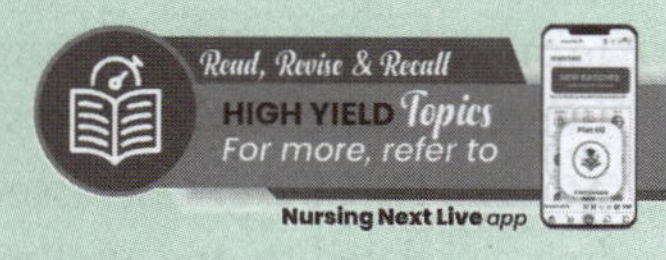

Definitions of Society

"As a collection of individuals united by certain relations or mode of behavior which mark them off from others who do not enter into these relations or who differ from them in behavior."

—**Morris Ginsberg**

"Society is the union itself, the organization, the sum of formal relations in which associating individuals are bound together."

—**Giddings**

"Society is complex of forms and processes each of which is living and growing by interaction with the others, the whole being so verified that what takes place in one form affects all the rest."

—**Cooley**

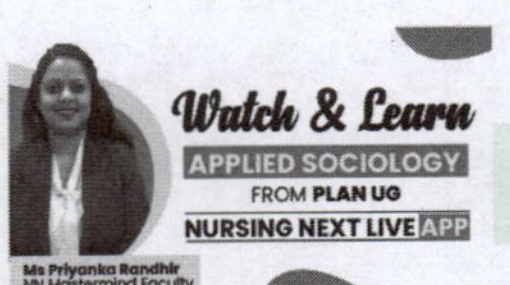

Characteristics of Society

- People
- Cooperation
- Mutual interaction and awareness
- Depends on likeness (in primitive society: mechanical solidarity) and differences (in modern society: Organic solidarity)
- Division of labor (Brought by Durkheim in Sociology) resulting in interdependence
- Dynamic
- Social control
- Culture
- Gregarious

Primitive versus Modern Society

Primitive society	Modern society
Societal conscience	Individual conscience
Mechanical solidarity (social interdependence based on commonly shared beliefs and strong group identity + simple division of labor)	Organic solidarity (social interdependence based on interdependence that appears among people from the specialization of work and complementarianism as result of more advanced (i.e., modern and industrial) societies.
Slow pace	Rapid pace
Limited scope	Global scope
Localized social activities	Activity extracted from social environment
Unity of time and space	Separation of time and space
Peripheral expert knowledge	Central expert knowledge
Threats from nature	Threats from reflexive modernity
Emphasis on fate	Emphasis on risk
External risk	Manufactured risks
Society is in individual	Individual is in the society
Similar to simple organisms/ machines (Individuals are functionally equivalent)	Same as complex organisms/ machines (organs not interchangeable)
Pre-industrial	Industrial

Definitions of Community

Community is "a social group with some degree of we-feeling and living in a given area." **—Bogardus**

Community is "the smallest territorial group that can embrace all aspects of social life." **—Kinsley Davis**

"A community is a group or collection of groups that inhabits a locality." **—Ogburn and Nimkoff**

Community is "any circle of people who live together and belong together in such a way that they do not share this or that particular interest only, but a whole set of interests". **— Manheim**

Characteristics of Community

- Defined locality
- Community sentiment
- Natural
- Stable
- Permanence
- Various goals
- Defined way of interaction (through culture, values, hierarchy, roles, expectation and behavior)
- Defined boundaries
- Sense of belongingness/identity
- Communication
- Provision of resources/skills
- Needs

Characteristics of Dysfunctional Community

Do not:

- Have goals
- Have shared beliefs, values or culture
- Have clearly defined boundaries
- Have ownership of their members
- Provide valued roles for their members
- Communicate effectively
- Have skills or resources they can depend upon
- Balance their own needs
- Share or draw on resources

Classification of Community

- Natural
- Man-made
- Cultural

Definitions of Association

- **RM MacIver:** An association is "an organization deliberately formed for the collective pursuit of some interest, or a set of interests, which its members share".
- **Morris Ginsberg:** An association is "a group of social beings related to one another by the fact that they possess or have instituted in common an organization with a view to securing a specific end or specific ends".

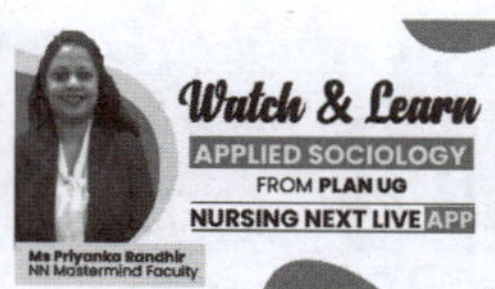

Characteristics of Association

- A human group
- Common interest or interests
- Cooperative spirit
- Organization
- Regulation of relations
- Association as agencies
- Durability of association

Definitions of Institutions

- **Moris Gins Berg:** Institutions may be described "as recognized and established usages governing the relations between individuals and groups".
- **HE Barnes:** Institutions represent "the social structure and the machinery through which human society organizes, directs and executes the multifarious activities required to satisfy human needs".

Characteristics of Institution

- Social in nature
- Universality
- Institutions are standardized norms
- Institution as means of satisfying needs
- Institutions are the controlling mechanisms
- Relatively permanent
- Abstract in nature
- Oral and written traditions
- Synthesis symbols
- Institutions are interrelated

Functions of Institutions

- Institutions cater to the satisfaction of needs
- Institutions control human behavior
- Institutions simplify actions for the individual
- Institutions assign roles and statuses to the individual
- Institutions contribute to unity and uniformity

Comparison of Society, Community, Association and Institution

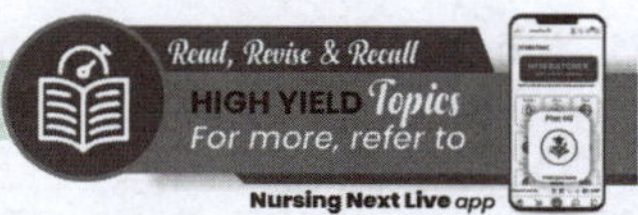

Society	Community	Association	Institution
Wider	Part of society	Part of society	Part of society
Membership voluntary	Involuntary membership	Membership voluntary	Membership voluntary
Heterogeneity	Homogeneity	Heterogeneity	Heterogeneity
Relationship not necessarily close	Face to face relationship	Relationship may or may not be close	Close relationship
Many goals	Less goals	Less goals	Less goals
Individual personality development in various ways	Individual personality development in narrow way	Individual personality development in narrow way	Individual personality development in narrow way
Natural/man-made	Natural/man-made	Man-made	Man-made
Norms may be written or unwritten	Unwritten norms	Written norms	Unwritten norms
Permanent, e.g., Indian society	Permanent, e.g., village	Temporary, e.g., industry	Temporary or permanent, e.g., family
Relationship not necessarily close	Face to face relationship	Relationship may or may not be close	Close relationship

INDIVIDUAL AND SOCIETY

The French sociologist Emile Durkheim is regarded as one of the founding fathers of sociology, along with Marx and Weber. Durkheim's analysis of how contemporary cultures may preserve social cohesion after the traditional ties of family and religion were supplanted by contemporary economic relationships was one of his principal objectives.

In the viewpoint of Durkheim, the interdependence of individual and society is summarized as:

- **Organic solidarity** is social cohesion that in more developed cultures is based on how dependent people are on one another.
- **Mechanical solidarity** is a phenomenon that frequently occurs in "traditional" and compact cultures. Solidarity is typically based on kinship relationships in smaller civilizations (like tribal ones).
- According to Durkheim, society has a significant impact on people. A collective consciousness, or a shared understanding

and manner of acting in the world, is made up, in Durkheim's view, of the norms, beliefs, and values of individuals.

- Individuals are connected to one another and become socially integrated through collective consciousness.
- As per Durkheim, the rise of modernity was significantly influenced by rising population density. A society becomes increasingly complicated as the population of a particular area grows together with the amount of interactions that take place there.
- The traditional ties of family, religion, and moral solidarity that had historically secured social integration start to wane as people do more commercial activity with nearby or distant traders. Durkheim was concerned that modernity could signal the breakdown of society.
- Mechanical solidarity, in which independent individuals are linked to one another by strong interpersonal relationships and traditions, is the foundation of simpler communities. Organic solidarity, or the dependence on one another for the division of labor, is the foundation of contemporary communities.
- Modern civilization may weaken the conventional mechanical solidarity ties, but it substitutes them with organic solidarity ties.
- Durkheim provided a hypothesis of the role of religion in indigenous and contemporary communities in The Elementary Forms of Religious Life, which also provided an explanation of the concepts of collective effervescence and collective awareness.
- Durkheim is referred to as a structural functionalist because his theories emphasize the role that particular institutions, such as religion, have in preserving social structure or cohesion.

PERSONAL DISORGANIZATION

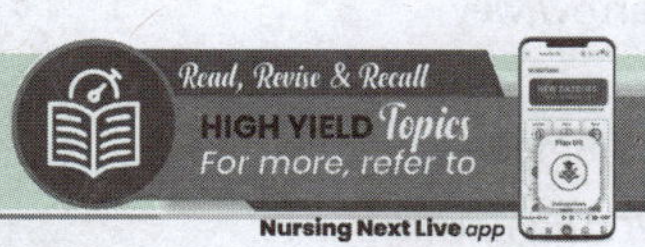

Definition: "The individual fails to meet the requirements of the society in which he lives, as a result, he develops personality problems and becomes disorganized."

Causes of Personal Disorganization

- Biological factors
- Environmental factors
- Status and role uncertainty
- Social crises
- Personality disorders

Implications of Personal Disorganization

The effects of personal disorganization on a person's personality can be seen in a number of ways. These are:

- Conflicting personality traits
- Personality traits related to family
- Insanity represents personal disorganization
- Mental illness or conflict
- Suicide is an extreme form

SOCIAL GROUP—MEANING, CHARACTERISTICS, AND CLASSIFICATION

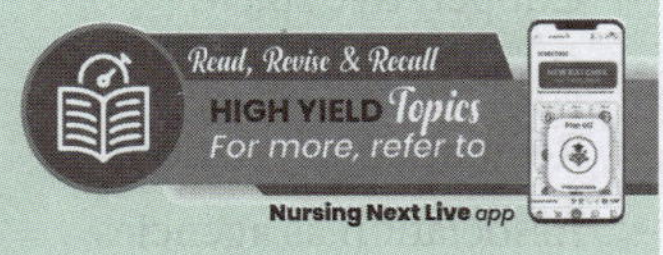

Definition: "Social group is a collection of two or more individuals who influence one another."

—Ogburn and Nimkoff

Or

"A social group may be thought of as a number of persons, two or more, who have some common objects of attention, who are stimulating to each other, who have common loyalty and participate in similar activities." **—Bogardus**

Meaning of Social Group

"A social group is a collection of human beings who are brought into social relationship with one another," according to **Maclver and Page**. A social relationship consists of some degree of reciprocity and mutual awareness among group members. Groups can form naturally or be organized to achieve certain goals and purposes.

As a result, a social group is made up of members who have reciprocal or mutual relationships. The members are united by a sense of belonging. Their interests are common, and their behavior is nearly identical. They are united by a shared awareness of interaction or relationships. A family, a village, a nation, a political party, the government, or a trade union are all examples of social groups.

Characteristics of Social Groups

- Mutual awareness
- Two or more persons
- Common interest
- Conscious interactions
- Reciprocal relations
- Collective behavior
- Feeling of unity
- Acceptance of common norms and values
- Definite structure

Classification of Social Group

- **By Charles Horton Cooley (1909-kind of contact)**
  - **Primary group:** A social group, large or small, that develops attitudes, values and orientations. Direct and personal relations.

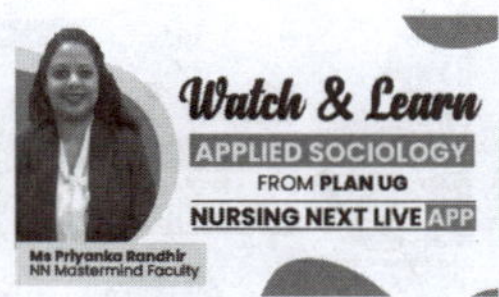

- **Secondary group:** A small close-knit group whose members interact because they value or enjoy one another as people. Indirect and formal.

DIFFERENCES BETWEEN PRIMARY AND SECONDARY GROUP

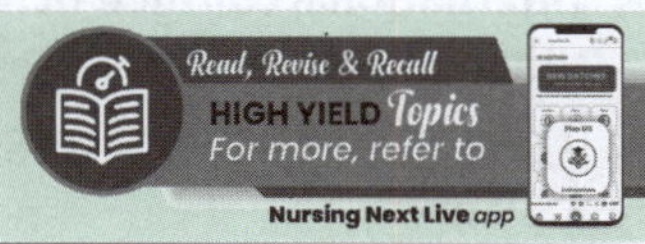

Primary group	Secondary group
Small in size	Large in size
Limited to a small area	Spread in large area
Durable	Temporary
Close, face to face relationship	Distant relationship
Spontaneous and natural relation	Artificial relationship
Relationship is not for any particular purpose	Relationship is to achieve definite purpose
Personal relationship	Impersonal, nominal relationship
The whole personality of the individual is involved in the relationship	Only limited aspects of the personality involved in the relationship
Play significant role in the process of socialization	Not very important in the socialization of an individual
Primary groups are as old as human society itself	Relatively new concern
Made of mostly blood relatives	Blood relatives are not involved

- **Simmel's classification of social group (as per size)**
  - Small size group
  - Large size group
  - Other classification:
    - **Dyad:** two persons in a group to form relationship
    - **Triad:** Three people unite to form three relationships
    - **Tetriad:** Four unite to form six relationships
    - **Pentad:** Includes five persons to form 10 relations

FH Giddings's classification of social groups—four types

1. **Genetic:** It is a group in which the man is born involuntarily. Example: Family.
2. **Congregate:** Is a voluntary group in which the individual moves or joins with his own will.
3. **Disjunctive:** Does not allow a person to be a member of another group at the same time. Example: College, nation.
4. **Overlapping:** Allows a person to be a member of another group at the same time. Example: INC, TNAI.

Miller's Classification of Social Groups

- **Horizontal:** They are large in size. For example, nation, political parties, international organization.
- **Vertical:** They are small in size. For example, family, peer groups, neighborhood, etc.

Sumner's Classification of Social Groups (Basis of Identification)

- **In-groups:** "There is a sense of solidarity, a feeling of brotherhood, loyalty, sacrifice, etc. Ethnocentrism is seen. Hostility and hatred for outsiders + sense of trust and respect
- **Out-groups:** Person feels a sense of competition or opposition

Sanderson's Classification of Social Groups (as per Structure)

- **Voluntary:** Based on one's own will or interest and is free to withdraw any time. For example, political party, trade union, religious association, youth organization, etc.
- **Involuntary:** Membership based on compulsion. For example, family, caste, race, community, state, etc.
- **Delegate:** People who elect or nominate their leaders. For example, legislative assembly or parliament.

Park and Burgess

- Territorial group
- Nonterritorial group

Other Classifications

Mob: An extremely emotional acting crowd that directs its violence against a specific target.

Public: It is a psychological group.

Audience: A group that sees, listens and thinks.

Rules and Regulations

- Formal
- Informal

Relation to Society

- Un-social
- Psuedo-social
- Pro-social
- Anti-social

Miscellaneous

- Clans
- Tribal group
- Crowd
- Reference group

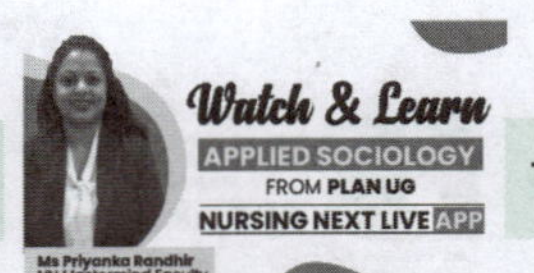

SOCIAL PROCESSES—DEFINITION AND FORMS, COOPERATION, COMPETITION, CONFLICT, ACCOMMODATION, ASSIMILATION, ISOLATION

Definition of Social Processes

"Social processes mean the various modes of interactions between individuals or groups." **—Ginsberg**

"Social processes are the manners in which the relations of the members of a group once brought together acquire a certain distinctive character." **—MacIver**

Forms of Social Processes

Social processes are:

1. Dissociative processes

Conflict

Introduction to conflict: It is an ever-present process in human relations. It is one of the forms of struggle between individuals or groups. When the interests of a person or a group are incompatible with those of the others and if they make an attempt to achieve their goals by applying sanctions and by using or by threatening to use violence, they can be considered to be in a situation of conflict.

Definitions of conflict:

AW Green: "Conflict is the deliberate attempt to oppose, resist or coerce the will of another".

Horton and Hunt: "Conflict may be defined as a process of seeking to monopolize rewards like eliminating or weakening the competitors".

Features of conflict:

- Conscious action
- Personal activity
- Lacks continuity
- Universal

Causes of conflict:

- Individual differences
- Cultural differences
- Clash of interests
- Social change
- Selfish and vested interest
- Limited resources

Types of conflicts:

- **Overt and latent:** (Openly)When hostile action is taken, the latent conflict becomes overt.
- **Corporate and personal conflict:** Between individuals or between society
- **Direct and indirect conflict:** If the people conflict directly (litigation, revolution or war) or create a situation
- **Caste and racial conflicts:** Between castes or between race, class conflict-Karl Marx (have and have-nots) and mutual hostility between strata
- **Group conflict:** Between two small groups based on differences in ideologies, interest or suppression. Political and religious conflicts
- **International conflict:** Between two nations on the basis of different political ideologies, economic, territorial.
- **Types of conflict by George Simmel**
  - War
  - Feud
  - Litigation
  - Impersonal idea

Isolation

Introduction to isolation: The absence of communicative interaction or social contact is isolation. It is a situation deprived of social contacts; both the individuals and the group can be isolated.

Types of isolation:

- Spatial
- Organic

2. Associative processes

Cooperation

Cooperation is one of the most basic, pervasive and continuous social processes. It is the very basis of social existence. Cooperation generally means working together for the pursuit of a common goal.

Definitions of Cooperation:

AW Green: "Cooperation is the continuous and common endeavor of two or more persons to perform a task or to reach a goal that is commonly cherished."

Fairchild: "Cooperation is the process by which the individuals or groups combine their effort, in a more or less organized way for the attainment of common objective".

Features of Cooperation:

- Universal
- Continuous process
- Has a motive of achieving goals
- Sharing of knowledge and skills
- Mutual
- Important for human survival
- Essential and urgent

Types of Cooperation:

By MacIver and Page

- Direct
- Indirect

By AW Green

- Primary
- Secondary
- Tertiary

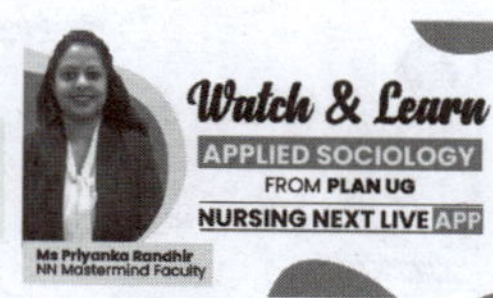

IMPORTANCE OF COOPERATION IN SOCIAL LIFE

- In times of various forms of natural calamities, such as floods, earthquakes, fires, and war, cooperation is required.
- Social existence is built on cooperation.
- Cooperation is required in the nature and socialization of individuals, particularly in the case of children.
- It is psychologically necessary to cooperate.
- Cooperation is necessary for growth.
- Division of labor and specialization are two examples of how cooperation is beneficial to the economy. Cooperation is crucial in all economic activities, including production, consumption, trade, and distribution.
- Cooperation from all parties is necessary for peace, harmony, and integration on a national or global scale.
- Numerous worldwide issues and conflicts have shown to be resolved through cooperation.

Competition

Introduction

Competition is a process, which occurs not only among human beings but also among all living beings. It is a struggle between two or more persons for a common end. Competition takes place whenever there is an insufficient supply of things that human beings commonly desire.

Definitions of competition:

Park and Burgess: "Competition is an interaction without social contact".

Sargent and Williamson: "Competition implies rivalry or struggle between two or more persons for the purpose of obtaining a nondivisible goal".

Accommodation

Introduction to accommodation: Accommodation is a form of social process. Professor JM Baldvin was the first to use the concept accommodation. Adjustments that people do continuously to pull on with other persons and situations can be called accommodation. It is a way of bringing social arrangement, which help people to work together.

Definitions of accommodation:

According to JM Baldvin: "Accommodation denotes acquired changes in the behavior of individuals which help them to adjust to their environment".

According to MacIver: "Accommodation is the process in which man attains a sense of harmony with his environment".

Features of accommodation:

- Conscious and unconscious
- Continuous
- Natural result of conflict
- Universal
- Consequences of it may vary with situation

Methods of Accommodation by Gillin and Gillin

- Yielding to coercion (by force)
- Compromise (equal in power)
- Role of 3rd party (arbitration, mediation, conciliation)
- Toleration (live and let live policy)
- Conversion (sudden rejection of one's belief)
- Sublimation (surrendering to love)
- Rationalization (explanation for one's behavior)

Assimilation

Introduction to assimilation: It is a type of social process like accommodation. Assimilation is also a form of social adjustment. Assimilation refers to the absorption of one culture by another person or assimilation requires more fundamental changes than accommodation. When individuals or different groups become similar and identify with the other groups, it is known as assimilation.

Definitions of assimilation:

According to Young and Mack: "Assimilation is a fusion of two distinct groups into one".

According to Ogburn and Nimkoff: "Assimilation is the process where by individuals or groups once dissimilar become similar, i.e., become identified in their interests and outlooks."

- **Features of assimilation:**
  - Unconscious
  - Two-way process
  - Slow and gradual process
  - Complex phenomenon
- **Factors favoring assimilation:**
  - Toleration
  - Intimate social relationship
  - Intercaste marriages
  - Cultural similarity
  - Education
  - Equal social and economic opportunity

Factors Hindering Assimilation

- **Isolation:** Groups are not in continuous contact
- **Racial differences:** Example: Negros and Whites
- **Cultural differences:** Striking cultural differences
- **Prejudice:** Dominant group has prejudice against a particular group

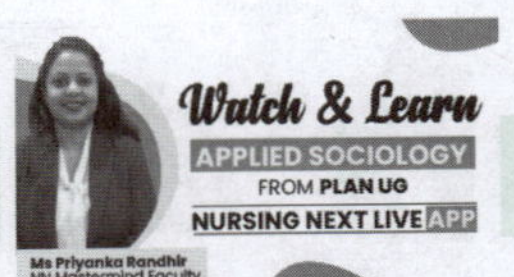

- **Dominants and subordination:** If the dominant group does not provide equal opportunities for the minority group

SOCIALIZATION—CHARACTERISTICS, PROCESS, AGENCIES OF SOCIALIZATION

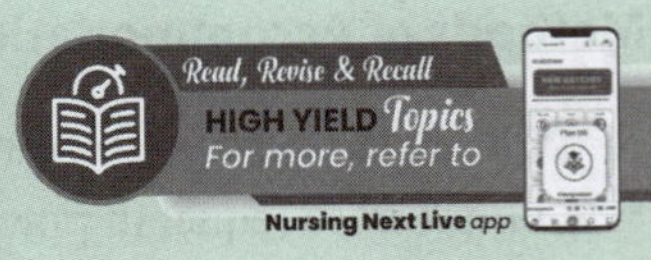

Definition of Socialization

- **Harry M Johnson:** "Socialization is a learning that enables the learner to perform social roles."
- **WF Ogburn:** "Socialization is the process by which the individual learns to conform to the norms of the group."
- **Bogardus:** "Socialization is the process of working together or developing group responsibility of being guided by the welfare needs of others."

Characteristics of Socialization

- **Inherited:** Physical and mental both.
- **Environment in which he lives:** Better then vironment, better is socialization: Good school, social equality.
- **Culture of group:** Cultural factor is responsible for his early or slow socialization process.

The Socialization Process

- **Imitation:** Copying the acts of others
- **Suggestion:** A child lacks the ability to think and reason and hence, he is highly susceptible.
- **Identification:** Child cannot make any distinction between himself and his environment. For instance, the legs with which he plays, the mother who feeds him, the brothers or sisters who play with him, are all identified.
- **Language:** In the beginning, the child utters meaningless sounds but gradually the skill of language is acquired. Thus, in the process of learning, language is important.

Forms of Socialization Process

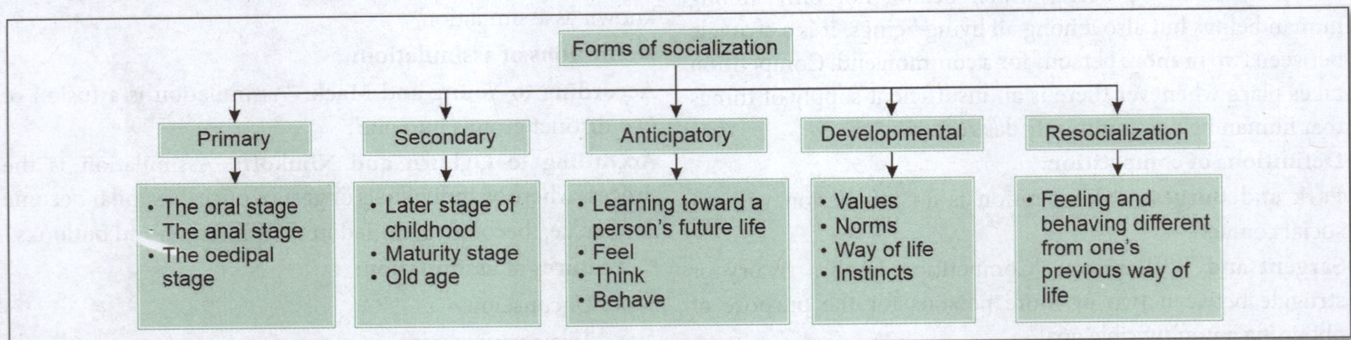

Six Agencies of Socialization

- Family
- School
- Peer group
- Mass media
- Workplace
- Religion

SOCIAL CHANGE—NATURE, PROCESS, AND ROLE OF NURSE

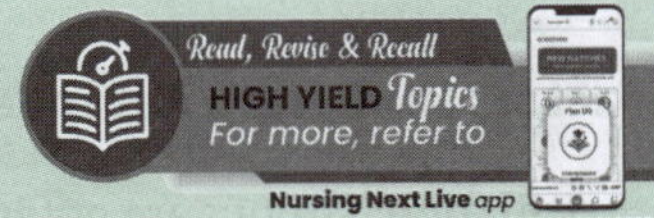

Definition of Social Change

- By "Social change is meant only such alterations as occur in social organization that is the structure and functions of society". —**Kingsley Davis**
- "Social change is change in the social relationships." – **MacIver**

Nature of Social Change

- Result of conscious or unconscious efforts
- Result of many factors
- Not necessary a progress
- Different in different societies
- Essential law
- Community change
- Change is not uniform
- Cannot be predicted
- Continous process
- Universal

Process of Social Change

- The process of social change is a complex process. Change must occur within the changing unit or thing as the manifestation of internal forces, rather than simply through the impact of external factors. The entire social system undergoes some alteration over time.

- All changes do not imply advancement.
- The concepts of "change," "evolution," "development," and "progress" are occasionally misunderstood or amalgamated into a single idea; in other circumstances, they are distinguished yet treated as logically related terms.
- Every culture makes every effort to connect its natural resources in its environment. A society's material and social prosperity is mostly determined by how well it uses its natural resources.
- The discrepancy between quickly growing technology and archaic aspects of beliefs and rigid social organization is a continual witness.
- People have changed their welfare practices, but not the sorts of political organizations that allow for recurring war.
- While technological advances are occurring at a rapid pace, the associated social system has failed to adapt.
- Technology has a variety of effects on society. It has an impact on social institutions and organizations. It alters the old social order. Technology has an impact on many elements of individual and society life.
- The Industrial Revolution brought about not only economic but also societal transformations.
- The way people lived, thought, and produced changed dramatically.
- Social change process works in the following ways:
  - Alteration in the experiences of people
  - Variation in the attitude of people
  - Diversification in thought process
  - Vagaries in social interactions
  - Deviations in social relations
  - Modifications in social structure
  - Social change

ROLE OF NURSE IN SOCIAL CHANGE

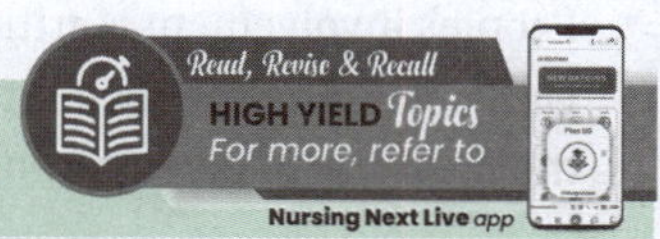

- The nurse can improve the health of a social person or a community member. The nurse can assess the health state of many domains such as schools, universities, and social institutions, among others.
- Nurses should practice good health habits.
- The nurse should have the ability to be a change agent in families, patients, and communities.
- A nurse's education can influence or improve social health. Nurses can help people in the community, handle social problems and accomplish their goals. As a result, the nurse is an important change agent.
- Nurses can establish a community research center where the community people will come and learn social development overseas. They can also learn how to prevent diseases and live a healthy lifestyle.

MAJOR HEALTH PROBLEMS IN URBAN, RURAL AND TRIBAL COMMUNITIES

Urban health problems: The health-related issues faced by people residing in urban areas are due to environmental, social and economic disturbances.

Major Health Issues in Urban Areas

- Communicable and noncommunicable diseases
- Environmental sanitation problem
- Problem of overpopulation
- Medical care problem
- Nutritional problem

Communicable and Noncommunicable Diseases

- Malaria or dengue
- Diarrhea and typhoid
- Hypertension
- Hepatitis
- HIV
- Problem of overpopulation
- Diabetes
- Nutritional problems
  - Protein-energy malnutrition
  - Nutritional Anemia
  - Low birth weight babies
  - Xerophathlmia
  - Iodine deficiency disease
- Other problems
- **Injuries/road traffic accidents**
  - Unplanned development, improper road and traffic infrastructure, mixed nature of vehicles and pedestrians, overuse and overloading of two-wheelers.
- **Occupational or residential injuries**
  - Living near construction site,/railways, unsafe poorly constructed housing, overcrowding, improper disposal of waste in children play areas.
- **Intentional/violence/crime**
  - For women, late working hours, improper lighting or inadequate support from police. Stress leading to alcoholism, drug abuse and domestic violence.
- **Uncertain livelihood**
  - Stability removes fear of uncertain livelihood leading to better participation in health care programs.
- **Psychological disorders**
  - Stress because of unemployment, competition, broken families, lack of support system, financial shortcomings, no place to live etc.
- Rural health or rural medicine is the interdisciplinary study of health and health care delivery in rural environments.

Urban versus Rural Health

- **Health indicators:** Almost all health indicators better than rural except in urban slums.
- **Health care facility:** Better in urban areas.
- **Levels of stress:** Less in rural area.
- **Social problems/health inequalities:** More in urban area.

Major Health Issues In Tribal Areas

- **Improper nutrition:** Deficiency of essential components in diet leads to malnutrition, protein calorie malnutrition and micronutrient deficiencies. Goiter of various grades is also endemic in some of the tribal areas.
- **Communicable diseases:** Water borne and communicable diseases: Gastrointestinal disorders are very common, leading to marked morbidity and malnutrition. Malaria and tuberculosis. Spectrum of viral and venereal diseases.
- **Genetic diorders:** High prevalence of genetic disorders mostly involving red blood cells: Genetically transmitted disorders like sickle cell anemia, G6PD deficiency and different forms of Thalassemia are also common.
- **Mental health issues:**
  - 20/1000 mental illness
  - 11/1000 depression
  - 3/1000 hysteria
  - 2/1000 phobia
  - 1/1000 schizophrenia
  - 0.4/1000 mania
- **Common diseases**
  - AIDS
  - Malnutrition
  - Malaria
  - Goiter
  - Sickle cell anemia
  - G6PD deficiency

IMPORTANCE OF SOCIAL STRUCTURE IN NURSING PROFESSION

- The phenomenon of social structure is abstract, speculative, hypothetical, and intangible.
- Social structure is important in society because it promotes order, command, and predictability.
- It refers to societal externalities. Individuals are members of organizations, associations, and groups.
- Social institutions, groups, statuses, roles, and norms all contribute to social structure.
- The permanent pattern of social ties that exists in a specific society or group is referred to as social structure. It offers the basis for our interactions with others.
- Social structure is significant in the nursing profession because it informs nurses about the general pattern of the group, such as the usual relationships between people and groups. This will assist nurses in assessing a person's behavior and attitude in regard to their social settings.
- Provision of information regarding social structure and its consequences, allowing health care personnel to use social structure knowledge to design more effective plans for specific actions. Evaluate intervention tactics and make necessary changes to the strategy.
- Knowledge of social structure is necessary in order to employ sociological principles and data to make people aware of parts of their social environment that they were previously unaware of.
- Individual/group members should be included in the planning process to increase the possibility that they will have an investment in the outcomes.
- Understanding of social structures in member selection. People's involvement is critical in community development.
- Understanding the social structure is necessary for making the most use of given resources.

CONCEPTUAL EXERCISES

LONG ANSWER QUESTIONS

1. "Community is a group within a society" Explain. (CCS)

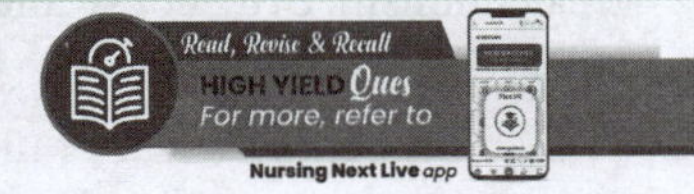

Answer

Community: A community "is a group or collection of groups that inhabits a locality." **—Ogburn and Nimkoff**

Community is a Group within a Society

- A community is a social group that resides in a certain location and has a strong sense of "we."
- A community is a social unit (a collection of living beings) that shares factors like geography, traditions, beliefs, values, or identity.
- Through communication platforms, communities may share a sense of place that is situated in a specific geographic location (for example, a country, hamlet, town, or neighborhood).
- Diverse contexts employ the idea of community.
- People frequently use the term "community" in a variety of contexts in informal conversation.
- A community is a focal point for group identification and a self-aware social entity.

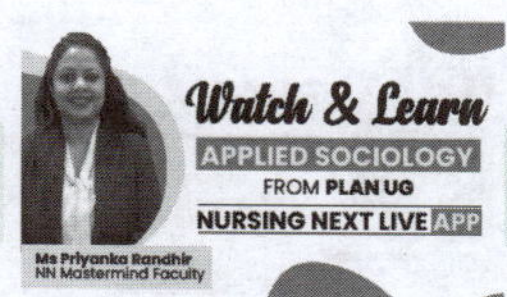

- A community serves as the local geographic and economic unit and offers its residents many of the essential goods and services.
- It is not always confined inside or defined by legal boundaries, such as those of a city or town, hence, it is not always a political entity.
- A collection of people with similar customs or interests, such as a community of academics or an ethnic group.
- The phrase in this sense is not associated with a specific physical region because the individuals who are considered to be a part of the community may be dispersed.
- A web of social ties makes up society. It encompasses every connection made between individuals. Direct, indirect, organized, unorganized, conscious, or unconscious social relationships are all possible. A community is made up of people.
- For society, a specific geographic location is not required. It is pervasive and universal; a community requires a specific geographic location.
- Community emotion, or a sense of "we feeling," is vital for a community but not necessary for a society. Without a feeling of community, there cannot be any community.
- A civilization can have multiple communities because society is larger than just one. smaller community than society. In a community, there can only be one society.
- Society is abstract. It is a web of social connections that cannot be seen or touched. Community is physical. It refers to a group of inhabitants of a specific location. This group is visible, and its location is known.
- Common goals and interests are essential in a community. In a community, residents work together to achieve shared goals and interests. There is no requirement for shared goals and interests in society.
- Similarity and diversity coexist throughout society. There are both common and distinct interests in society. But in a community, similarity is more significant than difference.

2. Write an essay on demographic characteristics of Indian society. (CCS)

Answer

Demography: The study of demographics, a population's social makeup, and statistics is known as demography. There are several uses of this research on the demographics, ages, and economics of various groups.

Demographic Characteristics of Indian Society

Sex composition: Number of females per thousand males comprises the sex composition/sex ratio. Finding the number of women in India and the gender ratio can be done with the help of the sex ratio. According to data from the 2011 Population Census, there are 940 girls for every 1000 males in India. From the census 2001 data, the Sex Ratio from 2011 shows an increased trend. According to the 2001 Census, there were 933 more girls than males, or 1000 total. India has had a decline in the sex ratio during the 1980s, but since the last two decades, there has been a minor uptick. The sex ratio has been shifting from 930 females to 1000 throughout the last five decades.

Age structure: A population's migration, birth rate, and mortality rate are all intimately correlated with its age structure. The percentage of children tends to be higher in areas with high birth rates, whereas the percentage of elderly people tends to be higher in areas with low birth and death rates. Approximately 25.69% of Indians were under the age of 14, 67.51% were between the ages of 15 and 64, and 6.8% were beyond the age of 65 in 2021.

Dependency ratio: It is the percentage of people who depend on those between the ages of 15 and 59 who are employed. Due to their lack of economic activity, persons over 60 and children between the ages of 0 and 14 are excluded.

Dependency ratio = (No. of persons in age group 0-14 years +No. of persons in age group 60 years or more) ÷ No. of persons in age group 15–59 years × 1000

- Dependency ratio comprises of two components:
- Older dependency ratio versus younger dependency ratio
  - The dependency ratio indicates the number of people that those in the economically active age group are responsible for supporting.
  - Reduced dependency ratios signify a stage of demographic transition where a bigger proportion of people are working age, which could result in increased per capita income for the country's economy.
  - This is sometimes referred to as the "Demographic Dividend Phase," during which a nation may profit. (Reference: 2011 Census of India)

Literacy ratio: India's social and economic development depends on literacy. According to the 2011 census, literacy increased by 97.2% between 2001 and 2011, which is less rapid than during the preceding ten years. According to an old analytical research from 1990, at the then-current rate of advancement, India wouldn't reach universal literacy until 2060.

Marital status: A person's marital status, which might include never married, married, widowed and not remarried, divorced and not remarried, married but legally separated, and de facto union, refers to civil status in respect to the country's marriage laws or customs.

Religion: India's religious landscape is characterized by a wide range of religious activities and beliefs.

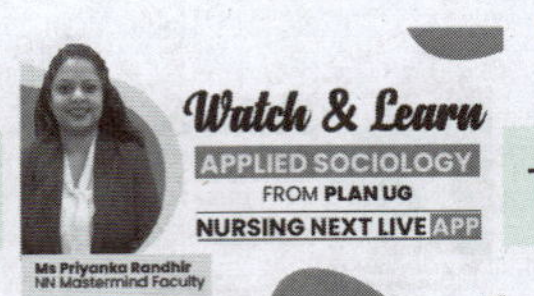

Hinduism, Buddhism, Jainism, and Sikhism are four of the world's major religions that originated in the Indian subcontinent. Religion has played a significant role in Indian culture. The right to freedom of religion has been proclaimed a fundamental right by the Indian Constitution, which also stipulates that India is a secular state.

In India, 79.8% of the population practices Hinduism, 14.2% follows Islam, 2.3% practices Christianity, 1.7% practices Sikhism, 0.7% practices Buddhism, and 0.4% practise Jainism, according to the 2011 census.

Income: India's financial situation is discussed in relation to income. India's income is increasing quickly along with the country's economic progress and prosperity. India's net national income, or NNI, per person was approximately 135 thousand rupees in 2020. [1] The gross measure of a nation's prosperity is its per-capita income. At constant prices, however, the gross national income was almost 128 trillion rupees.

Occupation: The country's occupational distribution of people, or occupational pattern, refers to the percentage of the working population that is employed in several significant economic sectors.

Family composition: In India, families and households have grown to be an important area of analysis due to the sheer number of people who live and work there, as well as the observed multilevel effects and variances among the country's multi-cultural and multi-ethnic population. Since 2001, the overall number of households has increased by 33%, from 25 crores to 33 crores, according to the 2011 Census. Out of these, roughly 22 crores were from rural areas and 11 crores were from metropolitan areas.

Race: The Negritos, Proto-Australoids, Mongoloids, and Mediterraneans make up the four racial groupings that currently make up the Indian subcontinent's population. The earliest racial group to arrive in India was the Negritos.

Language: There isn't a national language in India. However, Hindi and English are designated as "Official Languages", "for Official Purposes of the Union," according to Rule 1976 (As Amended, 1987) of the Indian Constitution. Both Hindi and English are used to conduct business in the Indian parliament. For official reasons, such as judicial proceedings, parliamentary sessions, and communications between the Central Government and a State Government, English is permitted.

Urban/rural population: With an estimate until 2022, this statistic shows India's population broken down by region for the year 2017. About 450 million people lived in rural areas of the nation in 2017, and that number was projected to rise to 506 million by 2022.

Growth rate of population: The current population of India in 2023 is 1,428,627,663, a 0.81% increase from 2022.

Birth rate: Birth rate is defined as the number of live births per thousand populations.

Death rate: Number of deaths per thousand populations. Also called mortality rate is called "death rate".

Infant mortality rate: IMR is the number of infants who have died below the age of one per thousand live births.

Maternal mortality rate: MMR is the number of women who die during child birth per thousand populations.

3. Describe meaning, characteristics of society, any four differences between community and society. (MGR)

Answer

Society: Talcott Parson says that society "may be regarded as the most general term referring to the whole complex of relations of man to his fellows".

Meaning of Society

- The word "society" refers to social ties; as social beings, men exhibit their nature by establishing and dismantling social structures that serve to direct and regulate their conduct in a variety of ways.
- Every human being must have society in order to live a full life. It both liberates and restricts men's activities.
- A person is born into a society, where he develops, matures, and ultimately passes away. Society can mean a variety of things in everyday language. For instance, the terms "high class," "poor class," and "middle class society" refer to distinct social classes.
- Societies are difficult to define. Society often relates to individuals and the local community.
- As man is a social animal, man is dependent on those around him to meet his basic requirements. Society is created by humans, who become more interdependent and connected through interaction.
- Thus, society can be characterized as a structured grouping of people who share common interests. Morris Ginsberg, a British sociologist, described society as "a group of people joined by particular interactions or modes of behavior that distinguish them from others who do not enter into these relations or who behave differently from them."
- R. M. MacIver, a renowned sociologist, defined society as "a network of social relationships."
- Society can be compared to a building, which, despite being made of bricks, nails, mortar, and pieces of wood, cannot be described just in terms of these components because it also has a form and has a purpose as a whole.
- A big social group that resides in the same physical or virtual territory, is referred to as a society or a

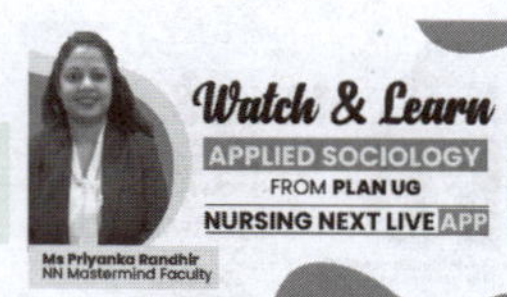

human society. This group of individuals is bound by the same political authority and prevailing cultural expectations.

Characteristics of Society

- **Interaction:** People engage with one another in society in order to meet their basic needs. Without humans, society is unimaginable. Man is a creature of social existence.
- **Group of groups:** There are many different groups and subgroups in society. This is why it is seen as a group of groups.
- **Likeness or dissimilarities:** In smaller societies, caste, family, and other social groups may have a role in the similarities. However, in contemporary society, similarities may only be based on a person's employment, interest, or hobby. The society needs diversity, and gender differences are the foundation of the family. People tend to live in groups and are unique in their appearance, personalities, skills, attitudes, tasks, intelligence, and religious beliefs, among other things.
- **Abstract:** The society is intangible and abstract. People make up society, and because people are aware of one another, there must be interactions and connections between them in order for society to function properly. Only by visualizing it can we comprehend its existence. According to Reuter, "Since society is not a thing but a process of association, just as life is not a thing but a process of living."
- **System of control:** The methods used by society to maintain social order are unique. All different social dynamics, including cooperation, accommodation, assimilation, competitiveness, and conflict, are present in society. Through both formal and informal methods of social control, the people's actions and behavior will be managed. For instance, laws, rules, regulations, legislation, and customs.
- **Complex:** Society is complex. Since society is a system of all human relationships, it is very complicated. Human behavior is extremely complicated and challenging to understand.
- **Non-human beings also have society:** There are well-functioning societies among animals, birds, and even insects. However, they follow their intuition. People are logical and driven by motivations. Sociology is the study of human society as a whole.
- **Cooperation and DOL:** Division of work is brought on by similarity and contrast. Cooperation is encouraged by the division of labor. In human society, the division of labor is determined by culture, whereas in other cultures, it is based on biological characteristics. The division of labor and cooperation are the foundations of society.
- **Culture:** A social inheritance includes culture. Culture, which is a monopoly of human society, is the one factor that distinguishes it from other societies. Culture and society are two sides of the same coin. They cannot be split apart.
- **Dynamic:** An ever-evolving aspect of human life is society. Change in social structure and functions of the society is one of the important characteristics of society. Man is very innovative, and change occurs organically.

Differences between Community and Society

Society	Community
Society is a large group.	As compared with society, community is limited group.
Web of relationship.	Consists of group of individuals.
Society composed of community.	Community exists in a society.
Society is a system of social relationships. It is abstract.	It is formed by group of human beings. It is concrete.

4. Describe the types of communities in India. Explain the features of the village community. (KUHS)

Answer

Community: MacIver defines community as "an area of social living, marked by some degree of social coherence.

Types of Community

Rural community: "The rural community comprises of the constellation of institutions and persons grouped about a small center and sharing common primary interest".

—Elridge and Merrill

Urban community: Town and cities: "City is a state of mind, a body of customs and traditions and the organized attitudes and sentiments that are inherent in these customs."

—Robert park

Tribal community: Tribal areas: **DN Majumdar** defines **tribe** as "a social group with territorial affiliation, endogamous with no specialization of functions ruled by **tribal** officers hereditary or otherwise, united in language or dialect recognizing social distance with other **tribes** or castes."

Features of the Village Community

Agricultural occupation: Agriculture, together with related industries including poultry, animal husbandry, and microbusinesses like apiculture and fishing, constitutes the principal occupation of the rural community.

Natural environment: Villages are built naturally. The village is home to a variety of animals, birds, rivers, ponds, and other natural features. There is a proverb that states that God or nature created the village. Rural residents can live a simple, natural existence because of the surrounding natural environment.

Small in size: The size of the local settlements is small. It could be a few households or a small population. In fact, there are hundreds of thousands of households in Indian villages.

Low density of population: The amount of people living in a given area per square mile or kilometre is referred to as population density. The communities have a lot of space available for farming, thus there aren't many people living there.

Homogeneity: There is a lot of uniformity in village life. A village's residents share a common occupation and way of life.

Low mobility: Mobility refers to the movement or transfer of individuals from one location to another or from one social rank to another; thus, both social and physical mobility exist. In villages, particularly in Indian communities, both are scarce. Village settlements are isolated as a result of the restricted transportation and communication options available there.

Less social differentiation and stratification: This holds true everywhere. But there is a lot of differentiation because of the caste-based stratification in our Indian villages.

Primary group relations: Rural communities, especially the smaller ones, have strong group relationships. The village resembles a big family. The people in the rural hamlet are friendly and directly acquainted with one another.

Large family: Families in the village are big. There are also combined or extended families in some circumstances. Agriculture requires greater manual labor. Hence, a sufficient number of kids are required.

Less education: Advanced education and specialty are not required because agriculture is the main occupation of the inhabitants. So, schooling is less prevalent in villages. In Indian villages, specifically, the literacy rate is low.

Less political consciousness: In villages, political awareness and involvement are lower. Politics is not something that the populace is involved in or interested in since they are too busy living their daily lives.

Less number of social problems: In villages, there are less social issues like crime, juvenile delinquency, prostitution, and murder. Nonetheless, it must be acknowledged that issues like illiteracy, ignorance, superstition, bad health, poverty, unemployment and underemployment, as well as disputes based on the caste system, are present in our Indian communities.

Stable public opinion: Due to the rigidity of customs, traditions, and values in villages, the public opinion is difficult to change. But new ideas and philosophies, along with communication, transportation, and education, are also altering public opinion in our villages.

Child marriages: In Indian villages, child marriage is still very common. Their inability to obtain education and the influence of traditions and values encourage child marriages.

Low status of women: Women are not thought to be capable of making decisions regarding their families. In various fields of employment, men consult with other male employees. Women have a lower than average rate of education and literacy.

Caste: In Indian communities, caste membership, caste-related social barriers, impairments, and even untouchability still exist.

Local self-government: Panchayat system is the form of local self-government.

5. Explain various implications of personal disorganization and ways to prevent it. (DU)

Answer

Personal disorganization: According to Allport (1961), "Personality is a dynamic organization, inside the person, of psychophysical systems that create the person's characteristic patterns of thoughts, feelings and behaviors."

Implications of Personal Disorganization

The effects of personal disorganization on a person's personality can be seen in a number of ways. These are:

- **Conflicting personality traits:** The result of personal disorganization that emerges at the first conception of the person that the family unit gives to him. Here, the person establishes personality and rises to popularity. He is no longer a biological being whose main interests are in meeting physiological needs; instead, he is a person whose actions generate acceptance or disapproval. He has gradually developed the ability to regard himself as a counterbalance to the regard that others have for him.
- **Personality traits related to family:** The child's birthplace has a big impact on deciding its place in the family. Being the only child at first and then having his position as the center of attention invaded by another is a unique experience for the first-born child. While initially he has a tendency to resist against this takeover, this distraction is quickly made up for by the responsibilities he is allowed to take on and the occasionally granted authority over his younger siblings.
- **Insanity represents personal disorganization:** Insanity is defined as cases in which the nervous system has been partially destroyed or impaired, as well as cases in which the disorder is functional. In general, functional insanity represents the peak of personal disorganization, but there are exceptions, particularly hereditary forms.

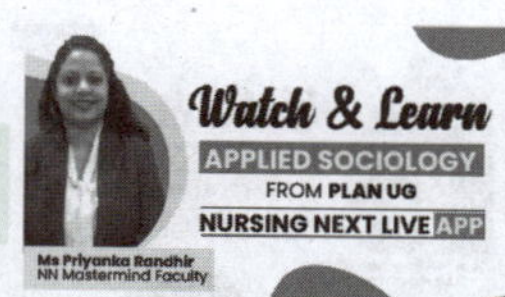

Alcoholism, and its related psychoses, for example, exhibit structural deterioration as a result of the use of alcohol as an escape mechanism. Drug addiction and the psychoses that result from excessive drug use are classified as the same thing.

- **Mental illness or conflict:** Mental illness is caused by biological and environmental factors. According to Queen and Mann, the majority of mental disorganization is caused by an inability to adjust to the stresses of modern life. The struggle for material possessions, job frustration, aggression threatened by competitors, migration involving significant cultural adjustment, the pervasive attempt to rise on the social scale, unhappy family relations, all of these factors combine to make modern life more difficult.
- **Suicide is an extreme form:** Suicide, according to Durkheim, is the term applied to all cases of death resulting directly or indirectly from a positive or negative act of the victim himself that he is aware will result in this result. If personal disorganization leads to insanity, the individual feels compelled to commit suicide.

Ways to Prevent Personal Disorganization

Personal disorganization can be prevented through:

- **Education and awareness:** Promoting education and awareness about personal organization skills and strategies can help individuals develop effective organizational habits. Providing resources, workshops, and training programs that teach time management, goal setting, and organization techniques can empower individuals to stay organized.
- **Community support and collaboration:** Providing resources, workshops, and training programs that teach time management, goal setting, and organization techniques can empower individuals to stay organized.
- **Public policies and infrastructure:** This can include measures such as efficient public transportation systems, accessible information management systems, and streamlined bureaucratic processes that minimize administrative burden.
- **Workplace organization and management:** Employers can promote effective organizational practices through clear communication, providing necessary resources and tools, establishing efficient workflows, and offering training on time management and prioritization.
- **Social and cultural norms:** Encouraging punctuality, emphasizing the importance of keeping commitments, and valuing proactive planning can foster a societal environment that prioritizes organization.
- **Mental health support:** Providing accessible mental health services, reducing stigma around seeking help, and promoting overall well-being can support individuals in maintaining mental clarity and organization.

6. What is the role of community in public health?

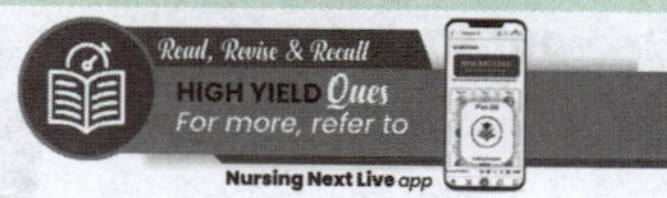

Answer

Role of Community in Public Health

The term "community" can refer to individuals, groups, organizations, associations, or informal networks that share common characteristics and interests based on location, issue, or identity.

Community engagement usually involves dynamic relationships and dialogue between community members and local health department staff, with varying degrees of involvement, decision-making, and control on the part of the community and the health department.

Community engagement in public health refers to efforts that promote the mutual exchange of information, ideas, and resources between community members and the health department.

Through this process, the health department shares its health expertise, services, and other resources with the community, but the community can also share its own wisdom and experiences to help guide public health program efforts. In addition to this, the role of community in public health includes:

- A community participation approach is a cost-effective way of extending a health care system to a country's geographical and social periphery, though it is far from free.
- Communities that begin to objectively understand their health status rather than fatalistically may be moved to take a series of preventive measures.
- Communities that invest in health-promoting activities with labor, time, money, and materials are more committed to using and maintaining the things they produce, such as water supplies.
- Health education is most effective when it is integrated into village activities.
- People trust community health workers if they are carefully selected. They may know the most effective techniques for achieving commitment from their neighbors and at the very least, are not likely to exploit them. They face intense social pressure to assist the community in carrying out its health-promoting activities. They must, however, have dependable supplies and support from higher levels of the health service.

These communities frequently share similar concerns, which can be shared with the health department to assist in the development of more relevant and effective health programs.

7. What is the role of social structure of hospital in our society?

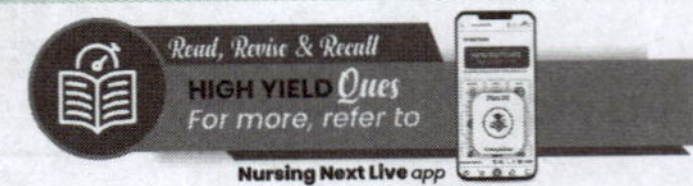

Answer

- Hospitals are complex social organizations that play a vital role in our society. The social structure of a hospital is essential for ensuring that these important functions are carried out effectively.
- Hospital word has been derived from the Latin word 'HOSPES' meaning 'a host or guest' or 'hotel', hostel.
- Some also believe that the origin of the hospital is from the word 'HOSPITUM' a rest house for travelers or night shelter showing 'hospitality' to the guests.
- The social structure of a hospital is defined by the interactions between the different groups of people who work there. These groups include doctors, nurses, other healthcare professionals, patients, and their families. The social structure of a hospital also includes the formal and informal rules and norms that govern these interactions.
- According to World Health Organization: "The 'hospital is an integral part of a social and medical organization, the function of which is to provide the population complete health care, both curative and preventive, and whose out-patient services reach out to the family in its home environment; the hospital is also a center for the training of health workers and for bio-social research."
  - As a social institution, the hospital delivers patient care through a multi-functional team made up of individuals with various levels of expertise.
  - A hospital is a structure that is designed, staffed, and equipped to diagnose diseases, treat the sick and injured with medical and surgical procedures, and provide shelter for patients while these procedures are being carried out. The contemporary hospital frequently functions as a place for research and teaching.
- The hospital organization is unique and distinct from other organizations. As a result, it is known as a 'MATRIX' organization.
- A hospital, as a 'MATRIX' organization, is a combination of product and function in which people with similar skills are grouped together to carry out activities to achieve organizational goals.
- Some parts of a hospital's organization have scalar functions, while others are more loosely structured.
- As a social organization, the hospital provides patient care through a multifunctional team of people with varying levels of knowledge and skill.
- A hospital is an institution that is built, staffed, and equipped for disease diagnosis, medical and surgical treatment of the sick and injured, and housing during this process. The modern hospital is also frequently used as a research and teaching facility.
- Here are some specific examples of the role of the social structure of a hospital in our society:
  - **The division of labor:** The social structure of a hospital is characterized by a division of labor. This means that different groups of people have different roles and responsibilities. For example, doctors are responsible for diagnosing and treating patients, nurses are responsible for providing care to patients, and administrative staff is responsible for managing the hospital.
  - **The hierarchy of authority:** The social structure of a hospital also includes a hierarchy of authority. This means that there is a clear chain of command, with some people having more power than others. For example, doctors have more authority than nurses, and nurses have more authority than administrative staff.
  - **The norms and values:** The social structure of a hospital is also characterized by norms and values. These are the unwritten rules that govern the behavior of people in the hospital. For example, there are norms about how to interact with patients and their families, and there are values about the importance of providing quality care.

SHORT NOTES

1. Characteristics of society.

Answer

For answer, refer to Long Question no. 3, pg. no. 1022

2. Interdependence of individual and society.

Answer

The French sociologist Emile Durkheim is regarded as one of the founding fathers of sociology, along with Marx and Weber. Durkheim's analysis of how contemporary cultures may preserve social cohesion after the traditional ties of family and religion were supplanted by contemporary economic relationships was one of his principal objectives.

In the viewpoint of Durkheim, the interdependence of individual and society is summarized as:

- **Organic solidarity** is social cohesion that in more developed cultures is based on how dependent people are on one another.

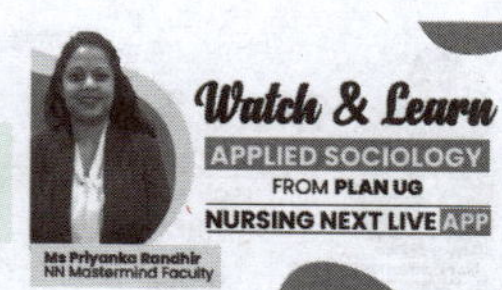

- **Mechanical solidarity** is a phenomenon that frequently occurs in "traditional" and compact cultures. Solidarity is typically based on kinship relationships in smaller civilizations (like tribal ones).
- According to Durkheim, society has a significant impact on people. A collective consciousness, or a shared understanding and manner of acting in the world, is made up, in Durkheim's view, of the norms, beliefs, and values of individuals.
- Individuals are connected to one another and become socially integrated through collective consciousness.
- As per Durkheim, the rise of modernity was significantly influenced by rising population density. A society becomes increasingly complicated as the population of a particular area grows together with the amount of interactions that take place there.
- The traditional ties of family, religion, and moral solidarity that had historically secured social integration start to wane as people do more commercial activity with nearby or distant traders. Durkheim was concerned that modernity could signal the breakdown of society.
- Mechanical solidarity, in which independent individuals are linked to one another by strong interpersonal relationships and traditions, is the foundation of simpler communities. Organic solidarity, or the dependence on one another for the division of labor, is the foundation of contemporary communities.
- Modern civilization may weaken the conventional mechanical solidarity ties, but it substitutes them with organic solidarity ties.
- Durkheim provided a hypothesis of the role of religion in indigenous and contemporary communities in The Elementary Forms of Religious Life, which also provided an explanation of the concepts of collective effervescence and collective awareness.
- Durkheim is referred to be a structural functionalist because his theories emphasize the role that particular institutions, such as religion, have in preserving social structure or cohesion.

3. Theories of society. (MGR)

Answer

Society: "Society is the complex of organized associations and institutions within a community." —**GDH Cole**

The theories of society are:

- Functionalist theory
- Conflict theory
- Interactionist theory
- Critical theories
- Feminist theories
- Figurational theory
- Social contract theory
- Organismic theory

4. Differentiate between community and society. (CCS, DU)

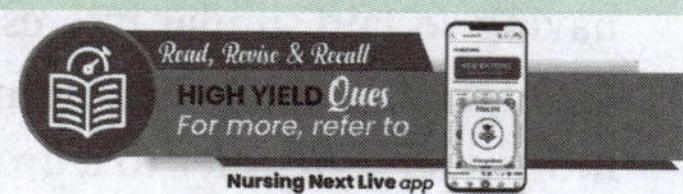

Answer

Differences between Community and Society

Society	Community
Society is a web of social relationships	Community consists of a group of individuals living in a particular area with some degree of "we-feeling"
A definite geographic area is not an essential aspect	It always denotes a definite locality/ geographical area
Society is abstract	Community is concrete
"We-feeling" may or may not be present	"Community sentiment" is an essential element
Society is wider. There can be more than one community in society	Community is smaller than society
The objectives and interest of society are more extensive and varied	Objectives and interests are comparatively less extensive and varied
Society involves both likeness and difference	Likeness is important than difference in community

5. Elements of community. (MGR)

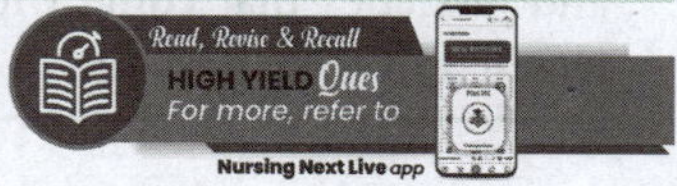

Answer

Community: Community is "the smallest territorial group that can embrace all aspects of social life." —**Kinsley Davis**

Elements of Community

- **Defined locality:** A territorial group is a community. It always takes up some physical space.
- The physical foundation of the community is locality. Living together makes it easier for people to form social bonds and provides security, safety, and protection. It aids the members in advancing and pursuing their shared interests. The locale includes physical elements including rich soil, minerals, forests, water resources, vegetation, weather, and climate. These elements have a variety of effects on how community people conduct their lives.

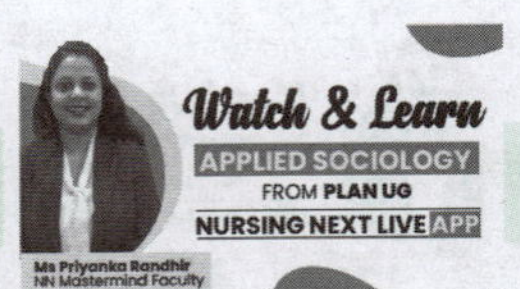

- **Community sentiment:** A community cannot be formed by a group of people alone. Sometimes people who live close to each other may not interact or communicate. A community is essentially a place where people all feel like they belong. Community spirit is defined as "a sense of unity." A sense of "we feeling" emerges from the members sticking together and sharing. It implies a certain level of group identification. There cannot be a community without a feeling of identification, awareness, living, and having certain similar interests.
- **Groups of people:** Community is an example of a group of individuals. We refer to a group of people as a community when they coexist in such a way that they share the necessities of daily living.
- **We feeling:** Wherever there are shared interests among men, "we feeling" is present. When our village, town, city, region, and especially our nation is attacked or threatened, it is rising within us, and we are frequently willing to sacrifice our personal interests.
- **Role feeling:** Each individual believes that he has a role to perform and personal responsibilities to complete in the mutual interactions of the social scene. This attitude, in which the individual feels subordinate to the total, is fostered by training and habituation in the everyday discipline of life.
- **Feeling of Dependency:** The individual's sense of dependence on the community as an essential condition of his own life is "closely related with role emotion." Due to the fact that it satisfies his material needs, this involves both a physical and psychological dependence. Since the community serves as his larger "home," it represents everything familiar, if not everything innate to his existence. The group serves as a haven from the loneliness and anxieties that come with individual isolation, which characterizes modern life.

6. Nature of society. (MGR, CCS)

Answer

Talcott Parson says that society "may be regarded as the most general term referring to the whole complex of relations of man to his fellows".

Nature of Society

The nature of society is as follows:

- **Abstract:** Human behavior and the resulting relationship and adjustment issues can be seen as society. The complex interrelations that exist between and among the group's members are implied by the term "society," according to Renter. In this sense, society can be found anywhere there are healthy or unhealthy, appropriate or inappropriate relationships between people. As these social ties are not obvious and without any tangible foundation, society is impersonal.
- **Not just a group of people:** Some sociologists have thought of society as a collection of individuals. Although society is a real thing, according to Wright, it is inherently an abstraction because it refers to a state, condition, or relationship.
- **Organization of relationships:** The totality of human relationships makes up society. It covers the full spectrum of human interactions.
- **Physical component in social interaction:** According to MacIver and Giddings and some other sociologists, social interactions always have a psychical component, such as knowledge of another person's existence, a shared goal or interest, etc.
- **Role feeling:** Each individual believes that he has a role to perform and personal responsibilities to complete in the mutual interactions of the social scene. This attitude, in which the individual feels subordinate to the total, is fostered by training and habituation in the everyday discipline of life.
- The definition of sociology continues to be up for debate. Some sociologists assert that it is a science, whereas others vehemently dispute this.

7. Concept of society. (DU)

Answer

Society

"As a collection of individuals united by certain relations or mode of behavior which mark them off from others who do not enter into these relations or who differ from them in behavior." —**Morris Ginsberg**

Concept of Society

- A concept is a broad description of all that surrounds us, including both physical and abstract experiences, such as things, people, events, etc.
- There is a type of phenomenon that all conceptions or thoughts reflect.
- The word "society," which implies "companionship or friendship," is derived from the Latin word "societus."
- Man is an expressive and social creature.
- To enjoy social or group life, humans need society.

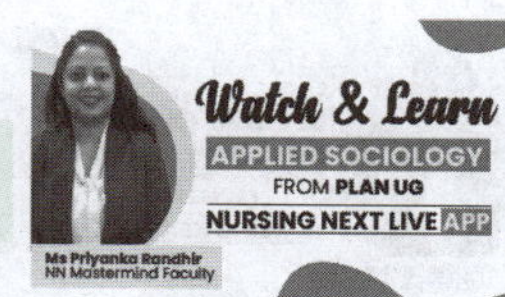

- One of the broadest definitions of "society" found in sociological literature.
- In actuality, the idea of society has become central to the entire discipline of sociology.
- The network of connections and the pattern of interactional rules that develop among society's members are crucial components of society.
- Thus, there are several intimate links or exchanges between people in society. Both are closely interlinked, interwoven, ordered, consistent, and interdependent.
- The word "society" refers to social ties; as social beings, men exhibit their nature by establishing and reconstructing social structures that serve to direct and regulate their conduct in a variety of ways.
- Every human being must have society in order to live a full life. It both liberates and restricts men's activities.
- A person is born into a society, where he develops, matures, and ultimately passes away.
- Society can mean a variety of things in everyday language. For instance, the terms "high class," "poor class," and "middle class society" refer to distinct social classes.
- Public distribution is the hallmark of a cooperative society. Yet, the term "global society" has a specific meaning in sociology.
- In actuality, the idea of "society" has grown to encompass the entire discipline of sociology.
- Nonetheless, the term "society" is employed in sociology to imply a certain connotation.

8. Write any two theories of society. (MGR)

Answer

Theory of Social Contract

The social contract idea sheds light on how society first came into being. This notion holds that everyone is born free and equal. Because of the agreements made by the individuals, society was born. Thomas Hobbes, John Locke, and Jean-Jacques Rousseau are considered the founding members of this school of thinking.

Organismic Theory of Society

This perspective, which is at least as old as the notion of a contract, sees society as a larger, more complex organism with similar structure and functions to a biological system. Even Plato and Aristotle may be traced back to this viewpoint.

9. Distinguish between social work and community work. (DU, MGR)

Answer

Social work	Community work
Not being forced onto people	Implementing the welfare program is required.
The consumer asks the social worker for assistance.	The social health worker approaches the client
Help is provided only if there is a dire need of the client	Drives change and looks for partnerships to do so
Concentrate on all categories of people	Focus on underprivileged group

10. Various causes of personal disorganization. (CCS)

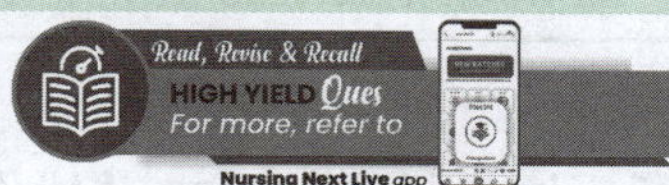

Answer

Personal Disorganization

Crime, prostitution, insanity, juvenile delinquency, alcoholism, drug addiction, gambling, and suicide are examples of personal or individual disorganization. These instances of personal disorganization show that some people struggle to coexist peacefully with society. Their inability to adapt to the shifting circumstances or ups and downs of society frequently leads to their personal disarray.

Causes of Personal Disorganization

When someone is angry, his normal daily activities may become disorganized. Elliott and Merrill identified four categories of elements or circumstances that frequently interfere with a person's way of life, and they are as follows:

- **Biological factors:** These are challenges brought on by functional disorders, such as physical ailments, injuries, mental impairments, or individual weaknesses that may necessitate restructuring in a person's life. The disabled person becomes maladjusted and unable to overcome his obvious disadvantages because of his biological makeup.
- **Environmental factors:** These include things like financial hardship, uncertainty, contradiction, and conflict in interpersonal relationships in the family, in the workplace, in religious settings, or in leisure activities that may cause a person's life to become disorganised.
- **Status and role uncertainty:** When a child or adult may look to society for security, it is important to remember that a child's sense of security is based on the fact that he is his parents' child and truly belongs to them. Disorganization is exacerbated when this sense is challenged, the person feels unappreciated and unaccepted by his family, friends, playmates, coworkers, and other associates, and when this feeling is shared by those around him. It is well

acknowledged that every person has a psychological desire to believe that he/she is an integral part of the cosmos.

- **Social crises:** These are sudden shocks that disrupt a person's daily routine, such as the death of a close relative, a job loss, a property loss, the death of a breadwinner, etc.
- **Personality disorders:** Some people have strong complexes that emerge early on and prevent them from integrating well into society. For instance, a man may be a compulsive homosexual, miser, or cheat as a result of some early events. Once more, some people have congenital defects that prevent them from making a suitable transition. Those who are extremely short or excessively tall have significant trouble in this area. Similar to men, some physical defects in women can lead them to become prostitutes.

11. Individualization. (KUHS)

Answer

Introduction

The term "individualization" was created to describe the process in which people are forced to make more complex decisions about their daily lives and to take greater personal responsibility for the results of those decisions as a result of the escalating pace of social change and growing uncertainty.

- The sociological viewpoints of Ulrich Beck and Anthony Giddens from the late modern period are most closely related to this idea.
- Comparing it to postmodern thought's notion of "individual freedom" makes it the most simple to comprehend.
- According to postmodernism, the destruction of conventional social norms and ways of life has increased people's freedom of choice. This is especially true since the 1980s, when people have had much more freedom to choose their careers, families (including whether or not they get married), religious beliefs, and even their sexual orientation.
- A postmodern society is one in which individuals have more flexibility to create their own unique identities.
- Beck and Giddens claim that postmodernists have oversold how free people are, that there is more going on.
- The transition to postmodernity has also increased social instability and uncertainty; careers last for a shorter time, relationships are more likely to end, the welfare state offers less security for us if we experience financial difficulty, and even experts (scientists/doctors) seem less able to provide us with clear-cut recommendations on how we should live.
- Hence, we are not so much given the freedom to live our lives as we like by postmodern culture as we are compelled to make hundreds or even thousands of decisions in order to survive. This is known as "individualization," which is not the same as being free.
- Individualization is 'compulsory' rather than being about genuine personal freedom, and is an integral part of self-hood in the neoliberal (dis) order.
- According to Ulrich Beck and Elisabeth Beck-Gernsheim (2001/2002), people are now forced to make antagonistic decisions throughout their lives because there may be no direction and they must bear full responsibility for the results of those decisions, whether they are made or not.
- The phenomenon of individualization is paradoxical, thrilling, and terrifying. In particular for women emancipated from patriarchal authority, it truly feels like freedom. But when anything goes wrong, nobody has an excuse. In a highly competitive and constantly hostile social context, the individual is punished severely for both personal failure and just plain poor luck. Even though the Beck disputed it, neoliberalism's cultivation of such a self—condemned to freedom and lone responsibility—combines unbridled consumer sovereignty with astute corporate acumen.

Individual as a Changing Agent

- A perfect mindset. I grow, we grow!
- People Inspire People!
- A Good Example Swacch Bharat Abhiyaan!
- Individuals create chain reactions, and other individuals join in.
- We are not alone, we just have to start what we have been thinking of doing.
- People will join us; we will join other people.
- Embrace other people egos, like you have embraced yours.
- This is how egos get sublimated and we focus more on work to do.
- We become more growth oriented.
- The societal change must begin NOW!

12. Write a short note on conflict. (CCSU)

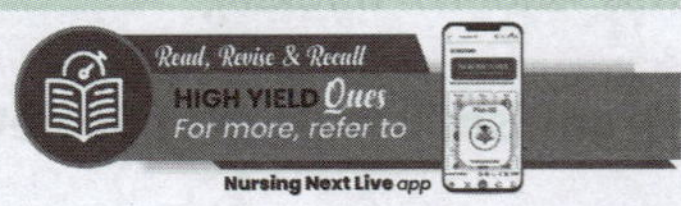

Answer

Definitions of Conflict

AW Green: "Conflict is the deliberate attempt to oppose, resist or coerce the will of another".

Horton and Hunt: "Conflict may be defined as a process of seeking to monopolize rewards like eliminating or weakening the competitors".

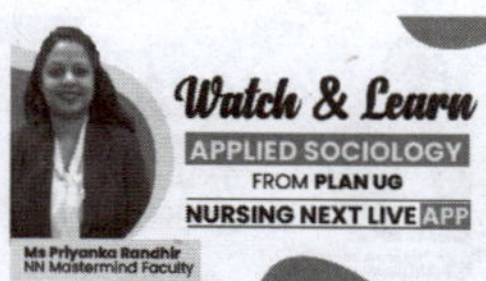

Features of Conflict

- Conscious action
- Personal activity
- Lacks continuity
- Universal

Causes of Conflict

- Individual differences
- Cultural differences
- Clash of interests
- Social change
- Selfish and vested interest
- Limited resources

Types of Conflicts

- **Overt and latent:** (Open) When hostile action is taken, the latent conflict becomes overt.
- **Corporate and personal conflict:** Between individuals or between society.
- **Direct and indirect conflict:** If the people conflict directly (litigation, revolution or war) or create a situation.
- **Caste and racial conflicts:** Between castes or between race, class conflict-karl marx (have and have-nots) and mutual hostility between strata.
- **Group conflict:** Between two small groups based on differences in ideologies, interest or suppression. Political and religious conflicts.
- **International conflict:** Between two nations on the basis of different political ideologies, economic, territorial.
- **Types of conflict by george simmel**
  - War
  - Feud
  - Litigation
  - Impersonal idea

Methods to Resolve Conflicts

- Recognize the conflict.
- Engage the opponent in conversation.
- Consider many solutions.
- Select the ideal resolution.
- Make use of a neutral arbitrator.
- Explore your options.
- Be able to handle pressure and difficult situations.

13. Write a short note on political groups. (CCSU)

Answer

Political Groups

A political group is a collection of independent individuals or political parties with similar beliefs.

Characteristics of Political Groups

A political party has the qualities listed below:

- **Obtaining power:** Political parties fight with one another for the same objective, and as long as the competition is fair, pursuing power is acceptable.
- **Pursuing an ideology:** A party's ideology can be summarized by the way it addresses specific societal issues. Today, the majority of political parties share similar ideologies, making it difficult for the typical voter to decide which party to support.
- **Possessing a common agenda:** Each party develops their agenda in accordance with their personal philosophies. They want to appeal to the masses in order to win elections and carry out their strategy.
- **Formation of government:** The political party with the most number of votes forms the government, while the parties with the lesser number votes make up the opposition.
- **To serve as a conduit between the populace and the executive branch of government:** Political parties serve as this conduit. The government uses political parties to garner support for its policies and programs from the general public, in return they communicate the concerns and requests of the general public to elected officials.

SHORT ANSWER QUESTIONS

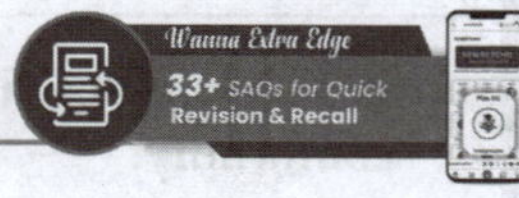

1. Define social structure.

Answer

- The term 'social structure' refers to the way in which society is organized into predictable relationships.
- According to Karl Mannheim, "Social structure refers to the web of interacting social forces from which have raised the various modes of observing and thinking. Social structure is an abstract and intangible phenomenon. Individuals are the units of association and institutions are the units of social structure".

2. Enlist agencies of socialization.

Answer

Socialization

Socialization is a comprehensive as well as complete process and through socialization, individual becomes a social person and attains his personality at maximum.

Agencies of Socialization

- Family
- School
- Playmates
- Religion
- Occupation/Work place
- State
- Political parties
- Mass media

3. Define conflict.

Answer

Conflict is an ever and constantly present process in human relation. According to Karl Marx, conflict is a process of economic development, a revolutionary change by class struggle between laborers and capitalists.

4. Define community.

Answer

Community has been derived from Latin words, namely 'com' and 'munis in which 'com' means together and 'munis' means to serve. Hence, community means to serve together.

According to **Lundeberg,** "Community means a human population living within a limited geographic area and carrying on a common interdependent life".

5. Mention any two differences between society and community.

Answer

Society	Community
Society is a large group.	As compared with society, community is limited group.
Society is a system of social relationships. It is abstract.	It is formed by group of human beings. It is concrete

CONCEPTUAL REVISION

MULTIPLE CHOICE QUESTIONS

1. Example of associative social process is:

a. Assimilation
b. Conflict
c. Isolation
d. None of these

Ans. a. Assimilation

2. Which among the following is not the cause of conformity?

a. Socialization
b. Insulation
c. Ideology
d. Weak sanction

Ans. d. Weak sanction

3. Which of the following is deliberately formed?

a. Community
b. Society
c. Association
d. None of these

Ans. c. Association

4. The theory which is essentially a morally justified agreement made amongst individuals through which an organized society is brought into existence is known as:

a. Organismic theory
b. Contingency theory
c. Trait theory
d. Social contract theory

Ans. d. Social contract theory

Golden Points

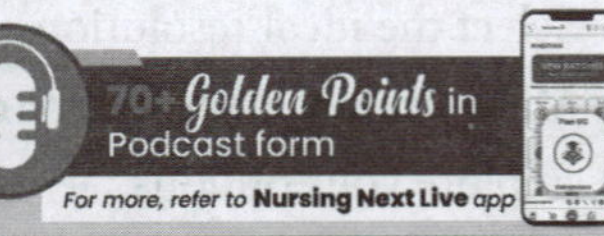

- In the view of Talcott Parson, social structure is the term applied to describe a particular arrangement of interrelated institutions, agencies and social patterns as well as the status and role which each person assumes in groups".
- Individual and society are inseparable.
- Social contract theory: According to the social contract hypothesis, everyone in a society must abide by a set of moral and political principles before they may coexist.

CHAPTER

3

Culture

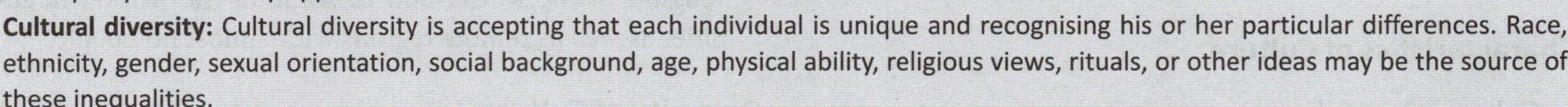

CONCEPTUAL THEORY

Terminology

Counterculture: Culture that is aberrant from society. A counterculture is a subculture that openly and actively opposes some characteristics of the wider culture.

Cultural diversity: Cultural diversity is accepting that each individual is unique and recognising his or her particular differences. Race, ethnicity, gender, sexual orientation, social background, age, physical ability, religious views, rituals, or other ideas may be the source of these inequalities.

Cultural evolutionism: Cultural evolutionism is described as the ongoing interaction between the evolution of social order, pattern, cultural achievements, and cognitive development.

Cultural lag: A phase of maladjustment in which the nonmaterial culture is still fighting to adapt to changing material conditions is referred to as cultural lag.

Cultural pattern: A cultural pattern is produced when traits and complexes are related to one other in functional functions.

Cultural relativism: Cultural relativism is the principle that a component of culture can only be evaluated or judged in terms of culture as a whole.

Cultural shock: Cultural shock can affect anyone who feels disoriented, uncertain, out of place, or even terrified while immersed in a strange society.

Cultural traits: Cultural traits are the sole ingredient, or smallest unit, of culture. They are the "units of observation" that, when combined, form culture. Culture's fundamental unit is traits. For example, shaking hands, touching feet, and so forth.

Culture: As per EB Taylor, "Culture is a complex whole, which includes knowledge, belief, art, morals, law, customs and any other capabilities and habits acquired by the man as a member of society."

Mores: Mores are rules that are judged extremely important to the wellbeing of a society, generally because they embody a people's most valued ideals. Each community expects conformity to its norms; failure to do so might result in harsh sanctions.

Nonmaterial culture: Nonmaterial culture refers to ways of employing material goods as well as conventions, beliefs, ideologies, governments, and communication patterns.

NATURE, CHARACTERISTIC AND EVOLUTION OF CULTURE

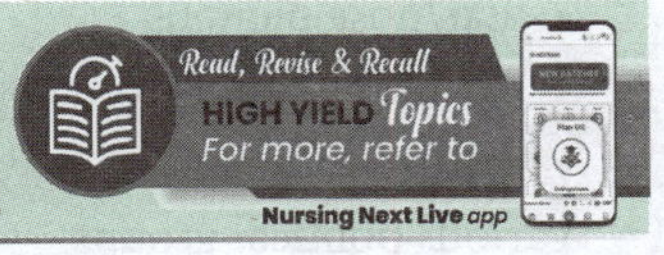

Introduction to Culture

A set of knowledge, beliefs, attitudes, and rules for behavior that are held commonly within a society.

- All the achievements of the group life
- If all these things are in an individual, he is "Cultured" as per sociology.

Important Definitions

Taylor: *"Culture is the complex whole which includes knowledge, belief, art, morals, law, customs and habits and any capabilities acquired by man as a member of society."*

Linton: *"Culture is social heredity, which is transmitted from one generation to another with the accumulation of individual experiences."*

John Beattie: "Culture is the way of life which is transmitted from generation to generation."

Ideal culture: The norms and beliefs that people in a society accept in principle.

Subculture: A set of knowledge, beliefs, attitudes, symbols, and norms held by a group sharing some common experience or situation within a larger society. Example: Hippies

"Culture is an organized body of conventional understanding manifest in art and artifact, which, persisting through tradition, characterizes a human group." **—Redfield**

Nature of Culture

Culture is:

- Acquired
- Not individual heritage
- Idealistic
- Total social heritage
- Fulfills some needs
- An integrated system
- Transferred through language
- Different in different society

Characteristics of Culture

- Culture is learned
- Culture is social
- Culture is shared
- Culture is idealistic
- Culture is transmitting
- Culture is gratifying
- Culture is dynamic
- Culture is integrated

Evolution of Culture

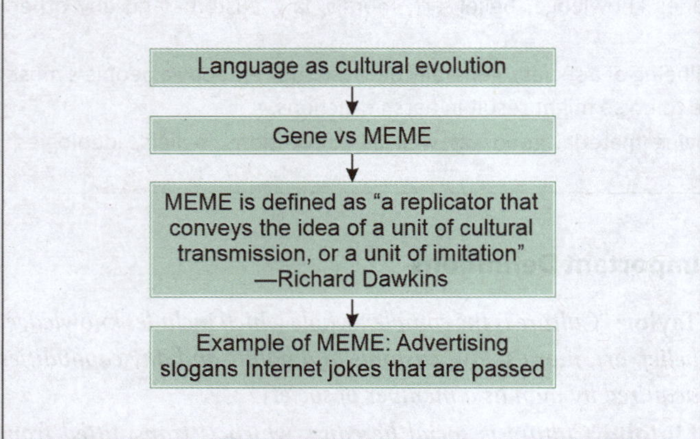

Also, cultural evolution compared with biological evolution is:

- Transfer of genes
- Idea or skill
  - Previous generations
  - Peers
  - Offspring brain
  - Next generations brains
  - Memes transmission
- Coined the word "meme" in 1976 and mentioned this in his book: *The Selfish Gene.* **—Richard Dawkins**
- "Just as genes propagate themselves in the gene pool by leaping from body to body via sperms or eggs, so, memes propagate themselves in the meme pool by leaping themselves from brain to brain via imitation.

DIVERSITY AND UNIFORMITY OF CULTURE

Introduction

- Culture diversity comprises various customs, ideas, social attributes and beliefs of people.
- India is a Kaleidoscope of cultures.
- Contemporary India stands as one of the most diverse countries in the world, a subcontinent that is home to over 100 languages, over 700 different tribes, every major religion in the world, and to some of the world's largest cities as well as remote regions with almost no people.

Diversity of Culture

Diversity of culture include:

- Religion/Social diversity
  - Hindus 85%
  - Muslim 13.4%
  - Christians 2.3%
  - Sikhs 1.9%
  - Buddhists 0.8%
  - Jains 0.4%
- Language
  - 22 Official languages
  - 1632 Languages
- Way of life
- Tradition
  - Joint families
  - Fasting
  - Martial arts
  - Vedic chanting
  - Ramlila
  - Kumbh mela
  - Ear/nose piercing
  - Drinking water from copper utentsils/silver cutkery
  - Eating with hands
- Various political groups
- Geographical area
- Racial diversity
- Historical accidents
- Mobility of human organism
- Invention and discoveries
- Individual habits
- Change in modes of production

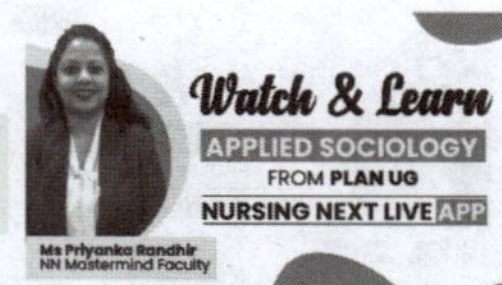

- Dominant cultural themes
- Unity is, all the culture has their fundamental approach to literature, philosophy, traditions and customs which are normally.
- Caste, religious rites, ceremonies are following all the culture.
- All the culture has music, dance, song, etc.
- Some festivals are celebrated as national and international festivals.

Cultural Uniformity

- Sharing of same cultural pattern by various groups of people.
- Members of a religious group exhibit cultural uniformity.
- Common health culture.

DIFFERENCES BETWEEN CULTURE AND CIVILIZATION

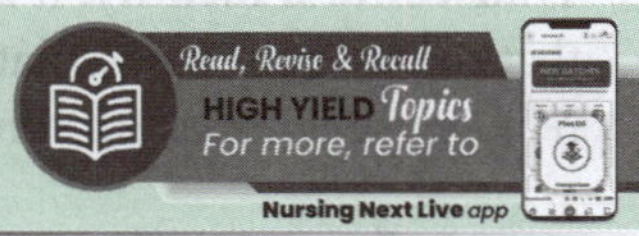

Ogburn and Nimkoff conceived of civilization as the latter phase of the super-organic culture but it needs to be remembered that is external civilization and mechanical whereas culture is internal and organic.

MacIver and Page noted the following differences between culture and civilization.

- Civilization is measurable quantitatively on the grounds of efficiency while culture is not.
- Civilization is a progressive one and culture is not.
- Civilization consists of external material things while culture is related to internal thoughts, feelings and values, etc.
- Civilization and the products of it could be easily transmitted not only from one country to another but also from one generation to another. On the other hand, culture and its products are transmitted by its assimilation by the votaries. Only those who are worthy of it, acquire it.

Other Differences Between Culture and Civilization

Civilization	Culture
Outward behavior	Inward behavior
External and mechanical, utilitarian (practical) and concerned only with means	Exclusively deals with ends and is internal, organic and final.
Interests are essentially competitive or exclusive	Interests are in general inclusive
Persistent or upward trend	Advances slowly, stagnation, retrogressive
Anybody can improve the work	Not possible here
Work easy to understand and communicate	Difficult in this case
Adopted without efforts	Depends on personality and nature
Less flexible in its elements	More flexible in its elements
Can be borrowed in its original form	Never borrowed in its original form
It is body	It is soul

CULTURE AND SOCIALIZATION

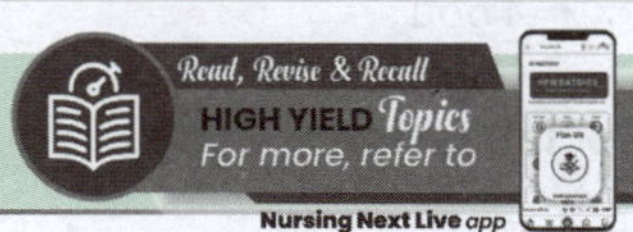

Introduction

- Culture is a way of life.
- **Culture:** The knowledge, language, values, customs and physical objects that are by the members of the society.
- **Culture changes for three reasons:** Discovery, invention and diffusion.
- Culture changes with time.
- Society is a specific territory inhabited by people who share a common culture and human behavior is based on the culture.
- Culture is learned.
- Culture and society are interwoven.
- Culture cannot exist without society and vice versa.
- Socialization is to be a member of society and follow its norms and be self-aware of the social role.
- Human infants are born without culture.
- They must be transformed by agents of socialization like family, parents, teachers, peers and mass media into culturally adapt human beings.
- This general process of acquiring culture is called "Socialization."
- Successful socialization can result in uniformity within society.
- Personality develops through socialization.
- Socialization helps us to perform specific role in society which is culturally bound.
- **Cultural socialization** refers to the manner by which parents address ethnic and racial issues within the family, specifically, the ways parents communicate or transmit cultural values (example: Namaste), beliefs, customs and behaviors to the child and the extent to which the child internalizes these messages, adopts to the cultural norms and expectations, and acquires the skills to become a competent and functional member of a racially diverse society.

—RM Lee, 2003

Culture

- Culture includes:
  - Art/drama/music

- Attitudes
- Language
- Faith! Religion
- Customs
- Behaviors
- Rituals
- Beliefs
- Food

Socialization

Socialization is the process by which new members of a society are taught to participate in that society learn their roles and develop a self-image.

Six Agents of Socialization

1. Family
2. School
3. Peer group
4. Mass media
5. Workplace
6. Religion

Types of Socialization

- Primary
- Secondary

Problems in Cultural Socialization

- Many factors lead to conflict between socializing agents.
- In the course of socialization, everyone develops, a self of self-identity and the capacity for independent thought and action.
- Cross cultural differences in social norms.

Ethnocentrism

Ethnocentric: Thinking your own culture is better than another culture.

TRANSCULTURAL SOCIETY

Introduction

- Transculturalism is defined as "seeing oneself in the other."
- Transcultural is a term described as "extending through all human culture" or "involving, encompassing, or combining elements of more than one culture.
- It is noncultural specific.
- Cultural traits invented or discovered in one society to another.
- Spreading directly and indirectly through radio and television.
- It is basically movement of traits through time (from generation to generation).
- **Example:** India, America and Rome.

Examples of Transculturation

- A well-known example of transculturation is "COLONIZATION" When Europeans colonized North America, South America and other territories, they took with them European values and traditions.
- **Current example:** Spreading of American cultural values in all parts of world.

Meaning of Transculturation

- Involving, encompassing or extending across two or more cultures
- **Transcultural identity:** It is a source of individual identity that draws from across national boundaries and cultural, religious, linguistic and ethnic backgrounds.

Factors Influencing Transcultural

- Transportation and communication
- Prestige of the transmitted culture and its people
- Migration
- **New element:** To meet crisis
- **Adaptibility:** Of the new culture by the recipients

CULTURE, MODERNIZATION AND ITS IMPACT ON HEALTH AND DISEASE

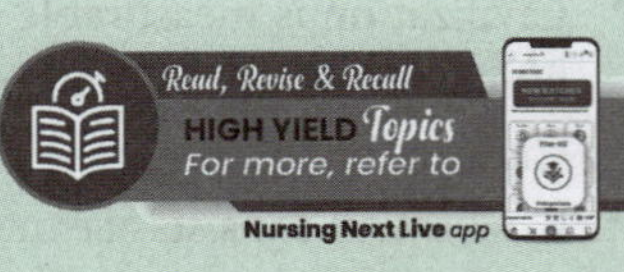

Introduction

Culture

"Culture is the complex whole which includes knowledge, belief, art, morals, law, customs and habits and any capabilities acquired by man as a member of society." —**Taylor**

Modernization

"Modernization refers to process in which society goes through industrialization, urbanization and other social changes that completely transform the lives of individuals."

Cultural Modernization

- A process of cultural transformation
    - It is the process of change and involving values, norms, institution and structure.
    - Transformation from a traditional to industrial society
    - A process of gradual change

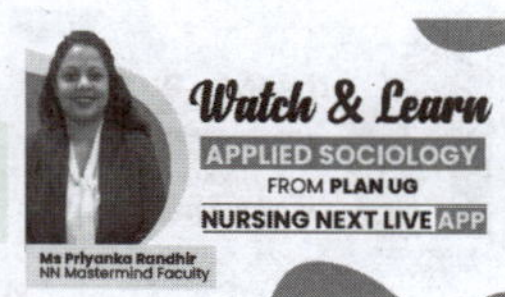

- Change in food habits, dresses, tastes, language, ideas, preferences, recreational activities, views, etc.
- A social change
  - **Growing differentiation:** Major elements of culture: Religion, philosophy and science
  - **Spread:** Expansion of media communication
  - **Development:** Development of new cultural element
  - **Expansion:** Expansion of media communication

CONCEPTUAL EXERCISES

LONG ANSWER QUESTIONS

1. Explain about culture and socialization. (CCS)

Answer

Culture

- Culture is a way of life.
- **Culture:** The knowledge, language, values, customs and physical objects that are by the members of the society.
- Culture changes for three reasons: Discovery, Invention and Diffusion.
- Culture changes with time.
- Society is a specific territory inhabited by people who share a common culture and human behavior is based on the culture.
- Culture is learned.
- Culture and society are interwoven.
- Culture cannot exist without society and vice versa.
- Socialization is to be a member of society and follow its norms and be self-aware of the social role.
- Human infants are born without culture.
- They must be transformed by agents of socialization like family, parents, teachers, peers and mass media into culturally adapt human beings.
- This general process of acquiring culture is called "Socialization."
- Successful socialization can result in uniformity within society.
- Personality develops through socialization.
- Socialization helps us to perform specific role in society which is culturally bound.
- Cultural socialization refers to the manner by which parents address ethnic and racial issues within the family, specifically, the ways parents communicate or transmit cultural values, (example: namaste) beliefs, customs and behaviors to the child and the extent to which the child internalizes these messages, adopts to the cultural norms and expectations, and acquires the skills to become a competent and functional member of a racially diverse society. —RM Lee, 2003
- Culture includes:
  - Art/Drama/Music
  - Attitudes
  - Language
  - Faith! Religion
  - Customs
  - Behaviors
  - Rituals
  - Beliefs
  - Food

Types of Culture

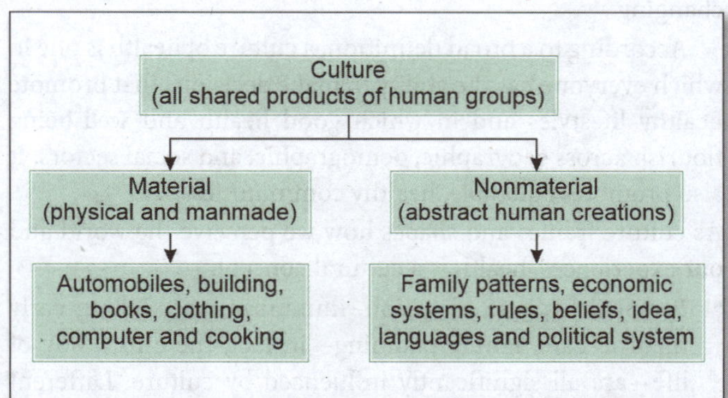

Dimensions of Culture

- **Cognitive:** Learning to process what we hear or see. Example: Ringtone of phone or cartoon of a politician.
- **Normative:** Rules of conduct. Example: Not to read other's messages or cremation.
- **Material:** Any activity done with the help of material. Example: Internet chatting.

Socialization

Socialization is the process by which new members of a society are taught to participate in that society learn their roles and develop a self-image.

Problems in Cultural Socialization

- Many factors lead to conflict between socializing agents.

- In the course of socialization, everyone develops, a self of self-identity and the capacity for independent thought and action.
- Cross cultural differences in social norms.

2. Describe the influence of culture on health and diseases. (CCS)

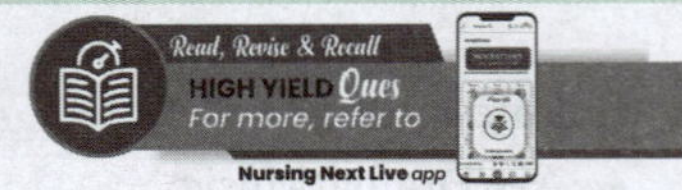

Answer

"Culture is the complex whole which includes knowledge, belief, art, morals, law, customs and habits and any capabilities acquired by man as a member of society." **—Taylor**

Influence of Culture on Health and Diseases

Health: WHO defines health as "it is a state of complete physical, mental and social well being, and note merely the absence of disease or infirmity."

Culture: Culture is a set of ideas, customs, and behaviors that are shared by a specific group of people or society. It is always changing.

According to a broad definition, a culture of health is one in which everyone has the ability to make decisions that promote healthy lifestyles and in which good health and well-being flourish across geographic, demographic, and social sectors. It also promotes equitable, healthy communities.

As culture frames and shapes how we perceive the world and our experiences, health is a cultural concept.

- Personal hygiene, nutrition, immunization, seeking early medical care, family planning—in fact, the entire way of life—are all significantly influenced by culture. Different cultures exist in many communities, which may or may not have a good impact on health.
- Some patients, for example, believe that their condition is caused by fatalism, the devil, or a demon. They may refuse to accept a diagnosis and may even believe they are powerless to change the course of events. Instead, they can only accept events as they unfold.
- Why are certain diseases or conditions stigmatized and rationalized. In many cultures, a mental illness is a common stigma and seeing a psychiatrist means a person is "crazy". Importantly, once the person's health issues are identified, communities tend to band together to provide the support structure needed to allow the person to function in a safe environment.
- Culture is learned and shared human behavior that includes health behavior and has a significant impact on our understanding of health and medicine.
- In other words, culture is a major determinant of personal health behaviors and medical professional practices.
- The concept of culture is thus fundamental to comprehending human population health conditions, allowing us to cope and protect ourselves from diseases or infirmities by implementing preventive and curative methods as a means of adjusting to the interaction of various physical and social environments.
- Culture has determined and impacted the multifaceted aspects of health, such as perception of disease cause, diagnosis, and subsequent treatment, as well as the use and selection of available resources as a preventative and protective measure for disease eradication.
- Health was regarded as an indicator of a person's usefulness or 'appropriacy' to their community.
- It was believed that if an individual's behavior was out of 'balance' with the needs of the community, it would lead to illness and suffering.
- Surprisingly, according to this belief system, the person who caused the imbalance was not always the one who suffered. Instead, another person or group of people may suffer as a result of an individual's wrong behavior.
- Health was a significant public concern in ancient society. Individual relationships can thus be understood as a common feature in ancient conceptions of culture, community, and health.
- Health care companies as well as patients stand to gain considerably from cultural competence.
- Increased patient safety can arise from increased patient engagement, which increases respect and understanding among patients.

3. List out the features of culture. Describe the relation between culture and health. (KUHS, DU, MGR)

Answer

Features of Culture

- Linked with society
- Culture is gratifying
- Culture is responsive
- Culture varies from society to society
- Culture is changing
- Culture is integrated
- Culture is accumulative
- Culture is continuous
- Culture is transmitted
- Culture is shared
- Culture is social
- Culture is learned

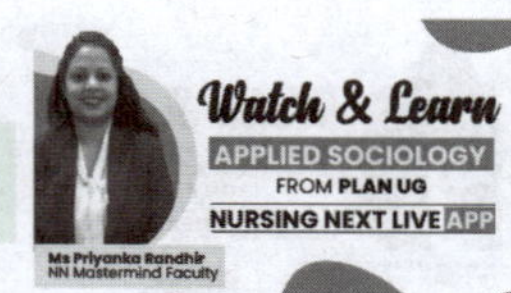

Relation between Culture and Health

- Culture influences individuals' beliefs, values, and practices related to health. Personal cleanliness, diet, immunization, getting early medical care, family planning are all significantly influenced by culture.
- There are several cultures in various societies, and these cultures may or may not be beneficial to health.
- A culture of health is one in which everyone has the ability to make decisions that promote healthy lifestyles and equitable, healthy communities.
- It is influenced by personal hygiene, nutrition, immunization, seeking early medical care, and family planning.
- Different cultures exist in many communities, which may or may not have a good impact on health.
- Stigma and Mental health: Cultural attitudes and beliefs can contribute to stigma around mental health. In some cultures, seeking help from a psychiatrist or acknowledging mental illness may be stigmatized, leading to delayed or inadequate treatment for mental health conditions.
- Culture is learned and shared human behavior that has a significant impact on our understanding of health and medicine.
- Culture is a major determinant of personal health behaviors and medical professional practices, allowing us to cope and protect ourselves from diseases or infirmities.
- Health disparities: Culture can contribute to health disparities, particularly among marginalized or minority populations. Socioeconomic, racial, ethnic, or religious differences embedded in culture can impact access to healthcare, quality of care, and health outcomes.
- Cultural Adaptation: As societies become more diverse and multicultural, healthcare systems need to adapt to the cultural needs and preferences of diverse populations.
- It is thought that when a person behaves in a way that is out of harmony with the demands of the community, it might result in illness and suffering.
- Ancient culture gave a high priority to health, so cultural sensitivity benefits both patients and health care providers.
- Increased patient engagement can lead to greater patient safety because it fosters greater patient understanding as well as respect.

SHORT NOTES

1. Define culture. Discuss its impact on health. (CCS)

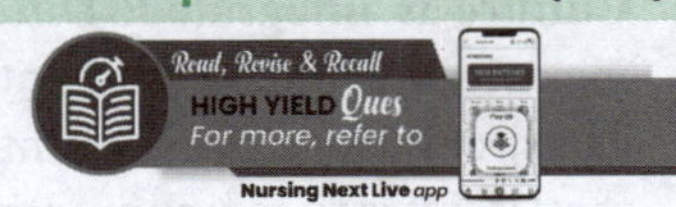

Answer

"Culture is the complex whole which includes knowledge, belief, art, morals, law, customs and habits and any capabilities acquired by man as a member of society."
—**Taylor**

"Culture is social heredity, which is transmitted from one generation to another with the accumulation of individual experiences."
—**Linton**

Impact of Culture on Health and Disease

Culture has a profound impact on health and disease.

- The impact of food culture on health is significant and can have both positive and negative effects.
- Nutritional pattern, cultural preferences on food choices (veg or nonveg), and food related rituals have impact on health.
  - **Example: North India versus South India:** Both have positive as well as negative impact on the health
  - **Example: Vegetarian versus nonvegetarians:** Nutrients like vitamin B_{12}, vitamin D, ω-3 fatty acids, calcium, iron, and zinc are low in vegetarian food. On the other hand, the north Indian diet is rich in fats.
- **Bad habits**
  - Chewing tobacco. Common in rural areas.
  - Considered as a taboo in ancient time
- **Occupational hazards:** Lung diseases, cervical spondylosis, arthritis in manual labor.
- **Consanguineous marriages:** More risk for development of physical and mental deformities.

Other Impacts on Health

- **Walking barefooted:** Walking barefoot enhances immunity as well as eyesight. On the other hand, it exposes the feet to bacteria and fungi that can cause skin and nail infections.
- **Using Datun in some culture:** Helps in improving dental health.
- **Oil bath—A Diwali ritual:** The oil bath is one of the oldest cultural practices in South India. Sesame oil reduces heat from body. Given to infants.
- **Early morning bath:** A bath during this time enables you to enjoy pleasure, good health, immunity from diseases, sharp intellect and concentration.
- **Drinking tulsi water:** Refreshens the senses and helps in relieving acidity.
- **Yoga:** Strengthens the body, relieves stress, provides flexibility, connects you with a supportive community.
- **Early to bed and early to rise:** For healthy life.
- **Neem leaves:** For chicken pox patients.
- Purdah system causes vitamin D deficiency.
- **Worshiping/pooja:** Physical and mental peace.
- **Superstitions:** Postpone health care services.
- **Polygamy:** Somatization, depression, anxiety, hostility, psychoticism and psychiatric disorder, unsatisfaction in marriage, conflicts.

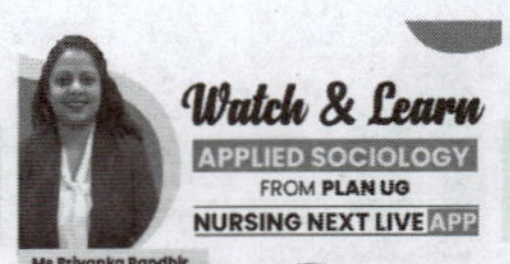

2. Define culture and socialization. Mention the components of culture. (CCS, MGR)

Answer

Definitions of Culture

"Culture is the complex whole which includes knowledge, belief, art, morals, law, customs and habits and any capabilities acquired by man as a member of society." **—Taylor**

"Culture is social heredity, which is transmitted from one generation to another with the accumulation of individual experiences." **—Linton**

"Culture is the way of life which is transmitted from generation to generation." **—John Beattie**

Definitions of Socialization

"Socialization is a learning that enables the learner to perform social roles." **—Harry M Johnson**

"Socialization is the process by which the individual learns to confirm to the norms of the group." **—WF Ogburn**

"Socialization is the process of working together or developing group responsibility of being guided by the welfare needs of others." **—Bogardus**

Components of Culture

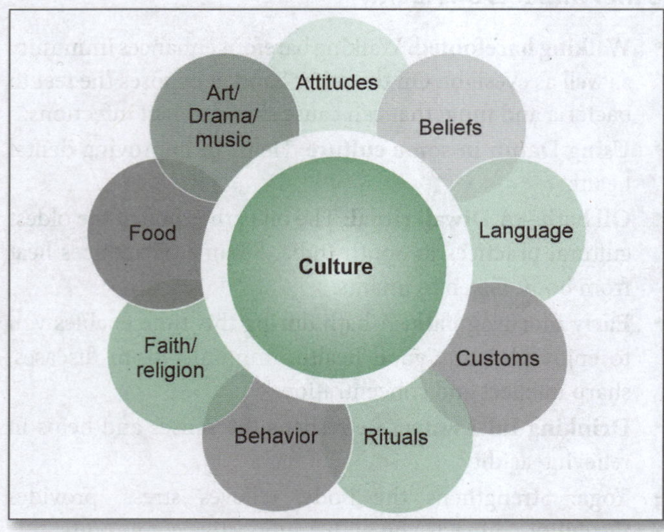

3. Write about culture. (CCS)

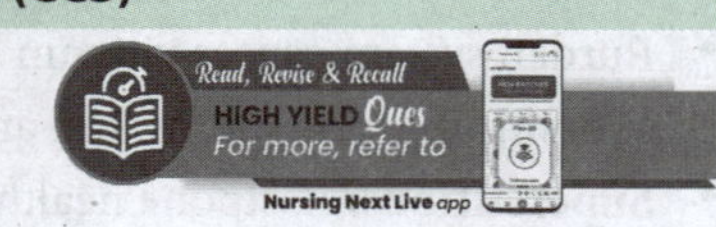

Answer

Introduction

- Sociologists and anthropologists use the term "culture" to refer to the symbolic and learned aspects of human society, such as languages, custom, and convention, that distinguish human behavior from that of other primates.
- The word "culture" is derived from the Latin word "colere," which means "to cultivate" or "to till the soil".
- Initially, the term alluded to agriculture. The term refers to any group's or society's beliefs, values, and expressive symbols.

Definition

"Culture is the expression of our nature in our modes of living and our thinking, intercourse in our literature, in religion in recreation and enjoyment." **—MacIver**

Characteristics of Culture

Each culture has its own distinct characteristics. Consider the following.

- **Culture is acquired:** It is not innate, and cultural characteristics can be acquired through socialization and habits. In other words, culture is acquired.
- **Culture is social:** Culture is social in the sense that it does not exist in isolation. It emerges and grows from social interaction. Man cannot develop human qualities unless he interacts with other men.
- **Culture is shared:** It is not individual, but rather collective. It includes the group's overall expectations. It is a social good. "Culture is the totality of group way, thought, and action duly accepted and followed by a group of people," writes Walter Paul.
- **Culture is idealistic:** It is true that what is included in culture is not all-encompassing. It is always idealized and strives to achieve these ideals. It reflects an ideal norm or group behavior. Culture has always been linked to the past. Customs and traditions are just two examples of how the past is transmitted to the present.
- **Culture is gratifying:** Culture is satisfying because each group has certain common goals that are met by culture. As a result, it meets the group's ethical and social needs.
- **Culture is dynamic:** Culture is dynamic rather than static. Culture is simply a way of life. Inventions, problems, planned changes, and so on all have an impact on culture. As a result, new ways of life emerge and are adopted in an attempt to adapt to changing circumstances. Every factor that has an impact on society will also have an impact on culture. As a result, culture is dynamic.
- **Culture is integrated:** Different aspects of culture are inextricably linked and integrated with one another. Thus, culture is not a disintegrated whole; any element that is introduced and accepted by the culture is also integrated.

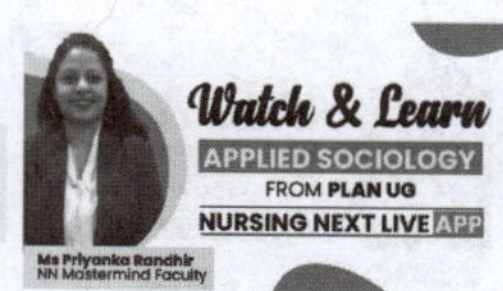

4. Nature of culture. (KUHS)

Answer

Culture

"Culture is the handwork of man and the medium through which he achieves his ends." —**Malinowski**

Nature of Culture

- Culture is founded on the uniquely human ability to classify experiences, symbolically encode such classifications, and teach such abstractions to others.
- The concept of culture is fundamental to the study of anthropology. Sir Edward Taylor, a British anthropologist, wrote in his book Primitive Culture that culture systems of human behavior and thought obey natural laws and can thus be studied scientifically.
- He defines culture as the complex whole of knowledge, belief, arts, morals, law, custom, and any other capabilities and habits acquired by man as a member of society.
- Tylor's definition focuses on characteristics that people acquire not through biological inheritance but by growing up in a specific society and being exposed to a specific cultural tradition.
- Enculturation is the process by which a child acquires knowledge of his or her culture.
- Culture teaches us how to express natural biological urges that we share with other animals in specific ways. People must eat, but culture teaches us what, when, and how to eat.
- Human nature is shaped in a variety of ways by cultural habits, perceptions, and inventions. For example, our bathroom habits, which include waste elimination, bathing, and dental care, are cultural traditions that have transformed natural acts into cultural customs.
- Our culture, and cultural changes, influence how we perceive nature, human nature, and the natural. Cultural advances have overcome many natural limitations through science, invention, and discovery.
- Man has prevented and cured diseases that afflicted his forefathers, such as polio and smallpox. Scientists have changed the way we think about biological identity and the meaning of life itself thanks to cloning.
- Natural threats have not been eliminated by culture. Hurricanes, floods, earthquakes, and other natural forces frequently force us to alter the environment through construction, development, and expansion.
- Cultures are not random assemblages of customs and beliefs. They are patterned integrated systems. When one component of the system changes, other components change as well.
- Culture, according to anthropologists, is much more than refinement, taste, sophistication, education, and appreciation of the fine arts.
- The most powerful cultural forces are those that influence people on a daily basis, particularly those that influence children during enculturation.
- Popular culture is an example of a feature that is sometimes considered trivial or unworthy of serious study.
- A rock star may be as interesting as a symphony conductor as a cultural manifestation, and a comic book may be as significant as a book award winner.
- Culture is an attribute of individuals as members of groups, not of individuals.
- Culture is passed down through society. We learn about other people's cultures by observing, listening, talking, and interacting with them. People who grow up in the same culture share common beliefs, values, memories, and expectations.
- Enculturation brings people together by providing us with shared experiences. People become agents in their children's enculturation, just as their parents were for them.
- Despite the fact that culture is constantly changing, certain fundamental beliefs, values, worldviews, and child rearing practices remain constant.
- Many other people share our thoughts and beliefs. We are more likely to agree with and feel comfortable with people who are socially, economically, and culturally similar to ourselves, demonstrating the power of shared cultural background.

5. Functions of culture. (KUHS)

Answer

Functions of Culture

- Culture gives us with living designs. It is always acquired and learned.
- Culture provides a system for meeting the biological and sociocultural needs of group members, such as food, housing, reproduction, and relationships with other groups and individuals.
- Culture establishes a system of principles to ensure that members in a community cooperate in adjusting to environmental changes.
- Culture equips an individual with a ready-made set of definitions about a circumstance.
- Culture aids in understanding and forecasting human behavior, as well as providing avenues for interaction among members of a society.

- Culture serves as a guidepost or map for all of our everyday activities. It defines an individual's behavior pattern so that he acts in accordance with the behavior pattern established and defined by culture.
- Culture exerts social control through norms, folkways, and moving laws.

Thus, culture serves to profoundly impact and steer the individual's and group's behavior and life. All of these functions are governed by societal standards or rules. These norms may be governed by penalties or punishment; therefore, studying norms, mores, folkways, laws, and so on is essential for understanding societal culture.

SHORT ANSWER QUESTIONS

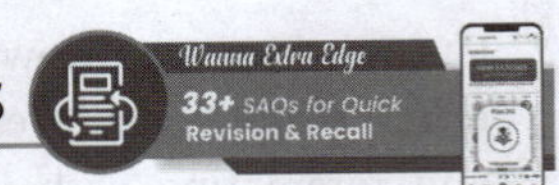

1. Define civilization.

Answer

According to William Ogburn, "Civilization is the material culture" and according to sociologist like MacIver, civilization is the things , techniques and material instruments which have been devised by man in his effort to control the conditions of his life.

2. What do you mean by culture?

Answer

According to The Center for Advance Research on Language Acquisition, culture is defined as shared patterns of behaviors and interactions, cognitive constructs and understanding that are learned by socialization.

William Ogburn has stated, "that culture has material and nonmaterial elements."

3. Define modernization.

Answer

Modernization symbolizes the advancement. According to S H Alatas, "Modernization is a process by which modern scientific knowledge is introduced in the society with the ultimate purpose of achieving a better and more satisfactory life in the broadest sense of the term accepted by the society concerned."

4. Point out two influences of culture on health.

Answer

Two influences of culture on health are:

1. **Nutritional factors:**
   - Pica, eating clay by pregnant women helps in normal development of baby.
   - Garlic increases milk production in lactating women.
   - Fruits like mango, eating in excessive amount causes boil formation.
   - Papaya in pregnancy causes abortion.
2. **Mother and child health:**
   - Certain foods such as eggs, meat and fish are forbidden during pregnancy.
   - In some part of India, baby is not breastfed during the first 3 days after birth because people think colostrum is harmful to the baby.

5. Mention the components of culture.

Answer

Components of culture are:

- **Cultural beliefs:** Belief is the component of culture. As an example, a cultural notion in a Christian culture would be that Christian missionaries should give medicine and recommend rest.
- While in ancient Indian society, the Indians believed that fasting was the best way to treat fever because it was thought to be brought on by poisoning or injury.
- **Cultural traits:** Cultural traits are the "units of observation" which when put together constitute culture.
- **Culture complex:** Folding hands, singing prayer song, touching feet of old person, and taking Prasad from the priest form a religious complex.
- **Culture pattern:** Traits and complexes converted into or related to each other in functional role form culture pattern.
- **Cultural area:** Communities with similar cultural traits and complexes constitute a cultural area.
- **Signs:** Include symbols and signals
- **Cognitive rudiments:** Culture of all societies whether preliterate carries a vast amount of knowledge about the physical and social world. The possession of this knowledge is referred to as a cognitive component.

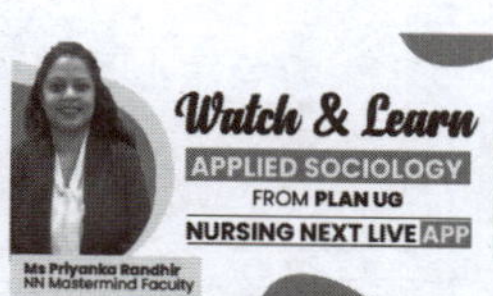

CONCEPTUAL REVISION

MULTIPLE CHOICE QUESTIONS

1. ________ is local self- government at village or small-town level in India.

a. Gram Panchayat
b. Zillah Parishad
c. Municipal Corporation
d. Panchayat Samiti

Ans. a. Gram Panchayat

2. All are included in the nature of social change; except:

a. Always progressive
b. Varies from society to society
c. Nonuniform
d. Cannot be predicted

Ans. a. Always progressive

3. Sex relations, marriage, social intermixture and the size of the family are included in ________ factors of social change.

a. Geographical b. Biological
c. Cultural d. Technological

Ans. b. Biological

4. Resisting social change because it comes from outside of one's group is called:

a. Diffusion b. Ethnocentrism
c. Cultural lag d. Self-fulfilment

Ans. b. Ethnocentrism

5. All of the following are sources of resistance to social change; except:

a. Vested interests b. Ethnocentrism
c. Cultural lag d. Wars and conquests

Ans. d. Wars and conquests

6. Which of the following statements is true?

a. Unlike other animals, human infants are born with a culture
b. Human infants come into the world ready to learn a culture but are not born with one
c. Socialization is another word for acculturation
d. b and c

Ans. b. Human infants come into the world ready to learn a culture but are not born with one

7. The general process of acquiring culture is referred to as ____________.

a. Socialization b. Acculturation
c. Semai d. None of these

Ans. a. Socialization

8. The chief vehicle of culture is:

a. Knowledge b. Beliefs and values
c. Language d. Law

Ans. c. Language

9. Meaning of ethnocentrism is:

a. Feeling of inferiority of their own culture
b. Feeling of superiority of their own culture
c. Feeling of disorientation of other culture
d. Process of introducing new ideas to a culture

Ans. b. Feeling of superiority of their own culture

10. Culture has influence on:

a. Social aspects of life b. Mental aspects of life
c. Political aspects of life d. Economic aspects of life

Ans. a Social aspects of life

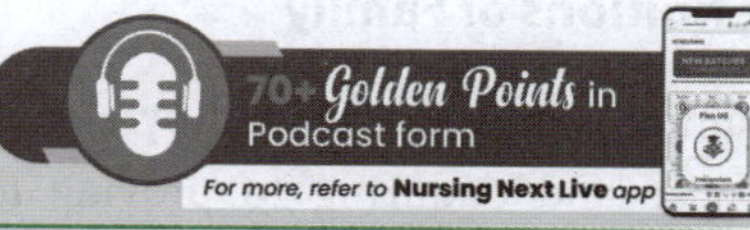

Golden Points

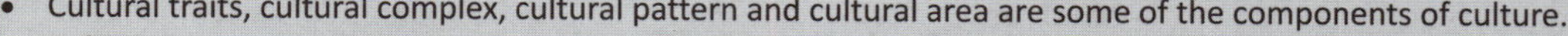

- Cultural traits, cultural complex, cultural pattern and cultural area are some of the components of culture.
- Culture is a symbolic, continuous, cumulative, adaptive, gratifying, dynamic, integrative, idealistic and manmade. —Leglic AY White
- Historical accidents, geographical environment and mobility of human beings, etc. contribute to cultural variations.

CHAPTER 4

Family and Marriage

CONCEPTUAL THEORY

Terminology

150+ key terminologies for Quick Recall & Revision

Blended family: A blended family is formed when two parents bring unrelated children from previous or foster parenting relationships into a new combined living situation. A family made up of a spouse, their children from previous partnerships, and their children from previous relationships.

Civil marriages: Civil marriages are contracted under state laws, which specify the conditions that must be followed for a marriage to be both official and valid.

Cohabitation: When a couple shares a residence but not a marriage, this is referred to as cohabitation.

Conjugal family: A conjugal family is a family system consisting of spouses and their dependent children.

Consanguine family: A consanguine family is made up of members who are related by blood or are related by blood.

Cross-cousin marriage: Cross-cousin marriage occurs when a person marries the daughter or son of their paternal uncle or the son or daughter of their paternal aunt.

Divorce: Divorce is the result of a couple's failure to fulfil their marital and familial responsibilities. It is the breakup of a family, and it distresses both the family and society.

Endogamy: A sort of marriage in which both partners are from the same caste, tribe, or race.

Exogamy: A sort of marriage in which the mate comes from a different caste, tribe, or race.

Extended family: A family formed by three or more generations living together. In addition to the nuclear family, it is a sort of family that includes relatives (aunts, uncles, grandparents, and cousins).

Family: Eliot and Merrill define family as "the biological, social unit composed of husband, wife, and children."

Isogamy: Isogamy refers to marriage between persons from two equal social level families.

Joint family: Dr Iravati Karve defines a joint family as "a group of people who generally live under one roof, eat food cooked at one hearth, hold property in common, participate in common family worship, and are related to each other."

Levirate marriage: A Levirate marriage occurs when a woman marries her husband's brother after his death.

FAMILY—CHARACTERISTICS, BASIC NEEDS, TYPES AND FUNCTIONS OF FAMILY

Definitions of Family

"Family is a group defined by a sex relationship sufficiently precise and enduring to provide for the procreation and upbringing of children." —**MacIver**

"Family is the logical social unit composed of husband, wife and children." —**Elliott and Merrill**

"Family is a group of people directly linked by kin connection, adult members of which assume responsibility of caring of children." —**Anthony Giddens**

Characteristics of Family (GP Murdock)

- Common residence
- Economic coordination
- Sexual reproduction
- Socially approved sexual relationships

(Exception: Blacks in southern USA)

Basic Needs of Family

- Sexual and reproductive needs
- Housing
- Food
- Security

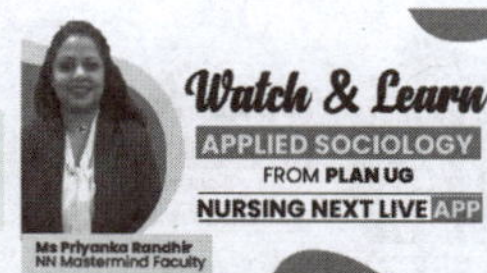

- Health
- Clothing
- Effective communication
- Education
- Access to information technology
- Entertainment

Types of Families

- **Based on authority**
  - Patriarchal
  - Matriarchal
- **Based on structure**
  - Nuclear
  - Joint or extended
- **Based on residence**
  - Patrilocal
  - Matrilocal
- **Based on marriage**
  - Monogamous
  - Polygamous
  - Polyandrous
- **Based on ancestry/descent**
  - Patrilineal
  - Matrilineal (Khasis in Meghalaya and Nayar in Kerala)
- **Based on in-groups and out-groups**
  - Endogamous
  - Exogamous
- **Based on blood relationships**
  - Conjugal family (based on marriage)
  - Consanguine family (based on blood)

Functions of Family (By MacIver)

- **Essential functions of family**
  - Satisfaction of sex needs
  - Production of children
  - Raring of children
  - Provision of home
- **Nonessential functions of family**
  - Economic
  - Religious health
  - Educational
  - Recreation
  - Civics
  - Social

MARRIAGE—FORMS OF MARRIAGE, SOCIAL CUSTOM RELATING TO MARRIAGE AND IMPORTANCE OF MARRIAGE

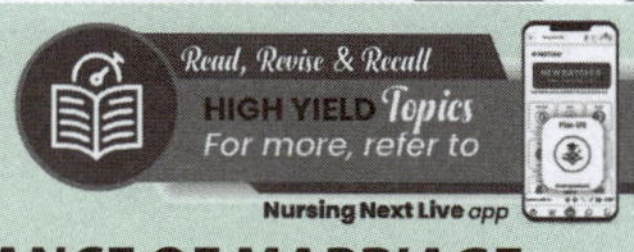

Definitions of Marriage

Marriage as "the more or less durable connection between male and female lasting beyond the mere act of propagation till after the birth of offspring." —**Edward Westermarck**

"Marriage is a relatively permanent bond between permissible mates." —**Robert H Lowie**

Elements of Marriage

- **Recognition:**
  - It is not an individual affair.
  - Some kind of recognition is must.
  - Recognition is in the form of: Cultural or legal recognition.
- **Individuals**
  - Marriage is between individuals but it results in the formation of much wider kin groups.
  - So, the marriage not only defines linkage between individuals, but also between groups.
- **Rights and obligations in marriage**
  - Implications for individual as well as groups
  - In most societies, these are defined culturally and also get legal recognition

Characteristics of Marriage

- Universality
- Relationship between man and woman and mutual obligations
- Marriage bond is enduring
- Marriage requires social approval
- Associated with civil/religious ceremony

Types of Marriages

A. Legitimate or accepted

B. Illegitimate or unaccepted

Forms of Marriage

- Based on number of life partners
- **Based on selection**
  - Love marriage
  - Arranged marriage

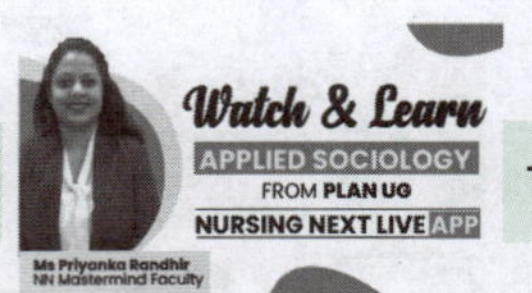

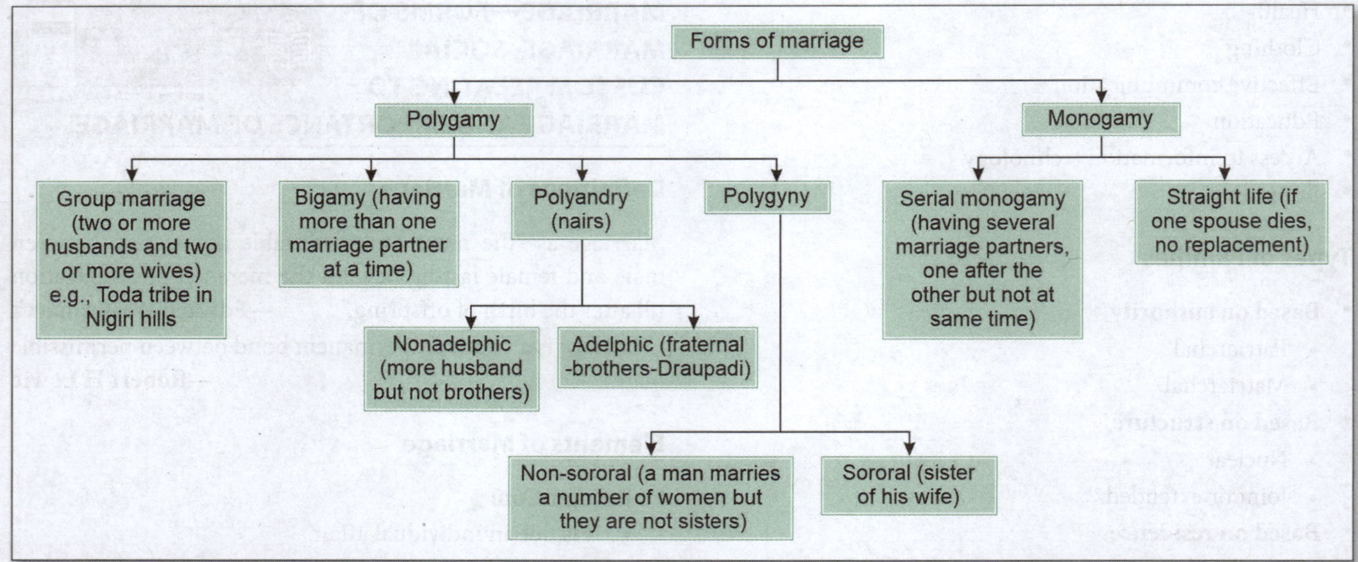

- **Based on priority of selection**
  - Exogamy marriage
  - Endogamy marriage
- **Based on status of couple**
  - Descending or odd marriage
  - Pratiloma or even marriage
- **Based on arrangement**
  - Closed (chosen from recommended categories)
  - Open marriage (no categories)

Marriage Classification by "Kapadia and Prabhu"

Endogamy

Endogamy refers to that exchange in which the selection of life made from own group is necessary.

Exogamy

- Exogamy refers to a social arrangement where marriage is allowed only outside a social group.
- It is usually defined through "KINSHIP" rather than ethnicity, religion and class.

Anuloma Marriage

- Man of higher class, subcaste, family or Gotra is married to such a girl which belongs to a comparatively lower class, caste, subcaste, family or gotra.

Pratiloma Marriage

- It is opposite of Anuloma marriage
- In this, the girl is from higher class, sub-caste and the man is from the lower class or caste.

- Hypogamy became popular (to marry girl of a higher caste or sub-caste)

Advantages	Disadvantages
Came to know about Shudra-Aryan connection	Origin of the practice of untouchability

Forms of Marriage

Based on the recognition type:

- Culturally recognized
- Civil marriage

Civil Marriage

- An application is filed to the registrar of court. As per the Christian Marriage Act, 1872, minimum age of groom should be 16 years and of bride is 13 years, also at the time of marriage none of the spouse of any party should be alive.
- Marriage can be registered under the Hindu Marriage Act, 1955 or under the Special Marriage Act, 1954

Mate Selection in India

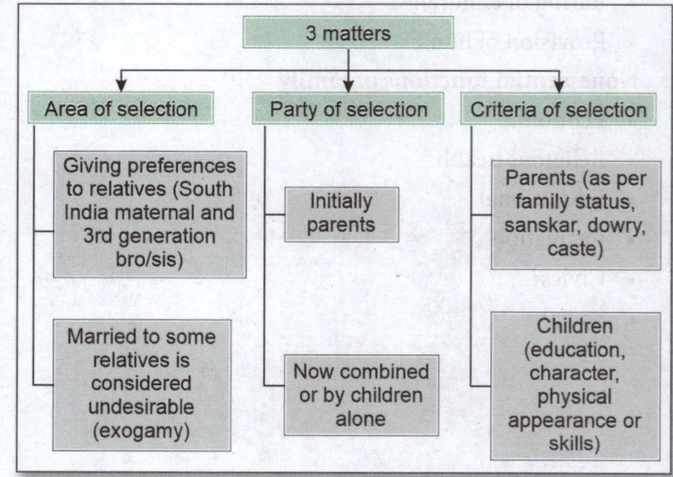

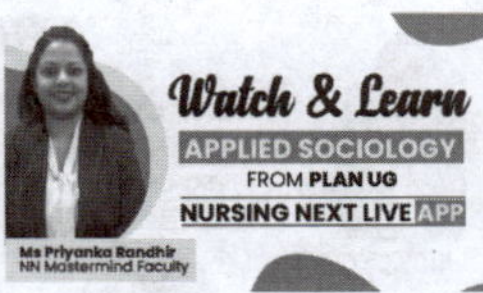

Mate Selection in West

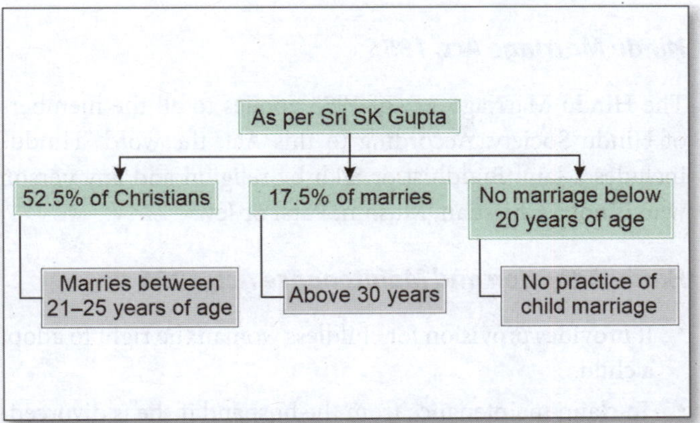

In Christians

- Marriage is done in all except blood relatives
- Can marry sister of deceased wife, widow of deceased brother, daughter of the brother/sister of deceased wife
- No prohibition of Widow remarriage
- No custom of dowry or bride-price
- Independent atmosphere
- Parents or girls or boys can decide from themselves
- In case of traditional marriage, the parents decide
- Love is given preference over religion or caste
- In the "Voice of Christ", it is said that our youths have to take help of their parents. In youth, the emotion of pride and sacrifice is abundant"

Marriages in India

- As per religion
- As per region
- Marriages as per religion
- Buddhist marriage
- Jain marriage
- Christian marriage
- Muslim marriage
- Sikh marriage
- Marriages as per region
- Bengali marriage
- Malyali marriage
- Assamese marriage
- Kannada marriage
- Gujarati marriage
- Kashmiri marriage
- Maharashtrian marriage
- Punjabi marriage
- Marwari marriage
- Pahari marriage

Changing Trends in Marriage

- Today, marriage is no longer a social ritual, it is perceived as "CONTRACT" which can be terminated.
- Inter-caste and love marriages are becoming common
- Cohabitation (Live-in relations)
- Living apart together
- Same-sex marriage (In March 2018, the Indian Supreme Court, in the case of Shakti Vahini vs. Union of India, held that an adult has the fundamental right to marry a person of their choice.)
- Late marriages
- Groom value system is growing
- Increased widow-remarriage
- No compulsion of marriage
- Changes in marriage rituals
- Changes in the way of selecting partners
- Religious type of marriages is becoming feeble
- More of civil marriages
- Romantic-based marriages are seen more because of western influence or due to independent environment.

Importance of Marriage

- Regulation of sex life
- Establishment of the family
- Economic cooperation
- Emotional and intellectual interest stimulation of the partners

LEGISLATION ON INDIAN MARRIAGE AND FAMILY

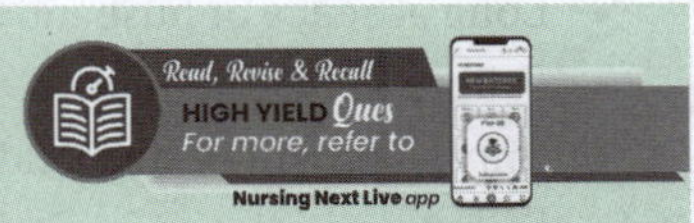

Before Independence

Prevention of Sati Act, 1829

Widows are often forced to make a vow or sankalpa to die after their husband's death.

Child Marriage Restraint Act, 1929

- According to this Act boys under 18 years of age, girls under 14 years of age, if get married is an offense.
- Later the Act was amended in 1978 to 21 years of age for boys and 18 years of age for girls.

Hindu Woman Right to Property Act, 1937

- The Hindu Women's Right to Properties Act, 1937, changed the doctrine of survivorship.
- Under this Act, the widow of a deceased coparcener (joint ownership) of a Mithakshara undivided family will have the same interest which her husband had while he was alive.

Hindu Widow Remarriage Act, 1856

- Salient features of the Hindu Widow Remarriage Act, 1856 are:
  - Widow re-marriage and the children born of such a marriage have been declared valid by section one of this Act.
  - By remarriage the widow loses her right over the property of her husband.
  - According to section 5 of this Act, after her remarriage the widows will enjoy all the rights which a married woman does.
  - If the widow is a minor, then for her remarriage the consent of her parents is necessary.

Christian Marriage Act, 1872

- Section 3 of the Indian Christian Act, 1872 defines the term 'Christian' as "a person professing Christian Religion". Under the Act, Indian Christians include native converts to Christianity and under their Christian descendants.

After Independence

Dissolution of Muslim Marriage Act, 1939

- Grounds of dissolution of marriage under provision of Section 2 of the Act:
  - Long absence of husband
  - Failure to maintain her
  - Imprisonment of husband
  - Failure to perform marital obligations
  - Impotence of husband
  - Insanity, leprosy or venereal diseases
  - Option of puberty
  - Cruelty
  - Other grounds
  - Zihar
  - Khula

Special Marriage Act, 1954

- The provisions of this Act are similar to those of the Hindu Marriage Act of 1955.
  - The special provisions under this Act are:
  - This Act fixed the minimum age of marriage at 21 years and 18 years for boys and girls respectively. And thereby this act is aimed at abolition of the practice of child marriage.
  - Divorce received the legal validity through this Act. This Act recognized the right of a wife and husband to divorce.
  - Through this Act inter-caste marriages received legal validity.

Hindu Marriage Act, 1955

The Hindu Marriage Act of 1955 applies to all the members of Hindu Society. According to this Act, the word "Hindu" includes a Jain, Buddhist or Sikh by religion and any person who is not a Christian, Muslim, Parsi or Jew.

Hindu Adoption and Maintenance Act, 1956

- It provides provision for childless woman the right to adopt a child.
- To claim maintenance from the husband if she is divorced.

Dowry Prohibition Act, 1961

- The main objective of this Act is to abolish the practice of giving and taking dowry at the time of marriage.
- The provisions of this Act were enforced since July 1, 1961.

Medical Termination of Pregnancy Act, 1971

Legalizes abortion conceding the right of a woman to undergo abortion on the ground of physical and mental health.

Muslim Women (Protection and Rights on Divorce) Act, 1986

- This act allegedly protects the rights of Muslim women who have been divorced by, or have obtained divorce from their husbands and to provide for matters connected therewith.
- The act was passed by Rajiv Gandhi government to nullify the decision in Shah Bano case.

Other Recent Acts in India

Recent Changes in Legislation Related to Marriage and Family

- Section 497 under IPC and Section 198 (2) the Criminal Procedure Code
- The triple talaq Act, 2019 or Muslim Women (Protection of Rights on Marriage) Bill, 2019
- Article 377-Homosexuality

New Law Related to Adultery

- **It was under Section 497** of the Indian Penal Code (IPC) a section dealing with adultery.
- Talaq-E-Sunnat
- Talaq-E-Biddat

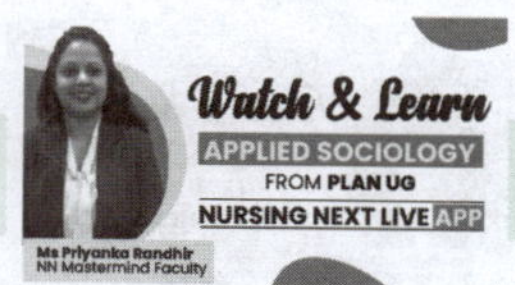

Muslim Women (Protection of Rights on Marriage) Bill, 2019

- Popularly known as "Triple Talaq"
- It was passed by the Indian Parliament as a law on July 30, 2019, to make instant Triple Talaq a criminal offense.
- Muslim men to instantly divorce their wives, to be unconstitutional

Section 377 of IPC: Homosexuality

- The court recognizes sexual orientation as **natural and inherent biological** phenomenon and not a matter of choice.
- The Supreme Court decriminalized consensual intercourse between persons of same sex which provided a huge boost to LGBTQ community
- They can marry each other

INFLUENCE OF MARRIAGE AND FAMILY ON HEALTH AND HEALTH PRACTICES

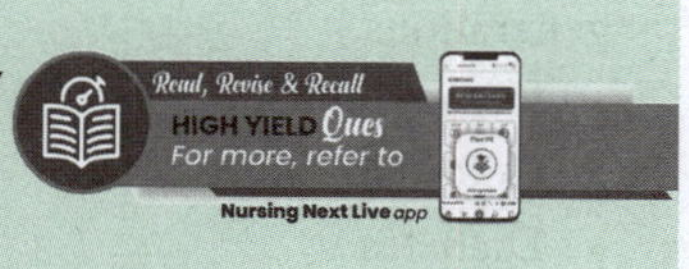

Effects of Marriage and Family on Health

Health Care

- Married people take more health insurance
- Married individuals occupy hospitals and health institutions less often than others (they get discharged sooner)
- Less likely to go to nursing home after hospital

Lifestyle

Married people have fair to good health than widowed, divorced or separated, never-married, or cohabiting persons

Severity of Illness

Married men and women have higher survival rates after being diagnosed with cancer, regardless of the stage of the cancer's progression, than do their unmarried counterparts.

Longevity

- Married couple live longer than others because of low mortality rate among them.
- They include low risk of death from accidents, disease, self-inflicted injuries, and suicide.
- The longer a person's marriage, the lower is their mortality risk, relative to that of the unmarried.
- Having children further reduces the risk of suicide.

Health of Children

- Children in family are more emotional and behavioral well-being than children in cohabiting or step families
- According to the National Survey of Children's Health, children who live with both biological parents score lower on the behavior problems scale (49.0) than those who live with a biological parent and a stepparent (51.8), and children who live with both biological parents or two adoptive parents are more socially developed than those who do not.
- Adolescents who live with both biological parents are less likely to use hard drugs than those living in step-families, those whose parents have divorced, or those raised by a cohabiting single parent
- Similarly, according to the National Longitudinal Study of Adolescent Health, children who live with both biological parents are less likely to get drunk
- Girls raised in intact married families have a later onset of puberty and thus are less likely to experience teenage pregnancy.

The secret of health lies in the homes of the people

—**Florence Nightingale**

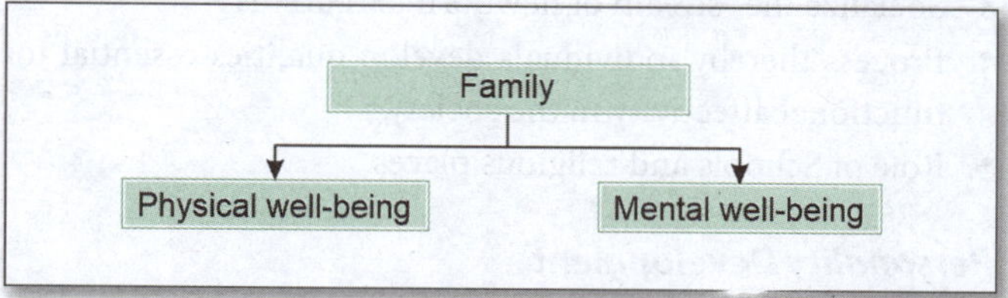

Role of Family in Health and Illness

- Somatic symptoms increase tension among the family members.
- Chronic illness and complicated illness are related to the family functioning.
- Family prestige is affected by mentally retarded child.
- The family will offer remedies and advice.
- To take over the role of the ill person when he/she is no longer capable of performing.
- It will provide care until recovery and long-term support.

Family

- Family is a primary source of many health beliefs and behaviors.
- Family is an important source of stress and social support.
- Physical symptoms may have an adaptive function within the family and be maintained by family patterns.
- Family has an influence on physical and "psychological health and well-being".

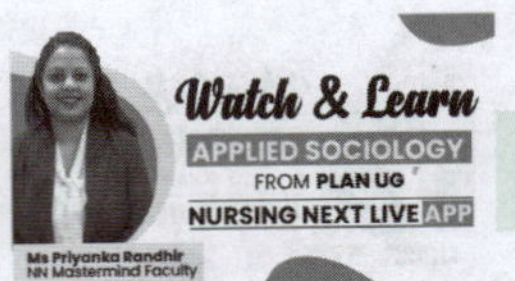

Family and Marriage

- Marriage and family relationships have powerful impact on health outcomes.
- Family members, not health professionals, provide most of health care of for patients.
- Family is a "primary social context" in which health issues are addressed.

Role of Marriage and Family in Health and Disease

Child Rearing

- Physical care of the dependent young
- Differs from society to society
- Capital resources, level of knowledge, state of technology and state of values
- Socially determined by the tradition
- Traditions act as hurdles.
- Patterns of child care: Feeding, nutrition, hygiene, sleep, clothing.

Socialization

- Socialize the "stream of newborn barbarians".
- Process thereby individuals develop qualities essential for functional affectivity in the society.
- Role of Schools and religious places.

Personality Development

- In this, sociology comes in contact with psychology.
- Capacity of an individual to withstand stress and strain is determined by the early experiences in the family.
- Family acts as a "PLACENTA" excluding various influences, modifying others that pass through it in laying foundation of physical, mental and social health of the child.

Care of Dependent

- Care of women during pregnancy and childhood
- Care of the aged
- Care of the handicapped
- Care of the Sick
- Care in Pregnancy
- Family does more nursing than hospital even in highly developed countries.
- Attitude of society to pregnant and childbearing may have an important bearing on the infant deaths, maternal morbidity and mortality

Stabilization of Adult Personality

- Family is like a "shock absorber" to the stress and strains.
- Family provides a basement for relieving the stress.
- Function in stabilization of personality of both adults and children in meeting their emotional needs.

Susceptibility of Family to Disease

- Genes act as a platform for carrying the disease over generations.
  - Hemophilia
  - Color blindness
  - Diabetes
  - Tuberculosis
  - Scabies
  - Measles, mumps, rubella
  - Diphtheria
  - Schizophrenia
  - Psychoneurosis
  - Congenital malformations

Coping with Stressors: Family Problems or Broken Family

- Whole family gets stressed.
- The way in which the family perceives the stressor explains the values and previous experiences of the family in meeting the crisis.
- Acts as a "shock absorber"

CONCEPTUAL EXERCISES

LONG ANSWER QUESTIONS

1. Define family. Explain in detail the role of family on individual's health. (MGR)

Answer

Family: "Family is a group defined by a sex relationship sufficiently precise and enduring to provide for the procreation and upbringing of children."
—**MacIver**

Or

"Family is the logical social unit composed of husband, wife and children."
—**Elliott and Merrill**

Role of Family on Individual's Health

The family is a collection of people who are related biologically. In most societies, this is a relatively common image. Families serve a variety of purposes. From a medical-sociology perspective, there are several activities that are significant and

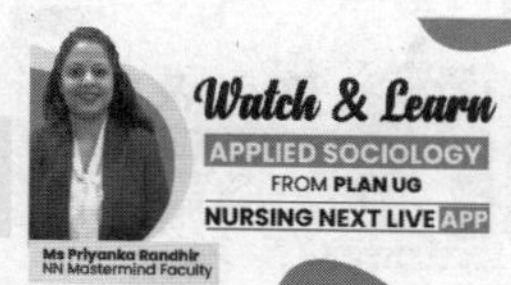

relevant to health and health behaviors. The family plays an important role in:

- **Raising children:** Family is responsible for proper rearing of children and to do so, it functions in different ways by focusing on:
  - Taking physical care of the dependent children in order for them to grow up and support the family.
  - Varying the raising of children depending on the society.
  - Providing financial resources, knowledge, technological conditions, and value system.
  - Incorporating values those are socially predetermined by custom.
  - Physical care for young people in need.
  - Child care routines, such as feeding, nourishment, cleanliness, sleep, and clothing.
- **Socialization:** Family acts as an institution of socialization. The family's second duty is to socialize the "stream of newly-born barbarians". It refers to the process by which people acquire traits necessary for thriving in the society in which they reside. With regard to socialization, it is aimed to impart knowledge, culture, beliefs, and general rules of behavior to children in order to prepare them for participation in the larger society, which includes their family.
- **Personality development:** The ability of a person to withstand stress and strain as well as the way in which he interacts with others are greatly influenced by his early experiences in the family, particularly with the father, mother, and siblings who provide the earliest and most immediate component of the child's external environment. The family acts as a "placenta", excluding various influences like changing those who pass through it and adding some of its own to establish a foundation for the child's physical, mental, and social wellness.
- **Caring for dependent adults:** Care for those who are ill or injured, care for expectant mothers and new mothers, and care for the elderly and handicapped.
  - Adults may become dependent in any type of culture, either intentionally or accidentally.
  - Sickness that results in a fundamental biological restriction on an individual's ability to undertake tasks that are typically expected of adults; the family is burdened with the duty of caring for such individuals.
  - The mother is expected to be the primary caregiver by the family.
  - How well she comprehends sickness and how much confidence she has in her ability to provide nursing care are key factors.
  - Studies have shown that even in highly developed nations, the family provides more nursing care than the hospital.
- **Stabilizing adult personalities:** The family acts as a "shock absorber" to the stresses and strains of life, which might include disruptive emotions, worry, anxiety, worry about the future and economic uncertainty. In these circumstances, the family offers an opportunity for tension release for both adults and children, allowing the person to regain mental equilibrium and work to preserve strong interpersonal connections.

  Alcoholism and drug addiction are other reflections of this trend, which has elevated the relevance of mental illness as a public health issue.

  The family plays a crucial role in the stabilization of the personality of both adults and children as well as in addressing their emotional needs. Certain chronic illnesses, such as peptic ulcer, high blood pressure, rheumatism, and skin diseases, are accepted as stress diseases and have a prominent emotional element in their development.
- **Illness susceptibility in families:** A family's genetic makeup and common surroundings work together to determine each member's susceptibility to disease.
  - It is well established that some illnesses, including mental illness, diabetes, color blindness, and hemophilia, run in families.
  - There is evidence that schizophrenia, psychoneurosis, and some types of mental illness can run in families.
  - Common cold, scabies, diphtheria, measles, mumps, rubella, chicken pox, dysentery, diarrhea, and enteric fever are just a few examples of communicable diseases that are known to spread quickly in families due to the shared environment that family members share.
  - It is also generally accepted that consanguineous children have a higher incidence of congenital malformation than nonconsanguineous children.
- **Broken families:** A broken family is one in which the parents have divorced or when one or both of the parents have passed away.
  - The development of a kid is influenced by both parental and dual-parental separation, both of which are known as paternal and dual-parental separation, respectively.
  - Early victims of broken families have been observed to occasionally exhibit later psychopathic behavior, immature personality, and even retardation in development, speech, and intelligence.
  - Children from these families may become involved in crime, prostitution, or vagrancy.
- **Family problems:** In these families, the standards of life are generally far below the accepted minimum and parents are unable to meet the physical and emotional needs of their children.
  - The home life is utterly unsatisfactory.

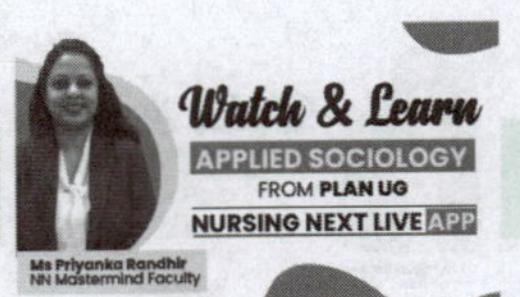

- The underlying factors in most family problems are usually those of personality and of relationship, backwardness, poverty, illness, mental and emotional instability, character defects and marital disharmony.

2. Define family. Explain its functions. (MGR, KUHS)

Answer

Family: "Family is a group defined by a sex relationship sufficiently precise and enduring to provide for the procreation and upbringing of children." —**MacIver**

Functions of Family

Due to the functional significance of the family, it serves as the foundation of all social organizations. The roles that families play are varied in kind.

According to MacIver, there are two categories of family functions:

1. Essential functions
2. Non-essential functions

Essential functions: Some family duties are essential to the unit's continuing survival; therefore, these functions are known as the essential of "primary" functions of the family. They are referred to as **"essential family functions"** and are explained below:

- **Stable satisfaction of sex need:** Satisfying sexual needs is the primary purpose of the family. Most societies recognize and approve of husband-and-wife's sexual encounters as acceptable. Families are created to give spouses a lifetime of companionship. Additionally, it prevents uncertainty and sex conflict. In a similar vein, families support improved personality development and sexual harmony.
- **Procreation and rearing:** The continuation of the family is yet another crucial family function. Consequently, procreation becomes crucial. A newborn human kid is unable to survive on its own. During its extended infancy, it needs its parents' assistance. As the children must be raised to have legal standing, the parents are required to provide for their basic needs such as care, education, and socialization. Family can efficiently create the fundamental foundation for a person's personality. Even the process of child rearing contributes to how an individual's personality develops in the family.
- **Provision of a home:** Families give their members a place to live. Both men and women have a great yearning for their own homes. Despite the fact that they are frequently delivered in hospitals or maternity homes, children are ultimately cared for and supported at home. Even parents who work outside rely on their house for comfort, security, and tranquilly. The comfort of home never changes.
- **Socialization:** The family acts as a socializing agent. Socialization is the process through which a person internalizes the norms of his community to become a separate, autonomous self. The values, morality, beliefs, and ideals of society are inculcated in the child through the family. It acquaints its children with a wider culture and prepares them for engagement in a greater world.
- **Affectional function:** Both physical and mental requirements are present in a man. Both of these must be met in order for the condition to be satisfied. Family is a social structure that offers its members protection and mental or emotional fulfillment. For all of its members, the family is the setting that fosters the closest and most precious relationships. The first time someone is shown affection is by his or her parents or siblings, who show them to that person. An infant's capacity to thrive is harmed by lack of affection. Never having been loved makes a person rarely joyful.

Nonessential functions: These functions are also known as the "secondary functions" and include:

- **Economic functions:** The needs of the family's members in terms of money are met. This has been the family's traditional role. In the past, the family served as an economic unit. The economic function of the modern family has significantly changed in recent years. Industrialization has had an impact on the family. The factory is now where most of the work is produced, rather than at home.
- **Educational functions:** The foundation for the child's formal education is provided by the family. Despite significant changes, the family continues to provide the child with the fundamental socialization that is necessary for an adult to participate in social life.
- **Religious functions:** The family serves as the children's primary place of religious instruction. The youngsters pick up religious qualities from their parents. The homes used to be placed of pilgrimage as well. The family used to instruct the kids on moral principles, religious beliefs, and methods of worship. Even now, the family is where the moral principles that will guide the children throughout their lives are established. With its members, the family satisfies spiritual requirements. The religious heritage is passed down to the following generation through the family.
- **Recreational functions:** In the past, recreation was mostly focused on the family. It encouraged a strong sense of unity. The whole family came together by reading aloud, visiting relatives, family reunions, church socials, singing, dancing, playing indoor games, etc. The organization of recreation

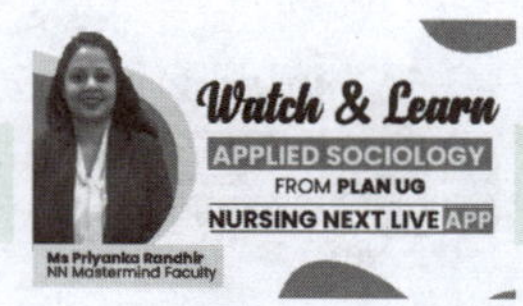

away from the family is growing. Modern leisure is not intended for involvement by the entire family.

3. Elaborate on: (MGR)

a. **What is marriage?**
b. **Write in detail about types and functions of marriage.**
c. **Discuss the family, marriage, and their influence on health and health practices.**

Answer

Marriage

"Marriage is a relatively permanent bond between permissible mates." **—Robert H Lowie**

Marriage is a "contract for the production and maintenance of children." **—Malinowski**

Types of Marriage

The main types of marriages are:

- **Polygyny:** Polygyny is a form of marriage in which one man married more than one woman at a given time. It was commonly practiced in ancient civilization. It is of two types:
  1. Sororal polygyny
  2. Non-sororal polygyny
- **Polyandry:** Polyandry is the marriage of one woman with several men. It is of two types:
  1. Fraternal polyandry
  2. Non-fraternal polyandry
- **Monogamy:**
  - Monogamy is a form of marriage in which one man marries the woman.
  - It is most common form of the marriage and it is universally practiced providing marital opportunity and satisfaction to all the individuals.
  - It is of two types:
    1. Serial monogamy
    2. Straight monogamy
- **Group marriage:** Group marriage means the marriage of two or more women with two or more men.

b. **Write in detail about types and functions of marriage.**

Answer

Functions of Marriage

- **Biological function:** The society gives recognition to children born out of wedlock and the children thus born are ascribed status as per the norms of the society. So, children are the most important aspect of marriage.
- **Economic cooperation:** Marriage results in an economic co-operation between men and women ensuring the survival of every individual in a society. It act as a protective measure wherein the men share their income with the wives
- **Social function:** A marriage provide the status to both husband and wife in a society and thus, they are also collectively accepted by society as husband and wife. Marriage is the foundation of a family.
- **Emotional and intellectual interest:** Marriage is responsible for enhanced emotional and intellectual interest not between individuals but also in their families and groups. Friendship between groups is increased through marriage

c. **Discuss the family, marriage, and their influence on health and health practices.**

Answer

Influence of Family and Marriage on Health and Health Practices

"Social Institutions are the structures devised to of a particular social group". **—MacIver and Page**

Family: "Family is a system of relationship existing between parents and children." **—Clare**

Marriage: "Marriage is a dividing line between the family of orientation and family of procreation in terms of the nature of roles one perform in the two families." **—Koos**

Family and marriage both influence the health and health practices as:

- **Health care:** Family unity has a negative (declining) impact on public health care and a good (rising) impact on the availability of private health care. Married people are more likely to have health insurance, frequent hospitals and other medical facilities, and stay in hospitals for shorter durations. Additionally, they are less likely to leave the hospital for a nursing home. The effects of marriage on one's health are also felt.
- **Lifestyle:** Compared to those who are widowed, divorced or separated, never married, or cohabit, married people have a reduced rate of bad health. Compared to cohabiters, married people are less likely to smoke or binge drink, but married men are more likely to do so. Young adults who are married are less likely to be alcoholics than those who are singles.
- **Severe diseases:** Regardless of the cancer's stage of development, married men and women had higher survival odds after receiving a cancer diagnosis. The way married people react to cancer therapy is better and on par with

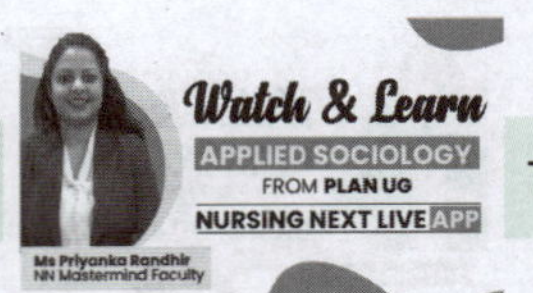

those who are 10 years younger. Married males experience higher three-year (breast cancer-specific) morbidity and survive longer after prostate cancer diagnosis. Compared to never-married, divorced, and widowed people, married people are less likely to pass away after being hospitalized for a heart attack and have higher stroke risks. A person's mental health can gain greatly from marriage as well.

- **Longevity:** People who are married live longer and are less likely to die from suicide, self-inflicted injuries, illness, and accidents. Divorced or separated people have an 83% greater risk of suicide, never-married people have a 48% higher risk, and bereaved people have a 41% higher risk. Marriages without children have a 33% lower suicide risk than adult singles, but those with kids have a 48% reduced risk.
- **Pregnancy and STIs:** Compared to single mothers, married mothers consistently avoid dangerous substances and practice superior prenatal care. Compared to mothers who live together permanently or mothers who have a romantic involvement with their child's father, married mothers are less likely to give birth to low birth weight babies. Women who are married have a lot less abortions than single woman.
- **Health of children:** Children and teenagers from intact marital families are better off emotionally and behaviorally than those from step families or cohabiting households. Children who live with both biological parents or two adoptive parents have more developed social skills than those who do not, according to the National Survey of Children's Health. Additionally, children who live with both biological parents or two adoptive parents have lower behavior problem scores than children who live with a biological parent and a stepparent. Adolescents who live with both of their biological parents are less likely to use hard drugs than those reared by a cohabiting single parent, stepfamilies, or stepparents. Children who live with both biological parents are less likely to develop behavioral problems. Similarly, kids who live with both of their biological parents are less likely to drink, according to the National Longitudinal Study of Adolescent Health.

4. Write an essay on family and its role in individual's health. (MGR)

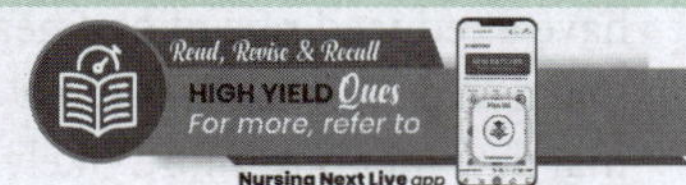

Answer

Families offer the encouragement and surroundings necessary for healthy living, disease prevention, and chances for early detection and treatment to avoid or delay problems. The socioeconomic determinants of health must always be taken into account for interventions to improve health to be effective.

- No matter how a family is structured—joint or nuclear—it will always be essential to a child's upbringing, socialization, and development. It can also act as a support system for other family members and have a profound impact on both positive and negative behaviors that have an impact on one's health as well as provide opportunities and role models for healthy living.
- Family circumstances affect early childhood development, particularly the social/emotional and language/cognitive domains, which in turn affects health. Adopting a life-course perspective focuses on how social determinants of health operate at every stage of development, including early childhood, childhood, adolescence, adulthood, and on age, to both directly influence health and serve as the foundation for health or illness in later stages of the life-course.
- Women traditionally have a significant impact on the health of the family. Their social standing, level of education, job, and cultural norms that support or restrict them from making family decisions all have an impact on how well they carry out this function.
- Family members can serve as role models for healthy behavior in addition to participating in health campaigns.
- Family members can encourage us in our efforts to adopt healthy habits.
- Teenagers who abstained from drug usage believed that their parents understood them more than teenagers who used drugs, according to research by Robert Coombs and his colleagues from 1991. Additionally, those who did not take drugs said that their parents had the biggest influence on them, but those who did said that their friends had the biggest impact.
- Families can alter children's access to healthy foods, in addition to modeling good habits. For instance, Michael Resnick and his colleagues (1997) discovered that the ease of access to cigarettes, alcohol, and marijuana among teenagers in the United States was related to their usage of these substances.
- Numerous studies have shown that during adolescence, one's views and behaviors toward their health are influenced by their family, friends, and school. In their longitudinal US study on adolescent health, Resnick and his colleagues (1997) discovered that, with the exception of prior pregnancies, parent-family connectedness and perceived school connectedness were barriers to every health risk behavior they had measured (emotional distress, suicidal thoughts and behaviors, violence, substance use, and sexual-risk behaviors).

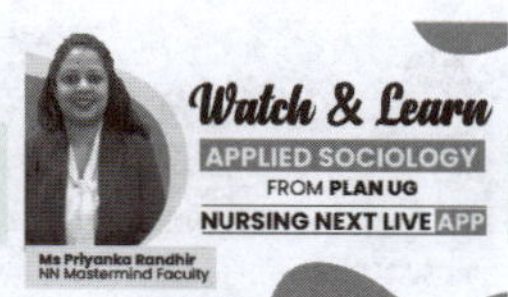

SHORT NOTES

1. Essential functions of family. (MGR)

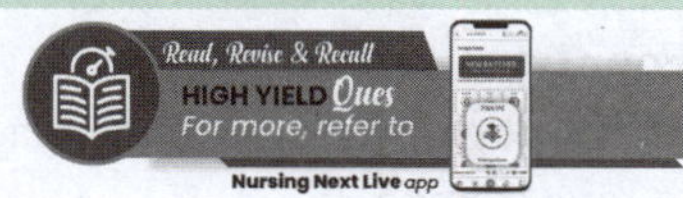

Answer

MacIver classifies the functions of family into two types—essential and nonessential functions.

Essential functions: Some family duties are essential to the unit's continuing survival; therefore, these functions are known as the essential of "primary" functions of the family. They are referred to as **"essential family functions" which are as follows:**

- **Stable satisfaction of sex need:** Satisfying sexual needs is the primary purpose of the family. Most societies recognize and approve of husband-and-wife's sexual encounters as acceptable. Families are created to give spouses a lifetime of companionship. Additionally, it prevents uncertainty and sex conflict. In a similar vein, families support improved personality development and sexual harmony.
- **Procreation and rearing:** The continuation of the family is yet another crucial family function. Consequently, procreation becomes crucial. A newborn human kid is unable to survive on its own. During its extended infancy, it needs its parents' assistance. As the children must be raised to have legal standing, the parents are required to provide for their basic needs such as care, education, and socialization. Family can efficiently create the fundamental foundation for a person's personality. Even the process of child rearing contributes to how an individual's personality develops in the family.
- **Provision of a home:** Families give their members a place to live. Both men and women have a great yearning for their own homes. Despite the fact that they are frequently delivered in hospitals or maternity homes, children are ultimately cared for and supported at home. Even parents who work outside rely on their house for comfort, security, and tranquilly. The comfort of home never change.
- **Socialization:** The family acts as a socializing agent. Socialization is the process through which a person internalizes the norms of their community to become a separate, autonomous self. The values, morality, beliefs, and ideals of society are inculcated in the child through the family. It acquaints its children with a wider culture and prepares them for engagement in a greater world.
- **Affectional function:** Both physical and mental requirements are present in man. Both of these must be met in order for the condition to be satisfied. Family is a social structure that offers its members protection and mental or emotional fulfillment. For all of its members, the family is the setting that fosters the closest and most precious relationships. The first time someone is shown affection is by his or her parents or siblings, who show them to that person. An infant's capacity to thrive is harmed by lack of affection. A person who has never been loved, can't be joyful.

2. Conditions of marriage. (MGR)

Answer

Marriage: "Marriage is the approved social pattern whereby two or more persons establish a family." **—Horton and Hunt**

Conditions of Marriage

Section 5 of the Hindu Marriage Act of 1955 stipulates five requirements for a legally binding Hindu marriage.

According to Section 5, a marriage between two Hindus may be ordained if the following requirements are met:

- Existing partner at the time of the marriage: Neither party to the marriage should have an existing spouse.
- Neither partner to the marriage should be unable to give a legally binding consent at the time of the wedding.
- At the time of marriage, despite being able to give a legally binding agreement, the person has a mental disorder of any kind or to any degree that renders them unfit for marriage or childbearing.
- Has experienced repeated episodes of lunacy at the time of marriage.
- The betrothed and groom must be at least 18 and 21 years old, respectively. (Now amended)
- The partners must not be in a relationship that is prohibited in any way. The only exception to this rule is given if the usage or tradition governing them permits such a union.
- There can be no sapinda relationships between the participants. The parties' ruling customs or usages permit an exception to this, though.

SHORT ANSWER QUESTIONS

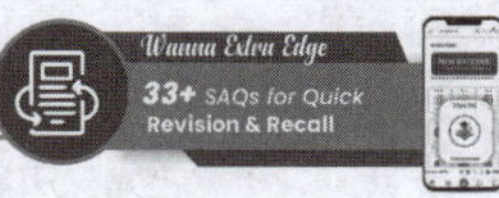

1. Define joint family.

Answer

Joint Family

According to Dr Irawati Karve, "a group of people who generally live under one roof, who eat food cooked at one hearth, who hold property in common, who participate in common family worship and who are related to each other."

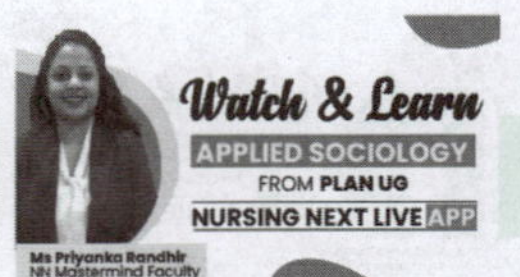

2. Meaning of polygamy marriage.

Answer

Polygamy is a form of marriage where one man marries more than one woman at a given time. In India, various religious and tribal communities follow this form of marriage.

It is further divided into two types:

1. **Polygamy:** Polygamy is a form of marriage in which men have more than one wife.
2. **Polyandry:** It is a form of marriage in which women have more than one husband.

3. What is extended family?

Answer

Extended family is a form of family that consists of three or more generations who live together. It is a type of family containing relatives (aunts, uncles, grandparents, and cousins) in addition to the nuclear family. The extended family is the most common type of family throughout the world. Extended families include at least three generations such as grandparents, married offspring, and grandchildren.

4. Mention any four types of marriage.

Answer

Four types of marriage are:

1. **Monogamy:** Form of marriage in which one man marries one woman.
2. **Isogamy:** Marriage takes place between the individuals of two equal social status families
3. **Anisogamy:** Marriage alliance or agreement is done between two individuals belonging to different social status families. It is further described in two forms—Hypergamy and Hypogamy.
4. **Levirate marriage:** Levirate marriage is a type of marriage in which the woman marries her husband's brother after his death.

5. List out two merits of joint family system.

Answer

Two merits of joint family system:

1. Greater support system as grandparents or other members are always there.
2. Greater bond of unity and affection and sharing and adjustment among members.

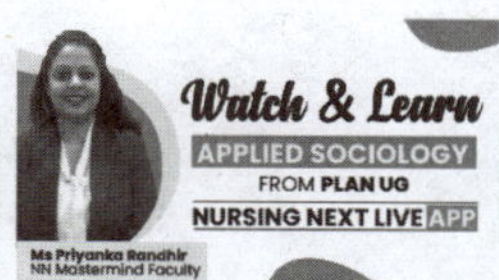

CONCEPTUAL REVISION

MULTIPLE CHOICE QUESTIONS

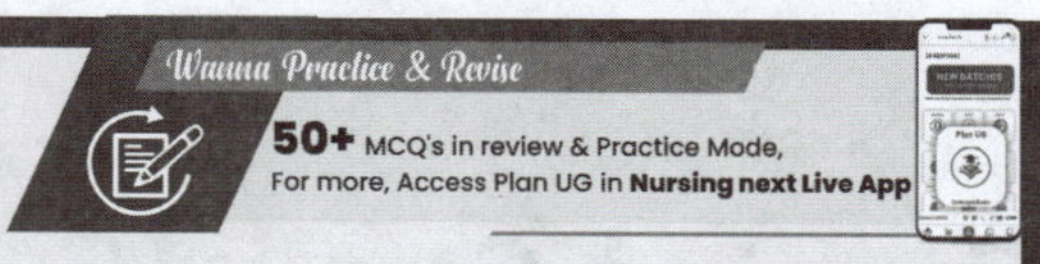

1. **"Family is the logical social unit composed of husband, wife and children". Who said this?**
   a. Clare   b. MacIver
   c. Elliott and Merrill   d. Anthony Giddens

Ans. c. Elliott and Merrill

2. **The system under which woman can marry more than one husband and keep all of them with herself is known as:**
   a. Polyandrous   b. Polygamous
   c. Patronymic   d. Procreation

Ans. a. Polyandrous

3. **MacIver argued that the two main functions of the modern family were:**
   a. Secondary socialization and strict discipline
   b. Emotional support and sexual gratification
   c. Primary socialization and personality stabilization
   d. Essential and nonessential

Ans. d. Essential and nonessential

4. **In some communities, the groom's family compensates the bride's family for her hand in marriage. This is the practice of:**
   a. Bride service   b. Bride wealth
   c. Dowry   d. Groom wealth

Ans. b. Bride wealth

5. **The Komachi are a patrilineal society. In patrilineal societies, inheritances:**
   a. Pass through the male line usually from father to son
   b. Pass through the male line usually from mother's brother to son
   c. Pass through the female line usually from mother to daughter
   d. Pass through the female line usually from mother to son

Ans. a. Pass through the male line usually from father to son

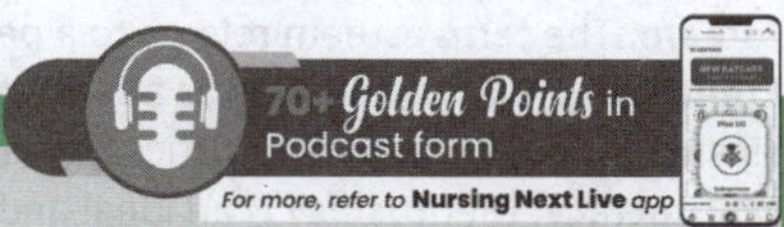

Golden Points

- Family is the most distinct primary group in the society.
- "Family is a group defined by a sex relationship sufficiently precise and enduring to provide for the procreation and upbringing of children." —**MacIver**
- Six basic functions of family by **William Ogburn** include:
  1. Reproduction
  2. Protection
  3. Socialization
  4. Regulation of sexual behavior
  5. Companionship
  6. Provision of social status
- Types of family are:
  - Family of orientation
  - Family of procreation
  - Monogamous family
  - Polygynous family
  - Polyandrous family
  - Matrilocal family
  - Patrilocal family
  - Matrilineal family
  - Patrilineal family
  - Matriarchy family
  - Patriarchy family
  - Conjugal family
  - Consanguine family
  - Nuclear family
  - Joint family
  - Extended family
- In addition to birth planning, family welfare also refers to the overall welfare of the family as a whole through comprehensive family health care.
- Marriage is very important institution which eventually leads to establishment of family.
- According to Gillin and Gillin, "Marriage is a socially approved way of establishing a family of procreation."
- Forms of marriage are:
  - Monogamy
  - Polygamy

CHAPTER

5

Social Stratification

CONCEPTUAL THEORY

Terminology

150+ key terminologies for Quick Recall & Revision

Achieved status: The class structure is not dependent on birth; as a person matures, the status must be earned on their own merits.

Ascribed social status: A position that is naturally granted and obtained by birth without any effort or hard work.

Capitalism: Capitalism is an economic system in which the means of production are predominantly held by private sector and the major motive for economic activity is profit accumulation.

Caste: Caste is a hereditary endogamous social group in which a person's rank and associated rights and obligations are determined by his birth into a certain social group.

Class: Max Weber defined a class as a group of people who have similar levels of wealth and income.

Class system: A class system is a social hierarchy that is mostly based on economic position, and achieved traits can impact social mobility.

Estate system: Peasants were compelled to work on land leased to them by nobility in exchange for military protection and other duties under the "estate" system, often known as feudalism.

Esteem: The term esteem relates to a person's reputation within an occupation or within a society.

Ethnicity: Ethnicity is defined as a sense of shared ancestry based on cultural attachments, linguistic heritage, religious affiliations, claimed kinship, or physical characteristics. Racial identities are commonly understood to include a variety of ethnic identities.

Meritocracy: Meritocracy is an ideal and another system of stratification based on the premise that social stratification is determined by personal effort or merit.

Open system: The open system is a social system in which each individual's position is influenced by his or her earned rank.

Power: Power is the ability to impose one's will on others.

Prestige: The phrase prestige refers to a profession's recognition and adoration in society.

Race: Biesanz defined race as "a large group distinguished by inherited physical characteristics."

Social group: According to Weber, a social group is a collection of people who share the same prestige or lifestyle. An individual obtains prestige through belonging to a desirable group, such as the engineering or medical professions.

Social stratification: According to Raymond W. Murray, "social stratification is a horizontal division of society into higher and lower social units."

SOCIAL STRATIFICATION

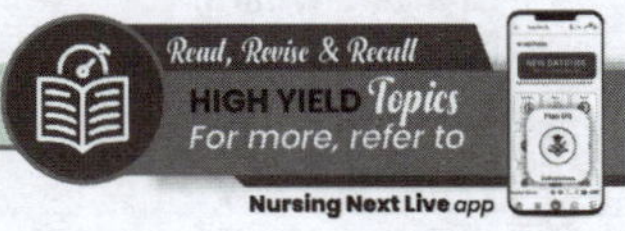

Introduction

- Every society is divided into more or less distinct groups.
- Even the most primitive societies had some form of social stratification.
- Stratification involves the distribution of unequal rights and privileges among the members of a society. Social stratification means division of society into social classes, therefore now, we shall examine the idea of a social class.

Definitions

- "The process by which the individuals and groups are ranked more or less enduring hierarchy of status is known as stratification." **—Ogburn and Nimkoff**
- "Social stratification is horizontal division of society into higher and lower social units." **—R W Murray**

Characteristics of Social Stratification

According to Malvin M. Tumin:

- Stratification is social

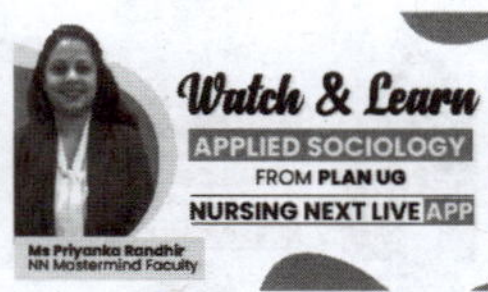

- Stratification is universal
- Stratification is consequential

Types of Social Stratification

- Open
- Closed

Forms of Social Stratification

- Primitive communism
- Slavery
- Caste
- Estate

By Max Weber

(Three Component Theory)

1. **Class**
   - As per the income of the person
   - His economic status in society
   - Set of people with similar accounts or wealth
2. **Party (power)**
   - When the person has the ability to make his way in spite of resistance.
   - A set of people with similar set of powers
3. **Status**
   - Social honor, prestige and popularity in society.
   - Set of people with similar social prestige or positive regard from members of the society

FUNCTIONS OF STRATIFICATION

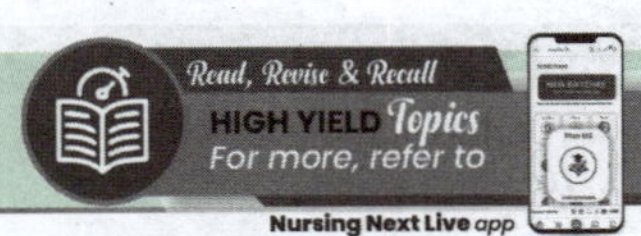

Functions of Social Stratification

- Hard work
- Values, talent
- Proper use of resources
- Economic satisfaction
- Social control

Dimensions of Social Stratification

- **Power:** Based on ability to achieve goals
- **Wealth:** Based on economic status
- **Prestige:** Approved and respected by the members of society

Process of Social Stratification

- **Differentiation of statuses:** Give social position/distinctive roles. E.g.,: mother, father
- **Ranking of statuses:** People having same characteristics
- **Evaluation:** Scale of value use (superior/inferior, better/worse, more/less)
- **Rewarding:** As per the social norms, rewards and punishments are given

Consequences of Social Stratification

Longevity

- Social disparity
- Unequal access to wealth, power and prestige

Family Life

Single-parent family-contributes to economical and social instability.

Health and Illness

High mortality, lower levels of health insurance

Childbearing

Lower class people have more children but poor rearing as compared to others.

Politics

Upper class individuals have greater **political** participation and greater **political** influence than those in lower positions.

Crime and Criminal Justice

Because certain populations are forced into positions of **social** inequality, **crime** becomes more common within those populations.

INDIAN CASTE SYSTEM

Read, Revise & Recall HIGH YIELD Topics For more, refer to Nursing Next Live app

Definitions

- "When a class is somewhat strictly hereditary we may call it as "caste". —**C H Cooley**
- "A caste is a closed group". —**Majumdar**
- "Caste status is wholly predetermined so that men are born to their lot without any hope of changing it, then class takes the extreme form of caste". —**A W GREEN**

Origin of Caste System

- Traditional theory
- Theory of cultural integration
- Occupational theory
- Political theory
- Evolutionary theory

Some other Theories of Caste System In India

- Abbe Dubois
- JH Hutton
- Herbert Risley

Characteristics of Caste System

- Segmental Division of the Society
- *Hierarchy of Status*
- Restrictions on food Habit
- Restrictions on Occupation
- Social and Religious Disabilities
- Restrictions on Marriage

POSITIVE AND NEGATIVE IMPACT OF CASTE IN SOCIETY

Positive Effects of Caste System

- Spirit of cooperation
- Provides a definite social environment
- Defines economic pursuit
- Racial purity
- Separation of social life from political life
- As constitution of Hindu society

Negative Effects of Caste System

- No scope for social mobility
- Untouchability
- Social disunity
- Wrong man in wrong occupation
- Social disunity
- Threat to national unity
- Scope for religious conversion

CLASS SYSTEM AND STATUS

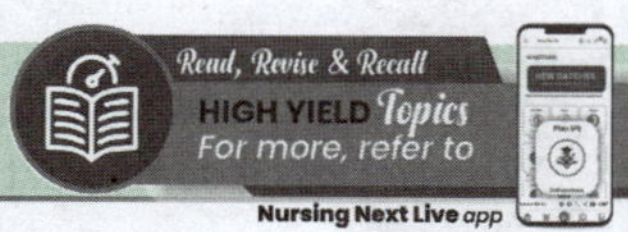

Definitions of Class System

- **Lapiere:** "A social class is a culturally defined group that is accorded a particular position or status within the population as a whole."
- **MacIver:** "A social class is a portion of community marked off from the rest by social status."

Characteristics of Class System

Hierarchy: Just like caste groups, classes also have a hierarchical order in relation to each other.

Open system: Class is an open system, because a person can change his status by his efforts.

Class is achieved: It is not based on birth like the caste but is achieved by individual qualities.

Common mode of life: People of same social class have usually a common mode of life and this may differentiate from other classes.

Social status determined by class: A person's status is more or less determined by the class to which he belongs.

Other Characteristics (On the Basis of Mode of Earning Livelihood)

- Business class
- Professional class
- Labor class

Other Characteristics (On the Basis of Economic Condition)

- Upper class
- Middle class
- Lower class

Other Characteristics (On the Basis of Educational Achievement)

- Educated
- Less educated
- Uneducated

Caste versus Class

Caste	Class
Particular: The caste system with all its peculiarities is unique to India, hence, it is not universal.	**Universal:** The class system is universal in nature. It is found in almost all the modern complex societies.
Ascribed status: Status is ascribed to the individual by birth. Birth is the criterion of the status and not achievement. Status can neither be changed nor be improved.	**Achieved status:** Status is achieved by the individual. There is scope for achievement. Hence status can be changed or improved.
Closed system: Caste system is a closed system. It restricts social mobility in the movement of people from one social status to that of others.	**Class is an open system:** It provides for social mobility. Individuals can move from the lower class to the upper class.
Endogamous group: Caste is an endogamous social group. Accordingly, every caste member has to marry within the group, select the life partner from his own caste system. Intercaste marriages are not allowed.	**A class is not an endogamous group:** The members are free to select their life partner from any one belonging to the class.
Divine origin: The caste system is believed to have a divine origin. It is closely associated with Hindu traditions.	**Secular:** The class system is secular. It has nothing to do with religion. It has been given no religious explanations.

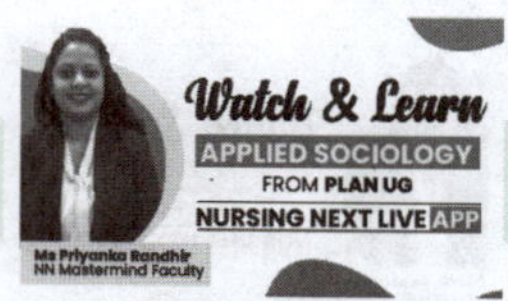

SOCIAL MOBILITY

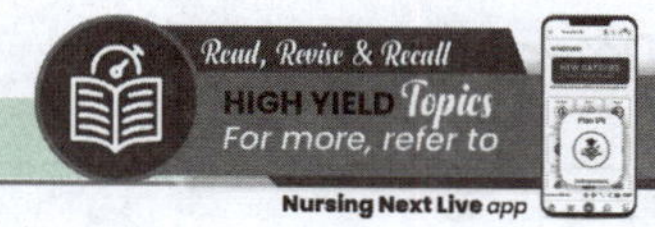

Definitions of Social Mobility

- Social mobility refers to movements up and down in social status. —**Hartone and Hunt**
- "Social mobility refers to the movement of a person from one social status to another." —**Wallace and Wallace**
- "Social mobility refers to the movement of an individual or group from one social position, class or social stratum to another." —**W P Scott**

Characteristics of Social Mobility

- Related to status of a person
- Related to change in status
- Change-multidirectional
- Mobility found in urban, industrial societies

Classification of Social Mobility—(Sorokin)

- **Horizontal:** Movement on the same level
  Example: A factory worker finds a new job in construction
- **Vertical:** Movement — upward and downward
  Example: A factory worker gets educated and becomes a business tycoon

Vertical Social Mobility

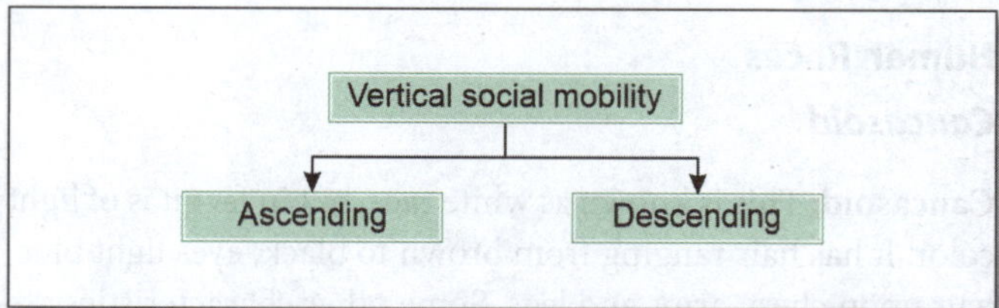

Figure 5.1: Classification of social mobility—(Sorokin)

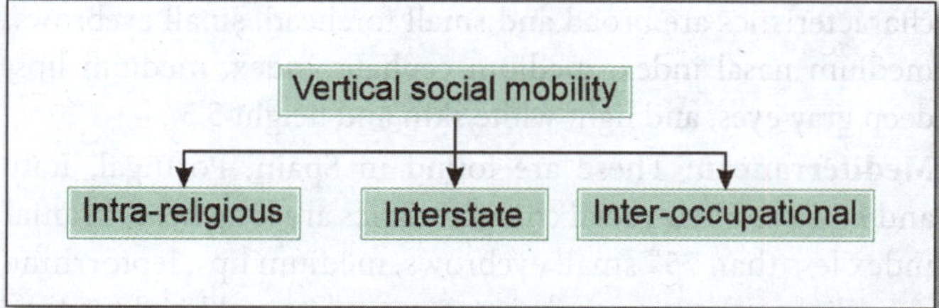

Figure 5.2: Classification of social mobility—(Lipset, Bondix)

Classification of Social Mobility-Lipset, Bondix

- **Intra-generational occupational mobility:** Change in occupation within one's life
- **Inter-generational occupational mobility:** Descending adoption of profession by next generation

Classification of Social Mobility—J H Kohl

- Productive mobility
- Migratory mobility
- Technical mobility

Factors Affecting Social Mobility

- Achievements and failures
- Motivation
- Education
- Skills and training
- Migration
- Industrialization
- Urbanization
- Politicization
- Legislation
- Modernization

Causes of Social Mobility

- Geographical causes
- Political, economic causes
- Desire to have better living standard
- Desire to have higher education
- Development of communication and media

Advantages of Social Mobility

- Betterment in living standards
- Increase in national unity
- Projection of different ideas
- Tendency to personal freedom
- End of obsolete customs

Disadvantages of Social Mobility

- Ethnic and cultural problems
- Unequal division of population
- Unemployment
- Increase in crime

RACE — CONCEPT, CRITERIA OF RACIAL CLASSIFICATION

Introduction to Race

- Race is a group, which has a common set of innate physical characteristics and a geographical origin within a certain area.

- Historically, three diagnostic traits have been used to divide the human species into races: Skin color, hair form, and various combinations of nose, face and lip shape.

Concept of Race

Historical Evidences of Race

14th to 18th Century

Monogenism: Racial classification by origin

18th to 19th Century

Polygenism: Emphasis on hierarchy of races/inheritance of traits

Early 19th Century

Evolutionism: Races evolved; dominance of Europeans seen

Late 19th Century

Race was considered a factor to determine social standing and culture.

19th to 20th Century

Race as ethnicity; determines political strategy.

Viewpoint of Other Sociologists

- **Skin color:** The Caucasian "race",
- **Religion:** The Jewish "race"
- **Nationality:** The British "race"
- **Entire human species:** The human "race"

Sociologist's Definition of Race

"A category of people who have been singled out as inferior or superior, often on the basis of real or alleged physical characteristics such as skin color, hair texture, eye shape, or other subjectively selected attributes."

Interracial Marriage in History

An interracial marriage in 1864.

Definitions of Race

- **J Biesanz and M Biesanz:** "A race is a large group of people distinguished by inherited physical differences."
- **A L Kroeber:** "A race is a valid biological concept. It is a group united by heredity, a breed or genetic strain or subspecies."

Determinants of Race

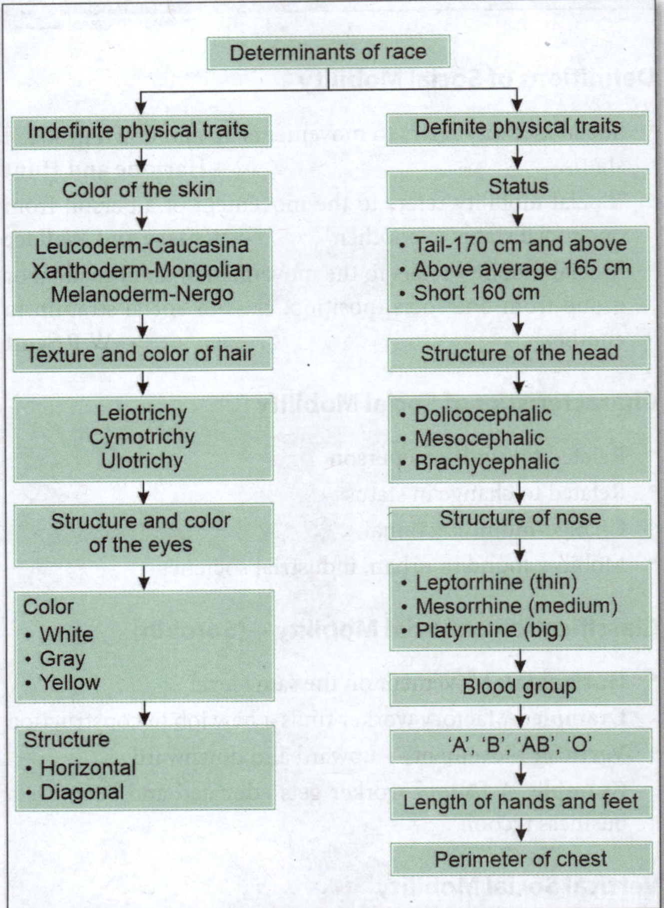

Human Races

Caucasoid

Caucasoid: This is known as white race, but in fact it is of light color. It has hair ranging from brown to black, eyes light blue, hair upon chest, arms and legs. Some other characteristics are medium to high structure, thin lips, etc.

Alpine: This race is found in Central Asia. Its important racial characteristics are broad and small forehead, small eyebrows, medium nasal index, medium cephalic index, medium lips, deep gray eyes, and light white skin and height 5'5".

Mediterranean: These are found in Spain, Portugal, Italy and France. Their racial characteristics are long head, cranial index less than 75", small eyebrows, medium lips, leptorrhine nose, light gray eyes, curly hairs, gray skin and height 5'4".

Nordic: The important characteristics of this race are high forehead, leptorrhine nose, thin lips, blue eyes, yellow hairs, white or red color of the skin, 5' 8" average height. The Nordic people are not only superior physically but also intellectually. They are mostly found in Scandinavia, Baltic and British Island.

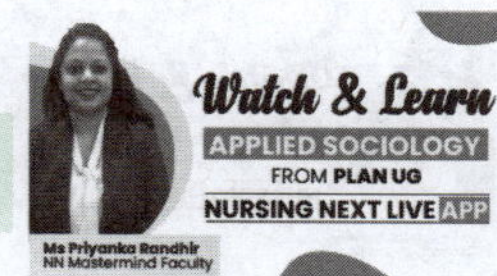

Mongoloid

Mongoloid: This race is mostly found in Asia particularly in Central Asia. Its physical characteristics are gray-eyes, yellow complexion, black hair on the body, flat nose, broad face and medium height. This group includes the following races.

Asian mongol: These are found in China, Japan, and East India.

Micronesian polynesian: These are found in the eastern islands of Melanesia. Their racial characteristics are highhead, thick lips, yellow or brown skin, few hairs on the head and the average height at 5 ft.

Negroid

The Negroid are found in Africa. Some scholars call it the first human race. Their important characteristics are black skin, wooly hair, broad nose, thick lips, high head and average height 5'6". These include the following races:

Negro: These are found in Africa.

Far eastern pygmy: These are found in Andaman and Philippines. Their average height is about 5 ft. only.

Melanesian: These are found in the South Pacific Islands. Their characteristics are as those of Negroes.

Bushman and Hottentots: These are found in Kalahari Desert of Africa. Their average height is less than 5 ft.

Australoid

Australoid: These are found in Australia. Their racial characteristics are: High head, low forehead, big and broad nose, medium lips, gray eyes, wavy hair and average height about India is often regarded as an "Ethnological museum." We find here people belonging to different ethnic groups.

Risley's Racial Classification

Sir Herbert Risley: A British ethnographer, attempted the first classification of Indian races in the census of 1901. On the basis of the census data, he tried to give a relatively scientific basis of racial classification in his work *"The peoples of India"*. According to him, the main ethnic groups at Indian population are:

- Indo Aryan
- Aryo Dravidian
- Mongolo Dravidian
- Scytho Dravidian
- Turko Iranian
- Mongoloid
- Jharkhand, Chhattisgarh, Odisha and West Bengal—the Pre-Dravidian
- Telangana, Andhra Pradesh and Tamil Nadu—Dravidian
- Punjab and Kashmir—the Indo-Aryans
- Uttar Pradesh and Rajasthan—Aryo-Dravidian
- Saurashtra, Coorg and hilly tracts of Madhya Pradesh. Scytho—Dravidian
- Assam and foothills of Himalaya—Mongoloid
- North Western Frontier province, Baluchistan and districts of Punjab and Sindh- **Turko-Iranians** (mixture of Indian Aryans, Persian Aryans and Mongolo-Asiatic people.

INFLUENCE OF CLASS, CASTE AND RACE SYSTEM ON HEALTH

Impact of Caste on Health

- Food habits
- Inferiority complex
- Cultural Practices and Superstitions
- Marriage and Religion

Food Habits

- Vegetarian vs nonvegetarian
- Food taboos
- Certain foods generate heat in body
- Certain foods cool the body
- Milk adulteration
- Fasting
- Consumption of alcohol, gaanja, bhaang
- Bathing before eating

Inferiority Complex

- Inferiority complex increases a person's tendency for risk taking, substance abuse, and aggressive behavior. Additionally, those who are impacted are more likely to struggle with depression and anxiety, among other mental health conditions.

Cultural Practices and Superstitions

Worshipping/Pooja: Physical and Mental Peace

Superstitions: Postpone Health Care Services,

Polygamy: Somatization, depression, anxiety, hostility, psychoticism and psychiatric disorder, dissatisfaction in marriage, conflicts.

Marriage and Religion

- Marriage gives resources and social support, and it is more likely to occur in people who are in better health, have more resources, and are less stressed. Marriage continues to have a positive impact on health even after selection factors are taken into account, proving that marriage is health-promoting.
- Compared to those who are less religious and spiritual, more religious and spiritual persons have better mental health and are quicker to adjust with health issues.

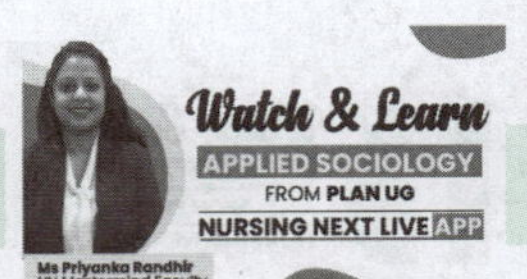

Impact of Class on Health

- Health is determined by class
- Lower class people have lower health and higher risk of communicable diseases and socioeconomic issues

Impact of Lower Class on Health

- Unemployment, poverty and illiteracy are prevalent
- Malnutrition, impaired physical & mental health are commonly seen

Impact of Upper Class on Health.

- Health is better in upper class
- Awareness of disease helps to access health care better
- Noncommunicable diseases are common in high class

Impact of Middle Class on Health

- Middle class people have socio-economic imbalance
- They suffer from both the Communicable, non-communicable disease and social disability

Influence of Class on Health

- **Education:** Lower class- more illiterate
  Higher class- level of literacy GOOD
- **Occupation:** Lower class- lack of autonomy at work that results in mental health issues
  Higher class-lots of stress again
- **Nutrition:** Lower class- poor nutrition
  Higher class-balanced diets
- **Residence:** In lower class- crowded places, lack of basic facilities
  In upper class –Pucca houses, access to luxurious life
- **Economic status:** Lower class-economically unstable
  Higher class-economically stable
- **Way of living:**
  - Eating balanced food
  - Proper sleep
  - Good company
  - Regular exercise
  - Positive thinking
  - Updated
  - Keep learning

Impact of Race on Health

- **Skin problems:** Caucasian- Acne
  African American: Melasma
- **Genetics:** Caucasians: Cystic fibrosis
  African Americans: Sickle cell anemia
- **Disease progression:** Differs from race to race and depends on the access to health services.
- **Geographical conditions:** In Negros occidental, a province in Philippines, people are more prone to foot and mouth diseases and bird flue.

Solution

The World Health Organization recommends three principles for action:

1. Improving the conditions of daily life;
2. Tackling the inequalities, distribution of power, money and resources
3. There is need to change social structures

CONCEPTUAL EXERCISES

LONG ANSWER QUESTIONS

1. a. Discuss the merits and demerits of caste system in India.

b. Discuss the social problems in India and their control measures. (CCSU)

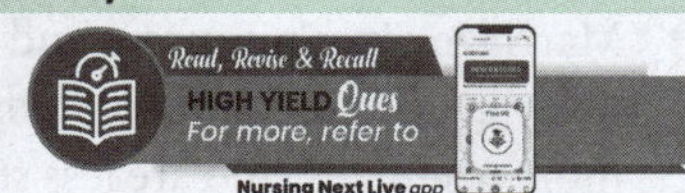

Answer

Caste System

The word "Caste" owes its origin to the Spanish word "Casta" which means breed, race or a complex of hereditary qualities. The Portuguese applied this term to the classes of people in India known by the name of "Jati". The English word caste is an adjustment of the original term.

The foundation of this form of classification is made up of deeply held conventional beliefs that are either unchangeable or exceedingly difficult to alter, including religious beliefs. This type of social stratification involves the division of individuals into various groups based on rigid, often religious, customs and practices that can be difficult to change.

Definitions of Caste System

- "When a class is somewhat strictly hereditary, we may call it as "caste." —**C H Cooley**
- "A caste is a closed group." —**Majumdar**

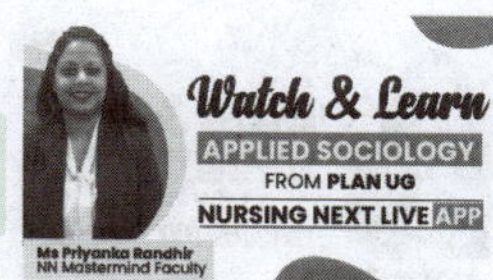

Merits of Caste System

- **Spirit of cooperation:** The caste structure encourages cooperation among its participants. Members of the group have a strong sense of community. This attitude is the reason that cooperation naturally arises.
- **Provides a definite social environment:** It offers its members a clear social atmosphere.

  Each group has a distinct culture from the others. Thus, the caste system improves one's quality of living by establishing a stable social environment.
- **Defines economic pursuit:** The members of a caste structure are assigned specific occupations. The parents and other older members of the family teach the young ones about caste.
- **Racial purity:** The caste structure preserves social purity by prohibiting marriages between castes. Each caste's tradition is preserved due to this.
- **Separation of social life from political life:** The caste structure clearly distinguishes between social life and political influence. Numerous foreign invaders, including Muslims and Westerners, attempted to convert Hindus to their own faith. However, the caste structure abstracts these efforts.
- **As constitution of Hindu society:** The caste system provides certain norms and rules that help in preventing antisocial behavior in the endogamous groups.

Demerits of Caste System

- **No scope for social mobility:** The caste structure discourages the movement of people. There is little chance to raise their social status as a result.
- **Untouchability:** Caste hierarchy fosters a sense of untouchability and supremacy. Higher caste individuals believe that even a Shudra's contact will contaminate them. They continue to receive subhuman treatment. Due to their numerous social impairments, they were prohibited from entering any public spaces like hotels, wells, and religious institutions.
- **Social disunity:** Thousands of caste and sub-caste groups have been created under the caste structure. The sense of respect and sympathy between members of upper and lower castes has been replaced by enmity and hatred as a result of this. This issue persists today in India just as it did a century ago.
- **Wrong man in wrong occupation:** Some specific professions are assigned to a caste under the system of caste. It is against the law for members of one caste to work in a position designated for a member of another caste. This has given the wrong guy, the wrong job.
- **Threat to national unity:** Only on the foundation of the principles of liberty, equality, and fraternity can a modern country grow strong. The caste structure, however, is the opposite. It has greatly decreased the interest in national unity. India was unable to cultivate a firm sense of national identity as a result.
- **Scope for religious conversion:** Due to the brutality of the higher caste, the people of the lower caste are converting to Islam and Christianity.

Social Problems in India and their Control Measures

Definitions of Social Problems

Fuller and Myers have defined a social problem as "a condition, which is defined by a considerable number of persons as a deviation from social norms which they cherish".

b. Discuss the social problems in india and its control measures

Answer

- **Poverty:** India has a significant population living below the poverty line. Poverty leads to lack of access to basic necessities such as food, clean water, education, and healthcare, resulting in a cycle of deprivation and limited opportunities.
  - **Control mesures:** Social welfare programs to provide financial assistance, education, healthcare, and skill development opportunities to the impoverished.
  - Inclusive economic growth through job creation and entrepreneurship development.
- **Gender inequality:** Issues such as female infanticide, dowry-related violence, unequal access to education and healthcare, limited economic opportunities for women, and gender-based violence are some of the challenges that India continues to grapple with.
  - **Control measures:** Enforce and strengthen laws against gender-based violence and discrimination.
  - Promote gender sensitization and awareness campaigns
  - Enhance access to education, healthcare, and economic opportunities for women through targeted approach. E.g., Beti Bachao Beti Padhao scheme.
- **Caste system and untouchability:** Discrimination based on caste limits social mobility, access to resources, and opportunities for marginalized communities.
  - **Control measures:** Implement affirmative action policies to promote social justice
  - Create awareness programs to challenge caste-based discrimination
  - Strengthen legal mechanisms
- **Child labor and exploitation:** India has a significant number of child laborers, who are forced to work in hazardous conditions, depriving them of education and a normal childhood. Child trafficking, child marriage, and child exploitation are also pressing issues.

- **Control measures:** Strengthen and enforce child labor laws.
- Enhance access to quality education and social support systems for children at risk
- **Religious and communal conflicts:** Religious and communal conflicts often arise from religious or sectarian differences, resulting in social divisions and challenges to peaceful coexistence.
  - **Control measures:** Foster interfaith dialogue, understanding, and cooperation to promote religious harmony.
  - Strengthen law enforcement to prevent and address communal violence
- **Education disparities:** Limited infrastructure, inadequate resources, and social barriers contribute to educational inequality and hinder social mobility.
  - **Control measures:** Improve infrastructure and resources in rural and marginalized areas.
  - Provide scholarships and financial assistance programs
  - Implement inclusive educational policies
- **Healthcare disparities:** Access to healthcare services is unequal in India, with rural areas and marginalized communities facing significant challenges in accessing quality healthcare.
  - **Control measures:**
  - Increase healthcare infrastructure and resources in rural and underserved areas
  - Implement universal healthcare initiatives
- **Environmental Degradation:** India faces environmental challenges such as air pollution, water pollution, deforestation, and improper waste management.
  - **Control measures:**
  - Implement and enforce stringent environmental regulations and policies.
  - Promote sustainable practices, renewable energy, and waste management systems.
  - Conduct awareness campaigns
- **Urbanization challenges:** Rapid urbanization has led to several social issues, including overcrowding, inadequate housing, slum proliferation, inadequate sanitation facilities, and insufficient access to basic services in urban areas.
  - **Control measures:**
  - Implement urban planning strategies that prioritize equitable access to housing
  - Develop affordable housing initiatives and slum improvement programs.
- **Corruption:** Corruption at various levels of society hinders economic development, erodes public trust, and perpetuates social inequalities.
  - **Control measures:**
  - Enact and enforce anti-corruption laws and establish independent oversight mechanisms.
  - Promote transparency and accountability in public administration

Specific Control Measures

- A few significant plans to reduce poverty include:
  - The **Indira Awaas Yojna (IAY)** was established to provide housing assistance to people from scheduled castes, scheduled tribes, freed bonded laborers, and rural impoverished people who are living below the poverty level.
  - In 2005, India as a whole adopted the **Mahatma Gandhi National Rural Employment Guarantee Scheme (MGNREGA).** Every rural family was promised 100 days of untrained manual labor work at a wage under this plan each fiscal year.
  - The 2003 **food security program** also provided priority and antyodya households with free distribution of certain quantities of food grains.
- The Indian administration is aware of the problem of unemployment there. They have made a lot of progress in the shape of employment creation plans. One important measure is the MGNREGA program.
- In order to encourage education among those between the ages of 15 and 35, the **National Adult Education (NAE) program** was launched in 1978. Launched in 1986, the **Rural Functional Literacy (RFL)** program is a division of the NAE. It was designed to educate people about various government programs from which they could gain access.
- The Scheduled Castes and Scheduled Tribes Prevention of Atrocities Act was enacted in 1989, and the Civil Rights Act was passed in 1976.

2. a. Define social stratification and its types in detail.
b. Explain the influence of class, caste and race on health and health practices. (CCSU)

Answer

Definitions of Social Stratification

- "The process by which the individuals and groups are ranked more or less enduring hierarchy of status is known as stratification." **—Ogburn and Nimkoff**
- "Social stratification is horizontal division of society into higher and lower social units." **—R W Murray**
- "Unstratified society with real equality of its members is a myth, that can never be realized in the history of mankind." **—P A Sorokin**

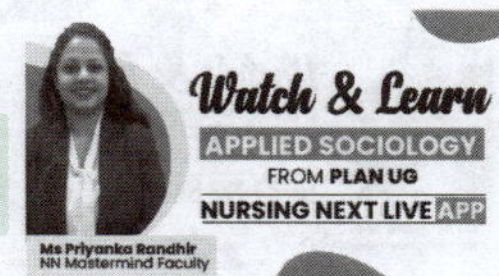

Types of Social Stratification

The major systems of stratification are slavery, estate systems, caste systems, and class systems.

- **Slavery:** A closed system of possession that has been prevalent throughout human history is slavery. It developed in agricultural communities 10,000 years ago and flourished in classical Greece and Rome. Europeans started exploring the Western Hemisphere in the 1500s, and by the 1800s, they had kidnapped and transported 10–12 million Africans to the New World, nearly 2 million of whom perished on the journey. Some figures place the number of slaves in the tens of millions, with slavery still existing in some areas of Africa, Asia, and South America. Men who are first taken as prisoners of war, women and girls who are caught during battle or abducted from their homes, kids who are sold by their parents to work as slaves, and people who are employed to pay off debts are all examples of modern-day slaves.
- **Estate system:** The landed nobility and the peasantry were the two main estates, and estate systems were widespread in Europe and Asia during the Middle Ages and into the 1800s. They were successful up until the French Revolution in 1789, when they gradually gave way to stratified class structures. After the American colonies gained their freedom from Britain, the South had at least one aspect of an estate system, where a small number of wealthy people and their families controlled sizable tracts of land, but the laborers were slaves rather than serfs. Many countries in Asia, particularly China and Japan, also used estate systems, which sparked peasant uprisings and political and economic unrest up until 1949, when the Communists seized power in China.
- **Caste system:** People are born into unequal groups according to the standing of their parents in India's caste systems. The "untouchables" were regarded as unclean and were not allowed to be around people of the higher castes, and they lived in utter poverty in rural regions. "Untouchables" were given equal rights under the constitution after India gained independence from Britain, and the caste system was further weakened by advances in communication and urban migration. Both India and South Africa, where a small group of white Afrikaners governed from 1950 to 1990, still struggle with caste prejudice. Jim Crow ruled the South in the US until the civil rights movement put a stop to legal segregation. Lynchings were frequent, and the Southern police apparatus supported racial supremacy.
- **Class system:** Class (which we will refer to as wealth), power, and prestige are the three stratification dimensions upon which class systems are founded. Max Weber argued that power and status are just as important as economic stratification in class systems. Power is the capacity to persuade people to do what you want, even if they don't want to, and prestige is the standing and respect that people enjoy among their peers. Wealth is the total worth of an individual or family. In the United States, social class is the most mobile vertically and is also the most open.

b. Explain the influence of class, caste and race on health and health practices.

Answer

- Class is a group of people having the same social status with respect to certain characteristics.
- These characteristics are not ascribed (given by birth) usually but are earned through individual efforts.
- "When a class is somewhat strictly hereditary, we may call it as "caste". **—C H Cooley**
- Race is a group, which has a common set of innate physical characteristics and a geographical origin within a certain area.
- **Class:** Based on economic status
- **Caste:** Ascribed in nature and inherited
- **Race:** Based on physical characteristics

Impact of Caste on Health

Caste influences health through food habits, perpetuating inferiority complexes, dictating cultural practices and superstitions, impacting marriage choices, and shaping religious affiliations. These factors collectively affect access to healthcare, well-being, and social determinants of health.

- Food habits
- Inferiority complex
- Cultural Practices and Superstitions
- Marriage and Religion

Food Habits

- Vegetarian vs nonvegetarian
- Food taboos
- Certain foods generate heat in body
- Certain foods cool the body
- Milk adulteration
- Fasting
- Consumption of alcohol, gaanja, bhaang
- Bathing before eating

Inferiority Complex

- Inferiority complex increases a person's tendency for risk taking, substance abuse, and aggressive behavior. Additionally, those who are impacted are more likely to struggle with depression and anxiety, among other mental health conditions.

Cultural Practices And Superstitions

Worshipping/Pooja: Physical and Mental Peace
Superstitions: Postpone Health Care Services

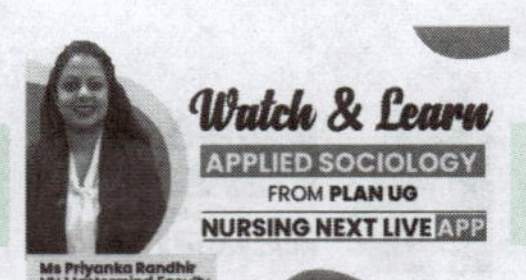

Polygamy: Somatization, depression, anxiety, hostility, psychoticism and psychiatric disorder, dissatisfaction in marriage, conflicts.

Marriage and Religion

- Marriage gives resources and social support, and it is more likely to occur in people who are in better health, have more resources, and are less stressed. Marriage continues to have a positive impact on health even after selection factors are taken into account, proving that marriage is health-promoting.
- Compared to those who are less religious and spiritual, more religious and spiritual persons have better mental health and are quicker to adjust with health issues.

Impact of Class on Health

- Health is determined by class
- Lower class people have lower health and higher risk of communicable diseases and socioeconomic issues

Impact of Lower Class on Health

- Unemployment, poverty and illiteracy are prevalent
- Malnutrition, impaired physical & mental health are commonly seen

Impact of Upper Class on Health

- Health is better in upper class
- Awareness of disease helps to access health care better
- Noncommunicable diseases are common in high class

Impact of Middle Class on Health

- Middle class people have socio-economic imbalance
- They suffer from both the Communicable, non-communicable disease and social disability

Influence of Class on Health

- **Education:** Lower class- More Illiterate-Poor health
  Higher class- higher level of literacy-Good health
- **Occupation:** Lower class- Lack of autonomy at work that results in mental health issues
  Higher class-Lots of stress again
- **Nutrition:** Lower class- Poor nutrition
  Higher class-Balanced diets
- **Residence:** In lower class- Crowded places, Lack of basic facilities
  In upper class –Pucca houses, Access to luxurious life
- **Economic status:** Lower class- Economically unstable
  Higher class-Economically stable

- **Way of living**
  - Eating balanced food
  - Proper sleep
  - Good company
  - Regular exercise
  - Positive thinking
  - Updated
  - Keep learning

All the above factors will help to maintain a good health.

Impact of Race on Health

- **Skin problems:** Caucasian- Acne
  African American: Melasma
- **Genetics:** Caucasians: Cystic fibrosis
  African Americans: Sickle cell anemia
- **Disease progression:** Differs from race to race and depends on the access to health services.
- **Geographical conditions:** In Negros occidental, a province in Philippines, people are more prone to foot and mouth diseases and bird flu.

3. Define social system and describe its types. (CCSU)

Answer

Definitions of Social System

"Social system is a network of interactions between actors."

—**Talcott Parsons**

"The term society refers not to group of people, but to the complex pattern of the norms of interaction that arises among and between them." —**Lapiere**

"It is constituted of the interaction of a plurality of individual actors whose relations to each other are mutually oriented through the definition of and mediation of a pattern of structured and shared symbols and expectations." —**Loomis**

Types of Social System

Parsons presents a classification of four major types on the basis of pattern variable:

1. **The particularistic ascriptive type**
   - According to Parsons, this type of social system is organized around kinship and sociality/roles are organized in terms of values. Parsons' view of the "Spanish Americans" in the USA exemplifies this type of social structure.
   - The normative patterns of such a system are traditional and are dominated by the elements of ascription.
   - Such type of system existed in preliterate societies (needs are limited to biological survival). Work, in this type "is considered a necessary evil just as morality is a necessary condition of minimum stability", says Talcott Parsons.

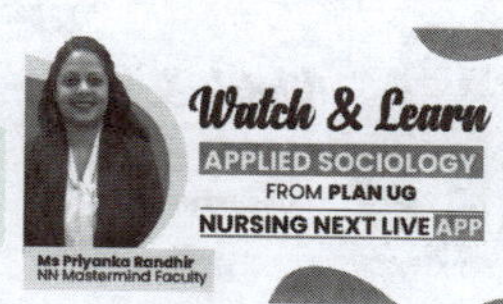

2. **The particularistic achievement type**
   - Role of religious ideas is emphasized as differentiating element in social life.
   - Seen in Chinese society.
   - This society was dominated by values of "familism".
   - 'Familism' means the notion of continuity with ancestors.
   - It has strong ties of kinship, but where the female line of descent is not favored (Particularistic-roles are not determined on the basis of universal principles).
   - On the other hand, entrances into services, based on examination or competition-Achievement type.
   - Seen in Chinese society.
3. **The universalistic achievement type**
   - Seen in American society, as per Parsons.
   - Value-orientations are dominant which encourage achievement based on legal rational methods among members of a society.
   - Societies have governing values of equality, democracy, freedom of enterprise, rationale management and openness in social interactions.
   - Division of society is not based on caste, religion, ethnicity or any particularistic values.
4. **The universalistic ascription type**
   - Under this social type, elements of value orientation are dominated by the elements of ascription
   - Therefore, emphasis is placed on status of the actor, rather than his performance.
   - Values of legal rationality are encouraged in performance of roles but the distribution of authority is not on the basis of equality or democracy. Parsons believed that Nazi in Germany had this society.

SHORT NOTE

1. Social stratification. (CCSU) (KUHS) (MGR)

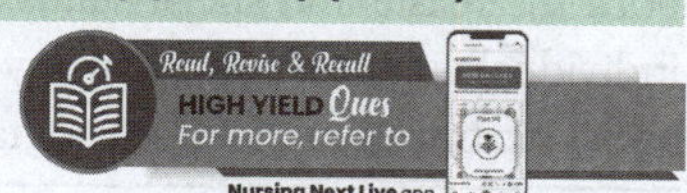

Answer

Definitions of Social Stratification

"The process by which the individuals and groups are ranked in more or less enduring hierarchy of status is known as stratification". —**Ogburn and Nimkoff**

"Social stratification is horizontal division of society into higher and lower social units." —**R W Murray**

"Unstratified society with real equality of its members is a myth, that can never be realized in the history of mankind." —**P A Sorokin**

Meaning of Social Stratification

- Not just reflection of individual differences, it is a characteristic of society.
- All societies arrange themselves in terms of superiority, inferiority and equality.
- Stratification ranks the society and places someone higher than others.

Origin of Social Stratification

General View

- **Natural inevitability:** Inequality exists because of natural differences in people's ability.
- **Structural-functionalist:** Stratification is useful in society as it enhances stability and makes people work hard.
- **Conflict:** Stratification occurs because of conflict between two classes as per the distribution of resources.
- **Evolutionary:** People will share enough resources to ensure the survival of the group until a surplus exists at which the those in power decides how surplus is distributed.
- **Symbolic interactionism:** Draws attention to the symbolic display of wealth and power for defining self and social situations.

Principles of Social Stratification

- Traits of society
- Generation to generation
- Not only inequality but beliefs (The inequality is not anybody's agenda but having beliefs different from others makes stratification come into account).
- Universal but variable

Characteristics of Social Stratification

According to Malvin M. Tumin

- **Stratification is social:** Social superiority and inferiority are not determined by biological traits before they are socially acknowledged and accorded significance. For instance, the manager of a bank achieves a dominant position not because of his physical prowess or age but rather by possessing the characteristics that are socially defined. It is determined that a person's education, training, abilities, experience, personality, etc. are more significant than biological qualities.
- **Stratification is universal:** The stratification system is a universal phenomenon. Difference between rich and poor is found everywhere. No society is unstratified.
- **Stratification is consequential:**

  Life chances and lifestyle
  - **Life chances:** Refer to such things as infant mortality, physical and mental illness, longevity, childlessness, divorce and desertion, etc. Life chances are more involuntary.

- **Lifestyle:** Includes such matters as the mode of housing, residential area, education, means of recreation, relationship between the parents and children, one's mode of conveyance and so on. Lifestyle reflects differences in preferences, tastes and values.

Types of Social Stratification

- **Open:** The stratification that promotes social mobility is an open class system, in which social rank is determined by individual accomplishment and personal merit. It takes effort for an individual to rise in the social hierarchy.
- **Closed:** There is little to no chance to move up social classes in a closed system of stratification. Based on a shared trait, social standing is inherited. Social mobility is the transition between different social statuses. (Individual, Collective)

Forms of Social Stratification

- **Primitive communism:** High degree of sharing and minimum social inequality.
- **Slavery:** Great social inequality and the ownership of some persons by others.
- **Caste:** This is ascribed which means an individual is permanently assigned to a status based on his or her parent's status.
- **Estate:** Peasants are required by law, to work on the land owned by the noble class in exchange for food and protection from outside attacks.

Functions of Social Stratification

The division of society into levels of authority and prestige serves several crucial purposes:

- Stratification enables the placement and motivation of people to influence how they carry out their necessary societal obligations.
- It offers a system of incentives and rewards to members for performing various tasks related to various roles.
- The rewards—typically monetary, prestigious, and leisure—are incorporated into the social positions, and because they are unequal, they lead to inequality of places.
- Societies are arranged into hierarchies of status levels in order to achieve the performance of the necessary social duties.
- Stratification divides a society's different positions into a hierarchy of status levels that governs how its members interact with one another.

SHORT ANSWER QUESTIONS

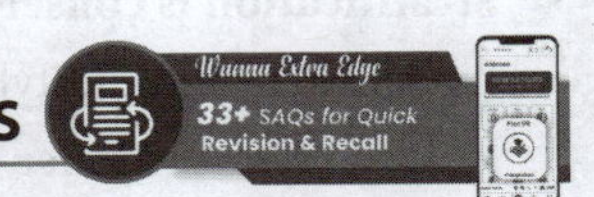

1. Enlist types of social stratification.

Answer

Types of Social Stratification

Slavery: Extreme or intense form of legalized social inequality for individuals or groups is slavery. Slavery is a system of enforced servitude in which some people are owned by other people.

Caste: Caste is a hereditary traditional endogamous social group in which a person's rank and its accompanying rights and obligations are ascribed on the basis of his birth into a particular group.

Estate: During Middle Ages, estates were associated with feudal societies. As the estate system developed, stratification became more differentiated. Gradually, estate system ended and a class of stratification came into existence.

Class: A class system is a social ranking based primarily on economic position or wealth of a person; in which achieved characteristics can influence social mobility.

2. What is race?

Answer

Race is defined as, "A category of humankind that shares certain distinctive physical traits."

Race is a socially constructed category of people who share biologically transmitted traits that members of a society consider important.

3. Define caste.

Answer

The caste system in India is an old and ancient system of social stratification. According to DN Mazumdar and TN Madan, "Caste is a closed group." Means there is no social mobility, an individual born in a caste and social status is determined by his caste. An individual's interest and talent have no meaning. Caste is a type of social stratification that does not facilitate vertical social mobility.

4. Give two differences between caste and class.

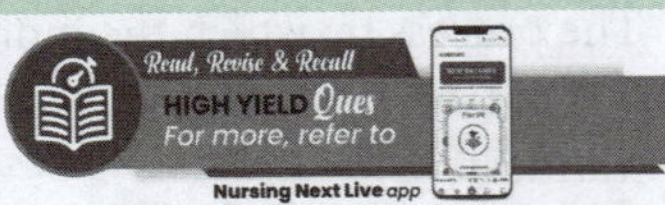

Answer

Caste	Class
Caste is a closed system. It confines social mobility.	Open system: Class is not confined; it is a bit flexible, anybody can move from higher class to lower class and vice versa
Caste system promotes endogamy. Marriage within the caste is well accepted.	Class system is exogamous; upper class people can marry lower class people and vice versa.

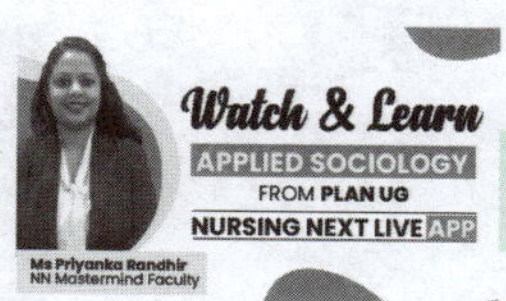

5. Define social mobility and vertical mobility.

Answer

Social mobility: Social mobility means transition of a person or social object from one social position to another. For example, a clerk becomes an officer.

Vertical mobility: Vertical mobility refers to the movement of people from one stratum to another or from one standing to another. Vertical mobility involves movement from lower position to higher or higher position to lower.

CONCEPTUAL REVISION

MULTIPLE CHOICE QUESTIONS

1. "Social stratification is horizontal division of society into higher and lower social units". Who said this?

a. PA Sorokin b. RW Murray
c. Ogburn and Nimkoff d. Weber

Ans. b. RW Murray

2. Natural inevitability in terms of social stratification means:

a. Draws attention to the symbolic display of wealth and power for defining self and social situations
b. Stratification occurs because of conflict between two classes as per the distribution of resources
c. Inequality exists because of natural differences in people's ability
d. Stratification is useful in society as it enhances stability and makes people work hard

Ans. c. Inequality exists because of natural differences in people's ability

3. Basis of social stratification as per the Conflict theory is:

a. Inequality in Economy b. Bourgeoisie Class
c. Proletariat Class d. Inequality of Caste

Ans. a. Inequality in Economy

4. As per Davis and Moore, the true statement regarding society is:

a. Positions and rewards are unrelated
b. Society is made up of positions
c. Society has class struggle
d. Future will be free of stratification

Ans. b. Society is made up of positions

5. According to Malvin M. Malvin, all are the characteristics of social stratification, except:

a. Stratification is universal
b. Stratification is diverse in its form
c. Stratification is modern concept
d. Stratification is social

Ans. c. Stratification is modern concept

6. The mode of housing, residential area, one's education, means of recreation etc. are categorized as:

a. Life chances b. Lifestyle
c. Material d. Non-material

Ans. b. Lifestyle

7. Status achieved through efforts and merit is a form of:

a. Closed social stratification
b. Open social stratification
c. Primitive communism
d. Caste

Ans. b. Open social stratification

8. The process of social stratification includes all, except:

a. Rewarding
b. Differentiation of statuses
c. Evaluation d. Follow-up

Ans. d. Follow-up

9. The deficiency of vitamin B12 causing anemia and blindness in a particular social group is primarily related to their:

a. Class system b. Caste system
c. Race d. Ethnicity

Ans. b. Caste system

CHAPTER 6

Social Organization and Disorganization

CONCEPTUAL THEORY

Terminology

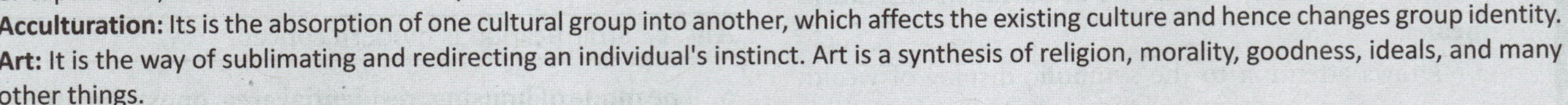

Accomplished status: When a person achieves a status via his or her own efforts or capabilities, it is referred to as accomplished status.

Acculturation: Its is the absorption of one cultural group into another, which affects the existing culture and hence changes group identity.

Art: It is the way of sublimating and redirecting an individual's instinct. Art is a synthesis of religion, morality, goodness, ideals, and many other things.

Ascribed status: It is when a person's status is given to them by birth without any effort on their part.

Association: An association is a group of social beings who are linked together by the fact that they share or have established a common organization to achieve a specified objective or set of goals.

Belief system: Man's behavior was profoundly influenced by his belief system. It fueled man's faith in benevolence.

Child laborer: According to the Indian Constitution, a child laborer is someone who is under the age of 14 and works for a living.

Community disorganization: A state of inadequacy and discord that allows for the forces of disintegration in community life to flourish.

Custom: It is defined as "a rule or norm of action." From one generation to the next, transfer or carry on.

Delinquency: "Delinquency consisted of socially unacceptable acts."

Dowry: "Dowry is the property which a woman brings with her or is given to her at the marriage."

Facility: A facility is described as a means, resources used to achieve purposes or specific goals within the system.

Folkway: It's a uniform and common way of living and helping in social control. A folkway describes or draws a line between right and wrong.

Formal organization: A formal organization has its own set of social standards or rules. Certain behaviors are acceptable in certain organizations. A formal organization establishes procedures for its members to follow.

Informal organization: An informal organization is a small group whose members are linked or connected to one another as individuals through primary relationships, such as family members. Individuals in the group have informal and face-to-face relationships, mutual aid, cooperation, and camaraderie.

Informal social control: Informal social control agencies have arisen in response to societal requirements. (Generally fundamental institution like family; exercises this form of social control).

Law: Law is society's most specialized and well-equipped engine or mechanism of social control.

Legislative process: The processes that must be taken in order for a proposed bill to become law. Parliament's primary role is to create, alter, or repeal legislation. The legislative process, or the process of establishing laws, is related to Parliament.

Literacy: Literacy is defined as the capacity or skill of a person to read and write.

Marginalized groups: "To be marginalized is to be placed on the margins, thus excluded from the privilege and power found at the center."

Mores: Mores, such as folkways, are moral judgments that are strongly ingrained in community life. Mores discriminate between what is right and what is bad.

Norms: Norms are the absolute norms that define what is right, incorrect, suitable, and improper in society. Every social structure has particular rules that members are required to obey or follow. In most societies around the world, for example, violence is immoral and peace is right.

Power: Depending on their social station, everyone has different levels of power in society.

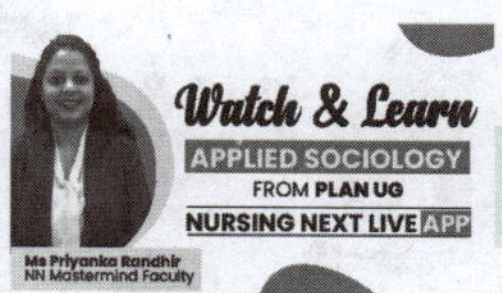

SOCIAL ORGANIZATION–MEANING, ELEMENTS AND TYPES

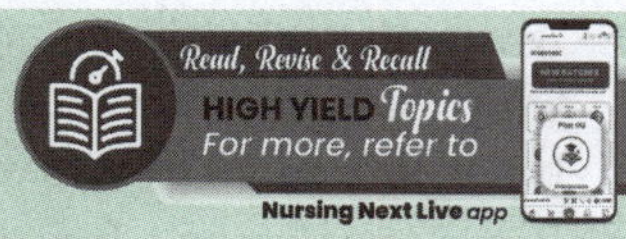

Introduction

- The term "social organization" and "disorganization" is relative.
- They represent two aspects of the whole functioning of the social system.
- As there may be various degrees of social organization, so is the case with social disorganization.
- No society can be in a state of either perfect organization or disorganization.

Meaning of Social Organization

- Social + organization
- The term organization means an arrangement of persons or parts.
- Thus, churches, colleges, play groups and political parties are examples of organization. In all these cases, there is an arrangement of persons or parts, which are interrelated or interdependent.
- We may take an example of educational institution or college.
- A college includes the principal, professors, clerks and students, etc. It is nothing but an arrangement of parts or persons.

Definitions of Social Organization

"Organization refers to an aspect of interaction system."

—**H M Johnson**

"An organization is a articulation of different parts which perform various functions, it is an active group device for gathering something done." —**Ogburn and Nimkoff**

Elements of Social Organization

- **Sanction**
  Sanction means condition which may be in form of punishments or warnings.
- **Goal**
  Members work together for the achievement of goal
- **Preparedness**
  To accept one's role. Every person has certain roles to perform
- **Control of society**
  Society exercises this control through the media of habits, customs, traditions, mores, rituals and institutions. It is this which creates unanimity in society.
- **Norms and mores**
  If norms are followed society will work smoothly

Types of Social Organization

- Political organizationww
- Economic organization
- Religious organization
- Financial organization
- Educational organization

Types of social organization: Authoritarian and Democratic

Authoritarian:
- Use of coercive power
- Greater dependency on leader
- Little input from group

Democratic:
- No use of coercive power
- Leader encourages group participation
- Leader offers guidance to group

Autocratic Mode of Participation

- One ruler or a small group of leaders have the real power in authoritarian political systems.
- Authoritarian governments may hold elections and they may have contact with their citizens, but citizens do not have any voice in how they are ruled.
- Their leaders do not give their subjects free choice. Instead, they decide what the people can or cannot have. Citizens, then, are subjects who must obey, and not participants in government decisions.
- Kings, military leaders, emperors, a small group of aristocrats, dictators, and even presidents or prime ministers may rule authoritarian governments.
- The leader's title does not automatically indicate a particular type of government.
- Authoritarian systems do not allow freedoms of speech, press, and religion, and they do not follow majority rule nor protect minority rights.
- Their leaders often come from one small group, such as top military officials, or from a small group of aristocratic families. Examples of such regimes include China, Myanmar, Cuba, and Iran.

Advantages of Autocratic Mode of Participation

- Quick decision-making
- Effective when workers are less skilled
- Control in one hand

Disadvantages of Autocratic Mode of Participation

- One-way communication
- Subordinates feel stressed
- "Them" and "us" attitude develops

Democratic Mode of Participation

- Many countries in the world today claim to be democratic. If the citizens are not involved in government and politics, they are democratic in name only.
- **Freedom of speech, press and religion:** Democracies in general respect these basic individual liberties. No government allows absolute freedom, but democracies do not heavily censor newspapers and public expression of opinions.
- **Majority rule with minority rights:** People accept decisions made by the majority of voters in a free election. Democracies try to avoid the "tyranny of the majority" by providing ways for minorities all kinds to have their voices heard as well.
- **Varied personal backgrounds of political leaders:** Democracies usually leave room for many different types of citizens to compete for leadership positions. In other words, presidents and legislators do not all come from a few elite families, the same part of the country, or the same social class
- **Free, competitive elections:** The presence of elections alone is not enough to call a country a democracy. The elections must be fair and competitive, and the government or political leaders cannot control the results. Voters must have real choices among candidates who run for public office.
- **Rule by law:** Democracies are not controlled by the whims of a leader, but they are governed by laws that apply to leaders and citizens equally.
- **Meaningful political participation by citizens:** By itself, a citizen's right to vote is not a good measure of democracy. The government must respond in some way to citizen demands. If they vote, the candidate they choose must actually take office. If they contact government in other ways—writing, protesting, phoning—officials must respond.

Advantages of Democratic Mode of Participation

- Solution for complex problems
- Promotes a creative environment
- Helps in building strong team

Disadvantages of Democratic Mode of Participation

- Becomes apologetic
- Time-consuming
- Delayed decision making

VOLUNTARY ASSOCIATIONS

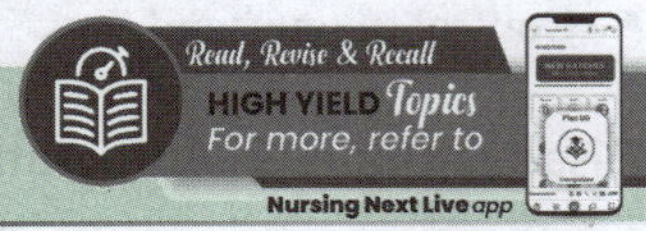

Introduction

- The term volunteerism is derived from the Latin word "voluntas" Which means "will" or "freedom"
- A voluntary association or union is a group of individuals who willingly enter into an agreement to form a body (or organization) so as to work together for a common goal.
- It performs various functions for the welfare, integration and solidarity of the society.
- As per Article 19 (1) (c) of the constitution of India confers on the Indian citizens the 'right to form association'.
- In UN voluntary organizations are called nongovernmental organizations (NGOs).

Definitions of Voluntary Associations

"Social system as a network of interactions between actors."

—Talcott Parsons

"Social system is composed of patterned interaction of visual actors whose relations to each other are mutually oriented through the definition of the mediation of pattern of structured and shared symbols and expectations" **Charles P Loomis**

List of Some Voluntary Health Associations in India

- Tuberculosis Association of India
- Indian Red Cross Society
- Bharat Sewak Samaj
- Indian Council for Child Welfare
- Hind Kusht Nivaran Sangh
- All India Women's Conference
- Kasturba Memorial Fund
- Professional Bodies
- Family Planning Association of India
- Central Social Welfare Board

Types of Voluntary Associations

On the basis of orientation:

- Empowering
- Service
- Charitable
- Participatory

On the basis of cooperation:

- City-wide organizations
- National NGO's
- International NGO's
- Community-based organizations

Characteristics of Voluntary Associations

- Method of formation, which is voluntary on the part of a group of people.
- Method of government, with self-governing organization to decide on its constitution, its servicing, its policy and clients.
- Method of financing, with at least some of its revenues drawn from voluntary sources.

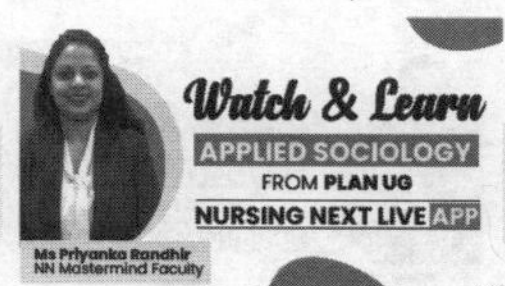

- Motives with the pursuit of profit extended.
- It has definite aims and objectives and programs for their fulfillment and achievement.
- It has an administrative structure and a duly constituted management and executive committee.
- It is an organization initiated and governed by its own members on democratic principles without any external control.
- It raises funds for its activities partly from the exchequer in the form of grants in aid and partly in the form of the contributions are subscription from the members of the local community and the beneficiaries of the programs.
- Imparts cultural values to individuals

Functions of Voluntary Associations

- Nonpartisan and nonpolitical function
- Imparting education
- Helping states
- Sustainable development
- Meeting needs of citizens
- Improve sociability
- Help groups and individuals
- Emphasis on individual learning
- Help in creating democratic system
- Meet health care requirements
- Create awareness
- Help in preventing diseases

SOCIAL SYSTEM – DEFINITION TYPES, ROLE AND STATUS AS STRUCTURAL ELEMENT OF SOCIAL SYSTEM

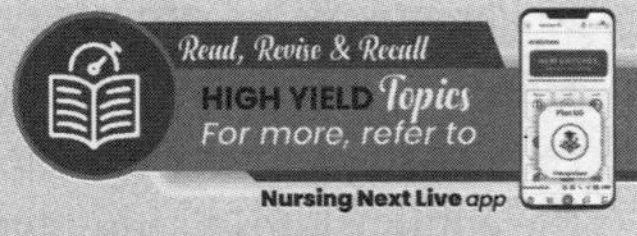

Introduction to Social System

- The term 'system' infers an orderly arrangement, or an interrelationship of different parts
- Similarly, society may be observed as a system of interrelated mutually dependent parts which cooperate to preserve a recognizable whole and to fulfil some purposes or goal
- Social system may be called an arrangement of social interactions grounded on shared norms and values
- A **social system** is an orderly and systematic arrangement of social interaction.
- Social system is made up of a plurality of individuals.
- They interact with others according to shared norms and meaning within the social system.
- There are various sub-systems of a social system (like political system, religious system, economic system, etc.).

Main Features of System

- A system is made up of different parts.
- There must be a systematic relationship between the parts.
- Arrangement of these parts should create a pattern.
- There is a functional relationship among the parts of a system.
- All the parts create a new entity when they are functionally related.
- They interact with each other according to shared norms and meanings within the social system.

Definitions of Social System

"Social system as a network of interactions between actors."

—Talcott Parsons

"The term society refers not to group of people, but to the complex pattern of the norms of interaction that arises among and between them." **—Lapiere**

Types of Social System

Parsons presents a classification of four major types on the basis of pattern variable

1. The Particularistic Ascriptive Type
   - Role of religious ideas are emphasized as differentiating element in social life
   - Seen in Chinese society
   - This society was dominated by values of "familism"
   - 'familism' means the notion of continuity with ancestors
   - It has strong ties of kinship, but where the female line of descent not favored (Particularistic-roles are not determined on the basis of universal principles)
2. The Particularistic-Achievement Pattern
   - On the other hand, Entrances into services, based on examination or competition is called Particularistic Achievement type
   - Seen in Chinese society
3. The Universalistic Achievement Type
   - Seen in American society, as per Parsons
   - Value-orientations are dominant which encourage achievement based on legal rational methods among members of a society
   - Societies have governing values of equality, democracy, freedom of enterprise, rationale management and openness in social interactions
   - Division of society is not based on caste, religion, ethnicity or any particularistic values.
4. The Universalistic Ascription Type
   - Under this social type, elements of value orientation are dominated by the elements of ascription

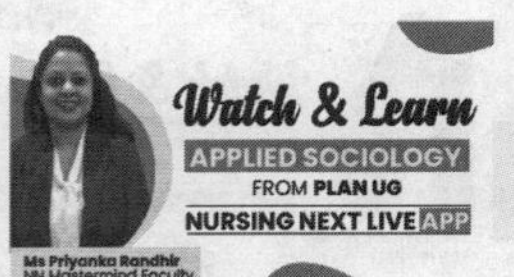

- Therefore, emphasis is placed on status of the actor, rather than his performance
- Values of legal rationality are encouraged in performance of roles but the distribution of authority is not on the basis of equality or democracy. Parsons believed that Nazis in Germany have this society

Functions of Social System

Agil Model by Talcott Parsons

- There are four main functions
- Four sets of Universal **Functional Requisites** are must for the survival of system
- Adaptation (resource generation, acquisition and distribution of resources-Economic System)
- GOAL (determination of goal, motivation, mobilizing, channelizing-political system)
- Integration (Consensus, solidarity, unity-Cultural System)
- Latency pattern maintenance and tension management: It is the hidden aspect for maintaining the motivation, tension management. This is the responsibility of the Family.

1. Adaptation

- Adaptability of social system to the changing environment is important
- A social system is the result of geographical environment and a long drawn historical process which by necessity gives it permanence and rigidity
- Economy for its maintenance, division of labor for better production of goods and effective services, and role differentiation for job opportunity is essential
- The British system, in the nineteenth century, when the continent was in the inferno of revolution, showed remarkable adaptability

2. Goal Attainment

- Goal attainment and adaptability are deeply interconnected
- Both contribute to the maintenance of social order
- Every social system has one or more goals to be attained through cooperative effort
- Adaptation to the social and nonsocial environment is, of course, necessary if goals are to be attained
- But in addition, human and nonhuman resources must be mobilized in some effective way, according to the specific nature of tasks
- The allocation of members and the allocation of scarce valuable resources are important, of course, for both adaptation and goal attainment

3. Integration

- Social system is essentially an integration system
- In the general routine of life, it is not the society but the group or the subgroup in which one feels more involved and interested
- An appeal in the name of society, culture, heritage, patriotism, national solidarity or social welfare invokes quick response
- When there is dispute concerning the interpretation of relational or regulative norms, or concerning the factual aspects of conflicts of interest, there is need for agreed-upon social arrangements for settling the dispute

4. Latent Pattern and maintenance

- Pattern maintenance and tension management is the primary function of social system
- In absence of appropriate effort in this direction maintenance and continuity of social order is not possible
- Every individual and subgroup learns the patterns in the process of the internalization of norms and values
- Society has the responsibility, like a family, to keep its members functional, to relieve them of anxiety, to encourage those who would be detrimental to the entire system

Equilibrium and Change in Social system

- The equilibrium condition is a "condition of integration and stability."
- Equilibrium can also be of moving sort, which according to Parsons, is "an orderly process of change of the system"
- Herbert Spencer introduced the cause and effect relationships to explain the changing nature of societies in the equilibrium/disequilibrium' analysis
- The structural-functional pattern of institutions which constitute a society would change in accordance with change it may encounter in its total external environment, and with changes in its internal conditions

Application in Nursing

- To promote health
- To restore health
- To prevent diseases
- To cure people
- To provide care
- To provide health education
- To provide stress management
- To plan for nursing management
- To make nursing diagnosis
- To assess patients

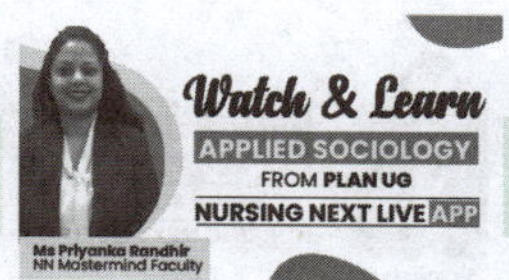

INTERRELATIONSHIP OF INSTITUTIONS

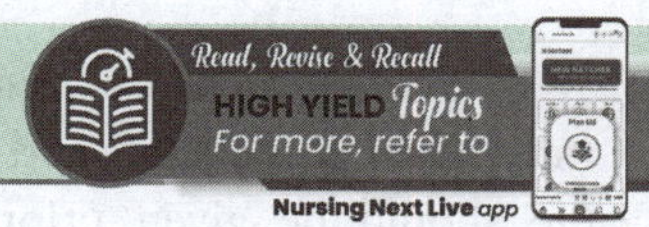

Social Institutions

Introduction to Social Institutions

- A social institution is an interrelated system of social roles and social norms arranged around the satisfaction of a social need or social function.
- These are patterns of beliefs and behavior.
- These are centered on basic social needs

Definitions of Institutions

- Morris Ginsberg: Institutions may be described "as recognized and established usages governing the relations between individuals and groups."

  "Institutions represent "the social structure and the machinery through which human society organizes, directs and executes the multifarious activities required to satisfy human needs" —HE Barnes

Types of Social Institutions

1. Familial institutions
2. Governmental institutions
3. Economic institutions
4. Educational institutions
5. Religious institutions

List of Social Institutions

- Family
- Religious institutions
- Marriage
- Educational institutes
- Economic institutes
- Welfare institutes
- Political institutes
- Government

Characteristics of Institutions

- Social in nature
- Universality
- Institutions are Standardized Norms
- Institutions as Means of Satisfying Needs
- Institutions are the Controlling Mechanisms
- Relatively Permanent
- Abstract in Nature
- Oral and Written Traditions
- Synthesis Symbols
- Institutions are Interrelated

Functions of Institutions

- Institutions cater to the Satisfaction of Needs
- Institutions control Human Behavior
- Institutions simplify Actions for the Individual
- Institutions assign roles and Statuses to the Individual
- Institutions Contribute to Unity and Uniformity
- Manifest Functions of Institutions
- The negative Functions of Institutions

Interrelationship between Social Institutions

1. All institutions created for human needs fulfillment.
2. Provide unity in human behavior.
3. Form of behaviors (culture) transfer from generation to generation.
4. Provide solution to social problem.
5. Every institution control the society.
6. Make cooperation among the people.

SOCIAL CONTROL – MEANING, AIMS AND PROCESS OF SOCIAL CONTROL

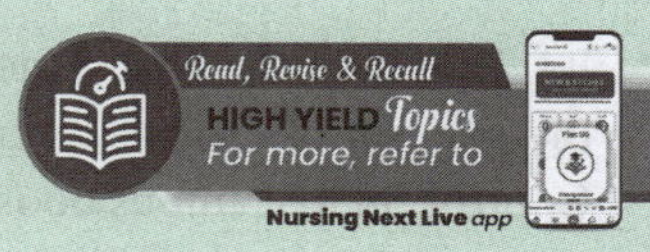

Introduction

- Peace and harmony are required in any social system.
- Unless individuals live up to the norms prescribed by the society, this harmonious living is not possible.
- In any society, at all times, there will be deviant elements, who fail to conform to the norms of the society.
- Methods by which these deviant elements are made to conform to the generally accepted pattern of behavior are called **social control.**

Historical Evidences

Early Prehistoric Days

Isolated Nomadic life, solitude, war with nature, so they wanted human association

In Neolithic Stage

Larger human congregations

Later

Group conflicts and clashes emerged

Then

Human became selfish individualistic, barbarous, hedonistic, power hungry and conflicting

Further

Regulations to restrain the undesirable human conduct and promote the desirable actions were established

Meaning of social control

- The term social control is used in various ways.
- It is commonly used to compel the individuals to conform to societal norms and standards
- But, it is a narrow meaning of social control.
- If seen comprehensively, social control involves the regulation of entire social order in order to achieve social ideals and objectives.
- In simpler terms, social control can be understood as any social or cultural means by which systematic and relatively consistent restraints are imposed upon individual's behavior.

Introduction

- EA Ross was the first American Sociologist to deal with the concept of "Social control in his famous book "Social Control" in his famous book "Social Control" in 1901.

Definitions of Social Control

- **EA Ross:** Social control refers to the "system of devices whereby society brings its members into conformity with the accepted standards of behavior."
- ***Mannheim:*** "Social control is the sum of those methods by which a society tries to influence human behavior to maintain a given order."

Aims of Social Control

1. **To form social solidarity:** When deviant elements are controlled, order is established in the group, and this brings about social solidarity
2. **To achieve social conformity:** Every group is prescribed
3. **Helps in socialization:** Socialization is meant that, the younger generation is taught to conform to the values and norms established by the older generation. Control is essential in this process.
4. **Maintaining social organization and order:** Agencies of control pressurize parts to fulfill their assigned functions.
5. ***Control over behavior of individuals:*** Human beings are characterized by extreme individualization traits. But if everybody is allowed to follow his own pattern of behavior, there will be utter chaos. Social control is essential to control the behavior of individuals so that individuality does not stand in the way of social life.
6. ***To provide procedure and prominence to group over individual:*** If social life and progress have to ensure, group life should be given priority over individual freedom. Agencies of social control assure that the group interest is maintained over individual interest.

Purposes of Social Control

- To establish stability in the social relations.
- Bringing desired modifications in the social environment
- Establishing primacy of social and humanitarian values over individualistic and separatist list ends.
- Tune the behavior
- To provide fair and equal chances
- To facilitate appreciation or punishment
- To exercise control over social tensions and conflicts.
- To bring solidarity and uniformity in the social organizations.

Types/Forms of Social Control

- Kimball Young—Classified social control into two types **"positive control"** and **"negative control"**
- Karl Mannheim has classified into "**direct control**" and "**indirect control**"

Overall Forms of Social Control

Conscious and Unconscious Control
Direct and Indirect Control
Positive and Negative Social Control
Organized, Unorganized and Automatic Social Control
Autocratic and Democratic Social Control
Some sociologists
Formal and Informal Social Control

1. **Conscious and Unconscious Control**

   The conscious behavior of human beings refers to such acts and actions as are done deliberately and in a planned way, e.g., a student does not sit in the chair of his teacher and also, while talking to his teacher he remains alert and attentive.

   On the other hand, some human actions are done unconsciously and the person himself does not know why he is doing so because repeated behavior pattern becomes a part off his personality, e.g., while putting I on our clothes, we follow a certain pattern (e.g., we put on our undergarments first and not after having put on upper garments)
2. **Direct and Indirect Control**
   - Control on human behavior is exercised by very close persons such as parents, friends, teachers, neighbors, etc. It is direct social control. It is more durable

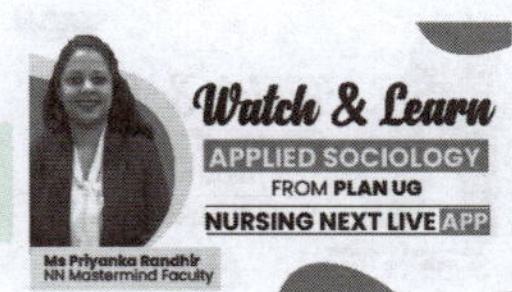

- Indirect social control is through social and physical environment, different groups and institutions. It is less durable.

3. Positive and Negative Social Control

- Positive social control depends on the positive motivation of the individual to conform
- In negative forms of social control, deviant behavior of individuals is discouraged and punished.

4. Organized, Unorganized and Automatic Social Control

- In organized social control, human behavior is influenced by a set of social agencies having clearly defined "do's and 'don'ts" for individuals, educational institutions, family, state, etc.
- In unorganized social control, influences the personality of human beings through the means of rites and rituals, customs and traditions, folkways and mores, etc.
- In the automatic social control, individuals are themselves motivated to act in order to meet their felt needs.

5. Autocratic and Democratic Social Control

- If administrative agency or the authority uses its force to attain the objectives other than those defined and recognized by society, it is autocratic form of social control.
- If the control is exercised by the agencies or authorities established by the people themselves and if their wishes are taken into consideration while framing rules and regulations, it is called democratic social control

6. Formal and Informal Social Control

- The classification of social control-organized and unorganized as given by Gurvitch and Moore can be termed formal and informal.
- The formal social control has the sanction of state whose authority is used to regulate, the human behavior. It has written rules and regulations.
- Informal social control influenced by belief, customs, traditions, criticism, public opinion, religion, etc. is exercised by society. Example: Primitive tribal society.

Broad Categorization of Social Control

1. Informal
2. Formal

Process and Means of Social Control

- Art
- Sanskars
- Social ideals
- Social suggestions
- Belief
- Leaders
- Humour and ridicule
- Fashion
- Nonviolence
- Language
- Punishment and rewards
- Mores
- Folkways
- Propaganda
- Law
- Religion and morality
- Public opinion

Role of Nurse

- The social control are to be followed by the individuals
- But no society completely succeeds in making all its members follow the social control
- Some of them fail to conform to the social control
- Failure of conform to the social control of society is called deviant behavior or deviance
- Social deviance disturbs life pattern of people and leads to many diseases
- As a nurse one should understand the patient's deviance behavior and treat the patient

SOCIAL NORMS, MORAL AND VALUES

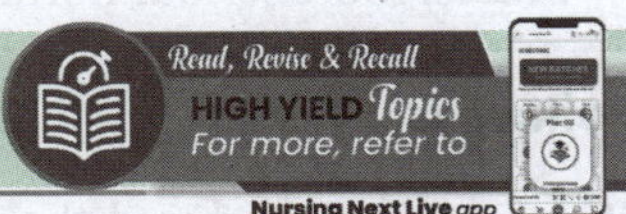

Introduction to Social Norms

- **M Sherif** in his book "The Psychology of Social, Norms" in 1936 used the term "Social norms" for the first time to describe the common standards or ideas which guide its members

Definitions

- **According to Buckman:** "A norm is a standard of behavior expectation shared by group members against which the validity of perceptions is judged and the appropriateness of feeling and behavior is evaluated."
- **According to Broom and Selznick:** "The norms are blueprints for behavior, setting limits within which individuals may seek alternate ways to achieve their goals"
- **According to Sherif and Sherif:** "Norms are standardized generalization concerning expected modes of behavior."

Importance of Social Norms

- The standards of behavior contained in the norms give order to social relations, interaction goes smoothly if the individuals follow the group norms

- Norms being accepted standards of social behavior regulate the behavior of the individual members of the society
- The normative order makes the factual order of human society
- The normative system gives to society a cohesion without which social life is not possible
- Norms regulate and control the individual as well as the social organization
- Norms help in maintenance of social aims and objectives
- Norms help the individual members of the society to fulfill his or her social needs properly
- Norms influence the individuals
- Norms influence the individual's attitude and his motives
- Norms determine and guide the members of society in initiating judgment of others and of his own

Types of Norms

- The expectations about behavior are called social norms.
- The four types of social norms are: folkways, mores, taboos, and laws
- **Folkways:** Informal norms used day to day
- **Law:** System of rules in society to maintain order
- **Taboos (Negative Mores):** Prohibition of social actions based on false beliefs
- **Mores:** More serious norms but informal

Folkways

WG Sumner introduced the concept "folkways" in his book Folkways (1906).

Definitions

- **WG Sumner:** "The folkways are habits of the individual and customs of the society which arise from efforts to satisfy needs"
- **Eldridge and Merrill:** "The folkways are literally the ways of the folk, that is social habits, and group expectations that have arisen in the daily life of the group"

Characteristics

- Folkways arise out of the efforts to satisfy needs
- They are popular habits and traditions
- They are wildly enforced in the sense that anybody who breaks the folkways are not strictly punished
- The punishment for not following the folkways is mainly social disapproval, may be, in the form of snubbing or gossip
- They are less essential as compared to mores
- They are considered as matters of good tastes and behavior in the society
- Folkways differ from place to place and also in different times at the same place

Examples of Folkways

- Manners
- Dressing sense
- Eating behavior
- Traffic rules
- Picking nose in public
- Rules of greeting
- Marriage ceremonies
- House decoration in festivals

Importance of Folkways

- Folkways help in the fulfillment of needs of the coming generation
- Folkways bring about homogeneity in social behavior
- Folkways are usually transmitted to the new generations
- Folkways are effective agencies of social control because breaking of folkways is punishable by social disapproval

Mores

- Mores develop from folkways and customs
- They are more stable, powerful and obligatory
- In smaller communities, mores are very important in social life and social control
- The must behavior is called Mores
- Unwritten customary ways of life
- Both formal and informal punishments can be given for its violation.

Definitions

- WG Sumner: "When the elements of truth and right are developed into the doctrines of welfare, the folkways are raised to another plane."
- MacIver and Page: "When the folkways have added to them conceptions of group welfare, standards of right and wrong, they are converted into mores."

Types of Mores: Positive and Negative

1. Positive
  - Prescribe behavior patterns
  - They represent the "do's"
  - Give instructions and provide guidance

2. Negative
  - Also prescribe behavior patterns
  - Also called "Taboos"
  - Prohibit/forbid certain behavior

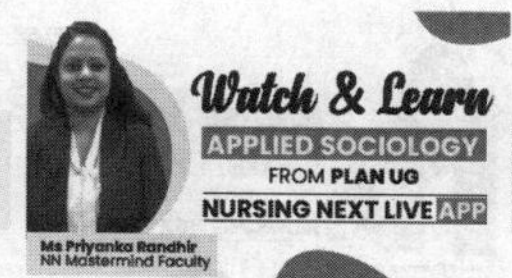

Characteristics of Mores

- Like folkways, mores also develop slowly, gradually and naturally
- The idea of group welfare is attached to the mores
- Mores carry with them a sense of right and wrong
- People who break the mores are severely punished
- Since the mores are very important for group welfare, they are included in the laws of the state also
- Mores are usually connected with the basic needs of the society
- Mores differ from place to place and time to time
- Mores are included in the normative system of the group

Examples of Mores

- Wearing clothes
- Respecting elders
- Students obeying educational norms
- No sexual relationship before marriage
- Entering someone's house without permission
- Drug abuse
- Abduction of children
- Loving one's country

Functions of the Mores

- Mores define a lot of our personal behavior
- Mores maintain the solidarity of the group
- Mores encourage behavior, which will keep up group welfare
- Mores are very important for social control because of the fear of punishment attached to mores, they are rigorously followed by the members of the society

Laws

- Laws are confined to modern societies
- In primitive societies, customs, traditions and folkways are sufficient agencies of control
- But in highly complex modern societies, customs become ineffective in maintaining order
- Law is the instrument of modern societies for maintaining social system

Definitions

- **MacIver and Page:** "Law is the body of rules which are recognized, interpreted and applied to particular situation by the courts of a state."
- **EA Ross:** "Law is the most specialized and highly finished engine of social control employed by the society."

Characteristics of Law

- Law is a body of rules and regulations
- Laws are made by the state or political power
- Laws are applied to and interpreted in different social situations and generally administered through agencies like police and court
- Laws are made from the existing customs, traditions, mores
- Laws are powerful agencies of social control
- When laws are broken, punishments are awarded by the state
- Laws differ from place to place and time to time

Examples of Laws

- Killing someone
- Dacoity
- Excessive drinking
- Rape

Morals and Values

Morals

- Morals are the rules which people use to direct their behavior and thinking.
- It enables the person to deal with, or become capable of distinguishing between, right and wrong.

Examples of Morals

- Do not cheat
- Always tell truth

Values

- A principle, standard, or quality considered worthwhile or desirable are the values.
- Values are broad ideas about what is good or desirable shared by people in a society.

Importance of Values

- It influences the social behavior
- It serves as the basis for norms

Values of Indian Society

- Diversity.
- Pride.
- Innovativeness.
- Adaptability.
- Harmony.
- Modesty.
- Lightheartedness.

Examples of Values

- Love animals
- Aim high and work hard for your dream

Social Sanctions

- Sanctions are the means of controlling human behavior
- They may take the form of both rewards and punishments
- Generally speaking, sanctions are understood to mean punishments or deprivations, but rightly understood sanctions refer to both rewards, gratification and punishments or deprivations.
- They are used to persuade or force an individual or group to conform to social expectations.

Aims of Social Sanctions

- The basic purposes of sanctions are to bring about conformity, solidarity and continuity of a particular group, community or larger group
- In primary groups and small societies, sanctions are not so much needed as in secondary groups and large societies
- As societies become heterogeneous not only complexity of interaction increases but also there are found cross currents of warring factions
- Sanctions control the individuals or groups who threaten solidarity

Types of Sanctions

- **Positive sanctions** are essentially pleasant or rewarding such as praise flattery, promotions, honor, medals, etc.
- **Negative sanctions** are essentially unpleasant. They inflict plain or threaten to do so such sanctions may vary from a mild expression of disapproval to fines and imprisonments or death.
- Sanctions can be **formal** or **informal.**
- The informal sanctions are illustrated by customs, the mores and public opinion.
- The formal sanctions are worded by a legally constituted authority. Such sanctions are physical torture, punishment, imprisonment or death.
- Sanctions can be symbolic or take the form of overt force.
- Symbolic sanctions are praise and flattery, promises, persuasion, propaganda, rewards, satire, commands, censure and threats.
- The form of overt force includes fines, punishment, imprisonment, torture and death.

Symbolic Sanctions

- Symbolic sanctions are in the form of words and gestures
- Praise is a reward in words especially from higher to lower strata
- Indoctrination, advertising and propaganda condition poisons to act along lines, which they like or imagine they like
- Satire employs wit and scorn as indirect criticism of actions feel to be socially harmful
- Threats are the most severe form of verbal sanctions

Social Conformity

- Society maintains its order through the normative system
- Normative system means the system of rules, regulations, practices, laws, etc. every individual has to accept and obey the system of norms
- In Merton's scheme, total conformity involves accepting both society's goals and the legitimate means of achieving them
- A young man or woman who gets a good education, finds a good job, and takes the "right" steps up the occupational ladder is conforming to both the goal of financial success and the legitimate means of achieving it

Definitions

- **William P Scott:** In his dictionary of sociology defines conformity as "Behavior that is in accord with the expectations of social group."
- It can also be defined as-"The endeavor to maintain a standard set by a group."

SOCIAL DISORGANIZATION – DEFINITIONS, CAUSES, CONTROL AND PLANNING

Meaning of Social Disorganization

- The concept was developed by **Thomas and Znaniecki** in their famous book "The Polish Peasant in Europe and America"
- According to them, the term "social disorganization" refers to the decrease in the influence of the existing social rules of behavior upon individual members.
- Will automatically and inevitably create social problems

Definition of Social Disorganization

- **Emile Durkheim:** "Social disorganization as a state of disequilibrium and a lack of social solidarity or consensus among the members of a society."

Causes of Social Disorganization

- Elliott and Merrill have given four causes:
  1. The social processes under the three main heads—cultural, political and economic
  2. Cultural lag
  3. Conflicting attitudes and values
  4. Social crisis

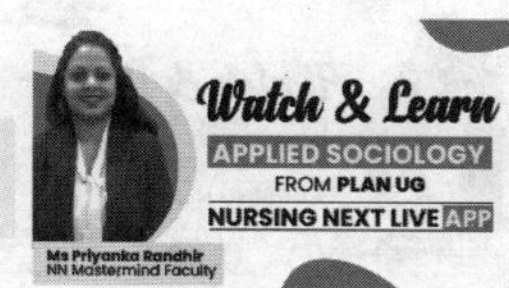

Social Problems

Social problems are behavior patterns or conditions that are considered objectionable or undesirable by many members of society

The problems of unmarried mothers, dowry system, prostitution, substance abuse (drug addiction, alcoholism), crime, handicapped, child abuse, child labor, women abuse, population explosion, corruption, poverty, housing, food supplies, illiteracy, prostitution, HIV/AIDS, unemployment, family disorganization, sexual deviance, etc. are considered social problems

Definitions of Social Problems

Fuller and Myers have defined a social problem as "a condition, which is defined by a considerable number of persons as a deviation from social norms which they cherish."

Horton and Leslie defined social problem as "a condition affecting significant number of people in ways considered undesirable; about which it is felt that something can be done through the collective social action."

Poverty in India

- The problem of poverty is the most formidable one faced by independent India
- It is a social as well as economic phenomenon in which a section of the society is unable to meet even its basic necessities of life
- When a substantial proportion of a society is deprived of the minimum level of living and continues at a base substantial level, the society is said to be living in poverty

Definitions of Poverty

According to Gillin and Gillin, "Poverty is that condition in which a person either because of inadequate income or unwise expenditure, does not maintain a scale of living high enough to provide for his physical and mental efficiency and to enable him and his natural dependents to function usefully according to the standards of the society to which he is a member."

According to Dr Smith, "Poverty is a socioeconomic phenomenon in which a section of the society is unable to fulfill even its basic necessities of life."

Thus, poverty has been defined as "that situation in which an individual fails to earn income sufficient to buy him, the barest means of subsistence."

Housing

- After the needs of food and clothing, a decent place of living is the third most basic need of a person.
- Homelessness is a growing. The world's homeless population is estimated to be around 1 billion people
- In India, the problem of housing is very acute.
- A number of housing clusters have mushroomed in and around various metropolitan centers in haphazard and unplanned manner, without a proper layout and devoid of service lines and other essential facilities.
- These unauthorized developments are encroachments on land parcels belonging to government bodies, public-private-institutions or areas meant to be green belts.
- The removal/resettlement of these overcrowded unhygienic clusters, commanding massive vote banks, is a serious challenge to correcting these aberrations for a planned growth of cities.
- So, massive concerted effort needs to be made with best of administrative actions and deft political handling for the sake of our future generations.
- There is a rise of homelessness in the urban and rural areas due to a number of factors.
- According to Census definition, houseless households are those which do not live in buildings but stay in open or roadside, railway platforms, under flyovers, etc. Urban population saw a rise in homeless population from 7.78 lakh people in 2001 to 9.38 lakh people in 2011, but rural areas witnessed a decline from 11.6 lakh people to 8.34 lakh people.

Food Supplies

- Food crisis often occurs in the poorest countries and even in communities of the most developed parts of the world. This crisis causes health problems related to lack of food, like malnutrition in children:
- Because of the technological means in place for planting and harvesting food, there are often surpluses, especially in richer countries, but food is often wasted
- After remaining a food deficit country for many years, India became largely self-sufficient in food grain production at the notable level

Problem of Illiteracy

- Illiteracy refers to the state of being unable to read or write
- Illiteracy is a great hurdle for the economic development India
- Millions of people in our country are still in the dark shadows of illiteracy and ignorance
- The problem of illiteracy in India will not be solved only by providing education for the children
- Illiteracy is rampant among the older generation of people, particularly in the rural areas

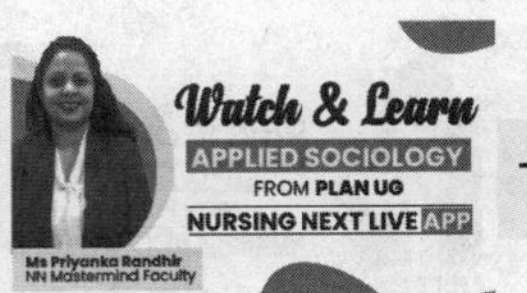

Prostitution

- There are many definitions of prostitution.
- The simplest definition says that it is an exchange of money for sexual purpose that is offering sexual intercourse for pay.
- In other words, it is an act of sexual intercourse in exchange for money
- Prostitution is a social problem not only in India but the world over and is said to be the oldest trade in the world.

Dowry

- In an ordinary sense dowry refers to money, gifts, goods or estate that wife brings to her husband in marriage
- Dowry is a major problem of marriage in India, especially in certain communities
- With the increasing importance of money, the amount of dowry is also increasing

Definitions of Dowry

- Encyclopedia: Britannica "Dowry is the property which a woman brings with her or is given to her at the marriage"
- Webster's New World Dictionary: "The money, goods or estate which a woman brings to her husband in marriage."
- Max Radin: Dowry is "the property which a man receives from his wife or her family at the time of marriage"

Child Labor

- The term "child labor" is considered equivalent to the term "working child" or "employed child"
- India has the largest number of child laborers in the world who are engaged in both organized and unorganized sectors
- A large majority of these child laborers are engaged in agriculture and allied sectors, while others are found in urban, semi-urban and industrial areas

Definitions

According to the Constitution of India—child laborer may be defined as a person who is below the age of 14 years and is working for an earning

According to the Concerned for Working Children of Bengaluru—a child laborer is "a person who has not completed his/her 15 year of age and is working with or without wages/income on a part-time or a full-time basis"

According to Home Folks, "child labor is any work by children that interfere with their full physical development, and their needed recreation"

A lot of companies look for juvenile labourers because they can get more work done by them while paying them less. Child laborer are primarily employed in the mining, glass, carpet, and leather industries because they lack a "labor union" of their own and "bargaining power" to do so.

Child Abuse/Neglect

Child neglect is the most common form of maltreatment. Neglect is generally defined as the failure of a parent or other person legally responsible for the child's welfare to provide for the child's basic needs and an adequate level of care. (Nester, 1998 and Kaplan and Labruna, 1999)

Definitions

A complex set of behaviors that include child neglect and the physical, emotional, and sexual abuse of children. (Medical dictionary)

Child abuse or child maltreatment is physical, sexual, and/or psychological maltreatment or neglect of a child or children, especially by a parent or a caregiver. Child abuse may include any act or failure to act by a parent or a caregiver that results in actual or potential harm to a child, and can occur in a child's home, or in the organizations, schools or communities the child interacts with. (Wikipedia)

Causes of Child Abuse

- Parents abused as child
- Unrealistic expectations
- Lack of effective parenting techniques
- Difficult children (hyperactive, demanding, mentally retarded)
- Social isolation, lack of support system or violent society

Effect of Child Abuse

1. Death/disability
   In severe cases
2. Behavior effects
   Affective and behavior disorders
3. Developmental effects
   Developmental delay and learning difficulties, failure to thrive and growth retardation
4. Psychological effects
   Predisposition to adult psychiatric disorders, abused becomes abuser

Juvenile Delinquency

- Juvenile delinquency is antisocial behavior committed by young people

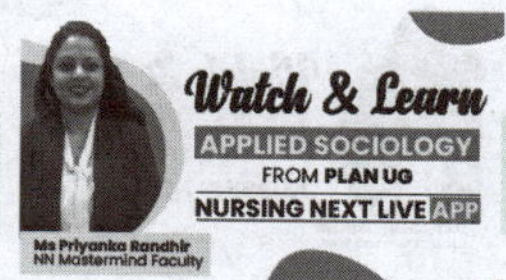

- Juvenile delinquents are simply under-age criminals that are, nonadult criminals, or Juveniles who engage in offenses that constitute crimes when committed by adults, and are between the age of 7 and 16 or 18 years, as prescribed by the law of the land.
- The maximum age today for Juvenile delinquents according to the Juvenile Justice Act of 1986 is 16 years for boys and 18 years for girls.

Definitions

Robinson: Juvenile delinquency is "Any behavior which a given community at a given time considers in conflict with its best interest, whether or not the offender has been brought to court"

Sethna: "Juvenile delinquency involves wrong doing by a child or young person who is under an age specified by the law of the place concerned"

Crime

Crime: As a Social Problem

- It is a form of deviance, specifically behavior that violates certain criminal laws
- The basic two types of crime are:
  1. Misdemeanor: A crime of lesser degree that typically involves punishment by paying a fine rendering community service or getting imprisoned for not more than one year.
  2. Felony: A serious crime such as killing, overthrowing the government, destroying other people's property, abusing minors, etc. in which a grave penalty is imposed ranging from more than a year of imprisonment to death penalty.

Classification of crime

- Crimes against person
- Crimes against property
- Crimes against chastity
- Crimes against public morals
- Crimes against the state

Causes of Crime

1. Unemployment forces many individuals to engage in illegal and immoral acts in order to provide for living.
2. Crimes like theft are committed due to poverty.
3. Crimes are committed due to behavioral disorders like kleptomania and pedophilia.
4. Crimes are committed by people who want to remain in power (politics) or protect their financial interests (businessman)
5. Crimes are a product of uncontrollable or involuntary behavior caused by excessive consumption of alcoholic beverages or addiction to drugs.
6. Crimes may arise from concupiscence (passion); too much infatuation sometimes leads to tragic death.
7. Crimes may be a product of individual ignorance (abandoning someone who is in danger is punishable under our penal code).
8. Crimes are sometimes caused by individual/group advocacy, political beliefs, or aspirations.
9. Crimes may be a result of an individual desire to gain profit using illegal means like prostitution, illegal recruitment, etc.
10. Crimes may be a product of one's failure to take precautionary measures, observe proper diligence and prudence that result in the death of another person or in the destruction of property

Substance Abuse

Drug Abuse and Drug Addiction

- "Drug abuse" is the use of illicit drug or misuse of legitimate drug resulting in the physical or psychological harm
- It includes smoking ganja or hashish, taking heroin or cocaine or LSD, injecting morphine, drinking alcohol, and so forth
- The word "addiction" is generally used to describe physical dependence

Characteristics of Drug Addiction

- An overpowering desires or need to continue taking the drug and to obtain it by any means
- A tendency to increase the dose
- A psychological and generally a physical dependence on the effects of the drugs
- An effect detrimental to the individual and to the society

Nature and Impact of Abusable Drugs

The abusable drugs may be divided into three categories: Alcohol, sedatives, stimulants, narcotics, hallucinogens, and nicotine

- **Alcohol:**
  - Alcohol is used by some people as a normal, pleasant and sociable activity, while others take it as a spur which enables them to work
  - It also acts as a sedative, which calms down nerves or a kind of an anesthetic which reduces the pain of living

Sedatives

- Sedatives or depressants relax the central nervous system, induce sleep and provide a calming effect

- Medically, these are used in high blood pressure, insomnia, epilepsy and to relax patients before and during surgery

Stimulants

- Activate the central nervous system and relieve tensions, treat mild depression, induce insomnia, increase alertness, minimize fatigue and expressive drowsiness, and lessen aggressive inhibitions
- The most widely known stimulants are amphetamines caffeine, and cocaine

Narcotics

- Like sedatives produce a depressant effect on the central nervous system
- They produce feeling of pleasure, strength, and superiority, reduce hunger, lessen inhibitions, and increase suggestibility
- Included in this category are opium, marijuana, heroin, Morphine, pethidine, cocaine and cannabis

Hallucinogens

- The well-known drug in this group is LSD, which is a man-made chemical
- It is so powerful that one ounce produces three lakh human doses

Nicotine

- It leads to relaxation, stimulates the central nervous system, increases wakefulness and removes boredom
- But frequent or heavy use of nicotine may cause heart attack, lung cancer, and bronchitis

Causes of Drug Addiction

- To get thrill or pleasure
- To relieve tension and to escape from situations of problem and anxiety
- Peer group
- To satisfy curiosity
- To express independence or hostility
- Broken homes, family disorganization, and history of addiction in the family
- Age—the use of drugs usually starts either in adolescence or early youth
- Easy availability of drugs
- Urban life with its anonymity, wide circle of contacts and easy means of transportation encourage the use of drugs
- Strenuous work or studies
- Affluent mode of life

Alcoholism

- Alcoholism and drug addictions are detrimental not only to the health and welfare of the individual, but of the family, community and society at large
- Alcoholism is condition in which an individual loses control over him
- Person is constantly unable to refrain from drinking once he begins
- According to Keller ad Efron, "alcoholism is characterized by the repeated drinking of alcoholic beverages to an extent that exceeds customary use or compliance with the social customs of the community and that adversely affects the drinker's health or interferes with his social or economic functioning."

Causes of Drinking

- Misery drinking: Men often start drinking in order to forget the miseries and problems of life
- Friendship: Many people are drawn into this habit by friends
- Fashion: Drinking has become a fashion among many people
- Occupational factors: Many men take to drinking because of physical exhaustion
- Ignorance: Many of the hard physical laborers are under the view that it relieves exhaustion
- Weak personality: A person whose moral fabric is weak and who gives way to temptations easily are led to drinking
- Unhealthy environment: People living in slums
- Sudden losses and frustration: Sudden loss of a dear one
- For business and professional reasons
- The new elites: Those people who become rich overnight
- Urbanization: Modern city life with its mechanical ways of life can lead to stress and alcohol serves as a stress reliever.
- Social inadequacy: Crisis in life may create a feeling of social inadequacy

Evil Effects of Drinking

- Drinking is a social evil and as far as possible every individual should keep himself away from it
- Drinks affect the health of the people adversely
- With long time use of alcohol, tremors, unsteady gait, lusterless eyes and haggard look may be observed
- Alcoholism is a root cause of family unhappiness, problems, tensions and even total disorganization
- Drinking is often associated with other social evils like gambling, prostitution, etc.

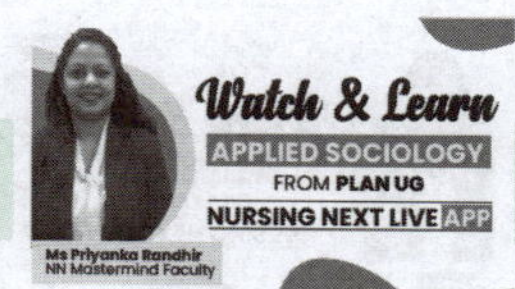

HIV/AIDS

- Acquired immunodeficiency syndrome (AIDS) is a sexually trans- mitted disease caused by the human immunodeficiency virus (HIV).
- It destroys the antibody producing white blood cells which are called T-cells and thus cripples the immune system
- The first case of AIDS was discovered at the Center for Disease Control in Atlanta, USA, in the year 1981
- The first case of AIDS reported in our country was from Tamil Nadu in 1986

Spread of HIV/AIDS

- Having sexual intercourse with infected person
- Intravenous drug abuse
- Using unsterilized needles and syringes
- Transfusion of HIV positive blood
- Using a common razor at the barber's shop or tonsuring at religious places
- Getting tattooed without sterilizing the needle
- An infected mother who passes on the infection to her unborn child
- Living with or caring for people with HIV or AIDS
- Using the same toilets as the infected people
- Swimming in pools used by infected persons
- Shaking hands, hugging or kissing infected persons
- Drinking water from the same glass used by an infected person
- Coughing, sneezing or from water, food, clothing, arid cutlery shared with infected persons
- By bites of a mosquito which has already bitten an infected person

Effects of AIDS

- Chronic pneumonia
- Chronic diarrhea
- Infections which block the throat, intestine and lungs
- Cancer of skin and bone
- Swelling in the brain
- Destruction of brain tissue causing loss of memory and personality changes

COVID-19

- This is a highly contagious disease caused by the novel Coronavirus (COVID-19) that spreads through sneezing and coughing droplets. This virus exhibits symptoms and signs similar to the common cold, but it is hazardous, and if not identified early and managed by health personnel, it can cause serious sickness and death in humans.
- **Impact of COVID-19 on Society:**
  - Increased poverty and inequality: The pandemic has led to widespread job losses and business closures
  - Increased mental health problems
  - Increased domestic violence
  - Increased school and college drop-outs

VULNERABLE GROUP – ELDERLY, HANDICAPPED, MINORITY AND OTHER MARGINAL GROUP

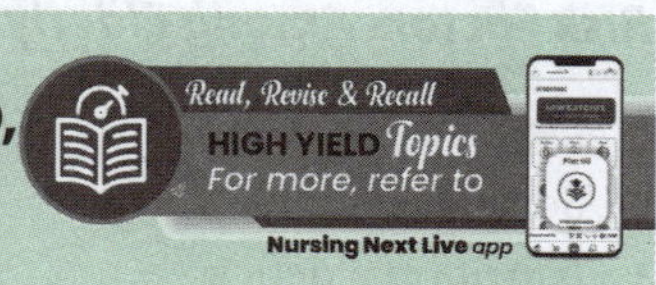

Vulnerability

- It is the function of sensitivity, exposure and the adaptive capacity.
- Sensitivity is the degree to which a system will be affected by, or responsive to climate stimuli (Smith et al., 2001).
- Exposure is the degree of climate stress upon a particular unit of analysis; it may be represented as either long-term changes in climate conditions, or by changes in climate variability, including the magnitude and frequency of extreme event (IPCC, 2001).
- Adaptive capacity: the potential or capability of a system to adjust to climate change, including climate variability and extremes, so as to moderate potential damages, to take advantage of opportunities, or to cope with consequences (Smit and Pilifosova, 2001)

Vulnerable Groups

- Elderly
- Persons with disabilities
- Minority groups
- Marginalized groups

Vulnerable Patients

- Infants
- Children
- Disabled individuals
- Elderly and frail
- Child abuse/Neglect
- Domestic violence
- Sexual assault/Abuse
- All SCBU/NICU, Comatose patients and patients on mechanical ventilation
- Elder abuse — dehydration, fearful at contact, bedsores
- Substance abuse
- Elderly — 70 years of age/older
- Mentally retarded individuals
- Patient in crisis

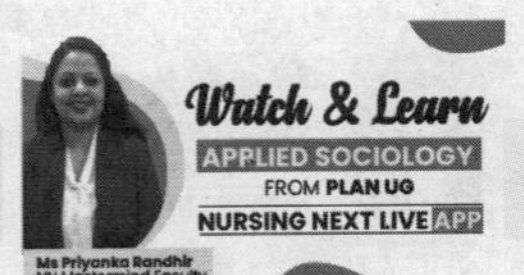

Elderly

Elderly are the people who are 65 or above.

They are considered vulnerable as they are at risk of injury through falls and other injuries due to impairment in physical and mental dimensions as the result of age.

Risk Factors Among Elderly

- Dementia
- Social isolation
- Nutritional deficit
- Muscle atrophy
- Impaired immune system
- Injury
  - Elderly 10 times more likely to be hurt from a fall
  - Fall prevention exercise programs appear to be useful
  - Cognitive functioning is a crucial factor
  - Most commonly the unexpected deaths are seen among the elderly
  - Vitamin D supplements are related with improved balance and walking
  - Vitamin D deficiency results in muscle weakness

Care of Elderly

Government Organizations

The problems of the aged can be mitigated by providing necessary welfare services to them by way of:

- Reasonable amount of old age pension
- Free medical care
- Housing facilities in the form of old age homes
- Recreational facilities to relative their loneliness
- Usual courtesies extended to them

Old Age Homes

The Central/State Governments Municipal Bodies Philanthropic Welfare Associations Old/Elderly Citizens Welfare Association have set up homes for the old/elderly citizens.

- At present there are only some 300 homes in the country mostly in urban areas.
- These demands are not really off-target, considering the hardship the senior citizens face to on retiring or when they have no means of livelihood and are ignored by the younger lot in their families.
- **Age-Care India (ACI)** was established in 1980.
- Providing educational, recreational, social, cultural and spiritual services.
- Arranging for medical services, part-time employment to supplement their income
- Organizing tours, trips and pilgrimages.

Persons with Disabilities

Introduction

- A disabled person is one who suffers from the loss or impairment of a limbs or deformity in physical or mental competence either naturally or due to an unexpected unfortunate accident.
- It is projected that about 12 million Indians about 1.8% of Indian population have at least one disability or the other.
- About 10% of the handicapped are having more than one type of physical disability.

Care of Persons with Disabilities

- Prevent falls
- Health education
- Additional safety tips
- District rehabilitation centers
- Loans are available from banks
- 3% vacancies in group "C" and "D" posts in government
- Ten years' age relaxation in reservation
- Special concerns while traveling
- Preference in allotment of government houses
- Scholarships from class 9th
- Sports competitions are held and winner is given prize
- Special devices made for assistance (braille wrist watches)
- Pensions to handicapped from state

Institutions for care of Disabled

- National Institute for the Orthopedically Handicapped at Calcutta.
- National Institute for the Visually Handicapped at Dehradun
- Ali Yavar Jung National Institute for the Hearing Handicapped at Mumbai
- National Institute for the Mentally Handicapped at Secunderabad

Minority Groups (SC, ST)

Definition of Minority Group

- Louis Wirth defined a minority group as "a group of people who, because of their physical or cultural characteristics, are singled out from the others in the society in which they live for differential and unequal treatment, and who therefore regard themselves as objects of collective discrimination."

Minority Groups

- The scheduled caste and scheduled tribe classes constitute under privileged who have been oppressed, suppressed,

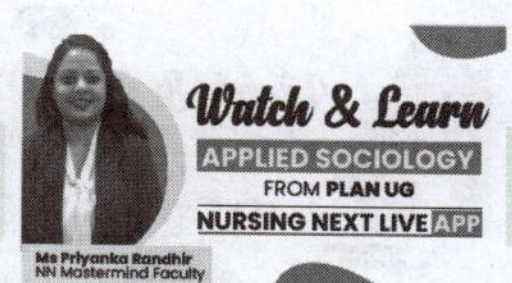

exploited humiliated and deprived equality liberty and justice in various field of life.

- The term scheduled caste appeared primarily in Government of India Act, 1935.
- In April 1936, the British Government had issued the Government of India (Scheduled Castes) order.
- The order stated certain castes, races and tribes as scheduled castes.

Care of Minority Groups

Constitutional Safeguards for Minority Groups Include

- The constitution prescribes protection and safeguards for the SCs and STs which protects the minority groups by:
  - The abolition of untouchability and the forbidding of its practices in any form (Art.17)
  - The throwing open by law of Hindu religious institutions of a public character to all classes and section of Hindus (Art.25 b)
  - Special representation in the Lok Sabha and the State Rajya Sabhas to SCs and STs till 25 January 2010 (Art. 330, 332 and 334).

Reservation in Services for minority groups:

- As per Article 16 (4) the groups are allowed for reservations in favor of citizens of backward classes, who may not be adequately represented in services.

Centrally Sponsored Schemes for Minority groups:

- Post-Matric Scholarships for SC and ST students.
- Pre-Matric Scholarships for the children of those engaged in unclean occupations.
- Book banks for SC/ST students who want to pursue degrees in Medical and Engineering colleges.
- Boys and Girls Hostels Scheme for SCs.
- Coaching and Allied schemes for SCs and STs.

Measures to Enhance Tribal Development

- Family oriented beneficiary program
- Prevent exploitation
- Human resource development
- Focus on infrastructure

Marginalized Groups (OBC)

- Marginalized groups are the groups and communities that experience discrimination and exclusion that could be in social, political and economic spheres.
- They experience this because of unequal power relationships across economic, political, social and cultural dimensions.

Examples of Marginalized Groups

- People with cognitive impairment
- SPMI (Serious and persistent mental illness)
- Physically challenged people
- People with below average intelligence
- Military combat veterns
- Racial/cultural minorities/OBC
- Senior citizens
- LGBT

Care of Marginalized Groups

- The Mandal Commission was established in 1979 to "identify the socially or educationally backward" and to consider the question of seat reservations and quotas for people to redress caste discrimination.
- The Mandal Commission covered more than 3,000 castes under Other Backward Class (OBC) category, regardless of their affluence or economic status

FUNDAMENTAL RIGHTS OF INDIVIDUAL, WOMEN AND CHILDREN

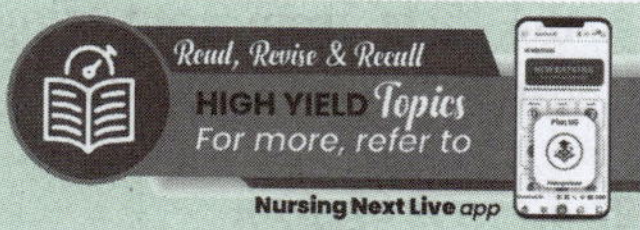

Introduction

- Human rights and sustainable human development are interdependent and mutually reinforcing
- While women's rights enrich the rights of children, children's rights can help promote the advancement of women's rights
- Human rights are enhanced when gender equity or poverty reduction programs empower people to claim their rights.

Rights can be in the form of:

- Human rights
- Civil rights
- Constitutional rights
- Civil liberties
- Privileges

Rights of Women

- Rights under constitutional Law
- Rights under family Law
- Rights under Muslim Law
- Rights against violence and indecency
- Rights of Maintenance under other laws
- Key NGO's working for women Rights

NGOs For Women

- Justice for Women
- Khushi Foundation
- Indraprashtha Sanjeevni NGO, Naraina
- Masum Zindagi, RK Puram
- Women's Political Watch, Hauz Khas
- Shuddhi NGO, Prashant Vihar

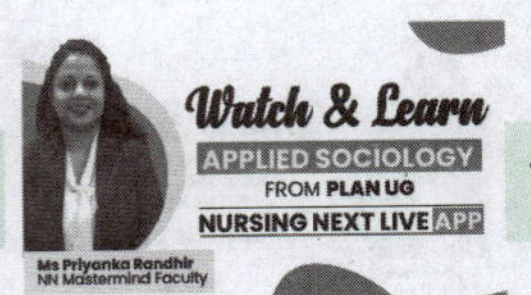

Basic Human Rights

Right to Equality

i. Equality before Law: Article 14 of the constitution guarantees that all citizens shall be equally protected by the laws of the country

ii. Social equality and equal access to public areas: Article 15 of the constitution states that no person shall be discriminated on the basis of caste, color, language, etc.

iii. Equality in matters of public employment: Article 16 of the constitution lays down that the State cannot discriminate against anyone in the matters of employment. All citizens can apply for government jobs.

iv. Abolition of untouchability: Article 17 of the constitution abolishes the practice of untouchability.

v. Abolition of Titles: Article 18 of the constitution prohibits the State from conferring any titles. Citizens of India cannot accept titles from a foreign State.

Right to Freedom

Following are the right to freedom subject to a reasonable restrictions by the state in the interest of public order

i. Freedom of Speech and expression, which enable an individual to participate in public activities.

ii. Freedom to assemble peacefully without

iii. Freedom to form associations or unions

iv. Freedom to move freely throughout the territory of India though reasonable restrictions can be imposed on this

v. Freedom to reside and settle in any part of the territory of India

vi. Freedom to practice any profession or to carry on any occupation, trade or business

Right Against Exploitation

The abolition of trafficking in human beings and Begar (forced labor). Abolition of child labour and human trafficking. Trafficking in humans for the purpose of slave trade or prostitution is also prohibited by law.

Right to Freedom of Religion

Citizens are free to preach, practice and propagate any religion of their choice.

Cultural and Educational Rights

Articles 29 and 30. Any community which has a language and a script of its own has the right to conserve and develop it. All minorities, religious or linguistic, can set up their own educational institutions to preserve and develop their own culture.

Right to Constitutional Remedies

Right to constitutional remedies empowers the citizens to move a court of law in case of any denial of the fundamental rights. This procedure of asking the courts to preserve or safeguard the citizen's fundamental rights can be done in various ways. The courts can issue various kinds of writs. These writs are habeas corpus, mandamus, prohibition, quo warranto and certiorari.

Rights of Women and Children

The Constitution not only grants equality to women, but also empowers the State to adopt measures of positive discrimination in favor of women.

Laws Related to Children

- Child Labor (Prohibition and Regulation) Act, 1986
- Child Marriage Restraint Act, 1929
- Children Act, 1960
- Children (Pledging of Labor) Act, 1933
- Commissions for the Protection of Child Rights Act, 2005
- Infant Milk Substitutes Act, 1992
- Infant Milk Substitutes Act, 2003
- Infant Milk Substitutes, Feeding Bottles and Infant Foods (Regulation of Production, Supply and Distribution) Act, 1992
- Infant Milk Substitutes, Feeding Bottles and Infant Foods (Regulation of Production, Supply and Distribution) Amendment Act, 2003
- Juvenile Justice (Care and Protection of Children) Act, 2000
- Infant Milk Substitutes, Feeding Bottles and Infant Foods (Regulation of Production, Supply and Distribution) Amendment Act, 2003
- Juvenile Justice (Care and Protection of Children) Amendment Act, 2006
- Prohibition of Child Marriage Act, 2006
- Reformatory Schools Act, 1897
- Role of nurse in reducing social problem and enhance coping

Role of Nurse in Alleviating the Effects of Poverty

- Helping families to maximize income levels (like helping families to claim benefits)
- Case advocacy (along with department of child and family welfare)
- Improving access to early childhood development services for families
- Minimizing the financial and emotional costs of using services (easily accessibility, less waiting time, etc.)

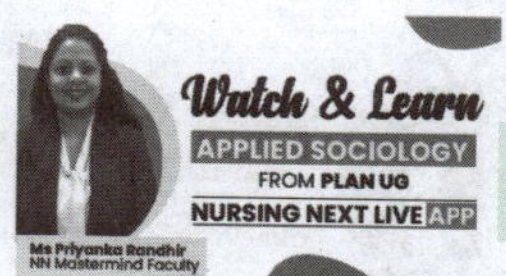

- Provide information about services (like low cost recreational or parent support program and how to get access to them)
- Targeting resources to those with greatest needs
- Providing support and working in partnership with individuals and groups
- Help in economic liberalization
- Assist in programs related to women empowerment
- Be a changing agent in capital, infrastructure and technology
- Provide health education
- Nurse should assist in poverty alleviation program

Poverty Alleviation Programs

- Swaranjayanti Gram Swarozgar Yojana (SGSY)
- National Food for Work Program
- Antyodya Ann Plan
- Legal Elimination of Bonded Labor
- Rural Employment Generation Program (REGP)
- Pradhan Mantri Gramodaya Yojana (PMGY)
- Rural Housing – Indira Awaas Yojana (IAY)
- Sampoorna Grameen Rozgar Yojana (SGRY)
- Prime Minister's Rozgar Yojana (PMRY)
- Pradhan Mantri Gram Sadak Yojana (PMGSY)
- Small Farmers Development Program
- Drought Area Development Program

Role of Nurse to Reduce Unemployment

- Integrated Rural Development Program
- Employment in Foreign Countries
- Jawahar Rozgar Yojana
- Training for Self-employment
- Training Programs
- Employment Guarantee Scheme
- Rural Employment Guarantee Program
- Liberalization of labor market
- Self-employment to educated unemployed youth
- Cottage industries
- Development of organized sectors
- Employment exchanges
- Prime Minister's Integrated Urban Poverty Program
- Employment Assurance Scheme

Role of Nurse to Control Prostitution

- Adequate legislation
- Social education and propaganda
- Job opportunities/rehabilitation
- Change of rigid social customs
- Sex education

Role of Nurse in Juvenile Delinquency

- Psychotherapy
- Reality therapy
- Behavior therapy
- Active therapy
- Env therapy
- Family counseling
- Individual counseling
- Vocational counseling

SOCIAL WELFARE PROGRAMS IN INDIA

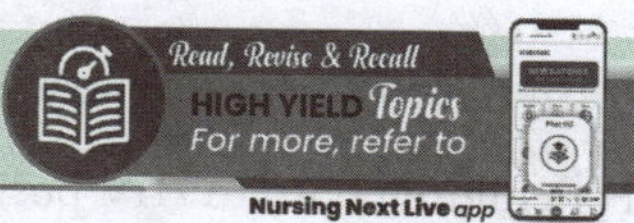

Introduction

Social welfare program is any type of governmental programs intended to protect citizens from the economic risks and insecurities of life. The most common types of programs provide benefits to the elderly or retired, the sick or invalid, dependent survivors, mothers, the unemployed, the work-injured, and families.

Target Groups

- Children
- Women
- Disabled
- Old people
- Under privileged and diseased

Principles of Welfare Programs

- Voluntary
- Comprehensive
- Services
- Effective for creating awareness, education and communication
- Easy accessibility

Welfare Program for Children

- Girl child Protection Scheme
- One female, undergone sterlization, <Rs. 50,000/pa
- Initial deposit of Rs. 22200/-for one or Rs 15,200/- each for 2 girls
- Monthly incentive of Rs 150/- from 5th year for educational purpose
- At 20 years lump sum amount given to girl, condition is that she should appear in 10th standard
- Cradle baby scheme
- Creches for working women

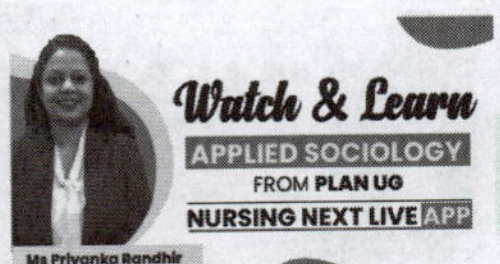

Child Protection (Nutrition and Care)

- ICDS Integrated Child Development Services Scheme
- Supplementary Nutrition
- Anganwadi Centers
- Parent education

Kasturba Gandhi Memorial Trust

For health care, education, and economic welfare of needy rural women and children

Indian Red Cross Society

For children born to HIV positive mothers

Central Social Welfare Board

It provides technical and financial assistance to the voluntary organizations for the general welfare of family, women and children.

Indian Council for Child Welfare

For children born to HIV positive mothers

- **UN support for primary education**
- **DPEP (District Primary Education Project)**
- **NPRPD:** National Program for Rehabilitation of Person with Disability
- **Sarva Shiksha Abhiyan**
- **Project for Integrated Education Development (PIED) and Integrated Education for Disabled Children (IEDC)**
- **National level practices on education of children with disability**

Welfare Program for Women

- Mahila mandals
- Legislative measures
- Family life institutes
- Hostels for working women
- Employment and income generation programs
- Educational programs
- Appointment of commission and committees
- Central Social Welfare Board

Central Social Welfare Board

- Central government gives financial assistance
- Establishing school and colleges for girls.
- Construction of women hostel building.
- Post — metric scholarship for ST/SC girls.
- Free clothing.
- Adult education centers.
- Nutrition child care and family planning.

Educational Programs

- Central government gives financial assistance
- Establishing school and colleges for girls.
- Construction of women hostel building.
- Post — metric scholarship for ST/SC girls.
- Free clothing.
- Adult education centers.
- Nutrition child care and family planning.

Employment and Income Generation Programs

Started in 1982-1983. 'ArTraining:- handloom weaving, food processing. Programs were implemented through public sector undertaking/corporations/autonomies bodies/ voluntary organization Rehabilitation of women in distress was launched in 1977. Women development corporation play important role in releasing loan for self employment.

Family Life Institutes

- Association for social health in India runs the family life institute in Delhi.
- Family life education.
- Training camp for social worker.

Hostels For Working Women

- Central government give financial assistance
- Establishing school and colleges for girls.
- Construction of women hostel building.
- Post — metric scholarship for ST/SC girls.
- Free clothing.
- Adult education centers.
- Nutrition child care and family planning.

Mahila Mandals

- Started in 1954
- Provide basic minimum services to women and children
- Compromise maternity health services, literacy and education service for women
- Social Welfare Board bears the expenditure up to 75%

Latest Programs or Schemes 2020

- Beti Bachao Beti Padhao
- One Stop Center Scheme
- Women Helpline Scheme
- Ujjawala Scheme

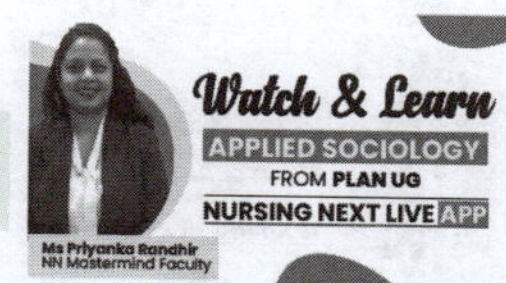

- Working women hostel
- Swadhar Greh (Women in difficulty)
- STEP (Support to Training and Employment Program for women)
- Nari shakti puraskar
- Stree shakti puruskar
- Rajya mahila samman
- Zila mahila samman
- Mahila shakti kendras (msk)
- Nirbhaya
- Mahila police volunteers
- Mahila e-haat
- Anganwadi service scheme
- Pradhan mantri matru vandana yojna
- National creche scheme
- Child protection scheme
- Poshan abhiyan
- Important milestones in family welfare
- Postpartum program, mtp
- Family welfare program
- Maternal child health and family planning integrated
- National family welfare program
- Mch, uip
- National health policy
- Cssm
- Creche scheme fof working mothersor the children

Role of Nurse

- Administrative role
- Supervisory role
- Functional role
- Educational role
- Evaluation and research

CONCEPTUAL EXERCISES

LONG ANSWER QUESTIONS

1. a. Explain the causes and concept of juvenile delinquency.

b. Discuss the measures to control juvenile delinquency. (CCS Uni)

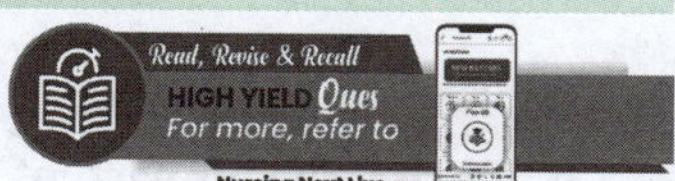

Answer

- Juvenile delinquency is antisocial behavior committed by young people.
- Juvenile delinquents are simply under-age criminals that are, nonadult criminals, or Juveniles who engage in offenses that constitute crimes when committed by adults, and are between the age of 7 and 16 or 18 years, as prescribed by the law of the land.
- The maximum age today for Juvenile delinquents according to the Juvenile Justice Act of 1986 is 16 years for boys and 18 years for girls.

Definitions

According to Sethna, "Juvenile delinquency involves wrong doing by a child or young person who is under an age specified by the law of the place concerned."

Characteristics of Juvenile Delinquency

- The delinquency rates are much higher among boys than girls.
- The delinquency rates tend to be highest during early adolescence (12–16 years).
- Juvenile delinquency is more of an urban than a rural phenomenon.
- Children not living with parents and guardians are found to be more involved in the Juvenile crimes.
- Low educational background is the prime attribute for delinquency.
- Poor economic background is another important characteristic of Juvenile delinquency in India.
- Though some delinquencies are committed in groups but the number of Juvenile gangs having support of organized adult criminals is not much in our country.
- More than four-fifths of the Juvenile delinquents are first offenders and only a little more than one-tenth are past offenders.

Forms of Juvenile Delinquency

- Delinquent action against property such as stealing, damaging, etc.
- Murder and suicide
- Assault
- Gambling
- Sexual offenses like rape and sodomy
- Ticket less travel especially in train, and
- Escape from custody

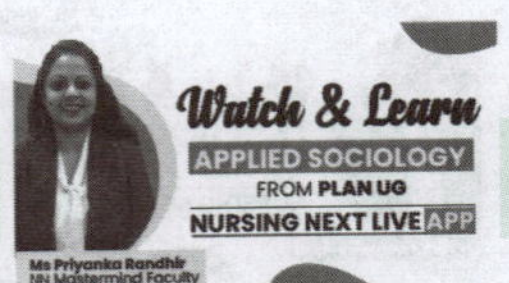

Causes of Juvenile Delinquency

- There are several causes that are responsible for Juvenile delinquency.
- According to ***Healy and Bronner***—Bad company, adolescent instability and impulses, early sex experiences, mental conflicts, extreme social stability, love for adventure, motion pictures, school dissatisfaction, poor recreation, street life, vocational dissatisfaction, sudden impulses and physical conditions of all sorts.

Causes of Juvenile Delinquency in India

- Poverty
- Breakdown of joint family
- Breakdown of caste
- Breakdown of traditional religion, morals and values
- Illiteracy and lack of proper education
- Lack of care by the government
- Industrialization and urbanization, together with large scale migration to the cities
- Absence of proper facilities for marriage and family counseling, so as to have responsible and mature parenthood
- Political problems
- Social change, etc.

Impact of Juvenile Delinquency

- Impact on victim
- Impact on juvenile delinquent
- Impact on families
- Impact on society

b. Measures to Control Juvenile Delinquency.

Answer

Some of the measures to prevent Juvenile delinquency are:

1. **Education:** It is necessary to undertake educational and awareness programs for parents on how to interact with their children, how their actions will affect them, and how important it is to do so. Additionally, social skills' education for kids in schools is necessary.
2. **Improving Parent-Child Relation:** Parenting techniques and the proper way for parents and children to interact should be covered in parenting education program. To adequately teach the child about the behavioral concerns, parents and children should have wholesome conversations. For the parents, there should be program on how to react to their child's behaviors.
3. **Prevent Bullying**: The majority of the time, peer groups or schoolyard bullies target youngsters in or near their neighborhood. The children's mental health may be impacted by the bullying. Sometimes young people may harbour resentments and unintentionally commit crimes.

   Early intervention and support services: Early intervention programs, such as counseling, mental health services, and substance abuse treatment, can help address underlying issues contributing to delinquency and prevent further involvement in criminal activities.

   Restorative justice practices: Implementing restorative justice practices that focus on repairing harm caused by delinquent behavior, promoting accountability, and fostering empathy can be more effective than traditional punitive measures in rehabilitating young offenders and reducing recidivism.
4. **Recreation:** Recreational programs give kids the chance to interact with both adults and other kids. They might develop a good friendship that will benefit them later. The personality and skills of the youngsters should be taken into consideration when designing these recreation program. The kids need access to extracurricular activities like music, dancing, sports, martial arts, painting, etc. to keep their minds stimulated and busy.

At some point, every nation in the world has dealt with—or is now dealing with—the issue of adolescent delinquency. However, developing nations are significantly more plagued by the issue of adolescent delinquency. There are numerous elements that can influence a child's growth in the developing world.

---

2. a. Explain child labor.

b. Write the impact of child labor on health and illness. (CCS Uni)

Answer

- The term "child labor" is considered equivalent to the term "working child" or "employed child."
- India has the largest number of child laborers in the world who are engaged in both organized and unorganized sectors.
- A large majority of these child laborers are engaged in agriculture and allied sectors, while others are found in urban, semi-urban and industrial areas.

Definitions

According to the Constitution of India—Child laborer may be defined as a person who is below the age of 14 years and is working for an earning.

Causes of Child Labor

Various factors have contributed to the problem of child labor among which the following may be noted:

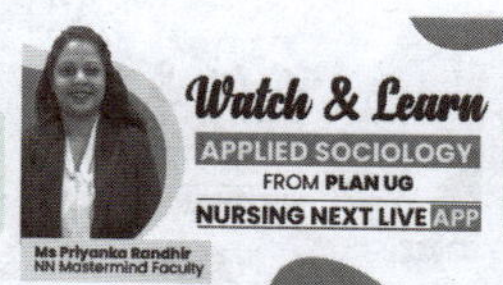

1. Economic factors
   - Poverty
     - Possibility of extracting more work for less wages
     - To secure more profit for factories
2. Familial factors
3. Other factors
   - Temptation of bad habits
   - Justification of employers of child laborers
   - Failure of government machinery and legislative system
   - Lack of public awareness
   - Kidnapping and blackmailing of children

Causes of Child Labor: Economic factors

- **Poverty:** Child labor is commonly found in all the developing countries where poverty is usually seen. India is a country in which more than 26% of the people are living below the conditions of poverty as per 2001 estimate.
- **Possibility of extracting more work for less wages:** Child labor is commonly found in all the developing countries where poverty is usually seen. India is a country in which more than 26% of the people are living below the conditions of poverty as per 2001 estimate.
- **To secure more profit for factories:** Some industrialists (owners of fireworks, match-box units, glass and brassware industries, etc.) believe that their units are able to maximize profits because of the appointment of child laborers whose labor is very cheap.

Causes of Child Labor: Familial factors

- **Family disorganization:** Divorce, desertion, rigid family relations, cruelty at home, parent too run away from the unpleasant family environment.

Causes of Child Labor: Other Factors

- **Temptation of bad habits:** Children belonging to the poor families often become the victims of certain bad and costly habits such as—smoking, gambling, purchasing lottery tickets, seeing the movies regularly, consuming alcoholic drinks, etc. When they don't get enough pocket money from home they often resort to outside work to earn money to satisfy their bad habits
- **Justification of employers of child laborers:** They argue that work keeps poor children away from starvation. They even say that they are rendering a service to the society by providing some jobs to the wandering children who would otherwise have become criminals or joined the rank of antisocial elements.
- **Failure of government machinery and legislative system:** Though the government has a constitutional obligation and a moral responsibility to promote the welfare of the children, it is not serious about the problem of child labor. The half-hearted legislations undertaken in this regard, are a bad failure. The government bureaucracy is also indifferent of the problems of the working children.
- **Lack of public awareness:** No organization has launched an effective movement at the all India level to rouse the consciousness of the public regarding its responsibility toward children.
- **Kidnapping and blackmailing of children:** There are some antisocial forces which often kidnap children and take them to a different place for selling them to some employers who are in search of cheap human labor.

b. Write the impact of child labor on health and illness. (CCS Uni)

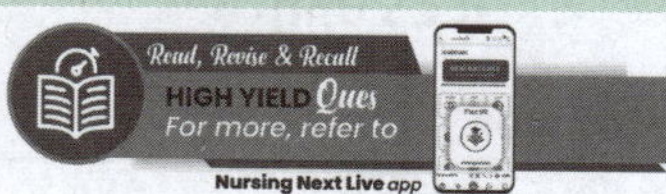

Answer

Impact of Child Labor on Health and Illness

- **Emotional conflicts**: It's important to consider how child labor affects children's mental health. Drug addiction, PTSD, depression, and other mental health conditions are widespread. Despite the paucity of research on child labor and health, the evidence that does exist points to detrimental consequences.
- **Human trafficking:** Trafficked children are subjected to prostitution, forced into marriage or illegally adopted; they provide cheap or unpaid labor, are forced to work as house servants or beggars and may be recruited into armed groups.
- **Increased mortality rates:** Due to workplace and equipment-related incidents, 10 minors between the ages of 14 and 18 and seven children under the age of 14 died.
- **Child abuse:** It suggests a lost or deprived childhood that results in child exploitation in a variety of ways, including mental, physical, social, and sexual.
- **Malnutrition:** Poor growth, malnutrition, skin infections, musculoskeletal disorders, and behavioral and mental disorders, which can result in a number of chronic diseases, are only a few of the detrimental health repercussions of child labor.
- **Unhygienic conditions**: Children are more vulnerable to infectious diseases such diarrhea, cholera, and dysentery due to poor personal hygiene, inadequate sanitation, and a lack of potable water.
- **Occupational diseases:** The wounds of children become more infected as a result of working with poisonous substances like coolants and grease. Tetanus risk is increased in cuts caused by sharp, rusted metal.
- **Horrible working conditions:** The working conditions of the children are poor which leads to various health problems.

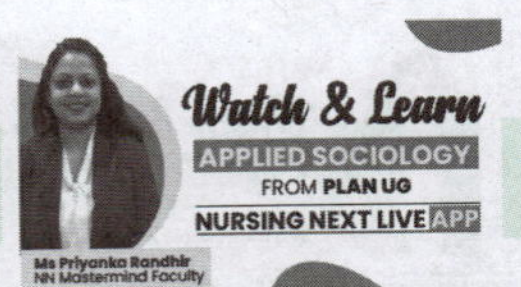

3. a. What is meant by population explosion?

b. Write down the consequences of overpopulation or discuss the impact of population explosion. (CCS Uni)

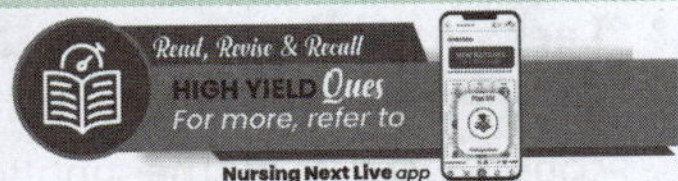

Answer

It is a sudden increase in the number of people in a particular location at a certain moment. We are all quite concerned about the population rise. Due to a quick rise in population, its effects can already be seen in many places.

b. Write down the consequences of overpopulation or discuss the impact of population explosion. (CCS Uni)

Answer

Impact of Population Explosion

The obvious consequence of a growing global population is that resources will be put under more stress. The need for food, water, housing, energy, health care, transportation, and other resources will rise as the population grows. And all that consumption increases the likelihood of major catastrophes like pandemics, increases conflicts, and degrades the environment.

Major consequences of overpopulation include:

- **Ecological degradation:** Population growth will unavoidably contribute to pressures that worsen climate change by increasing deforestation, reducing biodiversity, and increasing pollution and emissions. In the end, many experts think that the added stress on the planet will cause ecological upheaval and collapse that is so severe that it threatens the survival of life on Earth.
- **Enhanced conflicts:** Overpopulation and environmental disruption-induced scarcity have the potential to intensify violence and political upheaval. Warfare over water, land, and energy resources is already taking place in the Middle East and other places, and as the world's population rises, the unrest is certain to get worse.
- **Risk for disasters:** Numerous recent new infections, such as COVID-19, Zika virus, Ebola, and West Nile virus, that have wreaked havoc on people all over the world have their origins in animals or insects before spreading to humans. The destruction of wildlife habitats and an increase in human-wildlife contact are two factors that contribute to the world entering "a period of increased outbreak activity." It is now abundantly evident how challenging it is to maintain social distance in a world where there are close to 8 billion people.
- **Depletion of resources:** The available resources will not be enough to meet the increased demand of the overpopulation, resulting in imbalance between the two.
- **Unemployment issues:** A huge population translates into a large labor force. However, it is challenging to offer productive employment to the entire working population due to a lack of financial resources. An underdeveloped nation like India typically has concealed unemployment in rural areas and open unemployment in metropolitan areas.
- **Urbanization and infrastructure challenges:** Population explosion often leads to rapid urbanization as people migrate from rural to urban areas in search of better opportunities. This urbanization can strain existing infrastructure, leading to inadequate housing, inadequate access to clean water and sanitation, increased pollution, traffic congestion, and inadequate healthcare and education facilities.
- **Economic challenges:** Rapid population growth can create economic challenges, including high unemployment rates, income inequality, and increased demands for public services. Meeting the needs of a growing population in terms of employment, healthcare, education, and social services can be a significant economic burden for governments and societies.

4. Define social disorganization. Explain the causes and controlling measures. (MGR)

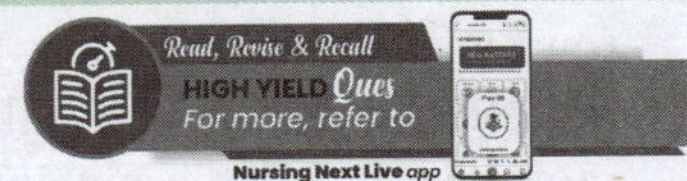

Answer

Definition of Social Disorganization

Elliott and Merrill: "Social disorganization represents a breakdown in the equilibrium of forces, a decay in the social structure, so that old habits and forms of social control no longer function effectively."

Causes of Social Disorganization

- A complex phenomenon such as social disorganization is caused by number of factors.
- These factors are so intermingled that it becomes difficult to say which out of these are predominant.
- Different writers have highlighted the importance of different factors.
- Elliott and Merrill have given four causes:
  1. The social processes under the three main heads—cultural, political and economic
  2. Cultural lag
  3. Conflicting attitudes and values
  4. Social crisis

Characteristics of Social Disorganization

Just as a disease is known by its symptoms, the nature of social disorganization can be understood by means of its characteristics. They are stated as follows:

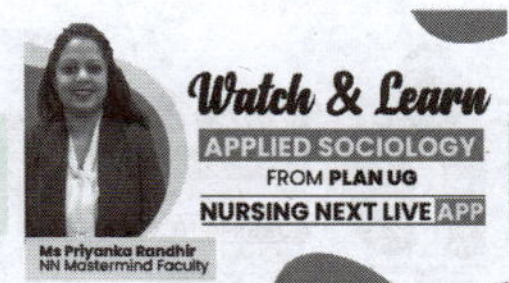

- Conflict of Mores and Institutions
- Transfer of functions from one group to another
- Individuation
- Inconsistency between expectations and achievements
- Inconsistency between status and role
- Diversity of opinion
- Heterogeneity of population
- Mutual distrust
- Uncertainty and insecurity
- Individuality and variety in interests and attitudes
- Emphasis on rights rather than on duties
- Contradictions between status and function
- Lack of clarity in status and roles
- Decreased social control
- Conflict between individual and society
- Disregard of values, norms and laws

Control Measures

- Based on theories
- **Social pathology approach:** Implement social welfare programs to address poverty, unemployment, and other socio-economic factors that contribute to social disorganization.
- **Value conflict approach:** Promote tolerance, understanding, and dialogue between different cultural, religious, and ethnic groups to reduce value conflicts and promote social cohesion.
- **Social disorganization approach:** Enhance community engagement and empowerment to strengthen social bonds and collective efficacy in communities.
- **Deviant behavior approach:** Implement effective law enforcement and crime prevention strategies to address deviant behaviors and maintain social order.
- Provide rehabilitation and reintegration programs for individuals involved in deviant behavior to promote their reintegration into society.
- **Cultural lag approach:** Promote education and awareness about the impacts of cultural lag on social disorganization. Encourage technological advancements and innovation to bridge the gap between cultural changes and societal structures.
- **Labeling approach:** Promote fair and unbiased labeling and avoid stigmatization of individuals and communities to prevent further marginalization and social disorganization.
- General Measures
- **End poverty:** Implement poverty reduction strategies, promote equitable distribution of resources, and provide economic opportunities for all members of society.
- **End hunger:** Implement food security programs, improve agricultural practices, and ensure access to nutritious food for all.
- **Health promotion:** Provide accessible healthcare services, promote preventive healthcare measures, and raise awareness about healthy lifestyles.
- **Equal and quality-based education for all:** Ensure access to education for all individuals and promote inclusive and quality education systems
- **Gender equality:** Promote gender equality, eliminate discrimination and violence against women and girls
- Sustainable development (water, energy for all): Implement sustainable development practices to ensure access to clean water, reliable energy sources, and environmental preservation.
- **Proper economic growth:** Foster inclusive economic growth, create employment opportunities, and promote fair trade practices.
- **Resilient infrastructure:** Invest in infrastructure development and supports the well-being and safety of communities.
- **Reduce inequality:** Address social and economic inequalities through policies and programs
- **Promote peace:** Foster peaceful and inclusive societies through conflict resolution, promoting dialogue, and addressing the root causes of violence and conflict.

SHORT NOTES

1. Write short note on Prostitution. (CCS Uni)

Answer

Prostitution

- The simplest definition says that it is an exchange of money for sexual purpose that is offering sexual intercourse for pay.
- In other words, it is an act of sexual intercourse in exchange for money.
- Prostitution is a social problem not only in India but the world over and is said to be the oldest trade in the world.
- In India, prostitutes are especially looked down upon by society which has designated it to the lowest rungs of the social ladder as they do not seem to offer any meaningful contributions to the society.
- According to Human Rights Watch report, 15 million prostitutes of varied groups, live and work in India.
- Every hour, four women and girls in India enter prostitution, three of them against their will.
- A large number of prostitutes in India are minors.
- Generally, we think only women are the victims of prostitution but even men and children are also victims of it.

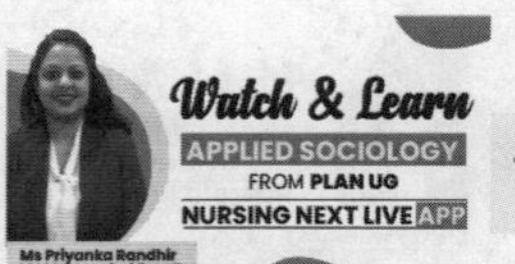

Causes of Prostitution in India

- Poverty
- Violence
- Debt
- Coercion
- Profits
- Promotion of tourism
- Social customs (Devadasi)
- Early marriage and desertion
- Ignorance and acceptance of prostitution
- Psychological factors (desire for physical pleasure and greed)
- Lack of sex education
- Prior incest or rape

Impact of Prostitution

On Society

- **Exploitation and Human Trafficking:** Prostitution is often associated with human trafficking, as individuals, including minors, may be coerced or forced into engaging in prostitution against their will.
- **Pornography and Objectification:** Prostitution can be connected to the pornography industry, as both involve the commodification and objectification of individuals for sexual purposes.
- **Family Conflicts:** Prostitution can lead to conflicts within families, including strained relationships, emotional distress, and breakdowns in trust.
- **Moral corruption:** Prostitution raises moral and ethical debates in society. This can lead to social divisions and debates about the rights and dignity of individuals involved in prostitution.
- **Health Risks and STDs:** Prostitution has been associated with increased risks of sexually transmitted infections (STIs), including HIV/AIDS.

On Individual

- **Emotional conflicts:** Engaging in prostitution can lead to emotional conflicts and psychological distress.
- **Unwanted pregnancies and abortions:** Individuals involved in prostitution may face a higher risk of unwanted pregnancies due to inconsistent or inadequate use of contraception.
- **Intimacy problems:** Engaging in prostitution may impact an individual's ability to form and maintain healthy intimate relationships.
- **Social isolation and stigma:** Individuals involved in prostitution often face social isolation and stigmatization.

2. Write short note on Poverty. (CCS, MGR)

Answer

Definitions of Poverty

According to Gillin and Gillin, "Poverty is that condition in which a person either because of inadequate income or unwise expenditure, does not maintain a scale of living high enough to provide for his physical and mental efficiency and to enable him and his natural dependents to function usefully according to the standards of the society to which he is a member."

According to Dr. Smith, "Poverty is a socioeconomic phenomenon in which a section of the society is unable to fulfill even its basic necessities of life."

Poverty in India

- The problem of poverty is the most formidable one faced by independent India.
- It is a social as well as economic phenomenon in which a section of the society is unable to meet even its basic necessities of life.
- When a substantial proportion of a society is deprived of the minimum level of living and continues at a base substantial level, the society is said to be living in poverty.

Meaning of Poverty

- The estimate of the minimum consumption expenditure necessary to meet the subsistence level of living and the population, whose level of income expenditure is below the mentioned figure, is called absolute poverty.
- According to Indian Planning Commission, the consumption of less than the required 2,400 nutritional calories per person per day for rural areas and 2,100 calories per person per day for urban areas is considered as the line of starvation or poverty line.
- Under relative poverty, we compare the different income groups in a country and their corresponding expenditure.
- For example, in USA poverty line is drawn at a level where the essential needs include all 20th century minimum conveniences such as electric lighting, indoor flush toilets, refrigerators, etc.

Causes of Poverty in India

The causes of poverty in India are as follows:

Rapid rise in population

Population in India during the last four decades has increased at the rate of 2.5% per annum. India's total population rose to 84 crores in 1991. On an average, India adds 1.4 crore every year to its population.

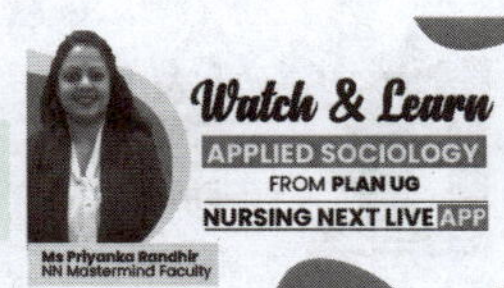

Low productivity in agriculture

In the absence of alternative occupations, the burden of increasing population falls upon the land. Land holdings are sub-divided and fragmented. Besides, cultivating methods are also primitive and outdated. It naturally results in low agricultural productivity and low level of income.

- Unutilized natural resources
- Growing unemployment and under-employment
- Inequalities of income
- Regressive tax structure
- Want of capital
- Low technological skill
- Social factors
- Political factors

Impact of Poverty

- Overutilization of natural resources
- Illegal land grabbing
- Anti-social behavior
- Reduced average lifetime
- Increased rate of crime

3. Dowry system. (CCS Uni)

Answer

Definitions of Dowry

"Dowry is the property which a woman brings with her or is given to her at the time of her marriage Encyclopedia: Britannica."

Causes of Dowry

1. Endogamy and the problem of getting a proper groom
2. Child marriage
3. Perception of people that the Dowry is a prestige symbol.
4. Ugly looking girls
5. For the stability of the marital bond
6. Aspiration to marry in high and rich family
7. Vicious circle
8. The custom of "Kanyadan"
9. Materialistic outlook in life
10. Weak enforcement of laws
11. The patrilocal system (the bride to move in with her husband's family after marriage)
12. Gender inequality
13. Lack of education

Negative Impact of Dowry on Society

1. Indebtedness
   - Often parents, especially of poor girls are forced to take loan in order to marry off the girls.
   - Such loans accumulate with interest, and the problem of indebtedness comes.
   - Things become worse if there are several girls to marry off.
2. Suicide of the young girls
   - Many young girls at the prime of their youth found they were burden on their parents as they were failing to find a suitable boy for them simply because they could not afford dowry.
   - Consequently, they decided to cut short their life by committing suicide.

4. Define 'Social control'. Mention the formal methods of social control.

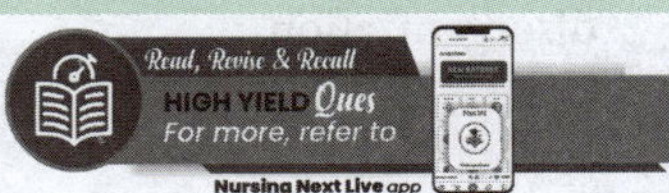

Answer

Social Control

Social control means to bring people of society within the limits and compel them to adopt conformity (standard rules or law) to social norms.

According to Ogburn and Nimkoff, the pattern of pressure that society exerts to maintain order, and establish rules is social control.

Formal methods of social control

- **Education:** Education inculcates moral, intellectual and social values in individual.
- **Law:** Law is for all practical purposes; as well as it is uniform and is meant for all.
- **Coercion:** Force as a means of social control to control the behavior of person.
- **State:** A state is an organized political community acting under a government.
- **Social administration:** Social administration is the study of social arrangements and policies aimed at meeting social needs—especially state welfare systems.
- **Legislative process:** Legislative process means the steps required for a proposed bill to become a law.
- **Judiciary:** The judiciary is that branch of the government that interprets the law, settles disputes and administers justice to all citizens.

SHORT ANSWER QUESTIONS

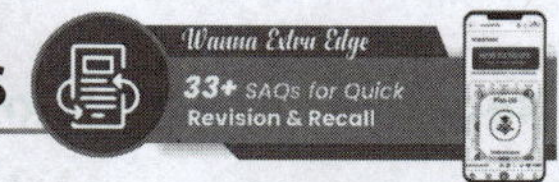

1. Mention four major causes of social disorganization.

Answer

Four major causes of social disorganization are:

1. **Violation of social rules:** According to WI Thomas and Znaniecki, when the rules and regulations of society fail to keep individuals under control, social disorganization arises.
2. **Industrialization:** Industrialization creates such circumstances or conditions leading to social disorganization
3. **Cultural lag:** Cultural lag is the concept or theory used by sociologists W E Ogburn, which refers to the imbalance in the rate and speed of change between the material aspects of cultural and non-material aspects.
4. **Division of labor:** According to Emile Durkheim, extreme division of labor are one of the important causes of social disorganization

2. Enlist types of poverty.

Answer

Poverty is the most important problem of rural people in India.

There are two types of poverty:

1. Abject poverty is a condition in which a person has nothing to eat, to put on or no proper housing.
2. Relative poverty means that compared with others in a particular society, a person is lacking certain things.

3. Mention any two social welfare measures for scheduled caste and other backward communities.

Answer

1. Pradhan Mantri Adarsh Gram Yojana (PMAGY): This scheme was launched in 2009–10 as a pilot project to develop those villages which had a higher ratio (above 50%) of scheduled castes.
2. National Scheduled Castes Finance and Development Corporation (NSFDC): NSFDC is the apex institution for financing, facilitating and mobilizing funds for the economic development activities of the persons belonging to the Scheduled Castes living below double the poverty line.

4. Define Child abuse.

Answer

As per POCSO Act 2012, Child Sexual Abuse is a violation of the child's body as well as of the child's trust and is against the law. It includes both contact and non-contact sexual behaviours. Child Sexual Abuse encompasses sexual assault, sexual harassment and use of a child for pornographic purposes.

5. Mention any four causes of dowry.

Answer

Four causes of dowry are:

1. Child marriage
2. Endogamy and the problem of getting a proper groom
3. The custom of kanyadan
4. For the stability of the marital bond

6. Write any two child welfare agencies.

Answer

Two child welfare agencies are:

- Indian Council for Child Welfare (ICCW): This council provides through a wide arrangement of programs from ameliorative to developmental support, protection and services to such children that are actually their birth right.
- Central Social Welfare Board: The Central Social Welfare Board was established in 1953 This welfare board is working for promoting voluntarism, providing technical and financial assistance to the voluntary organizations for the general welfare of society; family, women and specially children.

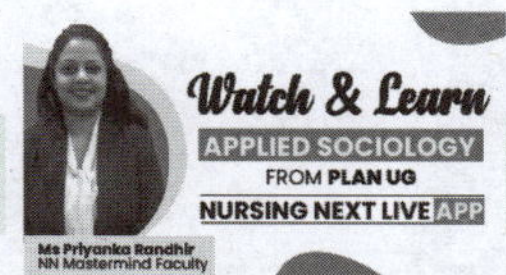

CONCEPTUAL REVISION

MULTIPLE CHOICE QUESTIONS

1. **"Social organization is the system by which the parts of society are related to each other and to the whole society in a meaningful way." Who said this?**
   a. Duncan Mitchell b. Philip Selznick
   c. Earnest Jones d. Leonard Broom

Ans. c. Earnest Jones

2. **Which among the following country has Democratic type of social organization?**
   a. China b. Myanmar
   c. Cuba d. Norway

Ans. d. Norway

3. **Which among the following is an advantage of authoritarian social organization?**
   a. Provides solution for complex problems
   b. Helps in making strong team
   c. Promotes a creative environment
   d. Quick decision making

Ans. d. Quick decision making

4. **Among the following which is not an Indian voluntary health agency?**
   a. Indian Red Cross Society
   b. Hind Kusht Nivaran Sangh
   c. TB Association of India
   d. Indian nursing council

Ans. d. Indian Nursing Council

5. **Like Socialization, ___________is also a system of measures by which society molds its members to conform with the approved pattern of social behavior:**
   a. Social role b. Social control
   c. Social change d. Social interaction

Ans. b. Social control

6. **The concept of "disorganization" was developed by**
   a. Schaefer
   b. Thomas and Znaniecki
   c. Giddens
   d. EA Ross

Ans. b. Thomas and Znaniecki

7. **All are the causes of social disorganization according to Elliott and Merrill, except:**
   a. Cultural lag
   b. Conflicting attitudes and values
   c. Social crisis
   d. Ecological factors

Ans. d. Ecological factors

8. **Delinquency is a kind of:**
   a. Abnormality
   b. Normality
   c. Illness
   d. All of these

Ans. a. Abnormality

9. **Dowry deaths, wife battering is an example of:**
   a. Criminal violence
   b. Domestic violence
   c. Social violence
   d. All of these

Ans. b. Domestic violence

10. **The function of sensitivity, exposure and the adaptive capacity is called:**
   a. Social problem
   b. Social injustice
   c. Vulnerability
   d. Delinquency

Ans. c. Vulnerability

CHAPTER

7

Clinical Sociology

CONCEPTUAL THEORY

Terminology

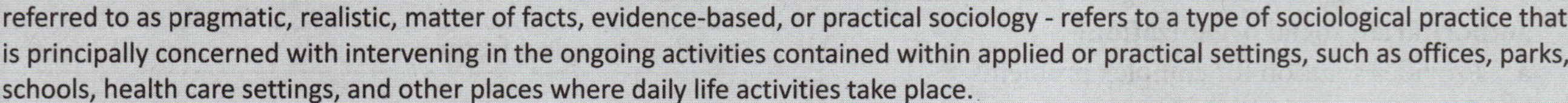

Applied sociology: Applied sociology is a branch of sociology that is sometimes referred to as pragmatic, realistic, matter of facts, evidence-based, or practical sociology - refers to a type of sociological practice that is principally concerned with intervening in the ongoing activities contained within applied or practical settings, such as offices, parks, schools, health care settings, and other places where daily life activities take place.

Case study: A method of analyzing a specific topic as if it were a case, spending more time and investigating a phenomenon in depth.

Client system: A client system, also known as a target group, is made up of people who require the direction and professional support of change agents.

Clinical analysis: It is the process of evaluating a condition. This comprises investigating the ideas, philosophies, policies, or practices of individuals as well as the groups or organizations to which they belong in order to improve the situation.

Clinical sociologists: They are also known as socio-therapists or life enrichment therapists, are usually members of another relevant profession, such as a medical doctor, psychiatrist, psychologist, nurse, social worker, criminologist, or activity and recreational professionals. They participate directly and honestly in case management and care planning.

Clinical sociology: Clinical sociology is a practice-oriented science that focuses on diagnoses and change. Clinical sociology is the analysis and creation of treatments for positive social change at any level of social organization using a sociological approach.

Clinical: A problem-solving perspective that focuses on the observation, assessment, intervention, and treatment of actual patients as opposed to theoretical or laboratory investigations.

Crisis intervention: It is a helping procedure that focuses on resolving an immediate or urgent crisis by utilizing personal, social, and environmental resources.

Crisis: A crisis is an acute emotional distress caused by situational, developmental, or social factors that results in a temporary incapacity to cope using one's normal problem-solving strategies.

Intervention: Action taken to improve a medical issue is referred to as intervention.

Social pathology: In general, social pathology refers to the pathos of society, such as societal diseases that impact the entire society.

Vulnerability: It is a sociological concept that refers to the characteristics of individuals and social groups (such as gender, age, ethnicity, occupation, and so on) that determine their ability to protect or guard themselves, withstand, and recover from disasters, including health hazards, based on their access to material and non-material resources.

CLINICAL SOCIOLOGY

Introduction

- **Applied sociology:** The use of the discipline of sociology with the specific intent of generating practical applications for human behavior and organizations.
- **Basic sociology:** Seeks a more insightful knowledge of the fundamental aspects of social phenomena.
- **Clinical sociology:** The use of the discipline of sociology with the particular intention to alter social relationships and facilitate change.
- The term "Clinical Sociology" was first used by Milton C. Winternitz (1885-1959), a physician who was dean of the Yale School of Medicine from 1920 through 1935.
- Clinical sociologists are change agents who use a sociological perspective as the basis for intervention. Many

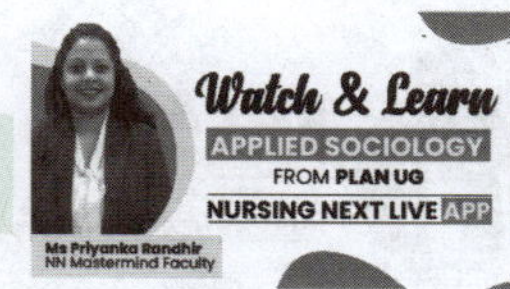

sociologists who teach are "clinicians" in that they try to foster change in students' attitudes and/or behavior as a result of classroom experiences. —Fritz

- Clinical sociology brings a sociological perspective to intervention and action for change. The clinical sociologist is essentially a change agent rather than a researcher or evaluator. Clients may be individuals, groups or organizations. The clinical task may involve, for example, a redefinition of the self, role, or situation. Clinical sociology uses a variety of techniques or methods for facilitating change. The field's value orientation is humanistic, holistic, and multi-disciplinary. —Glass

Meaning of Clinical Sociology

- Clinical sociology is the application of a sociological perspective to the analysis and design of interventions for positive social change at any level of social organization.
- Clinical sociologists have different areas of specialization, such as: Health promotion, aging, organizational development, or addressing social conflict.

Definition

Clinical sociology is the application of a variety of critically applied practices which attempt sociological diagnosis and treatment of groups and group members in the community

—Glassner and Freedman

Features of Clinical Sociology

- Uses insights derived from immersion in the critical sociological tradition.
- Uses sociological imagination
- Leads to behavior change and growth
- Tends to have a liberal/cynical or radical ideological cast
- Can move beyond the client's formulation of the problem to consider other factors that affect functioning, especially broad social trends
- Change-oriented
- Humanistic
- Diagnostic
- Works with individuals, groups, organizations, and communities
- Practice oriented
- Focuses on case studies

Role of Clinical Sociologist

- Individual counseling
- Family counseling
- System intervention
- Acts as an educator in clinical area
- As a changing agent in medical practice by developing, implementing and evaluating various health care programs
- Social world interventions

Application of Clinical Sociology

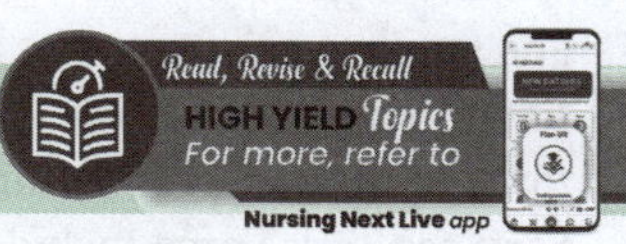

To improve individual and collective well-being.

Promotion of effective and holistic approaches to health and wellness through interventions

Help in development of deeper sense of understanding of social dynamics and its impact on health outcomes

Development of strategies to enhance overall societal and individual health.

SOCIOLOGICAL STRATEGIES FOR DEVELOPING SERVICES FOR THE ABUSED

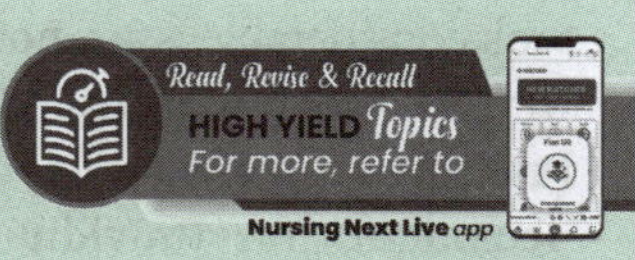

- In the social service fields and in the general public, there has been a growing awareness of the need for the development of services for victims of domestic abuse (Roy, 1977; Campbell, 1984).
- Social science principles and data were brought to bear in the design and implementation of a social service plan for abused wives in a major metropolitan area.
  (Reference: Clinical Sociology review, volume 5, issue 1, Article 13)

Intervention Strategies in a Committee Setting

- Throughout the process of selection of committee members, establishment of committee goals and objectives, and determination of methods for accomplishing these tasks, three major clinical strategies were employed:
  1. Provision of information about social structure and its consequences, enabling individuals and groups to use knowledge of social structure to develop more effective plans for group action;
  2. Use of sociological principles and data to make people aware of aspects of the social situation of which they had previously been unaware;
  3. Involvement of the individuals/group members in the planning process, to maximize the likelihood that they will have an investment in the outcomes.
- In reality, all three processes occur at once. Principles and data relating to the social structure are provided to key individuals in a manner designed to integrate them into the planning process.
- Social Structural Analysis is done to develop effective plan of action.

- **Use of Social Structural Factors** in Member Selection (police department and prosecutor's office, an attorney active in women's rights, and individuals who worked in mental health and family service agencies and educational institutes)
- **Establishment of Task Forces** (key figures in the police force and the prosecutor's office, and the Specialized Services Task Force included directors and representatives from family services and counseling agencies, as well as central figures from the county offices of the state department of social services.)
- **The Use of Hearings** (single meeting covering critical service needs for battered wives, and the individuals invited to appear were persons whose position in the community structure was key to the attainment of such services.
- **Avoiding the Pitfalls** (For example, one task force member took considerable issue, not with the goals of the group, but with the program plans it developed.)
- **Providing Knowledge of Sociological Principles and Data: Techniques for Providing Information:** It is important that the clinical sociologist be alert to the expression of such inaccuracies, for these incidents offer an opportune occasion for providing new information to correct the inaccuracies. This must be done with sensitivity, not that members and guests be insulted or offended. One effective technique for providing new information is to invite members of the group to check the literature and report back to the group
- **Developing Personal Commitment through Individual Involvement**
  - The role of group relationships in attitude stability and change has formed an important part of social psychological theory for some time (Asch, 1948; Newcomb, 1943; Lewin, 1951).
  - Include key members of these agencies in the planning process, and to obtain their commitment to the group and its goals

Role of Nurse

- Uses humanistic, multidisciplinary specialization that seeks to improve the quality of people's lives. (social scientist +active social change agent)
- Assesses situation
- Seeks solution
- Searches for alternatives
- Implementation
- Evaluates the quality of life

CRISIS AND ITS INTERVENTION

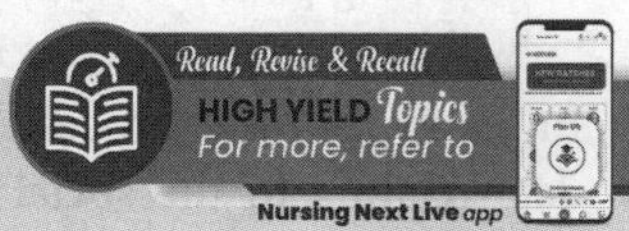

Definition

A crisis is any situation in which individual perceives a sudden loss of his or her ability to use effective problem-solving and coping skills.

Types of Crisis

Maturational/developmental crisis

Situational crisis

Adventitious crisis/social crisis

Crisis Interventions

Definition

Crisis intervention involves the methods used to render immediate, short-term help to individual who experiences an event that produces emotional, mental, physical and behavioral distress or problems.

Aims of Crisis Management

- **Prevention:** Minimizing the likelihood of crises
- **Preparedness:** Developing strategies, protocols, and resources
- **Response:** Swiftly addressing crises
- **Communication:** Providing clear, accurate, and timely information
- **Recovery:** Restoring normalcy post-crisis
- Learning and Improvement

Goal of Crisis Management

- To decrease emotional stress and protect the crisis victim from additional stress
- To assist the victim in organizing and mobilizing resources or support system to meet unique needs and reach a solution for a particular situation that precipitated the crisis.
- To assist the individual in recovery from the crisis and to prevent serious long-term problem.
- To reduce the intensity of an individual's emotional, mental, physical and behavioral reaction to a crisis
- To help the individuals return to their level of functioning before the crisis.

Steps in Crisis Intervention

Aguilera (1982)

- **Assessment:** What, when, how
- **Planning:** Therapeutic interventions
- **Implementation:** Intervention techniques
- **Resolution:** Along with anticipatory planning

ABC Model of Crisis Interventions

- Appropriate rapport
- Buliding measures to identify the nature and altering perceptions of crisis
- Coping skills use

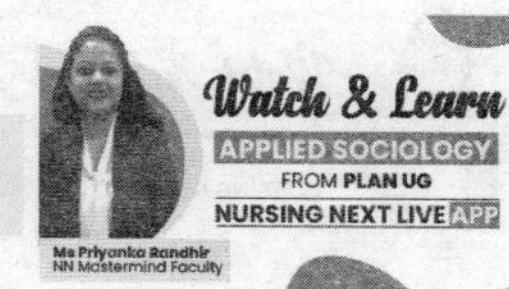

- **ABC method:**
  - Supported by scientific methods with evidence-based practice
  - Treat crisis situation
  - Used to change behavior and reduce suicidal ideations
  - Reframing of perception of events
  - Example: Death of Third Phase
  - A younger family member (crisis); one might ask themselves why this had to happen and why were they taken away when they were so young, It's not fair (perception) and the crisis begins with resistance of acceptance.
  - Use age old maxims: Life must go on....They are in better place... We might just don't know God's planning, etc. (cognitive disputation)
- **Recent perspective on crisis management**
  - MF Lechat gave five processes:
    1. Step reconstruction and rehabilitation (rehabilitation) (lechat, 1990: 3)
    2. Stage of release and relief of suffering and the normalization (relief phase)
    3. Rescue phase
    4. Alarm phase
    5. Stage of expectations or predictions (anticipatory phase)

Role of Clinical Sociologists or Use of Clinical Sociology in Crisis Intervention

- The role of clinical sociologists and the use of clinical sociology in crisis intervention are as follows:
- **Holistic Assessment:** Clinical sociologists analyze the social, cultural, and psychological aspects of a crisis, understanding its broader context and impact on individuals and communities.
- **Understanding Vulnerabilities:** They identify vulnerable populations affected by crises, considering factors such as socioeconomic status, cultural backgrounds, and systemic inequalities.
- **Cultural Sensitivity:** Clinical sociologists recognize cultural nuances, helping design interventions that respect diverse beliefs and practices to ensure effective communication and support.
- **Community Engagement:** They engage with local communities to understand their needs, strengths, and resources, fostering collaboration for more relevant and sustainable interventions.
- **Stigma Reduction:** Clinical sociologists address stigma associated with crises, promoting understanding and empathy to reduce discrimination and enhance social cohesion.
- **Psychosocial Support:** They offer psychosocial assistance to individuals and groups, addressing emotional and mental health needs, and mitigating long-term trauma.
- **Policy Advocacy:** Clinical sociologists advocate for policy changes based on their understanding of systemic issues revealed by crises, aiming to prevent future incidents and improve response systems.
- **Public Awareness:** They contribute to public education and awareness campaigns, disseminating accurate information and empowering individuals to navigate crises effectively.
- **Collaboration with Stakeholders:** Clinical sociologists work with healthcare providers, first responders, NGOs, and government agencies, ensuring a coordinated and comprehensive response.
- **Evaluation and Improvement:** They assess the effectiveness of crisis interventions, identifying successes and challenges, and recommending adjustments to enhance future crisis management strategies.

Nurse as a Clinical Sociologist Should Use the Following Techniques

- Catharsis
- Clarification
- Suggestions
- Reinforcement of behavior
- Support of defenses
- Raising self-esteem
- Exploration of solutions

CONCEPTUAL EXERCISES

LONG ANSWER QUESTIONS

1. **'Sociology is useful in understanding health problems'. Comment in detail. (CCSU)**

Answer

Sociology

Auguste Comte, the founding father of sociology, defines sociology as the science of social phenomena "subject to natural and invariable laws, the discovery of which is the object of investigation".

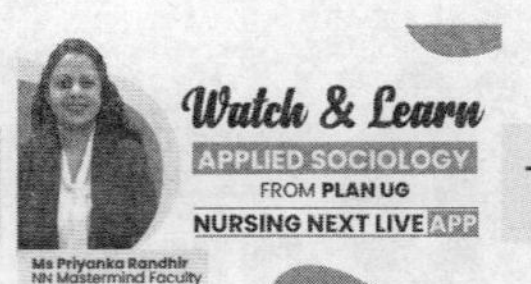

Sociology is useful in understanding health problems in the following ways:

- The field of sociology encompasses a wide range of topics, including those related to the social and scientific sciences. Being the study of society and its health, sociology deals with many social concerns that, in one way or another, affect a person's health, whether it be physically or mentally.
- A person is believed to be physically, psychologically, and mentally well when the person is healthy, and when either of these aspects is missing, they are thought to be sick.
- Sociologists take part in social context activities that, in one way or another, have an impact on people's wellbeing. One of these is health, and significant progress has been made in this area.
- Although the ideas of health and illness were formerly thought to be exclusively medical in nature, they have now found use in other disciplines, such as sociology.
- In a way, this has made it simpler to deal with the issue of health and illness through the use of diverse concepts and tactics that are not a part of the medical community. Through the treatment of health as a social issue and its perception, sociology has made significant contributions to our knowledge of health-related issues.
- Numerous social elements have been linked to contributing to health patterns in terms of how health issues arise and how they might be resolved in a social setting, such as through the offering of psychological counseling.
- Health and illness fall under a variety of disciplines, including sociology and medicine. The classification of this feature or the fields that should address the problem that affects every person on the planet has been the subject of considerable debate.
- Majority of medical illnesses are accompanied by social stigma and may take a long time to get better. The majority of sexually transmitted diseases, like HIV and AIDS, are a clear example of this. Because of how they influence the affected people and others around them, diseases cause far more social problems than medical ones.
- The consequences that health and sickness have on interpersonal relationships make obvious the social value that is attached to them. From minor health problems like various types of disability to serious ones like HIV and AIDS, which cause social bonds to be disrupted either deliberately or involuntarily, this can be witnessed.
- The affected people typically don't carry out their social obligations, such as their regular work or professional tasks, learning obligations related to school, as well as church and other community-based activities.
- In light of this, it becomes more of a social than a health problem. Both the affected person's own perception and that of other members of social group alter naturally as a result of the event.
- Numerous solutions have been implemented in an effort to address issues related to health since it is seen as a societal issue. Reducing poverty is one illustration.
- Numerous illnesses and sufferings are caused by poverty. It could also result in early deaths. People's health is influenced by a variety of social issues, including inequality, which is why sociologists are interested in this area. You might think of the delivery systems for health care as part of a social system. This is due to the fact that they focus more on social concerns that have an impact on people's health.
- Diseases or illnesses have an impact on the specific person who has the ailment, his/her family, and society as a whole. Sickness interferes with a person's ability to function normally, which limits the person's capacity to make significant personal and society contributions.
- In the majority of the world, and especially in the United States of America, illness is seen as a factor contributing to some sort of incapacity. The sick people are viewed as a burden on society because they don't make any good contribution and instead require the expenditure of economic resources in an effort to ameliorate their situation, which can never be done.
- Different diseases impact different bodily areas and individuals differently depending on their health status and level of resistance, which is influenced by factors including age and the environment.
- A person's disease not only affects physical and psychological well-being, but also social well-being and the well-being of those in the surroundings, such as family members.

2. Explain the application of sociology in Nursing. (CCSU)

Answer

In particular, sociology is a particularly useful subject for nursing education, practice, and profession.

- Sociology will assist medical professionals in understanding the social and cultural backgrounds of their patients.
- It is crucial to understand the patients' cultures in a place like India where individuals belong to many castes, tribes, faiths, and communities. To provide better medical and nursing services, cultural background must be known before treating patients, and study of sociology is required for this.
- Sociology's knowledge will assist doctors and nurses deal with the scenarios that arise in the hospital setting, such as the doctor-nurse-patient interaction, the doctor-nurse-administration relationship, and the doctor-nurse-public relations relationship.

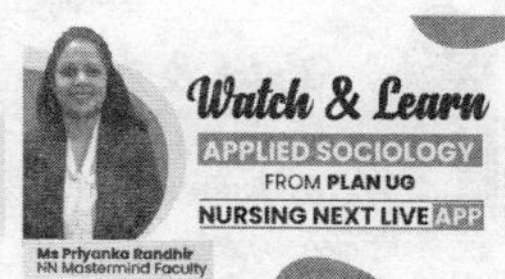

- The entire health care system can benefit greatly from medical sociology.
- An understanding of the importance of social factors on health, such as changes in cognitive function.
- It is necessary to address social processes like motivation and health values, i.e., changes to effective processes.
- Such forces are taken into consideration when planning and managing public health initiatives that aim to change behavioral processes.
- In addition to providing patient care, nurses should aid in disease prevention.
- In other words, they ought to encourage neighborhood health.
- The study of sociology will aid nurses in determining the patients' social backgrounds.
- The study of sociology enables nurses to recognize patients' sociopsychological issues, which enhances the effectiveness of care.
- The study of sociology enables nurses to comprehend how many facets of social life—such as those that are economic, political, moral, religious, and intellectual—relate to one another and to particular disorders.
- Nursing students can support the government in a variety of social planning initiatives by studying sociology. For instance, the family health program and government welfare schemes can only be implemented successfully with the active involvement of nurses.
- The study of sociology aids nurses in providing better care to vulnerable populations such as children, the elderly, persons with physical or mental disabilities, those living with HIV/AIDS, etc.
- Only by having a thorough understanding of the patients' varied cultural origins can these diseases be effectively treated.
- The study of sociology aids nurses in raising the standard of the government's Family Welfare Programs and Community Health Services.
- A wide range of people with diverse behaviors must be interacted with by nurses, including patients, doctors, other family members, management, the government, and society at large. Understanding these behavioral tendencies will be made easier through the study of sociology, which will enhance health care.
- The implementation of preventative, curative, and promotional components of health in the community benefits from the development of interpersonal relationships between patients, medical staff, and paramedical staff that are facilitated by sociological study.
- In order to be responsible citizens in the advancement of health education in the nation, nurses must have a good understanding of sociology.

3. Health problems associated with industrialization. (CCSU)

Answer

Industrialization

- Industrialization is the process of moving a country or region's economy away from reliance on agriculture and toward one that is driven by industry.

Health problems associated with industrialization

- Industrialization has had a profound impact on society, including on health.
- Some of the health problems associated with industrialization include:
- **Occupational hazards:** Industrial work can expose workers to a variety of hazards, including noise, dust, fumes, chemicals, and radiation. These hazards can lead to a number of health problems, including respiratory diseases, cancer, and reproductive problems.
- **Air pollution:** Industrial activity can release pollutants into the air, which can cause respiratory problems, heart disease, and cancer.
- **Water pollution:** Industrial activity can also pollute water, which can lead to a variety of health problems, including gastrointestinal problems, neurological problems, and reproductive problems.
- **Chemical exposure:** Industrial production involves the use and release of numerous chemicals. Workers and nearby communities may be exposed to toxic substances, leading to adverse health effects.
- **Nutritional deficiencies:** Industrialization can lead to changes in diet, which can lead to nutritional deficiencies. This is especially a problem in developing countries, where people may not have access to adequate food.
- **Work-related stress:** The pace of life in an industrialized society can be stressful, which can lead to a variety of health problems, including heart disease, high blood pressure, and depression.
- **Urbanization and lifestyle changes:** Industrialization is closely linked to urbanization, which brings changes in lifestyle, including sedentary behavior, unhealthy diets, and increased prevalence of non-communicable diseases (NCDs) such as obesity, diabetes, and cardiovascular diseases
- **Industrial accidents:** Industrial settings can be prone to accidents, including explosions, fires, and chemical spills, which can result in severe injuries, fatalities, and long-term health consequences for workers and nearby communities.

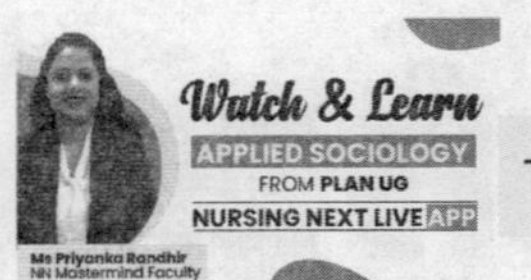

SHORT NOTES

1. Write a short note on Social stress. (CCSU)

Answer

Social Stress

A scenario that compromises one's relationships, self-worth, or sense of belonging within a relationship, group, or larger social environment is generally referred to as social stress.

Causes of Social Stress

- Failure, according to Vors, is one of the two primary sources of social stress since it lowers one's self-esteem and social standing. He explains that because failure plays a significant role in our sense of self and how people perceive other people, it raises our social stress levels.
- Feeling uncontrollable is the second psychosocial stressor. According to Vors, uncontrollability fosters a sense of failure in the brain since the person is unable to take the necessary steps to achieve his goal, which raises cortisol levels and lowers self-esteem.
- The final outcome of both stressors is always a decline in self-esteem, which significantly contributes to social stress. This is a continuity that can be found in both stressors.

Effect of Social Stress

- Stankiewicz outlines the negative consequences of persistent social stress.
- When under social stress for extended periods of time, the brain releases particular chemicals that lead to serious mental health disorders including sadness and anxiety.
- Many frequent and unusual mental diseases that adolescents experience are caused by excessive social stress that is experienced at school or at home.
- According to Stankiewicz, bodily ailments like heart disease, cancer, and ulcers are brought on by too much social stress.

Methods to Overcome Social Stress

- Social stress cannot be cured completely. However, there are numerous techniques to lessen the social stress.
- Communication is the key to mending strained connections. One can reduce some tension by discussing social anxiety with a close friend or by just using dialogue to mend a healthy relationship.
- Eliminating toxic relationships from one's life is another strategy to reduce emotional stress.
- Learn about your personality and abilities.
- Recognize interpersonal compatibility.
- Reduce friction and tension in relationships.
- Help groups collaborate more efficiently, from families and friends' groups to work teams and academic clubs.
- Encourage communication and collaboration.
- Find your stressors and reduce them.

2. Write a short note on Conflict. (CCSU)

Answer

Definitions of Conflict

AW Green: "Conflict is the deliberate attempt to oppose, resist or coerce the will of another".

Horton and Hunt: "Conflict may be defined as a process of seeking to monopolize rewards like eliminating or weakening the competitors".

Features of Conflict

- Conscious action
- Personal activity
- Lacks continuity
- Universal

Causes of Conflict

- Individual differences
- Cultural differences
- Clash of interests
- Social change
- Selfish and vested interest
- Limited resources

Types of Conflicts

- **Overt and latent:** (Open) When hostile action is taken, the latent conflict becomes overt.
- **Corporate and personal conflict:** Between individuals or between society.
- **Direct and indirect conflict:** If the people conflict directly (litigation, revolution or war) or create a situation.
- **Caste and racial conflicts:** Between castes or between race, class conflict-karl marx (have and have-nots) and mutual hostility between strata.
- **Group conflict:** Between two small groups based on differences in ideologies, interest or suppression. Political and religious conflicts.
- **International conflict:** Between two nations on the basis of different political ideologies, economic, territorial.
- **Types of conflict by george simmel**
  - War

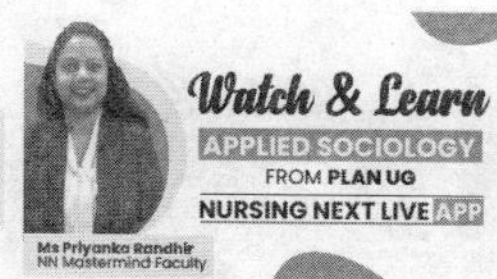

- Feud
- Litigation
- Impersonal idea

Methods to Resolve Conflicts

- Recognize the conflict.
- Engage the opponent in conversation.
- Consider many solutions.
- Select the ideal resolution.
- Make use of a neutral arbitrator.
- Explore your options.
- Be able to handle pressure and difficult situations.

SHORT ANSWER QUESTIONS

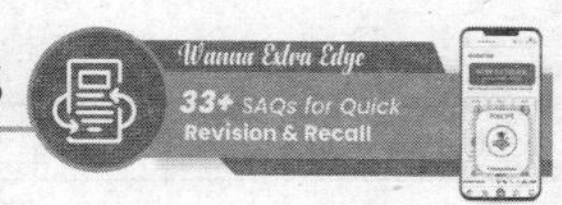

1. Define clinical sociology.

Answer

Clinical sociology is the application of sociological theories, research, modalities, methods, techniques, and interventions to social issues and problems presented by clients.

According to Fritz 2001, "Clinical sociology is a humanistic, multidisciplinary specialization that seeks to improve the quality of people's lives. Clinical sociologists assess situations and reduce problems through analysis and intervention. Clinical analysis is the critical assessment of beliefs, policies and or practices with an interest in improving the situation. Intervention, the creation of new systems as well as the change of existing systems, is based on continuing analysis."

2. Define crisis. Enlist steps of crisis intervention.

Answer

Crisis

"Crisis" is an acute emotional upset arising from situational, developmental, or social sources and resulting in a temporary inability to cope by means of one's usual problem-solving mechanisms.

Steps of Crisis Intervention

1. Assessment
2. Establish rapport
3. Identify major problem or crisis precipitants
4. Deal with feelings and emotions
5. Generate and explore alternatives
6. Implement an action plan
7. Follow-up and referral

3. Enlist two differences between clinical sociology and applied sociology.

Answer

Clinical sociology	Applied sociology
Clinical sociology is the application of a sociological perspective to the analysis and design of interventions for positive social change at any level of social organization.	Applied sociology is sometimes referred to as pragmatic, realistic, matter of facts, evidence- based or practical sociology that refers to a form of sociological practice that is primarily concerned with using sociological theories and research.
Clinical sociologists can work in a variety of different areas or settings. For instance, they can be employed as community organizers, socio-therapists, mediators, social policy implementers, and action researchers.	Applied sociologists use sociological theory, techniques, methods, expertise, competence and skills to collect information and analyze data and to communicate their findings.

4. Enlist characteristics of clinical sociology.

Answer

Characteristics of clinical sociology are:

- Practice oriented
- Collaborative practice
- Diagnostic approach
- Focuses on case studies
- Change-oriented
- Humanistic
- Sociological conception of personality
- Employs insight
- Theoretical and methodological grounding
- Leads to behavior change and growth
- Ideological cast

CONCEPTUAL REVISION

MULTIPLE CHOICE QUESTIONS

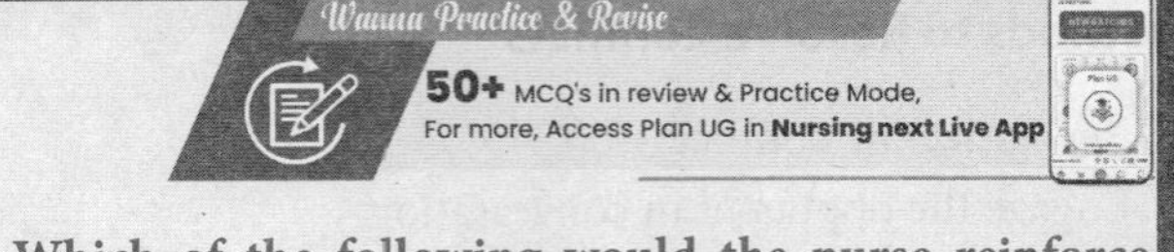

1. The use of the discipline of sociology with the particular intention to alter social relationships and facilitating change is called:

a. Clinical sociology
b. Psychosociology
c. Applied sociology
d. None of these

Ans. a. Clinical sociology

2. The term "Clinical Sociology" was first used by:

a. Karl Marx
b. Milton C. Winternitz
c. Kapadia
d. Lenski

Ans. b. Milton C. Winternitz

3. Which among the following is the model of crisis intervention?

a. XYZ
b. ABC
c. CDE
d. CIM

Ans. b. ABC

4. Identify the types of crisis:

a. Adventitious crisis/social crisis
b. Situational crisis
c. Maturational/developmental crisis
d. All of the above

Ans. d. All of the above

5. As per Aguilera (1982), how many steps are there in the crisis intervention?

a. 4 b. 6
c. 3 d. 5

Ans. a. 4

6. Which of the following would the nurse reinforce after a teaching session as the most important lifestyle modification for the patient whose age is 59, height is 5'11", weight is 280 pounds, and is hypertensive?

a. Reduce weight
b. Restrict salt intake
c. Increase potassium intake
d. Decrease alcohol intake

Ans. a. Reduce weight

7. A method used for individual health education in the community is:

a. Demonstration
b. Counseling and interview
c. Role play
d. Workshop

Ans. b. Counseling and interview

8. Averting the transition of disability into handicap relates to which level of prevention?

a. Primary b. Primordial
c. Secondary d. Tertiary

Ans. d. Tertiary

9. Work of clinical sociologists mainly focuses on:

a. Investigation
b. Case management and care planning
c. Case management
d. Care planning

Ans. b. Case management and care planning

10. The clinical analysis means:

a. Rehabilitative services
b. Sociocultural analysis
c. Preventive services
d. Assessing a situation

Ans. d. Assessing a situation

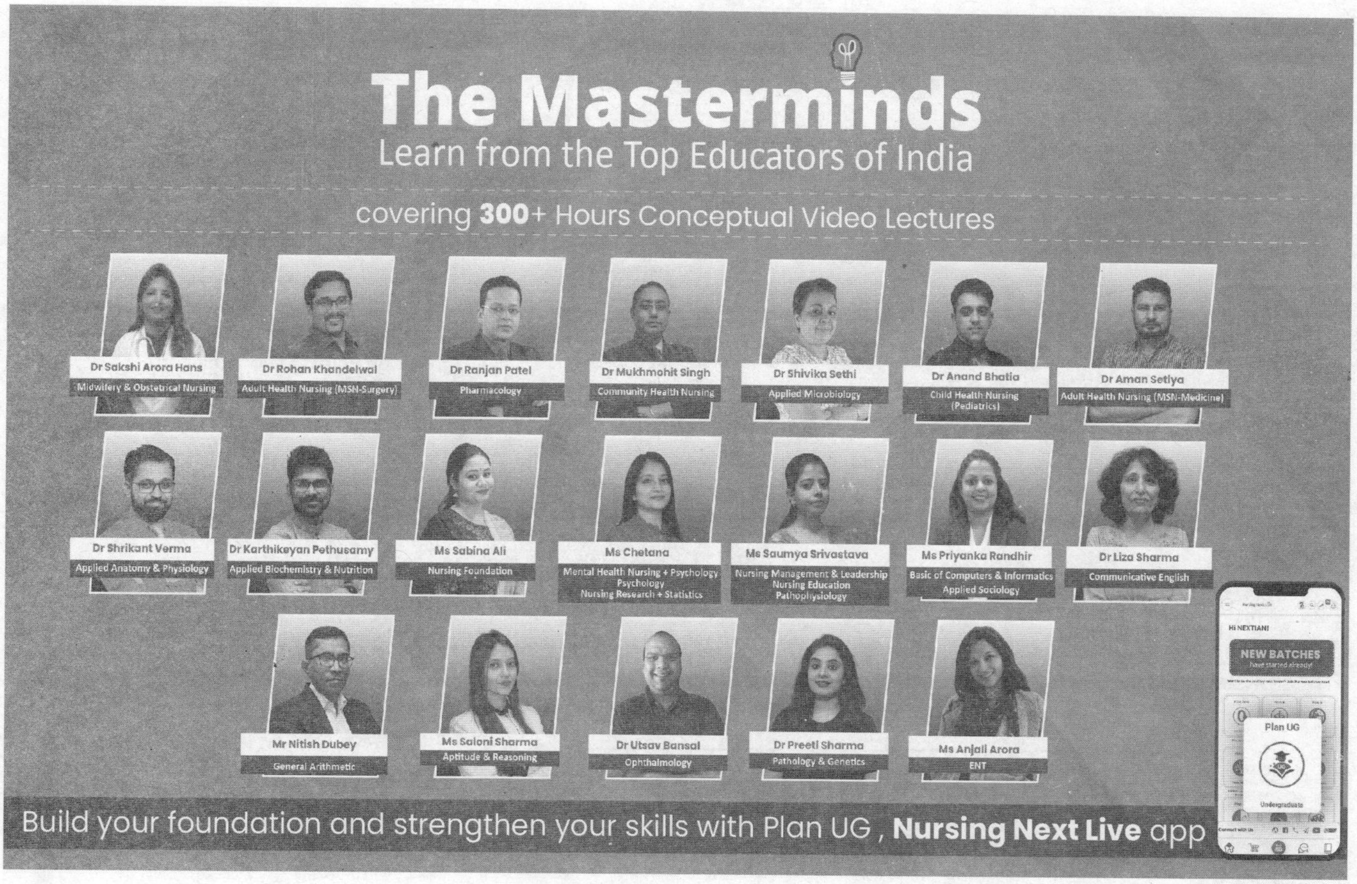

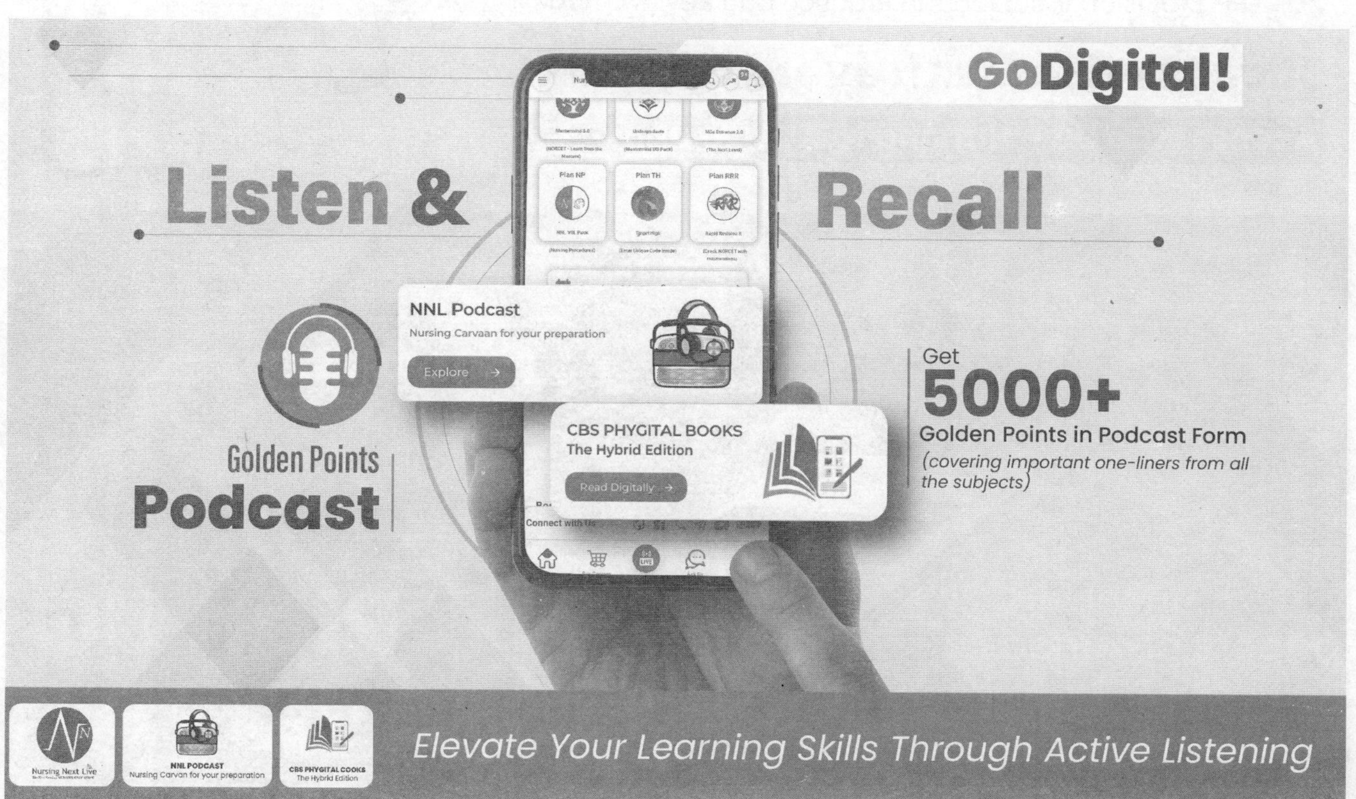

GoDigital!
Listen &
Recall
NNL Podcast
Nursing Carvaan for your preparation
Explore
CBS PHYGITAL BOOKS
The Hybrid Edition
Read Digitally
Golden Points
Podcast
Get
5000+
Golden Points in Podcast Form
(covering important one-liners from all the subjects)
Nursing Next Live
NNL PODCAST
Nursing Carvan for your preparation
CBS PHYGITAL BOOKS
The Hybrid Edition
Elevate Your Learning Skills Through Active Listening

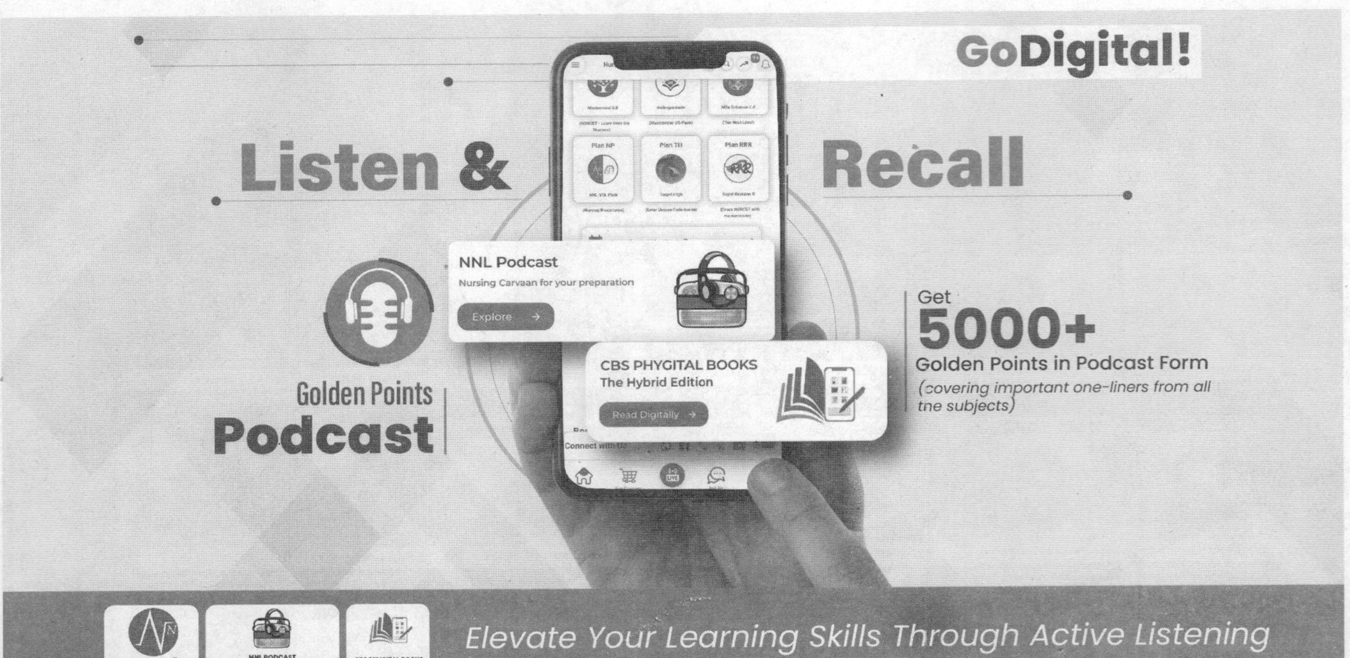
GoDigital!
Listen & Recall
NNL Podcast
Nursing Carvaan for your preparation
Explore
Golden Points
Podcast
CBS PHYGITAL BOOKS
The Hybrid Edition
Read Digitally
Get
5000+
Golden Points in Podcast Form
(covering important one-liners from all the subjects)
Elevate Your Learning Skills Through Active Listening

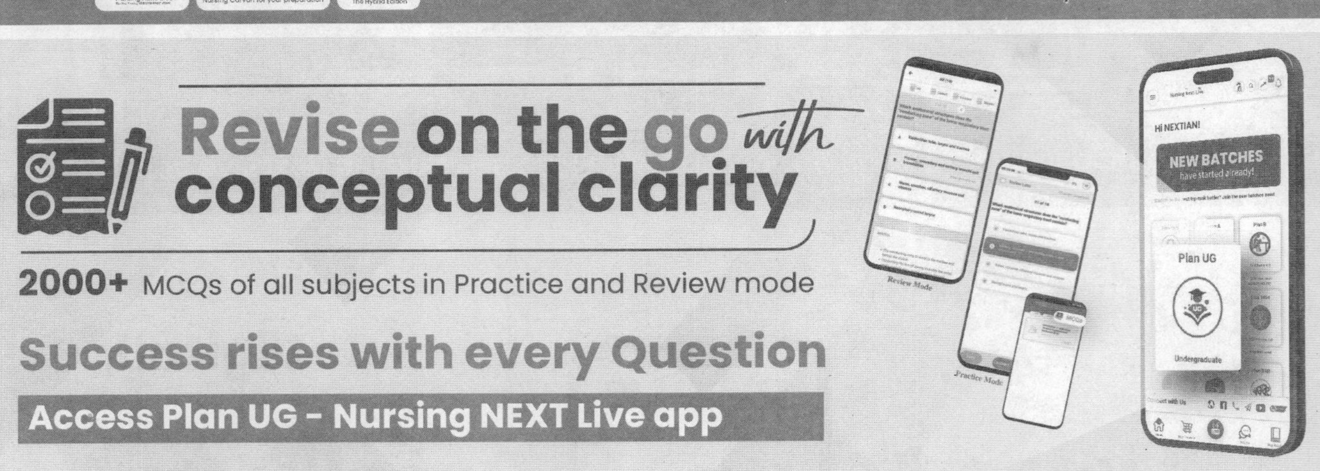
Revise on the go with conceptual clarity
2000+ MCQs of all subjects in Practice and Review mode
Success rises with every Question
Access Plan UG - Nursing NEXT Live app
HI NEXTIAN!
NEW BATCHES
have started already!
Plan UG
Undergraduate
Review Mode
Practice Mode

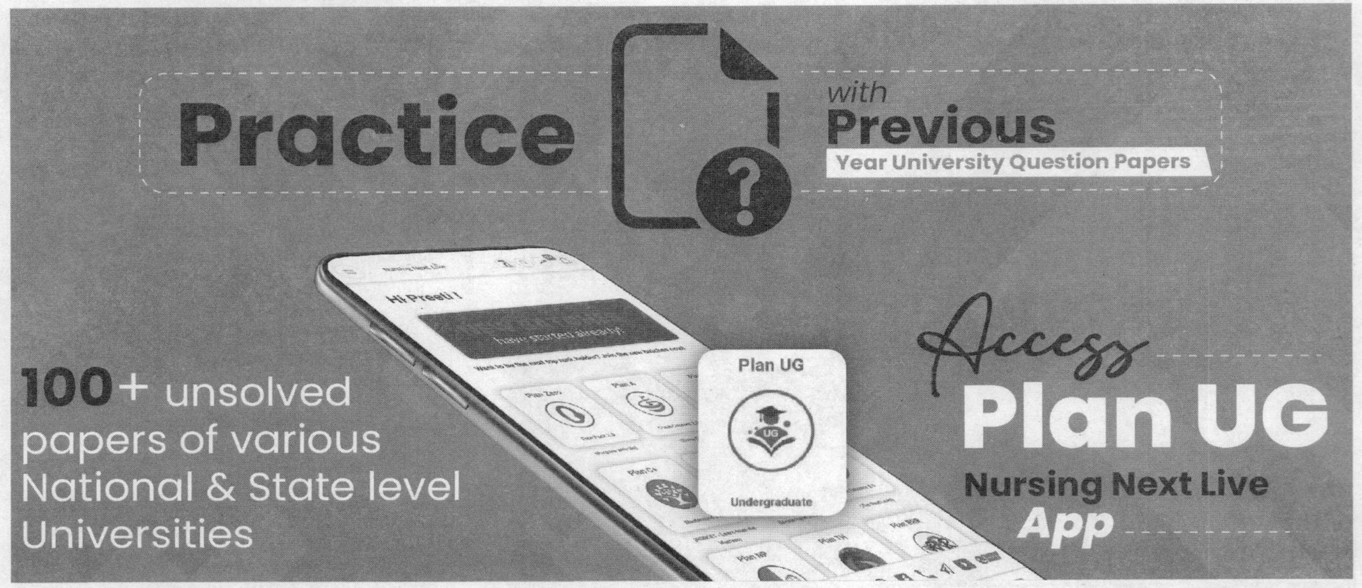
Practice
with
Previous
Year University Question Papers
100+ unsolved papers of various National & State level Universities
Plan UG
Undergraduate
Access
Plan UG
Nursing Next Live
App

What's Inside
The Booklet

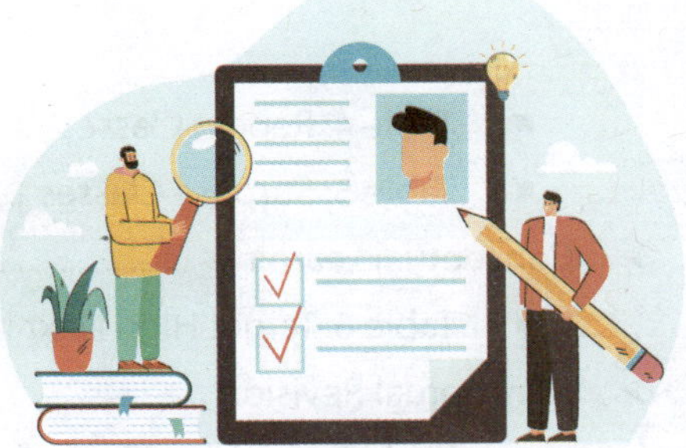

SEMESTER I

SEMESTER II

Director's Message

Dear Nextian,

I extend my warmest congratulations to you for embarking on the noble journey of nursing. Your decision marks the first step towards dedicating yourselves to the service of humanity. After completing your 12th-grade examinations, the two most esteemed paths in the medical field are those of Doctors and Nurses, both equally important in strengthening a country's health system.

Nursing used to be an underrated profession in the medical field, but over time, these perceptions have changed. Nurses now hold a more organized and esteemed role in healthcare and provide services on par with Physicians. We firmly believe that Nursing is a service that goes beyond self-interest, and you are among the fortunate individuals chosen by Almighty God for this purpose. Always keep in mind that to achieve excellence and noteworthy accomplishments, you must uphold certain principles and embody specific qualities, including:

1. A profound love for the profession you have chosen
2. Hard work
3. Sincerity in your actions
4. Faith in your abilities

At Nursing Next Live, we consider it a privilege to provide you with our academic services. Over the past six years, we have been wholeheartedly dedicated to enhancing nursing education. As part of our commitment, we have published several renowned resources for nursing undergraduates, including BD Chaurasia's Anatomy & Physiology for Nurses and Clinical Nursing Procedures, all under the banner of Nursing Knowledge Tree and CBS Publishers & Distributors.

In alignment with our dedication to offering top-notch education, we have introduced Digital Learning in the field of nursing. Over the past three years, we have revolutionized digital education for nursing students across India, an initiative that has been warmly embraced by those preparing for nursing competitive examinations like NORCET and other nationally esteemed Nursing Officers' exams. Now, we have extended our digital offerings to undergraduate students like yourselves. Our mission is to bring learning to you, wherever you are.

With Plan UG, we have streamlined your educational journey by granting you the freedom to study at your own convenience and pace. In your second year of study, we offer Video Lectures covering all subjects, presented by the top educators in India. Additionally, we provide well-researched content through Long & Short Q/As and voiceover-based Golden Points. We also grant access to Phygital Books to offer a comprehensive approach to your preparation.

We firmly believe in the adage, "One Day or Day One." So, why wait for that 'one day' to start your preparations? Let today be your 'Day One.' To excel in your undergraduate examinations and aspire to become a Nursing Officer or pursue further higher studies, and others, you must embrace a Dual Approach to Preparation. This approach focuses on both university exam patterns and next level preparation. Our aim is not only to help you succeed in your university exams but also to equip you for a future that holds immense potential. Without a doubt, Plan UG will lay a robust academic foundation for you with a futuristic perspective.

May you thrive and succeed in all your future endeavors!

With warm regards,

Bhupesh Aarora

Bhupesh Aarora
Project Director
Nursing Next Live

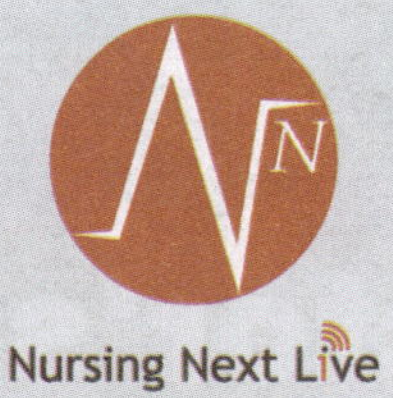

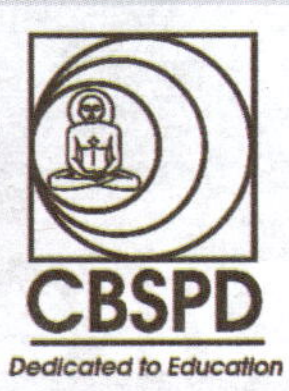

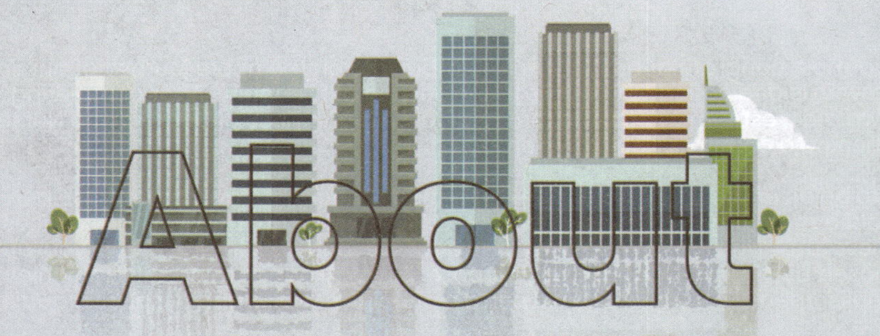

Nursing Next Live & CBS Publishers Pvt. Ltd.

Nursing Next Exam Prep Private Limited is an affiliated company of CBS Publishers & Distributors Pvt. Ltd., a renowned pioneer in Health Sciences Publishing known for its innovative ideas and progressive initiatives. CBS, having made a mark in the field of book publishing, ventured into the Nursing EdTech sector with the vision of delivering high-quality Nursing Education at the click of a button through its platform, Nursing Next Live (NNL) as an independent entity.

The idea was conceptualized in August 2019 and launched in August 2020, driven by the recognition of the need to bridge the gap between Medical and Nursing Education. It is an all-encompassing platform designed with a futuristic approach to cater to the learning needs of Nursing Students, covering everything from undergraduate studies to exams such as NORCET/NCLEX/MSc. The platform offers a variety of learning modules based on the latest INC Syllabus, meticulously curated by Top Medical & Nursing Educators.

With an ideology of Bringing learning to people instead of people going for learning, this one-stop platform includes

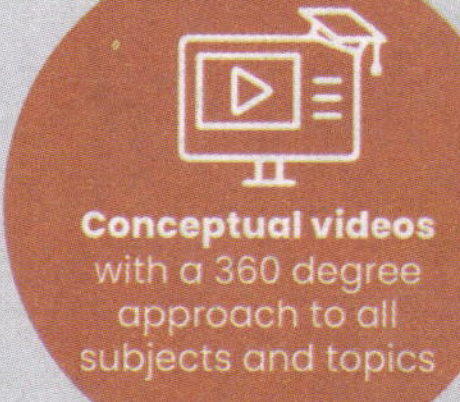

Conceptual videos with a 360 degree approach to all subjects and topics

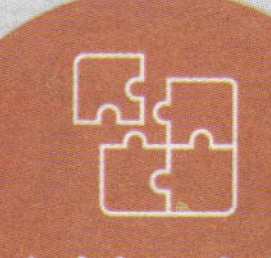

An **Integrated Approach** to learning as per the New CBME pattern.

Dual learning approach through both subjective and MCQ-based methods

Smart Approach with Digital Books,

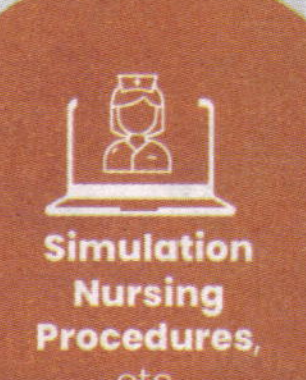

Simulation Nursing Procedures, etc.

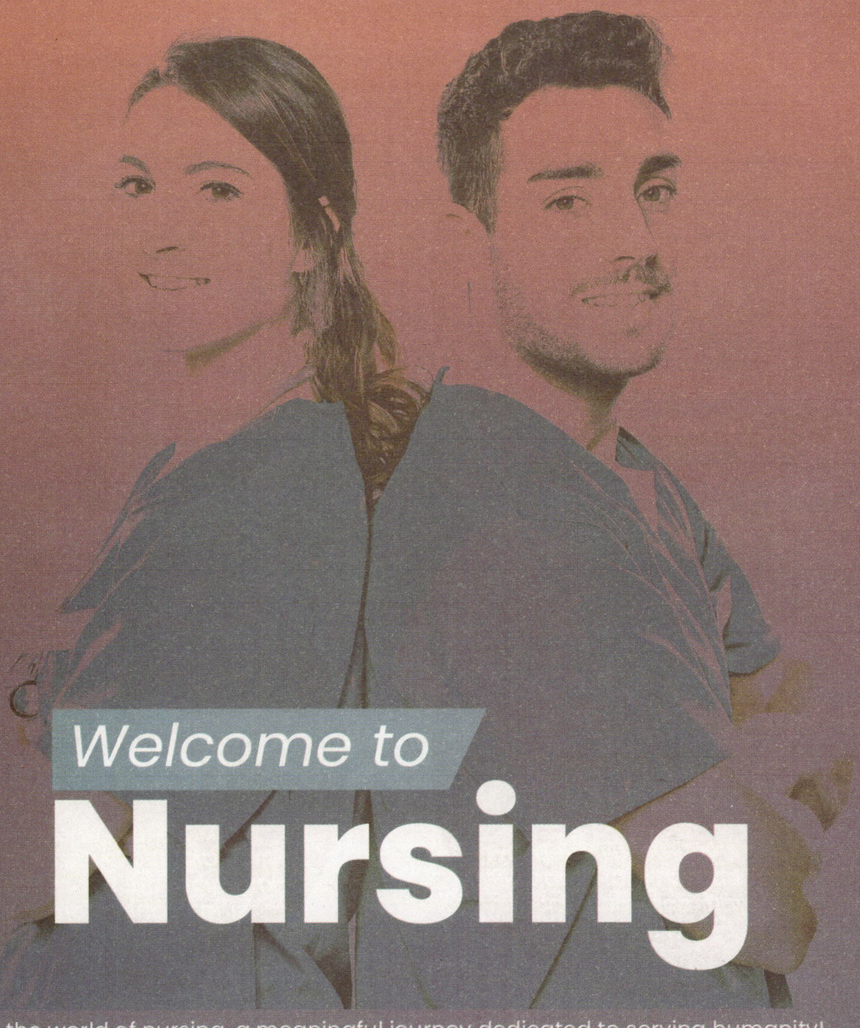

Welcome to Nursing

Welcome to the world of nursing, a meaningful journey dedicated to serving humanity!

Nurses are often referred to as the "heart" of healthcare for a good reason. They provide essential care and support to patients across the lifespan, whether it's assisting during surgery, managing chronic conditions, or offering comfort to those in their final moments.

With the changing healthcare landscape, nurses are increasingly recognized for their vital role in patient care and public health. As history has shown during the COVID-19 pandemic, nurses are the backbone of healthcare, and your decision to enter this field is commendable. Your education and dedication will contribute to reshaping the healthcare narrative.

Many nursing students find that it's not just a career choice but a calling. Nursing is about more than treating illnesses; it's about providing comfort, compassion, and healing. Your studies will empower you to care for others with empathy and healing. While nursing can be challenging and demanding, it's also highly rewarding. You've been chosen for this calling, and you're fortunate to be on this path.

As a nursing student, you're at the beginning of an exciting journey with numerous career opportunities. Your education will provide the foundation to set and adjust your goals based on your interests and experiences. Whether you aim to specialize in a specific nursing field, become an educator, or pursue advanced practice, your career path is adaptable to your passions and aspirations.

The sense of fulfillment from helping others and making a positive impact on lives is immeasurable. Nursing offers job stability, competitive salaries, and opportunities for career advancement. Consider these essential values to guide you through your career:

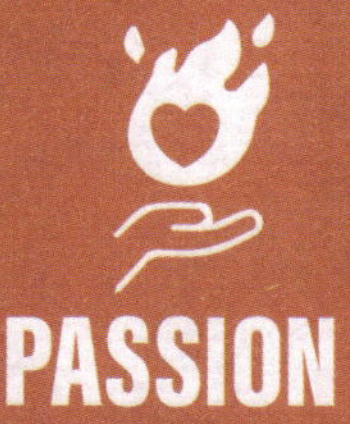

PASSION

Love what you do, as deep love for your chosen profession will drive your commitment to excellence.

HARD WORK

Working hard and staying dedicated is important, knowing your efforts make a significant difference in people's lives.

INTEGRITY

Love what you do, as deep love for your chosen profession will drive your commitment to excellence.

CONFIDENCE

Working hard and staying dedicated is important, knowing your efforts make a significant difference in people's lives.

You already possess these qualities, which have brought you here. However, this is just the beginning of an amazing journey. As you embark on this new chapter in your career, we are here to be your guiding light throughout the journey.

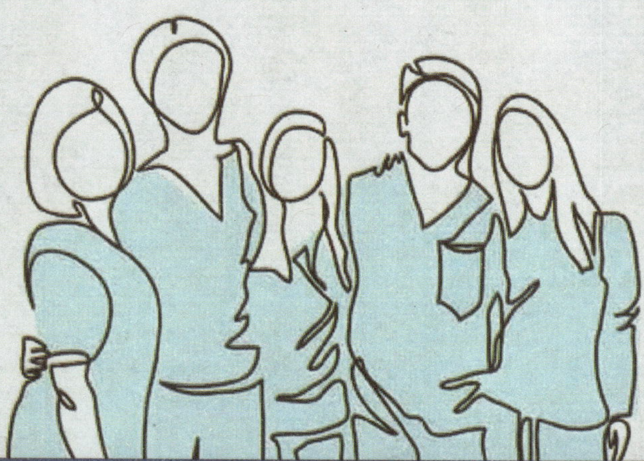

Welcome to the world of nursing, where you can be a hero every day!

Scope Of NURSING

Nursing is a versatile profession that extends beyond traditional hospital settings. Nurses can be found in various roles, including assessing astronauts' health at NASA. The field is continuously evolving, so when considering career options, remember that the sky's the limit! Scope of nursing practice includes **health protection, promotion, restoration, palliation, and rehabilitation.**

After completing your undergraduate, you have several higher education options to consider. Here are some of the common paths:

Master of Science in Nursing (MSc Nursing)

If you're looking to advance your career and clinical skills, MSc can be a great choice. Specializations can include Nurse Practitioner, Nurse Anesthetist, Nurse Educator, Nurse Administrator, and more. Upon successful completion, this degree can open up leadership positions and specialized nursing roles.

Nurse Practitioner in Critical Care (NPCC)

The NPCC program is a nursing residency program with main focus on competency- based training. The duration of the course is two years with the curriculum consisting of theory that includes core courses, advanced practice courses and clinical courses besides clinical practicum which is a major component. NPCC at Masters Level is intended to prepare registered graduate Nurses to provide advanced nursing care to Patients who are critically ill.

Doctor of Philosophy in Nursing (PhD Nursing)

A PhD in Nursing is a research-focused degree that allows you to conduct in-depth research in the field of nursing. Suitable for those interested in academia, research, and policy development, PhD programs can take several years to complete and often require a dissertation or thesis. However, this degree can lead to roles in academia, research institutions, healthcare policy, and advanced clinical practice.

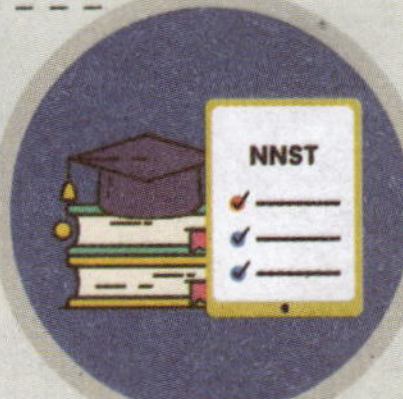

NORCET (Nursing Officer Recruitment Common Eligibility Test)

NORCET is an exam conducted by the All India Institute of Medical Sciences (AIIMS) for the recruitment of Nursing Officers in AIIMS and other central government hospitals. It's a competitive exam that requires preparation, and success can lead to a nursing career in prestigious institutions. It can be a viable choice if you are seeking immediate employment and a stable career in the nursing field.

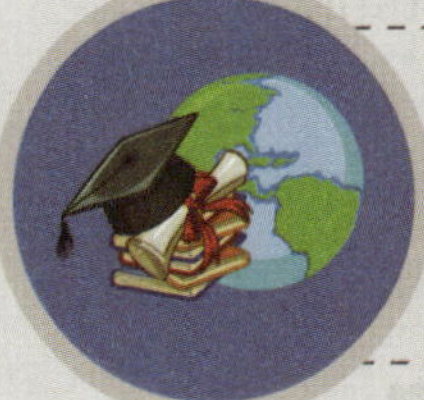

NCLEX (National Council Licensure Examination)

The NCLEX is an exam used for the licensure of nurses in the United States and some other countries. If you plan to work as a nurse in the U.S. or a country that recognizes the NCLEX, you will need to pass this exam. Preparing for the NCLEX often involves rigorous review and may include taking preparatory courses.

Before deciding on your path, it's essential to consider your career goals, interests, and the specific requirements for each option.

HOW TO

Ace UG Exams?

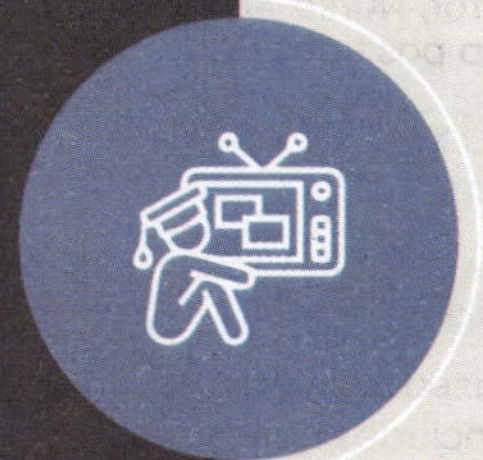

Watch & Learn

Watch & learn from the best in class hybrid lectures by the top educators, live doubt sessions, nursing procedures and add- on videos

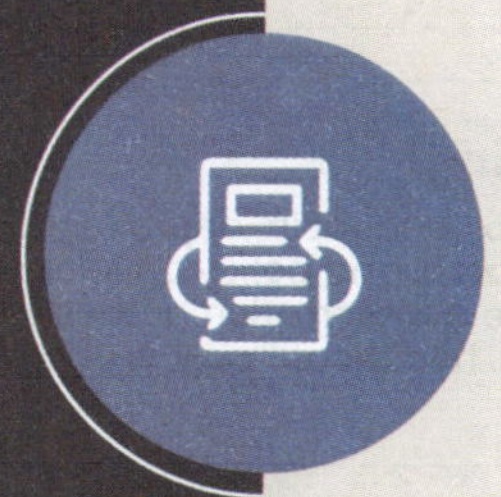

Revise & Retain

Do regular revision with live sessions and retain the concepts to sustain a strong foundation.

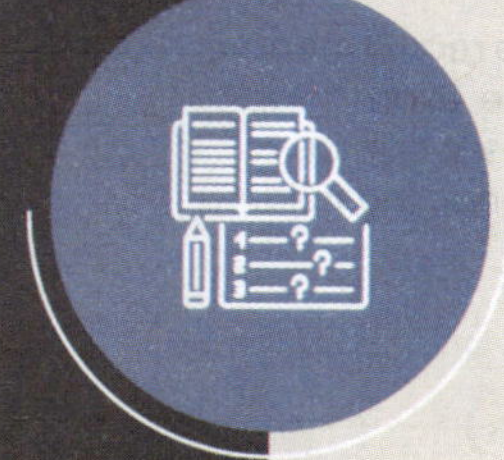

Read & Practice

Get better at understanding concepts with Target High Decode and Phygital books. Stay on top of your progress with Subject-wise/Topic-wise tests and monthly reviews.

Guidance & Counseling

We're here for you throughout your academic journey from Subscription Se Success tak. Our experienced counselors can help with personalized study tips and much more.

Introducing PLAN UG

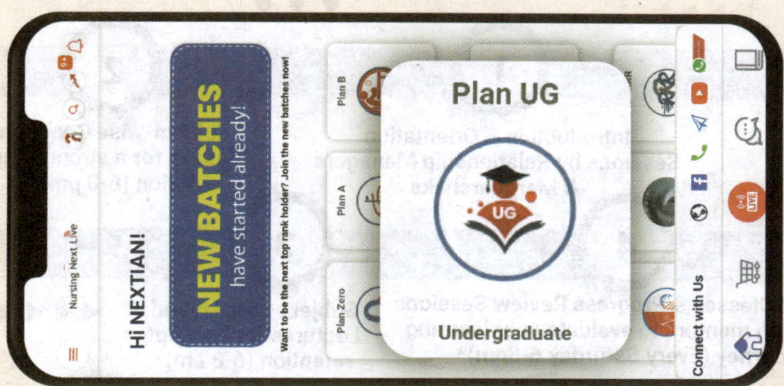

For Nursing students, the first year can present significant challenges, as it marks a huge step in your journey towards becoming a competent nurse. Everything in this phase is fresh and new, which can be quite frightening. However, we have some good news for you: NNL is here to support and guide undergraduates like yourself through this academic journey with Plan UG.

Plan UG is not just a curriculum; it's a holistic approach to nursing education, combining faculty expertise and student feedback, that aims to empower you with the knowledge, skills, and confidence to excel in your academic journey and beyond. With the constantly evolving education patterns, it's important to enhance your preparedness from the very beginning. While you can decide on your next steps later, the determination to take that first step should be made in the early stages of your education.

Our extensive research ensures that regardless of your college or university, you'll benefit from our comprehensive lectures by the Top Educators, Various Solved & Unsolved Exercises, well-researched study materials, and innovative "Phygital" books. We also prepare you for NORCET/NCLEX/M.Sc level success from the start.

Understanding *Your Needs*

At NNL, we recognize that the first year of nursing school is an important phase in your transformation into a proficient and compassionate nurse. We are well-aware of the unique set of challenges that nursing students face during this critical period. That's why Plan UG has been meticulously developed to address these challenges and provide you with the tools and resources needed to excel.

Our approach to nursing education goes beyond conventional teaching methods. We understand that the traditional approach to education may not always align with the dynamic and evolving field of healthcare. Therefore, we have adopted an innovative pedagogy that simplifies complex concepts and adapts to the ever-changing healthcare landscape, all based on the latest INC syllabus. Our educators are dedicated to creating an engaging and interactive learning environment that fosters a deep understanding of nursing concepts.

In our commitment to staying at the forefront of nursing education, we continually research and evaluate the effectiveness of our teaching methods. This dedication to research ensures that you receive the most up-to-date and evidence-based education available, equipping you with the knowledge and skills needed to thrive in the healthcare sector.
Indeed, Plan UG is designed to lay a strong foundation for your academic journey, guiding you towards a successful career in nursing. It will help you build the knowledge and skills you need for a bright future in the nursing field.

Roadmap of I & II Year

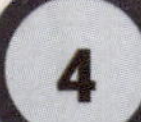

1. Introduction & Orientation Sessions by Relationship Managers & Margdarshaks

2. Subject-wise Conceptual Classes for a strong foundation (6-8 pm)*

3. Subject-wise Hybrid Lectures for concept retention (6-8 am)*

4. Special Classes & Progress Review Sessions by batch mentors to evaluate your learning journey (Every Saturday 6-8pm)*

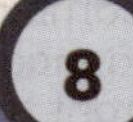

5. Weekly MCQ based Tests, Monthly Revision Tests, Bimonthly Unit Tests (Subjective) and Assignments for regular practice

6. Practical exam preparation session and OSCE introduction

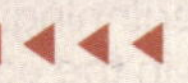

7. Selected Nursing Procedure Videos from the NNL-VSL Pack

8. Interaction with Toppers and discovering their secrets to success

9. Revision with Conceptual Classes, Model Tests and Decode book discussion sessions

10. E-workbooks & Pre Assessment Tests for ongoing learning

Special Classes may include:

Interactive learning sessions with Dr. Shrikant Verma

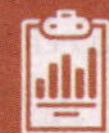

Progress Evaluation by Batch Mentor

Live Doubt Sessions

Understanding Nursing Procedures using simulation videos

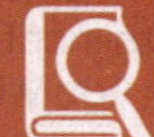

Discussions on E-workbooks for thorough knowledge and concept clarity

APPROACH

UG- I Year

THOROUGH CONCEPT BUILDING

(Basic Learning)

UG- II Year

CONCEPT STRENGTHENING & FUTURE SCOPE

(Advanced Learning)

**Schedule is subject to change*

Roadmap of III & IV Year

1 Introduction & Orientation Sessions

2 Subject Module–wise Conceptual Learning Classes for a Strong Foundation (Dec'23-Sep'25)

3 NORCET- Focused Weekly Live Interactive Sessions (Every Saturday 4-5 pm)

4 Topic Assessment Tests to Monitor Progress (Every Sunday)

5 Practical Sessions by Simulation-based Nursing Procedures and Viva-Voice Exercises

6 Subject-wise Conceptual Classes for a Strong Foundation of 1st & 2nd Year (Oct'25-Dec'25)

7 Revision Sessions for NORCET Preparation Including 1st to 4th Year Subjects (Jan'26-Mar'26)

8 Interaction with Toppers and Discovering their Secrets to Success

9 NORCET Preparation with Live Discussions on the Most Probable Q/A (Apr'26-May'26)

10 NORCET Preparation with Clinical Scenario-based Tests and Skill Assessment Tests comprising of Basic to Advance Level Qs

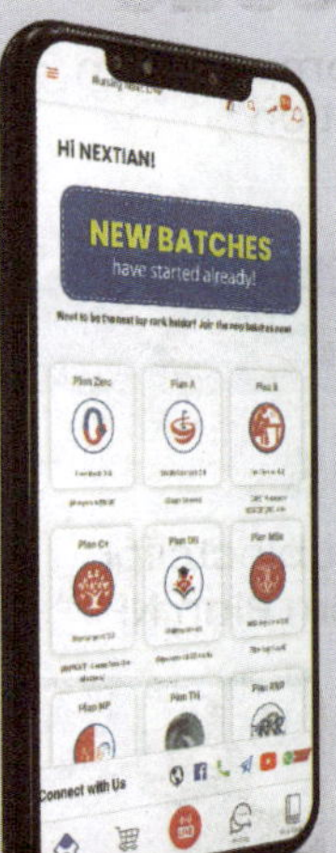

3-Phase 30-Months Strategy *to Success*

UG & NORCET Preparation (20 Months)

Modules covering 10 Major Subjects:

- Nursing Foundations
- Adult Health Nursing (Medical)
- Adult Health Nursing (Surgery)
- Midwifery/ Obstetrics & Gynecology Nursing
- Child Health Nursing
- Community Health Nursing
- Mental Health Nursing & Psychology
- Nursing Education
- Nursing Management & Leadership
- Introduction to Forensic Nursing and Indian Laws

+

Focus on NORCET (4 Months)

Emphasis on Basic/Non-Clinical Subjects:

- Applied Anatomy & Physiology
- Applied Biochemistry & Nutrition
- Applied Microbiology
- Pharmacology
- Nursing Information & Technology
- General Aptitude & Reasoning
- English

+

Intensive 6-month Revision:

Rapid review of major, basic, and non-clinical subjects

= ACING **NORCET** IN FIRST ATTEMPT**

*Schedule is subject to change

CORE ELEMENTS

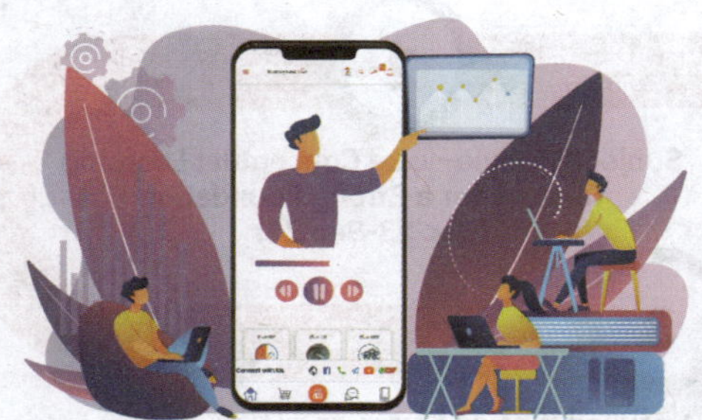

Conceptual Classes

Experience advanced learning with India's Top Educators (The Masterminds)

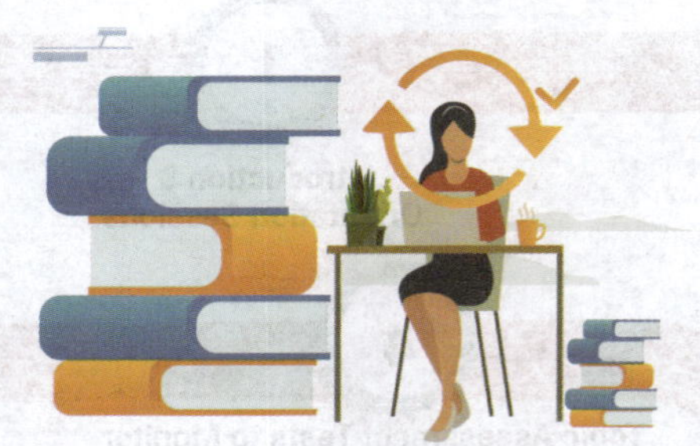

Conceptual Exercises

Solved Exercises of Long & Short Qs and Unsolved Exercises for practice

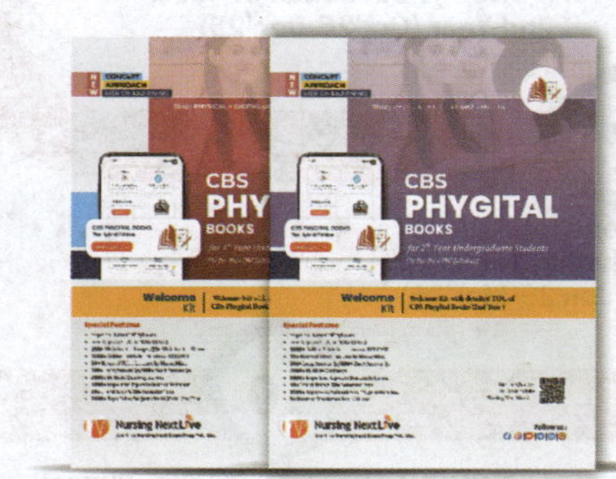

Phygital Books

Read from the Book and Practice Digitally

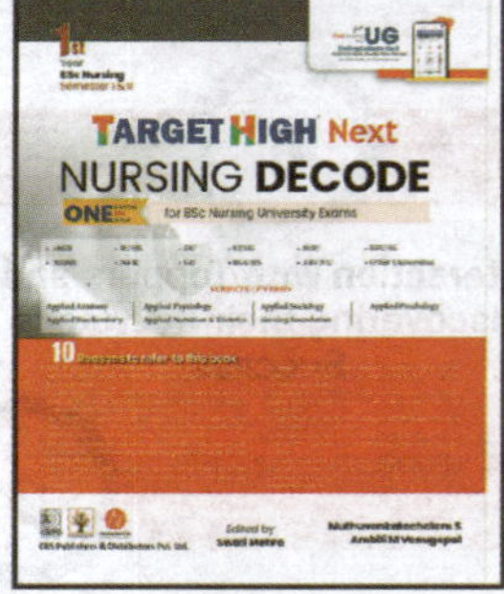

Target High Next Nursing Decode

From the Author of Target High a compendium to your last minute preparation

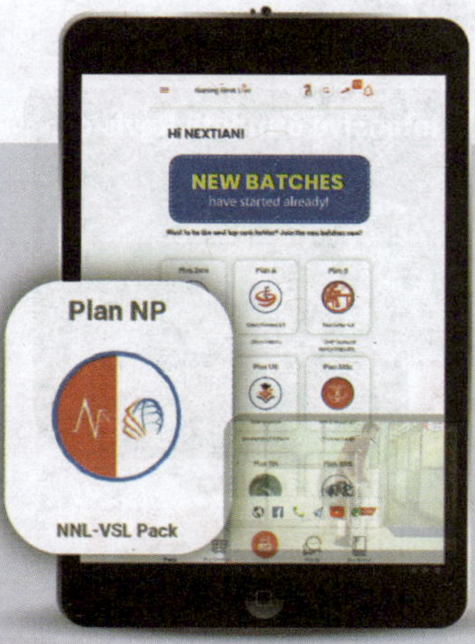

BONUS CONTENT

Clinical Procedure Videos

Selected Simulation Videos covering six core Nursing subjects for enhanced Clinical, Behavioral and Leadership Skills from Plan NP

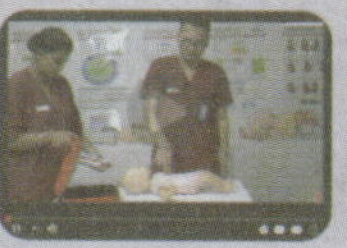
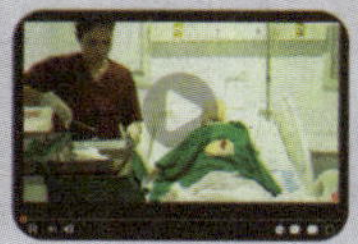
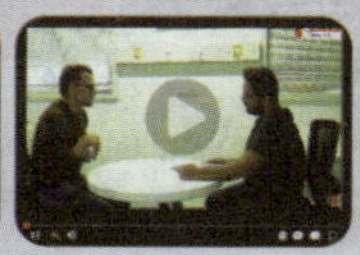
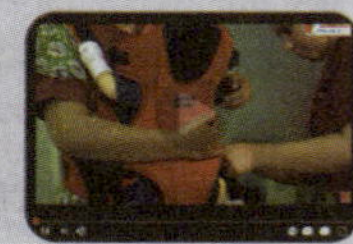
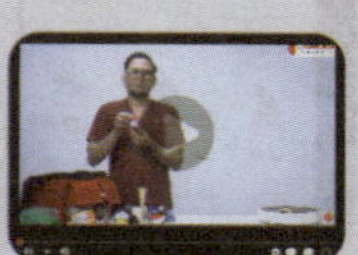

PLAN UG

Core Features

Hybrid Live Teaching by Top Educators

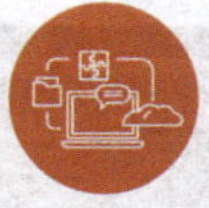

Subjective Exercises (Long & Short Q&A)

Phygital Books

Target High Next Nursing Decode

Live Doubt Sessions

Daily Live Classes

Special Classes for Nursing Procedure Demos

National Scholarship Tests

Weekly Tests & E-workbooks Assignments

Monthly Revision Tests

Progress Review Classes

Express Query Support

Orientation Programs for Thorough Guidance

OUR PEDAGOGY

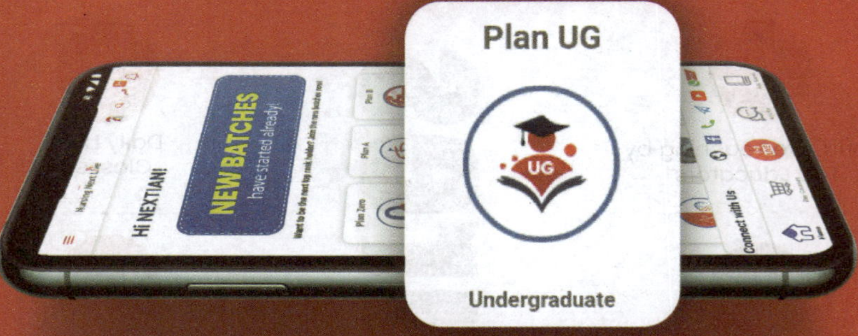

01 UG- I Year

THOROUGH CONCEPT BUILDING

(Basic Learning)

In the first year of your undergraduate preparation, our primary goal is to lay a strong foundation for your nursing education. We focus on clarifying fundamental concepts and simplifying the learning process, with an **exclusive focus of 100% on preparing you for your UG exams.** Our aim is to help you excel in your nursing examinations.

02 UG- II Year

CONCEPT STRENGTHENING & FUTURE SCOPE

(Advanced Learning)

During the second year, we take your learning to the next level by introducing advanced concepts. Approximately **80% of our focus remains on ensuring your success in UG exams, while the remaining 20% involves introducing you to the NORCET** (Nursing Officer Recruitment Common Eligibility Test) level. This year is crucial for making informed decisions about your future career path, whether it's pursuing a Master of Science (MSc), preparing for NORCET, or taking steps towards NCLEX (National Council Licensure Examination).

03 UG- III & IV Year

SECURING FUTURE

(Futuristic)

In your final years of undergraduate studies, our approach evolves to further prepare you for your future career options. We place a balanced emphasis on both advanced concepts and exam preparation, with a **50% focus on excelling in your UG exams.** Simultaneously, we allocate the **remaining 50% to introduce you comprehensively to the NORCET level.** We are dedicated to guiding you towards a successful and fulfilling nursing career

Our USPs

Unique Content & Expert Educators

for an unparalleled learning experience...

Smart Teaching Methodology

for empowering excellence...

Proactive Guidance/ Mentorship

for paving your path to success...

Our Salient Features

Pre-recorded INC Syllabus Lectures

Subject-wise Hybrid Conceptual Classes

E-workbooks/ Pre-Assessment Tests

Target High Next Nursing Decode

Weekly, Monthly and Unit Tests

Clinical Procedure Videos

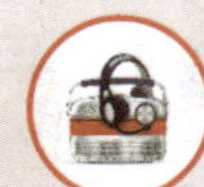

Podcast-Golden Points Revision

Customized Study Plans

Orientation, Guidance & Counseling

Doubt Sessions & Progress Evaluation

Our Batch Mentors

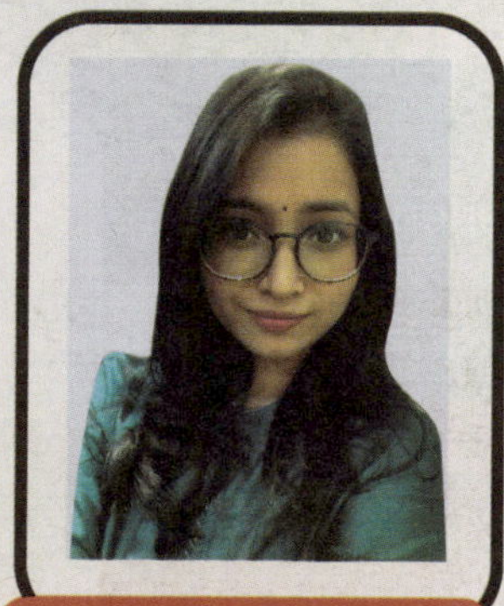

Ms. Chitra Pandey

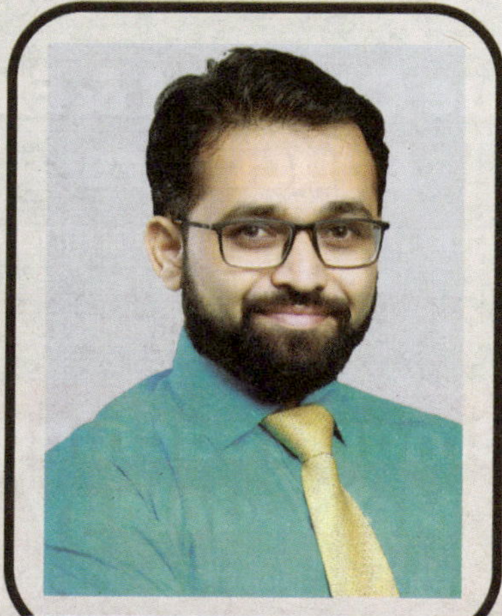

Dr. Shrikant Verma

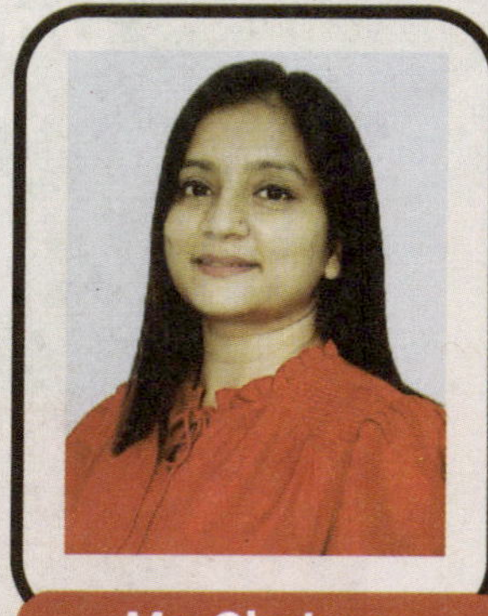

Ms. Chetana

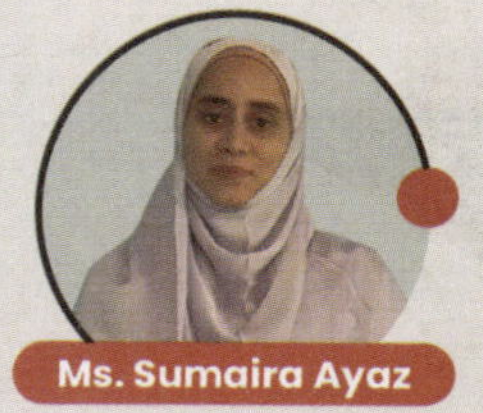

Ms. Sumaira Ayaz

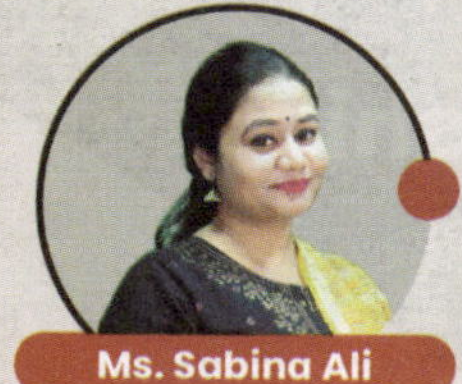

Ms. Sabina Ali

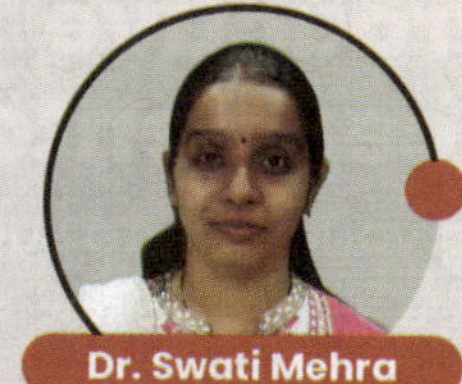

Dr. Swati Mehra

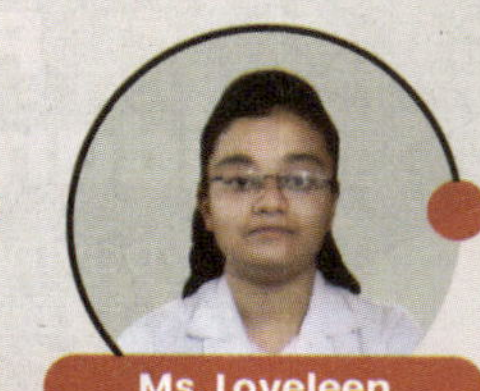

Ms. Loveleen

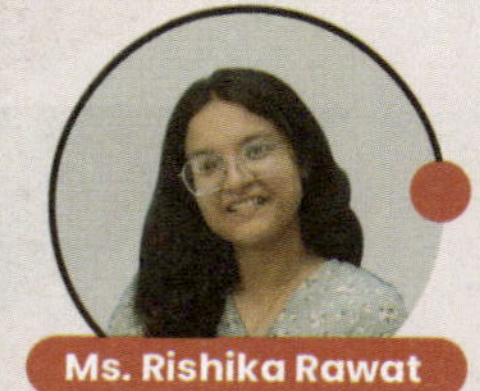

Ms. Rishika Rawat

Free Study Material with

Plan UG

(For Paid Subscribers)

Plan UG TOC

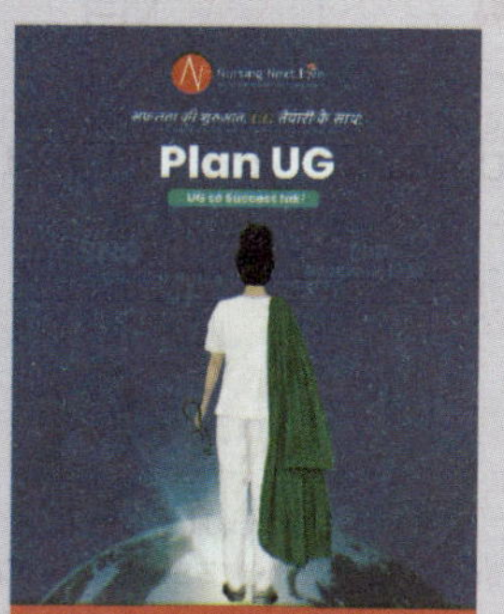

CBS Phygital Books

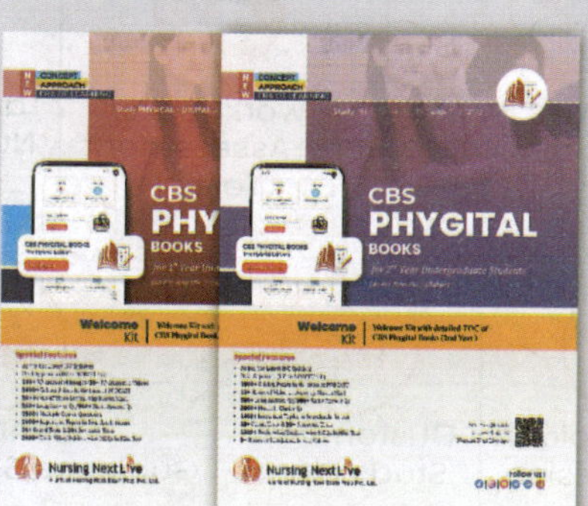

Target High Next Nursing Decode Book

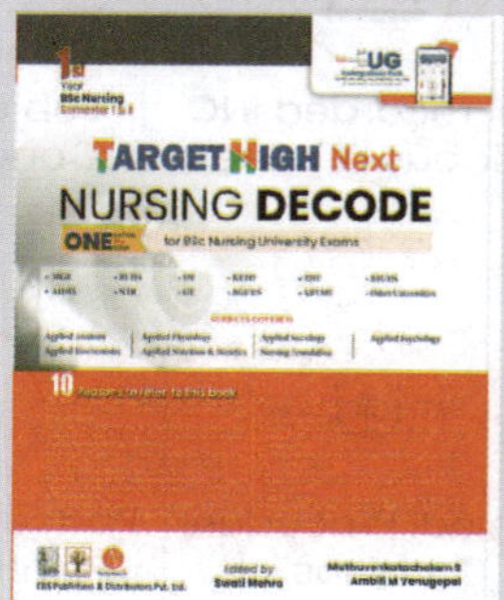

When you choose Nursing Next Live
you're not just choosing an educational platform

When you choose NNL, you're not just choosing an educational platform– you're choosing the expertise, guidance and mentorship of this exceptional faculty, each with their own strengths and wisdom.

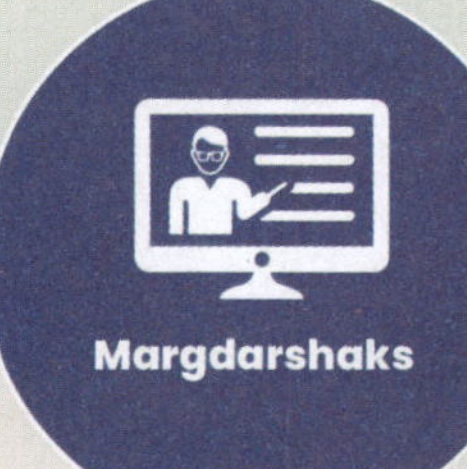

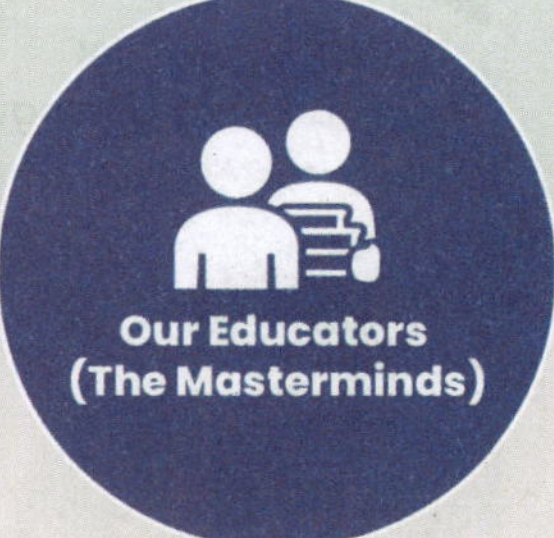

The Masterminds

UG I Year

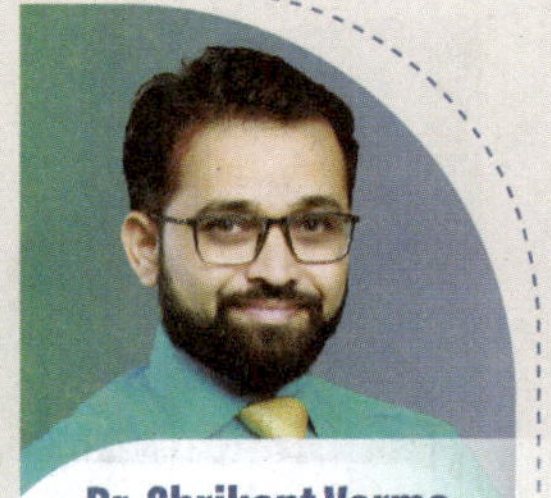

Dr. Shrikant Verma
Applied Anatomy & Physiology

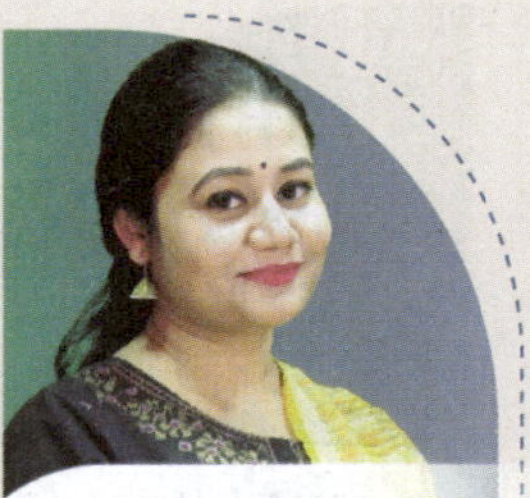

Ms. Sabina Ali
Nursing Foundations

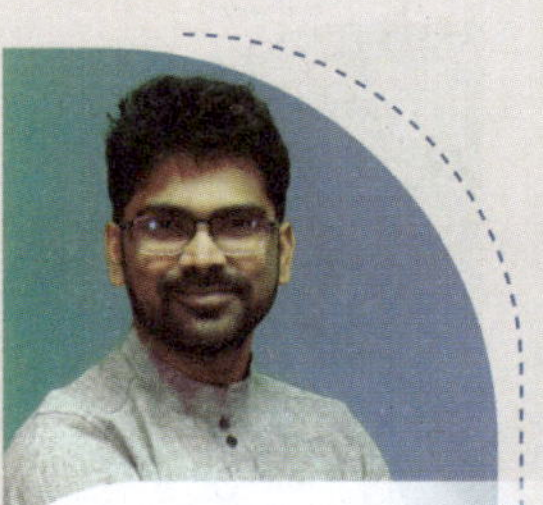

Dr. Karthikeyan Pethusamy
Applied Biochemistry & Nutrition

Ms. Chetana
Applied Psychology

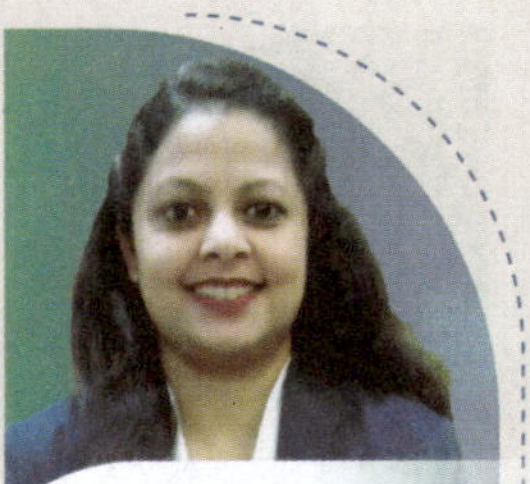

Ms. Priyanka Randhir
Applied Sociology & Nursing Informatics

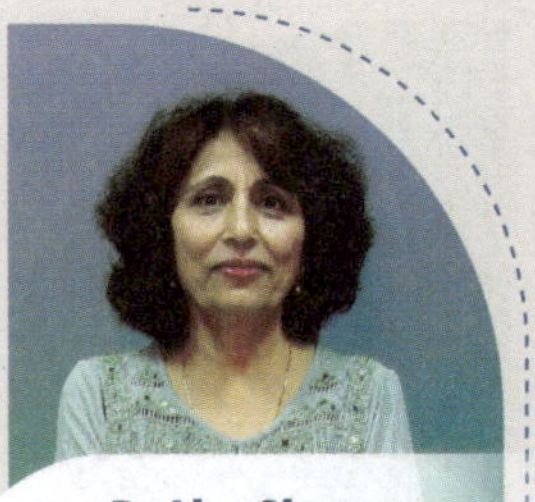

Dr. Liza Sharma
Communicative English

UG II Year

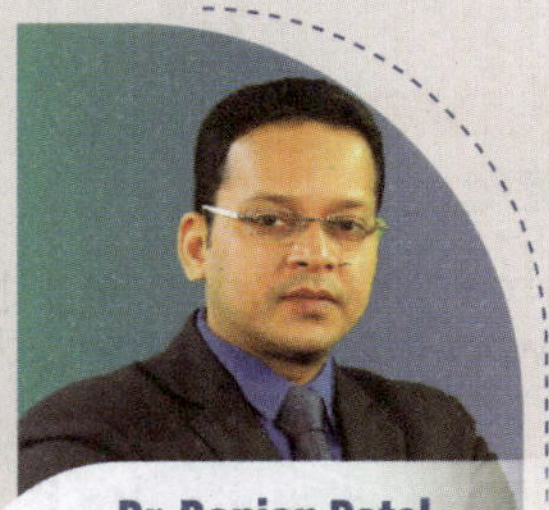

Dr. Ranjan Patel
Applied Pharmacology

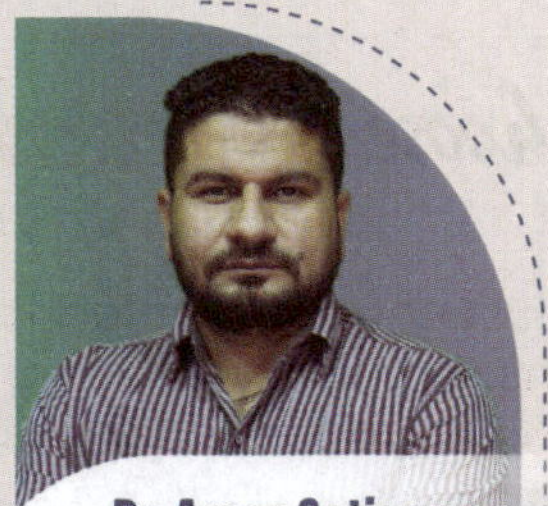

Dr. Aman Setiya
Adult Health Nursing (Medicine)

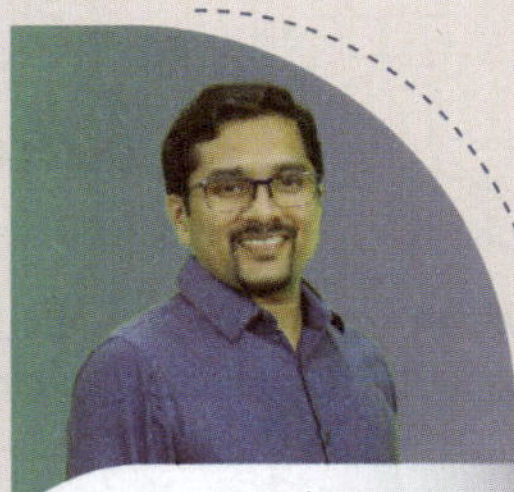

Dr. Rohan Khandelwal
Adult Health Nursing (Surgery)

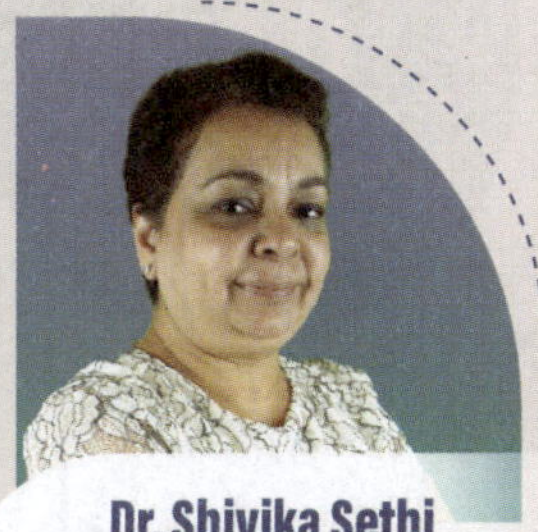

Dr. Shivika Sethi
Applied Microbiology

Dr. Preeti Sharma
Pathology & Genetics

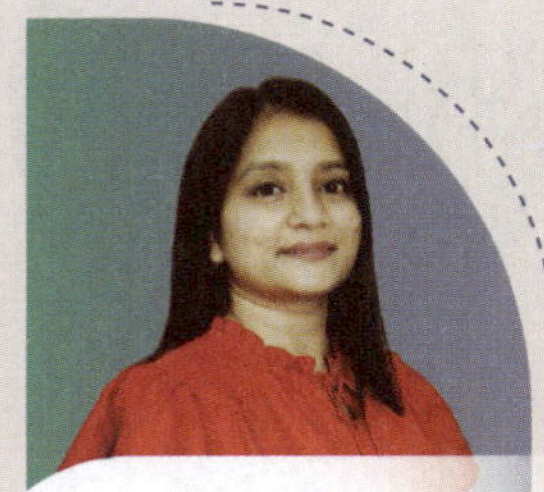

Ms. Chetana
Professionalism & Ethics

UG III & IV Year

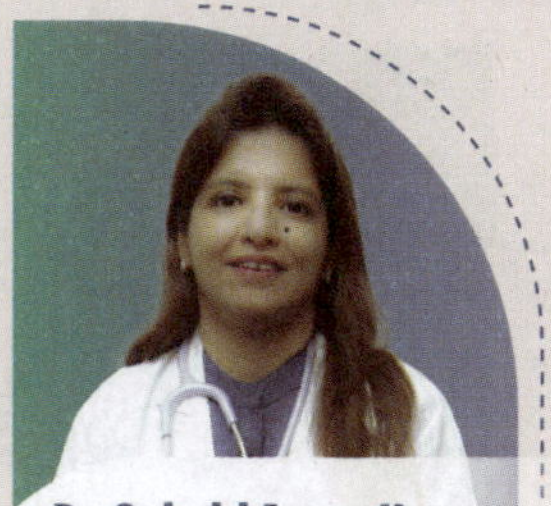

Dr. Sakshi Arora Hans
Midwifery & Obstetrical Nursing

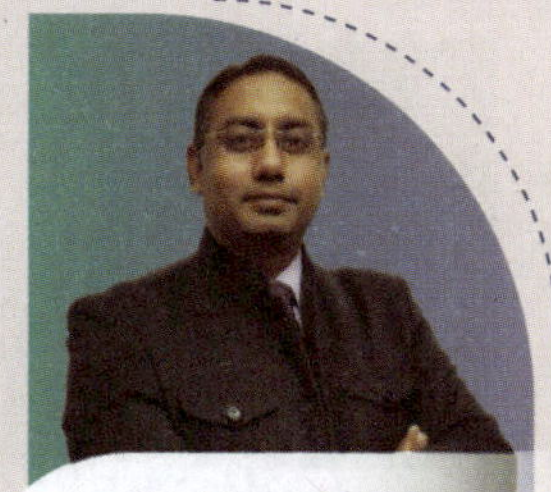

Dr. Mukhmohit Singh
Community Health Nursing

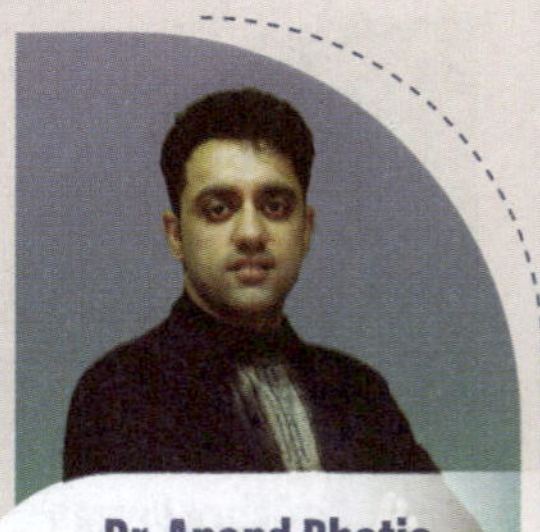

Dr. Anand Bhatia
Child Health Nursing

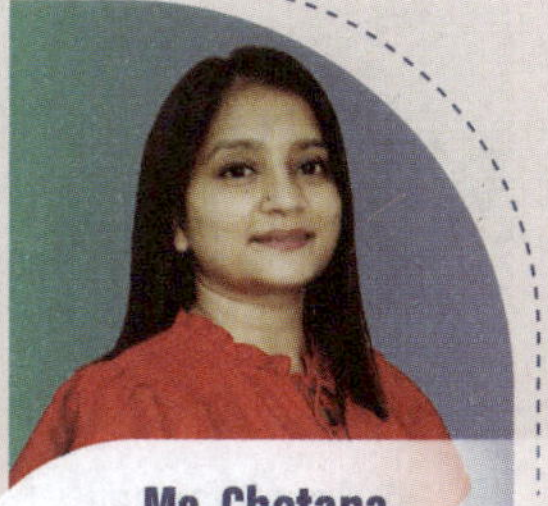

Ms. Chetana
Mental Health Nursing & Nursing Research

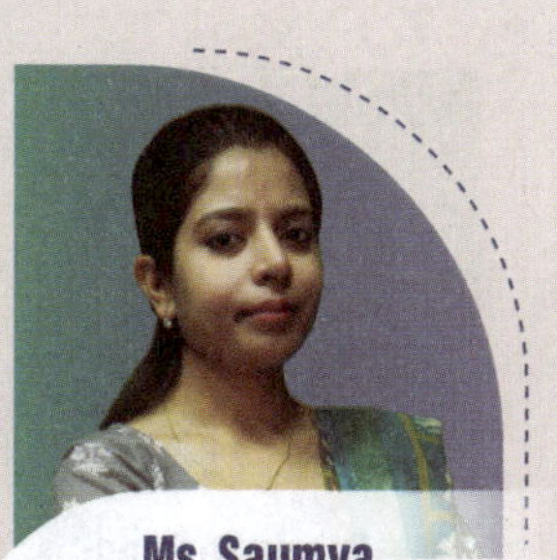

Ms. Saumya
Nursing Education & Management

Exclusive Add-ons

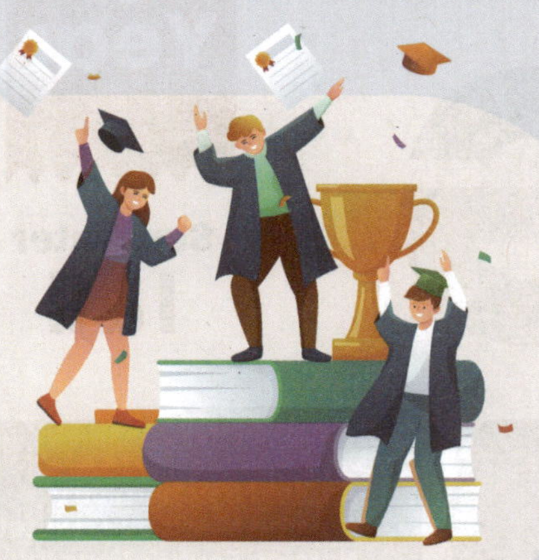

Scholarships:

Unlock significant savings with discounts of up to 80%. First-year students can qualify for discounts based on their Class 12th percentage, while second-year students can avail discounts based on their first-year university exam scores.

KYS Forms:

These all new 'Know Your Student' forms are here to help us get to know you better along with your preferences, weaknesses and requirements, so that we can create a study plan that's just right for you amd your dreams.

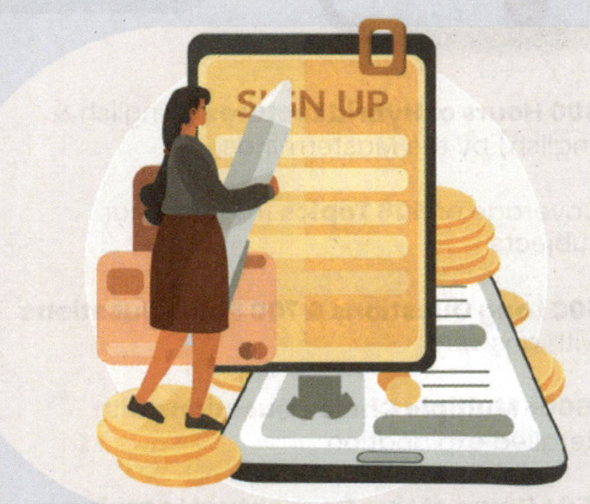

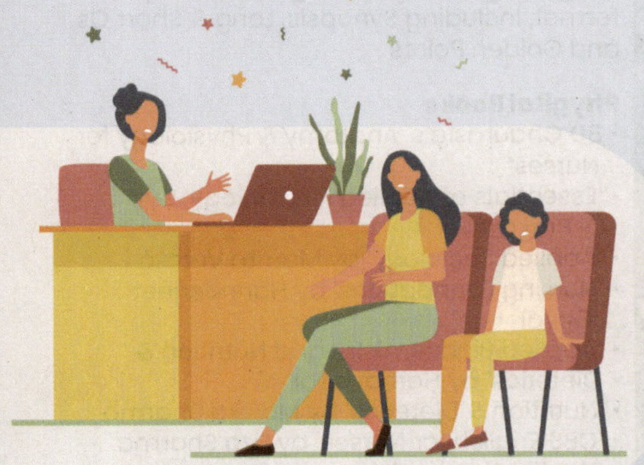

Parent/Student-Faculty Meeting:

Stay connected with your educational journey through our optional PTM sessions, offered twice every three months. It's an opportunity to discuss progress and stay informed about your child's development.

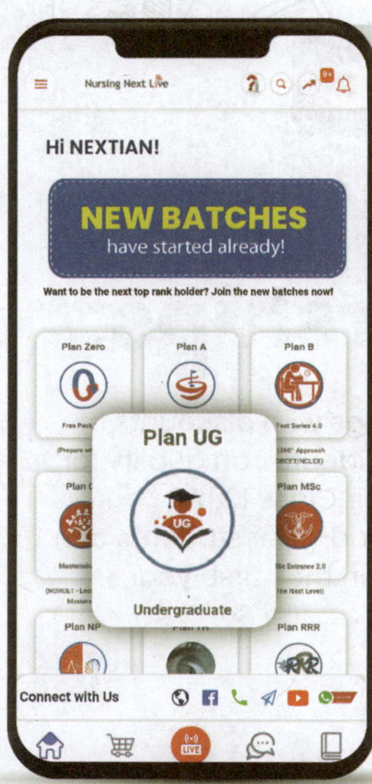

What's Included in

Plan UG

1st Year

Semester I & II

Semester- I

1. Communicative English
2. Applied Anatomy
3. Applied Physiology
4. Applied Sociology
5. Applied Psychology
6. Nursing Foundations I

Semester-II

1. Applied Biochemistry
2. Applied Nutrition & Dietetics
3. Nursing Foundations II
4. Health/ Nursing Informatics & Technology

1. **400 Hours of Hybrid Lectures** (Hinglish & English) by the Masterminds
2. Coverage of **508 Topics** from 1st year subjects
3. **500 Long Questions & 700 Short Questions** with answers
4. **1500+ Multiple Choice Questions** with detailed explanation
5. **150+ Hours of Live Conceptual Learning** by the Masterminds & Session Mentors
6. **10+ Progress Analysis Sessions** & **Student Faculty Meetings**
7. **50+ Hours of Live Revision Sessions,** discussing 100+ Qs from Target High Next Nursing Decode
8. **16 Weekly Test (MCQs)** covering 400 Qs with detailed Explanation
9. **30 Subject-wise Unit Tests** (Topic-wise) covering 300 Qs
10. **8 Revision Tests** based on the University Pattern examination, covering High Yield Topics
11. **4 Model Tests** reflecting Real-time University Examination Patterns, covering 50 FAQs
12. **30+ Previous Year Papers** from Top National Universities across India
13. **10+ Bedside Practical Preparation Sessions & Viva Voce**
14. **Analysis & Evaluation Sessions** for Unit & Model Tests
15. **Target High Next Nursing Decode** in printed format, including Synopsis, Long & Short Qs and Golden Points
16. **Phygital Books**
    - BD Chaurasia's 'Anatomy & Physiology for Nurses'
    - 'Essentials of Applied Psychology' by P Prakash
    - 'Applied Sociology' by Mamta Verma
    - 'Nursing Foundations' by Harinderjeet Goyal
    - 'Applied Biochemistry and Nutrition & Dietetics' by Harbans Lal
    - 'Nutrition & Dietetics' by Monika Sharma
    - 'CBS English for Nurses' by Liza Sharma
    - 'Health-Nursing Informatics and Technology' by Priyanka Randhir
17. **Express Query Support**

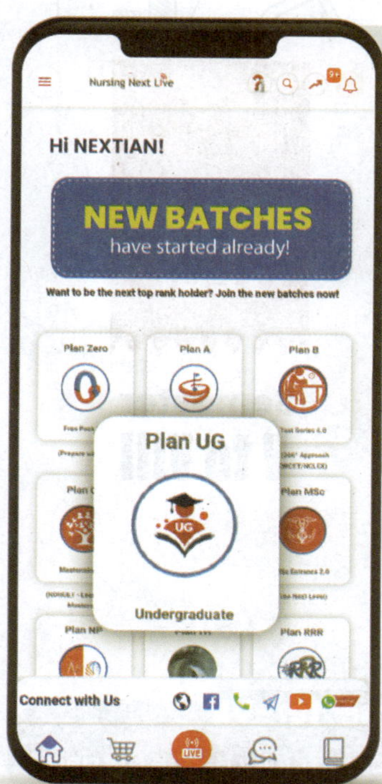

What's Included in

Plan UG

2nd Year

Semester III & IV

Semester-III

1. Applied Microbiology & Infection Control including Safety
2. Pharmacology I
3. Pathology I
4. Adult Health Nursing I with integrated Pathophysiology

Semester-IV

1. Pharmacology II
2. Pathology II & Genetics
3. Adult Health Nursing I with integrated Pathophysiology including Geriatric Nursing
4. Professionalism, Professional Values & Ethics including Bioethics

1. **300 Hours of Hybrid Lectures** (Hinglish & English) by the Masterminds
2. Comprehensive Coverage of **330 Topics** from all 2nd-year Subjects
3. **150 Long Questions & 430 Short Questions** with Answers
4. **2000+ MCQs** with Detailed Explanations
5. **Over 200 Hours of Live Conceptual Classes** by Masterminds & Session Mentors
6. **10+ Progress Analysis Sessions & Student-Faculty Meetings**
7. **60+ Hours of Live Revision Sessions,** discussing 100+ Questions from Target High Next Nursing Decode
8. **6 Live Doubt Resolution Sessions,** integrated with Progress Analysis
9. **20 Weekly Test (MCQs)** covering 400Qs with Detailed Explanations
10. **8 Subject-wise Unit Tests (Topic-wise),** covering 100 Subjective Pattern Questions
11. **4 Revision Tests** based on University Pattern Examinations, covering High Yield Topics
12. **19 Model Tests** reflecting Real-time University Examination Patterns, covering 50 FAQs
13. Access to **30+ Previous Year Papers** from Top National Universities across India
14. **10+ Bedside Practical Preparation Sessions & Viva Voce**
15. **Analysis & Evaluation Sessions** for Unit & Model Tests
16. **Target High Next Nursing Decode** in printed format, including Synopsis, Long & Short Qs and Golden Points
17. **Phygital Books**
    - 'Adult Health Nursing' by Usha Ukande
    - 'Applied Microbiology' by Dr. Anju Dhir
    - 'Applied Pharmacology' by Jogendar Pathania
    - 'Pathology & Genetics' by Vandana Puri
    - 'Essentials of Professionalism, Professional Values & Ethics' by Varinder Kaur
18. **Express Query Support**

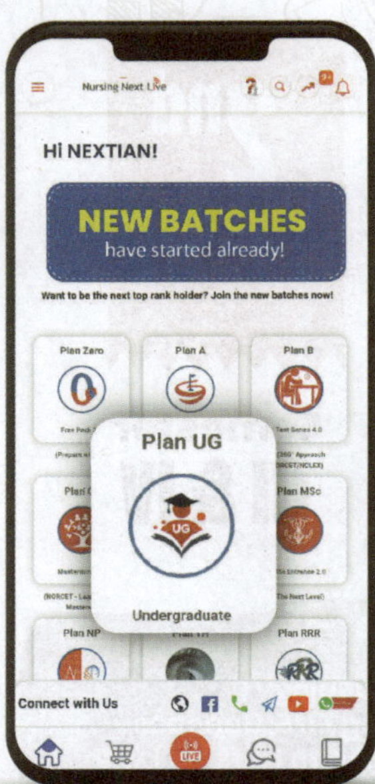

What's Included in

Plan UG

3rd & 4th Year

Semester V to VIII

Semester-V

1. Child Health Nursing I
2. Mental Health Nursing I
3. Community Health Nursing I including Environmental Science & Epidemiology
4. Educational Technology/ Nursing Education
5. Introduction to Forensic Nursing and Indian Laws

Semester-VI

1. Child Health Nursing II
2. Mental Health Nursing II
3. Nursing Management & Leadership
4. Midwifery/ Obstetrics & Gynecology (OBG) Nursing I

Semester-VII

1. Community Health Nursing II
2. Nursing Research & Statistics
3. Midwifery/ Obstetrics & Gynecology (OBG) Nursing II

ELEMENTS	UG FOCUSED	NORCET FOCUSED
Watch and Learn with Comprehensive Video Lectures	**900+** Hours of Recorded Video Lectures for Concept Building by India's Top Medical and Nursing Faculty	**520+** Hours of Video Sessions involving: • **174+** Hours of Fastrack PQD Sessions • **55+** Hours of Golden Points Chanting Sessions • **300+** Hours of Rapid Revision Sessions
Revise and Practice	**520+** Hours of Video Sessions involving: • **80** Topic Assessment Tests • **20** Subject Assessment Tests (Pre & Post)	**30,000+** Practice Questions • Grand Tests • Subject-Specific Tests • Clinical Scenario-based Tests • Super 30 Practice Tests • PYQs • IBQs
Read and Practice with Strong Study Material	• Target High Next Nursing Decode Book • Phygital Books	• NNL Revision Book-Vol 1, 2, &3 • 250+ Flashcards
Live Classes	300 + Hours of Live Interactive Sessions covering High Yield Topics, Missing Gaps for UG students	170+ Hours of Live Interactive Probable Q/A Discussion Sessions covering High Yield Topics for NORCET

SUMMARY PLAN UG

S.No	Year	Subjects	Guided Lectures by the Mastermind Faculty	Live Lectures by the Special Faculty	Videos	Short Qs	Long Qs	MCQs	Phygital Books
1	FIRST YEAR	Applied Anotomy	Dr. Shrikant Verma	Dr. Shrikant Verma	110	105	23	463	BD Chaurasia - Anatomy & Physiology 1/e 2021 (AVAILABLE)
2		Applied Physiology	Dr. Shrikant Verma	Dr. Shrikant Verma	123	85	9	527	
3		Applied Biochemistry & Nutrition	Dr. Karthikeyan Pethusamy	Dr. Shrikant Verma	88	NA	11	391	Textbook of Applied Biochemistry & Nutrition & Dietetics, Monica Sharma (NA)
4		Nursing Foundations I, II	Ms. Sabina Ali	Ms. Sabina Ali	173	74	3	413	Comprehensive Textbook of Nursing Foundation, Harinderjeet Goyal & Sabina Ali (NA)
5		Applied Psychology	Ms. Chetana	Ms. Chetana	20	31	51	135	Essentials of Applied Psychology for BSc Nursing Students, P Prakash (NA)
6		Applied Sociology	Ms. Priyanka Randhir	Ms. Priyanka Randhir	41	79	5	171	Essentials of Applied Sociology for BSc Nursing Students, Mamta Verma (NA)
7		Health Informatics and Technology	Ms. Priyanka Randhir	Ms. Priyanka Randhir	24	NA	NA	82	Textbook of Health/Nursing Informatics & Technology for BSc Nursing Students, Priyanka Randhir (NA)
8		Communicative English	Dr. Liza Sharma	Ms. Princy Jain	16	NA	NA	NA	NA
		Total			**595**	**387**	**102**	**2182**	
1	SECOND YEAR	Applied Microbiology and Infection Control including Safety	Dr. Shivika Sethi	Dr. Shrikant Verma *(Excluding Infection Control)*	31	NA	NA	170	Textbook of Microbiology for Nursing Students, Dr. Anju Dhir (NA)
2		Adult Health Nursing (Medicine)	Dr. Aman Setiya	Dr. Shrikant Verma	100	NA	NA	NA	Textbook of Adult Health Nursing, Usha Ukande (NA)
3		Adult Health Nursing (Surgery)	Dr. Rohan Khandelwal	Dr. Shrikant Verma					
4		Pharmacology I & II	Dr. Ranjan Patel	Dr. Ranjan Patel	47	NA	NA	638	Applied Pharmacology, Joginder Pathaniya (NA)
5		Pathology & Genetics	Dr. Preeti Sharma	Dr. Shrikant Verma	7	NA	NA	213	Pathology & Genetics, Vandana Puri & Kavita Gaur (NA)
6		Professionalism, Professional Values & Bioethics	Ms. Chetana	Ms. Chetana	NA	NA	NA	NA	NA
		Total			**185**	**0**	**0**	**1021**	
1	THIRD & FOURTH YEAR	Pediatric Nursing I & II	Dr. Anand Bhatia	Ms. Chitra Pandey	103	NA	NA	37	Textbook of Child Health Nursing, Panchali Pal (NA)
2		Mental Health Nursing I & II	Ms. Chetana	Ms. Chetana	53	NA	NA	92	Textbook of Mental Health Nursing, Deepika Khakha (NA)
3		Community Health Nursing I & II	Dr. Mukhmohit Singh	Ms. Manoranjini	89	NA	NA	NA	Community Health Nursing, Shyamala Manivanan (NA)
4		Nursing Education	Ms. Saumya P Srivastava	Ms. Manoranjini	34	NA	NA	NA	Essentials of Communiation & Educational Technology, L Gopichandran (NA)
5		Nursing Management and Leadership	Ms. Saumya P Srivastava	Ms. Manoranjini	24	NA	NA	NA	Textbook of Nursing Management & Leadership, JJ Kutty (NA)
6		Introduction to Forensic & Indian Laws	Dr Shrikant Verma	Dr. Shrikant Verma	NA	NA	NA	NA	NA
7		Midwifery & Obstetrical Nursing I & II	Dr. Sakshi Arora Hans	Dr. Shrikant Verma	140	NA	NA	NA	Textbook of Midwifery & Obstetrical Nursing, Sandeep Kaur (NA)
8		Nursing Research & Statistics	Ms. Chetana	Ms. Chetana	25	NA	NA	NA	Nursing Research in 21st Century, Sukhpal Kaur (NA)
		Total			**468**	**0**	**0**	**129**	

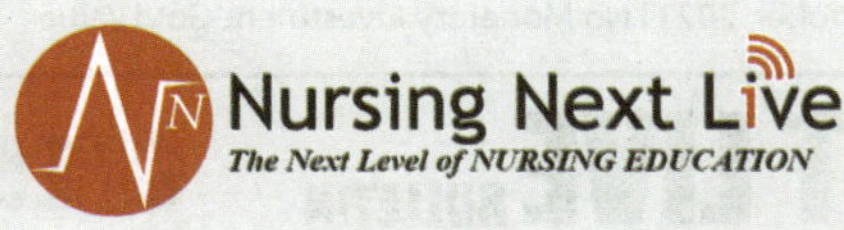

SEMESTER

I

Nursing Next Live Exam Prep Pvt Ltd | Patparganj Industrial Area, New Delhi | Vol 3 | 18th October, 2023 | No Monetary Investment Gold Value

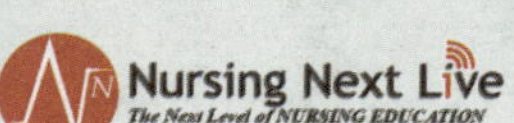

THE NURSING NEXT LIVE BULLETIN

18th October, 2023

The Next Level of Nursing Education

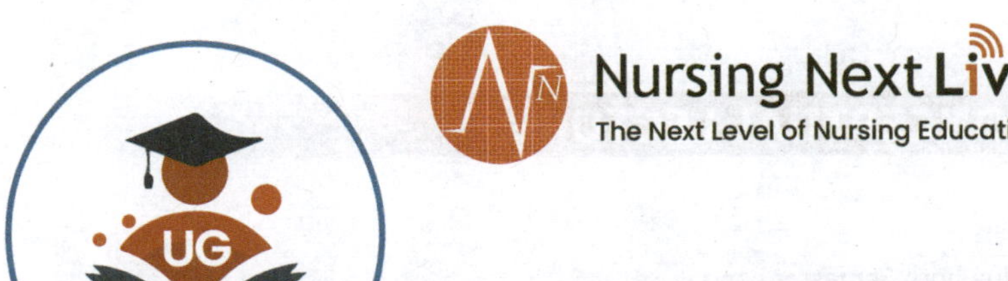

PLAN UG 1st YEAR

WHAT ALL YOU WILL GET

1. **400 Hours of Recorded Lecture** (Hinglish & English) by the Masterminds
2. **150+ Hours of Live Conceptual Learning** by the Masterminds & Session Mentors
3. Coverage of **508 Topics** from 1st year subjects
4. **Target High Next Nursing Decode** in printed format, including Synopsis, Long & Short Qs and Golden Points
5. **Phygital Books**
   - BD Chaurasia's 'Applied Anatomy & Physiology for Nurses'
   - 'Essentials of Applied Psychology' by P Prakash
   - 'Applied Sociology' by Mamta Verma
   - 'Nursing Foundations' by Harinderjeet Goyal
   - 'Applied Biochemistry and Nutrition & Dietetics' by Harbans Lal
   - 'Nutrition & Dietetics' by Monika Sharma
   - 'CBS English for Nurses' by Liza Sharma
   - 'Health-Nursing Informatics and Technology' by Priyanka Randhir
6. **50+ Hours of Live Revision Sessions,** discussing 100+ Qs from Target High Next Nursing Decode
7. **10+ Bedside Practical Preparation Sessions & Viva Voce**
8. **500 Long Questions & 700 Short Questions** with answers
9. **1500+ Multiple Choice Questions** with detailed explanation
10. **40 Weekly Test (MCQs)** covering 800 Qs with detailed Explanation
11. **20 Subject-wise Unit Tests** (Topic-wise) covering 300 Qs
12. **8 Revision Tests** based on the University Pattern examination, covering High Yield Topics
13. **4 Model Tests** reflecting Real-time University Examination Patterns, covering 50 FAQs
14. **30+ Previous Year Papers** from Top National Universities across India
15. **20+ Progress Analysis Sessions & Student Faculty Meetings**
16. **Analysis & Evaluation Sessions** for Unit & Model Tests
17. **Express Query Support**

CONCEPTUAL LECTURES

TABLE 1: All Subjects all Topics Covering both Semester I and II

S. No.	Subject	Faculty	Video Lectures Durations	Topics Covered	Long Qs	Short Qs	MCQs	Golden Points
1.	Applied Anatomy & Physiology	Dr Shrikant Verma	78	142	100	150	500	
2.	Applied Psychology	Ms Chetana	20	17	50	70	100	
3.	Applied Biochemistry & Applied Nutrition & Dietetics	Dr Karthik Pethusamy	48	102	100	150	250	
4.	Fundamentals of Nursing I	Ms Sabina Ali	150	159	100	150	600	
5.	Applied Sociology	Ms Priyanka Randhir	39	41	80	100	100	
6.	Health/Nursing Informatics Technology	Ms Priyanka Randhir	32	30	50	70	50	
7.	Communicative English	Dr Liza Sharma	33	17	NA	NA	NA	
	Grand Total		**400**	**508**	**480**	**690**	**1600**	

TABLE 2: Live Teaching All Subjects Important Topics Covering 30% content from Semester I

S.No.	Subject	Days	Faculty	Live Classes	Duration
1.	Applied Anatomy & Physiology	Monday & Tuesday	Dr Shrikant Verma	24	48 hours
2.	Applied Psychology	Friday & Saturday	Ms Chetana	18	30 hours
3.	Applied Sociology	Friday & Saturday	Ms Priyanka Randhir	12	24 hours
4.	Fundamentals of Nursing I	Wednesday & Thursday	Ms Sabina Ali	24	48 hours
	Total			**78**	**150 hours**

TABLE 3: Conceptual Lecture Hybrid Live Teaching All Subjects Important Topics Covering 70% content from Semester I

S.No.	Subject	Days	Faculty	Hybrid Live Classes	Duration
1.	Applied Anatomy & Physiology	Monday & Tuesday	Dr Shrikant Verma	26	52 hours
2.	Applied Psychology	Friday & Saturday	Ms Chetana	20	30 hours
3.	Applied Sociology	Friday & Saturday	Ms Priyanka Randhir	16	30 hours
4.	Fundamentals of Nursing I	Wednesday & Thursday	Ms Sabina Ali	30	60 hours
	Total			**92**	**172 hours**

TABLE 4: Repeat Live Classes

S.No.	Date	Subjects	Topics Covered	Timing
1.	09 December 2023	Applied Anatomy & Physiology	Topics Covered till 19th November	6 – 8 pm
2.	23 December 2023	Applied Sociology	Topics covered till 30th November	6- 8 pm
3.	24 December 2023	Applied Psychology	Topics covered till 17th December	9 am to 12 noon
4.	13 January 2024	Nursing Foundations I	Topics covered till 31st December	6- 8 pm
5.	27 January 2024	Applied Anatomy & Physiology	Topics covered till 14th January	6- 8 pm
6.	28 January 2024	Applied Psychology	Topics covered till 28th January	9 am to 12 noon
7.	10 February 2024	Nursing Foundations I	Topics covered till 11th February	6- 8 pm
8.	24 February2024	Applied Sociology	Topics covered till 25th February	6- 8 pm
9.	25 February 2024	Nursing Foundations	Topics covered till 25th February	9 am to 12 noon

TABLE 5: Surprise Classes

S. No	Date	Day	Faculty	Surprise Class	Durations
1.	05 November 2023	Sunday	Dr Shrikant Verma	Topic to be disclosed a day before the session	2 hours
2.	12 November 2023	Sunday	Dr Shrikant Verma	Topic to be disclosed a day before the session	2 hours
3.	19 November 2023	Sunday	Dr Shrikant Verma	Topic to be disclosed a day before the session	2 hours
4.	10 December 2023	Sunday	Dr Shrikant Verma	Topic to be disclosed a day before the session	2 hours
5.	24 December 2023	Sunday	Dr Shrikant Verma	Topic to be disclosed a day before the session	2 hours
6.	31 December 2023	Sunday	Dr Shrikant Verma	Topic to be disclosed a day before the session	2 hours
7.	14 January 2024	Sunday	Dr Shrikant Verma	Topic to be disclosed a day before the session	2 hours
8.	28 January 2024	Sunday	Dr Shrikant Verma	Topic to be disclosed a day before the session	2 hours
9.	11 February 2024	Sunday	Dr Shrikant Verma	Topic to be disclosed a day before the session	2 hours
10.	18 February 2024	Sunday	Dr Shrikant Verma	Topic to be disclosed a day before the session	2 hours
	Total				**20 hours**

CONCEPTUAL LEARNING

TABLE 6: Target High Next Nursing Decode

S. No	Over All Summary	Total no. of Synopsis	Total no. of Long Question	Total no. of Short Notes	Total no. of Short Answers	Total no. of MCQs	Total no. of Golden Point
1.	Applied Anatomy	41	27	102	51 (50+)	99 (100+)	188 (200+)
2.	Applied Physiology	40	24	56	86 (80+)	111 (100+)	222 (200+)
3.	Nursing Foundations I	121	56	181	107 (100+)	258 (200+)	301 (300+)
4.	Applied Psychology	31	45	62	75 (70+)	99 (100+)	80 (100+)
5.	Applied Sociology	58	28	28	33 (33+)	69 (50+)	71 (70+)
	Total	**291+**	**180+**	**400+**	**350+**	**650 +**	**900+**

CONCEPTUAL REVISION

TABLE 7: Revision through Target High Next Nursing Decode

Date	Day	Subject	Faculty	Sessions	Paper
01 March 2024	Friday	Applied Psychology	Ms Chetana	Decode Revision Session 1 with PQD	Model Test-1 Applied Psychology Set-1
02 March 2024	Saturday	Applied Psychology	Ms Chetana	Doubt Session	Model Test-2 Applied Psychology Set-2
05 March 2024	Tuesday	Applied Psychology	Ms Chetana	Decode Revision Session 3 with PQD	Model Test-3 Applied Psychology Set-3
06 March 2024	Wednesday	Applied Anatomy & Physiology	Dr Shrikant Verma/ Deepshikha	Decode Revision Session 3 with PQD	Model Test-4 Applied Anatomy & Physiology Set-1
09 March 2024	Saturday	Applied Anatomy & Physiology	Dr Shrikant Verma/ Deepshikha	Decode Revision Session 3 with PQD	Model Test-5 Applied Anatomy & Physiology Set-2
11 March 2024	Monday	Applied Anatomy & Physiology	Dr Shrikant Verma/ Deepshikha	Decode Revision Session 3 with PQD	Model Test-6 Applied Anatomy & Physiology Set-3
12 March 2024	Tuesday	Applied Anatomy & Physiology	Dr Shrikant Verma/ Deepshikha	Decode Revision Session 3 with PQD	Model Test-7 Applied Anatomy & Physiology Set-4
13 March 2024	Wednesday	Applied Anatomy & Physiology	Dr Shrikant Verma/ Deepshikha	Doubt Session	Model Test-8 Applied Anatomy & Physiology Set-5
18 March 2024	Monday	Applied Sociology	Ms Priyanka Randhir	Decode Revision Session 1 with PQD	Model Test-9 Applied Sociology Set-1
19 March 2024	Tuesday	Applied Sociology	Ms Priyanka Randhir	Decode Revision Session 2 with PQD	Model Test-10 Applied Sociology Set-2
20 March 2024	Wednesday	Applied Sociology	Ms Priyanka Randhir	Decode Revision Session 1 with PQD	Model Test-11 Applied Sociology Set-3
21 March 2024	Thursday	Nursing Foundations I	Ms Sabina Ali	Decode Revision Session 1 with PQD	Model Test-12 Nursing Foundations I Set-1
22 March 2024	Friday	Nursing Foundations I	Ms Sabina Ali	Decode Revision Session 1 with PQD	Model Test-13 Nursing Foundations I Set-2
25 March 2024	Monday	Nursing Foundations I	Ms Sabina Ali	Doubt Session	Model Test-14 Nursing Foundations I Set-3
27 March 2024	Wednesday	Nursing Foundations I	Ms Sabina Ali	Decode Revision Session 1 with PQD	Model Test-15 Nursing Foundations I Set-4
28 March 2024	Thursday	Nursing Foundations I	Ms Sabina Ali	Decode Revision Session 1 with PQD	Model Test-16 Nursing Foundations I Set-5
29 March 2024	Friday	Nursing Foundations I	Ms Sabina Ali	Decode Revision Session 1 with PQD	Model Test-17 Nursing Foundations I Set-6
30 March 2024	Saturday	Nursing Foundations I	Ms Sabina Ali	Decode Revision Session 1 with PQD	Model Test-18 Nursing Foundations I Set-7
31 March 2024	Sunday	Nursing Foundations I	Ms Sabina Ali	Decode Revision Session 1 with PQD	Model Test-19 Nursing Foundations I Set-8

CONCEPTUAL PRACTICE

TABLE 8: Overview of Practice Tests and Assignments

S. No	Test	Total No. of Tests	No of Qs
1.	Weekly Tests (Objective Type)	20	400
2.	10+ E-workbook	–	–
3.	Self-review Golden Points	–	–
4.	Subject-wise Unit Tests (Topic-wise)	8	40
5.	Revision Tests After Completion of Batch (Based on University Pattern)	08	800
6.	Model Tests (Based on University Pattern)	19	228
7.	Previous Years' Papers (Unsolved University Papers)	30+	350
	Total	**85+**	**1818**

TABLE 9: Weekly Tests Scheduled

S. No	Dates	Subjects	Tests	No. of Questions
1.	12 November 2023	Applied Anatomy & Physiology Applied Psychology, Fundamentals of Nursing	Weekly Test 1	20
2.	19 November 2023	Applied Anatomy & Physiology Applied Psychology, Nursing Foundations I	Weekly Test 2	20
3.	26 November 2023	Applied Anatomy & Physiology Applied Psychology, Nursing Foundations I	Weekly Test 3	20
4.	3 December 2023	Applied Anatomy & Physiology Applied Psychology, Nursing Foundations I	Weekly Test 4	20
5.	10 December 2023	Applied Anatomy & Physiology Applied Psychology, Nursing Foundations I	Weekly Test 5	20
6.	24 December 2023	Applied Anatomy & Physiology Applied Sociology, Nursing Foundations I	Weekly Test 6	20
7.	18 November 2023	Applied Anatomy & Physiology Applied Sociology	Weekly Test 7	20
8.	31 December 2023	Applied Anatomy & Physiology Applied Sociology, Nursing Foundations I	Weekly Test 8	20
9.	14 January 2024	Applied Anatomy & Physiology Applied Sociology, Nursing Foundations I	Weekly Test 9	20
10.	21 January 2024	Applied Anatomy & Physiology Applied Sociology, Nursing Foundations I	Weekly Test 10	20
11.	28 January 2024	Applied Anatomy & Physiology Nursing Foundations I	Weekly Test 11	20
12.	04 February 2024	Applied Anatomy & Physiology Nursing Foundations I	Weekly Test 12	20
13.	11 February 2024	Applied Anatomy & Physiology Nursing Foundations I	Weekly Test 13	20
14.	18 February 2024	Applied Anatomy & Physiology Nursing Foundations I	Weekly Test 14	20
15.	25 February 2024	Applied Anatomy & Physiology Nursing Foundations I	Weekly Test 15	20
		Total		**300**

TABLE 10: Subject-wise Unit Tests

S. No.	Dates	Subjects	Tests	No. of Questions	Duration (in Hours)
1.	12 November 2023	Mental Health Nursing	Unit Test-1	10	2
2.	26 November 2023	Applied Anatomy & Physiology	Unit Test-2	10	2
3.	17 December 2023	Mental Health Nursing	Unit Test-3	10	2
4.	31 December 2023	Applied Anatomy & Physiology	Unit Test-4	10	2
5.	14 January 2024	Nursing Foundations I	Unit Test-5	10	2
6.	28 January 2024	Applied Sociology	Unit Test-6	10	2
7.	11 February 2024	Nursing Foundations I	Unit Test-7	10	2
8.	25 February 2024	Applied Sociology	Unit Test-8	10	2
		Total		**80**	**16**

TABLE 11: Revision Tests

S. No	Dates (Yet to be decided)	Subjects	Subjects to be covered
1.	December 2023	Revision Test-1	Applied Anatomy & Physiology Applied Psychology
2.	January 2024	Revision Test-2	Applied Anatomy & Physiology Applied Sociology
3.	February 2024	Revision Test-3	Nursing Foundations I
	Total		

TABLE 12: Model Tests

S. No	Dates	Days	Tests
1.	1 March 2024	Friday	Model Test Applied Psychology Set-1
2.	2 March 2024	Saturday	Model Test Applied Psychology Set-2
3.	5 March 2024	Tuesday	Model Test Applied Psychology Set-3
4.	6 March 2024	Wednesday	Model Test Applied Anatomy & Physiology Set-1
5.	9 March 2024	Saturday	Model Test Applied Anatomy & Physiology Set-2
6.	11 March 2024	Monday	Model Test Applied Anatomy & Physiology Set-3
7.	12 March 2024	Tuesday	Model Test Applied Anatomy & Physiology Set-4
8.	13 March 2024	Wednesday	Model Test Applied Anatomy & Physiology Set-5
9.	18 March 2024	Monday	Model Test Applied Sociology Set-1
10.	19 March 2024	Tuesday	Model Test Applied Sociology Set-2
11.	20 March 2024	Wednesday	Model Test Applied Sociology Set-3
12.	21 March 2024	Thursday	Model Test Nursing Foundations I Set-1
13.	22 March 2024	Friday	Model Test Nursing Foundations I Set-2
14.	25 March 2024	Monday	Model Test Nursing Foundations I Set-3

Contd...

S. No	Dates	Days	Tests
15.	27 March 2024	Wednesday	Model Test Nursing Foundations I Set-4
16.	28 March 2024	Thursday	Model Test Nursing Foundations I Set-5
17.	29 March 2024	Friday	Model Test Nursing Foundations I Set-6
18.	30 March 2024	Saturday	Model Test Nursing Foundations I Set-7
19.	31 March 2024	Sunday	Model Test Nursing Foundations I Set-8
20.	01 April 2024	Monday	Model Test Nursing Foundations I Set-9

TABLE 13: Previous Years Papers

S. No.	Subjects	No of Tests	No. of Questions
1.	Applied Anatomy & Physiology	10	10–12
3.	Applied Psychology	10	10–12
4.	Applied Sociology	10	10–12
5.	Nursing Foundations I	10	10–12
	Total	**40**	**400+**

TABLE 14: Progress Analysis + Student Faculty Meet

S. No	Date	Progress Evaluation Class	Batch Mentor	Duration (Hours)	Topic/ Agenda
1.	15 October 2023	Class 1	Ms Chetana	1	How to make the effective use of Plan UG?
2.	25 October 2023	Class 2	Ms Chetana	1–2	• Benefits of taking Weekly Tests • Guiding new students
3.	7 November 2023	Class 3	Ms Chetana	1–2	• Tips and tricks for effective learning and memorizing • Guiding new students
4.	21 November 2023	Class 4	Ms Chetana	1–2	• Tips and tricks for attempting subjective questions • Guiding new students
5.	December 2023	Class 8	Ms Chetana	1–2	To be disclosed later
6.	December 2023	Class 9	Ms Chetana	1–2	To be disclosed later
7.	January 2024	Class 10	Ms Chetana	1–2	To be disclosed later
8.	January 2024	Class 11	Ms Chetana	1–2	To be disclosed later
9.	February 2024	Class 12	Ms Chetana	1–2	To be disclosed later
	Total			**15+**	

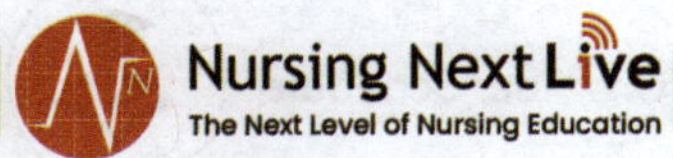

GUIDANCE & COUNSELLING

S. No	Schedule	Sessions	Total no. of Sessions
1.	At the Time of Joining	Welcome Call	1
2.	Orientation Sessions Every Week for Batch I after that Biweekly	Orientation Program by RM's	17–18
3.	Twice in a Month (1 and 3 Saturday) Tentative Dates	Progress Review by Batch Mentor	9
4.	1st Week of Every Month	Updates on Upcoming Classes & Important Tests	6–7
5.	Within 1 Week of Attempting the Subject-wise Unit Test	Analysis on Subject-wise Unit Tests	31
6.	Within 1 Week of Attempting Model Test	Analysis and Discussion on Model Test	4
7.	Within 1 Week of Attempting Revision Test	Analysis and Discussion on Revision Test	
8.	Throughout the Semester	Express Query Resolution	On a Regular Basis
9.	December 2023, February 2024, March 2024 (Dates to be Decided)	Interaction with Students (High Performers)	4–5
10.	After Completing 1st Month of all the Batches	Feedbacks & Surveys	3–4

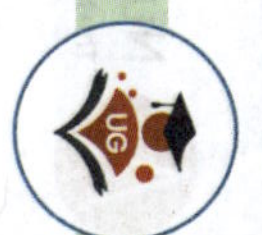

DAY WISE PLAN FOR UG 1st YEAR-SEMESTER I (1st NOVEMBER ONWARDS)

Date	Day	Subject	Faculty	Morning Session (HLT) (Recorded Video of MM Faculty) 6 am – 8 am	Evening Session (LIVE) (High Yield Topics/Missing Topics/ High Yield Subjective Q Discussion, Nursing implication) 6 pm – 8 pm	Tests	Doubt Session/ Progress Analysis	Assignments (Phygital & E-workbook + TH Decode) Golden Points + Solved Exercise (Self-study After Class)
1. Nov. 2023	Wednesday	Applied Psychology	Ms Chetana	**Unit 1: Introduction** Introduction of Applied Psychology Part 1–2	**Unit 1: Introduction** • Branches, Scopes, Methods • Significance of Applied Psychology in Nursing • Applied Psychology to Solve Everyday Issues			E-work Book Before the Week Schedule Start
2. Nov. 2023	Thursday	Applied Anatomy & Physiology	Dr Shrikant Verma	**Unit 1: Introduction to Anatomical Terms and Organization of the Human Body** • Anatomical Introduction and Terminology • Plan and Movement • Body Organization and Surface Anatomy	**Unit 1: Introduction to Anatomical Terms and Organization of the Human Body** • Recapitalization • Tissue • Features of Smooth, Skeletal, Cardiac Muscle			
3. Nov. 2023	Friday	Applied Psychology	Ms Chetana	**Unit 2: Biological Basis of Behavior –Introduction** Biology of Behavior Part 1–3	Unit 2: Biological Basis of Behavior –Introduction **Body Mind Relationship** Applied Psychology and Sensation – Sensory process – Normal and Abnormal			
4. Nov. 2023	**Saturday**	Applied Sociology	Ms Priyanka Randhir	Unit I: Introduction Definition, Nature and Scope of Applied Sociology Paradigm of Applied Sociology	Discussion on E-workbook/ Assignment/Tests (How to use/ Submit/Attempt)			
5. Nov. 2023	**Sunday**	Applied Anatomy & Physiology	Dr Shrikant Verma	SPL Class Nursing Procedure 2–4 procedures	Surprise Class Live	Week Test 1 (MCQ)		

Contd...

Date	Day	Subject	Faculty	Morning Session (HLT) (Recorded Video of MM Faculty) 6 am – 8 am	Evening Session (LIVE) (High Yield Topics/Missing Topics/ High Yield Subjective Q Discussion, Nursing implication) 6 pm – 8 pm	Tests	Doubt Session/ Progress Analysis	Assignments (Phygital & E-workbook + TH Decode) Golden Points + Solved Exercise (Self-study After Class)
6. Nov. 2023	Monday	Applied Anatomy & Physiology	Dr Shrikant Verma	**Unit 1: Introduction to Anatomical Terms and Organization of the Human Body** • Anatomical Spaces • Cell Structure • Cell Membrane	**Unit 1: Introduction to Anatomical Terms and Organization of the Human Body** • Recapitalization • Cell Organelles: Nucleus and Nucleolus • Cell Physiology • Cell Division • Body Fluid Compartments			
7. Nov. 2023	Tuesday	Applied Anatomy & Physiology	Dr Shrikant Verma	**Unit 1: Introduction to Anatomical Terms and Organization of the Human Body** Cytoplasm, ER, GA, Mito., Lysosome, Peroxisome, RB, Cytoskeleton and Centrioles Cartilage	Unit 1: General Physiology • Recapitalization • Cell Cycle • Membrane and Glands: Applied Anatomy & Physiology			
8. Nov. 2023	Wednesday	Nursing Foundations I	Ms Sabina Ali	Unit 1: Introduction to Health and Illness • Concept of Health • Concept of Health and Illness Part 1, 2, 3	Unit 1: Introduction to Health and Illness • Recap • Maslow'S Hierarchy • Health-Illness Continuum • Illness			
9. Nov. 2023	Thursday	Nursing Foundations I	Ms Sabina Ali	Unit 1: Introduction to Health and Illness • Concept of Health and Illness part 3 • Illness-wellness Continuum • Level of Prevention	Unit 1: Introduction to Health and Illness • Factors Influencing Health Causes and Risk Factors for Developing Illnesses • Illness – Types, Illness Behavior Impact of Illness on Patient and Family			

Contd...

Date	Day	Subject	Faculty	Morning Session (HLT) (Recorded Video of MM Faculty) 6 am – 8 am	Evening Session (LIVE) (High Yield Topics/Missing Topics/ High Yield Subjective Q Discussion, Nursing implication) 6 pm – 8 pm	Tests	Doubt Session/ Progress Analysis	Assignments (Phygital & E-workbook + TH Decode) Golden Points + Solved Exercise (Self-study After Class)
10. Nov. 2023	Friday	Applied Psychology	Ms Chetana	**Unit 1: Introduction** • Introduction of Applied Psychology Part 1–2	**Unit 1: Introduction** • Branches, Scopes, Methods • Significance of Applied Psychology in Nursing • Applied Psychology to Solve Everyday Issues			
11. Nov. 2023	Saturday	Applied Psychology	Ms Chetana	Unit 2: Biological basis of Behavior –Introduction **Biology of Behavior Part 1-3**	HYQ Discussion (Decode) Applied Anatomy & Physiology			
12. Nov. 2023	**Sunday**	Surprise Class	Dr Shrikant Verma	NP Class • 2–4 Procedures	Surprise Class	Week Test 2 (MCQ) Unit Test-1 (Subjective)		E-workbook for the Next Week
13. Nov. 2023	Monday	Applied Anatomy & Physiology	Dr Shrikant Verma	Unit 2: **Respiratory system (Anatomy)** • Nose, Nasal Cavity, Septum • Pharynx • Larynx	Unit 2: **Respiratory system (Anatomy)** • Recap • Trachea • Lungs • Functions of Respiratory Organs • Physiology of Respiration			
14. Nov. 2023	Tuesday	Applied Anatomy & Physiology	Dr Shrikant Verma	Unit 2: **Respiratory system (Anatomy)** Bronchial Tree, BP Segment Respiration and resp. unit Res. Movements Ventilation and Gaseous Exchange	Unit 2: **Respiratory system (Anatomy)** • Pulmonary Circulation – Functional Features • Pulmonary Ventilation, Exchange of Gases			
15. Nov. 2023	Wednesday	Nursing Foundations I	Ms Sabina Ali	Unit 1: Introduction to Health and Illness • Concept of Health • Concept of Health and Illness part 1, 2, 3	Unit 1: Introduction to Health and Illness • Recap • Maslow's Hierarchy • Health-Illness Continuum • Illness			

Contd...

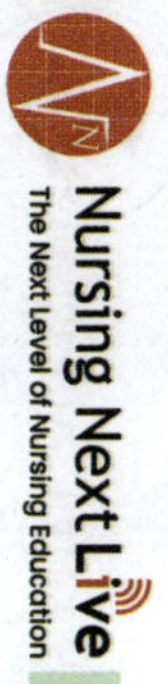

Date	Day	Subject	Faculty	Morning Session (HLT) (Recorded Video of MM Faculty) 6 am – 8 am	Evening Session (LIVE) (High Yield Topics/Missing Topics/ High Yield Subjective Q Discussion, Nursing implication) 6 pm – 8 pm	Tests	Doubt Session/ Progress Analysis	Assignments (Phygital & E-workbook + TH Decode) Golden Points + Solved Exercise (Self-study After Class)
16. Nov. 2023	Thursday	Nursing Foundations I	Ms Sabina Ali	Unit 1: Introduction to Health and Illness • Concept of Health and Illness part 3 • Illness-wellness Continuum • Level of Prevention	Unit 1: Introduction to Health and Illness • Factors Influencing Health Causes and Risk Factors for Developing Illnesses • Illness – Types, Illness Behavior Impact of Illness on Patient and Family			
17. Nov. 2023	Friday	Applied Psychology	Ms Chetana	**Unit 3:** Mental Health and Mental Hygiene • **Mental Health and Mental Hygiene Part 1-2**	Unit 2: Biological Basis of Behavior –Introduction • **Body Mind Relationship** • Applied Psychology and Sensation – Sensory Process – Normal and Abnormal			
18. Nov. 2023	**Saturday**	Applied Psychology	Ms Chetana	Unit 4: Developmental psychology • Developmental Applied Psychology	Discussion on E-workbook/ Assignment		Progress Analysis/ Doubt/E-workbook Discussion	
19. Nov. 2023	**Sunday**	Surprise Class	Dr Shrikant Verma	• SPL Class Nursing Procedure • 2-4 procedures per session	Surprise Class Live	Week Test 3 (MCQ)		E-workbook for the nextweek
20. Nov. 2023	Monday	Applied Anatomy & Physiology	Dr Shrikant Verma	**Unit 2: Respiratory system (Anatomy)** • Regulation of Respiration • Lung Volumes and Capacities	**Unit 2: Respiratory system (Anatomy)** • Carriage of Oxygen and Carbon-dioxide, Exchange of Gases in Tissue • Hypoxia, Cyanosis, Dyspnea, Periodic Breathing • Respiratory Changes During Exercise • Application and Implication in Nursing			

Contd...

Date	Day	Subject	Faculty	Morning Session (HLT) (Recorded Video of MM Faculty) 6 am – 8 am	Evening Session (LIVE) (High Yield Topics/Missing Topics/ High Yield Subjective Q Discussion, Nursing implication) 6 pm – 8 pm	Tests	Doubt Session/ Progress Analysis	Assignments (Phygital & E-workbook + TH Decode) Golden Points + Solved Exercise (Self-study After Class)
21. Nov. 2023	Tuesday	Applied Anatomy & Physiology	Dr Shrikant Verma	Unit 3: Digestive system • Introduction, Oral Cavity, Salivary Glands • Esophagus • Stomach	Unit 3: Digestive system • Composition and Function of Gastric Juice, Mechanism and regulation of Gastric Secretion • Composition of Pancreatic Juice, Function, Regulation of Pancreatic Secretion			
22. Nov. 2023	Wednesday	Nursing Foundations I	Ms Sabina Ali	Unit 3: History of Nursing and Nursing as a Profession • Values – Introduction – meaning and Importance • Code of Ethics and professional Conduct for Nurses – Introduction (Need to be Recorded)	Unit 3: History of Nursing and Nursing as a profession • Nursing – Definition – Nurse, Nursing, Concepts, Philosophy, Objectives, Characteristics, Nature and Scope of Nursing/ Nursing practice, Functions of Nurse, Qualities of a nurse, Categories of Nursing Personnel			
23. Nov. 2023	Thursday	Nursing Foundations I	Ms Sabina Ali	Unit 3: History of Nursing and Nursing as a Profession • Values – Introduction – Meaning and Importance • Code of Ethics and Professional Conduct for Nurses – Introduction (Need to be Recorded)	Unit 3: History of Nursing and Nursing as a profession • Nursing – Definition – Nurse, Nursing, Concepts, Philosophy, Objectives, Characteristics, Nature and Scope of Nursing/ Nursing Practice, Functions of Nurse, Qualities of a Nurse, Categories of Nursing Personnel			
24. Nov. 2023	Friday	Applied Psychology	Ms Chetana	Unit 4: Developmental psychology • Developmental psychology	Unit 3: Mental Health and Mental Hygiene • Promotive and Preventive Mental Health Strategies and Services • Defence Mechanism and its Implication			

Contd...

Date	Day	Subject	Faculty	Morning Session (HLT) (Recorded Video of MM Faculty) 6 am – 8 am	Evening Session (LIVE) (High Yield Topics/Missing Topics/ High Yield Subjective Q Discussion, Nursing implication) 6 pm – 8 pm	Tests	Doubt Session/ Progress Analysis	Assignments (Phygital & E-workbook + TH Decode) Golden Points + Solved Exercise (Self-study After Class)
25. Nov. 2023	Saturday	Applied Psychology	Ms Chetana	Unit: Personality Personality Part 1- 2	High Yield QD Nursing Foundations I			
26. Nov. 2023	Sunday	Surprise Class	Dr Shriknat	SPL Class Nursing Procedure 2–4 procedures per session	Surprise Class Live	Week Test 4 (MCQ) Unit Test-2 (Subjective)		E-workbook for the Next Week
27. Nov. 2023	Monday	Applied Anatomy & Physiology	Dr Shrikant Verma	Unit 3: Digestive System Small and Large Intestine Tongue, Teeth Palate and Swallowing	Unit 3: Digestive System • Functions of Liver, Gall Bladder and pancreas • Composition of Bile and Function			
28. Nov. 2023	Tuesday	Applied Anatomy & Physiology	Dr Shrikant Verma	Unit 4: The Circulatory and Lymphatic System • Pericardium and Heart • Blood Supply of Heart	Unit 3: Digestive System • Movements of Alimentary Tract • Digestion in Mouth, Stomach, Small Intestine, Large Intestine, Absorption of Food • Application and Implications in Nursing			
29. Nov. 2023	Wednesday	Nursing Foundations I	Ms Sabina Ali	Unit 4: Communication and Nurse Patient Relationship Part 1-3	Unit 3: History of Nursing and Nursing as a Profession Nursing – Definition – Nurse, Nursing, Concepts, Philosophy, Objectives, Characteristics, Nature and Scope of Nursing/ Nursing Practice, Functions of Nurse, Qualities of a Nurse, Categories of Nursing Personnel			
30. Nov. 2023	Thursday	Nursing Foundations I	Ms Sabina Ali	Unit 4: Communication and Nurse Patient Relationship Part 4-6	Unit 4: Communication and Nurse Patient Relationship • Factors Influencing • Barriers • Effective Communication with Patient, Family • Helping Relationships	Revision Test-1 (Based on Complete Month Teaching)	Progress Analysis/ Doubt/E-workbook Discussion	

Contd...

Date	Day	Subject	Faculty	Morning Session (HLT) (Recorded Video of MM Faculty) 6 am – 8 am	Evening Session (LIVE) (High Yield Topics/Missing Topics/ High Yield Subjective Q Discussion, Nursing implication) 6 pm – 8 pm	Tests	Doubt Session/ Progress Analysis	Assignments (Phygital & E-workbook + TH Decode) Golden Points + Solved Exercise (Self-study After Class)
1. Dec. 2023	Friday	Applied Psychology	Ms Chetana	**Unit 3:** Mental Health and Mental Hygiene • Promotive and Preventive Mental Health Strategies and Services Defense Mechanism and Its Implication (Repetition of This Lecture)	**Unit 3:** Mental Health and Mental Hygiene Frustration and Conflict Role of Nurse in Reducing Frustration and Conflict and Enhancing Coping • Dealing with EGO			
2. Dec. 2023	Saturday	Applied Psychology	Ms Chetana	**Unit 3:** Mental Health and Mental Hygiene Repetition of Eve. Lecture	Discussion on E-workbook/ Assignment			
3. Dec. 2023	**Sunday**			Special Sundays	Surprise Class			
4. Dec. 2023	Monday	Applied Anatomy & Physiology	Dr Shrikant Verma	Unit 4: The Circulatory and Lymphatic System • Blood Pressure and Pulse • ECG	Unit 4: The Circulatory and Lymphatic System • Functions of Heart, Conduction System, Cardiac Cycle, Stroke Volume and Cardiac Output			
5. Dec. 2023	Tuesday	Applied Anatomy & Physiology	Dr Shrikant Verma	• Unit 4: The Circulatory and Lymphatic System • Thoracic Cage • Branches of Aorta • RBCS	Unit 4: The Circulatory and Lymphatic System • Circulation – Principles, Factors Influencing Blood Pressure, Pulse			
6. Dec. 2023	Wednesday	Nursing Foundations I	Ms Sabina Ali	Unit 4: Communication and Nurse Patient Relationship Part 7-8	Unit 4: Communication and Nurse Patient Relationship Communicating Effectively with Patient, Families and Team Members Maintaining Effective Human Relations and Communication with Vulnerable Groups			

Contd...

Date	Day	Subject	Faculty	Morning Session (HLT) (Recorded Video of MM Faculty) 6 am – 8 am	Evening Session (LIVE) (High Yield Topics/Missing Topics/ High Yield Subjective Q Discussion, Nursing implication) 6 pm – 8 pm	Tests	Doubt Session/ Progress Analysis	Assignments (Phygital & E-workbook + TH Decode) Golden Points + Solved Exercise (Self-study After Class)
7. Dec. 2023	Thursday	Nursing Foundations I	Ms Sabina Ali	Unit 5: Documentation and Reporting Part 1-2	Unit 5: Documentation and Reporting Confidentiality Guidelines For Documentation			
8. Dec. 2023	Friday	Applied Sociology	Ms Priyanka Randhir	Unit 1: Introduction Definition, Nature and Scope of Applied Sociology Significance of Applied Sociology in Nursing	Unit 1: Introduction • Introduction of Subject • Revision of Morning Class			
9. Dec. 2023	Saturday	Applied Sociology	Ms Priyanka Randhir	Unit 2: Social Structure Part 1-3	High Yield QD			
10. Dec. 2023	**Sunday**	Surprise Class	Dr Shrikant Verma	Unit 2: Social Structure Part 4-6	Special Class on ECG by Dr Shrikant Verma			
11. Dec. 2023	Monday	Applied Anatomy & Physiology	Dr Shrikant Verma	Unit 4: The Circulatory and Lymphatic System • Hemoglobin • Hematopoiesis and Erythropoiesis	Unit 4: The Circulatory and Lymphatic System Coronary Circulation, Pulmonary and Systemic Circulation			
12. Dec. 2023	Tuesday	Applied Anatomy & Physiology	Dr Shrikant Verma	Unit 4: The Circulatory and Lymphatic System • Blood Groups • Blood Disorders	Unit 4: The Circulatory and Lymphatic System Coronary Circulation, Pulmonary and Systemic Circulation (Cont.)			
13. Dec. 2023	Wednesday	Nursing Foundations I	Ms Sabina Ali	Unit 5: Documentation and Reporting Part 3-6	Unit 5: Documentation and Reporting • Do's and Don'ts			
14. Dec. 2023	Thursday	Nursing Foundations I	Ms Sabina Ali	Unit 6: Vital Signs Part 1-2	Unit 6: Vital Signs Temperature Pulse			
15. Dec. 2023	Friday	Applied Sociology	Ms Priyanka Randhir	Unit 2: Social Structure Part 7-8	Unit 2: Social Structure Socialization Social Change			

Contd...

Date	Day	Subject	Faculty	Morning Session (HLT) (Recorded Video of MM Faculty) 6 am – 8 am	Evening Session (LIVE) (High Yield Topics/Missing Topics/ High Yield Subjective Q Discussion, Nursing implication) 6 pm – 8 pm	Tests	Doubt Session/ Progress Analysis	Assignments (Phygital & E-workbook + TH Decode) Golden Points + Solved Exercise (Self-study After Class)
16. Dec. 2023	Saturday	Applied Sociology	Ms Priyanka Randhir	Unit 2: Social Structure Part 9-10	Discussion on E-workbook/ Assignment			
17. Dec. 2023	**Sunday**	Surprise Class	Dr Shrikant Verma	Surprise Class				
18. Dec. 2023	Monday	Applied Anatomy & Physiology	Dr Shrikant Verma	Unit 4: The Circulatory and Lymphatic System • Anemia • Wbcs and Leucopoiesis • Arterial Supply	Unit 5: Blood (Physiology) • Blood – Functions, Physical Characteristics • Formation of Blood Cells			
19. Dec. 2023	Tuesday	Applied Anatomy & Physiology	Dr Shrikant Verma	Unit 4: The Circulatory and Lymphatic System • Anemia • Wbcs and Leucopoiesis • Arterial Supply (Cont.)	Unit 5: Blood (Physiology) • Platelets – Function and Production of Platelets • Clotting Mechanism of Blood, Clotting Time, Bleeding Time, PTT			
20. Dec. 2023	Wednesday	Nursing Foundations I	Ms Sabina Ali	Unit 6: Vital Signs Part 3-4 Hot and Cold App. Part 1	Unit 6: Vital Signs BP			
21. Dec. 2023	Thursday	Nursing Foundations I	Ms Sabina Ali	Unit 6: Vital Signs Heat and Cold Part 3-5	Unit 6: Vital Signs Respiration			
22. Dec. 2023	Friday	Applied Sociology	Ms Priyanka Randhir	Unit 3: Culture Part 1-3	Unit 2: Social Structure Structure and Characteristics of Urban, Rural and Tribal Community. Major Health Problems in Urban, Rural and Tribal Communities			
23. Dec. 2023	Saturday	Applied Sociology	Ms Priyanka Randhir	Unit 3: Culture Part 4-5	High Yield QD			
24. Dec. 2023	**Sunday**	Surprise Class	Dr Shriknat	NP 2-3/ Special Sunday	Surprise Class			

Contd...

Date	Day	Subject	Faculty	Morning Session (HLT) (Recorded Video of MM Faculty) 6 am – 8 am	Evening Session (LIVE) (High Yield Topics/Missing Topics/ High Yield Subjective Q Discussion, Nursing implication) 6 pm – 8 pm	Tests	Doubt Session/ Progress Analysis	Assignments (Phygital & E-workbook + TH Decode) Golden Points + Solved Exercise (Self-study After Class)
25. Dec. 2023	Monday	Applied Anatomy & Physiology	Dr Shrikant Verma	Unit 5: Endocrine System • Structure of Hypothalamus	Unit 5: Endocrine System Anatomy and Physiology of Pineal Gland, Pituitary Gland, Thyroid			
26. Dec. 2023	Tuesday	Applied Anatomy & Physiology	Dr Shrikant Verma	Repetetion of Important Lecture	Unit 5: Endocrine System Anatomy and Physiology of Parathyroid, Thymus, Pancreas and Adrenal Glands			
27. Dec. 2023	Wednesday	Nursing Foundations I	Ms Sabina Ali	Unit 7: Equipment and Linen Part 1	Unit 7: Equipment and Linen Linen, Rubber Goods, Glassware, Metal, Plastics, Furniture			
28. Dec. 2023	Thursday	Nursing Foundations I	Ms Sabina Ali	Unit 7: Equipment and Linen Part 2	Unit 7: Equipment and Linen Introduction – Indent, Maintenance, Inventory			
29. Dec. 2023	Friday	Applied Sociology	Ms Priyanka Randhir	Unit 4: Family and Marriage Part 1-3	Unit 3: Culture • Difference Between Culture and Civilization • Culture and Socialization			
30. Dec. 2023	Saturday	Applied Sociology	Ms Priyanka Randhir	Unit 4: Family and Marriage Part 4-5	High Yield QD			
31. Dec. 2023	**Sunday**			Special Sundays/NP 2-3	Surprise Class			
1. Jan. 2024	Monday	Applied Anatomy & Physiology	Dr Shrikant Verma	Unit 6: The Sensory Organs • Tongue • Taste • Smell • Eye	Unit 6: The Sensory Organs Structure and Function			
2. Jan. 2024	Tuesday	Applied Anatomy & Physiology	Dr Shrikant Verma	Unit 6: The Sensory Organs Vision Ear	Unit 6: The Sensory Organs Structure and Function (Cont.)			

Contd...

Date	Day	Subject	Faculty	Morning Session (HLT) (Recorded Video of MM Faculty) 6 am – 8 am	Evening Session (LIVE) (High Yield Topics/Missing Topics/ High Yield Subjective Q Discussion, Nursing implication) 6 pm – 8 pm	Tests	Doubt Session/ Progress Analysis	Assignments (Phygital & E-workbook + TH Decode) Golden Points + Solved Exercise (Self-study After Class)
3. Jan. 2024	Wednesday	Nursing Foundations I	Ms Sabina Ali	Unit 8: Introduction to Infection Control in Clinical Setting Infection Part 1-2	Unit 8: Introduction to Infection Control in Clinical Setting Infection Medical & Surgical Asepsis Hand Hygiene			
4. Jan. 2024	Thursday	Nursing Foundations I	Ms Sabina Ali	Unit 8: Introduction to Infection Control in Clinical Setting Infection Hand Hygiene Part 1- 3	Unit 8: Introduction to Infection Control in Clinical Setting Infection BMW			
5. Jan. 2024	Friday	Applied Psychology	Ms Chetana	Unit 4: Developmental Applied Psychology Review	Unit 4: Developmental Applied Psychology Review			
6. Jan. 2024	Saturday	Applied Psychology	Ms Chetana	Unit 5: Personality	Discussion on E-workbook/ Assignment			
7. Jan. 2024	Sunday			Special Sundays/NP 2–3	Surprise Class			
8. Jan. 2024	Monday	Applied Anatomy & Physiology	Dr Shrikant Verma	Unit 7: The Musculoskeletal System • Classification of Muscle • Bones and Classifications • Joints	Unit 7: The Musculoskeletal System • Functions of Bones • Joints • Properties and Functions of Skeletal Muscles – Mechanism of Muscle Contraction			
9. Jan. 2024	Tuesday	Applied Anatomy & Physiology	Dr Shrikant Verma	Unit 7: The Musculoskeletal System Classification of Muscle Bones and Classifications Joints	Unit 7: The Musculoskeletal System Structure and Properties of Cardiac Muscles and Smooth Muscles			
10. Jan. 2024	Wednesday	Nursing Foundations I	Ms Sabina Ali	Unit 9: Comfort, Rest & Sleep and Pain Bed Making Part 1-3	Unit 9: Comfort, Rest & Sleep and Pain Comfort			

Contd...

Date	Day	Subject	Faculty	Morning Session (HLT) (Recorded Video of MM Faculty) 6 am – 8 am	Evening Session (LIVE) (High Yield Topics/Missing Topics/ High Yield Subjective Q Discussion, Nursing implication) 6 pm – 8 pm	Tests	Doubt Session/ Progress Analysis	Assignments (Phygital & E-workbook + TH Decode) Golden Points + Solved Exercise (Self-study After Class)
11. Jan. 2024	Thursday	Nursing Foundations I	Ms Sabina Ali	Unit 9: Comfort, Rest & Sleep and Pain Pain Part 1-3	Unit 9: Comfort, Rest & Sleep and Pain Sleep and Rest			
12. Jan. 2024	Friday	Applied Psychology	Ms Chetana	Unit 5: Personality	Unit 5: Personality Meaning Classification			
13. Jan. 2024	Saturday	Applied Psychology	Ms Chetana	Unit 5: Cognitive Processes	High Yield QD			
14. Jan. 2024	Sunday			Special Sundays/NP 2–3	Surprise Class			
15. Jan. 2024	Monday	Applied Anatomy & Physiology	Dr Shrikant Verma	Unit 9: Renal System Introduction and Kidney Anatomy Nephron	Unit 9: Renal System • Functions • GFR • Mechanism			
16. Jan. 2024	Tuesday	Applied Anatomy & Physiology	Dr Shrikant Verma	Unit 10: The Reproductive System Male External Genitalia Anatomy	Unit 10: The Reproductive System Functions of Male and Female Reproductive System			
17. Jan. 2024	Wednesday	Nursing Foundations I	Ms Sabina Ali	Unit 9: Comfort, Rest & Sleep and Pain Pain Part 4-5	Unit 9: Comfort, Rest & Sleep and Pain Pain			
18. Jan. 2024	Thursday	Nursing Foundations I	Ms Sabina Ali	Unit 10: Promoting Safety in Health Care Environment Fall Risk Prevention Part 1-3	Unit 10: Promoting Safety in Health Care Environment Reduction of Physical Hazards – Fire, Accidents			
19. Jan. 2024	Friday	Applied Psychology	Ms Chetana	Unit 6: Cognitive Processes	Unit 6: Cognitive Processes Attention, Perception, Intelligence			
20. Jan. 2024	Saturday	Applied Psychology	Ms Chetana	Unit 6: Cognitive Processes	Discussion on E-workbook/ Assignment			

Contd...

Date	Day	Subject	Faculty	Morning Session (HLT) (Recorded Video of MM Faculty) 6 am – 8 am	Evening Session (LIVE) (High Yield Topics/Missing Topics/ High Yield Subjective Q Discussion, Nursing implication) 6 pm – 8 pm	Tests	Doubt Session/ Progress Analysis	Assignments (Phygital & E-workbook + TH Decode) Golden Points + Solved Exercise (Self-study After Class)
21. Jan. 2024	Sunday			Special Sundays/NP 2-3	Surprise Class			
22. Jan. 2024	Monday	Applied Anatomy & Physiology	Dr Shrikant Verma	Unit 10: The Reproductive System Menstrual Cycle	Unit 10: The Reproductive System Functions of Male and Female Reproductive System			
23. Jan. 2024	Tuesday	Applied Anatomy & Physiology	Dr Shrikant Verma	Unit 11: Nervous System Introduction Meninges	Unit 11: Nervous System Structure and Function Nerve Impulse			
24. Jan. 2024	Wednesday	Nursing Foundations I	Ms Sabina Ali	Unit 10: Promoting Safety in Health Care Environment Restraints Crutch Walking	Unit 10: Promoting Safety in Health Care Environment Safety Devices			
25. Jan. 2024	Thursday	Nursing Foundations I	Ms Sabina Ali	Unit 11: Hospital Admission and Discharge Part 1-3	Unit 11: Hospital Admission and Discharge Admission			
26. Jan. 2024	Friday	Applied Psychology	Ms Chetana	Unit 7: Motivation and Emotion	Unit 7: Motivation and Emotion Stress Adaptation			
27. Jan. 2024	Saturday	Applied Psychology	Ms Chetana	Unit 8: Psychological Assessment	Unit 8: Psychological Assessment Types, Clasifictaions			
28. Jan. 2024	Sunday			Special Sundays/NP 2-3	Surprise Class			
29. Jan. 2024	Monday	Applied Anatomy & Physiology	Dr Shrikant Verma	Unit 11: Nervous System Tracts Part 1-2 Cerebellum Hypothalamus	Unit 11: Nervous System PNS, Ans Limbic System Cranial Nerves			
30. Jan. 2024	Tuesday	Applied Anatomy & Physiology	Dr Shrikant Verma	Unit 11: Nervous System Parts of Brain, Bbb Blood Sypply to Brain	Unit 11: Nervous System Autonomic Functions Reflexes CSF			

Contd...

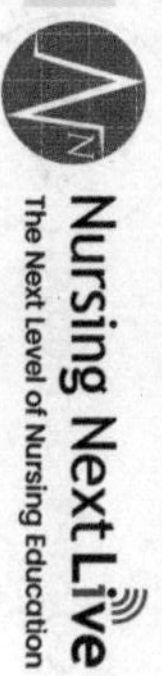

Date	Day	Subject	Faculty	Morning Session (HLT) (Recorded Video of MM Faculty) 6 am – 8 am	Evening Session (LIVE) (High Yield Topics/Missing Topics/ High Yield Subjective Q Discussion, Nursing implication) 6 pm – 8 pm	Tests	Doubt Session/ Progress Analysis	Assignments (Phygital & E-workbook + TH Decode) Golden Points + Solved Exercise (Self-study After Class)
31. Jan. 2024	Wednesday	Nursing Foundations I	Ms Sabina Ali	Unit 11: Hospital Admission and Discharge Repetition of Previous Lecture	Unit 11: Hospital Admission and Discharge • Discharge			
1. Feb. 2024	Thursday	Nursing Foundations I	Ms Sabina Ali	Unit 13: Patient Education Part 1–2	Unit 12: Mobility and Immobility • Normal Movement, Alignment • Principles of Body Mechanics • Alteration in Body Alignment and Mobility			
2. Feb. 2024	Friday	Applied Psychology	Ms Chetana	Unit 9: Soft Skill	Unit 9: Soft Skill			
3. Feb. 2024	Saturday	Applied Psychology	Ms Chetana	Unit 10: Self-Empowerment	Unit 10: Self-Empowerment			
4. Feb. 2024	Sunday			Special Sundays/NP 2-3	Surprise Class			
5. Feb. 2024	Monday	Applied Anatomy & Physiology	Dr Shrikant Verma	Unit 1: Revision	Unit 1: Revision			
6. Feb. 2024	Tuesday	Applied Anatomy & Physiology	Dr Shrikant Verma	Unit 1: Revision	Unit 1: Revision			
7. Feb. 2024	Wednesday	Nursing Foundations I	Ms Sabina Ali	Unit 14: First Aid Part 1-3	Unit 12: Mobility and Immobility Nursing Interventions For Impaired Body Alignment and Mobility – Assessment, Types, Devices Used, Method			
8. Feb. 2024	Thursday	Nursing Foundations I	Ms Sabina Ali	Unit 14: First Aid Part CPR 1-2	First Aid: Module • First Aid • Introduction • General Principles			
9. Feb. 2024	Friday	Applied Sociology	Ms Priyanka Randhir	Unit 5: Social Stratification	Unit 5: Social Stratification			

Contd...

Date	Day	Subject	Faculty	Morning Session (HLT) (Recorded Video of MM Faculty) 6 am – 8 am	Evening Session (LIVE) (High Yield Topics/Missing Topics/ High Yield Subjective Q Discussion, Nursing implication) 6 pm – 8 pm	Tests	Doubt Session/ Progress Analysis	Assignments (Phygital & E-workbook + TH Decode) Golden Points + Solved Exercise (Self-study After Class)
10. Feb. 2024	Saturday	Applied Sociology	Ms Priyanka Randhir	Unit 5: Social Stratification	High Yield QD			
11. Feb. 2024	Sunday			Special Sundays/NP 2-3	Surprise Class			
12. Feb. 2024	Monday	Applied Anatomy & Physiology	Dr Shrikant Verma	Unit 2: Revision	Unit 2: Revision			
13. Feb. 2024	Tuesday	Applied Anatomy & Physiology	Dr Shrikant Verma	Unit 2: Revision	Unit 2: Revision			
14. Feb. 2024	Wednesday	Nursing Foundations I	Ms Sabina Ali	Unit 14: First Aid	Ii. First Aid Techniques			
15. Feb. 2024	Thursday	Nursing Foundations I	Ms Sabina Ali	Unit 14: First Aid	Iii. First Aid Management of Common Emergencies			
16. Feb. 2024	Friday	Applied Sociology	Ms Priyanka Randhir	Unit 6: Social Organization and Disorganization	Unit 6: Social Organization and Disorganization			
17. Feb. 2024	Saturday	Applied Sociology	Ms Priyanka Randhir	Unit 6: Social Organization and Disorganization	Discussion on E-workbook/ Assignment			
18. Feb. 2024	Sunday			Special Sundays/NP 2-3	Surprise Class			
19. Feb. 2024	Monday	Applied Anatomy & Physiology	Dr Shrikant Verma	Unit 3: Revision	Unit 3: Revision			
20. Feb. 2024	Tuesday	Applied Anatomy & Physiology	Dr Shrikant Verma	Unit 3: Revision	Unit 3: Revision			
21. Feb. 2024	Wednesday	Applied Sociology		Unit 7: Clinical Applied Sociology	Unit 7: Clinical Applied Sociology			
22. Feb. 2024	Thursday	Nursing Foundations I	Ms Sabina Ali	Unit 14: First Aid	Iii. First Aid Management of Common Emergencies			

Contd...

Date	Day	Subject	Faculty	Morning Session (HLT) (Recorded Video of MM Faculty) 6 am – 8 am	Evening Session (LIVE) (High Yield Topics/Missing Topics/ High Yield Subjective Q Discussion, Nursing implication) 6 pm – 8 pm	Tests	Doubt Session/ Progress Analysis	Assignments (Phygital & E-workbook + TH Decode) Golden Points + Solved Exercise (Self-study After Class)
23. Feb. 2024	Friday	Nursing Foundations I	Ms Sabina Ali	Unit 14: First Aid	Iv. Selected First Aid Techniques V. First Aid Kit			
24. Feb. 2024	Saturday	Nursing Foundations I	Ms Sabina Ali	Unit 14: First Aid	High Yield QD			
25. Feb. 2024	Sunday				Surprise Class			
26. Feb. 2024	Monday	Applied Anatomy & Physiology	Dr Shrikant Verma	Unit 4: Revision	Unit 4: Revision			
27. Feb. 2024	Tuesday	Applied Anatomy & Physiology	Dr Shrikant Verma	Unit 5: Revision	Unit 5: Revision			
28. Feb. 2024	Wednesday	Applied Anatomy & Physiology	Dr Shrikant Verma	Unit 6: Revision	Unit 6: Revision			
29. Feb. 2024	Thursday	Nursing Foundations I						
1. March 2024	Friday	Applied Psychology	Ms Chetana		Decode Revision Session 1 with PQD	Model Test Applied Psychology Set-1		
2. March 2024	Saturday	Applied Psychology	Ms Chetana		Doubt Session	Model Test Applied Psychology Set-2		
3. March 2024	Sunday				Surprise Class			
5. March 2024	Tuesday	Applied Psychology	Ms Chetana		Decode Revision Session 3 with PQD	Model Test Applied Psychology Set-3		

Contd...

Date	Day	Subject	Faculty	Morning Session (HLT) (Recorded Video of MM Faculty) 6 am – 8 am	Evening Session (LIVE) (High Yield Topics/Missing Topics/ High Yield Subjective Q Discussion, Nursing implication) 6 pm – 8 pm	Tests	Doubt Session/ Progress Analysis	Assignments (Phygital & E-workbook + TH Decode) Golden Points + Solved Exercise (Self-study After Class)
6. March 2024	Wednesday	Applied Anatomy & Physiology	Dr Shrikant Verma/ Deepshikha		Decode Revision Session 3 with PQD	Model Test Applied Anatomy & Physiology Set-1		
9. March 2024	Saturday	Applied Anatomy & Physiology	Dr Shrikant Verma/ Deepshikha		Decode Revision Session 3 with PQD	Model Test Applied Anatomy & Physiology Set-2		
11. March 2024	Monday	Applied Anatomy & Physiology	Dr Shrikant Verma/ Deepshikha		Decode Revision Session 3 with PQD	Model Test Applied Anatomy & Physiology Set-3		
12. March 2024	Tuesday	Applied Anatomy & Physiology	Dr Shrikant Verma/ Deepshikha		Decode Revision Session 3 with PQD	Model Test Applied Anatomy & Physiology Set-4		
13. March 2024	Wednesday	Applied Anatomy & Physiology	Dr Shrikant Verma/ Deepshikha		Doubt Session	Model Test Applied Anatomy & Physiology Set-5		
14. March 2024	Thursday					Surprise Class		
18. March 2024	Monday	Applied Sociology	Ms Priyanka Randhir		Decode Revision Session 1 with PQD	Model Test Socio. Set-1		

Contd...

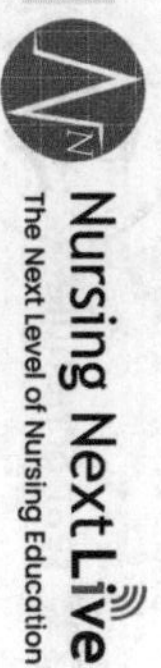

Date	Day	Subject	Faculty	Morning Session (HLT) (Recorded Video of MM Faculty) 6 am – 8 am	Evening Session (LIVE) (High Yield Topics/Missing Topics/ High Yield Subjective Q Discussion, Nursing implication) 6 pm – 8 pm	Tests	Doubt Session/ Progress Analysis	Assignments (Phygital & E-workbook + TH Decode) Golden Points + Solved Exercise (Self-study After Class)
19. March 2024	Tuesday	Applied Sociology	Ms Priyanka Randhir		Decode Revision Session 2 with Pqd	Model Test Socio. Set-2		
20. March 2024	Wednesday	Applied Sociology	Ms Priyanka Randhir		Decode Revision Session 1 with PQD	Model Test Socio. Set-3		
21. March 2024	Thursday	Nursing Foundations I	Ms Sabina Ali		Decode Revision Session 1 with PQD	Model Test Nursing Foundations I Set-1		
22. March 2024	Friday	Nursing Foundations I	Ms Sabina Ali		Decode Revision Session 1 with PQD	Model Test Nursing Foundations I Set-2		
25. March 2024	Monday	Nursing Foundations I	Ms Sabina Ali		Doubt Session	Model Test Nursing Foundations I Set-3		
27. March 2024	Wednesday	Nursing Foundations I	Ms Sabina Ali		Decode Revision Session 1 with PQD	Model Test Nursing Foundations I Set-4		
28. March 2024	Thursday	Nursing Foundations I	Ms Sabina Ali		Decode Revision Session 1 with PQD	Model Test Nursing Foundations I Set-5		
29. March 2024	Friday	Nursing Foundations I	Ms Sabina Ali		Decode Revision Session 1 with PQD	Model Test Nursing Foundations I Set-6		

Contd...

Date	Day	Subject	Faculty	Morning Session (HLT) (Recorded Video of MM Faculty) 6 am – 8 am	Evening Session (LIVE) (High Yield Topics/Missing Topics/ High Yield Subjective Q Discussion, Nursing implication) 6 pm – 8 pm	Tests	Doubt Session/ Progress Analysis	Assignments (Phygital & E-workbook + TH Decode) Golden Points + Solved Exercise (Self-study After Class)
30. March 2024	Saturday	Nursing Foundations I	Ms Sabina Ali		Decode Revision Session 1 with PQD	Model Test Nursing Foundations I Set-7		
31. March 2024	Sunday	Nursing Foundations I	Ms Sabina Ali		Decode Revision Session 1 with PQD	Model Test Nursing Foundations I Set-8		
1. April 2024	Monday	Nursing Foundations I	Ms Sabina Ali		Doubt Session	Model Test Nursing Foundations I Set 9		
3. April 2024	Wednesday	Nursing Foundations I	Ms Sabina Ali		Practical Prep Session			
4. April 2024	Thursday	Nursing Foundations I	Ms Sabina Ali		Practical Prep Session			
5. April 2024	Friday	Nursing Foundations I	Ms Sabina Ali		Practical Prep Session			
6. April 2024	Saturday	Nursing Foundations I	Ms Sabina Ali		Practical Prep Session			
8. April 2024	Monday	Nursing Foundations I	Ms Sabina Ali		Practical Prep Session			
9. April 2024	Tuesday	Nursing Foundations I	Ms Sabina Ali		Practical Prep Session			

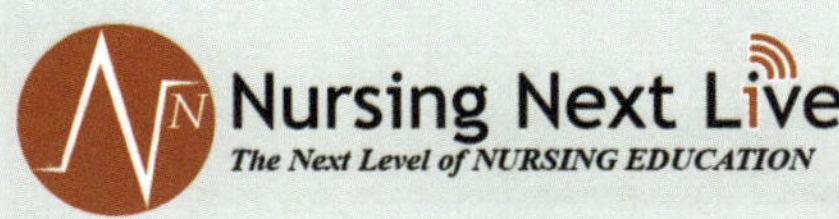

SEMESTER

II

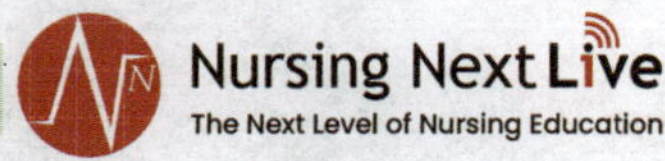

CONCEPTUAL LECTURES

TABLE 1: All Subjects Imp Topics Covering 30% of the content from Semester II

S.No.	Subject	Days	Faculty	Live Classes	Duration
1.	Applied Biochemistry & Applied Nutrition & Dietetics	Monday & Tuesday	Dr Neha Sethi	35	50+ Hours
2.	Fundamentals of Nursing	Friday & Saturday	Ms Sabina Ali	50	60+ Hours
	Total			**85**	**110+ Hours**

TABLE 2: All Subjects Imp Topics Covering 70% of the content from Semester II

S.No.	Subject	Days	Faculty	Live Classes	Duration
1.	Applied Biochemistry & Applied Nutrition & Dietetics	Monday & Tuesday	Dr Shrikant Verma	40	50 hours
2.	Nursing of Foundations	Friday & Saturday	Ms Sabina Ali	50	60 hours
	Total			**90**	**110 hours**

TABLE 3: Progress Analysis + Student Faculty Meet (Semester II)

S. No	Date	Progress Evaluation Class	Batch Mentor	Duration (Hours)	Topic/ Agenda
1.	16 May 2024	Class 1	Ms Chetana/Session Mentor	1–2	Discussion on e-workbook, assignment, tests/Progress review/ NP/Surprise class
2.	01 June 2024	Class 2	Ms Chetana/ Session Mentor	1–2	Discussion on e-workbook, assignment, tests/Progress review/ NP/Surprise class
3.	22 June 2024	Class 3	Ms Chetana/Session Mentor	1–2	Discussion on e-workbook, assignment, tests/Progress review/ NP/Surprise class
4.	06 July 2024	Class 4	Ms Chetana/Session Mentor	1–2	Discussion on e-workbook, assignment, tests/Progress review/ NP/Surprise class
5.	20 July 2024	Class 5	Ms Chetana/Session Mentor	1–2	Discussion on e-workbook, assignment, tests/Progress review/ NP/Surprise class
6.	10 August 2024	Class 6	Ms Chetana/Session Mentor	1–2	Discussion on e-workbook, assignment, tests/Progress review/ NP/Surprise class
7.	24 August 2024	Class 7	Ms Chetana/Session Mentor	1–2	Discussion on e-workbook, assignment, tests/Progress review/ NP/Surprise class
	Total			**7–14**	

TABLE 4: Surprise Class

S. No	Date	Day	Faculty	Surprise Class	Durations
1.	05 November 2023	Sunday	Dr Shrikant Verma	Topic to be disclosed a day before the session	2 Hours
2.	12 November 2023	Sunday	Dr Shrikant Verma	Topic to be disclosed a day before the session	2 Hours
3.	19 November 2023	Sunday	Dr Shrikant Verma	Topic to be disclosed a day before the session	2 Hours
4.	26 November 2023	Sunday	Dr Shrikant Verma	Topic to be disclosed a day before the session	2 Hours
5.	10 December 2023	Sunday	Dr Shrikant Verma	Topic to be disclosed a day before the session	2 Hours
6.	17 December 2023	Sunday	Dr Shrikant Verma	Topic to be disclosed a day before the session	2 Hours
7.	24 December 2023	Sunday	Dr Shrikant Verma	Topic to be disclosed a day before the session	2 Hours
8.	31 December 2023	Sunday	Dr Shrikant Verma	Topic to be disclosed a day before the session	2 Hours
9.	07 January 2024	Sunday	Dr Shrikant Verma	Topic to be disclosed a day before the session	2 Hours
10.	14 January 2024	Sunday	Dr Shrikant Verma	Topic to be disclosed a day before the session	2 Hours
11.	21 January 2024	Sunday	Dr Shrikant Verma	Topic to be disclosed a day before the session	2 Hours
12.	28 January 2024	Sunday	Dr Shrikant Verma	Topic to be disclosed a day before the session	2 Hours
13.	04 February 2024	Sunday	Dr Shrikant Verma	Topic to be disclosed a day before the session	2 Hours
14.	11 February 2024	Sunday	Dr Shrikant Verma	Topic to be disclosed a day before the session	2 Hours
15.	18 February 2024	Sunday	Dr Shrikant Verma	Topic to be disclosed a day before the session	2 Hours
16.	25 February 2024	Sunday	Dr Shrikant Verma	Topic to be disclosed a day before the session	2 Hours
	Total				**32 Hours**

TABLE 5: Repeat Class

S. No	Date	Subjects	Topics Covered	Timing
1.	27 May 2024	Applied Biochemistry & Applied Nutrition & Dietetics	Repeat Session of the Topics Covered in May	9 am to 12 pm 2 pm to 6 pm
2.	28 May 2024	Applied Biochemistry & Applied Nutrition & Dietetics	Repeat Session of the Topics Covered in May	9 am to 12 pm 2 pm to 6 pm
3.	29 May 2024	Applied Biochemistry & Applied Nutrition & Dietetics	Repeat Session of the Topics Covered in May	9 am to 12 pm 2 pm to 6 pm
4.	30 May 2024	Fundamentals of Nursing	Repeat Session of the Topics Covered in May	9 am to 12 pm 2 pm to 6 pm
5.	31 May 2024	Fundamentals of Nursing	Repeat Session of the Topics Covered in May	9 am to 12 pm 2 pm to 6 pm
6.	01 June 2024	Fundamentals of Nursing	Repeat Session of the Topics Covered in May	9 am to 12 pm 2 pm to 6 pm
7.	24 June 2024	Applied Biochemistry & Applied Nutrition & Dietetics	Repeat Session of the Topics Covered in June	9 am to 12 pm 2 pm to 6 pm
8.	25 June 2024	Applied Biochemistry & Applied Nutrition & Dietetics	Repeat Session of the Topics Covered in June	9 am to 12 pm 2 pm to 6 pm
9.	26 June 2024	Applied Biochemistry & Applied Nutrition & Dietetics	Repeat Session of the Topics Covered in June	9 am to 12 pm 2 pm to 6 pm

Contd...

S. No	Date	Subjects	Topics Covered	Timing
10.	27 June 2024	Fundamentals of Nursing	Repeat Session of the Topics Covered in June	9 am to 12 pm 2 pm to 6 pm
11.	28 June 2024	Fundamentals of Nursing	Repeat Session of the Topics Covered in June	9 am to 12 pm 2 pm to 6 pm
12.	29 June 2024	Fundamentals of Nursing	Repeat Session of the Topics Covered in June	9 am to 12 pm 2 pm to 6 pm
13.	22 July 2024	Applied Biochemistry & Applied Nutrition & Dietetics	Repeat Session of the Topics Covered in July	9 am to 12 pm 2 pm to 6 pm
14.	23 July 2024	Applied Biochemistry & Applied Nutrition & Dietetics	Repeat Session of the Topics Covered in July	9 am to 12 pm 2 pm to 6 pm
15.	24 July 2024	Applied Biochemistry & Applied Nutrition & Dietetics	Repeat Session of the Topics Covered in July	9 am to 12 pm 2 pm to 6 pm
16.	25 July 2024	Fundamentals of Nursing	Repeat Session of the Topics Covered in July	9 am to 12 pm 2 pm to 6 pm
16.	26 July 2024	Fundamentals of Nursing	Repeat Session of the Topics Covered in July	9 am to 12 pm 2 pm to 6 pm
17.	27 July 2024	Fundamentals of Nursing	Repeat Session of the Topics Covered in July	9 am to 12 pm 2 pm to 6 pm
18.	02 September 2024	Fundamentals of Nursing	Repeat Session of the Topics Covered in July	9 am to 12 pm 2 pm to 6 pm
19.	03 September 2024	Fundamentals of Nursing	Repeat Session of the Topics Covered in July	9 am to 12 pm 2 pm to 6 pm
20.	04 September 2024	Fundamentals of Nursing	Repeat Session of the Topics Covered in July	9 am to 12 pm 2 pm to 6 pm
21.	05 September 2024	Fundamentals of Nursing	Repeat Session of the Topics Covered in July	9 am to 12 pm 2 pm to 6 pm

CONCEPTUAL REVISION

TABLE 6: Revision Through Target High Next Nursing Decode

S. No	Date	Days	Subjects	Faculty	Sessions	Paper
1.	16 September 2024	Monday	Applied Biochemistry & Applied Nutrition & Dietetics	Dr Neha Sethi	Decode Revision Session 1 with PQD	Model Test Applied Biochemistry & Applied Nutrition & Dietetics Set-1
2.	17 September 2024	Tuesday	Applied Biochemistry & Applied Nutrition & Dietetics	Dr Neha Sethi	Decode Revision Session 2 with PQD	
3.	18 September 2024	Wednesday	Applied Biochemistry & Applied Nutrition & Dietetics	Dr Neha Sethi	Decode Revision Session 3 with PQD	Model Test Applied Biochemistry & Applied Nutrition & Dietetics Set-2

Contd...

S. No	Date	Days	Subjects	Faculty	Sessions	Paper
4.	19 September 2024	Thursday	Applied Biochemistry & Applied Nutrition & Dietetics	Dr Neha Sethi	Decode Revision Session 4 with PQD	
5.	20 September 2024	Friday	Applied Biochemistry & Applied Nutrition & Dietetics	Dr Neha Sethi	Decode Revision Session 5 with PQD	Model Test Applied Biochemistry & Applied Nutrition & Dietetics Set-3
6.	21 September 2024	Saturday	Applied Biochemistry & Applied Nutrition & Dietetics	Dr Neha Sethi	Decode Revision Session 6 with PQD	
7.	22 September 2024	Sunday				
8.	23 September 2024	Monday	Nursing Foundations II	Ms Sabina Ali	Decode Revision Session 1 with PQD	Model Test Applied Biochemistry & Applied Nutrition & Dietetics Set-1
9.	24 September 2024	Tuesday	Nursing Foundations II	Ms Sabina Ali	Decode Revision Session 2 with PQD	Model Test Applied Biochemistry & Applied Nutrition & Dietetics Set-2
10.	25 September 2024	Wednesday	Nursing Foundations II	Ms Sabina Ali	Decode Revision Session 3 with PQD	Model Test Applied Biochemistry & Applied Nutrition & Dietetics Set-3
11.	26 September 2024	Thursday	Nursing Foundations II	Ms Sabina Ali	Decode Revision Session 4 with PQD	Model Test Applied Biochemistry & Applied Nutrition & Dietetics Set-4
12.	27 September 2024	Friday	Nursing Foundations II	Ms Sabina Ali	Decode Revision Session 1 with PQD	Model Test Applied Biochemistry & Applied Nutrition & Dietetics Set-5
13.	28 September 2024	Saturday	Nursing Foundations II	Ms Sabina Ali	Decode Revision Session 1 with PQD	Model Test Applied Biochemistry & Applied Nutrition & Dietetics Set-6

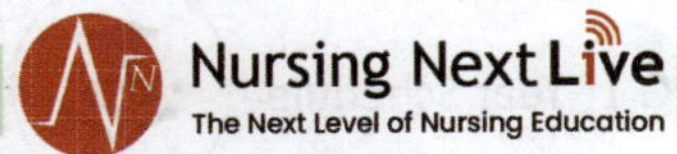

CONCEPTUAL PRACTICE

TABLE 7: Tests Summary

S. No	Test	Total No. of Tests	No. of Qs
1.	Weekly Test (Objective Type)	20	400
2.	Subject wise Unit Tests (Topic wise)	11	100
3.	Revision Tests After Completion of Batch (Based on University Pattern)	05	500
4.	Model Tests (Based on University Pattern)	05	60
5.	Previous Years' Papers (Unsolved University Papers)	30+	350
	Total	**71+**	**1410**

TABLE 8: Weekly Tests

S. No	Dates	Subjects	Tests	No. of Qs
1.	09 May 2024	Nursing Foundations II+ Applied Biochemistry & Applied Nutrition & Dietetics	Weekly Test-1	20
2.	16 May 2024	Nursing Foundations II+ Applied Biochemistry & Applied Nutrition & Dietetics	Weekly Test-2	20
3.	23 May 2024	Nursing Foundations II+ Applied Biochemistry & Applied Nutrition & Dietetics	Weekly Test-3	20
4.	01 June 2024	Nursing Foundations II+ Applied Biochemistry & Applied Nutrition & Dietetics	Weekly Test-4	20
5.	08 June 2024	Nursing Foundations II+ Applied Biochemistry & Applied Nutrition & Dietetics	Weekly Test-5	20
6.	15 June 2024	Nursing Foundations II+ Applied Biochemistry & Applied Nutrition & Dietetics	Weekly Test-6	20
7.	22 June 2024	Nursing Foundations I+ Applied Biochemistry & Applied Nutrition & Dietetics	Weekly Test-7	20
8.	29 June 2024	Nursing Foundations I+ Applied Biochemistry & Applied Nutrition & Dietetics	Weekly Test-8	20
9.	06 July 2024	Nursing Foundations I+ Applied Biochemistry & Applied Nutrition & Dietetics	Weekly Test-9	20
10.	13 July 2024	Nursing Foundations I+ Applied Biochemistry & Applied Nutrition & Dietetics	Weekly Test-10	20
11.	20 July 2024	Nursing Foundations I+ Applied Biochemistry & Applied Nutrition & Dietetics	Weekly Test-11	20
12.	27 July 2024	Nursing Foundations I+ Applied Biochemistry & Applied Nutrition & Dietetics	Weekly Test-12	20
13.	03 August 2024	Nursing Foundations I+ Applied Biochemistry & Applied Nutrition & Dietetics	Weekly Test-13	20

Contd...

S. No	Dates	Subjects	Tests	No. of Qs
14.	10 August 2024	Nursing Foundations I+ Applied Biochemistry & Applied Nutrition & Dietetics	Weekly Test-14	20
15.	17 August 2024	Nursing Foundations I+ Applied Biochemistry & Applied Nutrition & Dietetics	Weekly Test-15	20
16.	24 August 2024	Nursing Foundations I+ Applied Biochemistry & Applied Nutrition & Dietetics	Weekly Test-16	20
17.	31 August 2024	Nursing Foundations I+ Applied Biochemistry & Applied Nutrition & Dietetics	Weekly Test-17	20
18.	07 September 2024	Nursing Foundations I+ Applied Biochemistry & Applied Nutrition & Dietetics	Weekly Test-18	20
19.	14 September 2024	Nursing Foundations I+ Applied Biochemistry & Applied Nutrition & Dietetics	Weekly Test-19	20
		Total	**Weekly Test-19**	**380**

TABLE 9: Subject-wise Unit Tests

S. No	Dates	Subjects	Tests	No. of Qs	Duration (in Hours)
1.	16 May 2024	Nursing Foundations II & Applied Biochemistry & Applied Nutrition & Dietetics	Unit Test-1	10	2
2.	01 June 2024	Nursing Foundations II & Applied Biochemistry & Applied Nutrition & Dietetics	Unit Test-2	10	2
3.	15 June 2024	Nursing Foundations II & Applied Biochemistry & Applied Nutrition & Dietetics	Unit Test-3	10	2
4.	29 June 2024	Nursing Foundations II & Applied Biochemistry & Applied Nutrition & Dietetics	Unit Test-4	10	2
5.	13 July 2024	Nursing Foundations II & Applied Biochemistry & Applied Nutrition & Dietetics	Unit Test-5	10	2
6.	27 July 2024	Nursing Foundations II & Applied Biochemistry & Applied Nutrition & Dietetics	Unit Test-6	10	2
7.	11 August 2024	Nursing Foundations II & Applied Biochemistry & Applied Nutrition & Dietetics	Unit Test-7	10	2
8.	17 August 2024	Nursing Foundations II & Applied Biochemistry & Applied Nutrition & Dietetics	Unit Test-8	10	2
		Total	**08**	**80**	**16**

TABLE 10: Revision Tests

S. No	Dates (Yet to be Decided)	Subjects	Subjects to be covered
1.	01 June 2024	Revision Test-1	Nursing Foundations II & Applied Biochemistry & Applied Nutrition & Dietetics
2.	29 June 2024	Revision Test-2	Nursing Foundations & Applied Biochemistry & Applied Nutrition & Dietetics
3.	27 July 2024	Revision Test-3	Nursing Foundations II & Applied Biochemistry & Applied Nutrition & Dietetics
4.	24 August 2024	Revision Test-4	Nursing Foundations & Applied Biochemistry & Applied Nutrition & Dietetics
5.	31 August 2024	Revision Test-5	Nursing Foundations II & Applied Biochemistry & Applied Nutrition & Dietetics
	Total	**05**	

TABLE 11: Model Tests

S. No	Dates	Days	Paper
1.	16 September 2024	Monday	Model Test 1 Applied Biochemistry & Applied Nutrition & Dietetics
2.	17 September 2024	Tuesday	Model Test 2 Nursing Foundations
3.	18 September 2024	Wednesday	Model Test 3 Applied Biochemistry & Applied Nutrition & Dietetics
4.	19 September 2024	Thursday	Model Test 4 Nursing Foundations II
5.	20 September 2024	Friday	Model Test 5 Applied Biochemistry & Applied Nutrition & Dietetics
6.	21 September 2024	Saturday	Model Test 6 Nursing Foundations II
7.	22 September 2024	Sunday	Model Test 7 Applied Biochemistry & Applied Nutrition & Dietetics
8.	23 September 2024	Monday	Model Test 8 Nursing Foundations II
9.	24 September 2024	Tuesday	Model Test 9 Applied Biochemistry & Applied Nutrition & Dietetics
10.	25 September 2024	Wednesday	Model Test 10 Nursing Foundations II
11.	26 September 2024	Thursday	Model Test 11 Applied Biochemistry & Applied Nutrition & Dietetics
12.	27 September 2024	Friday	Model Test 12 Nursing Foundations II
13.	28 September 2024	Saturday	Model Test 13 Nursing Foundations II

TABLE 12: Previous Years Papers

S. No.	Subjects	No of Tests	No. of Questions
1.	Applied Biochemistry & Applied Nutrition & Dietetics	10	10–12
2.	Nursing Foundations I	10	10–12
	Total	**20**	**200+**

GUIDANCE & COUNSELLING

S. No	Schedule	Sessions	Total No. of Sessions
1.	At the time of joining	Welcome Call	1
2.	Orientation sessions every week for Batch I after that biweekly	Orientation Program by RM's	17-18
3.	Twice in a month (1 and 3 Saturday) Tentative dates	Progress Review by Batch Mentor	9
4.	1st Week of every month	Updates on Upcoming Classes & Important Tests	6-7
5.	Within 1 week of attempting the Subject wise Unit test	Analysis on Subject wise Unit Tests	31
6.	Within 1 week of attempting Model Test	Analysis and discussion on Model Test	4
7.	Within 1 week of attempting Revision test	Analysis and discussion on Revision Test	
8.	Throughout the Semester	Express Query resolution	On a regular basis
9.	December 2023, February 2024, March 2024 (Dates to be decided)	Interaction with Students (High performers)	4-5
10.	After completing 1st month of all the Batches	Feedbacks & Surveys	3-4

DAY WISE PLAN FOR UG 1st YEAR-SEMESTER II (MAY–SEPTEMBER 2024)

Date	Day	Subject	Faculty	Morning Session (HLT) (Recorded Video of MM Faculty) 6 am – 8 am	Evening Session (Live) (High Yield Topics/ Missing Topics/High Yield Subjective Q Discussion, Nursing Implication) 6 pm – 8 pm	Tests	Doubt session/ Progress Analysis	Assignments (Phygital & E-workbook + TH Decode) Golden Points + Solved Exercise (Self-study After class)
02 May 2024	Thursday			Introduction Session				
03 May 2024	Friday							
04 May 2024	Saturday	Applied Biochemistry & Applied Nutrition & Dietetics	Dr Neha Sethi	Unit 1: Carbohydrates • Carbs-composition, Rda, Dietary Sources • Digestion	Introduction of Applied Biochemistry & Applied Nutrition & Dietetics Significance of Applied Biochemistry & Applied Nutrition & Dietetics in Nursing Introducing the INC Syllabus of Applied Biochemistry & Applied Nutrition & Dietetics			E-workbook-1 before the week schedule start
05 May 2024	**Sunday**	Applied Biochemistry & Applied Nutrition & Dietetics	Dr Neha Sethi	Unit 1: Carbohydrates Carbohydrate Metabolism Gluconeogenesis	Unit 1: Carbohydrates Review of Morning Class Introduction of Carbs Regulation of Blood Glucose			
06 May 2024	Monday	Applied Biochemistry & Applied Nutrition & Dietetics	Dr Neha Sethi	Unit 1: Carbohydrates Fructose Metabolism and Disorders Metabolism of Galactose Von Geirke Disease	Unit 1: Carbohydrates Review of Morning Class Dm			
07 May 2024	Tuesday	Fundamentals of Nursing-II	Ms Sabina Ali	Unit 1: Health Assessment Part 1, 2	A. Introduction • Purposes of Health Assessment • Preparation for Health Assessment Methods of Health Assessment			

Contd...

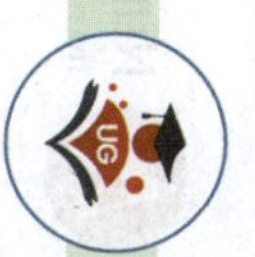

Date	Day	Subject	Faculty	Morning Session (HLT) (Recorded Video of MM Faculty) 6 am – 8 am	Evening Session (Live) (High Yield Topics/ Missing Topics/High Yield Subjective Q Discussion, Nursing Implication) 6 pm – 8 pm	Tests	Doubt session/ Progress Analysis	Assignments (Phygital & E-workbook + TH Decode) Golden Points + Solved Exercise (Self-study After class)
08 May 2024	Wednesday	Fundamentals of Nursing-II	Ms Sabina Ali		B. Comprehensive Health Assessment • Nursing Health History Physical Assessment			
09 May 2024	Thursday	Fundamentals of Nursing-II	Ms Sabina Ali		High Yield Topics Discussion from Target High Next Nursing DECODE	Week Test-1 (Combined MCQ)		
10 May 2024	Friday			Orientation Session				
11 May 2024	Saturday	Applied Biochemistry & Applied Nutrition & Dietetics	Dr Neha Sethi	Unit 2: Lipids Lipids Classifications Oils Phospholipids	Unit 1: Carbohydrates Review of Morning Class Investigations Hypoglycemia			E-workbook-2 before the week schedule start
12 May 2024	**Sunday**	Applied Biochemistry & Applied Nutrition & Dietetics	Dr Neha Sethi	Unit 2: Lipids Fatty Acid Oxidation Fatty Acid Synthesis Cholesterol Metabolism	Unit 2: Lipids • Review of Morning Class • Introduction • Fatty Acids – Definition, Classification • Definition & Clinical Significance of Mufa & Pufa, Essential Fatty Acids, Trans Fatty Acids			
13 May 2024	Monday	Applied Biochemistry & Applied Nutrition & Dietetics	Dr Neha Sethi	Unit 2: Lipids Lipoproteins Ketone Bodies	Unit 2: Lipids • Review of Morning Class • Digestion, Absorption & Metabolism of Lipids & Related Disorders • Ketone Bodies • Lipoproteins • Lipid Profile			

Contd...

Date	Day	Subject	Faculty	Morning Session (HLT) (Recorded Video of MM Faculty) 6 am – 8 am	Evening Session (Live) (High Yield Topics/ Missing Topics/High Yield Subjective Q Discussion, Nursing Implication) 6 pm – 8 pm	Tests	Doubt session/ Progress Analysis	Assignments (Phygital & E-workbook + TH Decode) Golden Points + Solved Exercise (Self-study After class)
14 May 2024	Tuesday	Fundamentals of Nursing-II	Ms Sabina Ali	Repetition of Important Videos	C. Guide in Performing Head-To-Toe Assessment • Integumentary System Head and Neck			
15 May 2024	Wednesday	Fundamentals of Nursing-II	Ms Sabina Ali	Repetition of Important Videos	• Anterior & Posterior Thorax (Breast & Axillae, Thorax, Lungs, Heart)			
16 May 2024	Thursday	Fundamentals of Nursing-II	Ms Sabina Ali	Repetition of Important Videos	**Special Class 1: Discussion on E-workbook, Assignment, Tests/ Progress Review/NP/ Surprise Class**	• Week Test-2 (Combined MCQ) • Subject-wise Unit Test-1 (Subjective)		
17 May 2024	Friday			Orientation Session				
18 May 2024	Saturday	Applied Biochemistry & Applied Nutrition & Dietetics	Dr Neha Sethi	Unit 3: Proteins • Amino Acids • Proteins • Protein Breakdown	Unit 3: Proteins • Review of Morning Class • Introduction • Classification • Digestion, Absorption, Metabolism		Progress Analysis/ Doubt/E-workbook Discussion	E-workbook-3 before the week schedule start
19 May 2024	**Sunday**	Applied Biochemistry & Applied Nutrition & Dietetics	Dr Neha Sethi	Unit 3: Proteins • Urea Cycle • Alkaptonuria and Tyrosinemia • Phenylketonuria	Unit 3: Proteins • Review of Morning Class • In Born Errors of Amino Acid Metabolism • Plasma Protein			

Contd...

Date	Day	Subject	Faculty	Morning Session (HLT) (Recorded Video of MM Faculty) 6 am – 8 am	Evening Session (Live) (High Yield Topics/ Missing Topics/High Yield Subjective Q Discussion, Nursing Implication) 6 pm – 8 pm	Tests	Doubt session/ Progress Analysis	Assignments (Phygital & E-workbook + TH Decode) Golden Points + Solved Exercise (Self-study After class)
20 May 2024	Monday	Applied Biochemistry & Applied Nutrition & Dietetics	Dr Neha Sethi	Unit 3: Proteins • Protein Digestion and Absorption • Inborn Errors	Unit 3: Proteins • Review of Morning Class • Causes of Proteinuria, Hypoproteinemia, Hyper-Gamma Globinemia • Principle of Electrophoresis, Normal & Abnormal Electrophoretic Patterns			
21 May 2024	Tuesday	Fundamentals of Nursing-II	Ms Sabina Ali	Repetition of Important Videos	• Abdomen • Male and Female Genitalia • Rectum and Anus • Extremities (Musculoskeletal System & Peripheral Vascular System)			
22 May 2024	Wednesday	Fundamentals of Nursing-II	Ms Sabina Ali	Repetition of Important Videos	• Neurological System • Assessment • Reflexes • Cranial Nerves • Gcs			
23 May 2024	Thursday	Fundamentals of Nursing-II	Ms Sabina Ali	Repetition of Important Videos	High Yield Topics Discussion from Target High Next Nursing DECODE	Week Test-3 (Combined MCQ)		
26 May 2024	Sunday			Orientation Session				

Contd...

Date	Day	Subject	Faculty	Morning Session (HLT) (Recorded Video of MM Faculty) 6 am – 8 am	Evening Session (Live) (High Yield Topics/ Missing Topics/High Yield Subjective Q Discussion, Nursing Implication) 6 pm – 8 pm	Tests	Doubt session/ Progress Analysis	Assignments (Phygital & E-workbook + TH Decode) Golden Points + Solved Exercise (Self-study After class)
27 May 2024	Monday	Applied Biochemistry & Applied Nutrition & Dietetics	Dr Neha Sethi	Revision Sessions of the Month	Revision Sessions of the Month			E-workbook-4 before the week schedule start
28 May 2024	Tuesday	Applied Biochemistry & Applied Nutrition & Dietetics	Dr Neha Sethi	Revision Sessions of the Month	Revision Sessions of the Month			
29 May 2024	Wednesday	Applied Biochemistry & Applied Nutrition & Dietetics	Dr Neha Sethi	Revision Sessions of the Month	Revision Sessions of the Month			
30 May 2024	Thursday	Fundamentals of Nursing-II	Ms Sabina Ali	Revision Sessions of the Month	Revision Sessions of the Month			
31 May 2024	Friday	Fundamentals of Nursing-II	Ms Sabina Ali	Revision Sessions of the Month	Revision Sessions of the Month			
01 June 2024	Saturday	Fundamentals of Nursing-II	Ms Sabina Ali	Revision Sessions of the Month	**Special Class 2: Discussion on E-workbook, Assignment, Tests/ Progress Review/Np/ Surprise Class**	Week Test-4 (Combined MCQ) Subject-wise Unit Test- 2 (Subjective) **Revision Test 1** (Based on complete month teaching)	Progress Analysis/ Doubt/E-workbook Discussion	
02 June 2024	**Sunday**			Orientation Session				

Contd...

Date	Day	Subject	Faculty	Morning Session (HLT) (Recorded Video of MM Faculty) 6 am – 8 am	Evening Session (Live) (High Yield Topics/ Missing Topics/High Yield Subjective Q Discussion, Nursing Implication) 6 pm – 8 pm	Tests	Doubt session/ Progress Analysis	Assignments (Phygital & E-workbook + TH Decode) Golden Points + Solved Exercise (Self-study After class)
03 June 2024	Monday	Applied Biochemistry & Applied Nutrition & Dietetics	Dr Neha Sethi	Unit 4: Clinical Enzymology Enzyme Inhibition Factors	Unit 4: Clinical Enzymology Review of Morning Class Introduction Isoenzymes – Definition & Properties			E-workbook-5 before the week schedule start
04 June 2024	Tuesday	Applied Biochemistry & Applied Nutrition & Dietetics	Dr Neha Sethi	Unit 4: Clinical Enzymology Regulation of Enzyme Isoenzymes and Enzymes	Unit 4: Clinical Enzymology Review of Morning Class Enzymes of Diagnostic Importance In: Liver Diseases – ALT, AST, ALP, GGT O Myocardial Infarction – CK, Cardiac Troponins, AST, LDH			
05 June 2024	Wednesday	Applied Biochemistry & Applied Nutrition & Dietetics	Dr Neha Sethi	Repetition of Important Topic Live Classes Till Now	Unit 4: Clinical Enzymology Review of Morning Class Enzymes of Diagnostic Importance in O Muscle Diseases – CL, Aldolase O Bone Diseases – ALP O Prostate Cancer – PSA, ACP			
06 June 2024	Thursday	Fundamentals of Nursing-II	Ms Sabina Ali	Unit 2: The Nursing Process Critical Thinking Part 1, 2	Unit 2: The Nursing Process Critical Thinking			
07 June 2024	Friday	Fundamentals of Nursing-II	Ms Sabina Ali	Unit 2: The Nursing Process Nursing Process Part 1	Unit 2: The Nursing Process Nursing Process Overview			

Contd...

Date	Day	Subject	Faculty	Morning Session (HLT) (Recorded Video of MM Faculty) 6 am – 8 am	Evening Session (Live) (High Yield Topics/ Missing Topics/High Yield Subjective Q Discussion, Nursing Implication) 6 pm – 8 pm	Tests	Doubt session/ Progress Analysis	Assignments (Phygital & E-workbook + TH Decode) Golden Points + Solved Exercise (Self-study After class)
08 June 2024	Saturday	Fundamentals of Nursing-II	Ms Sabina Ali	Unit 2: The Nursing Process Part 2, 3	Unit 2: The Nursing Process Assessment Diagnosis (With Example)	Week Test-5 (Combined MCQ)		
09 June 2024	Sunday			Orientation Session				
10 June 2024	Monday	Applied Biochemistry & Applied Nutrition & Dietetics	Dr Neha Sethi	Repetition of Important Topic Live Classes Till Now	Unit 5: Acid Base Maintenance • Ph – Definition, Normal Value • Regulation of Blood Ph – Blood Buffer, Respiratory & Renal			E-workbook-6 before the week schedule start
11 June 2024	Tuesday	Applied Biochemistry & Applied Nutrition & Dietetics	Dr Neha Sethi	Repetition of Important Topic Live Classes till Now	Unit 5: Acid Base Maintenance • Abg – Normal Values • Acid Base Disorders – Types, Definition & Causes			
12 June 2024	Wednesday	Applied Biochemistry & Applied Nutrition & Dietetics	Dr Neha Sethi	Unit 6: Heme Catabolism • Heme Synthesis • Porphyrias • Heme Breakdown • Jaundice	Unit 6: Heme Catabolism • Review of Morning Class • Introduction • Heme Degradation Pathway • Jaundice – Type, Causes, Urine & Blood Investigations (Van Den Berg Test)			
13 June 2024	Thursday	Fundamentals of Nursing-II	Ms Sabina Ali	Unit 2: The Nursing Process Part 4, 5	Unit 2: The Nursing Process Planning (With Example)			

Contd...

Date	Day	Subject	Faculty	Morning Session (HLT) (Recorded Video of MM Faculty) 6 am – 8 am	Evening Session (Live) (High Yield Topics/ Missing Topics/High Yield Subjective Q Discussion, Nursing Implication) 6 pm – 8 pm	Tests	Doubt session/ Progress Analysis	Assignments (Phygital & E-workbook + TH Decode) Golden Points + Solved Exercise (Self-study After class)
14 June 2024	Friday	Fundamentals of Nursing-II	Ms Sabina Ali	Unit 2: The Nursing Process Part 6	Unit 2: The Nursing Process Implementation, Evaluation (With Example)			
15 June 2024	Saturday	Fundamentals of Nursing-II	Ms Sabina Ali	Unit 2: The Nursing Process Part 7, 8	High Yield Topics Discussion from Target High Next Nursing DECODE	Week Test-6 (Combined MCQ) Subject-wise Unit Test-3 (Subjective)		
16 June 2024	**Sunday**			Orientation Session				
17 June 2024	Monday	Applied Biochemistry & Applied Nutrition & Dietetics	Dr Neha Sethi	Unit 7: Organ Function Tests (Biochemical Parameters & Normal Values Only) Blood Collection Tube LFT	Unit 7: Organ Function Tests (Biochemical Parameters & Normal Values Only) Review of Morning Class • Renal			E-workbook-7 before the week schedule start
18 June 2024	Tuesday	Applied Biochemistry & Applied Nutrition & Dietetics	Dr Neha Sethi	Unit 8: Immunochemistry Antibody-Structure, Function	Unit 7: Organ Function Tests (Biochemical Parameters & Normal Values Only) Review of Morning Class • Liver • Thyroid			
19 June 2024	Wednesday	Applied Biochemistry & Applied Nutrition & Dietetics	Dr Neha Sethi	Repetition of Imp Live Class	Unit 8: Immunochemistry • Structure & Functions of Immunoglobulin • Investigations & Interpretation – Elisa			

Contd...

Date	Day	Subject	Faculty	Morning Session (HLT) (Recorded Video of MM Faculty) 6 am – 8 am	Evening Session (Live) (High Yield Topics/ Missing Topics/High Yield Subjective Q Discussion, Nursing Implication) 6 pm – 8 pm	Tests	Doubt session/ Progress Analysis	Assignments (Phygital & E-workbook + TH Decode) Golden Points + Solved Exercise (Self-study After class)
20 June 2024	Thursday	Fundamentals of Nursing-II	Ms Sabina Ali	Unit 3: Nutritional Needs NG Part 1, 3	Unit 3: Nutritional Needs Factors Affecting Care of Patient With Dysphagia, Anorexia, Nausea, Vomiting Meeting Nutritional Needs			
21 June 2024	Friday	Fundamentals of Nursing-II	Ms Sabina Ali	Unit 3: Nutritional Needs Ng Intubation Part 1, 2	Unit 3: Nutritional Needs • Introduction to Other Enteral Feeds – Types, Indications, • Gastrostomy, Jejunostomy • Parenteral – Tpn (Total • Parenteral Nutrition)			
22 June 2024	Saturday	Fundamentals of Nursing-II	Ms Sabina Ali	Unit 3: Nutritional Needs NG Tube Removal and Feeding	**Special Class 3: Discussion on E-workbook, Assignment, Tests/ Progress Review/Np/ Surprise Class**	Week Test-7 (Combined MCQ)		
23 June 2024	**Sunday**			Orientation Session				
24 June 2024	Monday	Applied Biochemistry & Applied Nutrition & Dietetics	Dr Neha Sethi	Revision Sessions of the Month	Revision Sessions of the Month			E-workbook-8 before the week schedule start
25 June 2024	Tuesday	Applied Biochemistry & Applied Nutrition & Dietetics	Dr Neha Sethi	Revision Sessions of the Month	Revision Sessions of the Month			

Contd...

Date	Day	Subject	Faculty	Morning Session (HLT) (Recorded Video of MM Faculty) 6 am – 8 am	Evening Session (Live) (High Yield Topics/ Missing Topics/High Yield Subjective Q Discussion, Nursing Implication) 6 pm – 8 pm	Tests	Doubt session/ Progress Analysis	Assignments (Phygital & E-workbook + TH Decode) Golden Points + Solved Exercise (Self-study After class)
26 June 2024	Wednesday	Applied Biochemistry & Applied Nutrition & Dietetics	Dr Neha Sethi	Revision Sessions of the Month	Revision Sessions of the Month			
27 June 2024	Thursday	Fundamentals of Nursing-II	Ms Sabina Ali	Revision Sessions of the Month	Revision Sessions of the Month			
28 June 2024	Friday	Fundamentals of Nursing-II	Ms Sabina Ali	Revision Sessions of the Month	Revision Sessions of the Month			
29 June 2024	Saturday	Fundamentals of Nursing-II	Ms Sabina Ali	Revision Sessions of the Month	High Yield Topics Discussion from Target High Next Nursing DECODE	Week Test-8 (Combined MCQ) Subject-wise Unit Test-4 (Subjective) **Revision Test 2** (Based on complete month teaching)		
30 June 2024	**Sunday**			Orientation Session				
01 July 2024	Monday	Applied Biochemistry & Applied Nutrition & Dietetics	Dr Neha Sethi	Unit 1: Introduction to Nutrition Classification of Nutrients	Unit 1: Introduction to Nutrition • Concepts • Nutrients			E-workbook-9 before the week schedule start
02 July 2024	Tuesday	Applied Biochemistry & Applied Nutrition & Dietetics	Dr Neha Sethi	Unit 2: Carbohydrates Replay of Previous Videos	Unit 1: Introduction to Nutrition • Food Unit 2: Carbohydrates • Review • Introduction • Composition – Starches, Sugar and Cellulose • Recommended Daily Allowance (Rda)			

Contd...

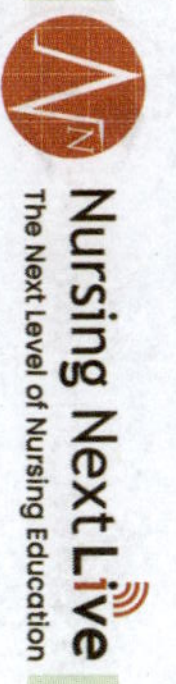

Date	Day	Subject	Faculty	Morning Session (HLT) (Recorded Video of MM Faculty) 6 am – 8 am	Evening Session (Live) (High Yield Topics/ Missing Topics/High Yield Subjective Q Discussion, Nursing Implication) 6 pm – 8 pm	Tests	Doubt session/ Progress Analysis	Assignments (Phygital & E-workbook + TH Decode) Golden Points + Solved Exercise (Self-study After class)
03 July 2024	Wednesday	Applied Biochemistry & Applied Nutrition & Dietetics	Dr Neha Sethi	Unit 2: Carbohydrates • Carbs-Composition, Rda, Dietary Sources Digestion Metabolism	Unit 2: Carbohydrates • Dietary Sources • Functions Energy • Unit of Energy Kcal • Basal Metabolic Rate (Bmr) • Factors Affecting Bmr			
04 July 2024	Thursday	Fundamentals of Nursing-II	Ms Sabina Ali	Unit 4: Hygiene Perineal Care Part 1, 2	Unit 4: Hygiene • Care of Pressure Points • Assessment of Pressure Ulcers Using Braden Scale and Norton Scale			
05 July 2024	Friday	Fundamentals of Nursing-II	Ms Sabina Ali	Unit 4: Hygiene Repetition of • Care of Pressure Points Assessment of Pressure Ulcers Using Braden Scale and Norton Scale	Unit 4: Hygiene Pressure Ulcers – Causes, Stages and Manifestations, Care and Prevention			
06 July 2024	Saturday	Fundamentals of Nursing-II	Ms Sabina Ali	Repetition of Unit 4: Hygiene Pressure Ulcers – Causes, Stages and Manifestations, Care and Prevention	**Special Class 4: Discussion on E-workbook, Assignment, Tests/ Progress Review/NP/ Surprise Class**	Week Test-9 (Combined MCQ)		
07 July 2024	**Sunday**			Orientation Session				
08 July 2024	Monday	Applied Biochemistry & Applied Nutrition & Dietetics	Dr Neha Sethi	Unit 3: Proteins • Amino Acids • Proteins • Protein Breakdown • Metabolism	Unit 3: Proteins • Composition • Eight Essential Amino Acids • Functions • Dietary Sources • Protein Requirements – Rda			E-workbook-10 before the week schedule start

Contd...

Date	Day	Subject	Faculty	Morning Session (HLT) (Recorded Video of MM Faculty) 6 am – 8 am	Evening Session (Live) (High Yield Topics/ Missing Topics/High Yield Subjective Q Discussion, Nursing Implication) 6 pm – 8 pm	Tests	Doubt session/ Progress Analysis	Assignments (Phygital & E-workbook + TH Decode) Golden Points + Solved Exercise (Self-study After class)
09 July 2024	Tuesday	Applied Biochemistry & Applied Nutrition & Dietetics	Dr Neha Sethi	Unit 4: Fats Lipids Classifications Oils Phospholipids Metabolism	Unit 4: Fats • Classification Saturated & Unsaturated • Calorie Value • Functions • Dietary Sources of Fats and Fatty Acids • Fat Requirements Rda			
10 July 2024	Wednesday	Applied Biochemistry & Applied Nutrition & Dietetics	Dr Neha Sethi	Unit 5: Vitamins Intro. Classification Vit A, D, E, K	Unit 5: Vitamins Classification Fat Soluble			
11 July 2024	Thursday	Fundamentals of Nursing-II	Ms Sabina Ali	Unit 5: Elimination Needs Urinary Catheterization Part 1, 2	Unit 5: Elimination Needs • Facilitating Urine Elimination • Providing Urinal/Bed Pan • Care of Patients With Condom Drainage Intermittent Catheterization Indwelling Urinary Catheter and Urinary Drainage			

Contd...

Date	Day	Subject	Faculty	Morning Session (HLT) (Recorded Video of MM Faculty) 6 am – 8 am	Evening Session (Live) (High Yield Topics/ Missing Topics/High Yield Subjective Q Discussion, Nursing Implication) 6 pm – 8 pm	Tests	Doubt session/ Progress Analysis	Assignments (Phygital & E-workbook + TH Decode) Golden Points + Solved Exercise (Self-study After class)
12 July 2024	Friday	Fundamentals of Nursing-II	Ms Sabina Ali	Unit 5: Elimination Needs Care of Patients With Ostomies Care of Ostomy Part 1, 2, 3	Unit 5: Elimination Needs • Care of Patients With Urinary Diversions Bladder Irrigation • Bowel Elimination Facilitating Bowel Elimination Enemas Suppository Care of Patients With Ostomies			
13 July 2024	Saturday	Fundamentals of Nursing-II	Ms Sabina Ali	Unit 5: Elimination Needs Bladder Irrigation Enema	High Yield Topics Discussion from Target High Next Nursing DECODE	Week Test-10 (Combined MCQ) Subject-wise Unit Test-5 (Subjective)		
14 July 2024	Sunday			Orientation Session				
15 July 2024	Monday	Applied Biochemistry & Applied Nutrition & Dietetics	Dr Neha Sethi	Unit 5: Vitamins • Vit B1, B2, B3, B5, B6, B7, B9, B12, C • Cooking Methods	Unit 5: Vitamins • Water Soluble Vitamins • Functions, Dietary Sources & Requirements – Rda of Every Vitamin			E-workbook-11 before the week schedule start
16 July 2024	Tuesday	Applied Biochemistry & Applied Nutrition & Dietetics	Dr Neha Sethi	Unit 6: Minerals • Intro • Ca, Phosphorus • Iron • Copper • Zinc	Unit 6: Minerals • Classification – Major Minerals (Calcium, Phosphorus, Sodium, Potassium and Magnesium) and Trace Elements			

Contd...

Date	Day	Subject	Faculty	Morning Session (HLT) (Recorded Video of MM Faculty) 6 am – 8 am	Evening Session (Live) (High Yield Topics/ Missing Topics/High Yield Subjective Q Discussion, Nursing Implication) 6 pm – 8 pm	Tests	Doubt session/ Progress Analysis	Assignments (Phygital & E-workbook + TH Decode) Golden Points + Solved Exercise (Self-study After class)
17 July 2024	Wednesday	Applied Biochemistry & Applied Nutrition & Dietetics	Dr Neha Sethi	Unit 6: Minerals • Iodine • Fluoride and Fluorosis • Mg • Selenium • Calcium	Unit 6: Minerals • Functions • Dietary Sources Requirements – RDA			
18 July 2024	Thursday	Fundamentals of Nursing-II	Ms Sabina Ali	Unit 6: Diagnostic Testing Blood Sampling Part 1, 2, 3	Unit 6: Diagnostic Testing CBC LFT GRBS			
19 July 2024	Friday	Fundamentals of Nursing-II	Ms Sabina Ali	Unit 6: Diagnostic Testing BT Part 1, 2, 3	Unit 6: Diagnostic Testing Urine Culture Stool Sputum			
20 July 2024	Saturday	Fundamentals of Nursing-II	Ms Sabina Ali	Unit 6: Diagnostic Testing LP Part 1-3	**Special Class 5: Discussion on E-workbook, Assignment, Tests/ Progress Review/Np/ Surprise Class**	Week Test-11 (Combined MCQ)		
21 July 2024	**Sunday**			Orientation Session				
22 July 2024	Monday	Applied Biochemistry & Applied Nutrition & Dietetics	Dr Neha Sethi	Revision Sessions of the Month	Revision Sessions of the Month			E-workbook-12 before the week schedule start
23 July 2024	Tuesday	Applied Biochemistry & Applied Nutrition & Dietetics	Dr Neha Sethi	Revision Sessions of the Month	Revision Sessions of the Month			

Contd...

Date	Day	Subject	Faculty	Morning Session (HLT) (Recorded Video of MM Faculty) 6 am – 8 am	Evening Session (Live) (High Yield Topics/ Missing Topics/High Yield Subjective Q Discussion, Nursing Implication) 6 pm – 8 pm	Tests	Doubt session/ Progress Analysis	Assignments (Phygital & E-workbook + TH Decode) Golden Points + Solved Exercise (Self-study After class)
24 July 2024	Wednesday	Applied Biochemistry & Applied Nutrition & Dietetics	Dr Neha Sethi	Revision Sessions of the Month	Revision Sessions of the Month			
25 July 2024	Thursday	Fundamentals of Nursing-II	Ms Sabina Ali	Revision Sessions of the Month	Revision Sessions of the Month			
26 July 2024	Friday	Fundamentals of Nursing-II	Ms Sabina Ali	Revision Sessions of the Month	Revision Sessions of the Month			
27 July 2024	Saturday	Fundamentals of Nursing-II	Ms Sabina Ali	Revision Sessions of the Month	Revision Sessions of the Month	Week Test-12 (Combined MCQ) Subject-wise Unit Test-6 (Subjective) **Revision Test 3** (Based on complete month teaching)		
28 July 2024	**Sunday**			Orientation Session				
29 July 2024	Monday	Applied Biochemistry & Applied Nutrition & Dietetics	Dr Neha Sethi	Unit 7: Balanced Diet Balanced Diet Calorific Value Rda	Unit 7: Balanced Diet • Review Or Morning Class • Definition, Principles, Steps • Food Guides – Basic Four Food Groups • Rda • Calculation of Nutritive Value of Foods			E-workbook-13 before the week schedule start

Contd...

Date	Day	Subject	Faculty	Morning Session (HLT) (Recorded Video of MM Faculty) 6 am – 8 am	Evening Session (Live) (High Yield Topics/ Missing Topics/High Yield Subjective Q Discussion, Nursing Implication) 6 pm – 8 pm	Tests	Doubt session/ Progress Analysis	Assignments (Phygital & E-workbook + TH Decode) Golden Points + Solved Exercise (Self-study After class)
30 July 2024	Tuesday	Applied Biochemistry & Applied Nutrition & Dietetics	Dr Neha Sethi	Unit 7: Balanced Diet Nutrition Across Life Part 1, 2	Unit 7: Balanced Diet • Nutrition Across Life Cycle • Meal Planning/Menu Planning – Definition, Principles, Steps • Infant and Young Child Feeding (Iycf) Guidelines			
31 July 2024	Wednesday	Applied Biochemistry & Applied Nutrition & Dietetics	Dr Neha Sethi	Repetition of Previous Important Live Videos	Unit 7: Balanced Diet • Diet Plan for Different Age Groups- Children, Adolescents and Elderly • Diet in Pregnancy • Anemia in Pregnancy • Nutrition in Lactation			
01 Aug. 2024	Thursday	Fundamentals of Nursing-II	Ms Sabina Ali	Unit 7: Oxygenation Needs Et Part 1-3	Unit 7: Oxygenation Needs Factors Alterations Nursing Interventions to Promote Oxygenation			
02 Aug. 2024	Friday	Fundamentals of Nursing-II	Ms Sabina Ali	Unit 7: Oxygenation Needs Suctioning Part 1-2	Unit 7: Oxygenation Needs Oxygen Adm Chest Pt			
03 Aug. 2024	Saturday	Fundamentals of Nursing-II	Ms Sabina Ali	Unit 7: Oxygenation Needs Oxygen Therapy Part 1, 2, 3	High Yield Topics Discussion from Target High Next Nursing DECODE	Week Test-13 (Combined MCQ)		
04 Aug. 2024	Sunday			Orientation Session				

Contd...

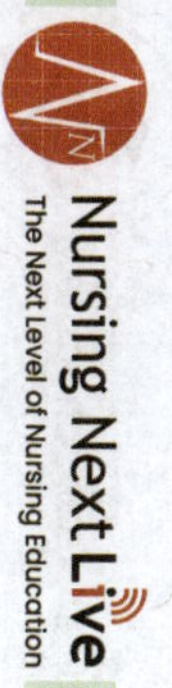

Date	Day	Subject	Faculty	Morning Session (HLT) (Recorded Video of MM Faculty) 6 am – 8 am	Evening Session (Live) (High Yield Topics/ Missing Topics/High Yield Subjective Q Discussion, Nursing Implication) 6 pm – 8 pm	Tests	Doubt session/ Progress Analysis	Assignments (Phygital & E-workbook + TH Decode) Golden Points + Solved Exercise (Self-study After class)
05 Aug. 2024	Monday	Applied Biochemistry & Applied Nutrition & Dietetics	Dr Neha Sethi	Unit 8: Nutritional Deficiency Disorders PEM	Unit 8: Nutritional Deficiency Disorders • Protein Energy Malnutrition			E-workbook-14 before the week schedule start
06 Aug. 2024	Tuesday	Applied Biochemistry & Applied Nutrition & Dietetics	Dr Neha Sethi	Repetition of Eve Class	Unit 8: Nutritional Deficiency Disorders • Childhood Obesity			
07 Aug. 2024	Wednesday	Applied Biochemistry & Applied Nutrition & Dietetics	Dr Neha Sethi	Repetition of Eve Class	Unit 8: Nutritional Deficiency Disorders • Vitamin Deficiency Disorders • Mineral Deficiency Diseases			
08 Aug. 2024	Thursday	Fundamentals of Nursing-II	Ms Sabina Ali	Unit 7: Oxygenation Needs Chest T Drain Pulse Oximeter Part 1, 2	Unit 7: Oxygenation Needs Suctioning Chest Drainage Pulse Oximeter Restorative & Continuing Care			
09 Aug. 2024	Friday	Fundamentals of Nursing-II	Ms Sabina Ali	Unit 8: Fluid, Electrolyte, and Acid –Base Balances	Unit 8: Fluid, Electrolyte, and Acid –Base Balances Disturbances in Fluid Volume: O Deficit Hypovolemia Dehydration			
10 Aug. 2024	Saturday	Fundamentals of Nursing-II	Ms Sabina Ali	Repetition of Important Videos	**Special Class 6: Discussion on E-workbook, Assignment, Tests/ Progress Review/Np/ Surprise Class**	Week Test-14 (Combined MCQ) Subject-wise Unit Test-7 (Subjective)		

Contd...

Date	Day	Subject	Faculty	Morning Session (HLT) (Recorded Video of MM Faculty) 6 am – 8 am	Evening Session (Live) (High Yield Topics/ Missing Topics/High Yield Subjective Q Discussion, Nursing Implication) 6 pm – 8 pm	Tests	Doubt session/ Progress Analysis	Assignments (Phygital & E-workbook + TH Decode) Golden Points + Solved Exercise (Self-study After class)
11 Aug. 2024	**Sunday**			Orientation Session				
12 Aug. 2024	Monday	Applied Biochemistry & Applied Nutrition & Dietetics	Dr Neha Sethi	Unit 9: Therapeutic Diets Repetition of Eve Class	Unit 9: Therapeutic Diets • Definition, Objectives, Principles • Modifications – Consistency, Nutrients,			E-workbook-15 before the week schedule start
13 Aug. 2024	Tuesday	Applied Biochemistry & Applied Nutrition & Dietetics	Dr Neha Sethi	Unit 9: Therapeutic Diets Repetition of Eve Class	Unit 9: Therapeutic Diets • Feeding Techniques. • Diet in Diseases – Obesity, Diabetes Mellitus, Cvd,			
14 Aug. 2024	Wednesday	Applied Biochemistry & Applied Nutrition & Dietetics	Dr Neha Sethi	Unit 9: Therapeutic Diets Repetition of Eve Class	Unit 9: Therapeutic Diets Diet in Diseases-Underweight, Renal Diseases, Hepatic Disorders Constipation, Diarrhea, Pre and Post-Operative Period			
15 Aug. 2024	Thursday	Fundamentals of Nursing-II	Ms Sabina Ali	Unit 8: Fluid, Electrolyte, and Acid –Base Balances Crystalloid and Colloids Iv Fluids	Unit 8: Fluid, Electrolyte, and Acid –Base Balances Excess • Fluid Overload • Edema • Electrolyte Imbalances (Hypo and Hyper) Acid-Base Imbalances • Metabolic – Acidosis & Alkalosis • Respiratory – Acidosis & Alkalosis			
16 Aug. 2024	Friday	Fundamentals of Nursing-II	Ms Sabina Ali	Repetition of Eve Class	Unit 8: Fluid, Electrolyte, and Iv Therapy			

Contd...

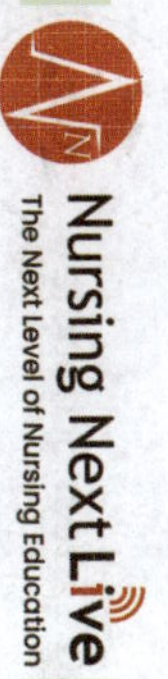

Date	Day	Subject	Faculty	Morning Session (HLT) (Recorded Video of MM Faculty) 6 am – 8 am	Evening Session (Live) (High Yield Topics/ Missing Topics/High Yield Subjective Q Discussion, Nursing Implication) 6 pm – 8 pm	Tests	Doubt session/ Progress Analysis	Assignments (Phygital & E-workbook + TH Decode) Golden Points + Solved Exercise (Self-study After class)
17 Aug. 2024	Saturday	Fundamentals of Nursing-II	Ms Sabina Ali	Repetition of Eve Class	High Yield Topics Discussion from Target High Next Nursing DECODE	Week Test-15 (Combined MCQ) Subject-wise Unit Test-8 (Subjective)		
18 Aug. 2024	Sunday			Orientation Session				
19 Aug. 2024	Monday	Applied Biochemistry & Applied Nutrition & Dietetics	Dr Neha Sethi	Unit 10: Cookery Rules and Preservation of Nutrients • Food Preservation • Safe Food Handling Food Fortification	Unit 10: Cookery Rules and Preservation of Nutrients Preservation of Nutrients Food Additives and Food Adulteration Prevention of Food Adulteration Act (Pfa) Food Standards			E-workbook-16 before the week schedule start
20 Aug. 2024	Tuesday	Applied Biochemistry & Applied Nutrition & Dietetics	Dr Neha Sethi	Unit 11: Nutrition Assessment and Nutrition Education Part 1, 2	Unit 11: Nutrition Assessment and Nutrition Education • Objectives of Nutritional Assessment Methods of Assessment –			
21 Aug. 2024	Wednesday	Applied Biochemistry & Applied Nutrition & Dietetics	Dr Neha Sethi	Unit12: National Nutritional Programs and Role of Nurse Nutritional Programs ICDS Poshan Abhiyan	Unit 11: Nutrition Assessment and Nutrition Education Nutrition Education – Purposes, Principles and Methods			
22 Aug. 2024	Thursday	Fundamentals of Nursing-II	Ms Sabina Ali	Unit 9: Administration of Medications Rights of Medication Part 1- 3	Unit 9: Administration of Medications Medication Dose Calculation Principles, 10 Rights of Medication Administration			

Contd...

Date	Day	Subject	Faculty	Morning Session (HLT) (Recorded Video of MM Faculty) 6 am – 8 am	Evening Session (Live) (High Yield Topics/ Missing Topics/High Yield Subjective Q Discussion, Nursing Implication) 6 pm – 8 pm	Tests	Doubt session/ Progress Analysis	Assignments (Phygital & E-workbook + TH Decode) Golden Points + Solved Exercise (Self-study After class)
23 Aug. 2024	Friday	Fundamentals of Nursing-II	Ms Sabina Ali	Unit 9: Administration of Medications IV Cannulation Part 1-3	Unit 9: Administration of Medications Oral, Sublingual and Buccal Routes: Equipment, Procedure • Introduction to Parenteral Administration of Drugs – Intramuscular, Intravenous, Subcutaneous, Intradermal			
24 Aug. 2024	Saturday	Fundamentals of Nursing-II	Ms Sabina Ali	Unit 9: Administration of Medications Care of CVP Line Part 1-2	**Special Class 7: Discussion on E-workbook, Assignment, Tests/ Progress Review/Np/ Surprise Class**	Week Test-16 (Combined MCQ) Subject-wise Unit Test-9 (Subjective) **Revision Test 4** (Based on complete month teaching)		
25 Aug. 2024	**Sunday**			Orientation Session				
26 Aug. 2024	Monday	Applied Biochemistry & Applied Nutrition & Dietetics	Dr Neha Sethi	• Repetition of Previous Important Classes	Unit12: National Nutritional Programs and Role of Nurse Nutritional Problems in India • National Nutritional Policy • National Nutritional Programs			E-workbook-17 before the week schedule start

Contd...

Date	Day	Subject	Faculty	Morning Session (HLT) (Recorded Video of MM Faculty) 6 am – 8 am	Evening Session (Live) (High Yield Topics/ Missing Topics/High Yield Subjective Q Discussion, Nursing Implication) 6 pm – 8 pm	Tests	Doubt session/ Progress Analysis	Assignments (Phygital & E-workbook + TH Decode) Golden Points + Solved Exercise (Self-study After class)
27 Aug. 2024	Tuesday	Applied Biochemistry & Applied Nutrition & Dietetics	Dr Neha Sethi	Repetition of Previous Important Classes	Unit 13: Food Safety • Definition, Food Safety Considerations & Measures • Food Safety Regulatory Measures in India – Relevant Acts • Five Keys to Safer Food • General Principles of Food Storage of Food Items (Ex. Milk, Meat) • Role of Food Handlers in Food Borne Diseases • Essential Steps in Safe Cooking Practices			
28 Aug. 2024	Wednesday	Fundamentals of Nursing-II	Ms Sabina Ali	Unit 9: Administration of Medications Care of CVP Line Part 3-4	Unit 9: Administration of Medications Prevention of Needle-Stick Injuries			
29 Aug. 2024	Thursday	Fundamentals of Nursing-II	Ms Sabina Ali	Unit 10: Sensory Needs Part 1-2	Unit 10: Sensory Needs Assessment of Sensory Alterations Unconsciousness			
30 Aug. 2024	Friday	Fundamentals of Nursing-II	Ms Sabina Ali	Unit 11: Care of Terminally Ill, Death and Dying Loss and Grief Part 1-3	Unit 11: Care of Terminally Ill, Death and Dying Theories of Grief & Loss – Kubler Ross 5 Stages of Dying Dying Patient's Bill of Rights Care of Dying Patient			

Contd...

Date	Day	Subject	Faculty	Morning Session (HLT) (Recorded Video of MM Faculty) 6 am – 8 am	Evening Session (Live) (High Yield Topics/ Missing Topics/High Yield Subjective Q Discussion, Nursing Implication) 6 pm – 8 pm	Tests	Doubt session/ Progress Analysis	Assignments (Phygital & E-workbook + TH Decode) Golden Points + Solved Exercise (Self-study After class)
31 Aug. 2024	Saturday	Fundamentals of Nursing-II	Ms Sabina Ali	Repetition of Previous Important Class	High Yield Topics Discussion from Target High Next Nursing DECODE	Week Test-17 (Combined MCQ) **Revision Test 5** (Based on complete month teaching)		
01 Sept. 2024	**Sunday**			Orientation Session				
02 Sept. 2024	Monday	Fundamentals of Nursing-II	Ms Sabina Ali	Revision of Important Topics	Psychosocial Needs A-Self-Concept			E-workbook-18 before the week schedule start
03 Sept. 2024	Tuesday	Fundamentals of Nursing-II	Ms Sabina Ali	Revision of Important Topics	Psychosocial Needs B- Sexuality			
04 Sept. 2024	Wednesday	Fundamentals of Nursing-II	Ms Sabina Ali	Revision of Important Topics	Psychosocial Needs C- Stress and Adaptation – Introductory Concepts			
05 Sept. 2024	Thursday	Fundamentals of Nursing-II	Ms Sabina Ali	Revision of Important Topics	Psychosocial Needs D- Concepts of Cultural Diversity and Spirituality			
06 Sept. 2024	Friday	Fundamentals of Nursing-II	Ms Sabina Ali	Unit 16: Nursing Theories: Introduction Part 1, 2	Unit 16: Nursing Theories: Introduction Meaning &Definition, Purposes, Types of Theories With Examples, Overview of Selected Nursing Theories – Nightingale, Orem, Roy			
07 Sept. 2024	Saturday	Fundamentals of Nursing-II	Ms Sabina Ali	Practical Prep Sessions	Practical Prep Sessions	Week Test-18 (Combined MCQ) Subject-wise Unit Test-10 (Subjective)		

Contd...

Date	Day	Subject	Faculty	Morning Session (HLT) (Recorded Video of MM Faculty) 6 am – 8 am	Evening Session (Live) (High Yield Topics/ Missing Topics/High Yield Subjective Q Discussion, Nursing Implication) 6 pm – 8 pm	Tests	Doubt session/ Progress Analysis	Assignments (Phygital & E-workbook + TH Decode) Golden Points + Solved Exercise (Self-study After class)
08 Sept. 2024	Sunday			Orientation Session				
09 Sept. 2024	Monday	Fundamentals of Nursing-II	Ms Sabina Ali	Practical Prep Sessions	Practical Prep Sessions			E-workbook-19 before the week schedule start
10 Sept. 2024	Tuesday	Fundamentals of Nursing-II	Ms Sabina Ali	Practical Prep Sessions	Practical Prep Sessions			
11 Sept. 2024	Wednesday	Fundamentals of Nursing-II	Ms Sabina Ali	Practical Prep Sessions	Practical Prep Sessions			
12 Sept. 2024	Thursday	Fundamentals of Nursing-II	Ms Sabina Ali	Practical Prep Sessions	Practical Prep Sessions			
13 Sept. 2024	Friday	Fundamentals of Nursing-II	Ms Sabina Ali	Practical Prep Sessions	Practical Prep Sessions			
14 Sept. 2024	Saturday	Fundamentals of Nursing-II	Ms Sabina Ali	Practical Prep Sessions	Practical Prep Sessions	Week Test-19 (Combined MCQ) Subject-wise Unit Test-11 (Subjective)		
15 Sept. 2024	Sunday							
16 Sept. 2024	Monday	Applied Biochemistry & Applied Nutrition & Dietetics	Dr Neha Sethi		Decode Revision Session 1 with PQD	Model Test Applied Biochemistry & Applied Nutrition & Dietetics Set-1		
17 Sept. 2024	Tuesday	Applied Biochemistry & Applied Nutrition & Dietetics	Dr Neha Sethi		Decode Revision Session 2 with PQD			

Contd...

Date	Day	Subject	Faculty	Morning Session (HLT) (Recorded Video of MM Faculty) 6 am – 8 am	Evening Session (Live) (High Yield Topics/ Missing Topics/High Yield Subjective Q Discussion, Nursing Implication) 6 pm – 8 pm	Tests	Doubt session/ Progress Analysis	Assignments (Phygital & E-workbook + TH Decode) Golden Points + Solved Exercise (Self-study After class)
18 Sept. 2024	Wednesday	Applied Biochemistry & Applied Nutrition & Dietetics	Dr Neha Sethi		Decode Revision Session 3 with PQD	Model Test Applied Biochemistry & Applied Nutrition & Dietetics Set-2		
19 Sept. 2024	Thursday	Applied Biochemistry & Applied Nutrition & Dietetics	Dr Neha Sethi		Decode Revision Session 4 with PQD			
20 Sept. 2024	Friday	Applied Biochemistry & Applied Nutrition & Dietetics	Dr Neha Sethi		Decode Revision Session 5 with PQD	Model Test Applied Biochemistry & Applied Nutrition & Dietetics Set-3		
21 Sept. 2024	Saturday	Applied Biochemistry & Applied Nutrition & Dietetics	Dr Neha Sethi		Decode Revision Session 6 with PQD			
22 Sept. 2024	Sunday							
23 Sept. 2024	Monday	Fundamentals of Nursing-II	Ms Sabina Ali		Decode Revision Session 1 with PQD	Model Test Applied Biochemistry & Applied Nutrition & Dietetics Set-1		
24 Sept. 2024	Tuesday	Fundamentals of Nursing-II	Ms Sabina Ali		Decode Revision Session 2 with PQD	Model Test Applied Biochemistry & Applied Nutrition & Dietetics Set-2		

Contd...

Date	Day	Subject	Faculty	Morning Session (HLT) (Recorded Video of MM Faculty) 6 am – 8 am	Evening Session (Live) (High Yield Topics/ Missing Topics/High Yield Subjective Q Discussion, Nursing Implication) 6 pm – 8 pm	Tests	Doubt session/ Progress Analysis	Assignments (Phygital & E-workbook + TH Decode) Golden Points + Solved Exercise (Self-study After class)
25 Sept. 2024	Wednesday	Fundamentals of Nursing-II	Ms Sabina Ali		Decode Revision Session 3 with PQD	Model Test Applied Biochemistry & Applied Nutrition & Dietetics Set-3		
26 Sept. 2024	Thursday	Fundamentals of Nursing-II	Ms Sabina Ali		Decode Revision Session 4 with PQD	Model Test Applied Biochemistry & Applied Nutrition & Dietetics Set-4		
27 Sept. 2024	Friday	Fundamentals of Nursing-II	Ms Sabina Ali		Decode Revision Session 1 with PQD	Model Test Applied Biochemistry & Applied Nutrition & Dietetics Set-5		
28 Sept. 2024	Saturday	Fundamentals of Nursing-II	Ms Sabina Ali		Decode Revision Session 1 with PQD	Model Test Applied Biochemistry & Applied Nutrition & Dietetics Set-6		
29 Sept. 2024	Sunday							

Notes

Notes

Notes